ACSM's
Sports Medicine
A COMPREHENSIVE REVIEW

Second Edition

ACSM's
Sports Medicine
A COMPREHENSIVE REVIEW

Second Edition

Senior Editor

Francis G. O'Connor, MD, MPH, FACSM
Uniformed Services University of the Health Sciences
Bethesda, Maryland

Editors

Brian A. Davis, MD, FACSM
Intermountain Healthcare
Las Vegas, Nevada

Korin B. Hudson, MD, FACSM
MedStar Health, Georgetown University
Washington, DC

Mary Lloyd Ireland, MD, FACSM
Ortho Sports Medicine, University of Kentucky
Lexington, Kentucky

Robert E. Sallis, MD, FACSM
Kaiser Permanente Medical Center
Fontana, California

Robert P. Wilder, MD, FACSM
University of Virginia
Charlottesville, Virginia

Jason L. Zaremski, MD, FACSM
University of Florida College of Medicine
Gainesville, Florida

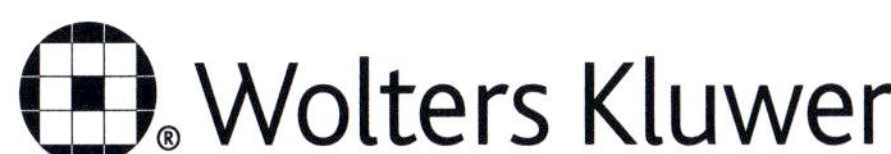

Philadelphia • Baltimore • New York • London
Buenos Aires • Hong Kong • Sydney • Tokyo

Acquisitions Editor: Lindsey Porambo
Senior Development Editor: Amy Millholen
Marketing Manager: Kirsten Watrud
Senior Production Specialist: Bridgett Dougherty
Manager, Graphic Arts & Design: Stephen Druding
Art Director, Illustration: Jennifer Clements
Manufacturing Coordinator: Margie Orzech-Zeranko
Prepress Vendor: TNQ Tech
ACSM Publications Committee Chair: Karyn L. Hamilton, PhD, RD, FACSM
ACSM Chief Executive Officer: Katie Feltman
ACSM Director of Publishing: Angie Chastain

Second edition

9 8 7 6 5 4 3 2 1

Printed in Mexico

Library of Congress Cataloging-in-Publication Data

ISBN-13: 978-1-975196-99-8

Cataloging in Publication data available on request from publisher.

DISCLAIMER

The opinions and assertions expressed herein are those of the author(s) and do not reflect the official policy or position of the Uniformed Services University of the Health Sciences or the Department of Defense.

Care has been taken to confirm the accuracy of the information present and to describe generally accepted practices. However, the authors, editors, and publisher are not responsible for errors or omissions or for any consequences from application of the information in this publication and make no warranty, expressed or implied, with respect to the currency, completeness, or accuracy of the contents of the publication. Application of this information in a particular situation remains the professional responsibility of the practitioner; the clinical treatments described and recommended may not be considered absolute and universal recommendations.

The authors, editors, and publisher have exerted every effort to ensure that drug selection and dosage set forth in this text are in accordance with the current recommendations and practice at the time of publication. However, in view of ongoing research, changes in government regulations, and the constant flow of information relating to drug therapy and drug reactions, the reader is urged to check the package insert for each drug for any change in indications and dosage and for added warnings and precautions. This is particularly important when the recommended agent is a new or infrequently employed drug.

Some drugs and medical devices presented in this publication have Food and Drug Administration (FDA) clearance for limited use in restricted research settings. It is the responsibility of the health care provider to ascertain the FDA status of each drug or device planned for use in their clinical practice.

shop.lww.com

QUADM1025

Dedication

This textbook is dedicated to the success of all students of sports medicine who are working hard to keep athletes, recreational, occupational, tactical, and elite, young and old, in the game!

With this second edition, we would additionally like to remember a true friend and fellow sports medicine colleague, as well as a prior contributor to this book, COL (Ret) John E. Glorioso, MD. His exemplary military leadership and healthcare mentorship inspired countless young men and women in their academic pursuits and community service through his enjoyment of sports medicine. He was a gentleman, scholar and soldier-physician. Rest in peace, JG. Job, well done.

Contents

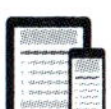
indicates online-only content

SECTION vii
Special Populations

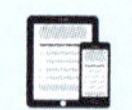

Additional Online Resources:

Preface

ACSM's Sports Medicine: A Comprehensive Review Second Edition had two guiding objectives — 1. To develop a premier educational primer for the clinician embarking on a career in sports medicine, and 2. To provide the foremost resource to assist clinicians preparing for their subspecialty sports medicine certification examination. We have carefully studied content identified by the medical specialties to identify what we believe to be the most important material to assist the reader with successfully passing their examination. The text is conveniently divided into seven sections to assist with your review: general considerations, evaluation of the injured athlete, medical problems in the athlete, musculoskeletal problems in the athlete, principles of rehabilitation, sports-specific populations, and special populations. The text is bulleted and well referenced. Where appropriate, tables, figures, and algorithms are provided to assist with important concepts. A quick review of the list of authors not only highlights the fact that we have compiled a "who's who" of sports medicine talent, but that we have members from nearly all medical specialties as well as leaders in athletic training and physical therapy.

Expanded to 136 chapters, the text is divided into the following seven sections, in addition to an online question bank:

- Section I. Foundational Considerations in Sports Medicine (Chapters 1–18), editor Robert P. Wilder, MD, FACSM
- Section II. Evaluation of the Injured Athlete (Chapters 19–30), editor Francis G. O'Connor, MD, MPH, FACSM
- Section III. Medical Problems in the Athlete (Chapters 31–47), editor Robert E. Sallis, MD, FACSM
- Section IV. Musculoskeletal Problems in the Athlete (Chapters 48–71), editor Mary Lloyd Ireland, MD, FACSM
- Section V. Rehabilitation (Chapters 72–87), editor Robert P. Wilder, MD, FACSM
- Section VI. Sports-Specific Considerations (Chapters 88–127), editor Korin B. Hudson, MD, FACSM
- Section VII. Special Populations (Chapters 128–136), editor Francis G. O'Connor, MD, MPH, FACSM
- Online. Question Bank (Chapters 1-136), editors Brian A. Davis, MD, CPT, FACSM and Jason L. Zaremski, MD, FACSM

Due to the comprehensive coverage provided by this text, several printed chapters include an online addendum with additional content and figures, and a handful of chapters are included in the online-only version of the text (noted in the table of contents, as well as in the text). Additionally, question editors Brian Davis and Jason Zaremski and their team refreshed and wrote new board-type questions for every chapter. Those questions, over 1,300, are available online as a resource for the reader. Each question provides an explanation on why the right answer is correct and the other items are incorrect. In addition, references are provided. To further support the text, the ancillaries include an online-only resource *Radiographic Lines and Angles* from authors Ryunosuke Hisatomi, MD; Ammar Husan, MD, MBA; and Peter H. Seidenberg, MD, MA, FACSM; and the Team Physician Consensus Conference (TPCC) Statements. Additional TPCC Statements are available at https://acsm.org/education-resources/pronouncements-scientific-communications/team-physician-consensus-statements/. Updates to the text, if needed, will be available at https://acsm.org/education-resources/books/acsm-book-updates/.

As the editors of *ACSM's Sports Medicine: A Comprehensive Review*, Second Edition, we sincerely believe we have produced the preeminent educational resource to guide your journey in sports medicine. We wish you all rewarding careers and academic success!

ADDITIONAL RESOURCES

Additional resources are available with purchase of this text:

- Online addenda to chapters
- Online-only chapters
- Refreshed and new extensive question bank
- *Radiographic Lines and Angles* resource
- TPCC Statements

See inside the front cover of this text for more details and access instructions.

Acknowledgments

The editors would like to collectively acknowledge the support of our families and teachers, who daily have both supported and inspired us through this effort. In addition, we would like to thank the teams from publisher Wolters Kluwer and the American College of Sports Medicine who supported this project.

Finally, and most importantly, we would like to acknowledge the feedback from our colleagues in reference to the first edition. We have done our best to address prior identified concerns and gaps to create what we believe to be the preeminent product with this second edition to guide new learners in the field of sports medicine and prepare clinicians, both novice and seasoned, for board preparation.

Contributors

Andre A. Abadin, DO
University of Washington
Seattle, Washington

Jeffrey S. Abrams, MD
Princeton Orthopaedic Associates
Princeton, New Jersey

Kathryn E. Ackerman, MD, MPH, FACSM
Women's Health, Sports & Performance Institute
Boston, Massachusetts

William B. Adams, MD
Dumfries Health Center
Dumfries, Virginia

Terry Adirim, MD, MPH, MBA
Uniformed Services University of the Health Sciences
Bethesda, Maryland

Stephanie F. Alessi-LaRosa, MD, MPH
Hartford Healthcare
Hartford, Connecticut

Joanne B. "Anne" Allen, MD, FACSM
Allen Spine and Sports Medicine
Wilmington, North Carolina

Robert A. Arciero, MD
UConn Health
Farmington, Connecticut

Elizabeth A. Arendt, MD
University of Minnesota Physicians
Minneapolis, Minnesota

Julia Arroyo
Universidad Complutense de Madrid
Madrid, Spain

Chad A. Asplund, MD, MPH, FACSM
Georgetown University
Washington, DC

Jared Astrow, DO
Brown University Health
East Providence, Rhode Island

Jonathan D. Bailey, MD
Uniformed Services University of the Health Sciences
Bethesda, Maryland

Wes Bailey, MD
Village Medical
Decatur, Georgia

Bjørn Bakken, MD
TRIA Orthopedic Specialists
Minneapolis, Minnesota

Guy Ball, DO
Rochester Hills Orthopaedics and Sports Medicine
Rochester Hills, Michigan

Kenneth P. Barnes, MD, MSc, FACSM
Barnes Sports Medicine Consulting PLLC
Burlington, North Carolina

Samuel I. Bartlett, DO
Uniformed Services University of the Health Sciences
Bethesda, Maryland

Kenneth B. Batts, DO
Naval Medical Center Portsmouth
Portsmouth, Virginia

Luke Bennett, MBBS, MSpMD
Hintsa Performance AG
Zug, Switzerland

Brandon Bentley, MD
Augusta University
Augusta, Georgia

Anthony I. Beutler, MD
Intermountain Health - Utah Valley Sports Medicine
Provo, Utah

Gitansh Bhargava, DO
University of Virginia Health System
Charlottesville, Virginia

Bradford Bindas, MD
BayCare Health Systems
Newport Richey, Florida

Zackary Birchard, DO
Licking Memorial Health Systems
Newark, Ohio

Chris Blaszka, MS
Georgia Football
Athens, Georgia

Barry P. Boden, MD
The Orthopaedic Center, a Division of CAO
Rockville, Maryland

Aaron Bolds, MD, MBA
Barbour Orthopaedics & Spine
Atlanta, Georgia

Joey Bonanno, MD Candidate
Hospital for Special Surgery
New York, New York

Elizabeth C. Bond, MD
Dunedin and Mercy Hospitals
Dunedin, New Zealand

Jacob Boomgaardt, DO
Ascent Medical Centre
Ottawa, Ontario, Canada

Naina Bouchereau-Lal, MD
Ochsner LSU Health
Shreveport, Louisiana

Fred H. Brennan Jr., DO, FACSM
University of South Florida
Clearwater, Florida

David L. Brown, MD
Olympia Orthopaedic Associates
Olympia, Washington

Linda L. Brown, MD
Dermatology and Allergy Specialists of Olympia
Olympia, Washington

Christopher M. Brusalis, MD
Hospital for Special Surgery
New York, New York

Brian Busconi, MD
Umass Memorial Health
Worcester, Massachusetts

Janus D. Butcher, MD, FACSM
Colonel, USA, Retired
Duluth, Minnesota

Malia Cali, MD
The Steadman Clinic
Frisco, Colorado

Dennis A. Cardone, DO
NYU Langone Health
New York, New York

Eduardo Carrera, MD
AdventHealth
Castle Rock, Colorado

Eric W. Carson, MD
Hospital for Special Surgery
New York, New York

Ellen Casey, MD, FACSM
Hospital for Special Surgery
New York, New York

Kristina M. Ceravolo, DMD
Family Dental
Morristown, New Jersey

Hannah C. Chen, MD
Alexander T. Augusta Military Medical Center
Fort Belvoir, Virginia

Marc A. Childress, MD
Inova Primary Care
Fairfax, Virginia

Brian J. Cole, MD, MBA
Midwest Orthopaedics at Rush - Chicago
Chicago, Illinois

Reid Collis, MD
University of Virginia School of Medicine
Charlottesville, Virginia

Alena Comella, DO
Maine Integrative Family Care
South Portland, Maine

Ron Courson, ATC, PT, CSCS
University of Georgia
Athens, Georgia

Katherine J. Coyner, MD, MBA
UConn Health
Farmington, Connecticut

Navya Dandu, MD
Allegheny Health Network
Pittsburgh, Pennsylvania

Brian A. Davis, MD, CPT, FACSM
Intermountain Healthcare
Las Vegas, Nevada

Brittany deCamp, MS, LAT, ATC
Georgia Football
Athens, Georgia

Preston DeHan, DO
Madigan Army Medical Center
Tacoma, Washington

Craig R. Denegar, PT, PhD
University of Connecticut
Storrs, Connecticut

Thea J. Dennis-Arends, MD
Oregon Health and Science University
Portland, Oregon

Patricia A. Deuster, PhD, MPH, FACSM
Uniformed Services University of the Health Sciences
Bethesda, Maryland

Kevin deWeber, MD, FACSM
SW Washington Sports Medicine Fellowship
Vancouver, Washington

Aman Dhawan, MD
Northwestern Medicine Regional Medical Group
Naperville, Illinois

Daniel Diaz, MD
The Ohio State University Wexner Medical Center
Columbus, Ohio

Jay Dicharry, MPT, SCS
MOBO, LLC
Bend, Oregon

Abby N. Diehl, PhD, ABPP
Uniformed Services University of the Health Sciences
Bethesda, Maryland

Robert J. Dimeff, MD
Texas Orthopaedic Associates
Dallas, Texas

Lindsay DiStefano, PhD, ATC
University of Connecticut
Storrs, Connecticut

Jonathan A. Drezner, MD
UW Medicine Center for Sports Cardiology
Seattle, Washington

James Dunlap, MD, FACSM
MaineGeneral Health
August, Maine

Matthew Eads, MD
Kentucky Bone and Joint Surgeons
Lexington, Kentucky

Samuel R. Engel, MA
UConn Health
Farmington, Connecticut

Scott Epsley, PT
Gotham FC
New York, New York

Yoram Epstein, PhD, FACSM
Tel Aviv University
Tel Aviv, Israel

Nathan P. Falk, MD
Florida State University
Winter Haven, Florida

Marcia Faustin, MD
University of California, Davis
Sacramento, California

Reginald S. Fayssoux, MD
Desert Orthopedic Center
Rancho Mirage, California

John F. Feller, MD
Desert Medical Imaging
Indian Wells, California

Karl B. Fields, MD
Cone Health System Sports Medicine Fellowship
Greensboro, North Carolina

Scott D. Flinn, MD
Palomar Health
Ramona, California

Jonathon M. Florance, MD
Duke University
Durham, North Carolina

Ryan Flowers, DO, MAS
UT Southwestern
Dallas, Texas

Michael P. Foy, MD
University of Illinois Chicago
Chicago, Illinois

Richard A. Francesco, DO
Main Line Health
Broomall, Pennsylvania

Michael Fredericson, MD, FACSM
Stanford Medicine
Redwood City, California

Jason Friedrich, MD
University of Colorado School of Medicine
Aurora, Colorado

Elizabeth Gannon, DO
One Medical
Reston, Virginia

Jennifer M. Garrison, DO
Houston Methodist
Katy, Texas

Peter Gerbino, MD, FACSM
Orthopedic Surgery
Monterey, California

Jeffrey L. Goodie, PhD, ABPP
Uniformed Services University of the Health Sciences
Bethesda, Maryland

Jordan S. Gross, MD
UCLA Health
Los Angeles, California

Jason Guo, MD
University of Virginia
Charlottesville, Virginia

F. Winston Gwathmey, MD
University of Virginia
Charlottesville, Virginia

Matthew Hall, DO
University of Connecticut
Storrs, Connecticut

John Hamilton, MD
Inova
Fairfax, Virginia

Kimberly G. Harmon, MD, FACSM
University of Washington School of Medicine
Seattle, Washington

Mark D. Harris, MD
MD Harris Institute, Inc.
Beckley, West Virginia

Joe M. Hart, PhD, ATC, FACSM
University of North Carolina at Chapel Hill
Chapel Hill, North Carolina

Gavin Santini Hautala, MD
TRIA Orthopaedics
Bloomington, Minnesota

Thomas Heckman, DO
Medstar National Rehabilitation Hospital
Washington, DC

Yuval Heled, PhD, LLB, FACSM
The Faculty of Sciences
Kibbutzim College, Tel Aviv

Curtis Henn, MD
MedStar Health, Georgetown University
Washington, DC

Stanley A. Herring, MD, FACSM
University of Washington
Seattle, Washington

Justin J. Hicks, MD
University of Pittsburgh
Pittsburgh, Pennsylvania

Ryunosuke Hisatomi, MD
LSU Science Center Shreveport
Shreveport, Louisiana

Garry W. K. Ho, MD, FACSM
OrthoVirginia
Fairfax, Virginia

R. Todd Hockenbury, MD
University of Louisville
Louisville, Kentucky

Thomas Hoke, MD
MaineGeneral Health
August, Maine

Mark Hopkins, MD
Emergency Medicine
Boise, Idaho

Thomas M. Howard, MD, FACSM
NC State Student Health
Raleigh, North Carolina

Melody R. Hrubes, MD, FACSM
Hospital for Special Surgery
New York, New York

Connie Hsia, MD
Uniformed Services University of the Health Sciences
Bethesda, Maryland

Yao-Wen Eliot Hu, MD, FACSM
University of Massachusetts
Boston, Massachusetts

Jeremy Huckleby, MD
Orthopedist
Saint Louis, Missouri

Shane Hudnall, MD
Cone Health Sports Medicine Center
Greensboro, North Carolina

Korin B. Hudson, MD, FACSM
MedStar Health, Georgetown University
Washington, DC

Chad D. Hulsopple, DO
Uniformed Services University of the Health Sciences
Bethesda, Maryland

Ammar Husan, MD, MBA, FAAFP
LSU Health Science Center Shreveport
Shreveport, Louisiana

Mark R. Hutchinson, MD, FACSM
University of Illinois
Chicago, Illinois

Christopher D. Ingersoll, PhD, ATC, FACSM
University of North Carolina at Chapel Hill
Chapel Hill, North Carolina

Benjamin J. Ingram, MD
Uniformed Services University of the Health Sciences
Bethesda, Maryland

Mary Lloyd Ireland, MD, FACSM
Ortho Sports Medicine, University of Kentucky
Lexington, Kentucky

Adriana Isacke, DO
MaineHealth
Portland, Maine

Haruki Ishii, MD
NYU Langone Health
New York, New York

Aeneas Janze, MD
Walter Reed National Military Medical Center
Bethesda, Maryland

Carrie A. Jaworski, MD, FACSM
Intermountain Healthcare
Park City, Utah

Jeffrey G. Jenkins, MD
University of Virginia
Charlottesville, Virginia

Jason E. Jesse, MD
Rush University Medical Center
Chicago, Illinois

Christopher E. Jonas, DO
Uniformed Services University of the Health Sciences
Bethesda, Maryland

Wayne B. Jonas, MD
Healing Works Foundation
Alexandria, Virginia

Lauren E. Juliano, MD
Steele Memorial Medical Center
Salmon, Idaho

Tyler Kalbac, MD
Orthopedic & Sports Medicine Center of Miami
Miami, Florida

Shawn F. Kane, MD, FACSM
University of North Carolina at Chapel Hill
Chapel Hill, North Carolina

Vasili Karas, MD
Rush University Medical Center
Chicago, Illinois

Kristine A. Karlson, MD, FACSM
Dartmouth Health
Lebanon, New Hampshire

Devin K. Kelly, PhD
University of North Carolina at Chapel Hill
Chapel Hill, North Carolina

Hamish A. Kerr, MD, FACSM
Albany Med Health System
Albany, New York

Khizer Khaderi, MD, MPH
Stanford Medicine
Palo Alto, California

Alexander R. Kheradi, MD
MedStar Health, Georgetown University
Washington, DC

Lee Kiefer, BS
KM Fencing, LLC.
Lexington, Kentucky

Matthew T. Kingery, MD
NYU Langone Orthopedic Hospital
New York, New York

Christian F. Klein, MD
University of Utah Health
Salt Lake City, Utah

John J. Klimkiewicz, MD
District Ortho
Chevy Chase, Maryland

Emma L. Klosterman, MD
University of Michigan
Ann Arbor, Michigan

Justine Ko, MD
Weill Cornell Medicine
New York, New York

Denver Kraft, MD
Medstar Georgetown University
Washington, DC

Roger Kruse, MD, FACSM
University of Toledo
Toledo, Ohio

Christopher M. Kuenze, PhD, ATC
University of Virginia
Charlottesville, Virginia

Anne M. Kuwabara, MD
Stanford University
Redwood City, California

Stephanie H. Lai, DO
Kaiser Permanente
Vacaville, California

Brent W. Lambson, DO
Intermountain Health - Cassia Sports Medicine
Burley, Idaho

Erek W. Latzka, MD
Boston Sports & Biologics
Wellesley, Massachusetts

Jacqueline Leemputte, DO
Northwestern Medical Group
Chicago, Illinois

Joshua E. Lider, DO
Helena Orthopedic Clinic
Helena, Montana

Christopher Lutrzykowski, MD
MaineGeneral Health
August, Maine

James Lynch, MD, LLC
All Star Pain Management & Regenerative Medicine
Annapolis, Maryland

Kevin Machino, DO
Intermountain Health
Los Vegas, California

John M. MacKnight, MD, FACSM
University of Virginia
Charlottesville, Virginia

Ryan Madaleno, LAT, ATC
UGA Football
Athens, Georgia

Scott A. Magnes, MD, FACSM
Department of Surgery, Uniformed Services University of the Health Sciences
Jacksonville, Florida

Eric M. Magrum, DPT, OCS
University of Virginia
Charlottesville, Virginia

Gretchen Mohney, PhD, ATC, CSCS
US Figure Skating
Colorado Springs, Colorado

Wyatt K. Maloy, MD
Alexander T. Augusta Medical Center
Fort Belvoir, Virginia

Lee A. Mancini, MD
U Mass Sports and Exercise Medicine
Worcester, Massachusetts

Michael R. Mancini, MD
University of Connecticut
Storrs, Connecticut

Sean N. Martin, DO
Transcend Performance & Lifestyle Institute
Montverde, Florida

Melissa Martinez, DO
Wellstar Health System
Marietta, Georgia

Ronica Martinez, MD
University of New Mexico
Albuquerque, New Mexico

Christina Master, MD, FACSM
Children's Hospital of Philadelphia
Philadelphia, Pennsylvania

Jason M. Matuszak, MD
Excelsior Orthopaedics
Amherst, New York

Augustus D. Mazzocca, MD
Massachusetts General Hospital
Boston, Massachusetts

Robert McCunney, MD
New England Baptist Hospital
Boston Massachusetts

Devin P. McFadden, MD
Womack Army Medical Center
Fort Bragg, North Carolina

James Alexander McIntyre, MD
Tufts Medical Center
Boston, Massachusetts

Katie J. McMorrow, BS
Rush University Medical Center
Chicago, Illinois

Gerek Meinhardt, BBA, MBA
KM Fencing, LLC.
Lexington, Kentucky

Brian F. Merrigan, MD
Alexander T. Augusta Military Medical Center
Fort Belvoir, Virginia

Christopher D. Meyering, DO
Orlando VA Medical Center
Orlando, Florida

Lindsey Migliore, DO
GamerDoc
Anchorage, Alaska

Erin Anne Miller, MD, MS
UW Medicine
Seattle, Washington

Mark D. Miller, MD
UVA Health
Charlottesville, Virginia

Melita N. Moore, MD
University of California Davis Health
Sacramento, California

Kambiz Motamedi, MD
UCLA Health
Los Angeles, California

Casey S. Mueller, MD
Eisenhower Army Medical Center
Fort Gordon, Georgia

Landon Mueller, MD
MedStar Health, Georgetown University
Washington, DC

Luke Mugge, MD
Inova
Fairfax, Virginia

Sean W. Mulvaney, MD
Uniformed Services University of the Health Sciences
Bethesda, Maryland

Bryan Murtaugh, MD
MedStar National Rehabilitation Network
Washington, DC

Michael Needham, MD
Uniformed Services University of the Health Sciences
Bethesda, Maryland

Bradley J. Nelson, MD
University of Minnesota
Minneapolis, Minnesota

Rochelle M. Nolte, MD
NTC Clinic
San Diego, California

Connor Norman, PT, DPT, SCS, ATC, CSCS
UGA Football
Athens, Georgia

Chad S. Norton, DO
Martin Army Community Hospital
Fort Benning, Georgia

Nathaniel Nye, MD
Intermountain Health
Cedar City, Utah

Elizabeth M. O'Connor, DDS
Advanced Family Dental Care
North Syracuse, New York

Francis G. O'Connor, MD, MPH, FACSM
Uniformed Services University of the Health Sciences
Bethesda, Maryland

Tracey O'Connor, MD
Moffitt Cancer Center
Tampa, Florida

Andrea L. Pana, MD, MPH
Serenity Medical Center and EviCore
Austin, Texas

Curtis Papenfuss, MD
Samaritan Healthcare
Moses Lake, Washington
Fort

Chris G. Pappas, MD
Colonel, US Army, Retired
Fort Walton Beach, Florida

Erika Parisi, MD
University of Michigan
Ann Arbor, Michigan

Paul F. Pasquina, MD
Uniformed Services University of the Health Sciences
Bethesda, Maryland

Robert B. Patton, MD
Jordan-Young Institute
Virginia Beach, Virginia

Evan Peck, MD
Cleveland Clinic Florida
West Palm Beach, Florida

Rebecca Peebles, DO
The University of Texas at Tyler
Tyler, Texas

Nicholas A. Piantanida, MD
UCHealth Primary Care and Sports Medicine Clinic
Colorado Springs, Colorado

Kinsley Pierre, BS
Stanford University
Stanford, California

Daniel Poole, MD
Ortho on Call
Richmond, Virginia

Jessica M. Poole, MEd, ATC
North Georgia College & State University
Dahlonega, Georgia

R. M. Barney Poole, PT, DPT
Confluent Health Physical Therapy
Stockbridge, Georgia

Salvador E. Portugal, DO, MBA
NYU Langone Orthopedic Center
New York, New York

William F. Postma, MD
MedStar Health, Georgetown University
Washington, DC

Jason Pothast, MD
MedStar Health
Baltimore, Maryland

Joel Press, MD
Hospital for Special Surgery
New York, New York

Scott W. Pyne, MD, FACSM
Family and Sports Medicine Physician
Annapolis, Maryland

Catherine R. Rainbow, MD
Atrium Health
Charlotte, North Carolina

Sara N. Raiser, MD
University of Virginia
Charlottesville, Virginia

Meghan F. Raleigh, MD
Carl R. Darnall Army Medical Center
Fort Hood, Texas

Naina Rao, MD
NYU Langone Health
New York, New York

Ravishankar E. Rao, MD
Sharp HealthCare
San Diego, California

Bradley A. Redick, MD
Uniformed Services University of the Health Sciences
Bethesda, Maryland

Ian R. Reynolds, MD
Carilion Clinic
Roanoke, Virginia

J. Logan Reynolds, MD
University of Kentucky
Lexington, Kentucky

Blair B. Rhodehouse, DO
Martin Army Community Hospital
Fort Benning, Georgia

John C. Richmond, MD
New England Baptist Hospital
Dedam, Massachusetts

Emily A. Ricker, MD
Uniformed Services University of the Health Sciences
Bethesda, Maryland

Nancy Rolnik, MD
Remedy Sports and Regenerative Medicine
Walnut Creek, California

Stephen Rossettie, MD, MBA
MedStar Georgetown University
Washington, DC

Elizabeth Rothe, MD
MaineGeneral Health
August, Maine

Aaron Rubin, MD, FACSM
Kaiser Permanente
Fontana, California

Kelly Ryan, DO, MD
MedStar Health
Baltimore, Maryland

Marc R. Safran, MD
Stanford Medicine
Stanford, California

Robert E. Sallis, MD, FACSM
Kaiser Permanente Medical Center
Fontana, California

Matthew J. Salzler, MD
Tufts Medical Center
Boston, Massachusetts

Jaron Santelli, MD
University of Utah, Intermountain Health
Park City, Utah

David Savin, MD
Desert Orthopedic Center - Eisenhower Health
Rancho Mirage, California

Allison Schafer, DO
UConn Health
Farmington, Connecticut

Michael B. Schwartz, MD
Princeton Longevity Center
Shelton, Connecticut

Matthew D. Sedgley, MD, FACSM
MedStar Health
Baltimore, Maryland

Peter H. Seidenberg, MD, MA, FACSM
LSU Health Shreveport School of Medicine
Shreveport, Louisiana

Ankit B. Shah, MD
Sports & Performance Cardiology
Chevy Chase, Maryland

Joel Shaw, MD
OhioHealth
Columbus, Ohio

Lauren Simon, MD, MPH, FACSM
Loma Linda University Health
Loma Linda, California

Jay Smith, MD, FACSM
Mayo Clinic
Rochester, Minnesota

Tawnee L. Sparling, MD
Uniformed Services University of the Health Sciences
Bethesda, Maryland

Arjun Srinath, MD, MPH
University of Miami
Miami, Florida

Patrick J. St. Martin, MD
Terrebonne General Sports Medicine
Houma, Louisiana

Patrick St. Pierre, MD
Desert Orthopedic Center - Eisenhower Health
Rancho Mirage, California

Taylor P. Stauffer, MD
Hospital for Special Surgery
New York, New York

Mark B. Stephens, MD, MS
Penn State College of Medicine
State College, Pennsylvania

Robert Stevens, DO
MaineGeneral Health
August, Maine

Genevra L. Stone, MD
Cambridge Health Alliance
Cambridge, Massachusetts

Eric J. Strauss, MD
NYU Langone Orthopedic Center
New York, New York

Steven J. Svoboda, MD
MedStar Health, Georgetown University
Washington, DC

Thomas Swaffield, MD
Children's Hospital of Philadelphia
Philadelphia, Pennsylvania

Michelle E. Szczepanik, MD
Veterans Health Administration
Winter Park, Florida

Dean C. Taylor, MD
Duke University
Durham, North Carolina

Ian Thomas, MD
Thomas Sports and Regenerative Orthopedics
Battle Creek, Michigan

Danielle Thornsberry
Kansas State University
Manhattan, Kansas

Denise Torbert, MD
Naval Hospital Camp Pendleton
Camp Pendleton, California

Courtney T. Tripp, DO
Evans U.S. Army Community Hospital
Colorado Springs, Colorado

Justin Tu, MD
Emory Healthcare, Department of Orthopedics
Atlanta Georgia

Aaron Tunison, JD, LLM-Tax
California Attorney
Rancho Mission Viejo, California

Brian K. Unwin, MD
Carilion Clinic
Roanoke, Virginia

Colin L. Uyeki, MD
University of Massachusetts
Worcester, Massachusetts

Raimundo Vial Irarrazal, MD
Pontifical Catholic University of Chile
Santiago, Chile

Heather K. Vincent, PhD, FACSM
United States Olympic and Paralympic Committee
Colorado Springs, CO and Gainesville, Florida

Kevin R. Vincent, MD, PhD, FACSM
The Orthopaedic Institute (TOI)
Alachua, Florida

Nicholas Walla, MD
UMass Memorial Health Center
Worcester, Massachusetts

Winston J. Warme, MD
University of Washington
Seattle, Washington

Michael Warwick, MD
University of Virginia
Charlottesville, Virginia

Micah K. Watson, DO
Martin Army Community Hospital
Fort Benning, Georgia

Charles W. Webb, DO
LSU Health
Shreveport, Louisiana

Rory B. Weiner, MD
Massachusetts General Hospital
Boston, Massachusetts

Alexander C. Weissman, MS
Rush University Medical Center
Chicago, Illinois

John H. Wilckens, MD
The Johns Hopkins Hospital University School of Medicine
Baltimore, Maryland

Robert P. Wilder, MD, FACSM
University of Virginia
Charlottesville, Virginia

Samantha C. Willer, DO, MA
PennState Health
Hershey, Pennsylvania

Erika Williams, MD
MedStar Health, Georgetown University
Washington, DC

Drew Willson
Youngstown State University
Youngstown, Ohio

Benjamin Wilson, MD
University of Kentucky
Lexington, Kentucky

Sean Wise, MD
U.S. Army
Fort Belvoir, Virginia

Jeffrey Wisinski, DO
Prisma Health - University of South Carolina
Columbia, South Carolina

Allen A. Yazdi, MD
University of Alabama at Birmingham
Birmingham, Alabama

Xiaoning (Jenny) Yuan, MD, PhD
Uniformed Services University of the Health Sciences
Bethesda, Maryland

Jacqueline Yurgil, DO
Alexander T. Augusta Military Medical Center
Ft. Belvoir, Virginia

Luke Zabawa, MD
University of Illinois
Chicago, Illinois

Kyle W. Zittel, MD
MedStar Georgetown University
Washington, DC

Reviewers

Andre A. Abadin, DO
University of Washington
Seattle, Washington

Jeffrey S. Abrams, MD
Princeton Orthopaedic Associates
Princeton, New Jersey

Kathryn E. Ackerman, MD, MPH, FACSM
Women's Health, Sports & Performance Institute
Boston, Massachusetts

William B. Adams, MD
Dumfries Health Center
Dumfries, Virginia

Stephanie F. Alessi-LaRosa, MD, MPH
Hartford Healthcare
Hartford, Connecticut

Joanne B. "Anne" Allen, MD, FACSM
Allen Spine and Sports Medicine
Wilmington, North Carolina

Elizabeth A. Arendt, MD
University of Minnesota Physicians
Minneapolis, Minnesota

Chad A. Asplund, MD, MPH, FACSM
Georgetown University
Washington, DC

Jonathan D. Bailey, MD
Uniformed Services University of the Health Sciences
Bethesda, Maryland

Bjørn Bakken, MD
TRIA Orthopedic Specialists
Minneapolis, Minnesota

Kenneth B. Batts, DO
Naval Medical Center Portsmouth
Portsmouth, Virginia

Luke Bennett, MBBS, MSpMD
Hintsa Performance, AG
Zug, Switzerland

Anthony I. Beutler, MD
Intermountain Health - Utah Valley Sports Medicine
Provo, Utah

Gitansh Bhargava, DO
University of Virginia Health System
Charlottesville, Virginia

Bradford Bindas, MD
BayCare Health Systems
Newport Richey, Florida

Zackary Birchard, DO
Licking Memorial Health Systems
Newark, Ohio

Aaron Bolds, MD, MBA
Barbour Orthopaedics & Spine
Atlanta, Georgia

Joey Bonanno, MD Candidate
Hospital for Special Surgery
New York, New York

Jacob Boomgaardt, DO
Ascent Medical Centre
Ottawa, Ontario, Canada

Naina Bouchereau-Lal, MD
Ochsner LSU Health
Shreveport, Louisiana

David L. Brown, MD
Olympia Orthopaedic Associates
Olympia, Washington

Janus D. Butcher, MD, FACSM
Colonel, USA, Retired
Duluth, Minnesota

Malia Cali, MD
The Steadman Clinic
Frisco, Colorado

Dennis A. Cardone, DO
NYU Langone Health
New York, New York

Hannah C. Chen, MD
Alexander T. Augusta Military Medical Center
Fort Belvoir, Virginia

Marc A. Childress, MD
Inova Primary Care
Fairfax, Virginia

Alena Comella, DO
Maine Integrative Family Care
South Portland, Maine

Katherine J. Coyner, MD, MBA
UConn Health
Farmington, Connecticut

Craig R. Denegar, PT, PhD
University of Connecticut
Storrs, Connecticut

Kevin deWeber, MD, FACSM
SW Washington Sports Medicine Fellowship
Vancouver, Washington

Daniel Diaz, MD
The Ohio State University Wexner Medical Center
Columbus, Ohio

Jay Dicharry, MPT, SCS
MOBO, LLC
Bend, Oregon

Lindsay J. DiStefano, PhD, ATC
University of Connecticut
Storrs, Connecticut

Matthew Eads, MD
Kentucky Bone and Joint Surgeons
Lexington, Kentucky

Yoram Epstein, PhD, FACSM
Tel Aviv University
Tel Aviv, Israel

Scott D. Flinn, MD
Palomar Health
Ramona, California

Jonathon M. Florance, MD
Duke University
Durham, North Carolina

Ryan Flowers, DO, MAS
UT Southwestern
Dallas, Texas

Michael Fredericson, MD, FACSM
Stanford Medicine
Redwood City, California

Jason Friedrich, MD
University of Colorado School of Medicine
Aurora, Colorado

Elizabeth Gannon, DO
One Medical
Reston, Virginia

Jeffrey L. Goodie, PhD, ABPP
Uniformed Services University of the Health Sciences
Bethesda, Maryland

Jordan S. Gross, MD
UCLA Health
Los Angeles, California

Jason Guo, MD
University of Virginia
Charlottesville, Virginia

Mark D. Harris, MD
MD Harris Institute, Inc.
Beckley, West Virgina

Gavin Santini Hautala, MD
TRIA Orthopaedics
Bloomington, Minnesota

Justin J. Hicks, MD
University of Pittsburgh
Pittsburgh, Pennsylvania

R. Todd Hockenbury, MD
University of Louisville
Louisville, Kentucky

Thomas M. Howard, MD, FACSM
NC State Student Health
Raleigh, North Carolina

Connie Hsia, MD
Uniformed Services University of the Health Sciences
Bethesda, Maryland

Shane Hudnall, MD
Cone Health Sports Medicine Center
Greensboro, North Carolina

Korin B. Hudson, MD, FACSM
MedStar Health, Georgetown University
Washington, DC

Chad D. Hulsopple, DO
Uniformed Services University of the Health Sciences
Bethesda, Maryland

Mark R. Hutchinson, MD, FACSM
University of Illinois
Chicago, Illinois

Benjamin J. Ingram, MD
Uniformed Services University of the Health Sciences
Bethesda, Maryland

Mary Lloyd Ireland, MD, FACSM
University of Kentucky
Lexington, Kentucky

Haruki Ishii, MD
NYU Langone Health
New York, New York

Aeneas Janze, MD
Walter Reed National Military Medical Center
Bethesda, Maryland

Carrie A. Jaworski, MD, FACSM
Intermountain Healthcare
Park City, Utah

Devin K. Kelly, PhD
University of North Carolina at Chapel Hill
Chapel Hill, North Carolina

Lee Kiefer, BS
KM Fencing, LLC.
Lexington, Kentucky

Christian F. Klein, MD
University of Utah Health
Salt Lake City, Utah

Emma L. Klosterman, MD
University of Michigan
Ann Arbor, Michigan

Justine Ko, MD
Weill Cornell Medicine
New York, New York

Denver Kraft, MD
Medstar Health, Georgetown University
Washington, DC

Roger Kruse, MD, FACSM
University of Toledo
Toledo, Ohio

Brent W. Lambson, DO
Intermountain Health - Cassia Sports Medicine
Burley, Idaho

Joshua E. Lider, DO
Helena Orthopedic Clinic
Helena, Montana

Christopher Lutrzykowski, MD
MaineGeneral Health
August, Maine

John M. MacKnight, MD, FACSM
University of Virginia
Charlottesville, Virginia

Scott A. Magnes, MD, FACSM
Department of Surgery, Uniformed Services University of the Health Sciences
Jacksonville, Florida

Wyatt K. Maloy, MD
Alexander T. Augusta Medical Center
Fort Belvoir, Virginia

Lee A. Mancini, MD, CSCSD, CSN
U Mass Sports and Exercise Medicine
Worcester, Massachusetts

Michael R. Mancini, MD
University of Connecticut
Storrs, Connecticut

Sean N. Martin, DO
Transcend Performance & Lifestyle Institute
Montverde, Florida

Ronica Martinez, MD
University of New Mexico
Albuquerque, New Mexico

Jason M. Matuszak, MD
Excelsior Orthopaedics
Amherst, New York

Devin P. McFadden, MD
Womack Army Medical Center
Fort Bragg, North Carolina

James Alexander McIntyre, MD
Tufts Medical Center
Boston, Massachusetts

Erin Anne Miller, MD, MS
University of Washington
Seattle, Washington

Melita N. Moore, MD
University of California Davis Health
Sacramento, California

Casey S. Mueller, MD
Eisenhower Army Medical Center
Fort Gordon, Georgia

Luke Mugge, MD
Inova
Fairfax, Virginia

Sean W. Mulvaney, MD
Uniformed Services University of the Health Sciences
Bethesda, Maryland

Nathaniel Nye, MD
Intermountain Health
Cedar City, Utah

Elizabeth M. O'Connor, DDS
Advanced Family Dental Care
North Syracuse, New York

Francis G. O'Connor, MD, MPH, FACSM
Uniformed Services University of the Health Sciences
Bethesda, Maryland

Andrea L. Pana, MD, MPH
Serenity Medical Centers and EviCore
Austin, Texas

Erika Parisi, MD
University of Michigan
Ann Arbor, Michigan

Paul F. Pasquina, MD
Uniformed Services University of the Health Sciences
Bethesda, Maryland

Robert B. Patton, MD
Jordan-Young Institute
Virginia Beach, Virginia

Evan Peck, MD
Cleveland Clinic Florida
West Palm Beach, Florida

Nicholas A. Piantanida, MD
UCHealth Primary Care and Sports Medicine Clinic
Colorado Springs, Colorado

Kinsley Pierre, BS
Stanford University School of Medicine
Redwood City, California

Daniel Poole, MD
Ortho on Call
Richmond, Virginia

R. M. Barney Poole, PT, DPT
Confluent Health Physical Therapy
Stockbridge, Georgia

Joel Press, MD
Hospital for Special Surgery
New York, New York

Scott W. Pyne, MD, FACSM
Family and Sports Medicine Physician
Annapolis, Maryland

Sara N. Raiser, MD
University of Virginia
Charlottesville, Virginia

Meghan F. Raleigh, MD
Carl R. Darnall Army Medical Center
Fort Hood, Texas

Ravishankar E. Rao, MD
Sharp HealthCare
San Diego, California

Ian R. Reynolds, MD
Carilion Clinic
Roanoke, Virginia

Blair B. Rhodehouse, DO
Martin Army Community Hospital
Fort Benning, Georgia

Emily A. Ricker, MD
Uniformed Services University of the Health Sciences
Bethesda, Maryland

Stephen Rossettie, MD, MBA
MedStar Georgetown University
Washington, DC

Aaron Rubin, MD, FACSM
Kaiser Permanente
Fontana, California

Kelly Ryan, DO, MD
MedStar Health
Baltimore, Maryland

Robert E. Sallis, MD, FACSM
Kaiser Permanente Medical Center
Fontana, California

David Savin, MD
Desert Orthopedic Center - Eisenhower Health
Rancho Mirage, California

Joel Shaw, MD
OhioHealth
Columbus, Ohio

Arjun Srinath, MD, MPH
University of Miami
Miami, Florida

Genevra L. Stone, MD
Cambridge Health Alliance
Cambridge, Massachusetts

Patrick St. Pierre, MD
Desert Orthopedic Center - Eisenhower Health
Rancho Mirage, California

Thomas Swaffield, MD
Children's Hospital of Philadelphia
Philadelphia, Pennsylvania

Michelle E. Szczepanik, MD
Veterans Health Administration
Winter Park, Florida

Denise Torbert, MD
Naval Hospital Camp Pendleton
Camp Pendleton, California

Justin Tu, MD
Emory Healthcare, Department of Orthopedics
Atlanta, Georgia

Heather K. Vincent, PhD, FACSM
United States Olympic and Paralympic Committee
Colorado Springs, CO and Gainesville, Florida

Kevin R. Vincent, MD, PhD, FACSM
The Orthopaedic Institute (TOI)
Alachua, Florida

Charles W. Webb, DO
LSU Health
Shreveport, Louisiana

Alexander C. Weissman, MS
Rush University Medical Center
Chicago, Illinois

Robert P. Wilder, MD, FACSM
University of Virginia
Charlottesville, Virginia

Luke Zabawa, MD
University of Illinois
Chicago, Illinois

Kyle W. Zittel, MD
MedStar Georgetown University
Washington, DC

Question Editors and Authors

SENIOR QUESTION EDITOR

Brian A. Davis, MD, CPT, FACSM
Intermountain Healthcare
Las Vegas, Nevada

ASSOCIATE QUESTION EDITOR

Jason L. Zaremski, MD, FACSM
University of Florida College of Medicine
Gainesville, Florida

ASSISTANT QUESTION EDITORS

Philip A. Blaney, MD
Franciscan Health
Indianapolis, Indiana

Robert L Bowers, DO, PhD
Emory University School of Medicine
Emory Sports Medicine Center

Pete Dawson, MD
Mosaic Life Care
Saint Joseph, Missouri

Steven K. Poon, MD
Mayo Clinic
Phoenix, Arizona

Allison N. Schroeder, MD
University Hospitals
Cleveland, Ohio

Alyssa Neph Speciale, MD
U.C. Davis Health
Sacramento, California

Naima Stennett, MD
University of South Florida
Tampa, Florida

QUESTION AUTHORS

Cedric Akau, MD, MS, MPH
Hawai'i Pacific Health Medical Group
Honolulu, Hawaii

Jared Astrow, DO
Brown University Health
East Providence, Rhode Island

Cyrus Bateni, MD
UC Davis Health
Sacramento, California

Joey Bonanno, MDCandidate
Hospital for Special Surgery
New York, New York

Kirra Borrello, MS-
University of Hawai'i at Manoa
Honolulu, Hawaii

Michael Brownstein, MD
Emory School of Medicine
Atlanta, Georgia

Eduardo Carrera, MD
AdventHealth
Castle Rock, Colorado

Ellen Casey, MD, CAQSM, FACSM
Hospital for Special Surgery
New York, New York

Spencer Chang, MD
Hawai'i Pacific Health Medical Group
Honolulu, Hawaii

Anthony F. Chen, MD
UC Davis Health
Sacramento, California

David S. Chen, MD
UC Davis Health
Sacramento, California

Marc A. Childress, MD
Inova Primary Care
Fairfax, Virginia

Brian A. Davis, MD, CPT, FACSM
Intermountain Healthcare
Las Vegas, Nevada

Daniel Diaz, DO
Essentia Health System
Duluth, Minnesota

Robert J. Dimeff, MD
Texas Orthopaedic Associates
Dallas, Texas

Nicholas C. DiSanti, MD
UC Davis Health
Sacramento, California

David M. Drozda, DO
University of Florida Health
Gainesville, Florida

James Dunlap, MD, FACSM
MaineGeneral Health
August, Maine

Marcia Faustin, MD
UC Davis Health
Sacramento, California

Nathan P. Falk, MD
Florida State University
Winter Haven, Florida

Ryan Flowers, DO, MAS
University of Texas Southwestern Medical Center
Dallas, Texas

Jason Friedrich, MD
University of Colorado School of Medicine
Aurora, Colorado

Mark D. Harris, MD
MD Harris Institute, Inc.
Beckley, West Virgina

R. Todd Hockenbury, MD
University of Louisville
Louisville, Kentucky

Thomas Hoke, MD
MaineGeneral Health
August, Maine

Thomas M. Howard, MD, FACSM
NC State Student Health
Raleigh, North Carolina

Carrie A. Jaworski, MD, FACSM, FAAFP
Intermountain Healthcare
Park City, Utah

Kristine A. Karlson, MD, FACSM
Dartmouth Health
Lebanon, New Hampshire

Daniel Kiehl, DO
University of Florida Health
Gainesville, Florida

Jennifer King, DO
Hawai'i Pacific Health Medical Group
Honolulu, Hawaii

Jacqueline Leemputte, DO
Northwestern Medical Group
Chicago, Illinois

Joshua E. Lider, DO
Helena Orthopedic Clinic
Helena, Montana

Christopher Lutrzykowski, MD
MaineGeneral Health
August, Maine

John M. MacKnight, MD
University of Virginia
Charlottesville, Virginia

Scott A. Magnes, MD, FACSM
Department of Surgery, Uniformed Services University of the Health Sciences
Jacksonville, Florida

Naveed Majd, DO
UC Davis Health
Sacramento, California

Lee A. Mancini, MD, CSCSD, CSN
U Mass Sports and Exercise Medicine
Worcester, Massachusetts

Sean N. Martin, DO
Transcend Performance & Lifestyle Institute
Montverde, Florida

Casey S. Mueller, MD
Eisenhower Army Medical Center
Fort Gordon, Georgia

Sean W. Mulvaney, MD
Uniformed Services University of the Health Sciences
Bethesda, Maryland

Francis G. O'Connor, MD, MPH, FACSM
Uniformed Services University of the Health Sciences
Bethesda, Maryland

Shammi Patel, DO
University of Florida Health
Gainesville, Florida

Scott W. Pyne, MD, FACSM, FAAFP
Family and Sports Medicine Physician
Annapolis, Maryland

Ravishankar E. Rao, MD
Sharp Grossmont Hospital
San Diego, California

Blair Rhodehouse, DO, CAQSM, ATC
Martin Army Community Hospital
Fort Benning, Georgia

Elizabeth Rothe, MD
MaineGeneral Health
August, Maine

Aaron Rubin, MD, FACSM
Kaiser Permanente
Fontana, California

Eli M. Snyder, BS, MS-
University of Hawai'i at Manoa
Honolulu, Hawaii

Mikayla Sonnleitner, MS-
University of Hawai'i at Manoa
Honolulu, Hawaii

Alyssa Neph Speciale, MD
U.C. Davis Health
Sacramento, California

Patrick St. Martin, MD
Terrebonne General Sports Medicine
Houma, Louisiana

Patrick St. Pierre, MD
Desert Orthopedic Center - Eisenhower Health
Rancho Mirage, California

Robert Stevens, DO
MaineGeneral Health
August, Maine

Ian Thomas, MD
Thomas Sports and Regenerative Orthopedics
Battle Creek, Michigan

Kiran Vadada, MD, RMSK
Hawai'i Pacific Health Medical Group
Honolulu, Hawaii

Sydnie Vo, MD
UCLA Health
Burbank, California

Alexandra E. Warrick, MD
University of California Davis School of Medicine
Sacramento, California

Charles W. Webb, DO
LSU Health
Shreveport, Louisiana

Michael Kenji Yamazaki, MD, MBA, RMSK
Hawai'i Pacific Health Medical Group
Honolulu, Hawaii

Justin Mark Young, MD
Hawai'i Pacific Health Medical Group
Honolulu, Hawaii

Jason L. Zaremski, MD, FACSM
University of Florida College of Medicine
Gainesville, Florida

SECTION I

Foundational Considerations in Sports Medicine

The Team Physician

1

Brent W. Lambson, Anthony I. Beutler, and John H. Wilckens

WHAT IS A TEAM PHYSICIAN?

- The team physician is one integral part of the larger group that provides care to athletes at all levels of sport. Properly understanding the team physician role optimizes the care and coordination of individual athletes and the entire team. Guidance from professional organizations can provide insight into this important role and how the team physician can aid in the safety and improved performance of those for whom they care.
- A valuable resource for the team physician is the Team Physician Consensus Conference (TPCC). This is a **project-based alliance** with partners including:
  - American Academy of Family Physicians;
  - American Academy of Orthopaedic Surgeons;
  - American Medical Society for Sports Medicine;
  - American Orthopaedic Society for Sports Medicine;
  - American Osteopathic Academy of Sports Medicine.
- The group meets to produce a consensus statement annually that addresses select medical issues in the care and treatment of athletes. The TPCC provides these documents to serve as guidance and teaching tools for physicians working in the field of sports medicine. Expert panel members formulate best practice statements that are supported by the literature using a format of **"essential" and "desirable"** information that the team physician is responsible for understanding.
  - **"Essential"** statements are information that every and any team physician must understand.
  - **"Desirable"** statements describe best practice in the settings where ample resources are available.
- All TPCC statements can be found on the ACSM website:
  - www.acsm.org/education-resources/pronouncements-scientific-communications/team-physician-consensus-statements;
  - The TPCC statements are additionally found in the online resources of this text, in Appendix A.
- Starting in 2000, with the last update in 2024, the TPCC issued a consensus statement on the duties and qualifications of a team physician (1). Since that time, the same conglomerate has published statements on sideline preparedness (2), concussion (3), conditioning (4), return to sport (5), and numerous other topics relevant to team physician care.
- The TPCC defines **required** educational qualifications for team physicians as follows:
  - Academic degree of M.D. or D.O. with unrestricted license in good standing
  - Board certification or eligibility in the core disciplines of emergency, family, or internal medicine; orthopedic surgery, pediatrics, PM&R, or osteopathic neuromuscular medicine
  - Training in fundamental aspects of on-field athlete and team care
  - Commitment to continuing medical education in sports medicine
- The TPCC lists **desirable** training and experiences as:
  - Board certification in the core disciplines listed above
  - Fellowship training and subsequent subspecialty certification (CAQ etc) in sports medicine
  - Active participation and membership in sports medicine professional associations
  - Continued contributions in sports medicine through education, research, advocacy activities
- Doctors from many specialties serve in the role of team physician, with primary care physicians comprising a majority. A recent survey from major U.S. men's and women's professional leagues shows that family medicine trained physicians occupy most primary care team physician roles. The breakdown of residency training for professional level primary care team physicians is: family medicine (55%), internal medicine (24%), emergency medicine (8%), PM&R (8%), pediatrics (4%), and other specialties (1%) (6).
- The team physician is part of a team of professionals that cares for the athletes and contributes to the athlete's success by maximizing training and competition preparation. They also assist by accurately diagnosing ailments and promptly, yet completely, rehabilitating injuries to return athletes to competition as quickly and safely as possible. In addition to expertise in the common medical conditions encountered in athletes, other necessary qualities include: flexibility and availability, good communication skills, a desire to educate, and an understanding of injury prevention principles (1). They also must be well prepared to respond to important issues such as sexual violence in sport; diversity, equity, and inclusion; and advocacy for athletes.

TIME REQUIREMENTS OF A TEAM PHYSICIAN

- The team physician must have an office schedule that can accommodate athletes with urgent and time-sensitive medical needs. Most team physicians have designated training room time each week, at least one to two evenings, where they can evaluate new and follow-up existing injuries of team members. Training room time is an especially important setting in which to communicate with the athletic trainer on the rehabilitation progress of athletes' injuries (4). An athlete's behavior and responses can vary widely, depending on the familiarity of the environment; therefore, training rooms should ideally be held in the athlete's "native environment," at a location convenient to the athletes and close to practice or training facilities.
- With the advent of the online medical record, the team physician must be decisive and quick to communicate, as patients often have diagnostic results promptly available to them. Patients, parents, and coaches often mistakenly assume that a lab test or an MRI image is the "ultimate truth" instead of appreciating that all clinical results have to be interpreted in a larger clinical context. A successful team physician prepares athletes and parents to receive uninterpreted results and then allow the medical team time to discuss and provide the best treatment plan.
- Although knowledge and ability are certainly important, the most valuable asset to the team physician is trust. Trust is earned by connecting to the athletes, coaches, and school officials.
- Team physicians often neglect team practices. Although it is not necessary that all practices be attended, occasional, brief appearances during practice allows the physician to gain insight into the environment and conditions in which the athletes train, the team's training regimen, and interactions between coaches and players. A better appreciation of all these factors can prove invaluable in the physician's medical decision making. In addition, brief appearances at practice help the physician build collegial relationships with coaches and players, establishing his or her role as a part of the team and distinguishing the physician from other officials, support staff, and media representatives who participate only in game-day activities.
- The amount of time spent at the actual competition depends on the team physician's role and availability, as well as on state laws and the regulations of the governing athletic association. Some laws mandate that a physician be in attendance for every game. Other laws allow nonphysician medical personnel, such as an athletic trainer, to cover an event with on-call physician backup (2).
- The clinician who is the team physician for an entire institution must decide whether to attend all the games for a few teams, or to attend a few games for every team. We recommend that team physicians attend at least part of one practice and at least one game for each team they supervise. Providing good "team medicine" is very difficult without observing the interactions and conditions of play and practice.

CORE KNOWLEDGE OF A TEAM PHYSICIAN

- To perform his or her duties effectively, a team physician needs an understanding of the medical conditions common to the athlete. This knowledge should encompass many areas of medicine, including but not limited to, orthopedics, cardiopulmonary medicine, neurology, dermatology, and rehabilitation (1).
- The team physician also needs expertise in pharmacology. Practical pharmacology for the team physician includes knowing how to treat illnesses, but also an understanding of performance-enhancing drugs and herbal medicines. Team physicians must be familiar with which substances are banned by the governing athletic association so that an athlete does not inadvertently lose eligibility to compete (6).
- A team physician must have a general knowledge of behavioral medicine and psychology. Mood disturbances and mental illnesses such as depression affect athletes and can be very common in injured athletes.
- Abuse, harassment, and bullying in sport remain serious issues at all levels of participation. Special training in these key issues can allow the team physician to respond appropriately and terminate any and all these practices. Team physicians must respond to and report any allegations of potential abuse. Prevention and effective treatment of abuse requires a multidisciplinary team of experts and professionals, not merely a single team physician. However, physicians should lead out in establishing and adhering to practices that promote athlete safety and in establishing a trusting atmosphere that facilitates open communication. For many abused athletes, the athletic medical team represents their only regular interaction with the medical community. Physicians should ensure that their medical team includes professionals who can support and treat athletes who have suffered abuse (5).
- A team physician's knowledge of exercise science and nutrition can help prevent injuries as well as maximize an athlete's performance (7). Disordered eating and overtraining can prove devastating if not recognized early and treated effectively (1).
- Perhaps the most critical element for the team physician, however, is leadership. Team physician leadership skills include effective communication, emotional intelligence, teamwork, selfless service, integrity, and critical thinking while utilizing an athlete-centered approach. These skills require development to lead an interdisciplinary sports medicine team (see Chapter 2, Leadership) (8).

MEDICAL RESPONSIBILITIES OF THE TEAM PHYSICIAN

- The first responsibility of a team physician is to determine whether an athlete is fit to participate. This evaluation most commonly occurs during the preparticipation physical. This examination may or may not be performed by the team physician, but the team physician should review its documentation so that he or she will be aware of any condition that may limit competition or predispose the athlete or other participants to injury. The preparticipation physical must be done before athletic training or participation — preferably 6–8 weeks before — so that all potentially disqualifying conditions can be fully evaluated without jeopardizing scheduled participation (2).
- Sideline and event coverage is the most obvious responsibility of the team physician. A physician should cover all collision and high-risk sports. Other athletic events can be covered by any allied health professional who is trained in recognition and initial treatment of athletic injuries (2). Team physicians must continually remind themselves that they are more than spectators. Each should be a "dispassionate observer," that is, the emotions of the competition must not affect medical decision making. Attention should be directed to the safety of the participants, not the immediate passions of the game.
- The team physician should focus attention on the aspects of play and the individuals who are prone to injury. In other words, the seasoned team physician will carefully follows the game, but not always follow the ball. For instance, in gridiron football, relatively little injury information can be gained by watching the flight of the ball on punts, kickoffs, and passes. Rather, injuries occur in — and attention should be focused on — lineman and quarterbacks after releasing the ball and wide receivers after catching the ball.
- The team physician must be prepared to handle nonparticipant emergencies because it is common for the team physician to be called on to treat an inadvertently involved coach, injured or sick referee, or emergently ill spectator. The team physician should verify that proper protocols and policies exist for medical emergencies involving spectators. The team physician may be the most qualified first responder, but he cannot assume final treatment responsibility for spectators because his first duty is toward the athletes on the field of play.
- The team physician maintains a sense of sideline awareness and encourages others to do the same. The team physician recognizes that the energy to play carries well beyond the field's sideline. The more advanced the athletic level, the greater the area of potential injury beyond the field of play. Many sideline personnel are distracted: cheerleaders, mascots, and photographers may be completely unaware of the action coming toward them. Even experienced coaches can be surprised and injured when the game suddenly "comes to them"(9,10). The individual who has a pass to the sidelines for the first time is often the most endangered person because he or she has very little concept of the speed of the game and the closeness of potential injury.
- The team physician ensures accurate diagnosis through the use of additional studies and specialty consults, communicates information regarding the player's condition clearly and confidentially to those who "need to know," coordinates the rehabilitation process, and determines when the athlete is able to compete again. This essential process involves active communication with athletes, parents, athletic trainers, physical therapists, coaches, administrators, and other medical specialists as necessary (11).
- Pursuing active follow-up with medical specialists is a critical duty. Team physicians may refer athletes to subspecialty providers to assist in treatment or with clearance for athletic participation; however, information from these visits does not naturally flow back to the team physician. Assuming that the specialty provider will call with any important information or that all pertinent information will flow back through the healthcare system will result in confusion for the team physician and danger for the athletes. Shadow files, "tickler lists," and other reminder systems can help team physicians actively and personally follow up on referrals, preventing the always embarrassing and often dangerous situations that result from incomplete medical communication between subspecialists and the team physician.
- Documentation of medical care is often mistakenly neglected in the team setting. The team physician needs to keep formal and confidential medical records that detail communication with consultants, give home treatment and follow-up instructions, and provide details for insurance and reimbursement purposes (11).
- The team physician should have the final say of when an athlete is initially cleared to begin competition and when a previously injured athlete may return to play (5). Although a detailed discussion of return-to-play criteria is beyond the scope of this chapter, several fundamental principles guide return-to-play decisions:
    - Injured athletes must have the muscular strength to perform adequately. Typically, the injured body part should have approximately 90% strength compared with the uninjured side or the player's normative strength. Athletes returned without adequate muscular strength rapidly revisit to the training room, often with a subsequent injury that is more severe than the first.
    - Before an athlete can return to play, he or she must demonstrate adequate agility. Contact athletes require full agility to protect themselves on the fields of friendly strife. Agility in noncontact athletes indicates the return of normal motor patterns that help protect against overuse injury. Strength and agility requirements vary widely between sports. An injured toe may be catastrophic to a basketball or football athlete and completely inconsequential to a rifle marksman.

- The returning athlete should pose no increased risk of injury to other players. Casts, splints, braces, and other protective equipment should be of a material suitable for safe competition.
- Finally, it should be recognized that clear thinking and intact cognition are required before any return to play or practice is considered. Further discussion on return to play is identified in Chapter 72, Principles of Rehabilitation and Return to Sport.

ADMINISTRATIVE RESPONSIBILITIES OF THE TEAM PHYSICIAN

- The team physician's primary concern is the coordination of medical supervision. This organization includes making sure qualified medical personnel are attending practices and competitions as needed, designing a plan for sideline evaluation, and having necessary medical equipment readily available. The team physician encourages defined roles and responsibilities for all involved in the medical care of the team, along with establishing a medical chain of command. The team physician may not make all the daily decisions but should have full authority concerning medical policy making.
- The team physician needs to lead the planning for and practicing of medical emergencies and urgencies. In addition to having an emergency treatment and transport plan, the team physician also must know the medical capabilities of surrounding hospitals — particularly around competition sites — so that injured athletes are brought to medical facilities that are best equipped to handle their specific medical problem (2).
- The team physician should become familiar and maintain familiarity with the rules and position statements established by the ACSM, the AMSSM, and other organizations. They should also maintain familiarity with regulations established by governing bodies of sport (*e.g.*, state high school athletic boards, the National Collegiate Athletic Association, Major League Baseball, and National Football League).
- The team physician should implement protocols that facilitate timely and quality medical care for situations when he or she is not immediately available. Preestablished guidelines for return to play are very helpful, especially when injuries to impact athletes result in high pressure for returning to competition before appropriate healing has occurred (1). The ACSM consensus statement on return-to-play issues more fully details the responsibilities of the team physician when returning athletes to competition (5).
- The team physician oversees the playing environment. He or she should evaluate both practice and game facilities for safety. A safe playing environment also involves appropriate and properly fitting protective equipment, available hydration, and an activity level appropriate for the climate.

MEDICOLEGAL CONCERNS FOR THE TEAM PHYSICIAN

- The team physician needs to consider the potential legal risks associated with team and event coverage. Through planning and awareness, they can ensure to protect themselves, the athlete, and the institution they represent (see Chapter 4, Medicolegal Considerations).
- Considerations for legal protection include the following:
  - Ensuring appropriate malpractice coverage. This can either come through their sponsoring institution or through self-funded insurance. A written contract or memorandum of understanding with the institution or team that defines responsibilities and expected level of coverage is essential — even if no compensation is to be received (11).
  - Team physicians routinely travel across state lines into other states where they do not have a license to practice medicine. Most state legislatures have passed an exemption for traveling team physicians, but some have not (12). Staying up to date on these laws is important to protect the physician from negative legal ramifications. Of note, the U.S. Congress has passed a bill allowing the physician to care for the team and the travel support group, within the scope of their practice.
  - If traveling across country lines with a team for coverage, it is best to check with your sponsoring institution to ensure their malpractice covers you in the country where the event is being held.
  - "Good Samaritan" laws exist in many states, but the exact law varies widely between different jurisdictions. Most such laws apply only if the physician is receiving no compensation for his or her services. Compensation may be defined by a specific dollar amount or be as little as receiving a team shirt to wear at games!
  - Medical Ethics: The team physician becoming an integral part of athletic culture has led to unique ethical dilemmas such as confidentiality, patient autonomy, informed consent, third parties, and advertising. Having legal protection and a team to help navigate these dilemmas is essential when ethical conflicts arise (see Chapter 3, Ethical Considerations in Sports Medicine) (13).

COMMUNICATION RESPONSIBILITIES OF A TEAM PHYSICIAN

- For a team to receive optimal medical care, the team physician and athletic trainer must communicate openly and clearly. Even before the season, they need to discuss medical treatment protocols, which preferably are documented in writing (11). When an injury occurs, there can be no confusion over who will go on the field for initial evaluation and who will communicate to the coach the extent of an athlete's injury and playing status.

- A potentially contentious area between team physicians, athletes, coaches, and school officials is the ordering of a magnetic resonance imaging (MRI) study. For physicians in nonsport settings, MRI scans are typically used as a diagnostic tool, to confirm a suspected diagnosis. In sports medicine, however, the MRI scan is more of a management tool. Although the team physician may not need an MRI study to make the diagnosis, an early MRI scan can allow team officials, coaches, and the athlete to get on the same page with the team physician. This shared unity results in management decisions that are timelier, better coordinated, and ultimately more appropriate for the athlete. Total player management includes not only medical management, but also administrative management. Administrative management may involve placing the player on injured reserves or the disabled list or beginning an application for a redshirt year. In addition to building unity among the management team, MRI often has mystical healing powers! For worried athletes, an MRI scan has not only diagnostic, but also mentally therapeutic effects. Early and timely MRI scans often require a strong working relationship with musculoskeletal radiologists and local radiology departments. Making them part of the medical team by providing them access to games or sideline passes can assist in developing this rapport.
- A team physician needs to develop good rapport with the coach. Offering injury prevention suggestions and player health education may demonstrate to the coach a shared desire to assist the team attaining their goals. Most importantly, a team physician must keep the coach informed of an injured player's ability to continue to compete safely. Without breaching player confidentially, the team physician should provide the coach with a time frame for further evaluation or the player's return. In general, this information should be communicated in terms of a sport-specific timeline, such as the player is out for a play, the player is out for a series, reassessment will be done at half-time or the game's end, or the player is likely out for the rest of the season.
- With technology advancements and patient access to the online medical record, the patient often has their test results almost in real time. As a result, the athlete will occasionally have the results of their diagnostic tests prior to the team physician. With this rapid dissemination of information, the team physician needs to stay apprised of the various tests being performed on their athletes and can quickly respond to questions regarding these tests if approached. This may include rapid consultation with specialists in regard to surgical decisions so the physician can provide a plan to the awaiting athlete and their supportive staff.
- Not all diagnostic, treatment, and return to play situations in sports medicine are clear cut. The healing or recovery process is dependent on multiple factors. This makes shared decision making an important principle for the team physician to master. It applies in all situations but is imperative when evidence is inadequate, or the clinical question is complex. Through these conversations, clinicians can help patients achieve greater autonomy and take ownership of the variable outcomes (14).
- The team physician may also be required to discuss a player's medical condition with school officials. Administrators often need to know specifics regarding physician recommendations, for example, how long the player will miss the class or be in the hospital. They seldom need to know medical or personal details of the athlete's situation. Remember that the athlete's confidentiality is the first concern.
- Members of the media rarely, if ever, need information from the team physician. Well-defined criteria for dealing with the media should be established. If a team physician is encouraged to participate in an interview, insist that written questions be submitted beforehand so that appropriate remarks can be constructed for the record. These planned responses can be reviewed with team coaches, athletic trainers, and administrators to ensure consistency, accuracy, and regard for the athlete's privacy.
- With social media readily accessible, the team physician and the athletic support staff must be cognizant of and committed to following the Health Insurance Portability and Accountability Act (HIPAA). They must strictly avoid discussing or reporting the condition of their athletes on social media platforms. They must also be aware that care of the athlete may be publicized by others through social media and so it is important to communicate the importance of confidentiality to all parties involved in the care of the athlete, including family and friends. Athletes, of course, have the legal right to share any of their health status they choose — but counseling from physicians, athletic trainers, and administrators can help ensure that this is done in a mature, thoughtful manner that shows respect for all members of the team.

OTHER CONSIDERATIONS FOR THE TEAM PHYSICIAN

- Sports medicine abounds with opportunities for research. Simply keeping accurate epidemiologic and injury data has the potential to impact training regimens, competition rules, or mandates for protective equipment (15). Injury surveillance is very important to preventative sports medicine and advances the safety of sport much better than any surgical technique or new prescription drug.
- The dedicated team physician uses his or her observations and recorded injury data to prevent future injuries on his or her teams. Observing a rise in concussions will prompt a review of the team's helmets or the tackling technique. An increase in acromioclavicular separations may trigger an inspection of shoulder pads. An outbreak of rashes, abscesses, or other skin conditions should prompt a review of sanitation, equipment, and laundry procedures.
- The astute team physician ensures that injury and outcome data are gathered, stored, and shared using methods that are HIPAA compliant. Sharing data across team, league, and state boundaries is essential to future efforts to prevent injury, but the privacy of the individual athlete must be protected.

- Judgment and good sense are required when evaluating new injury prevention programs. Team physicians must be open and responsive to proven changes that will benefit and protect their athletes, but they cannot afford to simply follow the latest fad. Judgment is also required when treating injuries to ensure that treatment decisions made for professional athletes are not automatically translated into other echelons of sport. Ulnar collateral surgery may be absolutely indicated in a 34-year-old major league pitcher. Does that make it right for a 16-year-old high school pitcher?
- Compensation as a team physician is variable. Almost all work with teams competing at lower than the collegiate level is voluntary. Deferring offers for nominal remuneration in favor of paying an athletic trainer's salary will likely benefit the athletes and the team physician (11). Almost all team physicians work with athletic teams solely for professional and personal satisfaction because of their interest in sports and athletes.
- Sponsorship and advertising are other considerations the team physician must be aware of. In many situations, a healthcare group or practice may sponsor a sporting event or team. Sponsorship is encouraged because there are many benefits to be gained that include but are not limited to: protection of the team physician through an extension of malpractice coverage, advertising for the sponsor and associated physician, opportunities for service within the community. Having a sponsoring institution also provides a separation between the athletic team and the medical decision makers. This separation provides protection for the athletes because it takes the decision to play from the confines of the team and puts it into the hands of a secondary group or physician that can objectively decide if an athlete is safe to return to play without fear of repercussions from team management. However, physicians who are employed by sponsoring entities need to be aware of potential pitfalls of privacy, perceived conflict of interest, Stark law, and other regulatory entanglements. Team sponsorship, such as team coverage, is a team sport (16).

REFERENCES

1. Herring SA, Putukian M, Leclere LE, et al. The team physician consensus statement 2024 update. *Med Sci Sports Exerc.* 2025;57(5):1067–75. doi:10.1249/MSS.0000000000003641
2. Herring SA, Bergfeld J, Boyd J, et al. Sideline preparedness for the team physician: a consensus statement. *Med Sci Sports Exerc.* 2001;33(5):846–9.
3. Herring S, Kibler WB, Putukian M, et al. Selected issues in sport-related concussion (SRC|mild traumatic brain injury) for the team physician: a consensus statement. *Br J Sports Med.* 202;55:1251–61.
4. Load, overload, and recovery in the athlete: select issues for the team physician—a consensus statement. *Med Sci Sports Exerc.* 2019;51(4):821–8. doi:10.1249/MSS.0000000000001910
5. Herring SA, Putukian M, Kibler WB, et al. Team physician consensus statement: return to sport/return to play and the team physician: a team physician consensus statement—2023 update. *Med Sci Sports Exer.* 2024;56(5):767–75. doi:10.1249/MSS.0000000000003371
6. Schultz EA, Durtschi MS, Oakes KG, Kussman A, Hwang CE. Training background and demographic characteristics of primary care team physicians in professional sports. *Orthop J Sports Med.* 2024;12(4). doi:10.1177/23259671241242412
7. Herring SA, Bergfeld JA, Bernhardt DT, et al. Selected issues for the adolescent athlete and the team physician: a consensus statement. *Med Sci Sports Exerc.* 2008;40(11):1997–2012.
8. Tayne S, Hutchinson MR, O'Connor FG, Taylor DC, Musahl V, Indelicato P. Leadership for the team physician. *Curr Sports Med Rep.* 2020 Mar;19(3):119–23.
9. Associated Press. *Paterno Fractured Leg Bone During Sideline Collision* [Internet]. 2011 [cited 2011 Jul 11]. Available from: http://sports.espn.go.com/ncf/news/story?id=2650560
10. Associated Press. *Weis Tears ACL and MCL on Sideline* [Internet]. 2011 [cited 2011 Jul]. Available from: http://nbcsports.msnbc.com/id/26690497
11. Rice SG. The high school athlete: setting up a high school sports medicine program. In: Mellion MB, Walsh WM, Madden C, Putukian M, Shelton GL, editors. *Team Physician's Handbook.* 3rd ed. Philadelphia (PA): Hanley & Belfus; 2002. p. 67–77.
12. Sports Medicine Practice Tools. *The American Medical Society for Sports Medicine*; 2022. https://www.amssm.org/PracticeTools.html
13. Testoni D, Hornik CP, Smith PB, Benjamin DK Jr, McKinney RE Jr. Sports medicine and ethics. *Am J Bioeth.* 2013;13(10):4–12. doi:10.1080/15265161.2013.828114
14. Epstein RM, Gramling RE. What is shared in shared decision making? Complex decisions when the evidence is unclear. *Med Care Res Rev.* 2013 Feb;70(1 suppl l):94S–112S.
15. Rice SG. Development of an injury surveillance system: results from a longitudinal study of high school athletes. In: Ashare AB, editors. *Safety in Ice Hockey.* West Conshohocken (PA): ASTM; 2000. p. 3–18.
16. American Academy of Family Physicians, American Academy of Orthopaedic Surgeons, American College of Sports Medicine, et al. Selected issues for the master athlete and the team physician: a consensus statement. *Med Sci Sports Exerc.* 2010;42(4):820–33.

Leadership in Sports Medicine

2

Jonathon M. Florance, Elizabeth C. Bond, Taylor P. Stauffer, and Dean C. Taylor

INTRODUCTION

- The definition of *Leadership in Health Care* is the ability to influence others for the benefit of patients and patient populations. *Leadership in Sports Medicine* shares an emphasis on the patient but includes the context of the athletic teams within which we work. Team physicians play an important leadership role in their organizations by the nature of this responsibility to athletes as patients (1).
- Leaders provide a vision and communicate it effectively. A sports medicine leader's vision aligns the team on the common goal of patient care while affording individual team members flexibility and autonomy commensurate with their training and aptitude. Providing purpose, direction, and motivation, while allowing team members the opportunity to demonstrate initiative, is the application of sports medicine leadership (2).
- Emotional intelligence (EI) is a foundational competency of leadership that includes the domains of self-awareness, self-management, social awareness, and relationship management (3). These elements allow leaders to influence groups by understanding themselves and how they interact with others. The relevance of EI to both leadership and medical competency has been endorsed consistently in medical literature, which demonstrates increased job satisfaction and decreased burnout with emphasis on EI skills (4,5).

HEALTH CARE MODELS OF LEADERSHIP

- Leadership models serve as a useful starting point, seeking to provide lasting comprehension by communicating concepts through simple structure (6).
- The structure of a model can help guide self-development or formal leadership curricula within an organization. This is important as leadership can be developed and improved through careful attention and training.
- Many leadership models exist, but few are both specific to health care and derived from an academically rigorous methodology. For these points, we favor the Duke Healthcare Leadership Model, created using a mixed qualitative-quantitative concept mapping approach where a diverse group of 92 faculty and trainees individually rank-sorted leadership competency statements. Combining the results from hierarchical cluster analysis with qualitative data led to the model seen in Figure 2.1 (7).

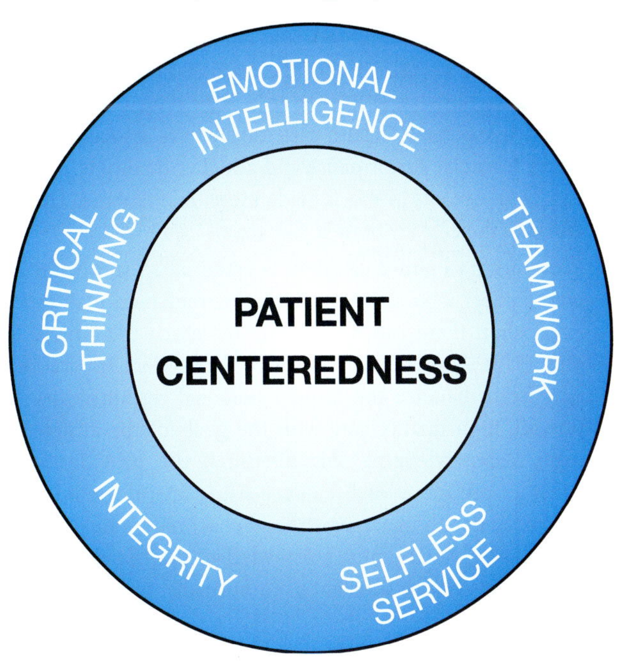

Figure 2.1: Duke Healthcare Leadership Model. (Used with permission from Dean C. Taylor, MD.)

- In the Duke Healthcare Leadership Model, patient-centeredness is intentionally positioned centrally as a core principle flanked with core competencies: emotional intelligence as the "keystone" at the top of the model, service and integrity positioned at the bottom as foundational competencies, and critical thinking and teamwork as pillars to provide structure (8).

LEADERSHIP CONSIDERATIONS IN PRACTICE

- Leaders in sports medicine function in a variety of locations and capacities, with the most common being in the clinic, in the operating room, and during sports team coverage. While these functions each have different facets, they have some of the following reoccurring elements.
- Mentorship allows leaders to develop team members as they work under a shared vision, while also enabling job satisfaction and potentially aiding in promoting a long-term career in academic medicine (9,10). Mentorship involves a senior individual counseling and guiding more junior individuals in growth and career development. While there can be different elements to being a good mentor, they often have a growth mindset, listen actively, promote trust, and help set goals (11).
- Coaching builds competency within the team while improving burnout and resiliency (12,13). Coaching is frequently confused with mentoring, but coaches do not give direction and instead help guide self-reflection. Coaches help others identify their strengths and weaknesses, and collaborate in idea generation (14). As a leader in sports medicine, you can benefit from coaching and foster a culture of coaching within the health care team.
- Fostering Diversity, Equity, and Inclusion (DEI) is a critical leadership tenet that serves to enhance the advancement of all people for the good of the organization (15). Beyond appeals to fairness, according to a 2019 review of diversity research specific to health care, diversity is associated with better financial performance and a higher quality of patient care (16). Leaders in sports medicine should embrace DEI to enhance the efficacy of their care teams.
- Promoting a culture of safety is essential to sports medicine leaders who are responsible for return-to-play guidance when there can be pressure to return the athlete to play (17). A particular challenge for leaders in practice may be to balance the leader's personal responsibility to provide high-quality care with the goals of the athlete or team. Acknowledging this dilemma, the provider may consider an operational balance using an integrated performance health management and coaching model (18). In such cases, leaders must acknowledge that the risk of too early return can be substantial emotionally, financially, and legally (19).

Leadership Considerations for the Clinic

- The clinic team is characterized by a small group of core members who work in parallel to accomplish a high number of short encounters. This environment is predicated upon efficiency and coordination of external resources.
- Empower team members to operate at the top of their scope of practice; however, a leader can only delegate authority, not responsibility. The leader is ultimately responsible for the conduct of the clinic.
- Communicating guidance and expectations among team members helps synchronize efforts.
- Early and repeated review of the schedule identifies friction points and enables the appropriate allocation of resources.
- With increasing demands on the time of each teammate, focusing the team on mission essential tasks can help streamline throughput and consolidate nonurgent tasks.
- Reinforcing through recognition or praise can be an especially powerful means of encouraging autonomy. In providing feedback, research suggests that focusing on the process instead of the person is more beneficial to enhancing development (20).
- High-reliability organizations have a preoccupation with failure (21). Observe for variance, carefully analyze why it occurs, and pursue systemic changes to prevent further occurrences.

Leadership Considerations for the Operating Room

- The operative room is a no-fail, high-stress environment where hierarchy in execution is balanced by highly trained team members each providing essential expertise.
- Establish collegiality at the morning huddle by encouraging open communication for safety issues. Encourage teammates to subside individual egos, and demonstrate deference to each teammate's expertise. Parallels have been drawn between surgical teams and aviation teams, specifically citing poor communication and interpersonal relations as behaviors that increase risk (22).
- Preoperative mental rehearsals that include alternate and subsequent courses of action can expedite execution in times of crisis and ensure availability of equipment (23).
- Utilize the preoperative timeout to role model sensitivity to operations, where organizations remain actively engaged in routine operations. Checklists and handover protocols, common in Formula 1 and aviation, have been shown to help avoid complacency and decrease technical errors (24).
- Clearly communicate setbacks or changes to plan, remaining calm while conveying gravitas of new developments.
- Demonstrate "extreme" ownership by accepting responsibility for everything that happens, a burden that can necessitate quick decision making from the leader and speedy execution from the team (25).

- After-action reviews instill a learning culture. Commit to resilience by accepting and openly discussing failures as opportunities to improve. This process enables reflection in real time and offers an ability for the team to improve during the next case.

Leadership Considerations for Team Coverage

- Sporting events can require substantial medical support, where the medical team can become large and complex. Leaders in this environment need to utilize extensive planning and decentralized teams.
- Clearly delineating and publishing tasks to empower individuals within broad guidance supports decentralized operations while ensuring unity of effort. Duties and responsibilities of physicians and athletic trainers in these settings have been described (26).
- Leaders demonstrate commitment with their presence, attend low-profile team events the same as larger game days. Check in with teammates often, demonstrating a commitment to servant leadership through trust and empowerment (27).
- When coordinating medical support for large events, carefully build and publish a responsive chain of command. Depending on responsibilities, ensure mid-level leaders are not overwhelmed by their "Span of Control," or the number of people directly reporting to them (28).
- Ensure a robust medical treatment and evacuation capability for emergencies, and then rehearse (29).
- Enlist a colleague to critique the medical support plan, working together to find scenarios that demonstrate gaps in planning. Leaders can ensure plan redundancy by covering these gaps.

LIFELONG DEVELOPMENT OF LEADERSHIP

- Developing as a leader follows many of the same principles as developing members of the team: seeking mentorship from other leaders, being open to coaching from peers, and affording time for self-reflection.
- Recognizing the underemphasis of leadership topics in traditional medical curricula, relying on a guiding leadership model can be helpful in focusing lifelong learning (30,31).
- Embracing new leadership roles and being open to opportunities can provide experience that helps build skills incrementally. Analyzing failure with careful attention to lessons learned can be a powerful source of improvement.
- Numerous external leadership development programs exist in orthopedic surgery including the American Orthopaedic Association (AOA) Emerging Leaders Program, Association of American Medical Colleges Early Career Women Faculty Leadership Development Seminar, Specialty Society Leadership Training, and the AOA North American Traveling Fellowship, among others (32).

THE CASE FOR SPORTS MEDICINE LEADERSHIP

- There is an incredible need for leadership in medicine. As the health care landscape continues to evolve in the 21st century, capable and adaptive leaders will be essential in maintaining the focus on patient-centered care.
- As a large multidisciplinary subspecialty, sports medicine offers an opportunity to meet this leadership need. The preeminence of team culture, where players are accustomed to sacrificing for each other, forms a welcoming environment for leaders who are committed to the development and success of their teammates. And benefiting from the proximity to incredible legends of elite athleticism, medical leaders can find inspirational examples of core translational values to serve as rallying points for others in the medical profession.

SUMMARY

- *Leadership in Health Care* is the ability to influence others for the benefit of patients and patient populations. *Leadership in Sports Medicine* shares an emphasis on the patient but includes the context of the athletic teams within which we work.
- Leaders in sports medicine function in a variety of locations and capacities with the most common being in the clinic, in the operating room, and during sports team coverage. While these functions each have different facets, they have reoccurring elements to include mentoring, coaching, DEI, and promoting a culture of safety.
- Leadership health care models can help guide self-development or formal leadership curricula within an organization. Individuals should seek to develop their leadership skills over their career.

REFERENCES

1. Herring SA, Kibler WB, Putukian M. Team physician consensus statement: 2013 update. *Med Sci Sports Exerc.* 2013 Aug;45(8):1618–22. doi:10.1249/MSS.0b013e31829ba437
2. *U.S. Department of the Army, Army Leadership and the Profession, Army Doctrine Publications (ADP)* 6-22. Washington (DC): U.S. Department of the Army. 2019 Jul.
3. White BAA, Quinn JF. Personal growth and emotional intelligence: foundational skills for the leader. *Clin Sports Med.* 2023 Apr;42(2):261–7. doi:10.1016/j.csm.2022.11.008

4. Abi-Jaoudé JG, Kennedy-Metz LR, Dias RD, Yule SJ, Zenati MA. Measuring and improving emotional intelligence in surgery: a systematic review. *Ann Surg.* 2022 Feb 1;275(2):e353–60. doi:10.1097/SLA.0000000000005022
5. Mintz LJ, Stoller JK. A systematic review of physician leadership and emotional intelligence. *J Grad Med Educ.* 2014 Mar;6(1):21–31. doi:10.4300/JGME-D-13-00012.1
6. Snook S, Nohria N, Khurana R, editors. *The Handbook for Teaching Leadership: Knowing, Doing, and Being.* Thousand Oaks (CA): Sage; 2012.
7. Hargett CW, Doty JP, Hauck JN, et al. Developing a model for effective leadership in healthcare: a concept mapping approach. *J Healthc Leadersh.* 2017 Aug 28;9:69–78. doi:10.2147/JHL.S141664
8. Taylor DC, Hettrich CM, Dickens JF, Doty J. Coaching, mentorship, and leadership in medicine: empowering the development of patient-centered care. *Clin Sports Med.* 2023 Apr;42(2):xv–xviii. doi:10.1016/j.csm.2023.01.001
9. Efstathiou JA, Drumm MR, Paly JP, et al. Long-term impact of a faculty mentoring program in academic medicine. *PLoS One.* 2018 Nov 29;13(11):e0207634. doi:10.1371/journal.pone.0207634
10. Jackson VA, Palepu A, Szalacha L, Caswell C, Carr PL, Inui T. “Having the right chemistry”: a qualitative study of mentoring in academic medicine. *Acad Med.* 2003 Mar;78(3):328–34. doi:10.1097/00001888-200303000-00020
11. West R. How to become a mentor and be good at it. *Clin Sports Med.* 2023 Apr;42(2):233–9. doi:10.1016/j.csm.2022.12.003
12. Theeboom T, Beersma B, van Vianen AE. Does coaching work? A meta-analysis on the effects of coaching on individual level outcomes in an organizational context. *J Posit Psychol.* 2014;9(1):1–18.
13. Dyrbye LN, Gill PR, Satele DV, West CP. Professional coaching and surgeon well-being: a randomized controlled trial. *Ann Surg.* 2023 Apr 1;277(4):565–71. doi:10.1097/SLA.0000000000005678
14. Lepre-Nolan M, Houde LD. Lessons from executive coaches: why you need one. *Clin Sports Med.* 2023 Apr;42(2):185–93. doi:10.1016/j.csm.2022.11.005
15. Coleman LR, Taylor ED. The importance of diversity, equity, and Inclusion for effective, ethical leadership. *Clin Sports Med.* 2023 Apr;42(2):269–80. doi:10.1016/j.csm.2022.11.002
16. Gomez LE, Bernet P. Diversity improves performance and outcomes. *J Natl Med Assoc.* 2019 Aug;111(4):383–92. doi:10.1016/j.jnma.2019.01.006
17. Kroshus E, Baugh CM, Daneshvar DH, Stamm JM, Laursen RM, Austin SB. Pressure on sports medicine clinicians to prematurely return collegiate athletes to play after concussion. *J Athl Train.* 2015 Sep;50(9):944–51. doi:10.4085/1062-6050-50.6.03
18. Dijkstra HP, Pollock N, Chakraverty R, Alonso JM. Managing the health of the elite athlete: a new integrated performance health management and coaching model. *Br J Sports Med.* 2014 Apr;48(7):523–31. doi:10.1136/bjsports-2013-093222
19. Sanders AK, Boggess BR, Koenig SJ, Toth AP. Medicolegal issues in sports medicine. *Clin Orthop Relat Res.* 2005 Apr;433:38–49. doi:10.1097/01.blo.0000159764.03919.33
20. Kamins ML, Dweck CS. Person versus process praise and criticism: implications for contingent self-worth and coping. *Dev Psychol.* 1999 May;35(3):835–47. doi:10.1037//0012-1649.35.3.835
21. Sutcliffe KM. High reliability organizations (HROs). *Best Pract Res Clin Anaesthesiol.* 2011 Jun;25(2):133–44. doi:10.1016/j.bpa.2011.03.001
22. Helmreich RL. On error management: lessons from aviation. *BMJ.* 2000 Mar 18;320(7237):781–5. doi:10.1136/bmj.320.7237.781
23. Eldred-Evans D, Grange P, Cheang A, et al. Using the mind as a simulator: a randomized controlled trial of mental training. *J Surg Educ.* 2013 Jul-Aug;70(4):544–51. doi:10.1016/j.jsurg.2013.04.003
24. Catchpole KR, De Leval MR, McEwan A, et al. Patient handover from surgery to intensive care: using Formula 1 pit-stop and aviation models to improve safety and quality. *Paediatr Anaesth.* 2007;17(5):470–8.
25. Willink J, Babin L. *Extreme Ownership: How US Navy SEALs lead and Win.* St. Martin's Press; 2017.
26. Courson R, Goldenberg M, Adams KG, et al. Inter-association consensus statement on best practices for sports medicine management for secondary schools and colleges. *J Athl Train.* 2014 Jan–Feb;49(1):128–37. doi:10.4085/1062-6050-49.1.06
27. Trastek VF, Hamilton NW, Niles EE. Leadership models in health care - a case for servant leadership. *Mayo Clin Proc.* 2014 Mar;89(3):374–81. doi:10.1016/j.mayocp.2013.10.012
28. Lucas V, Laschinger HK, Wong CA. The impact of emotional intelligent leadership on staff nurse empowerment: the moderating effect of span of control. *J Nurs Manag.* 2008 Nov;16(8):964–73. doi:10.1111/j.1365-2834.2008.00856.x
29. Andersen J, Courson RW, Kleiner DM, McLoda TA. National athletic trainers' association position statement: emergency planning in athletics. *J Athl Train.* 2002 Mar;37(1):99–104.
30. Doty J, Taylor D. Developing physician leaders. *Curr Sports Med Rep.* 2019 Feb;18(2):45. doi:10.1249/JSR.0000000000000561
31. Tayne S, Hutchinson MR, O'Connor FG, Taylor DC, Musahl V, Indelicato P. Leadership for the team physician. *Curr Sports Med Rep.* 2020 Mar;19(3):119–23. doi:10.1249/JSR.0000000000000696
32. Clark SC, Miskimin C, Mulcahey MK. Leadership in orthopaedic surgery: a survey of the value of leadership development for orthopaedic surgery faculty. *J Am Acad Orthop Surg Glob Res Rev.* 2021 Oct 27;5(10):e21.00119. doi:10.5435/JAAOSGlobal-D-21-00119

3

Ethical Considerations in Sports Medicine

Korin B. Hudson, Francis G. O'Connor, and Christopher E. Jonas

INTRODUCTION

- Ethical challenges are present for all clinicians, including the team physician (1).
- Ethics in general terms may be defined as conforming to accepted standards or principles of conduct.
  - No one achieves ethical perfection, but most sports medicine physicians are good by nature and guided by high ethical standards.
  - Sports are considered to reflect values generally thought to be important to the society: character building, health promotion as well as pursuit of competitive excellence and enjoyment (2).
- Ethical considerations in the area of sports medicine are similar to those in medicine in general, including basic concepts (3–5):
  - *Beneficence*: the principle of only performing acts and making recommendations that are potentially beneficial to an athlete. This is the overriding principle.
  - *Nonmaleficence*: "first do no harm," this principle prohibits clinicians from providing recommendations that may be detrimental to an athlete's short-term and long-term health. This should be considered with every action taken in the training room or medical setting when tending to an injured athlete.
  - *Justice*: maximizing benefit to patients and society while emphasizing equality, fairness, and impartiality.
  - *Autonomy*: respecting the individual patient and their rights and ability to make decisions with regard to their own health and future; a right to self-determination. This is inherent in informed consent.

PHYSICIAN RESPONSIBILITIES

- The sports physician's primary duty is to maintain or restore athlete health and functional ability whenever possible (6).
  - The health and welfare of the athlete must guide all efforts; the physician should not be influenced or encumbered by desires or requests by athletes, coaches, or other third parties that may not be in the athlete's best interest (6).
  - Special care must be given to the protection of athletes (7).
  - Whether a decision involves a diagnostic test, medical treatment, or the athlete's eligibility, the end result should be maintenance of good health with the least risk to the athlete.
- Inherent in the ethical relationship between athlete and physician are confidentiality, truthfulness, and shared decision making. These are essential in sports-related medical decision making.
  - Although autonomy is respected, athletes can and should rely on their sports physician to lead them in the shared decision-making process.
  - To make informed decisions and participate in decision-making processes, the injured athlete must understand the diagnosis, comprehend its implications, be able to weigh risks and benefits of treatments, and participate in all therapeutic decisions.
- Conflict between physician and athlete should always be minimized. Should conflict or difference of opinions arise, the physician should use all reasonable means to resolve any conflicts that arise (8).
- A good sports physician must have a genuine appreciation for the importance of athletics in an athlete's life and must recognize that harm may result equally from unnecessary or excessive restriction from activity as it can from failure to restrict activity when appropriate.
- All sports medicine physicians gain knowledge, wisdom, and better judgment with experience, recognizing that nearly all interventions have risks as well as benefits.
- Recognizing the wide range of opinions and expertise, as well as individual fallibility, athlete-patients can (and should) assert their right to a second opinion. And the sports physician should accept this request and provide these referrals without personal affront.
  - The referred patient should not be abandoned. The consultant may gain insight from the referring physician, and this affords the athlete continuing support from their primary sports physician.

- Although sports physicians will ideally be able to treat most patients, they must be aware of their own level of competence and know when and where to provide additional referral for specialized consultation or therapy. It is essential to know colleagues' ability, personality, and empathy for athletes to make appropriate referrals (9).
- There is no obligation to accept, without question, recommendations of consultants, especially if recommendations are incongruent with the referring physician's knowledge of the patient.

- The sports physician does not work in isolation. To make sports-oriented medical decisions, one must be well versed in current recommendations for eligibility and continued participation and not depend on their own limited personal experience or nonscientific reasoning (6).
- Continuing education of sports physicians' aids in the development of a suitable skill level, knowledge, and their maintenance (10). It is the responsibility of physicians to maintain knowledge and technical skills associated with their specialty.
- Those conducting research in sports medicine must follow the highest ethical standards (11).
- Adherence to these principles and fulfilling these responsibilities help foster trust between athletes and physicians, allowing a more comfortable decision-making process (12).

POTENTIAL FOR DUAL AGENCY

- Dual agency, also identified as mixed agency, refers to the conflicts and potential for unethical breaches that may occur when a clinician has duties to different entities that may come into conflict (13).
- It is increasingly common for physicians to be employed by a school system, club, or team, and not directly by athletes.
- An employed sports physician must always continue to respect the athlete's autonomy in medical decision making, while advising against any decision that could compromise the athlete's health and athletic career.
- If a sports physician is employed by a school, team, or similar entity, the sports physician's primary role remains advocating for the athlete's welfare, while simultaneously protecting team or school interests.
- This dual role may lead an athlete to question whether the physician prioritizes the best interests of the team or the athlete.
  - A salaried physician indeed has a potential conflict of interest that may interfere with the traditional doctor-patient relationship. Objective professional duties may be compromised by personal interests (*e.g.*, financial reward of a professional team association, as well as publicity and high visibility one may get from such a position).
  - Athletes may feel that their care is secondary to the physician's obligation to team owners and/or coaches (14). Although less common in high school or collegiate sports, this may lead to distrust between athletes and team physicians, particularly at the professional level (15).
- At times, athlete welfare may appear to be in conflict with wishes of parents, spouse, coaches, or team management, but the sports physician's priority should remain to the continued well-being of the athlete including fostering a healthy physician-patient relationship.
  - Medical decisions should be based on sound clinical judgment. If any third party (*e.g.*, a university or professional team) does not follow reasonable recommendations, there may be cause for the physician to cease providing services for that party (14).
- If the athlete's wishes/demands conflict with what the physician believes to be in the athlete's best interest and the conflict cannot be resolved, the physician should consider a second opinion, or the athlete should be reassigned to another physician (15).
- In professional sports, the unfavorable mix of high salaries and short careers can precipitate risky decision making by both athletes and physicians.
  - The physician must take great care to avoid becoming overly concerned with the team's record or athlete's statistics, rather remaining most concerned with the athlete's health.
  - Coaches may seek to encourage physicians to allow players to return earlier than they would otherwise be permitted to do so, and players themselves may desire to return to the field of play too quickly (16).
  - The team physician's actions should demonstrate a primary responsibility to the players' safety and well-being, and the physician should not allow players to be on the field who are not truly medically qualified (17).
- Furthermore, any athlete with a poor or unexpected outcome or any untimely death may undermine trust in the team physician.

DRUG USE

- Therapeutic medications are common in sports medicine. Used appropriately, they may control pain and inflammation, speed recovery, and hasten return to function.
- Sports physicians are obligated to know each drug thoroughly, especially efficacies, potential side effect(s), and any effects on safety or on the athlete's performance.
- Appropriate reference to World Anti-Doping Agency (WADA), United States Anti-Doping Agency (USADA), and

other applicable banned substance listings is of utmost importance for the sports medicine physician.

- The sports physician must not expose athletes to potential disqualification by prescribing a medication(s) known to be on the prohibited list (*e.g.*, as in the prevention of exercise-induced asthma) when an effective alternative and legal option is available.

CONFIDENTIALITY

- All athletes have a right to confidentiality, despite the fact that many may lead public lives (14).
  - Despite claims regarding the public's "right to know," right to privacy remains with the athlete-patient (4).
  - All inquiries made of sports physicians by the press or other interested parties should go unanswered or be referred to the athlete or their representative, unless specific comment has been permitted/requested by the athlete.
  - Great care must be taken regarding social media (18).
  - Permission to discuss medical information should be in writing and explicitly outline information that can be revealed.
- On occasion, a sports physician may advise an athlete regarding the amount and type of information to release to coaches (considering here the athlete's private sports physician, not one employed by a school or professional team). This is important when restriction from practice or competition is necessary.

RELATIONSHIP WITH COLLEAGUES

- Sports medicine is often multidisciplinary.
  - In elite and professional sports, the number of healthcare and sports performance professionals involved in athlete care is ever increasing.
  - It is critical to include the athlete in determining which professionals should be included in medical discussions.
  - Conflict can arise between a team physician and other medical professionals participating in care of the athlete. Sports physicians must insist all adhere to high ethical standards.
- The sports physician should never criticize the actions of another medical professional.
  - Private discussions with other medical professionals should occur regarding recommended therapy.
  - The sports physician is in a position to positively influence knowledge of other medical professionals by providing positive, collegial input.
- If inappropriate playing restrictions or early return have been recommended by another physician, the sports physician should perform an individual assessment of the athlete's return-to-play status.
- The sports medicine physician has an obligation to expose unproven, unethical, non–evidence-based or potentially dangerous practices, thus protecting athletes and their careers.

FEAR OF LEGAL ENTANGLEMENT

- Simply put, physicians should never allow fear of litigation to affect their medical decision making or clinical recommendations. When faced with a life-threatening situation or a potentially disabling condition, the physician should always have foremost consideration for the athlete's health and safety while allowing the athlete to share in decision-making.
- While maintaining highest ethical standards and practicing evidence-based medicine, poor or unexpected outcomes should not adversely affect a physician's role in care of other athletes.
  - A sports physician who is not afraid to make correct recommendations in a difficult medical situation should be sought out by other physicians and athletes.

SUMMARY

- Sports medicine requires ethical treatment of athletes in all situations (19).
- The physician must be devoted to confidentiality, informed consent, and truthfulness.
- The physician must be aware there is uncertainty in some decisions, and at times there may be no right/wrong answer. Decisions should be based on the literature and experience. Shared decision-making with the athlete and other stakeholders is critical.
- The physician must be familiar with unethical means of enhancing performance and should discourage and/or disallow these (16,20).
- The overriding principle for the team physician in managing ethical issues is to provide care solely focused on what is best for the patient-athlete (1).

All opinions and information in this represent the authors work as individuals. Nothing provided is intended, nor should it be understood to, represent any official policy, opinion or position of the U.S. Government, Department of Defense, U.S. Air Force, Air Force Surgeon General, and Uniformed Service University of the Health Sciences.

REFERENCES

1. Herring SA, Putukian M, Leclere LE, et al. The team physician consensus statement 2024 update. *Med Sci Sports Exerc.* 2025 May;57(5):1067–75.
2. Ghildiyal R. Role of sports in the development of an individual and role of psychology in sports. *Mens Sana Monogr.* 2015 Jan–Dec;13(1):165–70.
3. Anderson L. Writing a new code of ethics for sports physicians: principles and challenges. *Br J Sports Med.* 2009;43(13):1079–82.
4. Howe WB, McKeag DB. Primary care sports medicine: a part-timer's perspective. *Phys Sportsmed.* 1988;16(1):102–14.
5. Beauchamp TL, Childress JF. *Principles of Bioethics.* 5th ed. Oxford University Press; 2001.
6. American College of Sports Medicine. *Code of Ethics* [Internet]. 2023. Available from: https://www.acsm.org/news-detail/2023/05/23/acsm-releases-updated-code-of-ethics-for-certified-professionals
7. Mountjoy M. "Only by Speaking Out Can We Create Lasting Change": what can we learn from the Dr Larry Nassar tragedy? *Br J Sports Med.* 2019;53(1):57–60.
8. Capozzi JD, Rhodes R, Gantsoudes G. Ethics in practice: terminating the physician-patient relationship. *J Bone Joint Surg Am.* 2008;90(1):208–10.
9. Rizvi AA, Thompson PD. Hypertrophic cardiomyopathy: who plays and who sits. *Curr Sports Med Rep.* 2002;1(2):93–9.
10. Giordano S. A new professional code in sports medicine. *BMJ.* 2010;341:c4931.
11. Stewart RJ, Reider B. The ethics of sports medicine research. *Clin Sports Med.* 2016 Apr;35(2):303–14.
12. Maron BJ, Mitchell JH. 26th Bethesda Conference: recommendations for determining eligibility for competition in athletes with cardiovascular abnormalities. *J Am Coll Cardiol.* 1994;24(4):845–99.
13. Ray L. The physician's role in modern warfare: an ethical accounting. *Virtual Mentor.* 2007 Oct 1;9(10):663–6.
14. Anderson L. Contractual obligations and the sharing of confidential health information in sport. *J Med Ethics.* 2008;34(9):e6.
15. George T. Care by team doctors raises conflict issue. *The New York Times*; 2002 Jul 28. section 8, column 5. Available at: http://www.nytimes.com/2002/07/28/sports/pro-football-care-by-team-doctors-raises-conflict-issue.html
16. Tucker AM. Ethics and the professional team physician. *Clin Sports Med.* 2004;23(2):227–41.
17. Salkeld LR. Ethics and the pitchside physician. *J Med Ethics.* 2008;34(6):456–7.
18. Ahmed OH, Weiler R, Schneiders AG, McCrory P, Sullivan SJ. Top tips for social media use in sports and exercise medicine: doing the right thing in the digital age. *Br J Sports Med.* 2015;49(14):909–10.
19. Dunn WR, George MS, Churchill L, Spindler KP. Ethics in sports medicine. *Am J Sports Med.* 2007;35(5):840–4.
20. Holm S, McNamee M. Ethics in sports medicine. *BMJ.* 2009;339:b3898.

Medicolegal Considerations

4

Aaron Rubin, Aaron Tunison, and Lauren Simon

INTRODUCTION

- This chapter is by no means meant to substitute for the advice of an attorney but is presented to draw attention to potential legal issues that may arise in the practice of sports medicine.
- Sports are a microcosm of society.
- There are rules of sports and society that must be created, interpreted, and, at times, debated.
- Medical practice in sports holds no exemption from any other medical practice.
- Legal issues present in the area include, but are not limited to, malpractice, contracts, licensure, insurance, "Good Samaritan" laws, and confidentiality issues (Health Insurance Portability and Accountability Act [HIPAA] and Family Educational Rights and Privacy Act [FERPA]).
- These issues may be complicated by the practice of sports medicine in the public arena and the traditions of team and game coverage.
- The advice of an attorney should be considered before making any legal decisions.

DEFINITIONS

- **Law:** A body of rules or standards of conduct promulgated or established by some authority.
  - That which is laid down, ordained, or established. A body of rules of action or conduct prescribed by controlling authority and having binding legal force. The law of a state is found in statutory and constitutional enactments as interpreted by its courts. The word "law" contemplates both statutory and case law (1).
- **Lawful:** That which is permitted or authorized by the law.
  - Legal, warranted, or authorized by the law. Not contrary to nor forbidden by the law; not illegal (1).
- **Contract:** An agreement between two or more parties that creates legally binding obligations. A valid contract must involve competent parties, proper subject matter, consideration, and mutuality of agreement and of obligation. Contracts are classified in many ways.
  - An agreement between two or more persons that creates an obligation to do or not to do a particular thing. A legal relationship consisting of the rights and duties of the contracting parties; a promise or set of promises constituting an agreement between the parties that gives each a legal duty to the other and also the right to seek a remedy for the breach of those duties. Its essentials are competent parties, subject matter, and mutuality of agreement (1).
  - **Expressed:** An expressed contract is an actual agreement in terms that are openly declared at the time of making it, being stated in distinct and explicit language either orally or in writing (1).
  - **Implied:** An implied contract is one inferred by law to exist because the parties' conduct or surrounding circumstances indicate a contractual relationship exists.
  - **Bilateral:** A bilateral contract is one involving mutual promises between parties.
    - Bilateral or reciprocal contracts are those by which the parties expressly enter into mutual engagements such as sale or hire (1).
  - **Unilateral:** A unilateral contract is a one-sided promise where one party undertakes an obligation without a reciprocal promise or obligation being made or undertaken.
- **Civil law:** Body of law that a nation or state has established for itself as distinguished from natural law. Law determining private rights and liabilities as distinguished from criminal law.
  - Civil law is a branch of law that regulates the noncriminal rights, duties of persons and equal legal relations between individuals, as opposed to criminal or administrative law (2).
- **Criminal law:** The branch of law that defines what public wrongs are considered crimes and assigns punishment for those wrongs.
  - Criminal law, as distinguished from civil law is a system of laws concerned with punishment of individuals who commit crimes (3).
- **Natural law:** The moral or ethical law, formulated in accordance with reason, natural justice, and the original state of nature (1).
- **Case law:** Law based on judicial precedent rather than legislative enactment. The body of law founded in adjudicated cases as distinguished from statute, common law.

- The aggregate of reported cases as forming a body of jurisprudence, or the law of a particular subject as evidenced or formed by the adjudged cases, in distinction to statutes and other sources of law. It includes the aggregate of reported cases that interpret statutes, regulations, and constitutional provisions (1).

- **Tort:** A wrongful injury; a civil wrong. A tort is an action or conduct by the defendant that results from a breach of legal duty owed to the plaintiff, which causes injury or damage to the plaintiff.
- Torts may be "intentional" (when the defendant intends to injure) or "negligent" (when the defendant fails to exercise the proper degree of care established by law).
  - A private or civil wrong or injury for which the court will provide a remedy in the form of an action for damages (1).
  - A legal wrong committed on the person or property. It may be (a) a direct invasion of some legal right of the individual; (b) the infraction of some public duty by which special damage accrues to the individual; or (c) the violation of some private obligation by which like damage accrues to the individual (1).
- **Negligence:** The inadvertent or unintentional failure to exercise that care that a reasonable, prudent, and careful person would exercise; conduct that violates certain legal standards of due care.
  - The omission to do something that a "reasonable man," guided by those ordinary considerations that ordinarily regulate human affairs, would do, or the doing of something that a "reasonable and prudent man" would not do.
- **Liability:** An obligation or mandate to do or refrain from doing something.
  - An obligation one is bound in law or justice to perform (1).
- **Plaintiff:** Person who brings a lawsuit; the complainant; the prosecution in a criminal case.
  - The party who complains or sues in a civil action and is so named on the record. A person who seeks remedial relief for an injury to rights; it designates a complainant (1).
- **Defendant:** The person accused in a criminal case or sued in a civil action.
  - The person defending or denying; the party against whom relief or recovery is sought in an action or suit or the accused in a criminal case (1).
- **Captain of the ship doctrine:** Doctrine that imposes liability on the surgeon in charge of the operation for negligence of his assistants during the period when those assistants are under the surgeon's control, although the assistants are also employees of the hospital (1).

DUTIES, ROLES, AND RESPONSIBILITIES OF THE TEAM PHYSICIAN (4–7)

- The duties of the team physician to a team may be outlined in a contract between the organization and physician.
- The duties to the individual athlete should be the same as with any other patient-physician relationship.
- Balancing the duty to team and athlete must be considered in every situation.
- A consensus statement on the duties of the team physician has been created by several organizations and is available in its entirety from the following groups (see Chapter 1, The Team Physician):
  - American College of Sports Medicine (ACSM)
  - American Academy of Family Physicians (AAFP)
  - American Academy of Orthopaedic Surgeons (AAOS)
  - American Medical Society for Sports Medicine (AMSSM)
  - American Orthopaedic Society for Sports Medicine (AOSSM)
  - American Osteopathic Academy of Sports Medicine (AOASM)
- Qualifications from this consensus statement include:
  - Medical or osteopathic degree with unrestricted license to practice medicine
  - Fundamental knowledge of emergency care regarding sporting events
  - Trained in cardiopulmonary resuscitation (CPR) and automated external defibrillator use
  - Working knowledge of trauma, musculoskeletal injuries, psychological and medical conditions affecting the athlete
- Medical duties from this statement stated that the team physician has ultimate responsibility to include coordination of the preparticipation screening; management of on-field injuries; medical management of injury and illness; coordination of rehabilitation and return to participation; coordination of medical care; education; and documentation and record keeping.
- Administrative duties include: establishing relationships; education; development of a chain of command; plan and train for emergencies; address equipment and supply issues (as needed to provide adequate medical coverage); provide for event coverage; and assess environmental concerns and playing conditions.
- Administrative duties should also include establishment of an Emergency Action Plan for all locations (competition venues, practice facilities, training rooms) with plans for travel included. These should include all involved in the plan with attention to communication, equipment, ambulance and emergency vehicle entrance and exit, security, and safety of all participants (7).
- Standard definitions of negligence generally apply. The physician is held to what a reasonable, prudent man would do, although may be held to higher standards as a physician.
- As guidelines become more established, these may become the basis for duties and responsibilities of the team physician.
- Medicolegal issues are present for all physicians, including team physicians. Some ethical issues may also be viewed in a medicolegal context. Medicolegal issues may have unique presentations in sports medicine. Some key areas of potential medicolegal liability include the following:

- Compliance with school and governing body guidelines, standards, policies, regulations, and rules
- Compliance with local, state, and/or federal rules, regulations, and laws
  - Compliance with privacy laws
    - HIPAA: Health Insurance Portability and Accountability Act of 1996
    - FERPA: Family Educational Rights and Privacy Act
- Decisions made as a result of the Preparticipation Evaluation (PPE), clearance to play, waivers, and return to play (RTP)
- Evaluation and management of significant on-field injuries and illnesses (*e.g.*, concussion, cervical spine, cardiac, and heat-related illness)
- Medical record documentation (4)

DUTIES, ROLES, AND RESPONSIBILITIES OF THE TEAM AND ATHLETES (4–7)

- The responsibilities of the team (organization, ownership, administration) should be outlined in a contract.
  - The team should provide a safe venue (including adequate security), appropriate safety equipment, supplies needed to treat injured or ill athletes (unless otherwise specified in the contract), and appropriate response for emergency situations.
  - The team (including coaching staff) should not interfere with the care of the athlete, including return-to-play issues.
  - The athlete should be prepared for participation and participate safely and according to the rules of the sport. If not, the athlete may share in responsibility for the injury.
  - The athlete or team has a duty to report conditions to the team physician and not conceal illnesses, injury, or symptoms that may occur as this may lead to worsening conditions and not allow the medical staff to properly care for the athlete. This could increase risk of liability for the team physician and other medical staff.

CONTRACTS

- Traditionally, many team physicians work with as little as a handshake or loose agreement; one should consider "putting it in writing" with the advice of a lawyer. Verbal contracts are enforceable.
- This contract should outline duties, responsibilities for providing supplies, compensation, travel expectations, provision of coverage in the team physician's absence, length of contract, responsibilities for providing preparticipation evaluations liability coverage, and game decision processes (such as who has the final word on return-to-play issues).
- An attorney can be extremely helpful in creating such a document.

LIABILITY

Malpractice Coverage

- Malpractice is defined as unreasonable lack of skill or professional misconduct (1).
  - Failure to render professional services under circumstances in the community by the "average, prudent reputable member of the profession" with resultant injury or damage to the recipient of those services.
- Negligence is the predominant theory of liability in medical malpractice suits. It requires all the following elements to occur:
  - Physician's **duty** to the plaintiff
  - **Breach** of applicable standard of care
  - **Injury** that can be compensated
  - **Connection** between the violation of care and harm
- A physician should have adequate insurance coverage to defend any case brought against the physician and to compensate any judgments decided against the physician.
- Coverage may not be in effect if one is practicing outside of his or her scope of practice or in an area where not licensed.
- Physicians traveling out of state (or country) with teams should be aware of this possibility and check with their malpractice carrier.
  - This has been addressed with the Sports Medicine Licensure Clarity Act of 2017 (see below), but always best to check with malpractice carrier (8).
- Malpractice insurance should include an adequate "tail" to cover the physician in the event the physician changes jobs or insurance carrier before a case is brought.

Fallacy of the Good Samaritan

- Good Samaritan doctrine: One who sees a person in imminent and serious peril through negligence of another cannot be charged with contributory negligence (worsening the injury due to their actions) as a matter of law, in risking his own life or serious injury in attempting to affect a rescue, provided the attempt is not recklessly or rashly made. Under this doctrine, negligence of a volunteer must worsen the position of the person in distress before liability will be imposed. This protection from liability is provided by statute in most states.
- Specifics of Good Samaritan Laws can vary from state to state.
- These can be used as a defense in a lawsuit and must be presented by your attorney as such. There still will be a financial cost to have an attorney defend your actions.
- A person expected to act, such as a team physician at a game, may not be covered by Good Samaritan doctrine, whether compensated or not.

- Good Samaritan doctrine should not be a substitute for adequate malpractice coverage.
- The doctrine should be adequate in most states to cover a physician who renders aid when an unexpected medical situation arises, such as at an auto accident or if, when a spectator at an event, another spectator has a cardiac arrest.
- Good Samaritan–type legislation generally covers emergent care in unexpected situations except where that care was rendered in an imprudent or grossly negligent or wanton manner.
- Event liability insurance may or may not cover the health care personnel providing services in the medical tent for an event, and a physician's personal or professional liability should be reviewed before one volunteers to determine the applicability and limits of coverage.
- Although waivers and preparticipation releases are routinely used for mass-participation or community athletic events, the documents are not very useful against medical malpractice suits.
- "Physicians who volunteer should take time to review all these options to determine the best coverage option and seek independent and individualized legal advice" (9).

PATIENT (ATHLETE)-PHYSICIAN RELATIONSHIP

- The patient (athlete)-physician relationship should be one of mutual trust and teamwork.
- The athlete (or parents or guardian if a minor) has rights to autonomy, self-determination, privacy, and appropriate medical care.
- Even if a minor, the athlete has certain rights to seek medical care in many jurisdictions for treatment related to pregnancy, drugs, and sexually transmitted disease. Check with local laws. This does not generally include most sports medicine issues, unless it is an emergency.
- HIPAA, FERPA, and Protected Health Information (PHI)
  - HIPAA
    - HIPAA of 1996
    - Defines PHI
    - *Individually identifiable health information* is information, including demographic data, that relates to the individual's past, present, or future physical or mental health or condition; the provision of health care to the individual; or the past, present, or future payment for the provision of health care to the individual, and that identifies the individual or for which there is a reasonable basis to believe it can be used to identify the individual.
      - Individually identifiable health information includes many common identifiers (*e.g.*, name, address, birth date, social security number) (10).
  - FERPA
    - Family Educational Rights and Privacy Act
    - Relates primarily to protected educational information; could raise issues if acting as a team physician at an educational facility.
    - Effects of both laws have been to legislate protection of information that was once a moral and ethical issue for health care providers.
- Privacy is a difficult issue due to the public nature of athletic events and evaluation done on the field or courtside. All attempts to maintain privacy must be attempted. Reporters, scouts, and others may be with the physician on the sidelines.
- Professional and college organizations may consider waivers to allow certain information regarding athletic injuries or illnesses to be discussed with press representatives.
- It is advisable to have an administrative person deal with the press, such as a sports information director or public information officer, to keep the physician from inadvertently releasing private issues.

DRUGS AND THE ATHLETE (4)

Medications: Prescribing and Dispensing

- Medications are generally divided into two groups, prescription and over-the-counter (OTC). Prescription medications are further divided into controlled substances (*e.g.*, narcotics, sedatives), which have a higher potential for abuse and misuse, and standard prescription drugs (*e.g.*, antibiotics, anti-inflammatory, blood pressure, diabetes medications).
- In most states, a special prescription is needed for dispensing of the highest level of controlled substances.
- Medication prescribing and dispensing falls under many laws including state medical laws, pharmacy laws, and consumer safety laws.
- The National Collegiate Athletic Association (NCAA) has well-referenced specific guidelines regarding dispensing in the training room that provides good direction if considering dispensing medication (11).
- In general, a physician may prescribe medication or provide medications under the state laws, which usually include evaluation of the patient.
- A licensed pharmacist may provide medication as prescribed by a licensed physician.
- There are generally strict labeling requirements often including the name of the patient, name and strength of the medication, directions for use, date dispensed, quantity dispensed, and warnings of common side effects. In addition, many states require the pharmacist to counsel the patient on the medication.
- Dispensing medications by individuals not licensed to do so, even if OTC, may not be allowed and could open those

doing so to prosecution under appropriate laws. This may also open the individuals to liability for negligence if a bad effect or outcome occurs.

Drug Testing (see Chapter 28)

- The team physician may be asked to participate in a drug-testing program for teams.
- Testing may include recreational as well as performance-enhancing drugs.
- Testing may be voluntary or mandated by certain organizations such as the NCAA or International Olympic Committee (IOC).
- Careful consideration regarding the physician's role as an "enforcer" of rules versus a counselor for medical care must be undertaken and should be included in the terms of the contract.
- Proper protection of rights, fairness, and "due process" of the athlete must be maintained.

"CAPTAIN OF THE SHIP"

- Although this doctrine relates to surgeons and assistants, the philosophy could be expanded to team physicians and those they work with.
- Choose your partners in sports medical care wisely to avoid being drawn into bad situations (12).

RISK MANAGEMENT (12)

- Manage risk by being prepared, documenting care, working with like-minded professionals, anticipating problems, and communicating with athletes and, where appropriate, their families and adequate insurance coverage
- Advice of legal counsel should be sought in planning team coverage, in writing contracts, and if any events occur.
- Bad outcomes or breaches of duty can lead to legal actions (lawsuits).

CASE LAW AND LEGISLATION OF INTEREST TO THE TEAM PHYSICIAN

- Knapp versus Northwestern 1996 (13).
  - A competent, intelligent adult with Division I basketball skills signs a letter of intent to play with a Division I school.
  - Athlete suffers sudden cardiac arrest, is resuscitated, and has implantable cardioverter-defibrillator implanted.
  - School's team physician declares him ineligible quoting Bethesda Guidelines.
  - School does provide scholarship, but will not allow him to play or practice.
  - Player sues under Rehabilitation Act.
  - District court states the school violated the Act and must allow him to participate.
  - U.S. Seventh Circuit Court of Appeals reversed, stating the school does have the right to refuse his participation.
  - ". . . medical determinations of this sort are best left to team doctors."
- Kleinknecht versus Gettysburg College, April 27, 1993 (3).
  - Athlete collapses, and the coach runs to his side (not trained in CPR).
  - Sends for trainer and calls for help.
    - Pre–cell phone era, pre–automated external defibrillator era.
  - Student trainer arrives (2) minutes after collapse, but did not start CPR because the student was breathing.
  - Certified Athletic Trainer arrives, notes athlete stopped breathing, and begins CPR with bystander emergency medical technician.
  - Athlete dies, and parents file wrongful death suit.
  - College filed a motion against, which was initially denied and then allowed.
  - District court found for the college:
    - *College had no duty to anticipate and guard against the chance of a fatal arrhythmia in a young and healthy athlete.*
    - *Actions taken by school employees were reasonable. . . . College did not negligently breach any duty that might exist.*
  - U.S. Court of Appeals overturned finding (14):
    - There is a duty of care.
    - There is a special relationship between athletes and the school.
    - Negligence should be determined by the jury.
    - Immunity (Good Samaritan law)
    - College did not assert defense, but the court found that would not have been allowed.
  - Commonwealth of Kentucky versus David Jason Stinson, September 17, 2009 (8).
    - A 15-year-old high school football player dies of heat stroke days after the coach had team run wind sprints on a hot August day.
    - Parents file a wrongful death lawsuit against the head coach and five assistants.
    - Reckless homicide charges are filed against the coach.
    - Coach also indicted by Grand Jury for wanton endangerment.
    - Coach found not guilty after a 2-week trial.
    - Jury deliberated 90 minutes.
    - Civil case settled out of court (15).

- National Collegiate Athletic Association Student-Athlete Concussion Injury Litigation (8).
  - The NCAA will provide $70 million for concussion testing and diagnosis of current and former NCAA student-athletes as a part of its agreement to settle claims in several consolidated concussion-related class actions; includes educational initiatives and $5 million in concussion research.
  - Baseline concussion testing of NCAA student-athletes.
  - Student-athletes with a diagnosed concussion will not be allowed to RTP or practice on the same day and must be cleared by a physician.
  - Medical personnel with training in the diagnosis, treatment, and management of concussions must be present for all games and available during all practices.
  - Establish a process for schools to report diagnosed concussions and their resolution.
- Sports Medicine Licensure Clarity Act of 2017 (16).
  - Extends the liability insurance coverage of a state-licensed medical professional to another state when the professional provides medical services to an athlete, athletic team, or team staff member pursuant to a written agreement.
  - Prior to providing such services, the medical professional must disclose to the insurer the nature and extent of the services.
  - This extension of coverage does not apply at a health care facility or while a medical professional licensed in the state is transporting the injured individual to a healthcare facility.
  - Medical services provided in the secondary state will be treated as having occurred in the primary state, if the secondary state's licensure requirements are "substantially similar" to those in the primary state.
- Constitutional Law: Equal Protection & Transgender Students (17).
  - On January 20, 2021, President Biden Executive Orders EO 13988 Preventing and Combating Discrimination on the Basis of Gender Identity or Sexual Orientation,
  - Reinstated protections against discrimination for LGBTQ individuals, students, and student-athletes.
  - The restoration of the policy that the definition of the word "sex" in Title IX refers to "gender identity" will likely affect the outcome of Office for Civil Rights (OCR) complaints, federal lawsuits, and proposed/enacted state laws related to the sports participation rights of transgender students.

EXCULPATORY WAIVERS

- An "exculpatory waiver" or "risk release" is sometimes requested if an athlete and/or parents or guardians want the athlete to participate if not deemed medically eligible during their preparticipation evaluation (18).
- Some consider this an "express assumption of risk" indicating that the participant fully understands and voluntarily chooses to assume the risk (19,20).
- They may also be requested to allow an athlete to return to activity when not deemed "fully cleared" after an injury or illness.
- It is a contract among the athlete, parent or guardian, physician, school, or sport sponsoring institution that the athlete (parent or guardian) understands the risks involved in return to activities and releases the physician, school, or organization from liability for an untoward outcome.
- These are often narrowly interpreted and may be voided by the courts if there has been negligence by the physician, school, or organization and may not provide any additional protections from liability (21).
- Minors have limited ability to enter into contracts. Parents/guardians have limited ability to enter into an agreement that waives the future rights of the minor if they have a serious outcome.
- Any exculpatory waivers or risk release should be carefully reviewed by legal counsel.
- Some legal authorities recommend that a better course of action would be a letter written by the athlete and guardian outlining the risks of continued participation, and their understanding of those risks (18).
- Best medical judgment, good communications, and excellent documentation should prevail as opposed to attempts to shift responsibility to the athlete.

REFERENCES

1. Nolan JR, Nolan-Haley JM. *Black's Law Dictionary with Pronunciations.* 6th ed. St Paul (MN): West Publishing; 1990:1657.
2. Legal information institute. *Civil Law Cornell Law School.* [Accessed 2022 Oct 1]. Available from: https://www.law.cornell.edu/wex/civil_law
3. Legal information institute. *Criminal Law Cornell Law School.* [Accessed 2022 Oct 1]. Available from: https://www.law.cornell.edu/wex/criminal_law
4. Team Physician Consensus Statement: 2013 Update. *Med Sci Sports Exerc.* Aug 2013;45(8):1618–22. doi:10.1249/MSS.0b013e31829ba437
5. Mitten MJ. Emerging legal issues in sports medicine: a synthesis, summary, and analysis. *St John's L Rev.* 2002;76(1):5–8.
6. Miller TL, Jones GL, Hutchinson M, Vyas D, Borchers J. Evolving expectations of the orthopedic team physician: managing the sidelines and landmines. *Curr Sports Med Rep.* 2021 Oct 1;20(10):553–61.
7. Kinderknecht J. Roles of the team physician. *J Knee Surg.* 2016 Jul;29(5):356–63.
8. National Collegiate athletic Association student-athlete concussion injury litigation (MDL No. 2494/Master Docket No. 1:13-cv-09116 (N.D. Ill.) (Arrington matter). https://www.collegeathleteconcussionsettlement.com/Content/Documents/dkt%20558-1.pdf. Accessed December 12, 2025.
9. Ross DS, Ferguson A, Herbert DL. Action in the event tent! Medical-legal issues facing the volunteer event physician. *Sports Health.* 2013 Jul;5(4):340–5. doi:10.1177/1941738112474226
10. United States Department of Health and Human Services. *Summary of the HIPAA Privacy Rule Content Created by Office for Civil Rights (OCR)*

Content Last Reviewed. 2022 Mar 31. [Accessed 2022 Sep 30] Available from: https://www.hhs.gov/hipaa/for-professionals/privacy/index.html

11. *NCAA Sports Medicine Handbook,* 2011-2012 [Internet]. 2011 [cited 2011 Sep 10]. Available from: http://www.ncaapublications.com/productdownloads/MD11.pdf
12. Birnie B. Legal issues for the team physician. In: Rubin AL, editors. *Sports Injuries and Emergencies, a Quick-Response Manual.* New York: McGraw-Hill; 2003.
13. Knapp versus Northwestern. *United States Court of Appeals for the Seventh Circuit; No.* 96-3450. *Knapp v. Northwestern University, 942 F. Supp. 1191 (N.D. III. 1996).*
14. Kleinknecht versus Gettysburg College. *United States Court of Appeals for the Third Circuit; 1993 Apr 27: 25 Fed.R.Serv.3d 65; 61 USLW 2606; 989 F.2d 1360. Kleinknecht v. Gettysburg College, 989 F.2d 1360*; 1993.
15. Riley J. *Stinson Found Not Guilty in PRP Player's Death* [Internet]. 2011 [cited 2011 Sep 10]. Available from: http://www.courier-journal.com/article/20090917/SPORTS05/909170320/Stinson-found-not-guilty-PRP-player-s-death
16. Congress gov. *S.*808-115*th Congress (*2017–2018*): Sports Medicine Licensure Clarity Act of 2017*; 2018 Jul 9. http://www.congress.gov/
17. Green L *Constitutional Law: Equal Protection & Transgender Students 2021 Sports Law Year-in Review National Federation of State High School Associations.* 2021 Dec 20. [Accessed 2022 Sep 30]. https://www.nfhs.org/articles/2021-sports-law-year-in-review/
18. *PPE: Preparticipation Physical Evaluation.* 5th ed. American Academy of Pediatrics; 2019.
19. Gallup EM. *Law and the Team Physician.* Champaign (IL): Human Kinetics; 1995.
20. Chen S, Esposito E. Practical and critical legal concerns for sport physicians and athletic trainers. In *The Sport Journal.* [Accessed 2023 Sep 19]. https://thesportjournal.org/article/practical-and-critical-legal-concerns-for-sport-physicians-and-athletic-trainers/
21. Quandt EF, Mitten MJ, Black JS. Legal liability in covering athletic events. *Sports Health.* 2009 Jan;1(1):84–90. doi:10.1177/1941738108327530

6 Basics in Exercise Physiology

Emily A. Ricker and Patricia A. Deuster

INTRODUCTION

- Exercise physiology is a basic and an applied science that studies and describes the body's responses to acute exercise and its adaptation to chronic training to maximize human physical performance.
- The sports medicine provider requires a broad knowledge of how the body adapts itself to the demands of physical activity to facilitate the prevention, diagnosis, management, and rehabilitation of sports-induced injury.
- This chapter reviews the basic constructs of muscle and cardiovascular physiology, and introduces core concepts and terminology of training.
- These concepts and their practical application are further expanded in Chapters 11 (Training and Conditioning), 12 (Nutrition), 13 (Exercise Prescription), and 24 (Exercise Stress Testing).

SKELETAL MUSCLE PHYSIOLOGY

Skeletal Muscle Fibers

Basic Structures

- The basic structures that make up a skeletal muscle, from smallest to largest, include sarcomeres, myofilaments, myofibrils (basic units of contraction), muscle fibers (cells), fascicles (bundles of about 150 muscle fibers each), and a muscle (Fig. 6.1). The entire muscle is surrounded by the epimysium, fascicles are surrounded by the perimysium, and each muscle fiber is surrounded by an endomysium.
- Sarcomeres are the functional, contractile units of myofibrils (Fig. 6.2), spanning between structural proteins that form "Z-lines." Sarcomeres contain two main types of myofilaments: thick (myosin) and thin (actin) myofilaments, which are repeated throughout muscle myofibrils.
- Regions of the sarcomere include I bands (lighter, primarily actin filaments), A bands (darker, actin and myosin filaments), H zones (center of sarcomere, only myosin filaments), and M bands (sarcomere's center within H zone).
- Transverse tubules (T tubules; see Excitation-Contraction Coupling), found at the A-I junction of sarcomeres, and the sarcoplasmic reticulum (SR) are the primary regulators of calcium influx into muscle units, which is vital for muscle contraction. The sarcolemma is the muscle cell membrane.
- Satellite cells are muscle "stem" cells. They are activated to a full cell cycle from the quiescent state in response to heavy resistance training and cell damage. Activation of satellite cells is necessary for normal growth and regeneration of tissue damage. Insulin growth factor-1 is a primary regulator of satellite cells (1–3).

Muscle Proteins

- Key muscle proteins include actin, myosin, troponin, and tropomyosin. Actin and myosin constitute myofilaments within myofibrils; myosin is the site of adenosine triphosphate (ATP) binding for use in muscle contraction. Troponin complexes on actin filaments are the calcium binding sites for initiating contraction. In the absence of calcium binding to troponin, tropomyosin, also found on actin filaments, blocks the myosin binding site on actin and inhibits contraction until modified through binding of calcium to troponin.

Skeletal Muscle Fiber Types

- Skeletal muscle fiber types are characterized by differences in morphology, histochemistry, enzyme activity, surface characteristics, and functional capacity (2,4–8) (Table 6.1).
- Human muscle fiber types exist as a spectrum of multiple types as determined by the expression of three myosin heavy chain (MHC) isoforms within a single fiber. Each MHC isoform operates at a different speed: MHC I is the slowest isoform, MHC IIa is categorized as fast, and MHC IIx is even faster ("ultra-fast"). Thus, Type I ("slow twitch"), IIa ("fast oxidative glycolytic"), and IIx ("fast glycolytic") (5,8–10,12).
- In addition to different contractile speed, fiber types also differ in their metabolic attributes, glycogen and lipid content, and number of mitochondria (9,10,12).
- Distribution of Type I (slow twitch) and Type II (fast twitch) fibers within skeletal muscle in normal populations depends on many factors and shows extraordinary adaptive potential in response to innervation/neuronal activity, hormones, neural signaling, training, functional demands, and aging (6,12,13).
- Muscle fiber types appear to change in response to these effectors in a sequential manner from either slow to fast or fast to slow (6,9,12,14,15).

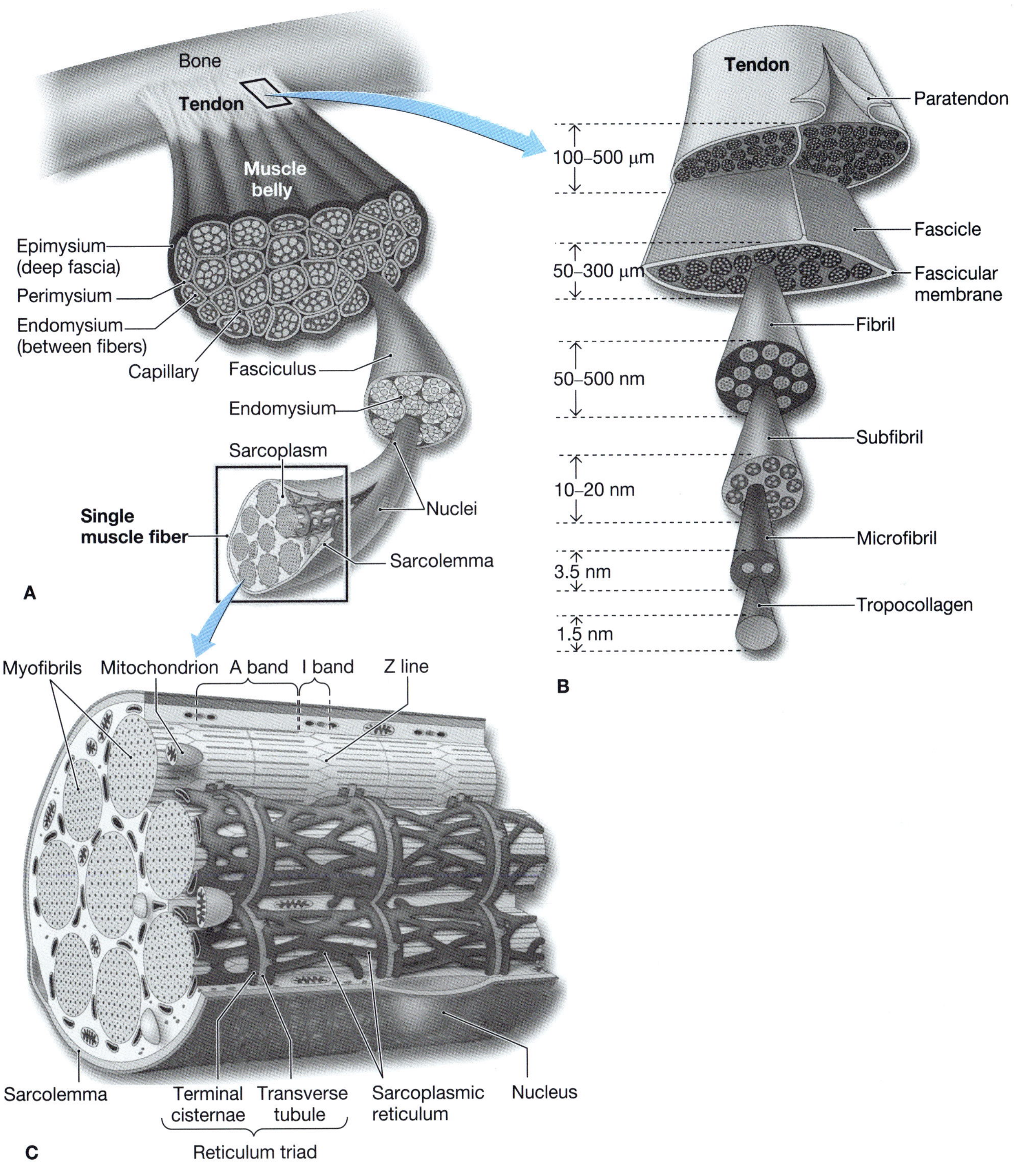

Figure 6.1: Organization of skeletal muscle. A: An entire skeletal muscle is enclosed within a dense connective tissue layer called the epimysium continuous with the tendon binding it to the bone. B: Each fascicle of muscle fibers is wrapped in another connective tissue layer called the perimysium. C: Individual muscle fibers (elongated multinuclear cells) are surrounded by a very delicate layer called the endomysium, which includes an external lamina produced by the muscle fiber (and enclosing the satellite cells) and ECM produced by fibroblasts. (Used with permission from McArdle WD, Katch FI, Katch VL. *Exercise Physiology: Nutrition, Energy, and Human Performance*. 9th ed. Wolters Kluwer; 2023.)

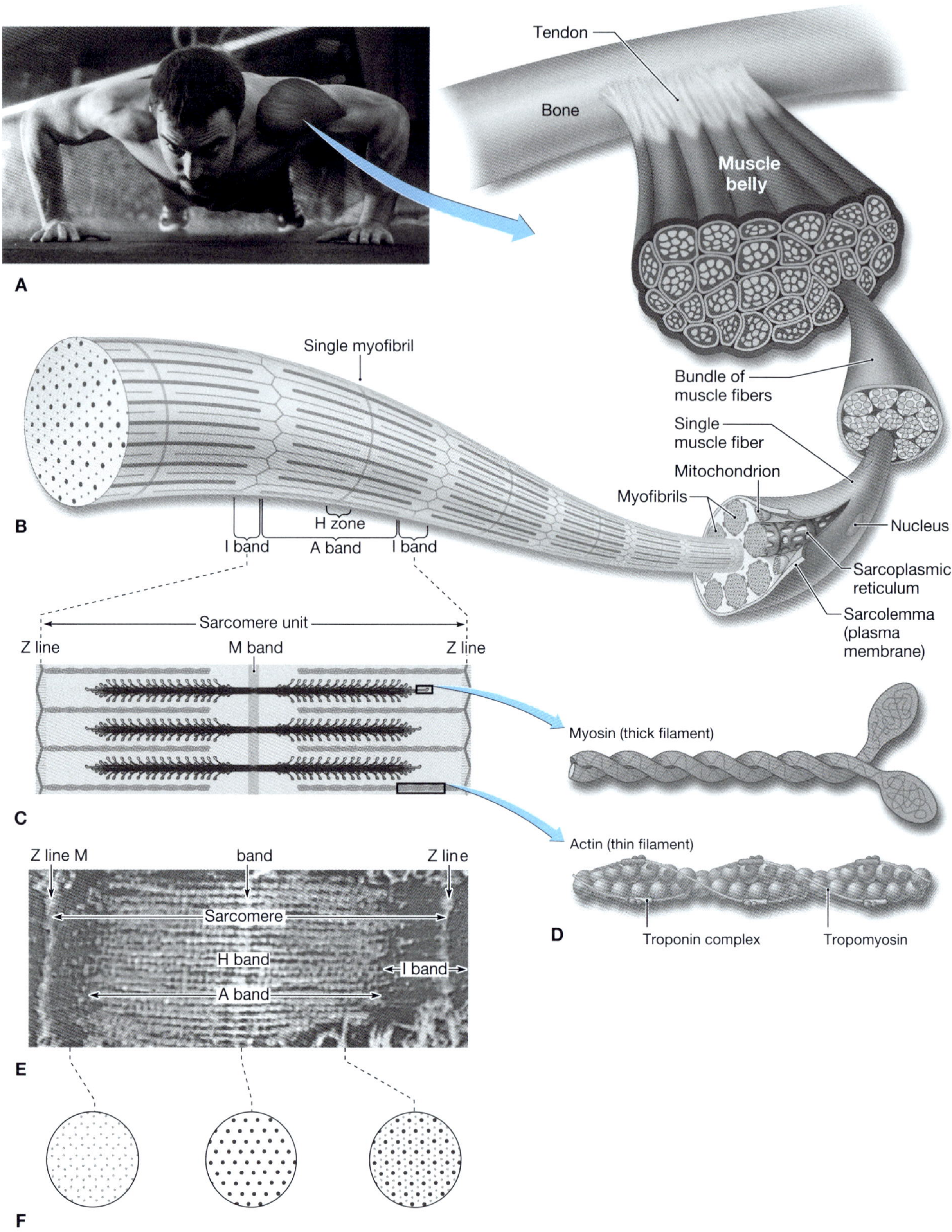

Figure 6.2: Structure of a myofibril: a series of sarcomeres. A: Diagram indicates that each muscle fiber contains several parallel bundles called myofibrils. B: Each myofibril consists of a long series of sarcomeres that contain thick and thin filaments and are separated from one another by Z discs. C: Thin filaments are actin filaments with one end bound to α-actinin, the major protein of the Z disc. Thick filaments are bundles of myosin, which span the entire A band and are bound to proteins of the M line and to the Z disc across the I bands by a very large protein called titin, which has spring-like domains. D: The molecular organization of the sarcomeres has bands of greater and lesser protein density, resulting in staining differences that produce the dark- and light-staining bands seen by light microscopy and TEM. (Used with permission from McArdle WD, Katch FI, Katch VL. *Exercise Physiology: Nutrition, Energy, and Human Performance*. 9th ed. Wolters Kluwer; 2023. E, Adapted with permission from Plowman SA, Smith DL. *Exercise Physiology for Health, Fitness, and Performance*. 5th ed. Baltimore: Wolters Kluwer; 2017.)

Table 6.1 Characteristics of Major Skeletal Muscle Fiber Types[a]

Fiber Characteristics	Slow Twitch	Fast Twitch	
	Type I	Type IIa	Type IIx
Other Terminology	Slow Oxidative (SO)	Fast Oxidative Glycolytic (FOG)	Fast Glycolytic (FG)
Aerobic capacity	High	Med/High	Low
Glycolytic capacity	Low	High	High
Myoglobin content	High	Med	Low
Color	Red	Red	Pink/White
Fatigue resistance	High	Med	Low
Glycogen content	Low	Med	High
Triglyceride content	High	Med	Low
Time to peak tension	Slow	Med	High
Myosin ATPase activity	Low	Med	Med
Myosin Heavy Chain (MHC)	MHCIβ	MHCIIa	MHCIIx
Tension cost[a]	Low	Med	Med
ATP/ADP	Low	Med	Med

ADP, adenosine diphosphate; ATP, adenosine triphosphate; Med, medium.
This chart represents current nomenclature for human skeletal muscle fiber types. Type IIb human muscle fibers are currently referred to as Type IIx because of the MHCIIx isoform found in human muscle. Type IIb muscle fibers are found in rodents and other species, with MHCIIb (5,6,9–11).
[a]Tension cost = ATPase activity to isometric tension ratio.

- All fibers innervated by a given alpha motor neuron (*i.e.*, one motor unit) are of the same fiber type; that is, all the fibers have similar characteristics (16).

Muscular Contraction

Motor Neurons

- Alpha and gamma motor neurons initiate and regulate muscle contraction. Alpha motor neurons initiate contractions in contractile (extrafusal) fibers, whereas gamma neurons innervate muscle spindle (intrafusal) fibers of muscle.

Motor Unit

- Motor units (basic functional unit of movement) consist of an alpha motor neuron, the synaptic junctions (motor endplate), and the muscle fibers the neuron innervates.
- One motor neuron can innervate 10 to several thousand muscle fibers. Release of acetylcholine by neurons initiates contraction, and degradation of acetylcholine by cholinesterase terminates action potentials and the resultant contraction.

Excitation-Contraction Coupling

- Muscle contraction is triggered by an action potential in a motor neuron, resulting in acetylcholine release. Acetylcholine binds to receptors on the motor endplate, relays the action potential down the transverse (T) tubules triggering calcium release from the sarcoplasmic reticulum (SR).
- Once calcium stores are released from the SR, an unstoppable contraction is initiated: Calcium binds to troponin that results in a conformational shift that moves tropomyosin away from the myosin binding sites on the actin filaments allowing myosin to bind to actin to form crossbridge linkages and contraction of sarcomeres via the sliding-filament theory.
- *Sliding-Filament Theory:* This theory states that muscle contraction occurs when two major myofilaments (actin and myosin) slide past one another through a series of crossbridge linkages. Driven by the binding, hydrolyzing, and releasing of ATP to myosin, myosin attaches to actin to form a crossbridge, changes conformation to pull actin toward the M line, detaches, and forms another crossbridge with the next myosin binding site. The continuous binding, pulling, detaching, and reattaching in oscillatory pattern causes the myosin and actin filaments to become more and more overlapping that shortens the muscle without the myofilaments themselves changing lengths. At any point in time about 50% of myosin heads are attached to actin binding sites.
- *All or None Law:* A motor neuron initiating an action potential will contract all muscle fibers innervated by that motor neuron simultaneously. Muscle fibers achieve gradation of contraction strength by recruiting fewer or more motor neurons to initiate contraction and/or by changing the frequency of action potentials to sustain contractions.
- *Length-Tension Relationship:* An optimal length of each muscle exists, at which point the overlap of actin and myosin

is ideal to produce the maximal force when a contraction is stimulated.

- *Force-Velocity Relationship:* The maximum velocity of muscle shortening is greatest at the lowest force and the greatest force of contraction is only possible at the lowest velocity of contraction.
- *Power-Velocity Relationship:* For each muscle, there is an optimum speed of movement to generate the greatest power output (around 200°–300° · s^{-1}).

Sensory Receptors

- *Muscle Spindles:* These specialized intrafusal muscle fibers are located between and among extrafusal fibers deep within the interior of muscles. These proprioceptors sense and relay the length of a muscle and rapid changes in length to initiate reflexive concentric contraction (*e.g.*, patellar reflex).
- *Golgi Tendon Organs:* These sensory organs detect muscle tension and can cause inhibitory reflexes when tension is too great to prevent muscle from contracting to the point of damage. Although quiescent during periods of slow to moderate muscle activity, they increase discharge when muscle load is excessive; they protect against injury due to excessive overloading.

Isometric/Static Contractions

- Isometric contractions refer to muscle fiber recruitment when no change in fiber length takes place, and no joint or limb motion occurs. Examples of isometric contractions include when a person is holding a weight still in a particular position and static postural stability, such as sitting up straight in a chair.

Isotonic/Dynamic Contractions

- Isotonic contractions occur when muscle fibers change length and movement at a joint(s) occurs. Specific types of dynamic contractions include *concentric*, *eccentric*, and *isokinetic.*
- *Concentric* contractions are movements where muscle fibers shorten as the muscle contracts, such as when bicep muscle fibers shorten during a bicep curl. This is also known as positive work.
- When the direction is reversed and the weight is lowered, the contraction becomes an *eccentric* contraction (negative work), where muscle fibers lengthen as the muscle contracts. More fast-twitch motor units are activated during eccentric contractions.

Isokinetic Contractions

- Isokinetic contractions occur when movement is performed at a constant speed against a variable resistance. Isokinetic machines make these contractions possible: the applied resistance during the contraction is increased or lowered at various points across the full range of motion so a constant speed of movement can be maintained. Diagnostic strength equipment uses isokinetic tension to make more accurate measurements of strength at varying joint angles.

CONCEPTS IN CARDIOPULMONARY PHYSIOLOGY

Pulmonary Ventilation

- Minute ventilation ($\dot{V}_e$) is the total volume of air moved into and out of the lungs each minute; it is a function of *tidal volume* (V_T, volume per breath) and *respiratory rate* (f_B, breaths per minute).
- At rest, $\dot{V}_e$ is between 5 and 7 L · min^{-1}, whereas during exercise it increases to between 60 and 180 L · min^{-1}, depending on the health of the person (Fig. 6.3). V_T increases by

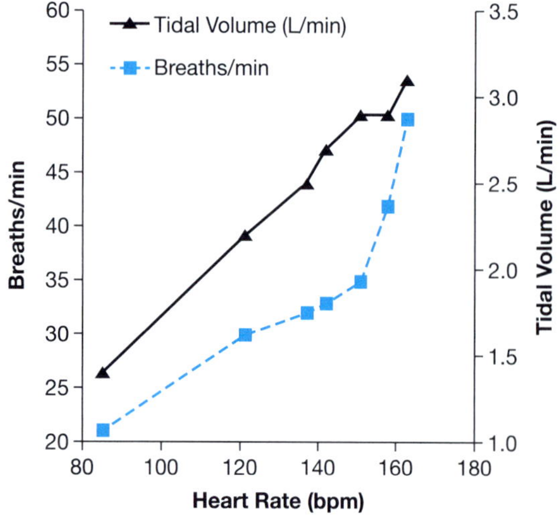

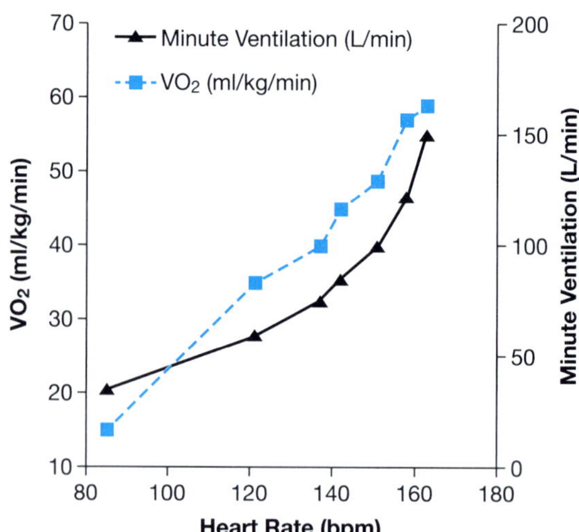

Figure 6.3: Breathing mechanics during progressive maximal exercise test. Left panel depicts breathing rate (dotted line) and tidal volume (solid line) as a function of heart rate. Right panel depicts $\dot{V}O_2$ (dotted line) and minute ventilation (solid line) as a function of heart rate.

expanding both inspiratory and expiratory volumes; these "extra" volumes are called inspiratory and expiratory reserve volumes (IRV and ERV), respectively. The increase in V_T allows $\dot{V}_e$ to increase 5- to 10-fold during exercise. An increase in f_B further augments $\dot{V}_e$ (17–19).

Maximal Voluntary Ventilation

- Maximal voluntary ventilation (MVV) is the volume of air exchanged during repeated maximal respirations in a specified time (10–15 seconds). It is expressed as $L \cdot min^{-1}$ and represents a measure of maximum breathing capacity.

Breathing Reserve

- Breathing reserve (BR) is the difference between MVV and $\dot{V}_e$ during maximal exercise ($\dot{V}_{emax}$), and is sometimes expressed as $\dot{V}_{emax}$/MVV; it is the additional ventilation available during maximal exercise. If a person achieves maximal work capacity prior to attaining MVV, the person has a normal BR, whereas if MVV = $\dot{V}_{emax}$, the person may have compromised pulmonary function. A typical BR is 11 $L \cdot min^{-1}$, with normal $\dot{V}_{emax}$/MVV ranging between 60% and 75%.
- BR may also be calculated by expressing the difference between MVV and $\dot{V}_{emax}$ as a percentage of MVV ($BR = 100 \times \left(MVV - \dot{V}_{emax}\right) / MVV$), in which case a healthy BR is 10%–40% of MVV.

Oxygen Uptake

- Oxygen uptake ($\dot{V}O_2$) is the product of cardiac output (CO, $L \cdot min^{-1}$) and arteriovenous O_2 content difference (a − vO_2), as expressed in the Fick equation: $\dot{V}O_2 = CO \times \left(a - vO_2\right)$. CO is a product of stroke volume (SV, $L \cdot beat^{-1}$) and heart rate (HR, beats $\cdot min^{-1}$). For an average 70-kg adult, CO is about 5 $L \cdot min^{-1}$ at rest and can increase to 20–30 $L \cdot min^{-1}$ during strenuous exercise.
- $\dot{V}O_2$, determined during exercise by measuring respiratory gases, is related to the fractional percent of O_2 in inspired and expired air and $\dot{V}_e$. Inspired air contains 20.93% O_2 and expired air around 17.0%.
- $\dot{V}O_2$ is usually expressed in absolute units ($L \cdot min^{-1}$) or relative to body weight ($mL \cdot kg^{-1} \cdot min^{-1}$). Resting $\dot{V}O_2$ ranges from 0.25 to 0.4 $L \cdot min^{-1}$, and maximal exercise $\left(\dot{V}O_{2max}\right)$ values can exceed 5.0 $L \cdot min^{-1}$ (15–70 $mL \cdot kg^{-1} \cdot min^{-1}$). Higher relative values indicate greater aerobic fitness.

Carbon Dioxide Production

- Carbon dioxide (CO_2) is produced metabolically in tissues, transported in blood by venous return to the lung, and eliminated from the lung on exhalation. Inspired air contains 0.03% CO_2 and expired air about 5% CO_2.
- Like $\dot{V}O_2$, $\dot{V}CO_2$ is usually expressed as $L \cdot min^{-1}$ or $mL \cdot kg^{-1} \cdot min^{-1}$. Resting and strenuous exercise values depend on metabolism and pulmonary function, but resting values are less than O_2.

Lactate

- Lactate serves a dual role as a metabolic intermediate and a signaling molecule within and between cells. It is an end-product of glycolytic metabolism but can also be taken up by other tissues as an oxidizable or gluconeogenic/glyconeogenic substrate (20–23).
- Lactate is formed from pyruvate in the recycling of nicotinamide adenine dinucleotide (NAD+), or when the rate of pyruvate formation in the cytosol exceeds its rate of use by mitochondria. Lactate formation depends on the availability of pyruvate and NADH.
- Blood lactate at rest is 0.8–1.5 mM, but can exceed 18 mM during intense exercise.
- Muscle cells release lactate into the circulation during exercise, where it becomes a fuel for the heart, nonexercising muscles, brain, and other tissues (20–23).
- Lactate released from the muscle can be converted into glucose in the liver by the Cori cycle.
- The cell-to-cell lactate shuttle underscores lactate as an energy intermediate, which is formed in tissues undergoing glycolysis and is subsequently distributed throughout the body to be taken up by tissues as an oxidizable or gluconeogenic/glyconeogenic substrate (23).

Oxygen Pulse (O_2 Pulse)

- O_2 pulse ($mL \cdot beat^{-1}$), or the ratio of $\dot{V}O_2$ ($mL \cdot min^{-1}$) to HR (bpm) when both measures are obtained simultaneously, is the product of stroke volume and a − vO_2 difference (see Fick equation under Oxygen Uptake [$\dot{V}O_2$]).
- O_2 pulse increases with increasing work effort (range 4–30 $mL \cdot beat^{-1}$) and is affected by various factors, including anemia and heart disease. A low value during exercise indicates HR is too high for O_2 and may suggest heart disease (19).

Respiratory Quotient and Respiratory Exchange Ratio

- Respiratory quotient (RQ), the ratio of CO_2 produced by cellular metabolism to O_2 used by *tissues* ($\dot{V}CO_2 / \dot{V}O_2$), is used to quantify the relative amounts of carbohydrate and fatty acids being oxidized for energy. The RQ cannot exceed 1.0; an RQ of 0.7 implies dependence on free fatty acids, and a value of 1.0 indicates dependence on carbohydrate.
- RER represents *pulmonary exchange* of CO_2 and O_2 ($\dot{V}CO_2 / \dot{V}O_2$) at rest and during exercise; it ranges between 0.7 and 1.0 during steady state exercise. RER often exceeds 1.0 during strenuous exercise when CO_2 production exceeds O_2 consumption, as CO_2 is a by-product of numerous mechanisms taking place to buffer hydrogen ion accumulation and maintain pH in the blood and working skeletal muscle.

- The terms RQ and RER are often used interchangeably, but their distinction is important.

Ventilatory Equivalents

- Ventilatory equivalents ($\dot{V}_e/O_2$ and $\dot{V}_e/CO_2$) are unitless numbers derived from the ratio of $\dot{V}_e$ to O_2 and CO_2. $\dot{V}_e/O_2$ indicates the volume (L) of air required to use 1 L of O_2, and $\dot{V}_e/CO_2$ indicates the volume of air required to remove 1 L of CO_2.
- During maximal exercise testing, $\dot{V}_e$ is linearly related to O_2 and CO_2, but at high exercise intensities, $\dot{V}_e$ increases more rapidly than $\dot{V}O_2$, and thus $\dot{V}_e/O_2$ begins to increase, which is followed by an increase in $\dot{V}_e/CO_2$. These increases reflect respiratory compensation for the corresponding rise in blood lactate (19).

Ventilatory Threshold

- The point where $\dot{V}_e$ begins to increase disproportionately to $\dot{V}O_2$ is known as the ventilatory threshold.

Maximal Heart Rate

- The highest HR achieved during a standardized maximal exercise test is the maximal HR (HRmax). If an exercise test is not possible, then age-predicted HR formulas can be used. Two formulas for predicting HRmax are: $HR = 208 - (0.7 \times age)$ and $HR = 220 - age$.
- The first formula, 208 − 0.7 × age, is being recommended by the American College of Sports Medicine (17) because it is more accurate for persons up to 80 years old and independent of gender and habitual physical activity (24).
- An estimated HRmax may be 5%–10% (10–20 bpm) higher or lower than the actual value.

Heart Rate Reserve

- The difference between HRmax during maximal exercise and resting HR is the heart rate reserve ($HRR = HRmax - HRrest$). For instance, if one's HRmax was 205 bpm and HRrest was 55 bpm, then HRR would be 150 bpm. The smaller the difference, the lower the reserve and the narrower the range for HR changes during exercise. HRR can be used to designate exercise intensity based on HR "zones" that reflect a percentage of HRR (see Target Training Heart Rate).

Target Training Heart Rate

- Exercise training programs can designate exercise intensity based on HR zones, or ranges of HR that one should aim for to achieve certain training outcomes. It is recommended that adults achieve at least 150 min · wk^{-1} of moderate intensity (40%–59% HRR or 64%–76% HRmax) or at least 75 min · wk^{-1} of vigorous intensity (60%–89% HRR or 77%–95% HRmax) aerobic physical activity (17). Therefore, to calculate the upper and lower limits of those target HR zones, the equations in Table 6.2 can be used.
- For example, in an individual with a resting HR of 60 bpm and a HRmax of 200 bpm, their moderate intensity target HR zone would be 116–143 bpm based on the Karvonen method or 128–152 bpm based on the HRmax method. Their vigorous intensity target HR zone would be 144–185 bpm based on the Karvonen method and 154–190 based on the HRmax method. The Karvonen method is thought to be more accurate, as it takes into account one's HRrest in addition to their HRmax.

Borg Scale or Rating of Perceived Exertion

- Exercise intensity can also be gauged by using a Rating of Perceived Exertion (RPE) scale, a scale used by an individual to rate their own "degree of physical strain." The original Borg RPE scale ranges from 6 to 20, with each number anchored by a simple verbal expression (no exertion at all to maximum exertion). RPE is also expected to approximate HR by multiplying the RPE by 10, such that a person reporting an RPE of 13 is expected to have an HR around 130 bpm, whereas a person exercising very strenuously and reporting an RPE of 19 is expected to have an HR around 190 bpm. This estimation is, of course, limited and would not be accurate for individuals of all ages.

Table 6.2 Calculating Target Heart Rate Training Zones

	Karvonen Method	HRmax
Lower limit moderate intensity	$HR = HRrest + (0.40 \times HRR)$	$HR = 0.64 \times HRmax$
Upper limit moderate intensity	$HR = HRrest + (0.59 \times HRR)$	$HR = 0.76 \times HRmax$
Lower limit vigorous intensity	$HR = HRrest + (0.60 \times HRR)$	$HR = 0.77 \times HRmax$
Upper limit vigorous intensity	$HR = HRrest + (0.89 \times HRR)$	$HR = 0.95 \times HRmax$

HR, heart rate; HRmax, maximal heart rate; HRrest, resting heart rate.

MEASUREMENTS OF ENERGY, WORK, AND POWER

Definitions of Energy, Work, and Power

- Physical exercise involves both mechanical and chemical work by the muscles; the degree of muscular effort depends on duration, frequency, and intensity of exercise. Together, these define energy, work, and power.
- *Energy:* The capacity to do work, with energy measured in kilojoules (kJ) or kilocalories (kcals): 1 kcal = 4.184 kJ.
- *Work:* When a force acts against resistance to produce motion: Work = Force × Distance. Work is often expressed in kilogram-meters or kgm, where 1 kcal = 426.85 kgm = 4.186 kJ.
- *Power:* Rate at which work is performed or the rate of energy transfer: Power = Work/Time. Power is usually expressed as watts (W), where $1\ W = 1\ J \cdot s^{-1}$; $6.12\ kgm \cdot min^{-1}$; and $0.01433\ kcal \cdot min^{-1}$.

Energy Expenditure

- Energy expenditure (EE) is usually determined by direct or indirect calorimetry. Direct calorimetry measures external work and heat output, and heat production is used as an estimate of metabolic rate. Indirect calorimetry uses either open or closed circuit spirometry.
- With open circuit spirometry, $\dot{V}O_2$ and $\dot{V}CO_2$ are measured and the RER is calculated. EE can be estimated with RER, $\dot{V}O_2$, and time: $EE(kcal) = \dot{V}O_2(L \cdot min^{-1}) \times (4 + RER) \times time(min)$.
- For example, if $\dot{V}O_2$ determined from gas analysis was $0.3\ L \cdot min^{-1}$ and RER was 0.75 at rest, EE would be $1.4\ kcal \cdot min^{-1}$. During exercise, if $\dot{V}O_2$ was $2.5\ L \cdot min^{-1}$ and RER was 0.95, EE would be $12.4\ kcal \cdot min^{-1}$, a difference of $11\ kcal \cdot min^{-1}$ compared to rest.
- EE can also be estimated from $\dot{V}O_2$ by assuming consumption of 1 L of O_2 has an energetic cost 5 kcal. If resting $\dot{V}O_2$ was $0.3\ L \cdot min^{-1}$, EE would be $1.5\ kcal \cdot min^{-1}$.

Work Efficiency

- Gross work efficiency is the ratio of mechanical work output to energy expended; it typically ranges between 15% and 30%.
- Net work efficiency is the ratio of mechanical work output to total energy expended minus resting EE.
- Example: A woman with a resting $\dot{V}O_2$ of $0.3\ L \cdot min^{-1}$ rides a cycle ergometer for 30 minutes at 150 W ($1\ W = 0.01433\ kcal \cdot min^{-1}$) and uses $2\ L\ O_2 \cdot min^{-1}$.
  - *Mechanical work output*: 64 kcal ($150\ W \times 0.01433\ kcal \cdot min^{-1} \times 30\ min$)
  - *Total energy expended:* 300 kcal ($2L \cdot min^{-1} \times 5\ kcal \cdot L^{-1} \times 30\ min$)
  - *Gross efficiency:* 64/300 = 21%
  - *Resting EE:* 45 kcal ($0.3\ L \cdot min^{-1} \times 5\ kcal \cdot L^{-1} \times 30\ min$)
  - *Net efficiency:* 64/(300 − 45) = 25%.
- Factors influencing exercise efficiency include work rate, speed of movement, muscle fiber composition, and various biomechanical factors, such as equipment and clothing.

Exercise Economy

- Economy of movement is the efficiency of converting metabolic power into mechanical power/velocity. It is defined in terms of $\dot{V}O_2$ (oxygen required) for a specific power output or velocity ($mL \cdot min^{-1} \cdot W^{-1}$ or $mL \cdot kg^{-1} \cdot min^{-1}$ to $km \cdot min^{-1}$ or $mile \cdot min^{-1}$). The more efficient a person is, the more power/velocity he or she can generate for the same O_2 cost.
- Selected factors affecting economy include age, body mass, HR, ventilatory rate, basal metabolic differences, leg length, stride frequency and other biomechanical variations, shoes for running, aerodynamic positioning for cycling, and velocity. Values may range from 200 to $350\ mL \cdot kg^{-1} \cdot km^{-1}$ for running and $10–15\ mL \cdot W^{-1}$ for cycling (25).

Metabolic Equivalents

- A metabolic equivalent (MET) is the energetic cost of rest (*i.e.*, resting metabolic rate) and the conventional value used for 1 MET is $3.5\ mL$ of $O_2 \cdot kg^{-1} \cdot min^{-1}$. Activities can then be expressed in terms of multiple of the MET unit. For instance, an activity requiring 3 METs would have an energetic cost of $10.5\ mL \cdot kg^{-1} \cdot min^{-1}$. These units are used by the Centers for Disease Control and Prevention to recommend exercise intensity and can also be used to estimate EE in the absence of indirect or direct calorimetry measurements.
- Energy expenditure for activities such as eating, dressing, and walking around the house range from 1 to 4 MET, whereas the cost of climbing a flight of stairs, walking on level ground, scrubbing floors, or playing a game of golf ranges from 4 to 10 MET. Strenuous sports, such as swimming, singles tennis, and football, often exceed 10 MET (26).
- See Table 6.3 for key equations and conversions.

BASIC CONCEPTS IN AEROBIC AND ANAEROBIC EXERCISE

Maximal Aerobic Power

- Maximal aerobic power, or Effeiciency = $\dot{V}O_{2max}$, is the greatest amount of O_2 a person can consume during physical exercise. It characterizes the functional capacity of the cardiovascular, pulmonary, and O_2 transport systems, and is considered "power" because it is a rate: L of $O_2 \cdot min^{-1}$.
- If two individuals had absolute $\dot{V}O_{2max}$ values of 4.2 and 3.2 $L \cdot min^{-1}$ and both weighed 70 kg, then normalizing for body weight would yield values of 60 and $45.7\ mL \cdot kg^{-1} \cdot min^{-1}$, respectively. If person 1 weighed 70 kg and person 2 weighed

Table 6.3 Key Equations and Conversions

Breathing Reserve (BR) (%)	$BR = \dot{V}_{emax} / MVV$ OR $BR = 100 \times (MVV - \dot{V}_{emax}) / MVV$
Fick Equation for $\dot{V}O_2$ ($L \cdot min^{-1}$, $mL \cdot kg^{-1} \cdot min^{-1}$	$\dot{V}O_2 = CO \times (a - vO_2)$
Cardiac Output (CO) (L)	$CO = HR(\text{bpm}) \times SV(\text{L} \cdot \text{beat}^{-1})$
O_2 Pulse ($mL \cdot beat^{-1}$)	$O_2\ pulse = \frac{\dot{V}O_2(\text{mL} \cdot \text{min}^{-1})}{HR(\text{bpm})}$
Respiratory Quotient (RQ)	$RQ = \dot{V}CO_2 / \dot{V}O_2$ (tissues level)
Respiratory Exchange Ratio (RER)	$RER = \dot{V}CO_2/\dot{V}O_2$ (pulmonary level)
Ventilatory equivalents	$\dot{V}_e/O_2$ $\dot{V}_e/CO_2$
Age-Predicted Maximal HR (bpm)	$HR = 220 - \text{age}$ OR $HR = 208 - (0.7 \times age)$
Energy (kcal, kJ)	1 kcal = 4.184 kJ
Work (kgm, kJ)	$Work = Force \times Distance$ 1 kcal = 426.85 kgm = 4.186 kJ
Power (W, $J \cdot s^{-1}$, $kgm \cdot min^{-1}$, $kcal \cdot min^{-1}$)	$Power = \frac{Work}{Time}$ $1\ W = 1\ J \cdot s^{-1}$ $= 6.12\ kgm \cdot min^{-1}$ $= 0.01433\ kcal \cdot min^{-1}$.
Energy Expenditure (EE) estimated with open circuit spirometry	$EE(\text{kcal}) = \dot{V}O_2(\text{L} \cdot \text{min}^{-1}) \times (4 + RER) \times time(\text{min})$ OR $1\ L\ O_2 = 5\ kcal$
Gross Work Efficiency (%)	$Efficiency = \frac{Work\ Output}{Energy\ Expended}$
Net Work Efficiency (%)	$Efficiency = \frac{Work\ Output}{(Energy\ Expended) - Resting\ EE}$
Metabolic Equivalent (MET)	$1\ MET = 3.5\ mL\ of\ O_2 \cdot kg^{-1} \cdot min^{-1}$

EE, energy expenditure; HR, heart rate; MVV, maximum voluntary reserve; SV, stroke volume.

53 kg, then normalized $\dot{V}O_{2max}$ values would be 60 $mL \cdot kg^{-1} \cdot min^{-1}$ for both persons. Normative values for $\dot{V}O_{2max}$ vary by age and sex, with older individuals and females expected to have lower $\dot{V}O_{2max}$ values than younger individuals and males. For instance, in adults 30–39 years of age, the 75th percentile $\dot{V}O_{2max}$ for males (considered the upper bound of good) is 49.2 $mL \cdot kg^{-1} \cdot min^{-1}$, whereas the 75th percentile for females is 36.1 $mL \cdot kg^{-1} \cdot min^{-1}$ (17).

Testing for Maximal Aerobic Power

- The best tests for measuring $\dot{V}O_{2max}$ are incremental and progressive exercise tests.
- $\dot{V}O_{2max}$ is measured by treadmill walking/running, cycle or arm ergometry, and step tests.
- Requirements for a valid maximal exercise test are as follows: standardized test conditions, involvement of large muscle groups, measurable and reproducible rates of work, little or no skill required, and tolerated by most people. Also, motivation should not be a major factor.
- Plateau in $\dot{V}O_{2max}$: During a progressive exercise test, when a step increase in work results in either no or a minimal increase in $\dot{V}O_{2max}$, the plateauing effect is considered the single best criterion for attaining a true $\dot{V}O_{2max}$.
- Criteria for achieving $\dot{V}O_{2max}$: If a leveling off or plateauing of $\dot{V}O_{2max}$ is not observed, then at least two of the following criteria should be met for a true $\dot{V}O_{2max}$ test: blood lactate levels above 7 or 8 mM; HR equal to or within 15 beats of the age-predicted HRmax; RER $\geq$ 1.15; and/or RPE $\geq$ 17 on the Borg 6–20 scale.
- $\dot{V}O_{2peak}$: When an exercise test is terminated and the criteria described are not met, the highest $\dot{V}O_2$ achieved is referred to as $\dot{V}O_{2peak}$.
- $\dot{V}O_{2peak}$ can be estimated by using the linear relation between HR and $\dot{V}O_2$. HRs at submaximal work rates can be plotted

against $\dot{V}O_2$, and then estimated HRmax can be used to extrapolate to $\dot{V}O_{2max}$ (Fig. 6.4). Walking tests, step tests, endurance runs, and nonexercise data can also be used to estimate $\dot{V}O_{2max}$. Potential errors exist for all these estimates, and care must be taken when interpreting these data.

Determinants of and Factors Affecting $\dot{V}O_{2max}$

- *Intrinsic and extrinsic factors:* Intrinsic factors affecting $\dot{V}O_{2max}$ include genetics, sex, body composition/lean mass, age, and existing pathologies. Extrinsic factors include training/activity levels, substance intake (alcohol, caffeine), nutritional and hydration status, and environmental conditions.
- *Determinants:* All systems serving a role in delivering O_2 can affect $\dot{V}O_{2max}$. Central factors include cardiac output, pulmonary ventilation, arterial pressure, hemoglobin (Hb) content, O_2 diffusion into and through the lungs, alveolar ventilation: perfusion ratio, and Hb-O_2 affinity. Peripheral determinants include muscle blood flow, capillary density, O_2 diffusion to and extraction by muscle cells, Hb-O_2 affinity, and properties of the skeletal muscle fibers. Such properties include the fiber type (type of myosin heavy chain), cross-sectional area, mitochondrial oxidative capacity, capillarization, myoglobin content, and glycogen storage (11).

Aerobic and Anaerobic Exercise

Exercise Domains

- Three specific exercise domains have been suggested by Gaesser and Poole (27): moderate, heavy, and severe. Figure 6.5 depicts the domains for an incremental exercise test and constant load tests at three workloads. In panel 1, lactate threshold (T_{Lac}) represents the boundary between the moderate and heavy domain, and critical power (W_a) represents the boundary for the severe domain. These concepts are described below.
- Lactate threshold: T_{Lac} represents the lowest exercise intensity that can be maintained where blood lactate appearance exceeds removal and is sustained at about 1 mM above pre-exercise levels. Also known as aerobic T_{Lac} (28–30).
- Maximal lactate at steady state (MLSS): MLSS is the highest intensity of exercise that can be maintained without blood lactate concentrations increasing greater than 1 mmol · L^{-1} between 10 and 30 minutes of exercise. At this intensity, blood lactate production is approximately equal to lactate clearance and a new steady state is achieved between 3 and 8 mM. This intensity is greater than the aerobic $T_{Lac.}$ Also known as anaerobic T_{Lac} (28,31,32). The MLSS has previously been said to demarcate the upper boundary of the heavy domain, although exercise at a higher intensity than that measured by a MLSS test may be possible without imminent fatigue (33).
- Critical power (W_a): W_a is the maximum power output that can be sustained without a continued and progressive anaerobic contribution; i.e., without imminent fatigue. Exercise above W_a will elicit VO_{2max}. W_a is greater than MLSS and has been proposed as the "gold standard" for demarcating the upper limit of the heavy exercise domain, rather than MLSS (33).
- Onset of blood lactate accumulation: At specific exercise intensity, muscle lactate production exceeds utilization and blood lactate begins to accumulate. An absolute blood lactate concentration of 4 mmol · L^{-1} has been used to define the onset of blood lactate accumulation threshold.
- Steady state exercise: When lactate production is balanced by the rate of oxidative removal and $\dot{V}O_2$ is stabilized within 3–6 minutes. Cardiac output, HR, and pulmonary gas exchange are in a steady state and exercise can continue for an extended period of time.

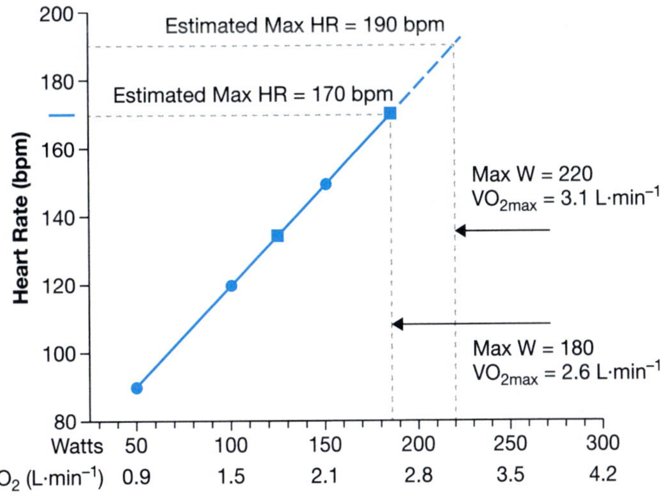

Figure 6.4: Extrapolation of $\dot{V}O_{2max}$ from heart rate and work load on a cycle ergometer test.

- Maximal accumulated oxygen deficit (MAOD): The difference between the accumulated oxygen demand and the accumulated oxygen uptake of the exercise bout. MAOD is considered an indicator of anaerobic capacity. Measurement of MAOD requires several submaximal exercise bouts and there are limitations in the ability to accurately capture the MAOD (34–36).
- Slow component of oxygen uptake: A continued rise in $\dot{V}O_2$ beyond the third minute when exercise is above the T_{Lac}. The rise in $\dot{V}O_2$ (see Fig. 6.5) usually stabilizes within 20 minutes when exercise is within the heavy domain or gradually increases to $\dot{V}O_{2max}$ when exercise is within the severe domain. The slow component may indicate additional recruitment of muscle fibers (27,37–40) and is believed to reflect a prolonged metabolic shift in energy sources and loss of locomotive efficiency (41).
- Velocity at $\dot{V}O_{2max}$ ($v\dot{V}O_{2max}$) is the minimal running velocity that elicits $\dot{V}O_{2max}$. It is considered the best indicator of endurance performance (42–45).

Oxygen Kinetics

- Oxygen deficit: When an individual begins to exercise, energy (ATP) is required that cannot immediately be met via aerobic mechanisms (oxidative phosphorylation). $\dot{V}O_2$ gradually increases until it reaches a steady state. The oxygen deficit refers to the difference between O_2 uptake in the first few minutes of exercise and an equal time period after steady state has been achieved (38).
- Oxygen debt: On termination of exercise, $\dot{V}O_2$ remains elevated to restore energy systems to their preexercise states. The term oxygen debt was coined by A.V. Hill in the early 1900s, when it was thought that the elevated $\dot{V}O_2$ following exercise was making up for "borrowed" ATP at the beginning of exercise when there is an oxygen deficit (*i.e.*, the body is replenishing the ATP, phosphocreatine, and tissue O_2 stores). However, evidence that the reason for the oxygen debt goes beyond replenishing body stores lead to the term falling out of use and favoring of the term excess post-exercise oxygen consumption (EPOC) instead (see below).
- EPOC: EPOC is the integral of $\dot{V}O_2$ during recovery after terminating exercise. It consists of a fast and slow component and is highly correlated with exercise intensity, with exercise bouts of greater intensity resulting in larger EPOC (46). The fast portion, lasting a couple of minutes, may indicate re-synthesis of stored phosphocreatine and restoration of muscle and blood O_2 stores. The slow component, lasting up to 30 minutes or more after exercise, may represent elevated breathing and HR, elevated body temperature, circulating catecholamines, accelerated metabolism (conversion of lactic acid to glucose/gluconeogenesis), and other hormonal/metabolic processes.

Resistance Exercise

- Resistance exercise is used to improve muscular strength, endurance, and power. Strength is the greatest force a muscle can exert in one effort. Muscle endurance is the muscle's ability to make repeated efforts. Power is a measure of how quickly muscular strength can be applied.

Weight Training Parameters

- When training with weights or using other resistance modalities (*e.g.*, bands), the magnitudes of increase in muscle strength and endurance depend on specific training parameters: repetitions, sets, volume, and intensity.
- *Repetition maximum (RM)* is the amount of force a person can lift a given number of times (repetitions). For example, 5-RM is the maximal force the person could lift five times.

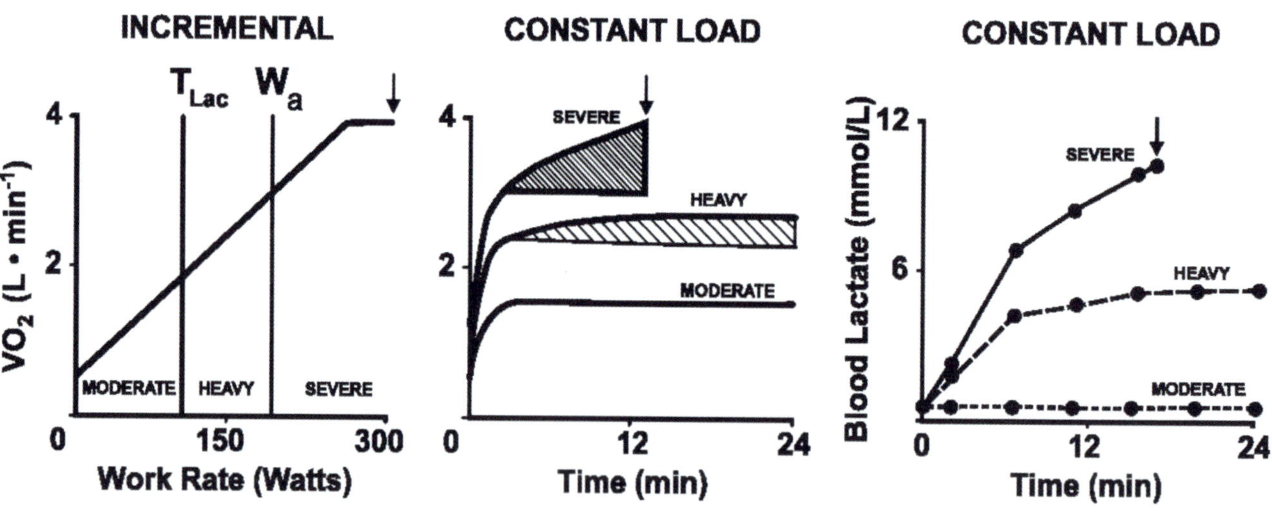

Figure 6.5: $\dot{V}O_2$ responses to incremental exercise (left panel), and $\dot{V}O_2$ (middle panel) and blood lactate (right panel) responses to constant load exercise as a function of exercise intensity domains. T_{Lac} represents the lactate threshold, and critical power approximate where maximal lactate at steady state occurs. (Used with permission from Gaesser GA, Poole DC. The slow component of oxygen uptake kinetics in humans. *Exerc Sport Sci Rev.* 1996;24:35–71.)

- *Repetitions* are the number of consecutive times a particular weight is lifted without a rest period. For examples, repetitions could be 5, 10, 12, 25, or 50 depending on the load and goals of the training session/program.
- *Sets:* The number of sets delineates how many times repetitions are repeated after a rest period. For example, a training session could consist of three sets of 12 repetitions for each exercise, for a total of 36 repetitions broken up by rest periods.
- *Volume* equates to the total number of times a weight was lifted (Sets × Repetitions). For example, for three sets of 12 repetitions with 50 lb, the volume would be 3 × 12 × 50, or 1800 lb. Volume indicates how much work was done: The greater the volume, the greater is the total work.
- *Intensity/Training Load* depends on the actual resistance lifted and is expressed as a percent of maximum weight (1-RM). If 1-RM for an exercise is 80 kg, then 60 kg would approximate 75% (10-RM) intensity. Conversely, if an individual can complete a maximum of 8 repetitions of an exercise with 80 kg, then their estimated 1-RM would be 100 kg.

Resistance Training Concepts

- *SAID (specific adaptation to imposed demand):* AKA, specificity. The specificity principle states that physiological, neurological, and psychological adaptations to training are specific to the "imposed demand." For example, to develop speed or power, the imposed demand must contain speed training (moving quickly) and power training (moving large loads quickly).
- *Strength-endurance continuum:* A weight training concept based on the premise that muscle strength and muscle endurance exist on a continuum, with muscle strength being the ability to exert force once (*i.e.*, 1-RM) and muscle endurance representing the ability to exert a lower force repeatedly over time. Performing low numbers of repetitions with higher weight (6- to 10-RM) are associated with increases in muscle strength, and high numbers with lower weight (20- to 100-RM) are associated with increases in muscle endurance. As repetitions increase, training focus transitions from strength to endurance, and the load must be adapted accordingly.
- *Muscle hypertrophy:* Compensatory growth in skeletal muscle in response to an imposed load.
- Muscle hypertrophy may take 2 months to begin, as the initial adaptation to an increased load is a neural response followed by an increase in muscle size. New contractile proteins appear to be incorporated into existing myofibrils, and there may be a limit to how large a myofibril can become; they may split at some point. Hypertrophy results primarily from growth of each muscle cell, rather than an increase in the number of cells.
- Muscle hypertrophy is observed in all three major fiber types (Types I, IIa, and IIx), most often when low numbers of repetitions with higher loads are performed. Physiological adaptations and performance are linked to both the volume and intensity of resistance training.

Biomechanical Factors in Muscle Strength

- Muscle strength is influenced by neural control, muscle cross-sectional area, arrangement of muscle fibers, muscle length, joint angle, velocity of muscle contraction, joint angular velocity, strength-to-mass ratio, body size, joint motion (joint mobility, dexterity, flexibility, limberness, range of motion), point of tendon insertion, and the interactions of these factors.

Delayed Onset Muscle Soreness

- Delayed Onset Muscle Soreness (DOMS) is a term used to describe temporary soreness that results primarily from eccentric exercise and resistance training. It is usually noted the day after the exercise and may last 3–4 days (47,48).
- Factors that may elicit DOMS include inflammation, osmotic changes within muscle tissue, microtrauma to the tissue, and/or alterations in calcium metabolism.

Plyometric Training

- Plyometric training is a specific method of training for power or explosiveness. Most plyometric exercises involve jumping, bounding, and hopping. Plyometric movements involve stimulating the stretch reflex as well as the elastic properties of muscles and tendons to create quick, powerful movements. In a plyometric movement, such as a rebound jump, the force generated by a lengthening contraction (eccentric, "loading the legs"), when quickly followed by a shortening contraction (concentric, "rebound"), results in a quick, powerful movement.

EXERCISE TRAINING

Principles of Training

- *FITT:* This is an acronym to describe physical training variables that can be altered to achieve various fitness goals. FITT stands for Frequency, Intensity, Time (duration), and Type of exercise. *ACSM's Guidelines for Exercise Testing and Prescription* describe FITT guidelines for endurance and resistance training (17).
- *Frequency:* It is recommended that aerobic (cardiovascular endurance) exercise be performed 3–5 $d \cdot wk^{-1}$. For resistance exercise, recommended frequency for novice exercisers is 2 $d \cdot wk^{-1}$, whereas recommendations for experienced exercisers can be more frequent and guided more so by preference and volume goals (17).
- *Intensity:* Recommended intensity for aerobic exercise is moderate (40%–59% HRR) and/or vigorous (60%–89% HRR) physical activity, and likely a combination of both. For resistance training, recommended intensity for novice exercisers is 60%–70% 1-RM for 8–12 repetitions; intensity can be varied for experienced exercisers based on fitness and performance goals (17).

- *Time:* Aerobic exercise of moderate intensity should be performed for 30–60 min · d^{-1}, accumulating ≥150 min · wk^{-1}, and/or 20–60 min · d^{-1} of vigorous intensity exercise, accumulating ≥75 min · wk^{-1}, or likely a combination of both (17). Time for resistance exercise will be dictated by the time it takes to meet the frequency/intensity and volume desired based on one's fitness and performance goals.
- *Type:* Aerobic exercise should be performed in a continuous or intermittent manner and should involve major muscle groups. Resistance training should involve multijoint exercises that affect more than one muscle group, targeting agonist and antagonist muscle groups. Single-joint and core exercise can also be included with the multijoint exercises. Resistance exercise can include a variety of equipment (*e.g.*, free weights, weight machines, resistance tubes) or use body weight (17).
- *Overload:* The overload principle states that gains in strength/endurance come about only when progressively greater demands are placed on musculoskeletal and cardiopulmonary systems.
- *Periodization:* The planned, systematic design of an exercise training program that varies exercise volume, intensity, frequency, density, and mode to achieve peak performance at the appropriate times (*e.g.*, for a major competition) (49).
- *Quantifying exercise intensity:* Exercise intensity can be estimated from METs, percent of HRmax, percent of $\dot{V}O_{2max}$, or RPE.
- *Absolute and relative intensity:* If two individuals have $\dot{V}O_{2max}$ values of 4.2 and 3.2 L · min^{-1}, respectively, and both work at 2.5 L · min^{-1}, they would be working at the same absolute power output, but at different relative intensities because of different $\dot{V}O_{2max}$ values. The individual with a $\dot{V}O_{2max}$ of 4.2 L · min^{-1} would be working at 2.5/4.2 or 60%, while the person with a $\dot{V}O_{2max}$ of 3.2 L · min^{-1} would be working at 2.5/3.2 or 78% of $\dot{V}O_{2max}$.

Adaptations to Training

Endurance Training

- Adaptations to endurance exercise include improvements in neuromuscular and cardiovascular function, respiratory muscle efficiency and cost of breathing, decreases in body mass/body fat, if appropriate, improvements in heat tolerance, increases in self-esteem, lower blood lactate accumulation at higher power outputs, and increased insulin sensitivity.

Resistance Training

- Resistance training induces a variety of adaptations, with clear increases in strength.
- Neural adaptations include increases in strength with or without hypertrophy, greater synchronicity in activating motor units, and increased density of presynaptic and postsynaptic neurotransmitter receptors.
- Contractile adaptations include muscle hypertrophy through increased synthesis and accretion of intracellular myofibrillar proteins and activation of local satellite cells to add new nuclei to existing myofibers.
- Fiber type–specific adaptations depend on exercise volume and intensity, but a common change is an increase in the percentage of Type IIa fibers, at the expense of Type IIx fibers.
- Resistance training is not usually associated with increases in $\dot{V}O_{2max}$, but may enhance cardiovascular function by improving strength and lessening the daily load.

ESTIMATING STRENGTH AND ENDURANCE

Aerobic and Anaerobic Power

- Simple in-office and field tests can be used to estimate $\dot{V}O_{2max}$. These include the 1-, 1.5-, or 2-mile run, 12-minute run, 3-minute step test, shuttle runs, and submaximal cycle ergometry. The vertical jump, Wingate anaerobic cycle, running-based anaerobic sprint (400 m), and 300-yd shuttle run tests are used for anaerobic power.

Muscular Strength and Endurance

- Tests to assess muscular strength include free weights (1-RM: back squats/bench presses), hand grip dynamometry (maximal strength), and isokinetic equipment (60°–120° × s^{-1}).
- Muscular endurance can be measured by maximal number of push-ups, pull-ups, and/or sit-ups, as well as hand grip dynamometry (sustained submaximal endurance) and isokinetic equipment (180°–300° × s^{-1}).

REFERENCES

1. Kok HJ, Barton ER. Actions and interactions of IGF-I and MMPs during muscle regeneration. *Semin Cell Dev Biol.* 2021;119:11–22.
2. Wilborn CD, Taylor LW, Greenwood M, Kreider RB, Willoughby DS. Effects of different intensities of resistance exercise on regulators of myogenesis. *J Strength Cond Res.* 2009;23(8):2179–87.
3. Zammit PS. All muscle satellite cells are equal, but are some more equal than others? *J Cell Sci.* 2008;121(pt 18):2975–82.
4. Pette D, Staron RS. Mammalian skeletal muscle fiber type transitions. *Int Rev Cytol.* 1997;170:143–223.
5. Pette D, Staron RS. Myosin isoforms, muscle fiber types, and transitions. *Microsc Res Tech.* 2000;50(6):500–9.
6. Pette D, Staron RS. Transitions of muscle fiber phenotypic profiles. *Histochem Cell Biol.* 2001;115(5):359–72.
7. Staron RS. Human skeletal muscle fiber types: delineation, development, and distribution. *Can J Appl Physiol.* 1997;22(4):307–27.
8. Staron RS, Hagerman FC, Hikida RS, et al. Fiber type composition of the vastus lateralis muscle of young men and women. *J Histochem Cytochem.* 2000;48(5):623–9.

9. Tobias IS, Galpin AJ. Moving human muscle physiology research forward: an evaluation of fiber type-specific protein research methodologies. *Am J Physiol Cell Physiol.* 2020;319(5):C858–76.
10. Schiaffino S, Reggiani C. Fiber types in mammalian skeletal muscles. *Physiol Rev.* 2011;91(4):1447–531.
11. van der Zwaard S, Brocherie F, Jaspers RT. Under the hood: skeletal muscle determinants of endurance performance. *Front Sports Act Living.* 2021;3:719434.
12. Sawano S, Mizunoya W. History and development of staining methods for skeletal muscle fiber types. *Histol Histopathol.* 2022;37(6):493–503.
13. Coletti C, Acosta GF, Keslacy S, Coletti D. Exercise-mediated reinnervation of skeletal muscle in elderly people: an update. *Eur J Transl Myol.* 2022;32(1):10416.
14. Demirel HA, Powers SK, Naito H, Hughes M, Coombes JS. Exercise-induced alterations in skeletal muscle myosin heavy chain phenotype: dose-response relationship. *J Appl Physiol (1985).* 1999;86(3):1002–8.
15. He ZH, Bottinelli R, Pellegrino MA, Ferenczi MA, Reggiani C. ATP consumption and efficiency of human single muscle fibers with different myosin isoform composition. *Biophys J.* 2000;79(2):945–61.
16. Scott W, Stevens J, Binder-Macleod SA. Human skeletal muscle fiber type classifications. *Phys Ther.* 2001;81(11):1810–6.
17. Liguori G. *ACSM's Guidelines for Exercise Testing and Prescription.* 11 ed. Philadelphia (PA): Wolters Kluwer; 2021.
18. Astrand PO, Rodahl K, Dalh HA, Stromme SB. *Textbook of Work Physiology: Physiological Bases of Exercise.* Champaign (IL): Human Kinetics; 2003.
19. Sietsema KE, Stringer WW, Sue DY, Ward S. *Wasserman & Whipp's: Principles of Exercise Testing and Interpretation—Including Pathophysiology and Clinical Applications.* Philadelphia (PA): Lippincott Williams & Wilkins; 2020.
20. Monsorno K, Buckinx A, Paolicelli RC. Microglial metabolic flexibility: emerging roles for lactate. *Trends Endocrinol Metab.* 2022;33(3):186–95.
21. Duraj T, Carrión-Navarro J, Seyfried TN, García-Romero N, Ayuso-Sacido A. Metabolic therapy and bioenergetic analysis: the missing piece of the puzzle. *Mol Metab.* 2021;54:101389.
22. Magistretti PJ, Allaman I. Lactate in the brain: from metabolic end-product to signalling molecule. *Nat Rev Neurosci.* 2018;19(4):235–49.
23. Ferguson BS, Rogatzki MJ, Goodwin ML, Kane DA, Rightmire Z, Gladden LB. Lactate metabolism: historical context, prior misinterpretations, and current understanding. *Eur J Appl Physiol.* 2018;118(4):691–728.
24. Tanaka H, Monahan KD, Seals DR. Age-predicted maximal heart rate revisited. *J Am Coll Cardiol.* 2001;37(1):153–6.
25. Hunter GR, Bamman MM, Larson-Meyer DE, et al. Inverse relationship between exercise economy and oxidative capacity in muscle. *Eur J Appl Physiol.* 2005;94(5-6):558–68.
26. Ainsworth BE, Haskell WL, Herrmann SD, et al. 2011 Compendium of Physical Activities: a second update of codes and MET values. *Med Sci Sports Exerc.* 2011;43(8):1575–81.
27. Gaesser GA, Poole DC. The slow component of oxygen uptake kinetics in humans. *Exerc Sport Sci Rev.* 1996;24:35–71.
28. Jamnick NA, Pettitt RW, Granata C, Pyne DB, Bishop DJ. An examination and critique of current methods to determine exercise intensity. *Sports Med.* 2020;50(10):1729–56.
29. Sales MM, Sousa CV, da Silva Aguiar S, et al. An integrative perspective of the anaerobic threshold. *Physiol Behav.* 2019;205:29–32.
30. Domínguez R, Maté-Muñoz JL, Serra-Paya N, Garnacho-Castaño MV. Lactate threshold as a measure of aerobic metabolism in resistance exercise. *Int J Sports Med.* 2018;39(3):163–72.
31. Ploszczyca K, Jazic D, Piotrowicz Z, Chalimoniuk M, Langfort J, Czuba M. Comparison of maximal lactate steady state with anaerobic threshold determined by various methods based on graded exercise test with 3-minute stages in elite cyclists. *BMC Sports Sci Med Rehabil.* 2020;12(1):70.
32. Beneke R, von Duvillard SP. Determination of maximal lactate steady state response in selected sports events. *Med Sci Sports Exerc.* 1996;28(2):241–6.
33. Jones AM, Burnley M, Black MI, Poole DC, Vanhatalo A. The maximal metabolic steady state: redefining the 'gold standard'. *Physiol Rep.* 2019;7(10):e14098.
34. Andersson EP, Björklund G, McGawley K. Anaerobic capacity in running: the effect of computational method. *Front Physiol.* 2021;12:708172.
35. Noordhof DA, de Koning JJ, Foster C. The maximal accumulated oxygen deficit method: a valid and reliable measure of anaerobic capacity? *Sports Med.* 2010;40(4):285–302.
36. Medbo JI, Mohn AC, Tabata I, Bahr R, Vaage O, Sejersted OM. Anaerobic capacity determined by maximal accumulated O2 deficit. *J Appl Physiol (1985).* 1988;64(1):50–60.
37. Billat VL, Richard R, Binsse VM, Koralsztein JP, Haouzi P. The V(O2) slow component for severe exercise depends on type of exercise and is not correlated with time to fatigue. *J Appl Physiol (1985).* 1998;85(6):2118–24.
38. Jones AM, Burnley M. Oxygen uptake kinetics: an underappreciated determinant of exercise performance. *Int J Sports Physiol Perform.* 2009;4(4):524–32.
39. Jones AM, Carter H, Doust JH. A disproportionate increase in VO2 coincident with lactate threshold during treadmill exercise. *Med Sci Sports Exerc.* 1999;31(9):1299–306.
40. Krustrup P, Soderlund K, Mohr M, Bangsbo J. The slow component of oxygen uptake during intense, sub-maximal exercise in man is associated with additional fibre recruitment. *Pflugers Arch.* 2004;447(6):855–66.
41. Colosio AL, Caen K, Bourgois JG, Boone J, Pogliaghi S. Bioenergetics of the VO_2 slow component between exercise intensity domains. *Pflugers Arch.* 2020;472(10):1447–56.
42. Hill DW, Rowell AL. Running velocity at VO2max. *Med Sci Sports Exerc.* 1996;28(1):114–19.
43. Lacour JR, Padilla-Magunacelaya S, Chatard JC, Arsac L, Barthelemy JC. Assessment of running velocity at maximal oxygen uptake. *Eur J Appl Physiol Occup Physiol.* 1991;62(2):77–82.
44. McLaughlin JE, Howley ET, Bassett DR Jr, Thompson DL, Fitzhugh EC. Test of the classic model for predicting endurance running performance. *Med Sci Sports Exerc.* 2010;42(5):991–7.
45. Denadai BS, Greco CC. Could middle- and long-distance running performance of well-trained athletes be best predicted by the same aerobic parameters? *Curr Res Physiol.* 2022;5:265–9.
46. Panissa VLG, Fukuda DH, Staibano V, Marques M, Franchini E. Magnitude and duration of excess of post-exercise oxygen consumption between high-intensity interval and moderate-intensity continuous exercise: a systematic review. *Obes Rev.* 2021;22(1):e13099.
47. Close GL, Ashton T, McArdle A, Maclaren DP. The emerging role of free radicals in delayed onset muscle soreness and contraction-induced muscle injury. *Comp Biochem Physiol Mol Integr Physiol.* 2005;142(3):257–66.
48. Dannecker EA, Hausenblas HA, Kaminski TW, Robinson ME. Sex differences in delayed onset muscle pain. *Clin J Pain.* 2005;21(2):120–6.
49. National Strength and Conditioning Association. *Essentials of Strength and Conditioning.* 4th ed. Chicago (IL): Human Kinetics; 2016.
50. Poole DC, Richardson RS. Determinants of oxygen uptake. Implications for exercise testing. *Sports Med.* 1997;24(5):308–20.

7 Articular Cartilage Injury

Alexander C. Weissman, Allen A. Yazdi, Katie J. McMorrow, Aman Dhawan, Vasili Karas, Jason E. Jesse
Christopher M. Brusalis, and Brian J. Cole

INTRODUCTION

- Articular cartilage is a complex structure lining the articulating surfaces of diarthrodial joints. It provides a smooth, low-friction surface, while minimizing peak stress on the underlying subchondral bone.
- Injuries to the chondral surfaces occur in all joints of the human body. Articular injury of the knee has received the most attention in the literature. This chapter will focus primarily on articular injury as it pertains to the knee joint; however, many of the principles of evaluation, grading, and management hold true for chondral injury in any anatomic joint.
- Injury to articular cartilage is very common; in one retrospective review of 31,516 knee arthroscopies, 63% of patients were found to have chondral injury (1). Cartilage injury of the knee affects approximately 900,000 Americans annually, resulting in over 200,000 surgical procedures (2). Notably, the literature analyzing the prevalence of articular cartilage pathology does not provide significant guidance or insight into the prevalence of lesions that are or become symptomatic and require treatment.
- Although nonsurgical management of articular cartilage injury has remained largely the same over the past decade, surgical treatment of chondral injuries continues to evolve. Reparative, restorative, and reconstructive techniques continue to be refined, giving surgeons more tools and options for biologic reconstruction of articular surfaces. In the last 2 decades, a decline in the volume of performed marrow stimulation techniques, such as microfracture, has occurred with a commensurate increase in more complex cartilage restoration procedures (3,4).

BASIC SCIENCE

- Articular cartilage is composed of water (65%–80% of wet weight), collagen (10%–20% of wet weight), proteoglycans (10%–15% of wet weight), and chondrocytes (5% of wet weight). The collagen in native cartilage is primarily type II, with smaller quantities of types V, VI, IX, X, and XI. Chondrocytes are the cells responsible for the production of the extracellular matrix. These cells differentiate from mesenchymal stem cells during skeletal morphogenesis and are subsequently a low turnover cell type. Chondrocytes receive their nutrition and oxygen from the surrounding synovial fluid via diffusion (5). In the intact, uninjured knee, the articular cartilage shares load-bearing responsibility with the menisci (up to 70% from the lateral meniscus), making the chondral surfaces significantly vulnerable to injury and degeneration with partial or complete injury or removal of the menisci.
- Four zones and the tidemark establish articular cartilage. Each zone is distinct and classified by the shape of the respective chondrocytes and the orientation of the type II cartilage. Superior to inferior, these zones are the superficial zone, intermediate zone, deep zone, tidemark, and calcified cartilage zone that lay above the subchondral bone. The superficial zone is composed of a high number of flattened chondrocytes and is packed tightly with collagen fibers aligned parallel to the surface. This structure aids in the protection and maintenance of the subsiding layers. Representing 40%–60% of the total cartilage volume, the intermediate zone provides resistance to compressive forces and is formed by a low density of spherical chondrocytes and thicker, more oblique layer of collagen. The third layer, the deep zone, is composed of vertical collagen fibrils, parallel columnar chondrocytes, and a high proteoglycan content that fulfill the role of providing the greatest resistance to impact. The tidemark is the distinguisher of the deep zone from the calcified layer. The chondrocytes here are hypertrophic and cell population is scarce (5,6).
- Cartilage being avascular, aneural, and alymphatic, relies heavily on diffusion for cell nutrition and waste removal. Chondrocyte division and migration is limited, resulting in the healing response being poor. Partial-thickness injury that does not penetrate the tidemark, the demarcation between the deep layer and calcified layer of cartilage, will result in cellular insult with decreased matrix production by the underlying and surrounding chondrocytes and ultimately little healing. In cartilage matrix and cell injuries, decreased proteoglycan concentration, increased hydration, and disorganization of the collagen network occur (1,5).
- Injury that penetrates the tidemark into the calcified cartilage layer and the subchondral bone (an osteochondral lesion)

will elicit an inflammatory response that includes an influx of marrow contents (undifferentiated mesenchymal stem cells, cytokines, and growth factors including transforming growth factor-β [TGF-β] and platelet-derived growth factor [PDGF]) triggered by hemorrhage and fibrin clot. The osteochondral injury has potential for a more robust healing response including a resultant repair that more closely resembles fibrocartilage, compared to native hyaline cartilage, and is composed of primarily type I collagen. This fibrocartilage-like repair is less stiff and more permeable than normal articular cartilage (1,5). Fibrocartilaginous repair tissue is far less durable than native hyaline cartilage and often begins to show evidence of depletion of proteoglycans, increased hydration, fragmentation and fibrillation, increased collagen content, and loss of chondrocytes within 1 year (7).

- Although the natural history of chondral injuries is not completely understood, it is postulated that defects, particularly larger, full-thickness injuries, can progress via edge loading and elevated contact pressures on the adjacent articular surfaces. This progression may lead to degradation of the surrounding chondral surfaces and ultimately osteoarthrosis. Symptoms of pain, swelling, stiffness, and locking or catching often accompany this progression that limits patient activities (8).

Patient Evaluation

- Articular cartilage injury can be caused by an acute injury that results in a focal chondral or osteochondral injury or chronic/subacute injuries or conditions that result in degenerative lesions. Damage to the chondral surfaces can occur in isolation or, as is often the case, in association with other intra-articular injury. The evaluating physician should maintain a high index of suspicion for chondral injury when evaluating the knee for any causes of pain, effusion, instability, or mechanical symptoms. Conversely, a comprehensive patient evaluation is paramount to establish a clear clinical correlation between imaging findings and a patient's symptoms, as a substantial number of focal chondral defects identified on imaging studies may be asymptomatic.
- A thorough history should include details related to the onset of symptoms (traumatic or insidious), mechanism of injury, previous injuries and surgery, and symptom-provoking activities. Importantly, symptoms from focal chondral defects within the knee must be distinguished from those of diffuse knee osteoarthritis, which often has a more severe presentation characterized by a dull, achy pain with recurrent knee swelling and pain when rising from a seated position (9).
- A thorough physical examination should evaluate formal alignment, abnormal gait, swelling, effusions, instability, meniscal symptoms, range of motion, strength, and neurovascular abnormalities. Crepitus, catching, locking, or grinding can occur with focal irregularities of the articular surfaces. Diagnosis of all concomitant pathology is critical to formulate a successful, global treatment plan.
- Radiographic workup should include posterior-anterior, weight-bearing, 45° plain films and patellofemoral, and non–weight-bearing lateral projections. Evaluation on plain films for joint space narrowing, subchondral sclerosis, osteophytes, and cysts should be performed. History and physical examination, along with these radiographs, are often all that is needed to make the appropriate diagnosis. Magnetic resonance imaging (MRI) can be valuable to assess the status of the knee ligaments and menisci but can underestimate the degree of cartilage abnormalities seen during arthroscopy (10). Use of 3.0-Tesla (T) magnets, cartilage imaging sequence techniques including fat-suppressed or fat-suppressed spoiled gradient-echo imaging, and balanced free precession steady-state sequences have improved detection and characterization of chondral injuries using MRI (11). Routine MRI sequences are typically sufficient to evaluate for subchondral abnormalities that may become useful findings during definitive decision making.

GRADING OF ARTICULAR CARTILAGE INJURY

- MRI provides excellent soft-tissue contrast and resolution for noninvasive evaluation of chondral injuries. MRI of cartilage is typically performed on high-field strength systems of at least 1.5 T, whereas 3 T systems are being increasingly used as well. Conventional MRI sequences can be used to detect discrete morphologic defects, whereas compositional studies can identify biochemical changes in water permeability before other lesions develop (12).
- Although MRI is being used with more frequency to evaluate chondral injuries, arthroscopic evaluation remains the most accurate way to assess the location, depth, size, shape, and stability of a chondral or osteochondral defect of the articular surface. The Outerbridge classification is most widely used to grade these injuries (Table 7.1) (13). More recently, the International Cartilage Repair Society has modified this to a more comprehensive description and grading system (see Table 7.1) (14,15). The International Cartilage Repair Society grading system can be used to describe lesions both arthroscopically and using advanced radiologic imaging techniques.

NONSURGICAL TREATMENT

- Nonsurgical techniques are often used to manage patients' symptoms and slow the progression of the injury or disease. They may be considered based on patient age, activity level, and extent of the injury. As with most joint pathology, initial treatment of articular cartilage injuries is typically

Table 7.1 Outerbridge Arthroscopic Grading System and Modified International Cartilage Repair Society (ICRS) Classification System for Chondral Injury (13–15)

Grade of Injury	Outerbridge Arthroscopic Grading System	Modified ICRS System
Grade 0	Normal cartilage	Normal cartilage
Grade I	Cartilage with softening and swelling	Nearly normal with superficial fissuring
Grade II	Partial-thickness defect with fissures on the surface that do not reach subchondral bone or exceed 1.5 cm in diameter	Lesions extending less than 1/2 of cartilage depth
Grade III	Fissuring to the level of subchondral bone in an area with a diameter more than 1.5 cm	Lesions extending greater than 1/2 of cartilage depth up to subchondral plate
Grade IV	Exposed subchondral bone	Through subchondral plate, exposing subchondral bone

conservative with recommendations that include activity modification, physical therapy, judicious use of nonsteroidal anti-inflammatory drugs (NSAIDs), glucosamine and chondroitin sulfate, corticosteroid or biologic injections, and consideration for viscosupplementation (16).

- See Chapters 76–79 for further discussion of nonoperative therapies (Medications and Ergogenic Aids, Prolotherapy, Orthobiologic Therapies, and Joint Injections/Aspiration.)
- Patients with mechanical symptoms (including catching, locking, sensation of loose body, or giving way), acute motion loss, or failed nonsurgical management with pain and loss of function should be considered for surgical intervention.

SURGICAL TREATMENT

Arthroscopic Debridement and Lavage

- Arthroscopic debridement and lavage can be a first-line surgical intervention in a patient with a symptomatic articular cartilage injury. This treatment modality allows the surgeon to perform a diagnostic arthroscopy to assess for chondral injury and for concomitant pathologies in the remainder of the joint. Patient expectations must be managed in that the results of this procedure can range from diagnostic to therapeutic due to the removal of degenerative debris, loose nonviable chondral fragments, and lavage of the associated inflammatory cytokines such as interleukin-1 and tumor necrosis factor-α (17). Care is taken to preserve intact, healthy articular cartilage. Irrigation and debridement alone has been proven to provide good to excellent short- and medium-term benefits in 60%–70% of patients (17–19). In a select group of highly active individuals, especially in-season when return-to-sport times are critical, debridement may be a first-line option to provide beneficial, temporary improvement. In general, however, the results of arthroscopic debridement and lavage are often not durable and deteriorate over time, and the primary benefit that remains is the diagnostic information obtained to help guide future treatment decisions (Table 7.2) (20–32).

Fragment Fixation

- Osteochondral lesions occur most frequently on the femoral condylar surface, and can include a breath of pathology including osteochondritis dissecans, osteochondral defects, osteochondral fractures, and osteonecrosis (33). Fixation of these lesions is predicated on the condition, size, shape, defect location, and adequacy of subchondral bone attached to the osteochondral fragment. Radiographic and MRI evaluation can help with the determination of many of these factors and appropriateness of this surgical option. Prior to fixation of the osteochondral fragment, both the fragment and defect must be prepared to create an adequate healing milieu. The fragment must be reduced anatomically into its bed, and fixation may then be completed using either absorbable or nonabsorbable implants. Occasionally, bone graft augmentation is required for deeper cavitating lesions. Treating osteochondral lesions with the same considerations as a fracture nonunion will lead to more predictable healing. These factors include debriding fibrocartilage at the base of the lesion, microfracture augmentation of the base to promote bleeding, and rigid fixation with compression. Fixation is accomplished with the use of metal or composite bioabsorbable pins and screws. Metallic implants removed at 6–8 weeks allow the opportunity to verify fragment healing and prevent the untoward effects of prominent hardware that can develop over time (17). Successful healing of the osteochondral fragment with the use of headless metallic cannulated screws has been reported in up to 90% of patients and has demonstrated positive clinical and imaging outcomes at 10 years post operatively (34). Arthroscopic fixation of osteochondral lesions with bioabsorbable pins has also shown excellent clinical and radiographic results. Further use of bioabsorbable and next-generation fixation material will likely continue to become more prevalent. Benefits of bioabsorbable fixation include fewer procedures for implant removal, and lessened interference with imaging (35).

Marrow-Stimulating Techniques

- The goal of marrow stimulation techniques (MST) is to deliver mesenchymal stem cell progenitors to the bed of a focal chondral defect, which can lead to the subsequent formation of a fibrocartilage-like repair tissue from these cells.

Table 7.2 Results of Arthroscopic Debridement and Lavage

Study	No. of Patients	Mean Follow-Up	Results
Acosta et al., 2020 (20)	485	26.9 mo (8–40 mo)	Systematic review: Stable meniscal lesions <2 cm in size were effectively treated with debridement alone and showed significantly increased Lysholm and IKDC scores ($P < 0.005$).
Weißenberger et al., 2019 (21)	126	12 mo	Case-control study: Focal cartilage defects treated with debridement had overall improvement with respect to the KOOS. Lesser improvement in defects >2 cm^2.
Anderson et al., 2017 (22)	53	31.5 ± 13.9 mo	Retrospective case series: Improvement in all patient-reported outcome measures (PROM) except the mental component of the VR-12.
Kirkley et al., 2008 (23)	163	2 y	Randomized controlled trial: Arthroscopy and PT vs. PT alone showed no difference in WOMAC, or SF-36 between groups ($P = 0.22$).
Jackson and Dieterichs, 2003 (24)	121	4–6 y	Retrospective case series: Stage I: 100% excellent/good Stage II: 90.6% excellent/good Stage III: 48.7% excellent/good Stage IV: 11.9% excellent/good
Moseley et al., 2002 (25)	180	2 y	Randomized controlled trial: Debridement, lavage, and placebo showed no difference in KSPS, AIMS2-P, and SF-36 scores.
Steadman et al., 2001 (26)	75	11.3 y	Retrospective case series: Lysholm 58.8 → 89 Tegner 3.1 → 5.8 Work 4.9 → 7.6 Sports 4.2 → 7.1
Timoney et al., 1990 (27)	109	48 mo	Retrospective case series: 63% good 37% fair/poor
Jackson, 1989 (28)	137	3.5 y (2–9 y)	Retrospective case series: 68% remained improved
Sprague, 1981 (29)	78	14 mo	Retrospective case series: 74% good 26% fair/poor

AIMS2-P, Arthritis Impact Measurement Scales; IKDC, International Knee Documentation Committee; KOOS, Knee Injury and Osteoarthritis Outcome Score; KSPS, Knee-Specific Pain Scale; PT, physical therapy; SF-36, Short Form-36; VR-12, Veteran RAND 12-item health survey; WOMAC, Western Ontario and McMaster Universities Arthritis Index.

This technique can be performed via drilling, abrasion, or microfracture and always involves penetration of the calcified cartilage layer into the subchondral bone to allow the migration of progenitor cells to the articular surface. In a 2021 retrospective comparative study of 68 patients, a battery-powered microdrilling technique demonstrated improved short-term outcomes compared to a traditional microfracture-and-awl technique (36). Microfracture can also be augmented with the local supplementation of chondrogenic growth factors to prolong the action of these mesenchymal stem cells (37). MST augmentation with a cartilage allograft extracellular matrix has recently been shown to improve outcomes with low complication rates at 2-year follow-up (38,39). Because of the limited fill that may occur in some lesions, particularly larger ones greater than 2 cm^2, and the different structural and biomechanical properties of this fibrocartilage-like repair tissue (see earlier Basic Science section), the best results are typically achieved with relatively small defects in a low-demand patient population (17). Results of microfracture technique are summarized in Table 7.3 (40–52).

Osteochondral Autograft

- An osteochondral autograft transfer system (OATS) harvests plugs of native cartilage and bone from load-sparing areas of the knee and transfers them into the area of a symptomatic chondral defect. It offers several advantages, including increased generation of hyaline-like cartilage, a relatively brief rehabilitation period, and the ability to perform the procedure in a single operation (53). Return to sports has been found to be as low as 90 days in some studies (54). Limitations include the availability of low-contact harvest areas, donor site morbidity, and the potential for surface

Table 7.3 Results of Microfracture

Study	No.	Mean Follow-Up[a]	Results
Wen et al., 2022 (40)	Systematic review (635 patients)	2 y (1–5 y)	Systematic Review: Augmented microfracture with orthobiologics showed minimal improvement over traditional microfracture
Kim et al., 2020 (41)	Systematic review (29 studies)	≥2 y	Systematic Review: Autologous matrix-induced chondrogenesis vs microfracture showed no significant difference in clinical outcomes, other than IKDC subjective score
Orth et al., 2020 (42)	Systematic review (1759 patients)	6.6 y (4.3–8.8 y)	Systematic Review: Failure rates at 5 y: 11%–27% Failure rate at 10 y: 6%–32%
Mithoefer et al., 2012 (43)	21 professional athletes	13 y	Retrospective case series: Return to professional sport at 12 mo: 95% Years of subsequent professional play: 5 y (1–13 y)
Solheim et al., 2010 (44)	110 patients	5 y (2-9 y)	Retrospective cohort: Lysholm 51 → 71 VAS function 41 → 74 VAS pain 52 → 30[b]
Mithoefer et al., 2009 (45)	Systematic review (3122 patients)	3.4 ± 0.4 y (1–3 y)	Systematic review: Short-term clinical improvement rate (≤24 mo): 75%–100% Long-term clinical improvement rate (≥24 mo): 67%–80%
Asik et al., 2008 (46)	90 patients	5.2 y (2–9 y)	Retrospective case series: Lysholm 52.4 → 84.6 Tegner 2.6 → 5.2
Bae et al., 2006 (47)	47 knees	1 y	Second look arthroscopy: Extent of cartilage healing >90% in 55% of cases; 80%–89% in 10% Radiographic evaluation: average joint space increase of 1.06 mm on anterior-posterior and 1.37 mm on lateral
Gobbi et al., 2005 (48)	25 competitive athletes	6 y (3–10 y)	Prospective cohort study: 30% improved Lysholm 56.8 → 87.2 Tegner 3.2 → 5
Steadman et al., 2002 (49)	71 knees Age ≤ 45 y	11 y (7–17 y)	Retrospective case series: 80% improved Lysholm 59 → 89 Tegner 6 → 9 Majority of improvement in first year Maximal improvement in 2–3 y Younger patients did better
Steadman et al., 2001 (26)	75 patients	11.3 y	Retrospective case series: Lysholm 58.8 → 89 Tegner 3.1 → 5.8 Work 4.9 → 7.6 Sports 4.2 → 7.1
Gill and Macgillivray, 2001 (50)	103 patients	6 y (2–12 y)	Retrospective case series: 86% rated knee as normal/nearly normal Acute (treated within 12 wk) did better
Blevins et al., 1998 (51)	140 recreational athletes Mean age, 38 y Mean defect size, 2.8 cm^2 38 high-level athletes Mean age, 26 y Mean defect size, 2.2 cm^2	3.7 y	Prospective cohort study: 77% returned to sports
Steadman et al., 1997 (52)	203 patients	3 y (2–12 y)	Retrospective case series: 75% improved, 19% unchanged, 6% worse, 60% improved sports Poor prognosis: joint space narrowing, age >30 y, no postoperative CPM

CPM, continuous passive motion; IKDC, International Knee Documentation Committee; VAS, visual analog scale.
[a]Represents median number of years as reported by study.
[b]Lower values denote improvement.

plug incongruity, although advances in computer modeling have improved donor site matching (55–57). Patient selection is critical and, in general, is recommended for lesions <2–3 cm^2 (58). Short- and mid-term results of this technique have been promising, showing greater than 90% good to excellent results and a 78% survival rate at 10 years (59–61).

Osteochondral Allograft

- Osteochondral allograft transplantation is a commonly used procedure used to treat lesions of the knee, shoulder, ankle, and hip. It involves transplantation of a prolonged, freshly preserved (at 4 or 37°C) cadaveric graft consisting of intact, viable hyaline cartilage, and its underlying subchondral bone into the articular cartilage defect. Because other preservation techniques such as fresh-freezing, freeze-drying, and cryopreservation have been shown to decrease chondrocyte viability and ultimate load and increase stiffness, fresh osteochondral allografts are typically used (62,63). This procedure is ideal for lesions that are large, multifocal, multicompartmental, or present with significant subchondral bone loss. It allows for a shorter operative time, replication of native knee anatomy, immediate transplantation of both cartilage and subchondral bone as a single-stage procedure, a lower incidence of postoperative arthrofibrosis, and no donor site morbidity (64).
- Limitations include concerns over insurance approval, graft availability, low but possible risk of immunologic rejection, potential for disease transmission, adequate graft healing, and technically demanding aspects of graft matching and sizing (62,64,65). Incorporation of graft preparation techniques prior to implantation have shown to have utmost importance in minimizing some of these concerns. Some recent advances include pulsed lavage, pressurized CO_2, biologic augmentation, and minimizing impaction loads during graft insertion (66–69).
- Use of osteochondral allografts (OAGs) in recent years have increased due to the ability to reliably improve patient-reported outcomes (PROs) and longevity after graft incorporation into host tissue (70). There are a number of well-demonstrated long-term clinical follow-up studies that demonstrate an average of 88% success at 5 years and 81% success at 10 years after surgery (59,64,71–74). In addition, a recent comprehensive review evaluating 205 patients demonstrated improvement in Lysholm scores (20,61–87), International Knee Documentation Committee (IKDC) scores (54–84), all five components of the Knee Injury and Osteoarthritis Outcome Score (KOOS) Pain, 57–76; Other Disease-Specific Symptoms, 55–73; Activities of Daily Living Function, 65–86; Sport and Recreation Function, 26–56; Knee-Related Quality of Life, 23–56), and Short Form-12 physical component scores (55–66,71). Literature outcomes on osteochondral allografts are included in Table 7.4.
- Although osteochondral allograft transplantation was popularized initially for focal articular cartilage injuries of the femoral condyles, the technique has proven efficacious for patellofemoral chondral injuries. In a systematic review of 129 patients across eight studies, OAGs conferred significant improvements in multiple patient-reported outcomes with a mean 77.2% survival at 10 years. OAG for patellofemoral defects was also associated with a higher rate of concomitant procedures, and therefore the relative contributions of individual procedures require further study (75).

Autologous Chondrocyte Implantation

- Autologous chondrocyte implantation requires a two-stage procedure including the biopsy of chondrocytes from the knee, culturing and expansion of the chondrocyte cell line, and reoperation for transplantation into the cartilage defect beneath a periosteal or collagen matrix patch. The potential advantages of this procedure include the ability to fill defects as large as 10 cm^2, the development of hyaline-like cartilage rather than fibrocartilage in the grafted defect, and possibly better long-term outcomes and longevity of the healing tissue. This procedure can be technically demanding, requiring the patient to undergo a relatively long rehabilitation in addition to a requirement for two surgical procedures. In addition, although the overall complication rate appears to be relatively low, the adverse events that do occur following autologous chondrocyte implantation can result in subsequent operative intervention.
- Peterson et al. (76,77) demonstrated that 92% of patients were satisfied and would have the autologous chondrocyte implantation (ACI) surgery again at 10–20 years after transplantation. In their cohort of 50 patients, Micheli et al. (78) demonstrated that 84% of patients had significant improvement in their symptoms at 3 years postoperatively. A recent multicenter cohort study evaluated outcomes of autologous chondrocyte transplantation after failed previous articular cartilage surgery (76). After 48 months of follow-up, 76% of the 154 patients had a successful outcome, whereas 24% were deemed as having treatment failure. Interestingly, 49% of the patients (n = 76) had a subsequent surgical procedure performed after the autologous chondrocyte implantation. These additional procedures, predominantly arthroscopic, were not predictive of failure. The use of type I/III bilayer collagen instead of a periosteal patch to cover the cells during the implantation procedure has been shown to decrease the reoperation rate significantly (80). A recent study evaluating 2- to 9-year outcomes of autologous chondrocyte implantation in a diverse patient population demonstrated that 75% of patients were completely or mostly satisfied with their outcomes and 83% would have the procedure done again (81,82).
- In 2016, matrix-induced autologous chondrocyte implantation (MACI; autologous cultured chondrocytes on porcine collagen membrane) received approval from the U.S. Food and Drug Administration for the treatment of symptomatic articular cartilage defects of the knee in adults with or

Table 7.4 Results of Osteochondral Allograft

Study	No.	Location	Mean Follow-Up	Results
Gilat et al., 2021 (71)	205	F	7.7 y	Case series: 86% success rate at 5 y 82% success rate at 10 y 21% failure
Familiari et al., 2018 (59)	1036	F, T, P	8.7 y	Systematic review: 87% success rate at 5 y 79% success rate at 10 y 73% success rate at 15 y 68% success rate at 20 y 18% failure
Frank et al., 2017 (64)	224	F	5 y	Case series: 87% success rate at 5 y 18% failure
Assenmacher et al., 2016 (65)	291	F, T, P	12.3 y	Systematic review: 75% success rate 25% failure
Cameron et al., 2016 (72)	28	F	7 y	Case series: 100% success rate at 5 y 92% success rate at 10 y 85% good/excellent
Briggs et al., 2015 (73)	55	F, T, P	>7.6 y	Case series: 90% success rate at 5 y 75% success rate at 10 y 85% good/excellent 6% fair/poor
Gracitelli et al., 2015 (74)	28	P	9.7 y	Case series: 78% success rate at 5 y 78% success rate at 10 y 56% success rate at 15 y 29% failure

F, femur; IKDC, International Knee Documentation Committee; P, patella; T, tibia.

without bone involvement (83). This approval was supported by the results of the European SUMMIT (Superiority of MACI Implant vs. Microfracture Treatment) trial, which found clinically and statistically significant improvements in MACI over microfracture treatment with regard to KOOS pain and function sub-scores (84). In addition, Ebert et al. (85) demonstrated significant improvements in MRI-based scores after 10 years postoperatively, as well as high patient satisfaction rates with the outcome of their surgery, improvement in knee pain relief, and ability to participate in sport again. Outcomes of autologous chondrocyte implantation from various studies over the years are summarized in Table 7.5 (76–78,82,84–89).

TREATMENT DECISION MAKING

- Management of articular cartilage injuries can be challenging, and there are multiple options available to treat similar lesions. Although there is no consensus on optimal treatment, certain guidelines can be followed. Decision making must consider patient goals, physical demands, expectations, and perceptions, as well as objective measurements such as defect size, depth, location, chronicity, previous treatments and responses, and concomitant pathology. Ligament insufficiency, meniscal pathology, and/or mechanical malalignment must be addressed, particularly in the treatment of articular cartilage injury of the femoral condyles. It is common for concomitant procedures to be performed, including meniscal allograft transplantation, distal femoral or high tibial osteotomy, and tibial tuberosity elevation. Our recommended primary treatment guideline is included in Figure 7.1.
- Articular cartilage surgical restoration allows for a high rate of return to high-impact sports, often at the preinjury competitive level. The time of return and durability can be variable and depend on repair technique and athlete-specific factors. Player age, competitive level, defect size, time to treatment, and repair tissue morphology all affect the ability and time to return-to-play. Sports participation after cartilage repair generally promotes joint restoration and functional recovery. Time to return to impact sports generally varies between 7 and 17 months, with the longest time after autologous chondrocyte transplantation.

Table 7.5 Results of Autologous Chondrocyte Transplantation

Study	No.	Location	Mean Follow-Up	Results
Ebert et al., 2020 (85)	70	F	>10 y, Range 10.5–11.5 y	Prospective randomized trial: Significant improvement in all clinical measures employed and MRI-based scores ($P < 0.05$) 88.3% patient satisfaction with the 10-y results of their surgery 93.3% patient satisfaction with the improvement in knee pain relief 88.3% patient satisfaction with the improvement in their ability to participate in sport
Saris et al., 2014 (84)	144	F	2 y	Prospective randomized trial: Statistically significant improvements in KOOS pain (11.76, $P < 0.001$) and function subscores (11.41, $P = 0.016$) over microfracture treatment Significant improvement for MACI over microfracture treatment observed in as early as 36 wk and maintained throughout study
Moseley et al., 2010 (86)	72	F	>5 y Mean, 9.2 y	Case series: 69% of patients improved from baseline 12.5% had no change 17% failed
Peterson et al., 2010 (76)	224	F, P, multiple	>10 y Mean, 12.8 y	Case series: 92% patient satisfaction
Bhosale et al., 2009 (87)	80	F, P, Tr, multiple	>2.7 y Mean, 5 y	Prospective cohort study: 81% clinical improvement 19% clinical decline
Peterson et al., 2002 (77)	18 14 17 11	F OCD P F/ACL	>5 y >5 y >5 y >5 y	Case series: 89% good/excellent 86% good/excellent 65% good/excellent 91% good/excellent
Micheli et al., 2001 (78)	50	F/Tr/P	>3 y	Prospective cohort study: 84% significant improvement 2% unchanged 13% declined
Peterson et al., 2000 (82)	25 19 16 16	F P F/ACL Multiple	>2 y >2 y >2 y >2 y	Case series: 92% good/excellent 62% good/excellent 75% good/excellent 67% good/excellent
Gillogly et al., 1998 (88)	25	F, P, T	>1 y	Case series: 88% good/excellent
Brittberg et al., 1994 (89)	16 7	F P	39 mo 36 mo	Prospective cohort study: 88% good/excellent 12% poor 29% good/excellent 71% fair/poor

ACL, anterior cruciate ligament; F, femur; KOOS, Knee Injury and Osteoarthritis Score; MACI, autologous cultured chondrocytes on porcine collagen membrane; MRI, magnetic resonance imaging; OCD, osteochondritis dissecans; P, patella; T, tibia; Tr, trochlea.

FUTURE DIRECTIONS

- Ongoing research in the area of articular cartilage continues. Indeed, it is one of the most studied topics in contemporary orthopedics. Additional treatments being evaluated include the incorporation of orthobiologic agents, including bone marrow aspirate concentrate (BMAC), platelet-rich plasma (PRP), cell-based therapies, amniotic suspension allografts, and adipose tissue with the above procedures.

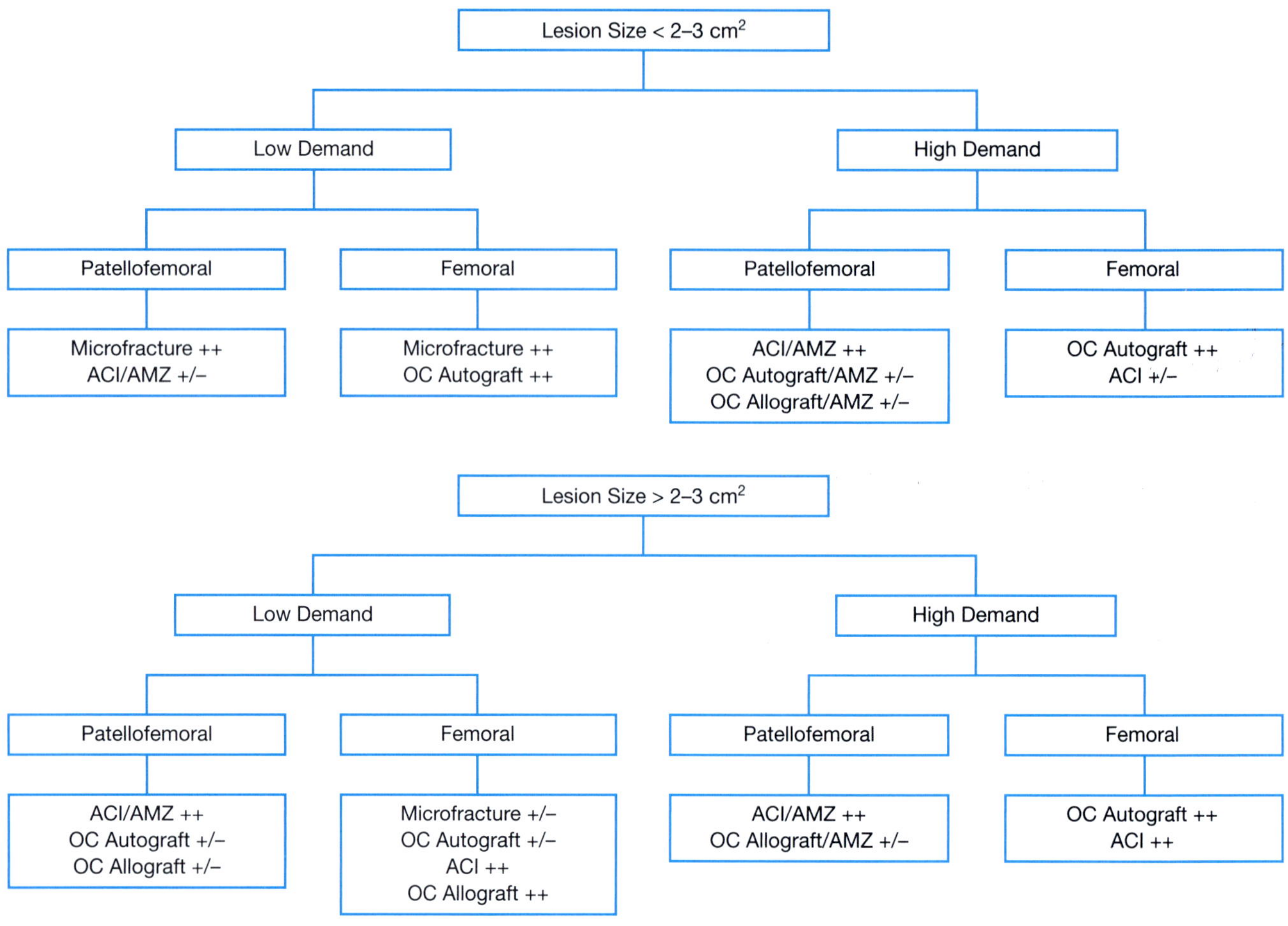

Figure 7.1: Surgical treatment algorithm of articular cartilage injuries. ACI, autologous chondrocyte implantation; AMZ, anteromedialization tibial tubercle osteotomy; OC, osteochondral.

These techniques involve delivery of growth factors, naturally derived blood components, and autologous tissue to the surgical site that have the potential to enhance healing and repair of the cartilage following the procedure. Human, animal, and basic science models have demonstrated early promise using these techniques; however, more rigorous, well-conducted human trials need be conducted to elucidate the scope of additional benefits associated with them (90–95).

REFERENCES

1. Curl WW, Krome J, Gordon ES, Rushing J, Smith BP, Poehling GG. Cartilage injuries: a review of 31,516 knee arthroscopies. *Arthroscopy*. 1997 Aug;13(4):456–60.
2. Cole B, Frederick R, Levy A, Zaslav K. Management of a 37-year old man with recurrent knee pain. *J Clin Outcomes Management*. 1999;6(6):46–57.
3. Frank RM, Cotter EJ, Hannon CP, Harrast JJ, Cole BJ. Cartilage restoration surgery: incidence rates, complications, and trends as reported by the American board of orthopaedic surgery Part II candidates. *Arthroscopy*. 2019 Jan;35(1):171–8.
4. Gowd AK, Cvetanovich GL, Liu JN, et al. Management of chondral lesions of the knee: analysis of trends and short-term complications using the national surgical quality improvement program database. *Arthroscopy*. 2019 Jan;35(1):138–46.
5. Buckwalter J, Rosenberg L, Hunziker E. Articular cartilage: composition and structure. In: *Injury and Repair of the Musculoskeletal Soft Tissues*; 1988:405–25.
6. Sophia Fox AJ, Bedi A, Rodeo SA. The basic science of articular cartilage: structure, composition, and function. *Sports Health*. 2009 Nov;1(6):461–8.
7. Buckwalter JA. Articular cartilage injuries. *Clin Orthop Relat Res*. 2002 Sep;402:21–37.
8. Krych AJ, Saris DBF, Stuart MJ, Hacken B. Cartilage injury in the knee: assessment and treatment options. *J Am Acad Orthop Surg*. 2020 Nov;28(22):914–22.
9. Gilat R, Haunschild ED, Patel S, et al. Understanding the difference between symptoms of focal cartilage defects and osteoarthritis of the knee: a matched cohort analysis. *Int Orthop*. 2021 Jul;45(7):1761–6.
10. Khanna AJ, Cosgarea AJ, Mont MA, et al. Magnetic resonance imaging of the knee. Current techniques and spectrum of disease. *J Bone Joint Surg Am*. 2001;83-A(suppl 2 pt 2):128–41.
11. Bauer JS, Barr C, Henning TD, et al. Magnetic resonance imaging of the ankle at 3.0 Tesla and 1.5 Tesla in human cadaver specimens with artificially created lesions of cartilage and ligaments. *Investig Radiol*. 2008 Sep;43(9):604–11.

12. Strickland CD, Ho CK, Merkle AN, Vidal AF. MR imaging of knee cartilage injury and repair surgeries. *Magn Reson Imaging Clin N Am*. 2022 May;30(2):227–39.
13. Outerbridge RE. The etiology of chondromalacia patellae. 1961. *Clin Orthop Relat Res*. 2001 Aug;389:5–8.
14. Brittberg M, Winalski CS. Evaluation of cartilage injuries and repair. *J Bone Joint Surg Am*. 2003;85-A(suppl 2):58–69.
15. Mainil-Varlet P, Aigner T, Brittberg M. International Cartilage Repair Society, et al. Histological assessment of cartilage repair: a report by the histology Endpoint Committee of the International cartilage repair Society (ICRS). *J Bone Joint Surg Am*. 2003;85-A(suppl 2):45–57.
16. Daher RJ, Chahine NO, Greenberg AS, Sgaglione NA, Grande DA. New methods to diagnose and treat cartilage degeneration. *Nat Rev Rheumatol*. 2009 Nov;5(11):599–607.
17. Alford JW, Cole BJ. Cartilage restoration, Part 2: techniques, outcomes, and future directions. *Am J Sports Med*. 2005 Mar;33(3):443–60.
18. Friedman MJ, Berasi CC, Fox JM, Del Pizzo W, Snyder SJ, Ferkel RD. Preliminary results with abrasion arthroplasty in the osteoarthritic knee. *Clin Orthop Relat Res*. 1984;182:200–5.
19. Totlis T, Marín Fermín T, Kalifis G, Terzidis I, Maffulli N, Papakostas E. Arthroscopic debridement for focal articular cartilage lesions of the knee: a systematic review. *Surgeon*. 2021 Dec;19(6):356–64.
20. Acosta J, Ravaei S, Brown SM, Mulcahey MK. Examining techniques for treatment of medial meniscal Ramp lesions during anterior cruciate ligament reconstruction: a systematic review. *Arthroscopy*. 2020 Nov;36(11):2921–33.
21. Weißenberger M, Heinz T, Boelch SP, et al. Is debridement beneficial for focal cartilage defects of the knee: data from the German Cartilage Registry (KnorpelRegister DGOU). *Arch Orthop Trauma Surg*. 2020 Mar;140(3):373–82.
22. Anderson DE, Rose MB, Wille AJ, Wiedrick J, Crawford DC. Arthroscopic mechanical chondroplasty of the knee is beneficial for treatment of focal cartilage lesions in the absence of concurrent pathology. *Orthop J Sports Med*. 2017 May;5(5):2325967117707213.
23. Kirkley A, Birmingham TB, Litchfield RB, et al. A randomized trial of arthroscopic surgery for osteoarthritis of the knee. *N Engl J Med*. 2008 Sep;359(11):1097–107.
24. Jackson RW, Dieterichs C. The results of arthroscopic lavage and debridement of osteoarthritic knees based on the severity of degeneration: a 4- to 6-year symptomatic follow-up. *Arthroscopy*. 2003 Jan;19(1):13–20.
25. Moseley JB, O'Malley K, Petersen NJ, et al. A controlled trial of arthroscopic surgery for osteoarthritis of the knee. *N Engl J Med*. 2002 Jul;347(2):81–8.
26. Steadman JR, Rodkey WG, Rodrigo JJ. Microfracture: surgical technique and rehabilitation to treat chondral defects. *Clin Orthop Relat Res*. 2001 Oct;391(suppl l):S362–9.
27. Timoney JM, Kneisl JS, Barrack RL, Alexander AH. Arthroscopy update #6. Arthroscopy in the osteoarthritic knee. Long-term follow-up. *Orthop Rev*. 1990 Apr;19(4):371–9.
28. Jackson RW. Meniscal and articular cartilage injury in sport. *J R Coll Surg Edinb*. 1989;34(6 suppl l):S15–7.
29. Sprague NF. Arthroscopic debridement for degenerative knee joint disease. *Clin Orthop Relat Res*. 1981 Oct;160:118–23.
30. Bernard J, Lemon M, Patterson MH. Arthroscopic washout of the knee-a 5-year survival analysis. *Knee*. 2004 Jun;11(3):233–5.
31. Hubbard MJ. Arthroscopic surgery for chondral flaps in the knee. *J Bone Joint Surg Br*. 1987 Nov;69(5):794–6.
32. Oliver-Welsh L, Griffin JW, Meyer MA, Gitelis ME, Cole BJ. Deciding how best to treat cartilage defects. *Orthopedics*. 2016 Nov;39(6):343–50.
33. Cordunianu MA, Antoniac I, Niculescu M, et al. Treatment of knee osteochondral fractures. *Healthcare (Basel)*. 2022 Jun;10(6):1061.
34. Ackermann J, Waltenspül M, Merkely G, et al. Association of subchondral changes with age and clinical outcome in patients with osteochondral fractures in the knee: MRI analysis at 1 to 10 Years postoperatively. *Orthop J Sports Med*. 2022 Jul;10(7):23259671221113234.
35. Komnos G, Iosifidis M, Papageorgiou F, Melas I, Metaxiotis D, Hantes M. Juvenile osteochondritis dissecans of the knee joint: midterm clinical and MRI outcomes of arthroscopic retrograde drilling and internal fixation with bioabsorbable pins. *Cartilage*. 2021 Dec;13(1 suppl):1228S–36S.
36. Beletsky A, Naveen NB, Tauro T, et al. Microdrilling demonstrates superior patient-reported outcomes and lower revision rates than traditional microfracture: a matched cohort analysis. *Arthrosc Sports Med Rehabil*. 2021 Jun;3(3):e629–38.
37. Strauss EJ, Barker JU, Kercher JS, Cole BJ, Mithoefer K. Augmentation strategies following the microfracture technique for repair of focal chondral defects. *Cartilage*. 2010 Apr;1(2):145–52.
38. Cole BJ, Haunschild ED, Carter T, Meyer J, Fortier LA, Gilat R, BC BioCartilage Study Group. Clinically significant outcomes following the treatment of focal cartilage defects of the knee with microfracture augmentation using cartilage allograft extracellular matrix: a multicenter prospective study. *Arthroscopy*. 2021 May;37(5):1512–21.
39. Brusalis CM, Greditzer HG, Fabricant PD, Stannard JP, Cook JL. BioCartilage augmentation of marrow stimulation procedures for cartilage defects of the knee: two-year clinical outcomes. *Knee*. 2020 Oct;27(5):1418–25.
40. Wen HJ, Yuan LB, Tan HB, Xu YQ. Microfracture versus enhanced microfracture techniques in knee cartilage restoration: a systematic review and meta-analysis. *J Knee Surg*. 2022 Jun;35(7):707–17.
41. Kim JH, Heo JW, Lee DH. Clinical and radiological outcomes after autologous matrix-induced chondrogenesis versus microfracture of the knee: a systematic review and meta-analysis with a minimum 2-year follow-up. *Orthop J Sports Med*. 2020 Nov;8(11):2325967120959280.
42. Orth P, Gao L, Madry H. Microfracture for cartilage repair in the knee: a systematic review of the contemporary literature. *Knee Surg Sports Traumatol Arthrosc*. 2020 Mar;28(3):670–706.
43. Mithoefer K, Steadman RJ. Microfracture in football (Soccer) Players: a case Series of Professional athletes and systematic review. *Cartilage*. 2012 Jan;3(1 suppl l):18S–24S.
44. Solheim E, Øyen J, Hegna J, Austgulen OK, Harlem T, Strand T. Microfracture treatment of single or multiple articular cartilage defects of the knee: a 5-year median follow-up of 110 patients. *Knee Surg Sports Traumatol Arthrosc*. 2010 Apr;18(4):504–8.
45. Mithoefer K, McAdams T, Williams RJ, Kreuz PC, Mandelbaum BR. Clinical efficacy of the microfracture technique for articular cartilage repair in the knee: an evidence-based systematic analysis. *Am J Sports Med*. 2009 Oct;37(10):2053–63.
46. Asik M, Ciftci F, Sen C, Erdil M, Atalar A. The microfracture technique for the treatment of full-thickness articular cartilage lesions of the knee: midterm results. *Arthroscopy*. 2008 Nov;24(11):1214–20.
47. Bae DK, Yoon KH, Song SJ. Cartilage healing after microfracture in osteoarthritic knees. *Arthroscopy*. 2006 Apr;22(4):367–74.
48. Gobbi A, Nunag P, Malinowski K. Treatment of full thickness chondral lesions of the knee with microfracture in a group of athletes. *Knee Surg Sports Traumatol Arthrosc*. 2005 Apr;13(3):213–21.
49. Steadman JR, Rodkey WG, Briggs KK. Microfracture to treat full-thickness chondral defects: surgical technique, rehabilitation, and outcomes. *J Knee Surg*. 2002;15(3):170–6.
50. Gill TJ, Macgillivray JD. The technique of microfracture for the treatment of articular cartilage defects in the knee. *Operat Tech Orthop*. 2001 Apr;11(2):105–7.

51. Blevins FT, Steadman JR, Rodrigo JJ, Silliman J. Treatment of articular cartilage defects in athletes: an analysis of functional outcome and lesion appearance. *Orthopedics.* 1998 Jul;21(7):761–8.
52. Steadman JR, Rodkey WG, Singleton SB, Briggs KK. Microfracture technique for full-thickness chondral defects: technique and clinical results. *Operat Tech Orthop.* 1997;7(4):300–4.
53. Riboh JC, Cvetanovich GL, Cole BJ, Yanke AB. Comparative efficacy of cartilage repair procedures in the knee: a network meta-analysis. *Knee Surg Sports Traumatol Arthrosc.* 2017 Dec;25(12):3786–99.
54. Werner BC, Cosgrove CT, Gilmore CJ, et al. Accelerated return to sport after osteochondral autograft plug transfer. *Orthop J Sports Med.* 2017 Apr;5(4):2325967117702418.
55. Bartz RL, Kamaric E, Noble PC, Lintner D, Bocell J. Topographic matching of selected donor and recipient sites for osteochondral autografting of the articular surface of the femoral condyles. *Am J Sports Med.* 2001;29(2):207–212.
56. Feczkó P, Hangody L, Varga J, et al. Experimental results of donor site filling for autologous osteochondral mosaicplasty. *Arthroscopy.* 2003 Sep;19(7):755–61.
57. LaPrade RF, Botker JC. Donor-site morbidity after osteochondral autograft transfer procedures. *Arthroscopy.* 2004 Sep;20(7):e69–73.
58. Dekker TJ, Aman ZS, DePhillipo NN, Dickens JF, Anz AW, LaPrade RF. Chondral lesions of the knee: an evidence-based approach. *J Bone Joint Surg Am.* 2021 Apr 7;103(7):629–45.
59. Familiari F, Cinque ME, Chahla J, et al. Clinical outcomes and failure rates of osteochondral allograft transplantation in the knee: a systematic review. *Am J Sports Med.* 2018 Dec;46(14):3541–9.
60. Hangody L, Feczkó P, Bartha L, Bodó G, Kish G. Mosaicplasty for the treatment of articular defects of the knee and ankle. *Clin Orthop Relat Res.* 2001 Oct;391(suppl l):S328–36.
61. Hangody L, Kish G, Kárpáti Z, Udvarhelyi I, Szigeti I, Bély M. Mosaicplasty for the treatment of articular cartilage defects: application in clinical practice. *Orthopedics.* 1998 Jul;21(7):751–6.
62. Beer AJ, Tauro TM, Redondo ML, Christian DR, Cole BJ, Frank RM. Use of allografts in orthopaedic surgery: safety, procurement, storage, and outcomes. *Orthop J Sports Med.* 2019 Dec;7(12):2325967119891435.
63. Wagner KR, DeFroda SF, Sivasundaram L, et al. Osteochondral allograft transplantation for focal cartilage defects of the femoral condyles. *JBJS Essent Surg Tech.* 2022;12(3):e21.00037.
64. Frank RM, Lee S, Levy D, et al. Osteochondral allograft transplantation of the knee: analysis of failures at 5 years. *Am J Sports Med.* 2017 Mar;45(4):864–74.
65. Assenmacher AT, Pareek A, Reardon PJ, Macalena JA, Stuart MJ, Krych AJ. Long-term outcomes after osteochondral allograft: a systematic review at long-term follow-up of 12.3 years. *Arthroscopy.* 2016 Oct;32(10):2160–8.
66. Sun Y, Jiang W, Cory E, et al. Pulsed lavage cleansing of osteochondral grafts depends on lavage duration, flow intensity, and graft storage condition. *PLoS One.* 2017;12(5):e0176934.
67. Yanke A, Dandu N, Bodendorfer B, et al. Paper 18: effect of bone marrow aspirate concentrate on osteochondral allograft transplantation incorporation – a prospective, randomized, single blind investigation. *Orthop J Sports Med.* 2022 Jul;10(7 suppl 5):2325967121S00582.
68. Meyer MA, McCarthy MA, Gitelis ME, et al. Effectiveness of lavage techniques in removing immunogenic elements from osteochondral allografts. *Cartilage.* 2017 Oct;8(4):369–73.
69. Kang RW, Friel NA, Williams JM, Cole BJ, Wimmer MA. Effect of impaction sequence on osteochondral graft damage: the role of repeated and varying loads. *Am J Sports Med.* 2010 Jan;38(1):105–13.
70. Wagner KR, Kaiser JT, DeFroda SF, Meeker ZD, Cole BJ. Rehabilitation, restrictions, and return to sport after cartilage procedures. *Arthrosc Sports Med Rehabil.* 2022 Jan;4(1):e115–24.
71. Gilat R, Haunschild ED, Huddleston HP, et al. Osteochondral allograft transplant for focal cartilage defects of the femoral condyles: clinically significant outcomes, failures, and survival at a minimum 5-year follow-up. *Am J Sports Med.* 2021 Feb;49(2):467–75.
72. Cameron JI, Pulido PA, McCauley JC, Bugbee WD. Osteochondral allograft transplantation of the femoral trochlea. *Am J Sports Med.* 2016 Mar;44(3):633–8.
73. Briggs DT, Sadr KN, Pulido PA, Bugbee WD. The use of osteochondral allograft transplantation for primary treatment of cartilage lesions in the knee. *Cartilage.* 2015 Oct;6(4):203–7.
74. Gracitelli GC, Meric G, Pulido PA, Görtz S, De Young AJ, Bugbee WD. Fresh osteochondral allograft transplantation for isolated patellar cartilage injury. *Am J Sports Med.* 2015 Apr;43(4):879–84.
75. Chahla J, Sweet MC, Okoroha KR, et al. Osteochondral allograft transplantation in the patellofemoral joint: a systematic review. *Am J Sports Med.* 2019 Oct;47(12):3009–18.
76. Peterson L, Vasiliadis HS, Brittberg M, Lindahl A. Autologous chondrocyte implantation: a long-term follow-up. *Am J Sports Med.* 2010 Jun;38(6):1117–24.
77. Peterson L, Brittberg M, Kiviranta I, Akerlund EL, Lindahl A. Autologous chondrocyte transplantation. Biomechanics and long-term durability. *Am J Sports Med.* 2002;30(1):2–12.
78. Micheli LJ, Browne JE, Erggelet C, et al. Autologous chondrocyte implantation of the knee: multicenter experience and minimum 3-year follow-up. *Clin J Sport Med.* 2001 Oct;11(4):223–8.
79. Zaslav K, Cole B, Brewster R, STAR Study Principal Investigators, et al. A prospective study of autologous chondrocyte implantation in patients with failed prior treatment for articular cartilage defect of the knee: results of the Study of the Treatment of Articular Repair (STAR) clinical trial. *Am J Sports Med.* 2009 Jan;37(1):42–55.
80. Gomoll AH, Probst C, Farr J, Cole BJ, Minas T. Use of a type I/III bilayer collagen membrane decreases reoperation rates for symptomatic hypertrophy after autologous chondrocyte implantation. *Am J Sports Med.* 2009 Nov;37(suppl 1):20S–3S.
81. McNickle AG, L'Heureux DR, Yanke AB, Cole BJ. Outcomes of autologous chondrocyte implantation in a diverse patient population. *Am J Sports Med.* 2009 Jul;37(7):1344–50.
82. Peterson L, Minas T, Brittberg M, Nilsson A, Sjögren-Jansson E, Lindahl A. Two- to 9-year outcome after autologous chondrocyte transplantation of the knee. *Clin Orthop Relat Res.* 2000 May;374:212–34.
83. Carey JL, Remmers AE, Flanigan DC. Use of MACI (autologous cultured chondrocytes on porcine collagen membrane) in the United States: preliminary experience. *Orthop J Sports Med.* 2020 Aug;8(8):2325967120941816.
84. Saris D, Price A, Widuchowski W, SUMMIT study group, et al. Matrix-applied characterized autologous cultured chondrocytes versus microfracture: two-year follow-up of a prospective randomized trial. *Am J Sports Med.* 2014 Jun;42(6):1384–94.
85. Ebert JR, Fallon M, Ackland TR, Janes GC, Wood DJ. Minimum 10-year clinical and radiological outcomes of a randomized controlled trial evaluating 2 different approaches to full weightbearing after matrix-induced autologous chondrocyte implantation. *Am J Sports Med.* 2020 Jan;48(1):133–42.
86. Moseley JB, Anderson AF, Browne JE, et al. Long-term durability of autologous chondrocyte implantation: a multicenter, observational study in US patients. *Am J Sports Med.* 2010 Feb;38(2):238–46.
87. Bhosale AM, Kuiper JH, Johnson WEB, Harrison PE, Richardson JB. Midterm to long-term longitudinal outcome of autologous chondrocyte

implantation in the knee joint: a multilevel analysis. *Am J Sports Med.* 2009 Nov;37(suppl 1):131S–8S.

88. Gillogly SD, Voight M, Blackburn T. Treatment of articular cartilage defects of the knee with autologous chondrocyte implantation. *J Orthop Sports Phys Ther.* 1998 Oct;28(4):241–51.
89. Brittberg M, Lindahl A, Nilsson A, Ohlsson C, Isaksson O, Peterson L. Treatment of deep cartilage defects in the knee with autologous chondrocyte transplantation. *N Engl J Med.* 1994 Oct 6;331(14):889–95.
90. Oladeji LO, Stannard JP, Cook CR, et al. Effects of autogenous bone marrow aspirate concentrate on radiographic integration of femoral condylar osteochondral allografts. *Am J Sports Med.* 2017 Oct;45(12):2797–803.
91. Enea D, Cecconi S, Calcagno S, Busilacchi A, Manzotti S, Gigante A. One-step cartilage repair in the knee: collagen-covered microfracture and autologous bone marrow concentrate. A pilot study. *Knee.* 2015 Jan;22(1):30–35.
92. Gigante A, Cecconi S, Calcagno S, Busilacchi A, Enea D. Arthroscopic knee cartilage repair with covered microfracture and bone marrow concentrate. *Arthrosc Tech.* 2012 Dec;1(2):e175–80.
93. Ow ZGW, Cheang HLX, Koh JH, et al. Does the choice of acellular scaffold and augmentation with bone marrow aspirate concentrate affect short-term outcomes in cartilage repair? A systematic review and meta-analysis. *Am J Sports Med.* 2023 May;51(6):1622–33.
94. Dávila Castrodad IM, Kraeutler MJ, Fasulo SM, Festa A, McInerney VK, Scillia AJ. Improved outcomes with arthroscopic bone marrow aspirate concentrate and cartilage-derived matrix implantation versus chondroplasty for the treatment of focal chondral defects of the knee joint: a retrospective case series. *Arthrosc Sports Med Rehabil.* 2022 Apr;4(2):e411–6.
95. Meng HYH, Lu V, Khan W. Adipose tissue-derived mesenchymal stem cells as a potential restorative treatment for cartilage defects: a PRISMA review and meta-analysis. *Pharmaceuticals.* 2021 Dec 8;14(12):1280.

8 Bone Injury and Fracture Healing

Casey S. Mueller

INTRODUCTION

- There are two modes of fracture healing: primary and secondary.
- Primary fracture healing occurs only with surgical fixation when bones are compressed together and held in a low-strain environment via rigid fixation, this healing occurs through Haversian bone remodeling.
- Secondary fracture healing is what this chapter will focus on and occurs through the endochondral ossification pathway.
- Secondary fracture healing involves multiple orchestrated events that are intimately linked to each other (1). The goal of fracture healing is to restore the injured bone to the pre-injury biologic and biomechanical state. To accomplish this, the body uses a stepwise sequence of inflammation, callous formation and ossification, and last remodeling. With normal fracture healing the cellular content within the fracture site, molecular signaling, and stability of the fracture change and evolve throughout these phases in a predictable and time-dependent manner.

BONE ANATOMY (2–4)

- See Figure 8.1.

Bone Cells

Osteoprogenitor Cells

- Present on all bone surfaces, make up the deep layer of the periosteum and the endosteum, and can migrate from surrounding tissue.
- Osteoprogenitor cells are marrow stromal cells that differentiate into osteoblasts (4).
- The periosteum contains two layers: an outer layer of fibrous tissue and an inner layer (cambium) that contains these osteoprogenitor cells.
- The endosteum is a single layer of osteogenic cells lacking a fibrous component.

Osteoblasts

- Mature, metabolically active bone-forming cells.
  - Secrete osteoid, the unmineralized matrix that subsequently undergoes mineralization.
  - Some osteoblasts become entrapped within the matrix and are converted into osteocytes, whereas others remain on the surfaces of bone and are active in baseline bone remodeling.
  - Act in a paracrine function through the release of receptor activator of nuclear factor κ-B ligand (RANKL) for the activation of bone resorption by osteoclasts.

Osteocytes

- Mature osteoblasts trapped within the bone matrix.
- Form a network of cytoplasmic processes extending through cylindrical canaliculi to blood vessels and other osteocytes.
- Involved in extracellular calcium and phosphorus homeostasis.
- Act as in a paracrine function on osteoblasts and osteoclasts.
- Act in endocrine function to aide in phosphate homeostasis and vitamin D metabolism (5).

Osteoclasts

- Multinucleated bone-resorbing cells controlled by hormonal and cellular mechanisms.
- Differentiate from hematopoietic cells from the monocyte/macrophage cell lines (4).
- Function in groups termed *cutting cones.*
- Attach to bare bone surfaces through the formation of ruffled border at bone-osteoclast interface leading to the breakdown of organic and inorganic matrices of bone and calcified cartilage through the use of hydrolytic enzymes (4).
- Process results in the formation of shallow pits on the bone surface called Howship lacunae (2).

Types of Bone (3)

Woven Bone (Primary Bone)

- Primary bone formed during embryonic development, during fracture healing, and in some pathologic states such as hyperparathyroidism and Paget disease (2,3).
- Composed of randomly arranged collagen bundles and irregularly shaped vascular spaces.

The author acknowledges the first edition work of Drs. Connor LaRose and Carlos Guanche.

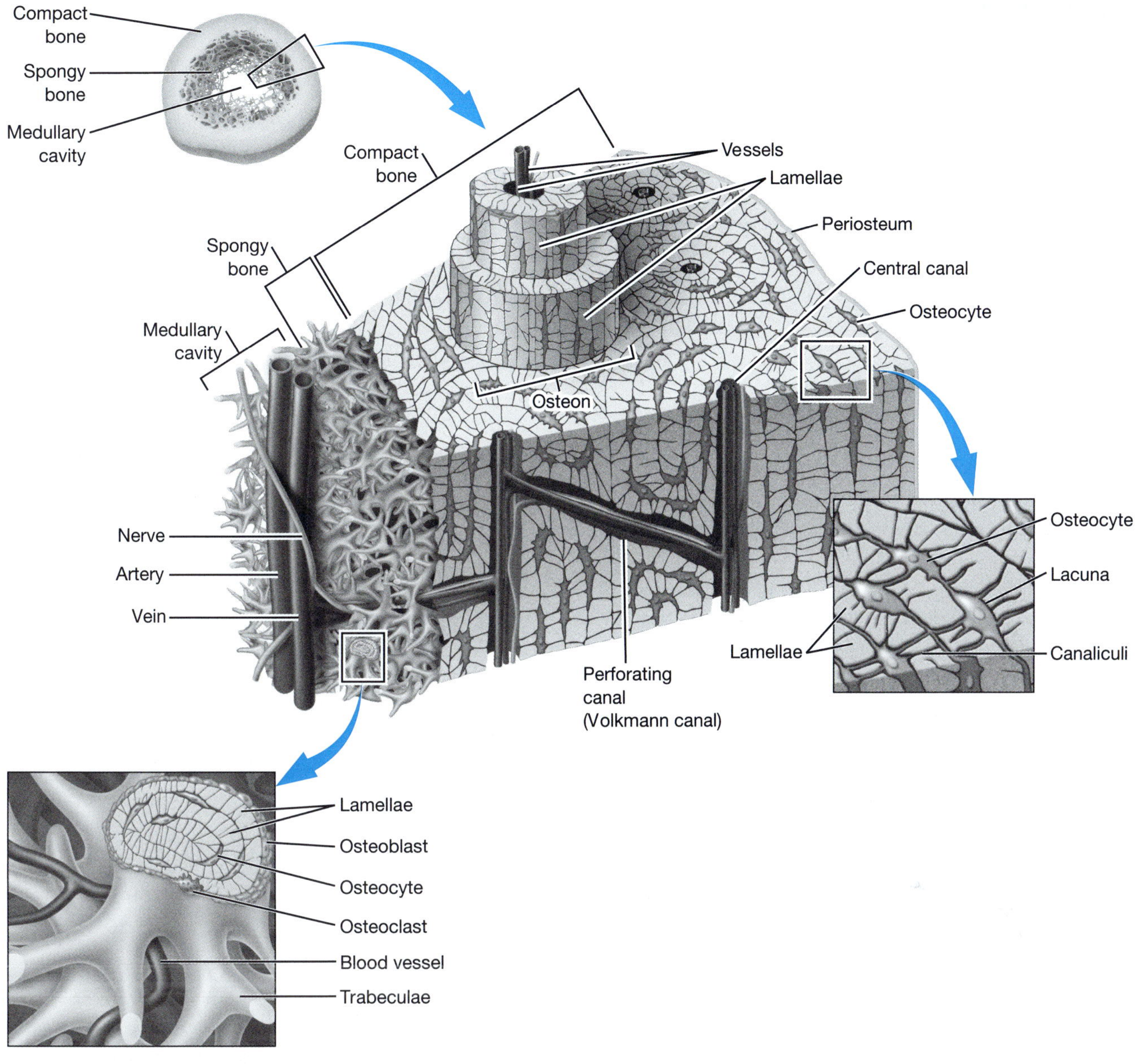

Figure 8.1: Bone anatomy.

- Higher cellularity than lamellar bone and is not organized according to mechanical stress.
- Weaker and more easily deformed compared to lamellar bone secondary to irregular collagen orientation.

Lamellar Bone (Secondary Bone)

- Highly organized with densely packed collagen fibrils that are organized according to stress lines via Wolff's Law.
- Behaves anisotropically; the mechanical properties of the bone change depending on the direction of the applied force.
- Woven bone present at a fracture site must be eventually replaced by lamellar bone to restore the normal mechanical properties of bone; this is done via bone remodeling.

Cortical Bone

- Dense compact bone that is primarily responsible for load bearing in the diaphysis of long bones.
- Remodeled from woven bone by means of vascular channels that invade the embryonic bone from its periosteal and endosteal surfaces.
- The primary structural unit of cortical bone is an osteon, also known as a Haversian system.
  - Consists of cylindrical-shaped lamellar bone that surrounds longitudinally oriented vascular channels called Haversian canals.
  - Horizontally oriented canals (Volkmann) connect adjacent osteons.
  - Mechanical strength of cortical bone is dependent on the concentration of the osteons.

Cancellous Bone (Trabecular)

- Lies between cortical bone surfaces and consists of a network of honeycombed interstices containing hematopoietic elements and bony trabeculae.
- Structurally important at epiphyseal-metaphyseal ends of long bones. Allows for absorption of loads across synovial joints.
- Trabeculae are oriented perpendicular to external forces to provide structural support (6).

BONE BIOCHEMISTRY (4)

- Bone is composed of organic matrix and mineral matrix.
  - Mineral matrix: Dry bone is made up of hydroxyapatite and tricalcium phosphate (65%–70% of the weight). Responsible for the compressive strength of bone.
  - Organic matrix: 90% type 1 collagen, 5% other collagen types, noncollagenous material, and growth factors (30%–35% of the weight).
  - Osteoid: Unmineralized organic matrix secreted by osteoblasts; composed of 90% type I collagen and 10% ground substance (noncollagenous proteins, glycoproteins proteoglycans, peptides, carbohydrates, and lipids). Mineralization of this substance by inorganic mineral salts provides bone with its strength and rigidity.
  - Inorganic bone contents: Primarily calcium phosphate and calcium carbonate with small quantities of magnesium, chloride, and sodium. Mineral crystals form hydroxyapatite, an orderly precipitate around the collagen fibers of the osteoid.

Regulators of Bone Metabolism (7–9)

- See Figure 8.2.
- Three of the calcitropic hormones that have the most effect on metabolism are parathyroid hormone, vitamin D, and calcitonin.
  - Parathyroid hormone is an amino acid made and secreted from the chief cells of the parathyroid gland. It is secreted in response to low plasma calcium. It directly activates osteoblasts to secrete RANKL, which stimulates osteoclastic development and resorption of bone.
  - Vitamin D stimulates intestinal and renal calcium-binding proteins aiding in calcium absorption and resorption, respectively, and facilitates active calcium transport.
  - Calcitonin is secreted by the parafollicular cells of the thyroid gland in response to rising plasma calcium level. Calcitonin serves to inhibit calcium-dependent cellular metabolic activity and also acts by directly inhibiting osteoclast activity.
- Miscellaneous proteins: Released from platelets, macrophages, and fibroblasts. Cause healing bone to vascularize, solidify, incorporate, and function mechanically. Induce mesenchymal-derived cells such as monocytes and fibroblasts to migrate, proliferate, and differentiate into bone cells (10,11).
- Proteins that enhance bone healing include the *bone morphogenic proteins* (BMPs), insulin-like growth factors, transforming growth factors (TGFs), platelet-derived growth factor, and fibroblast growth factor, among others (12–14).

Bone Morphogenic Proteins (15,16)

- Unique group of biologically active proteins that belong to the TGF-β superfamily.

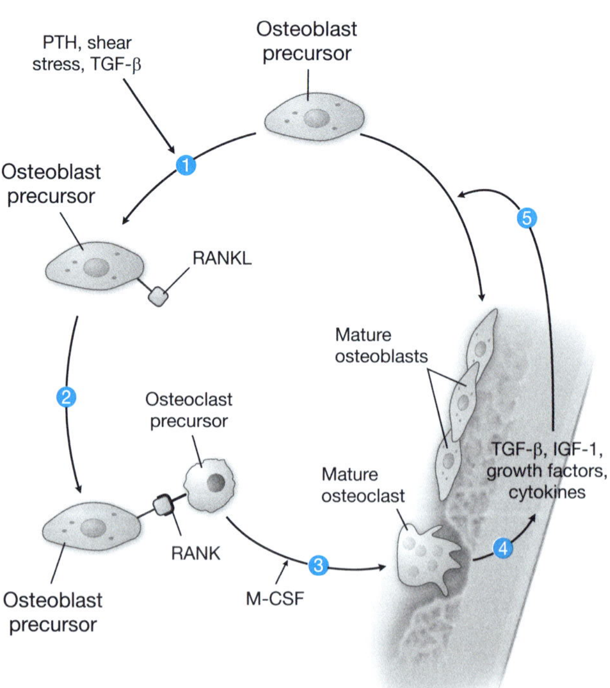

Figure 8.2: Regulators of bone metabolism.

- Over 20 different BMPs have been discovered, but only BMP-2, -4, -6, -7, and -9 have been shown to have osteogenic properties.
- In vivo, different BMPs act at different times and at differing concentrations during bone formation.
- Currently, BMP-2 and BMP-7 have been approved for use in the treatment of open tibial fractures and lumbar anterior spinal fusion (15–18).

BONE-HEALING PROCESS

- See Figure 8.3.
- Fracture healing restores the tissue to its original biological and mechanical properties and is influenced by a variety of systemic and local factors (19,20). Healing occurs in four distinct but overlapping stages (21,22).

Hematoma Development

- A hematoma develops within the fracture site during the hours after injury and is present for several days.

Inflammatory Stage

- Inflammatory cells and fibroblasts infiltrate the hematoma under prostaglandin mediation. This transforms the hematoma into granulation tissue, causing ingrowth of vasculature and migration of mesenchymal cells (8).
- Osteoblast proliferation occurs at the fracture site from the surrounding osteoprogenitor cells.
- Anti-inflammatory or cytotoxic medications during this first week can be detrimental to the initial inflammatory response to healing (23).

Repair Stage – Callous Formation and Ossification

- Fibroblasts begin to lay down a stroma that helps support vascular ingrowth.
- At this stage, nicotine can inhibit capillary ingrowth (24,25).
- As vascular ingrowth progresses, a collagen osteoid matrix is laid down known as soft callous.
    - Subsequently, the osteoid is mineralized with inorganic calcium and phosphate, this is the woven bone.
    - Soft callus is very weak in the first 4–6 weeks and requires adequate protection to allow correct strain environment for progression of healing (26).
    - Eventually, ossified callus (hard callus) forms a bridge of woven bone between the fracture fragments. If proper immobilization is not employed, failure of ossification results in a nonunion/fibrous union (27).

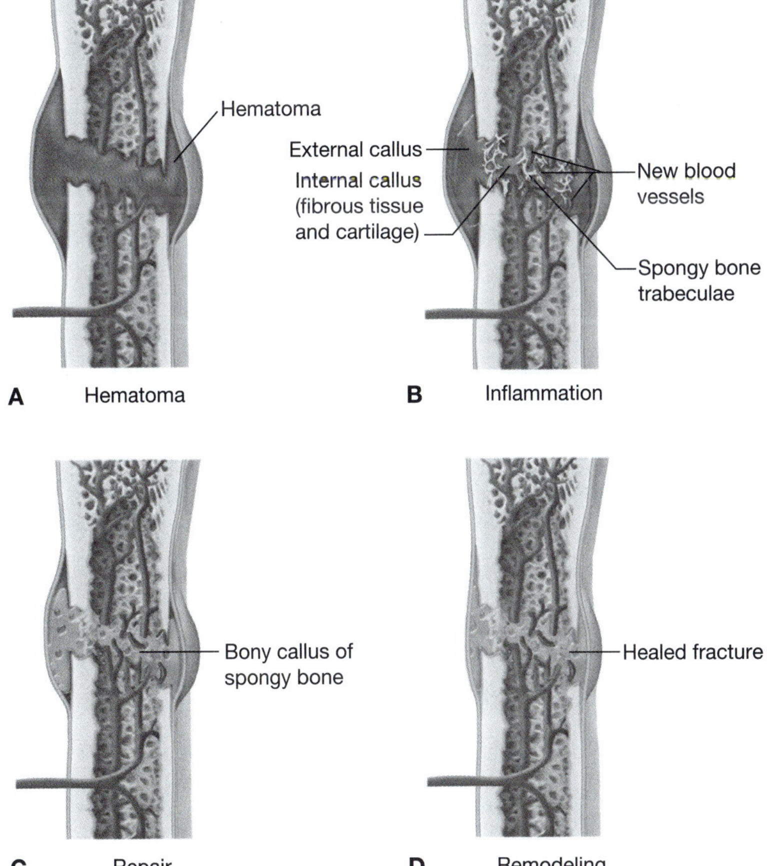

Figure 8.3: Four stages of bone repair. A: Hematoma. B: Inflammation. C: Repair. D: Remodeling.

Remodeling Stage

- Healing bone is restored to its original shape, structure, and mechanical strength via Haversian remodeling.
- Remodeling is a long-term process facilitated by mechanical stresses placed on the bone.
  - Bone remodels in response to loading where increased loading causes bone formation and decreased or lack of loading causes bone resorption — Wolff's law. Axial loading across the fracture site leads to bone being deposited where it is required for stability and reabsorbed where it is not (19). Adequate strength is typically achieved in 3–6 months; tibial shaft fractures can often take longer to heal.

BIOMECHANICS OF FRACTURES

Stress Fractures (28–30)

- Cyclic loading repeated over a long period of time may cause disruption of the bony architecture.
- The susceptibility of bone to fracture under stresses of low magnitude is related to its crystalline structure and collagen orientation.
- Under each cycle of loading, a small amount of strained energy may be lost through microscopic cracks along the cement lines of bone.
- Fatigue load under certain strain rates can cause progressive accumulation of microdamage in cortical bone.
  - Prolonged loading may eventually lead to catastrophic failure of the bone through propagation of these cracks to a complete fracture.
  - Bone may be created near the microscopic cracks through periosteal callus formation, thus arresting propagation.
- Fractures can be classified into low-risk and high-risk fracture types (28).
  - Low-risk fractures are typically treated without surgery with relatively quick healing. Includes femoral shaft, medial tibia, ribs, ulna shaft, and first through fourth metatarsals.
  - High-risk fractures can be very difficult to treat and may require surgical intervention because they are at high risk for progression to displaced fractures or have poor healing potential as a result of relative avascularity at the fracture site. These include tension-sided femoral neck, patella, anterior tibial diaphysis, medial malleolus, talus, tarsal navicular, proximal fifth metatarsal, and first metatarsal phalangeal sesamoids.

Acute Fractures (13,31)

- Classified according to the magnitude and area of distribution of the force applied and the rate at which the force acts.
  - Soft-tissue injury and fracture comminution are directly proportional to the loading rate and force applied (32).
- Typically, force is applied to bone in many directions and generates compressive, tensile, or torsional forces, or combination of these forces.
- The combination of the bone's material strength, anisometric properties, and forces applied dictates where, how, and along which path a fracture will occur.
  - Cortical bone is generally weakest in tension.
  - Area where tensile stresses arise fails first.
- Transverse fractures are the result of pure tensile forces or bending.
- Fractures from pure tensile force occur progressively across the bone, creating a transverse break without comminution.
- Bone undergoing rapid loading must absorb more energy than bone loaded at a slower rate.
  - At low speed, bending with tensile stress will cause a fracture with a single butterfly fragment.
  - High-speed bending will cause several butterfly fragments.
- The pattern of bone injury also impacts healing capacity (33).
  - Time to union is greatly prolonged in fractures with more soft-tissue stripping especially surgical soft-tissue stripping.
  - Larger load under bending failure may cause the surrounding soft tissues and periosteum to sustain more damage and thus may affect the fracture healing time and potential.

FACTORS INFLUENCING FRACTURE REPAIR

- Systemic factors can inhibit bone healing, including the following (34):
  - Cigarette smoking (35)
  - Malnutrition (36)
  - Diabetes (37)
  - Rheumatoid arthritis
  - Osteoporosis (38)
  - Steroid medications (39)
  - Nonsteroidal anti-inflammatory medications
  - Obesity (40)

Nutrition

- A typical diet including all food groups in proper amounts is enough to effect healing in a healthy individual.
  - Calcium usage is limited by absorption.
    - Preinjury calcium levels are predictive.
    - Intake of about 1 g of calcium and 1000 IU vitamin D daily is optimal for bone health. Increased doses of Vitamin D may be required in those that are deficient
  - True vegans with no alternative proteins are at risk for nonunion.

AUGMENTATION OF FRACTURE HEALING (13,41,42)

- See Figure 8.4.
- In augmenting fracture healing, three basic components are required to enhance skeletal repair: osteogenesis, osteoconduction, and osteoinduction. Every bone graft used to enhance healing must incorporate one or more of these components (1).

Osteogenesis (31,42,43)

- The ability of the graft to produce new bone. This process is dependent on the presence of live bone cells in a graft material.
- Contains viable cells with the ability to form bone (osteoprogenitor cells) or the potential to differentiate into bone-forming cells.
- Osteogenesis is a property found only in fresh autogenous bone and in bone marrow cells.

Osteoinduction (11,40,42)

- The ability of graft material to induce pluripotent mesenchymal stem cells from the surrounding tissues to develop into osteoprogenitor cells (1).
- Typically associated with the presence of bone growth factors within the graft material.
- Growth-promoting proteins. Several factors are known to be associated with healing:
    - TGF-β
    - IGFs
    - BMPs
        - Glycoproteins known to induce bone.
        - Several BMPs are known to exist. BMP-3 (osteogenin) induces rapid differentiation of mesenchymal tissue to bone. BMPs induce endochondral bone formation in segmental defects (14).
- Systemic factors: Injury to bone marrow enhances osteogenesis at distant skeletal sites.
    - Factors thought to be responsible: (a) IGF-1 and IGF-2, (b) parathyroid hormone, and (c) prostaglandins.
    - Isolation and clinical development of these factors may lead to systemic treatment of fractures.

Osteoconduction (25,42,44)

- The physical property of the graft to serve as a scaffold for viable bone healing.
- Allows for the ingrowth of neovasculature and the infiltration of osteogenic precursor cells into a graft site.
- Osteoconductive properties are found in cancellous autografts and allografts, demineralized bone matrix, hydroxyapatite, collagen, and calcium phosphate.

TYPES OF BONE GRAFT

Autologous Bone Graft (1,6,42)

- Graft is harvested from the patient, typically from a different site in the body, and used to augment fracture healing.
- Remains the gold standard of bone graft. Contains all properties (osteogenic, osteoconductive, and osteoinductive) required to help form bone.
- Donor site morbidity remains the biggest problem with autologous bone graft.

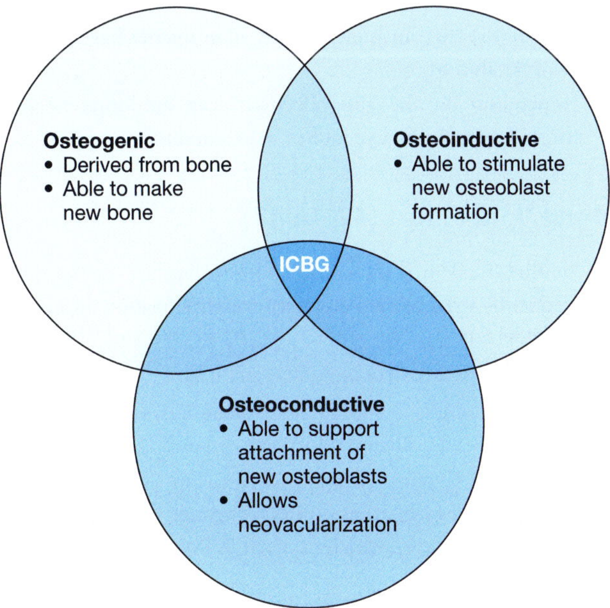

Figure 8.4: Three basic components are required to enhance skeletal repair: osteogenesis, osteoconduction, and osteoinduction.

Types of Autologous Bone Graft

Autologous Cancellous Bone Graft (1,42)

- Cancellous autografts effect vascular ingrowth and progenitor mesenchymal cell invasion, osteoblastic appositional new bone formation, and ultimately, remodeling of the trabecular structure.
- Does not provide any initial structural support.
- Typical harvest sites: iliac crest, distal radius, distal femur, proximal tibia, and calcaneus

Autologous Cortical Bone Graft (42)

- Slow to revascularize when compared to cancellous autograft.
- Primarily functions in osteoconductive manner with a lesser osteoinductive contribution.
- Must undergo osteoclastic resorption prior to osteoblastic new bone formation in a process called creeping substitution — an integrated process in which old necrotic bone is slowly reabsorbed and simultaneously replaced with new viable bone, thus incorporating bone grafts.
- Healing process begins at host-graft cortical junction.
- Provides initial structural support.

Autogenous Bone Marrow (42,45)

- Independent of cancellous or cortical bone.
- Undifferentiated progenitor cells aid in fracture healing by differentiation into various cells required for bone healing.
- Typically can be harvested from iliac crest bone marrow.

Allograft Bone Grafting (41,42,45)

- Cadaveric tissue bank bone is used to augment fracture healing.
- Comes in several different preparations: cancellous graft, cortical grafts, osteochondral grafts, and demineralized bone matrix (DBM).
- Readily available in the United States.
- No harvest site morbidity.
- Risk of disease transmission is small but varies based on tissue preparation.
- Depending on the allograft used, can aid bone healing through osteoinductive and/or osteoconductive properties.

Bone Void Fillers (42,46,47)

- Synthetic calcium phosphate bone fillers are being more frequently used to help augment fracture fixation and/or fill bone defects.
- Act as synthetic osteoconductive scaffold.
- Various products including hydroxyapatites, solid tricalcium phosphates, and calcium phosphate cements (CPCs), calcium sulfate, and bioactive glass.
- The body resorbs these fillers through an osteoclastic mediated process, which is then followed by new bone formation.
- Most commonly used to fill bone defects in subchondral bone to add mechanical strength to the fracture fixation as well as an osteoconductive scaffold.
- Most common areas of use: tibial plateau, distal radius, calcaneus, and spine.

PHYSICAL STIMULATION THERAPIES (48)

- Although most fracture healing therapies are applied during surgical interventions, there are several noninvasive technologies that are being used to help fractures unite.

Electromagnetic Fields (49)

- Bone has a piezoelectric potential that is load induced due to two factors.
  - Current is induced by deformation of collagen.
  - Electrokinetic current is produced by the strain-induced flow of charged extracellular fluids.
- *Pulsed electromagnetic fields* (PEMFs) are intended to noninvasively induce electrical currents to replace endogenous currents in the absence of loading.
- Mollon et al. (50) published a meta-analysis that concluded a trend toward improved healing in delayed unions.

Low-Intensity Pulsed Ultrasound (34,51,52)

- Low-Intensity Pulsed Ultrasound (LIPUS) has been shown to be effective in the treatment of acute, delayed, and nonunion of bone (52).
- LIPUS has been shown in animal models to improve all phases of fracture healing.
- There is evidence that it can modulate gene expression, influence second messenger activity of chondroblasts and osteoblasts, enhance blood flow, and accelerate and augment fracture healing.
- In a study of distal radius fractures, the LIPUS-treated group had a 34%–38% decrease in time to union compared to controls (34,53).

Extracorporeal Shock Wave Therapy (54)

- Single high-amplitude sound waves propagate through tissue to create a change in tissue pressure.
- In vivo animal models have shown increased callus formation, decreased healing time, and improved mechanical properties (34,54).
- Wang et al. (55) demonstrated higher union rates in femur and/or tibia fractures treated with surgery and ESWT than surgery alone.
- The clinical efficacy of ESWT is still not fully understood secondary to limited randomized clinical trials available to evaluate efficacy.

REFERENCES

1. Kakar S, Einhorn AE. Biology and enhancement of skeletal repair. In: Jupiter J, Browner BD, Levine AM, Trafton PG, Krettek C, editors. *Skeletal Trauma: Basic Science, Management, and Reconstruction*. 4th ed. Philadelphia (PA): Expert Consult: Online and Print; 2008.
2. Buckwalter JA, Glimcher MJ, Cooper RR, Recker R. Bone biology. I: structure, blood supply, cells, matrix, and mineralization. *Instr Course Lect*. 1996;45:371–86.
3. Buckwalter JA, Glimcher MJ, Cooper RR, Recker R. Bone biology. II: formation, form, modeling, remodeling, and regulation of cell function. *Instr Course Lect*. 1996;45:387–99.
4. Clohisy JC, Lindskog D, Abu-Amer Y. Bone and joint biology. In: Lieberman JR, editor. *AAOS Comprehensive Orthopaedic Review*. Rosemont (IL): American Academy of Orthopaedic Surgeons; 2009. Chapter 5.
5. Simic P, Babitt JL. Regulation of FGF23: beyond bone. *Curr Osteoporos Rep*. 2021;19(6):563–73.
6. White AA III, Hirsch C. An experimental study of the immediate load bearing capacity of some commonly used iliac bone grafts. *Acta Orthop Scand*. 1971;42(6):482–90.
7. Boden SD, Kaplan FS. Calcium homeostasis. *Orthop Clin North Am*. 1990;21(1):31–42.
8. Brinker MR, O'Connor DP. Bone. In: Miller MD, Hart JA, editors. *Review of Orthopaedics*. Philadelphia (PA): Saunders Elsevier; 2008. p. 1–43.
9. Reichel H, Koeffler HP, Norman AW. The role of the vitamin D endocrine system in health and disease. *N Engl J Med*. 1989;320(15):980–91.
10. Hynes RO. Integrins: versatility, modulation, and signaling in cell adhesion. *Cell*. 1992;69(1):11–25.
11. Mohan S, Baylink DJ. Bone growth factors. *Clin Orthop Relat Res*. 1991;263:30–48.
12. Connolly JF. Clinical use of marrow osteoprogenitor cells to stimulate osteogenesis. *Clin Orthop Relat Res*. 1998;355:S257–66.
13. Einhorn TA. Enhancement of fracture-healing. *J Bone Joint Surg Am*. 1995;77(6):940–56.
14. Yasko AW, Lane JM, Fellinger EJ, Rosen V, Wozney JM, Wang EA. The healing of segmental bone defects, induced by recombinant human bone morphogenetic protein (rhBMP-2). A radiographic, histological, and biomechanical study in rats. *J Bone Joint Surg Am*. 1992;74(5):659–70.
15. Garrison KR, Shemilt I, Donell S, et al. Bone morphogenetic protein (BMP) for fracture healing in adults. *Cochrane Database Syst Rev*. 2010;2010(6):CD006950.
16. Giannoudis PV, Dinopoulos HT. BMPs: options, indications, and effectiveness. *J Orthop Trauma*. 2010;24(suppl 1):S9–16.
17. Boden SD, Zdeblick TA, Sandhu HS, Heim SE. The use of rhBMP-2 in interbody fusion cages. Definitive evidence of osteoinduction in humans: a preliminary report. *Spine*. 2000;25(3):376–81.
18. Geesink RG, Hoefnagels NH, Bulstra SK. Osteogenic activity of OP-1 bone morphogenetic protein (BMP-7) in a human fibular defect. *J Bone Joint Surg Br*. 1999;81(4):710–8.
19. Kalfas IH. Principles of bone healing. *Neurosurg Focus*. 2001;10(4):E1.
20. Perlman MH, Thordarson DB. Ankle fusion in a high risk population: an assessment of non-union risk factors. *Foot Ankle Int*. 1999;20(8):491–6.
21. McKibbin B. The biology of fracture healing in long bones. *J Bone Joint Surg Br*. 1978;60-B(2):150–62.
22. Perren SM. Physical and biological aspects of fracture healing with special reference to internal fixation. *Clin Orthop Relat Res*. 1979;138:175–96.
23. Phillips AM. Overview of the fracture healing cascade. *Injury*. 2005;36(suppl 3):S5–7.
24. Daftari TK, Whitesides TE Jr, Heller JG, Goodrich AC, McCarey BE, Hutton WC. Nicotine on the revascularization of bone graft. An experimental study in rabbits. *Spine*. 1994;19(8):904–11.
25. Riebel GD, Boden SD, Whitesides TE, Hutton WC. The effect of nicotine on incorporation of cancellous bone graft in an animal model. *Spine*. 1995;20(20):2198–202.
26. Kenwright J, Gardner T. Mechanical influences on tibial fracture healing. *Clin Orthop Relat Res*. 1998;355:S179–90.
27. Burchardt H, Enneking WF. Transplantation of bone. *Surg Clin North Am*. 1978;58(2):403–27.
28. Diehl JJ, Best TM, Kaeding CC. Classification and return-to-play considerations for stress fractures. *Clin Sports Med*. 2006;25(1):17–28.
29. White AA III, Panjabi MM, Southwick WO. The four biomechanical stages of fracture repair. *J Bone Joint Surg Am*. 1977;59(2):188–92.
30. Young AJ, McAllister DR. Evaluation and treatment of tibial stress fractures. *Clin Sports Med*. 2006;25(1):117–28.
31. Brighton CT. The biology of fracture repair. *Instr Course Lect*. 1984;33:60–82.
32. Karladani AH, Granhed H, Kärrholm J, Styf J. The influence of fracture etiology and type on fracture healing: a review of 104 consecutive tibial shaft fractures. *Arch Orthop Trauma Surg*. 2001;121(6):325–8.
33. Carter DR, Blenman PR, Beaupré GS. Correlations between mechanical stress history and tissue differentiation in initial fracture healing. *J Orthop Res*. 1988;6(5):736–48.
34. Aifantis ID, Ampadiotaki MM, Pallis D, Tsivelekas KK, Papadakis SA, Chronopoulos E. Biophysical enhancement in fracture healing: a review of the literature. *Cureus*. 2023 Apr 17;15(4):e37704.
35. Glassman SD, Anagnost SC, Parker A, Burke D, Johnson JR, Dimar JR. The effect of cigarette smoking and smoking cessation on spinal fusion. *Spine*. 2000;25(20):2608–15.
36. Mankin HJ. Rickets, osteomalacia, and renal osteodystrophy. An update. *Orthop Clin North Am*. 1990;21(1):81–96.
37. Macey LR, Kana SM, Jingushi S, Terek RM, Borretos J, Bolander ME. Defects of early fracture-healing in experimental diabetes. *J Bone Joint Surg Am*. 1989;71(5):722–33.
38. Kelsey JL, Hoffman S. Risk factors for hip fracture. *N Engl J Med*. 1987;316(7):404–6.
39. Jones JP Jr. Concepts of etiology and early pathogenesis of osteonecrosis. *Instr Course Lect*. 1994;43:499–512.
40. Nicholson JA, Makaram N, Simpson AHRW, Keating JF. Fracture nonunion in long bones: a literature review of risk factors and surgical management. *Injury*. 2021;52(suppl 2):S3–11.
41. Giannoudis P, Psarakis S, Kontakis G. Can we accelerate fracture healing? A critical analysis of the literature. *Injury*. 2007;38(suppl 1):S81–9.
42. Prolo DJ. Biology of bone fusion. *Clin Neurosurg*. 1990;36:135–46.
43. Rodham PL, Giannoudis VP, Kanakaris NK, Giannoudis PV. Biological aspects to enhance fracture healing. *EFORT Open Rev*. 2023;8(5):264–82.
44. Hollinger JO, Brekke J, Gruskin E, Lee D. Role of bone substitutes. *Clin Orthop Relat Res*. 1996;324:55–65.
45. Khan SN, Cammisa FP Jr, Sandhu HS, Diwan AD, Girardi FP, Lane JM. The biology of bone grafting. *J Am Acad Orthop Surg*. 2005;13(1):77–86.
46. Kirkpatrick JS, Cornell CN, Hoang BH, et al. Bone void fillers. *J Am Acad Orthop Surg*. 2010;18(9):576–9.
47. Larsson S. Calcium phosphates: what is the evidence? *J Orthop Trauma*. 2010;24(suppl 1):S41–5.
48. Marsell R, Einhorn TA. Emerging bone healing therapies. *J Orthop Trauma*. 2010;24(suppl 1):S4–8.
49. Goldstein C, Sprague S, Petrisor BA. Electrical stimulation for fracture healing: current evidence. *J Orthop Trauma*. 2010;24(suppl 1):S62–5.
50. Mollon B, da Silva V, Busse JW, Einhorn TA, Bhandari M. Electrical stimulation for long-bone fracture-healing: a meta-analysis of randomized controlled trials. *J Bone Joint Surg Am*. 2008;90(11):2322–30.
51. Day SM, Ostrum RF, Chao EY. Bone injury, regeneration and repair. In: Buckwalter JA, Einhorn TA, Simon SR, editors. *Orthopaedic Basic Science*. Rosemont (IL). American Academy of Orthopaedic Surgeons Press; 1999. p. 392–8.

52. Pounder NM, Harrison AJ. Low intensity pulsed ultrasound for fracture healing: a review of the clinical evidence and the associated biological mechanism of action. *Ultrasonics*. 2008;48(4):330–8.
53. Watanabe Y, Matsushita T, Bhandari M, Zdero R, Schemitsch EH. Ultrasound for fracture healing: current evidence. *J Orthop Trauma*. 2010;24(suppl 1):S56–61.
54. Zelle BA, Gollwitzer H, Zlowodzki M, Bühren V. Extracorporeal shock wave therapy: current evidence. *J Orthop Trauma*. 2010;24(suppl 1):S66–70.
55. Wang CJ, Liu HC, Fu TH. The effects of extracorporeal shockwave on acute high-energy long bone fractures of the lower extremity. *Arch Orthop Trauma Surg*. 2007;127(2):137–42.

Nerve Injury

9

Jacob Boomgaardt, Justin Tu, and Jeffrey G. Jenkins

INTRODUCTION

- Trauma to peripheral nerves is a rare but important cause of sport-related injuries in the athlete (1).
- The segment of the peripheral nervous system affected by injury may include the nerve root, plexus, or peripheral nerve. The segment injured is based on numerous factors including the type of sport, level of competition, and age of the athlete (2).
- It is important for the physician to be aware of the presentation, diagnosis, prognosis, and treatment of common peripheral nerve injuries associated with certain sports and athletic participation in general.
- This chapter will provide an overview of peripheral nerve anatomy and nerve injury diagnosis, classification, and prognosis, and identify common peripheral nerve injuries that will likely be encountered in the athletic population. Chapter 23 details the principles of electrodiagnosis, whereas Chapters 61 and 71 further discuss upper and lower nerve entrapments in more detail.

PERIPHERAL NERVE ANATOMY (see Fig. 9.1)

- Cell body: Located in the anterior horn of the spinal cord for motor neurons and in the dorsal root ganglion for sensory neurons.
- Axon: Projection from the cell body involved in propagation of an action potential and transport of cell nutrients. Axons may be myelinated or unmyelinated.
- Myelin: Substance produced by Schwann cells, layered to form a myelin sheath around axons, which acts as insulation for the conduction of current.
- Epineurium: Loose connective tissue that surrounds the entire nerve and protects it from compression.
- Perineurium: Strong layer of connective tissue surrounding fascicles or bundles of nerve fibers.
- Endoneurium: Connective tissue that surrounds an individual axon.

NERVE INJURY

- Etiology of peripheral nerve injury includes stretch or traction, compression, vibration, laceration, and ischemia
- Most traumatic peripheral nerve injuries occur in the upper extremity, with the ulnar nerve most frequently injured (3).

Seddon Classification of Nerve Injury

- Neurapraxia denotes injury to myelin alone, with electrodiagnostic findings of conduction block and, later, conduction velocity slowing along the involved segment of nerve.
- Axonotmesis describes injury to axons resulting in Wallerian degeneration. Early electrodiagnostic findings include loss of nerve conduction across the site of the injury (indistinguishable from neurapraxia in the acute setting).
- Once Wallerian degeneration sets in (approximately 7 days post injury for motor responses, 11 days for sensory responses), there is a decrease or absent evoked potential distal to the site of injury (4).
- Neurotmesis is complete disruption of the nerve. There is injury to axons with associated Wallerian degeneration as well as disruption of the supporting connective tissue. This type of injury carries a poor prognosis for recovery and usually requires urgent surgical intervention.
- Electrodiagnostic testing cannot differentiate between complete axonotmetic lesions and neurotmesis because the difference between these types of lesions is in the integrity of the supporting structures, which have no electrophysiologic function.

Sunderland Classification of Nerve Injury

- Organizes injury type based on the nerve anatomy involved.
- Class 1: Injury to myelin alone (*i.e.*, neurapraxia). Prognosis for recovery is excellent.
- Class 2: Axonotmesis with injury to axons with intact endoneurium, perineurium, and epineurium. Prognosis is good in general but varies depending on percentage of axons injured and distance of lesion from muscle.

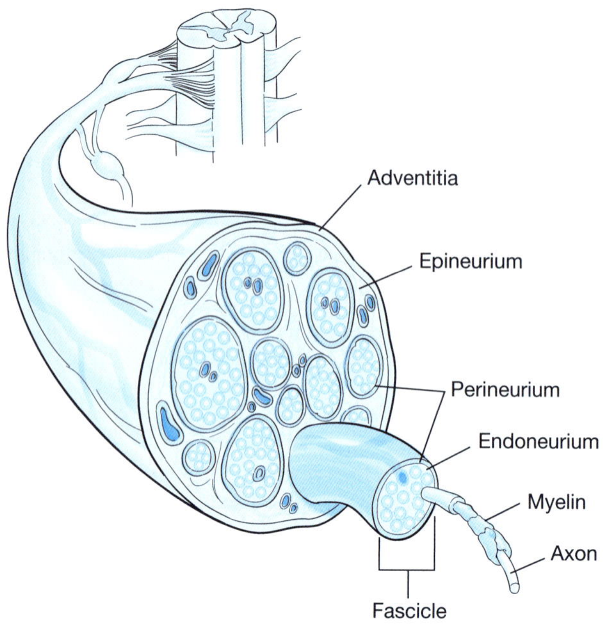

Figure 9.1: Anatomy of the peripheral nerve.

- Class 3: Axonotmesis with injury to the endoneurium and sparing of the perineurium and epineurium. Prognosis is variable. Surgery may be required (5).
- Class 4: Axonotmesis with injury to the endoneurium and perineurium and sparing of the epineurium. Prognosis is poor. Surgery is required to restore nerve continuity.
- Class 5: Neurotmesis. Complete transection of the peripheral nerve. Surgery is required to restore nerve continuity. Prognosis for recovery is particularly poor (6).

DIAGNOSIS OF PERIPHERAL NERVE INJURY

- Electrodiagnostic testing with nerve conduction studies (NCS) and electromyography (EMG) is necessary to determine location, severity, and prognosis of nerve injury (see Chapter 23, Principles of Electrodiagnosis).

Timing of Electrodiagnostic Testing

- Timing of testing depends on the question being asked.
- Immediate to 7 days: Localization of injury with NCS. Cannot reliably distinguish neurapraxia from axonotmesis at this stage (4,7).
- 1–2 weeks: Distinguishes complete lesions from incomplete lesions. May also distinguish axonal from demyelinating lesions (axonotmesis and neurotmesis from neurapraxia) (4).
- 3–4 weeks: Able to better characterize lesion as EMG may now show evidence of denervation. A single study at this point will yield the most information (7). Although EMG cannot accurately quantify axonal damage, it is the most sensitive indicator that axonal damage has occurred.
- 3–4 months: Detects reinnervation of previously denervated muscles (6,7).

Prognosis

- Prognosis is based on severity and type of damage to the nerve. Although purely neurapraxic (demyelinating) lesions have an excellent prognosis for fast and complete recovery, axonometric and neurotmetic lesions have variable outcomes based on the number of axons injured.
- Axon loss results in reduction in the amplitude of the compound muscle action potential (CMAP) or the sensory nerve action potential (SNAP) amplitudes. The percent of amplitude loss of the distal CMAP is an important prognostic feature and may be used to estimate the degree of axon loss.
- Classically, prognostication for motor recovery after peripheral nerve injury was extrapolated from a study of injured facial nerve compound motor action potential amplitudes in comparison with the asymptomatic contralateral side (8). Results indicated:
  - 0%–10% amplitude of contralateral side: poor prognosis
  - 10%–30% amplitude of contralateral side: good prognosis
  - >30% amplitude of contralateral side: excellent prognosis
- A 2015 review by Robinson identified the factors listed in Table 9.1 below as the most useful measures for prognostication in peripheral nerve lesions (9).

Table 9.1 Generally Useful Prognostic Measures for Focal Peripheral Nerve Lesions[a]

Useful Prognostic Factors	Good Prognosis	Poor Prognosis
Recruitment of muscle distal to lesion	Normal or mildly reduced	Discrete or absent
Distal CMAP	Normal or mildly reduced	Absent
Conduction block or slowing	Present	Absent
Distal SNAP (for injuries distal to DRG)	Present	Absent
Distal SNAP (for root avulsions)		Absent

CMAP, compound muscle sction potential; DRG, dorsal root ganglion; SNAP, sensory nerve action potential.

Reprinted from Robinson LR. How electrodiagnosis predicts clinical outcome of focal peripheral nerve lesions. *Muscle Nerve*. 2015 Sep;52(3):321–33. doi:10.1002/mus.24709. Table 1.

[a]These factors are most useful after 7 days, but within the first 2–3 months after injury, before reinnervation by collateral sprouting.

- Distance from the injury site to the muscle will impact prognosis in peripheral nerve injuries. With preservation of the endoneurial tubes, axons can traverse the injured segment in 8–15 days and regenerate along the distal nerve segment at 1–5 mm · d^{-1} (6).
- Mechanism of injury also contributes to prognosis, with avulsion-type injuries having the worst prognosis and compression injuries having the best prognosis (6).

Treatment of Nerve Injury

Pain Management

- Early treatment is focused on pain control to allow for passive range of motion of the affected joint and limb.
- Neuropathic pain is best managed with anticonvulsants, such as gabapentin, tricyclic antidepressants, and selective norepinephrine and serotonin reuptake inhibitors. Topical anesthetics and transcutaneous electrical nerve stimulation are good adjunct therapies (3,10,11).
- Pain refractory to these medications and modalities can be managed with opioids, nonsteroidal anti-inflammatory medications, or in severe cases, a peripheral nerve or spinal block (3,11).
- Desensitization techniques are important to reduce hypersensitivity and allodynia.
- Function and range of motion are also preserved with static or dynamic splinting.

Surgical Management

- Surgical management of nerve injury is dependent on the nerve injured, the type of injury, and the timing of injury (3,12,13).
- Acute surgery (within 72 hours of injury) is indicated when there is a sharp nerve transection or laceration, or a hematoma or pseudoaneurysm is compressing the nerve (6).
- Early surgery (within several weeks of injury) is indicated when there was blunt transection or avulsion of the nerve or when complete nerve lesions are noted during initial vascular repair surgery or on imaging (6).
- Delayed surgery (3–6 months from injury) is indicated in most cases when degree of nerve damage is uncertain. Because patients with incomplete nerve lesions have better outcomes without surgery, appropriate management involves watching and waiting for clinical or electrodiagnostic evidence of recovery (3).
- Surgical techniques for nerve repair include external neurolysis, which involves removal of the damaged epineurium, end-to-end nerve anastomosis, and nerve transfer or grafting (3,13).
- Repair to reinnervate the muscle must be performed before 12–18 months after injury, when irreversible damage to the denervated muscle occurs (3).
- Procedures such as tendon and muscle transfer can restore function when the primary muscle is irreversibly damaged.

PERIPHERAL NERVE INJURY IN NONCONTACT SPORTS

- Peripheral nerve injuries make up a small percentage of all sport-related traumas. However, there are certain relatively safe sports in which peripheral nerve injuries comprise a large proportion of all injuries incurred. These are volleyball, cycling, and racquet sports.

Volleyball (see Chapter 124, Volleyball)

- Peripheral nerve injuries are unfortunately common in volleyball, with the most common being suprascapular nerve entrapment at the spinoglenoid notch. Other common peripheral nerve injuries include axillary and long thoracic neuropathy (2).
- Suprascapular neuropathy typically presents as painless weakness and atrophy of the infraspinatus in the dominant serving arm of the player.
- Prevalence has been documented to range from 33% to 45% of symptomatic international-level players and to be 12% in asymptomatic players at the same level (14–16).
- EMG reveals isolated infraspinatus denervation and motor unit loss (16,17). Possible etiologies of this specific nerve entrapment related to volleyball serving include increased shoulder range of motion and impingement of the infraspinatus branch of the suprascapular nerve between the edge of the spine of the scapula and the medial tendinous margin between the infraspinatus and supraspinatus muscles (17–19).
- With regard to axillary mononeuropathy in volleyball players, there have been cases of quadrilateral space syndrome noted (20,21).

Cycling (see Chapter 99, Cycling)

- Cycling is commonly associated with two peripheral nerve injuries: ulnar neuropathy at the wrist, or "cyclist's palsy," and pudendal neuropathy.
- Other associated nerve injuries include ulnar neuropathy at the elbow, median neuropathy at the wrist (as seen in carpal tunnel syndrome), posterior cutaneous nerve of the thigh neuropathy, and sciatic nerve palsies among unicyclists (2).
- Cyclist's palsy presents as numbness and paresthesias in the ulnar distribution of the hand (small finger and ulnar half of the ring finger) and weakness of hand intrinsic muscles (22).
- Ulnar neuropathy at the wrist is highly prevalent in long-distance cyclists and is independent of handlebar design (22,23).
- Injury is due to compression of the ulnar nerve at the wrist. NCSs have demonstrated significantly increased distal motor latencies in the deep branch of the ulnar nerve after a long-distance cycling event, suggesting the possibility of acute trauma (22,24).

- Treatment is usually conservative, including temporary rest from cycling, use of gloves and padded handlebars, and hand position changes during long rides (22,25,26). Conservative management leads to resolution of symptoms in the majority of cases, and surgical decompression of Guyon canal is rarely indicated (22,27).
- Pudendal neuropathy presents as genital numbness affecting the penis, scrotum, and/or perineal area and erectile dysfunction. The area of sensory loss is dependent on the location of nerve compression, with more distal compression being associated with penile anesthesia alone.
- The pudendal nerve can be compressed proximally as the nerve crosses between the sacrospinal and sacrotuberous ligaments, within Alcock canal, or distally between the perineum and pubic symphysis (7,28).
- Pudendal neuropathy is highly prevalent in both competitive and recreational long-distance cyclists, with sensory symptoms present in 61% and impotency symptoms present in 24% of male cyclists riding more than 400 km · wk^{-1} (22,29–32).
- Treatment is usually conservative, including temporary rest from cycling; change of saddle design to shift weight from the perineum to the buttocks; switching to a wider, padded saddle with a flexible nose; positioning the saddle nose downward; decreasing height difference between seat and handlebar; and implementing riding breaks and position changes during longer rides (22,30). These modifications can prevent the need for surgical pudendal nerve decompression.

Racquet Sports (see Chapter 122, Racquet Sports)

- Injuries in racquet sports are almost exclusively peripheral nerve injuries to the dominant arm (16).
- The posterior interosseous nerve can become entrapped with the arcade of Frohse. This presents as wrist and finger extensor weakness (16,33,34).
- Suprascapular neuropathy can also occur due to repetitive overhand serving. The pathology of nerve compression is similar to that in volleyball players, as discussed earlier (16,35).
- The use of constrictive wrist bands can cause superficial radial neuropathy (16,36).
- Prolonged serving and excessive use of the forearm swing have been thought to contribute to long thoracic neuropathy and compression of the lateral antebrachial cutaneous nerve (37,38).
- Neurogenic thoracic outlet syndrome has been diagnosed in the serving arm of tennis players (16,39,40).

SPORTS AND PERIPHERAL NERVE INJURY

- Sports in general can put peripheral nerves at risk for injury, due to the susceptibility of anatomy used to play the sport or the contact nature required for play.
- The nerves of the upper extremity are involved the majority of the time, with the most common injury being the "stinger" or "burner" (1).
- Case series describing peripheral nerve injuries in athletes have findings that are culture and country specific; thus, numbers reflect different levels of participation in various sports. However, studies done in the United States and Canada indicate that most peripheral nerve injuries are sustained playing football (1,2,16). Wrestling and throwing sports are also more highly associated with peripheral nerve injuries.

CONTACT SPORTS AND NERVE INJURY

Stingers and Burners

- Stingers, also referred to as "burners," are thought to be the result of compression, distraction, or direct blow injuries of the C5 and C6 cervical nerve roots or the upper trunk of the brachial plexus. This causes acute, temporary pain and paresthesias in the upper extremity (1,7,41,42).
- Studies that have employed electrodiagnostic testing of athletes with stingers have demonstrated lesions to the cervical nerve roots and brachial plexus (1,7,43,44).
- This is the most common nerve injury encountered in football players, particularly defensive players, and in wrestlers (2,16,45,46).
- The current recommendation for diagnostic evaluation and return to play is based on number of stingers, whether or not stinger recurrence occurred in the same season, and degree of clinical sequelae. Players with one stinger and no lasting sequelae are able to return to play the same day. Those with two or more stingers need a diagnostic evaluation, including magnetic resonance imaging and electrodiagnostic testing, before returning to play. Those with three stingers in the same season or three stingers in different seasons with persistent symptoms are out for the season (47).

Peroneal Nerve Injury

- The peroneal nerve is the most frequently injured lower extremity nerve in athletes (1,48).
- Injury at the fibular head is most common, followed by at the ankle. Mechanism of injury is direct blow to the knee or ankle sprain.
- Concomitant peroneal nerve injury with ligamentous trauma (involving the anterior cruciate, posterior cruciate, or lateral collateral ligament) and knee dislocation has also been described in athletes.
- Compartment syndrome in the lower leg can also put the peroneal nerve at risk for damage (1).

Axillary Nerve Injury

- Axillary nerve injury in athletes has been associated with anterior shoulder dislocation or direct shoulder trauma (1).

- The axillary nerve is rarely injured in throwers, but when affected is usually due to the quadrilateral space syndrome. The syndrome involves compression of the axillary nerve in the quadrilateral space, due to a fibrous band or ganglion cyst within the space or decreased space between teres major and minor during the late cocking phase of pitch (49,50).
- Clinical presentation is often subtle, with the athlete reporting symptoms of arm fatigue ("dead arm") with overhead activities as well as dull posterior shoulder pain. Although there may be weakness in abduction and external rotation, due to the dynamic nature of this injury in the throwing athlete these findings may be absent (51).
- Treatment of nerve injury in the throwing arm is usually conservative, consisting of throwing rest, physical therapy focusing on shoulder and trunk flexibility and strength, and correction of altered throwing mechanics. Given the subtle presentation, ultrasound guided injection to the quadrilateral space may play an important role in both diagnosis as well as symptomatic management (52,53).
- Surgery is indicated if there is no improvement with nonoperative management, if there is a mass lesion causing the symptoms, or if the neuropathy is severe (50).

THROWING SPORTS AND NERVE INJURY (SEE CHAPTER 55, THE THROWING SHOULDER)

- Several upper extremity nerves, including the suprascapular, axillary, and ulnar nerves, are frequently injured in baseball and softball players due to the torque force that occurs during overhead throwing (16,50,51,54,55).

Ulnar Nerve Injury

- Ulnar neuropathy is the most common peripheral mononeuropathy in throwing athletes. Ulnar neuropathy is most common in baseball pitchers, whereas radial neuropathy is common in softball pitchers due to the biomechanics of underhand or "windmill" pitching (51,54,56,57).
- Throwing athletes are particularly susceptible to ulnar neuropathy due to excessive valgus forces and rapid elbow extension placing high tensile stress along the medial side of the elbow (51).
- Flexor carpi ulnaris contraction with the elbow flexed in the throwing motion has been found to increase pressure in the cubital tunnel 6–20 times baseline, which can further contribute to ulnar nerve compression and dysfunction (58).
- The initial clinical presentation is often subtle, including decreased performance and durability rather than typical nerve symptoms such as paresthesias. Once symptoms develop, it usually presents with medial elbow pain with numbness and tingling in the fourth and/or fifth fingers (59).
- As symptoms progress initially they will occur with throwing alone, most commonly in the late cocking and early acceleration phases. If untreated, symptoms will usually progress to the point where symptoms will be present at rest.
- With ulnar neuropathy at the elbow, electrodiagnostic studies will show slowed conduction velocity across the elbow and, in more severe cases, will demonstrate denervation in ulnar-innervated muscles. The ulnar innervated forearm muscles (flexor carpi ulnaris and flexor digitorum profundus) are not infrequently spared in cases of ulnar neuropathy at the elbow (60,61).
- Management of ulnar neuropathy at the elbow can include conservative treatment including activity modification, elbow pads, elbow extension braces, and ulnar nerve hydrodissections, but surgical decompression is usually most successful. Anterior subcutaneous transposition and submuscular transposition have demonstrated favorable outcomes when compared to simple decompression or medial epicondylectomy in the overhead-throwing athlete (3,16,36,50,54,56,62,63).

Suprascapular Nerve Injury

- The suprascapular nerve can be compressed in two different anatomic locations, producing different symptoms in the thrower:
  - In the suprascapular notch underneath the superior transverse scapular ligament (50,64). Injury at this location results in denervation of both the supraspinatus and infraspinatus muscles. Patients typically complain of posterior shoulder weakness and pain.
  - At the spinoglenoid notch. Patients classically present with painless shoulder weakness. The infraspinatus muscle alone is involved because the branch to the supraspinatus has been spared. Posterior shoulder pain is not usually present due to the nerve injury being distal to the suprascapular sensory nerve fibers (15,50). A ganglion cyst can also compress the suprascapular nerve, with the most common location for a cyst to develop at the spinoglenoid notch (50,65,66). There is case report–level evidence to suggest that ultrasound-guided aspiration ± corticosteroid injection of the paralabral cyst may be an efficacious treatment option to relieve suprascapular nerve compression (67).
  - Although the precise incidence of this injury is unknown, a retrospective analysis of professional baseball pitchers found isolated infraspinatus atrophy in 4.4% of pitchers, with a higher incidence associated with increased throwing volume (51,68).
- Electrodiagnostic studies can localize the suprascapular nerve injury, as well as rule out cervical radiculopathy and brachial plexopathy. NCSs can demonstrate increased compound motor action potential latency, whereas EMG determines whether there is denervation of the supraspinatus, infraspinatus, or both.

9.1 The Budapest Criteria for Complex Regional Pain Syndrome (CRPS)

1. Continuous pain disproportional to the inciting event
2. At least one symptom in ≥3 of the following categories:
   - Sensory (hyperesthesia, allodynia)
   - Vasomotor (temperature asymmetry, skin color changes, skin color asymmetry)
   - Sudomotor/Edema (edema, sweating changes, sweating asymmetry)
   - Motor/Trophic (decreased range of motion, weakness, tremor, dystonia, trophic changes affecting the skin, nails, hair)
3. At least one sign present upon evaluation in ≥2 of the following categories
   - Sensory (Evidence of hyperalgesia and/or allodynia)
   - Vasomotor (Evidence of temperature asymmetry and/or skin color changes/asymmetry)
   - Sudomotor/Edema (Evidence of edema and/or sweating changes/asymmetry)
   - Motor/Trophic (Evidence of decreased range of motion and/or weakness, tremor, dystonia and/or trophic changes affecting the skin, nails, hair)
4. Absence of another diagnosis that would better explain the symptoms and signs

Adapted from Harden, RN, Bruehl, S, Stanton-Hicks, M, et al. Proposed new diagnostic criteria for complex regional pain syndrome. *Pain Med.* 2007;8(4):330. Table 3.

CARPAL TUNNEL SYNDROME IN ATHLETES

- Cases of carpal tunnel syndrome (CTS) are usually found incidentally in asymptomatic athletes who undergo electrodiagnostic testing for other nerve injuries (1).
- Symptomatic CTS is most common in sports that require repetitive wrist maneuvers, such as weight lifting, cycling, and racquet sports (1,7,36,44,69–71).

NEUROMUSCULAR IMAGING

- MRI and ultrasound are the main modalities used in the evaluation of suspected peripheral nerve injuries.
- On ultrasound in short-axis images, nerves exhibit a rounded or ovoid shape with a honeycomb appearance. In long axis they appear as alternating hypoechoic and hyperechoic bands. Short-axis views are generally superior to long-axis views in the evaluation of suspected peripheral nerve pathology (72,73).
- Pathology is most commonly recognized by enlargement of the cross-sectional area of the affected nerve. Other common findings include changes in the echogenicity of the nerve as well as intraneural vascularization (74,75).
- A study by Padua and colleagues found that neuromuscular ultrasound altered either the diagnosis or therapeutic decision making in 42.3% of cases studied (76).
- A recent study by Zaidman et al. compared MRI to neuromuscular ultrasound in the evaluation of peripheral nerve lesions. Ultrasound was found to be more sensitive than MRI (93% vs. 67%) with equivalent specificity (86%) and is better at identifying multifocal lesions. As such they recommend ultrasound as the initial imaging modality for evaluation of peripheral nerve lesions (77).

CRPS

- Complex regional pain syndrome (CRPS) is a chronic pain disorder affecting the upper or lower extremities. It is characterized by severe neuropathic pain, with vascular, autonomic, and trophic dysfunction (78).
- There is no single gold standard diagnostic test for CRPS and the diagnosis is clinical based on the Budapest Criteria (79) (see Box 9.1).
- There are two subtypes: type I, formerly known as reflex sympathetic dystrophy, and type II, formerly known as causalgia. Type I occurs in the absence of nerve trauma, whereas type II occurs in the setting of known nerve trauma. Clinically they are indistinguishable and follow a regional rather than dermatomal or peripheral nerve distribution.
- Although there is no single diagnostic test to confirm CRPS, triple phase bone scan, particularly increased uptake in phase 3, has been proposed by some authors to be a sensitive and specific test for diagnosis (80,81). Recent work evaluating the utility of bone scans in patients diagnosed using the Budapest criteria revealed relatively poor sensitivity, drawing into question its clinical utility (82).
- Medication treatment options include anti-inflammatories such as NSAIDs or corticosteroids (potential efficacy largely early in the course of the condition), neuropathic pain medications, or opioids. Other treatment options include physical and occupational therapy as well as various procedural interventions notably sympathetic nerve blocks (83).

CONCLUSION

- Peripheral nerve trauma is a rare but potentially debilitating occurrence in sports.

- Nerves of the upper extremity are more often affected than those in the lower extremity.
- Sports in general put nerves at risk, but certain sports are more highly associated with peripheral nerve injury than others.
- Diagnosis of nerve injury is achieved by combining clinical findings, appropriate imaging, and electrodiagnostic studies.
- Treatment can be conservative or surgical, depending on the type and severity of nerve injury.
- Prognosis of nerve injury is dependent on injury severity, mechanism of injury, and location of injury.

REFERENCES

1. Krivickas LS, Wilbourn AJ. Peripheral nerve injuries in athletes: a case series of over 200 injuries. *Semin Neurol.* 2000;20(2):225–32.
2. Toth C. Peripheral nerve injuries attributable to sport and recreation. *Neurol Clin.* 2008;26(1):89–113.
3. Campbell WW. Evaluation and management of peripheral nerve injury. *Clin Neurophysiol.* 2008;119(9):1951–65.
4. Chaudry V, Cornblath DR. Wallerian degeneration in human nerves: a serial electrophysiologic study. *Muscle Nerve.* 1992;15:687–93.
5. Olivo R, Tsao B. Peripheral nerve injuries in sport. *Neurol Clin.* 2017 Aug;35(3):559–72. doi:10.1016/j.ncl.2017.03.010
6. Robinson LR. Traumatic injury to peripheral nerves. *Muscle Nerve.* 2000;23(6):863–73.
7. Aldridge JW, Bruno RJ, Strauch RJ, Rosenwasser MP. Nerve entrapment in athletes. *Clin Sports Med.* 2001;20(1):95–122.
8. Sillman JS, Niparko JK, Lee SS, Kileny PR. Prognostic value of evoked and standard electromyography in acute facial paralysis. *Otolaryngol Head Neck Surg.* 1992;107(3):377–81.
9. Robinson LR. How electrodiagnosis predicts clinical outcome of focal peripheral nerve lesions. *Muscle Nerve.* 2015 Sep;52(3):321–33. doi:10.1002/mus.24709
10. Dworkin RH, Backonja M, Rowbotham MC, et al. Advances in neuropathic pain: diagnosis mechanisms and treatment recommendations. *Arch Neurol.* 2003;60(11):1524–34.
11. Kingery WS. A critical review of controlled clinical trials for peripheral neuropathic pain and complex regional pain syndromes. *Pain.* 1997;73(2):123–39.
12. Siemionow M, Sari A. A contemporary overview of peripheral nerve research from the Cleveland Clinic microsurgery laboratory. *Neurol Res.* 2004;26(2):218–25.
13. Spinner RJ, Kline DG. Surgery for peripheral nerve and brachial plexus injuries or other nerve lesions. *Muscle Nerve.* 2000;23(5):680–95.
14. Eggert S, Holzgraefe M. Compression neuropathy of the suprascapular nerve in high performance volleyball players. *Sportverletz Sportschaden.* 1993;7(3):136–42. [in German].
15. Ferretti A, Cerullo G, Russo G. Suprascapular neuropathy in volleyball players. *J Bone Joint Surg Am.* 1987;69(2):260–3.
16. Treihaft MM. Neurologic injuries in baseball players. *Semin Neurol.* 2000;20(2):187–93.
17. Montagna P, Colonna S. Suprascapular neuropathy restricted to the infraspinatus muscle in volleyball players. *Acta Neurol Scand.* 1993;87(3):174–80.
18. Sandow MJ, Ilic J. Suprascapular nerve rotator cuff compression syndrome in volleyball players. *J Shoulder Elb Res.* 1998;7(5):516–21.
19. Witvrouw E, Cools A, Lysens R, et al. Suprascapular neuropathy in volleyball players. *Br J Sports Med.* 2000;34(3):174–80.
20. Distefano S. Neuropathy due to entrapment of the long thoracic nerve. A case report. *Ital J Orthop Traumatol.* 1989;15(2):259–62.
21. Paladini D, Dellantonio R, Cinti A, Angeleri F. Axillary neuropathy in volleyball players: report of two cases and literature review. *J Neurol Neurosurg Psychiatry.* 1996;60(3):345–7.
22. Kennedy J. Neurologic injuries in cycling and bike riding. *Neurol Clin.* 2008;26(1):271–9.
23. Patterson JM, Jaggars MM, Boyer MI. Ulnar and median nerve palsy in long-distance cyclists. A prospective study. *Am J Sports Med.* 2003;31(4):585–9.
24. Akuthota V, Plastaras C, Lindberg K, Tobey J, Press J, Garvan C. The effect of long-distance bicycling on ulnar and median nerves: an electrophysiologic evaluation of cyclist palsy. *Am J Sports Med.* 2005;33(8):1224–30.
25. Munnings F. Cyclist's palsy making changes brings relief. *Phys Sportsmed.* 1991;19(9):113–9.
26. Richmond DR. Handlebar problems in bicycling. *Clin Sports Med.* 1994;13(1):165–73.
27. Bachoura A, Jacoby SM. Ulnar tunnel syndrome. *Orthop Clin North Am.* 2012;43(4):467–74.
28. Leibovitch I, Mor Y. The vicious cycling: bicycling related urogenital disorders. *Eur Urol.* 2005;47(3):277–87.
29. Andersen KV, Bovim G. Impotence and nerve entrapment in long distance amateur cyclists. *Acta Neurol Scand.* 1997;95(4):233–40.
30. Schrader SM, Breitenstein MJ, Clark JC, Lowe BD, Turner TW. Nocturnal penile tumescence and rigidity testing in bicycling patrol officers. *J Androl.* 2002;23(6):927–34.
31. Schwarzer U, Wiegand W, Bin-Saleh A, et al. Genital numbness and impotence rates in long distance cyclists. *J Urol.* 1999;161(4 suppl):178.
32. Sommer F, König D, Graft C, et al. Impotence and genital numbness in cyclists. *Int J Sports Med.* 2001;22(6):410–3.
33. Kaplan PE. Posterior interosseous neuropathies: natural history. *Arch Phys Med Rehabil.* 1984;65(7):399–400.
34. Lorei MP, Hershman EB. Peripheral nerve injuries in athletes. Treatment and prevention. *Sports Med.* 1993;16(2):130–47.
35. Romeo AA, Rotenberg DD, Bach BR Jr. Suprascapular neuropathy. *J Am Acad Orthop Surg.* 1999;7(6):358–67.
36. Rettig AC. Neurovascular injuries in the wrists and hands of athletes. *Clin Sports Med.* 1990;9(2):389–417.
37. Pasternack JS, Veenema KR, Callahan CM. Baseball injuries: a Little League survey. *Pediatrics.* 1996;98(3 pt 1):445–8.
38. Felsenthal G, Mondell DL, Reischer MA, Mack RH. Forearm pain secondary to compression syndrome of the lateral cutaneous nerve of the forearm. *Arch Phys Med Rehabil.* 1984;65(3):139–41.
39. Karas SE. Thoracic outlet syndrome. *Clin Sports Med.* 1990;9(2):297–310.
40. Strukel RJ, Garrick JG. Thoracic outlet compression in athletes: a report of four cases. *Am J Sports Med.* 1978;6(2):35–9.
41. American College of Sports Medicine. Selected issues in injury and illness prevention and the team physician: a consensus statement. *Med Sci Sports Exerc.* 2007;39(11):2012–6.
42. Levitz CL, Reilly PJ, Torg JS. The pathomechanics of chronic, recurrent cervical nerve root neurapraxia. The chronic burner syndrome. *Am J Sports Med.* 1997;25(1):73–6.
43. Bergfeld JA, Herschman EB, Wilbourn AJ. Brachial plexus injury in sports: a five-year follow-up. *Orthop Trans.* 1988;12:743–4.
44. Sicuranza MJ, McCue FC III. Compressive neuropathies in the upper extremity of athletes. *Hand Clin.* 1992;8(2):263–73.
45. Diamond PT, Gale SD. Head injuries in men's and women's lacrosse: a 10 year analysis of the NEISS database. National Electronic Injury Surveillance System. *Brain Inj.* 2001;15(6):537–44.

46. Kline DG, Judice DJ. Operative management of selected brachial plexus lesions. *J Neurosurg.* 1983;58(5):631–49.
47. Standaert CJ, Herring SA. Expert opinion and controversies in musculoskeletal and sports medicine: stingers. *Arch Phys Med Rehabil.* 2009;90(3):402–6.
48. Hirasawa Y, Sakakida K. Sports and peripheral nerve injury. *Am J Sports Med.* 1983;9(4):244–6.
49. Cahill BR, Palmer RE. Quadrilateral space syndrome. *J Hand Surg Am.* 1983;8(1):65–9.
50. Cummins CA, Schneider DS. Peripheral nerve injuries in baseball players. *Neurol Clin.* 2008;26(1):195–215.
51. Bowers RL, Cherian C, Zaremski JL. A review of upper extremity peripheral nerve injuries in throwing athletes. *Pharm Manag PM R.* 2022 May;14(5):652–68. doi:10.1002/pmrj.12762
52. Feng SH, Hsiao MY, Wu CH, Ozcakar L. Ultrasound-guided diagnosis and management for quadrilateral space syndrome. *Pain Med.* 2017;18(1):184–6.
53. Zhang J, Zhang T, Wang R, Wang T. Musculoskeletal ultrasound diagnosis of quadrilateral space syndrome: a case report. *Medicine (Baltimore).* 2021;100(10):e24976.
54. Andrews JR, Timmerman LA. Outcome of elbow surgery in professional baseball players. *Am J Sports Med.* 1995;23(4):407–13.
55. Bennett G. Elbow and shoulder lesions of baseball players. *Am J Surg.* 1959;98:484–92.
56. Del Pizzo W, Jobe FW, Norwood L. Ulnar nerve entrapment syndrome in baseball players. *Am J Sports Med.* 1977;5(5):182–5.
57. Sinson G, Zager EL, Kline DG. Windmill pitcher's radial neuropathy. *Neurosurgery.* 1994;34(6):1087–90.
58. Werner CO, Ohlin P, Elmqvist D. Pressures recorded in ulnar neuropathy. *Acta Orthop Scand.* 1985;56(5):404–6.
59. Harris JD, Lintner DM. Nerve injuries about the elbow in the athlete. *Sports Med Arthrosc Rev.* 2014;22(3):e7–15.
60. Campbell WW, Pridgeon RM, Riaz G, Astruc J, Leahy M, Crostic EG. Sparing of the flexor carpi ulnaris in ulnar neuropathy at the elbow. *Muscle Nerve.* 1989 Dec;12(12):965–7. doi:10.1002/mus.880121203
61. Landau ME, Campbell WW. Clinical features and electrodiagnosis of ulnar neuropathies. *Phys Med Rehabil Clin N Am.* 2013 Feb;24(1):49–66. doi:10.1016/j.pmr.2012.08.019
62. Aoki M, Kanaya K, Aiki H, Wada T, Yamashita T, Ogiwara N. Cubital tunnel syndrome in adolescent baseball players: a report of six cases with 3- to 5-year follow-up. *Arthroscopy.* 2005;21(6):758.
63. Glousman RE. Ulnar nerve problems in the athlete's elbow. *Clin Sports Med.* 1990;9(2):365–77.
64. Rengachary SS, Neff JP, Singer PA, Brackett CE. Suprascapular entrapment neuropathy: a clinical, anatomical and comparative study. Part 1—clinical study. *Neurosurgery.* 1979;5(4):441–6.
65. Chochole M, Senker W, Meznik C, Breitenseher MJ. Glenoid-labral cyst entrapping the suprascapular nerve: dissolution after arthroscopic debridement of an extended SLAP lesion. *Arthroscopy.* 1997;13(6):753–5.
66. Fehrman D, Orwin J, Jennings R. Suprascapular nerve entrapment by ganglion cysts: a report of six cases with arthroscopic findings and review of the literature. *Arthroscopy.* 1995;11(6):727–34.
67. Wee TC, Wu CH. Ultrasound-guided aspiration of a paralabral cyst at the spinoglenoid notch with suprascapular nerve compressive neuropathy. *J Med Ultrasound.* 2018;26(3):166–7.
68. Cummins CA, Messer TM, Schafer MF. Infraspinatus muscle atrophy in professional baseball players. *Am J Sports Med.* 2004 Jan–Feb;32(1):116–20. doi:10.1177/0363546503260731
69. Cabrera JM, McCue FC III. Nonosseous athletic injuries of the elbow, forearm, and hand. *Clin Sports Med.* 1986;5(4):681–700.
70. Kulund DN, McCue FC, Rockwell DA, Gieck JH. Tennis injuries: prevention and treatment. A review. *Am J Sports Med.* 1979;7(4):249–53.
71. Szabo RM, Madison M. Carpal tunnel syndrome. *Orthop Clin North Am.* 1992;23(1):103–9.
72. Bignotti B, Tagliafico A, Martinoli C. Ultrasonography of peripheral nerves: anatomy and pathology. *Ultrasound Clin.* 2014;9:525–36.
73. Tagliafico A. Peripheral nerve imaging: not only cross-sectional area. *World J Radiol.* 2016;8:726–8.
74. Ghasemi-Esfe AR, Khalilzadeh O, Vaziri-Bozorg SM, et al. Color and power Doppler US for diagnosing carpal tunnel syndrome and determining its severity. A Quantitative Image Processing Method. *Radiology.* 2011;261(2):499–506.
75. Choi SJ, Ahn JH, Ryu DS, et al. Ultrasonography for nerve compression syndromes of the upper extremity. *Ultrasonography.* 2015;34(4):275–91.
76. Padua L, Liotta G, Di Pasquale A, et al. Contribution of ultrasound in the assessment of nerve diseases. *Eur J Neurol.* 2012 Jan;19(1):47–54. doi:10.1111/j.1468-1331.2011.03421.x
77. Zaidman CM, Seelig MJ, Baker JC, Mackinnon SE, Pestronk A. Detection of peripheral nerve pathology: comparison of ultrasound and MRI. *Neurology.* 2013 Apr 30;80(18):1634–40. doi:10.1212/WNL.0b013e3182904f3f
78. AlMakadma Y, Eirale C, Chamari K. Neuropathic pain in athletes: basics of diagnosis and monitoring of a hidden threat. *Biol Sport.* 2022 Oct;39(4):943–9. doi:10.5114/biolsport.2022.110744
79. Harden R, Bruehl S, Stanton-Hicks M, Wilson P. Proposed new diagnostic criteria for complex regional pain syndrome. *Pain Med.* 2007;8(4):326–31.
80. Cappello ZJ, Kasdan ML, Louis DS. Meta-analysis of imaging techniques for the diagnosis of complex regional pain syndrome type I. *J Hand Surg Am.* 2012;37(2):288–96.
81. Wuppenhorst N, Maier C, Frettloh J, Pennekamp W, Nicolas V. Sensitivity and specificity of 3-phase bone scintigraphy in the diagnosis of complex regional pain syndrome of the upper extremity. *Clin J Pain.* 2010;26(3):182–9.
82. Wertli M, Brunner F, Steurer J, Held U. Usefulness of bone scintigraphy for the diagnosis of complex regional pain syndrome 1: a systematic review and Bayesian meta-analysis. *PLoS One.* 2017;12(3):e0173688.
83. Harden RN, McCabe CS, Goebel A, Massey M, Suvar T, Grieve S, Bruehl S. Complex regional pain syndrome: practical diagnostic and treatment guidelines. *Pain Med.* 2022 May;23(suppl 1):S1–53. doi:10.1093/pm/pnac046

Muscle and Tendon Injury and Repair

10

Jonathon M. Florance, Bradley J. Nelson, and Dean C. Taylor

SKELETAL MUSCLE INJURY AND REPAIR

- Muscle injury is the most common musculoskeletal complaint in the athlete. Common muscle injuries include muscle strains, delayed muscle soreness, contusions, and cramps. The incidence of muscle injuries in sports depends on the sport, gender, and level of competition, but account for 15%–50% of all injuries sustained in sports with a majority presenting as muscle strains (1–6).

Anatomy and Physiology

- Primary components of skeletal muscle include contractile proteins (myosin and actin), regulatory proteins (tropomyosin and troponin), and a connective tissue matrix (7).
- The muscle fiber is the basic structural element of skeletal muscle. Muscle is a syncytium of multinucleated fibers (7). The functional unit of muscle is the sarcomere. Within each sarcomere are light and dark bands. The dark bands are made up of both the thick myosin and thin actin filaments, whereas the light bands are made up of just the thin actin filaments that connect to the Z lines (see Figs. 6.1 and 6.2).
- A muscle fiber originates via a tendon from bone, traverses one or more joints, and joins with a tendon that inserts to bone. Fiber arrangement can be parallel or oblique (unipennate, bipennate, multipennate) in orientation. Fibers can be classified as type I (slow-twitch oxidative) and type II (fast-twitch). Type II fibers are further classified into type IIa (fast-twitch oxidative glycolytic) and type IIb (fast-twitch glycolytic).
- Satellite cells are separate cells along the periphery of the muscle fiber that are important in cellular regeneration in response to injury. Satellite cells proliferate and transform into myotubes in response to growth factors and cytokines that mediate the repair process (8,9).

The authors acknowledge Donald T. Kirkendall for his assistance in preparing the revision of this chapter.

- The musculotendinous junction is a specialized region of highly folded membranes that increase the cross-sectional area for force transmission (7). Most muscle strain injuries occur in this region.
- The sarcoplasmic reticulum is a specialized cellular organelle that is responsible for calcium movement across the cell membrane and electrical transmission within the cell.
- A motor unit is a motor neuron and all the muscle fibers it innervates. The motor neuron innervates each of its muscle fibers at a motor end plate. The number of myofibers in a motor unit and the number of motor units in a skeletal muscle are determined by the function of the muscle (7). The fewer the fibers in a motor unit, the finer is the control (*e.g.*, ocular muscles), whereas many fibers in a motor unit lead to gross movements (*e.g.*, quadriceps).
- A muscle contraction begins when an electrical impulse travels down a motor neuron's axon to its motor end plates. This electrical impulse triggers the release of acetylcholine that migrates to receptors on the myofiber and causes a depolarization of the sarcolemma. The depolarization travels deep into the muscle by the transverse tubule, triggering the release of calcium from the sarcoplasmic reticulum. Calcium binds to troponin, which results in a conformational change in the tropomyosin, opening actin's active site and allowing the crossbridges of the myosin head to interact. The crossbridges then undergo their own conformational change that pulls the thin actin filament to slide past the myosin toward the center of the sarcomere. The process of sarcolemma depolarization and the resulting sliding of the filaments is referred to as excitation-contraction coupling. The physical process of muscle contraction is the sliding of the actin filament past the myosin filament toward the center of the sarcomere pulling the ends of the sarcomere (the Z lines) toward each other. The whole muscle shortens when the process is multiplied over thousands of sarcomeres, thousands of conformational changes at the myosin crossbridge heads, and all the activated fibers. This process is powered by the hydrolysis of adenosine triphosphate (ATP) to both bind and break the connection of the crossbridge with the actin filament (7,9).

- Muscle contraction can be isometric, concentric, or eccentric. Isometric contraction is when the force by the muscle is equal to the load, and although there is no visible joint movement, the muscle does shorten. By recruiting more muscle fibers to overcome the external load, a concentric (or shortening) contraction can occur, and there is visible joint movement. Eccentric contraction is when the external load is greater than the force generated by the muscle and the muscle lengthens (9). For example, raising the weight in an arm curl is a concentric contraction of the elbow flexors, and lowering the weight is an eccentric contraction of the same flexors. Isometric strength measurements are strongly predictive of functional capacity and are sensitive in detecting changes in muscle strength (10).
- Muscle physiology is further detailed in Chapter 6, Exercise Physiology.

Reparative Process

- The pathophysiology of the healing muscle is similar regardless of the type of injury. Healing occurs in three distinct phases: (a) degeneration and inflammation; (b) muscle regeneration; and (c) development of fibrosis (9). The reparative process involves both inflammatory cells (neutrophils, macrophages) and myogenic (satellite) cells.
- Acute hemorrhage and inflammatory cell infiltration of the damaged muscle tissue occurs shortly after injury (11).
  - Initially, neutrophils infiltrate the injury site via cellular chemotaxis. Mediators such as *basic fibroblast growth factor* (BFGF), *platelet-derived growth factor* (PDGF), and *interleukin-1* (IL-1) regulate myoblast proliferation and differentiation to foster regeneration and repair of the muscle, as well as stimulation of macrophages and fibroblasts within the muscle tissue (7,9).
  - Macrophages are the most prevalent inflammatory cells present in injured muscle. Distinct subclasses of macrophages have been identified and play specific roles in the healing process. One subclass of macrophages is involved in the phagocytosis of damaged tissue and further stimulation of the inflammatory response. A second subclass of macrophages helps modulate the reparative process (12).
- Satellite cells are myogenic mononuclear cells responsible for muscle fiber repair and regeneration processes. They are located beneath the basal lamina of skeletal muscle fibers. Mechanical or chemical insults stimulate quiescent satellite cells through hepatocyte growth factor (HGF)/nitric oxide radical–dependent pathways (13,14). The activated satellite cells enter the cycle cell and differentiate into myoblasts, which fuse together and develop into multinucleated muscle fibers. Typically, these repaired myofibers attach to the extracellular matrix of the newly formed scar (15).
- Fibroblast proliferation and collagen matrix synthesis occur along with the inflammatory response and muscle regeneration. This connective tissue scar formation may inhibit the complete repair of injured muscle (15). Muscle degeneration and inflammation occur during the first few days after the injury. Regeneration then starts after 1 week, peaks at 2 weeks, and is typically complete by 3–4 weeks. Scar tissue starts to form 2–3 weeks after the injury and increases.
- There has been considerable excitement investigating stem cell therapy in the past 20 years, incited by research demonstrating that stem cells participate in myofiber regeneration. In addition, these pluripotent stem cells can differentiate into endothelial and neural lineages, which may be beneficial in vascular and neural supply to the regenerating muscle (16). Continued research is necessary but early human trials demonstrate potential reparative effect of adipose-derived mesenchymal stem cells in tendinopathies (17).

Muscle Strain Injury

- Muscle strain is the most common injury sustained in sports. Muscle can be functionally limited from delayed muscle soreness (discussed later), partial muscle strain, or complete muscle disruption (18).
- A common feature in muscle tissue injury is muscle stretch in combination with a strong contraction in two-joint muscles (*e.g.*, rectus femoris, biceps femoris, gastrocnemius) or muscles with a complex architecture (*e.g.*, adductor longus). The injury occurs when selected muscles restrict the range of motion of the joint they cross and a significant amount of tension is placed on that muscle (11).
- Clinically, muscle injury (strain/contusion) is classified depending on the level of damage generated: *mild* when the loss of strength and movement is minimal or nonexistent, *moderate* with the inability to contract, and *severe* for absolute loss of function (19).

Mechanism of Injury

- Although a concentric muscle contraction alone is insufficient to create muscle strain injury, the force per fiber is higher in the relatively few muscle fibers needed during eccentric muscular contraction. The combination of passive stretch of the muscle past its resting length, eccentric loads, and the subsequent concentric contraction is required to injure the muscle (20). This overextension and tension development can then disrupt the myofibers near the myotendinous junction (21).
- Cellular disruption results in the hydrolysis of structural proteins and inflammation that further damages the muscle tissue (22).
- Animal studies reveal that muscle tissue sustaining a nondisruptive strain injury demonstrates decreased load to failure when subjected to stress (23,24). In addition, these partially injured muscles generate significantly less contractile force, which contributes to the clinical observation that significant muscle strain injuries are frequently preceded by a minor injury. These studies also underscore the importance of rest and complete recovery prior to the resumption of athletic activities.

Diagnosis and Imaging

- Although reviewing the athlete's history is essential, tenderness to palpation at the myotendinous junction is hallmark. When a complete rupture is present, a defect may be palpated, and weakness should be expected.
- Ultrasound, due to its lower costs and portability, is sometimes the first diagnostic modality. Evaluation of superficial structures such as the patellar tendon is easier with ultrasound; however, in athletes with a voluminous musculature, the evaluation of deep structures may be difficult due to dissipation of the sound waves and the lack of reflection over long distances (18).
- Magnetic resonance imaging is typically unnecessary for the diagnosis of muscle strain, but it may help determine the severity of the strain, continuity of the myotendinous junction, and possible convalescent time, which is crucial for elite athletes. T1-weighted images show excellent anatomic detail such as the myotendinous junction disruption, whereas T2-weighted images are fluid-sensitive and reveal pathologic processes involved in edema, making muscle strains easy to visualize (11,18).

Reparative Response

- Similar to the general reparative response of muscle described earlier.
- The presence of inelastic fibrotic tissue (scar) may make the muscle more susceptible to additional injury.

Treatment and Prevention

- Reduced activity is key in the treatment of muscle strain injuries. This helps control inflammation and prevents further tissue damage.
- The RICE (rest, ice, compression, and elevation) principle should be implemented immediately after skeletal muscle injury. Immobilization can diminish pain, reduce inflammation, and allow torn muscle ends to reapproximate. Prolonged muscle immobilization (>7–14 days) results in lower loads to failure and should be avoided. Early motion also limits adhesions and provides quicker proprioceptive recovery (11).
- Therapeutic ultrasound is thought to relieve pain and promote muscle regeneration during the initial phase of muscle injuries. Its recommendation and use is promoted although the results from animal studies have not been encouraging. In addition, its effectiveness in the complete healing process is questionable (25,26).
- Clinical trials have failed to demonstrate the benefits of hyperbaric oxygen therapy in the treatment of mild muscle injuries in athletes (27).

Nonsteroidal Anti-inflammatory Drugs

- Animal studies demonstrate that nonsteroidal anti-inflammatory drugs (NSAIDs) reduce the inflammatory response associated with muscle strain injury, providing more complete functional recovery by 1 week. A certain level of inflammation is necessary, however, to remove necrotic tissue and permit healing; thus, NSAIDs may delay complete healing of the damaged muscle tissue (22,23). The indication for the use of these drugs in muscle strain injury is unclear, and many physicians recommend only a short course of NSAIDs immediately after the acute strain (11).
- Cryotherapy provides a short-term analgesic effect, but its effect on inflammation is also unclear (28). Some authors state that icing on injured skeletal muscle should be applied for 6 hours to limit the hemorrhage and tissue necrosis formation (29).

Muscle Strengthening

- Muscle strengthening is an important factor in the recovery of injured muscle and the prevention of reinjury. Eccentric muscle strengthening exercises have been shown to decrease the rate of hamstring injuries in studies that compare conventional and eccentric strengthening exercises (30–34).
- The gradual return to training activity should be considered when the athlete is able to stretch the injured muscle as far as the contralateral muscle and denies pain with basic movements (35). One prospective randomized study on hamstring strains highlighted that exercises of progressive agility and trunk stabilization resulted in fewer reinjuries and accelerated the return to practice of the athlete when compared to a stretch and strength protocol (36).

Muscle Stretching and Warm-Up

- Muscle is viscoelastic material, and passive stretching can reduce stress for a given muscle length (37). In addition, preconditioned muscle and warm muscle fail at higher loads than control muscle (38). Earlier literature stated that a warm-up and stretching protocol implemented within the 15 minutes prior to starting physical activity results in better performance scores and fewer muscle injuries (39).
- A number of subsequent systematic reviews, however, questioned this conclusion, showing that an intense period of stretching prior to exercise does not decrease muscle injuries. However, there have been reviews demonstrating the beneficial effect of strength, balance, and psychological programs (40).
- A clinical study at the U.S. Military Academy examined the effects of dynamic warm-up versus a static stretching warm-up in running performance, underhand medicine ball throw for distance, and the five-step jump. The study concluded that dynamic warm-up enhanced the athlete's performance, whereas static stretching warm-up showed almost no effect and should be reassessed (41).

Delayed Muscle Soreness

- Delayed muscle soreness is defined as skeletal muscle pain 24–72 hours after unaccustomed physical activity. The pain lasts approximately 5–7 days and can range from mild soreness to severe discomfort (42). Loss of both muscle strength and joint range of motion, tenderness, and elevated muscle enzymes are also present.

- Strength loss can be explained by both the presence of pain and a decrease in the inherent force-producing capacity of the muscle fibers (42).
- Reduced range of motion and elevated levels of creatine kinase are common 1–2 days after the strenuous exercise; however, peak creatine kinase levels have not been shown to be correlated with the temporal aspects of pain or degree of tissue injury (43).
- No permanent muscle injury occurs, and complete muscle recovery is seen within 14 days. The adaptation to the unaccustomed exercise (*i.e.*, less soreness with successive bouts of the exercise) is rapid (44).
- Delayed muscle soreness occurs most commonly in fast-type muscle fibers when performing eccentric activity and is related to both the intensity and duration of activity.
- The symptoms of delayed muscle soreness can coincide with the signs of exertional rhabdomyolysis. Given the severity of exertional rhabdomyolysis, this condition is covered thoroughly in Chapter 40.

Pathophysiology

- High tension over a small cross-sectional area (seen in eccentric muscular contraction) results in cytoskeletal disruption.
- Sarcolemma (cell membrane) and other myofibrillar disruption results in an influx of intracellular Ca^{2+} that induces proteolytic enzyme-mediated myoprotein degradation (42,43,45).
- Cellular damage results in the activation of the inflammatory process. This stimulates nociceptors within the muscle, resulting in the production of pain (42,43).

Treatment and Prevention

- A recent meta-analysis determined several modalities that are effective in decreasing pain related to delayed muscle soreness, including massage, active exercises, compression, cryotherapy, phototherapy, contrast baths, vibration, and ultrasound. The authors suggest the primary driver to be changes in blood flow that evacuate inflammatory mediators and vasoconstriction to limit local edema (40). In the case of active exercise, other authors credit the therapeutic effect to production of endorphins, a stronger cytoskeleton, or alterations in neural pathways (42).
- There is still continued muscle tissue damage following therapeutic intervention, but to a progressively lesser extent. Perceptual discomfort associated with this tissue damage, however, is greatly diminished.
- NSAIDs demonstrate similar effects in an exercise-induced muscle injury model as they do in other muscle injury models. There is early benefit to the muscle by limiting inflammation, but the later negative effects on maximum muscle function discussed earlier persist (46).

Muscle Contusion Injury

- Muscle contusions are common injuries in collision and contact sports. These soft-tissue injuries are frequently caused by impact with a blunt, nonpenetrating object. In most cases, contusions involve the lower extremity muscle groups such as the quadriceps, gastrocnemius, or anterior muscles of the leg (6).
- The initial clinical presentation includes pain, swelling, loss of joint range of motion, and the possibility of a palpable muscle defect. This can be followed by persistent swelling and warmth, a firm mass, and continued loss of motion.
- Animal studies of muscle contusion injury demonstrate muscle fiber rupture, resulting in hematoma formation, edema, and inflammation (47).

Reparative Response

- The process of muscle contusion healing is similar to the general process of muscle healing, involving a combination of the formation of scar tissue by fibroblasts and the regeneration of normal muscle by migrating myoblasts (10). There appears to be less scar formation from a contusion than with a muscle strain injury.

Diagnosis and Treatment

- RICE principle is usually the first treatment option for the athlete immediately after the injury.

Immobilization Versus Mobilization of Contused Muscle

- Brief immobilization (<5 days) leads to faster healing without further tissue damage, whereas prolonged immobilization results in muscle atrophy and delayed muscle activity (in a rat model) (31,48). In addition, early mobilization results in increased tensile stiffness of contused muscle and more rapid resolution of the contusion injury (49).
- Clinical studies from the U.S. Military Academy demonstrate that a brief period of immobilization (24–48 hours), with the involved muscle in a lengthened position, followed by mobilization results in earlier recovery than prolonged muscle immobilization (19,50).
- Ultrasound has been useful in distinguishing swelling and edema from hematoma formation. This helps when considering surgical evacuation of the hematoma and when electing a less aggressive approach using compression and early mobilization (51).

Pharmacologic Treatment

- Animal studies have demonstrated that both corticosteroids and NSAIDs cause a decrease in the early inflammatory response (52); however, there is delayed muscle regeneration and a decrease in the later tensile properties of the healed muscle. Although the clinical use of anabolic steroids and growth factors has not been approved, recent animal studies show these can produce beneficial effects in the healing of contused muscle (51).
- Myositis ossificans is a complication of concern from muscle contusion injury. In the West Point study, 9% of the contusion injuries developed myositis ossificans as a complication (19,51). The etiology of this abnormal bone formation is unclear, but this diagnosis is related to the

degree of muscle injury, the region injured (quadriceps and brachialis), and the number of times the muscle is subjected to trauma (51). Clinically, there is tenderness, swelling, loss of motion, persistent warmth, and a firm mass in the area of the bone formation. By 4 weeks, abnormal bone is evident on radiographs that resembles mature bone by 6 months (6). There are three forms of myositis ossificans: (a) a thin stalk of bone that connects the ossified muscle to the bone; (b) a broad-based ossification that has contact with the bone lying beneath; and (c) an ossification that originates entirely in the muscle and does not have connection with the underlying bone (51). Frequently, the calcium deposits are spontaneously reabsorbed after several months. Surgical resection, if necessary, should be delayed until the osteoblast activity has ceased (6 months–1 year) and there is no evidence of increased tracer uptake on a bone scan.

Muscle Cramps

- Muscle cramps affect both athletes and nonathletes. The gastrocnemius, hamstrings, and quadriceps muscles are most commonly involved, but cramping can involve nearly any muscle group. Cramps begin with the muscle in a shortened position.
- The development of muscle cramps usually starts with a twitching of the muscle due to skeletal muscle fatigue ("cramp-prone state"), followed by spasmodic spontaneous contractions and pain. Electrical evidence suggests that the source of the abnormal activity originates from the nerve within the muscle (6). Relief from cramping and pain is achieved with complete cessation of the activity.
- The etiology of muscle cramping is unclear. Historically, muscle cramps were thought to be associated with systemic electrolyte abnormalities (hyponatremia, hypokalemia, hypocalcemia, and hypomagnesemia), hydration status, metabolic abnormalities, and environmental factors (53).
- Passive stretching is the most reliable immediate treatment to alleviate the cramped muscle group. Fluids and sodium replacement are still considered, but their use is controversial, and the effect is equivocal (53).
- A comprehensive and detailed assessment, including endocrine disorders, is needed for athletes who suffer from frequent cramps.

Muscle Laceration

- Muscle laceration is seen more often in trauma than sports. When a muscle is completely lacerated, 50% of its strength and 80% of its ability to shorten can be expected to be lost (11).
- In a murine model, immediate suturing of the fascia of the lacerated muscle has been shown to favor healing and to suppress the formation of deep scars, whereas with immobilization, the regeneration time of the injured muscle was longer and the scar was considerably larger (9).

TENDON INJURY REPAIR

- Tendon injuries are secondary to direct trauma (lacerations) or tensile overload.
- Tensile overload injuries are very common athletic injuries and can occur acutely or as a result of chronic overload.
- Acute tendon overload usually results in injury to the musculotendinous junction or a bony avulsion as tendons can withstand high tensile loads. A normal tendon does not rupture midsubstance.
- Chronic tendon overload is a common overuse injury and will be the focus of this section.

Anatomy and Physiology

- Tendons consist primarily of type I collagen fibrils, a proteoglycan matrix, and relatively few fibroblasts. A fibroblast is a contractile cell that produces procollagen that is secreted to the extracellular compartment as a soluble tropocollagen molecule, which after noncovalent cross-links results in insoluble collagen. The aggregation of this molecule forms collagen fibrils.
  - Type I collagen consists of two α-1 polypeptide chains and one α-2 chain that are organized into a triple helix stabilized by hydrogen and covalent bonds (54).
  - The collagen triple-helix molecules are aligned in quarter-staggered arrangement to make up the collagen microfibril. This alignment of oppositely charged amino acids contributes to a tendon's strength.
  - The microfibrils are then arranged in a parallel, well-ordered, and densely packed fashion. This organization also contributes to the tendon's tensile strength. The microfibrils are combined with a proteoglycan and water matrix to form collagen fascicles. The tendon consists of groupings of these fascicles surrounded by connective tissue that contains blood vessels, nerves, and lymphatics (54). Tendons receive blood through the surrounding tissues, which reaches the cells through the paratenon, mesotenon, or vincula. The nervous supply is picked up through mechanoreceptors located near the musculotendinous junction.
- The insertion of tendons onto bone is usually via four zones: tendon, fibrocartilage, mineralized fibrocartilage, and bone.
- Tendons that bend at acute angles (*e.g.*, flexor tendons in the hands) are enclosed in a distinct sheath that acts as a pulley (54). Synovial fluid within the sheath assists in tendon gliding. Tendons that are not enclosed in a sheath (*e.g.*, Achilles tendon) are covered by a paratenon.
- Mechanical forces affect the characteristics of the tendon. Tendons subjected to tensile loads have smaller densely packed collagen fibrils, increased collagen synthesis, smaller proteoglycan (decorin), and a higher collagen-to-proteoglycan ratio. Tendons sustaining compressive loads exhibit increased proteoglycan molecules and larger less dense collagen fibrils (55).

- Aging also affects the material characteristics of tendon. The decreased collagen synthesis, increased collagen fibril diameter, decreased proteoglycan content, decreased water content, and decreased vascularity of the aging tendon leads to a stiffer and weaker tendon (55).

Chronic Tensile Overload Injuries

Terminology

- There has been significant confusion regarding the terminology of chronic tendon injuries. Tendinitis (or tendonitis) and tendinosis are frequently used terms to describe the clinical picture of pain, swelling, and stiffness in a tendon but there is infrequent consensus on their meaning (56).
- The following terminology are proposed based on corroborating literature (57,58).
  - Tendinopathy: Persistent tendon pain and loss of function related to mechanical loading.
  - Tendon Tear: Macroscopic discontinuity of a load-bearing tendon.
  - Tendinitis/Tendonitis: Inflammation of the mid-substance of the tendon.
  - Paratenonitis: Inflammation of the paratenon or tendon sheath. Peritendinitis and tenosynovitis are included in this category.

Etiology

- The etiology of chronic tendon injuries is multifactorial and involves a combination of intrinsic and extrinsic factors.
- Important intrinsic factors include *anatomic abnormalities* (*e.g.*, malalignment, muscle weakness/imbalance, decreased flexibility, and joint laxity), age, gender, weight, and predisposing diseases (59–61).
- Important extrinsic factors include excessive mechanical load (frequency, duration, and intensity), training, errors (overtraining, rapid progression, fatigue, running surface, and poor technique), and equipment problems (footwear, racquets, and seat height) (59–61).
- There are very few well-controlled studies that examine the etiologic factors involved in chronic tendon injuries.

Pathophysiology

- Repetitive load on a tendon that results in 4%–8% strain causes microscopic tendon fiber damage. Continued load on the tendon at this level overwhelms the tendon's ability for repair. Damage occurs to the collagen fibrils, the noncollagenous matrix, and microvasculature (55).
- Multiple models for tendon pathology have been proposed that include mechanisms related to cellular response, collagen disruption, and inflammation (62). Important factors include tissue hypoxia, free radical–induced tendon damage, and tissue hyperthermia (61). Evidence shows that tendon overuse results in matrix metalloproteinase production, tendon cell apoptosis, chondroid metaplasia of the tendon, and release of protective factors such as insulin-like growth factor 1 and nitric oxide synthetase (15,63).
- A progressive link between initial inflammation of the enveloping tissue and tendon degeneration is unclear. Chronic paratenonitis can result in tendon degeneration in an animal model (64); however, a large clinical study showed no previous evidence of paratenonitis in over 60% of patients who sustained an Achilles tendon rupture (65). The initial paratenonitis may be a causative factor for tendon degeneration or it may coexist independently.
- Intrinsic tendon damage may occur with continued tendon overload. Tendon degeneration may appear as a number of histologic entities (*e.g.*, hypoxic degeneration, mucoid degeneration, fiber calcification) (61). The paratenon becomes thickened as fibroblast proliferation and fibrotic adhesions develop. This results in decreased tendon gliding and snapping.

Diagnosis

- The history often reveals repetitive mechanical overload. The athlete will usually be involved in either an endurance sport (*e.g.*, running, cycling, or swimming) or a sport that requires repetition of a specialized skill (*e.g.*, tennis, basketball, or baseball) (66). The athlete frequently will describe an increase in the duration, frequency, or intensity of the training regimen. The pain may be worse after a period of rest following the training period. Changes in footwear, equipment, or training surface may be present.
- The physical examination may reveal swelling or crepitation along the tendon sheath. The degenerative tendon may be tender to palpation or painful with compression (impingement signs). Range of motion may be restricted (60).
- Diagnostic tests include radiographs to exclude stress fractures or osteoarthritis. Ultrasound or magnetic resonance imaging can be useful in tendons that are not easily palpated (*e.g.*, the rotator cuff).

Treatment

- Removing or modifying the mechanical overload (relative rest) is the most important component in the treatment of chronic tendon injuries. Training errors and equipment problems should also be corrected.
- Prolonged immobilization should be avoided. Immobilization results in deceased tendon strength and stiffness due to proteolytic degradation of collagen (55).
- Physical therapy is often prescribed for chronic tendon disorders with a slow and progressive loading program as the primary evidence-based recommendation (56,62,67). An umbrella review of systematic reviews also found moderate evidence that modalities including low-level laser therapy and shockwave therapy are beneficial (68).
- NSAIDs are frequently taken for chronic tendon disorders. A review stated that five of nine placebo-controlled studies demonstrated the efficacy of NSAIDs in the treatment of tendinopathy (60). There is no evidence that NSAIDs improve healing processes in tendon degeneration, and there is evidence in muscle injury that NSAIDs may actually be harmful to tissue healing (46). Short-term use of NSAIDs may be indicated to provide analgesia for the athlete.

- The use of corticosteroid injections in the treatment of tendinopathy is controversial. The rationale of using a local anti-inflammatory medication for a disease process that involves tissue degeneration is questionable. Corticosteroids may decrease inflammation in the paratenon, reduce adhesions between the tendon and the peritendinous tissue, or block nociceptors in the damaged tendon (69); however, efficacy data are limited and there are accompanying risks (60). Direct injections into the tendon substance should be avoided because they result in elevated tissue pressure and tissue damage. The use of corticosteroid injections around weight-bearing tendons, such as the Achilles tendon and patellar tendon, remains controversial. There have been case reports of tendon rupture, but there are no controlled studies, and the tendon rupture may have occurred without injection. It is difficult to make recommendations on the use of corticosteroid injections because of the paucity of scientific evidence regarding their use.
- Platelet-rich plasma (PRP) is the plasma portion of autologous blood with a concentration of platelets above the baseline. PRP contains a high concentration of growth factors that upregulate numerous modulators involved in muscle and tendon regeneration. It is thought that PRP interrupts macrophage proliferation and IL-1 production, which would prevent fibrous scar (70). Outcomes of PRP injections have been mixed with beneficial results demonstrated for patellar tendinopathy (71), lateral epicondylitis (72), and rotator cuff tears (73), but systematic reviews having demonstrated no benefit for chronic Achilles tendinopathy (74). Overall, although PRP remains a hopeful treatment option for some chronic tendon injuries, its efficacy compared to traditional treatment remains in question.
- The surgical treatment of chronic tendon injury is usually reserved for those cases that do not resolve within 4–6 months of nonsurgical treatment. The surgical procedures usually involve debridement of the degenerative tendon tissue. Occasionally, grafting or complete resection and repair is required (59). Occasionally, removal of the involved paratenon or release of the tendon sheath is necessary. Bony prominences, osteophytes, or deformities may require removal (*e.g.*, Haglund tuberosity, around the acromion). There are case series reported in the literature that demonstrate the success of surgical management, but there are very few controlled studies.

REFERENCES

1. Rebella G. A prospective study of injury patterns in collegiate pole vaulters. *Am J Sports Med.* 2015 Apr;43(4):808–15. doi:10.1177/0363546514564542
2. Baugh CM, Weintraub GS, Gregory AJ, Djoko A, Dompier TP, Kerr ZY. Descriptive epidemiology of injuries sustained in National Collegiate Athletic Association men's and women's Volleyball, 2013-2014 to 2014-2015. *Sports Health.* 2018 Jan/Feb;10(1):60–9. doi:10.1177/1941738117733685
3. Dakic JG, Smith B, Gosling CM, Perraton LG. Musculoskeletal injury profiles in professional Women's Tennis Association players. *Br J Sports Med.* 2018 Jun;52(11):723–9. doi:10.1136/bjsports-2017-097865
4. Toohey LA, Drew MK, Finch CF, Cook JL, Fortington LV. A 2-year prospective study of injury epidemiology in elite Australian rugby sevens: exploration of incidence rates, severity, injury type, and subsequent injury in men and women. *Am J Sports Med.* 2019 May;47(6):1302–11. doi:10.1177/0363546518825380
5. Zuckerman SL, Wegner AM, Roos KG, Djoko A, Dompier TP, Kerr ZY. Injuries sustained in National Collegiate Athletic Association men's and women's basketball, 2009/2010-2014/2015. *Br J Sports Med.* 2018 Feb;52(4):261–8. doi:10.1136/bjsports-2016-096005
6. Best TM. Soft-tissue injuries and muscle tears. *Clin Sports Med.* 1997;16(3):419–34.
7. Garrett WEJ, Best TM. Anatomy, physiology, and mechanics of skeletal muscle. In: Buckwalter JA, Einhorn TA, Sheldon S, editors. *Orthopaedic Basic Science.* Chicago (IL): American Academy of Orthopaedic Surgeons; 2000.
8. Ulibarri JA, Mozdziak PE, Schultz E, Cook C, Best TM. Nitric oxide donors, sodium nitroprusside and S-nitroso-N-acetylpencillamine, stimulate myoblast proliferation in vitro. *In Vitro Cell Dev Biol Anim.* 1999;35(4):215–8.
9. Huard J, Li Y, Fu FH. Muscle injuries and repair: current trends in research. *J Bone Joint Surg Am.* 2002;84(5):822–32.
10. Maffiuletti NA. Assessment of hip and knee muscle function in orthopaedic practice and research. *J Bone Joint Surg Am.* 2010;92(1):220–9.
11. Noonan TJ, Garrett WE Jr. Muscle strain injury: diagnosis and treatment. *J AM Acad Orthop Surg.* 1999;7(4):262–9.
12. Tidball JG. Inflammatory cell response to acute muscle injury. *Med Sci Sports Exerc.* 1995;27(7):1022–32.
13. Anderson JE. The satellite cell as a companion in skeletal muscle plasticity: currency, conveyance, clue, connector and colander. *J Exp Biol.* 2006;209(Pt 12):2276–92.
14. Sheehan SM, Tatsumi R, Temm-Grove CJ, Allen RE. HGF is an autocrine growth factor for skeletal muscle satellite cells in vitro. *Muscle Nerve.* 2000;23(2):239–45.
15. Lehto MU, Järvinen MJ. Muscle injuries, their healing process and treatment. *Ann Chir Gynaecol.* 1991;80(2):102–8.
16. Gates CB, Karthikeyan T, Fu FH, Huard J. Regenerative medicine for the musculoskeletal system based on muscle-derived stem cells. *J Am Acad Orthop Surg.* 2008;16(2):68–76.
17. Itro A, Trotta MC, Miranda R, et al. Why use adipose-derived mesenchymal stem cells in tendinopathic patients: a systematic review. *Pharmaceutics.* 2022 May 27;14(6):1151. doi:10.3390/pharmaceutics14061151
18. Armfield DR, Kim DH, Towers JD, Bradley JP, Robertson DD. Sports-related muscle injury in the lower extremity. *Clin Sports Med.* 2006;25(4):803–42.
19. Jackson DW, Feagin JA. Quadriceps contusions in young athletes. Relation of severity of injury to treatment and prognosis. *J Bone Joint Surg Am.* 1973;55(1):95–105.
20. Garrett WE Jr, Nikolaou PK, Ribbeck BM, Glisson RR, Seaber AV. The effect of muscle architecture on the biomechanical failure properties of skeletal muscle under passive extension. *Am J Sports Med.* 1988;16(1):7–12.
21. Järvinen TA, Järvinen TL, Kääriäinen M, et al. Muscle injuries: optimising recovery. *Best Pract Res Clin Rheumatol.* 2007;21(2):317–31.
22. Nikolaou PK, Macdonald BL, Glisson RR, Seaber AV, Garrett WE Jr. Biomechanical and histological evaluation of muscle after controlled strain injury. *Am J Sports Med.* 1987;15(1):9–14.
23. Obremsky WT, Seaber AV, Ribbeck BM, Garrett WE Jr. Biomechanical and histologic assessment of a controlled muscle strain injury treated with piroxicam. *Am J Sports Med.* 1994;22(4):558–61.

24. Taylor DC, Dalton JD Jr, Seaber AV, Garrett WE Jr. Experimental muscle strain injury. Early functional and structural deficits and the increased risk for reinjury. *Am J Sports Med.* 1993;21(2):190–4.
25. Rantanen J, Thorsson O, Wollmer P, Hurme T, Kalimo H. Effects of therapeutic ultrasound on the regeneration of skeletal myofibers after experimental muscle injury. *Am J Sports Med.* 1999;27(1):54–9.
26. Wilkin LD, Merrick MA, Kirby TE, Devor ST. Influence of therapeutic ultrasound on skeletal muscle regeneration following blunt contusion. *Int J Sports Med.* 2004;25(1):73–7.
27. Huang X, Wang R, Zhang Z, Wang G, Gao B. Effects of pre-post- and intra-exercise hyperbaric oxygen therapy on performance and recovery: a systematic review and meta-analysis. *Front Physiol.* 2021 Nov 23;12:791872. doi:10.3389/fphys.2021.791872
28. Hohenauer E, Taeymans J, Baeyens JP, Clarys P, Clijsen R. The effect of post-exercise cryotherapy on recovery characteristics: a systematic review and meta-analysis. *PLoS One.* 2015 Sep 28;10(9):e0139028. doi:10.1371/journal.pone.0139028
29. Schaser KD, Disch AC, Stover JF, Lauffer A, Bail HJ, Mittlmeier T. Prolonged superficial local cryotherapy attenuates microcirculatory impairment, regional inflammation, and muscle necrosis after closed soft tissue injury in rats. *Am J Sports Med.* 2007;35(1):93–102.
30. Arnason A, Andersen TE, Holme I, Engebretsen L, Bahr R. Prevention of hamstring strains in elite soccer: an intervention study. *Scand J Med Sci Sports.* 2008;18(1):40–8.
31. Lehto M, Duance VC, Restall D. Collagen and fibronectin in a healing skeletal muscle injury. An immunohistological study of the effects of physical activity on the repair of injured gastrocnemius muscle in the rat. *J Bone Joint Surg Br.* 1985 Nov;67(5):820–8.
32. Brooks JHM, Fuller CW, Kemp SPT, Reddin DB. Incidence, risk and prevention of hamstring muscle injuries in professional rugby union. *Am J Sports Med.* 2006;34(8):1297–306.
33. Croisier JL, Ganteaume S, Binet J, Genty M, Ferret JM. Strength imbalances and prevention of hamstring injury in professional soccer players: a prospective study. *Am J Sports Med.* 2008;36(8):1469–75.
34. van Dyk N, Behan FP, Whiteley R. Including the Nordic hamstring exercise in injury prevention programmes halves the rate of hamstring injuries: a systematic review and meta-analysis of 8459 athletes. *Br J Sports Med.* 2019 Nov;53(21):1362–70. doi:10.1136/bjsports-2018-100045
35. Petersen J, Hölmich P. Evidence based prevention of hamstring injuries in sport. *Br J Sports Med.* 2005;39(6):319–23.
36. Sherry MA, Best TM. A comparison of 2 rehabilitation programs in the treatment of acute hamstring strains. *J Orthop Sports Phys Ther.* 2004;34(3):116–25.
37. Taylor DC, Dalton JD Jr, Seaber AV, Garrett WE Jr. Viscoelastic properties of muscle-tendon units. The biomechanical effects of stretching. *Am J Sports Med.* 1990;18(3):300–9.
38. Safran MR, Garrett WE Jr, Seaber AV, Glisson RR, Ribbeck BM. The role of warmup in muscular injury prevention. *Am J Sports Med.* 1988;16(2):123–9.
39. Woods K, Bishop P, Jones E. Warm-up and stretching in the prevention of muscular injury. *Sports Med.* 2007;37(12):1089–99.
40. Nahon RL, Silva Lopes JS, Monteiro de Magalhães Neto A. Physical therapy interventions for the treatment of delayed onset muscle soreness (DOMS): systematic review and meta-analysis. *Phys Ther Sport.* 2021 Nov;52:1–12. doi:10.1016/j.ptsp.2021.07.005
41. McMillian DJ, Moore JH, Hatler BS, Taylor DC. Dynamic vs. static-stretching warm up: the effect on power and agility performance. *J Strength Condit Res.* 2006;20(3):492–9.
42. Armstrong RB. Mechanisms of exercise-induced delayed onset muscular soreness: a brief review. *Med Sci Sports Exerc.* 1984;16(6):529–38.
43. Lieber RL, Friden J. Morphologic and mechanical basis of delayed onset muscle soreness. *J Am Acad Orthop Surg.* 2002;10(1):67–73.
44. Balnave CD, Thompson MW. Effect of training on eccentric exercise-induced muscle damage. *J Appl Physiol.* 1993;75(4):1545–51.
45. Proske U, Morgan DL. Muscle damage from eccentric exercise: mechanism, mechanical signs, adaptation and clinical applications. *J Physiol.* 2001;537(Pt 2):333–45.
46. Mishra DK, Fridén J, Schmitz MC, Lieber RL. Anti-inflammatory medication after muscle injury. A treatment resulting in short-term improvement but subsequent loss of muscle function. *J Bone Joint Surg Am.* 1995;77(10):1510–9.
47. Walton M, Rothwell AG. Reactions of thigh tissues of sheep to blunt trauma. *Clin Orthop Relat Res.* 1983;176:273–81.
48. Järvinen M. Healing of a crush injury in rat striated muscle. Part 2. A histological study of the effect of early mobilization and immobilization on the repair processes. *Acta Pathol Microbiol Scand (A).* 1975;83(3):269–82.
49. Järvinen M. Healing of a crush injury in rat striated muscle. Part 4. Effect of early mobilization and immobilization on the tensile properties of gastrocnemius muscle. *Acta Chir Scand.* 1976;142(1):47–56.
50. Ryan JB, Wheeler JH, Hopkinson WJ, Arciero RA, Kolakowski KR. Quadriceps contusions. West Point update. *Am J Sports Med.* 1991;19(3):299–304.
51. Beiner JM, Jokl P. Muscle contusion injuries: current treatment options. *J Am Acad Orthop Surg.* 2001;9(4):227–37.
52. Beiner JM, Jokl P, Cholewicki J, Panjabi MM. The effect of anabolic steroids and corticosteroids on healing of muscle contusion injury. *Am J Sports Med.* 1999;27(1):2–9.
53. Schwellnus MP, Drew N, Collins M. Muscle cramping in athletes—risk factors, clinical assessment, and management. *Clin Sports Med.* 2008;27(1):183–94.
54. Wood SL, An KN, Frank CB, et al. Anatomy, biology, and biomechanics of tendon and ligament. In: Buckwalter JA, Einhorn TA, Sheldon S, editors. *Orthopaedic Basic Science.* Chicago (IL): American Academy of Orthopaedic Surgeons; 2000.
55. Hyman J, Rodeo SA. Injury and repair of tendons and ligaments. *Phys Med Rehabil Clin N Am.* 2000;11(2):267–88.
56. Everhart JS, Cole D, Sojka JH, et al. Treatment options for patellar tendinopathy: a systematic review. *Arthroscopy.* 2017 Apr;33(4):861–72.
57. Järvinen M, Józsa L, Kannus P, Järvinen TL, Kvist M, Leadbetter W. Histopathological findings in chronic tendon disorders. *Scand J Med Sci Sports.* 1997;7(2):86–95.
58. Scott A, Squier K, Alfredson H, et al. ICON 2019: international scientific tendinopathy symposium consensus—clinical terminology. *Br J Sports Med.* 2020 Mar;54(5):260–2. doi:10.1136/bjsports-2019-100885
59. Almekinders LC. Tendinitis and other chronic tendinopathies. *J Am Acad Orthop Surg.* 1998;6(3):157–64.
60. Almekinders LC, Temple JD. Etiology, diagnosis, and treatment of tendonitis: an analysis of the literature. *Med Sci Sports Exerc.* 1998;30(8):1183–90.
61. Kannus P. Etiology and pathophysiology of chronic tendon disorders in sports. *Scand J Med Sci Sports.* 1997;7(2):78–85.
62. Cardoso TB, Pizzari T, Kinsella R, Hope D, Cook JL. Current trends in tendinopathy management. *Best Pract Res Clin Rheumatol.* 2019 Feb;33(1):122–40. doi:10.1016/j.berh.2019.02.001
63. Jones GC, Corps AN, Pennington CJ, et al. Expression profiling of metalloproteinases and tissue inhibitors of metalloproteinases in normal and degenerate human Achilles tendon. *Arthritis Rheum.* 2006;54(3):832–42.
64. Backman C, Boquist L, Friden J, Lorentzon R, Toolanen G. Chronic Achilles paratenonitis with tendinosis: an experimental model in the rabbit. *J Orthop Res.* 1990;8(4):541–7.

65. Kannus P, Józsa L. Histopathological changes preceding spontaneous rupture of a tendon. A controlled study of 891 patients. *J Bone Joint Surg Am.* 1991;73(10):1507–25.
66. Hess GP, Cappiello WL, Poole RM, Hunter SC. Prevention and treatment of overuse tendon injuries. *Sports Med.* 1989;8(6):371–84.
67. van der Vlist AC, Winters M, Weir A, et al. Which treatment is most effective for patients with Achilles tendinopathy? A living systematic review with network meta-analysis of 29 randomised controlled trials. *Br J Sports Med.* 2021 Mar;55(5):249–56. doi:10.1136/bjsports-2019-101872
68. Girgis B, Duarte JA. Physical therapy for tendinopathy: an umbrella review of systematic reviews and meta-analyses. *Phys Ther Sport.* 2020 Nov;46:30–46. doi:10.1016/j.ptsp.2020.08.002
69. Paavola M, Kannus P, Järvinen TA, Järvinen TL, Józsa L, Järvinen M. Treatment of tendon disorders. Is there a role for corticosteroids injection? *Foot Ankle Clin.* 2002;7(3):501–13.
70. Woodall JJr, Tucci M, Mishra A, Asfour A, Benghuzzi H. Cellular effects of platelet rich plasmainterleukin1 release from prp treated macrophages. *Biomed Sci Instrum.* 2008;44:489–94.
71. Filardo G, Di Matteo B, Kon E, Merli G, Marcacci M. Platelet-rich plasma in tendon-related disorders: results and indications. *Knee Surg Sports Traumatol Arthrosc.* 2018 Jul;26(7):1984–99. doi:10.1007/s00167-016-4261-4
72. Peerbooms JC, Sluimer J, Bruijn DJ, Gosens T. Positive effect of an autologous platelet concentrate in lateral epicondylitis in a double-blind randomized controlled trial: platelet-rich plasma versus corticosteroid injection with a 1-year follow-up. *Am J Sports Med.* 2010;38(2):255–62.
73. Chen X, Jones IA, Togashi R, Park C, Vangsness CT Jr. Use of platelet-rich plasma for the improvement of pain and function in rotator cuff tears: a systematic review and meta-analysis with Bias assessment. *Am J Sports Med.* 2020 Jul;48(8):2028–41. doi:10.1177/0363546519881423
74. Nauwelaers AK, Van Oost L, Peers K. Evidence for the use of PRP in chronic midsubstance Achilles tendinopathy: a systematic review with meta-analysis. *Foot Ankle Surg.* 2021 Jul;27(5):486–95. doi:10.1016/j.fas.2020.07.009

11 Basic Principles of Exercise Training and Conditioning

Kevin R. Vincent and Heather K. Vincent

INTRODUCTION

- Participation in exercise and physical activity are critical components of healthful living, disease prevention, and reduced all-cause mortality. Moderate-intensity physical activity is related to numerous health benefits, including muscle strength, endurance and power, bone and joint health, increased circulatory capacity, brain functioning, and improvements in metabolism and body composition. Regular exercise induces neuromotor benefits, reduces stress, manages pain, and improves quality of life (1–5).
- The Centers for Disease Control and Prevention (CDC) and the American College of Sports Medicine (ACSM) recommend that every U.S. adult accumulate 30 minutes or more of moderate-intensity physical activity on most — and preferably all — days of the week (1,6). Those who follow these recommendations will experience many of the health-related benefits of physical activity, and if they are interested in achieving higher levels of fitness, will be ready to do so (6). Recommendations also include participation in aerobic, strengthening, flexibility, and neuromotor components of activity and exercise (6).
- This chapter integrates and complements Chapters 6 (Exercise Physiology), 12 (Nutrition), and 13 (Exercise Prescription), by specifically identifying appropriate principles for effective training to achieve the aforementioned fitness goals.

EXERCISE PRESCRIPTION AND TRAINING PROGRAM

Recommendations for Cardiorespiratory Endurance Training

- Chapter 13 details current guidelines from the ACSM; this chapter elaborates on those recommendations and outlines the integration of these guidelines into a sequenced exercise program.

Mode

- The greatest improvements in cardiorespiratory endurance occur when large muscle groups are engaged in rhythmic aerobic activity.
- Variety facilitates enjoyment and motivation, and enhances adherence (7).
- Examples of activities include walking, running, cycling, rowing, stair climbing, aerobic dance (aerobics), water exercise, and cross-country skiing (6,8).

Intensity

- ACSM defines exercise intensities for both moderate and vigorous exercise using multiple methods including heart rate reserve (HRR), HR_{max}, VO_{2max}, and the rating of perceived exertion (RPE) scale (*e.g.*, moderate 40%–59% HRR/64%–76% HR_{max}/46%–63% VO_{2max}/12–13 RPE), and vigorous (60%–89% HRR/77%–95% HR_{max}/64%–90% VO_{2max}/RPE 14–17). Although ACSM recognizes the dose response with increasing intensity, intensity must be uniquely selected based on the individual's baseline fitness and risk factors (6).
  1. Because there is variability with the HR_{max} from age, the use of an actual HR from a graded exercise test can improve the accuracy of HR targets.
  2. Lower intensities (40%–50% of VO_{2max}) elicit a favorable response in low-fit individuals, inpatient populations, and individuals with musculoskeletal pain.
- **Calculating intensity:** The most common methods of setting the intensity of exercise to improve or maintain cardiorespiratory fitness use HR and RPE (see Table 11.1).
- **Heart rate methods:** HR is used as a guide to set exercise intensity because of the relatively linear relationship between HR and *percentage of VO_{2max}* (%VO_{2max}). It is best to measure HR_{max} during a progressive exercise test whenever possible as HR_{max} declines with age. HR_{max} can be estimated by using the following equation: (HR_{max} = 220 − age).
- **HR_{max} method:** Using 70%–85% of an individual's HR_{max} approximates 55%–75% VO_{2max}. Example: If HR_{max} = 180 bpm then target HR (70%–85% HR_{max}) would range 126–152 bpm. Given that there is variance around the HR of ±15 beats · min^{-1}, the target HR should be calculated 10%–15% higher than VO_2 max (8).
- **HRR method:** The HRR method is also known as the Karvonen method. Target HR range = $[(HR_{max} - HR_{rest}) \times 0.60 \text{ and } 0.85] + HR_{rest}$. Using the HR method allows a more direct correlation between HR and % VO_2 max and accounts for the resting HR (9).

Table 11.1 Oxygen Consumption, Heart Rate, Perceived Effort, MET Level Ranges, and Blood Lactate Accumulation at Progressive Aerobic Exercise Intensities

	Low Intensity	Moderate Intensity	Vigorous Intensity
VO_2 reserve (%)	30–39	40–59	≥60
HR reserve (%)	30–39	40–59	≥60
METs (#)	2–2.9	3–5.9	≥6
RPE (points)	9–11	12–13	≥14
Blood lactate accumulation	No	Yes	Yes

HR, heart rate; MET, multiples of resting VO_2 (3.5 mL · kg^{-1} · min^{-1}); RPE, rating of perceived exertion, Borg 6- to 20-point scale; VO_2, rate of oxygen consumption.

- **RPE:** The use of the RPE scale to guide exercise intensity is common across research, training, and clinical settings. RPE may be used with HR for regulating intensity, or alone if HR monitoring is not available. The RPE scales can be used to track exercise intensity and muscle fatigue during the session. One of two scales can be used: a 6- to 20-point scale (6 = no exertion, 20 = maximal exertion) and 0–10 (0 = no exertion, 10 = maximal exertion).
  - For aerobic exercise, the onset of blood lactate generally occurs between 12 and 16 on the 6- to 20-point category scale, and between 4 and 5 on the 0- to 10-point category-ratio scale (9).
  - RPE is considered a reliable indicator of exercise intensity and is particularly useful when a participant is unable to monitor their pulse or when HR response to exercise has been altered by medications such as β-blockers (6,8).
- The average RPE range associated with physiologic adaptation to exercise is 12–16 ("somewhat hard" to "hard") on the Borg category scale, or moderate to vigorous intensity. One should suit the RPE to the individual on a specific mode of exercise and not expect an exact matching of the RPE to a $\%HR_{max}$ or %HRR. It should be used only as a guideline in setting the exercise intensity.

Duration

- The ACSM recommends 30–60 minutes of continuous activity per session for fitness, and an accumulation of >30 minutes of activity per day for general health (9).
- Daily duration may be modified based on the intensity of accumulated activity:
  - Participation in 75 minutes of weekly vigorous aerobic activity produces similar health benefits as 150 minutes of moderate intensity activity, or an equivalent mix of vigorous and moderate activity at least 3 days a week (1).
- Individuals with chronic pain, joint disease, severe deconditioning or late-stage pregnancy may benefit from multiple, short-duration exercise sessions <10 minutes with frequent interspersed rest periods to accumulate the duration for health benefits.

Frequency

- The CDC and ACSM recommend that aerobic exercise be performed 3–5 d · wk^{-1} for fitness, and physical activity be performed on most if not all days per week for general health (1,9).

Recommendations for Resistance Training

- Overload and specificity are precepts of resistance training.
- **Overload** occurs when a greater than normal physical demand is placed on muscles or muscle groups. Strength and endurance are developed by increasing the resistance load, the frequency, or the duration of activity to levels above those normally experienced.
- A training intensity of approximately 40%–60% of one repetition maximum (1RM) appears sufficient to develop muscle strength (6) in most normally active individuals (6,8). Lift intensity can be increased to near maximal if the goal is to increase muscle strength (9).
- **Specificity** relates to the structural and functional, systemic and local changes that occur as a result of training. These adaptations occur only in the overloaded muscle groups or muscles (6).
- **Unilateral and Bilateral Strengthening:** Bilateral contractions induce less muscle individual limb activation than unilateral contractions, with greater cross activation at the motor cortex occurring at higher force output (10). Unilateral resistance exercise induces bilateral training effects in the unexercised limb ("cross-transfer"), which has health benefits even among challenging conditions such as degenerative joint disease (11) and stroke (12).
- **Concurrent Endurance and Resistance Exercise:** Combined endurance and resistance exercise programs can effectively increase muscle strength, power, and cardiorespiratory endurance than each exercise type alone, and may help maintain/improve functional capacity over the long term (13).

ACSM Guidelines for Resistance Training

- A 5–10-minutes warm-up period with aerobic activity (treadmill walking, stationary cycling) or a light set (50%–75% of training weight) of the specific resistance exercise should precede the resistance exercise session (6,8).

- Exercising with a partner enhances program success.

- **Mode:** At least 8–10 separate single and multijoint exercises that target major muscle groups (arms, shoulder, chest, abdomen, back, hips, and legs) is important for general strengthening. Exercises may be performed using free weights, weight machines, resistance bands, and electronic devices. Choose different exercises for each training day.
- **Intensity/Duration:** For strength gains in healthy adults, perform 2–4 sets of 8–12 repetitions, with a resistance that results in volitional fatigue. About 2–3 minutes of rest is recommended between sets. For developing muscular endurance and for those who are older or very deconditioned, ≥1 set of 10–15 repetitions is recommended.
    - High numbers of weekly sets of multijoint and single joint exercises produces greater gains in strength than low numbers of weekly sets (14).
    - Higher resistance loads (>75% of 1RM) produce greater strength effects than moderate intensity (55%–75% 1RM) or low intensities (>55% 1RM). Explosive resistance movements performed quickly at 40%–60% 1RM increase muscle power and strength, an important benefit for older adults (15) at risk for mobility limitation and falls.
- **Frequency:** These exercises should be performed 2–3 $d \cdot wk^{-1}$, with a rest day in between. Exercises may also be alternated between upper and lower intensities over consecutive days.
- **Progression:** Progressive overload can be accomplished by increasing the resistance, the repetitions for the current load, decreasing the rest period or increasing the rest period with high loads (for strength and power development) (8).
- Progression can occur when the target repetition number is completed with good technique and moderate effort (RPE < 15).
- **Safety considerations:**
    - Exercise should be performed in a controlled manner through a full range of motion using proper technique during both concentric and eccentric phases.
    - Maintain a normal breathing pattern and avoid breath-holding (*Valsalva maneuver*).
    - The Council on Sports Medicine and Physical Fitness and American Academy of Pediatrics (AAP) indicate that children can safely participate in resistance exercise using sets of 8–15 repetitions, 20–30 minutes, for 1–3 sets using both open and closed chain exercises 2–3 times a week. Volume may progress over time, to higher intensities (>80% of maximum) and lower repetition ranges if the skill competency is high (16) (see Chapter 128, The Pediatric Athlete, for further discussion).
    - Further specific considerations with weight training are discussed in Chapter 126, Weight Lifting.

Recommendations for Flexibility Training

- Static stretching involves slowly stretching a muscle to the point of mild discomfort and then holding that position usually 10–30 seconds. It can be active (*e.g.*, as with yoga) or passive (*e.g.*, using elastic bands or barre).
- Proprioceptive neuromuscular facilitation (PNF) involves isometric muscle contraction followed by a static stretch of the same muscle/tendon group. A 6-second contraction followed by a static stretch of 10–30 seconds repeated 3–4 times is a sample exercise.
- Stretching is more effective after a light dynamic warm-up or after an exercise session, and stretching preresistance exercise may actually decrease force producing ability of muscle (9).

ACSM Recommendations for Flexibility Training

- A stretching routine should use a variety of exercises for the major muscle and/or tendon groups.
- Stretching should be performed ≥2–3 $d \cdot wk^{-1}$ (9), accumulating 60 seconds stretching about each joint per session.
- In older individuals, each stretch duration may need to increase up to 60 seconds (6).
- Progression should target a goal of performing stretches up to 5–7 days a week and hold for 30–90 seconds for each stretch (9).

GENERAL COMPONENTS OF AN EXERCISE PROGRAM

- Each session of a comprehensive exercise conditioning program should contain:
    - **Warm-up** (10 minutes): Warm-up phase facilitates the transition from rest to exercise, stretches postural muscles, augments blood flow, and increases the metabolic rate from the resting level (1 MET) to the aerobic requirements for endurance training.
    - **Conditioning** (20–60 minutes): Aerobic conditioning commonly includes 20–60 minutes of continuous or intermittent activity (or minimum of 10-minutes bouts accumulated throughout the day).
    - **Cool-down** (5–10 minutes): A period of gradual recovery from the endurance phase and includes exercises of diminishing intensities. It permits appropriate circulatory adjustments and return of the HR and BP to near resting values (2,17).

Rate of Progression

- The recommended progression rate depends on functional capacity, medical and health status, age, individual activity preferences and goals, and an individual's tolerance to the current level of training. The exercise prescription has three stages of progression: initiation, improvement, and maintenance (6,8).

Initiation

- Initiation includes light muscular strengthening exercises and moderate-level aerobic activities and exercises that are compatible with minimal muscle soreness, discomfort, and injury. If applicable, disease symptoms should be monitored during the exercise.
- Exercise session duration depends on the starting point of the individual (healthy adults 15–20 minutes, fit adults 20–30 minutes, older, obese, very sedentary adults 10–20 minutes). The content of the sessions can be modified to account for symptoms. For example, increased stretching time or warm-up time can occur to minimize pain or breathing discomfort in individuals with osteoarthritis or pulmonary disease, respectively.
- It is recommended that individuals who are starting a moderate-intensity conditioning program should exercise 3–4 times · wk^{-1} (6,8).
- Focus on proper form, technique, and perceptual responses.

Improvement and Progression

- Gradual increases in exercise intensity and volume occur here to allow safe physiological improvements in cardiorespiratory fitness, musculoskeletal adaptation and circulatory capacity to occur (termed **progressive overload**). This process typically lasts 2–5 months.
- About 10%–30% increases in aerobic capacity typically occur following these guidelines.
- Progression that occurs too quickly contributes to musculoskeletal injury, loss of interest and motivation, and discontinuation of training.

Maintenance

- During maintenance, fitness is sustained over the long term. Once preestablished fitness goals are achieved, performing the same workout routine enables individuals to maintain their fitness (8).
- For general health, it is recommended that the weekly caloric expenditure should exceed 1000 kcal.
- **Cross training** adds variety to the program. Adaptations achieved by one mode may be maintained with the substitution of other modes. For example, replacing a session of running with cycling or swimming at similar relative intensities can maintain the cardiorespiratory status and reduce the risk of fatigue and overuse of body parts used in the typical exercise plan (8).

Concept of Periodization

- **Periodization:** Planned sequencing of increased training loads and recovery periods within a training program, which facilitates peak performance compared to nonperiodized programs, especially among trained individuals (18).
- Periodization consists of a series of microcycles, mesocycles, and macrocycles designed to keep proving new stimuli for persistent training adaptations (18).
  - Microcyle: several sessions separated by recovery days, lasting 1–2 weeks.
  - Mesocycle: two or more microcycles last 3–6 weeks. A mesocycle emphasizes one aspect of training such as endurance or speed. A number of mesocycles, arranged to produce physiologic adaptation, are known as a phase.
  - Macrocycle: three to four mesocycles comprise a macrocycle. Each macrocycle contains a preparatory phase, a first transition period, a competition phase, and finally a second transition period.
  - The periods or phases balance volume, intensity, and sports-specific training. The preparatory phase concentrates on volume and endurance with lower intensities, progressing ultimately through the first transition phase with more emphasis on sports specificity, moderate volume, and intensity, to the competition phase where volume is significantly decreased, and there is a concentration on sports-specific high-intensity exercise.
  - The final phase of a macrocycle is the second transition period or phase that allows for restoration/recovery. This phase should allow for complete recovery from the physiologic and psychological elements of training and competition.

Mind-Body Exercise

- Additional exercise forms that involve mind and body, balance, muscle strengthening, and stretch include yoga, T'ai Chi, and Qigong. These modes can be performed daily and are low impact.
- Yoga provides benefits on cardiovascular disease risk factors (body mass index, blood pressures, lipid profiles, and HbA_1c) and mental well-being additional to physical conditioning (17,19).
- T'ai Chi and Qigong provide significant positive adaptations to physical function (aerobic capacity, strength, balance, mobility, speed), cognitive ability, neuroplasticity, and mental clarity among older adults (20).
- These techniques may improve physical and mental health through down-regulation of the hypothalamic-pituitary-adrenal axis and the sympathetic nervous system, cerebral blood flow, and increased levels of brain-derived neurotrophic factor (BDNF) (20).

Rest Periods During Training

- The likelihood of injury increases and performance may decline with excessive volume (or overload) (21). Irrespective of age, rest is a necessary part of exercise programming. Varying the intensity of exercise sessions throughout the week and including 1–2 days of rest can improve performance and reduce injury risk, including overtraining syndrome.

Detraining

- The changes induced by regular exercise training generally are lost after 4–8 weeks of detraining. If training is reestablished, the rate at which the training effects occur do not appear to be faster.
- Overtraining syndrome (OTS) involves high-intensity, prolonged training that stimulates subclinical immunological changes and autonomic disturbances (sympathetic/parasympathetic) that may lower systemic resilience and increase the risk of illness in active people (21,22). Diagnosis is challenging due to variation in presentation, the complex systemic nature of the condition and biomarkers collected (23) (see Chapter 45, Overtraining Syndrome/Chronic Fatigue).
- Symptoms are highly variable and may include decline in exercise performance, extreme fatigue, immunological changes, elevated HR_{rest}, early onset of blood lactate accumulation, altered mood states, insomnia, and injuries related to overuse (21,23).
- Overtraining may require weeks to months of complete rest to recover.
- Although definitive treatment of OTS is not yet clear (22), the following may be useful: 1 week of complete rest, followed by limited weekly training of one to three sessions (10–20 minutes of easy pace); progress to longer sessions over a 6- to 12-week period.
- Daily monitoring of exercise training volume, mood state, and well-being may assist the individual with moderating the return to full performance.

MEDICAL CLEARANCE AND EXERCISE TESTING

- Exercise testing is not routinely recommended as part of medical clearance and the decision to pursue testing is at the clinical judgment of the healthcare provider. Details and an algorithm that includes symptoms and known presence of preexisting cardiovascular, metabolic or renal disease are provided in Chapter 24 (24).
- Based on the preparticipation results and algorithm, a tailored physical activity program can be designed using prescriptive guidelines (see Chapters 18, Preparticipation Examination, and 31, Cardiology, for further discussion).

TRAINING EFFECTS OF AEROBIC EXERCISE

Cardiovascular System

Changes at Rest

- HR decreases likely secondary to decreased sympathetic tone, increased parasympathetic tone, and a decreased intrinsic firing rate of the sinoatrial node.
- Stroke Volume (SV) increases secondary to increased myocardial contractility and increased heart size.
- Cardiac output is unchanged.
- Rate of oxygen consumption is unchanged.
- Total blood volume increases, due to an increased number of red blood cells and expansion of the plasma volume.

Adaptations During Submaximal Work

- At a submaximal, steady state workload, a stable rate of oxygen use is achieved.
  - HR is lower at any given workload due to the increased SV, decreased sympathetic drive, and improved metabolic and aerobic capacity of skeletal muscle.
  - SV increases due to increased myocardial contractility.
  - Cardiac output does not change significantly for a fixed workload; however, the same cardiac output is generated with a lower HR and higher SV.
  - The rate of oxygen consumption does not change significantly as oxygen requirement is similar for a fixed workload.
  - Arteriovenous oxygen difference (AVO_2 Diff) increases during submaximal work.
  - Lactate levels are decreased due to metabolic efficiency and increased lactate clearance rates.
  - Vascular reactivity improves for dilation during exercise (25).

Adaptations at Maximal Work

- *Maximal heart rate* (HR_{max}) does not change with exercise training.
- SV increases due to increased contractility and/or increased heart size, and this contributes to increased maximal cardiac output.
- Maximal rate of oxygen consumption (VO_{2max}) increases due to increased cardiac output, SV and a-VO_2 Diff.
- AVO_2 Diff. is improved due to mitochondrial proliferation and increased mitochondrial function (26).

Blood Pressure

- In normotensive individuals, regular exercise may reduce resting and exercise blood pressure by 3–4 mm Hg.
- Hypertensive individuals demonstrate a more marked reduction in resting blood pressure as a result of regular exercise.

Blood Lipids

- Total cholesterol may be decreased in individuals with hypercholesterolemia.
- *High-density lipoprotein cholesterol* (HDL) levels increase with exercise training (25).
- *Low-density lipoprotein cholesterol* (LDL) may remain the same or decrease with regular exercise.
- Triglycerides levels may decrease (25), and this change is facilitated by weight loss.

Body Composition

- Total body mass usually decreases with regular exercise, the magnitude of which is directly dependent on the weekly exercise volume and caloric expenditure.
- Fat-free mass may increase or decrease, depending on the exercise mode, volume, and amount of body mass lost.
- Percent body fat is generally reduced, with more fat loss with greater volumes of exercise.

Skeletal Muscle Adaptations

- Skeletal muscle glycogen and triglycerides levels increase.
- Aerobic exercise increases the number of type I fibers and reduces type II fibers, with small changes in cross-sectional area.
- The level of type I myosin heavy chain content increases, whereas the content of type IIa and IId/x decrease after aerobic training.

Nervous System Adaptations

- Exercise training may induce brain neuroplasticity, improve cognition, and memory, and reduce neuroinflammation (27).
- Exercise can improve psychological health and resilience (depression, anxiety, stress) (5,27).

Anti Inflammatory Adaptations

- Regular aerobic exercise can increase the production and release of anti-inflammatory cytokines and decrease the production of inflammatory cytokines and proteins such as C-reactive protein.
- Exercise can reduce the number of circulating proinflammatory monocytes, and can inhibit monocyte and macrophage infiltration into adipose tissue.

Adaptations to Resistance Exercise

- Numerous health adaptations occur irrespective of age and presence of comorbid illness; muscle strength gains can be very large; bone density may increase, especially in the hip, lumbar spine, and lower extremities.
- Resistance training induces a fiber type shift that increases the number of type I fibers and reduces type II fibers (26).
- Improved coordination of muscle activation patterns, reduced antagonist muscle coactivation. Functional ability (*e.g.*, stair climb, walking endurance, chair rise, sit to stand) and balance can be improved after resistance training.
- Blood pressure responses are lower for the same physical workload; HR and blood pressure recover more quickly after cessation of exercise; at rest, evidence is equivocal for improvement in these parameters.
- Increased ability to recruit high threshold motor units.
- Bone density, insulin sensitivity, and comorbidities associated with obesity can be effectively managed with resistance training (4).

SUMMARY

- Irrespective of age, sex, physical condition, significant health benefits can be achieved with moderate amounts of physical activity on most, if not all, days of the week. With a modest increase in daily activity, most individuals improve multiple health domains.
- Prescription components (time, mode, frequency, intensity, duration, and progression) can be adjusted to achieve specific fitness goals.
- Incorporation of aerobic, resistance, and flexibility components provide an overall exercise stimulus for health improvement and maintenance.
- Body systems are plastic and able to adapt to exercise stimuli throughout the lifespan.

REFERENCES

1. Centers for Disease Control. *Physical Activity Guidelines for Americans.* 2nd ed; 2018. Available from: https://health.gov/sites/default/files/2019-09/Physical_Activity_Guidelines_2nd_edition.pdf
2. Šarabon N, Kozinc Ž. Effects of resistance exercise on balance ability: systematic review and meta-analysis of randomized controlled trials. *Life Basel Switz.* 2020;10(11):284. doi:10.3390/life10110284
3. El-Kotob R, Ponzano M, Chaput JP, et al. Resistance training and health in adults: an overview of systematic reviews. *Appl Physiol Nutr Metab.* 2020;45(10 (suppl 2)):S165–79. doi:10.1139/apnm-2020-0245
4. Deschenes MR, Kraemer WJ. Performance and physiologic adaptations to resistance training. *Am J Phys Med Rehabil.* 2002;81(11 suppl 1):S3–16. doi:10.1097/00002060-200211001-00003
5. Jemni M, Zaman R, Carrick FR, et al. Exercise improves depression through positive modulation of brain-derived neurotrophic factor (BDNF). A review based on 100 manuscripts over 20 years. *Front Physiol.* 2023;14:1102526. doi:10.3389/fphys.2023.1102526
6. Lipouri G, American College of Sports Medicine. *ACSM's Guidelines for Exercise Testing and Prescription.* 11th ed. Philadelphia: Lippincott Williams & Wilkins; 2021.
7. Eather N, McLachlan E, Sylvester B, Beauchamp M, Sanctuary C, Lubans D. The provision and experience of variety in physical activity settings: a systematic review of quantitative and qualitative studies. *J Sport Exerc Psychol.* 2023;45(3):148–65. doi:10.1123/jsep.2020-0355
8. American College of Sports Medicine. *ACSM's Resource Manual for Guidelines for Exercise Testing and Prescription.* 7th ed. Philadelphia: Wolters Kluwer; 2013.
9. Garber CE, Blissmer B, Deschenes MR, et al. American College of Sports Medicine position stand. Quantity and quality of exercise for developing and maintaining cardiorespiratory, musculoskeletal, and neuromotor fitness in apparently healthy adults: guidance for prescribing exercise. *Med Sci Sports Exerc.* 2011;43(7):1334–59. doi:10.1249/MSS.0b013e318213fefb

10. Hendy AM, Chye L, Teo WP. Cross-activation of the motor cortex during unilateral contractions of the quadriceps. *Front Hum Neurosci.* 2017;11:397. doi:10.3389/fnhum.2017.00397
11. Bowen W, Frazer AK, Tallent J, Pearce AJ, Kidgell DJ. Unilateral strength training imparts a cross-education effect in unilateral knee osteoarthritis patients. *J Funct Morphol Kinesiol.* 2022;7(4):77. doi:10.3390/jfmk7040077
12. Ehrensberger M, Simpson D, Broderick P, Monaghan K. Cross-education of strength has a positive impact on post-stroke rehabilitation: a systematic literature review. *Top Stroke Rehabil.* 2016;23(2):126–35. doi:10.1080/10749357.2015.1112062
13. Markov A, Hauser L, Chaabene H. Effects of concurrent strength and endurance training on measures of physical fitness in healthy middle-aged and older adults: a systematic review with meta-analysis. *Sports Med.* 2023;53(2):437–55. doi:10.1007/s40279-022-01764-2
14. Ralston GW, Kilgore L, Wyatt FB, Baker JS. The effect of weekly set volume on strength gain: a meta-analysis. *Sports Med.* 2017;47(12):2585–601. doi:10.1007/s40279-017-0762-7
15. Fragala MS, Cadore EL, Dorgo S, et al. Resistance training for older adults: position statement from the National Strength and Conditioning Association. *J Strength Cond Res.* 2019;33(8):2019–52. doi:10.1519/JSC.0000000000003230
16. Stricker PR, Faigenbaum AD, McCambridge TM, Council on Sports Medicine and Fitness. Resistance training for children and adolescents. *Pediatrics.* 2020;145(6):e20201011. doi:10.1542/peds.2020-1011
17. Isath A, Kanwal A, Virk HUH, et al. The effect of yoga on cardiovascular disease risk factors: a meta-analysis. *Curr Probl Cardiol.* 2023;48(5):101593. doi:10.1016/j.cpcardiol.2023.101593
18. Moesgaard L, Beck MM, Christiansen L, Aagaard P, Lundbye-Jensen J. Effects of periodization on strength and muscle hypertrophy in volume-equated resistance training programs: a systematic review and meta-analysis. *Sports Med.* 2022;52(7):1647–66. doi:10.1007/s40279-021-01636-1
19. Kelley GA, Kelley KS. Yoga, health-related quality of life and mental well-being: a re-analysis of a meta-analysis using the quality effects model. *J Gerontol A Biol Sci Med Sci.* 2020;75(9):1732–6. doi:10.1093/gerona/glz284
20. Park M, Song R, Ju K, et al. Effects of tai chi and qigong on cognitive and physical functions in older adults: systematic review, meta-analysis, and meta-regression of randomized clinical trials. *BMC Geriatr.* 2023;23(1):352. doi:10.1186/s12877-023-04070-2
21. Load, overload, and recovery in the athlete: select issues for the team physician-A consensus statement. *Med Sci Sports Exerc.* 2019;51(4):821–8. doi:10.1249/MSS.0000000000001910
22. Schwellnus M, Soligard T, Alonso JM, et al. How much is too much? (Part 2) International Olympic Committee consensus statement on load in sport and risk of illness. *Br J Sports Med.* 2016;50(17):1043–52. doi:10.1136/bjsports-2016-096572
23. Armstrong LE, Bergeron MF, Lee EC, Mershon JE, Armstrong EM. Overtraining syndrome as a complex systems phenomenon. *Front Netw Physiol.* 2021;1:794392. doi:10.3389/fnetp.2021.794392
24. Riebe D, Franklin BA, Thompson PD, et al. Updating ACSM's recommendations for exercise preparticipation health screening. *Med Sci Sports Exerc.* 2015;47(11):2473–9. doi:10.1249/MSS.0000000000000664
25. Nystoriak MA, Bhatnagar A. Cardiovascular effects and benefits of exercise. *Front Cardiovasc Med.* 2018;5:135. doi:10.3389/fcvm.2018.00135
26. Coffey VG, Hawley JA. The molecular bases of training adaptation. *Sports Med.* 2007;37(9):737–63. doi:10.2165/00007256-200737090-00001
27. Mahalakshmi B, Maurya N, Lee SD, Bharath Kumar V. Possible neuroprotective mechanisms of physical exercise in neurodegeneration. *Int J Mol Sci.* 2020;21(16):5895. doi:10.3390/ijms21165895

Nutrition

12

Lee A. Mancini and Patricia A. Deuster

INTRODUCTION

- This chapter focuses on the basic concepts of nutrition and sports.
- Topics include basics in energy, metabolism, nutritional needs of athletes, hydration and fluid replacement, nutrient timing, selected nutritional issues, and information on ergogenic agents and nutritional supplements, which include sports drinks, bars, and energy drinks.

BASICS IN ENERGY METABOLISM

General Energy Needs

- Energy balance is critical for all athletes and demands matching energy intake to total energy expenditure (TEE).
- There are four components of TEE — resting metabolic rate (RMR, often referred to as resting energy expenditure (REE), diet induced. thermogenesis (DIT, also often referred to as the thermic effect of food or TEF), Non-exercise activity thermogenesis (NEAT), and Exercise Energy Expenditure (EEE) (1).
- The breakdown of TEE for each of these is TEF (8%–15%), EEE (15%–30%), NEAT (15%–30%), and RMR (60%–70%) (2).
- Energy Availability (EA) is defined as the amount of dietary energy remaining for other body functions after the energy cost of exercise is covered and normalized to fat-free mass (FFM) (or lean body mass). EA (kcal/kg FFM/day) = [Energy Intake (EI) (kcal/day) – EEE (kcal/day)]/FFM kg (1).
- A better equation for EA has been proposed that considers both NEAT and EEE. When NEAT + EEE are combined into the Activity-Induced Energy Expenditure (AEE).

  EA = [EI – AEE]/FFM (1)
- REE, or RMR, is the biggest contributor to TEE, and FFM is the biggest contributor to REE (3).
- REE or RMR can be estimated for men and women by using several different equations (4):

$$\text{Men}: \quad 9.99\times\text{Weight}(\text{kg})+6.25\times\text{Height}(\text{cm})-4.92\times\text{Age}(\text{yrs})+5, \text{or } 4.54\times\text{Weight}(\text{lbs})+15.875\times\text{Height}(\text{in})-4.92\times\text{Age}(\text{yrs})+5$$

$$\text{Women}: \quad 9.99\ \text{Weight}(\text{kg})+6.25\times\text{Height}(\text{cm})-4.92\times\text{Age}(\text{yrs})-161, \text{or } 4.54\times\text{Weight}(\text{lbs})+15.875\times\text{Height}(\text{in})-4.92\times\text{Age}(\text{yrs})-161$$

- Physical activity levels (PAL) vary, but a factor can be applied to REE (RMR) to estimate TEE. Table 12.1 presents suggested ranges for PAL factors. However, TEE may be overestimated in the low range of activity.
- The Institute of Medicine (IOM) (5) also proposes formulas for TEE as follows:

$$\text{Men}: \quad 662-9.53\times\text{Age}(\text{yrs})+\text{PAL}\times[15.91\times\text{Weight}(\text{kg})+539.6\times\text{Height}(\text{m})]$$
$$662-9.53\times\text{Age}(\text{yrs})+\text{PAL}\times[7.232\times\text{Weight}(\text{lbs})+13.71\times\text{Height}(\text{in})]$$
$$\text{Women}: \quad 354-6.9\times\text{Age}(\text{yrs})+\text{PAL}\times[9.36\times\text{Weight}(\text{kg})+726\times\text{Height}(\text{m})]$$
$$354-6.9\times\text{Age}(\text{yrs})+\text{PAL}\times[4.255\times\text{Weight}(\text{lbs})+18.44\times\text{Height}(\text{in})]$$

- Comparison of the two formulas at the same PAL values reveals that the TEE estimated by the IOM formula is higher by 600–1200 kcal $\cdot$ d^{-1} for both men and women.
- Failure to maintain energy balance can result in loss of muscle mass; menstrual disturbances; compromised bone density; decreased testosterone levels, increased risk of fatigue, injury, and illness; and overtraining (6).

Energy Sources and Stores

- The universal source of metabolic fuel for energy is adenosine triphosphate (ATP) and the fuel sources to produce ATP are carbohydrates (CHO), fats (fatty acids), protein (amino acids), and alcohol. One gram of CHO (glucose, glycogen, etc.) yields 4 kcal; 1 g of protein yields 4 kcal; 1 g of fat provides 9 kcal; and 1 g of alcohol yields 7.4 kcal. These fuel sources are converted into energy.
- The thermic effect of food (TEF) is the amount of energy it takes your body to digest, absorb, and metabolize the food you eat. This affects how many actual calories an athlete can

Table 12.1 Suggested Ranges for Physical Activity Factors Based on Activity

Level of Physical Activity	PAL
Sedentary	1.2
Minimal regular physical activity	1.4–1.5
Some regular activity	1.6–1.7
Moderate physical activity	1.8–1.9
Strenuous physical activity	2.0–2.4

PAL, physical activity level.

Table 12.2 Energy Stores for a 60-kg Person With 15% Body Fat

Energy Source	Energy (g)	Energy (kcal)
Liver and muscle glycogen	400–750	500–1000
Glucose in body fluids	15–20	60–80
Total Carbohydrate Stores	**415–770**	**560–1080**
Subcutaneous adipose triglycerides	9000	81,000
Intramuscular triglycerides	150	1350
Total Triglyceride Stores	**9150**	**82,350**
Total Energy Stores	**9565–9920**	**82,910–83,430**

utilize from a meal (7). Protein has a TEF of 25%–30%, CHO (6%–8%), and Fat (2%–3%) (2).

- TEF is also affected by the size of a meal (larger meals have a higher TEF) and by type of protein (whey is higher than casein, casein is higher than soy) (2).
- ATP, glucose, and free fatty acids are stored in various amounts: ATP storage is sufficient for only 10–15 seconds of activity.
- Glycogen, the storage form of CHO and a polymer of glucose, is found in both liver and muscle tissue.
- Triglycerides, the storage form of lipids, consist of three fatty acids and a glycerol backbone.
- Energy yields for glycogen (4 kcal $\cdot$ g^{-1}) in liver and skeletal muscle and triglycerides (9 kcal $\cdot$ g^{-1}) in skeletal muscle and adipose tissues are shown in Table 12.2.
- Storing 1 g of glycogen requires 2.7–4 g of water; thus, the energy yield is less than half of what would be expected: if 120 g of glycogen were stored, at least 80 g would be water, and the energy yield would be 160 rather than 480 kcal (8).
- The breakdown of glycogen to form glucose for energy is called *glycogenolysis*.
- The process of converting amino acids or lactate into glucose is called *gluconeogenesis*.

Energy Systems

- Table 12.3 presents the length of time exercise that can be maintained for the three different energy systems used in muscular activity.
- The *immediate, or phosphagen, system* consists of ATP and creatine phosphate (PC or phosphocreatine) and allows for very short bursts of maximal power. It does not rely on oxygen.
- The *short-term, or glycogen-lactic acid, system* consists of glucose entering the glycolytic pathway and subsequent oxidation of pyruvate to lactate. The energy formed allows for only 1–1.6 minutes of maximal muscle activity at a reduced power output as compared to the phosphagen system. This often can happen in the absence of oxygen, but lactate can be both formed and used under fully aerobic conditions (9).
- The *aerobic, or long-term, system* involves glucose entering the glycolytic pathway through to pyruvate and its subsequent oxidation to acetyl-coenzyme A (acetyl-CoA) for entry into the tricarboxylic acid (TCA) cycle. Free fatty acids (FFAs) from triglycerides can be broken down into two-carbon acetyl fragments to form acetyl-CoA. This process, known as β-oxidation, can only occur under aerobic conditions (10).
- Amino acids can enter the TCA cycle after deamination/transamination and conversion into acetyl-CoA and/or acetoacetate. NADH and $FADH_2$, the reduced coenzymes formed during glycolysis and the TCA cycle, are shuttled to the electron transport chain within the mitochondria to be oxidized to NAD and FAD, respectively. ATP is regenerated from adenosine diphosphate (ADP) with 2.5 ATP per NADH and 1.5 ATP per $FADH_2$. The O_2 used for oxidation is tightly linked to aerobic ATP production.
- One molecule of glucose going through the glycolytic pathway to lactate yields 2 ATP, whereas one molecule of glucose going through the aerobic pathway yields 30 ATP.

Table 12.3 Comparison of the Maximal Rates of Power and Length of Time Exercise Can Be Maintained for the Immediate, Short-Term, and Long-Term Energy Systems

Energy Systems	Mole of ATP/min	Time to Fatigue
Immediate: phosphagen (phosphocreatine and ATP)	4	5–10 s
Short term: glycolytic (glycogen-lactic acid)	2.5	1.0–1.6 min
Long term: aerobic (glucose, fatty acids)	1	Unlimited time

ATP, adenosine triphosphate.

Determinants of Fuel Utilization

- The primary determinant of substrate preference is exercise intensity. The higher the intensity, the greater the demand on the immediate and short-term glycolytic energy system. Low-intensity exercise uses the aerobic system almost exclusively.
- The crossover point for metabolism is the power output (hard to maximal) at which an individual switches from a predominant reliance on FFA to a primary reliance on CHO utilization (glycogen; blood glucose; and blood, muscle, and liver lactate). Moreover, further increases in power elicit relative increments in CHO utilization and relative decrements in lipid oxidation (11).
- Use of FFA increases in proportion to the energy demand until the exercise intensity approaches 60% of $\dot{V}O_{2max}$, after which glucose becomes the dominant fuel source (12–14). Figure 12.1 shows the contributions of fat and CHO as substrate for various exercise intensities.
- Trained athletes can oxidize fatty acids as fuels at higher exercise intensities than untrained persons.
- During exercise and recovery from the exercise at altitude, CHO utilization is increased compared with conditions at sea level (15).

NUTRITIONAL REQUIREMENTS OF ATHLETES

- Athletes have increased energy needs, as well as increased protein needs (16,17). Although many athletes can meet their nutritional needs by consuming whole food sources, there are several instances where a food-only approach may not always be optimal for athletes.

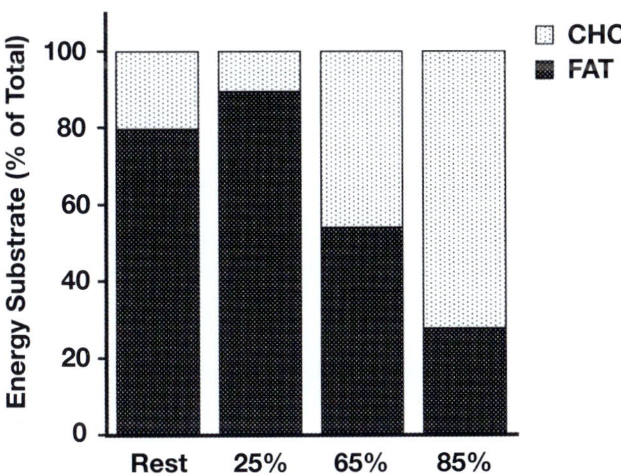

Figure 12.1: Relative contributions of fat and carbohydrate (CHO) to energy at rest and during exercise at 25%, 65%, and 85% of maximal aerobic capacity.

- A whole food-only approach may not always be optimal for athletes — (1) some nutrients are difficult to obtain in sufficient quantities or may require excessive energy intake, (2) some nutrients are abundant only in foods athletes do not eat/like, (3) the nutrient content of some foods is highly variable, (4) concentrated doses of some nutrients are required to correct deficiencies and/or promote immune tolerance, (5) some foods may be difficult to consume pre-, during, and post-exercise (17,18).
- A whole food first, but not always food-only approach maximizes athletes choosing whole foods, but also recognizes supplements may be useful in specific circumstances.

Carbohydrates

- CHO intake is necessary to maintain blood glucose levels during exercise and restore muscle glycogen after exercise. CHOs provide dietary fiber, vitamins, and minerals to athletes.
- Total intake will depend on TEE, with increasing exercise volume determining a greater intake of CHOs, so there is a range of CHO intake. Low to moderate volume of activity (30–60 min · d^{-1}, 3–4 times per week) 3–5 g kg^{-1} body wt (~1.3–2.3 g · lb^{-1} body wt · d^{-1}), higher volume of activity of 6–10 g · kg^{-1} body wt · d^{-1} (1–3 h · d^{-1}) (~2.7–4.5 g · lb^{-1} body wt · d^{-1}), depending on energy needs, are currently recommended (19,20).
- The percentage of kilocalories in the diet from CHO varies based on the sport, volume of training, and body composition goals. Thereby CHO intake has a wide range between 40% and 65% of total energy intake
- The CHO source and quality should be considered for athletes, as not all CHO sources are created equally. Athletes should focus on whole foods, vegetables, fruits, and legumes, while minimizing processed and added sugars (19,21).

Protein

- Athletes need protein to prevent muscle breakdown, for muscle growth, and for tissue repair. Approximately 10%–35% of the total energy should come from protein, depending on the actual energy intake (22).
- It is well established that athletes have a higher requirement for protein than the RDA (0.8 g · kg^{-1} body wt · d^{-1}) (16,20,23,24).
- The recommended range of intake for strength athletes is 1.4–2.0 g · kg^{-1} body wt · d^{-1} (0.64–0.91 g · lb^{-1} body wt · d^{-1}). This equates to a protein intake of 98–140 g · d^{-1} for a 70-kg (154-lb) person.
- The recommended protein intake for endurance athletes is 1.2–1.7 g · kg^{-1} body wt · d^{-1} (0.55–0.77 g · lb^{-1} body wt · d^{-1}). This equates to a protein intake of 84–119 g · d^{-1} for a 70-kg (154-lb) person (16,20,22).
- There is evidence that athletes trying to lose body fat or athletes on a hypocaloric diet should increase protein intake

further (2.3–3.1 g · kg^{-1} body wt · d^{-1}) to maintain lean muscle mass (22,23,25–28).

- Essential amino acids (EAA) are not synthesized by the body and must be provided in the diet; they include leucine, isoleucine, valine, histidine, lysine, methionine, phenylalanine, threonine, and tryptophan (29,30).
- Protein intake needs to be spread throughout the day, 0.25–0.3 g · kg^{-1} body wt every 3–4 hours (20–40 g per meal), to optimize MPS (muscle protein synthesis). Higher doses of protein >40 g per meal have not shown to augment MPS further. MPS peaks between 20 and 40 g per meal (16,20,22).
- The goal should be for athletes to meet the daily protein requirement through whole food sources. However, athletes may need to take protein powders or amino acid supplements to achieve their daily needs in certain instances (20,23).

Fat

- Fat is essential for cell membrane formation, absorption of fat-soluble vitamins, hormone regulation, brain health, and energy for metabolism (31).
- It is recommended that athletes not have fat intake be below 20% of total energy — as it puts them at risk for low intake of fat-soluble vitamins and essential fatty acids such as the omega-3 fatty acids, DHA, and EHA (16,19).
- Dietary fat intake should provide between 20% and 35% of the total energy. For example, a 70-kg (154-lb) person who consumes 3750 kcal · d^{-1} would ingest between 83 and 146 g of fat (750–1312 kcal from fat).
- Endurance athletes in training may have a lower percentage of fat intake, closer to 20%–25% of the total energy because of a higher consumption of adequate amounts of CHO.
- Ingestion of a high-fat, low-CHO diet is associated with lower resting muscle glycogen content and higher rates of fat oxidation during exercise as compared to a CHO-rich diet (10,32–34).
- There is evidence that ultra-endurance athletes may benefit from keto-adaptation — becoming fat-adapted or training low with a high fat, low CHO diet, which upregulates lipid oxidation (16,35,36).
- Athletes should choose healthier fat sources such as nuts, seeds, nut butters, avocadoes, wild caught fish such as salmon, coconut oil, and extra virgin olive oil. Trans fats should be avoided, as well as highly processed oils (19).
- The ratio between n-3 (omega-3) and n-6 (omega-6) fatty acids is also important, as n-6 fatty acids are proinflammatory, whereas n-3 are anti-inflammatory (16,37,38).
- Omega-3 fatty acids (DHA and EPA) have been shown to decrease delayed onset muscle damage, increase anabolic sensitivity to amino acids and protein synthesis, and decrease inflammation of tissues (39–43).

Vitamins and Minerals

- Vitamins and minerals are of fundamental importance for biochemical processes within our bodies. Active individuals should consume adequate vitamins and minerals to achieve the most recent Dietary Reference Intakes (DRIs) based on their life stage, gender, and activity level. Athletes have a higher rate of turnover of key vitamins and minerals. Active individuals want to maximize their performance and should make sure to consume adequate vitamins and minerals to do this (17,44).
- Athletes who perspire heavily or engage in physical activity in hot conditions may be prone to increased losses of minerals in their sweat.
- The gut microbiome affects the absorption and bioavailability of vitamins and minerals — which can impact the nutritional status of athletes. This is an area of further research within sports nutrition (45,46).

HYDRATION AND FLUID REPLACEMENT

- Water is the most important nutrient for regulating hydration status in individuals.
- Water losses during exercise occur primarily through sweat and can be considerable during prolonged exercise, particularly in warm or hot weather. Electrolyte losses in sweat can also be substantial.
- Sweat rate is influenced by ambient temperature, humidity, exercise intensity, training status, and rate of fluid intake.
- Fluid replacement is important for sustaining exercise performance and the current American College of Sports Medicine (ACSM) guidelines note that the goal of fluid replacement is to prevent dehydration in excess of 2% weight loss and extreme changes in electrolyte balance to avoid performance decrements (47).
- ACSM recommends that people take personal responsibility for sustaining their hydration and develop fluid replacement programs to suit their individual needs (47).

Effects of Dehydration

- Dehydration in an athlete is affected by the environment, such as the WBGT (Wet Bulb Globe Temperature), the intensity of training, and the availability and accessibility of fluids to the athlete (48,49).
- Dehydration (loss of body fluids) in excess of >1% of body mass loss (BML) (>0.7 L of water for a 70-kg person) has been shown to compromise thermoregulation (48,49).
- Dehydration in excess of >2% of BML (>1.4 L of water for a 70-kg person) has been shown to decrease cardiac output, decrease cognitive awareness, and decrease time to exhaustion (16,50).

- Dehydration between 3% and 5% of BML (2.1–3.5 L of water for a 70-kg person) has been shown to decrease agility and sports-specific skills (50).
- Dehydration has been shown to have negative effects on performance with exercise lasting longer than 30 seconds, and has little to no effect on exercise lasting less than 15 seconds (51).
- Dehydration can increase the perceived effort of the task, decrease time to exhaustion, decrease anaerobic power, impair balance control, and is a risk factor for exertional heat illness, including heat stroke. The greater the level of dehydration, the more severe the effect (48,51,52).
- Dehydration also is a risk factor for an exertional sickling episode and exertional rhabdomyolysis. Special attention should be paid for athletes with known sickle cell disease or sickle cell trait (49).

Monitoring Hydration

- Calculating body mass change is a quick and effective way to track hydration status. The method is most valid when compared with at least 3 consecutive days of euhydrated baseline average (53–55).
- Nude body mass should be measured before and after exercise is the most effective way to evaluate the adequacy of a hydration program. Measuring body mass before and after practices or training sessions provides an objective measure to quantify weight loss (49,52).
- If body mass loss is greater than 2%, the individual is drinking too little; if body mass is greater than preexercise, the individual is drinking too much.
- Assessment of the first morning urine void increases the validity of hydration-status measurement. Health care professionals can test the first morning urine for urine specific gravity, when feasible, to evaluate hydration status (49,56,57).
- Personal cues are also important for each athlete to gauge their own hydration status — thirst sensation, void frequency, and urine color are valuable indicators that can aid in assessing hydration status (58,59).
- Drinking in excess of sweat rate should be avoided.

Hydration Recommendations

- Fluid intake prior to exercise is necessary to increase the likelihood of starting the activity well hydrated. Consuming 400–600 mL (14–22 oz) of fluid 2 hours prior to exercise is recommended (47,60).
- Fluid intake during exercise is necessary to replace the fluid lost through sweat; fluid intake should approximate fluid losses. For exercise lasting less than 1 hour — water is the best fluid and the practical recommendation is to consume 150–350 mL (5–12 oz) of water every 15–20 minutes of exercise (61).
- Exercise that lasts more than 1 hour, a beverage containing 6%–8% CHO (glucose, sucrose, fructose, glucose polymers, and the like) and/or electrolytes can be beneficial (47,60,62). This amount of CHO with the addition of electrolytes ensures maximal stimulation of fluid absorption because of increased palatability and promotes gastric emptying.
- With excessive dehydration, persons should drink approximately 1.5 L of fluid for each kilogram of body weight lost, and the fluid should contain more sodium than usual: A concentration of approximately 50 mmol · L^{-1} or 1 g of sodium per 1 L of fluid will stimulate thirst and fluid retention to enhance a more rapid and complete recovery (47,61,63,64).

ELECTROLYTES

- Electrolyte (sodium, potassium, chloride) and mineral (calcium, zinc, magnesium, iron) losses from sweating can be substantial, depending on training status, workout length, workout intensity, fluid intake, genetics, sweat rate, prior heat exposure, and may lead to severe medical problems (47).
- Sodium should be ingested during exercise when large sweat sodium losses occur. The average sodium concentration in sweat is 50 mmol · L^{-1} or 1 g of sodium per 1 L (20). ACSM recommends starting with 300–600 mg · h^{-1} (1.7–2.9 g salt) during prolonged exercise (16).
- Sodium losses, which have been associated with muscle cramps, can range from 60 to 5000 mg · L^{-1} · d^{-1}, with higher values noted in heavy sweaters and those unaccustomed to working in the heat.
- Potassium losses may range from 25 to 2000 mg (47).
- Electrolytes lost through sweating can be replaced by fluid replacement beverages and foods. Dried fruits are good food choices for potassium, and pretzels and pickles are good sources of sodium. A small box of raisins provides 322 mg of potassium, and a snack of 10 small, plain, hard salted pretzels (60 g) provides about 814 g of sodium. In addition, one small dill or kosher cucumber pickle provides about 569 g of sodium.
- Adding ½ teaspoon of table salt to food provides 1200 mg of sodium.

NUTRIENT TIMING

- Nutrient timing is a concept developed by Drs. John Ivy and Robert Portman to indicate that when food is eaten is as important as what is eaten (65).
- Considerations around nutrient timing around workouts, training, and exercise can be divided into — pre-, during, and post-workout. Athletes should also consider the nutrient timing needs of the first post-exercise meal, nutrient timing at bedtime, and nutrient timing differences around training and nontraining days (66) (Fig. 12.2).

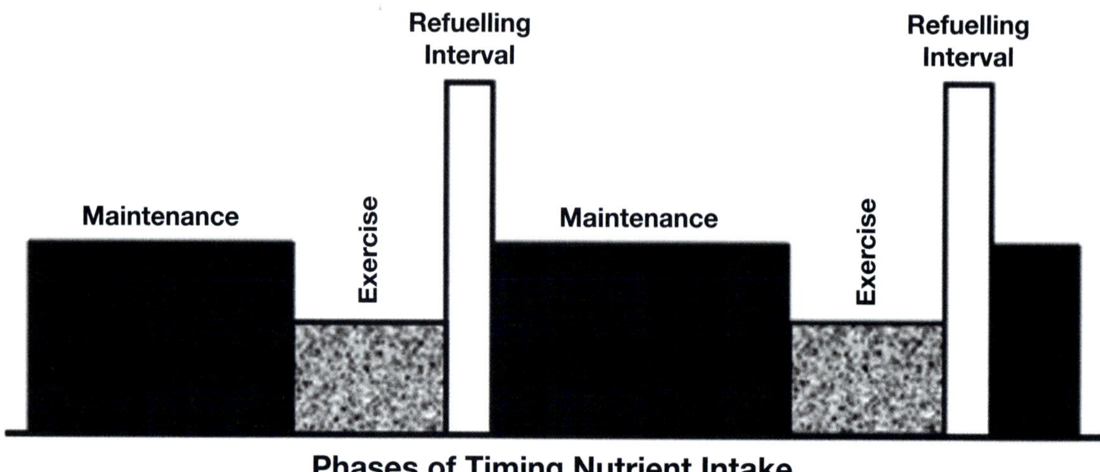

Figure 12.2: Three major phases for nutrient timing: maintenance and growth, exercise, and the refueling interval for recovery.

Preexercise Nutrition

- The intensity of the exercise may dictate the preexercise meal. Foods consumed before low-intensity exercise may have adverse gastrointestinal effects at a higher intensity level. Try different foods to see what works best based on exercise intensity levels (67).
- Eating prior to exercise, as compared to exercising after an overnight fast, may improve performance (68–70).
- Fluid intake prior to exercise is necessary to increase the likelihood of starting the activity well hydrated. Consuming 400–600 mL (14–22 oz) of fluid 2 hours prior to exercise is recommended (47,60).
- Prior to training, athletes should look to easily digestible CHOs, and protein sources that are quickly broken down and absorbed such as whey protein (16,20).
- CHO consumed in meals and/or snacks during the 1–4 hours prior to exercise help increase glycogen stores as well as provide gut glucose release during exercise (20).
- Consume a meal or snack 1–4 hours before heavy training or competition to minimize hunger, ensure food digestion and gastric emptying, and maximize endogenous glycogen stores. Table 12.4 presents several light preexercise meals.
- Ingesting a small meal less than 1 hour before heavy training or competition does not appear to benefit performance (20).

Exercise Nutrition

- Fluid, CHO, and protein ingestion during exercise depends on the duration and intensity.
- During exercise (training or competition), energy-providing beverages and foods are usually consumed only when the exercise is of sufficient duration to demand additional fuel (*e.g.*, marathons, triathlons, ultra-endurance events).
- The individual should consume what is familiar; no new fluids or foods should be consumed during competition. During practice sessions is the best time to try new fluids, foods, or supplements to see how the body reacts.
- For endurance activities longer than 1 hour, fluids should be consumed at regular intervals to replace fluid losses, and CHO (approximately 30–60 $g \cdot h^{-1}$) should be ingested to maintain blood glucose levels.

Table 12.4 Suggested Foods for Preexercise Meal or Snack

Type of Food	kcal	Carbohydrate (g)	Fat (g)	Protein (g)
2 slices whole-wheat bread, 2 oz turkey, lettuce, and 1 medium orange	289	40	4	23
1 baked potato w/yogurt	201	41	1	7
8 oz low-fat yogurt w/fruit	255	47	3	11
½ cup low-fat granola w/½ cup skim milk	241	46	3	8
Bagel w/2 tbsp low-fat cream cheese	330	55	6	13
8 oz low-fat chocolate milk and 1 medium apple	264	51	3	9

- The above recommendations are particularly important when the exercise is under extreme environmental (heat, cold, or high altitude) conditions, in particular at high altitude.
- For resistance training, team sport practices, and speed and power activities — consuming protein in the form of EAA and leucine has been shown to help adaptations to training as well as muscle growth and recovery (66).

Postexercise Nutrition

- The goals post-exercise are to provide adequate fluids, electrolytes, protein, and CHO to promote recovery, ensure tissue repair, and maximize muscle growth.
- Fluids should be replenished with 1–1.5 L · kg^{-1} body weight loss (16–24 oz · lb^{-1}) (16).
- Protein that is easily digested should be consumed after training. Whey protein is ideal as it is high in EAAs, especially leucine, is easily absorbed, leads to greater lean muscle gains, and has maximal MPS compared to other protein sources (22,71–74).
- The combination of protein with CHO leads to greater increase in glycogen restoration (40%–100%) (16), greater increase in insulin levels, greater increase in growth hormone release, better post-exercise rehydration, and reduced post-exercise muscle damage(66,75–79).
- Athletes should ingest 0.8 g · kg^{-1} CHO and 0.4 g · kg^{-1} protein post-exercise. This has been shown to maximize MPS and glycogen resynthesis (16,20,66).
- Ingestion of protein (20–40 g) with the CHO during recovery can increase muscle protein synthesis and improve nitrogen balance compared with consuming only CHO (20,80–83).
- Presleep nutrition is important for recovery to help athletes prevent protein catabolism and improve recovery. Casein is a slow-release protein that clots in the presence of gastric acid, which delays digestion and elevates MPS for a prolonged time period. Casein also maintains overnight lipolysis and fat oxidation (66,84).

Maintenance Nutrition

- During the maintenance and growth phase of nutrient timing, a high daily intake of CHO, in combination with adequate protein and fat, should be consumed.
- CHO intake should match energy intensity and expenditure. As exercise intensity and/or workload increases, CHO intake should increase to ensure glycogen stores (20,71).
- The recommended amounts of vitamins and minerals should be consumed through proper choice of foods to meet nutritional demands of strenuous training (71).
- During the maintenance phase, it is important to develop nutritional strategies that consider nutrient timing as a function of training schedule and competitive events. In particular, the time it takes to digest certain foods, what types of foods best meet the needs of the athlete, and ensuring snacks are available to provide protein and CHO at regular intervals should be considered.
- CHO intake should be different between training and non-training days — with training days having an increased CHO intake. CHO intake should be adjusted based on the duration and intensity of the training.

NUTRITIONAL ISSUES

Glycemic Index

- The glycemic index (GI), a concept proposed by Jenkins et al. (85), describes how rapidly a particular food raises blood glucose levels after eating.
- CHOs come in different forms. Some contain dietary fiber, and the time required for digestion and absorption differs.
- High GI foods are usually digested and absorbed rapidly and release glucose into the circulation, whereas low GI foods take longer to digest and absorb (85). Figure 12.3 presents a comparison of blood glucose changes after the ingestion of a high and low GI food.
- On a scale of 0–100, foods with a GI > 70 are classified as high, whereas foods with a GI < 55 are considered low GI foods (85).
- High GI foods may be most effective in restoring glycogen post-exercise because they produce a rapid rise in blood glucose (85,86).
- Preexercise meals should consist of low GI foods to minimize a rapid rise in blood glucose (86).

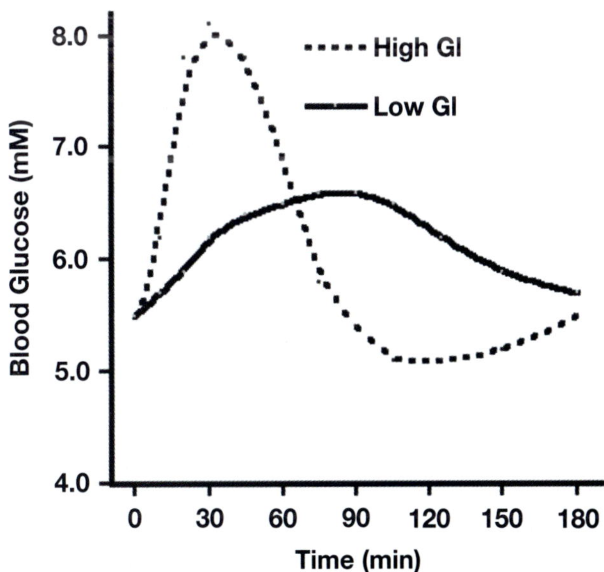

Figure 12.3: Patterns of change in blood glucose in response to high and low glycemic index (GI) foods.

Carbohydrate Macronutrient Manipulations

- Although protein intake usually remains consistent in an athlete's nutritional plan, CHO intake and fat intake can fluctuate based on an athlete's goals, training volume, and sport.
- Reduced CHO intake defined by CHO consisting of 25%–40% of the Total daily intake (TDI), around 125–200 g · d^{-1}.
- Low CHO intake is when CHO make up 10%–25% of the TDI, around 50–125 g · d^{-1}.
- Ketogenic diet, also known as a Very Low CHO Diet (VLCD) is when CHO make up < 10% of TDI, usually less than 50 g · d^{-1} (36).
- Consuming a high-CHO diet creates a greater reliance on CHO as the fuel of choice: CHO loading decreases oxidation of fatty acids (87,88).
- One method of CHO manipulation termed "train low, compete high" has emerged. Train low means training with glycogen stores low (89–92). This is accomplished by ingesting a high-fat, low-CHO diet; having two training sessions daily and consuming no CHO between training sessions; and training after an overnight fast.
- Training with low glycogen induces a variety of metabolic and training adaptations, but they do not benefit athletic performance (61,89,92,93).

Fat Macronutrient Manipulations

- Consuming a high-fat diet (>65% of energy as fat) for at least 5 days enhances fatty acid oxidation and spares glycogen (10,32,33,93) (Fig. 12.4). Such a practice will reduce muscle and liver glycogen stores, which can compromise exercise performance, particularly high-intensity exercise.
- High-fat diets may be useful for ultra-endurance events where the intensity is typically low. A fat-adapted endurance athlete can oxidize fat at 1.5 g · min^{-1} (810 cal · h^{-1}) (35).
- Higher fat, lower CHO nutrition plans have been shown to decrease body fat, decrease waist circumference, and less lean muscle loss when compared to higher CHO plans (36,94).

ERGOGENIC AGENTS AND NUTRITIONAL SUPPLEMENTS

- Dietary supplements can be found in various forms: pills, powders, liquids, beverages, and bars.
- In 1994, the Dietary Supplement Health and Education Act (DSHEA) was passed. It placed dietary supplements in the special category of foods. The law defines a "dietary supplement" as a product intended to supplement the diet and contains a "dietary ingredient." Dietary ingredients may include vitamins, minerals, herbs, amino acids, and substances such as enzymes, organ tissues, and glandular extracts (95).
- In the United States dietary supplements are classified as food products, not drugs, and there is no mandate to register products with the FDA or obtain FDA approval.
- In Canada, under the Natural Health Product (NHP) Regulations enacted in 2004 — supplements must be reviewed, approved, and registered with Health Canada (95).
- Manufacturers of dietary supplements often make claims that sound appealing, but many are not legal. No claims of preventing disease or improving health are allowed unless the Food and Drug Administration approves the claim. Claims related to structure and function can be made. For

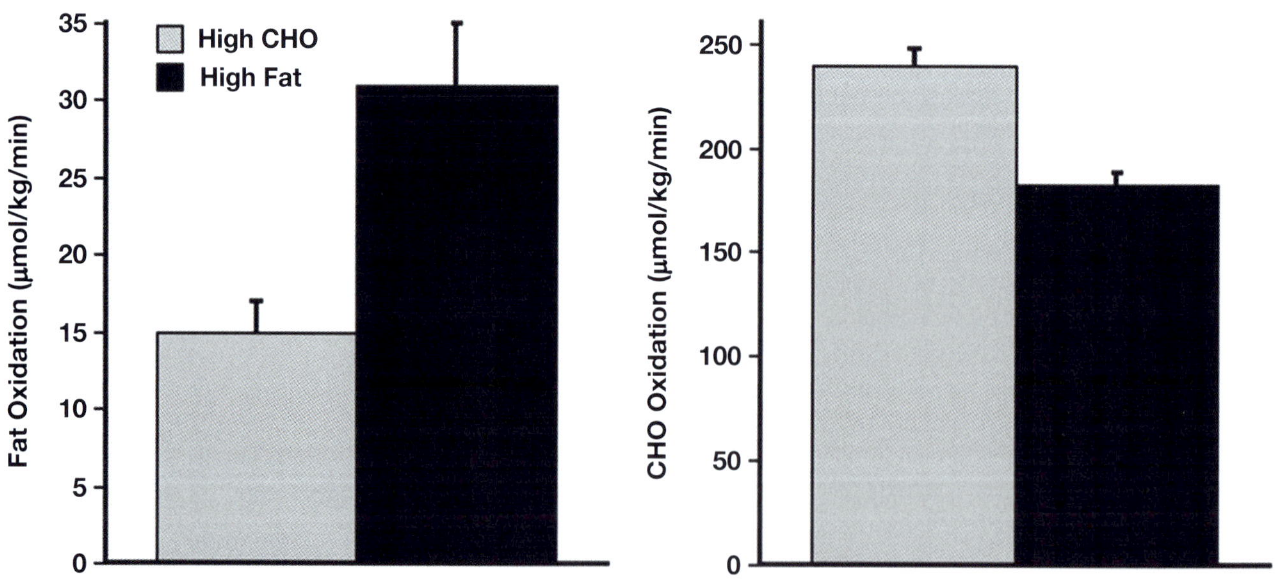

Figure 12.4: Amounts of fat and carbohydrate (CHO) oxidized during exercise at 70% of maximal capacity after 5 days of a high-fat diet (~68% of energy), followed by 1 day of rest with a high-CHO diet (~70% of energy).

example, the statement "calcium promotes bone health" is legal because it relates to a structure — bone — but does not claim to improve health or disease.

- Vitamin-mineral supplements may be necessary for athletes who restrict energy intake, engage in severe weight-loss practices, or eliminate food group(s) from their diet.
- When choosing supplements, look for a seal that demonstrates participation in a third-party verification program, such as U.S. Pharmacopeia (USP), National Sanitation Foundation International, or Informed-Choice, which ensures quality and purity.
- Athletes should consider the tolerable upper intake levels (ULs) for nutrients when selecting dietary supplements. The UL is the maximum level of total chronic intake of a nutrient from all sources judged to be unlikely to pose a risk of adverse health effects in humans (96).
- ULs for nutrients can be found at: https://www.efsa.europa.eu/sites/default/files/assets/UL_Summary_tables.pdf
- No supplements should provide more than 150% of the DRI of the nutrient.
- When an athlete is considering taking a supplement — they should consider whether it is legal and safe, and does it work based on the literature.
- Athletes should think of supplements more as "complements," as athletes should be obtaining the majority of their nutrition from whole foods, and using supplements to fill in the gaps to "complement" their nutritional plan.
- Athletes should refer to their sport's governing bodies to determine whether a supplement or ergogenic aid if legal.
- WADA (World Anti-Doping Agency) List: https://www.usada.org/athletes/substances/?gad=1&gclid=EAIaIQobChMIxuyqyIyggQMVAvXjBx0u6wQnEAAYASAAEgKHHPD_BwE
- NCAA List: https://www.ncaa.org/sports/2015/6/10/ncaa-banned-substances.aspx
- Chapter 76, Medications and Ergogenic Aids, further elaborates selected dietary supplements.

Protein Powders

- The bioavailability of amino acids from various sources of protein is influenced by the source/type of protein and purification methods (22,97).
- Casein and whey are high-quality proteins but differ markedly in their digestion and absorption. Ingestion of whey protein produces a rapid, but transient (1–2 hours) peak in serum amino acids, whereas casein produces a more prolonged, modest increase (over 7 hours), which results in casein having a greater anabolic effect compared to whey (98).
- Protein hydrolysates are produced from purified proteins by hydrolysis with acid or by adding proteolytic enzymes (99).
- Hydrolysates are absorbed more rapidly than free-form amino acids and intact proteins, and whey hydrolysates are absorbed more rapidly than those of soy; both are absorbed more rapidly than casein hydrolysates (100).
- Whey protein has been shown to enhance MPS and aid in recovery post-exercise (22,72).

Caffeine

- Caffeine is one of the substances most commonly used by athletes to enhance their performance.
- Caffeine can be ingested in capsule or powder form, in gum, in gel, or in beverages such as tea, coffee, and energy drinks.
- Caffeine's ergogenic mechanism of action is its blocking effect on adenosine receptors A_1, A_2, and A_{2B} due to the similar structure between caffeine and adenosine.
- The optimal dose of caffeine for performance improvements is between 3 and 6 $mg \cdot kg^{-1}$ (101,102); higher doses may impair performance (102,103).
- Caffeine has been shown to improve cognitive functions, improve reaction time, decrease fatigue, and improve mood (102,104).
- Preexercise caffeine consumption (greater than 3 $mg \cdot kg^{-1}$) has been shown to enhance fat oxidation during exercise. This effect was dose-dependent and greater in untrained individuals versus trained athletes (102,105).
- Caffeine has been shown to increase strength, power, anaerobic effort, and speed (102,106).
- Caffeine has been shown to increase aerobic performance for endurance athletes and decrease time to exhaustion (102,107–110).
- Caffeine supplements are typically consumed 60 minutes preexercise. The source of the caffeine can affect optimal timing. Gels, mouth washes, and chews may require a shorter time period (102).
- Responses to caffeine differ among individuals due to varying abilities to metabolize caffeine: A single substitution in the CYP1A2 gene that codes for the protein, cytochrome P450 1A2, causes those persons to be slow caffeine metabolizers (102,111).
- Side effects from caffeine intake are dose-related, greater than 6 $mg \cdot kg^{-1}$ can cause multiple side effects, including insomnia, headaches, restlessness, nervousness, agitation, muscle twitching, tremors, gastric irritation, nausea, vomiting, heart palpitations, and tachycardia. Above 9 $mg \cdot kg^{-1}$ leads to even greater side effects (102).
- Tolerance to caffeine appears after 4–5 days of consecutive use.
- The Food and Drug Administration approved the addition of caffeine to soft drinks and limited the maximum caffeine content of cola-type soft drinks to 0.02% caffeine, or 71 mg per 12 oz of fluid (112).

Creatine

- Creatine is one of the supplements most widely used by athletes to increase muscle mass and enhance energy and athletic performance. Creatine monohydrate is the most commonly studied form of creatine (113).

- Creatine is a naturally occurring non–protein amino acid compound and member of the guanidine phosphagen family that is found in red meat and seafood (113).
- Approximately 95% of the body's total creatine content is located in skeletal muscles; a greater concentration is found in fast-twitch compared to slow-twitch muscle fibers (114–118).
- The other 5% is found in the brain and testes (113).
- Creatine exists in one of two forms in the body: free creatine (~33%), and a phosphorylated form, creatine phosphate (~67%) (115,117).
- The upper limit of creatine storage is about 160 mmol · kg^{-1} of dry muscle mass (113).
- The body needs to take about 1–3 g of creatine per day to maintain normal creatine stores. Supplementation with creatine serves to increase muscle creatine and creatine phosphate by 20%–40% (113).
- Creatine phosphate (CP) is the energy reservoir that provides rapid phosphate-bond energy to resynthesize ATP from ADP and phosphate.
- Literature shows 0.3 g · kg^{-1} of creatine is a safe and effective dose to maximize muscle creatine levels (119).
- Creatine has been shown to not cause renal dysfunction, muscle cramping, or gastrointestinal distress (113).
- Creatine in combination with carbohydrates and protein appears to increase muscular uptake of creatine (113).
- Creatine has been shown to increase lean muscle mass, anaerobic performance, and strength.
- Creatine has been shown to improve short-term memory (120).
- The typical washout period for creatine is 28–36 days (121).

Carnosine and β-Alanine

- Carnosine is one of the most abundant dipeptides found in skeletal muscle; it is synthesized from the amino acids L-histidine and β-alanine by carnosine synthase (122). β-Alanine is the rate-limiting factor, so increasing β-alanine increases the carnosine content of skeletal muscle (123).
- Carnosine is a major contributor to H^+ buffering during high-intensity exercise (124).
- Increasing muscle carnosine content (via β-alanine supplementation) can improve high-intensity exercise performance probably by reducing contractile fatigue or enhancing muscle-buffering capacity (122).
- Consuming 3.2 or 6.4 g of β-alanine (regardless of weight) has been shown to elevate muscle carnosine content by 42% and 64%, respectively (125).
- Discontinuation of β-alanine supplementation causes carnosine to washout at a rate of 2.5%–3.5% per week; an increase of 55% would require a washout period of about 15 weeks (126).
- β-alanine been shown to improve high-intensity exercise performance for exercise lasting over 60 seconds (124).

Branched Chain Amino Acids

- Branched-chain amino acids (BCAAs), which consist of the EAAs leucine, isoleucine, and valine, are metabolized in the muscle, rather than in the liver (127,128).
- BCAAs serve as precursors for the synthesis of other amino acids and proteins and as an energy substrate during exercise and periods of stress (22,127,129).
- BCAAs, in particular leucine, have anabolic effects on human skeletal muscle under resting conditions and during recovery from endurance events (22,130–132).
- BCAAs have been shown to aid in recovery by decreasing post-exercise muscle damage and soreness (22,132–134).
- Leucine, out of the 3 BCAAs, literature has shown to increase MPS, even without isoleucine and valine (22,134).

Antioxidants

- Antioxidants are substances that can slow down the oxidation of proteins, carbohydrates, lipids, and DNA. They are capable of inhibiting the oxidation of other molecules or delaying, preventing, or protecting cells from oxidative damage (135).
- There are 3 main categories. The first line of defense include substances such as superoxide dismutase, catalase, glutathione reductase, and minerals (selenium, copper, and zinc). The second line of defense include glutathione, Vit C, albumin, Vit E, carotenoids, and flavonoids. The third line of defense comprise enzymes that repair damaged DNA (21,136).
- Reactive oxygen species (ROS) are natural byproducts of cellular processes. During exercise, metabolism speeds up due to increased need for oxygen. This causes the release of highly reactive oxygen species from the mitochondria.
- Increased ROS can harm cells and contribute to muscle damage, fatigue, and immune problems. However, ROS also can have positive effects such as aiding in glycogen resynthesis, reducing risk of infection, and enhancing athletic performance through adaptive responses to training. Whether ROS are harmful or helpful depends on factors such as exercise duration, intensity, fitness level, and nutrition (21,137).
- There is some evidence that specific supplemental antioxidants, vitamin C, vitamin E, resveratrol, selenium, coenzyme Q10, Omega-3 fatty acids (DHA/EHA), and curcumin may decrease the damaging effects by scavenging ROS (21).

Sports Drinks

- Sport drinks are noncarbonated flavored liquids containing added sugars, minerals, and electrolytes to help maintain hydration and replenish the body during exercise. After exercise, they promote rehydration, replace electrolytes lost from sweating, and maximize muscle glycogen repletion (63,67,138–140).

- Excessive consumption of sports drinks has been associated with obesity, diabetes, cardiovascular disease, and dental caries — similar to other sweetened beverages such as fruit juices and soda (138–140).
- Sport drinks are not needed during exercise lasting less than 1 hour, and water should be the first choice in this case. Sports drinks are more important when exercising for extended periods of time, at high levels of intensity, particularly in hot and humid conditions (139).
- The ideal commercial fluid replacement beverage provides sodium, potassium, and CHO; recommended ranges for sodium and potassium are 20–30 mEq · L^{-1} (460–700 mg · L^{-1}) and 5–10 mEq · L^{-1} (200–390 mg · L^{-1}), respectively, to offset sweat losses and promote fluid absorption; the anion, chloride, is recommended because it optimizes fluid absorption. The optimal CHO range is 5%–10%, or 50–100 g · L^{-1} of fluid (47).

Energy Drinks

- Energy drinks are beverages promoted as being able to increase alertness, improve cognitive tasks, enhance athletic performance, and promote weight loss; they are not fluid-replacement beverages (141).
- Most energy drinks contain caffeine and a combination of other ingredients, including taurine, sucrose, guarana, ginseng, niacin, pyridoxine, glucuronolactone, and cyanocobalamin (141–143).
- Doses of caffeine in energy drinks range from 50 to 505 mg per can or bottle as compared to only 100 mg in a 6-oz cup of coffee (112).
- Some energy drinks are also sold in combination with a 10%–12% alcohol content; thus, it is essential to read the nutrition label before purchasing and/or consuming such products.
- Weekly or daily energy drink use is strongly associated with alcohol dependence (144).
- Consistent use of energy drinks can lead to tolerance and dependence due to the caffeine content. Because of the high glycemic carbohydrate content in energy drinks, they can lead to weight gain and negative impact on metabolic health (145,146).

Sport Bars

- Sport bars originated when it was shown that ultra-marathoners and other endurance athletes performed better when provided concentrated sources of easily absorbable CHO during long training and competitive events.
- Athletes use sport bars during training and competition to provide CHO and as recovery snacks to replete glycogen and restore protein balance.
- Athletes may also use carbohydrate gel, goo, and mouth rinses to provide CHO during long training endurance events.
- Sport bars should be ingested with fluids to enhance digestion and absorption of nutrients and should provide less than 100% of the DRI for vitamins and minerals.
- The CHO from sports bars is effectively oxidized during exercise and is a practical form of supplementation with other CHO forms (147).

SPECIAL POPULATION CONSIDERATIONS

Nutrition Considerations for the Vegetarian or Vegan Athlete

- 3.3% of Americans report being vegetarian. About 5% of high school students (grades 9–12) report being vegetarian. The overall prevalence of vegetarian athletes is unknown (148).
- There are several subsets of vegetarianism.
  - Lacto-vegetarian — eats dairy, but no red meat, poultry, fish, or eggs
  - Ovo-vegetarian — eats eggs, but no red meat, poultry, fish, or dairy
  - Pesco-vegetarian — eats fish, but no red meat, poultry, dairy, or eggs
  - Lacto-ovo-vegetarian — eats dairy and eggs, but no red meat, poultry, or fish
  - Vegan — eats only plant-based foods — no red meat, poultry, fish, dairy, or eggs
- Athletes who perform a vegetarian diet are at risk for having low intakes of iron, zinc, calcium, vitamin B12, and vitamin D (149–152).
- Athletes who perform a vegetarian diet are also at risk for deficiencies in protein, creatine, carnitine, EPA/DHA omega-3 fatty acids (148,152).
- Creatine has been shown to improve exercise performance in vegetarians to a greater extent than omnivores (153).
- Vegetarian and vegan athletes may need to supplement to meet their micronutrient needs of specific vitamins and minerals.
- Vegans within the general population consume 30% less protein when compared with omnivores (151).
- Females who follow a vegetarian diet may be at greater risk for lower BMD compared to female athletes who are omnivores (154).
- Female athletes who follow a vegetarian diet are at greater risk for low energy availability (155).
- Athletes following a vegan or vegetarian diet can meet their macronutrient needs with a carefully well thought out plan. They will just have to make smart food choices (150–152).

- With any sports nutrition plan, the quality of the macronutrient intake matters as much as the quantity of the macronutrient consumption, whether an omnivore or a vegetarian, because the quality affects nutrient density and micronutrient consumption.

Nutrition Considerations for the Athlete with Celiac Disease

- Approximately 1% of the population has active celiac disease. Females are 2.5 times more likely to have celiac disease (156).
- Athletes with celiac disease should seek CHO sources from beans, rice, nuts, potatoes, corn flour, and quinoa, as well as fruits and vegetables.
- Athletes with celiac disease should also increase caloric intake to balance the malabsorption issues (156).
- Supplementation in iron, calcium and vitamin D are important as athletes with celiac disease may be deficient in these (156).
- Other deficiencies in athletes with celiac disease can include vitamin B12, folic acid, zinc, and copper (156).

Nutrition Considerations for and the Injured Athlete

- Athletes recovering from injuries have greater protein requirements to aid in tissue repair and maintenance of lean body mass (LBM). Studies have shown an increased protein need of 2.0–3.0 mg · kg^{-1} to enhance recovery. Protein intake should be ingested every 3–4 hours throughout the day (38,39,157).
- Leucine, an EAA, has been shown to be an anabolic stimulus for MPS. Injured recovering athletes should aim for 2–3 g daily (38,39,157).
- HMB (hydroxy-methylbutyrate) supplementation has been shown to attenuate muscle breakdown in injured athletes (38,39).
- Supplementation with 2000–4000 mg of Omega-3 fatty acids has been shown to stimulate upregulation of MPS. Omega-3 fatty acids also increase anabolic sensitivity to amino acids and improve MPS (38,39).
- Creatine has been found to increase muscle mass recovery following injuries and to enhance bone remodeling for skeletal injuries (38,39,157).

REFERENCES

1. Taguchi M, Manore MM. Reexamining the calculations of exercise energy expenditure in the energy availability equation of free-living athletes. *Front Sports Act Living.* 2022;4:885631–5.
2. Aragon AA, Schoenfeld BJ, Wildman R, et al. International society of sports nutrition position stand: diets and body composition. *J Int Soc Sports Nutr.* 2017;14(14):16–9.
3. Schofield KL, Thorpe H, Sims ST. Resting metabolic rate prediction equations and the validity to assess energy deficiency in the athlete population. *Exp Physiol.* 2019;104(4):469–75.
4. Frankenfield D, Roth-Yousey L, Compher C. Comparison of predictive equations for resting metabolic rate in healthy nonobese and obese adults: a systematic review. *J Am Diet Assoc.* 2005;105(5):775–89.
5. Institute of Medicine. *Dietary Reference Intakes: Water, Potassium, Sodium, Chloride, and Sulfate.* Washington (DC): The National Academies Press; 2005. p. 618.
6. Gould RJ, Ridout AJ, Newton JL. Relative energy deficiency in sport (RED-S) in adolescents. a practical review. *Int J Sports Med.* 2023;44(4):236–46.
7. Calcagno M, Kahleova H, Alwarith J, et al. The thermic effect of food: a review. *J Am Coll Nutr.* 2019;38(6):547–51.
8. Sherman WM, Plyley MJ, Sharp RL, et al. Muscle glycogen storage and its relationship with water. *Int J Sports Med.* 1982;3(1):22–4.
9. Brooks GA. Cell-cell and intracellular lactate shuttles. *J Physiol.* 2009;587(pt. 23):5591–600.
10. Helge JW, Watt PW, Richter EA, Rennie MJ, Kiens B. Fat utilization during exercise: adaptation to a fat-rich diet increases utilization of plasma fatty acids and very low-density lipoprotein-triacylglycerol in humans. *J Physiol.* 2001;537(pt. 3):1009–20.
11. Brooks GA, Mercier J. Balance of carbohydrate and lipid utilization during exercise: the "crossover" concept. *J Appl Physiol.* 1994;76(6):2253–61.
12. Horowitz JF, Mora-Rodriguez R, Byerley LO, Coyle EF. Substrate metabolism when subjects are fed carbohydrate during exercise. *Am J Physiol.* 1999;276(5):E828–35.
13. Romijn JA, Coyle EF, Sidossis LS, Rosenblatt J, Wolfe RR. Substrate metabolism during different exercise intensities in endurance-trained women. *J Appl Physiol.* 2000;88(5):1707–14.
14. Sahlin K, Harris RC. Control of lipid oxidation during exercise: role of energy state and mitochondrial factors. *Acta Physiol.* 2008;194(4):283–91.
15. Katayama K, Goto K, Ishida K, Ogita F. Substrate utilization during exercise and recovery at moderate altitude. *Metabolism.* 2010;59(7):959–66.
16. Vitale K, Getzin A. Nutrition and supplement update for the endurance athlete: review and recommendations. *Nutrients.* 2019;11(1289):1–20.
17. Larson-Meyer DE, Woolf K, Burke L. Assessment of nutrient status in athletes and the need for supplementation. *Int J Sport Nutr Exerc Metab.* 2018;28(2):139–58.
18. Close GL, Kasper AM, Walsh NP, Maughan RJ. Food first but not always food only: recommendations for using dietary supplements in sport. *Int J Sport Nutr Exerc Metab.* 2022;32(5):371–386.
19. Bytomski JR. Fueling for performance. *Sports Health.* 2018;10(1):47–53.
20. Thomas DT, Erdman KA, Burke LM, American College of Sports Medicine. Joint position statement: nutrition and athletic performance. *Med Sci Sports Exerc.* 2016;48(3):543–68.
21. Clemente-Suarez VJ, Mielgo-Ayuso J, Martin-Rodriguez A, Ramos-Camp DJ, Redondo-Florez L, Tornero-Aguilera JF. The burden of carbohydrates in health and disease. *Nutrients.* 2022;14:1–28.
22. Jager R, Kerksick CM, Campbell BI, et al. International Society of Sports Nutrition position stand: protein and exercise. *J Int Soc Sports Nutr.* 2017;14(14):20–5.
23. Phillips SM. Dietary protein requirements and adaptive advantages in athletes. *Br J Nutr.* 2012;108(suppl 2):S158–67.
24. Bagheri R, Shakibaee A, Camera DM, et al. Effects of 8 weeks of resistance training in combination with a high protein diet on body composition, muscular performance, and markers of liver and kidney function in untrained older ex-military men. *Front Nutr.* 2023;10:1205310–4.

25. Longland TM, Oikawa SY, Mitchell CJ, Devries MC, Phillips SM. Higher compared with lower dietary protein during an energy deficit combined with intense exercise promotes greater lean mass gain and fat mass loss: a randomized trial. *Am J Clin Nutr.* 2016;103(3):738–46.
26. Hector AJ, Phillips SM. Protein recommendations for weight loss in elite athletes: a focus on body composition and performance. *Int J Sport Nutr Exerc Metab.* 2018;28(2):170–7.
27. Antonio J, Ellerbroek A, Silver T, Vargas L, Peacock C. The effects of a high protein diet on indices of health and body composition – A crossover trial in resistance-trained men. *J Int Soc Sports Nutr.* 2016;13(3):3–7.
28. Antonio J, Candow DG, Forbes SC, Ormsbee MJ, Saracino PG, Roberts J. Effects of dietary protein on body composition in exercising individuals. *Nutrients.* 2020;12(6):1890.
29. Børsheim E, Tipton KD, Wolf SE, Wolfe RR. Essential amino acids and muscle protein recovery from resistance exercise. *Am J Physiol Endocrinol Metab.* 2002;283(4):E648–E57.
30. Fujita S, Dreyer HC, Drummond MJ, et al. Nutrient signalling in the regulation of human muscle protein synthesis. *J Physiol.* 2007;582 (Pt 2):813–23.
31. Potgieter S. Sport nutrition: a review of the latest guidelines for exercise and sport nutrition for the American College of Sport Nutrition, the International Olympic Committee and the International Society of Sports Nutrition. *South Afr J Clin Nutr.* 2013;26:6–16.
32. Burke LM, Hawley JA. Effects of short-term fat adaptation on metabolism and performance of prolonged exercise. *Med Sci Sports Exerc.* 2002;34(9):1492–8.
33. Helge JW. Adaptation to a fat-rich diet: effects on endurance performance in humans. *Sports Med.* 2000;30(5):347–57.
34. Helge JW. Long-term fat diet adaptation effects on performance, training capacity, and fat utilization. *Med Sci Sports Exerc.* 2002;34(9):1499–504.
35. Noakes T, Volek JS, Phinney SD. Low-carbohydrate diets for athletes: what evidence? *Br J Sports Med.* 2014;48(14):1077–8.
36. Macedo RCO, Santos HO, Tinsley GM, Reischak-Oliveira A. Low-carbohydrate diets: effects on metabolism and exercise – A comprehensive literature review. *Clin Nutr ESPEN.* 2020;40(40):17–26.
37. Jeromson S, Gallagher IJ, Galloway SDR, Hamilton DL. Omega-3 fatty acids and skeletal muscle health. *Mar Drugs.* 2015;13(11):6977–7004.
38. Smith-Ryan AE, Hirsch KR, Saylor HE, Gould LM, Blue MNM. Nutritional considerations and strategies to facilitate injury recovery and rehabilitation. *J Athl Train.* 2020;55(9):918–30.
39. Papadopoulou SK. Rehabilitation nutrition for injury recovery of athletes: the role of macronutrient intake. *Nutrients.* 2020;12(8):2449.
40. Kyriakidou Y, Wood C, Ferrier C, Dolci A, Elliott B. The effect of omega-3 polyunsaturated fatty acid supplementation on exercise-induced muscle damage. *J Int Soc Sports Nutr.* 2021;18(1):9.
41. Thielecke F, Blannin A. Omega-3 fatty acids for sports performance – are they equally beneficial for athletes and amateurs? A narrative review. *Nutrients.* 2020;12:1–28.
42. Gammone MA, Riccioni G, Parrinello G, D'Orazio N. Omega-3 polyunsaturated fatty acids: benefits and endpoints in sport. *Nutrients.* 2018;11(1):46.
43. Rawson ES, Miles MP, Larson-Meyer DE. Dietary supplements for health, adaptation, and recovery in athletes. *Int J Sport Nutr Exerc Metab.* 2018;28(2):188–99.
44. Peeling P, Sim M, McKay AK. Considerations for the consumption of vitamin and mineral supplements in athlete populations. *Sports Med.* 2023;53(suppl 1):15–24.
45. Bielik V, Kolisek M. Bioaccessibility and bioavailability of minerals in relation to a healthy gut microbiome. *Int J Mol Sci.* 2021;22(13):6803–18.
46. Barone M, D'Amico F, Brigidi P, Turroni S. Gut microbiome-micronutrient interaction: the key to controlling the bioavailability of minerals and vitamins?. *Biofactors.* 2022;48(2):307–14.
47. American College of Sports Medicine, Sawka MN, Burke LM, Eichner ER, Maughan RJ, Montain SJ, Stachenfeld NS. American College of Sports Medicine position stand. Exercise and fluid replacement. *Med Sci Sports Exerc.* 2007;39(2):377–90.
48. Ayotte D Jr, Corcoran MP. Individualized hydration plans improve performance outcomes for collegiate athletes engaging in in-season training. *J Int Soc Sports Nutr.* 2018;15(1):27.
49. McDermott BP, Anderson SA, Armstrong LE, et al. National athletic Trainers' association position statement: fluid replacement for the physically active. *J Athl Train.* 2017;52(9):877–95.
50. Nuccio RP, Barnes KA, Carter JM, Baker LB. Fluid balance in team sport athletes and the effect of hypohydration on cognitive, technical, and physical performance. *Sports Med.* 2017;47(10):1951–82.
51. Carlton A, Orr RM. The effects of fluid loss on physical performance: a critical review. *J Sport Health Sci.* 2015 Dec;4(4):357–63.
52. Belval LN, Hosokawa Y, Casa DJ, et al. Practical hydration solutions for sports. *Nutrients.* 2019;11(7):1550.
53. Munoz CX, Johnson EC, Demartini JK, et al. Assessment of hydration biomarkers including salivary osmolality during passive and active dehydration. *Eur J Clin Nutr.* 2013;67(12):1257–63.
54. Cheuvront SN, Ely BR, Kenefick RW, Sawka MN. Biological variation and diagnostic accuracy of dehydration assessment markers. *Am J Clin Nutr.* 2010;92(3):565–73.
55. Widjaja A, Morris RJ, Levy JC, Frayn KN, Manley SE, Turner RC. Within- and between-subject variation in commonly measured anthropometric and biochemical variables. *Clin Chem.* 1999;45(4):561–6.
56. Perrier E, Demazieres A, Girard N, et al. Circadian variation and responsiveness of hydration biomarkers to changes in daily water intake. *Eur J Appl Physiol.* 2013;113(8):2143–51.
57. McKenzie AL, Munoz CX, Armstrong LE. Accuracy of urine color to detect equal to or greater than 2% body mass loss in men. *J Athl Train.* 2015;50(12):1306–9.
58. Armstrong LE, Ganio MS, Klau JF, Johnson EC, Casa DJ, Maresh CM. Novel hydration assessment techniques employing thirst and a water intake challenge in healthy men. *Appl Physiol Nutr Metabol.* 2014;39(2):138–44.
59. Burchfield JM, Ganio MS, Kavouras SA, et al. 24-h void number as an indicator of hydration status. *Eur J Clin Nutr.* 2015;69(5):638–41.
60. American Dietetic Association, Dietitians of Canada, American College of Sports Medicine, Rodriguez NR, Di Marco NM, Langley S. American College of Sports Medicine position stand. Nutrition and athletic performance. *Med Sci Sports Exerc.* 2009;41(3):709–31.
61. Burke L. Fasting and recovery from exercise. *Br J Sports Med.* 2010;44(7):502–8.
62. von Duvillard SP, Arciero PJ, Tietjen-Smith T, Alford K. Sports drinks, exercise training, and competition. *Curr Sports Med Rep.* 2008;7(4): 202–8.
63. Montain SJ. Hydration recommendations for sport 2008. *Curr Sports Med Rep.* 2008;7(4):187–92.
64. Noakes TD. Hydration in the marathon: using thirst to gauge safe fluid replacement. *Sports Med.* 2007;37(4–5):463–6.
65. Ivy J, Portman R. *Nutrient Timing: The Future of Sports Nutrition.* Laguna Beach, CA: Basic Health Publications, Inc; 2004. 224 p.
66. Kerksick CM, Arent S, Schoenfeld BJ, et al. International Society of Sports Nutrition position stand: nutrient timing. *J Int Soc Sports Nutr.* 2017;14(14):33–21.
67. Mondazzi L, Arcelli E. Glycemic index in sport nutrition. *J Am Coll Nutr.* 2009;28(suppl l):455S–63S.

68. Jentjens RL, Cale C, Gutch C, Jeukendrup AE. Effects of pre-exercise ingestion of differing amounts of carbohydrate on subsequent metabolism and cycling performance. *Eur J Appl Physiol.* 2003;88(4–5):444–52.
69. Moseley L, Lancaster GI, Jeukendrup AE. Effects of timing of pre-exercise ingestion of carbohydrate on subsequent metabolism and cycling performance. *Eur J Appl Physiol.* 2003;88(4–5):453–8.
70. Rodriguez NR, DiMarco NM, Langley S, American Dietetic Association, Dietitians of Canada, American College of Sports Medicine: Nutrition and Athletic Performance. Position of the American Dietetic Association, Dietitians of Canada, and the American College of Sports Medicine: nutrition and athletic performance. *J Am Diet Assoc.* 2009;109(3):509–27.
71. Wilkinson K, Koscien CP, Monteyne AJ, Wall BT, Stephens FB. Association of postprandial postexercise muscle protein synthesis rates with dietary leucine: a systematic review. *Physiol Rep.* 2023;11(15):e15775.
72. Lam FC, Bukhsh A, Rehman H, et al. Efficacy and safety of whey protein supplements on vital sign and physical performance among athletes: a network meta-analysis. *Front Pharmacol.* 2019 April;10(10):317.
73. West DWD, Sawan SA, Mazzulla M, Williamson E, Moore DR. Whey protein supplementation enhances whole body protein metabolism and performance recovery after resistance exercise: a double-blind crossover study. *Nutrients.* 2017;9(735):1–18.
74. Phillips SM, Hartman JW, Wilkinson SB. Dietary protein to support anabolism with resistance exercise in young men. *J Am Coll Nutr.* 2005;24(2):134S–9S.
75. Kreider RB, Earnest CP, Lundberg J, et al. Effects of ingesting protein with various forms of carbohydrate following resistance-exercise on substrate availability and markers of anabolism, catabolism, and immunity. *J Int Soc Sports Nutr.* 2007;4(18):18–11.
76. Li L, Wong SHS, Sun FH. Effects of protein addition to carbohydrate-electrolyte solutions on post-exercise rehydration. *J Exerc Sci Fit.* 2015;13(1):8–15.
77. Saunders MJ, Kane MD, Todd MK. Effects of a carbohydrate-protein beverage on cycling endurance and muscle damage. *Med Sci Sports Exerc.* 2004;36(7):1233–8.
78. Fedewa MV, Spencer SO, Williams TD, Becker ZE, Fuqua CA. Effect of branched-chain amino acid supplementation on muscle soreness following exercise: a meta-analysis. *Int J Vitam Nutr Res.* 2019;89(5–6):348–56.
79. Kreider RB. Dietary supplements and the promotion of muscle growth with resistance exercise. *Sports Med.* 1999;27(2):97–110.
80. Howarth KR, Moreau NA, Phillips SM, Gibala MJ. Coingestion of protein with carbohydrate during recovery from endurance exercise stimulates skeletal muscle protein synthesis in humans. *J Appl Physiol.* 2009;106(4):1394–402.
81. Hulmi JJ, Lockwood CM, Stout JR. Effect of protein/essential amino acids and resistance training on skeletal muscle hypertrophy: a case for whey protein. *Nutr Metab.* 2010;7(7):51–11.
82. Koopman R, Wagenmakers AJ, Manders RJ, et al. Combined ingestion of protein and free leucine with carbohydrate increases postexercise muscle protein synthesis in vivo in male subjects. *Am J Physiol Endocrinol Metab.* 2005;288(4):E645–53.
83. Nielsen LLK, Lambert MNT, Jeppesen PB. The effect of ingesting carbohydrate and proteins on athletic performance: a systematic review and meta-analysis of randomized controlled trials. *Nutrients.* 2020;12(1483):1–19.
84. Reis CEG, Loureiro LMR, Roschel H, da Costa THM. Effects of pre-sleep protein consumption on muscle-related outcomes – A systematic review. *J Sci Med Sport.* 2021;24(2):177–82.
85. Jenkins DJ, Wolever TM, Taylor RH, et al. Glycemic index of foods: a physiological basis for carbohydrate exchange. *Am J Clin Nutr.* 1981;34(3):362–6.
86. Wong SH, Chan OW, Chen YJ, Hu HL, Lam CW, Chung PK. Effect of preexercise glycemic-index meal on running when CHO-electrolyte solution is consumed during exercise. *Int J Sport Nutr Exerc Metab.* 2009;19(3):222–42.
87. Andrews JL, Sedlock DA, Flynn MG, Navalta JW, Ji H. Carbohydrate loading and supplementation in endurance-trained women runners. *J Appl Physiol.* 2003;95(2):584–90.
88. McLay RT, Thomson CD, Williams SM, Rehrer NJ. Carbohydrate loading and female endurance athletes: effect of menstrual-cycle phase. *Int J Sport Nutr Exerc Metab.* 2007;17(2):189–205.
89. Burke LM. New issues in training and nutrition: train low, compete high?. *Curr Sports Med Rep.* 2007;6(3):137–8.
90. Burke LM. Fueling strategies to optimize performance: training high or training low? *Scand J Med Sci Sports.* 2010;20(suppl 2):48–58.
91. Havemann L, West SJ, Goedecke JH, et al. Fat adaptation followed by carbohydrate loading compromises high-intensity sprint performance. *J Appl Physiol.* 2006;100(1):194–202.
92. Hulston CJ, Venables MC, Mann CH, et al. Training with low muscle glycogen enhances fat metabolism in well-trained cyclists. *Med Sci Sports Exerc.* 2010;42(11):2046–55.
93. Yeo WK, Lessard SJ, Chen ZP, et al. Fat adaptation followed by carbohydrate restoration increases AMPK activity in skeletal muscle from trained humans. *J Appl Physiol.* 2008;105(5):1519–26.
94. Volek JS, Quann EE, Forsythe CE. Low-carbohydrate diets promote a more favorable body composition than low-fat diets. *Strength Cond J.* 2010;32(1):42–7.
95. Kerksick CM, Wilborn CD, Roberts MD, et al. ISSN exercise & sports nutrition review update: research and recommendations. *J Int Soc Sports Nutr.* 2018;15(1):1–57.
96. European Food Safety Authority. *Overview on Tolerable Upper Intake Levels as Derived by the Scientific Committee on Food (SCF) and the EFSA Panel on Dietetic Products, Nutrition and Allergies*; 2018. Version 4. September 2018.
97. Campbell B, Kreider RB, Ziegenfuss T, et al. International Society of Sports Nutrition position stand: protein and exercise. *J Int Soc Sports Nutr.* 2007;4:8.
98. Lemon PW, Berardi JM, Noreen EE. The role of protein and amino acid supplements in the athlete's diet: does type or timing of ingestion matter? *Curr Sports Med Rep.* 2002;1(4), 214–21.
99. Manninen AH. Protein hydrolysates in sports nutrition. *Nutr Metab.* 2009;6(6):38.
100. Tang JE, Moore DR, Kujbida GW, Tarnopolsky MA, Phillips SM. Ingestion of whey hydrolysate, casein, or soy protein isolate: effects on mixed muscle protein synthesis at rest and following resistance exercise in young men. *J Appl Physiol.* 2009;107(3):987–92.
101. Ganio MS, Klau JF, Casa DJ, Armstrong LE, Maresh CM. Effect of caffeine on sport-specific endurance performance: a systematic review. *J Strength Cond Res.* 2009;23(1):315–24.
102. Guest NS, VanDusseldorp TA, Nelson MT, et al. International society of sports nutrition position stand: caffeine and exercise performance. *J Int Soc Sports Nutr.* 2021;18(1):1–37.
103. Burke LM. Caffeine and sports performance. *Appl Physiol Nutr Metabol.* 2008;33(6):1319–34.
104. Calvo JL, Fei X, Dominguez R, Pareja-Galeano H. Caffeine and cognitive functions in sports: a systematic review and meta-analysis. *Nutrients.* 2021;13(3):1–17.
105. Collado-Mateo D, Lavin-Perez AM, Merellano-Navarro E, Coso JD. Effect of acute caffeine intake on the fat oxidation rate during

exercise: a systematic review and meta-analysis. *Nutrients.* 2020; 12(12):3603.

106. Grgic J, Trexler ET, Lazinica B, Pedsic Z. Effects of caffeine intake on muscle strength and power: a systematic review and meta-analysis. *J Int Soc Sports Nutr.* 2018;15(11):1–10.
107. Wang Z, Qiu B, Gao J, Del Coso J. Effects of caffeine intake on endurance running performance and time to exhaustion: a systematic review and meta-analysis. *Nutrients.* 2022;15(1):148–65.
108. Costill DL, Dalsky GP, Fink WJ. Effects of caffeine ingestion on metabolism and exercise performance. *Med Sci Sports.* 1978;10(3):155–8.
109. Graham TE, Hibbert E, Sathasivam P. Metabolic and exercise endurance effects of coffee and caffeine ingestion. *J Appl Physiol.* 1998;85(3):883–9.
110. Graham TE. Caffeine and exercise: metabolism, endurance, and performance. *Sports Med.* 2001;31(11):785–807.
111. Astorino TA, Roberson DW. Efficacy of acute caffeine ingestion for short-term high-intensity exercise performance: a systematic review. *J Strength Cond Res.* 2010;24(1):257–65.
112. Reissig CJ, Strain EC, Griffiths RR. Caffeinated energy drinks — A growing problem. *Drug Alcohol Depend.* 2009;99(1–3):1–10.
113. Kreider RB, Kalman DS, Antonio J, et al. International Society of Sports Nutrition position stand: safety and efficacy of creatine supplementation in exercise, sport, and medicine. *J Int Soc Sports Nutr.* 2017;14(14):18.
114. Bemben MG, Lamont HS. Creatine supplementation and exercise performance: recent findings. *Sports Med.* 2005;35(2):107–25.
115. Buford TW, Kreider RB, Stout JR, et al. International Society of Sports Nutrition position stand: creatine supplementation and exercise. *J Int Soc Sports Nutr.* 2007;4(6):6–8.
116. Clarkson PM. Antioxidants and physical performance. *Crit Rev Food Sci Nutr.* 1995;35(1–2):131–41.
117. Dechent P, Pouwels PJ, Wilken B, Hanefeld F, Frahm J. Increase of total creatine in human brain after oral supplementation of creatine-monohydrate. *Am J Physiol.* 1999;277(3):R698–704.
118. Demant TW, Rhodes EC. Effects of creatine supplementation on exercise performance. *Sports Med.* 1999;28(1):49–60.
119. Poortmans JR, Rawson ES, Burke LM, Stear SJ, Castell LM. A-Z of nutritional supplements: dietary supplements, sports nutrition foods and ergogenic aids for health and performance. Part 11. *Br J Sports Med.* 2010;44(10):765–6.
120. Avgerinos KI, Spyrou N, Bougioukas KI, Kapogiannis D. Effects of creatine supplementation on cognitive function of healthy individuals: a systematic review of randomized controlled trials. *Exp Gerontol.* 2018;108:166–73.
121. Hultman E, Söderlund K, Timmons JA, Cederblad G, Greenhaff PL. Muscle creatine loading in men. *J Appl Physiol.* 1996;81(1):232–7.
122. Derave W, Everaert I, Beeckman S, Baguet A. Muscle carnosine metabolism and beta-alanine supplementation in relation to exercise and training. *Sports Med.* 2010;40(3):247–63.
123. Derave W, Ozdemir MS, Harris RC, et al. beta-Alanine supplementation augments muscle carnosine content and attenuates fatigue during repeated isokinetic contraction bouts in trained sprinters. *J Appl Physiol.* 2007;103(5):1736–43.
124. Hobson RM, Saunders B, Ball G, Harris RC, Sale C. Effects of β-alanine supplementation on exercise performance: a meta-analysis. *Amino Acids.* 2012;43(1):25–37.
125. Harris RC, Tallon MJ, Dunnett M, et al. The absorption of orally supplied beta-alanine and its effect on muscle carnosine synthesis in human vastus lateralis. *Amino Acids.* 2006;30(3):279–89.
126. Baguet A, Reyngoudt H, Pottier A, et al. Carnosine loading and washout in human skeletal muscles. *J Appl Physiol.* 2009;106(3):837–42.
127. Platell C, Kong SE, McCauley R, Hall JC. Branched-chain amino acids. *J Gastroenterol Hepatol.* 2000;15(7):706–17.
128. Khemtong C, Kuo C, Chen C, Jaime SJ, Condello G. Does BCAAs supplementation attenuate muscle damage markers and soreness after resistance exercise in trained males? A meta-analysis of randomized controlled trials. *Nutrients.* 2021;13(6):1–14.
129. Foure A, Bendahan D. Is branched-chain amino acids supplementation an efficient nutritional strategy to alleviate skeletal muscle damage? A systematic review. *Nutrients.* 2017;9(10):1047.
130. Blomstrand E, Saltin B. BCAA intake affects protein metabolism in muscle after but not during exercise in humans. *Am J Physiol Endocrinol Metab.* 2001;281(2):E365–74.
131. Burke LM, Castell LM, Stear SJ, et al. BJSM reviews: A-Z of nutritional supplements. Dietary supplements, sports nutrition foods and ergogenic aids for health and performance. Part 4. *Br J Sports Med.* 2009;43(14):1088–90.
132. Tipton KD, Wolfe RR. Protein and amino acids for athletes. *J Sports Sci.* 2004;22(1):65–79.
133. Martinho DV, Nobari H, Faria A, Field A, Duarte D, Sarmento H. Oral branched-chain amino acids supplementation in athletes: a systematic review. *Nutrients.* 2022;14(19):4002–4016.
134. Plotkin DL, Delcastillo K, Van Every DW, Tipton KD, Aragon AA, Schoenfeld BJ. Isolated leucine and branched-chain amino acid supplementation for enhancing muscular strength and hypertrophy: a narrative review. *Int J Sport Nutr Exerc Metab.* 2021;31(3): 292–301.
135. Halliwell B. Biochemistry of oxidative stress. *Biochem Soc Trans.* 2007;35(pt. 5):1147–50.
136. Pisoschi AM, Pop A. The role of antioxidants in the chemistry of oxidative stress: a review. *Eur J Med Chem.* 2015;97(97):55–74.
137. De Sousa CV, Sales MM, Rosa TS, Lewis JE, de Andrade RV, Simões HG. The antioxidant effect of exercise: a systematic review and meta-analysis. *Sports Med.* 2017;47(2):277–93.
138. Galemore CA. Sports drinks and energy drinks for children and adolescents – are they appropriate? A summary of the clinical report. *NASN Sch Nurse.* 2011;26:320–1.
139. Munoz-Urtubia N, Vega-Munoz A, Estrada-Munoz C, Salazar-Sepulveda G, Contreras-Barraza N, Castillo D. Healthy behavior and sports drinks: a systematic review. *Nutrients.* 2023;15(13):1–14.
140. Schneider MB, Benjamin HJ, Bhatia JJS, Committee on Nutrition and the Council on Sports Medicine and Fitness, et al. Sports drinks and energy drinks for children and adolescents. Are they appropriate? *Pediatrics.* 2011;127:1182–9.
141. Duchan E, Patel ND, Feucht C. Energy drinks: a review of use and safety for athletes. *Phys Sportsmed.* 2010;38(2):171–9.
142. Ballard SL, Wellborn-Kim JJ, Clauson KA. Effects of commercial energy drink consumption on athletic performance and body composition. *Phys Sportsmed.* 2010;38(1):107–17.
143. O'Brien MC, McCoy TP, Rhodes SD, Wagoner A, Wolfson M. Caffeinated cocktails: energy drink consumption, high-risk drinking, and alcohol-related consequences among college students. *Acad Emerg Med.* 2008;15(5):453–60.
144. Arria AM, Caldeira KM, Kasperski SJ, Vincent KB, Griffiths RR, O'Grady KE. Energy drink consumption and increased risk for alcohol dependence. *Alcohol Clin Exp Res.* 2011;35(2):365–75.
145. Jagim AR, Harty PS, Tinsley GM, et al. International society of sports nutrition position stand: energy drinks and energy shots. *J Int Soc Sports Nutr.* 2023;20(1):1–72.
146. Gutierrez-Hellin J, Varillas-Delgado D. Energy drinks and sports performance, cardiovascular risk, and genetic associations; future prospects. *Nutrients.* 2021;13(3):715–28.

147. Pfeiffer B, Stellingwerff T, Zaltas E, Jeukendrup AE. Oxidation of solid versus liquid CHO sources during exercise. *Med Sci Sports Exerc.* 2010;42(11):2030–7.
148. Vitale K. Update on vegetarian and vegan athletes: a review. *J Phys Fit Sports Med.* 2021;10(1):1–11.
149. Rosdiana DS. Vegetarian diet among athletes on nutrient adequacy and performance: literature review. *J Appl Food Nutr.* 2022;3(1):1–11.
150. Rogerson D. Vegan diets: practical advice for athletes and exercisers. *J Int Soc Sports Nutr.* 2017;14(14):36.
151. West S, Monteyne AJ, van der Heijden I, Stephens FB, Wall BT. Nutritional considerations for the vegan athlete. *Adv Nutr.* 2023;14(4):774–95.
152. Pohl A, Schunemann F, Bersiner K, Gehlert S. The impact of vegan and vegetarian diets on physical performance and molecular signaling in skeletal muscle. *Nutrients.* 2021;13(11):3884.
153. Kaviani M, Shaw K, Chilibeck PD. Benefits of creatine supplementation for vegetarians compared to omnivorous athletes: a systematic review. *Int J Environ Res Public Health.* 2020;17(9):3041–54.
154. Ma X, Tan H, Hu M, He S, Zou L, Pan H. The impact of plant-based diets on female bone mineral density. *Medicine.* 2021;100(46):1–10.
155. Cialdella-Kam L, Kulpins D, Manore M. Vegetarian, gluten-free, and energy restricted diets in female athletes. *Sports.* 2016;4(4):50–61.
156. Mancini LA, Trojian T, Mancini AC. Celiac disease and the athlete. *Curr Sports Med Rep.* 2011;10(2):105–8.
157. Tipton KD. Nutritional support for exercise-induced injuries. *Sports Med.* 2015;45(suppl 1):S93–104.

Exercise Prescription

13

Ravishankar E. Rao, Jeffrey Wisinski, and Mark B. Stephens

INTRODUCTION

- Nearly three-quarters (74%) of all Americans are either overweight or obese, an explosive increase that has unfolded over the last 30 years (1). Physical inactivity and obesity are correlated with increases in coronary heart disease, diabetes, certain cancers, and all-cause mortality. Lack of physical activity is also associated with osteoporosis, falls, and behavioral health issues, including depression (2). Sufficient physical activity protects against these conditions. Furthermore, obesity and physical activity are considered possible U.S. national security threats, with a lower percentage of the population meeting BMI and physical activity standards for eligibility (3) for military service.
- Guidelines from the Department of Health and Human Services (DHHS) and the American College of Sports Medicine (ACSM) recommend a minimum of 150 minutes of moderate activity per week (4) or 75 minutes of vigorous activity per week to obtain substantial health benefits (5). Guidelines further suggest that more extensive health benefits can be obtained with 300 minutes of moderate or 150 minutes of vigorous activity per week and explicitly recommend that adults also engage in muscle-strengthening activities on 2 or more days a week while spreading aerobic activity throughout the week. The ACSM guidelines additionally recommend flexibility exercises on 2 $d \cdot wk^{-1}$ to maintain joint range of motion, and neuromotor exercise training 2 to 3 $d \cdot wk^{-1}$ (coordinated exercises involving motor skills including balance, agility, and coordination) (4).
- Estimates from 2020 found that only 54% of U.S. adults meet the minimum recommendations from the DHHS for aerobic activity. These updated findings reflect benefits of all activity (however brief) by removing minimum duration of activity and focusing on cumulative physical activity time (6).
- From 1999 to 2016, obesity rates in adults went from 30% to 39%, and youth from 13% to 18% showing a sustained linear trend (6).
- Physical activity is one of the critically important Objective Topic Areas for Healthy People 2030 (7) the national effort to define public health priorities and goals for the United States. Multidisciplinary targets include the DHHS guidelines for physical activity (5) and the ACSM Position Stand on the Quantity and Quality of Exercise for Developing and Maintaining Cardiorespiratory, Musculoskeletal, and Neuromotor Fitness in Apparently Healthy Adults: Guidance for Prescribing Exercise (4).
- Health care professionals do a poor job recognizing, addressing, and documenting the physical activity needs of patients. National data show just 29% of patients with obesity are formally diagnosed with this medical condition, and just 18% receive weight loss counseling. Women and individuals with higher income and educational levels are more likely to receive counseling than others (8). Some physicians fail to include physical activity counseling as part of their routine practice, citing limitations in time, reimbursement, knowledge, and lack of practical tools (9).
- The 2022 U.S. Preventive Services Task Force (USPSTF) guidelines recommend that clinicians individualize the decision to refer adults without risk factors for cardiovascular disease to behavioral counseling as a way to promote a healthy diet and physical activity ("C" recommendation). In adult patients with risk factors for cardiovascular disease, the USPSTF recommends offering a referral for interventions to promote healthy diet and physical activity ("B" recommendation) (10).
- The ACSM strongly endorses interventions to increase physical activity for prevention of weight gain, for weight loss, and to maintain weight after previous weight loss (4,11).
- The American Medical Association calls for primary care physicians to assess lifestyle "vital signs" (including physical activity) and to collaboratively develop appropriate exercise prescriptions based on individual patient responses (12).
- The collaborative Exercise Is Medicine initiative (http://www.exerciseismedicine.org) encourages physicians to specifically include physical activity as part of their prescribing practices for the treatment and prevention of chronic disease (13). Guidelines for preexercise graded exercise testing are discussed in Chapter 24 (Exercise Stress Testing).

BENEFITS OF PHYSICAL ACTIVITY (5)

- Strong evidence indicates that physical activity decreases adult risk for:
  - Early death
  - Coronary heart disease

  - Stroke
  - Hyperlipidemia
  - High blood pressure
  - Type 2 diabetes
  - Cancer
  - Osteoporosis
- Strong evidence also suggests that physical activity helps with:
  - Prevention of weight gain
  - Weight loss (especially when combined with lower calorie intake)
  - Improved cardiorespiratory and muscular fitness (adults and children/adolescents)
  - Prevention of falls
  - Reduced depression
  - Better cognitive function in older adults
- Strong evidence links physical activity with favorable body composition, improved bone health, and improved cardiovascular and metabolic health markers in children and adolescents.
- Other benefits of physical activity for which there is moderate evidence include improved sleep quality and reduced risk for cancer, hip fracture, and abdominal obesity.
- Recent literature in light of the novel SARS-CoV-2 pandemic highlights the importance of exercise in overall immune response (beyond its significant role in reducing risk posted by metabolic syndrome). Active populations show increased immune response and immunovigilance as well as reduced pulmonary and tissue inflammatory damage during and post infection. In addition, improvements in immune competence and reduction in age-related senescence are seen in those who obtain adequate regular physical activity (14). Meeting basic physical activity guidelines on a regular basis was strongly associated with a reduced risk of severe COVID-19 outcomes among infected adults (15).

EXERCISE PRESCRIPTION: WHAT TO INCLUDE

- An exercise prescription (also referred to as an activity prescription) should include clear descriptions of the frequency, intensity, type, and duration (time) of activities that individuals should engage in to maximize health benefits. Providing these recommendations as a written prescription (as with other medical treatments) may help patient adherence.
- The mnemonic "FITT" (frequency, intensity, type, time) is a useful guide for clinicians working with patients to develop an individualized exercise prescription.
- Each exercise prescription should include specific recommendations for different physical activities (aerobic and muscle-strengthening) in the context of patient goals and preexisting health conditions.

Frequency

- Patients should accumulate a minimum of 150 minutes of moderate or 75 minutes of vigorous exercise every week to optimize health (5). For most patients, this can be accomplished with at least 30 minutes of moderate-intensity walking most (preferably all) days of the week (16,17). Newer activity guidelines emphasize the value of physical activity that accumulated throughout the week. Activity sessions that spread across the week may also help reduce the risk of injury. The ACSM Position Stand (4) recommends 30 minutes of moderate-intensity cardiorespiratory exercise 5 $d \cdot wk^{-1}$ (totaling 150 $min \cdot wk^{-1}$). An alternative is 20 or more minutes of vigorous-intensity exercise at least 3 $d \cdot wk^{-1}$ (totaling 75 $min \cdot wk^{-1}$).
- Adults should perform muscle-strengthening activities of moderate or high intensity involving all major muscle groups at least 2 $d \cdot wk^{-1}$ for additional health benefits (4,5).

Intensity

- There are many ways to prescribe exercise intensity. The intensity of each exercise session should be tailored to the individual's preexisting health and individual goals.
- Patients wishing to improve health and lower disease-specific risk should be aware that sufficient levels of physical activity can be accumulated through small bouts of activity throughout the day. A dedicated activity or training session is not necessary.
- The target heart rate is the most common method of prescribing exercise intensity. The training heart rate is based on an age-predicted maximal heart rate (APMHR; 220-patient age). Patients are instructed to exercise at a range of 40%–80% of the APMHR based on their specific goals.
- A modification of the target heart rate includes calculation of the heart rate reserve (HRR). This method takes into account the patient's resting heart rate (RHR). Moderate activities typically are performed at 40%–60% of the HRR, whereas vigorous activities are performed at 60%–90% of HRR. To calculate the target HR based on this method:

$$HRR = \{(220 - \text{patient age}) - HR_{resting}\}$$

$$HR_{target} = \{(HRR \times \text{training intensity}) + HR_{resting}\}$$

- The *talk test* is another safe and easy way to counsel individuals about exercise intensity. Patients should exercise at an intensity that allows them to carry out a conversation without undue shortness of breath.

Type

- The type of activity should be based on the individual's fitness level and interests.
- Activities involving repetitive movement of large muscle groups are most often recommended. Walking is the easiest activity for an exercise prescription. Non–weight-bearing

activities, such as swimming, rowing, and cycling, should be considered for individuals with orthopedic concerns.

- Engaging in activities that are enjoyable increases the likelihood of long-term adherence to an exercise routine.
- Examples of vigorous-intensity activities include running, jogging, swimming, tennis (singles), aerobic dancing, bicycling (>10 mph), jumping rope, and heavy gardening.
- Examples of typically moderate-intensity activities include walking briskly (>3 mph), water aerobics, bicycling (<10 mph), tennis (doubles), and ballroom dancing.

Duration (Time)

- Each individual bout of moderate- and vigorous-intensity exercise were initially recommended to be at least 10 minutes in duration; however, recent data have shown cumulative smaller bouts provide similar health benefits. A "move more, sit less" mindset is encouraged (5).
- One approach to meet the activity guidelines is to recommend 30 to 60 minutes of walking most if not all days of the week.
- It is important to help patients understand that while all activity is good, increasing levels of activity to 300 min · wk^{-1} or more has additional health benefits (colon and breast cancer risk reduction and prevention of unhealthy weight gain are two specific examples) (5).

EXERCISE PRESCRIPTION: BEYOND CARDIOVASCULAR ENDURANCE

- An exercise prescription should also include advice regarding muscular strength and endurance.
- The same FITT principle used to guide aerobic exercise prescriptions can be applied to muscular conditioning.
- **Frequency:** Activities focused on muscular strength should be performed at least two times per week (4,5).
- **Intensity:** To develop muscular strength, individuals should perform exercises using 60%–70% of the one-repetition maximum (1-RM) level of resistance (1-RM is the maximum amount of weight that an individual can lift one time using proper technique). To develop muscular endurance, an individual should perform exercises using lower resistance, typically 50% of the 1-RM. Increases in the amount of weight will result in stronger muscles (5).
- **Sets/repetitions:** For strength, two to three sets of 8–12 repetitions are recommended. For muscular endurance, two sets of 15–20 repetitions are recommended.
- **Type:** Muscular strength and endurance can be developed using either free weights or dedicated resistance machines. Household items such as rubber tubing can be used creatively as resistance training tools.
- **Duration (time):** Typically, two sets are performed for each muscular group. Rest for 2–3 minutes between sets. Rest for 48 hours between strength training sessions.

EXERCISE PRESCRIPTION: OVERCOMING BARRIERS TO ACTIVITY

- **Time:** Patients commonly cite lack of time as a significant barrier to physical activity. Small bouts of physical activity scattered through the day help overcome this barrier.
- **Convenience:** Lack of convenience is also cited as a common obstacle. Efforts to incorporate physical activity and exercise into normal routines help eliminate this barrier. Walking or biking to work is one example. Using public transportation in combination with walking or bicycling is another. Using available public facilities (parks, trails, courts, fields), particularly with an exercise partner, can also be helpful. Walking around the house (or office) and up/down stairs is convenient and can be done frequently throughout the day in most settings.
- **Family Responsibilities:** Serving as the primary caregiver and caring for children or grandchildren is a common activity that interferes with time for physical activity (18).
- **Poor Environmental Conditions:** Weather, poor physical conditions in neighborhoods, access to facilities, and crime are other obstacles (18).
- **Fatigue:** Although it is common for patients to suggest that they are "too tired to exercise," regular physical activity improves energy levels and can become self-sustaining.
- **Boredom:** Exercising with a friend or family member increases social support and accountability and reduces boredom. Choosing activities that are intrinsically fun can also help people overcome boredom.
- All these common barriers may be addressed by both creating environments where it is physically and socially easier for people to exercise and by allowing patients to come up with creative ways to overcome the barriers themselves (see motivational interviewing).

EXERCISE PRESCRIPTION: ASSESSING READINESS TO CHANGE

- Not all patients are immediately ready to engage in a program of increased physical activity. The likelihood of sustaining an active lifestyle can be quickly assessed using the stages-of-change (transtheoretical) model (19).

Precontemplation

- Individuals who are in the precontemplative stage have not seriously considered participating in regular physical activity. They perceive that the disadvantages of engaging in regular activity outweigh the benefits. These patients are unlikely to change their current pattern of behavior (19). Inform these patients about the risks associated with physical inactivity and encourage them to be more active.

Contemplation

- Patients who are in the contemplative stage are ready for an exercise prescription. They are actively thinking about making healthy changes. Steady encouragement with suggestions to overcome predictable barriers often helps move individuals in the contemplative stage toward action.

Preparation/Action

- Patients in this stage particularly benefit from an individualized exercise prescription. Set a start date for engaging in regular activity and discuss how to overcome day-to-day challenges. Offer encouragement and support and set specific follow-up dates to assess patient progress.

Maintenance

- Individuals in the maintenance stage have incorporated physical activity into their regular routine. The exercise prescription should be revised and updated periodically to ensure patients continue to maintain physically active behaviors. Offer ongoing praise and support.
- Most individuals who are successful at incorporating an exercise prescription into their routine lifestyle note progressing through predictable phases of *acclimation*, *improvement*, and *maintenance*.
  - **Acclimation:** This is the phase when patients are "getting used to" their new habits of activity. Acclimation typically lasts several weeks and can be the most psychologically challenging phase. Dropout rates are highest during the acclimation phase. Encourage patients to commit to the frequency of activity first, then to duration, and finally to intensity.
  - **Improvement:** Improvement occurs after patients have acclimated to regular activity. Patients experience predictable improvements in self-efficacy, physical fitness, and mood. The exercise prescription can be modified during the improvement phase to meet modified patient goals.
  - **Maintenance:** As patients establish patterns of regular physical activity, normal adaptations in heart rate, and exercise tolerance take place. This is a good time to update (or modify) the exercise prescriptions account for changes in cardiovascular conditioning and muscular performance.

EXERCISE PRESCRIPTION: RESOLVING AMBIVALENCE ABOUT CHANGE

- Motivational interviewing is a helpful technique to resolve ambivalence around health-related behaviors (20). Motivational interviewing is also helpful and effective for improving physical activity levels (4). Even brief motivational interviewing interventions in primary care clinics have a positive effect on exercise efforts (21). The key questions in motivational interviewing are: (a) Are you interested in making a behavioral change? (b) Are you able to make a behavioral change? (c) How important is the behavioral change to you? (d) How confident are you that you can make the necessary change? (e) What type of behavioral change do you think would work best for you? Patients who perceive behaviors as important and who are confident that they are able to make necessary changes are most likely to succeed (19).
- Other helpful tips for motivational counseling include (19,20):
  - Agenda Setting (asking permission to discuss)
  - Providing an accurate and empathetic style
  - Being collaborative (rather than authoritarian)
  - Listening to patient's reaction and then summarizing for them
  - Evoking the patient's own motivation (rather than trying to instill it)
  - Honoring patient autonomy

SUMMARY

- Exercise prescription is a cornerstone skill of the sports medicine provider.
- The American College of Sports Medicine (ACSM) has recently updated their signature resource on exercise testing and prescription. The updated 12th Edition provides authoritative summaries of recommended procedures for exercise testing and exercise prescription in both healthy populations and individuals with conditions or special considerations (22).

REFERENCES

1. Fryar CD, Carroll MD, Afful J. *Prevalence of Overweight, Obesity, and Severe Obesity Among Adults Aged 20 and over: United States, 1960–1962 Through 2017-2018*. NCHS Health E-Stats; 2020.
2. Remington PL, Brownson RC, Wegner MV. *Chronic Disease Epidemiology and Control*. 3rd ed. Washington (DC): American Public Health Association; 2010. 659 p.
3. Webber BJ, Bornstein DB, Deuster PA, et al. BMI and physical activity, military-aged U.S. Population 2015-2020. *Am J Prev Med*. 2023 Jan;64(1):66–75.
4. Garber CE, Blissmer B, Deschenes MR, et al. American College of Sports Medicine position stand. Quantity and quality of exercise for developing and maintaining cardiorespiratory, musculoskeletal, and neuromotor fitness in apparently healthy adults: guidance for prescribing exercise. *Med Sci Sports Exerc*. 2011;43(7):1334–59.
5. U.S. Department of Health and Human Services. *Physical Activity Guidelines for Americans*, 2nd ed [Internet]. Washington (DC): U.S. Department of Health and Human Services; 2018. [cited 2022 Nov 22]. 118 p. Available from: https://health.gov/sites/default/files/2019-09/Physical_Activity_Guidelines_2nd_edition.pdf.

6. Singh R, Pattisapu A, Emery MS. US Physical Activity Guidelines: current state, impact and future directions. *Trends Cardiovasc Med.* 2020;30(7):407–12.
7. *Healthy People 2030 Web site* [Internet]. Washington (DC): U.S. Department of Health and Human Services; [cited 2022 Nov 22]. Available from: http:www.healthypeople.gov
8. Greaney ML, Cohen SA, Xu F, Ward-Ritacco CL, Riebe D. Healthcare provider counselling for weight management behaviours among adults with overweight or obesity: a cross-sectional analysis of National Health and Nutrition Examination Survey, 2011–2018. *BMJ Open.* 2020;10(11):e039295. doi:10.1136/bmjopen-2020-039295
9. Meriwether RA, Lee JA, Lafleur AS, Wiseman P. Physical activity counseling. *Am Fam Physician.* 2008;77(8):1029–136, 1138.
10. *U.S. Preventive Services Task Force Web site* [Internet]. Rockville (MD): U.S. Preventive Services Task Force; [cited 2022 Nov 22]. Available from: http://www.uspreventiveservicestaskforce.org/draftrec.htm
11. Donnelly JE, Blair SN, Jakicic JM, et al. Position Stand: appropriate physical activity intervention strategies for weight loss and prevention of weight regain for adults. *Med Sci Sports Exerc.* 2009;41(2):459–71.
12. Lianov L, Johnson M. Physician competencies for prescribing lifestyle medicine. *JAMA.* 2010;304(2):202–3.
13. *Exercise Is Medicine Web site* [Internet]. Indianapolis (IN): American College of Sports Medicine; [cited 2022 Nov 22].Available from: http://www.exerciseismedicine.org
14. da Silveira MP, da Silva Fagundes KK, Bizuti MR, Starck É, Rossi RC, de Resende E Silva DT. Physical exercise as a tool to help the immune system against COVID-19: an integrative review of the current literature. *Clin Exp Med.* 2021 Feb;21(1):15–28. doi:10.1007/s10238-020-00650-3
15. Sallis R, Young DR, Tartof SY, et al. Physical inactivity is associated with a higher risk for severe COVID-19 outcomes: a study in 48 440 adult patients. *Br J Sports Med.* 2021 Oct;55(19):1099–l05.
16. Haskell WL, Lee IM, Pate RR, et al. Physical activity and public health: updated recommendation for adults from the American College of Sports Medicine and the American Heart Association. *Med Sci Sports Exerc.* 2007;39(8):1423–34.
17. U.S. Department of Health and Human Services. *Physical Activity and Health: A Report of the Surgeon General* [Internet]. Atlanta (GA): U.S. Department of Health and Human Services, Centers for Disease Control and Prevention, National Center for Chronic Disease Prevention and Health Promotion. 1996 [cited 2022 Nov 22]. 300 p. Available from: http://www.cdc.gov/nccdphp/sgr/pdf/sgrfull.pdf
18. Gothe NP, Kendall BJ. Barriers, motivations, and preferences for physical activity among female African American older adults. *Gerontol Geriatr Med.* 2016;2:2333721416677399.
19. Searight RH. Realistic approaches to counseling in the office setting. *Am Fam Physician.* 2009;79(4):277–84.
20. Miller WR, Rose GS. Toward a theory of motivational interviewing. *Am Psychol.* 2009;64(6):527–37.
21. Ang D, Kesavalu R, Lydon JR, Lane KA, Bigatti S. Exercise-based motivational interviewing for female patients with fibromyalgia: a case series. *Clin Rheumatol.* 2007;26(11):1843–9.
22. Ozemek C. *ACSM's Guidelines for Exercise Testing and Prescription,* 12th ed. Lippincott Williams and Wilkins; 2025 https://acsm.org/education-resources/books/guidelines-exercise-testing-prescription/

14 Playing Surface and Protective Equipment

Sara N. Raiser

PLAYING SURFACE

- In many sports, the athlete or event organizer has no choice with regard to playing surface as only one option exists; however, in some sports, different options offer their own advantages and disadvantages. These are addressed below.

Turf Sports

- Turf sports (*e.g.*, football, soccer, field hockey) may be played on either artificial turf or natural grass.
- First-generation artificial turf, AstroTurf, was introduced in the late 1960s and consisted of a dense short nylon fiber (<1.25 mm) carpet on top of the foam padding over soil. Second-generation artificial turf was developed in 1976 and incorporated a pad beneath a carpet of longer polyethylene fibers (40–70 mm) as well as silica sand infill. Third-generation artificial turf came about in 1997, layered with a base of gravel, asphalt, or concrete, an overlying shock-absorbing pad up to 25 mm thick, and the polyethylene fiber carpet with a rubber or combination of rubber and silica sand infill (1).
- Multiple studies have demonstrated no significant difference in overall injury incidence for soccer players when third-generation artificial turf is compared with natural grass (2–6).
- Evidence is sparse and less conclusive when comparing injury rates on third-generation artificial turf versus natural grass in American football. A 5-year study comparing injury rates in high school football players found a higher rate of injuries occurring during games played on third-generation turf (7). By contrast, a study involving National Collegiate Athletic Association (NCAA) Division I-A football players found a significantly lower overall incidence of injury on artificial turf (8).
- Although overall injury incidence may be comparable between third-generation turf and natural grass, injury patterns do differ. Injuries due to twisting or shearing mechanisms tend to occur more often on artificial turf, presumably due to the lack of ability to "divot" or damage the artificial turf to release a cleat in a potentially injurious situation (9–12).
- In a study evaluating NCAA American football players, artificial turf was associated with higher rates of posterior collateral ligament (PCL) injury. And specifically in lower divisions, there were higher rates of anterior collateral ligament (ACL) injury on artificial turf (13).
- Ankle ligament injuries in soccer players tend to be more prevalent and have been shown to be the most common season-ending injury on artificial turf (3). Two studies showed that ligamentous knee injuries are the most common season-ending injury for soccer players on natural grass (3,4), whereas a systematic review in 2022 revealed no difference in ACL injury rate in male soccer players when comparing artificial turf and natural grass, but an increased ACL injury rate in female soccer players on artificial turf (6).
- Concussion tends to occur more often on natural grass surfaces in competitive contact sports, most notably with rugby and American football (7,14).
- Certain types of minor injuries are exclusive to artificial turf. These include turf burns, abrasions associated with the surface. Artificial turf is slightly more likely to cause abrasions as compared to grass (7). In one study, college football players were seven times more likely to have a methicillin-resistant *Staphylococcus aureus* infection after acquiring turf burn (15).
- Temperatures on artificial turf can be significantly higher than grass (1).

Tennis

- Tennis is another sport with playing surface options, which include clay (slow), hard court (medium), and grass (fast).
- Hard courts are associated with greater stress on the lower extremities as a result of the reduced shock-absorption and increased traction between the shoe and court, which results in increased peak loads related to shorter stopping distances (16).
- With its energy-absorbing properties, clay is more forgiving to the upper extremities due to reduced ball speed (17).
- One study of recreational tennis players conducted by Pluim et al in the Netherlands demonstrated similar overall injury rates when several tennis court surfaces were compared: clay,

hard court, and artificial grass. Prevalence of lower extremity injuries related to overuse was higher on hard courts. And athletes who played on multiple court surfaces were more likely to experience overuse injuries (18).

Running

- When harder running surfaces such as asphalt or concrete are compared with softer surfaces such as grass or woodchips, increased forces on the lower extremity are associated with the harder surfaces (19–22), potentially contributing to increased impact-related overuse injury risk.
- Cambered surfaces affect joint kinetics and ground reaction forces and should be considered with regard to injury risk in athletes running on asphalt roads or concrete sidewalks (23).
- Treadmills provide the greatest shock absorption when mechanical properties are compared to other surfaces such as artificial turf, rubber track, concrete, and asphalt (24).

PROTECTIVE EQUIPMENT

- The purpose of protective equipment is to prevent injury and to protect injured areas from further injury. Sanctioning bodies (*e.g.*, the NCAA) of various sports have rendered certain protective equipment mandatory.

Football

- The NCAA mandates the use of a helmet, facemask, four- or six-point chin strap, mouthguard, shoulder pads, and hip, coccyx, thigh, and knee pads during football competition.
- The outer shell consists of polymer plastic, whereas the inner shell consists of pads, air- or fluid-filled cells, or a combination thereof.
- All football helmets in use at the high school or college level must meet National Operating Committee on Standards for Athletic Equipment (NOCSAE) specifications and, as of 2015, are certified through the third-party Safety Equipment Institute (SEI). This ensures that each helmet has been tested to withstand repeated blows of high mass and low velocity. A study by Cantu and Mueller attributed in large part a dramatic reduction in brain injury–related fatalities from football to the adoption of NOCSAE helmet standards (25). These standards went into effect in 1978 for colleges and in 1980 for high schools.
- Proper fitting of a helmet is ensured by the following criteria: the frontal crown of the helmet should sit approximately one to two fingerbreadths above the eyebrows; the back edge of the helmet should not impinge on the neck as it extends; when the head is held straight forward, an attempt to turn the helmet on the head should result in only a slight movement; jaw pads should fit the jaw area snugly to prevent lateral rocking of the helmet; the chin strap should fit snugly with equal tension on both sides; the hair should be cut as desired prior to fitting and kept the same length throughout the season.
- Mouthguards include stock, mouth-formed ("boil and bite"), and custom-made types. Ready-made stock mouthguards are the least comfortable and least protective type (26). Mouthguards have been required equipment for high school football players since 1962 and for their collegiate counterparts since 1973. Orofacial injuries have been reduced by more than half since the adoption of mouthguards for use in sport (27,28). There may be a role for mouthguards in concussion prevention; however, evidence has been conflicted (28,29).
- Two types of shoulder pads are in use: flat and cantilevered. Flat pads allow greater glenohumeral motion and are appropriate for limited contact positions, such as quarterbacks, receivers, and kickers. Cantilevered pads are named for the cantilever bridge that extends over the shoulder, dispersing impact force over a wider area. These pads offer greater protection to the shoulder area and are appropriate for the majority of players.
- A proper shoulder pad fit is achieved when the tip of the inner pad extends just past the lateral edge of the shoulder. The sternum and clavicles should be covered, and the flaps or epaulets should cover the deltoid.
- Controversy exists regarding the use of prophylactic knee braces in football. A study carried out at West Point (30) and another from the Big Ten Conference (31) showed a consistent trend toward a reduction of medial collateral ligament (MCL) injuries with the use of prophylactic braces. But a systematic review by Salata et al in 2010 reported that prophylactic knee bracing in American football has not successfully reduced MCL injuries (32). A systematic review by Tuang et al in 2023 suggested that ACL injury risk may be mitigated by the use of prophylactic bracing (33) although studies have had mixed results. Due to these inconsistent findings and the lack of demonstrated proof of efficacy, both the American Academy of Pediatrics and the American Academy of Orthopedic Surgeons have recommended against the routine use of prophylactic knee bracing in football as well as functional ACL bracing after primary isolated ACL reconstruction (34,35).
- Custom-fit functional ACL braces have not been shown to perform better or offer more protection than off-the-shelf braces (36,37).

Baseball/Softball

- The NCAA mandates the use of a double earflap helmet for all batters and base runners as well as a face mask and throat guard for catchers.
- Little League Baseball requires protective helmets for batters, catchers, base runners, first and third base coaches, and on-deck hitters.
- All helmets should meet NOCSAE standards to ensure strength and safety and bear a NOCSAE standard seal.

- Eye protection to reduce the risk of eye injury should be utilized. This includes helmet-mounted faceguards/visors for batters and base runners and protective eyewear for fielders. Baseball is a leading cause of sports-related eye injuries in youth.
- Breakaway bases are available, which can decrease sliding-associated injuries (38).

Ice Hockey

- The NCAA mandates the use of helmets with fastened chin straps, face masks, and a mouthguard.
- Shoulder pads, elbow pads, protective gloves, padded pants, athletic cup, and shin guards are also standard equipment.
- Neck or throat guard is also recommended for goalies.
- The use of full-face shields results in a significantly decreased risk of facial or dental injury (39). A systematic review found that face shields offer these protective benefits without increasing the incidence of head and neck injury (40). Full-face shields have been required for youth and high school since 1975 and mandated by the NCAA since 1980.
- It has been shown that prophylactic knee braces do not significantly reduce the incidence of knee injury among hockey players (41).

Lacrosse

- The NCAA requires the use of a helmet that meets NOCSAE specifications with full-face mask, chin pad, and cupped four-point chin strap, as well as mouthguard, protective gloves, athletic cup, and shoulder, elbow, and arm pads for all men's lacrosse players.
- Goalies are additionally required to wear chest protectors meeting NOCSAE specifications and throat protectors.
- For the NCAA women's lacrosse players, goalies must wear a helmet with a full-face mask and a chest protector and throat protector that meet NOCSAE standards; gloves and leg pads are also standard equipment. Field players must wear American Society for Testing and Materials (ASTM) women's lacrosse eye protectors. And, all players must wear a mouthguard.
- Although not a contact sport, headgear for high school girls' lacrosse field players was made available in 2017. This headgear is not required equipment in girls' lacrosse at this time, although it has been shown to reduce head impact severity (42).
- Many players also wear rib protector vests.

Racquet Sports

- Players are required to wear eye protection in any USA Racquetball or US Squash sanctioned event. Some clubs also require eye protection during racquet sports.
- Protective eyewear should meet ASTM and American National Standards Institute (ANSI) standards. Lenses should be composed of at least a 3-mm-thick polycarbonate plastic, which is shatter resistant.
- Lenses should be mounted in a nylon sports frame with a steep posterior lip and temples that rotate about 180°. When a lens in a sports frame is struck, it projects forward rather than backward and toward the eye.

Basketball

- Mouthguards are recommended, but not mandatory, to reduce the risk of dental trauma.
- Sport-related traumatic eye injuries are commonly seen in basketball players. Protective eyewear with shatterproof polycarbonate lenses should be considered; however, protective eyewear is currently not mandatory.
- High top basketball shoes have been shown not to reduce the incidence of ankle sprains during play based on one study (43).
- The use of a semirigid ankle stabilizing brace in basketball players does seem to reduce the incidence of ankle injury, but not the severity of such injuries (44,45).

Wrestling

- High school and the NCAA require the use of ear protectors, which protect wrestlers against the formation of auricular hematomas and the cosmetic deformity of cauliflower ear.
- It is recommended that all wrestlers use mouthguards.

Soccer

- Shin guards should be worn to reduce incidence of tibia and fibula fractures, as well as compartment syndrome from anterior leg contusions. Shin guards should protect the entire length of the tibia. They are mandated by the NCAA and must meet NOCSAE standards.
- Use of a semirigid ankle orthosis has been shown to decrease the incidence of recurrent ankle sprains in soccer players with history of sprains (45,46).
- Mouthguards are recommended, especially for goalkeepers.

SUMMARY

- Overall injury incidence appears to be similar when comparing natural grass and artificial turf; however, injury patterns do differ. Ligamentous injuries tend to be more common on artificial turf whereas concussions are more frequent on natural grass.
- Injury rates in tennis players tend to be higher on hard courts when compared to clay.
- Sports-related eye injuries are most common in basketball, baseball, and softball. Eye protection should be considered in these sports but is not mandatory. Eye protection is mandatory with play for sports such as ice hockey, both men's and women's lacrosse, racquetball, and squash.

- Helmets are required in sports such as football, ice hockey, and men's lacrosse. As of 2017, protective headgear is available for use in women's lacrosse but is not mandatory at this time.
- Mouthguards should be worn in any sport where orofacial trauma is common; however, mouthguards are only mandatory in some sports such as football, ice hockey, and men's lacrosse. There is inconsistent evidence that mouthguards may protect against concussion.

REFERENCES

1. Jastifer JR, McNitt AS, Mack CD, et al. Synthetic turf: history, design, maintenance, and athlete safety. *Sports Health.* 2019 Jan;11(1):84–90.
2. Aoki H, Kohno T, Fujiya H, et al. Incidence of injury among adolescent soccer players: a comparative study of artificial and natural grass turfs. *Clin J Sport Med.* 2010 Jan;20(1):1–7.
3. Ekstrand J, Timpka T, Hagglund M. Risk of injury in elite football played on artificial turf versus natural grass: a prospective two-cohort study. *Br J Sports Med.* 2006;40(12):975–80.
4. Fuller CW, Dick RW, Corlette J, Schmalz R. Comparison of the incidence, nature and cause of injuries sustained on grass and new generation artificial turf by male and female football players. Part 1: match injuries. *Br J Sports Med.* 2007 Aug 1;41(suppl 1):i20–6.
5. Steffen K, Andersen TE, Bahr R. Risk of injury on artificial turf and natural grass in young female football players. *Br J Sports Med.* 2007 Aug 1;41(suppl 1):i33–7.
6. Xiao M, Lemos JL, Hwang CE, Sherman SL, Safran MR, Abrams GD. Increased risk of ACL injury for female but not male soccer players on artificial turf versus natural grass: a systematic review and meta-analysis. *Orthop J Sports Med.* 2022 Aug 1;10(8):23259671221114353.
7. Meyers MC, Barnhill BS. Incidence, causes, and severity of high school football injuries on FieldTurf versus natural grass: a 5-year prospective study. *Am J Sports Med.* 2004 Oct;32(7):1626–38.
8. Meyers MC. Incidence, mechanisms, and severity of game-related college football injuries on FieldTurf versus natural grass: a 3-year prospective study. *Am J Sports Med.* 2010 Apr;38(4):687–97.
9. Dragoo JL, Braun HJ, Harris AHS. The effect of playing surface on the incidence of ACL injuries in National Collegiate Athletic Association American Football. *Knee.* 2013 Jun;20(3):191–5.
10. Hershman EB, Anderson R, Bergfeld JA, et al. An analysis of specific lower extremity injury rates on grass and FieldTurf playing surfaces in National Football League Games: 2000-2009 seasons. *Am J Sports Med.* 2012 Oct;40(10):2200–5.
11. Hunt KJ, George E, Harris AHS, Dragoo JL. Epidemiology of syndesmosis injuries in intercollegiate football: incidence and risk factors from National Collegiate Athletic Association injury surveillance system data from 2004-2005 to 2008-2009. *Clin J Sport Med.* 2013;23(4):278–82.
12. Kent R, Forman JL, Crandall J, Lessley D. The mechanical interactions between an American football cleat and playing surfaces *in-situ* at loads and rates generated by elite athletes: a comparison of playing surfaces. *Sports Biomech.* 2015 Jan 2;14(1):1–17.
13. Loughran GJ, Vulpis CT, Murphy JP, et al. Incidence of knee injuries on artificial turf versus natural grass in National Collegiate Athletic Association American Football: 2004-2005 through 2013-2014 seasons. *Am J Sports Med.* 2019 May;47(6):1294–301.
14. O' Leary F, Acampora N, Hand F, O' Donovan J. Association of artificial turf and concussion in competitive contact sports: a systematic review and meta-analysis. *BMJ Open Sport Exerc Med.* 2020 May;6(1):e000695.
15. Begier EM, Frenette K, Barrett NL, et al. A high-morbidity outbreak of methicillin-resistant *Staphylococcus aureus* among players on a college football team, facilitated by cosmetic body shaving and turf burns. *Clin Infect Dis.* 2004 Nov 15;39(10):1446–53.
16. Girard O, Eicher F, Fourchet F, Micallef JP, Millet GP. Effects of the playing surface on plantar pressures and potential injuries in tennis. *Br J Sports Med.* 2007 Nov 1;41(11):733–8.
17. Nicola T. Tennis. In: *The Team Physician's Handbook.* 2nd ed. Philadelphia (PA): Hanley & Belfus; 1997. p. 816–27.
18. Pluim BM, Clarsen B, Verhagen E. Injury rates in recreational tennis players do not differ between different playing surfaces. *Br J Sports Med.* 2018 May;52(9):611–5.
19. Boey H, Aeles J, Schütte K, Vanwanseele B. The effect of three surface conditions, speed and running experience on vertical acceleration of the tibia during running. *Sports Biomech.* 2017 Apr 3;16(2):166–76.
20. Hollis CR, Koldenhoven RM, Resch JE, Hertel J. Running biomechanics as measured by wearable sensors: effects of speed and surface. *Sports Biomech.* 2021 Jul 4;20(5):521–31.
21. Tessutti V, Trombini-Souza F, Ribeiro AP, Nunes AL, Sacco IDCN. In-shoe plantar pressure distribution during running on natural grass and asphalt in recreational runners. *J Sci Med Sport.* 2010 Jan;13(1):151–5.
22. Tessutti V, Ribeiro AP, Trombini-Souza F, Sacco ICN. Attenuation of foot pressure during running on four different surfaces: asphalt, concrete, rubber, and natural grass. *J Sports Sci.* 2012 Oct;30(14):1545–50.
23. Willwacher S, Fischer KM, Benker R, Dill S, Brüggemann G. Kinetics of cross-slope running. *J Biomech.* 2013 Nov;46(16):2769–77.
24. Colino E, Felipe JL, Van Hooren B, et al. Mechanical properties of treadmill surfaces compared to other overground sport surfaces. *Sensors.* 2020 Jul 9;20(14):3822.
25. Cantu RC, Mueller FO. Brain injury-related fatalities in American football, 1945-1999. *Neurosurgery.* 2003 Apr;52(4):846–53.
26. Newsome PRH, Tran DC, Cooke MS. The role of the mouthguard in the prevention of sports-related dental injuries: a review. *Int J Paediatr Dent.* 2001 Nov;11(6):396–404.
27. Knapik JJ, Marshall SW, Lee RB, et al. Mouthguards in sport activities: history, physical properties and injury prevention effectiveness. *Sports Med.* 2007;37(2):117–44.
28. Knapik JJ, Hoedebecke BL, Rogers GG, Sharp MA, Marshall SW. Effectiveness of mouthguards for the prevention of orofacial injuries and concussions in sports: systematic review and meta-analysis. *Sports Med.* 2019 Aug;49(8):1217–32.
29. Chisholm DA, Black AM, Palacios-Derflingher L, et al. Mouthguard use in youth ice hockey and the risk of concussion: nested case–control study of 315 cases. *Br J Sports Med.* 2020 Jul;54(14):866–70.
30. Sitler M, Ryan J, Hopkinson W, et al. The efficacy of a prophylactic knee brace to reduce knee injuries in football: a prospective, randomized study at West Point. *Am J Sports Med.* 1990 May;18(3):310–5.
31. Albright JP, Powell JW, Smith W, et al. Medial collateral ligament knee sprains in college football. Effectiveness of preventive braces. *Am J Sports Med.* 1994 Jan-Feb;22(1):12–8.
32. Salata MJ, Gibbs AE, Sekiya JK. The effectiveness of prophylactic knee bracing in American football: a systematic review. *Sports Health.* 2010 Sep;2(5):375–9.
33. Tuang BHH, Ng ZQ, Li JZ, Sirisena D. Biomechanical effects of prophylactic knee bracing on anterior cruciate ligament injury risk: a systematic review. *Clin J Sport Med.* 2023 Jan;33(1):78–89.
34. Martin T. American academy of pediatrics committee on sports medicine: knee brace use by athletes. *Pediatrics.* 1990;85(2):228.
35. American Academy of Orthopaedic Surgeons.*Management of Anterior Cruciate Ligament Injuries. Evidence-Based Clinical Practice Guideline* [Internet]. 2022. Available from: www.aaos.org/aclcpg

36. Wojtys E, Huston L. "Custom fit" versus "off the shelf" ACL functional braces. *Am J Knee Surg*. 2001;14(3):157–62.
37. Beynnon BD, Pope MH, Wertheimer CM, et al. The effect of functional knee-braces on strain on the anterior cruciate ligament in vivo. *J Bone Joint Surg Am*. 1992 Oct;74(9):1298–312.
38. Janda DH, Bir C, Kedroske B. A comparison of standard vs. breakaway bases: an analysis of a preventative intervention for softball and baseball foot and ankle injuries. *Foot Ankle Int*. 2001 Oct;22(10):810–6.
39. Benson BW, Mohtadi NG, Rose MS, Meeuwisse WH. Head and neck injuries among ice hockey players wearing full face shields vs half face shields. *JAMA*. 1999 Dec 22;282(24):2328–32.
40. Asplund C, Bettcher S, Borchers J. Facial protection and head injuries in ice hockey: a systematic review. *Br J Sports Med*. 2009 Dec 1;43(13):993–9.
41. Tegner Y, Lorentzon R. Evaluation of knee braces in Swedish ice hockey players. *Br J Sports Med*. 1991 Sep 1;25(3):159–61.
42. Caswell SV, Kelshaw PM, Lincoln AE, et al. The effects of headgear in high school girls' lacrosse. *Orthop J Sports Med*. 2020 Dec 1;8(12):2325967120969685.
43. Barrett JR, Tanji JL, Drake C, Fuller D, Kawasaki RI, Fenton RM. High-versus low-top shoes for the prevention of ankle sprains in basketball players: a prospective randomized study. *Am J Sports Med*. 1993 Jul;21(4):582–5.
44. Sitler M, Ryan J, Wheeler B, et al. The efficacy of a semirigid ankle stabilizer to reduce acute ankle injuries in basketball: a randomized clinical study at West Point. *Am J Sports Med*. 1994 Jul;22(4):454–61.
45. Handoll H, Rowe B, Quinn K, de Bie R. WITHDRAWN: interventions for preventing ankle ligament injuries. *Cochrane Database Syst Rev*. 2011;2011(5):CD000018.
46. Surve I, Schwellnus MP, Noakes T, Lombard C. A fivefold reduction in the incidence of recurrent ankle sprains in soccer players using the sport-stirrup orthosis. *Am J Sports Med*. 1994 Sep;22(5):601–6.

Sideline Emergencies

Korin B. Hudson and Matthew D. Sedgley

15

INTRODUCTION

- Although most sports injuries are not emergencies and are musculoskeletal in nature, there are certain life- and limb-threatening injuries that the sideline physician must be prepared to handle immediately. The so-called "sideline" emergencies may be field-side, court-side, pool-side, rink-side, at the finish-line, or anywhere else that athletes participate in sport, both for training or competition.
- The most important step in the management of sideline emergencies is the preparation, development, and rehearsal of appropriate Emergency Action Plans (EAPs).
  - Depending on the setting, resources may be limited, although the EAP must at a minimum have ready access to appropriate health care personnel, appropriate medical supplies and emergency equipment, immediate access to a telephone, and the ability to transport an athlete to a medical facility.
- All health care providers working with athletes should be familiar with basic life support (BLS), and should be certified in cardiopulmonary resuscitation (CPR) and the use of an automated external defibrillator (AED) (1). Physicians providing sideline care should be at least familiar with advanced cardiac life support (ACLS), basic trauma care, and comfortable with the care of both common and rare but serious injuries specific to the event being covered.

GENERAL APPROACH TO THE COLLAPSED ATHLETE (2)

- When approaching the collapsed athlete, the initial evaluation should be both rapid and focused with a goal of evaluating for immediate life threats.
- The age of the athlete, his/her general conditioning, and any specific medical conditions should be considered, as should the general characteristics of the sport, such as the amount of contact (*i.e.*, collision, limited contact, and noncontact), the degree of speed involved, and the duration of the event. Finally, the environmental conditions must be considered as both a potential causative and/or exacerbating factor in the injury.
- Depending on the sport, circumstances, and whether the collapse was witnessed, trauma may or may not be suspected. However, in general the "primary survey" should follow the "CAB" (Circulation, Airway, Breathing) approach and should occur where the athlete is found.
  - If deficits are found, they must be corrected before moving on. For example, if no pulse is found then an AED should be applied immediately. Likewise, if inadequate respirations are noted, the airway should be opened using a jaw thrust maneuver and an AED should be applied, recalling that agonal respirations are often a sign of cardiac dysrhythmia and that respirations need not be absent, especially in the earliest moments of witnessed cardiac arrest.
- If the athlete is prone, s/he should be quickly, but carefully transitioned to a supine position using an inline spinal motion control with a logroll maneuver (3,4).
  - The logroll should ideally be a four-person technique in which the team leader is at the athlete's head maintaining in-line stabilization of the head and neck, while the other three members of the team control the torso, hips, and legs.
  - The athlete should be turned in the direction of the three assistants according to the count of the leader and then directly onto a rigid transfer device such as a long spine board, scoop stretcher, or similar that has been placed under the athlete.
- The supine athlete is best transferred using a six- to eight-person lift.
  - With one person maintaining the control of the cervical spine, two to three assistants (depending on the size of the patient) kneel at the chest, hips, and legs, respectively, on each side of the patient with a final assistant at the foot of the patient with the immobilization device ready to slide from foot toward the head.
  - The four to six assistants on each side of the patient slide their arms under the patient such that they cross underneath.
  - On a coordinated count provided by the leader at the head of the patient, all lift only about 6 in off the ground.
  - The assistant at the foot of the patient slides the immobilization device toward the head of the patient until it stops at the knees of the leader at the head.
  - On a coordinated count provided by the leader at the head, the patient is slowly lowered onto the device.

- After the primary survey is complete and the patient is stabilized, a more detailed secondary survey should be performed either on the field or on the sideline, depending on the status of the athlete and the environmental conditions.
- After the initial examination of the patient is completed, any additional concerns should be categorized as being of either an immediate or potentially life-threatening, disabling nature, and treated accordingly. Frequent reevaluation of the injured athlete is required.

IMMEDIATE LIFE-THREATENING INJURIES

Cardiac Arrest

- Sudden cardiac arrest death is relatively rare, with incidence varying depending on the age of the athlete and the sporting event (5). Although in the United States there is a cardiac arrest in a high school or college athlete approximately once every 3 days (6).
  - The most common cause of sudden cardiac death in young athletes include congenital structural abnormalities, such as hypertrophic cardiomyopathy and anomalous coronary arteries, and arrhythmias such as long QT and channelopathies (7).
  - The most common cause in middle-aged athletes (over age 35) is atherosclerotic heart disease causing acute ischemic events.
  - The field-side treatment of any cause of cardiac arrest should focus on early high-quality CPR and early access to AED with defibrillation as indicated.
  - An equally important task for the sideline physician is identification of potentially at-risk athletes through the preparticipation exam, which is described in detail in Chapter 18 of this text (6,7).
  - *Commotio cordis* is a specific type of cardiac arrest in which a localized traumatic force to the anterior chest occurs during a specific phase of the cardiac cycle. This leads to the so-called "R-on-T phenomenon" leading to ventricular dysrhythmia.
    - The most successful intervention has been immediate high-quality CPR and application/use of an AED.
    - Better protection from direct blows to the chest may be the best way to prevent this rare but often lethal injury (8).

Respiratory Compromise

- *Upper Airway Obstruction* (UAO): Although rare in organized sports, respiratory arrest can result from upper airway obstruction (UAO). Principles of trauma airway management can help in the evaluation and treatment of these emergency situations (9).
  - Signs include respiratory distress with little or no air movement, significant accessory muscle use, wheezing, and stridor or snoring breath sounds.
  - If the athlete is unconscious, the airway should be opened with a jaw-thrust maneuver to keep the tongue from occluding the airway, and an airway adjunct such as an oropharyngeal or nasopharyngeal (OP or NP) airway should be inserted as necessary. A jaw thrust may be required. The head-tilt/chin-lift is not recommended in situations where trauma may have occurred.
  - The oropharynx should be inspected for foreign bodies, which should be removed if visualized; however, blind finger sweeps are not recommended.
  - Significant facial or mandibular trauma may lead to blood, secretion, and even teeth, which can lead to UAO, particularly in the athlete with depressed level of consciousness who has lost protective airway reflexes.
  - Other causes of UAO, such as airway edema from anaphylaxis, inhalation burn injuries (seen in motorsports), or an expanding neck hematoma from neck trauma (as seen in hockey, lacrosse, and martial arts, among other sports) should be considered, with early intubation a priority.
  - In high-risk sports, it is prudent to consider the capabilities of the sideline physician to perform a surgical airway. This is outside the scope of many primary sports physicians, and early access to emergency services and an emergency department with surgical airway capabilities is critical in these situations.
- *Laryngeal Fracture*: is an injury that occurs after direct trauma to the anterior neck.
  - Signs include stridor, hoarseness, subcutaneous emphysema, and perhaps bony crepitus and a palpable fracture.
  - Although airway obstruction may not be immediate, symptoms may rapidly progress due to edema.
  - Similar to the other causes of UAO listed above, early intubation is a priority; surgical airway may be required.
- *Pneumothorax*: the presence of air in the pleural space, between the lung and the chest wall, causing collapse of the lung parenchyma.
  - A *simple pneumothorax* may be either spontaneous or traumatic, with spontaneous pneumothoraxes occurring more often in tall, thin, young men, and in sports that involve changes in intrathoracic pressure (*e.g.*, scuba diving and weightlifting). By contrast, traumatic pneumothoraxes occur secondary to rib fractures.
    - Symptoms may include unilateral chest pain, dyspnea, and cough.
    - Diagnosis is suspected when lung sounds are noted on the affected side; oxygen saturation may or may not be altered. Chest radiographs are the diagnostic gold standard, but bedside ultrasound may be useful in making the diagnosis as well and may be more readily available in the sideline or athletic training room setting.

- Immediate treatment is rarely needed unless the patient is severely dyspneic, or the pneumothorax is open or under tension (see below). Patients with a stable simple pneumothorax should be given oxygen and transported to a medical facility for further evaluation and management.

- An *open pneumothorax* is a pneumothorax that is accompanied by, and often caused by, an open wound to the chest wall. This may be due to an open fracture of a rib, or due to penetrating trauma from a foreign object. In athletics, open pneumothoraxes are more common in high energy and extreme sports such as mountain biking, motocross, and so on.
  - Treatment consists of placing an occlusive dressing over the open wound and taping it down on three sides to create a one-way valve that allows air to exit without reentering until a definitive thoracostomy tube can be placed.
- A *tension pneumothorax* occurs when a pneumothorax is accompanied by progressive accumulation of air in the pleural space that leads to increased intrathoracic pressure, causing a shift of mediastinal structures away from the pneumothorax and decreased venous return and decreased cardiac output.
  - In addition to the previously listed symptoms, these athletes may have tracheal deviation away from the affected side with jugular venous distention and hypotension.
  - This is a true medical emergency that requires immediate treatment by needle decompression of the chest with a large (3-in, 14 gauge) needle or angiocatheter inserted in the anterior chest wall, ideally in the second intercostal space at the midclavicular line, followed by transport to the hospital by placement of an appropriate thoracostomy tube.

Anaphylaxis

- *Anaphylactic reactions* are acute systemic hypersensitivity reactions that although typically allergen induced, can also be exercise induced or idiopathic. In athletics, food and drug allergies are common, and insect (especially *Hymenoptera*) stings.
  - By definition, anaphylaxis requires involvement of two or more organ systems. These symptoms may include: urticaria, angioedema and/or upper airway edema, dyspnea, wheezing, flushing of skin, dizziness, hypotension, syncope, gastrointestinal symptoms, rhinitis, and/or headache.
  - Symptom onset is typically rapid (within 5–30 minutes of exposure), and in its most severe form, anaphylaxis can progress to severe bronchospasm, airway edema, and fatal cardiovascular collapse.
  - Following a primary assessment, 0.3–0.5 mg of intramuscular epinephrine in adults (or 0.01 $mg{\cdot}kg^{-1}$ in children, not to exceed 0.3 mg) may be administered and may be repeated every 10–15 minutes as needed. Intravenous (IV) fluids should be considered in the hypotensive patient, β-agonists may be given if bronchospasm is present. Antihistamines (H_1 and H_2 blockers) may be considered part of supportive care as well. Routine use of steroids is no longer recommended (10).
  - The athlete should be rapidly transported to a medical facility for further evaluation and care.

Severe Hemorrhage

- *Severe Hemorrhage* in the athlete may be the result of lacerations, fractures, vascular disruptions, or visceral organ or muscle disruptions.
  - Hemorrhage may manifest as either massive external bleeding or insidious and occult internal bleeding. Severe bleeding can lead to hypovolemia, hypotension, and death.
  - Signs and symptoms of hypovolemic shock include altered sensorium; pale and cool extremities with a decreased capillary refill; weak, thready, and rapid pulses; hypotension; tachycardia; and tachypnea.
  - Injuries that may lead to occult blood loss include hemorrhage into the thoracic and abdominal cavities (*i.e.*, splenic or hepatic injuries), long bone fractures leading to hemorrhage into surrounding soft tissues, and hemorrhage into the retroperitoneal space secondary to a pelvic fracture (11).
    - Occult bleeding may produce delayed signs and symptoms, and what may at first appear to be an atraumatic incident may have been caused by recent unnoticed or unwitnessed trauma (12).
    - Scalp lacerations may be a source of significant bleeding and often go unnoticed if the athlete is lying on his back or is strapped to a spine board.
  - Control of external bleeding should follow the basic principles of hemostasis, which include steady direct pressure over the bleeding site, elevation of the affected body part, and application of a tourniquet for limb wounds. Hemostatic gauze and packing of large wounds may be appropriate. Blind clamping of bleeding vessels is generally not recommended.

POTENTIAL LIFE-THREATENING/ DISABLING INJURIES: SPINE AND HEAD INJURIES

Neck Injuries

- *Neck injuries*, although relatively uncommon and usually self-limited (13), represent one of the most feared and potentially catastrophic injuries in sports.
  - The sideline physician must promptly recognize the potential for spine injury based on the mechanism of

injury and presenting signs/symptoms and should adhere strictly to spinal precautions (discussed previously in this chapter), while determining whether an athlete requires emergency transfer to a medical facility, or whether s/he simply requires further sideline observation and when the athlete may return to play.

- Indications for spinal stabilization and transport for emergency care include: severe neck pain, midline bony tenderness on examination, post-traumatic loss of consciousness (LOC) or mental status changes, peripheral neurologic abnormalities, or significant mechanism of injury (3,4,14).
- Usually minor, *burners* or *stingers* are nerve injuries resulting from trauma to the neck and/or shoulder that cause either a compressive or a traction injury to the cervical nerve roots or the brachial plexus itself (6,14).
  - Symptoms include burning pain radiating down the arm, usually unilateral in distribution, often associated with numbness, paresthesia, and muscle weakness or paresis.
  - This is typically self-limited, with most cases resolving in a matter of minutes, although some symptoms may persist for weeks to months.
  - A burner should *not* be considered as an initial diagnosis if an athlete has any of the following:
    Bilateral upper extremity involvement
    Any lower extremity involvement
    Neck pain or tenderness

- Although there are no definitive guidelines regarding which athletes with neck injuries may safely return to play, it is generally agreed on that only those players with no neck pain and no neurologic symptoms and with a completely normal examination may return to play safely, with repeated evaluation being necessary (13–15).

Head Injuries

- *Head Injuries* in sports are quite common and often provoke anxiety and uncertainty. The most common head injury in sports is a concussion, and 90% or more of concussions do not involve an LOC (13,15). The sideline physician should be confident in performing an assessment for concussion on the sidelines with a low threshold for transfer to an emergency facility if needed. Head Injuries are discussed in depth in Chapter 48 of this text.
  - When approaching the fallen athlete with a suspected head injury, the sideline physician should perform a rapid primary assessment and should next determine the level of consciousness as well as note any spontaneous movement and speech. Assessment for potential spine injury should be performed, and if no concern for life threats or spine injury exists, the player may be moved to the sidelines and a focused neurologic examination may be performed.
    - This should include a thorough sensory, motor, and cranial nerve examination as well as assessment of vestibular, oculomotor, cognitive, and memory function.
  - Evaluate for signs of skull fracture or intracerebral bleeding, such as: pupil asymmetry, postauricular or periorbital ecchymosis, clear otorrhea, rhinorrhea, or hemotympanum, and any depression in the skull.
    - Frequent reassessment is mandatory because victims of head injury may rapidly deteriorate; abnormal findings may be delayed.

ABDOMINAL/PELVIC INJURY

- Abdominal/Pelvic Injury: generally result from rapid deceleration, direct blunt trauma to the abdomen, or indirect trauma from a displaced lower rib fracture. And although potentially serious and even life-threatening, most abdominal injuries can be managed nonoperatively with close observation.
  - *Splenic/Hepatic Injury*: The spleen and liver comprise two common organs injured in blunt abdominal trauma. There may be left or right upper quadrant and/or shoulder pain (Kehr sign), respectively, as well as signs of hypotension if bleeding is significant. All athletes with significant pain and/or appropriate mechanism of injury may require urgent ultrasound, computed tomography (CT) imaging, and/or observation.
  - Injuries to the abdominal wall include simple contusions and rectus sheath hematomas, both of which are benign and usually managed conservatively, although the latter can occasionally require surgical intervention. It is critical however that the sideline physician remains vigilant in evaluating for and excluding associated intra-abdominal injuries.
  - *Exercise-related transient abdominal pain* (ETAP) or "stitch" is an intense stabbing subcostal pain usually occurring early in the conditioning of the athlete and goes away as the athlete gets in shape. It may be due to diaphragmatic ischemia and is benign (16).
  - Injuries to the genitourinary system should be suspected based on the mechanism of injury as well as the presence and degree of hematuria. However, one must keep in mind that injury to the kidney may be present without hematuria and that hematuria does not always signify significant renal injury.
    - Examination is often difficult because of pain and swelling; however, severe scrotal or testicular swelling or a nonpalpable testicle warrants further evaluation. And, in the absence of direct trauma, testicular torsion must be ruled out in the athlete presenting with acute onset of testicular pain. In either case, removal from the field of play and transfer to an emergency department for color flow is recommended.

- Gross blood may occur at the urethral meatus because of blunt trauma to the scrotal region or other significant injury to the GU system.
  - Doppler ultrasound studies may define the nature or extent of the problem and retrograde urethrogram or CT pyelogram may be required if blood is noted at the urethral meatus. Urology consultation is recommended.

MUSCULOSKELETAL INJURIES

- Musculoskeletal Injuries: are the most encountered injuries in sports. Most are minor and self-limited and are discussed extensively throughout this text. However, a few specific high-risk extremity injuries are reviewed here.
  - When considering the emergency sideline evaluation of severe musculoskeletal injuries, it is important that the neurovascular status of the affected limb is evaluated for any suspected fracture, dislocation, or other severe extremity injury.
    - If there is vascular compromise, reduction of dislocations and/or fractures should be attempted in the field with gentle traction. Otherwise, fractures should be splinted in the position in which they are found, unless some degree of reduction is required because of neurovascular compromise. Finally, no athlete should return to play if there is a question of a fracture, no matter how minor the injury may seem, because this may transform a nondisplaced or a closed fracture into a displaced or open one.
  - The following injuries represent a potential threat to a limb:
    - *Open Fracture*: previously known as a compound fracture, this is a fracture associated with overlying soft-tissue injury with communication between the fracture site and the skin. These are at high risk for subsequent infection and osteomyelitis and require washout in the operating room.
      - On the field, the open wound should be covered with moist sterile gauze and the extremity splinted with no attempts made to push extruding bone or soft tissue back into the wound or to reduce the fracture, unless neurovascular compromise is present.
    - *Traumatic Amputations*: are very rare and dramatic injuries that are easy to recognize.
      - The proximal stump should be irrigated with a sterile solution and a sterile pressure dressing applied, with a tourniquet used only for severe, uncontrolled bleeding and the amputated portion should be irrigated, wrapped in a sterile fashion, placed in a bag, and put on ice with rapid transport to an appropriate medical facility.
    - *Compartment Syndrome*: is a state of increased pressure within a closed tissue compartment that compromises blood flow through nutrient capillaries supplying muscles and nerves within that compartment. The potential causes of compartment syndrome are numerous, although in terms of athletes, this is typically an injury with the most common site being the anterior and/or lateral compartment of the lower leg.
      - Presentation typically occurs within a few hours after injury and will consist of severe and constant pain over the involved compartment and an increase in pain with both active contraction and passive stretching of the involved muscles. There may also be significant dysesthesias as well as an absent or diminished pulse, pallor, and/or paralysis of the affected neuromuscular group, although these are late findings that indicate that significant myoneural ischemia has already occurred. This acute compartment syndrome which is a medical emergency contrasts with chronic exertional compartment syndrome that is atraumatic and resolves after a few minutes of rest from running.
      - Treatment is an emergent fasciotomy and requires rapid transport of the athlete to a medical facility.
    - *Knee Dislocation*: is rare and usually associated with a high-velocity/high-energy mechanism of injury, this is a very serious injury that may require a high index of suspicion because many dislocations will have spontaneously reduced prior to evaluation.
      - The knee will typically be very swollen and painful and will often demonstrate severe instability in multiple directions on examination. The seriousness of the injury lies in the high rate of associated complications, specifically popliteal artery injury and peroneal nerve injury (which may occur despite spontaneous reduction and normal pulses).
      - Early reduction of a visible dislocation is important. Rapid transport of the patient with a known or suspected dislocation to a medical facility for orthopedic and vascular consultation is essential.
    - *Hip Dislocation*: also rare in sports and usually involves a high-velocity/high-energy mechanism of injury. Posterior dislocations are by far the most common type, and the seriousness of this injury lies in the risk for avascular necrosis (AVN) of the femoral head as circulation is disrupted. This occurs in a matter of hours, with the incidence of AVN reported at 2%–10% and rates increasing significantly if the dislocation is not reduced within 6 hours (17). Sciatic nerve injuries may also be seen with this injury.
    - Other dislocations, such as digits, patellae, shoulders, and so on, rarely result in limb-threatening conditions, and most sideline physicians are both familiar with the injuries and are capable of recognition and

reduction. However, there will be the occasional unreducible event that necessitates prompt referral. All dislocations should have some form of splinting and follow-up care to ensure appropriate and successful outcomes.

OTHER SERIOUS INJURIES

- Severe injuries to the eye and orbit may occur in sports and often require prompt attention by ophthalmologic specialists. The sideline physician is frequently called on to stabilize and triage these injuries to determine which injuries require same day, emergency evaluation rather than in-office consultation. Chapter 35 of this text describes ocular injuries in athletics in detail.
- Likewise, there are many auricular and nasal injuries that may occur including nasal fractures, epistaxis and auricular hematomas, and lacerations. Chapter 36 of this text describes the evaluation and management of ear, nose, and throat conditions commonly seen in athletics.

ENVIRONMENTAL EMERGENCIES

- Environmental Emergencies are described in Chapter 47 but will be briefly described here as well.
    - *Hypothermia*: Defined as core body temperature <95°F (<35°C), usually occurs because of prolonged exposure to cold environmental conditions. When approaching the hypothermic athlete, the sideline physician should keep the following points in mind:
        - Treatment should routinely start with passive external rewarming (*i.e.*, moving the athlete from a cold to a warm environment, removing all wet clothing, and covering with dry blankets).
        - Active external rewarming and core rewarming should usually be deferred until the hospital environment because patients with moderate to severe hypothermia are at high risk of having significant electrolyte, acid-base, and cardiovascular changes associated with rewarming.
        - Significantly hypothermic patients are at very high risk of fatal cardiac arrhythmias.
        - Assessment for pulse/breathing may take a little longer than usual due to the difficulty of palpation in cold tissue as well as the bradycardia, but if none is detected in 30–60 seconds, CPR will be required. And if started, CPR should continue until the patient's temperature reaches 92°F (32°C); the phrase "they are not dead until they are warm and dead" still applies (1).
    - *Hyperthermia*: Heat-related illnesses are a spectrum of diseases ranging from heat cramps and edema to heat exhaustion to heat stroke and death (18–21).
        - *Heat stroke* is a true medical emergency, with high mortality rates if unrecognized (6). It typically presents in warm, humid conditions with elements of overexertion on the part of the athlete, but has been documented in temperatures <60°F.
        - A core body temperature >104°F (>40°C) and prominent central nervous system (CNS) changes make the diagnosis in the field. These signs and symptoms may be accompanied by multisystem organ dysfunction including renal and liver dysfunction.
        - Treatment includes removing athlete from activity and from the warm environment if possible and gold standard care is cold water immersion or a method whereby they are actively doused by cold water while simultaneously massaged with ice bags (see Fig. 15.1).
    - *Lightning Injury*: although rare, lightning injury is one of the more frequent injuries by a natural phenomenon, with the largest number of injuries occurring in golf and

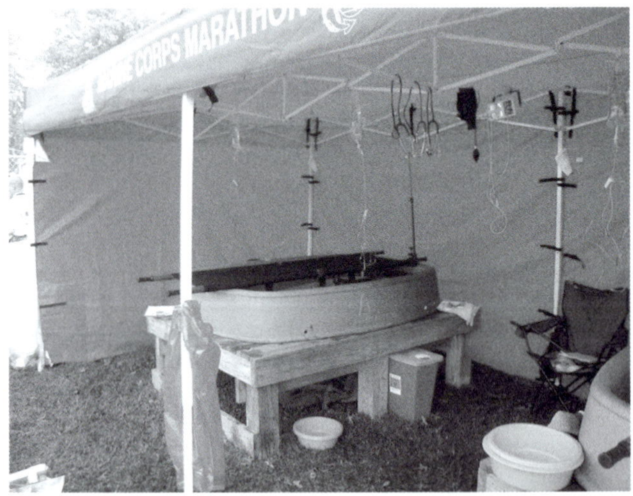

Figure 15.1: Heat deck used at Marine Corps Marathon for management of exertional heat stroke.

water sports. Most injuries occur during the months of June through September.

- Although the voltage of lightning is extraordinarily high, it is usually an instantaneous contact that tends to flash over the outside of a victim's body, often creating superficial burns, but sparing extensive damage to internal organs and structures.
- Lightning may injure a person by striking either the person directly or something they are holding, or by splashing over from a nearby person or object that has been struck. It may also strike the ground and spread circumferentially, often creating multiple victims.
- Although it can potentially affect any organ system, injuries to the cardiovascular and neurologic systems tend to be the most serious, primarily due to asystole, with the immediate cause of death most commonly being cardiopulmonary arrest.
- Minor injuries include dysesthesias, minor burns, temporary LOC, confusion, amnesia, tympanic membrane perforation, and ocular injury.
- Long-term sequelae include peripheral neuropathies and mental impairment (22).
- The sideline physician should keep the following points in mind when approaching a victim of lightning injury:
  - Triage should occur in "reverse" order, that is, approach and treat the pulseless patients first, rather than triaging them to an "unsalvageable" category and moving on.
  - In lightning victims with cardiopulmonary arrest, cardiac automaticity, and contractions will often resume spontaneously in a short period of time, whereas respiratory arrest from paralysis of the medullary respiratory center may be prolonged. Therefore, unless the victim is ventilated quickly, the victim will progress to a secondary hypoxic cardiac arrest despite normal cardiac activity. If promptly resuscitated and supported, full recovery may ensue.
  - Standard ACLS protocols should be followed.
  - Victims do not "retain charge" and are not dangerous to touch, so CPR should not be delayed for this reason.
  - Contrary to popular belief, lightning can and often does strike the same place twice, so personal safety must be taken into consideration.
  - Hypotension in a lightning victim should prompt a search for occult hemorrhage or fractures because of blunt trauma; spinal precautions are required.
  - Pupils may become "fixed and dilated" because of the nature of lightning injuries, and this should not preclude resuscitation attempts as these changes do not necessarily indicate brain death in lightning victims.
  - Long bone fractures, vertebral injuries, and dislocations are common, so a secondary survey for concomitant injuries is appropriate once the patient is stabilized.

EQUIPMENT MANAGEMENT (2,3)

- In many sports athletes wear protective equipment that may hinder access to both the airway and to the chest for AED placement and performance of high-quality CPR.
- Removal of this equipment requires several highly trained providers who have rehearsed the procedure together. However, if the equipment maintains appropriate neutral spinal alignment, it may remain in place as long as appropriate airway access is secured and access to the chest can be quickly obtained if needed.
- In American Football, the helmet and shoulder pads should typically be considered a single unit — the removal of either one necessitates the removal of the other, as leaving only one of them in place forces the neck out of a neutral position.
  - The same is not always true for other sports including ice hockey, lacrosse, BMX, or equestrian sports.
- Regardless of the sport, if an athlete is wearing an appropriately fitted helmet, any facemask should be removed to guarantee airway access and spinal motion control should be maintained using an extrication device such as a scoop stretcher, long spine board, or vacuum mattress.
  - If the facemask cannot be removed, the helmet should be removed entirely to assure that the airway can be accessed in the event of apnea or cardiopulmonary arrest.
  - In this case, neutral spinal alignment should be maintained either by removing shoulder pads or by padding behind the occiput as appropriate.

EMERGENCY ACTION PLANNING

- Emergency Action Planning: as important as it is to respond appropriately in the event of an emergency, that response is generally more effective and more efficient when preparations are made in advance in the form of an EAP.
  - EAPs should be developed for each sporting venue and may need to be adapted or updated for specific events (23).
  - EAPs should include:
    - A list of the key personnel including contact phone numbers.
    - The ingress and egress routes for EMS.
    - Locations for all critical emergency equipment including AEDs, hemorrhage control kits, and items such as cooling tubs, oxygen, and/or epinephrine auto injectors, if appropriate.

- Any specific plans related to athletes with unique medical needs, *i.e.*, diabetic emergency plans, asthma plans.
- EAPs should be reviewed and revised at least annually.
  - For most organizations this is the responsibility of the head athletic trainer and/or the supervising team physician.
- EAPs should be rehearsed at least annually, although some jurisdictions require more frequent review.
  - These reviews should involve all key personnel including: coaches, athletic trainers, team physicians, administrators, EMS, security, and anyone else who may be involved in a practice time or game day emergency
  - It is important to review scenarios for both practice and game time as staffing/personnel likely vary significantly
  - It is important to consider how emergency scenarios will be managed at both home and away venues as well as at "neutral site" venues
- The EAP should be shared with visiting teams and their medical staff in advance of their arrival.
- A preevent "time-out" should include members of the medical staff from each participating team as well as EMS, Police/Security, Operations/Command Center, and any other key participants.
  - This brief meeting serves as an opportunity for medical staff and emergency responders to meet, for each to understand and define their respective roles should an emergency occur and for the EAP to be reviewed
  - This is the appropriate time to make sure that everyone knows where all key members of the response team will be located during the event, where the emergency equipment is stored/located, and where the ingress/egress routes will be
  - This meeting can also help establish incident command so that there is no question who is in charge if and when an emergency occurs
  - Finally, this is an opportunity for "just-in-time" training and/or review of key protocols and algorithms for the most critical procedures or situations

MASS CASUALTY INCIDENTS

- Mass Casualty Incidents (MCIs): although mass casualty events at sporting venues are thankfully rare, weather events, structural collapse, crowd stampede, or man-made mass disruption events such as shooting/bombing events can threaten public safety at sporting events at any large gathering (24).
  - In such cases, the sideline physician is not likely to become the incident command for the event. However, as a trained medical professional on scene, s/he may choose to provide initial care until additional help arrives.
  - It is important to recall that all medical staff should wait until the scene is determined to be safe by police before attempting to render aid, as there is little value in becoming additional victims.
  - Once cleared to enter the scene, a triage — or sorting — process can begin according to any one of a number of predetermined algorithms.
  - It is likely that local EMS responders will assume command of the scene and the sideline physician can offer to support their efforts or can return to the care of the athlete group or to their initial staffing assignment.

SUMMARY

- Although most sports-related injuries are minor, for the few emergency events the sideline physician will encounter, planning and practice is paramount.
  - Medical equipment appropriate for the event and knowledge of life support techniques are essential.
  - Development, review, and rehearsal of emergency action plans (EAPs) are critical.
  - A preevent time-out will help guarantee that all key stakeholders are aware of, and agree on, the key components of the emergency plan before an emergency event occurs.

REFERENCES

1. American Heart Association. [Accessed 2023 May 30]. Available from: www.heart.org
2. Mills BM, Conrick KM, Anderson S, et al. Consensus recommendations on the prehospital care of the injured athlete with a suspected catastrophic cervical spine injury. *J Athl Train*. 2020 Jun 1;55(6):563–72.
3. Courson R, Boden BP, Ellis J, Henry G, Rehberg R. Acute and emergent spinal injury assessment and treatment. *Clin Sports Med*. 2023;42(3):491–514.
4. Sanchez AR II, Sugalski MT, LaPrade RF. Field-side and pre-hospital management of the spine injured athlete. *Curr Sports Med Rep*. 2005;4(1):50–5.
5. Maron BJ, Doerer JJ, Haas TS, Tierney DM, Mueller FO. Sudden deaths in young competitive athletes: analysis of 1866 deaths in the United States, 1980-2006. *Circulation*. 2009;119(8):1085–92.
6. Maron BJ, Doerer JJ, Haas TS, et al. Profile and frequency of sudden death in 1463 young competitive athletes: from a 25-year U.S. national registry—1980-2005. *Circulation*. 2006;114:830.
7. Peterson DF, Kucera K, Thomas LC, et al. Aetiology and incidence of sudden cardiac arrest and death in young competitive athletes in the USA: a 4-year prospective study. *Br J Sports Med*. 2021;55(21):1196–203.
8. Weinstock J, Maron BJ, Song C, Mane PP, Estes NA, Link MS. Failure of commercially available chest wall protectors to prevent sudden cardiac death induced by chest wall blows in an experimental model of commotio cordis. *Pediatrics*. 2006 Apr;117(4):e656-62.
9. James D, Pennardt AM. *Trauma Care Principles*. [Updated 2022 Apr 21]. In: *StatPearls* [Internet]. Treasure Island (FL): StatPearls Publishing; 2023 Jan.
10. Fischer D, Vander Leek TK, Ellis AK, Kim H. Anaphylaxis. *Allergy Asthma Clin Immunol*. 2018 Sep 12;14(suppl 2):54.

11. Yumoto T, Kosaki Y, Yamakawa Y, et al. Occult sources of bleeding in blunt trauma: a narrative review. *Acta Med Okayama*. 2017 Oct;71(5):363–8.
12. Blue JG, Pecci MA. The collapsed athlete. *Orthop Clin North Am*. 2002;33(3):471–8.
13. McAlindon RJ. On field evaluation and management of head and neck injured athletes. *Clin Sports Med*. 2002;21(1):1–14.
14. Haight RR, Shiple BJ. Sideline evaluation of neck pain: when is it time for transport? *Phys Sportsmed*. 2001;29(3):45–62.
15. Patricios JS, Schneider KJ, Dvorak J, et al. Consensus statement on concussion in sport: the 6th International Conference on Concussion in Sport-Amsterdam, October 2022. *Br J Sports Med*. 2023 Jun;57(11):695–711.
16. Atkins JM, Taylor JC, Kane SF. Acute and overuse injuries of the abdomen and groin in athletes. *Curr Sports Med Rep*. 2010;9(2):115–20.
17. Kellam P, Ostrum RF. Systematic review and meta-analysis of avascular necrosis and posttraumatic arthritis after traumatic hip dislocation. *J Orthop Trauma*. 2016 Jan;30(1):10–6.
18. Li Z, McKenna ZJ, Kuennen MR, Magalhães FC, Mermier CM, Amorim FT. The potential role of exercise-induced muscle damage in exertional heat stroke. *Sports Med*. 2021;51(5):863–72.
19. Casa DJ, DeMartini JK, Bergeron MF, et al. National athletic trainers' association position statement: exertional heat illnesses. *J Athl Train*. 2015 Sep;50(9):986–1000. Erratum in: *J Athl Train*. 2017 Apr;52(4):401.
20. Roberts WO, Armstrong LE, Sawka MN, Yeargin SW, Heled Y, O'Connor FG. ACSM expert consensus statement on exertional heat illness: recognition, management, and return to activity. *Curr Sports Med Rep*. 2023 Apr;22(4):134–49.
21. McDermott BP, Casa DJ, O'Connor FG, et al. Cold-water dousing with ice massage to treat exertional heat stroke: a case series. *Aviat Space Environ Med*. 2009;80(8):720–2.
22. Bauer AK, Golden KG, Colvin CM, Lammlein KP, Wise SR. When lightning strikes: sports and recreational activities safety. *Curr Sports Med Rep*. 2023 Apr;22(4):126–31.
23. Herring S, Putukian M, Kibler B, et al. Sideline preparedness for the team physician: a consensus statement—2012 update. *Med Sci Sports Exerc*. 2012;44(12):2442–5.
24. Sedgley M, Hudson K, Hulsopple C. Prepare for the unexpected: a new look at trauma triage and care in mass participation sporting events. *Curr Sports Med Rep*. 2023 Jan 1;22(1):4–9.

16 Mass Participation Events

Scott W. Pyne

GOALS

- Mass participation events are those sporting events in which many people participate and are generally spread out over several miles and variable terrain. These most commonly involve running events, but may include multidiscipline events such as triathlons, obstacle course races, and team sport tournaments.
- Advanced planning and preparation are critical to successfully accommodate the medical needs of the event participants.
- The medical director has numerous responsibilities as planner, communicator, and organizer in addition to the care of injured athletes (1).

Medical Coverage

- The needs of the athletes competing must be considered prior to the event.
- Specific considerations of the type of event, number of participants, course peculiarities, and environmental predictions are all very important in determining the medical coverage required.
- The formation and implementation of an emergency action plan have proven successful in numerous situations (2).

Safe Environment

- As a key advisor to the event director, the medical director must ensure that the event is conducted with the safety of the competitors being of utmost importance. Often, this is furthest from the minds of race organizers especially with competing priorities of sponsor, financial, and community concerns.
- In extreme conditions, such as environmental temperature, adverse weather events, illness outbreaks or threats, or acts of terrorism, the event may need to be canceled or rescheduled. It is best that these possibilities and contingency plans be discussed and prepared prior to the scheduled event.
- Wet bulb globe temperature (WBGT) index factoring temperature/dry bulb (Tdb), humidity/wet bulb (Twb), wind, and solar radiation/black globe (Tbg) in a formula $WBGT = 0.7\ Twb + 0.2\ Tbg + 0.1\ Tdb$ is an environmental heat stress index often used to gauge the risk of heat injury (3,4). The WBGT index has been used to modify, postpone, or cancel road running events, as increased medical casualties, potentially exceeding the event and community medical capabilities, have been demonstrated under high WGBT loads (5). The WGBT's utility may not be equally applicable across sports for different athletes (6,7).
- It is often necessary to review the course for any potential trouble spots and hazards that could cause injury. The start and finish are common sites of medical concern. The start area should be on a large level surface devoid of obstacles, thereby allowing the athletes to more easily accommodate the surge that invariably occurs. The finish area should also be large enough to prevent the athletes from bunching up and being forced to stand in one place. It should also have necessary facilities and resources to allow the athletes to properly cool down and recover after the event and easily access medical treatment areas as required.
- Biking, swimming, skiing and extreme events carry additional risk elements, such as water safety and trauma potential associated with high speeds. Water temperature; sea conditions; road conditions; transition, acceleration, and deceleration zones; and protective equipment must be carefully scrutinized (8–11).
- Safety, security, and comfort of medical support staff should not be overlooked.

MEDICAL ENCOUNTER DOCUMENTATION

- The documentation of medical team interactions with ill or injured participants is important in providing information to higher levels of care as needed, for medical legal purposes, and to be used to predict future event requirements.
- Regarding mass community-based endurance sport events, an international consensus statement has been developed to standardize definitions of (1) sports event, (2) medical encounters, (3) severity and timing of medical encounters, (4) diagnostic categories of medical encounters, and (5) standardizing research methods (10). If implemented, this will allow data from events to be more easily compared and aggregated.

EPIDEMIOLOGY

Injury Rate

- Running (42 km), 1%–20%; running (<21 km), 1%–5%; triathlon (225 km), 15%–30%; Nordic skiing (55 km), 5%; triathlon (51 km), 2%–5%; cycling (variable), 5% (12–22).
- Injury rate increases with increased distance and environmental temperature (23–25).

Predicting Injury Rate

- Previous years' experience is very helpful in planning for subsequent years. This also stresses the importance of a reliable medical documentation and injury data tracking system.
- Similar events in similar elements can be used in the initial planning and preparation stages.
- Fortunately, the risk for cardiac arrest and sudden exertional death in marathons is quite small (26–29).

MEDICAL PHILOSOPHY

Level of Care

- The level of medical care that will be available on the course must be defined and agreed on between the medical director and the event director early in the planning stage.
- This may differ among the aid stations throughout the course with the most robust resources usually being provided at the finish area.
- It is essential to provide on-site basic first aid and cardiopulmonary resuscitation (CPR). It is desirable to provide on-site early defibrillation, advanced cardiac life support (ACLS), and advanced trauma life support (ATLS) (1).
- The usage and type of intravenous fluids and availability of oxygen, medications, and advanced cardiac and trauma life support equipment are all areas requiring discussion.
- Coordination with the local emergency medical system (EMS) and emergency rooms and hospitals is absolutely required.
- Mobile medical assets in the form of bike, golf cart, all-terrain vehicle, canoe/kayak teams, and EMS units provide an excellent means to access injured competitors throughout the course (30,31).

Medication Plan

- A decision must be made as to the provision of medication on the race course and in the medical aid stations. It is recommended that these medications be tightly controlled and kept to a minimum if dispensed at all.
- In longer events, it is common for athletes to carry and take their own medication during the competition. This must be anticipated to best treat the competitor and prevent overprescribing.
- The availability of urgent or emergency medication, such as aspirin, epinephrine auto injector, albuterol metered-dose inhaler, glucose, and ACLS medications, should be considered.

Laboratory Plan

- Medical aid stations may or may not have basic laboratory capability. The ability to assess an athletes' blood glucose and sodium levels will assist with their rapid evaluation and allow for the appropriate treatment of a collapsed athlete (32,33).
- Hand-held glucose and electrolyte monitors are readily available and have become part of the standard medical kit for many endurance events (34).

Communication Plan

- It is vital that medical support assets have the ability to communicate with each other, EMS assets, local hospitals, and the event director before, during, and after the competition.
- Various communication networks have been used to include cellular phones, computer networks, ham radio, and hand-held radios. These systems should be tested well before the event, and a backup plan should be established in the case of failure of the primary means of communication.
- Awareness of who has access to the communication network is required to avoid unauthorized disclosure of medically sensitive information to those without a need to know.
- A communication plan outlining how EMS will be requested and dispatched, where injured athletes will be taken, and when to contact the medical director will increase the efficiency of the medical care provided.
- The advent of medical record mobile phone applications has provided a convenient mechanism to communicate the number of casualties, diagnoses, location, and disposition while maintaining control of network access.

MEDICAL CHAIN OF COMMAND

- An individual must be identified to serve as the medical director. Their responsibilities include advanced planning, event day medical decision making, and medical troubleshooting. The medical support staff, event director, and media all benefit from having one identified contact, rather than a committee, to oversee all medical issues.
- As event coordination increases in complexity, it may be advisable to establish a medical committee structure with delegated and assigned tasks, such as medical volunteers, nonmedical volunteers, local emergency medical services, local hospital, and local law enforcement, to appropriate teams under the supervision of the medical director (35).

- It is also recommended that each aid station have an assigned medical leader well versed in the event medical philosophy. This medical leader can organize the support staff and coordinate medical care provided at their site.

MEDICAL TRAINING

Medical Staff

- It is common that the medical support for mass participation events is gathered from diverse backgrounds and experience levels. Most are more comfortable providing medical care within a clinical or hospital facility than in the field environment. As such, the best leaders may not be those with the most advanced degrees or time in practice, but rather those most experienced and at ease with medical management in circumstances similar to the event.
- The medical plan, chain of command, and level of care provided must be reviewed with the medical staff. It is helpful, although not always practical, to provide a didactic session prior to race day.
- Triage plan, treatment guidelines, and medical management protocols specific for the event provided in writing are useful, as well as administration information to include the course map, parking, proximity to water, food, and facility stations, and communication and transportation plans (36).

Competitors

- Preevent and on-site education may reduce injury risk and improve event safety (1). This is most easily provided with the race information and can be coordinated through the event director. Additions to event websites, handouts to accompany the race packet pick-up, and information posters displayed in common areas are several examples.
- Common medical conditions and injury prevention, location of medical aid stations on the course, and available services at these areas assist the participants in their planning and preparation for a safe event.
- Medical presentations to the athletes and interest groups are often well received.
- Race day information regarding weather conditions and health warnings has been used with success at numerous events (37).

STAFFING

Medical and Nonmedical Support

- The appropriate staffing of medical treatment areas with both medical and nonmedical staff is important in the safe conduct of the medical aid station. The composition and number of this staff will vary depending on the location and nature of the event.
- The number of staff can be best derived from previous experience or through comparison with similar events in similar conditions. Organizations such as the International Institute for Race Medicine and individual event medical directors are excellent resources in establishing baseline staffing requirements for new events (38,39).
- Nonmedical staff can assist with the transport of injured athletes, documentation, medical tracking, and provide information within the medical aid station and to event staff.
- Medical support staff should be easily identifiable to competitors and other event support. Different color shirts, vests, hats, and identification badges are a few suggestions.

Staff Feedback

- After the event, it is most important to elicit feedback from both medical and nonmedical staff. This often identifies areas that had not been considered in the initial planning and execution phases of the event.
- The follow-up of these comments in a written after-action report is highly recommended because it allows the documentation of areas of concern, develops solutions, and prepares for subsequent events.

TRIAGE AND TREATMENT GUIDELINES

- The majority of the medical conditions presenting at a given event can be predicted well in advance. Preparing, training, and practicing for these conditions are important in the evaluation, treatment, and disposition of injured participants.
- Protocols and algorithms can assist in standardizing race day medical care delivery (40).

Serious Life-Threatening Versus Nonserious

- The initial evaluation of an athlete in the medical aid station should focus on the severity of their injury (24). Fortunately, most complaints are nonserious in nature and can be quickly treated and released.
- Serious life-threatening medical conditions include cardiac events, exertion heat stroke, exercise-associated hyponatremia, hypothermia, near-drowning, and head and neck trauma. These can be quickly differentiated from nonserious conditions by the evaluation of mental status, core temperature (41), blood pressure, and pulse. Serum glucose and sodium levels may also aid in the diagnosis.
- Depending on the medical care plan of the event, some of these serious conditions may be treated at the medical aid station or transported via EMS to the most appropriate medical treatment facility.

Illness Versus Injury

- Illness conditions, such as exercise-associated collapse, heat stroke, chest pain, and hyponatremia, can be triaged from injuries, muscle cramps, blisters, and extremity pain, in the treatment areas.
- This separation of care allows the assignment and preparation of support staff in the area of care for which they are most experienced. It also allows those with more serious conditions to be treated in the same area where they can be more closely monitored.
- The establishment of a medical holding area has proven successful (36). This area is reserved for athletes who are waiting for transportation for nonserious conditions or who are not prepared to leave the medical area, but do not require further care. This group is continuously observed and encouraged to make their way back to the after-event areas.

Evaluation of Exercise-Associated Collapse

- The majority of cases of exercise-associated collapse are the result of predictable physiologic events associated with exertion and respond rapidly to positioning with the head down and legs and pelvis in an elevated position (24,36,42). These athletes generally have normal mental status.
- Individuals with altered mental status should be rapidly evaluated with a core temperature for hyperthermia or hypothermia (3). Persistent altered mental status with relatively normal core temperatures should be treated as suspected hyponatremia until proven otherwise (24).
- Hyperthermic individuals should be rapidly cooled onsite, preferably with ice water immersion (9,24).

FINANCE AND LOGISTICS

Financial Planning

- The conduct of mass participation events both requires and has the potential to generate money. Medical directors must ensure that the safety of the participants and the support staff is not compromised by decisions to increase revenue for the event. The medical director must be involved in any plans affecting the event that may have medical implications.
- Planning for the costs of medical supplies, transportation, and personnel compensation must be made and agreed on early in the event-planning process.

Medical Aid Station Location

- The spacing of medical aid stations throughout the course is determined by many variables. The course must be previewed and the location of medical aid stations established based on anticipated need, appropriate location, and course-specific considerations (37).
- Increased staffing at the finish areas of endurance events is critical to address the larger number of participating medical requirements at the end of the event.
- Medical aid stations must be easily identifiable to competitors and EMS units.
- Medical evacuation routes must be established to avoid conflict with the event in progress and ensure the most efficient transport requirements.
- Adequate (unlimited) fluid must be available throughout the event, at all aid stations and the finish. Runners should also be educated regarding the risk of hyponatremia associated with overhydration.

Transportation Plan

- It is not unusual for participants to decide that a medical treatment area is a good place to end their participation in the event. If this decision is realized in the middle of the course, a plan for the removal of these athletes must be used.
- Many races have a "sweep" vehicle that follows the last competitor and can transport these participants to the finish area. Other transport arrangements may be available depending on the nature of the competition, but must be anticipated prior to the event.

MEDICAL LEGAL

- An additional responsibility of the medical director is the assurance of medical staff liability coverage (43).
- General event insurance packages usually exclude medical coverage (44).
- Options for medical liability coverage should be discussed with legal representation in advance of the event and include individual or group policies and Good Samaritan laws.

MASS PARTICIPATION AND INFECTIOUS DISEASE

- The COVID-19 pandemic, in causing a severe health crisis, led to significant social distancing as a main preventative measure for person-to-person transmission of SARS CoV-2. This action put a halt to many mass participation endurance sporting events with some being indefinitely postponed or canceled. As infectious disease outbreaks will continue to represent a future threat, medical risk stratification and planning are required.
- In 2020, the International Institute for Race Medicine and World Athletics published an Infectious Diseases Outbreak Management Tool (https://idom.worldathletics.org/) for endurance mass participation sporting events organizers and should help by:

- Assessing the risk level of the event in both quantitative and qualitative manner.
- Determining the public health and sport event's mitigation preparedness.
- Proposing the steps to take to further mitigate and reduce the risk (45).

CONCLUDING COMMONSENSE PRINCIPLES

- Medical planning and preparation are absolute requirements for the successful conduct of mass participation events.
- Following established medical plans and treatment guidelines and remembering limitations with a focus on competitor and staff safety invariably result in a fulfilling experience for everyone involved.

REFERENCES

1. Herring SA, Kibler WB, Putukian M, et al. Mass participation and tournament event management for the team physician: A consensus statement (2022 Update). *Med Sci Sports Exerc*. 2024;56(4):575–89. doi: 10.1249/MSS.0000000000003325
2. Courson R. Preventing sudden death on the athletic field: the emergency action plan. *Curr Sports Med Rep*. 2007;6(2):93–100.
3. American College of Sports Medicine, Armstrong LE, Casa DJ, et al. American College of Sports Medicine position stand. Exertional heat illness during training and competition. *Med Sci Sports Exerc*. 2007;39(3):556–72.
4. Yaglou CP, Minard D. Control of heat casualties at military training centers. *AMA Arch Ind Health*. 1957;16(4):302–16.
5. Roberts WO. Determining a "do not start" temperature for a marathon on the basis of adverse outcomes. *Med Sci Sports Exerc*. 2010;42(2):226–32.
6. Budd GM. Wet-bulb globe temperature(WBGT)—its history and its limitations. *J Sci Med Sport*. 2008;11(1):20–32.
7. Racinais S, Alonso JM, Coutts AJ, et al. Consensus recommendations on training and competing in the heat. *Sports Med*. 2015;45(7):925–38.
8. Greenland K. Medical support for adventure racing. *Emerg Med Australas*. 2004;16(5-6):465–8.
9. Mayers LB, Noakes TD. A guideline to treating ironman triathletes at the finish line. *Phys Sportsmed*. 2000;28(8):33–50.
10. Schwellnus M, Kipps C, Roberts WO, et al. Medical encounters (including injury and illness) at mass community-based endurance sports events: an international consensus statement on definitions and methods of data recording and reporting. *Br J Sports Med*. 2019;53(17):1048–55.
11. Young CC. Extreme sports: injuries and medical coverage. *Curr Sports Med Rep*. 2002;1(5):306–11.
12. Breedt M, Janse van Rensburg DC, Fletcher L, Grant CC, Schwellnus MP. The injury and illness profile of male and female participants in a 94.7 km cycle race: a cross-sectional study. *Clin J Sport Med*. 2019;29(4):306–11.
13. Breslow RG, Giberson-Chen CC, Roberts WO. Burden of injury and illness in the road race medical tent: a narrative review. *Clin J Sport Med*. 2021;31(6):e499–505.
14. Breslow RG, Shrestha S, Feroe AG, Katz JN, Troyanos C, Collins JE. Medical Tent Utilization at 10-km road races: injury, illness, and influencing factors. *Med Sci Sports Exerc*. 2019;51(12):2451–7.
15. Feletti F, Saini G, Naldi S, et al. Injuries in medium to long-distance triathlon: a retrospective analysis of medical conditions treated in three editions of the ironman competition. *J Sports Sci Med*. 2022;21(1):58–67.
16. Gosling CM, Forbes AB, McGivern J, Gabbe BJ. A profile of injuries in athletes seeking treatment during a triathlon race series. *Am J Sports Med*. 2010;38(5):1007–14.
17. Krabak BJ, Waite B, Schiff MA. Study of injury and illness rates in multiday ultramarathon runners. *Med Sci Sports Exerc*. 2011;43(12):2314–20.
18. Pasquina PF, Griffin SC, Anderson-Barnes VC, Tsao JW, O'Connor FG. Analysis of injuries from the Army Ten Miler: a 6-year retrospective review. *Mil Med*. 2013;178(1):55–60.
19. Roberts WO. A 12-yr profile of medical injury and illness for the Twin Cities Marathon. *Med Sci Sports Exerc*. 2000;32(9):1549–55.
20. Schwabe K, Schwellnus M, Derman W, Swanevelder S, Jordaan E. Medical complications and deaths in 21 and 56 km road race runners: a 4-year prospective study in 65 865 runners—SAFER study I. *Br J Sports Med*. 2014;48(11):912–8.
21. Sewry N, Schwellnus M, Boulter J, Seocharan I, Jordaan E. Medical encounters in a 90-km ultramarathon running event: a 6-year study in 103 131 race starters-SAFER XVII. *Clin J Sport Med*. 2022;32(1):e61–7.
22. Tan CM, Tan IW, Kok W, Lee MC, Lee VJ. Medical planning for mass-participation running events: a 3-year review of a half-marathon in Singapore. *BMC Public Health*. 2014;14:1109.
23. Hiller WD, O'Toole ML, Fortess EE, Laird RH, Imbert PC, Sisk TD. Medical and physiological considerations in triathlons. *Am J Sports Med*. 1987;15(2):164–7.
24. Holtzhausen LM, Noakes TD. Collapsed ultraendurance athlete: proposed mechanisms and an approach to management. *Clin J Sport Med*. 1997;7(4):292–301.
25. Roberts WO. Heat and cold: what does the environment do to marathon injury? *Sports Med*. 2007;37(4-5):400–3.
26. Day SM, Thompson PD. Cardiac risks associated with marathon running. *Sports Health*. 2010;2(4):301–6.
27. Kim JH, Malhotra R, Chiampas G, et al. Cardiac arrest during long-distance running races. *N Engl J Med*. 2012;366(2):130–40.
28. Maron BJ, Poliac LC, Roberts WO. Risk for sudden cardiac death associated with marathon running. *J Am Coll Cardiol*. 1996;28(2):428–31.
29. Webner D, DuPrey KM, Drezner JA, Cronholm P, Roberts WO. Sudden cardiac arrest and death in United States marathons. *Med Sci Sports Exerc*. 2012;44(10):1843–5.
30. Laird RH. Medical care at ultraendurance triathlons. *Med Sci Sports Exerc*. 1989;21(5 suppl):S222–5.
31. Martinez JM. Medical coverage of cycling events. *Curr Sports Med Rep*. 2006;5(3):125–30.
32. Davis DP, Videen JS, Marino A, et al. Exercise associated hyponatremia in marathon runners: a two-year experience. *J Emerg Med*. 2001;21(1):47–57.
33. Jaworski CA. Medical concerns of marathons. *Curr Sports Med Rep*. 2005;4(3):137–43.
34. Speedy DB, Noakes TD, Holtzhausen LM. Exercise-associated collapse: postural hypotension, or something deadlier? *Phys Sportsmed*. 2003;31(3):23–9.
35. Adams WM, Hosokawa Y, Troyanos C, Jardine JF. Organization and execution of on-site health care during mass participation events. *Athl Train Sports Health Care*. 2018;10(3):101–4.
36. O'Connor FG, Pyne SW, Brennan FH, Adirim TA. Exercise-associated collapse: an algorithmic approach to race day management part I of II. *Am J Med Sports*. 2003;5:221–7, 229.

37. Cianca JC, Roberts WO, Horn D. Distance running: organization of the medical team. In: O'Connor FG, Wilder RP, editors. *Textbook of Running Medicine*. New York: McGraw-Hill; 2001. p. 489–503.
38. *International Institute of Race Medicine Web site* [Internet]. Plymouth (MA): International Institute of Race Medicine; [cited 2022 Dec 14]. Available from: https://racemedicine.org/
39. Roberts WO. *Preparation and Management of Mass-Participation Endurance Sporting Events*. Up-to-date [Internet]. 2022 [cited 2022 Dec 1]. Available from: https://www.uptodate.com/contents/preparation-and-management-of-mass-participation-endurance-sporting-events
40. Sedgley MD, Hudson K, Madsen CM, O'Connor FG. Something old, something new, something for the marathon for the red, white, and blue. *Curr Sports Med Rep*. 2020 Oct;19(10):393–5.
41. Roberts WO. Assessing core temperature in collapsed athletes: what's the best method? *Phys Sportsmed*. 2000;28(9):71–6.
42. Asplund CA, O'Connor FG, Noakes TD. Exercise-associated collapse: an evidence-based review and primer for clinicians. *Br J Sports Med*. 2011;45(14):1157–62.
43. Roberts WO. Administration and medical management of mass participation endurance events. In: Mellion MB, Walsh WM, Madden C, Putukian M, Shelton GL, editors. *Team Physician's Handbook*. Philadelphia (PA): Hanley & Belfus; 2002. p. 748–56.
44. Ross DS, Ferguson A, Herbert DL. Action in the event tent! Medical-legal issues facing the volunteer event physician. *Sports Health*. 2013;5(4):340–5.
45. Adami PE, Cianca J, McCloskey B, et al. Infectious Diseases Outbreak Management Tool for endurance mass participation sporting events: an international effort to counteract the COVID-19 spread in the endurance sport setting. *Br J Sports Med*. 2021 Feb;55(3):181–2.

17 Catastrophic Sports Injuries

Barry P. Boden

INTRODUCTION

- In the United States, approximately 10% of all brain injuries and 7% of all new cases of paraplegia and quadriplegia are related to athletic activities (1).
- Information on catastrophic injuries in athletes is collected by the National Registry of Catastrophic Sports Injuries (NRCSI), the National Center for Catastrophic Sports Injury Research (NCCSIR), the U.S. Consumer Product Safety Commission (CPSC), and the professional league data registries.
- The NRCSI and NCCSIR define catastrophic sports injury as "any severe spinal, spinal cord, or cerebral injury incurred during participation in a school- or college-sponsored sport." Concussions are not classified as catastrophic injuries.
- Catastrophic injuries are categorized as direct/traumatic, resulting from participating in the skills of a sport (*i.e.*, trauma from a collision), or indirect/nontraumatic, resulting from systemic failure due to exertion while participating in a sport.
- Catastrophic injuries are divided into three subtypes: fatal, nonfatal, and serious. A nonfatal injury is any injury where the athlete suffered a permanent, severe, functional disability. A serious injury is a severe injury with no permanent functional disability (*e.g.*, a fractured cervical vertebra without paralysis) (2).
- The CPSC operates a statistically valid injury and review system known as the National Electronic Injury Surveillance System (NEISS). The NEISS estimates are calculated using data from a sample of hospitals that are representative of emergency departments in the United States. The CPSC does not provide data on injury specifics nor does it include information on injuries that initially presented to physician offices.
- The National Collegiate Athletic Association (NCAA) and the National Federation of State High School Associations (NFHS) review injury epidemiology annually and publish rules with the intent of promoting safe play.

EPIDEMIOLOGY

- The total direct and indirect incidence of catastrophic injuries is approximately 1 per 100,000 high school (HS) athletes and 4 per 100,000 college athletes (2).
- The combined fatality rate for direct and indirect injuries in HS is 0.40 for every 100,000 HS athletes and 1.42 for every 100,000 college participants (2).
- Football is associated with the greatest number of catastrophic injuries for all major team sports followed by cheerleading, baseball, wrestling, and track and field (2).
- Cheerleading is associated with the highest number of direct/traumatic catastrophic injuries for all female sports (2).
- Sports with the highest incidence of catastrophic injuries are female cheerleading, gymnastics, football, male ice hockey, skiing, and female equestrian (2).
- Football fatalities: The most common causes of combined traumatic and nontraumatic football fatalities (1990–2010) were cardiac failure (41%), brain injury (25%), exertional heat stroke (EHS, 16%), and exertional collapse associated with sickle cell trait (ECAST, 11.5%) (3). The average annual combined fatality rate was 12 with the overall fatality risk 3 times higher in college, compared with HS, football players (3).
- From 1998 to 2018 there were an average of 9.4 nontraumatic football fatalities per year (4). The most common causes of death were cardiac (57.7%), EHS (23.6%), ECAST (12.1%), asthma (4.9%), and hyponatremia (1.6%) (3). The risk of a nontraumatic fatality was 4 times higher in NCAA compared to HS athletes (3). Less common causes of nontraumatic deaths include rhabdomyolysis and electrocution caused by lightning (3).
- Since the 1960s, the annual incidence of traumatic fatalities in football has declined four (college)- to five (HS)-fold (4). Conversely, the annual incidence of nontraumatic fatalities has remained constant (4).

INDIRECT INJURIES

Cardiac Conditions

- Most nontraumatic deaths in athletes are caused by cardiovascular conditions such as hypertrophic cardiomyopathy (HCM), cardiac artery anomalies, myocarditis, aortic stenosis, and dysrhythmias (5,6).
- The most common etiology of sudden cardiac death is HCM for those under age 35 and coronary artery disease for those over age 35 (5).

- Athletes with HCM typically have prodromal symptoms such as pre-syncope or syncope with or without exercise prior to the fatal event. A systolic murmur is often appreciated only in the standing position or with a Valsalva maneuver.
- Congenital coronary artery anomalies are a frequent cause of sudden cardiac death (5). These athletes may or may not have symptoms of syncope or chest pain with exercise, making diagnosis difficult.
- Athletes with aortic stenosis and mitral valve prolapse have abnormal auscultatory findings that should lead to the suspected diagnosis.

Prevention

- Prevention strategies for sudden cardiac arrest include detecting cardiac abnormalities during the pre-participation physical examination (PPE), developing and rehearsing an emergency action plan, and immediate application of an automated external defibrillator (AED) (7).
- Due to the difficulties in detecting covert cardiovascular conditions during the PPE, priority should be placed on identifying athletes with previous exertion-related symptoms.
- Sudden cardiac arrest has a high survival rate when an AED is applied within 3 minutes (7,8).

Heat Illness

Epidemiology

- Heat illness is the third most common cause of death in football athletes and the second most common cause of nontraumatic deaths (3,4).
- The greatest risk factor for EHS is being a lineman (9). Linemen are predisposed to heat illness due to larger size and lower baseline aerobic fitness (10), which both contribute to higher core temperature during physical activity.
- From 1998 to 2018 all HS and college heat fatalities occurred during conditioning sessions, not during games (9).
- The primary cause of EHS is intense physical exertion and/or punishment drills during conditioning sessions supervised by the football coach or strength and conditioning coach (9).
- These conditioning sessions often lack exercise science to include consideration of body habitus (obesity), position played (lineman vs. skill player), and acclimation (9). Common scenarios are repetitive sprints where all players are asked to exercise as a unit despite varying baseline conditioning levels (10).
- Environmental conditions such as severe heat and humidity, hydration, and practicing in full pads may contribute to heat illness but are secondary risk factors compared to intense physical exertion.
- Proper hydration does not eliminate the risk for heat illness and excessive hydration can lead to fatality from hyponatremia (9).
- Transition periods (first 10 days of a new conditioning cycle), such as preseason, start of offseason practices, or return from illness are also secondary risk factors.
- In football, an inadequate medical response was documented in most cases in which distressed athletes were ignored, signs and symptoms were missed or misinterpreted, and/or medical treatment was not enacted properly. Athletic trainers were often under the authority of the coaching staff and did not have independent authority for medical decisions (9).

Clinical Features

- Heat cramps is a misnomer and should be termed exercise cramps. Muscle cramping is triggered by fatigue and can occur at any temperature (11).
- Heat syncope is associated with an abrupt loss of consciousness in a heat-exposed athlete, whose core temperature is normal or mildly elevated. The condition often occurs toward the completion of exercise due to reduced cardiac return and postural hypotension. Heat syncope usually occurs during the first few days of heat exposure before the body has acclimatized.
- Heat exhaustion is defined as the inability to continue to exercise in the heat as the cardiovascular system fails to respond to workload. The condition occurs at core or rectal temperatures between 100.4 and 104 °F. Symptoms of heat exhaustion can include muscle cramping, mild confusion, headache, dizziness, chills, nausea, and often collapse.
- Heatstroke is exercise-associated collapse with thermoregulatory failure and central nervous system dysfunction. Heatstroke and mental status changes begin at temperatures in excess of 104 °F. The athlete may or may not be sweating. The condition may result in a variety of life-threatening problems, such as rhabdomyolysis, renal failure, disseminated intravascular coagulopathy, liver failure, and brain injury (11).
- The athlete with repeated heat illness requires a workup for a muscle enzyme deficiency.

Diagnosis and Treatment

- A correct diagnosis is based on the history, physical examination, core body temperature, and differential including hyponatremia and cardiac conditions.
- Treatment involves rapid cooling; moving to a cooler environment; removing clothing; tepid water spray; fans; and ice to the neck, groin, and axilla. Hydration should include both oral intake and intravenous fluids. Rehydration with sports drinks containing electrolytes is preferred over water.
- Athletes with core temperatures greater than 104 °F require cold water immersion. Emergency medical services (EMS) should be contacted for athletes with heat exhaustion and heat stroke (11).

Prevention

- The 2003 NCAA EHS policy has not significantly reduced the risk of heat fatalities in football players because it focuses on the first 5 days of preseason, football equipment worn, number of practices, and the duration of practice sessions, with no regard for intensity of conditioning drills.

- New recommendations encourage a shift from heat and uniform to an emphasis on preventing overexertion, all 365 days of the year, which is the primary component of EHS and most nontraumatic fatalities (9).
- Exercise regimens should be science based, dependent on baseline fitness level, specific for body habitus and position played, allow for acclimation, hold coaches accountable for the conditioning programs that should be publicly available, ensure compliance with current athlete health and welfare policies, and establish independent medical care to allow healthcare providers' authority over athlete medical care (9).
- Leadership is key to educating coaches, strength and conditioning coaches, athletic trainers, physicians, and administrators on risk factors and proper training programs based on position and baseline fitness levels.
- Punishment drills should never be employed (9).
- The culture in football needs to change from teaching mental toughness, which may be associated with risk for overexertion and adverse medical events, to rational training based on exercise science.
- Positions specific training designed to prepare athletes for game requirements with appropriate work to rest ratios is critical. Linemen rarely run more than 30–40 yards during each game play and typically have 35–55 seconds to recover between plays (12).
- Performance tests, such as timed mile runs, should be avoided.
- Overexertion training in sports, especially football can also lead to rhabdomyolysis. The condition is usually caused by repetitive eccentric exercises performed to failure (13). The same conditioning flaws as described with EHS are usually responsible. Although the condition is rarely fatal it can have significant sequelae.

Exertional Sickling With Sickle Cell Trait

- Exertional sickling (ES) with sickle cell trait (SCT) predominantly occurs in African American athletes due to one abnormal sickle gene. Athletes with SCT have a 10- to 37-fold higher risk of sudden death compared with athletes without SCT (14).
- ES with SCT can result in fatality due to overexertion during conditioning sessions (9).
- In 2010, the NCAA mandated rules to prevent Division I football ES with SCT fatalities to include SCT screening, documentation of previous screening, or declination of testing with a signed written release. The policy also promotes targeted education of SCT status inclusive of signs and symptoms of ES with SCT. Precautions allow athletes with SCT to train at their own pace and avoid serial sprints (4).
- Since 2010, the NCAA bylaw has successfully reduced the risk (0.83–0.13 fatalities) and incidence (3.34–0.40 per 100,000 athletes) of ES with SCT deaths in Division I football athletes (4).
- Based on the success of the NCAA SCT bylaw, the author recommends similar laws be mandated at the HS and youth levels.

DIRECT INJURIES

Football

Epidemiology

- Football has the highest number of catastrophic head and neck injuries per year for all HS and college sports (1).

Cervical Injuries

- From 1989 through 2002, the average number of quadriplegic events for HS and college football players was 6 per year (15). The number of quadriplegic events has averaged less than 5 cases · yr^{-1} over the past 20 years (2,16).

Mechanisms

- Spearing or tackling a player with the top of the head is the primary cause of permanent cervical quadriplegia. When the neck is flexed 30°, the cervical spine becomes straight, and the forces are transmitted directly to the spinal structures (17).
- The majority of quadriplegia injuries occur in defensive backs, while making a tackle (17). Special teams' players are also vulnerable to quadriplegia from spear tackling (15).
- Cervical cord neurapraxia (CCN) is an acute, transient neurologic episode associated with sensory changes with or without motor weakness or complete paralysis in the arms, legs, or both (17).
- As opposed to a stinger/burner, which only involves one extremity, CCN diagnosis requires involvement of at least two extremities.
- Complete recovery from CCN usually occurs within 10–15 minutes but may take up to 2 days. The *pincer* mechanism involves cord compression either through hyperflexion or hyperextension of the neck (17). Axial compression also may cause CCN via shear forces on the cervical spine (15).
- An episode of CCN is not an absolute contraindication to return to football (17). It is unlikely that athletes who experience CCN are at risk for permanent neurologic sequelae with return to play.
- The overall risk of a recurrent CCN episode with return to football is approximately 50% and is correlated with the canal diameter size (17). The smaller the canal diameter, the greater is the risk of recurrence (17).

Prevention

- In 1976, spear tackling was banned, and the rate of catastrophic cervical injuries dramatically dropped from an initial average of 30–35 per year to an average of less than 5 per year over the past 20 years (17).
- In addition to the ban on spear tackling, players are taught to play "heads up" ball avoiding contact on the top of the helmet (17).
- Due to the persistent, albeit low rate of quadriplegia due to spear tackling (15), the football rules committees strengthened the spear tackling rule, effective in the 2005–2006

academic year, by removing the word "intentional" from the rule, making it easier for referees to call the spear tackling penalty.

- In response to the number of catastrophic cervical (15) and brain (18) injuries reported during special team plays, the NFL (2011) moved the kickoff spot 5 yards closer to the opponent's end zone to reduce the number of kickoff returns and injuries. Similar kickoff rule changes have been mandated at the nonprofessional levels of football.

Traumatic Brain Injury

Epidemiology

- From 1945 to 1975, there was an average of 9.5 brain fatalities annually at the HS and college levels (19). This number decreased to approximately 5 per year in the 1980s and 3 per year in the 1990s and 2000s (18).
- From 1989 through 2002, there was an average of seven traumatic brain injury (TBIs) per year (0.67 per 100,000) for HS and college football participants (18).
- Between 2002 and 2019 the number of HS and college TBI cases increased to 10 per year (0.8 per 100,000).

Mechanisms

- The majority of catastrophic head injuries are subdural hematomas (18).
- Injuries are 3–4 times more common in a game than a practice session with a disproportionate number of catastrophic brain injuries in special teams' players (18).
- The most common positions played at the time of TBI are defensive backs, linebackers, running backs, and special team players.
- Return to football prior to full recovery from a prior concussion may predispose to a TBI event (18).
- In May 2009, Washington State passed legislation requiring any HS athlete with a suspected concussion to be removed from play and allowed to return to sports (game or practice) only with written permission from a licensed health care provider trained in the evaluation and management of concussion (20). By 2014, similar legislation, referred to as the 'Lystedt laws,' was passed in all 50 states.

Prevention

- The development of a safety standard for the football helmet by the National Operating Committee on Standards for Athletic Equipment (NOCSAE) has been a significant factor in reducing catastrophic head injuries since the 1970s (18,19).
- Enhanced coverage at games and advances in diagnosis and treatment of major brain injuries have also likely reduced the number of fatalities since the 1970s (18).
- Careful surveillance for concussions and referral to medical personnel before return to play is recommended.
- Younger athletes often have a protracted recovery from concussion and may require delayed return to play compared to college and professional athletes (18,21).
- Training medical personnel to understand on-field management of athletic head and neck injuries and guidelines for return to contact or collision sport after an injury may help reduce injuries.
- While the Lystedt laws have demonstrated an increased concussion diagnosis rate and a decline in recurrent concussion rate, there is no evidence that the laws have reduced TBI rates.

Pole Vaulting

Epidemiology

- Pole vaulting is a unique sport in that athletes often land from heights ranging from 10 to 20 ft. Prior to 2003, pole vaulting had one of the highest rates of direct, catastrophic injuries per 100,000 participants for all sports monitored by the NCCSIR and the second highest number of traumatic fatalities for all HS and college sports (22).
- The vast majority of catastrophic pole vaulting injuries are head injuries in male athletes. From 1982 to 1998 there was an average of two catastrophic pole vault injuries per year, and one fatality per year. Most injuries occurred at the HS level (22).

Mechanisms

- Two common mechanisms of injury have been described (22). The most common mechanism was when a pole vaulter completely or partially missing the side or the back of the landing pad and his head strikes the surrounding hard surface (in most cases, either concrete or asphalt).
- The second most common mechanism occurs when the vaulter releases the pole prematurely or does not have enough momentum and lands in the vault or planting box.

Prevention

- As of January 2003, both the NCAA and NFHS increased the minimum pole vault landing pad size from 16′ × 12′–19′8″ × 16′5″.
- Any hard or unyielding surfaces such as concrete, metal, wood, or asphalt around the landing pad must be padded or cushioned with a minimum of 2 in. of dense foam.
- A new rule was adopted placing the crossbar farther back over the landing pad.
- A coach's box or painted square in the middle of the landing pad was recommended. This zone would help train athletes to instinctively land near the center of the landing pad. Other safety measures include marking the runway distances so athletes can better gauge their takeoff and prohibiting the practice of tapping or assisting the vaulter at takeoff.
- Pole vaulting is a complicated sport requiring extensive training. Certification by coaches is encouraged.
- The value of helmets in reducing head injuries in HS pole vaulters is controversial. Without conclusive data as to their protective effect, the use of helmets is optional for athletes at this time.

- Since the rule changed in 2003, the number of catastrophic pole-vaulting injuries reported from athletes missing the sides or back of the landing pad has dramatically dropped by 68%, from 1.38 before to 0.44 after the rule change (23).
- More importantly, the annual fatality rate has dropped from 0.90 before to 0.13 after the rule changes. The rule changes have saved an estimated 12 lives from 2003 to 2019 and there have been no pole vault fatalities over the last 9 years (23).
- Despite the dramatic reduction in fatalities after the 2003 rule changes, the annual number of catastrophic injuries from athletes landing in the vault box (plant box) area has persisted (23).
- In a survey of 5840 vaulters, 80% reported landing in or directly around the vault box during their career, indicating the vault box area is currently the most dangerous landing zone (24,25).
- In another study, 533 vault boxes were inspected and 97% were estimated to result in a fatal injury with an unprotected fall from a height of 12′5″ (25).
- Based on these findings new vault boxes and the perimeter surfaces are being developed with improved shock absorption properties. In addition, the new plant boxes have features ensuring the front lip is flush or lower than the runway.

Soccer

Epidemiology

- Injuries to the head, neck, and face in soccer account for between 5% and 15% of all injuries. Most head and neck injuries occur when two players collide, especially when jumping to head the ball.
- Direct fatalities in soccer are usually associated with either movable goalposts falling on a victim or player impact with the goalpost (26). The CPSC identified at least 21 deaths over a 16-year period associated with movable goalposts (27).
- The incidence of concussions in college soccer athletes is approximately one per team per season (28). There is a 50% chance for a professional athlete to sustain a concussion over a 10-year span. Most concussions occur as a result of contact with an opposing player, not with the soccer ball.
- There is no evidence that an isolated episode of heading a soccer ball can cause any head injury; however, there is controversy over whether repetitive soccer heading over a prolonged career can lead to neuropsychological deficits.

Prevention

- Children should never be allowed to climb on the net or goal framework. Soccer goalposts should be secured at all times.
- During the off-season, goals should be either disassembled or placed in a safe storage area. Goals should be moved only by trained personnel and should be used only on flat fields (1,27).
- The use of padded goalposts may also reduce the incidence of impact injuries with the goalposts (26).
- Children should use smaller soccer balls to reduce the risks of repetitive heading. Leather or water-soaked soccer balls should never be used.
- Proper heading techniques should be employed: contact on the forehead with the neck muscles contracted. Soccer players should be trained to hit the ball, not to be hit by the ball.
- New rules are beginning to limit heading in youth soccer.

Wrestling

Epidemiology

- Indirect catastrophic wrestling injuries are often the result of rapid weight loss, which causes dehydration and potential cardiovascular compromise (29,30).
- There are approximately two direct catastrophic wrestling injuries per year at the HS and college levels (31). The direct catastrophic injury rate in HS and college wrestlers is approximately 1 per 100,000 participants.

Mechanisms

- The majority of injuries occur in match competitions, where intense, competitive situations place wrestlers at a higher risk (31–33).
- There is a trend toward more direct injuries in the low- and middle-weight classes.
- Cervical fractures or major cervical ligament injuries constitute the majority of direct catastrophic wrestling injuries (31).
- There is no clear predominance of any one type of takedown hold that contributes to wrestling injuries.
- The position most frequently associated with injury is the defensive posture during the takedown maneuver, followed by the down position (kneeling) and the lying position (31).
- The athlete is typically injured by one of three scenarios: (a) The wrestler's arms are in a hold such that he or she is unable to protect his head when thrown to the mat. (b) The wrestler attempts a roll but is landed on by the full weight of his opponent, causing a twisting, usually hyperflexion, neck injury. (c) The wrestler lands on the top of his head, sustaining an axial compression force to the cervical spine (31).

Prevention

- A minimum body fat for HS and college wrestlers has been established to reduce weight loss injuries. The NFHS also instituted a rule that competitors cannot lose more than 1.5% body weight per week. Both the NCAA and NFHS have banned the use of laxatives, diuretics, and other rapid weight loss techniques such as rubber suits.
- Referees should strictly enforce penalties for slams and gain more awareness of dangerous holds (31). There is particular vulnerability for the defensive wrestler who may be off balance, have one or both arms held, and then have his opponent land on top of him.
- Stringent penalties for intentional slams or throws are encouraged. The referee should have a low threshold of

tolerance to stop the match during potentially dangerous situations.

- Coaches can prevent serious injuries by emphasizing safe, legal wrestling techniques. Coaches should teach wrestlers to keep their head up during any takedown maneuver to prevent axial compression injuries to the cervical spine. Proper rolling techniques, with avoidance of landing on the head, need to be emphasized in practice sessions (31).

Cheerleading

Epidemiology

- Cheerleading has evolved into an activity demanding high levels of skill, athleticism, and complex gymnastics maneuvers.
- Cheerleading is one of the most popular organized sports activities for HS girls (34).
- Cheerleaders in college and HS account for more than half of the catastrophic injuries that occur in female athletes (35). From 1982 to 2002 there were approximately two direct catastrophic cheerleading injuries per year. The catastrophic injury rate is 0.4 per 100,000 in HS cheerleaders, 2 per 100,000 college participants, or an overall rate of 0.6 per 100,000 cheerleaders (35).
- In 2000, the CPSC estimated a total of 1258 head injuries in cheerleaders, of which 604 were recorded as concussions and six as skull fractures. In the same year, there were 1814 neck injuries with 76 fractures in cheerleaders that initially presented to an emergency department in the United States (27).
- Compared with other sports, cheerleading has a low overall incidence of injuries (34) but a high risk of catastrophic injuries (35).
- The most frequent catastrophic cheerleading injuries are brain injuries followed by cervical fractures or major ligament injuries.
- The majority of injuries occur in female athletes because there are more female than male cheerleaders and the women are usually at the top of the pyramid or being thrown into the air during basket tosses (BTs). The majority of injuries occur during the winter months because cheerleaders perform on indoor hard surfaces.
- College athletes are five times more likely to sustain a catastrophic injury than their HS counterparts due to the increased complexity of stunts at the college level (35). Catastrophic head injuries are twice as common as cervical injuries.

Mechanisms

- The most common stunts resulting in catastrophic injury are the pyramid or the BT (35). The cheerleader at the top of the pyramid is most frequently injured. A BT is a stunt where a cheerleader is thrown into the air, often between 6 and 20 ft, by either three or four tossers. Poor judgment or inadequate training of the spotter is often the main problem leading to injury.
- Less common mechanisms include advanced floor tumbling routines, participating on a wet surface, or performing a mount. The majority of injuries occur when an athlete lands on an indoor hard gym surface (35).

Prevention

- Height restrictions on pyramids are limited to two levels in HS and 2.5 body lengths in college (35). The top cheerleaders are required to be supported by one or more individuals (base) who are in direct weight-bearing contact with the performing surface. The base cheerleaders must remain stationary and maintain constant contact with the suspended or top athlete. Spotters must be present for each person extended above shoulder level. The suspended person is not allowed to be inverted (head below horizontal) or to rotate on the dismount. Limiting the total number of cheerleaders in a pyramid as well as the quick transitions between pyramids and other complex stunts may also help reduce injuries.
- BT rules limit the stunt to four tossers, starting the toss from the ground level (no flips) and having one of the tossers behind the top person during the toss. The top person (flyer) must be directed vertically and not allow the head to drop backward out of alignment with the torso or below a horizontal plane with the body.
- All stunts should be restricted when wet conditions are present.
- Injuries from floor tumbling routines can be prevented by proper supervision, progression to complex tumbling only when simple maneuvers are mastered, and using spotters as necessary.
- Mini trampolines, springboards, and any apparatus used to propel a participant have been prohibited since the late 1980s.
- Cheerleading coaches need to place equal time and attention on the technique and attentiveness of spotters in practice compared with the athletes performing the stunts.
- Pyramids and BTs should be limited to experienced cheerleaders who have mastered all other skills and should not be performed without qualified spotters or landing mats.
- The governing bodies implemented several safety measures after the 2005–6 academic year. The most important new rule mandated that cheerleaders be prohibited from BT stunts on any hardwood court unless it is on a mat (minimum thickness 1⅝"), and it had to be performed during halftime or postgame in an area free of obstruction.
- In the same year college teams were required to have two spotters for each individual at the 2.5 person height, and outline the allowable surfaces for the pyramid.
- The NCAA also adopted a policy that all cheerleading teams be supervised by a certified coach.
- Since the rule changed in 2006, there has been a 70% (HS) and 66% (college) reduction in the annual number of all catastrophic cheerleading injuries (36). There have been no BT injuries reported at the collegiate level since the 2006

rule change. At the HS level there was a lag effect with the number of BT injuries being reduced between 2007 and 2010 and no injuries over the last 9 years of data collection (2010–2019) (36).

Baseball

Epidemiology

- Baseball has a low rate of noncatastrophic injuries but a high incidence of catastrophic injuries.
- Head injuries constitute the majority of catastrophic injuries.
- There are approximately two direct catastrophic injuries reported to the NCCSIR per year or 0.6 injuries per 100,000 participants (37). The total incidences of catastrophic injuries and fatalities are 5 and 13 times higher, respectively, at the college level than at the HS level (37).

Mechanisms

- The most common catastrophic injury mechanism is a pitcher hit by a batted ball, followed by a collision of two fielders and a collision of a runner and a fielder (37). Head first diving by the runner, especially at home plate, can place the runner at risk for an axial compression cervical injury potentially resulting in quadriplegia (37).
- An area of controversy in baseball is the safety of aluminum or enhanced bats. Non-wood bats are typically lighter than wood bats and can be swung faster with greater ball velocity off the bat. In addition, the non-wood bats are more compliant than wood bats, so the ball recoils at a greater speed, compared to a wood bat, where the ball loses much of its energy on impact.
- Commotio cordis is arrhythmia or sudden death from low-impact blunt trauma to the chest in subjects with no preexisting cardiac disease (38–40). The proposed mechanism is impact just prior to the peak of the T wave on an electrocardiogram, which induces ventricular fibrillation. The pediatric population may be more susceptible because of a thinner layer of soft tissue to the chest wall, increased compliance of the immature rib cage, and slower protective reflexes.

Prevention

- Protecting pitchers from a batted ball may be accomplished by requiring pitchers to wear helmets, using protective screens during batting practice, and regulating the bat and ball (37).
- In 2003, the NCAA and NFHS placed new regulations on bats. All bats must be certified as having a ball exit speed that cannot exceed 97 miles · h^{-1} as measured by the Baum hitting machine. In addition, certified bats may not weigh more than 3 oz less than the length of the bat (*e.g.*, a 34-in. long bat cannot weigh less than 31 oz) (37).
- The NHFS (Jan. 2012) strengthened the bat rules replacing the ball-exit-speed-ratio with the Bat-Ball-Coefficient of Restitution (BBCor). The BBCor more accurately measures the trampoline effect of the ball off the bat, ensuring non-wood bats perform comparably to wood bats in an attempt to improve player safety.
- Decreasing the ball's hardness and weight may significantly reduce injury severity. The coefficient of restitution or the measure of rebound that a ball has off a hard surface cannot exceed 0.555 at the HS and college levels.
- Preventive strategies for commotio cordis include teaching youth baseball players to turn their chest away from a batted ball. The use of chest protectors is controversial.
- AEDs are the most effective current method for preventing fatalities from commotio cordis (39,40).

Ice Hockey

Epidemiology

- Although the number of catastrophic injuries in ice hockey is low compared with other sports, the incidence per 100,000 participants is high (2,41).
- The majority of catastrophic injuries occur to the cervical spine.

Mechanisms

- Most injuries occur when an athlete is struck from behind by an opponent and contacts another object, especially the boards, with the crown of the head (42,43).
- Head and facial injuries are common from collisions or being hit by the puck or stick.
- Catastrophic accidents from collisions with goalposts were common before the advent of displaceable goalposts.

Prevention

- Cervical quadriplegia in ice hockey can be prevented by enforcing current rules against pushing or checking from behind, especially near the boards (43).
- Ice hockey players are encouraged to use helmets and full-face masks.
- Padding the boards and developing a potential space between the boards and the Plexiglass extension may reduce the frequency and severity of head and neck injuries.
- Goals should not be fixed so they can slide out of position to protect athletes from colliding against an immovable object.
- Fighting should be discouraged in ice hockey.

Swimming

Mechanisms

- Most catastrophic swimming injuries are caused by diving into the shallow end of pools and contacting the bottom of the pool with the top of the head (41).
- Hyperventilating just prior to swimming can rid the body of carbon dioxide. This fools the brain into thinking it doesn't need to breathe, even when its oxygen stores are dangerously low, which may lead to loss of consciousness and drowning.

Prevention

- At the HS level, swimmers must start the race in the water if the water depth at the starting end is less than 3.5 ft. If the water depth is 3.5 ft to less than 4 ft at the starting end, the swimmer may start from the deck or in the water. If the water depth at the starting end is 4 ft or more, the swimmer may start from a platform up to 30 in. above the water surface.

- The NFHS mandates that swimmers break the surface of water to breathe at or before 15 m to prevent shallow water blackout.

Rugby

Mechanisms

- Cervical spine injuries occur most frequently during a scrum, when the opposing sides of tightly bound players come forcibly together (engagement) (44).
- The hooker or central player on the front row of the scrum suffers the most injuries. If engagement does not occur properly or the hooker employs the top of the head as a weapon with the neck flexed during contact, an axial compression injury with quadriplegia may result (44).

Prevention

- Preventative methods include avoiding a mismatch in physical size of the hookers, not allowing unskilled players to participate on the front row, and restricting tackling with the top of the head (43).
- Sequential engagement or having the front rows engage separately from the pack is encouraged (43). A new international rugby rule in 2007 requires a "crouch, touch, pause, and engage" maneuver during the scrum. Front row players are not allowed to be more than an arm's length away from the opponent before engagement.

Gymnastics

- Most injuries are associated with a missed vault, a fall from the parallel bars or horizontal bar, or a faulty dismount (41).

GENERAL PREVENTION TIPS

- Preparticipation physicals
- Qualified coaches
- Proper strength and conditioning programs that avoid irrational overexertion
- Supervision of athletes at all times
- EMS protocols in place at all times
- Continued research concerning catastrophic injuries and methods to prevent these injuries

REFERENCES

1. Boden BP. Direct catastrophic injury in sports. *J Am Acad Orthop Surg.* 2005;13(7):445–54.
2. Kucera K, Cantu R. *NCCSIR Thirty-Eighth Annual Report. National Center for Catastrophic Sports Injury Research: Fall 1982–Spring 2020. Sept 24, 2021 Ed.* Chapel Hill (NC): National Center for Sports Injury Research; 2021.
3. Boden BP, Breit I, Beachler JA, Williams A, Mueller FO. Fatalities in high school and college football players. *Am J Sports Med.* 2013;41(5):1108–16. doi:10.1177/0363546513478572
4. Boden BP, Fine KM, Breit I, Lentz W, Anderson SA. Nontraumatic exertional fatalities in football players, part 1: epidemiology and effectiveness of National Collegiate Athletic Association bylaws. *Orthop J Sports Med.* 2020;8(8):2325967120942490. doi:10.1177/2325967120942490
5. Maron BJ, Haas TS, Ahluwalia A, Murphy CJ, Garberich RF. Demographics and epidemiology of sudden deaths in young competitive athletes: from the United States National Registry. *Am J Med.* 2016;129(11):1170–7. doi:10.1016/j.amjmed.2016.02.031
6. Maron BJ, Doerer JJ, Haas TS, Tierney DM, Mueller FO. Sudden deaths in young competitive athletes: analysis of 1866 deaths in the United States, 1980-2006. *Circulation.* 2009;119(8):1085–92. doi:10.1161/circulationaha.108.804617
7. Casa DJ, Almquist J, Anderson SA, et al. The inter-association task force for preventing sudden death in secondary school athletics programs: best-practices recommendations. *J Athl Train.* 2013;48(4):546–53. doi:10.4085/1062-6050-48.4.12
8. Drezner JA, Toresdahl BG, Rao AL, Huszti E, Harmon KG. Outcomes from sudden cardiac arrest in US high schools: a 2-year prospective study from the National Registry for AED Use in Sports. *Br J Sports Med.* 2013;47(18):1179–83. doi:10.1136/bjsports-2013-092786
9. Boden BP, Fine KM, Spencer TA, Breit I, Anderson SA. Nontraumatic exertional fatalities in football players, part 2: excess in conditioning kills. *Orthop J Sports Med.* 2020;8(8):2325967120943491. doi:10.1177/2325967120943491
10. Boden BP, Ahmed AE, Fine KM, Craven MJ, Deuster PA. Baseline aerobic fitness in high school and college football players: critical for prescribing safe exercise regimens. *Sports Health.* 2022;14(4):490–9. doi:10.1177/19417381211058458
11. Howe AS, Boden BP. Heat-related illness in athletes. *Am J Sports Med.* 2007;35(8):1384–95. doi:10.1177/0363546507305013
12. Hoffman JR. The applied physiology of American football. *Int J Sports Physiol Perform.* 2008;3(3):387–92.
13. Boden BP, Isaacs DJ, Ahmed AE, Anderson SA. Epidemiology of exertional rhabdomyolysis in the United States: analysis of NEISS database 2000 to 2019. *Phys Sportsmed.* 2022;50(6):486–93. doi:10.1080/00913847.2021.1956288
14. Harmon KG, Drezner JA, Klossner D, Asif IM. Sickle cell trait associated with a RR of death of 37 times in National Collegiate Athletic Association football athletes: a database with 2 million athlete-years as the denominator. *Br J Sports Med.* 2012;46(5):325–30. doi:10.1136/bjsports-2011-090896
15. Boden BP, Tacchetti RL, Cantu RC, Knowles SB, Mueller FO. Catastrophic cervical spine injuries in high school and college football players. *Am J Sports Med.* 2006;34(8):1223–32. doi:10.1177/0363546506288306
16. Kucera K, Klossner D, Colgate B, Cantu R. *Annual Survey of Football Injury Research*, 1931-2019; 2020. National Center for Sports Injury Research.
17. Torg JS, Guille JT, Jaffe S. Injuries to the cervical spine in American football players. *J Bone Joint Surg Am.* 2002;84(1):112–22.
18. Boden BP, Tacchetti RL, Cantu RC, Knowles SB, Mueller FO. Catastrophic head injuries in high school and college football players. *Am J Sports Med.* 2007;35(7):1075–81. doi:10.1177/0363546507299239
19. Cantu RC, Mueller FO. Brain injury-related fatalities in American football, 1945-1999. *Neurosurgery.* 2003;52(4):846–53; discussion 852-3.
20. Bompadre V, Jinguji TM, Yanez ND, et al. Washington State's Lystedt law in concussion documentation in Seattle public high schools. *J Athl Train.* 2014;49(4):486–92. doi:10.4085/1062-6050-49.3.30

21. Field M, Collins MW, Lovell MR, Maroon J. Does age play a role in recovery from sports-related concussion? A comparison of high school and collegiate athletes. *J Pediatr.* 2003;142(5):546–53. doi:10.1067/mpd.2003.190
22. Boden BP, Pasquina P, Johnson J, Mueller FO. Catastrophic injuries in pole-vaulters. *Am J Sports Med.* 2001;29(1):50–4.
23. Boden BP, Boden MG, Peter RG, Mueller FO, Johnson JE. Catastrophic injuries in pole vaulters: a prospective 9-year follow-up study. *Am J Sports Med.* 2012;40(7):1488–94. doi:10.1177/0363546512446682
24. Boden BP, Johnson J. Pole vault landings and injury. In: *Track Coach 221.* Indianapolis (IN): USATF; 2017. p. 6991–8.
25. Johnson J, Boden B. Causes and effects of pole vault plant box landings and potential improvements. In: *Track Coach.* Indianapolis (IN): USATF; 2017. p. 7015–22.
26. Janda DH, Bir C, Wild B, Olson S, Hensinger RN. Goal post injuries in soccer. A laboratory and field testing analysis of a preventive intervention. *Am J Sports Med.* 1995;23(3):340–4. doi:10.1177/036354659502300316
27. Consumer Product Safety Commission. *National Electronic Injury Surveillance System* 2000-2019 *on NEISS Online Database*; April 2020.
28. Boden BP, Kirkendall DT, Garrett WE Jr. Concussion incidence in elite college soccer players. *Am J Sports Med.* 1998;26(2):238–41.
29. Kiningham RB, Gorenflo DW. Weight loss methods of high school wrestlers. *Med Sci Sports Exerc.* 2001;33(5):810–3. doi:10.1097/00005768-200105000-00021
30. Oppliger RA, Case HS, Horswill CA, Landry GL, Shelter AC. American College of Sports Medicine position stand. Weight loss in wrestlers. *Med Sci Sports Exerc.* 1996;28(10):135–8.
31. Boden BP, Lin W, Young M, Mueller FO. Catastrophic injuries in wrestlers. *Am J Sports Med.* 2002;30(6):791–5.
32. Pasque CB, Hewett TE. A prospective study of high school wrestling injuries. *Am J Sports Med.* 2000;28(4):509–15. doi:10.1177/0363546500 0280041101
33. Jarret GJ, Orwin JF, Dick RW. Injuries in collegiate wrestling. *Am J Sports Med.* 1998;26(5):674–80. doi:10.1177/03635465980260051301
34. Currie DW, Fields SK, Patterson MJ, Comstock RD. Cheerleading injuries in United States high schools. *Pediatrics.* 2016;137(1). doi:10.1542/peds.2015-2447
35. Boden BP, Tacchetti R, Mueller FO. Catastrophic cheerleading injuries. *Am J Sports Med.* 2003;31(6):881–8.
36. Yau RK, Dennis SG, Boden BP, Cantu RC, Lord JA III, Kucera KL. Catastrophic high school and collegiate cheerleading injuries in the United States: an examination of the 2006-2007 basket toss rule change. *Sports Health.* 2019;11(1):32–9. doi:10.1177/1941738118807122
37. Boden BP, Tacchetti R, Mueller FO. Catastrophic injuries in high school and college baseball players. *Am J Sports Med.* 2004;32(5):1189–96. doi:10.1177/0363546503262161
38. Maron BJ, Shirani J, Poliac LC, Mathenge R, Roberts WC, Mueller FO. Sudden death in young competitive athletes. Clinical, demographic, and pathological profiles. *JAMA.* 1996;276(3):199–204.
39. Janda DH, Bir CA, Viano DC, Cassatta SJ. Blunt chest impacts: assessing the relative risk of fatal cardiac injury from various baseballs. *J Trauma.* 1998;44(2):298–303. doi:10.1097/00005373-199802000-00011
40. Maron BJ, Poliac LC, Kaplan JA, Mueller FO. Blunt impact to the chest leading to sudden death from cardiac arrest during sports activities. *N Engl J Med.* 1995;333(6):337–42. doi:10.1056/nejm199508103330602
41. Mueller FO, Cantu RC, Van Camp SP. *Catastrophic Injuries in High School and College Sports.* Human Kinetics; 1996.
42. Tator CH, Edmonds VE, Lapczak L, Tator IB. Spinal injuries in ice hockey players, 1966-1987. *Can J Surg.* 1991;34(1):63–9.
43. Morrissette C, Park PJ, Lehman RA, Popkin CA. Cervical spine injuries in the ice hockey player: current concepts in epidemiology, management and prevention. *Global Spine J.* 2021;11(8):1299–306. doi:10.1177/2192568220970549
44. Wetzler MJ, Akpata T, Laughlin W, Levy AS. Occurrence of cervical spine injuries during the rugby scrum. *Am J Sports Med.* 1998;26(2):177–80. doi:10.1177/03635465980260020501

18

Preparticipation Physical Examination

Robert E. Sallis and Stephanie H. Lai

INTRODUCTION

- It is estimated that approximately 10–15 million or more athletes from grade school to college require preparticipation examinations (PPEs) annually in the United States (1).
- No defined national standard exists for PPEs and each state has differing laws and statutes regarding how they are done.
- The utility, effectiveness, and accessibility of the PPE have been areas of debate and controversies. There is currently limited evidence to support the PPEs effectiveness for detecting conditions that predisposed athletes to injury or illness. Areas of lower socioeconomic class may have affordability or availability barriers that may prevent them from having access to PPEs (2).

GOALS

- Ensure that athletes of all ages and skill levels can safely compete.
- Detect any condition, medical or musculoskeletal, that may limit an athlete's participation or require treatment, rehabilitation, or adequate control prior to participation.
- Detect any condition that may predispose an athlete to injury or lead to sudden death during competition.
- Meet legal or insurance requirements (all 50 states require yearly examinations).
- Determine general health of the athlete.
- Assess fitness level for specific sports.
- Counsel on lifestyle issues and high-risk behaviors.
- Answer health-related questions, and update vaccines.

QUALIFIED PROVIDERS

- It is recommended by the American Heart Association (AHA) that providers who perform screening PPEs have adequate medical training, particularly in cardiovascular auscultation (3).
- Currently, however, 18 states allow chiropractors and naturopathic practitioners to screen athletes (3).

FORMAT

- Private office with primary care provider
  - Advantages: privacy, controlled environment, access to medical records, better continuity of care, and easier to perform counseling and routine preventive care.
  - Disadvantages: higher cost, less communication with school athletic staff, and potential for providers who have insufficient knowledge and skills necessary for a complete and appropriate evaluation.
- Group examination (usually done as a station-based examination)
  - Advantages: more cost-effective, more time-efficient, usually done at school with athletic staff present, so easier to communicate.
  - Disadvantages: lack of privacy, loud and chaotic environment thereby impairing proper cardiac auscultation, and poor follow-up.

FREQUENCY AND TIMING OF EXAMINATION

- Most states require an examination to be done yearly for high school–aged and younger athletes. However, a comprehensive exam every 2 years with yearly updates as needed is recommended by the AHA.
- The National Collegiate Athletic Association (NCAA) requires an initial complete PPE prior to participation in intercollegiate athletics, with interim annual updates of the athlete's history. Further PPEs are not deemed necessary unless indicated by the updated history (4).
- Optimal timing for the examination is at least 6 weeks before the season starts to allow sufficient time for further evaluation, treatment, and/or rehabilitation of any problems that may be uncovered.

CONTENT

- Because the stress of sports and exercise falls primarily on the cardiovascular and musculoskeletal systems, these areas are essential for assessment as part of the PPE. This evaluation should begin with a thorough history, followed by a focused physical examination.
- Close attention should also be paid to the neurologic history to specifically address concussions, stingers, and other neurologic issues.
- In 1992, representatives from several national physician groups assembled to develop a comprehensive PPE tool for use among providers who perform athletic screening. Since then, there have been periodic updates.
  - *Preparticipation Physical Examination*, 6th Edition (PPE Monograph), is the most recent iteration of this work, which has been established through the collaboration of the American College of Sports Medicine, American Academy of Family Physicians (AAFP), American Academy of Pediatrics (AAP), American Medical Society for Sports Medicine (AMSSM), American Orthopaedic Society for Sports Medicine (AOSSM), and American Osteopathic Academy of Sports (AOASM) (5).
  - It is recommended that all providers use this monograph as the primary resource and template for the PPE.

MEDICAL HISTORY

- A thorough personal and family medical history has been shown to identify up to 75% of all medical problems affecting athletes (6).
- The easiest method for obtaining an athlete's history is to use a preprinted questionnaire (such as the one available in the PPE monograph) that the parent(s) of the athlete completes prior to the examination (Fig. 18.1). The history portion of these forms is best filled out by the parents and the athlete together, because the athlete may not be fully aware of his or her complete personal and/or family history.
- Key questions include asking about any major preexisting medical problems or injuries; if the athlete is taking any medicines or supplements; if the athlete has any significant environmental and/or medication allergies; and about the athlete's current state of health, including mental health.
- Assess for cardiovascular risk. Because most sudden death episodes in sports are due to cardiovascular causes, thorough cardiovascular screening is extremely important.
  - The relative risk for sudden cardiac death (SCD) has been found to be 2.5 times higher in athletes than in the general population (7).
  - The AHA has recommended 10 history questions as the initial screening for cardiovascular risk. The PPE Monograph uses those questions (see Fig. 18.1).
  - Positive answers to critical history questions such as "Have you ever passed out or nearly passed out DURING or AFTER exercise?" and "Have you ever had discomfort, pain, tightness, or pressure in your chest during exercise?" (Questions 1 and 2) may signal the presence of a structural heart problem.
  - It is also important to assess for family history of unexplained death before the age of 50, cardiovascular abnormalities, or concerning signs and symptoms that may suggest possible undiagnosed cardiac abnormalities in family members.
  - Universal mandatory electrocardiograms are not recommended given cost-efficacy in the setting of false-negative and false-positive results that may be influenced by observer variability in ECG interpretation (8).
- Assess for symptoms of exercise-induced bronchospasm (EIB):
  - Symptoms include coughing, wheezing, and/or chest tightness during or immediately after exercise, especially in those with a personal or family history of allergic rhinitis, eczema, or asthma.
  - Improvement of symptoms after using an inhaled bronchodilator is highly suggestive.
- Assess for concussion history:
  - It is important to ask about the symptoms of concussion because those who have had one may not have sought medical attention and been diagnosed.
  - Common symptoms include headache, nausea, dizziness, blurred vision, getting "dinged" or your "bell rung," fatigue, either hypersomnolence or insomnia, retrograde amnesia, emotional lability, inability to concentrate in school or with homework, irritability, confusion, "not feeling right," and "feeling like in a fog" (9,10).
  - If the patient can recall one or more of these symptoms in association with an impact to the head or body (possibly denoting a contrecoup injury), then he or she likely had a concussion.
- Assess for history of repeated "stingers" and/or "burners," which are symptoms of numbness and/or pain radiating down an arm after a blow to the head, neck, or ipsilateral shoulder; if present, they may indicate cervical stenosis or a similar condition.
- Assess for history of recent COVID-19 infection:
  - Severity of symptoms will guide return to physical activity and clearance. If an athlete has already returned to exercise, it is important to assess for any cardiovascular symptoms and to educate athletes on reporting new onset of cardiovascular symptoms during exercise (11).
  - Use the opportunity to determine vaccination status and facilitate administration if not vaccinated.
  - Becoming fully vaccinated not only decreases the risk of infection and the safe resumption of sport activities, but it also allows for reduction in loss of time due to outbreak,

This form should be placed into the athlete's medical file and should *not* be shared with schools or sports organizations. The Medical Eligibility Form is the only form that should be submitted to a school or sports organization.

Disclaimer: Athletes who have a current Preparticipation Physical Evaluation (per state and local guidance) on file should not need to complete another History Form.

PREPARTICIPATION PHYSICAL EVALUATION (Interim Guidance)

HISTORY FORM

Note: Complete and sign this form (with your parents if younger than 18) before your appointment.

Name: ______________________ Date of birth: ______________

Date of examination: ______________ Sport(s): ______________________

Sex assigned at birth (F, M, or intersex): ________ How do you identify your gender? (F, M, non-binary, or another gender): ________

Have you had COVID-19? (check one): ☐ Y ☐ N

Have you been immunized for COVID-19? (check one): ☐ Y ☐ N If yes, have you had: ☐ One shot ☐ Two shots ☐ Three shots ☐ Booster date(s) ______________

List past and current medical conditions. ______________________

Have you ever had surgery? If yes, list all past surgical procedures. ______________________

Medicines and supplements: List all current prescriptions, over-the-counter medicines, and supplements (herbal and nutritional).

____

Do you have any allergies? If yes, please list all your allergies (ie, medicines, pollens, food, stinging insects).

____

Patient Health Questionnaire Version 4 (PHQ-4)

Over the last 2 weeks, how often have you been bothered by any of the following problems? (Circle response.)

	Not at all	Several days	Over half the days	Nearly every day
Feeling nervous, anxious, or on edge	0	1	2	3
Not being able to stop or control worrying	0	1	2	3
Little interest or pleasure in doing things	0	1	2	3
Feeling down, depressed, or hopeless	0	1	2	3

(A sum of ≥3 is considered positive on either subscale [questions 1 and 2, or questions 3 and 4] for screening purposes.)

GENERAL QUESTIONS (Explain "Yes" answers at the end of this form. Circle questions if you don't know the answer.)	Yes	No
1. Do you have any concerns that you would like to discuss with your provider?		
2. Has a provider ever denied or restricted your participation in sports for any reason?		
3. Do you have any ongoing medical issues or recent illness?		
HEART HEALTH QUESTIONS ABOUT YOU	**Yes**	**No**
4. Have you ever passed out or nearly passed out during or after exercise?		
5. Have you ever had discomfort, pain, tightness, or pressure in your chest during exercise?		
6. Does your heart ever race, flutter in your chest, or skip beats (irregular beats) during exercise?		
7. Has a doctor ever told you that you have any heart problems?		
8. Has a doctor ever requested a test for your heart? For example, electrocardiography (ECG) or echocardiography.		

HEART HEALTH QUESTIONS ABOUT YOU (*CONTINUED*)		Yes	No
9. Do you get light-headed or feel shorter of breath than your friends during exercise?			
10. Have you ever had a seizure?			
HEART HEALTH QUESTIONS ABOUT YOUR FAMILY	**Unsure**	**Yes**	**No**
11. Has any family member or relative died of heart problems or had an unexpected or unexplained sudden death before age 35 years (including drowning or unexplained car crash)?			
12. Does anyone in your family have a genetic heart problem such as hypertrophic cardiomyopathy (HCM), Marfan syndrome, arrhythmogenic right ventricular cardiomyopathy (ARVC), long QT syndrome (LQTS), short QT syndrome (SQTS), Brugada syndrome, or catecholaminergic polymorphic ventricular tachycardia (CPVT)?			
13. Has anyone in your family had a pacemaker or an implanted defibrillator before age 35?			

Figure 18.1: Preparticipation physical examination forms. (© 2019 American Academy of Family Physicians, American Academy of Pediatrics, American College of Sports Medicine, American Medical Society for Sports Medicine, American Orthopaedic Society for Sports Medicine, and American Osteopathic Academy of Sports Medicine. Permission is granted to reprint for noncommercial, educational purposes with acknowledgment.) *(continued)*

BONE AND JOINT QUESTIONS		Yes	No
14. Have you ever had a stress fracture or an injury to a bone, muscle, ligament, joint, or tendon that caused you to miss a practice or game?			
15. Do you have a bone, muscle, ligament, or joint injury that bothers you?			
MEDICAL QUESTIONS		**Yes**	**No**
16. Do you cough, wheeze, or have difficulty breathing during or after exercise?			
17. Are you missing a kidney, an eye, a testicle, your spleen, or any other organ?			
18. Do you have groin or testicle pain or a painful bulge or hernia in the groin area?			
19. Do you have any recurring skin rashes or rashes that come and go, including herpes or methicillin-resistant *Staphylococcus aureus* (MRSA)?			
20. Have you had a concussion or head injury that caused confusion, a prolonged headache, or memory problems?			
21. Have you ever had numbness, had tingling, had weakness in your arms or legs, or been unable to move your arms or legs after being hit or falling?			
22. Have you ever become ill while exercising in the heat?			
23. Do you or does someone in your family have sickle cell trait or disease?	Unsure		
24. Have you ever had or do you have any problems with your eyes or vision?			

MEDICAL QUESTIONS (*CONTINUED*)		Yes	No
25. Do you worry about your weight?			
26. Are you trying to or has anyone recommended that you gain or lose weight?			
27. Are you on a special diet or do you avoid certain types of foods or food groups?			
28. Have you ever had an eating disorder?			
MENSTRUAL QUESTIONS	**N/A**	**Yes**	**No**
29. Have you ever had a menstrual period?			
30. How old were you when you had your first menstrual period?			
31. When was your most recent menstrual period?			
32. How many periods have you had in the past 12 months?			

Explain "Yes" answers here.

____

____

____

____

____

____

____

____

____

____

____

____

I hereby state that, to the best of my knowledge, my answers to the questions on this form are complete and correct.

Signature of athlete: ____

Signature of parent or guardian: ____

Date: ______________________________

Figure 18.1: *(continued)*

This form should be placed into the athlete's medical file and should *not* be shared with schools or sports organizations.

■ PREPARTICIPATION PHYSICAL EVALUATION

ATHLETES WITH DISABILITIES FORM: SUPPLEMENT TO THE ATHLETE HISTORY

Name:______________________________ Date of birth: ______________

1. Type of disability:
2. Date of disability:
3. Classification (if available):
4. Cause of disability (birth, disease, injury, or other):
5. List the sports you are playing:

	Yes	No
6. Do you regularly use a brace, an assistive device, or a prosthetic device for daily activities?		
7. Do you use any special brace or assistive device for sports?		
8. Do you have any rashes, pressure sores, or other skin problems?		
9. Do you have a hearing loss? Do you use a hearing aid?		
10. Do you have a visual impairment?		
11. Do you use any special devices for bowel or bladder function?		
12. Do you have burning or discomfort when urinating?		
13. Have you had autonomic dysreflexia?		
14. Have you ever been diagnosed as having a heat-related (hyperthermia) or cold-related (hypothermia) illness?		
15. Do you have muscle spasticity?		
16. Do you have frequent seizures that cannot be controlled by medication?		

Explain "Yes" answers here.

____

____

____

Please indicate whether you have ever had any of the following conditions:

	Yes	No
Atlantoaxial instability		
Radiographic (x-ray) evaluation for atlantoaxial instability		
Dislocated joints (more than one)		
Easy bleeding		
Enlarged spleen		
Hepatitis		
Osteopenia or osteoporosis		
Difficulty controlling bowel		
Difficulty controlling bladder		
Numbness or tingling in arms or hands		
Numbness or tingling in legs or feet		
Weakness in arms or hands		
Weakness in legs or feet		
Recent change in coordination		
Recent change in ability to walk		
Spina bifida		
Latex allergy		

Explain "Yes" answers here.

____

____

____

I hereby state that, to the best of my knowledge, my answers to the questions on this form are complete and correct.

Signature of athlete: ______________________________

Signature of parent or guardian: ______________________________

Date: ______________________________

Figure 18.1: *(continued)*

This form should be placed into the athlete's medical file and should *not* be shared with schools or sports organizations. The Medical Eligibility Form is the only form that should be submitted to a school or sports organization.

Disclaimer: Athletes who have a current Preparticipation Physical Evaluation (per state and local guidance) on file should not need to complete another examination.

PREPARTICIPATION PHYSICAL EVALUATION (Interim Guidance)

PHYSICAL EXAMINATION FORM

Name: ______________________________ Date of birth: ______________

PHYSICIAN REMINDERS

1. Consider additional questions on more-sensitive issues.
   - Do you feel stressed out or under a lot of pressure?
   - Do you ever feel sad, hopeless, depressed, or anxious?
   - Do you feel safe at your home or residence?
   - Have you ever tried cigarettes, e-cigarettes, chewing tobacco, snuff, or dip?
   - During the past 30 days, did you use chewing tobacco, snuff, or dip?
   - Do you drink alcohol or use any other drugs?
   - Have you ever taken anabolic steroids or used any other performance-enhancing supplement?
   - Have you ever taken any supplements to help you gain or lose weight or improve your performance?
   - Do you wear a seat belt, use a helmet, and use condoms?
2. Consider reviewing questions on cardiovascular symptoms (Q4–Q13 of History Form).

EXAMINATION		
Height: Weight:		
BP: / (/) Pulse: Vision: R 20/ L 20/ Corrected: ☐ Y ☐ N		
COVID-19 VACCINE		
Previously received COVID-19 vaccine: ☐ Y ☐ N Administered COVID-19 vaccine at this visit: ☐ Y ☐ N If yes: ☐ First dose ☐ Second dose ☐ Third dose ☐ Booster date(s) ________		
MEDICAL	**NORMAL**	**ABNORMAL FINDINGS**
Appearance • Marfan stigmata (kyphoscoliosis, high-arched palate, pectus excavatum, arachnodactyly, hyperlaxity, myopia, mitral valve prolapse [MVP], and aortic insufficiency)		
Eyes, ears, nose, and throat • Pupils equal • Hearing		
Lymph nodes		
Heart[a] • Murmurs (auscultation standing, auscultation supine, and ± Valsalva maneuver)		
Lungs		
Abdomen		
Skin • Herpes simplex virus (HSV), lesions suggestive of methicillin-resistant *Staphylococcus aureus* (MRSA), or tinea corporis		
Neurological		
MUSCULOSKELETAL	**NORMAL**	**ABNORMAL FINDINGS**
Neck		
Back		
Shoulder and arm		
Elbow and forearm		
Wrist, hand, and fingers		
Hip and thigh		
Knee		
Leg and ankle		
Foot and toes		
Functional • Double-leg squat test, single-leg squat test, and box drop or step drop test		

[a] Consider electrocardiography (ECG), echocardiography, referral to a cardiologist for abnormal cardiac history or examination findings, or a combination of those.

Name of health care professional (print or type): ______________________ Date: ____________

Address: ______________________ Phone: ____________

Signature of health care professional: ______________________, MD, DO, NP, or PA

Figure 18.1: *(continued)*

The Medical Eligibility Form is the only form that should be submitted to a school or sports organization.

■ PREPARTICIPATION PHYSICAL EVALUATION

MEDICAL ELIGIBILITY FORM

Name: ______________________________ Date of birth: ______________

□ Medically eligible for all sports without restriction

□ Medically eligible for all sports without restriction with recommendations for further evaluation or treatment of

____

____

□ Medically eligible for certain sports

____

____

□ Not medically eligible pending further evaluation

□ Not medically eligible for any sports

Recommendations: ______________________________

____

____

I have examined the student named on this form and completed the preparticipation physical evaluation. The athlete does not have apparent clinical contraindications to practice and can participate in the sport(s) as outlined on this form. A copy of the physical examination findings are on record in my office and can be made available to the school at the request of the parents. If conditions arise after the athlete has been cleared for participation, the physician may rescind the medical eligibility until the problem is resolved and the potential consequences are completely explained to the athlete (and parents or guardians).

Name of health care professional (print or type): ______________________ Date: ______________

Address: ______________________________ Phone: ______________

Signature of health care professional: ______________________________, MD, DO, NP, or PA

SHARED EMERGENCY INFORMATION

Allergies: ______________________________

____

____

Medications: ______________________________

____

____

Other information: ______________________________

____

____

Emergency contacts: ______________________________

____

____

Figure 18.1: *(continued)*

frequency of testing, and secondary conditions associated with social isolation (12).

- Screen females for signs and symptoms related to the "female athlete triad" (low energy availability with or without disordered eating, menstrual dysfunction, and low bone mineral density).
- Screen for mental health disorders that include depression, anxiety, and attention-deficit/hyperactivity disorder. Use the opportunity to provide education on bullying, sleep disorder, substance abuse, or sexual abuse (5).

PHYSICAL EXAMINATION

Cardiovascular Assessment

- Cardiac auscultation should be done both standing and supine.
- Benign systolic murmurs are common in athletes. If a murmur is grade III or louder, or diastolic, further evaluation is recommended.
- The murmur associated with hypertrophic cardiomyopathy (HCM) is best heard while upright and may disappear with supine position as well as squatting.
- If there is a potentially concerning murmur, having the patient perform a Valsalva maneuver can provide additional information. Typically, Valsalva will accentuate murmurs due to outflow obstruction abnormalities such as HCM.
- Twenty-five percent of patients with HCM with left ventricular outflow obstruction have a murmur on a physical exam (13).
- Ectopic beats are also common. Those that disappear with exercise are usually benign, whereas those brought on with exercise are more worrisome. Ventricular ectopy in young athletes should also raise suspicion for possible use of stimulants (*e.g.*, cocaine).
- Simultaneous palpation of the radial and femoral pulses for asymmetry is a simple screen for coarctation of the aorta.

Blood Pressure

- Readings that indicate hypertension vary for different age ranges and between genders (14). Three separate elevated blood pressure (BP) readings are needed to diagnose hypertension (14,15).
- Hypertension in children and adolescents is based on percentiles for each age according to gender and height (14,16).
  - Preadolescents:
    - Normal BP: <90th percentile
    - Elevated BP: >90th percentile to <95th percentile or 120/80 mm Hg to <95th percentile (whichever is lower)
    - Stage 1 HTN: ≥95th percentile to <95th percentile + 12 mm Hg or 130/80–139/89 mm Hg (whichever is lower)
    - Stage 2 HTN: ≥95th percentile + 12 mm Hg or ≥140/90 mm Hg (whichever is lower)
  - Adolescent:
    - Normal BP: <120/<80 mm Hg
    - Elevated BP: 120/<80–129/<80 mm Hg
    - Stage 1 HTN: 130/80–139/89 mm Hg
    - Stage 2 HTN: ≥140/90 mm Hg
  - In people age 18 and higher, the definitions of hypertension are as follows (17):
    - Normal BP: <130/<85 mm Hg
    - High-normal BP: Systolic (130–139 mm Hg) and/or diastolic (85–89 mm Hg)
    - Grade 1 hypertension: Systolic (140–159 mm Hg) and/or diastolic (90–99 mm Hg)
    - Grade 2 hypertension: Systolic (≥160 mm Hg) and/or diastolic (≥100 mm Hg)
- Those who have stage 1 hypertension without evidence of end-organ damage do not be restricted from competitive sports, however, should have BP surveillance every 2–4 months (18).
- Stage II hypertensives without evidence of end-organ damage should be restricted from high static sports (*e.g.*, weightlifting) until their BP is controlled (18).
- Systolic hypertension in young athletes is frequently related to anxiety or inappropriate cuff size in husky individuals.
- If the initial measurement is high, it is recommended that another reading be taken after resting for 5 minutes.

Musculoskeletal Assessment

- It is not necessary to perform a comprehensive joint-by-joint musculoskeletal exam on all PPEs.
- The "2-minute musculoskeletal examination" can be a useful screen (Table 18.1).
- Look for preexisting injuries because they are likely to recur. The knees, shoulders, and ankles are most at risk.
- Focus more of your examination on problem areas if they exist.
- Keep in mind the demands of the particular sport the athlete will be playing and focus more on areas of the body that will be under stress and prone to injury from that sport.
- Musculoskeletal problems found during the PPE should be treated with appropriate rehabilitation and conditioning programs prior to returning to activity.

Other Areas for Assessment

- Height/weight
  - Eating disorders, ideal body weight
- General appearance
  - Stigmata of Marfan disease: kyphoscoliosis

Table 18.1 Two-Minute Musculoskeletal Examination for Screening Athletes During the Preparticipation Examination

Instructions	Observation
Stand facing the examiner	Acromioclavicular joints, general habitus
Look at ceiling, floor, over both shoulders; touch ears to shoulders	Cervical spine motion
Shrug shoulders (examiner resists at 90°)	Trapezius strength
Abduct shoulders 90° (examiner resists at 90°)	Deltoid strength
Full external rotation of arms	Shoulder motion
Flex and extend elbows	Elbow motion
Arms at sides, elbows 90° flexed; pronate and supinate wrists	Elbow and wrist motion
Spread fingers; make fist	Hand or finger motion and deformities
Tighten (contract) quadriceps	Symmetry and knee effusion; ankle effusion
"Duck" walk four steps (away from examiner with buttocks on heels)	Ability to perform this rules out significant hip and knee abnormalities
Back to examiner	Shoulder symmetry, scoliosis
Knees straight, touch toes	Scoliosis, hip motion, hamstring tightness
Raise up on toes, raise heels	Calf symmetry, leg strength

Source: Smith NJ. *Sports Medicine: Health Care for Young Athletes.* Evanston (IL): American Academy of Pediatrics; 1983. 1 p.

- Eyes
  - Vision
  - Pupils for the presence of anisocoria, which may be present in up to 10% of patients.
- Ears/nose/throat
- Lungs
- Abdominal
  - Hepatosplenomegaly, masses
- Skin
  - Infectious diseases, acne
- Neurologic
  - As guided by history
- Genitourinary
  - Male genitourinary exam is only indicated if there is a history of undescended testicle, hernia, testicular or groin pain (5).
  - Tanner staging to assess physical maturity is no longer recommended.

DIAGNOSTIC TESTS

Laboratory Tests

- Consensus is that laboratory tests should not be done routinely during the PPE.
- Consider routine hematocrit in female athletes, especially those involved in endurance sports.
- Perform cholesterol testing if indicated by history.

Sickle Cell Trait

- The NCAA now requires testing for SCT with sickle cell solubility test for all athletes in which the presence of SCT is unknown. Individual athletes can no longer opt out of testing (19).

Concussion

- Consider baseline sports concussion asssessment tool (SCAT 6) and/or formal neuropsychological testing if there is a history of concussion, prolonged post-concussion symptoms, or inconsistent or significantly diminished school performance (see Chapter 26).

Exercise-Induced Bronchospasm

- EIB appears to be much more prevalent in endurance athletes (20).
- If there is concern for EIB, it is recommended to perform testing to confirm or rule out the condition, because it has been shown that the correlation between symptoms and actual disease is poor (21–23) (see Chapter 24).
- Although this testing may be difficult to accomplish and simply prescribing a trial of an inhaled β_2 agonist is much easier and more time efficient, one must be aware not only of misdiagnosis and subsequent unnecessary treatment, but also of the potential for doping infractions for athletes competing at the collegiate or elite levels (20).
- There are NCAA restrictions regarding the use of inhaled β_2 agonists and the International Olympic Committee (IOC) has them on the banned substances list except for the long-acting versions (24).

Cardiac Testing

- There has been considerable debate recently regarding the inclusion of routine screening electrocardiogram (ECG) as a part of the PPE in the United States (see Chapters 23 ECG Screening in Athletes and 31 Cardiology).
- Routine ECG is being performed in Europe and is recommended by the European Society of Cardiology (ESC) and the IOC as part of their baseline screening programs. The recommendations are based on data out of Italy that showed including ECG in regular screening resulted in an 89% reduction in SCD (25).
- It has been shown that for HCM (the most common identifiable cause of SCD in the United States), ECG abnormalities

are present in 75%–95% of those with the condition (26–28). However, most of the ECG findings are subtle and require added expertise to detect.

- In addition, the sensitivity and specificity of history and physical in detecting cardiac abnormalities responsible for SCD are quite low, and often SCD is the first manifestation of the underlying disorder (4,10,14,27,29–33).
- In a recent consensus statement (3), the AHA concluded that implementing a nationwide screening program that would include ECG for athletes in the United States is not viable for the following reasons:
  - Lack of medical resources and infrastructure to perform this testing on the large number of athletes in this country (estimated to be 10–12 million), when the incidence of sudden death is low (range of 1 in 80,000 to 1 in 200,000).
  - The need to enact federal statutes to establish mandatory compliance with the screening process and nationwide consensus regarding the disqualification standards in the face of more pressing public health care issues.
  - Lack of financial resources for this kind of endeavor within our current healthcare system.
  - The relatively large percentage of false-positives that result from these screening programs, mostly related to ECG interpretation. This leads to subsequent testing, further increasing the cost in addition to causing additional anxiety for the athlete and his or her family.
  - The detrimental effect of unnecessary disqualification from sport and activity of children and adolescents within the context of our current epidemic of inactivity and obesity.

SCREENING TO PREVENT EXERCISE-RELATED SUDDEN DEATH

- The cause of sudden death during exercise is usually cardiac: under 35 years, usually structural heart problem; over 35 years, usually coronary artery disease.
- The overall prevalence of cardiac abnormalities responsible for SCD is approximately 0.3% (13). The leading cause of sudden cardiac death is unexplained, with autopsy revealing no structural or identifiable abnormality.
- Preparticipation screening is the primary preventive tool. Exercise-related SCD in the United States is rare, but its actual incidence is still in question. Estimates range from 0.3 to 3 per 100,000 athletes per year (14,15,21,29,34–41).
- The official recommendation of the AHA is to perform a thorough personal and family history, with questions specific for cardiac conditions (as noted earlier), and focused physical examination to detect cardiovascular abnormalities. Proceed with further testing only as indicated.
- Including routine screening ECG and/or echocardiogram would be the individual choice of certain communities and would be considered optional. However, it is warned that including these additional baseline tests brings with it added liability and increased (and likely unsustainable) financial and medical resource needs.
- If there are any concerning findings on history or physical exam, further evaluation is warranted. The subsequent workup will depend on the suspected abnormality.
- ECGs can usually be performed in most primary care offices but should also be interpreted by a cardiologist or someone well versed in ECG findings associated with young healthy athletes as well as those conditions known to cause SCD. As mentioned later, there are many ECG changes associated with normal adapted ("athletic") hearts, as well as very subtle findings that can alert one to concerning cardiac abnormalities.
- In the adult athlete, however, a resting ECG and/or exercise stress test may be indicated in males over the age of 45 and females over the age of 55 with one or more cardiac risk factors, prior to starting an exercise program(42).
- Causes of SCD in sports include the following.

Hypertrophic Cardiomyopathy

- Leading identifiable cause of SCD in athletes confirmed on autopsy.
- Symptoms: may exhibit palpitations, syncope, chest pain, and dyspnea on exertion. Most are asymptomatic until an episode of sudden death.
- Examination: may have high-frequency systolic ejection murmur at the left lower sternal border while standing, increased with Valsalva, decreased with supine position and squatting.
- Diagnosis: echocardiogram (ventricular septum >15-mm thick); cardiac magnetic resonance imaging (MRI) with enhancement. The presence of the "athletic heart syndrome" (see Chapter 23) may complicate screening.

Congenital Coronary Artery Anomalies

- Types:
  - Origin of left coronary artery from right sinus of Valsalva
  - Single coronary artery
  - Origin of coronary artery from the pulmonary artery
  - Coronary artery hypoplasia
  - Coronary bridging
- Symptoms: vast majority are asymptomatic; may have exertional chest pain or syncope.
- Diagnosis: angiogram; cardiac MRI.

Marfan Syndrome

- Quick screen for stigmata:
  - Tall stature, arachnodactyly (positive Walker and Steinberg signs), significant pectus carinatum or excavatum, arm span to height ratio greater than 1.05, reduced upper body to lower body ratio of 0.85 or lower, ectopic lens, significant pes planus, scoliosis >20°, systolic murmur, known family history of Marfan.
- If some characteristics are noted or there is a documented family history, patient should be referred for genetic and cardiovascular screening (including echocardiogram).

- Useful website to assist providers with screening and diagnosing connective tissue disorders: https://marfan.org/dx/

Coronary Artery Disease

- Consider exercise stress testing for the following:
  - Those with two or more risk factors: hyperlipidemia, hypertension, smoking, diabetes, personal history of stroke and/or peripheral vascular disease, and family history of heart attack or SCD in a first-degree relative younger than 60 years. An alternative approach might be to select patients with a Framingham risk score consistent with at least a moderate risk of serious cardiac events within 5 years (42).
  - Anyone with angina, syncope, or palpitations, exertional or otherwise.
- Those with a prior history of heart disease should be evaluated by their physician before initiating an exercise program (see Chapters 12 and 21).

Valvular Disorders

- Aortic stenosis:
  - Usually a result of a congenital bicuspid valve.
  - This often results in sudden death, with or without exercise.
- Mitral valve prolapse: uncommon cause of SCD.

Cardiac Conduction System Abnormalities

- Idiopathic long QT syndrome: QT_c interval >440 ms.
- Wolff-Parkinson-White syndrome (accessory pathway disorder leading to tachyarrhythmias).
- Brugada syndrome (sodium channelopathy).
- Catecholaminergic polymorphic ventricular tachycardia.
- All must be suspected in cases of sudden death in which no structural heart problems are found, and all may produce symptoms of palpitations, syncope, or near syncope.

Arrhythmogenic Right Ventricular Cardiomyopathy

- Condition in which normal myocardium is replaced by fibrofatty tissue, leading to arrhythmias that are potentially fatal.
- More common in Mediterranean populations than in the United States; most common cause of SCD in Italy.
- Cause of SCD in 4% of athletes in the United States in a recent study (13).

CLEARANCE

- If a problem is found, the following factors should be considered in deciding whether to clear an athlete to participate:
  - Does the problem place the athlete at increased risk of injury?
  - Is any other participant at risk of injury or illness because of the problem?
  - Can the athlete safely participate with treatment (medication, rehabilitation, bracing, or padding)?
  - Can limited participation be allowed while evaluation is being completed or treatment is being initiated?
  - If clearance is denied only for certain activities, in what activities can the athlete safely participate?
- "Medical Conditions Affecting Sports Participation," a policy statement released by the AAP, is a useful guide to help make decisions about clearance (Tables 18.2 and 18.3) (40).

Table 18.2 Classification of Sports by Contact

Contact/Collision	Limited Contact	Noncontact
Basketball	Baseball	Archery
Boxing	Bicycling	Badminton
Diving	Cheerleading	Body building
Field hockey	Canoeing/kayaking (white water)	Bowling
Football (flag or tackle)	Fencing	Canoeing/kayaking (flat water)
Ice hockey	Field events	Crew/rowing
Lacrosse	High jump	Curling
Martial arts	Pole vault	Dancing
Rodeo	Floor hockey	Field events
Rugby	Gymnastics	Discus
Ski jumping	Handball	Javelin
Soccer	Horseback riding	Shot put
Team handball	Racquetball	Golf
Water polo	Skating	Orienteering
Wrestling	Ice	Power lifting
—	In-line	Race walking
—	Roller	Riflery
—	Skiing	Rope jumping
—	Cross country	Running
—	Downhill	Sailing
—	Water	Scuba diving
—	Softball	Strength training
—	Squash	Swimming
—	Ultimate frisbee	Table tennis
—	Volleyball	Tennis
—	Windsurfing/surfing	Track
—	—	Weightlifting

Source: Rice SG; American Academy of Pediatrics Council on Sports Medicine and Fitness. Medical conditions affecting sports participation. *Pediatrics.* 2008 Apr;121(4):841–8. doi: 10.1542/peds.2008-0080.

Table 18.3 Recommendations Regarding Sports Participation With Common Medical Conditions

Condition	May Participate
Atlantoaxial instability (instability of the joint between cervical vertebrae 1 and 2)	Qualified yes
Explanation: Athlete needs evaluation to assess risk of spinal cord injury during sports participation.	
Bleeding disorder	Qualified yes
Explanation: Athlete needs evaluation.	
Cardiovascular disease	No
Carditis (inflammation of the heart)	
Explanation: Carditis may result in sudden death with exertion.	
Hypertension (high blood pressure)	Qualified yes
Explanation: Those with significant essential (unexplained) hypertension should avoid weight and power lifting, body building, and strength training. Those with secondary hypertension (hypertension caused by a previously identified disease) or severe essential hypertension need evaluation. The National High Blood Pressure Education Working Group defined significant and severe hypertension.	
Congenital heart disease (structural heart defects present at birth)	Qualified yes
Explanation: Those with mild forms may participate fully; those with moderate or severe forms or who have undergone surgery need evaluation. The 2025 Scientific Statement from the American Heart Association and American College of Cardiology defined sports participation consideration based on the anatomy and physiology of specific congenital heart disease (43).	
Dysrhythmia (irregular heart rhythm)	Qualified yes
Explanation: Those with symptoms (chest pain, syncope, dizziness, shortness of breath, or other symptoms of possible dysrhythmia) or evidence of mitral regurgitation (leaking) on physical examination need evaluation. All others may participate fully.	
Heart murmur	Qualified yes
Explanation: If the murmur is innocent (does not indicate heart disease), full participation is permitted. Otherwise, the athlete needs evaluation (see congenital heart disease and mitral valve prolapse).	
Cerebral palsy	Qualified yes
Explanation: Athlete needs evaluation.	
Diabetes mellitus	Yes
Explanation: All sports cart be played with proper attention to diet, blood glucose concentration, hydration, and insulin therapy. Blood glucose concentration should be monitored every 30 min during continuous exercise and 15 min after completion of exercise.	
Diarrhea	Qualified no
Explanation: Unless disease is mild, no participation is permitted, because diarrhea may increase the risk of dehydration and heat illness (see fever).	
Eating disorders	Qualified yes
Anorexia nervosa	
Bulimia nervosa	
Explanation: Patients with these disorders need medical and psychiatric assessment before participation.	
Eyes	Qualified yes
Functionally one-eyed athlete	
Loss of an eye	
Detached retina	
Previous eye surgery or serious eye injury	
Explanation: A functionally one-eyed athlete has a best-corrected visual acuity of less than 20/40 in the eye with worse acuity. These athletes would suffer significant disability if the better eye were seriously injured, as would those with loss of an eye. Some athletes who previously have undergone eye surgery or had a serious eye injury may have an increased risk of injury because of weakened eye tissue. Availability of eye guards approved by the American Society for Testing and Materials and other protective equipment may allow participation in most sports, but this must be judged on an individual basis (Kurowski and Chandran (6) and Maron et al. (31)).	

Table 18.3 Recommendations Regarding Sports Participation With Common Medical Conditions (*Continued*)

Condition	May Participate
Fever	No
Explanation: Fever can increase cardiopulmonary effort, reduce maximum exercise capacity, make heat illness more likely, and increase orthostatic hypertension during exercise. Fever may rarely accompany myocarditis or other infections that may make exercise dangerous.	
Heat illness, history of	Qualified yes
Explanation: Because of the increased likelihood of recurrence, the athlete needs individual assessment to determine the presence of predisposing conditions and to arrange a prevention strategy.	
Hepatitis	Yes
Explanation: Because of the apparent minimal risk to others, all sports may be played that the athlete's state of health allows. In all athletes, skin lesions should be covered properly, and athletic personnel should use universal precautions when handling blood or body fluids with visible blood.	
Human immunodeficiency virus infection	Yes
Explanation: Because of the apparent minimal risk to others, all sports may be played that the athlete's state of health allows. In all athletes, skin lesions should be covered properly, and athletic personnel should use universal precautions when handling blood or body fluids with visible blood.	
Kidney, absence of one	Qualified yes
Explanation: Athlete needs individual assessment for contact, collision, and limited contact sports.	
Liver, enlarged	Qualified yes
Explanation: If the liver is acutely enlarged, participation should be avoided because of risk of rupture. If the liver is chronically enlarged, individual assessment is needed before collision, contact, or limited contact sports are played.	
Malignant neoplasm	Qualified yes
Explanation: Athlete needs individual assessment.	
Musculoskeletal disorders	Qualified yes
Explanation: Athlete needs individual assessment.	
Neurologic disorders	
History of serious head or spine trauma, severe or repeated concussions, or craniotomy.	Qualified yes
Explanation: Athlete needs individual assessment for collision, contact, or limited contact sports and also for noncontact sports if deficits in judgment or cognition are present. Research supports a conservative approach to management of concussion.	
Seizure disorder, well-controlled	Yes
Explanation: Risk of seizure during participation is minimal.	
Seizure disorder, poorly controlled	Qualified yes
Explanation: Athlete needs individual assessment for collision, contact, or limited contact sports. The following noncontact sports should be avoided: archery, riflery, swimming, weight or power lifting, strength training, or sports involving heights. In these sports, occurrence of a seizure may pose a risk to self or others.	
Obesity	Qualified yes
Explanation: Because of the risk of heat illness, obese persons need careful acclimatization and hydration.	
Organ transplant recipient	Qualified yes
Explanation: Athlete needs individual assessment.	
Ovary, absence of one	Yes
Explanation: Risk of severe injury to the remaining ovary is minimal.	
Respiratory conditions	
Pulmonary compromise, including cystic fibrosis	Qualified yes
Explanation: Athlete needs individual assessment, but generally, all sports may be played if oxygenation remains satisfactory during a graded exercise test. Patients with cystic fibrosis need acclimatization and good hydration to reduce the risk of heat illness.	

(*continued*)

Table 18.3 Recommendations Regarding Sports Participation With Common Medical Conditions (*Continued*)

Condition	May Participate
Asthma	Yes
Explanation: With proper medication and education, only athletes with the most severe asthma will need to modify their participation.	
Acute upper respiratory infection	Qualified yes
Explanation: Upper respiratory obstruction may affect pulmonary function. Athlete needs individual assessment for all but mild disease (see fever).	
Sickle cell disease	Qualified yes
Explanation: Athlete needs individual assessment. In general, if status of the illness permits, all but high exertion, collision, and contact sports may be played. Overheating, dehydration, and chilling must be avoided.	
Sickle cell trait	Yes
Explanation: It is unlikely that persons with sickle cell trait have an increased risk of sudden death or other medical problems during athletic participation, except under the most extreme conditions of heat, humidity, and possibly increased altitude. These persons, like all athletes, should be carefully conditioned, acclimatized, and hydrated to reduce any possible risk.	
Skin disorders (boils, herpes simplex, impetigo, scabies, molluscum contagiosum)	Qualified yes
Explanation: While the patient is contagious, participation in gymnastics with mats; martial arts; wrestling; or other collision, contact, or limited contact sports is not allowed.	
Spleen, enlarged	Qualified yes
Explanation: A patient with an acutely enlarged spleen should avoid all sports because of risk of rupture. A patient with a chronically enlarged spleen needs individual assessment before playing collision, contact, or limited contact sports.	
Testicle, undescended or absence of one	Yes
Explanation: Certain sports may require a protective cup.	

Those listed with a "qualified" yes or no require individual assessment.
Source: Rice SG; American Academy of Pediatrics Council on Sports Medicine and Fitness. Medical conditions affecting sports participation. *Pediatrics*. 2008 Apr;121(4):841–8. doi: 10.1542/peds.2008-0080.

- The AHA/ACC produced a scientific statement in 2015 that addressed issues that were not addressed in the 36th Bethesda Conference. The scientific statement identified 15 Task Forces, of which nine are diseases related with specific recommendations for clearance guidelines for athletes. In 2025, the task force issued updated recommendations, revising those released in 2015 that included 11 sections to help guide shared decision making on participation for athletes with cardiovascular disease (43).
- A clearance form (see Fig. 18.1) is a useful tool to clearly express recommendations regarding clearance.

REFERENCES

1. Maron BJ, Doerer JJ, Haas TS, Tierney DM, Mueller FO. Sudden deaths in young competitive athletes: analysis of 1866 deaths in the United States, 1980-2006. *Circulation*. 2009;119(8):1085–92.
2. MacDonald J, Schaefer M, Stumph J. The preparticipation physical evaluation. *Am Fam Physician*. 2021 May 1;103(9):539–46.
3. Maron BJ, Levine BD, Washington RL, et al. Eligibility and disqualification recommendations for competitive athletes with cardiovascular abnormalities. Task force 2: preparticipation screening for cardiovascular disease in competitive athletes. A scientific statement from the American Heart Association and American College of Cardiology. *Circulation*. 2015;132(22):e267–72.
4. The National Collegiate Athletic Association. *NCAA Sports Medicine Handbook 2014–2015* [Internet]. 25th ed. Indianapolis (IN): The National Collegiate Athletic Association; 2014 [cited 2022 Sep 1]. Available from: https://www.ncaapublications.com/productdownloads/MD15.pdf
5. American Academy of Family Physicians, American Academy of Pediatrics, American Medical Society for Sports Medicine, American Orthopedic Society for Sports Medicine, and American Osteopathic Academy of Sports Medicine: *Preparticipation Physical Evaluation*. 5th ed. Elk Grove Village (IL): American Academy of Pediatrics; 2019. 240 p.
6. Kurowski K, Chandran S. The preparticipation athletic evaluation. *Am Fam Physician*. 2000;61(9):2683–98.
7. Corrado D, Basso C, Rizzoli G, Schiavon M, Thiene G. Does sports activity enhance the risk of sudden death in adolescents and young adults? *J Am Coll Cardiol*. 2003;42(11):1959–63.
8. Maron BJ, Levine BD, Washington RL, et al. Eligibility and disqualification recommendations for competitive athletes with cardiovascular abnormalities. Task force 2: preparticipation screening for cardiovascular disease in competitive athletes. A scientific statement from the American Heart Association and American College of Cardiology. *Circulation*. 2015;132(22):e267–72.
9. McCrory P, Meeuwisse W, Johnston K, et al. Sport concussion assessment tool 2, adapted from the 3rd International Consensus Meeting on concussion in sport held in Zurich, Switzerland in November 2008. *Br J Sports Med*. 2009;43(2).

10. Valovich McLeod TC, Bay RC, Heil J, McVeigh SD. Identification of sport and recreational activity concussion history through the preparticipation screening and a symptom survey in young athletes. *Clin J Sport Med*. 2008;18(3):235–40.
11. Baggish AL, Chang CJ, Drezner JA, et al. ACSM-AMSSM call to action: adapting preparticipation cardiovascular screening to the COVID-19 pandemic. *Curr Sports Med Rep*. 2022 May 1;21(5):159–62.
12. Narducci DM, Diamond AB, Bernhardt DT, Roberts WO. COVID vaccination in athletes & updated interim guidance on the preparticipation physical examination during the SARS-CoV-2 pandemic. *Curr Sports Med Rep*. 2021 Nov 1;20(11):608–13.
13. Maron BJ. Hypertrophic cardiomyopathy. *Lancet*. 1997;350(9071):127–33.
14. U.S. Department of Health and Human Services, National Institutes of Health, National Heart, Lung, and Blood Institute. *The Fourth Report on the Diagnosis, Evaluation, and Treatment of High Blood Pressure in Children and Adolescents* [Internet]. Revised May 2005. 2011 [cited 2011 Feb 3]. Available from: http://www.nhlbi.nih.gov/health/prof/heart/hbp/hbp_ped.pdf
15. Chobanian AV, Bakris GL, Black HR, et al. The seventh report of the Joint National Committee on prevention, detection, evaluation, and treatment of high blood pressure: the JNC 7 report. *JAMA*. 2003;289(19):2560–72.
16. Flynn JT, Kaelber DC, Baker-Smith CM, et al. Clinical practice guideline for screening and Management of high blood pressure in children and adolescents. *Pediatrics*. 2017;140(3):e20171904. *Pediatrics*. 2018 Sep;142(3):e20181738.
17. Unger T, Borghi C, Charchar F, et al. 2020 International Society of Hypertension Global Hypertension practice guidelines. *J Hypertens*. 2020;38(6):982–1004.
18. Black HR, Sica D, Ferdinand K, White WB. Eligibility and disqualification recommendations for competitive athletes with cardiovascular abnormalities. Task force 6: hypertension. A scientific statement from the American Heart Association and the American College of Cardiology. *J Am Coll Cardiol*. 2015 Dec 1;66(21):2393–7.
19. NCAA. *Various Bylaws — Sickle Cell Solubility Test – Elimination of Written Release*. Legislative Services Database – LSDBI. [Accessed 2022 Oct 28]. https://web3.ncaa.org/lsdbi/search/proposalView?id=105737
20. McKenzie DC, Fitch KD. The asthmatic athlete: inhaled beta-2 agonists, sport performance, and doping. *Clin J Sport Med*. 2011;21(1):46–50.
21. Capão-Filipe M, Moreira A, Delgado L, Rodrigues J, Vaz M. Exercise-induced bronchoconstriction and respiratory symptoms in elite athletes. *Allergy*. 2003;58(11):1196.
22. Hammerman SI, Becker JM, Rogers J, Quedenfeld TC, D'Alonzo GE Jr. Asthma screening of high school athletes: identifying the undiagnosed and poorly controlled. *Ann Allergy Asthma Immunol*. 2002;88:380–4.
23. Rundell KW, Im J, Mayers LB, Wilber RL, Szmedra L, Schmitz HR. Self-reported symptoms and exercise-induced asthma in the elite athlete. *Med Sci Sports Exerc*. 2001;33(2):208–13.
24. *World Anti-Doping Agency Web Site* [Internet]. Montreal, Canada: World Anti-Doping Agency; 2022 [cited 2022 Sep 1]. Available from: http://www.wada-ama.org
25. Corrado D, Basso C, Pavei A, Michieli P, Schiavon M, Thiene G. Trends in sudden cardiovascular death in young competitive athletes after implementation of a preparticipation screening program. *JAMA*. 2006;296(13):1593–601.
26. Maron BJ, Roberts WC, Epstein SE. Sudden death in hypertrophic cardiomyopathy: a profile of 78 patients. *Circulation*. 1982;65(7):1388–94.
27. Maron BJ, Seidman JG, Seidman CE. Proposal for contemporary screening strategies in families with hypertrophic cardiomyopathy. *J Am Coll Cardiol*. 2004;44(11):2125–32.
28. Pelliccia A, Di Paolo FM, Corrado D, et al. Evidence for efficacy of the Italian national pre-participation screening programme for identification of hypertrophic cardiomyopathy in competitive athletes. *Eur Heart J*. 2006;27(18):2196–200.
29. Atkins DL, Everson-Stewart S, Sears GK, et al. Epidemiology and outcomes from out-of-hospital cardiac arrest in children: the resuscitation outcomes consortium epistry-cardiac arrest. *Circulation*. 2009;119(11):1484–91.
30. Baggish AL, Hutter AM, Wang F, et al. Cardiovascular screening in college athletes with and without electrocardiography: a cross-sectional study. *Ann Intern Med*. 2010;152(5):269–75.
31. Maron BJ, Shirani J, Poliac LC, Mathenge R, Roberts WC, Mueller FO. Sudden death in young competitive athletes. Clinical, demographic, and pathological profiles. *JAMA*. 1996;276(3):199–204.
32. Pelliccia A, Maron B: Preparticipation cardiovascular evaluation of the competitive athlete: perspectives from the 30-year Italian experience. *Am J Cardiol*. 1995;75(12):827–9.
33. Wilson MG, Basavarajaiah S, Whyte GP, Cox S, Loosemore M, Sharma S. Efficacy of personal symptom and family history questionnaires when screening for inherited cardiac pathologies: the role of electrocardiography. *Br J Sports Med* 2008;42(3):207–11.
34. American Academy of Pediatrics Committee on Sports Medicine and Fitness. Medical conditions affecting sports participation. *Pediatrics*. 1994;94(5):757–60.
35. Borjesson M, Pelliccia A. Incidence and aetiology of sudden cardiac death in young athletes: an international perspective. *Br J Sports Med*. 2009;43(9):644–8.
36. Chugh SS, Reinier K, Balaji S, et al. Population-based analysis of sudden death in children: the Oregon sudden Unexpected death study. *Heart Rhythm*. 2009;6(11):1618–22.
37. Eckart RE, Scoville SL, Campbell CL, et al. Sudden death in young adults: a 25-year review of autopsies in military recruits. *Ann Intern Med*. 2004;141(11):829–34.
38. Maron BJ. Sudden death in young athletes. *N Engl J Med*. 2003;349(11):1064–75.
39. Maron BJ, Gohman TE, Aeppli D. Prevalence of sudden cardiac death during competitive sports activities in Minnesota high school athletes. *J Am Coll Cardiol*. 1998;32(7):1881–4.
40. Rice SG, American Academy of Pediatrics Council on Sports Medicine and Fitness. Medical conditions affecting sports participation. *Pediatrics*. 2008;121(4):841–8.
41. Van Camp SP, Bloor CM, Mueller FO, Cantu RC, Olson HG. Nontraumatic sports death in high school and college athletes. *Med Sci Sports Exerc*. 1995;27(5):641–7.
42. Gibbons RJ, Balady GJ, Beasley JW, et al. *ACC/AHA 2002 update for exercise testing: a report of the American College of Cardiology/American Heart Association Task Force on practice guidelines (Committee on exercise testing)* [Internet]. 2011 [cited 2011 Feb 3]. Available from: http://www.americanheart.org/downloadable/heart/1032279013658exercise.pdf
43. Kim JH, Baggish AL, Levine BD, et al. Clinical considerations for competitive sports participation for athletes with cardiovascular abnormalities: a scientific statement from the American Heart Association and American College of Cardiology. *J Am Coll Cardiol*. 2025 Mar 18;85(10):1059–108.

SECTION ii

Evaluation of the Injured Athlete

Diagnostic Imaging

19

Jordan S. Gross and Kambiz Motamedi

INTRODUCTION

- There are several imaging modalities available in the assessment and evaluation of sports injuries. The strengths and weaknesses of each modality with their specific indications are discussed in this chapter. The choice of the imaging modality depends on several factors, including the anatomic location of interest, chronicity of the symptoms, suspected pathology, and potential treatment alternatives.
- Guidelines for "what to use when" can be found on the American College of Radiology Web site "ACR Appropriateness Criteria" at: https://www.acr.org/Clinical-Resources/ACR-Appropriateness-Criteria. On this Web site, these criteria can be searched by topic, scenario, or procedure.
- There are least 25 different clinical vignettes within the ACR Appropriateness Criteria, ranging from "Acute Hip Pain — Suspected Fracture" to "Stress (Fatigue/Insufficiency) Fracture, Including Sacrum, Excluding Other Vertebrae."

IMAGING MODALITIES

- Imaging tools that are commonly available and will be discussed include (1) plain radiography (with or without applied stress); (2) conventional arthrography; (3) computed tomography (CT), which may be combined with arthrography; (4) magnetic resonance imaging (MRI), which may be combined with arthrography; (5) ultrasonography (US); and (6) radionuclide bone scans.
- Over the past several years, US has gained substantial popularity in sports medicine imaging.
- Radionuclide bone scans have diminished in popularity, having been largely replaced by MRI.
- MRI and US are further discussed in Chapters 20 and 21, respectively.

MODALITY DESCRIPTION, STRENGTHS, AND WEAKNESSES

- *Plain radiography* is widely available, is relatively inexpensive, and provides excellent detail of bony structures and soft-tissue calcifications. Although resolution has improved with digital radiography, the ability of radiography to depict soft-tissue pathology remains far inferior to more advanced imaging (MRI, CT, and US). Plain radiography imaging can be augmented by stress and arthrography.
- *Stress radiography* (*e.g.*, varus or valgus) reveals abnormal laxity of joints and can indirectly diagnose soft-tissue injury. Stress must be applied by the referring health care provider (*i.e.*, MD, PA-C, NP) or technologist who is readily available and knowledgeable about *how* to provide the needed stress image. Disadvantages include availability of the health care provider, radiation exposure, and subjectivity of the amount of stress needed. In some cases, it may exacerbate underlying pathology. For subtle cases, comparison with the contralateral side may be needed. Consequently, indirect evaluation of soft-tissue injury with stress radiography has been replaced by MRI and US.
- *Arthrography* delineates the synovial space and intra-articular structures by joint distention. Although invasive, there are few inherent risks. Arthrography requires patient preparation and cooperation, informed consent, and the availability of a radiology provider. Prior to the advent of cross-sectional imaging (MRI and CT), conventional arthrography was popular, consisting of a fluoroscopically guided injection of iodinated contrast and/or air, followed by spot imaging during provocative maneuvering. This procedure is now rarely done in isolation, having been supplanted with injection of dilute gadolinium for magnetic resonance arthrography, or less commonly, dilute iodinated contrast for CT arthrography when there is a contraindication to MRI (*e.g.*, cardiac pacemaker). For both procedures, coordination is needed for scheduling scanner time to immediately follow the procedure.

- *CT* is superior to other modalities for fine bone detail and is an important tool for depicting the anatomy of complex fractures such as around the shoulder, elbow, hip, and knee. Newer generation multislice scanners have significantly diminished acquisition time and artifact and are capable of submillimeter slice thickness. CT is often used as a surrogate for MRI, in cases where MRI is contraindicated. Volumetric image acquisition enables rapid data reconstruction into not only standard axial, sagittal, and coronal planes, but also any obliquity desired to optimize depiction of anatomy. Reconstruction artifact commonly encountered with older scanners is far less of a problem with newer generation scanners. Two of the main limitations/disadvantages of CT include (1) limited soft-tissue contrast and (2) radiation dose. To minimize radiation, scanning should be coned as tightly as possible to the area of interest.
- *MRI* provides unparalleled soft-tissue and bone marrow contrast. It has become the premiere imaging modality for sports-related injuries, but also has a role in evaluating nondisplaced fractures, infection, inflammatory conditions, and neoplastic disease. Although there are many pulse sequences that can be used with MRI, four are the mainstay of musculoskeletal imaging: T1-weighted (T1W), T2-weighted (T2W) and short tau inversion recovery (STIR), proton density (PD), and gradient-echo (GRE) sequences.
  - T1W imaging is most useful for looking at and evaluating the patient's anatomy (and anatomical variants). Fat (including fatty bone marrow) appears with high signal intensity, or bright; muscles appear with intermediate signal intensity; and cortex, tendons, and ligaments appear with low signal intensity, or dark.
  - T2W (usually undertaken with fat suppression) and STIR imaging highlights tissues with increased water content, displaying them as bright. By suppressing fat signal (turning it dark), T2W and STIR imaging obscures normal anatomy, but highlights edema and tears of muscles, tendons, and ligaments. If tears are complete, this sequence can help assess the associated degree of tendon retraction.
  - PD imaging takes advantage of both of these techniques by demonstrating anatomy but highlighting certain types of pathology. Each of these different sequences plays a role in the comprehensive evaluation of a joint. For instance, T1W imaging is a mainstay sequence in looking for a fracture line or avascular necrosis. PD-weighted imaging is superior in the evaluation of articular cartilage, particularly useful in the shoulder and knee. It also proves to be a workhorse for evaluating meniscal tears at the knee.
  - GRE sequences are generally faster sequences, obtained by using "gradients" instead of the traditional radiofrequency pulses used in other sequences. GRE sequences are not efficient at reducing magnetic inhomogeneity; therefore, they are poor at reducing metallic susceptibility artifact. This artifact can be used to the radiologists' advantage — specifically, these sequences can be useful in evaluating hemorrhage (*i.e.*, hemosiderin deposition). GRE sequences have also been shown to highlight cartilage and labral pathologies, particularly after intra-articular gadolinium administration.
  - There are several relative and absolute contraindications to MRI, including claustrophobia, cardiac pacemakers, certain kinds of neurosurgical aneurysmal clips, and inner ear implants.
- Musculoskeletal *ultrasound* (US) has dramatically gained popularity over the past 2 decades. Portable US equipment is now common at sporting events to provide a rapid assessment of injury severity and clearly competes with MRI in evaluation of muscle, tendon, and ligament injuries. One of the strengths of US lies in its ability to perform dynamic imaging, depicting soft-tissue structures while in motion. A normal control is readily available by acquiring images from the contralateral side. There is direct patient contact with the sonographer, facilitating immediate customization of the examination to the patient's symptoms. The major disadvantage is that US is operator dependent, requiring appropriate training with hands-on experience for competency. One of the main disadvantages of ultrasound is also its inability to scan past bone due to its impedance ("stiffness of tissue"). Therefore, ultrasound is limited in its evaluation of bony abnormalities (*e.g.*, bone stress injury) and joint pathologies (*e.g.*, labrum abnormalities).
- *Radionuclide bone scanning* with technetium-99m methylene diphosphonate is extremely sensitive for detecting areas of increased bone turnover. However, it is nonspecific, and traumatic lesions cannot be differentiated from inflammation or neoplasia. Any abnormality on a bone scan needs to be correlated with radiography, CT, or MRI. In addition, radionuclide bone scans also have poor spatial resolution. This can be improved by either obtaining oblique projections or using *single photon emission computed tomography* (SPECT). In addition, the triple-phase (three-phase) bone scan can be additionally performed; often to evaluate for musculoskeletal infection (particularly in the setting of joint replacement or hardware), or for hardware loosening or complication.
  - SPECT imaging produces multiplanar tomographic slices similar to CT and MRI, allowing precise localization of foci of abnormal tracer activity. A major consideration for the use of radionuclide bone scan or SPECT is in the evaluation of osseous metastatic disease.
  - The triple-phase bone scan is performed by acquiring an angiogram at the time of tracer injection, a blood-pool phase within 5 minutes of injection, and 3-hour delayed (static) images. This technique assists in differentiating soft tissue from bone pathology. Soft-tissue abnormalities generally show preferential uptake on the first two phases, whereas bone pathology should show increased activity on all three phases. For single- or triple-phase bone scans, pinhole collimation should be used for small parts such as hands and feet to provide magnification and increased spatial resolution. Over the past years, MRI has largely replaced radionuclide bone scans.

SPECIFIC UTILIZATION OF DIFFERENT MODALITIES

- *Plain radiography* should usually be used for the initial assessment of an acute traumatic event to assess for fracture and/or alignment abnormality. It is also a key resource for trauma follow-up — *i.e.*, to evaluate for fracture healing or to evaluate after the reduction of a joint dislocation. Radiographs are also important in the initial evaluation for arthritis, inflammatory processes/infection, and musculoskeletal tumors.
- *Stress radiography* may find its niche in cases of chronic trauma with instability and suspected soft-tissue injury. It has, however, been widely replaced by MRI and/or US.
- *Arthrography* is used when joint distention is required to evaluate intra-articular pathology. This may include cases of cartilage or labral injury, meniscal re-tears, capsular tears, and joint bodies.
- *CT* is indicated for demonstrating the extent and anatomy of fractures. It is particularly valuable when evaluating complex trauma, particularly at the shoulder, elbow, bony pelvis, and knee. At the bony pelvis, many fractures can be obscured on radiography due to overlapping bone and soft-tissue structures. CT with multiplanar reconstruction and 3D reformations provide an excellent road map for the surgeon in planning the appropriate operation. Other uses for CT include the evaluation of mineralization of bone or soft-tissue lesions, the quick assessment for deep soft-tissue infection (*i.e.*, deep soft-tissue gas), and follow-up studies with certain types of cancers (*i.e.*, melanomas).
- *MRI* is used for suspected bone or soft-tissue injury, especially when plain radiographs are normal. As mentioned earlier, MRI can be performed in conjunction with arthrography to look for cartilage or labral abnormalities, meniscal injuries (particularly in the setting of prior surgery and suspected re-injury), or joint bodies. Of note, MRI arthrography of the shoulder is considered by many providers the preferred initial imaging choice to evaluate for SLAP tears (superior labral anterior to posterior), which are common in collegiate athletes.
- *US* has many uses in musculoskeletal imaging, and the list of indications continues to grow. It is considered the ***first-choice*** imaging modality to evaluate for the presence of superficial foreign bodies and peripheral nerves. It is also highly considered in the evaluation for focal superficial ligament or tendon pathologies, fluid collections, and muscle strains. In fact, certain academic societies have deemed ultrasound to be equal with MRI in evaluating for rotator cuff pathology. However, ultrasound's best advantage is the ability to perform dynamic imaging — *e.g.*, evaluating for snapping tendons or impingement syndromes. In the sports imaging world, mobile units allow immediate field-side evaluation of injured athletes for tendon tears, muscle strains, and hematomas. Finally, US is also gaining popularity as a device to guide diagnostic and therapeutic interventional procedures, including cyst aspiration and steroid and/or anesthetic injections within joints and around tendons.
- *Radionuclide bone scans* are useful primarily for localizing the site of bone pathology in cases where symptoms may be focal, generalizable, or diffuse. They have previously been used in the evaluation of bone stress injuries, due to their ability to capture the bone turnover that happens in the acute phase of injury. If a lesion or injury is chronic, there will not be much tracer accumulation. Other uses for radionuclide bone scans include osseous metastatic disease, musculoskeletal infection, and hardware loosening/complications.

CLINICAL CONSIDERATIONS

- Considering that different modalities have differing sensitivity to demonstrate certain pathology, it becomes evident that clinical information is paramount in not only deciding which method to use, but also in tailoring the imaging study to the patient's specific needs.
- Clinical information also helps to choose the correct modality for acute versus overuse injury. In both cases, one should usually begin with plain radiography. In cases of normal radiographs and suspected acute bone injury, one may choose to obtain a CT or MRI to evaluate for a possible nondisplaced fracture. CT is more useful when fractures are complex or multipartite. MRI is more useful in detecting concomitant soft-tissue injuries.
- MRI is also useful for more chronic injuries or internal derangement of a joint, including cartilage, labrum, meniscal, ligament, or tendon injuries.
- The choice of imaging modality also depends on the level of the patient's activity. In the case of an elite athlete where the decision of "**return to play**" is important, one may choose to obtain MRI or US immediately after obtaining radiographs.

TISSUE OF INTEREST

- Due to its superior contrast resolution and its ability to perform a "comprehensive" examination, MRI has become a workhorse in musculoskeletal imaging, particularly in the world of sports imaging. Interpreting radiologists often evaluate MRI based on tissues of interest, with a search pattern that includes (1) bone/marrow, (2) cartilage, (3) joint-stabilizing ligaments/tendons and muscle units, and (4) bursae.
- *Bone* is the fundamental scaffolding of the musculoskeletal system and plays a central role in diagnostic imaging. Looking at the bone marrow pattern is an important tool for radiologists, particularly in the setting of trauma. On MRI, marrow edema in the context of an injury indicates trabecular microtrauma and contusion. Specific patterns of marrow edema may prompt a closer search for injury to specific soft-tissue structures. For example, at the knee, a bone contusion

pattern at the intercondylar sulcus of the lateral femoral condyle and posterior lateral tibial plateau is highly associated with anterior cruciate ligament tear.

- *Cartilage* is a highly specialized connective tissue that outlines the bony surfaces of the joints. As a shock absorber, it is prone to chronic wear and tear. However, cartilage is also susceptible to acute injury in the setting of high-impact trauma. Acute chondral fractures, often with an adjacent bone fragment (osteochondral fracture), are not entirely uncommon in the athlete. In the more chronic phases of wear and tear, MRI can also evaluate cartilage for focal areas of thinning, fissuring, and ulceration. With high-field MRI scanners (specifically 3T), detailed evaluation of joint surfaces rarely requires arthrography.
- Joint-stabilizing *ligaments* and *tendons* and the dynamic *muscle* and tendon units are prone to injuries. Certain sports are associated with specific injury patterns. The examples are innumerable; however, a few include tennis or golfer's elbow (collateral ligament), jumper's knee (patellar tendon), and tennis leg (plantaris tendon and/or gastrocnemius muscle). If plain films are normal or equivocal, MRI will provide the necessary soft-tissue resolution for diagnosis. The spectrum of findings ranges from mild edema, partial tear, and complete disruption (and associated hematoma). With experience, US is a viable alternative for evaluation of the more superficial tendons and muscles.
- *Bursae* are fluid-filled structures with synovial linings that act as cushions at areas of increased motion or friction. They are classically found between bones and tendons or muscles and skin, but can form anywhere (albeit without a synovial lining) where protection is needed (adventitious bursa). Inherent to their function, bursae are prone to inflammation, especially in cases with overuse. MRI is excellent for demonstrating inflamed and fluid-filled bursal structures. US is suitable for detecting superficial fluid collections and possibly hyperemia in an inflamed superficial bursa. US may also provide guidance for therapeutic aspirations or injections.

ACUTE INJURY VERSUS OVERUSE

- As mentioned earlier, plain radiography is usually the first step in evaluating for acute fracture. Plain films are also used to evaluate fracture healing, by evaluating for periosteal new bone formation, bone sclerosis, and callus formation.
- Plain films may be helpful in demonstrating acute or chronic joint effusions (*e.g.*, at the elbow or knee) by demonstrating a joint effusion (soft-tissue density) displacing radiolucent normal fat planes. In cases of chronic injuries, patients may develop soft-tissue mineralization(s), which can be easily seen with radiography.
- If plain films are deemed to be normal and symptoms warrant, MRI is usually the next modality undertaken. When the suspicion of an acute fracture is high and plain films are normal, MRI will detect radiographically occult fractures. This is especially important in weight-bearing bones such as the proximal femur and the tibial plateau. Early diagnosis can prevent fragment displacement. With chronic or overuse disorders, stress reaction or fracture will appear on MRI as bone marrow edema, possibly with immature periosteal new bone formation. Focal abnormalities are also evident in muscles, tendons, and ligaments.
- If a patient's symptoms persist after adequate conservative treatment or seem out of proportion to the clinical setting, additional imaging is warranted. It is not uncommon for bone and soft-tissue tumors to be initially diagnosed as a hematoma or muscle strain. *Any palpable mass diagnosed as a hematoma should be followed with imaging and/or clinically to maturation or resolution.*

CHRONIC SEQUELAE TO TRAUMA

- Areas of prior hemorrhage, hematoma, or inflammation may undergo transformation into mature bone. This phenomenon is called heterotopic ossification. The term myositis ossificans has fallen out of favor, because this is not an inflammatory process of the muscles. Plain radiography and CT play a crucial role in recognizing this entity. Over time, as this matures, it will appear as a masslike focus in the traumatized muscle with peripheral mineralization (and more centrally lucent). This is contrary to mineralized tumors such as osteosarcoma, where the osteoid matrix is situated centrally. Unfortunately, these two entities may be confused histologically. With maturation, the mineralization of heterotopic ossification will often completely ossify with marrow induction centrally and cortex peripherally.
- An area of heterotopic ossification immediately adjacent to bone may result from an avulsion injury. This is termed periostitis ossificans.
- Calcific deposits may be seen not only in tendons and ligaments, but also in chronic inflammation of a bursa (calcific bursitis). These calcifications are composed of calcium hydroxyapatite and have a "toothpaste"-like appearance. They may be linear or globular. Depending on the location of the symptoms, radiographs, CT or US may be used for diagnosis.

SITE-SPECIFIC PLAIN RADIOGRAPHY: STANDARD AND SPECIAL VIEWS

- Each institution has its own set of plain film series, and as such, it is useful to know what views are included in each radiologic examination. The referring physician may request a specific view that may be useful for the diagnosis of the suspected pathology, or the radiologist may suggest additional views depending on the initial findings and/or pathology suspected.

- As mentioned earlier, radiography is essential after acute traumatic injury. Most acute traumatic events require at least two orthogonal views for satisfactory evaluation. Some may require three views, depending on the queried injury. It should always be noted by the technologist when the patient has a difficult time cooperating with a position due to the level of trauma. That information can be invaluable to the radiologist in helping make an appropriate diagnosis.
- Fractures can often be followed-up with just two orthogonal views.
- In addition to plain film selection, there are numerous classification systems and angular measurements utilized in musculoskeletal medicine that assist the radiologist and sports medicine physician in both diagnosis and management. These measurements are beyond the scope of this chapter; while several measurements are discussed in Section IV Musculoskeletal Problems in the Athlete, the interested reader is referred to definitive radiographic resources listed in suggested reading at the conclusion of this chapter.

Shoulder

- Internal and external rotation views in the anteroposterior (AP) projection are included in most shoulder series. Axillary and trans-scapular Y views are common third projections obtained and are needed for a perpendicular view of the glenoid. Grashey, outlet (caudally angulated trans-scapular), and West Point views may be obtained for evaluation of the glenohumeral joint space, anterior acromial shape and subacromial space, and anteroinferior glenoid rim, respectively.

Elbow

- AP and lateral views are standard. The lateral view should be obtained with the elbow in 90° of flexion to allow detection of an elbow joint effusion. Elbow effusions are detected by looking for displacement of the anterior and posterior fat pads of the elbow joint. The presence of an elbow effusion can often be the first radiographic sign of a nondisplaced fracture (often, a fracture of the radial head in skeletally mature patients). Other views, such as oblique or angulated radial head views, can be obtained to look for a fracture line; however, if no fracture line is seen, repeat radiographs can be performed in 7–10 days to evaluate for fracture healing. In addition, oblique views are often helpful to look for calcifications, enthesopathy and joint space narrowing, and/or erosive-type changes at the radiocapitellar and ulnotrochlear articulations.

Hand/Wrist

- Posteroanterior (PA), lateral, and oblique views usually constitute a hand series. The basic wrist series consists of four projections, those above coned to the wrist, as well as a scaphoid view to lay the bone out on its long axis. Similar to radial head fractures, scaphoid waist fractures can sometimes be radiographically occult. Repeat radiographs can be performed in 7–10 days to evaluate for fracture healing. A carpal tunnel view will show fractures of the hook of the hamate or the pisiform bone, and ulnar and radial deviation views may reveal widening of the scapholunate or lunotriquetral space, implying a ligament tear.

Cervical Spine

- AP and lateral views are the basic series for the cervical spine. Oblique views can be obtained to evaluate the neural foramina and assess for any neural foraminal narrowing/impingement. Lateral flexion and extension views may be added to evaluate for instability. When obtaining flexion/extension images, the patient should provide range of motion independently and never be forced into position. This is especially true in the setting of acute trauma. Additional cervical spine views that can be added to the series include an open-mouth view, a Fuchs view, and a swimmer's view. The open-mouth view shows alignment of the first two vertebral segment lateral masses and the odontoid base. This is a helpful view in the setting of a dens fracture, not entirely uncommon in the setting of cervical spine trauma. The Fuchs view shows the odontoid tip. The swimmer's view shows the lower cervical and upper thoracic segments that may be obscured by shoulder soft tissues on the conventional lateral projection.

Thoracic Spine

- AP and lateral views are standard. A swimmer's view is frequently obtained to evaluate the upper thoracic segments. Oblique views of the thoracic spine add no useful information. The thoracic facets are best assessed with CT.

Lumbar Spine

- AP and lateral views are the basic series for the lumbar spine. Similar to the cervical spine, oblique views can be obtained, as necessary. The oblique views allow for the evaluation of facet joints; these can nicely show pars interarticularis defects. Lateral flexion and extension views may also be added to evaluate for instability. A coned lateral view of the L5-S1 disc is often useful, as this level is subject to distortion from beam angulation on the standard lateral lumbar film.

Pelvis

- The most common view of the pelvis is the AP projection. Inlet/outlet and bilateral Judet (lateral oblique) views may also be obtained, but these are usually reserved for significant pelvic trauma. Judet views, for instance, are beneficial to evaluate complex acetabular fractures.
- The PA view is preferred over an AP projection for imaging the sacroiliac (SI) joints because of the oblique orientation

of the joints. This allows the X-ray beam to travel down the axis joint and minimizes overlap of the cortices of the lower synovial portion of the articulation. It should be coned to the SI joints and sacrum. The PA projection of both joints may be combined with oblique views of each side, oriented down the long axis of the joint.

Hip

- AP and frog-leg lateral views are standard. Although these provide two views of the proximal femur, they show the acetabulum in only one projection. A true acetabular lateral may be obtained with an axial lateral view. A lateral view may also be helpful in the setting of hip dislocation/subluxation evaluation. The lateral Dunn view, in addition to the frog-leg lateral, may additionally assist in the assessment of femoral-acetabular impingement.

Knee

- AP, lateral, and patellar views are standard for the plain radiographic series. Except in the setting of acute trauma where fracture is of clinical concern, these should be obtained in the upright position. In acute trauma, the lateral view should be positioned in a cross-table manner to allow demonstration of a lipohemarthrosis, a sign of an intra-articular fracture. The patellar view (also referred to as the sunrise view or Merchant view) is obtained with the knee flexed, usually oriented superior-to-inferior. This shows the patellofemoral compartment to best advantage. Additional options for knee imaging include the flexed PA view. This gives insight into the intercondylar notch and may be more sensitive than the fully extended upright position for detecting early joint space narrowing. The flexed PA view can also be used to look for acute or chronic osteochondral lesions of the femoral condyles. Oblique views can be helpful to demonstrate a nondisplaced tibial plateau fracture.

Ankle/Foot

- AP, lateral, and oblique views are usually obtained. As with the knee, the images should be taken upright except when an acute fracture is suspected. In the setting of acute trauma at the ankle, stress radiographs may be needed to evaluate for medial or lateral ankle clear space widening at the tibiotalar joint. If widening exists, this could be indicative of ligamentous injury and can have an impact on overall treatment strategy. At the foot, alignment can only truly be assessed on a weight-bearing study. This is particularly true in the setting of Lisfranc injury. Weight-bearing views are needed to evaluate for subtle offset at the Lisfranc joint proper. Additionally, AP standing views with the contralateral foot can be performed for direct comparison.
- With respect to the calcaneus, Harris views can be performed to evaluate the calcaneus in its longitudinal plane. This is a good view to evaluate the alignment of complex calcaneus fractures.

CLINICALLY CHALLENGING CASES IN SPORTS MEDICINE AND THE USE OF MULTIMODAL IMAGING

- Popliteal artery entrapment syndrome
  - Popliteal artery entrapment syndrome (PAES) can be a difficult clinical and imaging diagnosis (1); this diagnosis often requires a high index of clinical suspicion.
  - There are six different types of PAES that were recognized by the Popliteal Vascular Entrapment Forum in 1998. A few of these types are anatomic variants that may predispose patients to popliteal vessel entrapment; the radiologist has the potential to make some of these diagnoses on routine MRI.
    - For instance, a Type III PAES occurs when there is an accessory slip of gastrocnemius muscle, which can be identified on routine MRI.
  - Other imaging modalities can be useful adjuncts; however, no imaging modality is diagnostic or has become the gold standard in making this diagnosis. Duplex ultrasound, angiography, CT angiography, and MRI angiography with provocative maneuvers (plantarflexion) have shown varying degrees of sensitivity in evaluating for popliteal artery compression.
- Effort-associated thrombosis
  - Effort-associated thrombosis (ET) is a subset or category of venous thoracic-outlet syndrome (2); ET most commonly presents in athletes who perform overhead motions, such as baseball players and weightlifters. This diagnosis requires a high index of clinical suspicion.
  - Imaging can act as a useful adjunct for this diagnosis:
    - Radiographs can be useful to evaluate for the presence of cervical ribs.
    - Other imaging modalities to assess vein patency, including duplex ultrasound, catheter-directed venography, CT venography (CTV), and/or MR venography, may also be indicated for full evaluation. Duplex ultrasound is the most appropriate of these modalities to assess for upper-extremity venous thrombosis.
    - Contrast venography is considered the gold standard for this diagnosis; however, there are no widespread studies assessing the diagnostic accuracy of CTV.
    - Catheter-directed venography may be highly considered in patient workup, because if positive, thrombosis can be directly treated at the same time as diagnosis.
- Groin pain
  - One of the most common causes of groin (inguinal) pain is hernia-related pain (3). These patients do not often present as a diagnostic dilemma, and if the hernia is large enough, the diagnosis can be made with an appropriate history and physical examination. However, if the hernia

is small, ultrasound or MRI might be helpful to document its presence and provide additional anatomic detail.

- Ultrasound is considered first-choice in patients who have not had prior surgery. Ultrasound is particularly useful in performing certain maneuvers that might exacerbate the hernia and/or the patient's symptomatology (*i.e.*, Valsalva maneuver).
- Either ultrasound or MRI could be considered in patients with a history of prior hernia surgery; the choice of which modality is often determined by the type of surgery performed.

- Musculoskeletal injury and/or overuse can be another important cause of groin pain. Common key areas to evaluate and consider include (1) the proximal adductors, (2) the pubic symphysis, (3) the iliopsoas muscle, and (4) the hip joint.
  - MRI is the most comprehensive and easiest way to evaluate these potential causes of groin pain. They can all be included in the field-of-view on standard MRI pelvis or MRI hip imaging.
  - MRI protocols can be tailored to evaluate for both hernia-related causes and musculoskeletal etiologies for pain.
  - If a very specific diagnosis is being considered, focused MRI protocols can be created. For instance, for a "sports hernia" (injury to the rectus abdominis-common adductor aponeurosis), the radiologist and MRI technologist can use a tailored field-of-view that focuses on the attachment site to the pubic symphysis.
  - The PLAC (pyramidalis-anterior pubic ligament-adductor longus complex) is an anatomical concept that was introduced in 2017 and can be a cause of groin pain in the athlete. Similar to "sports hernia" MRI protocols, PLAC injuries can be diagnosed with a focused (or "coned-in") MRI.

SUMMARY

- When dealing with the athlete, plain radiography is usually the first imaging study that should be performed. This holds true whether dealing with an acute injury or overuse.
- CT is preferred for complex bone trauma.
- MRI is preferred for the diagnosis of radiographically occult bone injury and soft-tissue trauma, be it acute or chronic. This is not an urgent examination unless one is dealing with an elite athlete where return to play is an issue or there is concern for a radiographically occult fracture in a weight-bearing bone.
- US is a viable alternative to MRI for evaluation of superficial soft tissues, but it requires an appropriately trained operator.
- The clinical history will affect both image acquisition and interpretation. Open communication between the clinician and radiologist is essential for optimal patient care.

REFERENCES

1. Burnham KJ, Poudel M. Diagnostic challenges in an athlete with popliteal artery entrapment syndrome: a case report. *Curr Sports Med Rep.* 2023;22(2):52–4.
2. Hollabaugh WL, Bowman EN. Effort-associated thrombosis: imaging is key when suspicion is high. A case report. *Curr Sports Med Rep.* 2022;21(11):395–7.
3. Plumb AA, Rajeswaran G, Abbasi MA, Masci L, Warren O, Wilson J. Contemporary imaging of inguinal hernia and pain. *Br J Radiol.* 2022;95(1134):20220163. doi:10.1259/bjr.20220163

SUGGESTED READING

Allen GM, Wilson DJ. Ultrasound in sports medicine—a critical evaluation. *Eur J Radiol.* 2007;62(1):79–85.

Brittenden J, Robinson P. Imaging of pelvic injuries in athletes. *Br J Radiol.* 2005;78(929):457–68.

Cubon VA, Putukian M, Boyer C, Dettwiler A. A diffusion tensor imaging study on the white matter skeleton in individuals with sports-related concussion. *J Neurotrauma.* 2011;28(2):189–201.

Delgado J, Jaramillo D, Chauvin NA. Imaging the injured pediatric athlete: upper extremity. *Radiographics.* 2016;36(6):1672–87.

Gonzalez FM, Morrison WB. Magnetic resonance imaging of sports injuries involving the ankle. *Top Magn Reason Imaging.* 2015;24(4):205–13.

Healy JC, Lee JC. Sports injury of the lower extremity: role of imaging in diagnosis and management. *Semin Musculoskelet Radiol.* 2011;15(1):1–2.

Hagezi TM, Belair JA, McCarthy EJ, Roedl JB, Morrison WB. Sports injuries about the hip: what the radiologist should know. *Radiographics.* 2016;36(6):1717–45.

Kijowski R, de Smet AA. The role of ultrasound in the evaluation of sports medicine injuries of the upper extremity. *Clin Sports Med.* 2006;25(3):569–90.

Khoury V, Guillin R, Dhanju J, Cardinal E. Ultrasound of ankle and foot: overuse and sports injuries. *Semin Musculoskelet Radiol.* 2007;11(2):149–61.

Liong SY, Whitehouse RW. Lower extremity and pelvic stress fractures in athletes. *Br J Radiol.* 2012;85(1016):1148–56.

Meyer NB, Jacobson JA, Kalia V, Kim SM. Musculoskeletal ultrasound: athletic injuries of the lower extremity. *Ultrasonography.* 2018;37(3):175–89.

O'Dell MC, Jaramillo D, Bancroft L, Varich L, Logsdon G, Servaes S. Imaging of sports-related injuries of the lower extremity in pediatric patients. *Radiographics.* 2016;36(6):1807–27.

Patel NB, Thomas S, Lazarus ML. Throwing injuries of the upper extremity. *Radiol Clin North Am.* 2013;51(2):257–77.

Parker BJ, Zlatkin MB, Newman JS, Rathur SK. Imaging of shoulder injuries in sports medicine: current protocols and concepts. *Clin Sports Med.* 2008;27(4):579–606.

Raissaki M, Apostolaki E, Karantanas AH. Imaging of sports injuries in children and adolescents. *Eur J Radiol.* 2007;62(1):86–96.

Robinson P. *Essential Radiology for Sports Medicine*. New York (NY): Springer; 2010. 268 p.

Sanchez TRS, Jadhav SP, Swischuk LE. MR imaging of pediatric trauma. *Radiol Clin North Am*. 2009;47(6):927–38.

Serhal A, Hinkel T, Adams B, Garg A, Omar IM, Younger J. Imaging of sports injuries of the upper extremity. *Adv Clin Radiol*. 2021;3:203–16.

Stoller DW. *Magnetic Resonance Imaging in Orthopaedics and Sports Medicine*. Philadelphia (PA): Lippincott Williams & Wilkins; 2007. 2045 p.

Torriani M, Kattapuram SV. Musculoskeletal ultrasound: an alternative imaging modality for sports-related injuries. *Top Magn Reson Imaging*. 2003;14(1):103–11.

Waldt S, Woertler K. *Measurements and Classifications in Musculoskeletal Radiology*. Stuttgart (Germany): Thieme Medical Publishers, Inc.; 2013.

Magnetic Resonance Imaging in the Upper and Lower Extremity

20

Hannah C. Chen, Courtney T. Tripp, and John F. Feller

INTRODUCTION

- Magnetic resonance imaging (MRI) provides unparalleled soft tissue and bone marrow contrast in musculoskeletal imaging; it has become the premiere imaging modality for sports-related injuries.
- MRI has multiple purposes in sports medicine, including: facilitating an accurate diagnosis, prognostication for return to play, and assessment of healing following injury or surgical intervention (1).
- Chapter 19 *Diagnostic Imaging*, discusses MRI imaging in context with other modalities, and describes the many pulse sequences that can be used with MRI, including: T1-weighted (T1W), T2-weighted (T2W) and short tau inversion recovery (STIR), proton density (PD), and gradient-echo sequences (GRE).
- This chapter details site-specific considerations, utilization, and interpretation of MRI in sports medicine for the provider. All figures identified in this chapter are found in the online addendum chapter 20.

SHOULDER

- Conventional noncontrast MRI and direct magnetic resonance arthrography (MRA) have demonstrated a high sensitivity and specificity for diagnosing osseous and soft tissue abnormalities in the shoulder to include the labrum, articular cartilage, long head biceps tendon (LHBT), and rotator cuff (RC) tendons (2–4).
- The glenoid labrum is an ovoid-shaped fibrocartilaginous structure attached to the margin of the glenoid and appears as a uniformly low-signal intensity triangular-shaped structure on MRI. The joint capsule and LHBT, along with multiple band-like regions of capsular thickening known as glenohumeral ligaments, attach directly to the glenoid labrum (5,6).
- A tear of the glenoid labrum is diagnosed on MRI as a detached or displaced labral fragment, and/or hyperintense fluid-like signal extending into the labrum, oriented away from the glenoid. There are several anatomic variants, predominantly in the anterosuperior labrum, which can mimic a labral tear; however, the presence of a paralabral cyst provides a clue that a labral tear is present (5).
- Superior labral pathology, specifically superior labrum anterior-posterior (SLAP) tears, is a clinically important cause of shoulder instability. SLAP lesions can extend in the anterior to posterior direction and are usually centered at the LHBT and can be referred to as the biceps labrum complex (Fig. 20.1). SLAP lesions were first described by Snyder et al. in 1990 with four distinct types. The original four types of SLAP lesions are described below and are accurately diagnosed on high-resolution noncontrast MRI (5,7–9) and MRA (10,11):
  - Type 1: Degenerative fraying of the free edge of the superior labrum
  - Type 2: Unstable with tears of the biceps labral complex
  - Type 3: Bucket-handle tear of the superior labrum with an intact biceps anchor
  - Type 4: Bucket-handle tear of the superior labrum with extension into the biceps anchor
- The classification of SLAP lesions has since been expanded into SLAP type 2a-c and additional SLAP types V-X, which are associated with other injuries of the labrum and capsular structures (5,12); however, the original Snyder classification remains the most widely used (13).
- The abduction-external rotation (ABER) sequence increases the anterior capsulolabral tension and aids in the detection of nondisplaced labral tears and anterior capsule pathology (14,15) (Fig. 20.2). Cvitanic et al. (16) found increased accuracy in the detection of anteroinferior labral injuries with imaging in the ABER position.
- Accurate assessment of the articular cartilage in the glenohumeral joint is important for clinical decision making and is optimally evaluated with MRI. Normal articular cartilage has a layered appearance, which is best evaluated with high-resolution imaging acquired on 1.5 and 3T scanners. The intermediate layer of the articular cartilage is the thickest layer and has an intermediate to hyperintense signal; however, this can vary depending on the imaging orientation and sequence parameters (17). The articular cartilage of the humeral head is thinner along the periphery and thicker centrally, whereas the cartilage along the glenoid is thicker

peripherally and thinner centrally (18). The glenoid cartilage is best evaluated on axial sequences and the humeral head cartilage is best evaluated on coronal sequences (19–21).

- LHBT pathology is a known cause of shoulder pain and functional impairment. Tendinosis of the intra-articular LHBT occurs frequently in association with impingement syndromes and RC tears, usually the subscapularis or far anterior leading edge of the supraspinatus. Biceps tendon tears are categorized as either partial or full-thickness and are accurately diagnosed on MRI.
- Biceps instability is a dynamic condition that can manifest on MRI as medial subluxation/dislocation of the biceps tendon. Injuries to associated structures in the rotator interval to include the coracohumeral ligament, superior glenohumeral ligament, superior subscapularis tendon, and anterior supraspinatus tendon can aid in the diagnosis of biceps instability on MRI (22–24).
- The RC tendons appear as uniformly hypointense curvilinear bands on all MRI sequences. Tendinosis is seen as either an abnormal morphology, such as tendon thickening and/or alterations in the signal of the tendon, such as intermediate to hyperintense signal; these findings are true for all tendons imaged on MRI.
- RC tears are described as partial or full-thickness discontinuity of the tendon that can be articular-sided, bursal-sided, or intrasubstance with hyperintense fluid-like signal. Several studies have evaluated the diagnostic accuracy of detecting partial and full-thickness RC tears on MRI and have a pooled sensitivity of 84% and specificity of 92% (25). In addition, Tirman et al. (26) found increased detection rates of partial-thickness articular-sided RC tears in overhead-throwing athletes with imaging in the ABER position. Fluid distention of the subacromial-subdeltoid bursa is a secondary sign often associated with bursal-sided or full-thickness RC tears.
- In the case of full-thickness RC tears, the degree of tendon retraction, fatty muscle infiltration, and muscle atrophy are important as these findings may portend a poor postsurgical functional outcome and can significantly influence clinical management (27,28). On MRI, fatty muscle infiltration is diagnosed as fatty streaks within the muscle belly (linear/streaky T1 hyperintense signal within the muscle), and muscle atrophy is diagnosed as an overall decrease in muscle bulk (29).
- Traumatic anterior glenohumeral dislocations are one of the most common upper extremity injuries in athletes, and MRI provides valuable information regarding the integrity of the labrum, capsule, cartilaginous, and osseous structures, which are likely to be injured.
- The most common injury associated with a traumatic anterior glenohumeral dislocation is a Bankart lesion, which is the detachment of the anteroinferior labrum and capsule from the glenoid rim, first described by Bankart in 1923 (30) (Fig. 20.3). It is called a "bony" Bankart lesion if the anteroinferior glenoid rim fractures along with the labrum or a reverse Bankart lesion in the setting of a posterior glenohumeral dislocation (Fig. 20.4). Several soft tissue Bankart variants have subsequently been described, which involve injury to the anteroinferior capsulolabral complex (5,31) (Fig. 20.5).
- A Hill-Sachs lesion is an osseous impaction injury at the posterolateral humeral head, which occurs during an anterior glenohumeral dislocation and is seen on MRI as a wedge-shaped defect in the humeral head at or above the level of the coracoid process (5) (Fig. 20.6).
- Bipolar bone loss in the humeral head and glenoid after an anterior glenohumeral dislocation is an important predictive factor for recurrent dislocations. The pattern of bone loss can be described as an on-track/non-engaging Hill-Sachs defect where the Hill-Sachs interval is greater than the glenoid track or as an off-track/engaging Hill-Sachs defect where the Hill-Sachs interval is less than the glenoid track. Determining on-track versus off-track lesions was initially described on CT but can also be assessed on MRI (32,33).
- Impingement syndrome of the shoulder is a clinical diagnosis and constitutes a range of pathology affecting the RC tendons to include tendinosis, partial and full-thickness tears, and calcific tendinitis. Impingement syndrome of the shoulder can be further divided into external and internal types.
- External impingement results from abnormal contact between the humeral head and extra-articular structures such as the acromion and/or coracoid process (34). Although this is a clinical syndrome, MRI can provide supportive diagnostic confidence by revealing several indirect findings to include a hooked type III acromion, a subacromial enthesophyte, a small lateral angle of the acromion, coracoacromial ligament thickening, a decreased acromiohumeral distance, an increased critical shoulder angle (CSA), subacromial bursitis, RC tendinosis, and/or partial- or full-thickness RC tears (34,35).
- Internal impingement syndrome (IIS) develops when the posterior glenoid labrum and RC tendons (posterior supraspinatus and anterior infraspinatus) are repeatedly wedged between the greater tuberosity and posterosuperior glenoid rim during maximal cocking of the arm in abduction and external rotation. MRI findings of IIS include partial-thickness articular-sided tears in the supraspinatus and infraspinatus tendons, posterosuperior labral tears, posterior capsular thickening, cystic changes in the posterosuperior humeral head, and degenerative changes in the posterosuperior glenoid (14,36).
- The clinical syndrome of adhesive capsulitis ("frozen shoulder") manifests as shoulder pain and stiffness and can be suggested on MRI and MRA with findings of coracohumeral ligament thickening, obliteration of the subcoracoid fat, capsular and synovial edema and thickening and reduced capsular volume, especially in the axillary recess (37) (Fig. 20.7).
- Injuries to the pectoralis major musculotendinous unit often occur in weightlifters and can be difficult to examine in the acute setting due to localized swelling and pain (38,39). MRI

can accurately identify high-grade partial and complete tears, which have better outcomes with surgical repair shortly after the time of injury.

- Acromioclavicular (AC) joint separations are classified into six types (Rockwood classification): Type I consists of partial disruption of the AC joint capsule. Type II consists of disruption of the AC joint capsule and partial disruption of the coracoclavicular (CC) ligament. Type III through VI injuries all result from double disruption of the suspensory ligaments of the shoulder (AC and CC ligaments) and may be treated surgically. MRI can help establish the integrity of these suspensory ligaments, especially in cases wherein radiographic and clinical findings are confounding (differentiating between types II and III) (40,41).

ELBOW

- Most sports-related elbow injuries are adequately evaluated with a noncontrast MRI. Triplanar imaging of the elbow is routinely performed with a combination of T1, T2, and/or water-sensitive STIR sequences. Imaging can be performed with the elbow either at the patient's side or with the arm positioned overhead (42). MRA is generally unnecessary, although it may be helpful for detecting cartilage injuries, intra-articular bodies, and collateral ligament tears (43).
- MRI is useful in evaluating partial or complete sprains of the collateral ligaments about the elbow.
- Injuries to the ulnar collateral ligament (UCL) are most common in throwing athletes, where there is repetitive and/or excessive valgus stress applied to the elbow. There are three bundles that comprise the UCL, the anterior, posterior, and transverse bundles. The anterior bundle of the UCL is the primary restraint to valgus stress and is the most commonly injured, resulting in valgus instability. The anterior bundle of the UCL is normally a thin dark band at the medial margin of the elbow joint. Complete full-thickness tears are easily detected on noncontrast MRI (Fig. 20.8), whereas more subtle abnormalities, such as attenuation, redundancy, or focal partial discontinuity of the ligament, which suggest a partial-thickness tear may be aided with the use of intra-articular contrast (43–45).
- Lateral ulnar collateral ligament (LUCL) tears are typically the result of an elbow dislocation in young individuals and caused by a varus extension stress injury without dislocation in adults. LUCL tears are often full-thickness, occurring at the proximal attachment to the lateral epicondyle, and manifest as a focal disruption on MRI. Disruption of the LUCL is closely associated with posterolateral rotary instability of the elbow (46,47).
- Imaging evaluation for epicondylitis, while typically a clinical diagnosis, is a common indication for MRI. The term epicondylitis implies that inflammation is present and is a misnomer. The preferred term of tendinosis (of the elbow) more accurately describes the histology of mucoid degeneration and vascular hyperplasia that exists within the diseased tendon (48). An advantage of MRI includes characterization of the severity of tendinosis, partial or full-thickness tendon tears, and evaluation and/or exclusion of other possible causes of elbow pain.
- Tendinosis of the common flexor-pronator tendons and extensor tendons about the elbow is seen as a thickening and abnormal intermediate to hyperintense signal within the tendon. Partial- or full-thickness tears can be seen as hyperintense fluid-like signals within the tendon, an important finding directing patient treatment (49) (Fig. 20.9).
- Lateral epicondylitis (tennis elbow) commonly affects tennis players, although it is more common in nonathletic populations; it occurs with activities involving repetitive pronation and supination of the forearm with the elbow in extension. The tendinosis principally affects the extensor carpi radialis brevis tendon portion of the common extensor tendon, with tenderness over the lateral epicondyle. When MRI is used to evaluate lateral epicondylitis, imaging findings of tendinosis and the degree of tear correlate well with surgical findings (49).
- Medial epicondylitis (golfer's elbow), although less common than lateral epicondylitis, is mainly seen in athletes. The tendinosis principally involves the flexor carpi radialis and pronator teres tendons at the medial condylar origin and shows MRI findings of tendinosis and/or tearing as described previously (50).
- Distal biceps tendon ruptures occur almost exclusively in men and are the result of a single traumatic event with sudden forceful extension. Tears typically occur at the insertion site of the tendon onto the radial tuberosity and can be characterized on MRI as partial or complete. The flexion-abduction-supination (FABS) sequence can be performed in challenging cases of a high-grade partial versus complete tear (51) (Fig. 20.10). Complete full-thickness distal biceps tendon tears are often associated with tendon retraction, which can be accurately assessed on MRI (Fig. 20.11).
- MRI is extremely useful for detecting occult fractures and osteochondral injuries of the elbow. Subtle nondisplaced fractures of the radial head and supracondylar/epicondylar regions in children are readily diagnosed on MRI with linear low-signal fracture lines and surrounding marrow edema.
- Osteochondral abnormalities, such as traumatic osteochondral injuries, osteochondritis dissecans in adolescents, and osteochondrosis of the capitellum (Panner disease) in children, are well characterized with MRI. Osteochondral lesions are characterized as stable or unstable. An unstable osteochondral lesion on MRI is characterized by a hyperintense fluid-like signal between the fragment and parent bone, overlying chondral irregularities, and subchondral bone plate disruption with or without cyst-like changes (42,52,53).
- An apophyseal stress injury of the medial epicondyle apophysis (little leaguer's elbow) can be seen in children involved

in throwing sports. MRI may aid in the diagnosis by revealing the widening of the epicondylar physis with an increased hyperintense fluid-like signal along both sides of the physis. If the physis is nearly closed, then MRI may show loss of the normal fatty marrow signal around the apophysis. Progression to a partial or complete avulsion of the apophysis can be seen if there is continued repetitive stress (42).

WRIST AND HAND

- Common indications for MRI of the wrist and hand include ganglion cysts, carpal tunnel syndrome, tears and/or degeneration of the intrinsic ligaments, triangular fibrocartilaginous complex (TFCC), and tendons.
- Conventional noncontrast MRI of the wrist and hand routinely includes triplanar sequences with a high-resolution and small field-of-view using dedicated surface coils. T1 and intermediate-weighted sequences provide excellent anatomic detail, whereas T2-weighted sequences are useful for visualizing most pathologic conditions. Coronal three-dimensional (3D) sequences are also routinely acquired to allow for improved contrast and higher spatial resolution of the intrinsic ligaments of the wrist (54–56).
- Tendons of the hand and wrist, as seen elsewhere in the body, are tubular-shaped structures with uniformly low-signal intensity.
- The flexor digitorum superficialis, flexor digitorum profundus, and flexor pollicis longus tendons are the main flexor tendons of the digits. These tendons pass within the carpal tunnel and are best evaluated on axial sequences.
- The median nerve also passes through the carpal tunnel and is seen as an intermediate-intensity tubular structure with visible internal fascicles. Compression of the median nerve within the carpal tunnel may occur due to space-occupying lesions such as soft tissue masses or ganglion cysts, which contribute to the clinical entity of carpal tunnel syndrome. The flexor retinaculum, which is superficial to the median nerve, is often bowed in the setting of carpal tunnel syndrome. MRI is useful in assessing the signal intensity of the nerve, the cross sectional area of the nerve proximal and distal to the carpal tunnel, and palmar retinacular bowing, which help determine the severity of carpal tunnel syndrome (57).
- Among the dorsal extensor tendons of the wrist, tenosynovial effusion (tenosynovitis) is most commonly seen in the extensor carpi ulnaris (ECU) tendon. ECU tenosynovitis can present with ulnar-sided wrist pain and is frequently associated with instability of the tendon due to abnormal subluxation/dislocation with wrist movement, particularly with supination (58,59).
- Tendinopathy and stenosing tenosynovitis of the first dorsal extensor compartment tendons, composed of the abductor pollicis longus and extensor pollicis brevis tendons, is referred to as de Quervain tenosynovitis. Although often idiopathic, de Quervain tenosynovitis can occur in athletes involved in racket sports and golfing. MRI findings include thickening and abnormal intermediate to hyperintense signals within the first compartment tendons, thickened and edematous retinaculum, tenosynovitis, and peritendinous edema (58,60).
- The intrinsic ligaments of the wrist are important stabilizers and can be accurately evaluated with high-resolution MRI. Scapholunate instability is the result of a full-thickness scapholunate ligament tear and is the most common type of carpal instability. The scapholunate ligament (SLL) comprises dorsal, membranous, and volar components. The dorsal component serves as the main scapholunate joint stabilizer and is band-like with a low-signal intensity. The volar component of the SLL has a more striated, heterogeneous appearance with increased signal (61,62). MRI is more sensitive in evaluating SLL tears than lunotriquetral ligament (LTL) tears due to the LTL having more variability in shape and internal signal intensity. Complete tears are seen as discontinuity of the ligament or complete absence of the ligament (Fig. 20.12). Some authors advocate for the use of MRA, which has shown a slightly increased sensitivity in the detection of intrinsic ligamentous tears. However, the superiority of MRA over MRI is debatable as per literature as there are more false positive results with MRA, which is also more invasive and costly compared to a conventional noncontrast MRI (58). Additionally, with advances in coil technology and pulse sequencing, noncontrast 3T MRI may have equivocal results, especially when MRA is not available (63).
- The TFCC is a complex structure composed of a central articular disk, volar and dorsal distal radioulnar ligaments, ulnocarpal collateral ligament, ulnotriquetral and ulnolunate ligaments, and the ECU tendon subsheath. TFCC tears and/or perforations are associated with ulnar-sided wrist pain and instability and may be traumatic or degenerative in etiology with the exact locations of tears identified on MRI, which can direct further treatment (64,65).
- Ulnar impaction syndrome is a clinical entity that results from abutment of the distal end of the ulna against the carpus. The associated imaging findings include positive ulnar variance, tears in the TFCC, and arthritic changes involving the distal ulna, ulnar side of the lunate, and radial side of the triquetrum. MRI can demonstrate these findings as well as lunotriquetral ligament tears and cartilage changes in the distal ulna, which is often a precursor to radiographic findings (66,67) (Fig. 20.13).
- "Gamekeeper's thumb" or "skier's thumb" is an injury of the ulnar collateral ligament of the metacarpophalangeal joint of the thumb that typically occurs in skiers, football players, and wrestlers. This is generally apparent on physical examination, but MRI allows for confirmation of the diagnosis and further evaluates for a possible complication termed a Stener lesion, which was first described by Dr. Stener in 1962. A Stener lesion occurs wherein the adjacent adductor pollicis

aponeurosis is interposed between the torn and retracted ulnar collateral ligament and the underlying bone, which may impede healing (68,69). On MRI, the retracted ligament appears as a tiny balled-up mass of tissue superficial to the aponeurosis (70). This is important as it would be an indication of surgical intervention (67).

- Traumatic finger injuries are common in both sports and work-related activities. With dedicated small surface coils and high-resolution imaging sequences, an MRI of the finger can accurately evaluate the integrity of the flexor and extensor tendons, collateral ligaments, and pulley system of the fingers. Lesions caused by hyperextension injuries are those most frequently seen in sports medicine practices. Commonly torn or avulsed structures include the volar plate, flexor tendons, and/or pulleys. Injuries common to the athletic population include both the "mallet finger" deformity resulting from avulsion of the terminal extensor tendon from the base of the distal phalanx and the "jersey finger" deformity resulting from avulsion of the flexor digitorum profundus tendon from the volar distal phalanx (71).
- MRI is extremely sensitive to bone marrow abnormalities and hence useful in the diagnosis of nondisplaced carpal bone fractures and avascular necrosis. STIR sequences are highly water-sensitive and easily detect bone marrow edema, which is particularly useful in identifying occult carpal bone fractures, especially in the scaphoid and hook of the hamate. Contrast-enhanced MRI with gadolinium-enhanced sequences can also assess the vascularity in osseous fragments and aid in the staging of Kienbock disease, which has significant clinical implications (56).

HIP

- MRI evaluation of the hip in the young athletic population is performed to optimize the assessment of both internal and external derangements of the hip. MRI evaluation routinely includes a combination of large field-of-view bilateral hip and pelvic structures that aid in the evaluation of extra-articular abnormalities (*i.e.*, musculotendinous injuries, osseous injuries, and bursitis) and high-resolution small field-of-view unilateral imaging for intra-articular abnormalities (*e.g.*, chondral injuries, acetabular-labral tears, intra-articular bodies, and femoral acetabular impingement (FAI)) (72,73). Intra-articular bodies are especially conspicuous in the presence of a joint effusion or joint distension with direct arthrography.
- The acetabular labrum is a fibrocartilaginous structure, which is uniformly hypointense on all sequences and appears as a triangular-shaped structure attached to the acetabular rim. Acetabular-labral tears most commonly occur in the anterior and anterosuperior locations, whereas labral variants, such as a labral sulcus, more commonly occur in the posteroinferior location.
- Labral tears are diagnosed on MRI as a linear or curvilinear hyperintense fluid-like signal traversing the labrum or extending to the acetabular-labral interface, labral fragmentation, and/or complete detachment of the labrum (72–74). MRA is superior to noncontrast MRI at detecting labral pathology; however, some studies have recently shown that high-resolution noncontrast 3T MRI may be equivocal to MRA in detecting labral tears (74,75).
- MRI assessment of the articular cartilage in the hip is notoriously difficult due to the curved morphology of the acetabulum and femoral head. The normal acetabular and femoral articular cartilage has an intermediate to high signal intensity on intermediate and T2 weighted sequences. Chondral abnormalities can initially appear as heterogeneous signal changes, fraying, fissuring, thinning and progress to partial- and full-thickness defects, chondral delamination, and chondral flaps.
- Several studies have shown that MRA has a higher diagnostic accuracy for detecting chondral abnormalities compared to a conventional noncontrast MRI, at both 1.5 and 3T. Additional MR techniques have been studied to assess the articular cartilage and include indirect MRA, delayed gadolinium-enhanced images, MRA with leg traction, T2 relaxation time mapping, and diffusion tensor imaging (74).
- Osteochondral lesions in the hip may occur secondary to an impaction injury, hip dislocations, and/or subclinical chondral shearing, which most commonly affects the superomedial femoral head.
- MRI is useful in evaluating injuries to the extra-articular regional musculotendinous structures that are common in athletes, especially to the hamstring and rectus femoris muscles. MRI findings of a muscle contusion and/or strain include abnormal high signal within the muscle, architectural distortion, fiber discontinuity, an intramuscular hematoma, and tendon retraction (76).
- Tendinosis is seen as a thickening and/or intermediate to hyperintense signal in the tendon, which is common in the hamstring tendon origin at the ischial tuberosity and in the gluteus medius and minimus tendon insertions at the greater trochanter.
- FAI is a dynamic phenomenon resulting from abnormal contact between the femur and acetabulum during hip motion, especially terminal movements, and may contribute to early onset osteoarthritis of the hip. The abnormal contact between the femur and acetabulum may occur at the femoral-neck junction (cam morphology), at the acetabular rim (pincer morphology), or both (mixed) (73,77).
- Several findings on MRI may suggest the clinical syndrome of FAI and include labral tears, especially at the labral-chondral transition zone, loss of articular cartilage, an os acetabulum, and a synovial herniation pit. A nonspherical shape of the femoral head with an osseous prominence at the femoral head-neck junction, decreased femoral head-neck offset, and anterosuperior chondral loss is characteristic of a cam morphology. Local or diffuse acetabular over-coverage, labral ossification, and posteroinferior acetabular chondral loss characterize a pincer morphology (73,78–81) (Fig. 20.14).

- In adductor avulsion syndrome ("thigh splints"), there is periosteal edema near the insertion of the adductor muscles of the femur (82).
- Athletic pubalgia ("sports hernia") is a non-specific term that refers to lower abdominal wall and peripubic pain. It encompasses soft tissue injuries involving the rectus abdominis tendon, adductor tendons, aponeurotic plate, and osteitis pubis. Athletic pubalgia-specific MRI protocols are useful in evaluating the relevant anatomy and aid in preoperative planning. MRI findings of rectus abdominis and adductor tendon injuries at their pubic bone insertion include tendon thickening with or without intermediate intrasubstance signal, partial or complete disruption of the fibers, and a cleft of fluid signal interposed between the aponeurosis and pubic bone (81,83).
- MRI is the imaging modality of choice to evaluate for osseous stress injuries, avascular necrosis, and occult fractures in the hip. Osseous stress reaction and stress fractures common to the athletic population involve the femoral neck, the pubic bones, and the sacrum, all of which demonstrate marrow edema, and in the case of stress fracture, a low-signal intensity line (Figs. 20.15 and 20.16).
- AVN and subchondral insufficiency fractures of the femoral head can be difficult to distinguish in the early stages as both demonstrate edema in the femoral head. Findings of AVN include a "double line sign," which may progress to a subchondral fracture and eventual femoral head collapse. Subchondral insufficiency fractures may demonstrate a low T2 signal line and/or band that parallels the subchondral surface (73).
- Inflammation of bursae around the hip can occur due to repetitive microtrauma and friction, which is seen on MRI as thickening and distension of the bursa with fluid. Commonly seen around the hip on MRI include the greater trochanteric, subgluteus medius, iliopsoas, obturator externus, and ischial bursae (84).

KNEE

- The knee is one of the most commonly evaluated joints by MRI, which provides superior evaluation for internal derangement compared to other imaging modalities. A conventional knee MRI includes triplanar imaging with both high-resolution T1, intermediate-weighted, and water-sensitive (T2 fat-suppressed or STIR) sequences to evaluate the osseous, intra-articular, and extra-articular soft tissues of the knee (85).
- The knee comprises two fibrocartilaginous menisci, a medial meniscus, and a lateral meniscus, which are C-shaped structures with a thicker peripheral portion and thinner central free edge. The menisci can be subdivided into the anterior root, anterior horn, body, posterior horn, and posterior root. As evaluated in the coronal plane, the menisci have a triangular-shaped appearance and a bow-tie configuration with opposing triangles in the sagittal plane (86). The posterior horn of the medial meniscus is larger than the anterior horn by almost 1.5 to 2 times. The lateral meniscus is smaller and more circular in shape than the medial meniscus, with the anterior and posterior horns nearly equal in size, except for a discoid variant, which has an enlarged central extension (Fig. 20.17).
- The menisci, like other fibrocartilaginous structures in the body, have a uniformly low-signal intensity on all sequences. Exceptions to this occur in children, where prominent vascularity can be reflected as an increased intrasubstance signal, or in adults with mucinous degeneration. It is important to know that an increased intrasubstance signal within a meniscus (grade 1 or 2) that does not extend to a meniscal articular margin does not represent a meniscal tear.
- Meniscal tears are diagnosed on MRI by an abnormal morphology, displaced or missing meniscal tissue, and/or hyperintense fluid-like signal in the meniscus, which contacts the articular surfaces (grade 3), typically seen on at least two slices (86). Meniscal tears can be accurately detected with high spatial resolution MRI as studies have shown MRI to have a sensitivity, specificity, and accuracy ranging from 85% to 95% (87). Short echo time, T1, or intermediate-weighted sequences are the most sensitive for identifying meniscal tears.
- On MRI, meniscal tears are categorized as horizontal, vertical, or radial in configuration (Fig. 20.18). Description of the location of the tear with respect to the periphery of the meniscus is important in determining the reparability of the tear. Typically, meniscal tears in the peripheral portion are repaired in the young athletic population because there is a greater likelihood of viability due to greater vascular supply to the peripheral meniscus.
- Longitudinal vertical meniscal tears deserve special note because they may become displaced within the joint and form a "bucket-handle tear," wherein the cleaved displaced inner meniscal fragment may be displaced into the intercondylar notch, anteriorly, posteriorly, or laterally. A bucket-handle tear of the medial meniscus may be displaced into the intercondylar notch adjacent and inferior to the PCL, a configuration termed the "double PCL sign" (Fig. 20.19). Bucket-handle tears of the lateral meniscus are hindered from displacement into the intercondylar notch to the level of the PCL due to be presence of an intact anterior cruciate ligament (ACL) and, therefore, typically displace anteriorly, forming the so-called "double anterior horn sign" (88,89) (Fig. 20.20).
- In the postoperative meniscus, the presence of a hyperintense fluid signal on noncontrast MRI is not definitive for a retear as this may reflect granulation tissue, which has been shown to persist up to 27 months after surgical repair (90). For this reason, evaluation of the postoperative meniscus with an MRA is recommended over a conventional noncontrast MRI. On MRA, a retear of the meniscus is defined as contrast extending into the meniscus.

- Various normal anatomic structures in close approximation to the meniscus can mimic tears on MRI, and therefore, an understanding of normal anatomy and variants is necessary for accurate diagnosis.
- MRI is well suited to assess chondral injuries of the knee, which in the athletic population is crucial for directing early treatment. The normal articular cartilage on conventional 2D intermediate and fluid-sensitive sequences demonstrates a layered appearance with relative uniform thickness and intermediate to hyperintense signal. Chondral injuries include focal abnormal signal, fibrillation/fissuring, partial- and full-thickness chondral defects, and chondral shear injuries (91) (Fig. 20.21).
- Over the past decade, several advanced cartilage-sensitive sequences have been evaluated (*i.e.*, T2 mapping, T1 mapping, diffusion-weighting, and spoiled gradient echo) and often employ 3D techniques (*i.e.*, 3D FSE, 3D SPGR, and 3D DESS). While cartilage-sensitive sequences have been shown to be more accurate in evaluating the articular cartilage, it is often at the expense of longer acquisition times (20,87).
- Various surgical repair techniques of articular cartilage defects are used, including subchondral microfracture, matrix-induced autologous chondrocyte implantation, osteochondral autograft transplant/mosaicplasty, and osteochondral allograft, all of which can be successfully imaged with MRI postoperatively (92).
- The normal ligamentous and tendinous structures of the knee have uniformly low-signal intensity on all MRI sequences. The cruciate ligaments are best seen on sagittal sequences, and the collateral ligaments are best seen on coronal sequences. However, correlation with orthogonal imaging planes is valuable in corroborating pathology because, occasionally, volume averaging of signal with adjacent soft tissue structures may falsely suggest pathology (86,93).
- The ACL comprises two bundles, an anteromedial bundle and a posteromedial bundle, which on MRI are thick, low-signal band-like structures that parallel the roof of the intercondylar notch.
- In athletes, the ACL is one of the commonly injured structures in the knee. Full-thickness ACL tears are diagnosed by observation of complete discontinuity of the ligament fibers (Fig. 20.22). Partial-thickness ACL tears are more difficult to diagnose on MRI but can be aided with a sequence specifically designed to evaluate the ACL, which is acquired in a coronal oblique plane (86). Direct MRI signs of an ACL disruption include focal discontinuity of the ligament fibers, abnormal slope of the ACL, and avulsion of the anterior tibial spine. Indirect MR signs of an ACL disruption include a deep sulcus sign, a Segond fracture (capsular avulsion fracture of lateral tibial plateau), anterior translation of the tibia relative to the femur, hyperextension bone contusion injuries involving the anterior tibia and femur, buckling of the posterior cruciate ligament (PCL) and pericruciate fat pad signal alterations (94,95).
- ACL tears are typically repaired in the athletic population to regain stability and to prevent chronic ACL deficiency, a condition associated with a higher risk of medial meniscal degenerative tearing.
- The posteroperative ACL can be evaluated with MRI and should parallel the roof of the intercondylar notch, without buckling, as seen in the sagittal plane. ACL graft tears are diagnosed by observing focal discontinuity of graft fibers, not unlike that seen in a native ACL tear. Postoperatively, non-fat-suppressed T2-weighted or PD sequences should be used as these are less susceptible to metallic artifacts, which can result in particle-magnetic field inhomogeneities (96).
- Arthrofibrosis ("cyclops lesion") may develop after an ACL reconstruction and is seen on MRI as scar tissue in the anterior intercondylar region, which may impede full joint extension (97).
- Tears of the PCL are much less common and are associated with significant trauma, such as "dashboard" injuries resulting in posterior translation of the tibia in relation to the femur. Direct signs of a PCL disruption include focal discontinuity and/or high signal traversing the fibers on fluid-sensitive images (95).
- Ligamentous sprains of the medial and lateral collateral ligaments of the knee are common injuries in the athletic population and can be seen in isolation or in conjunction with other injuries to the knee. Ligamentous sprains are graded on MRI as follows: grade 1: intact fibers with high signal within the ligament; grade 2: partial tearing of the ligament; and grade 3: complete disruption of the ligament with discontinuity of fibers (Fig. 20.23).
- Proximal patellar tendinosis, as diagnosed on MRI, demonstrates localized hyperintensity and thickening of the proximal patellar tendon near its origin at the inferior pole of the patella. Reactive marrow edema in the inferior pole of the patella can also be seen.
- Partial and complete tears of the patellar and quadriceps tendons can be confirmed on MRI and are diagnosed as either focal or complete tendinous discontinuity, as seen elsewhere in the body.
- MRI has a high sensitivity for diagnosing bone marrow edema, the causes of which are varied and include trauma, AVN, subchondral stress reaction, and/or insufficiency fractures due to altered biomechanics or arthritic changes (Fig. 20.24). Subchondral stress fractures and osteochondral injuries typically occur on weight-bearing articular surfaces. Classic osteochondritis dissecans; however, it is more commonly seen in the posterior non–weight-bearing aspect of the medial femoral condyle. MRI is important in determining the size, location, and stability characteristics of osteochondral lesions. Signs of an unstable lesion include a fluid-like signal surrounding the fragment, a fluid-like signal extending into the overlying articular cartilage, cystic changes undermining the lesion, and/or complete detachment of the fragment (98–101).

- Several sports-related knee injuries have a common mechanism of injury and present with characteristic bone marrow contusion patterns on MRI.
- The "pivot shift injury" is a common contusion pattern with bone marrow edema in the posterolateral tibial plateau and in the midportion of the lateral femoral condyle (Fig. 20.25). Invariably torn with this mechanism of injury is the ACL. There are often other associated soft tissue injuries to the knee that can be seen in this pattern, which include medial collateral ligament sprains, longitudinal tears in the peripheral aspect of the posterior menisci, and posterior capsular injuries (85,86).
- A transient lateral patellar dislocation is common in the young athletic population and is associated with bone contusions in the anterolateral femoral condyle and inferomedial patella, osteochondral injuries, and disruption of the medial patellofemoral ligament and medial patellar retinaculum (Fig. 20.26).

ANKLE AND FOOT

- Conventional noncontrast MRI of the ankle and foot adequately evaluates the articular cartilage, ligaments, tendons, muscles, and osseous structures. Although ankle and foot MRI protocols vary by institution, it is standard practice to include triplanar imaging with T1 and T2-weighted sequences. Due to incomplete fat saturation that often occurs when imaging the foot, inversion recovery sequences are preferred as this results in less regional field inhomogeneities (102).
- The ankle is one of the most frequently injured joints in the athletic population. The use of MRI in evaluating ankle and foot injuries allows simultaneous evaluation of both the soft tissue and osseous structures. Although less indicated in the acutely injured ankle, MRI evaluation of chronic ankle pain is useful for determining causes of pain or instability that are not readily apparent on clinical exam, including osteochondral, ligamentous, and tendinous injuries, osseous stress injuries, occult fractures, or bone contusions.
- Osteochondral lesions of the talus (OLTs) occur due to impaction injuries at the articular surface and typically affect the talar dome because of ankle inversion injuries. OLTs, especially lower-stage lesions, are often not well detected with conventional radiographs but are rather well depicted with MRI, which also allows accurate staging of OLTs into stable and unstable groups (103) (Fig. 20.27).
- Ligaments are seen as smooth, low-signal bands or thin strands with continuity from bone to bone on all MRI sequences. Sprains of the ankle ligaments are common and involve the distal syndesmotic ligaments, the lateral collateral ligamentous complex, and the medial deltoid ligament complex. Direct signs of an acute ligament injury on MRI include abnormal morphology and increased signal abnormality within the ligament. Ligament discontinuity implies a complete tear (Fig. 20.28). Chronic sprains/tears may demonstrate ligamentous thickening or thinning (104).
- In the ankle, there are four main functional tendon groups that are best evaluated in the axial plane or perpendicular to the long axis of the tendon. Tendinosis is characterized by variable tendinous thickening and increased intermediate signal intensity. Tendon tears are diagnosed by observing fluid signal intensity within the tendon or tendon fiber discontinuity. Tenosynovitis is inflammation of the tendon sheath characterized on MRI by excessive fluid distention of the tendon sheath. Tendons commonly injured among athletes include the peroneus brevis and tibialis posterior tendons (TPT).
- Longitudinal split tears of the peroneal tendons, especially the peroneus brevis tendon, are increasingly recognized and are well depicted with MRI (Fig. 20.29). Dislocation of the peroneal tendons from the retromalleolar groove can also occur if there is disruption of the superior peroneal retinaculum.
- TPT tears generally occur in older athletes and are categorized as either partial tears (hypertrophic or atrophic types) or complete tears with tendon discontinuity. Injury of the TPT is important to recognize because insufficiency of the TPT can contribute to and is associated with abnormalities of the sinus tarsi and plantar fascia and can lead to loss of the longitudinal arch of the foot (adult-acquired flatfoot deformity) (105).
- As the largest tendon in the body, the Achilles tendon is normally seen as a thick low-signal intensity band inserting into the calcaneus. Tendinosis of the Achilles tendon manifests on MRI as a thickening and abnormally increased signal. Achilles tendon injuries may be divided by location into insertional and noninsertional. Most sports-related Achilles tendon injuries consist of tendinosis, peritendinitis, and/or paratenonitis, often near the insertional region. Most Achilles tendon tears occur approximately 2–6 cm proximal to the calcaneal enthesis. MRI is useful to differentiate between partial and complete tears and between myotendinous versus distal insertional tears. Dystrophic calcifications and ossification within the tendon can be seen in cases of a healed partial-thickness tear and/or chronic tendinosis (106).
- Stress and insufficiency fractures of the ankle and foot are common in athletes who have undergone a change in their training routines, wherein normal bone is exposed to repeated excessive stress. Stress fractures in the ankle and foot can be divided into low risk and high risk depending on their propensity to heal and likelihood to progress to nonunion. High-risk stress fractures include the tarsal navicular, medial malleolus, talus, hallux sesamoid, and proximal fifth metatarsal (107). In a report of 320 cases of stress fractures in athletes, the most commonly injured bones included the tibia, followed by the tarsals, metatarsals, fibula, and sesamoids (108). Exercise- and sports-related stress fractures

(and their common associated activity) include those of the metatarsals and calcaneus (military recruits), tarsal navicular (runners), sesamoids (ballet dancers/runners and sprinters), and the fibula (ballet dancers/runners) (109–111). Initial radiographs of stress fractures are often negative, and because of their high sensitivity and specificity, even exceeding that of bone scintigraphy, MRI is considered the preferred imaging modality of choice (103). MRI findings of stress fractures typically demonstrate periosteal and intramedullary bone marrow edema with a low-signal intensity fracture line (112) (Fig. 20.30).

- Occult nondisplaced fractures are often difficult to diagnose on conventional radiographs, such as calcaneal and talar fractures. MRI can help detect radiographically occult fractures of the ankle and foot by demonstrating a low-signal intensity fracture line associated with cortical disruption and marrow hyperintensity.
- Various ankle impingement syndromes can be evaluated with MRI. In anterior impingement, marginal osteophytes at the anterior margin of the tibiotalar joint may be seen in association with focal bone marrow edema. Posterior ankle impingement (PAI) refers to a group of pathologic entities resulting from repetitive forced plantarflexion of the foot (classically in ballet dancers) with the most common causes including an os trigonum, elongated lateral tubercle (Stieda process), or prominent posterior process of the calcaneus. MRI findings of PAI typically show marrow edema and cystic changes within these osseous structures (113) and thickening and degeneration of the posterior ligaments (114). Anterolateral impingement may be implicated with a history of chronic anterolateral ankle pain and manifests on MRI as an abnormal soft tissue mass and/or fibrous band in the anterolateral gutter (114,115).
- Sinus tarsi syndrome (STS) is a clinical condition characterized by pain along the lateral aspect of the foot with associated hindfoot instability. STS may develop after an inversion injury and can be suggested on MRI when low-signal intensity fibrous scarring or inflammatory tissue replaces the normal fat signal intensity within the tarsal sinus and/or when there is disruption of the sinus tarsi ligaments.
- Plantar fasciitis is a common overuse injury seen in athletes involved in running and jumping sports. Although essentially a clinical diagnosis, MRI may be helpful in clinically equivocal or refractory cases. Imaging findings in plantar fasciitis include focal fascial thickening with intrafascial hyperintensity and perifascial edema, most commonly near the calcaneal attachment. Partial and complete fascial tears can also be diagnosed on MRI.
- The term "turf toe" refers to a sprain of the plantar capsuloligamentous complex of the metatarsophalangeal joint of the great toe, which is due to severe dorsiflexion at the joint. With high-resolution small field-of-view MRI sequences, the osseous and capsuloligamentous structures can be evaluated to help direct treatment and avoid further morbidities such as hallux rigidus and osteoarthrosis of the joint (116).

SUMMARY

- MRI is the premiere imaging modality for sports-related injuries.
- Core to the utilization of MRI for diagnosis is the selection of the appropriate sequencing strategy; optimal imaging is achieved when there is active communication between the sports medicine provider and the musculoskeletal radiologist.

REFERENCES

1. Sneag DB, Lim WY, Potter HG. The role of MRI in sports medicine. In: Guermazi A, Roemer F, Crema M, editors. *Imaging in Sports-Specific Musculoskeletal Injuries*. Cham: Springer; 2016. DOI:10.1007/978-3-319-14307-1_4
2. Ajuied A, McGarvey CP, Harb Z, Smith CC, Houghton RP, Corbett SA. Diagnosis of glenoid labral tears using 3-tesla MRI vs. 3-tesla MRA: a systematic review and meta-analysis. *Arch Orthop Trauma Surg*. 2018;138(5):699–709.
3. Arirachakaran A, Boonard M, Chaijenkij K, Pituckanotai K, Prommahachai A, Kongtharvonskul J. A systematic review and meta-analysis of diagnostic test of MRA versus MRI for detection superior labrum anterior to posterior lesions type II–VII. *Skelet Radiol*. 2017;46(2):149–60.
4. Mardani-Kivi M, Alizadeh A, Asadi K, Izadi A, Leili EK, Arzpeyma SF. Can indirect magnetic resonance arthrography be a good alternative to magnetic resonance imaging in diagnosing glenoid labrum lesions?: A prospective study. *Clin Shoulder Elb*. 2022;25(3):182–7.
5. De Coninck T, Ngai SS, Tafur M, Chung CB. Imaging the glenoid labrum and labral tears. *Radiographics*. 2016;36(6):1628–47.
6. Jung JY, Jee WH, Park MY, Lee SY, Kim YS. SLAP tears: diagnosis using 3-T shoulder MR arthrography with the 3D isotropic turbo spin-echo space sequence versus conventional 2D sequences. *Eur Radiol*. 2013;23(2):487–95.
7. Amin MF, Youssef AO. The diagnostic value of magnetic resonance arthrography of the shoulder in detection and grading of SLAP lesions: comparison with arthroscopic findings. *Eur J Radiol*. 2012;81(9):2343–7.
8. Gusmer PB, Potter HG, Schatz JA, et al. Labral injuries: accuracy of detection with unenhanced MR imaging of the shoulder. *Radiology*. 1996;200(2):519–24.
9. Snyder SJ, Karzel RP, Del Pizzo W, Ferkel RD, Friedman MJ. SLAP lesions of the shoulder. *Arthroscopy*. 1990;6(4):274–9.
10. Magee T, Williams D, Mani N. Shoulder MR arthrography: which patient group benefits most? *AJR Am J Roentgenol*. 2004;183(4):969–74.
11. Waldt S, Burkart A, Lange P, Imhoff A, Rummeny E, Woertler K. Diagnostic performance of MR arthrography in the assessment of superior labral anteroposterior lesions of the shoulder. *AJR Am J Roentgenol*. 2004;182(5):1271–8.
12. Mohana-Borges AV, Chung CB, Resnick D. Superior labral anteroposterior tear: classification and diagnosis on MRI and MR arthrography. *AJR Am J Roentgenol*. 2003;181(6):1449–62.
13. Woertler K, Waldt S. MR imaging in sports-related glenohumeral instability. *Eur Radiol*. 2006;16(12):2622–36.
14. Fessa CK, Peduto A, Linklater J, Tirman P. Posterosuperior glenoid internal impingement of the shoulder in the overhead athlete: pathogenesis, clinical features and MR imaging findings. *J Med Imaging Radiat Oncol*. 2015;59(2):182–7.

15. Tian CY, Cui GQ, Zheng ZZ, Ren AH. The added value of ABER position for the detection and classification of anteroinferior labroligamentous lesions in MR arthrography of the shoulder. *Eur J Radiol.* 2013;82(4):651–7.
16. Cvitanic O, Tirman PF, Feller JF, Bost FW, Minter J, Carroll KW. Using abduction and external rotation of the shoulder to increase the sensitivity of MR arthrography in revealing tears of the anterior glenoid labrum. *AJR Am J Roentgenol.* 1997;169(3):837–44.
17. Markhardt BK, Huang BK, Spiker AM, Chang EY. Interpretation of cartilage damage at routine clinical MRI: how to match arthroscopic findings. *Radiographics.* 2022;42(5):1457–73.
18. Kadi R, Milants A, Shahabpour M. Shoulder anatomy and normal variants. *J Belg Soc Radiol.* 2017;101(suppl 2):3.
19. Potter HG, Black BR, Chong LR. New techniques in articular cartilage imaging. *Clin Sports Med.* 2009;28(1):77–94.
20. Shindle M, Foo L, Kelly B, et al. Magnetic resonance imaging of cartilage in the athlete: current techniques and spectrum of disease. *J Bone Joint Surg Am.* 2006;88(suppl 4):27–46.
21. VanBeek C, Loeffler BJ, Narzikul A, et al. Diagnostic accuracy of noncontrast MRI for detection of glenohumeral cartilage lesions: a prospective comparison to arthroscopy. *J Shoulder Elb Surg.* 2014;23(7):1010–16.
22. Baptista E, Malavolta EA, Gracitelli ME, et al. Diagnostic accuracy of MRI for detection of tears and instability of proximal long head of biceps tendon: an evaluation of 100 shoulders compared with arthroscopy. *Skelet Radiol.* 2019;48(11):1723–33.
23. Malavolta EA, Assunção JH, Guglielmetti CL, de Souza FF, Gracitelli ME, Ferreira Neto AA. Accuracy of preoperative MRI in the diagnosis of disorders of the long head of the biceps tendon. *Eur J Radiol.* 2015;84(11):2250–4.
24. Petchprapa CN, Beltran LS, Jazrawi LM, Kwon YW, Babb JS, Recht MP. The rotator interval: a review of anatomy, function, and normal and abnormal MRI appearance. *AJR Am J Roentgenol.* 2010;195(3):567–76.
25. Liu F, Cheng X, Dong J, Zhou D, Han S, Yang Y. Comparison of MRI and MRA for the diagnosis of rotator cuff tears: a meta-analysis. *Medicine.* 2020;99(12):e19579.
26. Tirman P, Bost F, Steinbach L, et al. MR arthrographic depiction of tears of the rotator cuff: benefit of abduction and external rotation of the arm. *Radiology.* 1994;192(3):851–6.
27. Gladstone JN, Bishop JY, Lo IK, Flatow EL. Fatty infiltration and atrophy of the rotator cuff do not improve after rotator cuff repair and correlate with poor functional outcome. *Am J Sports Med.* 2007;35(5):719–28.
28. Williams MD, Lädermann A, Melis B, Barthelemy R, Walch G. Fatty infiltration of the supraspinatus: a reliability study. *J Shoulder Elb Surg.* 2009;18(4):581–7.
29. Kuzel BR, Grindel S, Papandrea R, Ziegler D. Fatty infiltration and rotator cuff atrophy. *J Am Acad Orthop Surg.* 2013;21(10):613–23.
30. Bankart AS. Recurrent or habitual dislocation of the shoulder-joint. *Br Med J.* 1923;2(3285):1132–3.
31. Murray PJ, Shaffer BS. Clinical update: MR imaging of the shoulder. *Sports Med Arthrosc.* 2009;17(1):40–8.
32. Di Giacomo G, Itoi E, Burkhart SS. Evolving concept of bipolar bone loss and the Hill-Sachs lesion: from "engaging/non-engaging" lesion to "on-track/off-track" lesion. *Arthroscopy.* 2014;30(1):90–8.
33. Gyftopoulos S, Beltran LS, Bookman J, Rokito A. MRI evaluation of bipolar bone loss using the on-track off-track method: a feasibility study. *AJR Am J Roentgenol.* 2015;205(4):848–52.
34. Pesquer L, Borghol S, Meyer P, Ropars M, Dallaudière B, Abadie P. Multimodality imaging of subacromial impingement syndrome. *Skelet Radiol.* 2018;47(7):923–37.
35. Rothenberg A, Gasbarro G, Chlebeck J, Lin A. The coracoacromial ligament: anatomy, function, and clinical significance. *Orthop J Sports Med.* 2017;5(4):2325967117703398.
36. Cowderoy GA, Lisle DA, O'Connell PT. Overuse and impingement syndromes of the shoulder in the athlete. *Magn Reson Imaging Clin N Am.* 2009;17(4):577–93.
37. Fields BK, Skalski MR, Patel DB, et al. Adhesive capsulitis: review of imaging findings, pathophysiology, clinical presentation, and treatment options. *Skelet Radiol.* 2019;48(8):1171–84.
38. Connell DA, Potter HG, Sherman MF, Wickiewicz TL. Injuries of the pectoralis major muscle: evaluation with MR imaging. *Radiology.* 1999;210(3):785–91.
39. Lee J, Brookenthal KR, Ramsey ML, Kneeland JB, Herzog R. MR imaging assessment of the pectoralis major myotendinous unit: an MR imaging-anatomic correlative study with surgical correlation. *AJR Am J Roentgenol.* 2000;174(5):1371–5.
40. Alyas F, Curtis M, Speed C, Saifuddin A, Connell D. MR imaging appearances of acromioclavicular joint dislocation. *Radiographics.* 2008;28(2):463–619.
41. Flores DV, Goes PK, Gómez CM, Umpire DF, Pathria MN. Imaging of the acromioclavicular joint: anatomy, function, pathologic features, and treatment. *Radiographics.* 2020;40(5):1355–82.
42. Chauvin NA, Gustas-French CN. Magnetic resonance imaging of elbow injuries in children. *Pediatr Radiol.* 2019;49(12):1629–42.
43. Joyner PW, Bruce J, Hess R, Mates A, Mills FB IV, Andrews JR. Magnetic resonance imaging–based classification for ulnar collateral ligament injuries of the elbow. *J Shoulder Elb Surg.* 2016;25(10):1710–16.
44. Kijowski R, Tuite M, Sanford M. Magnetic resonance imaging of the elbow. Part II: abnormalities of the ligaments, tendons, and nerves. *Skelet Radiol.* 2005;34(1):1–18.
45. Lee RK, Griffith JF, Yuen BT, Ng AW, Yeung DK. Elbow MR arthrography with traction. *Br J Radiol.* 2016;89(1064):20160378.
46. O'Driscoll SW, Bell DF, Morrey BF. Posterolateral rotatory instability of the elbow. *J Bone Joint Surg.* 1991;73(3):440–6.
47. Potter HG, Weiland AJ, Schatz JA, Paletta GA, Hotchkiss RN. Posterolateral rotatory instability of the elbow: usefulness of MR imaging in diagnosis. *Radiology.* 1997;204(1):185–9.
48. Kraushaar BS, Nirschl RP. Tendinosis of the elbow (tennis elbow). Clinical features and findings of histological, immunohistochemical, and electron microscopy studies. *J Bone Joint Surg Am.* 1999;81(2):259–78.
49. Tuite MJ, Kijowski R. Sports-related injuries of the elbow: an approach to MRI interpretation. *Clin Sports Med.* 2006;25(3):387–408.
50. Van Hofwegen C, Baker CL III, Baker CL Jr. Epicondylitis in the athlete's elbow. *Clin Sports Med.* 2010;29(4):577–97.
51. Tiegs-Heiden CA, Frick MA, Johnson MP, Collins MS. Utility of the FABS MRI sequence in the evaluation of distal biceps pathology. *Skelet Radiol.* 2021;50(5):895–902.
52. Nguyen JC, Degnan AJ, Barrera CA, Hee TP, Ganley TJ, Kijowski R. Osteochondritis dissecans of the elbow in children: MRI findings of instability. *AJR Am J Roentgenol.* 2019;213(5):1145–51.
53. Rosenberg ZS, Blutreich SI, Schweitzer ME, Zember JS, Fillmore K. MRI features of posterior capitellar impaction injuries. *AJR Am J Roentgenol.* 2008;190(2):435–41.
54. Chang AL, Yu HJ, Von Borstel D, et al. Advanced imaging techniques of the wrist. *AJR Am J Roentgenol.* 2017;209(3):497–510.
55. Shahabpour M, Staelens B, Van Overstraeten L, et al. Advanced imaging of the scapholunate ligamentous complex. *Skelet Radiol.* 2015;44(12):1709–25.
56. Zanetti M, Saupe N, Nagy L. Role of MR imaging in chronic wrist pain. *Eur Radiol.* 2007;17(4):927–38.
57. Ng AW, Griffith JF, Tong CS, et al. MRI criteria for diagnosis and predicting severity of carpal tunnel syndrome. *Skelet Radiol.* 2020;49(3):397–405.
58. Bencardino JT, Rosenberg ZS. Sports-related injuries of the wrist: an approach to MRI interpretation. *Clin Sports Med.* 2006;25(3):409–32.

59. Petchprapa CN, Meraj S, Jain N. ECU tendon "dislocation" in asymptomatic volunteers. *Skelet Radiol*. 2016;45(6):805–12.
60. McBain B, Rio E, Cook J, Grabinski R, Docking S. Diagnostic accuracy of imaging modalities in the detection of clinically diagnosed de Quervain's syndrome: a systematic review. *Skelet Radiol*. 2019;48(11):1715–21.
61. Burns JE, Tanaka T, Ueno T, Nakamura T, Yoshioka H. Pitfalls that may mimic injuries of the triangular fibrocartilage and proximal intrinsic wrist ligaments at MR imaging. *Radiographics*. 2011;31(1):63–78.
62. Lee RK, Ng AW, Tong CS, et al. Intrinsic ligament and triangular fibrocartilage complex tears of the wrist: comparison of MDCT arthrography, conventional 3-T MRI, and MR arthrography. *Skelet Radiol*. 2013;42(9):1277–85.
63. Cherian BS, Bhat AK, Rajagopal KV, Maddukuri SB, Paul D, Mathai NJ. Comparison of MRI & direct MR arthrography with arthroscopy in diagnosing ligament injuries of wrist. *J Orthop*. 2020;19:203–7.
64. Ng AW, Griffith JF, Fung CS, et al. MR imaging of the traumatic triangular fibrocartilaginous complex tear. *Quant Imaging Med Surg*. 2017;7(4):443–60.
65. Skalski MR, White EA, Patel DB, Schein AJ, RiveraMelo H, Matcuk GR Jr. The traumatized TFCC: an illustrated review of the anatomy and injury patterns of the triangular fibrocartilage complex. *Curr Probl Diagn Radiol*. 2016;45(1):39–50.
66. Sachar K. Ulnar-sided wrist pain: evaluation and treatment of triangular fibrocartilage complex tears, ulnocarpal impaction syndrome, and lunotriquetral ligament tears. *J Hand Surg Am*. 2012;37(7):1489–500.
67. Zlatkin M, Rosner J. MR imaging of ligaments and triangular fibrocartilage complex of the wrist. *Magn Reson Imaging Clin N Am*. 2004;12(2):301.
68. Beutel BG, Melamed E, Rettig ME. The Stener lesion and complete ulnar collateral ligament injuries of the thumb: a review. *Bull Hosp Jt Dis*. 2019;77(1):11–20.
69. Hirschmann A, Sutter R, Schweizer A, Pfirrmann CW. MRI of the thumb: anatomy and spectrum of findings in asymptomatic volunteers. *AJR Am J Roentgenol*. 2014;202(4):819–27.
70. Stener B. Skeletal injuries associated with rupture of the ulnar collateral ligament of the metacarpophalangeal joint of the thumb. A clinical and anatomical study. *Acta Chir Scand*. 1963;125:583–6.
71. Clavero JA, Alomar X, Monill JM, et al. MR imaging of ligament and tendon injuries of the fingers. *Radiographics*. 2002;22(2):237–56.
72. Boutin R, Newman JS. MR imaging of sports-related hip disorders. *Magn Reson Imaging Clin N Am*. 2003;11(2):255–81.
73. Mak MS, Teh J. Magnetic resonance imaging of the hip: anatomy and pathology. *Pol J Radiol*. 2020;85(1):489–508.
74. Linda DD, Naraghi A, Murnaghan L, Whelan D, White LM. Accuracy of non-arthrographic 3T MR imaging in evaluation of intra-articular pathology of the hip in femoroacetabular impingement. *Skelet Radiol*. 2017;46(3):299–308.
75. Petchprapa CN, Rybak LD, Dunham KS, Lattanzi R, Recht MP. Labral and cartilage abnormalities in young patients with hip pain: accuracy of 3-Tesla indirect MR arthrography. *Skelet Radiol*. 2015;44(1):97–105.
76. Isern-Kebschull J, Mechó S, Pruna R, et al. Sports-related lower limb muscle injuries: pattern recognition approach and MRI review. *Insights Imaging*. 2020;11(1):108–17.
77. Heerey JJ, Srinivasan R, Agricola R, et al. Prevalence of early hip OA features on MRI in high-impact athletes. The femoroacetabular impingement and hip osteoarthritis cohort (FORCe) study. *Osteoarthr Cartil*. 2021;29(3):323–34.
78. James SL, Ali K, Malara F, Young D, O'Donnell J, Connell DA. MRI findings of femoroacetabular impingement. *AJR Am J Roentgenol*. 2006;187(6):1412–9.
79. Pfirrmann CW, Mengiardi B, Dora C, Kalberer F, Zanetti M, Hodler J. Cam and pincer femoroacetabular impingement: characteristic MR arthrographic findings in 50 patients. *Radiology*. 2006;240(3):778–85.
80. Silva MS, Fernandes AR, Cardoso FN, Longo CH, Aihara AY. Radiography, CT, and MRI of hip and lower limb disorders in children and adolescents. *Radiographics*. 2019;39(4):1232–794.
81. Varada S, Moy MP, Wu F, Rasiej MJ, Jaramillo D, Wong TT. The prevalence of athletic pubalgia imaging findings on MRI in patients with femoroacetabular impingement. *Skelet Radiol*. 2020;49(8):1249–58.
82. Anderson MW, Kaplan PA, Dussault RG. Adductor insertion avulsion syndrome (thigh splints): spectrum of MR imaging features. *AJR Am J Roentgenol*. 2001;177(3):673–5.
83. Zoland MP, Maeder ME, Iraci JC, Klein DA. Referral patterns for chronic groin pain and athletic pubalgia/sports hernia: magnetic resonance imaging findings, treatment, and outcomes. *Am J Orthop*. 2017;46(4):E251–6.
84. Yukata K, Nakai S, Goto T, et al. Cystic lesion around the hip joint. *World J Orthop*. 2015;6(9):688–704.
85. Sanders TG, Medynski MA, Feller JF, Lawhorn KW. Bone contusion patterns of the knee at MR imaging: footprint of the mechanism of injury. *Radiographics*. 2000;20:S135–51.
86. Nguyen JC, De Smet AA, Graf BK, Rosas HG. MR imaging–based diagnosis and classification of meniscal tears. *Radiographics*. 2014;34(4):981–99.
87. Nacey NC, Geeslin MG, Miller GW, Pierce JL. Magnetic resonance imaging of the knee: an overview and update of conventional and state of the art imaging. *J Magn Reson Imaging*. 2017;45(5):1257–75.
88. Rosas HG, De Smet AA. Magnetic resonance imaging of the meniscus. *Top Magn Reson Imaging*. 2009;20(3):151–73.
89. Wright DH, De Smet AA, Norris M. Bucket-handle tears of the medial and lateral menisci of the knee: value of MR imaging in detecting displaced fragments. *AJR Am J Roentgenol*. 1995;165(3):621–5.
90. Baker JC, Friedman MV, Rubin DA. Imaging the postoperative knee meniscus: an evidence-based review. *AJR Am J Roentgenol*. 2018;211(3):519–27.
91. Alatakis S, Naidoo P. MR imaging of meniscal and cartilage injuries of the knee. *Magn Reson Imaging Clin N Am*. 2009;17(4):741–56, vii.
92. Krych AJ, Saris DB, Stuart MJ, Hacken B. Cartilage injury in the knee: assessment and treatment options. *J Am Acad Orthop Surg*. 2020;28(22):914–22.
93. Roychowdhury S, Fitzgerald SW, Sonin AH, Peduto AJ, Miller FH, Hoff FL. Using MR imaging to diagnose partial tears of the anterior cruciate ligament: value of axial images. *AJR Am J Roentgenol*. 1997;168(6):1487–91.
94. Draghi F, Torresi M, Urciuoli L, Gitto S. Magnetic resonance signal abnormalities within the pericruciate fat pad: a possible secondary sign for acute anterior cruciate ligament tears. *Can Assoc Radiol J*. 2017;68(4):438–44.
95. Sanders T, Miller M. A systematic approach to magnetic resonance imaging interpretation of sports medicine injuries of the knee. *Am J Sports Med*. 2005;33(1):131–48.
96. Viala P, Marchand P, Lecouvet F, Cyteval C, Beregi JP, Larbi A. Imaging of the postoperative knee. *Diagn Interv Imaging*. 2016;97(7–8):823–37.
97. Bradley DM, Bergman AG, Dillingham MF. MR imaging of cyclops lesions. *AJR Am J Roentgenol*. 2000;174(3):719–26.
98. Accadbled F, Vial J, de Gauzy JS. Osteochondritis dissecans of the knee. *J Orthop Traumatol Surg Res*. 2018;104(1):S97–105.
99. Collins JA, Beutel BG, Strauss E, Youm T, Jazrawi L. Bone marrow edema: chronic bone marrow lesions of the knee and the association with osteoarthritis. *Bull Hosp Jt Dis*. 2016;74(1):24–36.
100. De Smet AA, Ilahi OA, Graf BK. Reassessment of the MR criteria for stability of osteochondritis dissecans in the knee and ankle. *Skelet Radiol*. 1996;25(2):159–63.

101. Gorbachova T, Amber I, Beckmann NM, et al. Nomenclature of subchondral nonneoplastic bone lesions. *AJR Am J Roentgenol.* 2019;213(5):963–82.
102. Ali M, Chen TS, Crues JV III. MRI of the ankle. *Appl Radiol.* 2006;35(8):27.
103. Narváez JA, Cerezal L, Narváez J. MRI of sports-related injuries of the foot and ankle: part 1. *Curr Probl Diagn Radiol.* 2003;32(4):139–55.
104. Perrich KD, Goodwin DW, Hecht PJ, Cheung Y. Ankle ligaments on MRI: appearance of normal and injured ligaments. *AJR Am J Roentgenol.* 2009;193(3):687–95.
105. Geideman WM, Johnson JE. Posterior tibial tendon dysfunction. *J Orthop Sports Phys Ther.* 2000;30(2):68–77.
106. Schweitzer ME, Karasick D. MR imaging of disorders of the Achilles tendon. *AJR Am J Roentgenol.* 2000;175(3):613–25.
107. Greaser MC. Foot and ankle stress fractures in athletes. *Orthopedic Clinics.* 2016;47(4):809–22.
108. Matheson GO, Clement D, McKenzie DC, Taunton JE, Lloyd-Smith DR, MacIntyre JG. Stress fractures in athletes. A study of 320 cases. *Am J Sports Med.* 1987;15(1):46–58.
109. Bergman A, Fredericson M. MR imaging of stress reactions, muscle injuries, and other overuse injuries in runners. *Magn Reson Imaging Clin N Am.* 1999;7(1):151–174, ix.
110. Khan K, Brown J, Way S, et al. Overuse injuries in classical ballet. *Sports Med.* 1995;19(5):341–57.
111. Niva MH, Sormaala MJ, Kiuru MJ, Haataja R, Ahovuo J, Pihlajamaki H. Bone stress injuries of the ankle and foot: an 86-month magnetic resonance imaging-based study of physically active young adults. *Am J Sports Med.* 2007;35(4):643–9.
112. Sofka CM. Imaging of stress fractures. *Clin Sports Med.* 2006;25(1):53–62, viii.
113. Sofka CM. Posterior ankle impingement: clarification and confirmation of the pathoanatomy. *HSS J.* 2010;6(1):99–101.
114. Berman Z, Tafur M, Ahmed SS, Huang BK, Chang EY. Ankle impingement syndromes: an imaging review. *Br J Radiol.* 2017;90(1070):20160735.
115. Narváez JA, Cerezal L, Narváez J. MRI of sports-related injuries of the foot and ankle: part 2. *Curr Probl Diagn Radiol.* 2003;32(5):177–93.
116. Crain JM, Phancao JP, Stidham K. MR imaging of turf toe. *Magn Reson Imaging Clin N Am.* 2008;16(1):93–103, vi.

Musculoskeletal Ultrasound

21

Sean W. Mulvaney and Sean N. Martin

INTRODUCTION

- Musculoskeletal ultrasound (MSK US) is an established modality in the field of sports medicine. It is a powerful tool in both the diagnosis and management of the injured athlete. MSK US is unique in that this modality provides previously unavailable point of care diagnostic imaging in the hands of the clinician with the patient in the examination room (1). This technology is the result of continued improvement of broadband high-frequency transducers and new developments in signal-processing software are improving the image quality for evaluating MSK structures (2). Given the rapid advancement in technology, availability, and acceptance of this newer imaging modality, standardized terminology has been adopted with expert consensus (3). In addition, the inclusion of MSK US education in specialty training programs, such as Sports Medicine Fellowships, have rapidly evolved from select few programs nationwide to the industry standard, guided by standardized curricula (4). Top-level support and guidance for wide adoption of MSK US by nonradiologist providers has been published by governing bodies — a testament of the recognized utility of this tool to the practice and advancement of sports medicine as a profession (5). These three critical documents, collectively, serve to provide robust and readily accepted governance on the training requirements and application parameters of MSK US to the modern sports medicine physician.
- Advantages of US imaging:
  - Portable, point of care imaging.
  - Direct, dynamic visualization of injured structure, aiding in a pathoanatomic diagnosis.
    - Many pathologic conditions are only apparent while a structure is in motion.
    - Magnetic resonance imaging (MRI) only allows the injured tissue to be viewed in one position.
  - Relatively inexpensive.
  - Established billing codes ultimately make MSK US a revenue generator in almost all practices.
  - Focus: Ability to focus on the area of interest to a degree not possible with MRI.
  - Side-to-side comparison views are simple to obtain for anatomic variants and growth plate comparison.
  - Lowest risk imaging modality for visualization of soft tissue and superficial bone:
    - No risk associated with iodinated contrast;
    - No risk associated with MRI contrast (gadopentetate dimeglumine contrast resulting in gadolinium-associated nephrogenic systemic fibrosis);
    - No risks associated with ionizing radiation.
  - Ability to accurately image soft-tissue structures despite metallic implants.
  - Immediate correlation of imaging with history and augmentation of the physical examination.
  - Superior imaging modality for peripheral nerve pathology (2,5) and for assessing injuries to fascia (6).
  - Ability to accurately guide percutaneous procedures directly to the joint of soft-tissue injury.
  - Using US-guided diagnostic injections, the exact pain-generator can be determined in cases when multiple pathologic structures are visualized.
- Disadvantages of US imaging:
  - Significant time, effort, and cost investment to become proficient.
  - Although US can rule in a fracture, it can neither rule out nor characterize a fracture.
  - Some intra-articular pathology may not be visible on US examination.
  - Labral pathology may be incompletely viewed on US (however, in many cases dynamic exams can ameliorate this shortfall.)
  - Even if a surgical lesion is identifiable on US, many orthopedic surgeons are more comfortable with MRI imaging to justify surgery, for presurgery planning and as a reference during surgery.
  - Becomes more limited with obese patients.

PHYSICS

- The US image is the product of sound waves that have been formed by a beam generator and emitted by the piezoelectric crystals of the US transducer, passed through tissues, some of which are reflected to the transducer for interpretation by the US processor and rendered into a real-time two-dimensional image.

- Echosignature of bone, ligaments, tendons, muscles, and other soft tissues is based on the degree of absorption versus reflection of the sound waves.
- The US image is a software interpretation of the reflected US waves.
- Attenuation is the name for all interactions that decrease the intensity of the US beam except reflection. Attenuation includes the effects of scattering and wave absorption that reduce the US wave amplitude.
- Constant = frequency × wavelength:
  - The constant used is the velocity of sound in tissue (dermis, adipose, muscle, tendon, cartilage, and ligament). It is approximately 1540 $m \cdot s^{-1}$.
  - As the position of any object measured with US can be determined only to an accuracy of about one wavelength, the limitation on image resolution is imposed by wavelength.
  - The resolution required in diagnostic US is 1 mm or less.
    - Therefore: frequency = constant/wavelength
      - Frequency = 1540 meters per second per .001 m
      - 1.54×10^6 $m \cdot s^{-1}$ = 1.54 mHz = the minimum usable frequency for MSK US applications; which will yield a resolution of about 1 mm before significant attenuation degrades this.
- US technology allows for a degree of lateral resolution; defined as the ability to visualize and differentiate structures parallel to the transducer footprint and determined by:
  - Hardware: Chiefly the number or character (including "single crystal" transducer design) of sound-emitting crystals on the transducer. This is a fixed number determined at the time the transducer is manufactured. The number of crystals determines the potential number of lines of sight (LOS) and is one of the primary quantitative indicators of the quality of a transducer.
  - Software: By sequencing the sound emission by the crystals the software is able to activate the sound-emitting crystals in different time sequences to generate multiple sound wave fronts. By having the computing power to process these multiple reflecting LOS, the software generates a significantly more detailed two-dimensional image on the display screen than if all the crystals fired all only in one sequence. This sequence processing is referred to as "multi-beam" or "cross-beam" imaging.
- Axial resolution allows for clearer visualization of structures at varying depths; in the same axis as the transducer. Axial resolution can be increased or decreased by adjusting the frequency.
  - Frequency refers to the time between emissions of sound waves.
  - Higher frequencies result in greater axial resolution resulting in a more detailed US image, however higher frequencies have less tissue penetration (the ability to see deeper structures clearly). High-frequency sound waves have less penetration because they are more subject to more rapid *attenuation* of sound waves by refraction and absorption of sound waves by tissues (reflectors).
  - Lower frequencies result in less axial resolution resulting in a less detailed US image; however, lower frequency sound waves have greater tissue penetration because they are less subject to attenuation by reflectors. This allows for visualization of structures at greater depths.
  - Higher frequency = higher resolution and less penetration (more attenuation). Use higher frequencies to view relatively shallow structures with greater detail.
  - Lower frequency = less resolution and higher penetration (less attenuation). Use lower frequencies to view deeper structures.
  - Contemporary transducer technology emits multiple (broadband) frequencies near simultaneously to generate the most useful real-time US image by maximizing potential resolution (using some higher frequencies) and penetration (using some lower frequencies). The mix of high and low frequencies may be manually or automatically selected depending on the particular US machine used. The mix of frequencies is based on the depth of the structure of interest, with the frequencies emitted for deeper structures viewed weighted toward lower frequencies and vice versa with superficial structures.

TERMINOLOGY

- Anisotropy
  - US best interprets echosignatures when the transducer is positioned directly perpendicular to a structure.
  - The artificial lack of signal (artifact) caused by loss of perpendicular positioning is termed *anisotropy* (root: anis: unequal + tropy: exhibiting a behavior or response) and is a significant and omnipresent challenge in MSK US.
  - The physical explanation for this phenomenon remains largely undetermined, however it is associated with viewing relatively fibrillar structures, and the effects of anisotropy are more pronounced as structures become more fibrillar.
  - Anisotropy is a commonly encountered artifact when visualizing bundles of fibers (ligaments, tendons, muscle) or fascicles (nerves) as they curve (with loss of perpendicular positioning of the transducer) and can be easily misinterpreted as a tear. With slight probe movement anisotropy will resolve, whereas a tear will remain hypoechoic. Anisotropy, it affects higher-density (more fibrillar) structures before less fibrillar structures.
    - Ligament > Tendon > Muscle > Nerve
  - Knowledge of the relative anisotropic nature of structures aids the scanner in identification of anatomy.

For example: When viewing the carpal tunnel in a transverse axis, as the operator tilts the probe the carpal ligament signal will drop out of the image first, followed in turn by the tendons, the muscle, with the median nerve as the last fibrillar structure in view.

- A tilt as small as three to seven degrees away from a perpendicular plane can produce anisotropy and can be seen in both the longitudinal and transverse planes.
- This affect is particularly evident when scanning a curved structure, such as a tendon insertion, and can be corrected by positioning the probe to remain perpendicular to the curvature.

- Volume Averaging
  - US transducers emit a shaft of sound approximately 1 mm thick. This 1 mm three-dimensional shaft of sound gradually spreads and becomes wider as it penetrates the tissue. The reflected sound waves from this three-dimensional shaft of sound are then processed by the computer to render a two-dimensional image.
  - The generated image is an *average* representation of the total volume of the reflected signal.
  - Disruption of normal echosignature of a structure is often not translated into the image until more than 50% of the 1 mm shaft is abnormal. Even if 75% of a tendon in an image is disrupted, it may still appear to be grossly intact although relatively hypoechoic compared to the other parts of the tendon.
    - This is a crucial concept when it comes to interpretation of partial thickness tears.
  - If a defect is suspected, the transducer should be turned orthogonally to assess for relative hypoechoic areas consistent with partial tears.
  - Aside from traditional longitudinal and transverse scanning axis, oblique approaches should be undertaken when attempting to delineate a partial thickness tear.
  - An understanding of volume averaging is crucial to successful visualization of US-guided needles in longitudinal axis.
    - Because needles are relatively narrow, if the needle is located within the outer 25% of the projected sound shaft, the signal from the needle will be "volume averaged out" and no needle will be seen on the generated image.
    - The needle must be in the middle 50% of the projected shaft of sound to be visible; this requirement becomes more exacting with deeper injections.
    - A clinicians' eye dominance needs to be accounted for when attempting to place a needle under a transducer. What looks to be the centerline of the probe may actually be slightly to the left or right of centerline.
- Through Transmission Enhancement
  - If a sound wave passes through relatively less echodense material, it will be less subject to attenuation and will result in a relatively stronger reflection back to the transducer. For example, if a sound wave passes through a fluid-filled cyst lying over a bone, the image of the bone beneath the fluid-filled cyst will appear brighter than the adjacent bone.
  - In the case of a defect in a tendon, the structure immediately deep to this defect exhibits a relatively hyperechoic echosignature. Through transmission enhancement is critical to help identify partial thickness tears, fluid interfaces, and tenosynovitis, as artificially hyperechoic structures provide a clue to a hypodense area immediately superficial to them.
  - In the same case of a defect in a tendon overlying bone, through transmission enhancement produces an artifact of relatively more intense hyperechoic area beneath the defect, which is referred to as "crescent sign" or "cartilage interface sign."
- Gain
  - Gain adjusts the intensity of the acoustic pulse emitted by the piezoelectric crystals with the result being a stronger echo return.
  - Increasing gain enhances the detection of weak reflectors.
- Artifacts are any visible structures in an image that do not correlate directly with the actual tissue.
- Sono-palpation: Placing a finger in view on the US image between the transducer and the patient's skin to specifically palpate the structure of interest.

MUSCULOSKELETAL US SIGNALS

- Echosignatures are based on density of tissue reflecting the US waves.
  - Anechoic (black): No or almost no reflection of sound waves: hyaline cartilage, fluid.
  - Hypoechoic (relatively darker): Scant reflection of sound waves OR *relatively* darker in appearance than other tissues within the viewed structure. A relatively reduced density (darker area) in a tendon.
  - Echoic: A structure of sufficient reflectiveness to be visible on a US image.
  - Mixed Echogenicity: An image made up of both hypoechoic and hyperechoic structures: muscle tissue.
  - Isoechoic: Similar reflectiveness relative to the compared tissue.
  - Hyperechoic: Relatively brighter (whiter) in appearance than comparative structures on the screen (*e.g.*, cortical surfaces, fascial layers, foreign bodies).
- Classic US Descriptions of Tissues
  - Muscle-loosely compact fibrillar pattern.
    - Transverse Axis: "Starry Night" appearance.
    - Longitudinal Axis: Pennate pattern.

- Tendon-compact fibrillar pattern in longitudinal and transverse axis.
- Ligaments
  - Transverse Axis: Very compact fibrillar pattern.
  - Longitudinal Axis: trilaminar appearance.
    - Intrasubstance appears dark compared to whiter, adjacent surfaces (white-black-white appearance).
- Nerves
  - Transverse Axis: fascicular pattern.
    - "Bundle of Grapes" appearance.
  - Longitudinal Axis: Striated fascicular appearance.

INDICATIONS FOR US IN SPORTS MEDICINE

- MSK US is a valuable tool in the evaluation and management of the injured athlete. The remainder of this chapter is devoted to highlighting the value of real-time US imaging in several common MSK injuries (7).
- Anterior Hip
  - Significant hip effusions are obvious on US imaging. Measure the distance from the anterior femoral head to the anterior capsule at its closest approach. Greater than 4 mm distance is considered abnormal and should be further evaluated for a hip effusion.
  - The anterior labrum is visible as a cartilage hyperechoic wedge at the boney contour of the femoral head and the anterior acetabulum. Dynamically view this area by both observing the anterior labrum while passively flexing the hip or moving the hip in internal external rotation.
  - Cortical anomalies on the femoral neck may be associated with femoral acetabular impingement.
  - A "snapping" iliopsoas tendon was commonly assumed to be due to the tendon "snapping" over the pectineal eminence with hip extension. However, with dynamic US exam while reproducing the patients "snapping," this can often be observed to be an internal "snapping" of the psoas portion of the tendon "snapping" around the iliacus portion of the iliopsoas tendon. Holding the transducer in position during this dynamic exam may be challenging but possible.
- Posterior hip pain
  - US allows the astute clinician to differentiate what appeared to be piriformis pain from an obturator internus tendinopathy as it sharply bends as it courses over the ileum. Sonopalpation or an US-guided diagnostic injection can quickly differentiate these two common sources of posterior hip pain.
- Lateral hip pain
  - Often what clinically appears to be "greater trochanteric bursitis" (GTB) is actually a tendinopathy in one or both of the gluteus medius tendons or the gluteus minimus tendon as they insert on to the superior aspect of the greater trochanter.
  - Insertional tendinopathy of the piriformis as it inserts onto the superior/lateral aspect of the greater trochanter or an insertional tendinopathy of the obturator internus as it inserts on the posterior medial border of the greater trochanter can also clinically present as GTB.
  - With diagnostic US and an US-guided diagnostic injection with a small amount (1 mL) of local anesthetic, an astute clinician can make a precise diagnosis of many painful conditions.
- Hamstring
  - Acute complete and partial hamstring tears and their associated hematomas are often obvious on US. US-guided aspiration, followed by a compressive wrap, significantly ease pain and may speed recovery.
  - Hamstring origin tendinopathies at the conjoined tendon can be differentiated from adductor magnus origin tendinopathy, but a precise diagnosis may require an US-guided diagnostic injection. The fascia around the hamstring tendon do not stop at their insertion onto the ischial tuberosity, but rather continue on as the sacrotuberous ligament, which should be part of the evaluation.
  - Whenever considering an injection of the hamstring origin area, the sciatic nerve as well as the posterior cutaneous nerve of the thigh (which often courses longitudinally along the dorsal surface of the hamstring insertion), should be clearly identified because it runs immediately lateral to these structures.
- Quadriceps
  - Quadriceps tendon partial and full-thickness tears are readily evident on US exam. Quadriceps muscle hematomas are obvious and can be safely aspirated under US guidance.
- Knee
  - MSK US can quickly assess many common chronic and acute knee injuries.
  - Knee effusions are obvious on US exam of the suprapatellar pouch, and are more obvious if the patient tenses the quadriceps muscle with the leg extended.
  - Baker's cysts (popliteal cysts) in the posterior knee can also be easily identified at the junction of the semimembranosus tendon and the medial gastrocnemius. They can be safely aspirated without puncture of the popliteal neurovascular structures, under US guidance.
  - US can rule in (but not rule out) tears in the outer menisci. Meniscal tears are often visible on US, and when combined positive sonopalpation and an effusion provide even stronger evidence of a tear.
  - Meniscal cysts are an indication of a meniscal tear and are readily viewed.

- Tears, partial tears, and tendinopathies of the patellar and quadriceps tendons are readily visible. Patellar tendon origin pathology, "jumper's knee" has a characteristic fusiform (cigar shaped) appearance and has mixed echogenicity and partial loss of the normal fibular pattern of tendons when viewed in long axis. Osgood-Schlatter has a similar appearance at the insertion, but also has an obvious cortical swelling.
- Pathologic plica capsular folds are visible and can be confirmed with a combination of sonopalpation, dynamic exam, and guided diagnostic injections.
- Injuries to the lateral and medial collateral ligaments are readily visible and gradable on a dynamic US exam.
- Cartilage thickness and some cartilage defects can be measured with US. The most common cartilage measurement is of the (anechoic) cartilage thickness of the trochlear groove view with the knee flexed, where 4 mm is considered a normal value.
- The common peroneal nerve, a potential source of lateral knee pain, can be additionally identified as it branches from the sciatic nerve and courses to the anterior lower leg just distal to fibular head.

- Calf
  - Partial and complete tears of the gastrocnemius and soleus are readily visible, as are their associated hematomas.
  - Achilles tendon partial tears, complete tears, and tendinopathies are readily viewed and measured with US. Achilles tendinopathy may be at the enthesis or the watershed area 3–4 cm proximal to the insertion. At the watershed area tendinopathy has a characteristic (tender) thickened fusiform shape with mixed echogenicity and loss of the normal fibular pattern of a tendon. The ability to definitively establish a diagnosis of a ruptured tendon may reduce the delay before surgical repair.
  - The os trigonum, in the posterior heel can be viewed and injected under ultrasound guidance.
  - Nerve injuries and neuromas within the lower leg are also readily viewed with ultrasound.
- Ankle
  - Ligament sprains, including high ankle sprains, can be dynamically evaluated and accurately graded to establish appropriate treatment and prognosis.
  - Ankle joint effusions are readily viewed.
  - Tenosynovitis, such as a posterior tibial tenosynovitis, can be viewed in any of the tendons as they course over the ankle joint.
  - Split tears in the peroneal and tibial tendons are often difficult to image with other modalities and are often only viewed in the oblique axis.
  - Entrapment with increase in nerve cross-sectional area (NCA) of the tibial and plantar nerves can be readily viewed at the tarsal tunnel.
- Foot
  - One of the more common running-related complaints is heel pain, with plantar fasciitis representing the "low back pain" of the runner.
  - The plantar fascia is readily measured; if it is thickened over 4 mm is considered enlarged and consistent with a diagnosis of plantar fasciosis (8).
- Shoulder
  - Rotator Cuff Tears: US is as accurate as MRI in the detection of rotator cuff tears (9).
  - Dynamic US exam of the shoulder can clearly show anterior and posterior impingement, as well as AC joint dysfunction and arthropathy (dynamic scarf testing).
  - The presence of a paralabral cyst in the posterior glenohumeral joint is an indirect sign of labral tear.
  - Diagnostic injections with as little as 1 mL of lidocaine can differentiate the pain generator where multiple pathologies can be seen.
  - Glenohumeral joint injections can be performed while sparing the articular cartilage surfaces and the labrum from needle trauma.
  - US can be used to guide AC joint injections, increasing confidence in accurate placement of the injectate.
- Elbow
  - Medial and lateral tendinopathies and partial tears can be assessed and accurately injected with US.
  - It is possible to readily assess other common sources of lateral elbow pain, such as anconeus tears, radial collateral ligament injuries, radial nerve entrapments, and annular ligament tears.
- Wrist
  - Scapholunate ligament injuries can be assessed by performing a dynamic exam by having the patient grip an object while observing for an instability and gapping between the scaphoid and lunate (Terry Thomas sign).
  - It is possible to assess TFCC injuries, including with dynamic exams while facilitating ulnar deviation.
  - Carpal dislocations and fractures can be ruled in (but not ruled out).
  - De Quervain tenosynovitis and intersection syndrome are readily assessed and accurately injected.
  - Median nerve entrapment and associated increased NCA, loss of normal "bundle of grapes" appearance and relative hypoechoic appearance are diagnostic for carpal tunnel syndrome (or any other peripheral nerve entrapment). The median nerve mean cross-sectional area was reported to be 11.5 mm^2 in a recent study of nonsymptomatic individuals (10,11).
- Hands
  - A potential gamekeeper's thumb can be assessed with a cautious dynamic exam.
  - Extensor and flexor tendons are readily assessed.
  - 1st CMC joints are easily assessed for arthropathies.

EVIDENCE FOR USE OF US IN SPORTS MEDICINE

- Although there are hundreds of studies in the peer-reviewed medical literature demonstrating the benefit of both US in diagnosis and for procedure guidance, included in the remaining section of this chapter are several studies that address clinical questions that are pertinent to the physician seeking to use US clinically.
- A retrospective care record review of 1012 patients treated by musculoskeletal and sports physician over a 10-month period by Sivan et al. concluded that the use of clinic-based MSK US enables a one-stop approach, reduces repeated hospital appointments, and improves quality of care in an outpatient musculoskeletal clinic (12).
- "Does US needle guidance affect the clinical outcomes" was addressed by Sibbet et al. in a randomized controlled study of 148 painful joints that were randomized to intra-articular corticosteroid injection by conventional palpation-guided or sonographic image-guided injection. Relative to conventional palpation-guided methods; sonographic guidance resulted in 43% reduction in procedural pain ($P > .001$), 58% reduction in absolute pain scores at the 2-week outcome ($P > .001$), 75% reduction in significant pain ($P > .001$), 62% reduction in nonresponder rate. Sonography also increased the detection of effusion by 200% and volume of aspirated fluid by 337%. They concluded that sonographic guidance significantly improved clinical outcomes (13).
- Naredo et al. concluded that US-guided subacromial injection resulted in improved VAS pain and Shoulder Function Assessment scores at 6 weeks versus clinically guided injections ($P < .001$) (14).
- The need for US guidance for standard injections such as knee injections has been questioned. In a prospective series of 240 consecutive injections in patients without clinical knee effusion Jackson et al. tested the accuracy of clinically guided intra-articular knee injections by an experienced orthopedic surgeon. Accuracy rates for needle placement were confirmed with fluoroscopic imaging to document the dispersion pattern of injected contrast material. Of 80 injections performed through an anterolateral portal, 57 were confirmed to have been placed in the intra-articular space on the first attempt (an accuracy rate of 71%). Investigators demonstrated the difficulty of accurately placing a needle into the intra-articular space of the knee when an effusion is not present. They concluded that their study highlights the need for clinicians to refine injection techniques for delivering intra-articular therapeutic substances that are intended to coat the articular surfaces of the knee joint (15).
- Curtiss et al. in their study of US-guided versus clinically guided injections into the supra-patellar pouch of the knee (an approach that does not risk injury to the cartilage surfaces by the needle), concluded the US-guided knee injections that use a superolateral approach are very accurate in a cadaveric model, whereas the accuracy of palpation-guided knee injections that use the same approach is variable and appears to be significantly influenced by clinician experience. Their findings suggest that US guidance should be considered when one performs knee injections with a superolateral approach that requires a high degree of accuracy (16).
- How does the US perform versus MRI in the detection of rotator cuff tears? In their prospective study of 124 patients, Teefey et al. compared the accuracy of the two tests (MRI vs. US) for detection and measurement of the size of rotator cuff tears, with arthroscopic findings used as the standard. They concluded that ultrasonography and magnetic resonance imaging had comparable accuracy for identifying and measuring the size of full-thickness and partial-thickness rotator cuff tears (9).
- Ziswiler et al. in their prospective study of 110 patients determined the largest cross-sectional area of the median nerve at the carpal tunnel and compared this to nerve conduction studies (NCS) and clinical signs and symptoms. They concluded that the nerve cross-sectional area was diagnostically as accurate as NCS and can be used to rule in or rule out carpal tunnel syndrome (10).
- Although the focus of US in the field of Sports Medicine has been on musculoskeletal maladies, recent inquiries have examined the potential use of US for other sports-related conditions beyond the musculoskeletal system. Examples of potential applications of this imaging modality in the sports medicine clinic include optic nerve sheath diameter in the case of increased intracranial pressure, limited echocardiographic screening during the preparticipation physical, sports-related vocal cord dysfunction, and assessment of muscle glycogen stores (17,18).

RESOURCES

- University of Michigan Musculoskeletal website: http://www.med.umich.edu/rad/muscskel/mskus/
- American Institute of Ultrasound in Medicine (AIUM) http://www.aium.org/
- RadiologyInfo.Org: http://www.radiologyinfo.org/en/info.cfm?pg=musculous
- American Medical Society for Sports Medicine: https://www.amssm.org/

REFERENCES

1. Bianchi S, Martinoli C. *Ultrasound of the Musculoskeletal System*. Berlin (Germany): Springer-Verlag; 2007.
2. Tagliafico AS, Michaud J, Marchetti A, Garello I, Padua L. US imaging of the musculocutaneous nerve. *Skeletal Radiol*. 2010;8:7701953.
3. Hall MM, Allen GM, Allison S, et al. Recommended musculoskeletal and sports ultrasound terminology: a Delphi-based consensus statement. *Br J Sports Med*. 2022 Mar;56(6):310–19.

4. Hall MM, Bernhardt D, Finnoff JT, et al. American Medical Society for Sports Medicine sports ultrasound curriculum for sports medicine fellowships. *Br J Sports Med.* 2022 Feb;56(3):127–37.
5. Finnoff JT, Hall MM, Adams E, et al. American Medical Society for Sports Medicine (AMSSM) position statement: interventional musculoskeletal ultrasound in sports medicine. *PM R.* 2015 Feb;7(2):151–68.e12.
6. Mulvaney S. Ultrasound guided percutaneous neuroplasty of the lateral femoral cutaneous nerve for the treatment of meralgia paresthetica: a case report and description of a new ultrasound guided technique. *Cur Sports Med Rep.* 2011;10(2):99–104.
7. Soares HR, Pinheiro AR, Crasto C, Barbosa P, Dias N, de Carvalho P. Diagnostic ultrasound assessment of deep fascia sliding mobility in vivo: a scoping review — part 1 — thoracolumbar and abdominal fasciae. *J Bodyw Mov Ther.* 2021;27:92–102.
8. Harmon KG, O'Connor FG. Musculoskeletal ultrasound: taking sports medicine to the next level. *Br J Sports Med.* 2010;44(16):1135–6.
9. McMillan M, Landorf KB, Barrett JT, Menz HB, Bird AR. Diagnostic imaging for chronic plantar heel pain: a systematic review and meta-analysis. *J Foot Ankle Res.* 2009;2:32. doi:10.1186/1757-1146-2-32
10. Teefey SA, Rubin DA, Middleton WD, Hildebolt CF, Leibold RA, Yamaguchi K. Detection and quantification of rotator cuff tears. Comparison of ultrasonographic, magnetic resonance imaging, and arthroscopic findings in seventy-one consecutive cases. *J Bone Joint Surg Am.* 2004;86(4):708–16.
11. Ziswiler HR, Reichenbach S, Vögelin E, Bachmann LM, Villiger PM, Jüni P. Diagnostic value of sonography in patients with suspected carpal tunnel syndrome: a prospective study. *Arthritis Rheum.* 2005; 52(1):304–11.
12. Jain N, Cortez-Garcia E, Cartwright MS. Cross-sectional area reference values of the median nerve at the palm using ultrasound. *Muscle Nerve.* 2020;62(3):389–92.
13. Sivan M, Brown J, Brennan S, Bhakta B. A one-stop approach to the management of soft tissue and degenerative musculoskeletal conditions using clinic-based ultrasonography. *Musculoskeletal Care.* 2011;9(2): 63–8.
14. Sibbet WL, Peisajovich A, Michael AA, et al. Does sonographic needle guidance affect the clinical outcome of intraarticular injections. *J Rheumatol.* 2009;36:9.
15. Naredo E, Cabero F, Beneyto P, et al. A randomized comparative study of short term response to blind injection versus sonographic-guided injection of local corticosteroids in patients with painful shoulder. *J Rheumatol.* 2004;31(2):308–14.
16. Jackson DW, Evans NA, Thomas BM. Accuracy of needle placement into the intra-articular space of the knee. *J Bone Joint Surg Am.* 2002;84(9):1522–7.
17. Curtiss HM, Finnoff JT, Peck E, Hollman J, Muir J, Smith J. Accuracy of ultrasound-guided and palpation-guided knee injections by an experienced and less-experienced injector using a superolateral approach: a cadaveric study. *PM R.* 2011;3(6):507–15.
18. Finnoff JT, Ray J, Corrado G, Kerkhof D, Hill J. Sports ultrasound: applications beyond the musculoskeletal system. *Sports Health.* 2016 Sep;8(5):412–7.

22 Electrodiagnostic Testing

Jason Friedrich and Eduardo Carrera

INTRODUCTION

- Electrodiagnostic (EDX) testing can be a valuable tool in the evaluation of athletes with neurological problems.
- Although clinical recognition of patterns of pain and sensory or motor abnormalities is the first step toward identifying a nerve problem, EDX testing can augment the clinical examination to better localize and characterize neuropathology (1,2).
- EDX testing involves both nerve conduction studies (NCS) and electromyography (EMG). Clinicians and patients will often informally describe the EDX study as EMG, although both components are almost always performed.
- A thorough EDX consultation integrates the history, physical examination, and selected nerve conduction and electromyographic studies into a meaningful diagnostic conclusion.
- Whereas imaging studies identify structural abnormalities, EDX studies evaluate the physiology and function of the peripheral nervous system.
- A negative EDX examination may not rule out the possibility of pathology because electrophysiologic studies are time- and severity-dependent (2,3).
- EDX studies depend on the proficiency of the electromyographer, as clinical judgment is often required (3–5).
- This chapter describes the pathophysiology of nerve injury, the associated chronology of electrophysiological findings, and the components of an EDX consultation.

ANATOMY

- EDX studies evaluate the large fibers of the peripheral nervous system (5).
- Standard EDX studies typically give limited information regarding central nervous system pathology.
- The components of the peripheral nervous system include afferent sensory nerves and efferent motor nerves.
- See Chapter 9, Nerve Injury, Figure 9.1, for an anatomical picture and description of peripheral nerve anatomy.

Sensory (Afferent) Pathway

- Cutaneous receptors → sensory axons → peripheral pure sensory or mixed sensorimotor nerve → ventral or dorsal rami → spinal nerve → cell bodies in the dorsal root ganglion (DRG) → sensory (dorsal) root → Spinal cord/CNS pathways.
- The sensory pathway from the cutaneous receptor to the DRG is evaluated during NCS of pure sensory or mixed nerves. The DRG is frequently located within the intervertebral foramina, with few exceptions (3).
- Sensory NCS can effectively evaluate pathology affecting the DRG and distal structures. Conversely, pathology proximal to the DRG often results in a normal sensory NCS.

Motor (Efferent) Pathway

- CNS pathways → Anterior horn cell (lower motor neuron, spinal cord) → ventral (motor) root → spinal nerve → ventral or dorsal rami → peripheral pure motor or mixed sensorimotor nerve → neuromuscular junction → muscle fibers.
- A motor unit is a single anterior horn cell and the muscle fibers it innervates.
- This pathway is evaluated during NCS of motor or mixed nerves, from the point of stimulation to the recording site. Pathology proximal to the point of stimulation may result in a normal motor NCS.
- Individual motor units can be evaluated during EMG with voluntary muscle activation.

PATHOPHYSIOLOGY OF NERVE INJURY

- Peripheral nerves can either be myelinated or unmyelinated.
- Myelinated fibers conduct faster by way of saltatory ("jumping") conduction, in which depolarization occurs only at interspersed nodes of Ranvier, allowing current to jump rapidly from node to node (5).

Seddon Classification

- Divides peripheral nerve injury into neurapraxia, axonotmesis, and neurotmesis (Table 22.1).

Table 22.1 Classification of Nerve Pathophysiology

Type	Pathology	EDX Correlation	Prognosis
Neurapraxia	Myelin injury	CV slowing across segment DL prolonged across segment Loss of amplitude proximal but not distal EMG normal	Recovery in weeks to months
Axonotmesis	Axonal injury with variable stromal disruption	Loss of amplitude distal and proximal EMG shows spontaneous activity EMG shows abnormal voluntary motor units	Longer recovery and more variable
Neurotmesis	Severance of entire nerve	No waveform with proximal or distal stimulation EMG shows spontaneous activity EMG shows no recruited motor units	Poor recovery, surgery required

CV, conduction velocity; DL, distal latency; EMG, electromyography.

Neurapraxia

- Neurapraxia is a comparatively mild injury that affects only the myelin sheath and causes focal conduction slowing or conduction block due to current leakage between the nodes of Ranvier. Although the myelin is injured, the nerve fibers remain in axonal continuity. This results in sensory or motor loss from impaired conduction across the demyelinated segment. However, impulse conduction is normal in the segments proximal and distal to the injury, where the myelin remains intact (6).
- Demyelination is typically seen with focal nerve entrapments (*e.g.*, carpal tunnel syndrome). It may also occur in peripheral polyneuropathies either as a patchy process (*e.g.*, Guillain-Barre syndrome) or a diffuse process (*e.g.*, diabetic peripheral neuropathy).

Axonotmesis and Neurotmesis

- Axonotmesis and neurotmesis refer to axonal injury with Wallerian degeneration of nerve fibers disconnected from their cell bodies. These types of injuries result in loss of nerve conduction at the site of injury and distally.
- Axonotmesis involves damage to the axon, with some preservation of the surrounding stroma (endoneurium, perineurium, and epineurium). This typically occurs with profound compression or nerve traction (5).
- Neurotmesis implies complete disruption of the enveloping nerve sheath, generally via nerve transection or severe traction injury (6).
- EDX studies typically cannot distinguish axonotmesis from neurotmesis.

SPECIFIC EDX STUDIES

- EDX studies typically consist of NCS and EMG.
- Each part of the evaluation has its strengths and shortcomings; therefore, it is imperative that a well-trained consultant performs EDX studies and can recognize sources of error during testing (7).

Nerve Conduction Studies

- There are numerous pitfalls associated with performing NCS (Box 22.1). Standard NCS tests only the fast, large, myelinated axons of a nerve (*e.g.*, Aα and Aβ fibers). Small, lightly myelinated (Aδ pain and temperature fibers) or unmyelinated fibers (C pain fibers) are not examined (5,8,9).
- NCS may be performed on motor, sensory, or mixed nerves.
- An appropriately trained technician may perform NCS, but a clinician must analyze and interpret the waveforms.
- Motor nerves are stimulated at accessible sites, and the *compound motor action potential* (CMAP) is recorded over the motor points of their target muscles. Motor points represent regions of high concentration of neuromuscular junctions, typically in the central muscle belly. Figure 22.1 provides an example of a median nerve CMAP.

22.1 Sources of Error With Nerve Conduction Studies

- Temperature (cold temperature leads to slower speed of conduction)
- Inadequate or excessive stimulation
- Improper placement of electrodes
- Distance measurement error
- Not adjusting values for age
- Anomalous innervation
- Volume conduction of impulse to nearby nerve
- Improper filter settings
- Improper electrode montage setup
- Involuntary muscle contractions

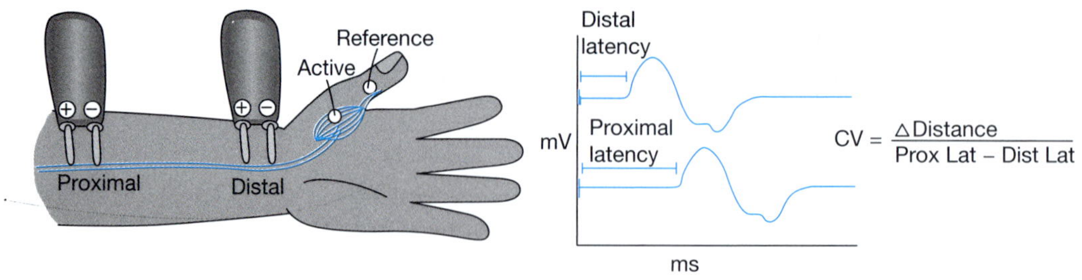

Figure 22.1: Compound motor nerve action potential (CMAP) recorded from the abductor pollicis brevis muscle. Stimulation of the median nerve at the wrist and elbow is demonstrated. For motor nerves, latency reflects time for nerve conduction, as well as neuromuscular junction depolarization and muscle fiber activation. Conduction velocity is measured between two points of stimulation. (Used with permission from Frontera WR, DeLisa JA, Gans BM, Robinson LR, Bockenek W, Chae J. *DeLisa's Physical Medicine and Rehabilitation: Principles and Practice*. 6th ed. Wolters Kluwer; 2019.)

- Deep motor nerves and proximal muscles are difficult to study and interpret using NCS (3). EMG has more utility for these deeper structures.
- A stimulated sensory nerve produces the recorded *sensory nerve action potential* (SNAP). Figure 22.2 provides an example of a median nerve SNAP.
- Frequently, sensory nerves are tested within mixed nerves, such as the plantar nerves, and produce a mixed nerve action potential (MNAP).
- CMAP, SNAP, and MNAP waveforms are analyzed and interpreted by the clinician.
- Waveform parameters include amplitude, latency, and conduction velocity.
- Amplitude evaluates the number of functioning axons in a given nerve, and the number of muscle fibers activated for motor nerves.
- Latency refers to the time (msec) from the stimulus to the recorded action potential.
- With sensory NCS, latency measures only the conduction time within the segment of the nerve stimulated. The sensory conduction velocity can be easily calculated by dividing the distance to the recording electrode by the latency.
- With motor NCS, latency accounts for nerve conduction distal to the site of stimulation, neuromuscular junction transition time, and muscle fiber activation time (3). The motor nerve conduction velocity must be calculated by dividing the distance between a distal and proximal stimulation site and the difference in latency between these two points.

Late Responses

- Whereas routine NCS typically evaluate distal nerve segments, late responses, such as the H reflex and F wave, evaluate the entire length of a nerve.
- Late responses can identify an injury somewhere on the pathway, but cannot distinguish exactly where it occurs.

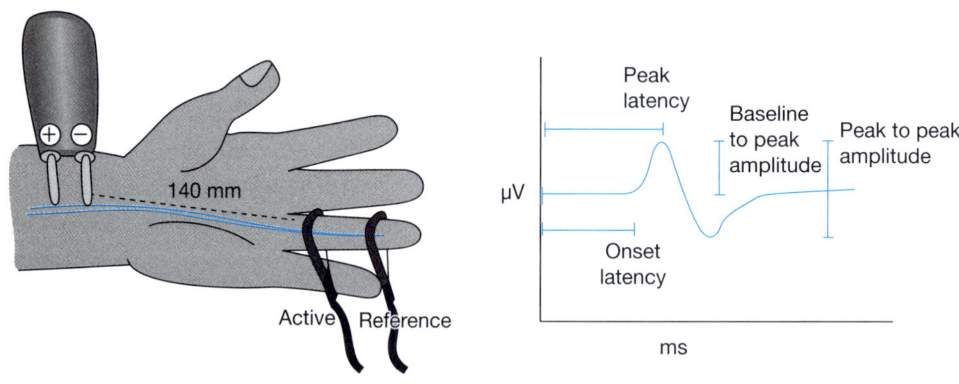

Figure 22.2: Sensory nerve action potential (SNAP) recorded from digital branches of the median nerve. Latency reflects the speed of conduction and amplitude reflects the number of functioning axons. (Used with permission from Frontera WR, DeLisa JA, Gans BM, Robinson LR, Bockenek W, Chae J. *DeLisa's Physical Medicine and Rehabilitation: Principles and Practice*. 6th ed. Wolters Kluwer; 2019.)

- The long pathway length means that the signal of smaller abnormalities may be washed out.

H Reflex

- The H reflex is the electrophysiological analog to the ankle stretch reflex. It measures afferent and efferent conduction along the S1 nerve root pathway.
- The H reflex evaluates the afferent and efferent pathway; thus, it gives information about the sensory pathway that is not tested on EMG.
- The S1 nerve injury can be due to S1 radiculopathy from a herniated disc or lumbar stenosis, peripheral neuropathy (usually with bilaterally abnormal H reflexes), or sciatic/tibial nerve injuries (5).

F Wave

- The F wave is a late muscle potential that results from a motor nerve volley created by supramaximally stimulated anterior horn cells. Thus, the F wave represents conduction up and down a motor nerve without any sensory afferent contribution (5).
- Unlike the H reflex, the F wave can be elicited at many spinal levels and from any muscle.

Needle Examination in EMG

- Evaluates the entire motor unit (lower motor neuron pathway), but not the sensory pathway.
- Assesses muscles at rest (to detect potential axonal injury) and with volitional activity (to evaluate voluntary motor unit morphology and recruitment).
- Needs to be timed such that abnormalities are optimally detected.
- If performed too early (*i.e.*, less than 3 weeks after the initial injury), spontaneous muscle fiber discharges (denervation potentials) may not have had time to develop. This can yield a false-negative result (6).
- If performed too late (*i.e.*, more than 6 months after the initial injury), reinnervation from collateral sprouting may have stabilized the muscle membrane and halted spontaneous muscle fiber discharges (3).
- At rest, the electrical activity of selected muscles is studied for abnormal spontaneous waveforms. Of these, the most common are fibrillation potentials and positive sharp waves. They are found when the muscle tested has been denervated or direct damage to the muscle has occurred, such as following direct trauma, procedures such as biopsies, and surgery (3,6). Figure 22.3 provides an example of fibrillations and positive sharp waves.
- Fibrillations and positive sharp waves are graded on a scale from 0 to 4+ (Table 22.2).
- Complex repetitive discharges (CRDs) are also common and represent ephaptic spread of spontaneous discharges ("cross-talk") from a single muscle fiber to neighboring fibers. CRDs may be present in the setting of longstanding cycles of denervation and reinnervation.
- Fasciculation potentials represent spontaneous discharges of an entire motor unit; thus, they are much larger than fibrillations and positive waves and can sometimes be grossly observed as muscle twitches. They can be found in a variety of benign or malignant conditions. Benign fasciculations may be found in runners following heavy exercise, dehydration, anxiety, fatigue, coffee consumption, or smoking (2).
- With muscle activation, motor unit action potentials (MUAPs) may be analyzed. Motor unit analysis provides an opportunity to distinguish between neuropathic and myopathic processes based on MUAP morphology and differences in recruitment pattern (3).
- EMG also may help differentiate acute from chronic neuropathic conditions.
- The amplitude of fibrillation potentials can grade nerve injury as occurring for less than or more than 1 year (with smaller potentials for the latter) (10). This can be particularly helpful in identifying an athlete's acute on chronic nerve injury.
- Chronic nerve injuries, without significant ongoing denervation, may additionally show large-amplitude, long-duration, polyphasic MUAPs (11).

Provocation EDX

- Some authors advocate performing EDX testing after exercise or with the limbs in provocative positions. These techniques are generally not well validated and are subject to significant measurement error; therefore should be interpreted with caution (2,3).
- The best data exist for piriformis syndrome. The H reflex is tested in the normal position and with the hip in flexion, adduction, and internal rotation (FAIR). Prolongation of the H reflex in the FAIR position is suggestive of piriformis syndrome (12). The use of this provocative test remains limited due to significant sources of measurement error and the need for further validation (3).
- Studies of other peripheral nerves have not supported the notion that EDX sensitivity is improved in dynamic positions (13). Spuriously slow and fast nerve conduction velocity can be recorded with the limb in various positions, most famously described with ulnar nerve studies around the elbow (14).

Dynamic or Quantitative Electromyography

- Demonstrates the sequence of muscle recruitment and muscle force for a given activity. In this capacity, only available in specialized gait laboratories (2).
- Employs surface or needle electrodes to record EMG signals through multiple channels. Fine wire electrodes may be used to record the signal from deeper muscles.

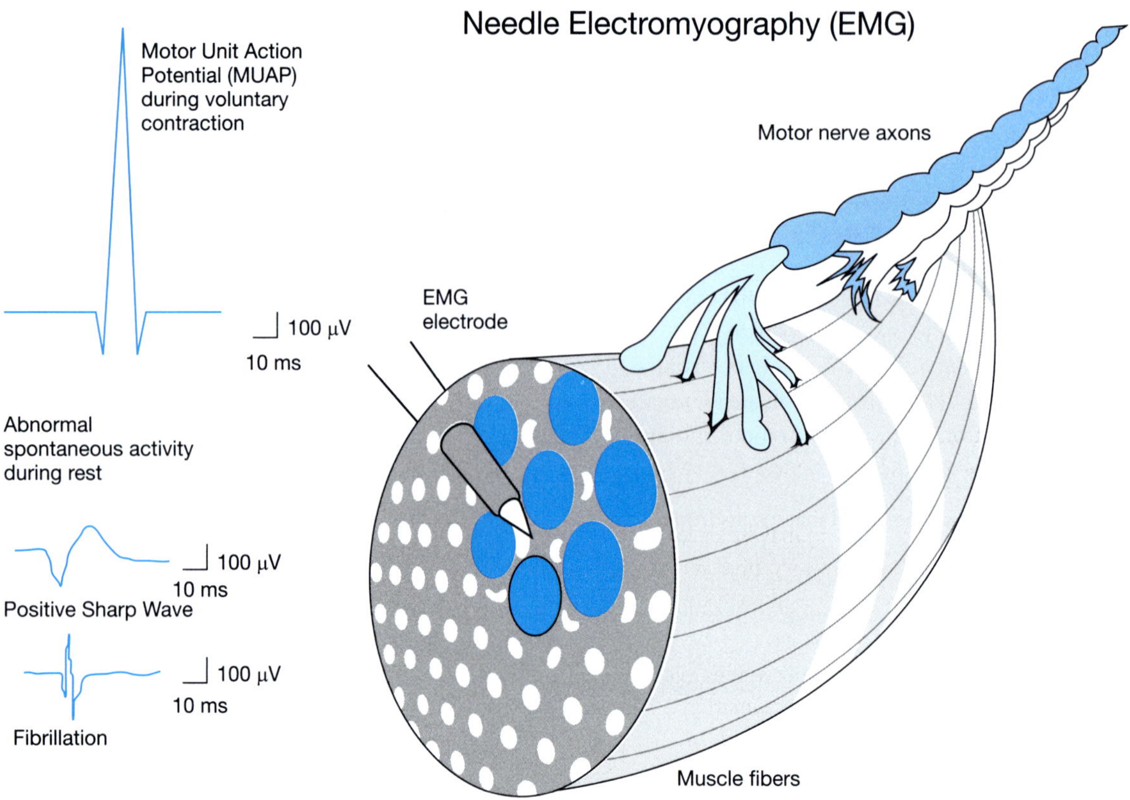

Figure 22.3: Needle electromyography 3–6 weeks after a partial axonal injury causing selective muscle fiber denervation. Terminal sprouting and axonal regrowth have not yet started. Note hypertrophy of muscle fibers with intact axon innervation (blue) and atrophy of denervated fibers (white). When the needle electrode is adjacent to innervated hypertrophied muscle fibers during voluntary contraction, a large-amplitude motor unit action potential is produced (as shown top left). When the needle electrode is adjacent to the denervated muscle fibers during rest, abnormal spontaneous activity is recorded in the form of positive sharp waves and fibrillation potentials (as shown bottom left). Recorded potentials will change in morphology over time throughout the denervation, terminal sprouting, and reinnervation process. (Reprinted and adapted from Kraft GH. The electromyographer's guide to the motor unit. *Phys Med Rehabil Clin N Am*. 2007;18(4):711–32, vi. doi:10.1016/j.pmr.2007.08.003; with permission from Elsevier.)

- Caution should be used in correlating EMG amplitude with muscle force generated because the relationship is not consistently linear (15).
- In research, quantitative EMG has also been used to assess the degree of muscle fatigue and biomechanics of sports activities or adaptations following injury (such as knee mechanics after ACL tear) (16,17).

Table 22.2 Grading of Fibrillations and Positive Waves

Grading	Characteristics
0	No activity
1+	Persistent (longer than 1 s) in two muscle regions
2+	Persistent in three or more muscle regions
3+	Persistent in all muscle regions
4+	Continuous in all muscle regions

INDICATIONS FOR ELECTRODIAGNOSTIC TESTING

- The utility of EDX testing in a given athlete can be estimated following a thorough history and physical examination, by a review of supplemental information (*e.g.*, imaging studies), and through an appreciation for the chronology of the electrophysiological changes that occur following nerve injury (2).
- Some useful generalizations about the indications for EDX testing are discussed here (3,4,6).
  1. Establish and/or confirm a clinical diagnosis:
     a. EDX study can rule in a suspected diagnosis or rule out a competing diagnosis.
     b. EDX may alert the examiner to the possibility of an unsuspected concomitant pathological process (*e.g.*, an athlete with tarsal tunnel syndrome and superimposed radiculopathy).

2. Localize nerve lesions:
   a. Nerve injury location often needs to be objectively confirmed prior to contemplating invasive or surgical treatment.
   b. For example, an athlete presenting with plantar surface numbness and tingling may have a sciatic nerve lesion anywhere along the course of the sciatic nerve or its branches.
   c. EDX studies can be used to localize the injury within the nerve roots, plexus, or peripheral nerves.
3. Determine the extent and chronicity of nerve injury:
   a. Properly timed EDX studies can differentiate a neurapraxic injury from axonal degeneration. This may significantly impact the aggressiveness of treatment for the nerve injury.
   b. The chronicity of a nerve lesion may be assessed using the combination of clinical history, fibrillation amplitude measurement, and motor unit analysis.
4. Correlate findings of anatomic studies:
   a. Because EDX studies examine nerve physiology, they can provide a correlate of nerve function within a region of structural pathology found on imaging studies.
   b. This may be particularly useful in the spine where structural pathology, such as disc herniations effacing nerve roots, can be seen in asymptomatic individuals.
5. Assist in prognosis and return to play (see below).

Nerve Recovery and Return to Play

- The clinician can predict nerve recovery by determining the degree of nerve injury.
- Neurapraxic injuries generally recover faster than axonal injuries (neurotmesis and axonotmesis) (2,6).
- Nerve conduction studies can determine if a neurapraxic injury is present.
- Motor (CMAP) amplitudes of weak muscles can be compared to the asymptomatic side to estimate the extent of the injury. A side-to-side difference of greater than 50% is likely significant (3).
- EMG of volitional motor units can also help predict prognosis.
- If no motor units are detected during the early stages, and NCS do not reveal a conduction block, a severe axonal injury is present and full recovery is unlikely.
- After a couple of months, motor unit analysis can indicate reinnervation by means of terminal reorganization or sprouting from preserved axons (6).
- EDX studies should not be a prerequisite for return to play because they may lag behind clinical recovery.
- The best determination of return to play remains the athlete's functional performance in simulated sports activities.

Timing of EDX Testing

- When ordering EDX studies, the timing of findings should be kept in mind (Table 22.3) (5).

Table 22.3 Timing of Wallerian Degeneration, Nerve Recovery, and EDX Findings With Axonal Injury

Time	Nerve Degeneration	Nerve Recovery	NCS Correlate	EMG
Day 0	None	None	Proximal-recorded segment abnormal; distal segment normal	Decreased recruitment
Day 3	NMJ impaired	Nodal and terminal sprouts		↓
Day 9	Motor axons lost	↓	Decreased distal segment CMAP	Increased insertional activity
Day 11	Sensory axons lost		↓	↓
Day 14	See nerve recovery		Decreased distal segment SNAP	Large denervation potentials in proximal muscles
Day 21		Increased fiber density	↓	Denervation potentials in distal muscles
Week 6–8		Axonal sprouting	CMAP/SNAP increasing back toward normal	Nascent reinnervation potentials
Week 16		Axonal regrowth 1 mm/d	↓	Maturing reinnervation proximal muscles
Week 20		↓		Maturing reinnervation distal muscles
Year 1				Smaller denervation potentials
Year 2		Muscle no longer viable		↓

CMAP, compound muscle action potential; EMG, electromyography; NCS, nerve conduction study; NMJ, neuromuscular junction; SNAP, sensory nerve action potential.

- EDX studies performed before day 9 post-injury may show normal distal segment motor nerve conduction parameters (or before day 11 post-injury in the case of sensory nerve conduction).
- EMG findings can take from 2 to 6 weeks to manifest.
- If considering surgical intervention, assessing with EDX 3 months post-injury is helpful. At this stage, neurapraxia should have been resolved. With traumatic injuries, serial EDX studies, including an immediate study, may be helpful in determining the extent of the injury.

LIMITATIONS OF ELECTRODIAGNOSTIC TESTING

- EDX testing has limitations and should not be performed in every athlete with neurologic signs and symptoms (2).
- Some diagnoses are unequivocal, and treatment should be initiated without delay. An example includes progressive neurological deficits, such as after traumatic posterior knee dislocation; the results of the EDX studies will not change management as the patient will require emergent care.
- The clinician must also understand that the probability of false-positive result increases with the number of tests performed (*e.g.*, the probability of obtaining one false-positive result out of five tests is 12%, which increases to 20% with nine tests) (5).
- EDX findings always need to be considered in the full clinical context. EDX impressions should emphasize patterns of abnormalities rather than isolated findings.
- Relative contraindications to EDX testing include pacemaker (no Erb's point stimulation), arteriovenous fistula, open wound, coagulopathy, lymphedema, anasarca, and pending muscle biopsy (3,5).
- EDX studies do not specifically evaluate pain fibers. An EDX study may prove unhelpful in a patient with pain without neurologic findings such as weakness and numbness.

ELECTRODIAGNOSTIC REPORT

- The EDX report should include several important pieces of data for the referring physician.
- The electrophysiologic findings should correlate with the physical findings and any discrepancies identified. Inconsistencies may have as much importance in the clinical treatment of the patient as consistent results (2).
- The degree of definitiveness of the findings needs to be conveyed to the referring physician. A diagnosis of S1 radiculopathy by H reflex alone will carry different weight than abundant spontaneous activity in the S1 myotomal distribution.
- One abnormal finding does not make the diagnosis if all other evidence is pointing to a different diagnosis (5).
- When possible, the report should include:
  - Sufficient evidence to rule out alternative possibilities and to identify superimposed conditions.
  - The degree of injury and chronicity.
  - Prognostic information.
  - Comparison with previous EDX data.

SUMMARY

- EDX studies (including NCS and EMG) serve as an extension of the physical exam to better characterize and localize nerve injury.
- EDX studies evaluate the physiology and function of the largest fibers of the peripheral nervous system (lower motor neuron pathway).
- NCSs attempt to localize peripheral entrapment neuropathies by identification of conduction block (focally decreased amplitude or conduction slowing) and can often differentiate demyelination (prolonged latency/slow conduction velocity) from axonal injury (low amplitude).
- Neurapraxic injuries are limited to the nerve myelin and tend to have more rapid recovery than axonal injuries.
- EMG can identify patterns of denervation from axonal injury, including information about chronicity. Acute denervation changes include abnormal spontaneous activity, such as fibrillations and positive sharp waves. Chronic changes may include long-duration, large-amplitude, or polyphasic MUAPs.
- The timing of EDX study is important. Although immediate study after a trauma can provide useful information (such as the presence of conduction block), some EMG abnormalities may take 2–6 weeks to manifest.
- Although EDX studies are considered reliable for detecting nerve pathology, they are dependent on the quality of the examiner.

REFERENCES

1. McKean KA. Neurologic running injuries. *Neurol Clin*. 2008 Feb;26(1):281–296; xii.
2. Akuthota V, Casey E. Diagnostic tests for nerve and vascular injuries. In: Herring SA, Akuthota V, editors. *Nerve and Vascular Injuries in Sports Medicine* [Internet]. New York, NY: Springer; 2009 [cited 2023 Jan 28]. pp. 17-26. Available from: doi:10.1007/978-0-387-76600-3_2
3. Preston DC. *Electromyography and Neuromuscular Disorders: Clinical-Electrophysiologic-Ultrasound Correlations* [Internet]. 4th ed. Philadelphia, PA: Elsevier, Inc.; 2021 [cited 2023 Jan 28]. Available from: https://www.clinicalkey.com/dura/browse/bookChapter/3-s2.0-C20150019335

4. Chémali KR, Tsao B. Electrodiagnostic testing of nerves and muscles: when, why, and how to order. *Cleve Clin J Med*. 2005 Jan;72(1):37–48.
5. Dillingham T, Andary M, Dumitru D. Electrodiagnostic medicine. In: *Braddom's Physical Medicine and Rehabilitation*. 6th ed.
6. Robinson LR. Traumatic injury to peripheral nerves. *Muscle Nerve*. 2022 Dec;66(6):661–70.
7. American Association of Electrodiagnostic Medicine. AAEM position statements. Who is qualified to practice electrodiagnostic medicine? *Muscle Nerve Suppl*. 1999;8:S263–5.
8. Gooch CL, Weimer LH. The electrodiagnosis of neuropathy: basic principles and common pitfalls. *Neurol Clin*. 2007 Feb;25(1):1–28.
9. Horowitz SH. The diagnostic workup of patients with neuropathic pain. *Med Clin*. 2007 Jan;91(1):21–30.
10. Kraft GH. Fibrillation potential amplitude and muscle atrophy following peripheral nerve injury. *Muscle Nerve*. 1990 Sep;13(9):814–21.
11. Campbell WW. Evaluation and management of peripheral nerve injury. *Clin Neurophysiol*. 2008 Sep 1;119(9):1951–65.
12. Fishman LM, Dombi GW, Michaelsen C, et al. Piriformis syndrome: diagnosis, treatment, and outcome—a 10-year study. *Arch Phys Med Rehabil*. 2002 Mar 1;83(3):295–301.
13. Mysiew WJ, Colachis SC. The pronator syndrome. An evaluation of dynamic maneuvers for improving electrodiagnostic sensitivity. *Am J Phys Med Rehabil*. 1991 Oct;70(5):274–77.
14. Won SJ, Yoon JS, Kim JY, Kim SJ, Jeong JS. Avoiding false-negative nerve conduction study in ulnar neuropathy at the elbow. *Muscle Nerve*. 2011;44(4):583–6.
15. Hug F, Hodges PW, Tucker K. Muscle force cannot Be directly inferred from muscle activation: illustrated by the proposed imbalance of force between the vastus medialis and vastus lateralis in people with patellofemoral pain. *J Orthop Sports Phys Ther*. 2015 May;45(5):360–5.
16. Feinberg JH. The role of electrodiagnostics in the study of muscle kinesiology, muscle fatigue and peripheral nerve injuries in sports medicine. *J Back Musculoskelet Rehabil*. 1999 Jan 1;12(2):73–88.
17. Hurd WJ, Snyder-Mackler L. Knee instability after acute ACL rupture affects movement patterns during the mid-stance phase of gait. *J Orthop Res*. 2007 Oct;25(10):1369–77.

23 ECG Interpretation in Athletes

Christian F. Klein and Jonathan A. Drezner

INTRODUCTION

- Sudden cardiac arrest (SCA) in a previously healthy athlete remains the leading cause of sudden death in athletes, resulting in an estimated 0.5–11 deaths per 100,000 athlete years (1–4).
- Studies indicate that the majority of SCA cases in young competitive athletes result from etiologies detectable by a 12-lead electrocardiogram (ECG) (5–7). As such, some preparticipation screening guidelines now recommend ECG screening prior to competition, either in higher-risk individuals (the American Medical Society for Sports Medicine) (8) or universally (the European Society of Cardiology) (9,10). (see Chapter 18, The Preparticipation Examination).
- Physiologic cardiac adaptations to regular, intensive training commonly produce structural and electrical changes in athletes (so-called 'athlete's heart') that may in other circumstances be considered abnormal. Thus, ECG interpretation in athletes requires the distinction of physiologic findings from ECG abnormalities that may indicate an underlying cardiac disease.
- Accurate ECG interpretation in athletes requires training and experience to avoid false-positive results and unnecessary testing or restriction from competition (8).
- This chapter reviews which electrocardiographic findings in athletes should be considered normal, borderline, or abnormal, as identified by international consensus criteria, as well as the recommended secondary investigations of ECG abnormalities to exclude underlying cardiac pathology (11).

NORMAL ECG FINDINGS IN ATHLETES

- Athletic training can result in distinct cardiac adaptive structural and physiologic changes, dependent on sports-specific demands, which may be reflected in the electrocardiogram (see Chapter 31, Cardiology).
- When reading an athlete's electrocardiogram knowledge of the athlete's sport and training regimen can provide context for interpretation. Electrocardiographic alterations are mostly identified in athletes engaged in high-intensity dynamic endurance sports (*e.g.*, running). Studies have demonstrated that cardiac adaptation generally necessitates at least 3 hours a week of training (12).
- In the absence of other signs or symptoms concerning for cardiac pathology, the following ECG findings should be considered normal physiologic adaptations to regular exercise (see Table 23.1).

Left Ventricular Hypertrophy/Right Ventricular Hypertrophy

- Enlarged cardiac chamber size represents a normal physiologic change in athletes after prolonged periods of intensive exercise.
- Isolated voltage criteria for left ventricular hypertrophy (SV1 + RV5 or RV6 >35 mV) or right ventricular hypertrophy (RV1 + SV5 or SV6 >11 mV), without other ECG or clinical abnormalities, is considered a normal response to athletic training. Some studies suggest that isolated voltage criteria for ventricular hypertrophy may not accurately predict increased LV or RV size (13–15).

Early Repolarization

- Early repolarization is defined as a ≥0.1 mV elevation at the QRS-ST junction, or J-point, often associated with QRS slurring or notching (J-wave) in the inferior and/or lateral leads (see Fig. 23.1) (16).
- Early repolarization is a common finding in highly trained athletes and does not carry elevated risk for adverse cardiac events (17).

Repolarization Variants in Athletes

- A common finding first described in Black athletes (specifically defined as athletes of Afro-Caribbean descent) is a repolarization variant characterized by J-point elevation and convex ST-segment elevation followed by T-wave inversion (TWI) confined to leads V1-V4 (see Fig. 23.2) (18–20).
- Evidence suggests this repolarization pattern is normal regardless of race or ethnicity when confined to leads V1-V4, and thus does not require further evaluation in the absence of other clinical concerns (21).

Table 23.1 Normal ECG Findings in Athletes

ECG Finding	Definition
LVH/RVH voltage criteria	LVH: SV1 + RV5 or RV6 >35 mV RVH: RV1 + SV5 or SV6 >11 mV
Early repolarization	≥0.1 mV elevation at the QRS-ST junction (J-point), often with QRS slurring or notching (J-wave) in the inferior and/or lateral leads
Athlete repolarization variant	J-point elevation and convex ST-segment elevation in leads V1-V4 followed by a T-wave inversion
Juvenile ECG pattern	T-wave inversions in leads V1-V3 in ages ≤16 year old
Physiologic arrhythmias	Sinus bradycardia >30 bpm Sinus arrhythmia: heart rate variation with respiration 1st degree AV block: PR interval 200–400 ms 2nd degree Mobitz type 1 AV block (Wenckebach): progressive PR interval lengthening followed by nonconducted P wave without associated QRS
Incomplete RBBB	rSR' in V1 and QRS in V6 with QRS <120 ms

AV, atrioventricular; ECG, electrocardiogram; LVH, left ventricular hypertrophy; RBBB, right bundle branch block; RVH, right ventricular hypertrophy.
Adapted from Drezner JA, O'Connor FG, Harmon KG, et al. AMSSM position statement on cardiovascular preparticipation screening in athletes: current evidence, knowledge gaps, recommendations, and future directions. *Clin J Sport Med.* 2016 Sep;26(5):347–61.

Juvenile ECG Pattern

- TWI when confined to the anterior precordial leads only (V1-V3) is considered a normal finding in athletes up to the age of 16. This so-called juvenile ECG pattern should not prompt further testing in the absence of other clinical findings (see Fig. 23.3) (22,23).

Physiologic Arrhythmias

- Increased vagal tone resulting from prolonged periods of intensive training can lead to sinus bradycardia, sinus arrhythmias (heart rate variation with respiration) and low-grade heart block (first-degree AV block or Mobitz type I second-degree AV block, also known as Wenckebach

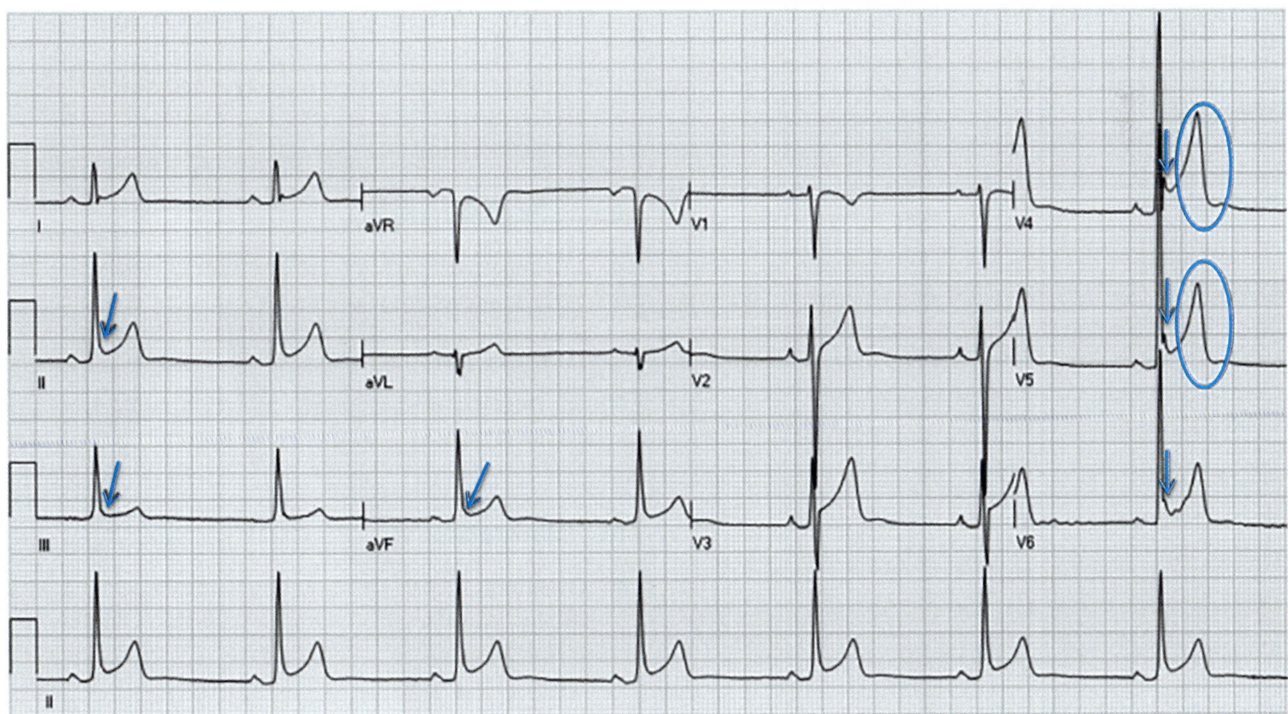

Figure 23.1: Early repolarization is a normal finding in athletes characterized by ≥0.1 mV elevation at the J-point (arrows). J-point notching and tall, peaked T-waves (circles) also may be present. (Reprinted from Figure 2 of Drezner JA, Sharma S, Baggish A, et al. International criteria for electrocardiographic interpretation in athletes: consensus statement. *Br J Sports Med.* 2017;51:704–31. Copyright © 2017 BMJ Publishing Group Ltd. Used with permission.)

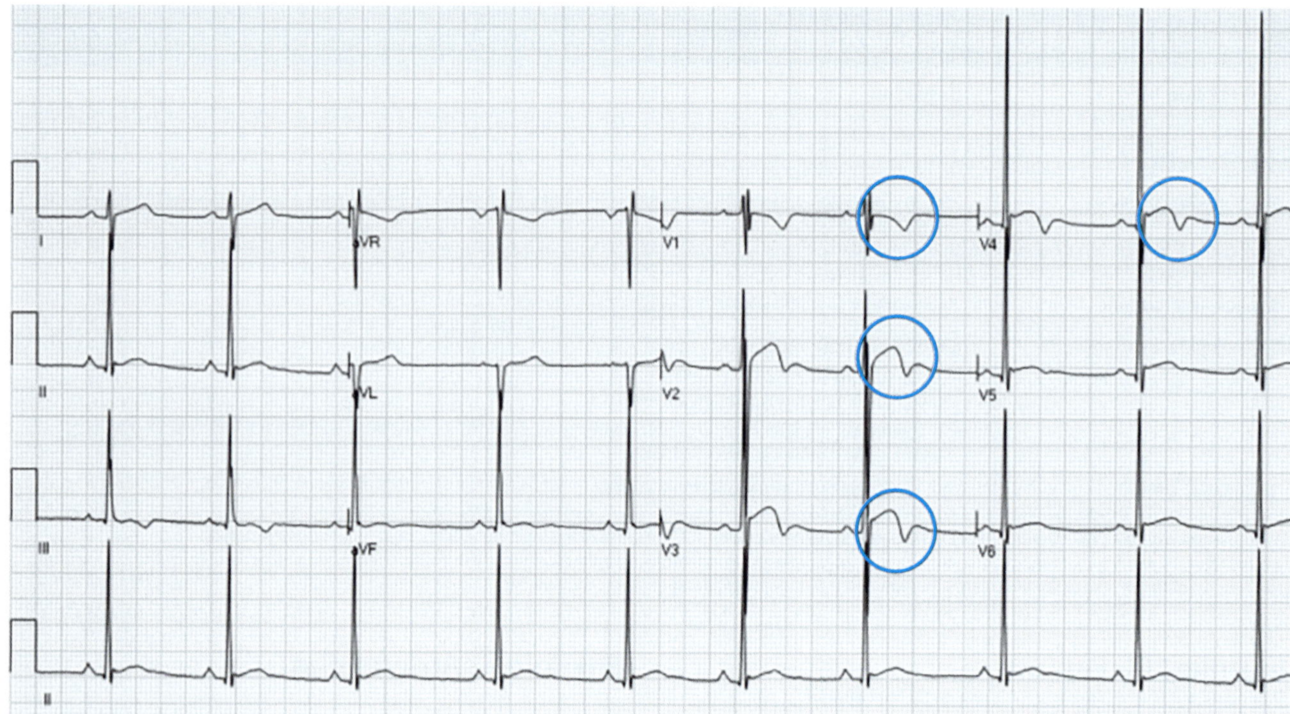

Figure 23.2: Athlete repolarization variant is a normal pattern consisting of J-point elevation, convex ST-segment elevation, and T-wave inversion confined to leads V1-V4 (circles). This variant is more commonly found in athletes of Afro-Caribbean descent and is likely benign regardless of race/ethnicity.

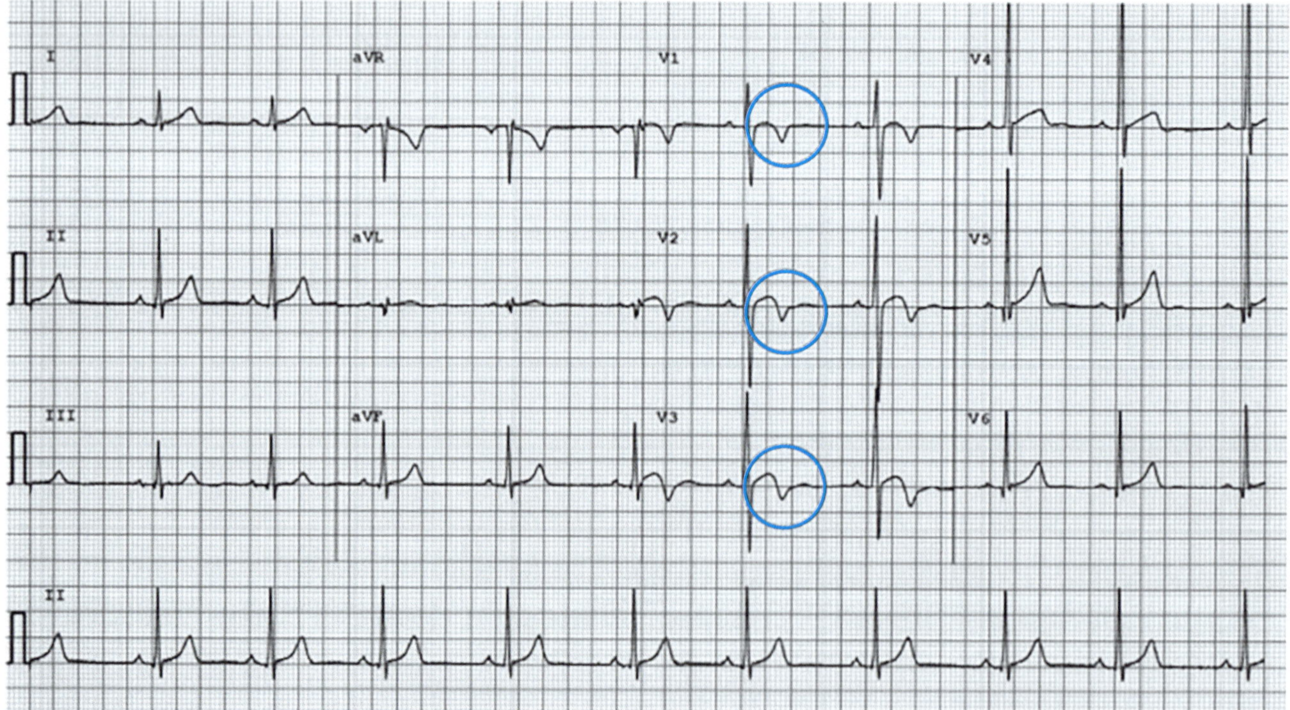

Figure 23.3: "Juvenile" T-wave inversion pattern consists of T-wave inversions confined to leads V1-V3, and is considered normal in athletes under 16 years.

phenomenon). These findings are common in junior and adult athletes and considered a normal physiologic response to regular training (22,24).

Right Bundle Branch Block

- Incomplete right bundle branch block (iRBBB) is defined as an rSR' pattern in V1 and QRS in V6 with QRS <120 ms. It is a common and benign finding in athletes and should not prompt further workup (8).
- Complete right bundle branch block (RBBB) is defined as QRS ≥120 ms with an rSR' pattern in V1 and slurred S wave in V6. Complete RBBB is associated with increased RV size and mildly reduced ejection fraction, but normal fractional area change and therefore preserved systolic function. It results from physiologic RV enlargement causing stretch of the Purkinje fibers. When found in isolation, complete RBBB is not associated with structural cardiac disease but may be further investigated in the appropriate clinical context (25,26).

BORDERLINE ECG FINDINGS IN ATHLETES

- The following ECG variants may represent normal adaptations to high-level training in athletes and do not require further testing if present in isolation and without other concerning findings.
- However, if more than one "borderline" finding is present, or if there are other concerning features on history or physical exam, then further workup is indicated (see Table 23.2).

Axis Deviation and Atrial Enlargement

- In one study, >40% of ECGs in athletes had left or right axis deviation or atrial enlargement by voltage criteria. When found in isolation, these ECG findings are typically not associated with structural pathology (27).

Table 23.2 Borderline ECG Findings in Athletes

ECG Finding	Definition
Atrial enlargement	Left atrial enlargement: P wave >120 ms in leads I or II with negative portion of P wave ≥1 mm and ≥40 ms in V1 Right atrial enlargement: P-wave amplitude ≥2.5 mm in II, III, or aVF
Axis deviation	Left axis deviation: −30° to 90° Right axis deviation: >120°
Complete RBBB	rSR' in V1 and slurred S in V6 with QRS ≥120 ms

ECG, electrocardiogram; RBBB, right bundle branch block.
Adapted from Drezner JA, O'Connor FG, Harmon KG, et al. AMSSM position statement on cardiovascular preparticipation screening in athletes: current evidence, knowledge gaps, recommendations, and future directions. *Clin J Sport Med.* 2016 Sep;26(5):347–61.

ABNORMAL ECG FINDINGS IN ATHLETES

- The following ECG findings should be considered abnormal and warrant further workup for electrical or structural cardiac pathologies. Restriction from training and competition is reasonable in these athletes until further investigation has been performed (see Table 23.3).

Abnormal TWI

- Abnormal TWI is defined as ≥1 mm inversions in two or more contiguous leads, excluding aVR, III, and V1 (excluding athlete repolarization variants and the juvenile TWI pattern discussed above) (see Fig. 23.4).
- Lateral and/or inferolateral TWI are commonly associated with hypertrophic cardiomyopathy (HCM) and dilated cardiomyopathy (DCM), and also may be found in left ventricular noncompaction (LVNC) cardiomyopathy, arrhythmogenic cardiomyopathy (AC), and myocarditis. Abnormal anterior TWI may suggest AC and less frequently HCM or DCM (28,29).
- Initial diagnostic testing should include transthoracic echocardiography (TTE). Cardiac MRI (CMR) is indicated for deep (>2 mm) lateral or inferolateral TWI or if TTE is nondiagnostic. CMR allows more accurate wall thickness measurements and tissue characterization (*i.e.*, late gadolinium enhancement [LGE] suggesting myocardial fibrosis/scar) and thus has improved the sensitivity to detect apical HCM, AC, and myocarditis.
- "Gray zone" findings on CMR, such as mid-range hypertrophy of 13–16 mm without LGE, may be followed by exercise ECG testing or ambulatory ECG monitoring ≥24 hours to evaluate for ventricular arrhythmias.
- In athletes with lateral and/or inferolateral TWI with unremarkable initial testing, serial (annual) cardiac imaging is recommended to monitor for the development of cardiomyopathy (30,31).

ST-Segment Depression

- Abnormal ST-segment depression (STD) is defined as ≥0.5 mm depression of the ST segment relative to the PR segment in two or more contiguous leads.
- STD is commonly found in patients with cardiomyopathy and should prompt workup with TTE and/or CMR.

Pathologic Q Waves

- Pathologic Q waves in athletes are defined as those ≥40 ms in duration in two or more contiguous leads (excluding III and aVR) or those with a Q/R ratio ≥0.25 (19).
- Pathologic Q waves isolated to V1-V2 may represent lead misplacement and can be first investigated by ensuring proper lead placement and repeating an ECG. If normal, no further testing is necessary (32).

Table 23.3 Abnormal ECG Findings in Athletes

ECG Finding	Definition	Differential Diagnosis	Recommended Evaluation
Abnormal TWI	≥1 mm TWI in 2 or more contiguous leads excluding aVF, III, V1	Lateral/inferolateral TWI: HCM, DCM, LVNC, AC, myocarditis Anterior TWI: AC, HCM, DCM Inferior TWI: HCM, myocarditis	TTE CMR Exercise ECG test Ambulatory ECG monitoring ≥24 h
ST-segment depression	≥0.5 mm ST segment depression in 2 or more contiguous leads	HCM, DCM, LVNC, AC, myocarditis	TTE CMR
Pathologic Q waves	Q wave ≥40 ms or Q/R ratio ≥0.25 in 2 or more contiguous leads excluding III, aVR	HCM, DCM, LVNC, myocarditis, CAD	TTE CMR Coronary evaluation (For V1-V2 Q waves: repeat ECG ensuring proper lead placement)
Complete LBBB	QRS ≥120 ms with predominantly negative QRS complex in V1 and upright notched or slurred R in I and V6	DCM, HCM, LVNC, CAD, Myocarditis, Sarcoidosis	TTE CMR with stress perfusion study
Profound IVCD	QRS ≥140 ms	DCM, HCM, LVNC	TTE
Epsilon wave	Small positive deflection or notch between the end of the QRS and beginning of the T wave in V1-V3	AC	TTE CMR Exercise ECG test Ambulatory ECG monitoring ≥24 h
Ventricular preexcitation	PR-interval <120 ms with slurred upstroke to the QRS complex (delta wave) and widened QRS ≥120 ms	Wolff-Parkinson-White	TTE EP referral for EP study and possible ablation of high-risk accessory pathways
Prolonged QTc	QTc ≥470 ms (male) or ≥480 ms (female) QTc ≥500 ms (marked prolongation)	Congenital long QT syndrome	Repeat ECG on separate day Evaluate for reversible factors (medications, electrolyte abnormalities) Detailed medical and family history Genetic testing EP referral for high-risk findings
Brugada type 1 pattern	Coved/downsloping rSr' with ST elevation ≥2 mm and TWI in V1-V3	Brugada syndrome	Evaluate for reversible factors EP referral
Profound sinus bradycardia Profound 1st-degree AV block	Sinus bradycardia <30 bpm PR interval ≥400 ms	Myocardial or electrical disease	Repeat ECG after aerobic activity to assess chronotropic competence Consider TTE, exercise ECG and/or ambulatory monitoring
High-grade AV block	2nd-degree Mobitz type II AV block: intermittently nonconducted P waves without PR prolongation 3rd-degree AV block: complete heart block	Myocardial or electrical disease	TTE Exercise ECG test Ambulatory ECG monitoring ≥24 h Consider CMR
Multiple PVCs	2 or more PVCs on 10-s ECG	AC, DCM, HCM, LVNC, Nonischemic LV scar, Myocarditis, Sarcoidosis	TTE Exercise ECG test Ambulatory ECG monitoring ≥24 h Consider CMR for >2000 PVCs per 24 h
Atrial tachyarrhythmias	Atrial fibrillation/flutter, SVT, resting sinus tachycardia >120 bpm	Myocardial or electrical disease	TTE Exercise ECG test Ambulatory ECG monitoring ≥24 h Evaluate for reversible causes of resting sinus tachycardia (anxiety, dehydration, fever, thyroid dysfunction, and anemia)
Ventricular arrhythmias	Couplets, triplets, nonsustained ventricular tachycardia	Myocardial or electrical disease	TTE CMR Exercise ECG test Ambulatory ECG monitoring ≥24 h Detailed family history Consider EP referral and genetic testing

AC, arrhythmogenic cardiomyopathy; AV, atrioventricular; CAD, coronary artery disease; CMR, cardiac MRI; DCM, dilated cardiomyopathy; ECG, electrocardiogram; EP, electrophysiology; HCM, hypertrophic cardiomyopathy; IVCD, intraventricular conduction delay; LBBB, left bundle branch block; LV, left ventricle; LVNC, left ventricular noncompaction; SVT, supraventricular tachycardia; TTE, transthoracic echocardiogram; TWI, T wave inversion.

Adapted from Drezner JA, O'Connor FG, Harmon KG, et al. AMSSM position statement on cardiovascular preparticipation screening in athletes: current evidence, knowledge gaps, recommendations, and future directions. *Clin J Sport Med.* 2016 Sep;26(5):347–61.

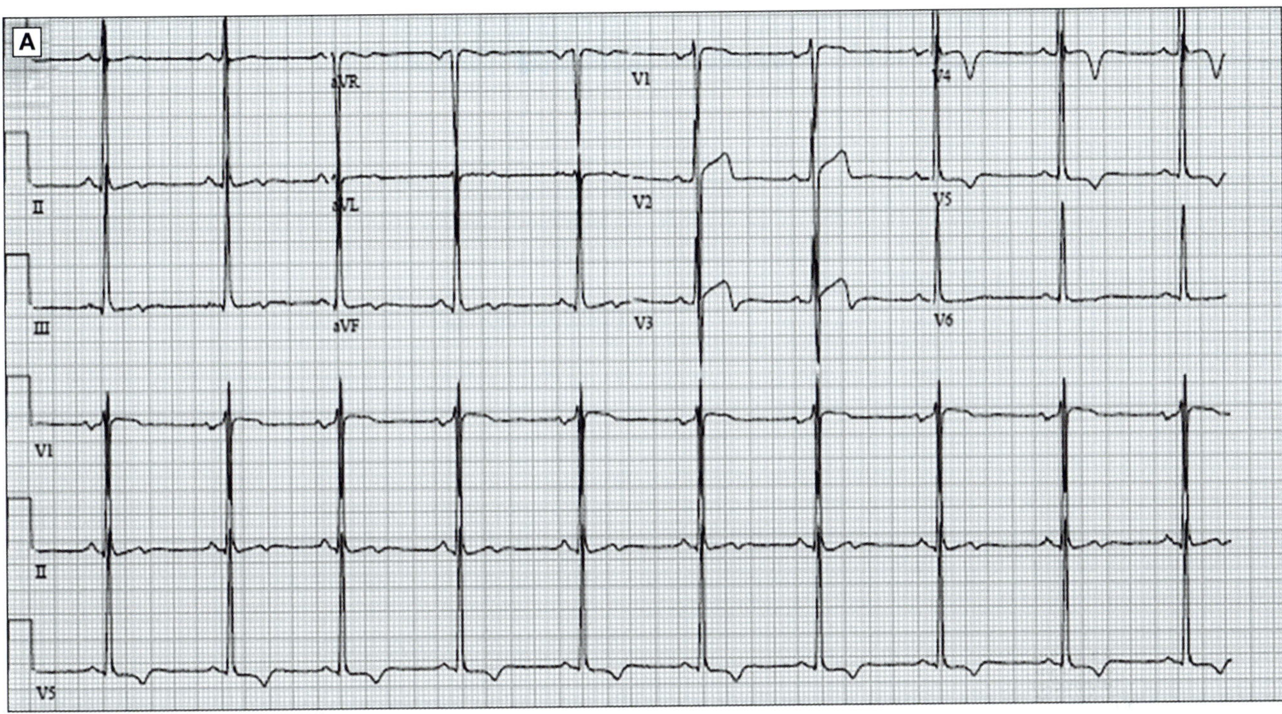

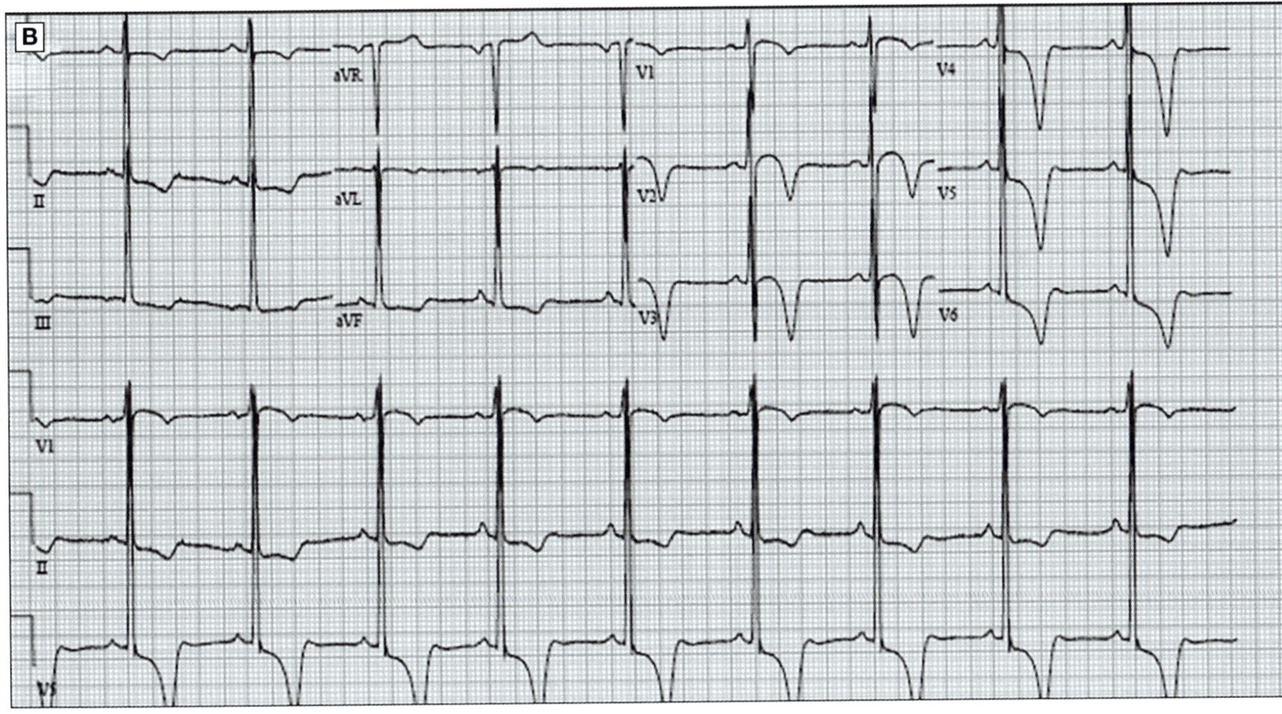

Figure 23.4: Abnormal T-wave inversions are defined as in two or more contiguous leads, excluding aVR, III, and V1 (excluding athlete repolarization variants and the juvenile TWI pattern discussed above). Lateral TWI (A) and inferolateral TWI (B) are considered abnormal and are commonly associated with hypertrophic and dilated cardiomyopathies. (Reprinted from Figure 12 of Drezner JA, Sharma S, Baggish A, et al. International criteria for electrocardiographic interpretation in athletes: consensus statement. *Br J Sports Med*. 2017;51:704–31. Copyright © 2017 BMJ Publishing Group Ltd. Used with permission.)

- Pathologic Q waves in other distributions may suggest cardiomyopathy, myocarditis, or coronary artery disease (CAD) (33,34). Initial evaluation should include TTE; if TTE is normal and clinical suspicion is low, no further testing is required, although increased clinical suspicion or other abnormal findings should prompt CMR and/or coronary evaluation to assess for ischemic heart disease.

Complete Left Bundle Branch Block

- Complete left bundle branch block (LBBB) is defined as QRS ≥120 ms with a predominantly negative QRS complex in lead V1 and upright notched or slurred R wave in I and V6.
- Contrary to RBBB, LBBB should always be considered abnormal and suggests the presence of cardiomyopathy, ischemic heart disease, myocarditis, or infiltrative diseases such as cardiac sarcoidosis. Studies have found a weak association of LBBB with an increased risk for arrhythmic sudden cardiac death (26,35).
- Workup of LBBB should include TTE and CMR with stress perfusion study to evaluate for myocardial diseases.

Profound Intraventricular Conduction Delay

- Profound intraventricular conduction delay (IVCD), defined as a QRS ≥140 ms, carries uncertain significance but may be found in cardiomyopathies and is weakly associated with an increased risk of arrhythmic SCD (35). In patients with an underlying cardiomyopathy such as HCM, a prolonged QRS is an independent and strong predictor of increased cardiovascular mortality (36).
- TTE is recommended in patients with IVCD ≥140 ms, with additional testing based on TTE findings or other clinical features.

Epsilon Wave

- An epsilon wave is a small positive deflection or notch present between the QRS complex and onset of the T wave in leads V1-V3.
- Epsilon waves are highly specific for AC. Similar to abnormal TWI, epsilon waves should prompt evaluation with TTE, CMR, and consideration of exercise ECG testing and/or ambulatory ECG monitoring.

Ventricular Preexcitation

- Ventricular preexcitation is marked by the Wolff-Parkinson-White (WPW) pattern, defined as a PR interval of <120 ms combined with a slurred upstroke to the QRS complex (delta wave) and a widened QRS ≥120 ms (Fig. 23.5).

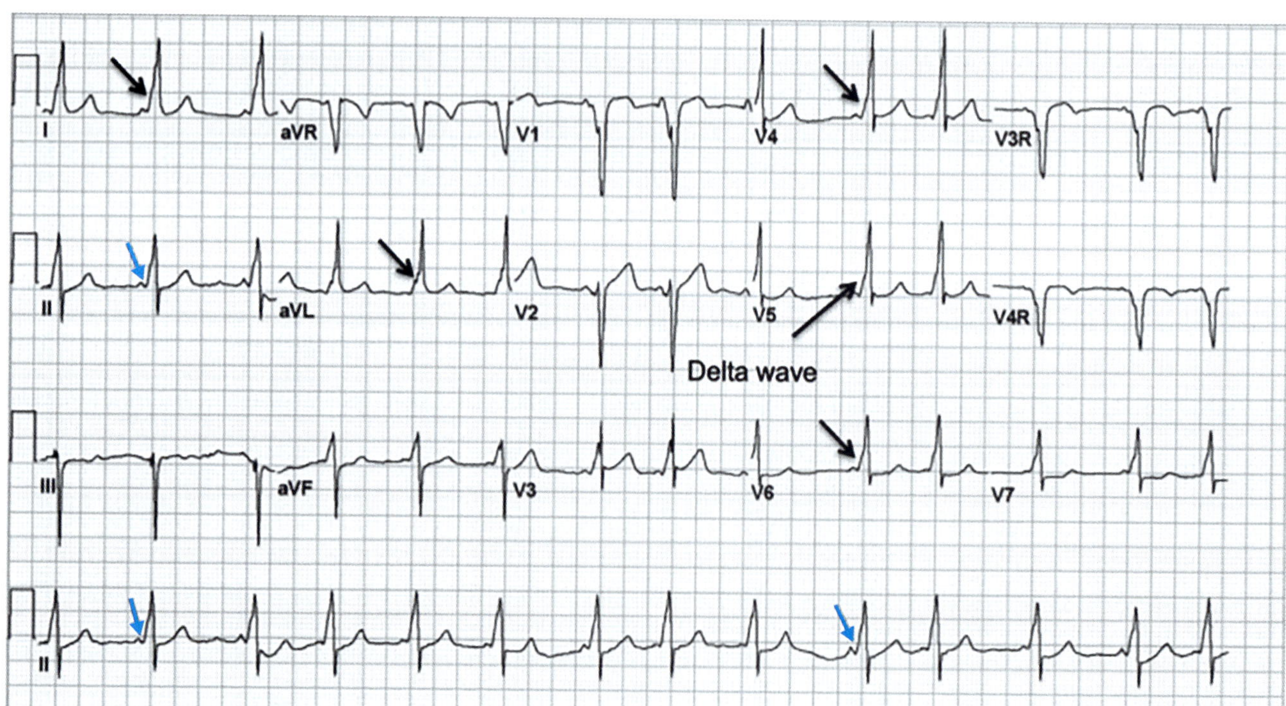

Figure 23.5: Ventricular preexcitation, also referred to as the Wolff-Parkinson-White (WPW) pattern, consists of a shortened PR interval <120 ms (red arrows) combined with a delta wave (slurred QRS upstroke, black arrows) and prolonged QRS complex ≥120 ms. (Reprinted from Figure 17 of Drezner JA, Sharma S, Baggish A, et al. International criteria for electrocardiographic interpretation in athletes: consensus statement. *Br J Sports Med.* 2017;51:704–31. Copyright © 2017 BMJ Publishing Group Ltd. Used with permission.)

- The WPW pattern results from an accessory electrical pathway that bypasses the AV node, which can lead to ventricular fibrillation and sudden cardiac death (37).
- Workup for ventricular preexcitation should include TTE to exclude coexistent cardiomyopathy. Young competitive athletes with ventricular preexcitation should be referred for electrophysiological study and possible ablation. An international registry of young patients with WPW found that risk stratification by stress ECG testing did not adequately distinguish low versus high-risk accessory pathways at risk of sudden cardiac death (38,39).

Prolonged QTc

- Prolonged QTc is defined as ≥470 ms in a male or ≥480 ms in a female athlete (using the Bazett formula), with a QTc ≥500 ms considered marked QT prolongation. Prolonged QTc, particularly in hereditary pathologies such as congenital long QT syndrome, may predispose athletes to lethal ventricular arrhythmias (40,41).
- Detection of a prolonged QTc should be confirmed with repeat ECG on a separate day, and if confirmed should prompt evaluation for other QT-prolonging factors including medications and electrolyte abnormalities. If persistent, athletes should be assessed for a high-risk medical history (*e.g.*, syncope, seizures) or family history of explained death at a young age. Screening of first-degree relatives and genetic testing should be considered.
- Persistent QTc prolongation >500 ms without other reversible causes should prompt referral to electrophysiology.

Brugada Type 1 Pattern

- Brugada syndrome is an inherited channelopathy carrying elevated risk for ventricular tachyarrhythmias and sudden cardiac death (Fig. 23.6). The diagnostic Type 1 Brugada pattern on ECG consists of a coved, or downsloping, rSr' with ST-segment elevation ≥2 mm followed by an inverted T wave in V1-V3. The downsloping nature of the ST-segment elevation distinguishes the type 1 Brugada pattern from the upsloping ST elevation in early repolarization (41).
- Suspected type 1 Brugada patterns can be confirmed by performing a high precordial lead ECG, with V1 or V2 placed in the 2nd or 3rd intercostal space. Patients with confirmed type 1 Brugada pattern should be evaluated for exacerbating factors such as electrolyte abnormalities or medications with sodium channel-blocking properties and should be referred to electrophysiology.

Profound Sinus Bradycardia or First-Degree AV Block

- Sinus bradycardia <30 bpm, or profound first-degree atrioventricular block with a PR interval ≥400 ms, may represent myocardial or electrical disease (8).
- Profound sinus bradycardia or first-degree AV block can first be evaluated by repeating an ECG after aerobic activity to assess for chronotropic competence. Continued abnormal results can be further investigated with TTE, exercise ECG, and/or ambulatory ECG monitoring.

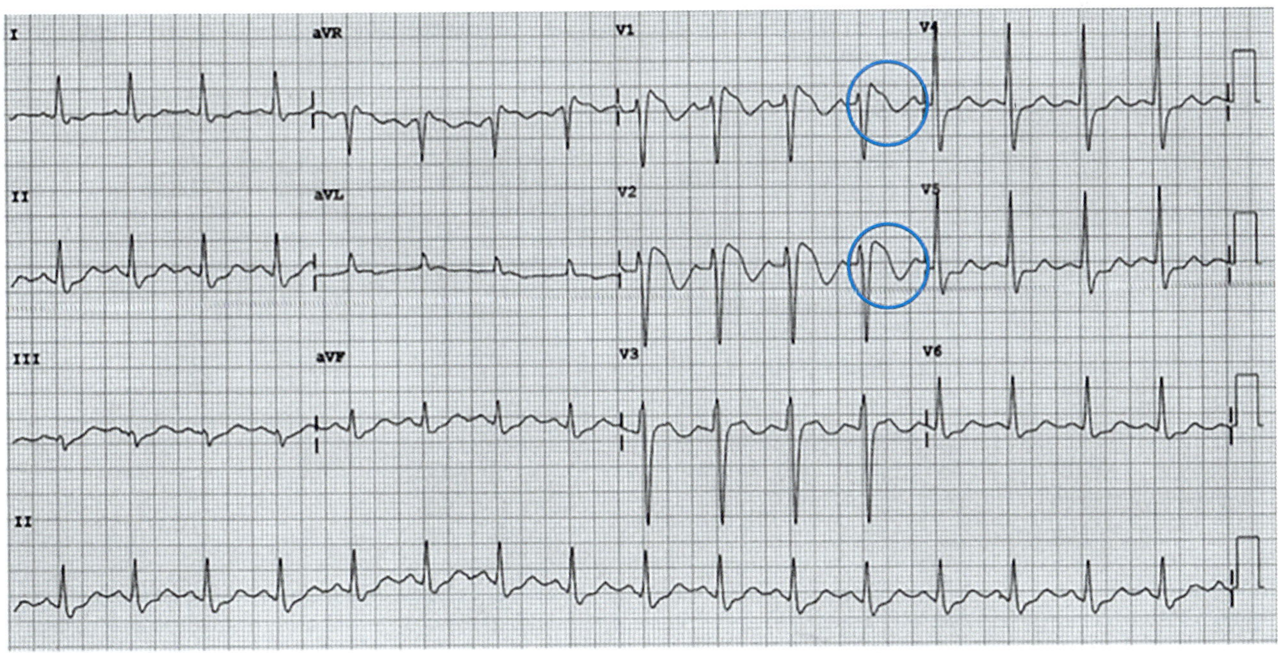

Figure 23.6: Type 1 Brugada pattern consists of a downsloping ("coved") rSr' with ST-segment elevation ≥2 mm followed by TWI in leads V1-V3 (circles).

High-Grade AV Block

- Second-degree Mobitz type II or third degree (complete) AV block may be signs of myocardial or electrical disease.
- High-grade AV block may be investigated with TTE, exercise ECG, ambulatory ECG monitoring, and potentially CMR.

Multiple PVCs

- Two or more PVCs present on a single 10-second ECG should be considered abnormal in athletes. Athletes with >2000 PVCs in a 24-hour period have been shown to be at higher risk of underlying structural disease (42).
- Emerging research has defined pathologic PVC patterns in which a single pathologic PVC may warrant more investigation.
- High PVC burden can be further investigated with TTE, exercise ECG, and/or ambulatory ECG monitoring. In athletes with >2000 PVCs per 24 hours, a CMR should be considered to investigate for myocardial disease.

Atrial Tachyarrhythmias

- Atrial tachyarrhythmias, including atrial fibrillation, atrial flutter, supraventricular tachycardias, or resting sinus tachycardia >120 bpm, may indicate underlying myocardial or electrical disease or a metabolic disorder.
- Patients with atrial fibrillation or flutter should be investigated according to standard guidelines including thyroid function testing, TTE, and consideration of ambulatory ECG monitoring.
- Patients with high resting tachycardia should undergo repeat ECG in the absence of exacerbating factors such as dehydration, recent exercise, or anxiety. Other contributing factors should be elucidated including fever, infection, anemia, or thyroid disease. Further testing can include appropriate laboratory studies, TTE, exercise ECG, and/or ambulatory ECG monitoring (43).

Ventricular Arrhythmias

- Ventricular arrhythmias, including couplets, triplets, and nonsustained ventricular tachycardia are abnormal and can suggest myocardial or electrical disease.
- Workup of ventricular arrhythmias should include a thorough family history for hereditary cardiac disease as well as TTE, CMR, ambulatory ECG monitoring, and/or exercise ECG. Electrophysiology studies and/or genetic testing should be considered based on initial results.

SUMMARY

- Electrocardiogram interpretation is a core skill for the sports medicine provider. The International Criteria for Electrocardiographic Interpretation in Athletes, endorsed by international cardiac and sports medical societies and sports governing bodies, provide a clear guide in interpreting ECGs of athletes to appropriately identify abnormal ECG findings.
- The screening physician must be trained in interpreting ECGs of athletes utilizing the most recent ECG criteria to optimize decision-making.

REFERENCES

1. Maron BJ, Gohman TE, Aeppli D. Prevalence of sudden cardiac death during competitive sports activities in Minnesota high school athletes. *J Am Coll Cardiol*. 1998 Dec;32(7):1881–4.
2. Maron BJ, Haas TS, Ahluwalia A, Rutten-Ramos SC. Incidence of cardiovascular sudden deaths in Minnesota high school athletes. *Heart Rhythm*. 2013 Mar;10(3):374–7.
3. Eckart RE, Scoville SL, Campbell CL, et al. Sudden death in young adults: a 25-year review of autopsies in military recruits. *Ann Intern Med*. 2004 Dec 7;141(11):829–34.
4. Harmon KG, Asif IM, Maleszewski JJ, et al. Incidence, cause, and comparative frequency of sudden cardiac death in national collegiate athletic association athletes: a decade in review. *Circulation*. 2015 Jul 7;132(1):10–9.
5. Maron BJ, Haas TS, Murphy CJ, Ahluwalia A, Rutten-Ramos S. Incidence and causes of sudden death in U.S. college athletes. *J Am Coll Cardiol*. 2014 Apr 29;63(16):1636–43.
6. Peterson DF, Siebert DM, Kucera KL, et al. Etiology of sudden cardiac arrest and death in US competitive athletes: a 2-year prospective surveillance study. *Clin J Sport Med*. 2020 Jul;30(4):305–14.
7. Peterson DF, Kucera K, Thomas LC, et al. Aetiology and incidence of sudden cardiac arrest and death in young competitive athletes in the USA: a 4-year prospective study. *Br J Sports Med*. 2021 Nov;55(21):1196–203.
8. Drezner JA, O'Connor FG, Harmon KG, et al. AMSSM position statement on cardiovascular preparticipation screening in athletes: current evidence, knowledge gaps, recommendations, and future directions. *Clin J Sport Med*. 2016 Sep;26(5):347–61.
9. Corrado D, Pelliccia A, Bjørnstad HH, et al. Cardiovascular preparticipation screening of young competitive athletes for prevention of sudden death: proposal for a common European protocol — consensus statement of the Study Group of Sport Cardiology of the Working Group of Cardiac Rehabilitation and Exercise Physiology and the Working Group of Myocardial and Pericardial Diseases of the European Society of Cardiology. *Eur Heart J*. 2005 Mar 1;26(5):516–24.
10. Pelliccia A, Sharma S, Gati S, et al. 2020 ESC guidelines on sports cardiology and exercise in patients with cardiovascular disease. *Eur Heart J*. 2021 Jan 1;42(1):17–96.
11. Drezner JA, Sharma S, Baggish A, et al. International criteria for electrocardiographic interpretation in athletes: consensus statement. *Br J Sports Med*. 2017 May 1;51(9):704–31.
12. Fagard R. Athlete's heart. *Heart*. 2003 Dec;89(12):1455–61.
13. Pelliccia A, Maron BJ, Culasso F, et al. Clinical significance of abnormal electrocardiographic patterns in trained athletes. *Circulation*. 2000 Jul 18;102(3):278–84.
14. Sathanandam S, Zimmerman F, Davis J, Marek J. Abstract 2484: ECG screening criteria for LVH does not correlate with diagnosis of hypertrophic cardiomyopathy. *Circulation*. 2009 Nov 3;120(suppl_18):S647.
15. Sohaib SMA, Payne JR, Shukla R, World M, Pennell DJ, Montgomery HE. Electrocardiographic (ECG) criteria for determining left ventricular mass in young healthy men; data from the LARGE Heart study. *J Cardiovasc Magn Reson*. 2009 Jan 16;11(1):2.

16. Macfarlane PW, Antzelevitch C, Haissaguerre M, et al. The early repolarization pattern: a consensus paper. *J Am Coll Cardiol.* 2015 Jul 28;66(4):470–7.
17. Quattrini FM, Pelliccia A, Assorgi R, et al. Benign clinical significance of J-wave pattern (early repolarization) in highly trained athletes. *Heart Rhythm.* 2014 Nov 1;11(11):1974–82.
18. Papadakis M, Carre F, Kervio G, et al. The prevalence, distribution, and clinical outcomes of electrocardiographic repolarization patterns in male athletes of African/Afro-Caribbean origin. *Eur Heart J.* 2011 Sep 1;32(18):2304–13.
19. Sheikh N, Papadakis M, Ghani S, et al. Comparison of electrocardiographic criteria for the detection of cardiac abnormalities in elite black and white athletes. *Circulation.* 2014 Apr 22;129(16):1637–49.
20. Sheikh N, Papadakis M, Carre F, et al. Cardiac adaptation to exercise in adolescent athletes of African ethnicity: an emergent elite athletic population. *Br J Sports Med.* 2013 Jun;47(9):585–92.
21. Calore C, Zorzi A, Sheikh N, et al. Electrocardiographic anterior T-wave inversion in athletes of different ethnicities: differential diagnosis between athlete's heart and cardiomyopathy. *Eur Heart J.* 2016 Aug 21;37(32):2515–27.
22. Papadakis M, Basavarajaiah S, Rawlins J, et al. Prevalence and significance of T-wave inversions in predominantly Caucasian adolescent athletes. *Eur Heart J.* 2009 Jul 1;30(14):1728–35.
23. Migliore F, Zorzi A, Michieli P, et al. Prevalence of cardiomyopathy in Italian asymptomatic children with electrocardiographic T-wave inversion at preparticipation screening. *Circulation.* 2012 Jan 24;125(3):529–38.
24. Sharma S, Whyte G, Elliott P, et al. Electrocardiographic changes in 1000 highly trained junior elite athletes. *Br J Sports Med.* 1999 Oct 1;33(5):319–24.
25. Kim JH, Noseworthy PA, McCarty D, et al. Significance of electrocardiographic right bundle branch block in trained athletes. *Am J Cardiol.* 2011 Apr 1;107(7):1083–9.
26. Kim JH, Baggish AL. Electrocardiographic right and left bundle branch block patterns in athletes: prevalence, pathology, and clinical significance. *J Electrocardiol.* 2015 May 1;48(3):380–4.
27. Gati S, Sheikh N, Ghani S, et al. Should axis deviation or atrial enlargement be categorised as abnormal in young athletes? The athlete's electrocardiogram: time for re-appraisal of markers of pathology. *Eur Heart J.* 2013 Dec 14;34(47):3641–8.
28. Sheikh N, Papadakis M, Schnell F, et al. Clinical profile of athletes with hypertrophic cardiomyopathy. *Circ Cardiovasc Imaging.* 2015 Jul;8(7):e003454.
29. Bent RE, Wheeler MT, Hadley D, et al. Systematic comparison of digital electrocardiograms from healthy athletes and patients with hypertrophic cardiomyopathy. *J Am Coll Cardiol.* 2015 Jun 9;65(22):2462–3.
30. Pelliccia A, Di Paolo FM, Quattrini FM, et al. Outcomes in athletes with marked ECG repolarization abnormalities. *N Engl J Med.* 2008 Jan 10;358(2):152–61.
31. Schnell F, Riding N, O'Hanlon R, et al. Recognition and significance of pathological T-wave inversions in athletes. *Circulation.* 2015 Jan 13;131(2):165–73.
32. MacAlpin RN. Clinical significance of QS complexes in V1 and V2 without other electrocardiographic abnormality. *Ann Noninvasive Electrocardiol.* 2004;9(1):39–47.
33. Rowin EJ, Maron BJ, Appelbaum E, et al. Significance of false negative electrocardiograms in preparticipation screening of athletes for hypertrophic cardiomyopathy. *Am J Cardiol.* 2012 Oct 1;110(7):1027–32.
34. Lakdawala NK, Thune JJ, Maron BJ, et al. Electrocardiographic features of sarcomere mutation carriers with and without clinically overt hypertrophic cardiomyopathy. *Am J Cardiol.* 2011 Dec 1;108(11):1606–13.
35. Aro AL, Anttonen O, Tikkanen JT, et al. Intraventricular conduction delay in a standard 12-lead electrocardiogram as a predictor of mortality in the general population. *Circ Arrhythm Electrophysiol.* 2011 Oct;4(5):704–10.
36. Bongioanni S, Bianchi F, Migliardi A, et al. Relation of QRS duration to mortality in a community-based cohort with hypertrophic cardiomyopathy. *Am J Cardiol.* 2007 Aug 1;100(3):503–6.
37. Surawicz B, Childers R, Deal BJ, et al. AHA/ACCF/HRS recommendations for the standardization and interpretation of the electrocardiogram: part III — intraventricular conduction disturbances—a scientific statement from the American Heart Association Electrocardiography and Arrhythmias Committee, Council on Clinical Cardiology; the American College of Cardiology Foundation; and the Heart Rhythm Society — endorsed by the International Society for Computerized Electrocardiology. *Circulation.* 2009 Mar 17;119(10):e235–40.
38. Pediatric and Congenital Electrophysiology Society PACESHeart Rhythm Society HRSAmerican College of Cardiology Foundation ACCF, et al. PACES/HRS expert consensus statement on the management of the asymptomatic young patient with a Wolff-Parkinson-White (WPW, ventricular preexcitation) electrocardiographic pattern: developed in partnership between the Pediatric and Congenital Electrophysiology Society (PACES) and the Heart Rhythm Society (HRS). Endorsed by the governing bodies of PACES, HRS, the American College of Cardiology Foundation (ACCF), the American Heart Association (AHA), the American Academy of Pediatrics (AAP), and the Canadian Heart Rhythm Society (CHRS). *Heart Rhythm.* 2012 Jun 1;9(6):1006–24.
39. Escudero CA, Ceresnak SR, Collins KK, et al. Loss of ventricular preexcitation during noninvasive testing does not exclude high-risk accessory pathways: a multicenter study of WPW in children. *Heart Rhythm.* 2020 Oct;17(10):1729–37.
40. Ackerman MJ, Zipes DP, Kovacs RJ, et al. Eligibility and disqualification recommendations for competitive athletes with cardiovascular abnormalities: task force 10 — the cardiac channelopathies — a scientific statement from the American Heart Association and American College of Cardiology. *Circulation.* 2015 Dec;132(22):e326–9.
41. Priori SG, Wilde AA, Horie M, et al. HRS/EHRA/APHRS expert consensus statement on the diagnosis and management of patients with inherited primary arrhythmia syndromes: document endorsed by HRS, EHRA, and APHRS in May 2013 and by ACCF, AHA, PACES, and AEPC in June 2013. *Heart Rhythm.* 2013 Dec 1;10(12):1932–63.
42. Biffi A, Pelliccia A, Verdile L, et al. Long-term clinical significance of frequent and complex ventricular tachyarrhythmias in trained athletes. *J Am Coll Cardiol.* 2002 Aug 7;40(3):446–52.
43. American College of Cardiology FoundationAmerican Heart Association European Society of Cardiology, et al. Management of patients with atrial fibrillation (compilation of 2006 ACCF/AHA/ESC and 2011 ACCF/AHA/HRS recommendations): a report of the American College of Cardiology/American Heart Association Task Force on practice guidelines. *Circulation.* 2013 May 7;127(18):1916–26.

24 Exercise Testing

Erika Parisi, Rory B. Weiner, and Ankit B. Shah

INTRODUCTION

- Exercise testing (ET) plays an important role in the evaluation of the symptomatic athlete given its utility in assessing chest pain, syncope, exertional intolerance, lightheadedness, aerobic capacity, chronotropic competence, arrhythmias, and formulation of an exercise prescription.
- ET is a cardiovascular stress test, most commonly on a treadmill or cycle ergometer, utilizing electrocardiographic and blood pressure monitoring. Incorporating gas exchange measurements through cardiopulmonary exercise testing (CPET) allows for a comprehensive assessment of the cardiovascular, pulmonary, and metabolic response to exercise.
- ET is a widely available and cost-effective, noninvasive tool that has been used for over 65 years for the identification of obstructive coronary artery disease (CAD) (1). The reported sensitivity (mean 68%, range 23%–100%) and specificity (mean 77%, range 17%–100%) are widely variable, highlighting the importance of appropriate patient selection (2).
- When warranted, physicians may couple physiologic ET with imaging techniques such as stress echocardiography or nuclear perfusion imaging to increase diagnostic accuracy compared to ET alone (3,4).
- Here, we will discuss the clinical significance, indications, contraindications, and interpretation for the ET to assist the primary care sports medicine clinician.

ET TERMINOLOGY

- Clinicians should be familiar with basic ET terminology prior to performing the test (see also Chapter 6 Exercise Physiology and Chapter 23 ECG Interpretation in Athletes):
  - **PR segment:** The isoelectric line on a resting ECG from which the ST segment and the J point are measured. With exercise, the PR segment shortens and slopes downward. Thereafter, the PQ junction replaces the PR segment as the baseline point of reference for ST segment measurements.
  - **J point:** The point that distinguishes the QRS complex from the ST segment and is the point at which the slope changes. This is the point against which the ST segment deviation (depression or elevation) is measured.
  - **ST segment:** ST segment level is measured relative to the PQ junction. If the baseline is depressed, the deviation from that level to the level during exercise or recovery is measured. The ST segment is measured at 60–80 ms after the J point. At ventricular rates >130 beats · min^{-1} (bpm), it is measured at 60 ms after the J point (5).
  - **VO_{2max}:** Represents a true measure of cardiorespiratory capacity for an individual at a given level of oxygen availability (6). Maximal oxygen uptake is a physiologic characteristic quantified by the Fick equation; VO_2 = cardiac output (heart rate [HR] × stroke volume [SV]) × maximal arteriovenous oxygen content difference (a- VO_2 difference).
    - The maximal achievable HR is unique to each patient and maximal HR is affected by many factors including activity type, body position, fitness level, presence of heart disease, medications, blood volume, and ambient environment and age. Maximal effort-limited ET is recommended to determine an individual's true maximal HR (HR_{max}). However, a person's age-predicted maximum HR (APMHR) has been traditionally estimated utilizing the formula; HR_{max} = (220 − age), which was derived from older studies performed primarily in middle-aged men (7). Since then, tremendous intersubject variability has been documented, with a standard deviation of ±12 bpm and even higher in those with CAD on beta-blockers, which has called into question the utility of this equation (5,8). Newer equations that more accurately predict maximal HR have been developed (for men HR_{max} = 208 − [0.7 × age] and for women, HR_{max} = 206 − [0.88 × age]) but have not been universally incorporated into ET standards (5).
    - One of the hallmarks of an endurance athlete is increased stroke volume, at rest and during exercise, which is caused by adaptive increases in left ventricular end-diastolic volume (9). During exercise, stroke volume (SV) augments due both to an increased ventricular end-diastolic volume (volume of blood in the ventricle immediately before it contracts) and decreased end-systolic volume (volume of blood in the ventricle at the immediate end of contraction). SV augmentation is most robust at lower intensities and increased SV works in parallel with increasing HR to maximize an athlete's ability to increase cardiac output.

- In normal individuals at sea level, the a-VO_2 difference is typically not a limiting factor in VO_{2max} and although a_VO_2 difference may be enhanced in the trained endurance athlete, it is not the major factor contributing to a robust VO_{2max} (6). Exercise-induced arterial hypoxemia can be seen at or near maximal exercise in about 50% of young, highly fit athletes. The absence of symptoms coupled with supranormal exercise capacity, normal cardiac structure/function, and normal cardiopulmonary physiology on CPET suggest that desaturations noted near peak exercise are not pathologic (10,11). Meanwhile, venous oxygen content is determined by the amount of blood flow directed to the muscle and by capillary density. Muscle blood flow increases with exercise due to increased cardiac output and due to preferential redistribution of the cardiac output to the exercising muscle. A decrease in local and systemic vascular resistance also facilitates greater skeletal muscle flow. Finally, there is an increase in the overall number of capillaries with ongoing physical training (12).

- **Metabolic equivalents (METs):** A measure for quantifying energy uptake required for a task when compared to rest. One MET is defined as the resting oxygen requirements or metabolic rate (1 MET = ~3.5 mL $O_2 \cdot kg^{-1} \cdot min^{-1}$). The level of METs achieved at peak exercise has consistently been shown to be inversely associated with mortality risk (13,14). Patients achieving ≥10 METS on ET have very low rates of cardiac death (0.1% per year) and nonfatal MI (0.7% per year) (15). Example activities at different intensity levels are as follows (16):
  - 1 MET = Basal O_2 requirements (*e.g.*, sitting, lying)
  - Light intensity (2–2.9 METS)
    - Slow walking (2 METS)
    - Light housework (*e.g.*, making the bed, ironing) (2.0–2.5 METS)
  - Moderate intensity (3–5.9 METS)
    - Sweeping floors, vacuuming, heavy cleaning (3.0–3.5 METS)
    - Brisk walking (5 METS)
  - Vigorous intensity (≥6 METS)
    - Running at 7 miles $\cdot$ h^{-1} (11.5 METS)
    - Shoveling sand, coal (7 METS)
    - Singles tennis (8 METS)
    - Young endurance athletes (>18 METS) (1)

- **Rate-Pressure Product:** Myocardial oxygen uptake is determined primarily by intramyocardial wall stress, contractility and HR, and an accurate assessment requires invasive approach. The rate-pressure product or double product, defined as the product of HR_{max} and peak systolic blood pressure, has been used as a surrogate noninvasive measure of myocardial oxygen uptake during ET (17). Standard values vary from 6000 at rest, to greater than 20,000 in most normal individuals with exercise and greater than 40,000 during high-intensity exercise (1). Myocardial ischemia (MI) usually occurs at the same rate-pressure product rather than at the same external workload (18).

- **Cardiopulmonary Exercise Testing (CPET):** involves integrative ET of the cardiovascular, pulmonary and musculoskeletal systems through the direct noninvasive measurement of individual organ system function. This form of testing allows for a more detailed analysis of unexplained dyspnea and exercise intolerance, and in athletes, may be utilized to improve performance. CPET testing involves measurements of respiratory oxygen uptake (VO_2), carbon dioxide production (VCO_2), and other ventilatory parameters during a symptom-limited exercise test (see Chapter 6, Exercise Physiology). CPET will not be reviewed in detail in this chapter; the interested reader is referred to dedicated papers on the topic (18,19).

PERFORMING THE ET

Indications

- The major indications for ET relate to diagnosis, prognosis, and therapeutic prescription for both CAD and non-CAD disease states. The ET is not helpful in diagnosing ischemic heart disease in patients with a left bundle branch block, ventricular-paced rhythm, or with persistent preexcitation.

ET COMMON USES

- Detection of CAD in patients with chest pain syndromes
- Evaluation of the anatomic and functional severity of CAD
- Prediction of cardiovascular (CV) events and all-cause death
- Evaluation of physical capacity and effort tolerance
- Evaluation of exercise-related symptoms
- Assessment of chronotropic incompetence, arrhythmias, and response to implanted device therapy
- Assessment of response to medical intervention
- Risk stratification in patients with Wolff-Parkinson-White (WPW) pattern (asymptomatic)
- Evaluation of peripheral artery disease
- Evaluation of valvular heart disease
- Evaluation in patients with congenital heart disease

PREPARTICIPATION SCREENING

- The most recent ACSM guidelines (20) no longer recommend ET as part of medical clearance and instead leave the decision to pursue ET up to the clinical judgment of the healthcare provider. This has been done to align with evidence that ET is not a uniformly recommended screening procedure as it is a poor predictor of acute cardiac events in asymptomatic individuals (21). There is a low risk of sudden cardiac death and acute myocardial infarction associated with light-to-moderate intensity exercise. In contrast, acute bouts of vigorous exercise in untrained susceptible individual are associated with the greatest risk, but this risk can be mitigated by gradually increasing the duration and intensity of exercise (22).

- Exercise intensity was previously defined in absolute terms with METs but use relative intensities may be beneficial to creating an individualized exercise plan:
  - Low Intensity: 30%–39% of heart rate reserve (HR_{max}-resting HR) or oxygen uptake reserve (VO_{2max} – basal VO_2, rate of perceived exertion 9–11
  - Moderate Intensity: 40%–59% HR reserve or oxygen uptake reserve, rate of perceived exertion 12–13
  - Vigorous Intensity: ≥60% HR reserve or oxygen uptake reserve, rate of perceived exertion ≥14
- The new guidelines use an algorithm (Fig. 24.1) that assesses for symptoms (Box 24.1 and Table 24.1) and if there is known underlying cardiovascular, metabolic, or renal disease (23).
  - Individuals without known disease who are asymptomatic, but do not routinely exercise are not required

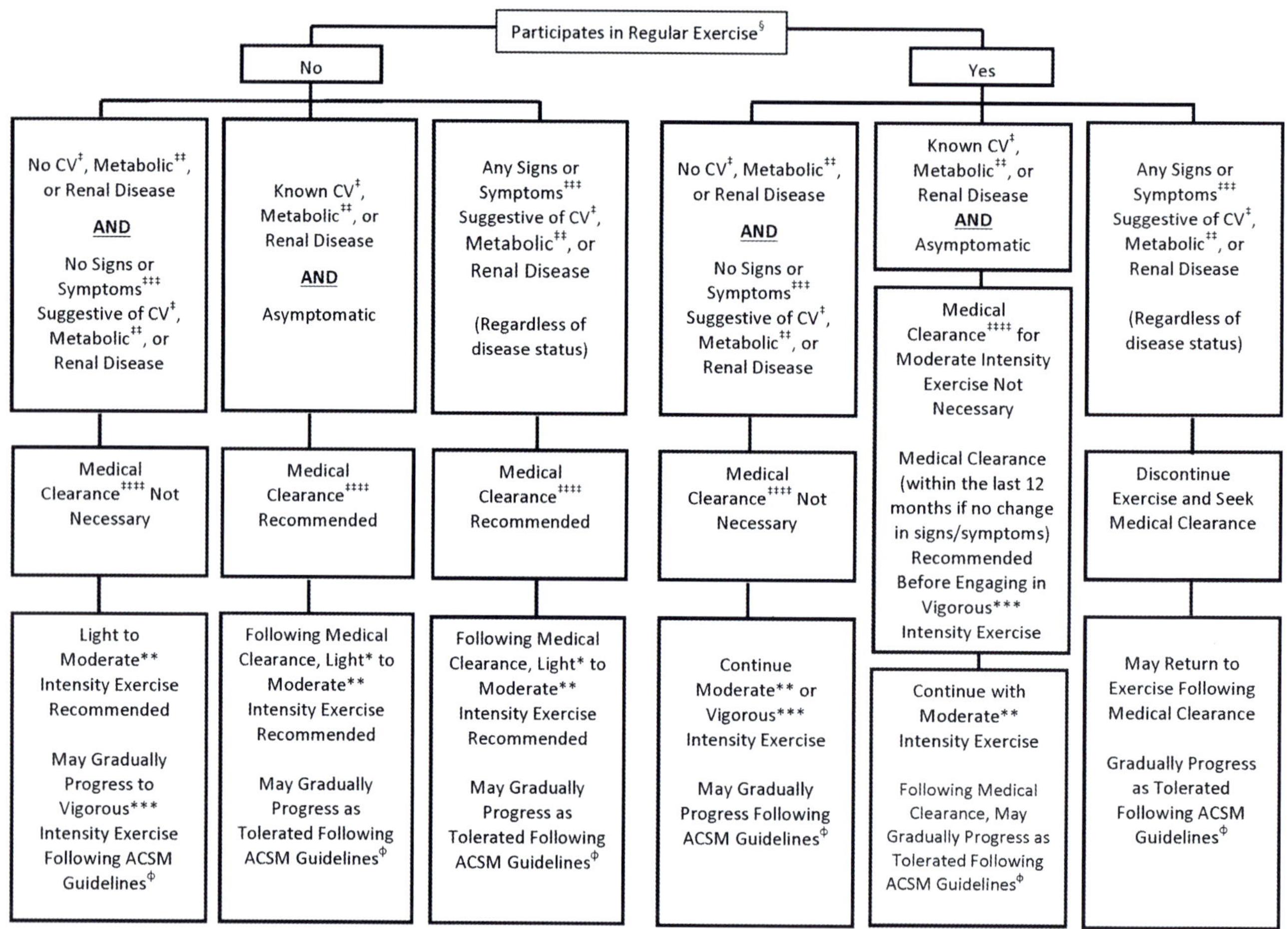

Figure 24.1: Exercise preparticipation health screening logic model for aerobic exercise participation. §Exercise participation, performing planned, structured physical activity at least 30 min at moderate intensity on at least 3 d · wk^{-1} for at least the last 3 mo. *Light-intensity exercise, 30%–G40% HRR or V˙ O2R, 2 to G3 METs, 9–11 RPE, an intensity that causes slight increases in HR and breathing. **Moderate-intensity exercise, 40%–G60% HRR or V˙ O2R, 3–G6 METs, 12–13 RPE, an intensity that causes noticeable increases in HR and breathing. ***Vigorous-intensity exercise Q60% HRR or V˙ O2R, Q6 METs, Q14 RPE, an intensity that causes substantial increases in HR and breathing. ‡CVD, cardiac, peripheral vascular, or cerebrovascular disease. ‡‡Metabolic disease, type 1 and 2 diabetes mellitus. ‡‡‡Signs and symptoms, at rest or during activity; includes pain, discomfort in the chest, neck, jaw, arms, or other areas that may result from ischemia; shortness of breath at rest or with mild exertion; dizziness or syncope; orthopnea or paroxysmal nocturnal dyspnea; ankle edema; palpitations or tachycardia; intermittent claudication; known heart murmur; or unusual fatigue or shortness of breath with usual activities. ‡‡‡‡Medical clearance, approval from a health care professional to engage in exercise. ΦACSM Guidelines, see the most current edition of ACSM's Guidelines for Exercise Testing and Prescription. (Reprinted from Figure 2 Riebe D, Franklin BA, Thompson PD, et al. Updating ACSM's recommendations for exercise preparticipation health screening. *Med Sci Sports Exerc.* 2015;47(11):2473–9. Copyright © 2015 American College of Sports Medicine. Used with permission.)

24.1 Major Signs or Symptoms Suggestive of Cardiovascular, Metabolic, and Renal Disease

1. Pain or discomfort (or other anginal equivalent) in the chest, neck, jaw, arms, or other areas that may result from ischemia
2. Shortness of breath at rest or with mild exertion
3. Dizziness or syncope
4. Orthopnea or paroxysmal nocturnal dyspnea
5. Ankle edema
6. Palpitations or tachycardia
7. Intermittent claudication
8. Known heart murmur
9. Unusual fatigue or shortness of breath with usual activities

Adapted from Table 2.1 Liguori G. *ACSM's Guidelines for Exercise Testing and Prescription.* 11th ed. Philadelphia: Wolters Kluwer; 2021. Copyright © 2021 American College of Sports Medicine. Used with permission. Originally in Gordon SMBS. Health appraisal in the non-medical setting. In: Durstine JL, editor. *ACSM's Resource Manual for Guidelines for Exercise Testing and Prescription.* 2nd ed. Philadelphia (PA): Lippincott Williams & Wilkins; 1993. p. 219–28.

to have medical clearance to engage in exercise but are advised to start with light-to-moderate intensity and gradually progress to vigorous exercise. If symptoms develop during light-to-moderate training, then the individual should stop and notify the healthcare provider.

- Individuals with any signs or symptoms or known CV, metabolic or renal disease are recommended to have medical clearance prior to initiating exercise regimen. Further need for risk stratification and/or use of ET is made by the individual provider.
- For individuals who routinely exercise but have signs or symptoms of CV, metabolic or renal disease should stop and be evaluated. For those who have no known disease and are asymptomatic, they can continue training without evaluation. For those who are asymptomatic but have known CV, metabolic, or renal disease, medical evaluation is recommended prior to participating in vigorous exercise.

Contraindications

- In some individuals, there may be contraindications to performing the procedure.

Absolute Contraindications (5)

- Acute MI (within 2 days)
- Ongoing unstable angina
- Uncontrolled ventricular or atrial arrhythmias with hemodynamic compromise
- Symptomatic, severe aortic stenosis
- Decompensated heart failure (HF)
- Acute aortic dissection (suspected or known)
- Active myocarditis or pericarditis
- Active endocarditis
- Acute pulmonary embolism or pulmonary infarction or deep venous thrombosis
- Physical disability that precludes safe and adequate testing

Table 24.1 Cardiovascular Disease (CVD) Risk Factors and Defining Criteria

Positive Risk Factors	Defining Criteria
Age	Male ≥45 y; female ≥55 y
Family history	Myocardial infarction, coronary revascularization, or sudden death before 55 y of age in father or other male first-degree relative, or before 65 y of age in mother or other female first-degree relative
Cigarette smoking	Current cigarette smoker or those who quit within the previous 6 mo or exposure to environmental tobacco smoke
Physical inactivity	Not meeting the minimum threshold of 500–1000 MET-min of moderate-to-vigorous physical activity or 75–150 min · wk^{-1} of moderate-to-vigorous intensity physical activity
Body mass index/waist circumference	Body mass index ≥30 kg · m^{-2} *or* waist girth >102 cm (40 inches) for men and ≥88 cm (35 inches) for women
Blood pressure	Systolic blood pressure ≥130 mm Hg and/or diastolic blood pressure ≥80 mm Hg, based on an average of ≥2 readings on at least two separate occasions, *or* on antihypertensive medication
Lipids	Low-density lipoprotein cholesterol ≥130 mg · dL^{-1} *or* high-density lipoprotein cholesterol <40 mg · dL^{-1} in men and <50 mg · dL^{-1} in women *or* on lipid-lowering medication. If total serum cholesterol is all that is available, use ≥200 mg · dL^{-1}
Blood glucose	Fasting plasma glucose ≥100 mg · dL^{-1}; or 2-h plasma glucose values in oral glucose tolerance test ≥140 mg · dL^{-1}; or HbA1C ≥ 5.7%
Negative Risk Factor	**Defining Criteria**
HDL-Cholesterol	≥60 mg · dL^{-1}

Adapted from Table 2.2 Liguori G. *ACSM's Guidelines for Exercise Testing and Prescription.* 11th ed. Philadelphia: Wolters Kluwer; 2021. Copyright © 2021 American College of Sports Medicine. Used with permission.

Relative Contraindications (1)

- Risks of performing procedure may outweigh benefits.
  - Tachyarrhythmias with uncontrolled ventricular rates
  - Moderate to severe aortic stenosis with uncertain relation to symptoms
  - Untreated severe pulmonary hypertension
  - Resting systemic blood pressure (BP) > 200/110
  - Recent stroke or transient ischemic attack
  - High-degree atrioventricular (AV) block
  - Uncorrected medical conditions (significant anemia, electrolyte imbalance, hyperthyroidism)
  - Known left main coronary artery stenosis
  - Hypertrophic obstructive cardiomyopathy with severe resting gradient
  - Mental or physical impairment leading to inability to cooperate/exercise safely

Special Considerations

- There are certain situations in which the physician must evaluate the patient carefully before undertaking ET or should consider an alternative test. For example, a patient with significant osteoarthritis may be unable to exercise to the diagnostic threshold required (HR_{max} > 85% APMHR), and thus require a pharmacologic test for evaluation. Other special situations include: medication effects (β-blockers, calcium channel blockers, digoxin), and certain clinical situations (unstable hypertension, previous MI, known severe CAD) (20).

Physician Responsibilities

- During ET, the physician's responsibilities include the following:

Pretest Patient Evaluation and Clearance

- Review the patient's medical history including recent symptoms, cardiac risk factors, medications, and previous exercise testing.
- Perform a pertinent physical exam, including evaluation for murmurs or gallops.
- Clarify indications for ET and confirm the patient does not meet any contraindications.
- Obtain a resting supine ECG and compare prior to assessing for changes.
- Consent patient and document risks versus benefits within the medical record.
- Educate the patient on what to expect during the ET to increase likelihood of high-quality and diagnostic data.

Protocol Selection

- If there are no contraindications to perform the ET, a protocol must then be selected. There are a number of protocols, each designed to increase the workload in stages, with the goal of achieving maximal effort at 8–12 minutes of exercise duration (24). Based on the clinical question, the physician must decide whether a maximal or submaximal test is required. The chosen protocol should be individualized based on the patient's age, exercise tolerance, and symptoms. Examples of exercise protocols include the following:
  - Bruce: This is the most commonly used and has the most extensive data, but the initial stage requires moderate aerobic capacity (~5METs) and has large (~3METs) increases between stages making it suboptimal for those with poor exercise capacity.
  - Modified Bruce: Allows for a more gradual increase in intensity with two stages prior to the standard Bruce protocol.
  - Balke and Naughton protocols provide more modest increases in workload between stages and can be useful in elderly, deconditioned patients.
  - Ramp protocols have a slow continuous increase in workload and have excellent correlation with VO_{2max} determinations.
  - Bicycle or arm ergometry may be beneficial when a treadmill is not appropriate but also to assess specific patients (such as a cyclist).
  - Custom protocols can and should be used to mimic speed/incline/duration that provoke symptoms for patients when they are exercising outside of the medical laboratory.

PERFORMING THE TEST

- A pretest checklist should include the following: an equipment safety check, consent and pretest assessment, supine and standing BP measurements, supine ECG, and protocol selection. During the ET, the patient and heart rhythm should be monitored continuously by trained personnel with ECG and BP readings at each stage. The patient should be alerted to stage changes, and in athletes and active people the test should be terminated when the patient reaches maximal effort *or* exhibits clinical signs requiring termination of the test and not a predetermined HR such as 85% of the APMHR (1). ET is safe, with death reported in 1 per 10,000 tests (25).
- Absolute indications for test termination:
  - ST elevations (>1.0 mm) in leads without preexisting Q waves (other than aVR, aVL, and V_1)
  - Moderate-severe angina or angina equivalents
  - Exertional drop in systolic BP (>10 mm Hg) from baseline when accompanied by any other evidence of ischemia
  - Serious arrhythmias (*e.g.*, ventricular tachycardia, second- or third-degree AV block)
  - Evidence of poor perfusion (*e.g.*, pallor, cyanosis, nausea or cold, clammy skin)

- Central nervous system symptoms (*e.g.*, ataxia, vertigo, visual or gait problems)
- Technical difficulties or equipment failure
- Patient's request to stop

- Relative indications for test termination:
  - Pronounced ECG changes from baseline (*e.g.*, >2 mm of horizontal or downsloping ST segment depression) in a patient with suspected ischemia
  - Arrhythmias including supraventricular tachycardia, atrial fibrillation, ventricular triplets, or nonsustained ventricular tachycardia that may interfere with hemodynamic stability
  - Exercise-induced bundle branch block that cannot be distinguished from ventricular tachycardia
  - Progressive or increasing chest pain
  - Pronounced fatigue, dyspnea, or wheezing
  - Leg cramps or claudication (grade 3)
  - Hypertensive response (systolic BP > 250 mm Hg or diastolic BP > 115 mm Hg)
  - Exertional drop in systolic BP (>10 mm Hg) from baseline in the absence of other evidence of ischemia
  - Oxygen saturation <80%
- After exercise cessation, the recovery stage begins. The patient may either be placed in the supine position immediately or allowed to perform a "cool-down walk." Because a "cool-down" period can delay or mask the appearance of ST depressions compared to abruptly returning the patient to supine, maximal test sensitivity is achieved with the patient supine after exercise. However, care should be taken as abrupt cessation of exercise can result in drop in venous return and hypotension. During the recovery phase, the clinician has the following responsibilities:
  - Auscultate for abnormal heart sounds (*e.g.*, new heart murmur or S3)
  - Auscultate lungs for any evidence of exercise-induced bronchospasm that might cause chest pain
  - Obtain BP and ECG 1-minute post-exercise and at subsequent 1-minute intervals until return to baseline (26).
  - Carefully monitor the patient for a minimum of 6 minutes or until clinically stable and ECG has returned to normal
  - Monitor carefully for any recovery-only ST segment depression and for ventricular arrhythmias in recovery (27,28).

INTERPRETATION OF THE TEST

- The ET report should outline the baseline ECG, HR, and BP as well as the presence of any arrhythmia during the study. Furthermore, the maximum BP, HR, METs, and stage achieved/total duration of exercise should be documented. Finally, the presence or absence of cardiopulmonary symptoms should be reported and the reason for ET termination should be included. Peak end-exercise of recovery-phase ST-segment deviation should be described, and the test should be defined as positive, negative, or equivocal (29). Prognostic information such as the Duke treadmill score, HR recovery, and chronotropic response are important parts of the ET report.
- A "normal" ET involves appropriate augmentation in HR and BP in response to graded exercise, no symptoms, and the absence of ECG changes suggestive of ischemia or arrhythmia. However, it is important to highlight that the diagnostic utility of the ET lies in the identification of obstructive CAD in an appropriately selected patient. A normal ET in a patient with a moderate to high pretest probability and typical CP symptoms may require ET with imaging or anatomic assessment to provide better accuracy for the assessment of obstructive CAD.

HR Response

- Physiologic increases in HR during aerobic exercise are in response to withdrawal of vagal tone and an increase in circulating catecholamines. The achieved HR_{max} during the maximal ET is often reported as a percentage of the APMHR. Chronotropic incompetence (CI) is the failure of the HR to appropriately augment during activity such that cardiac output cannot match metabolic demand (30). Several cutoffs have been proposed but <80% of the chronotropic index ([HR_{max}-resting HR]/[APMHR-resting HR] × 100) is typically used to diagnose CI (30). CI is a proven and independent predictor of mortality in the general population and may suggest underlying CAD (31).
- Before CI is considered, patient effort and medications (antiarrhythmics, AV nodal blockers) should be reviewed. Confirming maximal effort can be difficult on ET and CPET can be used to help objectively assess patient effort by assessing the respiratory exchange ratio (RER).
- Abnormal HR recovery, defined as the failure of the HR to decrease by 12 bpm during the first minute of the recovery period, portends an increased mortality (32).

Blood Pressure Response

- As workload increases, there is a corresponding increase in the systolic BP, which should peak at maximum exercise. A decrease in systolic BP during exercise is highly concerning and suggestive of underlying myocardial dysfunction (5). During exercise, the diastolic BP remains the same or decreases. An absolute increase in systolic BP ≥ 210 mm Hg (for men) and ≥190 (for women) is abnormal and an increase in diastolic BP of >10 mm Hg from baseline and/or absolute value > 90 mm Hg is abnormal (33). These findings are classified as a hypertensive response to exercise.
- The BP response during the recovery phase also has prognostic utility. A 3-minute post-exercise systolic BP/peak systolic BP > 0.90 is considered abnormal and equivalently predictive of CAD (75% positive predictive value) when compared to ST segment depressions during ET (26,34).

Signs and Symptoms

- The presence or absence of symptoms during ET, such as chest pain, claudication, wheezing, and dyspnea, should be mentioned in the report. Patients with exercise-induced typical angina are predictive of CAD and are even more concerning when associated with ST-segment depression (35). Signs of poor perfusion and new gallop or murmur on examination suggest LV dysfunction resulting from exercise (36).

Arrhythmias/Conduction Disturbances

- Ventricular ectopic activity is seen in up to 20% of patients during ET; however, frequent ventricular ectopy is seen in only 2%–3% (5). The physiologic response in the healthy individual is for PVCs to suppress with increasing work. If exercise results in an increased PVC burden or nonsustained ventricular tachycardia (NSVT) then further consideration should be given to underlying CVD. Recent data have shown that in asymptomatic individuals, high-grade PVCs occurring during the recovery period were associated with long-term risk of cardiovascular mortality, whereas PVCs only during exercise were not (28).
- Exercise-induced supraventricular arrhythmias are not predictive of ischemia or any cardiovascular endpoint.
- Exercise-induced advanced AV block (Mobitz type II and higher) are abnormal and require further investigation.
- Bundle branch blocks occur infrequently with exercise and require further evaluation, especially left bundle branch block, which may portend an increased mortality if structural heart disease is present (37).

Aerobic Capacity

- The ET can either measure the maximal functional aerobic capacity (VO_{2max}) by direct gas analysis as part of a CPET or estimate it from workload performed in a maximal ET. A nomogram is used to convert minutes (or METs) into VO_{2max}. The results can then be compared with standard tables of fitness levels for age and sex (20).

Electrocardiographic Responses to Exercise Testing

- ST segment changes are the most common signs of ischemia. ST segment *depression* represents subendocardial ischemia but does not localize ischemia to a precise coronary territory. Conversely, ST segment *elevation* represents transmural ischemia and the location of the anatomic ischemia does correlate with associated ECG changes.

Normal Responses With Exercise (1)

- The PR segment shortens and slopes downward in the inferior leads. The QRS complex may show increased Q wave magnitude in lateral leads, a decrease in R wave amplitude with an increased S wave depth in inferior leads. The J point may become depressed with exercise. If already elevated at rest, it will commonly normalize. The T wave decreases in amplitude early in exercise but normalizes at higher workloads and may have increased amplitude in early recovery, and the ST segment can develop a positive upslope that returns to baseline within 60–80 ms.

Abnormal Responses With Exercise

- ST segment depression: The traditional hallmark of exercise-induced ischemia (see next section). ST-segment depression has been shown to be the strongest predictor of both cardiac death and a composite of cardiac death and nonfatal MI in a Duke study of 2842 patients (38). Three of more consecutive beats in the same lead with stable baseline should be identified to assess for magnitude of ST segment depression. Clinicians should visually verify computer-averaged complexes. ST segment depression may be upsloping, horizontal, or downsloping.
- ST segment normalization: T-wave inversion or ST-segment depression that are present at rest may normalize (pseudonormalization) during exercise and may reflect significant underlying CAD. However, in normal subjects with resting J-point elevation because of early repolarization, the ST level normalization with exercise should be considered a normal finding and not be considered equivalent to ST depression in relation to the elevated baseline.
- ST segment elevation: In patients without a prior history of MI, consider acute MI (especially if accompanied by chest pain) or transmural ischemia involving proximal high-grade stenosis. Less often, this may be seen with severe coronary artery spasm (Prinzmetal angina) in otherwise nonobstructive or normal coronary arteries (14). ST elevations, in the presence of Q waves may represent areas of peri-infarct ischemia, abnormal ventricular wall motion, or ventricular aneurysm (18).
- U-wave inversion: U-wave inversion during exercise is suggestive of single-vessel ischemia of the left anterior descending artery, but U-wave changes are typically seen with ST segment changes (39).

Final Determination for MI

- Positive
  - Horizontal ST segment depression ≥1 mm at 60–80 ms past the J point
  - Downsloping ST segment depression ≥1 mm at the J point *or* J + 20 ms
  - ST segment elevation >1 mm at 60 ms after the J point
- Negative
  - Above criteria are not met and the patient achieved at least 85% of APMHR
- Equivocal
  - Above criteria are not met and the patient DOES NOT achieve at least 85% of APMHR
  - ≥1 mm upsloping ST segment depression
  - ST segment depression in the setting of preexistent preexcitation

CLINICAL DECISION MAKING

- The results of the ET should be used to help inform further management of the patient. This approach should include a probability statement of CAD and a prediction of CAD severity, prognosis of the likelihood of future adverse events based on prognostic indicators such as the Duke Treadmill Score (DTS) (40), the functional capacity of the patient, HRR. The strongest predictor of prognosis from the ET is functional capacity (5).

Pretest Probability of Coronary Artery Disease

- Meta-analyses have demonstrated the mean sensitivity and specificity of the ET are 68% and 77%, respectively (2). The diagnostic value of the ET for the detection of ischemia heart disease is influenced depending largely on the patient's overall pretest probability of having CAD.
- In the assessment of ischemic heart disease, the ET is less accurate in those with very low, low or high pretest probability of ischemic heart disease and should not be routinely used for this indication (1). Pretest probability has traditionally been assessed using the Diamond/Forrester score, which includes age, sex, and clinical symptoms (41). However, more recent data suggest that this score may overestimate CAD prevalence given all patients had diagnostic coronary angiography and thus subject to work-up bias.
- The CAD consortium clinical score (42), which is derived from data that use CT coronary angiography and includes age, sex, type of pain, presence of atherosclerotic risk factors, has been shown to have greater predictive accuracy for obstructive CAD than the Diamond/Forrester score (43).

Prediction of Severity of CAD

- At present, a validated calculator is not available to assess the post-test likelihood of obstructive CAD but in a given patient this can be estimated using exercise ST-segment criteria couple with knowledge of the sensitivity and specific of the ET. ET findings that increase concern for significant CAD include severe ST segment depression, ST segment depression beginning at low workloads, diffuse ST depression, prolonged ST segment depression in recovery, ST elevation, and exercise induced hypotension (1).
- In asymptomatic patients, ST depression exclusively at high workloads generally correlates with a low mortality and good overall prognosis. In fact, the ability to exercise at >10 METs has a good prognosis regardless of the ECG changes (44,45).

Duke Exercise Treadmill Score

- The DTS is a validated prognostic tool that assists with risk assessment in those undergoing ET by using standard Bruce protocol exercise duration, maximal ST segment deviation, and exercise-induced angina to assign a weighted index score to estimate average annual cardiovascular mortality risk, 5-year survival, and categorizes individuals into low-, moderate-, and high-risk groups (38,40).
- The DTS is calculated by the equation: exercise duration (minutes) – [5 × maximal ST deviation (mm)] – [4 × treadmill angina index]. Treadmill angina index = 0 if no exercise-associated angina, 1 for exercise-associated angina, and 2 for exercise-limiting angina) with a range of −25 to +15. However, this scoring system does not include known CAD risk factors including age, HR, and BP. It works equally well in males and females and has been validated in those with diabetes but has not been extensively studied in the elderly, or those with congenital heart disease, prior cardiac surgery, or uninterpretable baseline ECG (46).
  - Low risk: score ≥ +5. The patient has a very good prognosis, with a survival rate of 97%.
  - Moderate risk: a score of −10 to +4 is associated with an intermediate prognosis.
  - High risk: score ≤ −11. The patient has a poor prognosis, with a 5-year survival rate of 65%.

Exercise Prescription

- The ET can assist in determination of the exercise prescription. A maximal ET establishes a baseline fitness level and individualized HR_{max}. All training sessions should incorporate warm-up and cool-down phases. The core components of the exercise prescription include defining the frequency, intensity, duration, and type of training for patients and should be tailored to each patient based on their goals, health status, physical ability, and fitness (20). Prior to initiating an exercise regimen, patients should be assessed by the preparticipation screening methods as previously discussed.

SPECIAL POPULATION CONSIDERATIONS

Exercise Stress Testing in Athletes

- Although exercise remains the cornerstone of maintaining health, it does not negate other risk factors and athletes are not immune from developing CAD, or other cardiovascular comorbidities. ET in athletes can be nuanced and ideally should try to reproduce the conditions that provoke symptoms during their training. CPET with ramp protocols to maximal volitional effort are routinely employed given better mimic exercise physiology and provides data on exercise physiology and maximal aerobic capacity. Certain techniques may enhance the diagnostic utility such as using a cycle ergometer for a cyclist or adding sprints/custom ET after the standard protocol to elicit symptoms (47).

- Athletes manifest many differences compared with the general population both clinically and on ECG. They commonly have increased ventricular volume and mass along with sinus bradyarrhythmias. It is common to see certain ECG findings such as first-degree AV blocks, right axis deviation, ventricular hypertrophy with repolarization abnormalities, or right bundle branch block. These findings are considered benign and part the electrical remodeling seen with vigorous training (48).
- The diagnostic criteria of the ET in athletes are the same as the general population but the interpretation can be nuanced. For example, a VO_{2max} of 100% predicted may be a concerning result in an endurance athlete with symptoms who trains vigorously 6 days a week. Knowing that the reference population is healthy but not athletic, we would expect this athlete's VO_{2max} to be well above 100% predicted.

Exercise Stress Testing in Females

- Historically, women with CAD are more likely to have a delay in diagnosis, worse prognosis, and incomplete and/or suboptimal therapy when compared to their male counterparts. Importantly, women with anginal symptoms or abnormal stress tests are less likely to be referred for further management (49).
- There are a number of differences between men and women, which may account for this including the fact that compared to men, women had more baseline ST- and T-wave changes (50,51), more ST depressions with exercise (52), and in recovery, as well as digoxin-like effects from natural and exogenous circulating estrogen seen in pre- and post-menopausal females, respectively (53).
- ST segment depressions occurring during an ET are thought to be less accurate in identifying CAD in women when compared to men (49). Based on two meta-analyses, sensitivity, and specificity of ST depressions in intermediate-risk women is lower compared to their male counterparts (61% vs. 68%) and (70% vs. 77%), respectively (54).
- The positive predictive value of a positive test is lower in women compared to men given the lower overall prevalence of CAD, 47% versus 77%, respectively (55).
- Although this is a multifaceted public health issue for which there is active work ongoing, current recommendations continue to endorse similar stress test selection algorithms when evaluating both men and women for CAD. Furthermore, the incorporation of the exercise capacity, chronotropic response, HRR, BP response, and DTS can all be used to further enhance diagnostic and prognostic utility of the ET.
- Exercise capacity remains an important prognostic marker in asymptomatic and symptomatic women with 17%–25% reduced in rate of all cause death for every 1 MET increase in exercise capacity (56,57).

Exercise Stress Testing in Black Patients

- There is a paucity of published data comparing ET among races, with the majority of data discussing racial differences in CRF between black and white patients. Data on Medicare beneficiaries show that despite similar physician visit frequency, black patients were less likely to have stress tests compared to nonblack men (58).
- Maximal exercise capacity has been shown to be significantly, albeit only modestly, higher in white males compared to black males (59). Black and white females had similar exercise capacities (60).
- Given the severe lack of data in this space, future studies are necessary to examine diagnostic and prognostic differences in ET among different races as well behavioral, cultural, socioeconomical, and physiological reasons for these differences.

SUMMARY

- ET has many applications that provide significant value in the evaluation and treatment of athletes. Primary care sports clinicians can utilize ET to help in clinical decision making.
- At the time of this manuscript submission, the ACSM was preparing an updated 12th edition of the *Guidelines for Exercise Testing and Prescription*. This text is currently published, and there are no substantive changes in the tables and figures that accompany this chapter on exercise testing. However, there is new guidance for using the results of exercise testing for prescribing exercise and the reader is referred to this new resource (61).

REFERENCES

1. Fletcher GF, Ades PA, Kligfield P, et al. Exercise standards for testing and training: a scientific statement from the American Heart Association. *Circulation*. 2013;128(8):873–934.
2. Gianrossi R, Detrano R, Mulvihill D, et al. Exercise-induced ST depression in the diagnosis of coronary artery disease. A meta-analysis. *Circulation*. 1989;80(1):87–98.
3. Geleijnse ML, Fioretti PM, Roelandt JR. Methodology, feasibility, safety and diagnostic accuracy of dobutamine stress echocardiography. *J Am Coll Cardiol*. 1997;30(3):595–606.
4. Pellikka PA, Nagueh SF, Elhendy AA, Kuehl CA, Sawada SG, American Society of Echocardiography. American Society of Echocardiography recommendations for performance, interpretation, and application of stress echocardiography. *J Am Soc Echocardiogr*. 2007;20(9):1021–41.
5. Libby P, Bonow RO, Mann DL, et al. *Exercise Physiology and Exercise Electrocardiographic Testing. Braunwald's Heart Disease*. 12th ed. Philadelphia, PA: Elsevier, 2022, p. 175–95.
6. Levine BD. VO_{2max}: what do we know, and what do we still need to know?. *J Physiol*. 2008;586(1):25–34.
7. Fox SM 3rd, Naughton JP, Haskell WL. Physical activity and the prevention of coronary heart disease. *Ann Clin Res*. 1971;3(6):404–32.
8. Arena R, Myers J, Kaminsky LA. Revisiting age-predicted maximal heart rate: can it be used as a valid measure of effort?. *Am Heart J*. 2016;173:49–56.
9. Martinez MW, Kim JH, Shah AB, et al. Exercise-induced cardiovascular adaptations and approach to exercise and cardiovascular disease: JACC state-of-the-art review. *J Am Coll Cardiol*. 2021;78(14):1453–70.

10. Dempsey JA, Sheel AW, Haverkamp HC, Babcock MA, Harms CA. The John Sutton Lecture: CSEP, 2002. Pulmonary system limitations to exercise in health. *Can J Appl Physiol.* 2003;28(suppl l):S2–24.
11. Powers SK, Williams J. Exercise-induced hypoxaemia in highly trained athletes. *Sports Med.* 1987;4(1):46–53.
12. Jensen L, Bangsbo J, Hellsten Y. Effect of high intensity training on capillarization and presence of angiogenic factors in human skeletal muscle. *J Physiol.* 2004;557(pt 2):571–82.
13. Kokkinos P, Myers J, Faselis C, et al. Exercise capacity and mortality in older men: a 20-year follow-up study. *Circulation.* 2010;122(8):790–7.
14. Blair SN, Haskell WL. Objectively measured physical activity and mortality in older adults. *JAMA.* 2006;296(2):216–8.
15. Bourque JM, Charlton GT, Holland BH, Belyea CM, Watson DD, Beller GA. Prognosis in patients achieving ≥10 METS on exercise stress testing: was SPECT imaging useful?. *J Nucl Cardiol.* 2011;18(2):230–7.
16. Ainsworth BE, Haskell WL, Herrmann SD, et al. 2011 Compendium of physical activities: a second update of codes and MET values. *Med Sci Sports Exerc.* 2011;43(8):1575–81.
17. Kitamura K, Jorgensen CR, Gobel FL, Taylor HL, Wang Y. Hemodynamic correlates of myocardial oxygen consumption during upright exercise. *J Appl Physiol.* 1972;32(4):516–22.
18. Balady GJ, Arena R, Sietsema K, et al. Clinician's guide to cardiopulmonary exercise testing in adults: a scientific statement from the American Heart Association. *Circulation.* 2010;122(2):191–225.
19. Husaini M, Emery MS. Cardiopulmonary exercise testing interpretation in athletes: what the cardiologist should know. *Cardiol Clin.* 2024;16(1):71–80.
20. Ozmel C. *ACSM's Guideline for Exercise Testing and Prescription.* 11 ed. Philadelphia: Wolters Kluwer, 2022.
21. van de Sande DA, Breuer MA, Kemps HM. Utility of exercise electrocardiography in pre-participation screening in asymptomatic athletes: a systematic review. *Sports Med.* 2016;46(8):1155–64.
22. Franklin BA. Preventing exercise-related cardiovascular events: is a medical examination more urgent for physical activity or inactivity?. *Circulation.* 2014;129(10):1081–4.
23. Riebe D, Franklin BA, Thompson PD, et al. Updating ACSM's recommendations for exercise preparticipation health screening. *Med Sci Sports Exerc.* 2015;47(11):2473–9.
24. Myers J, Froelicher VF. Optimizing the exercise test for pharmacological investigations. *Circulation.* 1990;82(5):1839–46.
25. Myers J, Voodi L, Umann T, Froelicher VF. A survey of exercise testing: methods, utilization, interpretation, and safety in the VAHCS. *J Cardiopulm Rehabil.* 2000;20(4):251–8.
26. Taylor AJ, Beller GA. Postexercise systolic blood pressure response: clinical application to the assessment of ischemic heart disease. *Am Fam Physician.* 1998;58(5):1126–30.
27. Lachterman B, Lehmann KG, Abrahamson D, Froelicher VF. Recovery only ST-segment depression and the predictive accuracy of the exercise test. *Ann Intern Med.* 1990;112(1):11–6.
28. Refaat MM, Gharios C, Moorthy MV, et al. Exercise-induced ventricular ectopy and cardiovascular mortality in asymptomatic individuals. *J Am Coll Cardiol.* 2021;78(23):2267–77.
29. Goldschlager N, Selzer A, Cohn K. Treadmill stress tests as indicators of presence and severity of coronary artery disease. *Ann Intern Med.* 1976;85(3):277–86.
30. Zweerink A, van der Lingen ALCJ, Handoko ML, van Rossum AC, Allaart CP. Chronotropic incompetence in chronic heart failure. *Circ Heart Fail.* 2018;11(8):e004969.
31. Lauer MS, Francis GS, Okin PM, Pashkow FJ, Snader CE, Marwick TH. Impaired chronotropic response to exercise stress testing as a predictor of mortality. *JAMA.* 1999;281(6):524–9.
32. Califf RM, McKinnis RA, McNeer JF, et al. Prognostic value of ventricular arrhythmias associated with treadmill exercise testing in patients studied with cardiac catheterization for suspected ischemic heart disease. *J Am Coll Cardiol.* 1983;2(6):1060–7.
33. Le VV, Mitiku T, Sungar G, Myers J, Froelicher V. The blood pressure response to dynamic exercise testing: a systematic review. *Prog Cardiovasc Dis.* 2008;51(2):135–60.
34. Taylor AJ, Beller GA. Postexercise systolic blood pressure response: association with the presence and extent of perfusion abnormalities on thallium-201 scintigraphy. *Am Heart J.* 1995;129(2):227–34.
35. Weiner DA, McCabe C, Hueter DC, Ryan TJ, Hood WB Jr. The predictive value of anginal chest pain as an indicator of coronary disease during exercise testing. *Am Heart J.* 1978;96(4):458–62.
36. Tavel ME. The appearance of gallop rhythm after exercise stress testing. *Clin Cardiol.* 1996;19(11):887–91.
37. Grady TA, Chiu AC, Snader CE, et al. Prognostic significance of exercise-induced left bundle-branch block. *JAMA.* 1998;279(2):153–6.
38. Mark DB, Hlatky MA, Harrell FE Jr, Lee KL, Califf RM, Pryor DB. Exercise treadmill score for predicting prognosis in coronary artery disease. *Ann Intern Med.* 1987;106(6):793–800.
39. Kodama K, Hiasa G, Ohtsuka T, et al. Transient U wave inversion during treadmill exercise testing in patients with left anterior descending coronary artery disease. *Angiology.* 2000;51(7):581–9.
40. Mark DB, Shaw L, Harrell FE Jr, et al. Prognostic value of a treadmill exercise score in outpatients with suspected coronary artery disease. *N Engl J Med.* 1991;325(12):849–53.
41. Diamond GA, Forrester JS. Analysis of probability as an aid in the clinical diagnosis of coronary-artery disease. *N Engl J Med.* 1979;300(24):1350–8.
42. Genders TS, Steyerberg EW, Hunink MG, et al. Prediction model to estimate presence of coronary artery disease: retrospective pooled analysis of existing cohorts. *BMJ.* 2012;344:e3485.
43. Bittencourt MS, Hulten E, Polonsky TS, et al. European society of cardiology-recommended coronary artery disease consortium pretest probability scores more accurately predict obstructive coronary disease and cardiovascular events than the Diamond and forrester score: the partners registry. *Circulation.* 2016;134(3):201–11.
44. Thompson CA, Jabbour S, Goldberg RJ, et al. Exercise performance-based outcomes of medically treated patients with coronary artery disease and profound ST segment depression. *J Am Coll Cardiol.* 2000;36(7):2140–5.
45. Bourque JM, Holland BH, Watson DD, Beller GA. Achieving an exercise workload of > or = 10 metabolic equivalents predicts a very low risk of inducible ischemia: does myocardial perfusion imaging have a role?. *J Am Coll Cardiol.* 2009;54(6):538–45.
46. Lakkireddy DR, Bhakkad J, Korlakunta HL, et al. Prognostic value of the Duke treadmill score in diabetic patients. *Am Heart J.* 2005;150(3):516–21.
47. Churchill TW, Disanto M, Singh TK, et al. Diagnostic yield of customized exercise provocation following routine testing. *Am J Cardiol.* 2019;123(12):2044–50.
48. Drezner JA, Sharma S, Baggish A, et al. International criteria for electrocardiographic interpretation in athletes: consensus statement. *Br J Sports Med.* 2017;51(9):704–31.
49. Kohli P, Gulati M. Exercise stress testing in women: going back to the basics. *Circulation.* 2010;122(24):2570–80.
50. Cumming GR, Dufresne C, Kich L, Samm J. Exercise electrocardiogram patterns in normal women. *Br Heart J.* 1973;35(10):1055–61.
51. Higgins JP, Higgins JA. Electrocardiographic exercise stress testing: an update beyond the ST segment. *Int J Cardiol.* 2007;116(3):285–99.

52. Weiner DA, Ryan TJ, McCabe CH, et al. Exercise stress testing. Correlations among history of angina, ST-segment response and prevalence of coronary-artery disease in the Coronary Artery Surgery Study (CASS). *N Engl J Med.* 1979;301:230–5.
53. Grzybowski A, Puchalski W, Zieba B, et al. How to improve noninvasive coronary artery disease diagnostics in premenopausal women? The influence of menstrual cycle on ST depression, left ventricle contractility, and chest pain observed during exercise echocardiography in women with angina and normal coronary angiogram. *Am Heart J.* 2008;156(5):e964.e1–5.
54. Kwok Y, Kim C, Grady D, Segal M, Redberg R. Meta-analysis of exercise testing to detect coronary artery disease in women. *Am J Cardiol.* 1999;83(5):660–6.
55. Barolsky SM, Gilbert CA, Faruqui A, Nutter DO, Schlant RC. Differences in electrocardiographic response to exercise of women and men: a non-Bayesian factor. *Circulation.* 1979;60(5):1021–7.
56. Roger VL, Jacobsen SJ, Pellikka PA, Miller TD, Bailey KR, Gersh BJ. Prognostic value of treadmill exercise testing: a population-based study in Olmsted County, Minnesota. *Circulation.* 1998;98(25):2836–41.
57. Gulati M, Pandey DK, Arnsdorf MF, et al. Exercise capacity and the risk of death in women: the St James women take heart project. *Circulation.* 2003;108(13):1554–9.
58. Lucas FL, Siewers AE, DeLorenzo MA, Wennberg DE. Differences in cardiac stress testing by sex and race among Medicare beneficiaries. *Am Heart J.* 2007;154(3):502–9.
59. Swift DL, Staiano AE, Johannsen NM, et al. Low cardiorespiratory fitness in African Americans: a health disparity risk factor?. *Sports Med.* 2013;43(12):1301–13.
60. Lavie CJ, Kuruvanka T, Milani RV, Prasad A, Ventura HO. Exercise capacity in adult African-Americans referred for exercise stress testing: is fitness affected by race?. *Chest.* 2004;126(6):1962–8.
61. Ozemek C. *ACSM's Guideline for Exercise Testing and Prescription.* 12 ed. Philadelphia: Wolters Kluwer; 2025.

Gait Analysis

Nathaniel Nye, Jacqueline Yurgil, and Francis G. O'Connor

25

INTRODUCTION

- The goal of gait analysis is to understand the complex relationships between an individual's capabilities/impairments and their gait pattern, thus providing a basis for gait modifications to enhance performance while reducing injury risk (1,2).
- Advancing technology allows providers to capture immense quantities of increasingly complex data on a patient's gait. However, analyzing such large quantities of data and integrating them into a rational treatment plan requires significant time and expertise, thus most high-level gait analysis is performed at specialized clinics with gait laboratories. Nevertheless, there is much that a sports medicine physician can do within the confines of a routine clinic visit (3).
- Modern gait analysis techniques enable the clinician to understand the effects of both intrinsic (*e.g.*, muscle strength, joint range of motion) and extrinsic (*e.g.*, footwear, orthoses) factors that influence an individual's biomechanics (3).
- An array of tools, from simple to highly sophisticated, can be utilized in gait analysis. Despite being simple and low-tech, visual gait observation and slow-motion video with markup software are powerful in experienced hands and remain the most common techniques in a sports medicine clinic. Additional tools include inertial measurement units (IMU), pressure-sensing mats or insoles, pressure-plated treadmills, force-plated treadmills and force platforms, 3-D motion capture (infrared stereophotogrammetric cameras), and surface electromyography (EMG).
- Gait analysis techniques are a key component of many rehabilitation protocols. A running-related overuse injury (*e.g.*, patellofemoral pain, iliotibial band syndrome, bone stress injury) is likely to recur if the underlying biomechanics are not addressed. Gait analysis also has important roles in rehabilitation following stroke or limb loss, children with cerebral palsy or individuals with disabilities, and for performance optimization (often with elite athletes) (4).

The authors acknowledge the work of Timothy L. Switaj, Brian R. Hoke, and Francis G. O'Connor, who skillfully authored the version of this chapter that appeared in the first edition of this textbook.

FUNDAMENTALS AND PRACTICAL ASPECTS OF GAIT ANALYSIS

Gait Analysis Terminology

- Step Length: the distance between one footfall and the next (left vs right) during walking or running gait, as measured from the same part of each foot.
- Stride Length: the distance between consecutive footfalls with the same foot (*e.g.*, left foot initial contact to the subsequent left foot initial contact) during walking or running gait.
- Cadence: the step rate or step frequency during gait (*e.g.*, 170 steps $\cdot$ min^{-1}).
- Pronation: a complex, triplanar movement of the foot and ankle that occurs during the stance phase, serving as a normal loading response and a necessary mechanism for shock absorption and elastic energy storage. The primary components of foot/ankle pronation include rearfoot (subtalar) eversion, forefoot abduction, ankle dorsiflexion, and tibial internal rotation. Pronation is not an isolated event but a coordinated movement of these interconnected segments. Maximum pronation is attained just after heel-off (transition from midstance to terminal stance), during maximum force application to the ground (3).
- Supination: simply put, supination is pronation in reverse. Supination occurs during the terminal stance phase and serves to return the foot to a more rigid lever for energy transfer during toe-off (transition from terminal stance to float phases). The foot and ankle also supinate in preparation for initial contact, at which point the foot/ankle again begins to pronate as the cycle continues.
- Ground reaction force (GRF): the force exerted by the ground on the foot during stance phase. Like all forces, GRF has a magnitude and vector (in 3 dimensions). In accordance with Newton's third law (for every force in nature there is an equal and opposite reaction), this can be thought of as "how hard the runner hits the ground." During heel strike gait, vertical GRF reaches a first peak at initial contact and a second peak (typically higher magnitude) during terminal stance as the runner pushes the ground away, propelling the body upward and forward. In contrast, midfoot and forefoot gait patterns typically exhibit a single vertical GRF peak, which occurs during terminal stance.

GAIT CYCLE

- The basic unit of walking and running is the gait cycle or stride. Perry et al. described various temporal and functional variables within the gait cycle, and this has become a standard paradigm to describe gait (5). The running gait cycle is depicted in Figure 25.1.
- The walking gait cycle is primarily divided into double support and single support phases (no float phase), whereas the running gait cycle is divided into stance and float phases. During the single support or stance phase, one lower extremity is in stance while the other is in a swing phase. While walking, stance and swing begin at initial and final contact of the foot, respectively. The percentages of time in stance and swing are reversed in walking and running: walking is made up of about 60% stance and 40% swing compared to about 40% and 60%, respectively, for running (4,6). During normal walking at an average speed, each double-limb support time comprises approximately 10% of the gait cycle. Walking gait is described as an inverse pendular motion, meaning the pendulum pivot point is at the ground as the body advances over the planted foot.
- When focusing on functional aspects of gait, the gait cycle can be divided into three functional tasks: weight acceptance, single limb support, and limb advancement, with the first two occurring during stance and the third occurring primarily during swing. The tasks are further subdivided into eight phases: weight acceptance comprises initial contact and loading response; single-limb support comprises midstance, terminal stance, and preswing; and limb advancement comprises initial swing, midswing, and terminal swing.
- There is no single "correct" way to walk or run. Every athlete is unique in many ways (age, limb length, foot structure, running experience/history, etc.), which will influence their current and optimal gait patterns. There is an art to running, and some variability is allowed as each runner uses their own strategies to accomplish the goals of movement. Nevertheless, there are several key fundamental principles that pertain to optimal human gait and can be assessed during gait analysis. In simple terms, these can be thought of as the runner's "hardware" (skeletal alignment, joint mobility, core strength and stability, large muscle strength, tendon stiffness) and "software" (posture, muscle activation patterns, movement coordination/skill).

CLINICAL EVALUATION

- Prior to evaluating an athlete's gait, a thoughtful and detailed clinical history and examination are vital to provide background, context, and direction for the gait analysis.
- A targeted running history should include the age at which the athlete began running regularly, competition history, periods off running (whether due to injury or other factors),

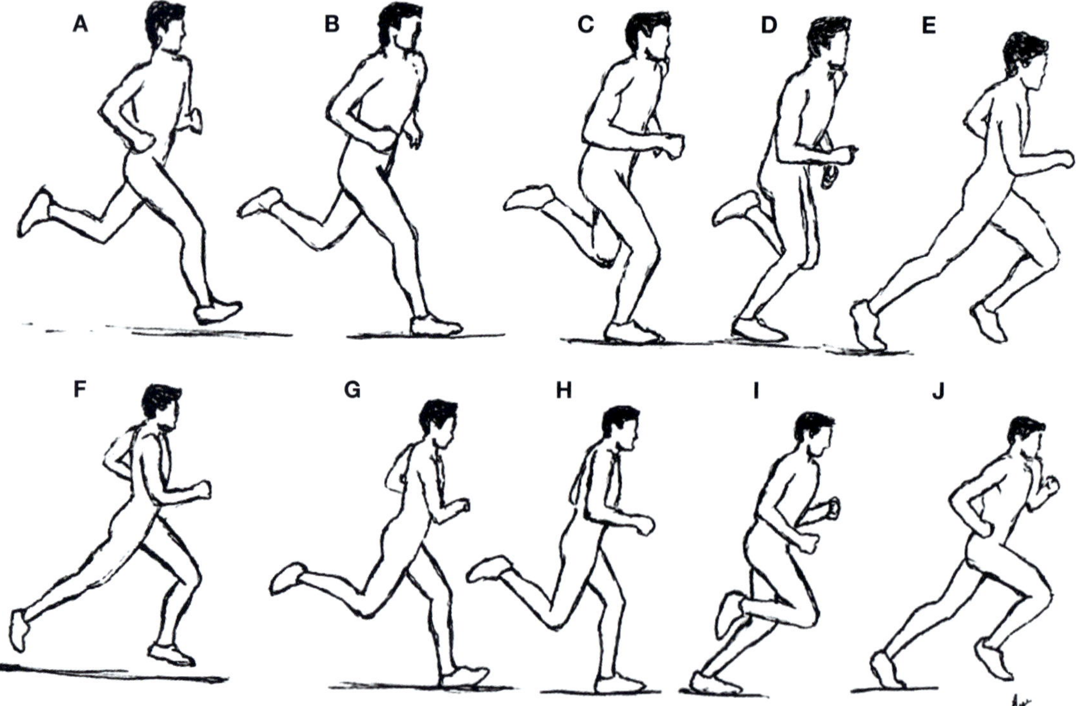

Figure 25.1: Biomechanical activity during various phases of the gait cycle, referring to the right lower extremity. A: Float, terminal swing right, B: Initial contact, C: Early stance, D: Midstance, E: Terminal stance or "toe-off", F: Float, early swing right, G: Early swing, H: Early swing, progressing to midswing, I: Midswing, J: Late swing. (From Prasanth H, Caban M, Keller U, et al. Wearable sensor-based real-time gait detection: a systematic review. *Sensors*. 2021 Apr 13;21(8):2727.)

history of running-related injuries, shoe history, other sports participation (How well-rounded is the athlete? What other demands are being placed on the body?), and importantly, their current goals with running.

- An astute physical examination can provide important data that sheds light on why a runner may display particular patterns during gait. The clinician should consider examining the following aspects:
  - Standing posture (cervical, scapulothoracic, lumbopelvic)
  - Hip mobility, in particular extension (essential during propulsive movements of late stance phase)
  - Knee mobility, in particular quadriceps and hamstring flexibility
  - Ankle mobility, particularly tibiotalar dorsiflexion (required for "ankle rocker" movement, which allows the foot to progress behind the runner during midstance to terminal stance phases without prematurely elevating the heel)
  - First metatarsophalangeal joint mobility, most importantly dorsiflexion (required during terminal stance)
  - Single leg balance (evaluated with eyes open and eyes closed)
  - Single leg squat, to evaluate quad/core/foot strength and stability, preferred muscle activation patterns (*e.g.*, quadricep dominance), balance/postural control during movement, and skill/coordination of movement.
    - See Chapter 72, Principles of Rehabilitation and Return to Sport, for further discussion.

GAIT EVALUATION

- Clinically meaningful information can be obtained from the wealth of data gathered from the instruments and analysis techniques available. Whether utilizing simple or more sophisticated tools, the clinician gets a glimpse into the athlete's movement patterns and then must integrate this information into a coherent rehabilitation and gait retraining plan. Stretching and strengthening key muscle groups is important but insufficient to alter gait mechanics. Gait retraining utilizing cues and feedback must be integrated to result in neuromuscular reeducation (1).
- In analyzing gait (in particular, an atypical gait pattern or an effect of a shoe type, brace, musculoskeletal injury, or impairment), at least two distinct qualities need to be considered (3).
- The first is energetics (*i.e.*, how does the pattern, shoe, etc., affect metabolic cost); this can be measured directly with oxygen consumption or indirectly with center of mass (CoM) calculations (paired with observing whether EMG activities are consistent with kinetic needs).
- The second is the risk for biomechanical injury (*i.e.*, how does the pattern affect risk over time for ligamentous, muscle, tendon, cartilage, or bone injury); this is best estimated with joint kinetics, in particular joint moments. When measured to be higher than normal, these may indicate a greater risk for injury (1).

Video Observational Gait Analysis

- Video observational gait analysis (VOGA) techniques can assist in the identification of minute discrepancies that are not visible in real-time analysis by clinical observation.
- VOGA typically starts with the placement of reflective tape, or other markers, on key landmarks of the human body. Commonly used landmarks are listed in Table 25.1 and depicted in Figure 25.2. VOGA can also be accomplished without reflective markers, but a degree of precision may be lost; when not using surface markers, the clinician measures angles based on the approximate location of joint centers.
- VOGA is conducted through protocols with differing views across all phases of gait during either walking, running, or both. Table 25.2 represents sample, simple and detailed video protocols.
- Provider analysis of videotaped results is variable based on the degree of training and experience in gait analysis (1,3). Modern tablets are convenient and effective tools for VOGA. Their large screens assist with analysis and education of patients, cameras with high resolution and high frame rates allow slow-motion analysis, and motion analysis applications aid in the detection of fine abnormalities.

Table 25.1 Reflective Surface Marker Landmarks — Sample Protocol

Body Part	Marker Position Landmark
Head	Zygomatic arch
Shoulder	Acromion
Elbow	Lateral epicondyle
Wrist	Ulnar styloid
Hip	Greater trochanter
Hip	Anterior superior iliac spine
Lower back	Posterior superior iliac spine
Knee	Lateral femoral condyle
Knee	Popliteal fossa
Knee	Patella midpoint
Lower leg	Tibial tuberosity
Lower leg	Bisection of distal third of tib/fib
Ankle	Lateral malleolus
Foot	Lateral border parallel to floor
Posterior foot	Calcaneal bisection (posterior heel)
Foot	Midline of second metatarsal

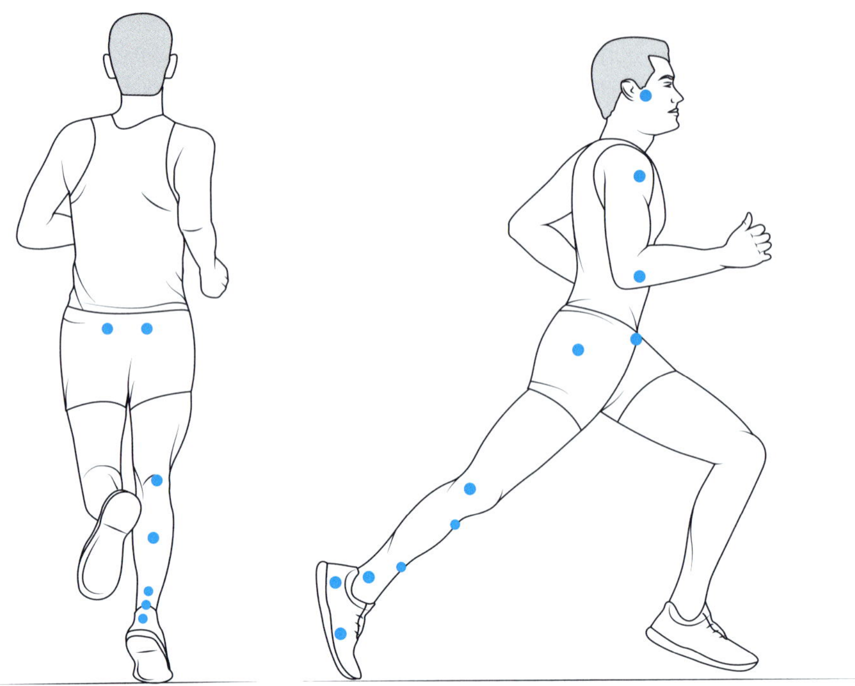

Figure 25.2: Placement of reflective surface markers over skeletal landmarks.

- VOGA protocols present a systematic approach to identify subtle pathology in runners. After marking surface landmarks and conducting the filming protocol, the trained provider must perform an analysis of the video footage. This is best performed by working through the footage from the head to the feet and in all phases of motion. Angles between reflective markers landmarks are the most common measurements needed and the most likely to yield relevant findings. The key is to identify the most relevant deficiencies or abnormalities and integrate these observations into a cohesive rehabilitation and gait retraining plan for the athlete.

Table 25.2 Video Gait Analysis Session — Detailed and Abbreviated Protocols

Camera Angle	Detailed Protocol	Abbreviated Protocol
Static Posture (head to feet)	Anterior: 10 s Lateral: 10 s Posterior: 10 s	Visual observation only
Lateral (sagittal plane) view	Head to feet: 30 s Hips to feet: 30 s	Head to feet: 10 s
Posterior (frontal plane) view	Head to feet: 30 s Hips to feet: 30 s Knee to feet: 30 s Shoes off (walking): 30 s Shoes off (running): 30 s	Head to feet: 10 s Shoes off (running): 10 s (optional)
Anterior (frontal plane) view	Head to feet: 30 s Hips to feet: 30 s Knees to feet: 30 s	Visual observation only

- A basic VOGA may include assessment of multiple variables in the sagittal plane including posture (craniocervical, scapulothoracic, lumbopelvic), torso orientation, tibial inclination angle, knee flexion angle (at initial foot contact and at midstance), and hip extension (at its maximum, during toe-off). Additional variables should be assessed in the frontal plane, including pelvic drop, hip adduction in midstance, dynamic knee valgus, degree and duration of foot/ankle pronation and supination, arm movement, step width (also called base of support), trunk lean, and trunk rotation. A depiction of basic sagittal and frontal plane measurements is shown in Figure 25.3. Finally, several important variables are not specific to any plane but should also be assessed, including cadence, ground contact time, and float time (or float ratio, which is calculated as the float time divided by the time/duration of one step cycle). When completing a clinical gait analysis report, additional notes should be made concerning shoe wear patterns and treadmill speed/incline.

Getting Started: Building Gait Analysis Capability Within a Clinic

- Many gait analysis systems are now available commercially, and it can be challenging to determine the gait analysis equipment that is the best solution for a clinician/clinic. Factors to consider are:
  - What type of information about gait would benefit the patient population. This depends on the degree of running experience among the typical patients, goals of the patients, and most importantly, the level of training of the clinician.

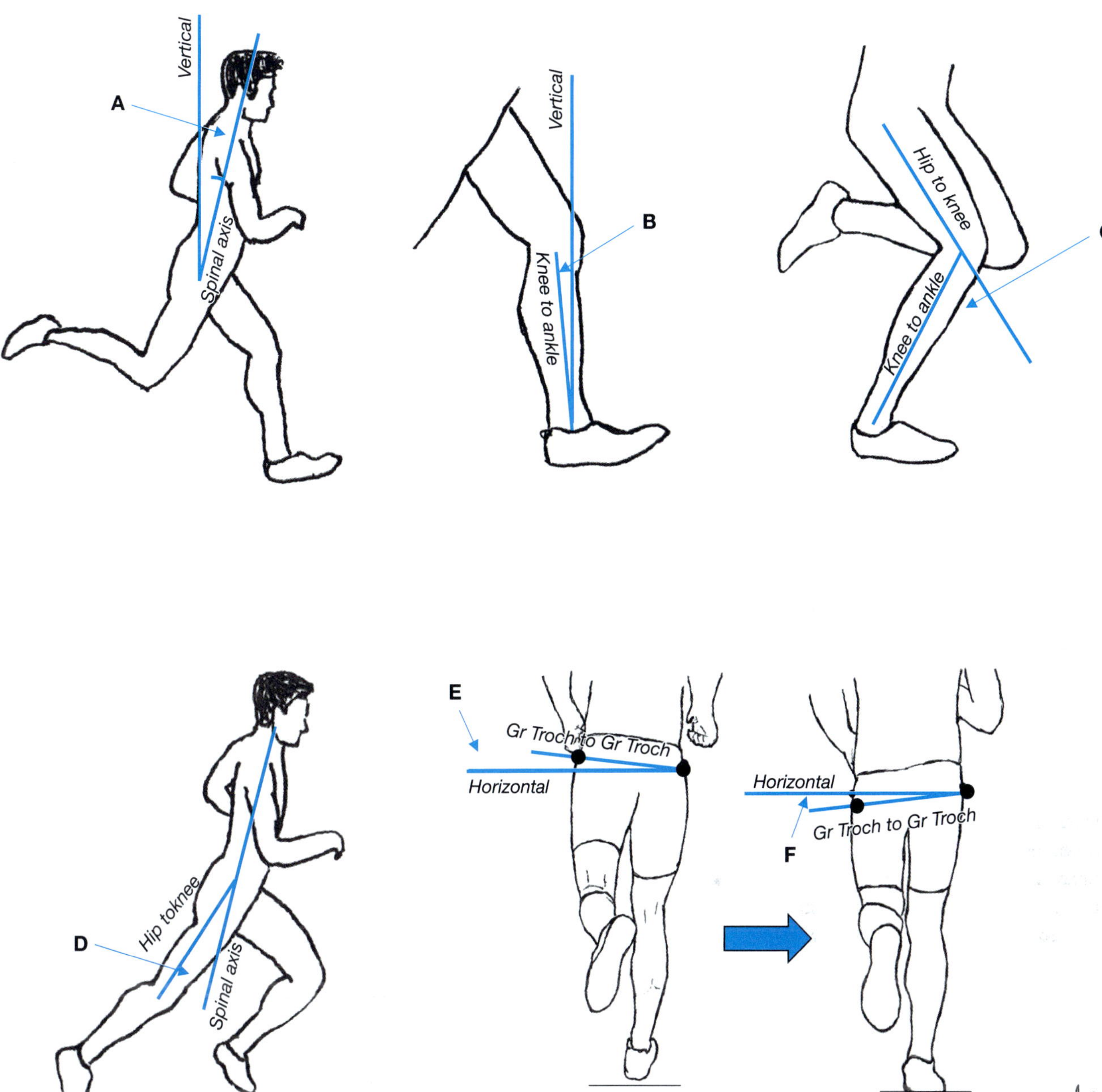

Figure 25.3: Measurement of several fundamental kinematic variables during a VOGA protocol. A: Torso orientation, B: Tibial inclination angle (measured at initial foot contact), C: Knee flexion angle (measured at initial foot contact and at midstance, as depicted here), D: Hip extension (measured at its peak, which occurs during toe-off), E and F: Pelvic drop is measured as the difference between pelvic angle (the angle created by a line between bilateral greater trochanters as referenced to the horizontal) during float phase versus at midstance. This must be measured bilaterally and compared.

The fact that a system is more expensive or captures more data does not necessarily mean it is a better solution.

- In addition, the clinician must understand the level of accuracy/precision of the data provided, the pitfalls inherent to a particular system, and how to interpret and apply the data into a meaningful treatment plan.
- A basic gait analysis set-up is sufficient for most sports medicine clinics, whereas highly sophisticated gait technology may be more appropriate for specialized running clinics with highly trained staff.

- A basic gait analysis set-up may include:
  - Environment: a motorized treadmill with stiff deck (mimics the ground), high horsepower motor (reduces drag or slippage of the belt with foot landing), minimally obstructing handles/rails, and enough space to capture video from the sagittal and frontal planes (from behind and in front of the treadmill).

Table 25.3 Typical Values of Some Temporal and Spatial Gait Variables (as Seen in Healthy Adults Walking or Running Comfortably on a Level Surface)

Temporal/Spatial Variable	Average Value — Walking	Average Value — Running
Velocity (m/min)	~80	~180
Cadence (steps/min)	110–120	160 (tall/heavy/novice runner) 180 (short/light/elite runner)
Stride length (m)	1.4	2.0–2.5
Stance (% of gait cycle)	60	40
Swing (% of gait cycle)	40	60
Double support (% of gait cycle)	10	N/A
Float (% of gait cycle)	N/A	10–20
Contact time (per step) (milliseconds)	630–680	270–310

- Video capability (tablet or dedicated cameras on tripods)
- Video gait analysis software package
- Wall-mounted grid background for reference measurements
- Reflective markers/tape
- Metronome

- With steadily improving wearable sensor technology, greater capabilities are becoming more accessible and practical, and these may become keystones to clinic-based gait analysis in the future (7).

EMERGING TECHNOLOGIES WITH PRACTICAL APPLICATION

- Gait analysis has historically been largely reliant on technologies that must be kept stationary, requiring the patient to run on a treadmill during gait analysis. Although treadmill running is a close approximation to overground running, studies have shown that they are not equivalent (8). Therefore, assessments and rehabilitation plans may be slightly inaccurate.
- IMU devices are rapidly gaining acceptance in sports medicine and physical therapy clinics, and a growing body of evidence supports their accuracy and validity (9–11). They are, however, susceptible to artifact (such as data drift) and some variables are measured more accurately than others when compared to sophisticated 3-D gait laboratories.
- The primary advantage of IMU devices is their small size and portability, allowing them to be worn while running on a trail or track outside of the clinic and collecting data during an entire workout. In this way, they can capture data that reflects true overground running mechanics (avoiding artifact of treadmill running) and shows the effects of fatigue on gait mechanics.

ADVANCED ASPECTS OF GAIT ANALYSIS

- Elastic recoil is a key element of optimal, efficient running gait and describes the cyclical storage and release of energy. This action is performed mainly by the elasticity of tendons, ligaments, and fascia, which behave as springs and are tensioned by the relevant muscles (6).
- There are important differences between kinetics versus kinematics. "Kinematics" describes how an individual moves. Kinematic variables involve time and space (angles, displacement, and velocities) and are observable with the eye/camera and a clock. However, "kinetics" refers to forces that create movement. Forces are typically measured in terms of Newtons and can be linear (measured with a vector or directionality) or angular/rotational (called a "moment," measured in Newton-meters). Kinetic variables can only be measured with advanced instruments such as force plates.

KINEMATICS

- Temporospatial parameters can be measured with 2-dimensional video, wearable sensors (*e.g.*, IMU), pressure mats or insoles, and 3-D motion analysis (using infrared cameras). 3-D motion analysis is considered the gold standard but is costly (both time and money).
- Typical values (3,4) of temporospatial gait parameters in healthy young adults, walking and running comfortably on a level surface, are summarized in Table 25.3.
- With quantitative three-dimensional gait analysis, joint angles throughout the gait cycle are described with respect to flexion/extension, abduction/adduction, and internal/external rotation (6). CoM position in time is expressed in vertical, anterior-posterior, and mediolateral time histories.
- During walking, the CoM trajectory reaches its highest point in stance (it is an inverse pendular gait pattern). During running, the CoM trajectory reaches its maximum height during the float phase.
- Double-limb support times are greater when walking slowly and decrease with faster walking speed. Walking becomes running when there is no longer an interval of time in which both feet are in contact with the ground.

KINETICS

- Kinetics is defined as the study of forces and moments that cause movement.
- GRF refers to the forces exerted by the ground on the foot during foot contact. They can be measured with force-plated treadmills or force platforms embedded in the ground. The center of the distribution of these forces is called the center

of pressure. The term "joint moment" refers to angular force applied at a distance from a joint.

- The vertical GRF typically demonstrates an initial impact peak at the very first contact of the heel during heel strike gait, as demonstrated in Figure 25.4, and then reaches a maximum during terminal stance. The slope of this GRF curve is termed the "loading rate." During running, the peak vertical GRF divides absorption from generation phases. Maximum and minimum values are dependent on the mass and speed of the runner. The amplitude of the pattern during running can be threefold the amplitude during walking (6).

MUSCLE ACTIVATION AND DYNAMIC ELECTROMYOGRAPHY

- Evaluation of muscle activation patterns during gait allows us to discriminate in time the muscle groups that are responsible for the observed joint moment (often due to relative weakness or inappropriate timing of contraction) (5).
- Surface EMG is the most common method for detecting muscle activity during gait.

EFFICIENCY AND OXYGEN CONSUMPTION

- The measurement of oxygen consumption provides information regarding the economy (or efficiency) of gait — defined as the energy expenditure per unit of distance. This can be measured using wearable pulmonary gas exchange devices.
- Many runners display efficient movement (lower rate of energy expenditure) at lower speeds and shorter distances, becoming less efficient as an athlete's form breaks down at higher speeds and/or with fatigue. The goal of improving performance and reducing injury risk is to develop efficient running form, beginning at low speeds, and maintaining efficient form at higher speeds and longer distances.

COMMON RUNNING GAIT ERRORS

- Two main error patterns include overstriding and overcompliance. Overstriding is identified by a combination of rearfoot strike, high tibial inclination angle (>5°) at initial contact/loading response, and limited knee flexion in early stance (12,13). This is observed as the athlete lands with their heel at an excessive distance in front of the CoM, causing high ground reaction forces (including high forward-directed or "braking" forces), high loading rates, and prolonged ground contact time. The result is high energy storage but poor elastic loading and recoil, which yields a poor running economy and higher injury risk (12–14). See Figure 25.5 for visual comparison with a more efficient running gait.
- Runners do not naturally land with their foot directly (vertically) below their CoM unless they are accelerating. While running at a steady cruising speed, the efficient runner will land with their foot/ankle directly below their knee, not their CoM.
- Overcompliance is a combination of excessive lateral pelvic tilt at midstance, a narrow base of support (foot placement in frontal plane — like "tightrope" running), resulting in increased hip adduction and internal rotation, CoM vertical excursion, and foot/ankle pronation (12,13). A variety of injury patterns, including medial tibial stress syndrome and patellofemoral pain syndrome, have been linked to an overcompliant gait pattern (15,16).
- As previously described, pronation is a complex and normal movement during the loading phases (early and midstance) of gait involving simultaneous tibiotalar dorsiflexion, rearfoot (subtalar) eversion, forefoot abduction relative to the midfoot, and tibial internal rotation. Because these cannot all be measured directly in a single measurement, many

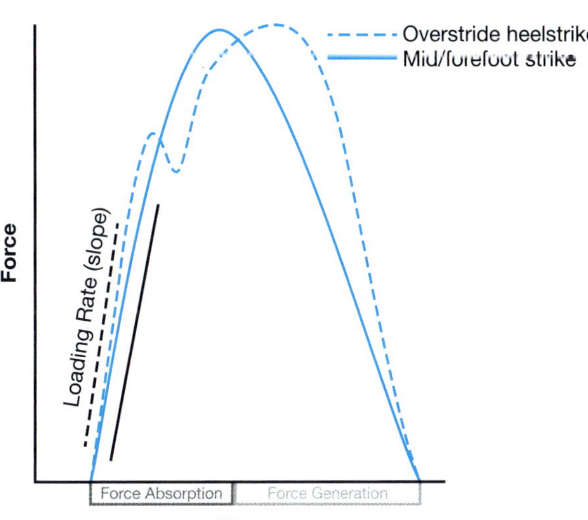

Figure 25.4: Vertical ground reaction force (GRF) curve, as would be typical of an overstride heel strike gait (dotted curve, compared to midfoot or forefoot strike depicted by the solid curve), evaluated on a force plate.

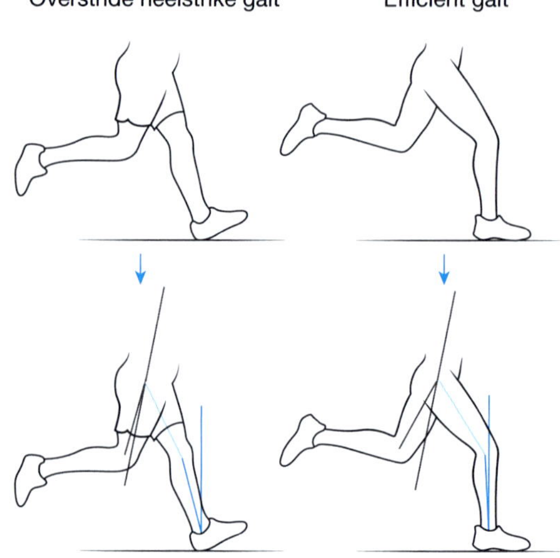

Figure 25.5: Comparison sagittal plane images depicting an overstride heel strike running gait (left) and a much more efficient midfoot strike gait (right). Special attention should be paid to differences in hip extension (diminished in overstride heel strike gait), knee flexion angle at initial foot contact (note nearly fully extended knee in overstride heel strike gait), and tibial inclination angle at initial foot contact (tibia approximately vertical at initial foot contact in efficient runners).

biomechanical studies measure rearfoot eversion as a surrogate marker of pronation. The term "overpronation" is often used inappropriately as there is no defined normal versus pathologic degree, duration, or velocity of pronation.

SUMMARY

- Walking and running gait are dynamic and complex movements that can be dissected by careful examination and evaluation to provide insight into an athlete's risks and injuries. A clinical gait analysis with practical applications for an athlete can be performed without extravagant technology, but research benefits the precision and extensive data provided by 3-D motion analysis. Finding representative visually identifiable angles and measurements, as described here, can be used to process the beautiful complexity into manageable data points. As there is no particular "correct" way to run, clinicians are encouraged to take the athletes' exam findings and gait patterns in context of their injury and movement history to develop a relevant treatment plan.

REFERENCES

1. Davis IS, Futrell E. Gait retraining: altering the fingerprint of gait. *Phys Med Rehabil Clin N Am.* 2016 Feb;27(1):339–55.
2. Birrer RB, Buzermanis S, DellaCorte MP, et al. Biomechanics of running. In: O'Connor F, Wilder R, editors. *The Textbook of Running Medicine.* New York: McGraw-Hill; 2001. p. 11–9.
3. Dicharry J. Kinematics and kinetics of gait: from lab to clinic. *Clin Sports Med.* 2010;29(3):347–64.
4. Kerrigan DC, Edelstein JE. Gait. In: Gonzalez EG, Myers SJ, Edelsteinet JE, et al., editors. *The Physiological Basis of Rehabilitation Medicine.* Boston: Butterworth-Heinemann; 2001. p. 397–416.
5. Perry J. *Gait Analysis: Normal and Pathological Function.* Thorofare (NJ): Slack. 1992. p. 556.
6. Novacheck TF. The biomechanics of running. *Gait Posture.* 1998;7(1):77–95.
7. Prasanth H, Caban M, Keller U, et al. Wearable sensor-based real-time gait detection: a systematic review. *Sensors.* 2021 Apr 13;21(8):2727.
8. Lafferty L, Wawrzyniak J, Chambers M, et al. Clinical indoor running gait analysis may not approximate outdoor running gait based on novel drone technology. *Sports Health.* 2022 Sep–Oct;14(5):710–16.
9. Benson LC, Clermont CA, Bošnjak E, Ferber R. The use of wearable devices for walking and running gait analysis outside of the lab: a systematic review. *Gait Posture.* 2018 Jun;63:124–38.
10. DeJong AF, Hertel J. Validation of foot-strike assessment using wearable sensors during running. *J Athl Train.* 2020 Dec 1;55(12):1307–10.
11. Hollis CR, Koldenhoven RM, Resch JE, Hertel J. Running biomechanics as measured by wearable sensors: effects of speed and surface. *Sports Biomech.* 2021 Aug;20(5):521–31.
12. Souza RB. An evidence-based videotaped running biomechanics analysis. *Phys Med Rehabil Clin N Am.* 2016;27(1):217–36. doi:10.1016/j.pmr.2015.08.006
13. Pipkin A, Kotecki K, Hetzel S, Heiderscheit B. Reliability of a qualitative video analysis for running. *J Orthop Sports Phys Ther.* 2016;46(7):556–61.
14. Sugimoto D, Kelly BD, Mandel DL, et al. Running propensities of athletes with hamstring injuries. *Sports.* 2019 Sep 12;7(9):210.
15. Daoud AI, Geissler GJ, Wang F, Saretsky J, Daoud YA, Lieberman DE. Foot strike and injury rates in endurance runners: a retrospective study. *Med Sci Sports Exerc.* 2012;44(7):1325–34.
16. Meardon SA, Derrick TR. Effect of step width manipulation on tibial stress during running. *J Biomech.* 2014;47(11):2738–44.

Compartment Syndrome Testing

26

Chad D. Hulsopple and Samuel I. Bartlett

INTRODUCTION

- Exertional leg pain is a common complaint in athletes with broad a differential diagnosis, including chronic exertional compartment syndrome (CECS), popliteal artery entrapment syndrome (PAES), bone stress injuries, and medial tibial stress syndrome (MTSS) (see Chapter 68 Soft Tissue Injuries of the Leg, Ankle, and Foot).
- CECS has predictable patterns of transient, sometimes severe, pain or cramping in muscle compartments with increased duration or intensity of exercise. On cessation of exercise, symptoms typically resolve in minutes to hours.
- CECS is a clinical diagnosis of exclusion based on the history and physical of the patient. However, intramuscular compartment pressure (IMCP) measurements are frequently utilized to guide management. Although IMCP is considered a gold standard, there is controversy around the validity of IMCP measurements to rule out or confirm CECS as the etiology of exertional leg pain or guide initial management.

COMPARTMENT SYNDROMES

- Compartment syndrome occurs when intracompartmental pressures (ICP) increase in an inelastic fascial space, resulting in decreased perfusion to the compartment (1–3).
- Compartment syndromes in the athlete can occur in two forms, acute and chronic. The distinction between the two forms is the mechanism of injury and reversibility.
- Acute compartment syndrome (ACS) most commonly occurs due to acute trauma (*i.e.*, fracture) or soft tissue or muscle injury (*i.e.*, crush injury, rhabdomyolysis), leading to an irreversible increase in ICP rapidly leading to tissue ischemia and necrosis unless emergently decompressed via fasciotomy.
  - The patient's history and physical examination assist in establishing the clinical diagnosis. Characteristic findings include pain out of proportion to the injury, paresthesias and sensory deficits, tense and swollen compartments on palpation decreased or loss of active motion, and severe pain with passive stretch. Clinical assessment, however, has been demonstrated to have limited sensitivity for identifying ACS (13%–64%) and a wide range of specificity (63%–98%) (4).
  - IMCP testing has been advocated prior to emergent fasciotomy if any doubt exists about the diagnosis. Currently it is recommended that an emergency fasciotomy be performed based on a delta pressure (delta pressure = diastolic blood pressure minus IMCP) with a differential pressure threshold of 30 mg Hg or less for more than 2 hours to confirm ACS, which reduces time to fasciotomy versus waiting for clinical signs and symptoms to occur. ICMP delta pressure of 30 mm Hg or less for more than 2 hours has sensitivity for ACS of 94% and specificity of 98% (4,5).
- CECS symptoms present in a predictable pattern with increased duration or intensity of exercise and reverse on cessation of the exercise, which is thought to be related to a transient increase in ICPs resulting in reversible hypoperfusion.
  - CECS can occur in any athlete. However, it is more common in repetitive activities such as running and skating (6).
  - CECS can occur in any muscle compartment, but the most common location is in the lower extremity, with rare reports in the upper extremity, foot, and trunk (6–9).
- Although IMCP testing can aid in diagnosing ACS, the following discussion applies to using IMCP for CECS.

Anatomy of Lower Extremity Compartments

- The lower leg contains four compartments supported by tibia and fibula. Each compartment is covered by a tight inelastic fascia that encloses specific muscle groups with a unique neurovascular supply creating distinct symptomology in compartment syndromes (Table 26.1).
- The anterior compartment contains the tibialis anterior, extensor hallucis longus, extensor digitorum longus muscles, and peroneus tertius, which extend the toes and dorsiflex the ankle. The neurovascular supply is from the deep peroneal nerve and anterior tibial artery.
- The lateral compartment contains the peroneus longus and the peroneus brevis muscles, which evert the ankle. The neurovascular supply is via the superficial peroneal nerve and branches of the anterior tibial and peroneal arteries.
- The superficial posterior compartment contains the gastrocnemius, soleus, and plantaris muscles, which plantarflex the foot. The neurovascular supply is via the penetrating branches of the tibial nerve and posterior tibial and peroneal arteries.

Table 26.1 Muscle Compartments

Compartment	Nerve	Muscles	Vascular
Anterior	Deep peroneal	Tibialis anterior Extensor hallucis longus Extensor digitorum longus Peroneus tertius	Anterior tibial artery and vein
Lateral	Superficial peroneal	Peroneus longus Peroneus brevis	Branches of the anterior tibial and peroneal arteries and veins
Superficial posterior	Penetrating branches of the tibial nerve	Gastrocnemius Soleus Plantaris	Penetrating branches of the posterior tibial and peroneal arteries and veins
Deep posterior	Tibial nerve	Tibialis posterior Flexor hallucis longus Flexor digitorum longus Popliteus	Posterior tibial artery and vein Peroneal artery and vein

- The deep posterior compartment contains the flexor hallucis longus, the flexor digitorum longus, the tibialis posterior, and popliteus muscles, which flex the toes and plantarflex the ankle. The neurovascular supply is via the tibial nerve and posterior tibial and peroneal arteries.
- When present, the fibular head of the flexor digitorum can create a separate and distinct subcompartment around the posterior tibialis within the deep posterior compartment (10).

PATHOPHYSIOLOGY

- The etiology of CECS is incompletely understood. The symptoms of CECS are believed to be a result of an exercise-induced transient increase in the ICP due to expansion of the muscle volume within noncompliant osseofascial compartments resulting in reversible hypoperfusion that leads to transient neuromuscular ischemia, pain, and impairment of muscular function (11).
- The increase in ICP seen during exertion is likely multifactorial, but four factors may contribute (12–14):
  - Fascial restriction from the enclosure of compartmental contents in an inelastic fascial sheath.
  - Increased skeletal muscle volume with exertion resulting from venous congestion and edema.
  - Muscle hypertrophy as a response to exercise.
  - Dynamic contraction factors due to the gait cycle

CLINICAL PRESENTATION

- In CECS, the characteristic complaint is recurrent, transient, exercise-induced muscle pain that occurs at predictable intensities and duration of exercise and increases if the training persists.
- The quality of pain is described as a tight, cramp-like, or squeezing ache over a specific compartment of the leg. Symptoms are relieved only on discontinuation of activity. Post-exercise soreness can resolve in minutes to hours after cessation of activity.
- Neurologic complaints such as paresthesias, and transient palsy, of the leg or foot with exertion, may indicate involvement of the nerve traversing the compartment.
  - Nerve entrapment syndromes of the lower extremity often present with similar complaints and should be included in the differential diagnosis.
- The physical examination is commonly unremarkable at rest, with a normal walking gait and lower extremity examination. A muscle herniation through a fascial defect can be identified in up to 45% of patients with CECS (15).
- An exercise challenge followed by a post-exercise clinical examination can help establish the diagnosis (16).
  - After reproducing discomfort with the exercise challenge, the athlete should be assessed for tenderness, tightness, swelling over the involved compartment, and pain with passive stretching.
  - The tenderness should involve the muscle mass, not the bone or muscle-tendon junction; symptoms can present bilaterally in 60% of cases (6,17).
  - A neurologic and vascular examination should be completed.
  - Fascial herniations that were not readily apparent during the exam at rest can be more apparent after exercise.
- Although the history may suggest CECS, no physical examination finding can firmly establish the diagnosis (18,19). Diagnosis based solely on a clinical presentation can lead to misdiagnosis, inappropriate therapy, and delay of proper therapy (20).

INDICATIONS FOR INTRAMUSCULAR COMPARTMENTAL PRESSURE MEASUREMENTS

- CECS is a clinical diagnosis. IMCP testing for CECS is a procedure that has demonstrated inconsistent and conflicting evidence. Evidence suggests that the patient's pain may not correlate to higher IMCPs (21–24). In addition, there is emerging evidence that initial pressure measurement may not be associated with predicting the clinical outcomes of an initial conservative treatment program, suggesting that surgical intervention can be safely postponed (25,26).

- An exercise challenge with a detailed physical examination immediately after the reproduction of symptoms will lead to more judicious use of invasive techniques (16).
- If the history and physical examination are consistent with CECS, IMCP can be considered to evaluate the patient further.
  - Significant historical features include recurrent, exercise-induced leg discomfort that increases as the training persists and dissipates on cessation of activity.
  - Pain quality is described as a tight, cramp-like, or squeezing ache over a specific leg compartment.
  - Paresthesias of the leg or foot can occur with exertion.

TECHNIQUES TO MEASURE COMPARTMENT PRESSURES

- Multiple techniques have been described for measuring static and dynamic intramuscular pressures. Techniques include the needle manometer (27), the wick catheter (28), the slit catheter (29), continuous infusion (30), and a solid-state transducer intracompartmental catheter (12).
- The solid-state transducer intracompartment Intra-Compartmental Pressure Monitor (Critical Care Diagnostic Inc., Schoolcraft, MI) is a battery-operated, hand-held, digital, fluid pressure monitor. This device is more accurate, versatile, convenient, and much less time-consuming in the clinical setting (31,32).
- The arterial line manometer and Intra-Compartmental Pressure Monitor are accurate in an in-vitro model (33).

PERFORMANCE OF THE PROCEDURE

- ICMP testing is an invasive procedure, and proper technical performance and patient safety demand a thorough knowledge of each compartment's anatomy to avoid damage to neurovascular structures.
- The athlete must be made aware of the indications of the procedure, and consent must be obtained with thorough counseling on the risk of infection, scarring, damage to the nerve and vascular structures, and reaction to local anesthesia.
- IMCP testing can be performed through a static or dynamic assessment.
  - To reproduce symptoms adequately, the athlete should perform the specific activity that causes pain or discomfort.
  - The most common procedure is testing IMCPs in a static position with a straight needle at rest and after exertion. This procedure allows the athlete to perform the activity that causes symptoms without an indwelling catheter in the compartment and the measuring device attached to the leg. A negative aspect of this technique is that IMCP testing is performed at rest (prior to exertion), immediately after (1-minute post-exertion) when the reproduction of symptoms occurs, and 5–10 minutes into rest, which results in multiple needle sticks for the patient and technical difficulties of performing all measurements in the recommended time, especially in the event bilateral lower extremity compartments are tested.
  - Dynamic monitoring of IMCPs is performed using a slit catheter inserted before exertion and attached to the athlete's leg. This technique allows continuous IMCP monitoring during exertion without halting activity and provides precise pressure monitoring during activity, potentially a better indicator of pathology (12). Several negative aspects of this technique include restricting the athlete to a treadmill to monitor continuous IMCPs, maintaining the catheter's placement in the compartment, keeping the device attached to the athlete during activity, and the ability only to monitor one compartment at a time. This technique makes the results inconsistent and difficult to obtain and interpret (34,35).
- Multiple factors may alter the pressure measurements:
  - Compartment pressure measuring techniques were compared using an in vitro model, and side port needles and slit catheters were found to be more accurate than straight needles, which tended to overestimate the pressure (33).
  - Patients with diabetes have been shown to have higher IMCPs (24).
  - Proper calibration of the monitor is essential for reliable readings. The monitor must be zeroed at the same angle used to penetrate the skin, and this angle must be maintained with repeated sticks.
  - Joint position at the knee and ankle affects pressures (36).
  - Compression or squeezing the leg can alter pressures. Externally applied pressure is additive to any pressure already existing within the compartment (30).

APPROACH TO EACH LEG COMPARTMENT

- Measurement of IMCPs is an invasive procedure. To avoid damage to neurovascular structures, each compartment should be approached with an understanding of the anatomic contents (37).
- In routine IMCP testing, the palpation-guided technique is as accurate as ultrasound-guided IMCP testing (38).

Anterior Compartment

- Identify the muscle belly of the anterior tibialis just lateral to the anterior tibial border. The approach should have the needle penetrate through the fascia and into the muscle belly of the anterior tibialis at the level of the mid-third of the tibia.

- The neurovascular bundle containing the deep peroneal nerve, anterior tibial artery, and veins are anatomic structures to avoid. The neurovascular bundle commonly sits just above the interosseous membrane at this level.

Lateral Compartment

- The muscle bellies of the peroneus longus and brevis are palpable on the lateral surface of the leg, just superficial to the shaft of the fibula.
- A helpful technique to enter this compartment involves palpating the head of the fibula and lateral malleolus and palpating the muscle bellies at the midpoint between these two bony landmarks.
- The superficial peroneal nerve innervates the lateral compartment as it transverses through the compartment, and vascular supply is through branches of the anterior tibial and peroneal arteries.

Posterior Superficial Compartment

- The muscle bellies of the gastrocnemius and soleus muscles are easily identified and palpated.
- Approach to this compartment just medial to the midline will avoid the small saphenous vein and the medial and lateral sural cutaneous nerves.
- Branches of the tibial nerve innervate this compartment, and the vascular supply is through penetrating branches of posterior tibial and peroneal arteries.

Posterior Deep Compartment

- The approach to the deep posterior compartment is technically more difficult because of the proximity of neurovascular structures.
- Two bundles are contained within this compartment that should be understood anatomically prior to needle insertion. A vascular bundle consisting of the peroneal artery and veins lies medial to the posterior aspect of the fibula. A neurovascular bundle consisting of the tibial nerve, posterior tibial artery, and veins lie in the posterior aspect of this compartment behind the mass of the tibialis posterior muscle.
- The posterior medial aspect of the mid-tibia must first be palpated. The needle should then be inserted just posterior to the tibia, closely approximating the posterior border of the bone. The needle first enters the flexor digitorum longus muscle and, if guided deeper, penetrates the posterior tibialis muscle. This approach keeps the needle anterior and medial to the neurovascular structures if not driven too deeply.

Diagnostic Criteria

- Compartment pressure must be obtained both preexercise and post-exercise. Post-exercise pressures should be performed immediately after an exercise challenge reproduces the patient's symptoms.
- For CECS, the diagnostic criteria described by Pedowitz et al. (20) are commonly used. One or more of the following criteria must be met in addition to appropriate history and physical examination:
    - Preexercise >15 mm Hg
    - 1-minute post-exercise >30 mm Hg
    - 5-minutes post-exercise >20 mm Hg

DIFFERENTIAL DIAGNOSIS

- CECS is a diagnosis of exclusion with a broad differential diagnosis with the potential of concomitant conditions, which include PAES, bone stress injuries, MTSS, tendinopathies, muscle strains, neuropathies, radiculopathy, infection, and malignancies.
- Nerve entrapment and compression may cause exertional leg pain.
    - Common peroneal nerve entrapment can present with activity-related pain, paresthesias, or numbness in the anterolateral aspect of the leg and dorsum of the foot, along with foot drop or a slapping gait with exertion.
    - Superficial peroneal nerve entrapment presents with distal lateral leg and dorsum of the foot paresthesias and peroneal muscle weakness.
    - Saphenous nerve entrapment presents as medial knee and medial leg paresthesias or pain.
    - Sural nerve entrapment can present with posterior calf pain and paresthesias.
    - Proximal tibial nerve entrapment also presents with pain and paresthesias in the posterior calf and plantar surface of the foot and weakness of foot and ankle muscles.
- Lumbosacral radiculopathy should be suspected in athletes with complaints of leg pain, especially if associated with back or buttock discomfort.
- Popliteal artery entrapment is often misdiagnosed as posterior CECS because of the ischemic etiology in the pathogenesis of symptoms in both syndromes (37).

OTHER DIAGNOSTIC OPTIONS

- IMCP testing assesses only one aspect of CECS. Altered tissue perfusion, neurologic and muscular ischemia, and increased interstitial fluid play a role in the pathophysiologic process.
- Recent attention has focused on noninvasive techniques that can detect these pathophysiologic alterations associated with or as a result of pressure elevations. These emerging diagnostic options offer an alternative to direct ICP measurements

in cases where the athlete is averse to invasive procedures or pressure monitoring results may be nondiagnostic.

- Magnetic resonance imaging (MRI): MRI has shown promising results but can be limited by the ability of medical facilities to perform specific MRI procedures to capture image sequences (24). MRI is sensitive to changes in water distribution in skeletal muscle. In CECS patients, edema is seen in the muscles for more extended periods than in patients without CECS, which has been shown to correspond to increased IMCPs (39,40). The MRI sequences, while having the patient perform active exercises, have demonstrated high sensitivity and specificity for the diagnosis of CECS (41).
- Near-infrared spectroscopy (NIRS): Focusing on the induced ischemia resulting from impaired perfusion, NIRS has been used as a noninvasive method to measure tissue oxygen saturation and thereby support the diagnosis of CECS. Compared to controls, patients with CECS display significant differences in peak exercise and post-exercise tissue oxygen saturation as measured by NIRS (42). Consistent with the induced ischemia theory, patients with CECS demonstrated greater deoxygenation with exercise than controls. Though some studies suggest sensitivity of NIRS is equivalent to IMCP measurements (43), a recent review highlights variable NIRS accuracy, with sensitivity and specificity dependent on the device and analysis (41).

Limitations of IMCP Measurement

- Diagnostic Unreliability: IMCP measurement, while considered the standard for the diagnosis of CECS, presents several limitations that warrant careful consideration. Studies consistently demonstrate conflicting evidence about the inconsistencies and unreliability of current IMCP criteria for CECS diagnosis, which stems from inconsistent testing protocols, significant variability in measurement techniques, and the absence of blinded, comparative studies (24,41,44,45).
- Complex Clinical Correlation: The relationship between IMCP values and the patient's exertional pain is not always linear suggesting that CECS pathophysiology may involve factors beyond elevated compartment pressures, complicating the interpretation of IMCP measurements as a sole diagnostic indicator (46).
- Risks of an Invasive Procedure: IMCP measurement carries inherent risks, including pain, hematoma formation, nerve damage, and infection. These potential complications limit the widespread applicability of IMCP, particularly in routine clinical practice (41).

REFERENCES

1. Baria MR, Sellon JL. Botulinum toxin for chronic exertional compartment syndrome: a case report with 14 month follow-up. *Clin J Sport Med.* 2016 Nov;26(6):e111–13. doi:10.1097/JSM.0000000000000289
2. Campano D, Robaina JA, Kusnezov N, Dunn JC, Waterman BR. Surgical management for chronic exertional compartment syndrome of the leg: a systematic review of the literature. *Arthroscopy.* 2016 Jul;32(7):1478–86. doi:10.1016/j.arthro.2016.01.069
3. Irion V, Magnussen RA, Miller TL, Kaeding CC. Return to activity following fasciotomy for chronic exertional compartment syndrome. *Eur J Orthop Surg Traumatol.* 2014 Oct;24(7):1223–8. doi:10.1007/s00590-014-1433-0
4. McQueen MM, Duckworth AD. The diagnosis of acute compartment syndrome: a review. *Eur J Trauma Emerg Surg.* 2014 Oct;40(5):521–8. doi:10.1007/s00068-014-0414-7
5. White TO, Howell GE, Will EM, Court-Brown CM, McQueen, MM. Elevated intramuscular compartment pressures do not influence outcome after tibial fracture. *J Trauma.* 2003 Dec;55(6):1133–8. doi:10.1097/01.TA.0000100822.13119
6. de Bruijn JA, van Zantvoort APM, van Klaveren D, et al. Factors predicting lower leg chronic exertional compartment syndrome in a large population. *Int J Sports Med.* 2018 Jan;39(1):58–66. doi:10.1055/s-0043-119225
7. Liu B, Barrazueta G, Ruchelsman DE. Chronic exertional compartment syndrome in athletes. *J Hand Surg Am.* 2017 Nov;42(11):917–23. doi:10.1016/j.jhsa.2017.09.009
8. Orta C, Petit J, Gremeaux V. Chronic exertional compartment syndrome in hands successfully treated with botulinum toxin-A: a case. *Ann Phys Rehabil Med.* 2018 May;61(3):183–5. doi:10.1016/j.rehab.2018.02.006
9. Sindhu K, Cohen B, Gil JA, Blood T, Owens BD. Chronic exertional compartment syndrome of the forearm. *Phys Sportsmed.* 2019 Feb;47(1):27–30. doi:10.1080/00913847.2018.1530577
10. Hislop M, Tierney P, Murray P, O'Brien M, Mahony N. Chronic exertional compartment syndrome: the controversial "fifth" compartment of the leg. *Am J Sports Med.* 2003 Sep-Oct;31(5):770–6. doi:10.1177/03635465030310052201
11. George CA, Hutchinson MR. Chronic exertional compartment syndrome. *Clin Sports Med.* 2012 Apr;31(2):307–19. doi:10.1016/j.csm.2011.09.013
12. McDermott AG, Marble AE, Yabsley RH, Phillips MB. Monitoring dynamic anterior compartment pressures during exercise. A new technique using the STIC catheter. *Am J Sports Med.* 1982 Mar-Apr;10(2):83–9. doi:10.1177/036354658201000204
13. McGinley JC, Thompson TA, Ficken S, White J. Chronic exertional compartment syndrome caused by functional venous outflow obstruction. *Clin J Sport Med.* 2022 Jul 1;32(4):355–60. doi:10.1097/JSM.0000000000000929
14. Styf J. Compartment syndromes: diagnosis, treatment, and complications. In: Campbell B, editor. *Compartment Syndromes: Diagnosis, Treatment, and Complications.* Boca Raton (FL): CRC Press LLC; 2004. p. 5–6.
15. Fraipont MJ, Adamson GJ. Chronic exertional compartment syndrome. *J Am Acad Orthop Surg.* 2003 Jul-Aug;11(4):268–76. doi:10.5435/00124635-200307000-00006
16. Glorioso JE, Wilckens JH. Compartment syndrome testing. In: O'Connor FG, Wilder RP, editors. *Textbook of Running Medicine.* New York: McGraw-Hill; 2001. p. 95–9.
17. Davis DE, Raikin S, Garras DN, Vitanzo P, Labrador H, Espandar R. Characteristics of patients with chronic exertional compartment syndrome. *Foot Ankle Int.* 2013 Oct;34(10):1349–54. doi:10.1177/1071100713490919
18. Kiuru MJ, Mantysaari MJ, Pihlajamaki HK, Ahovuo JA. Evaluation of stress-related anterior lower leg pain with magnetic resonance imaging and intracompartmental pressure measurement. *Mil Med.* 2003 Jan;168(1):48–52.

19. Styf JR, Körner LM. Diagnosis of chronic anterior compartment syndrome in the lower leg. *Acta Orthop Scand.* 1987 Apr;58(2):139–44. doi:10.3109/17453678709146460
20. Pedowitz RA, Hargens AR, Mubarak SJ, Gershuni DH. Modified criteria for the objective diagnosis of chronic compartment syndrome of the leg. *Am J Sports Med.* 1990 Jan-Feb;18(1):35–40. doi:10.1177/036354659001800106
21. Hislop M, Tierney P. Intracompartmental pressure testing: results of an international survey of current clinical practice, highlighting the need for standardised protocols. *Br J Sports Med.* 2011 Sep;45(12):956–8. doi:10.1136/bjsports-2011-090368
22. Mohler LR, Styf JR, Pedowitz RA, Hargens AR, Gershuni DH. Intramuscular deoxygenation during exercise in patients who have chronic anterior compartment syndrome of the leg. *J Bone Joint Surg Am.* 1997 Jun;79(6):844–9. doi:10.2106/00004623-199706000-00007
23. Tsintzas D, Ghosh S, Maffulli N, King JB, Padhiar N. Ayak bileği pozisyonunun bacakta kompartman içi basinca etkisi [The effect of ankle position on intracompartmental pressures of the leg]. *Acta Orthop Traumatol Turcica.* 2009 Jan-Feb;43(1):42–8. doi:10.3944/AOTT.2009.042
24. Velasco TO, Leggit JC. Chronic exertional compartment syndrome: a clinical update. *Curr Sports Med Rep.* 2020 Sep;19(9):347–52. doi:10.1249/JSR.0000000000000747
25. Vogels S, Bakker EWP, O'Connor FG, Hoencamp R, Zimmermann WO. Association between intracompartmental pressures in the anterior compartment of the leg and conservative treatment outcome for exercise-related leg pain in military service members. *Arch Rehabil Res Clin Transl.* 2021 Dec 4;4(1):100171. doi:10.1016/j.arrct.2021.100171
26. van der Wee MJL, Vogels S, Bakker EWP, O'Connor FG, Hoencamp R, Zimmermann WO. Association between intracompartmental pressures in the deep posterior compartment of the leg and conservative treatment outcome for exercise-related leg pain in military service members. *Arch Rehabil Res Clin Transl.* 2022 Sep 14;4(4):100232.
27. Whitesides TE Jr, Haney TC, Harada H, Holmes HE, Morimoto K. A simple method for tissue pressure determination. *Arch Surg.* 1975 Nov;110(11):1311–3. doi:10.1001/archsurg.1975.01360170051006
28. Mubarak SJ, Hargens AR, Owen CA, Garetto LP, Akeson WH. The wick catheter technique for measurement of intramuscular pressure. A new research and clinical tool. *J Bone Joint Surg Am.* 1976 Oct;58(7):1016–20.
29. Rorabeck CH, Castle GS, Hardie R, Logan J. Compartmental pressure measurements: an experimental investigation using the slit catheter. *J Trauma.* 1981 Jun;21(6):446–9.
30. Matsen FA III, Mayo KA, Sheridan GW, Krugmire RB Jr. Monitoring of intramuscular pressure. *Surgery.* 1976 Jun;79(6):702–9.
31. Awbrey BJ, Sienkiewicz PS, Mankin HJ. Chronic exercise-induced compartment pressure elevation measured with a miniaturized fluid pressure monitor. A laboratory and clinical study. *Am J Sports Med.* 1988 Nov-Dec;16(6):610–5. doi:10.1177/036354658801600610
32. Hutchinson MR, Ireland ML. Chronic exertional compartment syndrome: gauging pressure. *Phys Sportsmed.* 1999 May;27(5):101–2. doi:10.3810/psm.1999.05.871
33. Boody AR, Wongworawat MD. Accuracy in the measurement of compartment pressures: a comparison of three commonly used devices. *J Bone Joint Surg Am.* 2005 Nov;87(11):2415–22. doi:10.2106/JBJS.D.02826
34. Rorabeck CH, Bourne RB, Fowler PJ, Finlay JB, Nott L. The role of tissue pressure measurement in diagnosing chronic anterior compartment syndrome. *Am J Sports Med.* 1988 Mar-Apr;16(2):143–6. doi:10.1177/036354658801600209
35. Rorabeck CH, Fowler PJ, Nott L. The results of fasciotomy in the management of chronic exertional compartment syndrome. *Am J Sports Med.* 1988 May-Jun;16(3):224–7. doi:10.1177/036354658801600304
36. Gershuni DH, Yaru NC, Hargens AR, Lieber RL, O'Hara RC, Akeson WH. Ankle and knee position as a factor modifying intracompartmental pressure in the human leg. *J Bone Joint Surg Am.* 1984 Dec;66(9):1415–20.
37. Glorioso JE, Wilckens JH. Exertional leg pain. In: O'Connor FG, Wilder RP, editors. *Textbook of Running Medicine.* New York: McGraw-Hill; 2001. p. 181–97.
38. Peck E, Finnoff JT, Smith J, Curtiss H, Muir J, Hollman JH. Accuracy of palpation-guided and ultrasound-guided needle tip placement into the deep and superficial posterior leg compartments. *Am J Sports Med.* 2011 Sep;39(9):1968–74. doi:10.1177/0363546511406235
39. Amendola A, Rorabeck CH, Vellett D, Vezina W, Rutt B, Nott L. The use of magnetic resonance imaging in exertional compartment syndromes. *Am J Sports Med.* 1990 Jan-Feb;18(1):29–34. doi:10.1177/036354659001800105
40. Ringler MD, Litwiller DV, Felmlee JP, et al. MRI accurately detects chronic exertional compartment syndrome: a validation study. *Skeletal Radiol.* 2013 Mar;42(3):385–92. doi:10.1007/s00256-012-1487-1
41. Ritchie ED, Vogels S, van Dongen TTCF, et al. Systematic review of innovative diagnostic tests for chronic exertional compartment syndrome. *Int J Sports Med.* 2023 Jan;44(1):20–8. doi: 10.1055/a-1866-5957
42. van den Brand JG, Verleisdonk EJ, van der Werken C. Near infrared spectroscopy in the diagnosis of chronic exertional compartment syndrome. *Am J Sports Med.* 2004 Mar;32(2):452–6. doi:10.1177/0363546503261733
43. van den Brand JG, Nelson T, Verleisdonk EJ, van der Werken C. The diagnostic value of intracompartmental pressure measurement, magnetic resonance imaging, and near-infrared spectroscopy in chronic exertional compartment syndrome: a prospective study in 50 patients. *Am J Sports Med.* 2005 May;33(5):699–704. doi:10.1177/0363546504270565
44. Roberts A, Franklyn-Miller A. The validity of the diagnostic criteria used in chronic exertional compartment syndrome: a systematic review. *Scand J Med Sci Sports.* 2012 Oct;22(5):585–95. doi: 10.1111/j.1600-0838.2011.01386.x
45. Aweid O, Del Buono A, Malliaras P, et al. Systematic review and recommendations for intracompartmental pressure monitoring in diagnosing chronic exertional compartment syndrome of the leg. *Clin J Sport Med.* 2012 Jul;22(4):356–70. doi: 10.1097/JSM.0b013e3182580e1d
46. Zimmermann WO, Ligthert E, Helmhout PH, et al. Intracompartmental pressure measurements in 501 service members with exercise-related leg pain. *Transl J ACSM.* 2018;3(14)107–12. doi: 10.1249/TJX.0000000000000065

27

Exercise-Induced Bronchoconstriction Testing

Meghan F. Raleigh and Fred H. Brennan Jr

EPIDEMIOLOGY

- Exercise-induced bronchoconstriction (EIB) is a common medical condition that affects at least 10%–15% of athletes (1,2). More common in certain elite athletes who participate in cold weather sports (3).
- Exercise-induced asthma (EIA) is the presence of similar symptoms in a patient with a known diagnosis of asthma (4). The prevalence of EIB in asthmatic patients is 80%–90% (5).
- Respiratory symptoms alone are insensitive in predicting bronchospasm in athletes (6).
- Common respiratory symptoms suggestive of asthma (coughing, wheezing, etc.) have only a 60%–70% positive predictive value for EIB (7,8).

INDICATIONS FOR EIB TESTING

- An athlete with signs or symptoms suggestive of EIB.
- An athlete with known chronic asthma may be tested for an exercise-triggering event.
- An athlete with exertional dyspnea, once cardiac etiologies have been clinically and/or diagnostically eliminated. May help distinguish from Exercise-Induced Laryngeal Obstruction (EILO) (5).

CONTRAINDICATIONS FOR EIB TESTING

- Active or recent pulmonary infection within the past 30 days.
- Ongoing or recent exacerbation of asthma.
- Known allergy to methacholine (methacholine challenge).
- An athlete using inhaled corticosteroids may still be tested; however, the provocation test may be falsely negative in up to 50% of patients (4,9).

EIB PROVOCATIVE TESTING

Exercise Challenge

- A baseline pulmonary function test (PFT) should be performed and results recorded prior to this and any provocative test (3). The PFT is a graphic representation of both inspiration and expiration (see Fig. 27.1A).
- The sensitivity and specificity of this test for identifying EIB in athletes are approximately 65% and 90%, respectively (1,2,10,11). The challenge should be sport-specific and conducted in the environment in which athletes most commonly experience their symptoms (12).
- An exercise challenge may be used as a first-line diagnostic study.

Conducting an Exercise Challenge

- Allow athletes to stretch, but do not allow them to exercise or warm up prior to the challenge. A warm-up period may result in a false-negative result.
- Obtain a baseline PFT or peak expiratory flow rate (PEFR). Record FEV_1 (forced expiratory volume in 1 second) and FEF_{25-75} (forced expiratory flow during the middle portion of expiration), or PEFR.
- The sport-specific exercise should be conducted for 8–10 minutes at 85%–90% of maximum calculated heart rate (220 − age in years = estimated maximum heart rate).
- After 10 minutes of exercise, allow a 1-minute rest. Check PFT or PEFR three times and record the best result.
- Repeat these measurements at 3, 5, 10, 15, and 20 minutes after termination of the exercise challenge.
- A decrease of >10% in the FEV_1 or PEFR and/or a decrease in FEF_{25-75} of >20% are diagnostic for EIB (11,13,14).

EUCAPNIC VOLUNTARY HYPERVENTILATION TEST

- Used by the International Olympic Committee–Medical Committee (IOC–MC) to verify EIB and the need for precompetition β-agonist (1,2,13,15).

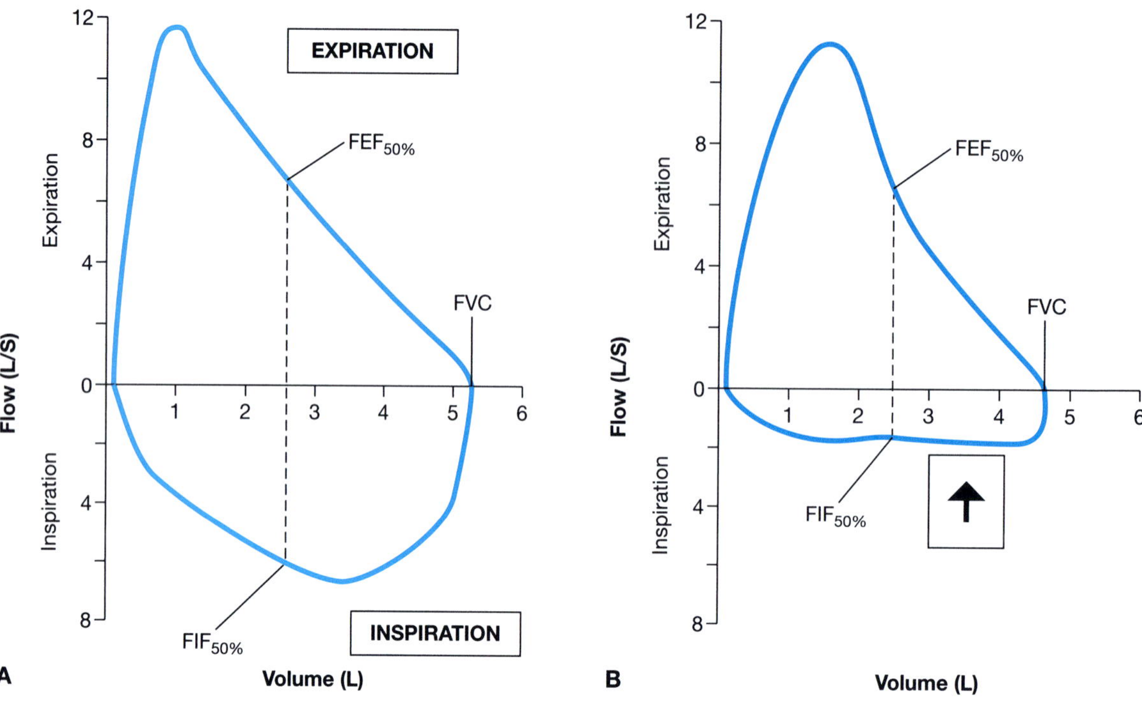

Figure 27.1: Example of a flow-volume loop in a normal subject (**A**) and in a patient with VCD (**B**). Note the blunting and flattening of the inspiratory loop of the flow-volume curve (*arrow*). (Adapted from Brooks SM. Vocal cord dysfunction after an inhalation exposure. *J Allergy Ther.* 2017;8:261. doi:10.4172/2155-6121.1000261.)

- Sensitivity and specificity in athletes have been shown to be 50% and up to 100%, respectively (1,2,16).
- Eucapnic voluntary hyperventilation (EVH) is a well-known and accepted provocative test for EIB (6,11).
- This test is more sensitive than an exercise challenge in the field or in the lab (6,11).
- EVH is more sensitive than methacholine in response to dry air hyperpnea (6).
- Negative test is highly likely to exclude EIB (16).

Conducting the Test

- Obtain a baseline PFT. Record the best FEV_1.
- The Argyros and colleagues (17) protocol, which is based on single-level ventilation of 85% of the maximum voluntary ventilation (MVV), is used. MVV is calculated as 35 times the best recorded pretest FEV_1 and is used to calculate the volume of dry gas ventilated per minute.
- The athlete inhales dry gas consisting of 5% carbon dioxide, 21% oxygen, and the remainder nitrogen gas. The volume of ventilated gas is measured by a metered instrument. The athlete gauges and adjusts the rate of ventilation based on the volume of dry gas ventilated.
- The athlete breaths at a rate of 85% MVV for 6 minutes.
- At the completion of the 6 minutes, the FEV_1 is measured twice at 1, 3, 5, 7, and 8 minutes post challenge. The best FEV_1 value is used.
- A drop in FEV_1 of at least 20% is diagnostic for EIB (6).
- A bronchodilator may be administered at the conclusion of the study to decrease the patient's symptoms and document reversibility of airway hyperresponsiveness.

METHACHOLINE CHALLENGE

- Methacholine stimulates muscarinic receptors located in the airway smooth muscle (12).
- The sensitivity and specificity of this test are estimated to be 55% and up to 100%, respectively (1,2).
- The positive predictive value may be as high as 100%, with a negative predictive value of 61% (6).
- Negative test in symptomatic patients is useful to exclude asthma, but does not exclude EIB (16).

Conducting the Methacholine Challenge

- Obtain a baseline PFT. Record the best FEV_1.
- Solutions of methacholine are prepared in the following concentrations: 0.025, 0.25, 2.5, 0, and 25 mg · mL^{-1}.
- The athlete inhales five breaths of the lowest concentration solution via nebulizer. A PFT is performed 3 minutes after inhalation of the methacholine.
- The concentration of methacholine solution is increased to the next highest concentration, and a PFT is performed 3 minutes after inhalation.

- This provocative test is concluded and considered positive if there is a decline in the FEV_1 of at least 20%. The test is concluded but considered negative if the maximum solution concentration of 25 mg · mL^{-1} is administered without the diagnostic drop in FEV_1 (1,2).
- Albuterol may be given 3 minutes after a positive test to demonstrate airway bronchospasm reversibility that is consistent with asthma.

EVALUATING ATHLETES WITH EXERCISE-INDUCED DYSPNEA

- As asthma has a higher prevalence rate, and assuming a low risk for cardiovascular disease, athletes with exertional dyspnea should first be evaluated for EIB.
- The most appropriate provocative test for identifying EIB remains controversial (3,8,9).
- EVH may be the preferred method of laboratory provocative testing because of its relative ease and excellent sensitivity. It is also more sensitive than an exercise challenge in a lab or field environment (6,11). EVH provocative testing is the preferred diagnostic study of the IOC–MC.
- If EVH testing is unavailable, a sport- and climate-specific exercise challenge is an acceptable alternative. A methacholine challenge is also an acceptable option.
- EILO is a condition where breathing is hampered by narrowing of the larynx with exercise, commonly presenting with inspiratory stridor. This may occur either in the form of vocal fold adduction (glottic EILO) or due to medial movement of the cuneiform tubercles and the aryepiglottic folds obstructing the laryngeal inlet (supraglottic EILO) (18).
- EILO has an estimated prevalence of 8.1% in the adolescent athletic population. The prevalence in the general adolescent population is 5.7%–7.5% (19).
- Athletes with disabling exercise-induced respiratory symptoms, who are either EIB negative or EIB positive and still symptomatic despite successful EIB treatment, should be considered for referral for Continuous Laryngoscopy Exercise (CLE) testing to assess for upper airway obstruction (EILO) (19).
- Although pulmonary function testing with a flow-volume loop assessment can demonstrate that the expiratory loop will be normal and the inspiratory loop can be flattened, this testing is often found to be unremarkable, with CLE testing recommended (19). See Figure 27.1B.

SUMMARY

- Exercise-induced bronchoconstriction testing is an important component of evaluating athletes with dyspnea.
- Avoid empirically treating for EIB without formal provocative testing. Classic symptoms alone are unreliable for both EIB and EILO and may lead to both over or under usage of the appropriate medical therapy (3,19).

REFERENCES

1. Carlsen KH, Anderson SD, Bjermer L, et al. Exercise-induced asthma, respiratory and allergic disorders in elite athletes: epidemiology, mechanisms and diagnosis — part I of the report from the Joint Task Force of the European Respiratory Society (ERS) and the European Academy of Allergy and Clinical Immunology (EAACI) in cooperation with GA2LEN. *Allergy*. 2008;63:387–403.
2. Eliasson AH. Blow dry your asthma. *Chest*. 1999;115(3):608–9.
3. Brennan FH, Alent J, Ross MJ. Evaluating the athlete with suspected exercise-induced asthma or bronchospasm. *Curr Sports Med Rep*. 2018;17(3):85–9.
4. Rundell KW, Im J, Mayers LB, Wilber RL, Szmedra L, Schmitz HR. Self-reported symptoms and exercise-induced asthma in the elite athlete. *Med Sci Sports Exerc*. 2001;33(2):208–13.
5. Rundell KW, Spiering BA. Inspiratory stridor in elite athletes. *Chest*. 2003;123(2):468–74.
6. Fitch KD, Sue-Chu M, Anderson SD, et al. Asthma and the elite athlete: summary of the International Olympic Committee's consensus conference, Lausanne, Switzerland, January 22–4, 2008. *J Allergy Clin Immunol*. 2008;122(2):254–60.e2607.
7. Provost-Craig MA, Arbour KS, Sestili DC, Chabalko JJ, Ekinci E. The incidence of exercise-induced bronchospasm in competitive figure skaters. *J Asthma*. 1996;33(1):67–71.
8. Rice SG, Bierman CW, Shapiro GG, Furukawa CT, Pierson WE. Identification of exercise-induced asthma among intercollegiate athletes. *Ann Allergy*. 1985;55(6):790–3.
9. Anderson SD, Argyros GJ, Magnussen H, Holzer K. Provocation by eucapnic voluntary hyperpnoea to identify exercise induced bronchoconstriction. *Br J Sports Med*. 2001;35(5):344–7.
10. Avital A, Godfrey S, Springer C. Exercise, methacholine, and adenosine 5'-monophosphate challenges in children with asthma: relation to severity of the disease. *Pediatr Pulmonol*. 2000;30(3):207–14.
11. Lin CC, Wu JL, Huang WC, Lin CY. A bronchial response comparison of exercise and methacholine in asthmatic subjects. *J Asthma*. 1991;28(1):31–40.
12. Brennan FH Jr. Exercise-induced asthma testing. In: O'Connor FG, Wilder R, editors. *Textbook of Running Medicine*. New York (NY): McGraw-Hill; 2001. p. 101–7.
13. Eliasson AH, Phillips YY, Rajagopal KR, Howard RS. Sensitivity and specificity of bronchial provocation testing. An evaluation of four techniques in exercise-induced bronchospasm. *Chest*. 1992;102(2):347–55.
14. Mannix ET, Manfredi F, Farber MO. A comparison of two challenge tests for identifying exercise-induced bronchospasm in figure skaters. *Chest*. 1999;115(3):649–53.
15. Anderson SD, Fitch K, Perry CP, et al. Responses to bronchial challenge submitted for approval to use inhaled beta2-agonists before an event at the 2002 Winter Olympics. *J Allergy Clin Immunol*. 2003;111(1):45–50.
16. Anderson SD. Provocative challenges to help diagnose and monitor asthma: exercise, methacholine, adenosine, and mannitol. *Curr Opin Pulm Med*. 2008;14(1):39–45.
17. Argyros GJ, Roach JM, Hurwitz KM, Eliasson AH, Phillips YY. The refractory period after eucapnic voluntary hyperventilation challenge and its effect on challenge technique. *Chest*. 1995;108(2):419–24.
18. Nordang L, Norlander K, Walsted ES. Exercise-induced laryngeal obstruction-an overview. *Immunol Allergy Clin North Am*. 2018;38(2):271–80.
19. Ersson K, Mallmin E, Malinovschi A, Norlander K, Johansson H, Nordang L. Prevalence of exercise-induced bronchoconstriction and laryngeal obstruction in adolescent athletes. *Pediatr Pulmonol*. 2020;55(12):3509–16.

28 Drug Testing

Aaron Rubin and Aaron Tunison

INTRODUCTION

- Drug testing of the athlete is an ethical, moral, legal, regulatory, and medical issue.
- Team physicians, athletic trainers, team psychologists, coaches, administrators, and others dealing with the care of the athlete may become involved with drug testing.
- Care should be exercised to keep the punitive aspect of drug testing separate from the therapeutic care for athlete's problems.
- Drug testing is performed for many reasons: (1–3)
  - To prevent "cheating" by use of drugs and chemicals
  - To "level the playing field" by keeping "clean" athletes from having to compete with anabolic using athletes
  - To prevent drug-induced illness and death
  - To prevent public relations problems for teams and organizations

SCOPE OF PROBLEM

- Olympic drug testing began in the 1968 Mexico City Olympics (1,4).
- Between the 1968 and 2020 Olympics, over 51,000 athletes (13,366 in the Winter Games and 38,083 in the Summer Games) were tested at competition (4).
- August 23, 2012 — Lance Armstrong was stripped of his seven Tour de France titles after declining to fight doping charges (1).
- December 9, 2019 — The World Anti-Doping Agency (WADA) banned Russia from global competition (1).
- September 14, 2021 — WADA announced it would review the status of marijuana as a prohibited drug (1).
- Various studies suggest that 5%–11% of high school males and 0.5%–2.5% of high school females have tried anabolic steroids (5,6).
- This is not merely a problem of athletes; of the high school students, 33% using anabolic steroids were not athletes (5,6).

REGULATING AGENCIES

- The United States Anti-Doping Agency (USADA) — http://www.usantidoping.org
  - Independent antidoping agency for Olympic sports in the United States (7)
- WADA — http://www.wada-ama.org
  - The mission of WADA is to promote and coordinate at international level the fight against doping in sport in all forms (8).
- International Testing Agency (ITA) — https://ita.sport
  - The ITA is an international organization constituted to manage antidoping programs, independent from sporting or political powers, for international federations, major event organizers, and all other antidoping organizations requesting support.
- National Collegiate Athletic Association (NCAA) — http://www.ncaa.org/drugtesting
  - Regulate and provide safety guidelines for student athletes from member colleges in the United States (9,10).

DRUGS, MEDICATIONS, AND OTHER SUBSTANCES (8,10)

- There are not inherently good, bad, dangerous, safe, legal, or illegal substances. This is often dependent on dosage, therapeutic use, and local laws that can be changed legislatively.
- In terms of athlete testing, it is best to consider permitted or prohibited (or allowed or not allowed) substances.
- Illegal substances are determined by law and may vary from jurisdiction to jurisdiction. The use of illegal substances can be punished by criminal law. (Marijuana and "crack" cocaine are illegal substances in most jurisdictions in the United States.)
- Components of these substances may be legal. (Dronabinol is a derivative of marijuana and legal under prescription of a licensed physician. Cocaine is a legal medicine for specific indications.)
- Some legal substances can be used illegally (anabolic steroids are legal substances but can be obtained and used illegally).
- Over-the-counter medications are theoretically legal but may be prohibited for athletic competitions (such as high-dose caffeine in NCAA testing and on the WADA Prohibited List).
- Some substances are legal but not allowed under certain circumstances (alcohol and β-blockers may not be allowed for some events).

- The ultimate decision regarding permitted or prohibited (allowed or not allowed) substances falls to the regulating agencies responsible for establishing the rules for the various sports teams, leagues, events, and organizations.
- Therapeutic drugs:
  - Prescribed drugs are those given to the athlete under the direction (prescription) of a licensed physician or dentist. Just because a medication is prescribed does not exempt an athlete from sanctions (see TUE below).
  - Over-the-counter medications may be taken by the athlete on their own or by the direction of a physician or other health care provider. Again, this does not exempt an athlete from sanctions if products are not allowed.
  - "Natural" products can be misleading. Many drugs (legal and illegal, prescription and nonprescription) are based on natural products. To complicate matters even more, many of these products may not be fully labeled with all ingredients. The athletes are ultimately responsible for what they put in their body.
- The use of banned substances for medical therapy requires that a process is followed by the athlete and medical provider (11).
- **WADA considers this process a Therapeutic Use Exemption (TUE):** (11)
  - TUE allows an athlete with a medical condition to use a prohibited substance or prohibited method. A TUE allows use of the medication or method as it will not afford a competitive advantage, but rather ensure one can compete in a proper state of health.
- **The NCAA has a Medical Exception Documentation Reporting Form** (10).
  - Exceptions may be granted for the following classes:
    - Stimulants, anabolic agents, β-blockers, diuretics, narcotics, peptide hormones, growth factors, hormone and metabolic modulators, and β_2-agonists
    - Special considerations and clearance are needed for treatment except for attention deficit hyperactivity disorder.
    - At the time of this writing, there are no medical exception review for substances in the class of cannabinoids (CBD) (see Below under Consequences).
    - The use of CBD products represents a risk for athletes resulting from the potential presence of other natural CBD such as tetrahydrocannabinol and other substance. These could cause an adverse analytical finding if detected at concentrations exceeding established thresholds (12).
- **Conditions to be considered for an exception or TUE**
  1. "The *Athlete* would experience a significant impairment to health if the *Prohibited Substance* or *Prohibited Method* were to be withheld in the course of treating an acute or chronic medical condition."
  2. "The therapeutic *Use* of the *Prohibited Substance* or *Prohibited Method* would produce no additional enhancement of performance other than that which might be anticipated by a return to a state of normal health following the treatment of a legitimate medical condition. The *Use* of any *Prohibited Substance* or *Prohibited Method* to increase 'low-normal' levels of any endogenous hormone is not considered an acceptable therapeutic intervention."
  3. "There is no reasonable therapeutic alternative to the *Use* of the otherwise *Prohibited Substance* or *Prohibited Method.*"
  4. "The necessity for the *Use* of the otherwise *Prohibited Substance* or *Prohibited Method* cannot be a consequence, wholly or in part, of prior nontherapeutic *Use* of any substance from the *Prohibited List.*"
- Recreational drugs
  - Alcohol is banned by the NCAA for rifle competition and by the Olympic movement "where the rules of the governing body so provide." The use of alcohol by minors is illegal (10).
  - Tobacco is generally not tested, although use of tobacco is not allowed at NCAA practice or competitions (10).
  - Marijuana is not allowed and is tested by the NCAA and WADA.
  - Stimulants such as amphetamine, cocaine, ephedrine, caffeine (at set concentrations for the NCAA), methylenedioxymethamphetamine (ecstasy), and related products are banned.
  - Hallucinogens such as lysergic acid diethylamide are listed as banned substances (as recreational drugs) and are illegal.
  - Many narcotics are generally banned as therapeutic or recreational substances (8).
- Performance enhancements
  - Sports characteristics may give clues to type of doping to be anticipated.
  - Aerobic and muscular endurance sports may lead to more methods and drugs to increase aerobic capacity such as blood doping or use of erythropoietin.
  - Sports high in strength and power may lead to increased use of anabolic agents and may be of most benefit in out-of-competition conditioning phase (13).
  - Stimulants as discussed earlier are prohibited.
  - Androgenic/anabolic agents such as anabolic steroids, testosterone, clenbuterol, and related compounds are banned by the NCAA and Olympic movement.
  - Recombinant erythropoietin and related compounds and blood doping are not allowed. Blood doping is the removal of one's own blood (or using donor blood) and later transfusing it to improve aerobic capacity.
  - In addition, techniques to mask drug testing or fool drug testers are not allowed. These include diuretics, urine substitution, masking agents, and other techniques.

- The NCAA publishes a list that bans classes of drugs and substances related chemically to the classes.
- In addition, NCAA has procedures subject to restrictions:
  - Blood doping
  - Local anesthetics (under some conditions)
  - Manipulation of urine samples
  - β_2-Agonists permitted only by prescription and inhalation
  - Caffeine if concentrations in urine exceed 15 μg · mL^{-1} (10)
- WADA publishes a prohibited list that is also available for handheld devices.
- WADA adds the following caveat:
  - "Any pharmacological substance which is not addressed by any of the subsequent sections of the List and with no current approval by any governmental regulatory health authority for human therapeutic use (i.e., drugs under preclinical or clinical development or discontinued) is prohibited at all times" (8).
- Warnings regarding use of nutritional supplements are prominent in NCAA materials, including the lack of regulation of the industry and inability for the athlete to know about contaminated or unlabeled ingredients (10).
- WADA gives similar precautions (8).

TESTING PROCEDURES (BASED ON THE NCAA DRUG TESTING PROGRAMS)

- Selection process must be fair and based on random testing, universal testing, or testing based on probable cause (evidence of drug use or previous positive test).
- Testing may be done out-of-competition (year-round) or in-competition (postseason championship) (10). In-competition is defined as the period commencing at 11:59 pm on the day before through the end of such competition.

POSTSEASON TESTING

- Facilities and procedures are fully outlined in the NCAA Drug-Testing Program Site Coordinators Manual (10).
- WADA urine testing procedures are similar, and WADA has procedures for blood testing as well as developing the Athlete Biological Profile, which attempts to set "normal" standards for an individual athlete as opposed to a population (such as baseline hemoglobin/hematocrit to try to determine blood doping or use of recombinant erythropoietin).
- The athlete is notified of testing by a drug testing courier and given a written notification form instructing the athlete to accompany the courier to the collection station. The athlete must report within 1 hour and remain in visual contact with the courier until the athlete signs in at the testing center. Only authorized agents for testing and the athletes are allowed in the testing center.
- A designated Doping Control Officer (DCO) or their designee confirms the athlete's identification and assures testing rules are followed.
- Sealed beverages without caffeine or other banned substances are allowed at the testing center.
- The athlete will select a sealed specimen collection container and attach a unique barcode to the collection container.
- If the specimen is not sufficient (usually about 90 mL), it is discarded, and the athlete is asked to provide another specimen. The athlete is not allowed to leave the test center until adequate specimen is provided unless approved by the DCO.
- Specific gravity and pH are checked. If the specific gravity is less than 1.005 (1.010 if checked with a reagent strip), the specimen is discarded. If the pH is greater than 7.5 or less than 4.5, the specimen is discarded (9).
- The specimen is processed if the specific gravity is above 1.005 (1.010 if using a reagent strip) and the pH is between 4.5 and 7.5 (9).
  - pH and specific gravity requirements were outlined in the 2011 NCAA drug testing guidance (9) but not specified in current (2022) document (10).
  - Doing these tests help determine if the specimen has been diluted or otherwise manipulated.
- Containers and unique bar-coded labels are selected by the athlete.
- The specimen is divided into the "A vial" and the "B vial" by the crew member. The vials are sealed, forms are filled out, and the specimens prepared for shipping. All is done in the presence of the athlete.
- Chain of evidence must be maintained. The specimen must be controlled, tracked, and signed for at every step in the process.
- The specimens are sent to an approved laboratory for testing. Specimen A is tested.
- Results of positive tests are reported to the National Center for Drug Free Sport who breaks the number code and identifies the athlete. The athletics director or designate is notified by overnight mail marked confidential, who in turn must notify the athlete.
- The athlete may be represented at the laboratory when testing specimen B. Different lab personnel will test specimen B.
- The results of specimen B are considered final (10).

INSTITUTIONAL DRUG TESTING (14)

- Extreme care must be taken to protect the rights of the athlete.
- Goals of testing, education program, punishment, selection process, procedures for testing, notification, confidentiality,

appropriate follow-up, and legal issues must be carefully thought out and put into writing.

- Multiple individuals may be involved in creating such a policy, including but not limited to administrators, legal counsel, medical advisors, psychologists, and representatives of the athletes.
- After notification, the athlete must present to a testing center within a set amount of time.
- Testing may be performed at an on-campus center or a designated industrial clinic for drug testing. If sent to an outside facility, the school or organization must assure that proper conduct and procedures are followed.
- Testing procedures should be similar to those discussed earlier under "Postseason Testing."
- Lists of substances that are not allowed must be published and the athletes educated regarding the substances, health risks, treatment options, and sanctions for positive tests.

TESTING TECHNIQUES

- Initial screening may be done by the relatively lower cost thin-layer chromatography or radioimmunoassay methods.
- Confirmation and definitive testing should be performed by gas chromatography and mass spectroscopy (8,14).

LEGAL ISSUES

- Expect legal challenges to testing procedures and especially to positive tests.
- Athletes must be afforded due process of law.
- Institutions and all organizations mandating testing should define rights of appeal.

PUBLIC RELATIONS

- Privacy of the athlete must be maintained.
- The public and press often feel they have a "right to know" about the dealings of "their" teams, schools, and athletes.
- The loss of an athlete from a team for "disciplinary" reasons is often assumed to be for positive drug tests.

CONSEQUENCES

- Student-athletes who test positive for a banned substance, or who breach NCAA testing protocol requirements, are subject to loss of eligibility. These student-athletes may be subject to additional testing for all NCAA-banned substances by the NCAA at any time.
- The NCAA Committee on Competitive Safeguards and Medical Aspects of Sports recommended removal of CBD from the NCAA list of banned substances awaiting each division of the NCAA to introduce and adopt legislation (15).
- WADA sanctions for Use or Attempted Use of Prohibited Substance or Prohibited Method and Possession of Prohibited Substance or Methods.
  - First violation: Two years' ineligibility
  - Second violation: Lifetime ineligibility
- If an athlete can establish the use was not intended to enhance performance, then the first violation consequences should result in the following:
  - Warning and reprimand and no ineligibility from future events
  - Up to a maximum of 1 year ineligibility
- There should be an opportunity for the athlete to establish basis for eliminating or reducing sanctions.

REFERENCES

1. Britannica. [Accessed September 30, 2022]. ProCon.org. https://sportsanddrugs.procon.org/historical-timeline/
2. Ritchie I. *Cops and Robbers? The Roots of Anti-Doping Policies in Olympic Sport February 2016.* [Accessed September 30, 2022]. https://origins.osu.edu/article/cops-and-robbers-roots-anti-doping-policies-olympic-sport?language_content_entity=en
3. Vlad RA, Hancu G, Popescu GC, Lungu IA. Doping in sports, a never-ending story? *Adv Pharm Bull.* 2018 Nov;8(4):529–34. doi:10.15171/apb.2018.062
4. International Olympic Committee. *Factsheet: Fight against doping and Health promotion update December 2021* [Internet]. [Accessed October 1 2022]. Available from: https://stillmed.olympics.com/media/Documents/Athletes/Factsheets/Fight-against-doping-and-health-promotion.pdf?_ga=2.106259909.732979760.1665711741-1487478262.1665711741
5. Greydanus DE, Patel DR. Sports doping in the adolescent athlete the hope, hype, and hyperbole. *Pediatr Clin North Am.* 2002;49(4):829–55.
6. Knopp WD, Wang TW, Bach BR. Ergogenic drugs in sports. *Clin Sports Med.* 1997;16(3):375–92.
7. United States Anti-Doping Agency (USADA). *Protocol for Olympic and Paralympic Movement Testing as Revised January 1, 2021.* [Accessed September 30, 2022]. https://www.usada.org/wp-content/uploads/USADA_protocol.pdf
8. World Anti-Doping Agency (WADA). *World Anti-Doping International Standard Prohibited List.* [Accessed October 1, 2022]. Available from: https://www.wada-ama.org/sites/default/files/2022-01/2022list_final_en_0.pdf
9. National Collegiate Athletic Association. *Drug testing program* 2010-11 *[Internet].* [cited 2022 Sep 27]. Available from: http://www.ncaapublications.com/productdownloads/dt11.pdf
10. National Collegiate Athletic Association. *Drug testing program* 2022-23 *[Internet].* [cited 2022 Sep 27]. Available from: https://ncaaorg.s3.amazonaws.com/ssi/substance/2022-23/2022-23SSI_DrugTestingProgram.pdf
11. World Anti-Doping Agency. *Therapeutic Use Exemption Guidelines 2022 [Internet].* [cited 2022 Sep 30]. Available from: https://www.wada-ama.org/en/athletes-support-personnel/therapeutic-use-exemptions-tues

12. Thevis M, Kuuranne T, Geyer H. Annual banned-substance review: Analytical approaches in human sports drug testing 2020/2021. *Drug Test Anal.* 2022 Jan;14(1):7–30.
13. Hayward G, Gaborini L, Sims D, et al. The athletic characteristics of Olympic sports to assist anti-doping strategies. *Drug Test Anal.* 2022 Sep;14(9):1599–613.
14. Moeller KE, Lee KC, Kissack JC. *Urine Drug Screening: Practical Guide for Clinicians Mayo Clinic Proceedings.* 2008 Jan 1;83(1):66–76, https://www.mayoclinicproceedings.org/action/showPdf?pii=S0025-6196%2811%2961120-8
15. *NCAA Committee on Competitive Safeguards and Medical Aspects of Sports Question and Answer Document Legislative recommendation to remove cannabinoids from list of NCAA Banned Substances.* [cited 2023 Nov 15]. https://ncaaorg.s3.amazonaws.com/committees/ncaa/safeguards/statements/SSI_RemoveCannabinoidsQandA.pdf

Thermotolerance Testing

29

Yoram Epstein and Yuval Heled

INTRODUCTION

- In a healthy individual, the balance between heat accumulation and heat dissipation dictates body-core temperature. Body temperature will be maintained within the physiological limits of 36.5–37.5 °C when heat dissipation equalizes heat accumulation. However, when heat accumulation overwhelms heat dissipation, heat is stored and consequently body temperature rises.
- In a physically fit individual wearing light clothing while exercising in moderate environmental heat, 1–2 °C increase in body-core temperature can be expected and can be sustained for relatively long durations (1). During vigorous exercise/work, metabolic heat production can be increased by 15–20 times compared to rest and consequently, under unfavorable environmental conditions of climate and clothing, body-core temperature can increase by 1 °C every 5 minutes (1). A rise of 4–5 °C in body-core temperature can prove to be catastrophic for human health (1,2).
- Exertional heat illness (EHI) is an array of syndromes (1,3). The more serious forms of heat illness are characterized by elevation in body-core temperature and collapse (1,3,4). In the spectrum of EHI, the most extreme form is exertional heatstroke (EHS) that can be a life-threatening injury (2–4); EHS is considered to be one of the three leading causes of death among athletes (5–7). EHI is further described in Chapter 47, Environmental Illness.
- Recovery from EHS and return to activity usually takes a few weeks, is straightforward, and is unremarkable, provided adequate time for clinical recovery is allowed (4,8,9). Nevertheless, some patients might experience long-term complications, such as a temporary condition of heat intolerance, and the recovery period may vary from 7 days to 15 months (10).
- Heat tolerance test (HTT) is a tool that has been developed to assist in assessing underlying heat tolerance and facilitating return-to-play and return-to-duty clinical decisions.

HEAT TOLERANCE/INTOLERANCE

- Heat tolerance is termed to describe the ability to sustain physical activity in warm to hot conditions. Thus, individuals in the population who are not able to sustain an exercise-heat stress and whose body temperature will start rising earlier and at a higher rate than that of others under the same conditions are regarded as "heat intolerant" (HI) (11,12). The cumulative experience, especially with soldiers who recovered from EHS, is that HI is in most cases a temporary phenomenon (13–16).
- In athletes, individual susceptibility to EHS is a consequence of intrinsic and extrinsic factors. A temporarily acquired cause underlies most EHS cases; however, some inherent conditions and genetic susceptibility may endanger an individual's tolerance to heat and expose them to a recurrent EHS (4,9,11,12,17) (Table 29.1).
- A major concern among athletes/soldiers is behavioral responses to perform beyond the level of acclimatization or fitness, *i.e.*, overmotivation of the individual from either extrinsic (peer-pressure) or intrinsic (the pursuit of excellence) pressures (1,2,18,19).
- While, for many years, body dimensions and especially body surface area-to-mass ratio have been mentioned as a risk factor (11,20), only recently they attained more attention. A low body surface area-to-mass ratio indicates a higher metabolic heat accumulation disproportional to the ability to dissipate heat (21–23). A former condition of heatstroke is also said to be a temporary or (rarely) permanent cause of heat intolerance (1,11).
- As EHI is a sporadic event with only the minority of trainees/competitors who are exposed to the same environmental and exercise conditions as their peers are impacted (4), it follows that an underlying inherent or acquired cause of the thermoregulatory ability of patients with EHS is clearly compromised at the time of collapse, limiting their ability to sustain an exercise-heat stress.

Table 29.1 Most Common Factors Underlying Heat Intolerance (9,11)

Functional	Congenital	Acquired
Low physical fitness	Chronic idiopathic anhidrosis	Viral/bacterial infection
Reduced BSA/mass	Ectodermal dysplasia	Dehydration
Lack of acclimatization	Malignant hyperthermia (?)	Large burn scarred area
Low work efficiency		Sweat gland dysfunction
		stimulating/illicit drugs
		Previous EHS

?, suspected but not verified; BSA, body surface area; EHS, exertional heatstroke.

The Heat Tolerance Test

- The heat tolerance test (HTT) is regarded as a functional (and not clinical) test that reflects the ability of the individual to thermoregulate properly and attain thermal balance under the test's conditions (13,14). Therefore, the test is based on standardized settings of exercise-heat stress that triggers the thermoregulatory response and that can adequately be observed and assessed.
- The rationale behind the test is that if an individual who recovered from EHS will sustain the test, then the interpretation is that their thermoregulatory ability is intact. Those who fail the test are regarded as HI and should be further evaluated for the reason of heat intolerance.
- Over the years, many modalities and protocols for the HTT have been suggested (3). To date, the most common HTT is the test suggested by the Israel Defense Forces (IDF), which is in use for over 4 decades (see 'conducting the test') (9,13). This is an exercise-heat stress test, which is performed under high environmental heat load that limits sweat evaporation (13). It is a simple-to-perform test, reproducible, and suited for athletes as well (9).
- Since full recovery from EHI might vary in time, it is advised to take the test after a few weeks post clinical recovery and allowing the transient state of deficient thermoregulatory ability to improve (9,13), although testing after 10–14 days of recovery has also been advocated (24).

HTT Indications

- The process of safely returning individuals to strenuous activity following recovering EHS is not well established and is a clinical challenge. Current guidance is based on subjective physician assessments and clinical blood biomarker findings to return to normal (4,9).
- The American College of Sports Medicine (ACSM) currently recommends consideration of a structured HTT as part of the decision-making process for athletes in whom return to vigorous activity and evidence of an athlete's ability or adapt to exercise-heat stress over several days is not accomplished within 4–6 weeks (4,9).
- Accordingly, the HTT is in use as an auxiliary tool for deciding when an athlete/soldier may return safely to physically demanding activities. ACSM's recommendation, however, does not specify a distinct protocol.

Conducting the HTT (the IDF Protocol) (9)

- The test is performed only after a complete clinical recovery.
- The subject should be instructed to avoid tobacco and caffeine before the test. They should not perform any exhaustive exercise, should not drink any alcohol for at least 24 hours before the test, and should sleep at least 7 hours during the night before the test. In the hour before the test, the subject should drink 0.5 L of water.
- The test is performed in a controlled climatic chamber under the conditions of 40 °C and 40% relative humidity while exercising for 120 minutes on a treadmill at a pace of 5 km · h^{-1} and 2% incline.
- During the exposure, men are dressed in shorts and no shirt (women wear a sports bra), and athletic shoes.
- At the morning of testing, the subject should undergo a general medical examination and assessment of their baseline core temperature, which should be <37.3 °C. Any manifestation of illness, including subclinical presentations, contraindicates performing the test.
- During the entire testing exposure, rectal temperature and heart rate are continuously monitored. Measurements of these two variables enable also to score the physiological strain (on a scale of 0–10) by calculating the physiological strain index (PSI) (16). Although the PSI is not an outcome criterion, it may assist when comparing results across tests.
- To calculate sweat rate, body weight is measured before and after the exposure and corrected for water intake and urine output. Sweat rate is measured to uncover a possible condition of hypo-anhidrosis (as this might be the cause of a positive test and the possible underlying cause of EHS).
- **Safety measures:** Test will be stopped if (a) rectal temperature exceeds 39.0 °C, (b) heart rate exceeds 200 beats · min^{-1}, (c) the individual is willing to cease the test, or (d) the attending physician decides to cease the test, according to the subject's clinical condition.

HTT Interpretation

- The HTT is interpreted in one of three categories: heat tolerant, heat intolerant, and borderline. (Fig. 29.1 demonstrates normal and abnormal graphs of HTT data.)
- **HI criteria:** (a) rectal temperature >38.5 °C with no tendency to plateau (the tendency to plateau is a requisite because it reflects a balance between heat gain and heat dissipation (13)); (b) heart rate >150 beats · min^{-1} with no tendency to plateau.
- Several supportive criteria assist in the decision on a positive (namely, HI) IDF HTT, especially in borderline cases such as when the rectal temperature tends to plateau somewhat above but close to 38.5 °C: (a) no tendency to plateau — the increase in rectal temperature during the 2nd hour of the test (60–120 minutes) is >0.45 °C (25); (b) the rectal temperature-to-heart rate ratio at the end of the test (the average of the last 5 minutes) is <0.279 °C · bpm^{-1} (26); (c) the probability of heat tolerance (PHT) (13).
- PHT is an algorithm that was developed based on the IDF HTT criteria (13). The PHT enables a standardized objective interpretation of the HTT results. A PHT value >0.9 is regarded as heat tolerance and PHT <0.5 as heat intolerance. The sensitivity, specificity, and accuracy of the index are 100%, 90%, and 92.06%, respectively.

HTT AND CLINICAL DECISION-MAKING

- The decision on return to activity after an individual has recovered from an EHI (especially EHS) is a challenging medical decision. Being a functional test that reflects the individual's ability to properly thermoregulate, the HTT is a supportive decision-making tool (9).
- A negative test result reflects an effective thermoregulatory response. In this case, the individual is considered 'heat tolerant' and can safely return to activity.
- If the thermoregulatory response is abnormal and the results point to 'heat intolerance', a second test should be scheduled to be performed 3 months after the first test (9,10,27). Based on the IDF experience, only 10% of individuals who perform the HTT fail on the first attempt, and less than 2% of individuals fail after the retest 3 months later (17).
- Only after the second test (and eventually a third test), a permanent state of heat intolerance can usually be assumed. Patients who do not achieve thermal balance at repeat assessments should be referred for further medical investigations to determine their underlying cause for HI.
- It should be emphasized that being a functional test the HTT's ability to predict a recurrent heatstroke is limited (anhidrosis is a risk factor that can be uncovered by the HTT). Even those who pass the test might be inflicted under uncompensable exercise-heat stress conditions. On the other hand, those who are regarded as HI should take further measures to eliminate exercising under harsh conditions, unless a temporary underlying cause for HI has been identified.
- The sensitivity, specificity, and diagnostic accuracy of the IDF HTT are high, and the current conclusion is that the risk of heatstroke recurrence is measurable and that a negative HTT result is associated with a substantial reduction of future heatstroke risk (27).

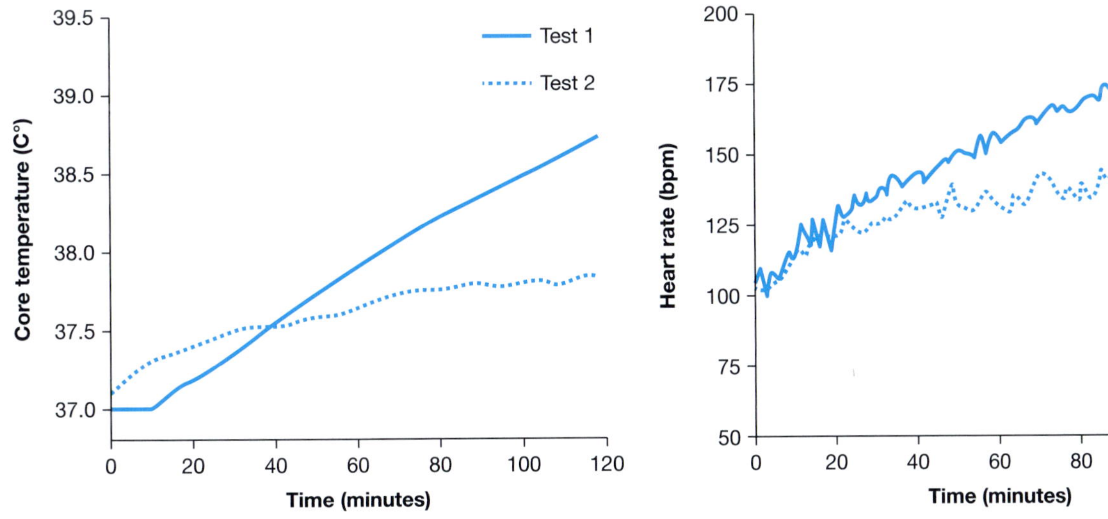

Figure 29.1: Rectal temperature and heart rate during two Israel Defense Forces heat tolerance tests. Test 1 is regarded as positive — heat intolerant (HI). A constant increase in rectal temperature and heart rate with no tendency to plateau. Test 2 is regarded as negative — heat tolerant (HT). Rectal temperature and heart rate tended to plateau within the permissible range (13,16).

REPORTED LIMITATIONS OF THE IDF HTT

- The IDF HTT is the most common test assisting the physician in the decision of returning a soldier/athlete to activity (3,9,11). The IDF uses the test on a regular basis with great clinical success (27). Others also advocate using this test as part of the challenging clinical decision on return to activity following the recovery from EHI (9). Nevertheless, the test is not applicable for everyone (9).
- The IDF HTT criteria were established for relatively young and moderately fit individuals. Therefore, individuals who are older, unfit, ill, and/or obese will probably fail the test and may need different criteria. In a recent review article, Mitchell et al. also questioned the test's external validity for tasks with high metabolic load (3).
- The HTT does not consider seasonal weather variations or acclimatization status, but a recent study from the IDF concluded that the season of testing has yielded no difference in results, and therefore acclimatization status does not alter the HTT responses (25).
- The data in regard to sex differences are lacking and inconclusive. When the standard IDF HTT criteria, which were developed based on men, are applied to women, women present higher physiological strain and are diagnosed more frequently as HI (28–30).

SUMMARY

- EHI is an array of syndromes, directly related to physical exercise, spanning from heat exhaustion to heatstroke. EHI is a sporadic event; only those individuals with a compromised thermoregulatory response due to intrinsic or extrinsic factors are inflicted.
- Under exercise-heat stress, the inability to efficiently dissipate heat as expected by normal average individuals under similar conditions is defined as heat intolerance. In those individuals, body temperature starts rising earlier and at a higher rate than others under the same conditions.
- Return to activity of an individual who sustained an EHI (especially EHS) is a complex medical decision, which should be taken by an attentive and astute clinician.
- A powerful tool that helps in uncovering a condition of heat intolerance is the HTT. The test is a functional test, which depicts the ability to thermoregulate effectively under a given structured exercise-heat stress. A negative result proves an intact, effective temperature-regulating mechanism and, thus, heat tolerance, while a positive result of the test corresponds to a condition of heat intolerance. The HTT result may, therefore, be a useful supportive tool in the decision of returning to activity following EHI.

REFERENCES

1. Leon LR, Bouchama A. Heat stroke. *Compr Physiol.* 2015;5(2):611–47.
2. Epstein Y, Yanovich R. Heatstroke. *N Engl J Med.* 2019;380(25):2449–59.
3. Mitchell KM, Cheuvront SN, King MA, Mayer TA, Leon LR, Kenefick RW. Use of the heat tolerance test to assess recovery from exertional heat stroke. *Temperature.* 2019;6(2):106–19.
4. Roberts WO, Armstrong LE, Sawka MN, Yeargin SW, Heled Y, O'Connor FG. ACSM expert consensus statement on exertional heat illness: recognition, management, and return to activity. *Curr Sports Med Rep.* 2021;20(9):470–84.
5. Yankelson L, Sadeh B, Gershovitz L, et al. Life-Threatening events during endurance sports: is heat stroke more prevalent than arrhythmic death? *J Am Coll Cardiol.* 2014;64(5):463–9.
6. Maron BJ, Doerer JJ, Haas TS, Tierney DM, Mueller FO. Sudden deaths in young competitive athletes: analysis of 1866 deaths in the United States, 1980-2006. *Circulation.* 2009;119(8):1085–92.
7. Howe AS, Boden BP. Heat-related illness in athletes. *Am J Sports Med.* 2007;35(8):1384–95.
8. Epstein Y, Moran DS, Shapiro Y, Sohar E, Shemer J. Exertional heat stroke: a case series. *Med Sci Sports Exerc.* 1999;31(2):224–8.
9. O'Connor FG, Heled Y, Deuster PA. Exertional heat stroke, the return to play decision, and the role of heat tolerance testing: a clinician's dilemma. *Curr Sports Med Rep.* 2018;17(7):244–8.
10. O'Connor FG, Williams AD, Blivin S, Heled Y, Deuster P, Flinn SD. Guidelines for return to duty (play) after heat illness: a military perspective. *J Sport Rehabil.* 2007;16(3):227–37.
11. Epstein Y. Heat intolerance: predisposing factor or residual injury? *Med Sci Sports Exerc.* 1990;22(1):29–35.
12. Hosokawa Y, Stearns RL, Casa DJ. Is heat intolerance state or trait? *Sports Med.* 2019;49(3):365–70.
13. Schermann H, Craig E, Yanovich E, Ketko I, Kalmanovich G, Yanovich R. Probability of heat intolerance: standardized interpretation of heat-tolerance testing results versus specialist judgment. *J Athl Train.* 2018;53(4):423–30.
14. House C, Stacey M, Woods D, Allsopp A, Roiz de Sa D. Procedure for assessing patients referred to the UK's military Heat Illness Clinic: a case series. *BMJ Mil Health.* 2023;169(4):310–15.
15. Epstein Y, Heled Y. Back to play of athletes after exertional heat stroke. *Curr Sports Med Rep.* 2013;12(5):346.
16. Kazman JB, Heled Y, Lisman PJ, Druyan A, Deuster PA, O'Connor FG. Exertional heat illness: the role of heat tolerance testing. *Curr Sports Med Rep.* 2013;12(2):101–5.
17. Westwood CS, Fallowfield JL, Delves SK, Nunns M, Ogden HB, Layden JD. Individual risk factors associated with exertional heat illness: a systematic review. *Exp Physiol.* 2021;106(1):191–9.
18. Abriat A, Brosset C, Brégigeon M, Sagui E. Report of 182 cases of exertional heatstroke in the French Armed Forces. *Mil Med.* 2014;179(3):309–14.
19. McDuff D, Stull T, Castaldelli-Maia JM, Hitchcock ME, Hainline B, Reardon CL. Recreational and ergogenic substance use and substance use disorders in elite athletes: a narrative review. *Br J Sports Med.* 2019;53(12):754–60.
20. Lisman P, Kazman JB, O'Connor FG, Heled Y, Deuster PA. Heat tolerance testing: association between heat intolerance and anthropometric and fitness measurements. *Mil Med.* 2014;179(11):1339–46.
21. Alele FO, Malau-Aduli BS, Malau-Aduli AEO, Crowe JM. Individual anthropometric, aerobic capacity and demographic characteristics

as predictors of heat intolerance in military populations. *Medicina (Kaunas)*. 2021;57(2):173.

22. Giersch GEW, Taylor KM, Caldwell AR, Charkoudian N. Body mass index, but not sex, influences exertional heat stroke risk in young healthy men and women. *Am J Physiol Regul Integr Comp Physiol.* 2023;324(1):R15–9.
23. Akavian I, Epstein Y, Rabotin A, Peretz S, Charkoudian N, Ketko I. The significance of body surface area to mass ratio for thermal responses to a standardized exercise-heat stress test. *Med Sci Sports Exerc.* 2025;57(1):88–93. doi:10.1249/MSS.0000000000003545
24. Schermann H, Hazut-Krauthammer S, Weksler Y, et al. When should a heat-tolerance test be scheduled after clinical recovery from an exertional heat illness? *J Athl Train.* 2020;55(3):289–94.
25. Druyan A, Ketko I, Yanovich E, et al. Redefining the distinction between heat tolerant and intolerant individuals during a heat tolerance test. *J Therm Biol.* 2013;38(8):539–42.
26. Ketko I, Eliyahu U, Epstein Y, Heled Y. The thermal-circulatory ratio (TCR): an index to evaluate the tolerance to heat. *Temperature.* 2014;1(2):101–6.
27. Schermann H, Heled Y, Fleischmann C, et al. The validity of the heat tolerance test in prediction of recurrent exertional heat illness events. *J Sci Med Sport.* 2018;21(6):549–52.
28. Druyan A, Makranz C, Moran D, Yanovich R, Epstein Y, Heled Y. Heat tolerance in women–reconsidering the criteria. *Aviat Space Environ Med.* 2012;83(1):58–60.
29. Yanovich R, Ketko I, Muginshtein-Simkovitch J, et al. Physiological differences between heat tolerant and heat intolerant young healthy women. *Res Q Exerc Sport.* 2019;90(3):307–17.
30. Gagge AP, Gonzalez RR. Mechanisms of heat exchange: biophysics and physiology. In: Blatteis CM, Fregly MJ, editors. *Handbook of Physiology: Environmental Physiology.* Bethesda (MD): American Physiological Society; 1996. p. 45–84.

30 Neuropsychological Testing in Concussion

Andrea L. Pana, Danielle Thornsberry, and Matthew Hall

INTRODUCTION

- The incidence of sport-related concussions varies depending on the sport and level of participation and is likely underestimated in epidemiologic studies due to lack of reporting (1). One source estimated that only one out of every nine concussions is captured in data collection in the United States (2).
- Diagnosis and management of concussion involves a careful assessment of the history of the injury and subsequent symptoms, a thorough clinical examination, as well as the consideration of advanced diagnostic testing. Neuropsychological assessment is one of several tools currently used in the evaluation and management of concussions and can include brief sideline assessments of memory and attention, computerized neuropsychological testing, and formal written neuropsychological testing with evaluation by a neuropsychologist.
- The Amsterdam Concussion in Sport Group concluded "Neurocognitive test batteries, where accessible, may add value to assessing SRC and its sequelae. Computer-based test batteries, especially in comparison of reaction times against patient baseline and community norms, may be useful. The results of these tests should be interpreted in the context of broader clinical findings and are not to be used in isolation to inform management or diagnostic decisions" (3).
- The Team Physician Consensus Statement on Concussion states that neuropsychological testing "is recommended as an aid to clinical decision-making but not a requirement for concussion management." The document also states, "the value of NP testing is enhanced when used as part of a multifaceted assessment and treatment program" and that it is "one component of the evaluation process and should not be used as a stand-alone tool to diagnose, manage or make RTP decisions in concussion" (4).
- The NCAA Consensus on Diagnosis and Management of Sport-Related Concussion Best Practices recommends a "one time, pre-participation baseline concussion assessment for all varsity student athletes," which should include a "cognitive assessment" but does not mandate or require specific neuropsychological testing (5).
- The NATA Position Statement on Management of Sport Concussion states, "neurocognitive testing should never be used in isolation but rather in conjunction with symptoms and motor-control assessments to support the clinical examination" (6).

WHY IS NEUROPSCHOLOGICAL TESTING USEFUL IN CONCUSSION?

- "Continuing to play immediately following a concussion is a risk for increased symptom burden, worsening of the injury and prolonged recovery. Athletes who return to sport prior to full recovery are at increased risk of repeat concussion" (1).
- Self-reported symptoms are not a reliable indicator of resolution of concussion. Athletes may underreport symptoms as they may mislabel or fail to identify symptoms when they occur or attribute them to something else such as stress, dehydration, a tight helmet, or another medical condition. They might blatantly deny symptoms due to internal or external pressures (fear of losing position, losing respect, seeming weak, letting the team down). Mild post-concussive symptoms such as fatigue or sleep issues may be viewed as their baseline level of functioning.
- "Although in most cases, cognitive recovery largely overlaps with the time course of symptom recovery, cognitive recovery may occasionally precede or lag behind clinical symptom resolution, suggesting that the assessment of cognitive function should be an important component in the overall assessment of SRC and, in particular, any return-to-play protocol" (7).

TYPES OF NEUROPSYCHOLOGICAL TESTING IN CONCUSSION

- Sideline Neuropsychological Assessment Tools: These are basic neuropsychological tests designed for sideline assessment of athletes with concussion. Specifically, they involve tests of orientation, memory, concentration, and delayed recall.

- Clinician Administered Neuropsychological Tests: Consist of paper-and-pencil neuropsychological tests to assess cognitive function. Concussion assessment batteries typically focus on cognitive function but additional tests assessing related psychological dysfunction can be added in cases where more extensive neuropsychological testing may be warranted in a patient.
- Computerized Neuropsychological Tests: These are computer-based neuropsychological tests, which measure various aspects of memory (new learning), cognitive processing speed, working memory, or executive functions.

STATISTICAL FACTORS NECESSARY IN CHOOSING A NEUROPSYCHOLOGICAL TEST

- For NP testing to be valuable in the evaluation and treatment of concussion, certain statistical parameters should be met to demonstrate that as a clinical tool it has added value to the clinical armamentarium. Ultimately, one would like to be able to say that using this tool changes outcomes in the individuals one is treating with concussion.
- In the literature, statistical parameters applied in assessing neuropsychological test batteries include reliability, validity, sensitivity, specificity, reliable change, and clinical utility.
- Additional information regarding statistical parameters in assessing neuropsychological testing is available in the online content of this chapter.

Reliability

- Reliability is a measure of the stability of a score or test over time. Test-retest reliability should ideally reflect clinically relevant intervals.

Change Scores

- Change scores measure the variability of a test over time. Variability is made up of the real or normal fluctuation of a test from one session to the next and an error variance or change in the test that is due to the flaws in the measurement technique.
- In the sports medicine/neuropsychology literature the two most common techniques for change scores are reliable change indices and regression analyses (10).
- Reliable Change Indices (RCI) provide a value above which an observed change can be said to be meaningful. A standard RCI does not correct for the effects of measurement error caused by practice effects or other confounding variables. A modified RCI controls for measurement errors and practice effects.
- The size of an RCI depends on the reliability of the test and the desired level of confidence (*e.g.*, 80%, 90%, 95%) (11).
- Simple and multiple regression techniques can be used to calculate or predict a subject's score after concussion. Multiple regression equations may include estimates of effects of variables such as age, education, socioeconomics, and prior concussion history. A significant change is said to occur when the difference between the observed and predicted score is greater than a certain criterion (10).

Validity

- Test validity is the degree to which a test accurately measures what it is supposed to measure.
- Concurrent validity is the degree to which a test in question correlates with an established test.
- Performance validity is the extent to which a cognitive test score reflects the examinee's true cognitive abilities.

Sensitivity and Specificity

- In concussion, sensitivity is the ability of the NP test to have a positive result in those athletes with concussion.
- In concussion, specificity refers to the ability of the test to correctly identify the athlete who does not have a concussion.

Clinical Utility

- A neuropsychological test can have high reliability and high sensitivity but not be clinically useful. For concussion, an NP test would be clinically useful if it is sensitive in detecting neurocognitive impairments once symptoms have resolved.
- A test is also clinically useful if the decision made from using it changes clinical outcomes. For example, does holding an athlete beyond the time they are asymptomatic until the time their NP tests return to baseline change the clinical outcome?

SIDELINE AND OFFICE ASSESSMENT: BRIEF NEUROPSYCHOLOGICAL TESTS

Historical Perspective

- Sideline neuropsychological assessment consists of brief tests of orientation, memory, concentration, and delayed recall used to assess an athlete's cognitive functioning and in determining if the athlete sustained a concussion.
- Maddocks questions, composed of questions of orientation and recent memory, were validated in a 1995 study. It was here that it was concluded that questions relating to orientation (person, date of birth, age, month) were not sensitive in discriminating between a concussed and nonconcussed athlete. Questions relating to recall of recently acquired events (ground, quarter, how far into quarter, last team to score, team played last, who won last) were sensitive in detecting concussion (12).

- Standardized Assessment of Concussion (SAC) was developed in 1996 in response to the need for a standardized concussion assessment tool. It is a validated tool assessing orientation, immediate and delayed memory, and concentration. It is a scored tool that is optimally utilized when compared to a preseason baseline (13).
- Sport Concussion Assessment Tool (SCAT) is a validated tool developed from the 2nd International Consensus Conference on Concussion in Sport (Prague). It was created by combining several existing assessment tools used by medical and sports organizations into a new standardized tool. SCAT consists of evaluation of signs, memory assessment, symptoms, cognitive assessment, and neurological screening (13).
- SCAT evolved into the SCAT2 in 2008 and into the SCAT3 in 2012. At this time, a Child SCAT was also introduced. The SCAT 5 was the result of a consensus process and systematic review completed at the 5th Concussion in Sport Group international meeting in Berlin in 2016. SCAT6 was published in June of 2023 and is just beginning to be used clinically. It was a product of the 6th International Conference on Concussion in Sport in Amsterdam, October 2022. Also at this meeting, a new standardized concussion office assessment tool, SCOAT6, and Child SCOAT6 were developed. These were developed with the goal to "better guide the evaluation and management in an office setting from 72 hours after injury and for serial evaluations in the following weeks" (3).
- Graded Symptom Checklist, SAC, and Balance Error Scoring System (BESS) were found to be most useful immediately post-injury in differentiating concussed from nonconcussed athletes (14).
- Diagnostic utility of SCAT and its components appear to decrease significantly after 3–5 days post injury (14).
- Symptoms Checklist does demonstrate utility in tracking recovery (14).
- Scoring on the SCAT5 should not be used as a stand-alone method to diagnose concussion, measure recovery, or make decisions about an athlete's readiness to return to competition after concussion (14).
- Further information regarding SCAT 5/6 and SCOAT 6 is available in the online content of this chapter.

COMPREHENSIVE (CLINICAL) NEUROPSYCHOLOGICAL TESTING

Paper-and-Pencil (Clinician-Administered) Neuropsychological Testing

- A variety of paper-and-pencil test batteries have been used for neurocognitive assessment. In patients with concussion, tests that measure various aspects of memory (new learning), cognitive processing speed, working memory, attention, or executive functions have been utilized the most. The rationale for choosing tests from these domains is that these are functions typically affected by traumatic brain injury, as opposed to language or visuospatial skills, which are more resistant to the effects of brain injury (18).
- Examples of Traditional Paper-and-Pencil Neurocognitive tests (18,19):
  - Hopkin Verbal Learning (Memory/Verbal learning)
  - Brief Visuospatial Memory test (Memory)
  - WAIS-III Digit Symbol subtest (Processing speed)
  - Symbol Digit Modalities test (Processing speed)
  - Trail Making test (Processing speed, executive)
  - Controlled Oral Word Association (Processing speed, executive)
  - Stroop Color Word test (Executive)
  - WAIS-III Digit Span test (Working memory)
  - WAIS-III Letter-Number Sequencing test (Working memory)
  - Paced Auditory Stimulation test (Working memory, speed of processing)
- Statistical support for use of paper-and-pencil testing
  - Paper-and-pencil tests have been used for years and have many studies looking at their validity. The validity of the tests has been well documented (18).
  - Reliability of individual tests have been documented through various studies. Reliability measures range from .39 to .93 for these individual tests with most being in the .63 to .75 ranges: almost all below the ideal of .90 but above the minimally acceptable .60 (20,21). There have been no attempts to combine several tests with similar cognitive domain measures into a composite score. This method is used with computer NP batteries and increases the reliability.
  - Randolph et al. reviewed seven studies involving paper-and-pencil NP testing with respect to sensitivity. They concluded that the studies demonstrated "some evidence that standard pencil and paper tests are sensitive to the effects of concussions, at least within the first five days of concussion" (18). However, others have noted sensitivities as low as 23 % within 2 days of concussion (19).
  - Clinical utility has not been demonstrated; most studies have not demonstrated that paper-and-pencil NP tests can detect concussion once players are asymptomatic.

Computerized Neuropsychological Testing

- Computerized batteries measure the domains of memory, attention, concentration, processing speed and reaction time, as well as symptoms. The rationale for choosing tests from these domains is that these are functions typically affected by traumatic brain injury, as opposed to language or visuospatial skills, which are more resistant to the effects of brain injury (20).

- Computerized NP tests have been around for more than 20 years. The ones used in Sports Medicine are listed below. A more thorough discussion of each is included in the online content of this chapter.
  - Automated Neuropsychological Assessment Metric (ANAM)
  - CogSport/Axon Sports CCAT
  - Concussion Vital Signs
  - C3 Logix
  - Headminder CRI (Concussion Resolution Index)
  - ImPACT

STATISTICAL SUPPORT FOR THE USE OF COMPUTERIZED NEUROPSYCHOLOGICAL TESTING IN CONCUSSION

Additional details regarding each aspect below are discussed further in the online content of this chapter.

Reliability

- Resch suggested the variety of methodological factors that may explain the difference in reliability in various studies. These include administration of multiple test platforms versus single test platform, use of different versions or iterations, variable age of participants, varied testing settings and test-retest intervals, and hardware and software variations. In addition to these, other factors include varying statistical models used, single versus average ICC as well as all known administrative and environmental factors known to affect NP tests (26).

Validity

- Concurrent validity of computerized NP tests has been well established (18,27,28).
- In recent years, there have been more studies on performance validity. Nelson looked at rates and predictors of invalid baselines of three NP tests to examine the rates and predictors of invalid baseline performance for three popular CNTs: Automated Neuropsychological Assessment Metrics (ANAM), Axon Sports, and Immediate Post-Concussion and Cognitive Testing (ImPACT). The overall percentage of tests flagged as of questionable validity was lowest for ImPACT (2.7%) and higher for ANAM and Axon (10.7% and 11.3%, respectively). It was noted that the validity criteria for these CNTs may not identify the same causes of invalidity or be equally sensitive to effort. The validity indicators also may not be equally appropriate for some athletes (*e.g.*, those with neurodevelopmental disorders) (29).
- Reasons for invalid baselines identified by predetermined criteria include: failure to read/understand instructions, distracting environment, sandbagging, or intentional effort to perform poorly (19).

Sensitivity and Specificity

- The sensitivity and specificity of these tools have been evaluated with mixed findings.
- In a 2007 study, Broglio compared computerized neuropsychological testing (CNTs) and paper-and-pencil (neuropsychological tests) within 24 hours of concussion and found CNTs had a sensitivity of 78%–79% in detecting concussion compared to 43.5% for paper-and-pencil tests (19).
- Sensitivity of a paper-and-pencil test battery has been reported to be as low as 23% within 2 days of concussion (19).

Clinical Utility

- Neuropsychological testing has shown that there can be cognitive deficits beyond the time that a patient exhibits symptoms.

CONSIDERATIONS IN NEUROPSYCHOLOGICAL TESTING

Administration of Testing

- Testing should be administered by a qualified health professional trained in the administration of that test. For computerized NP testing in the collegiate, professional, and high school setting, this role has largely been delegated to the athletic trainer.
- Testing environment should be quiet and free of distractions.
- Testing can be done in an individual or group setting. Evidence suggests no significant difference in validity between either modality (38,39).
- NP tests can be administered preinjury to establish baseline neurocognitive functioning or postinjury to identify neurocognitive changes or deficits.
- NP tests can be administered serially to track recovery of concussion. However, there are no evidence-based guidelines on frequency of serial NP testing.
- In clinical practice, NP tests are commonly administered when the athlete is asymptomatic to assess whether it is safe to begin an exercise progression. However, some practitioners choose to start an exercise progression when asymptomatic and use the NP test at the end of the progression before clearance to full-contact sports.
- It is common for an athlete to take two or more NP tests before return to sport. One must be careful not to administer too many tests in a short span of time because factors of learning, interference (of word groups, card numbers, etc.), and decreased motivation may affect test scores.

- Although there is no standardized baseline testing guidelines, a recent study suggests that administering baseline computerized NP testing first, prior to balance testing and symptom score, improves overall performance on baseline NP testing (40).

Factors Affecting Testing (13,41)

- Psychological: anxiety, depression, ADHD, performance anxiety, fear, stress, or other emotional states
- Physiological: sleep, alertness, pain, medication, nutrition, hormonal changes, concussion severity
- Cultural: education, language, previous exposure to NP testing, comfort with computers
- Premorbid conditions: learning disorders (attention-deficit hyperactivity disorder, etc.), developmental disorders, history of concussion or traumatic head/brain injury, substance abuse
- Genetic: age, sex, race, IQ, visual acuity, auditory acuity, hand dominance
- Methodological: test setting/atmosphere, time of day, computer screen visibility, practice/learning effects, administrator expertise
- Other: random variance/chance, motivation, effort (unintentional or intentional poor performance), testing frequency

Interpretation of Testing

- Paper-and-pencil should be administered and interpreted by a neuropsychologist or other trained practitioner.
- Computerized NP testing batteries offer training in their use and interpretation. On completion, they generate clinical reports summarizing the results of the test. These reports can include derived composite scores for each testing category, percentile and raw data scores, and a relative change comparison if baseline or previous testing is available. Some reports provide comparison to acceptable normative data. The ability to analyze the results of individual categories allows the clinician to interpret the results with respect to an individual patient's situation and use their clinical judgment to incorporate the NP testing results with findings of other tools in their armamentarium for concussion assessment.
- Interpretation of NP testing results requires an understanding of patient symptoms, psychometric properties of the test, complex interactions of test data, sources of error, extra-test variables, and intraindividual variables (42).
- Interpretation should always consider the previously described factors affecting testing.

Baseline Comparison Data

- Baseline data are used for comparison to an athlete's neurocognitive functioning after concussion to evaluate for neurocognitive deficit. Baseline data may be obtained from individual preparticipation baseline neurocognitive testing or by utilizing normative values (specific to age, gender, and infrequently sport) for comparison (43).
- There is insufficient evidence to recommend the frequency of baseline testing. Options include annually, bi-annually, or one-time. Current NCAA guidelines require cognitive testing as a component of a one-time preparticipation baseline concussion assessment (5).
- Arguments against widespread baseline testing include the potential financial cost, lack of resources, and poor test-retest reliability of neuropsychological test batteries (8,44,45).
- Some studies suggest that cognitive changes from baseline can be reliably observed in comparison to age and gender-matched normative data (46,47).
- The primary argument for individualized baseline testing is the individualistic approach, that comparing postinjury testing to an individual's preinjury baseline is the most accurate. Using one's own data comparison controls for a variety of the factors (psychological, physiological, genetic, premorbid conditions) that could affect scores.
- Walton et al. compared institutionally based normative values to manufacturer provided data and found that the institutionally derived data demonstrated above-average performance for verbal memory, visual memory, and visual motor speed and slightly below average performance for reaction time compared to the manufacturer norms (48).
- Multiple studies have shown significantly worse performance on baseline computerized NP testing among athletes who self report ADHD or learning disorder, which also supports the importance of baseline testing for some individuals or groups (49–53).
- In a recent systematic review, relating to SCAT and NP testing, Echemendia et al. concluded that "the need for baseline neurocognitive testing, whether using computer-administered or examiner-administered, neuropsychological tests and/or the SCAT tools, remains a topic of discussion. Generally, when well-developed normative data are available, the absolute need for individual neuro-cognitive baseline data is less supported. Quality normative data, however, may not be available for a broad range of athletes, and particularly those with psychiatric/neurologic history, learning disabilities (LD)/attention deficit hyperactivity disorder (ADHD), giftedness, cultural/linguistic differences, or para athletes" (16).
- The 2017 Concussion in Sport Group (CISG) consensus statement did not recommend mandatory baseline testing. Instead, they stated "baseline testing may be useful, but it is not necessary for interpreting post-injury scores" (7).
- The 2018 AMSSM consensus statement on concussion in sport stated that there is utility in one-time initial baseline testing, "but is not necessary, required or an accepted standard of care for the appropriate management of [sport-related concussion]" (1).

Factors Affecting Baseline or Post-Injury Scores and Recovery Course

Effort

- Current research has revealed "sandbagging" or intentional poor performance of baseline testing to be a challenge to the validity of NP testing (29–31,33).
- As athletes have incentive to play, sandbagging baseline NP testing allows them to mask cognitive deficits on postinjury NP testing and return to play as quickly as possible.
- Computerized NP testing batteries have internal validity indicators that may detect sandbagging. Despite this, evidence shows that these indicators may not consistently flag all invalid NP test results (30,31,33).

Age

- Age may affect concussion recovery for a variety of reasons including differences in head-to-body ratio, neck strength, brain size and degree of myelination, and developmental maturity. Younger brains may be more susceptible to injury because of their developmental immaturity (21,25).
- Most studies suggest clinical recovery from SRC with *average* time to begin return-to-play as 5–7 days, decreasing with increasing age. Most children and young adults will clinically recover within 4 weeks (25,45,54,55).
- There is conflicting evidence to support the age group with the highest incidence of concussion (56).
- A study by French et al. found that younger age groups performed relatively worse in verbal and visual memory, visual motor processing speed, and reaction time categories (39).
- Many studies find lower total symptom reporting among younger age groups, suspected to be due to their differences in brain development affecting symptom recognition (21,39,54,57).
- Although French et al found no statistical difference in validity between age groups, a study by Lichtenstein et al does support increased frequency of invalid test results in younger age groups (39,45).
- To account for age as a factor affecting NP testing, computerized testing batteries often have age-specific versions.

Sex

- Females have been shown to have a higher incidence of concussion than their male counterparts. They also tend to report higher total symptom scores and different symptomatology (39,58,59).
- Although there is some evidence that females may exhibit prolonged recovery times in comparison to males, studies are conflicting (58–62).
- Females have been found to perform better on some categories in NP baseline testing (verbal memory, visual motor speed, and reaction time) compared to their male counterparts (37,63–65).
- The study by French et al. corroborates that there may be domain-specific differences in NP baseline testing between females and males (39).

History of Prior Concussion

- A retrospective study including 6075 high school athletes found a correlation between history of multiple concussions and symptom burden, but not NP testing baseline performance (66).
- A meta-analysis utilizing 17 datasets from 13 studies found no significant differences in baseline performance on ImPACT neuropsychological testing battery between subjects with and without a history of previous concussion (67).
- Despite conflicting evidence regarding the correlation between concussion history and symptom burden or recovery time, most recent evidence does not support a difference in computerized NP testing performance between athletes with and without concussion history (54,61,62,66,67).

History of Mental Health and Learning Disorders

- Most recent studies do not consistently find a correlation between learning disorders or ADHD and clinical recovery from SRC (54,68,69). However, in their systematic review on ADHD and outcome after concussion, Cook et al. noted that "there are major methodological weaknesses and limitations that preclude definitive conclusions" (69).
- Multiple studies have found athletes with ADHD to have consistently increased symptom scores on both baseline and post-concussion testing (49,50,63,70–72). The overlap of concussion symptoms with daily ADHD symptoms such as fatigue, concentration difficulty, irritability, disturbed sleep may make assessment of concussion more difficult. It is also important to note that recovery from concussion in an athlete with ADHD may not mean complete symptom resolution.
- Self-reported history of ADHD or learning disorder has also been shown to correlate with increased frequency of invalid NP testing results (25,29,32,52). However, "repeating baselines on those with ADHD/LD may not improve scores and may impede the utility and accuracy of post injury score comparisons" (52). Separate invalidity indices may be needed for each of these populations.
- Athletes who self-report ADHD or learning disorders have been shown to have significantly lower performance on baseline and/or postinjury computerized NP testing (49–53,63,71). Although most of these studies showed decreased performance in all components of the testing (verbal memory, visual memory, visual motor speed, reaction time, impulse control), a few studies only noted declines in a few of the scores (53,71). In studies where they controlled for stimulant use, the use of stimulants resulted in only the visual motor speed and reaction time differing from that of controls (51,63,72).
- In a study of baseline neurocognitive testing in athletes with ADHD, LD, or ADHD + LD by Zuckerman et al., young athletes with ADHD had significantly lower verbal memory, visual memory, and visual motor processing speed scores, along with significantly higher reaction time, impulse control, and symptom scores compared with those without LD or ADHD. Participants with LD had similar results, with significantly lower verbal memory, visual memory,

and visual motor processing speed scores, higher reaction time and symptom score, but did not differ in their impulse control score compared with those without LD or ADHD. Participants with both LD and ADHD had a significantly lower visual motor speed score and a significantly higher reaction time and symptom score than those without LD or ADHD but did not differ with regard to the other composite scores (50). This difference in results among LD, ADHD, and ADHD + LD highlights the importance of baseline testing for individuals with ADHD and LD or the need for normative data that accounts for each of these factors.

- A systematic review performed by Iverson and his colleagues found that 9 out of 12 included studies showed a correlation between preinjury mental health disorders (anxiety, depression, bipolar disorder, etc.) and either prolonged clinical recovery or worse clinical outcome (73).
- Studies show a particularly high prevalence of prolonged concussion recovery in pediatric patients with a preinjury history of anxiety or depression (74,75).
- There is limited research comparing NP testing performance and specific mental health disorders. One review found contradicting evidence as to whether anxiety disorders have any significant effect on NP testing performance in athletes (76).

Symptomatology and Recovery

- Headache is the most often reported symptom associated with concussion and may be tension or cluster type. A review of evidence found the presence of subacute postinjury headache to be associated with overall worse clinical outcomes (54).
- Posttraumatic headaches may be tension or cluster-type, however posttraumatic migraines, associated with symptoms of photophobia, phonophobia, nausea, vomiting, or vision changes, are indicative of increased severity in concussion and prolonged recovery time (77).
- Concussed athletes with posttraumatic migraine were found to have significant decreases in visual memory, verbal memory, and reaction time on NP testing (77).
- Although historical evidence suggests average return-to-play time of 5–7 days, Wasserman et al. found post-SRC return-to-play times of greater than 1 week was increasing, likely due to the widespread implementation of concussion return-to-play protocols (55,77).

FUTURE DIRECTIONS AND CONCLUSIONS

- The landscape of concussion assessment utilizing NP testing has changed over the past 2 decades, overwhelmingly favoring computerized over paper-and-pencil testing. Many brands of computerized NP tests have been marketed, each with similar testing domains, however no single iteration has been proven or accepted as a gold standard.
- Improvements to Computerized NP tests that should be considered are reevaluating and/or replacing subtests that contribute to outcome scores with lower reliability (*i.e.*, verbal and visual memory) and focusing more on measures with greater reliability such as visual motor speed and reaction time to improve the over-reliability as well as clinical utility of the test. Ultimately, creating an integrated multimodal assessment that incorporates NP tests along with other tests to increase the sensitivity, reliability, and clinical utility for the diagnosis and management of concussion would be ideal.
- It is important to realize that neuropsychological testing is not meant to be and has not been proven to be the gold standard single test in the evaluation of concussion and should not replace clinical judgment. It is one of several tools along with history, symptoms, physical exam, VOMS, and balance testing that together can provide information that can assist the treating physician in decision making for the treatment and return-to-play decisions in athletes with concussion.

REFERENCES

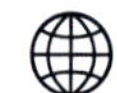 *These references are cited only in the online content of the chapter.*

1. Harmon KG, Clugston JR, Dec K, et al. American Medical Society for Sports Medicine position statement on concussion in sport. *Br J Sports Med.* 2018;53:213–25.
2. Pierpoint LA, Collins C. Epidemiology of sport-related concussion. *Clin Sports Med.* 2021;40:1–18.
3. Patricios JS, Schneider KJ, Dvorak J, et al. Consensus statement on concussion in sport: the 6th international conference on concussion in sport-Amsterdam, October 2022. *Br J Sports Med.* 2023;57(11):695–711. 
4. Herring SA, Cantu RC, Guskiewicz KM, et al. Concussion (mild traumatic brain injury) and the team physician: a consensus statement—2011 update. *Med Sci Sports Exerc.* 2011;43(12):2412–22.
5. *NCAA Sport Science Institute Interassociation Consensus: Diagnosis and Management of Sports Related Concussion Best Practices.* 2016. Initially accessed on NCAA SSI resource page. Now Available from: https://www.brainandlife.org/siteassets/disorders/featured-disorders/concussion/17ncaaconcussion_tr.pdf
6. Broglio SP, Cantu RC, Gioia GA, et al. National athletic trainers' association position statement: management of sport concussion. *J Athl Train.* 2014;49(2):245–65.
7. McCrory P, Meeuwisse W, Dvorak J, et al. Consensus statement on concussion in sport—the 5th international conference on concussion in sport held in Berlin, October 2016. *Br J Sports Med.* 2018;51:838–47.
8. Broglio SP, Ferrara MS, Macciocchi SN, Baumgartner TA, Elliott R. Test-retest reliability of computerized concussion assessment programs. *J Athl Train.* 2007;42(4):509–14. 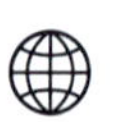
9. Schatz P. Long-term test-retest reliability of baseline cognitive assessments using ImPACT. *Am J Sports Med.* 2010;38(1):47–53. 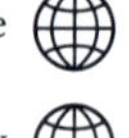
10. Collie A, Maruff P, Makdissi M, McStephen M, Darby DG, McCrory P. Statistical procedures for determining the extent of cognitive change following concussion. *Br J Sports Med.* 2004;38(3):273–8. 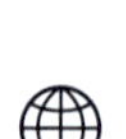
11. Farnsworth JL, Dargo L, Ragan BG, Kang M. Reliability of computerized neurocognitive tests for concussion assessment: a meta-analysis. *J Athl Train.* 2017;52(9):826–33. 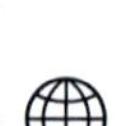
12. Maddocks DL, Dicker GD, Saling MM. The assessment of orientation following concussion in athletes. *Clin J Sport Med.* 1995;5(1):32–5. 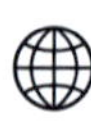

13. Patel DR, Shivdasani V, Baker RJ. Management of sport-related concussion in young athletes. *Sports Med.* 2005;35(8):671–84.

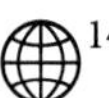
14. Echemendia RJ, Meeuwisse W, McCrory P, et al. The sport concussion assessment tool 5th edition (SCAT5): background and rationale. *Br J Sports Med.* 2017;51(11):848–50.

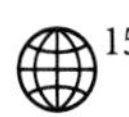
15. Hanninen T, Parkkari J, Howell DR, et al. Reliability of the sport concussion assessment tool 5 baseline testing: a 2-week test–retest study. *J Sci Med Sport.* 2021;24(2):129–34.

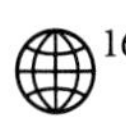
16. Echemendia RJ, Burma JS, Bruce JM, et al. Acute evaluation of sport-related concussion and implications for the Sport Concussion Assessment Tool (SCAT6) for adults, adolescents and children: a systematic review. *Br J Sports Med.* 2023;57(11):722–35.

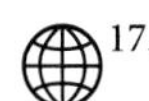
17. Echemendia RJ, Brett BL, Broglio S, et al. Introducing the sport concussion assessment tool 6 (SCAT6). *Br J Sports Med.* 2023;57(11):619–21.

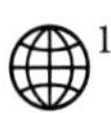
18. Randolph C, McCrea M, Barr WB. Is neuropsychological testing useful in the management of sport-related concussion? *J Athl Train.* 2005;40(3):139–52.

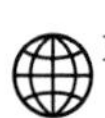
19. Kontos AP, Sufrinko A, Womble M, Kegel N. Neuropsychological assessment following concussion: an evidence-based review of the role of neuropsychological assessment pre- and post-concussion. *Curr Pain Headache Rep.* 2016;20(6):38.

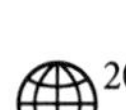
20. Ellemberg D, Henry LC, Macciocchi SN, Guskiewicz KM, Broglio SP. Advances in sport concussion assessment: from behavioral to brain imaging measures. *J Neurotrauma.* 2009;26(12):2365–82.

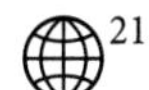
21. Hunt TN, Ferrara MS. Age-related differences in neuropsychological testing among high school athletes. *J Athl Train.* 2009;44(4):405–9.

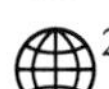
22. Alsalaheen B, Stockdale K, Pechumer D, Broglio SP. Measurement error in the immediate postconcussion assessment and cognitive testing (ImPACT): systematic review. *J Head Trauma Rehabil.* 2016;31(4):242–51.

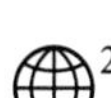
23. Elbin RJ, Fazio-Sumrok V, Anderson MN, et al. Evaluating the suitability of the Immediate Post-Concussion Assessmentand Cognitive Testing (ImPACT) computerized neurocognitive battery forshort-term, serial assessment of neurocognitive functioning. *J Clin Neurosci.* 2019;62:138–41.

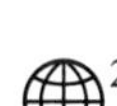
24. Brett BL, Solomon S. The influence of validity criteria on Immediate Post-Concussion Assessment and Cognitive Testing (ImPACT) test-retest reliability among high school athletes. *J Clin Exp Neuropsychol.* 2017;39(3):286–95

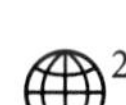
25. Nelson LD, LaRoche AA, Pfaller AY, et al. Prospective, head-to-head study of three computerized neurocognitive assessment tools (CNTs): reliability and validity for the assessment of sport-related concussion. *J Int Neuropsychol Soc.* 2016;22(1):24–37.

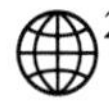
26. Resche JE, Schneider MW, Cullum CM. The test-retest reliability of three computerized neurocognitive tests used in the assessment of sport concussion. *Int J Psychophys.* 2018;132:21–38.

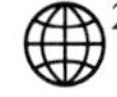
27. Schatz P, Putz BO. Cross-validation of measures used for computer-based assessment of concussion. *Appl Neuropsychol.* 2006;13(3):151–9.

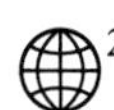
28. Segalowitz SJ, Mahaney P, Santesso DL, MacGregor L, Dywan J, Willer B. Retest reliability in adolescents of a computerized neuropsychological battery used to assess recovery from concussion. *NeuroRehabilitation.* 2007;22(3):243–51.

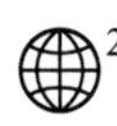
29. Nelson LD, Pfallar AY, Rein LE, McCrea MA. Rates and predictors of invalid baseline test performance in high school and collegiate athletes for 3 computerized neurocognitive tests, ANAM, Axon sports, and ImPACT. *Am J Sports Med.* 2015;43(8):2018–26.

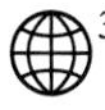
30. Abeare C, Messa I, Whitfield C, et al. Performance validity in collegiate football athletes at baseline neurocognitive testing. *J Head Trauma Rehabil.* 2019;34(4):E20–31.

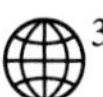
31. Schatz P, Glatts C. "Sandbagging" baseline test performance on ImPACT, without detection, is more difficult than it appears. *Arch Clin Neuropsychol.* 2013;28(3):236–44.

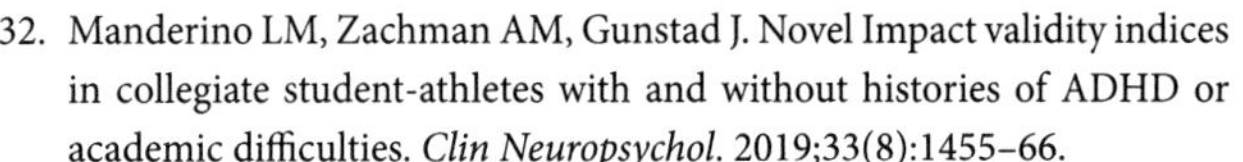
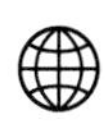
32. Manderino LM, Zachman AM, Gunstad J. Novel Impact validity indices in collegiate student-athletes with and without histories of ADHD or academic difficulties. *Clin Neuropsychol.* 2019;33(8):1455–66.

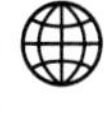
33. Tsushima WT, Yamamoto MH, Ahn HJ, Siu AM, Choi SY, Murata NM. Invalid baseline testing with ImPACT: does sandbagging occur with high school athletes? *Appl Neuropsychol Child.* 2021;10(3):209–18.

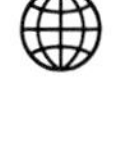
34. Czerniak LL, Liebel SW, Garcia GG, et al. Sensitivity and specificity of computer based neurocognitive tests in sport related concussion: findings from the NCAA DoD CARE consortium. *Sports Med.* 2021;51(2):351–65.

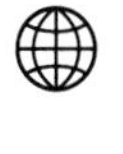
35. Czerniak LL, Liebel SW, Zhou H, et al. Sensitivity and specificity of the ImPACT neurocognitive test in collegiate athletes and US Military Service Academy Cadets with ADHD and/or LD: findings from the NCAA DoD CARE consortium. *Sports Med.* 2023;53(3):747–59.

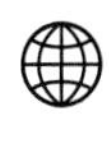
36. Masterson C, Tuttle J, Maerlender AC. Confirmatory factor analysis of two computerized neuropsychological test batteries: immediate post-concussion assessment and cognitive test (ImPACT) and C3 logix. *J Clin Exp Neuropsychol.* 2019;41(9):925–32.

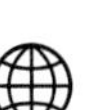
37. Lempke LB, Howell DR, Eckner JT, Lynall RC. Examination of reaction time deficits following concussion: a systematic review and metaanalysis. *Sports Med.* 2020;50(7):1341–59.

38. Vaughn CG, Gerst EH, Sady MD, Newman JB, Gioia GA. The relation between testing environment and baseline performance in Child and adolescent concussion assessment. *Am J Sports Med.* 2014;42(7):1716–22.

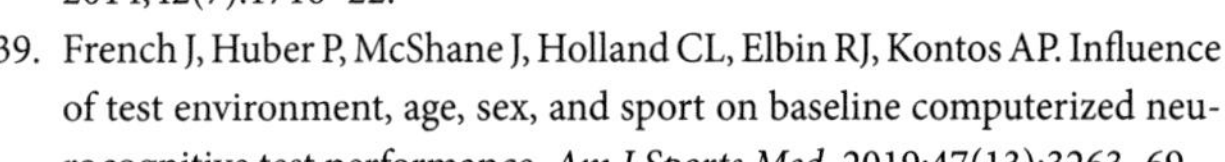
39. French J, Huber P, McShane J, Holland CL, Elbin RJ, Kontos AP. Influence of test environment, age, sex, and sport on baseline computerized neurocognitive test performance. *Am J Sports Med.* 2019;47(13):3263–69.

40. Lempke LB, Lynall RC, Anderson MN, et al. Optimizing order of administration for concussion baseline assessment among NCAA student athletes and military cadets. *Sports Med.* 2022;52(1):165–76.

41. McCrory P, Makdissi M, Davis G, Collie A. Value of neuropsychological testing after head injuries in football. *Br J Sports Med.* 2005;39(suppl 1):i58–i63.

42. Echemendia RJ, Herring S, Bailes J. Who should conduct and interpret the neuropsychological assessment in sports-related concussion? *Br J Sports Med.* 2009;43(suppl 1):i32–5.

43. Merritt VC, Meyer JE, Cadden MH, et al. Normative data for a comprehensive neuropsychological test battery used in the assessment of sports-related concussion. *Arch Clin Neuropsychol.* 2017;32(2):168–83.

44. Echemendia RJ, Iverson GL, McCrea M, et al. Advances in neuropsychological assessment of sport-related concussion. *Br J Sports Med.* 2013;47(5):294–8.

45. Lichtenstein JD, Moser RS, Schatz P. Age and test setting affect the prevalence of invalid baseline scores on neurocognitive tests. *Am J Sports Med.* 2014;42(2):479–84.

46. Schmidt JD, Register-Mihalik JK, Mihalik JP, Kerr ZY, Guskiewicz KM. Identifying impairments after concussion: normative data versus individualized baselines. *Med Sci Sports Exerc.* 2012;44(9):1621–8.

47. Echemendia RJ, Bruce JM, Bailey CM, Sanders JF, Arnett P, Vargas G. The utility of post-concussion neuropsychological data in identifying cognitive change following sports-related MTBI in the absence of baseline data. *Clin Neuropsychol.* 2012;26(7):1077–91.

48. Walton SR, Broshek DK, Freeman JR, et al. Institutionally based ImPACT Test® normative values may differ from manufacturer-provided normative values. *Arch Clin Neuropsychol.* 2020;35(3):275–82.

49. Elbin RJ, Kontos AP, Kegel N, Johnson E, Burkhart S, Schatz P. Individual and combined effects of LD and ADHD on computerized neurocognitive concussion test performance: evidence for separate norms. *Arch Clin Neuropsychol.* 2013;28(5):476–84.

50. Zuckerman SL, Lee YM, Odom MJ, Solomon GS, Sills AK. Baseline neurocognitive scores in athletes with attention deficit-spectrum disorders and/or learning disability. *J Neurosurg Pediatr.* 2013;12(2):103–9.
51. Gardner RM, Yengo-Kahn A, Bonfield CM, Solomon GS. Comparison of baseline and post-concussion ImPACT test scores in young athletes with stimulant-treated and untreated ADHD. *Phys Sportsmed.* 2017;45(1):1–10.
52. Manderino L, Gunstad J. Collegiate student athletes with history of ADHD or academic difficulties are more likely to produce an invalid protocol on baseline ImPACT testing. *Clin J Sport Med.* 2018;28(2):111–6.
53. Maietta JE, Kuwabara HC, Cross CL, et al. Influence of autism and other neurodevelopmental disorders on cognitive and symptom profiles: considerations for baseline sport concussion assessment. *Arch Clin Neuropsychol.* 2021;36(8):1438–49.
54. Iverson GL, Gardner AJ, Terry DP, et al. Predictors of clinical recovery from concussion: a systematic review. *Br J Sports Med.* 2017;51(12):941–8.
55. Wasserman EB, Kerr ZY, Zuckerman SL, Covassin T. Epidemiology of sports-related concussions in National Collegiate Athletic Association athletes from 2009–2010 to 2013–2014: symptom prevalence, symptom resolution time, and return-to-play time. *Am J Sports Med.* 2016;44(1):226–33.
56. Tsushima WT, Siu AM, Ahn HJ, Chang BL, Murata NM. Incidence and risk of concussions in youth athletes: comparisons of age, sex, concussion history, sport and football position. *Arch Clin Neuropsychol.* 2019;34(1):60–9.
57. Murdaugh DL, Ono KE, Morris SO, Burns TG. Effects of developmental age on symptom reporting and neurocognitive performance in youth after sports-related concussion compared to control athletes. *J Child Neurol.* 2018;33(7):474–81.
58. Solomito MJ, Reuman H, Wang DH. Sex differences in concussion: a review of brain anatomy, function, and biomechanical response to impact. *Brain Inj.* 2019;3(2):105–10.
59. O'Connor KL, Baker MM, Dalton SL, Dompier TP, Broglio SP, Kerr ZY. Epidemiology of sport-related concussions in high school athletes: National Athletic Treatment, Injury and Outcomes Network (NATION), 2011-2012 through 2013-2014. *J Athl Train.* 2017;52(3):175–85.
60. Aggarwal SS, Ott SD, Padhye NS, Meininger JC, Armstrong TS. Clinical and demographic predictors of concussion resolution in adolescents: a retrospective study. *Appl Neuropsychol Child.* 2019;8(1):50–60.
61. Aggarwal SS, Ott SD, Padhye NS, Schulz PE. Sex, race, ADHD, and prior concussions as predictors of concussion recovery in adolescents. *Brain Inj.* 2020;34(6):809–17.
62. Putukian M, Riegler K, Amalfe S, Bruce J. Preinjury and postinjury factors that predict sports-related concussion and clinical recovery time. *Clin J Sport Med.* 2021;31:15–22.
63. Cottle JE, Hall EE, Patel K, Barnes KP, Ketcham CJ. Concussion baseline testing: preexisting factors, symptoms, and neurocognitive performance. *J Athl Train.* 2017;52(2):77–81.
64. Covassin T, Elbin R, Kontos A, Larson E. Investigating baseline neurocognitive performance between male and female athletes with a history of multiple concussion. *J Neurol Neurosurg Psychiatry.* 2010;81(6):597–601.
65. Tanveer S, Zecavati N, Delasobera EB, Oyegbile TO. Gender differences in concussion and postinjury cognitive findings in an older and younger pediatric population. *Pediatr Neurol.* 2017;70:44–9.
66. Mannix R, Iverson GL, Maxwell B, Atkins JE, Zafonte R, Berkner PD. Multiple prior concussions are associated with symptoms in high school athletes. *Ann Clin Transl Neurol.* 2014;1(6):433–8.
67. Alshaheen B, Stockdale K, Pechumer D, Giessing A, He X, Broglio SP. Cummulative effects of concussion history on baseline computerized neurocognitive test scores: systematic review and meta-analysis. *Sports Health.* 2017;9(4):324–32.
68. Cook NE, Iaccarino MA, Karr JE, Iverson GL. Attention-deficit/hyperactivity disorder and outcome after concussion: a systematic review. *J Dev Behav Pediatr.* 2020;41(7):571–82.
69. Cook NE, Iverson GL, Maxwell B, Zafonte R, Berkner PD. Adolescents with ADHD do not take longer to recover from concussion. *Front Pediatr.* 2020;8:606879.
70. Poysophon P, Rao AL. Neurocognitive deficits associated with ADHD in athletes: a systematic review. *Sports Health.* 2018;10(4):317–26.
71. Kaye S, Sundman MH, Hall EE, Williams E, Patel K, Ketcham CJ. Baseline neurocognitive performance and symptoms in those with ADHD and history of concussion with previous loss of consciousness. *Front Neurol.* 2019;10:1–5.
72. Littleton AC, Schmidt JD, Register-Mihalik JK, et al. Effects of attention deficit hyperactivity disorder and stimulant medication on concussion symptom reporting and computerized neurocognitive test performance. *Arch Clin Neuropsychol.* 2015;30(7):683–93.
73. Iverson GL, Williams MW, Gardner AJ, Terry DP. Systematic review of preinjury mental health problems as a vulnerability factor for worse outcome after sport-related concussion. *Orthop J Sports Med.* 2020;8(10):2325967120950682.
74. Corwin DJ, Zonfrillo MR, Master CL, et al. Characteristics of prolonged concussion recovery in a pediatric subspecialty referral population. *J Pediatr.* 2014;165(6):1207–15.
75. Zemek R, Barrowman N, Frredman SB, et al. Clinical risk score for persistent postconcussion symptoms among the children with acute concussion in the ED. *JAMA.* 2016;315(10):1014–25.
76. Tomczyk CP, Shaver G, Hunt TN. Does anxiety affect neuropsychological assessment in college athletes? *J Sport Rehabil.* 2020;29(2):238–42.
77. Kontos AP, Elbin RJ, Lau B, et al. Posttraumatic migraine as a predictor of recovery and cognitive impairment after sport-related concussion. *Am J Sports Med.* 2013;41(7):1497–504.

SECTION iii

Medical Problems in the Athlete

Cardiology

Marc A. Childress and Francis G. O'Connor

31

INTRODUCTION

- Exercise is clearly associated with improved cardiovascular health. In addition to a direct conditioning effect, physical activity is critical in the management and prevention of many chronic medical conditions that impact overall health. Cardiovascular fitness improves mortality risk, regardless of age or gender (1,2). While a high level of physical activity is associated with an overall reduced risk for sudden cardiac arrest (3), vigorous exercise also can be a trigger for sudden cardiac arrest in individuals with underlying cardiovascular disease (4).
- Sudden death in athletes is most often attributable to an underlying cardiovascular disorder. Sudden cardiac death represents 75% of fatalities in National Collegiate Athletic Association (NCAA) athletes during training or competition; more than deaths related to blunt trauma, heat stroke, and sickle cell trait combined (5).
- A high index of suspicion must be maintained during screening to detect conditions associated with sudden death, including appropriate individual assessments as well as reasonable measures to evaluate large populations. Cardiovascular remodeling to exercise can create changes that require careful scrutiny to delineate normal adaptation from intrinsic pathology (6).
- When a serious cardiovascular condition is identified, appropriate treatment and activity modification may decrease the risk of sudden death. The American Heart Association and the American College of Cardiology scientific statements provide clinical considerations and guidance for shared decision making for sports participation in athletes with cardiovascular disorders (7).

CARDIOVASCULAR BENEFITS OF EXERCISE

- The lack of regular physical activity has clearly been associated with an increase in coronary heart disease and the incidence of adverse cardiac events (8–10). Multiple studies have confirmed the benefit of aerobic exercise with a reduction in the number of cardiac events and a reduction in mortality (11–14).
- Exercise, in particular heavy exercise, has been demonstrated to be a risk factor for both myocardial infarction (MI) and sudden cardiac arrest. Mittleman et al., demonstrated that while exercise is a trigger for MI in all adults, regardless of fitness status, the relative risk of an event is inversely related to fitness level. Among people who usually exercised less than one, one to two, three to four, or five or more times per week, the respective relative risks were 107 (95% confidence interval, 67–171), 19.4 (9.9–38.1), 8.6 (3.6–20.5), and 2.4 (1.5–3.7). Thus, increasing levels of habitual physical activity were associated with progressively lower relative risks (15).
- Therefore, although there is an increased risk for adverse cardiac events during activity, there is overwhelming evidence that the net benefits of consistent and regular physical exercise outweigh these risks in the primary prevention of cardiovascular disease (16).

THE ATHLETIC HEART SYNDROME

- Vigorous athletic training is associated with specific physiologic and structural cardiovascular changes, often referred to as the athletic heart syndrome (AHS) (17). These changes represent normal adaptations to physical conditioning and have recently been identified as exercise-induced cardiac remodeling (6).
- Studies demonstrate a constellation of morphologic changes that vary depending on the type of training (6,18). In endurance-trained athletes, a chronic volume overload results in an increase in both LV end-diastolic diameter and LV wall thickness. This eccentric hypertrophy allows a larger stroke volume and thus a greater overall cardiac output at faster heart rates. Biatrial enlargement and right ventricular dilation can also be seen. Strength-trained athletes develop concentric hypertrophy with an increase in absolute and relative wall thickness without significant changes in end-diastolic diameter. Right-sided and atrial dimensions typically remain unchanged.
- It is important to remember that the adaptive structural and physiologic response of the normal athletic heart does not rule out the presence of an underlying pathologic condition. In fact, it makes the task of diagnosing that condition more

challenging for the primary care physician, sports medicine physician, and cardiologist (19).

- The phenotypic overlap between normal adaptation and structural pathology has been further identified by the Maron Gray Zone (LV wall thickness of 13–15 mm; LV cavity 56–70 mm) (20). Criteria for distinguishing the characteristics of AHS from significant underlying pathology have been further defined and, in some circumstances, may require detraining for 2–3 months (6,20). In benign cases, full resolution should be observed, whereas residual hypertrophic changes may suggest underlying concerns (21). Advanced imaging, to include the use of cardiac MRI to assess for late gadolinium enhancement seen in hypertrophic cardiomyopathy (HCM), is one of many tools that can assist the sports cardiologist in delineating challenging cases (6).

Physical Examination

- The heart rate of well-conditioned athletes is usually between 40 and 60 bpm, secondary to enhanced vagal tone, decreased sympathetic tone, and a larger stroke volume. Thus, sinus bradycardia is a common finding, and sinus arrhythmia may be more noticeable.
- The physiologic splitting of S2 may be slightly delayed during inspiration due to the larger stroke volume. An S3 may be noted in endurance-trained athletes secondary to the increased rate of LV filling associated with the relative LV dilatation (22,23). Although an S4 may be noted in strength-trained athletes secondary to concentric hypertrophy, its presence always warrants clinical evaluation.
- Functional (flow) murmurs characterized by a soft 1–2/6 ejection murmur often present when supine and diminished with standing or Valsalva may be noted in 30%–50% of athletes on careful examination (17).

Electrocardiographic Changes

- Several electrocardiographic changes can be seen in well-conditioned athletes. In most cases, these changes are benign reflections of structural and functional changes. However, some findings are abnormal and may suggest underlying pathology. It can be challenging to distinguish adaptive versus pathologic changes in trained athletes, and modern electrocardiogram (ECG) criteria should be used to assist in interpretation (24). Electrocardiography interpretation in athletes is further detailed in Chapter 24.
- Similar to nonathletes, ECG is helpful in the initial evaluation of cardiac conditions in athletes who present with cardiovascular symptoms or have abnormal findings on physical examination.
- The role of ECG in the preparticipation screening of athletes is controversial. Opponents of ECG screening are concerned about false-positive results, cost-effectiveness, and unnecessary disqualifications in athletes (25–27). Proponents of ECG screening recognize that the sensitivity of a history and physical examination alone to detect potentially lethal cardiovascular disorders in athletes is very low, that the addition of an ECG increases the sensitivity, and that it can be accomplished with a low and acceptable false-positive rate when performed by experienced physicians guided by modern ECG criteria (28).
- In 2017, the American Medical Society for Sports Medicine published a position stand recognizing this controversy. The statement presented a new paradigm to assist the individual physician in assessing the most appropriate cardiovascular screening strategy unique to their athlete population, community needs and resources. The decision to implement a cardiovascular screening program, with or without the addition of ECG, necessitates careful consideration of the risk of SCA/D in the targeted population and the availability of cardiology resources and infrastructure (29).

SUDDEN CARDIAC DEATH IN EXERCISE

- The overall risk of sudden death during exercise varies depending on age, gender, and sport. Estimates from studies in runners range from 1:15,000 joggers per year to 1:50,000 marathon participants per race (4,30). For high school and college-aged athletes, studies have reported ranges from 1:35,000 to 1:160,000 per year, and sudden deaths occur disproportionally more often in males, African Americans, and basketball and football players (4,31,32). Recent evaluations have suggested that these numbers may reflect significant underreporting (33).
- The specific etiologies contributing to sudden cardiac death are strongly related to age. For sudden death in persons over age 35, more than 75% are associated with coronary artery disease (CAD). This association increases with age, consistent with the rising prevalence of atherosclerosis (10).
- In younger athletes, sudden cardiac death is most often the result of intrinsic structural or electrical abnormalities, accounting for nearly two-thirds of reported deaths (32). Based on cases of sudden death in athletes over a 26-year period in the United States, HCM was identified as the most common cause of sudden cardiac death, followed by coronary artery anomalies, myocarditis, and arrhythmogenic right ventricular cardiomyopathy (ARVC). Other etiologies include genetic conductive system abnormalities such as ion channel disorders (long QT syndrome), aortic rupture from Marfan syndrome, premature CAD, idiopathic LV hypertrophy, substance abuse (cocaine or steroids), aortic stenosis, mitral valve prolapse, sickle cell trait, blunt chest trauma (commotio cordis) and autopsy negative sudden death (31,32). Petek et al, in fact, recently identified in a twenty year retrospective review of NCAA athletes that autopsy negative sudden unexplained death was the most common postmortem examination finding (34).
- The category of sudden arrhythmic death syndrome (SADS) has recently been introduced and includes long QT syndrome (LQTS) and Brugada syndrome, catecholaminergic polymorphic ventricular tachycardia (CPVT), and

conduction abnormalities such as Wolff-Parkinson-White Syndrome, which may not be diagnosed premortem. SADS may have been previously underrepresented in earlier studies that relied on an autopsy diagnosis, as morphologically normal hearts were sometimes excluded (32).

- It is important to note that the relative prevalence of many of these conditions is variable, based on regional, ethnic and age differences. For example, ARVC is the leading cause of sudden cardiac death in the Veneto region of Italy (35). A recent study additionally noted that coronary anomalies may be more common in middle school-aged athletes (36).

Screening for Sudden Death

- The American Heart Association (AHA), Science and Advisory Committee (ACC) published consensus guidelines for preparticipation cardiovascular screening for high school and college athletes in 1996, updated in 2007 (36,37). A 12-element history and physical examination was moved to 14 with the addition of questions on prior evaluations and restrictions (37). A complete personal and family history and physical examination should be done for all athletes. It should focus on identifying those cardiovascular conditions known to cause sudden death (Table 31.1). Evaluations are recommended prior to training and competition, with interval evaluation every 2 years in high school, and annually for collegiate athletes (38).
- Family history should include a specific inquiry for a family history of premature CAD, diabetes mellitus, hypertension, sudden death, syncope, death or significant disability from cardiovascular disease in relatives younger than age 50, or the presence of inherited cardiac disorders such as HCM, ARVC, Marfan syndrome, and LQTS.
- Personal history should include specific inquiries on the detection of a heart murmur; risk factors for CAD, such as diabetes mellitus, hypertension, hyperlipidemia, and smoking; and a history of syncope, near syncope, exercise intolerance, exertional chest pain, dyspnea, or excessive fatigue.
- Physical examination should specifically address blood pressure, heart rhythm, cardiac auscultation, and the physical stigmata associated with Marfan syndrome (39) (Table 31.2).
- Cardiac auscultation should be performed in the supine and standing positions. The classic murmur of obstructive HCM increases with maneuvers that decrease venous return, such as Valsalva or moving from squatting to standing. In contrast, innocent flow murmurs and the murmur of aortic stenosis intensify with squatting and decrease with Valsalva (40).
- Simultaneous radial and femoral artery pulses should be assessed to exclude coarctation of the aorta. Brachial blood pressure should be measured with the appropriately sized cuff in the sitting position, and in the pediatric population, normative values should be adjusted for age, gender, and height (41).
- The use of ECG as a screening tool for conditions associated with sudden cardiac death continues to be the subject of much debate. An increasing number of governing bodies have endorsed the use of ECG screening for athletes, including the International Olympic Committee, European Society for Sports Medicine, Fédération Internationale de Football (FIFA), and all of the major U.S. professional sports leagues. However, as previously discussed, concerns remain as to the feasibility of widespread ECG screening in younger or amateur populations (27). False-positive rates, high relative costs, limited availability, and low prevalence of disease have all been cited as concerns for using ECG as a broad-based screening tool. The AHA/ACC Task Force has previously recommended against mandatory, universal screening of athletes with 12-lead EKGs in large, general populations for these reasons (42). Current recommendations stress the need for appropriately trained clinicians in the interpretation of EKGs if they are to be included in a screening PPE, as well as the challenges/limitations of implementing screening EKGs (7).

Table 31.1 The 14-Element AHA Recommendations for Preparticipation Cardiovascular Screening of Competitive Athletes

Medical History[a]
Personal History
1. Exertional chest pain/discomfort
2. Unexplained syncope/near syncope[b]
3. Excessive exertional and unexplained dyspnea/fatigue, associated with exercise
4. Prior recognition of a heart murmur
5. Elevated systemic blood pressure
6. Prior restriction from participation in sports.
7. Prior testing for the heart, ordered by a physician.
Family History
8. Premature death (sudden and unexpected, or otherwise) before age 50 years due to heart disease, in ≥1 relative
9. Disability from heart disease in a close relative <50 years of age
10. Specific knowledge of certain cardiac conditions in family members: HCM, long QT syndrome, or other ion channelopathies, Marfan syndrome, or clinically important arrhythmias
Physical Examination
11. Heart murmur[c]
12. Femoral arterial pulses to exclude aortic coarctation
13. Physical stigmata of Marfan syndrome
14. Brachial blood pressure (sitting position)[d]

AHA, American Heart Association; HCM, hypertrophic cardiomyopathy.
Source: Reproduced with permission from Maron BJ, Thompson PD, Ackerman MJ. Recommendations and considerations related to preparticipation screening for cardiovascular abnormalities in competitive athletes: 2007 update—a scientific statement from the American Heart Association Council on Nutrition, Physical Activity, and Metabolism—endorsed by the American College of Cardiology Foundation. *Circulation.* 2007;115(12):1643–55; Adapted from Maron BJ, Levine BD, Washington RL, et al. Eligibility and disqualification recommendations for competitive athletes with cardiovascular abnormalities—Task Force 2: preparticipation screening for cardiovascular disease in competitive athletes—a scientific statement from the American Heart Association and American College of Cardiology. *Circulation*, 2015;132:e267.
[a]Parental verification is recommended for high school and middle school athletes.
[b]Judged not to be neurocardiogenic (vasovagal); of particular concern when related to exertion.
[c]Auscultation should be performed in both supine and standing positions (or with Valsalva maneuver), specifically to identify murmurs of dynamic left ventricular outflow tract obstruction.
[d]Preferably taken in both arms.

Table 31.2 Features of Marfan Syndrome on Physical Examination

Musculoskeletal
Tall stature
Thin body habitus (arm span to height ratio >1.05)
Arachnodactyly (long, thin fingers; able to wrap hand around opposite wrist and overlap thumb and small finger)
Pectus deformity
High-arched palate
Kyphoscoliosis
Joint laxity
Cardiovascular
Systolic murmur (mitral valve prolapse)
Diastolic murmur (aortic regurgitation)
Ocular
Myopia
Retinal detachment
Lens subluxation

Source: Adapted from De Paepe A, Devereux RB, Dietz HC, Hennekam RC, Pyeritz RE. Revised diagnostic criteria for the Marfan syndrome. *Am J Med Genet.* 1996;62(4):417–26.

- Exercise testing may be advisable prior to beginning an exercise program in older athletes with risk factors for CAD. See Chapters 13 (Exercise Prescription) and 25 (Exercise Testing) for further discussion and recommendations.
- Many conditions that cause sudden death in young athletes are familial (HCM — autosomal dominant defect in sarcomere formation; LQTS — autosomal dominant sodium channel defect; Marfan syndrome — autosomal dominant mutation of *FBN1* fibrillin gene; Brugada syndrome — autosomal dominant SCN5A channelopathy; ARVC — autosomal dominant defect). Although genetic testing is not routinely recommended for screening, it may be helpful in the evaluation of athletes or family members when a relative is identified with an inherited cardiac disease (43).

SYNCOPE AND EXERCISE-ASSOCIATED COLLAPSE

- Syncope is defined as a sudden loss of consciousness for a brief duration, in the absence of head trauma. Syncope occurs secondary to a sudden drop in cerebral blood flow or metabolic change (*e.g.*, hypoglycemia or hypoxemia). Athletes who present with a history of exercise-related syncope (ERS) require a careful history and physical to differentiate benign from life-threatening etiologies (44) (Table 31.3).
- Exercise-associated collapse (EAC) refers to athletes who are unable to stand or walk unaided after exertion because of weakness, lightheadedness, faintness, or dizziness (45,46).
- Although ERS and EAC are not mutually exclusive, they demonstrate the spectrum of adverse events that can occur in the context of exercise. The history in each case becomes critical in the appropriate evaluation and treatment. The occurrence of collapse or syncope *during* exertion is an ominous sign of potential underlying pathology, whereas events occurring immediately *after* stopping exertion are more often associated with benign etiology (47).
- The presence of prodromal symptoms may help to identify specific conditions. Careful attention should be paid to any history of palpitations (arrhythmia), chest pain (ischemia or aortic dissection), nausea (ischemia or vagal activity), wheezing, or pruritus (anaphylaxis). Patients who suffer vasovagal reflex syncope often experience brief prodromal symptoms such as lightheadedness, tunnel vision, diaphoresis, and nausea. In contrast, abrupt syncope is concerning for ventricular arrhythmia.
- A detailed physical examination should include a careful assessment of orthostatic vital signs, precordial auscultation attentive to the murmurs of HCM and aortic stenosis, and a careful search for any morphologic features of Marfan syndrome. An ECG should be obtained in all cases and should be evaluated closely for conditions that predispose to sudden death. This includes careful ECG assessment of rate, rhythm, QT interval, repolarization abnormalities (T wave inversion, ST depression), left or right ventricular hypertrophy, preexcitation pattern, and complications of ischemic heart disease (Q waves) (48).
- Initial blood test and additional ancillary evaluation should be directed by clinical suspicion based on the history and physical. In cases where no clear noncardiac cause is identified, it is recommended that an echocardiogram and stress testing be completed.
- Advanced cardiac imaging, including cardiac MRI and coronary CT angiography, may be advisable in cases of suspected cardiac etiology when the preceding evaluation has been nondiagnostic (49). These advanced imaging modalities provide detailed morphologic assessments to further evaluate for cardiomyopathy or coronary artery anomalies.
- The AHA/ACC Scientific Statement recommends that athletes with exercise-induced syncope or syncope associated with high-risk features (sudden/unheralded collapse, abrupt palpitations, exertional dyspnea, or excessive dyspnea) should be restricted from all competitive athletics until evaluated by a qualified medical professional. Evaluation for structural or electrical heart disease must be completed before the athlete is allowed to return to sports (7).
- Figure 31.1 provides a suggested algorithm for the primary care evaluation of exertional syncope in the athlete.

HYPERTENSION IN ATHLETES

- Systemic hypertension remains one of the most common cardiovascular disorders in the United States and affects athletes of all ages and sports. The diagnosis, workup, and initial

Table 31.3 Clinical Clues to Common Etiologies Presenting With Exertional Syncope

Diagnosis	Clinical Clues	ECG	Suggested Diagnostic Testing
Neurocardiogenic syncope	Noxious stimulus, prolonged upright position	Normal	Exercise testing
Supraventricular tachyarrhythmias	Palpitations, response to carotid sinus pressure	Preexcitation	Electrophysiologic study and definitive therapy
HCM	Grade III/VI systolic murmur, louder with Valsalva (when present)	Deep inverted T waves, Q waves, pseudoinfarction pattern, LV hypertrophy with strain	Echocardiography with Doppler, consider cardiac MRI with gadolinium
Myocarditis	Prior upper respiratory tract infection, pneumonia, exertional fatigue, shortness of breath, and recreational drug use	Simulating a myocardial infarction with ectopy	Viral studies, echocardiogram, and drug screening
Aortic stenosis	Exertional syncope, grade III/VI harsh systolic crescendo-decrescendo murmur	LV hypertrophy	Echocardiography with Doppler
Mitral valve prolapse	"Thumping heart," midsystolic click with or without a murmur	Normal	Echocardiography with Doppler
Prolonged QT syndrome	Recurrent syncope with a family history of sudden death	Prolonged corrected QT interval (>0.47 males, >0.48 females)	Family history; exercise stress test with ECG after exercise
Coronary anomalies	Syncope, exertional chest pain	Normal resting ECG	Cardiac MRI or CT angiography
Acquired coronary artery diseases	Acute coronary syndrome (chest pain), family history	Ischemia, may be normal	Exercise testing with or without perfusion or contractile imaging
ARVC	Syncope, tachyarrhythmias	T wave inversion V1-V3 PVCs with LBBB configuration	Echocardiography with Doppler study, cardiac MRI

ARVC, arrhythmogenic right ventricular cardiomyopathy; CT, computed tomography; ECG, electrocardiogram; HCM, hypertrophic cardiomyopathy; LBBB, left bundle branch block; MRI, magnetic resonance imaging; PVC, premature ventricular contraction.

Source: Adapted from Giese EA, O'Connor FG, Brennan FH, Depenbrock PJ, Oriscello RG. The athletic preparticipation evaluation: cardiovascular assessment. *Am Fam Physician.* 2007;75(7):1008–14, and O'Connor FG, Levine BD, Childress MA, Asplundh CA, Oriscello RG. Practical management: a systematic approach to the evaluation of exercise-related syncope in athletes. *Clin J Sport Med.* 2009;19(5):429–34.

nonpharmacologic approach to treatment does not differ between athletes and nonathletes. This approach is consistent with current recommendations. (Joint National Committee on Prevention, Detection, Evaluation, and Treatment of High Blood Pressure, 2014) (50) and the International Society of Hypertension (51).

- Care must be taken not to overdiagnose the condition in young athletes and to use proper fitting cuffs with three different measures on 3 different days, adjusting for norms for age, gender, and height (41) (Table 31.4).
- Blood pressure tables are published by the American Academy of Pediatrics. These tables reflect age, gender, and height, with listed ranges for *elevated BP*: ≥90th percentile; *stage 1 HTN*: ≥95th percentile; and *stage 2 HTN*: ≥95th percentile +12 mm Hg) (41).
- An appropriate search for secondary etiologies and assessment for target end-organ damage should guide the history, physical, laboratory evaluation, and ancillary testing.
- History should inquire about substances that may affect blood pressure (*e.g.*, nonsteroidal anti-inflammatory drugs, stimulants, anabolic steroids), and testing should include ECG, urinalysis, complete blood count, electrolytes, fasting glucose, lipid profile, blood urea nitrogen, and creatinine. An echocardiogram should be considered in athletes with stage 2 hypertension, abnormal ECG findings, or laboratory evidence of end-organ damage (52).
- Nonpharmacologic treatment should be initiated, including engagement in moderate physical activity, maintenance of ideal body weight, limitation of alcohol, reduction in sodium intake, maintenance of adequate potassium intake, and consumption of a diet high in fruits and vegetables and low in total and saturated fat (53).
- When indicated, pharmacologic treatment should be initiated. Generally, angiotensin-converting enzyme inhibitors, calcium channel blockers, and angiotensin-II receptor blockers are excellent choices for athletes with hypertension. Their low side effect profile and favorable physiologic hemodynamics make them generally safe and effective. It is preferable to avoid diuretics and β-blockers in young athletes. Volume and potassium balance issues limit diuretic use, and β-blockers adversely impact maximum cardiovascular performance (50,53). Additional care must be taken in prescribing antihypertensives in elite athletes because some may be prohibited by sport governing bodies, including the NCAA, International Olympic Committee, and the World Anti-Doping Agency (http://www.wada-ama.org).

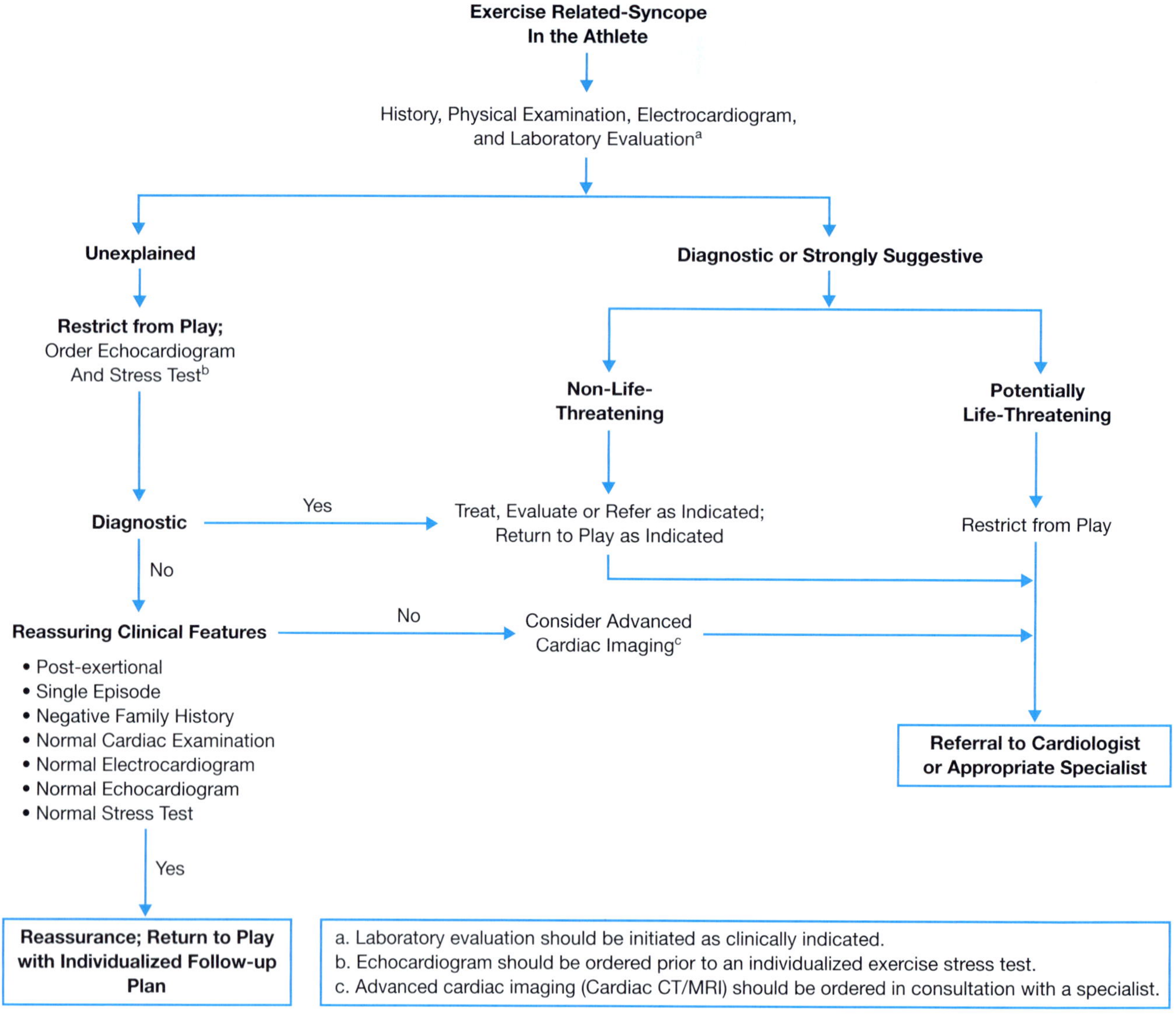

Figure 31.1: Algorithm for the evaluation of exercise-related syncope in the athlete. (Reproduced with permission from O'Connor FG, Levine BD, Childress MA, Asplundh CA, Oriscello RG. Practical management: a systematic approach to the evaluation of exercise-related syncope in athletes. *Clin J Sport Med.* 2009;19(5):429–34.)

- The presence stage 1 or stage 2 hypertension without end organ damage or concomitant heart disease should not limit eligibility for competitive sports. Athletes with hypertensive emergency (defined as SBP > 180 mm Hg or DBP > 120 mm Hg in conjunction with evidence of new or worsening end organ damage) should be restricted until their hypertension is controlled. When hypertension coexists with other cardiovascular diseases, eligibility for competitive sports is usually based on the severity of the other associated condition (7).
- In children and adolescents, the presence of severe hypertension (stage 2) or target organ disease warrants restriction until hypertension is under adequate control. The presence of mild to moderate hypertension (stage 1) should not limit a young athlete's eligibility for competitive athletics (41).

CORONARY ARTERY DISEASE IN ATHLETES

- Individuals diagnosed with CAD require careful risk stratification prior to continuing or initiating exercise. This evaluation can vary based on the underlying risk and the desired activity. Such an evaluation may require procedures for LV assessment and careful interpretation of treadmill testing to determine functional capacity and inducible ischemia (54).
- The American Heart Association and the American College of Cardiology scientific statement defines clear recommendations for athletes with CAD (Table 31.5) (7).

Table 31.4 Classification of Hypertension in Children and Adolescents, With Measurement Frequency and Therapy Recommendations[a]

	SBP or DBP Percentile	Interval BP Measurement (if Elevation Persists)	Upper/Lower Extremity BP	Ambulatory BP Measurement	Further Diagnostic Evaluation[b]	Pharmacologic Therapy
Normal	<90th	Annual				
Elevated Blood Pressure	≥90th percentile to <95th percentile or 120/80 mm Hg to <95th percentile (whichever is lower)	Initial				None unless compelling indications such as chronic kidney disease, diabetes mellitus, heart failure, or LVH exist.
		2nd (in 6 mo)	Y			
		3rd (in 12 mo)		Y	Y	
Stage 1 hypertension	≥95th percentile to <95th percentile + 12 mm Hg, or 130/80 to 139/89 mm Hg (whichever is lower)	Initial				None unless compelling indications.
		2nd (in 1–2 wk)	Y			None unless compelling indications.
		3rd (in 3 mo)		Y	Y	Y
Stage 2 hypertension	≥95th percentile + 12 mm Hg, or ≥140/90 mm Hg (whichever is lower)[c]	Initial	Y			Not immediate unless compelling indications
		2nd (in 1 wk) Consider specialist eval within 1 wk		Y	Y	Y

Source: Adapted from Flynn JT, Kaelber DC, Baker-Smith CM, et al. Clinical practice guideline for screening and management of high blood pressure in children and adolescents. Subcommittee on Screening and Management of High Blood Pressure in Children. *Pediatrics.* 2017 Sep;140(3):e20171904.

[a]At all stages, lifestyle interventions are warranted to include diet change, safe progressive exercise, and avoidance of provocative substances.

[b]Diagnostic evaluation to include consideration of urinalysis, blood chemistries, lipids, and renal imaging, with additional studies per age and comorbidities.

[c]If symptomatic or BP is 30 mm Hg above 95th percentile, emergent evaluation is warranted at any time.

Table 31.5 Summary of scientific statement from the American Heart Association and American College of Cardiology scientific statement recommendations for athletes with coronary artery disease

High cardiorespiratory fitness and regular exercise reduce the overall risk of cardiovascular disease and death, but vigorous exercise is associated with a transient increase in acute cardiac events in those with underlying cardiovascular disease.

Cardiovascular risk scores derived from the general population have not been validated in masters athletes and may overestimate risk when applied to masters athletes (risk scores do not account for physical activity).

Low-risk (<7.5% ASCVD risk) masters athletes should not undergo routine cardiac risk stratification testing, including imaging for CAC.

Clinicians should consider further risk stratification with options including CAC, maximal-effort exercise stress testing, functional stress imaging (with maximal-effort exercise), or imaging (coronary CT angiography), for presumed intermediate* and high-risk* masters athletes.

The benefits of competitive sports participation likely outweigh risks for asymptomatic masters athletes with chronic stable CAD, and if all of the following criteria are met:

- Normal LV systolic function
- Absence of inducible ventricular arrhythmias
- No regional wall motion abnormalities
- No ischemic ECG changes or exertional symptoms during maximal-effort exercise stress testing

The risks likely outweigh the benefits of competitive sports participation for masters athletes with chronic stable CAD and any of the following criteria:

- Reduced LV systolic function inconsistent with exercise-induced cardiac remodeling (in this population generally <45% in the absence of LV dilation)
- The presence of inducible complex ventricular arrhythmias
- Regional wall Motion abnormalities
- Ischemia as Manifest by ECG changes or Exertional symptoms during Maximal-effort Exercise stress testing
- The presence (including magnitude) of ischemic scar identified by CMR associated with any of the above risk factors
- Among masters athletes with any of the above risk factors, limited participation in competitive sports can be considered with SDM using individualized intensity thresholds

Revascularization, in addition to aggressive guideline-based lifestyle modifications and optimal medical therapy, can be considered with SDM for masters athletes with evidence of obstructive CAD associated with ischemic symptoms.

Routine surveillance stress testing for asymptomatic masters athletes with stable CAD, who have incorporated appropriate lifestyle modifications and are compliant with guideline-based medical therapy, should not be performed.

AMI, acute myocardial infarction; ASCAD, atherosclerotic coronary artery disease.

Source: Adapted from Kim JH, Baggish AL, Levine BD, et al. Clinical considerations for competitive sports participation for athletes with cardiovascular abnormalities: A scientific statement from the American Heart Association and American College of Cardiology. *J Am Coll Cardiol.* 2025 Mar 18;85(10):1059–1108.

ARRHYTHMIAS IN ATHLETES

- Lethal cardiac arrhythmias ultimately represent the most serious cause of sudden death in athletes. Arrhythmias are often secondary to those conditions discussed above as culprits in sudden cardiac death. If not manifested in a lethal episode, symptoms of a potential ventricular arrhythmia may include syncope, near syncope, palpitations, exertional chest discomfort, severe dyspnea, or uncommon exertional fatigue.
- Importantly, it is increasingly recognized higher levels of prolonged vigorous activity are associated with an increased risk of developing atrial fibrillation compared with control subjects (6).
- This will include a meticulous history, physical examination, and ECG, and in many circumstances, an echocardiogram, stress test, and possibly advanced cardiac imaging. These investigations should be pursued in conjunction with appropriate specialty consultation (37).
- Various supraventricular arrhythmias may be compatible with competitive sports once they are diagnosed and controlled. The AHA/ACC Scientific Statement offers explicit details as to the recommended evaluations and allowed return-to-play considerations for most encountered arrhythmias (7).

REFERENCES

1. Lavie CJ, Sanchis-Gomar F, Ozemek C. Fit is it for longevity across populations. *J Am Coll Cardiol.* 2022 Aug 9;80(6):610–12.
2. Villeneuve PJ, Morrison HI, Craig CL, Schaubel DE. Physical activity, physical fitness, and risk of dying. *Epidemiology.* 1998;9(6):626–31.
3. Aune D, Schlesinger S, Hamer M, Norat T, Riboli E. Physical activity and the risk of sudden cardiac death: a systematic review and meta-analysis of prospective studies. *BMC Cardiovasc Disord.* 2020 Jul 6;20(1):318.
4. Siscovick DS, Weiss NS, Fletcher RH, Lasky T. The incidence of primary cardiac arrest during vigorous exercise. *N Engl J Med.* 1984 Oct 4; 311(14):874–877.
5. Asif I, Harmon K, Drezner J, Klossner D. Incidence and etiology of sudden death in NCAA athletes. *Clin J Sports Med.* 2010;20:136.
6. Martinez MW, Kim JH, Shah AB, et al. Exercise-induced cardiovascular adaptations and approach to exercise and cardiovascular disease: JACC state-of-the-art review. *J Am Coll Cardiol.* 2021 Oct 5;78(14):1453–70.
7. Kim JH, Baggish AL, Levine BD, et al. Clinical considerations for competitive sports participation for athletes with cardiovascular abnormalities: a scientific statement from the American Heart Association and American College of Cardiology. *J Am Coll Cardiol.* 2025 Mar 18;85(10):1059–108.
8. Warren TY, Barry V, Hooker SP, Sui X, Church TS, Blair SN. Sedentary behaviors increase risk of cardiovascular disease mortality in men. *Med Sci Sports Exerc.* 2010;42(5):879–85.
9. Wei M, Kampert JB, Barlow CE, et al. Relationship between low cardiorespiratory fitness and mortality in normal-weight, overweight, and obese men. *JAMA.* 1999;282(16):1547–53.
10. Richardson CR, Kriska AM, Lantz PM, Hayward RA. Physical activity and mortality across cardiovascular disease risk groups. *Med Sci Sports Exerc.* 2004;36(11):1923–9.
11. Blair SN, Kohl HW III, Barlow CE, Paffenbarger RS Jr, Gibbons LW, Macera CA. Changes in physical fitness and all-cause mortality. A prospective study of healthy and unhealthy men. *JAMA.* 1995;273(14): 1093–8.
12. Kohl HW III, Powell KE, Gordon NF, Blair SN, Paffenbarger RS Jr. Physical activity, physical fitness, and sudden cardiac death. *Epidemiol Rev.* 1992;14(1):37–58.
13. Paffenbarger RS Jr, Hyde RT, Wing AL, Lee IM, Jung DL, Kampert JB. The association of changes in physical-activity level and other lifestyle characteristics with mortality among men. *N Engl J Med.* 1993;328(8):538–45.
14. Pate RR, Pratt M, Blair SN, et al. Physical activity and public health. A recommendation from the Centers for Disease Control and Prevention and the American College of Sports Medicine. *JAMA.* 1995;273(5): 402–7.
15. Mittleman MA, Maclure M, Tofler GH, Sherwood JB, Goldberg RJ, Muller JE. Triggering of acute myocardial infarction by heavy physical exertion. Protection against triggering by regular exertion. Determinants of Myocardial Infarction Onset Study Investigators. *N Engl J Med.* 1993 Dec 2;329(23):1677–83.
16. Maron BJ. The paradox of exercise. *N Engl J Med.* 2000;343(19):1409–11.
17. Huston TP, Puffer JC, Rodney WM. The athletic heart syndrome. *N Engl J Med.* 1985;313(1):24–32.
18. Pluim BM, Zwinderman AH, van der Laarse A, van der Wall EE. The athlete's heart. A meta-analysis of cardiac structure and function. *Circulation.* 2000;101(3):336–44.
19. Maron BJ. Sudden death in young athletes. *N Engl J Med.* 2003;349(11): 1064–75.
20. Maron BJ. Distinguishing hypertrophic cardiomyopathy from athlete's heart physiological remodelling: clinical significance, diagnostic strategies and implications for preparticipation screening. *Br J Sports Med.* 2009;43(9):649–56.
21. Pelliccia A, Maron BJ, De Luca R, Di Paolo FM, Spataro A, Culasso F. Remodeling of left ventricular hypertrophy in elite athletes after long-term deconditioning. *Circulation.* 2002;105(8):944–9.
22. Giese EA, O'Connor FG, Brennan FH, Depenbrock PJ, Oriscello RG. The athletic preparticipation evaluation: cardiovascular assessment. *Am Fam Physician.* 2007;75(7):1008–14.
23. Mukerji B, Alpert MA, Mukerji V. Cardiovascular changes in athletes. *Am Fam Physician.* 1989;40(3):169–75.
24. Sharma S, Drezner JA, Baggish A, et al. International recommendations for electrocardiographic interpretation in athletes. *Eur Heart J.* 2018 Apr 21;39(16):1466–80.
25. Roberts WO, Asplund CA, O'Connor FG, Stovitz SD. Cardiac preparticipation screening for the young athlete: why the routine use of ECG is not necessary. *J Electrocardiol.* 2015 May–Jun;48(3):311–5.
26. Thompson PD, Levine BD. Protecting athletes from sudden cardiac death. *JAMA.* 2006;296(13):1648–50.
27. Van Brabandt H, Desomer A, Gerkens S, Neyt M. Harms and benefits of screening young people to prevent sudden cardiac death. *BMJ.* 2016;353:i1156.
28. Drezner J, Berger S, Campbell R. Current controversies in the cardiovascular screening of athletes. *Curr Sports Med Rep.* 2010;9(2):86–92.
29. Drezner JA, O'Connor FG, Harmon KG, et al. AMSSM position statement on cardiovascular preparticipation screening in athletes: current evidence, knowledge gaps, recommendations and future directions. *Br J Sports Med.* 2017 Feb;51(3):153–67.

30. Maron BJ, Poliac LC, Roberts WO. Risk for sudden cardiac death associated with marathon running. *J Am Coll Cardiol.* 1996;28(2):428–31.
31. Maron BJ, Doerer JJ, Haas TS, Tierney DM, Mueller FO. Sudden deaths in young competitive athletes: analysis of 1866 deaths in the United States, 1980-2006. *Circulation.* 2009;119(8):1085–92.
32. Harmon KG. Incidence and causes of sudden cardiac death in athletes. *Clin Sports Med.* 2022 Jul;41(3):369–88.
33. Asif IM, Harmon KG. Incidence and etiology of sudden cardiac death: new updates for athletic departments. *Sports Health.* 2017 May/Jun;9(3):268–79.
34. Petek BJ, Churchill TW, Moulson N, et al. Sudden cardiac death in National Collegiate Athletic Association athletes: A 20-year study. *Circulation.* 2024 Jan 9;149(2):80–90.
35. Firoozi S, Sharma S, Hamid MS, McKenna WJ. Sudden death in young athletes: HCM or ARVC?. *Cardiovasc Drugs Ther.* 2002;16(1):11–7.
36. Peterson DF, Kucera K, Thomas LC, et al. Aetiology and incidence of sudden cardiac arrest and death in young competitive athletes in the USA: a 4-year prospective study. *Br J Sports Med.* 2021 Nov;55(21):1196–203.
37. Maron BJ, Thompson PD, Ackerman MJ, et al. Recommendations and considerations related to preparticipation screening for cardiovascular abnormalities in competitive athletes: 2007 update—a scientific statement from the American Heart Association Council on Nutrition, Physical Activity, and Metabolism—endorsed by the American College of Cardiology Foundation. *Circulation.* 2007;115(12):1643–55.
38. Maron BJ, Thompson PD, Puffer JC, et al. Cardiovascular preparticipation screening of competitive athletes: addendum—an addendum to a statement for health professionals from the sudden death Committee (Council on Clinical Cardiology) and the Congenital Cardiac Defects Committee (Council on Cardiovascular Disease in the Young), American Heart Association. *Circulation.* 1998 Jun 9;97(22):2294.
39. De Paepe A, Devereux RB, Dietz HC, Hennekam RC, Pyeritz RE. Revised diagnostic criteria for the Marfan syndrome. *Am J Med Genet.* 1996;62(4):417–26.
40. Lammlein KP, Stoddard JM, O'Connor FG. Preparticipation screening of young athletes: identifying cardiovascular disease. *Prim Care.* 2018 Mar;45(1):95–107.
41. Flynn JT, Kaelber DC, Baker-Smith CM, et al. Clinical practice guideline for screening and management of high blood pressure in children and adolescents. *Pediatrics.* 2017;140(3):e20171904. *Pediatrics.* 2018 Sep;142(3):e20181739.
42. Maron BJ, Friedman RA, Kligfield P, Levine BD, Viskin S, on behalf of the American Heart Association Council on Clinical Cardiology, Advocacy Coordinating Committee, Council on Cardiovascular Disease in the Young, Council on Cardiovascular Surgery and Anesthesia, Council on Epidemiology and Prevention, Council on Functional Genomics and Translational Biology, Council on Quality of Care and Outcomes Research, and American College of Cardiology, Chaitman BR, Okin PM, Saul JP, Salberg L, Van Hare GF, Soliman EZ, Chen J, Matherne GP, Bolling SF, Mitten MJ, Caplan A, Balady GJ, Thompson PD, American Heart Association Council on Clinical Cardiology, Advocacy Coordinating Committee, Council on Cardiovascular Disease in the Young, Council on Cardiovascular Surgery and Anesthesia, Council on Epidemiology and Prevention, Council on Functional Genomics and Translational Biology, Council on Quality of Care and Outcomes Research, and American College of Cardiology. Assessment of the 12-lead ECG as a screening test for detection of cardiovascular disease in healthy general populations of young people (12-25 Years of Age): a scientific statement from the American Heart Association and the American College of Cardiology. *Circulation.* 2014;130(15):1303–34.
43. Webster G, Puckelwartz MJ, Pesce LL, et al. Genomic autopsy of sudden deaths in young individuals. *JAMA Cardiol.* 2021 Nov 1;6(11):1247–56.
44. O'Connor FG, Levine BD, Childress MA, Asplundh CA, Oriscello RG. Practical management: a systematic approach to the evaluation of exercise-related syncope in athletes. *Clin J Sport Med.* 2009;19(5):429–34.
45. Asplund CA, O'Connor FG, Noakes TD. Exercise-associated collapse: an evidence-based review and primer for clinicians. *Br J Sports Med.* 2011 Nov;45(14):1157–62.
46. Roberts WO. Exercise-associated collapse care matrix in the marathon. *Sports Med.* 2007;37(4-5):431–3.
47. Colivicchi F, Ammirati F, Santini M. Epidemiology and prognostic implications of syncope in young competing athletes. *Eur Heart J.* 2004;25(19):1749–53.
48. Childress MA, O'Connor FG, Levine BD. Exertional collapse in the runner: evaluation and management in fieldside and office-based settings. *Clin Sports Med.* 2010;29(3):459–76.
49. Prakken NH, Cramer MJ, Olimulder MA, Agostoni P, Mali WP, Velthuis BK. Screening for proximal coronary artery anomalies with 3-dimensional MR coronary angiography. *Int J Cardiovasc Imaging.* 2010;26(6):701–10.
50. James PA, Oparil S, Carter BL, et al. 2014 evidence-based guideline for the management of high blood pressure in adults: report from the panel members appointed to the Eighth Joint National Committee (JNC 8). *JAMA.* 2014;311(5):507–20.
51. Buelt A, Richards A, Jones AL. Hypertension: new guidelines from the International Society of hypertension. *Am Fam Physician.* 2021 Jun 15;103(12):763–5.
52. Ghasem W, Abouzeid C, Toresdahl BG, Shah AB. Updated blood pressure guidelines: implications for athletes. *Curr Hypertens Rep.* 2022;24(10):477–84.
53. Schweiger V, Niederseer D, Schmied C, Attenhofer-Jost C, Caselli S. Athletes and hypertension. *Curr Cardiol Rep.* 2021;23(12):176.
54. Rao P, Shipon D. Exercise recommendations for the athlete with coronary artery disease. *Curr Treat Options Cardiovasc Med.* 2019 Dec 9;21(12):82.

32 Dermatology

Kenneth B. Batts

INTRODUCTION

- Skin serves as a protective barrier against mechanical, environmental, and infective forces.
- Sport-specific dermatoses may incapacitate or disqualify an athlete or expose a teammate to a potential infection, placing him or her at risk for disqualification or impaired performance.

MECHANICAL INJURY

Abrasions

- Commonly known as *rug burn*, *strawberry*, or *road rash*, abrasion may occur on any surface, but primarily artificial turf, floor mats, synthetic courts, and asphalt roads.
- Treatment consists of cleaning and debriding the tissue with warm, soapy water and applying a topical antibacterial ointment.
- Topical anesthesia facilitates easier exploration and debridement and may be achieved with 2% lidocaine jelly or one of several commercially available anesthetics (lidocaine, epinephrine, tetracaine [LET]; eutectic mixture of local anesthetics [EMLA]; Ela-Max) (1).
- A thin covering of antibacterial ointment (mupirocin) or an adhesive hydrocolloid dressing (DuoDERM, OpSite) promotes healing (1).
- Because of the risk of bloodborne pathogens and subsequent disease transmission, all wounds should be covered with an occlusive dressing during participation.
- The National Collegiate Athletic Association (NCAA) mandates that an athlete with active bleeding must be removed from competition, the bleeding stopped, and a dressing applied to withstand the rigors of competition prior to continued participation (2).

Acne Mechanica

- An occlusive obstruction of the follicular pilosebaceous units.
- The pustular eruption commonly occurs in a warm, moist environment occluded by protective equipment across the back and shoulders or on the chin (3).
- Wearing sweat-wicking underclothing, good personal hygiene, and regular cleaning of equipment help prevent outbreaks of lesions.
- Acne mechanica in dark-skinned athletes may evolve into acne keloidalis on the nape of the neck (4).
- The condition can be treated with various topical keratolytics with astringents (3% salicylic acid, 70% resorcinol) and antibiotics (tetracycline, clindamycin) (5).
- Athletes should be clearly informed of side effects including muscle soreness, joint pain, and lethargy prior to the use of isotretinoin for severe pustular acne (5).

Athletic Nodules

- Fibrotic connective tissue (collagenomas) formed as a result of repetitive pressure, friction, or trauma over bony prominences.
- Commonly located on knuckles (boxers, football players), tibial tuberosity (surfers), or dorsal feet (hockey "skate bites," runners, hikers) (4).
- Treatment includes intralesional steroids, protective taping and padding, and excision (4).
- Resolve after the discontinuation of causal activity.

Black Heel

- Black heel, or talon noir, refers to bluish-black petechiae within the stratum corneum on the posterior or posterolateral aspect of the heel caused by shearing forces between epidermis and dermis (6).
- Commonly occurs in basketball, tennis, track, and similar events requiring sudden changes in direction.
- A similar condition, black palm or tache noir, has been described in baseball players, golfers, gymnasts, mogul skiers, mountain climbers, and weightlifters (4).
- Self-limiting and will resolve spontaneously once the season ends.
- The use of heel cups, felt pads, cushioned athletic socks, and properly fitted footwear may help prevent black heel formation.

Black Toenail

- Rapid deceleration of the forefoot against the shoe toe box may produce painful subungual hemorrhages of the first and second toenail beds.

- The condition occurs with greater frequency in sports requiring quick stops, such as tennis, skiing, hiking, and rock climbing (4).
- The hematoma can be drained by carefully boring a hole through the nail with an 18-gauge needle or an electrocautery unit.
- Appropriate running shoes (2 cm from the longest toe to the end of the shoe), lacing shoes tightly enough to prevent the foot from sliding forward, and properly trimming the distal nail to its shortest length in a straight cut line will reduce the likelihood of developing this condition (7).
- Notable exceptions are the persistence of a linear black band or streak running the entire length of the nail representing a melanocytic nevus or the more serious involvement of the proximal nail fold as in malignant melanoma (8).

Blisters

- Vesicles or bullae filled with serosanguinous fluid or blood.
- Repeated pressure or friction over bony prominences associated with excessive perspiration and improperly fitted equipment leads to the formation of blisters (9).
- Treat early blisters with moleskin donuts and nylon foot stockings to decrease friction, talcum powder or antiperspirant to keep feet dry, and benzoin to harden the epidermis (3,10).
- Bullous blisters should be drained at the edge with a small needle leaving the roof of the blister as a protective layer.
- Ruptured and deroofed blisters may require the application of a hydrocolloidal dressing (DuoDERM) or an adhesive polyurethane dressing (OpSite) as a second-skin layer to reduce discomfort and enhance healing (11).
- Primary prevention includes wearing properly fitted and broken-in footwear, use of absorbent socks or two pairs of socks of different materials, and applying petrolatum jelly or commercial antichafing preparations (Body Glide) over bony prominences (12,13).

Corns and Calluses

- Corns are small, soft or hard, deep, and painful conical lesions with a translucent central core in the web spaces of the toes and the plantar surface over the distal heads of the metatarsals (4).
- Calluses tend to be larger, hyperkeratotic, nonpainful lesions that serve as a protective skin layer and are considered an advantage in gymnastics, racquet sports, and rowing.
- The development of small black dots representing thrombosed capillaries implies the presence of plantar warts, compared to calluses that display a thickened epidermis with intact dermatoglyphics.
- The most important factor for successful recovery and prevention of the condition is redistributing pressure away from the lesion.
- The shaping of a metatarsal pad to the plantar surface, creating a wider shoe toe box, adding cotton or foam padding between the toes, and applying moleskin will all aid in decreasing the pressure over the existing lesion and prevent further injury.
- Keratolytic agents (5%–10% salicylic acid in colloid, 40% salicylic acid plaster, 12% lactic acid) soften the stratum corneum (keratin layer) and a pumice stone or emery board will then remove the lesion by rubbing the overlying skin or by paring with a scalpel blade (14,15).

Follicular Keloiditis

- An inflammatory proliferation of fibrous tissue that is usually painless and is more prevalent in dark-skinned athletes.
- Multiple, small keloids commonly develop where the headgear comes in contact with the forehead, cheeks, and posterior neck or where the undergarment pads cover the thighs, knees, and shoulders.
- Treatment involves gradual reduction of the lesion with intralesional steroid injections or topical application of a steroid-impregnated adhesive tape (16).

Ingrown Toenail

- This condition is caused by distal nail bed pressure forcing the lateral edge of the nail plate into the lateral nail fold.
- The distal nail should be trimmed straight across, and at least one thumbnail in distance should exist from the longest distal toenail to the end of the shoe to prevent recurrence.
- Acute treatment options include soaks in an Epsom salt or soapy water bath followed by application of topical antibiotic or a mid-to high-potency topical steroid, gentle manual nail elevation, placing a small piece of cotton or dental floss under the corner of the nail to elevate the lateral margin, use of oral antibiotics, and excision of the lateral one-third of the nail with electrodessication or chemical matricectomy using 80%–88% phenol (17–19).

Jogger's Nipples

- Irritation and friction from coarse, cotton fabrics on an unprotected nipple and areola leading to pain and bleeding.
- The majority of jogger's nipples occur in male athletes, especially long-distance runners and triathletes (5).
- Preventive measures include wearing of soft, natural, silk fiber shirts or no shirt, or application of breast padding, electrocardiographic lead pads, band-aids, or a double coat of fingernail polish over the nipples prior to running to prevent chafing.
- Treat by washing and gently drying and applying petroleum jelly, antibiotic ointment, or topical steroid cream to alleviate inflammation (7,20).

Piezogenic Papules

- Flesh-colored papules noticeable only on weight-bearing are found in up to 20% of the general population.
- Herniations of subdermal fat into the dermis visibly evident on either side of the heel (21).
- Typically asymptomatic, but may become painful, possibly due to herniation of nerve fibers with subdermal fat (22).
- More common in endurance athletes.
- Padding, compression stockings, taping for support, heel cups, and steroid injections may help reduce the pain (22).

Rower's Rump

- Rower's rump develops in the gluteal cleft of rowers training on small, unpadded scull seats, and metal rowing machines (23).
- Repeated friction produces a lichen simplex chronicus of the buttocks.
- Treatment consists of padding the rowing seat and the use of potent, fluorinated topical steroids.

Runner's Rump

- A collection of ecchymotic lesions on the superior portion of the gluteal cleft of long-distance runners (5,7).
- Results from constant friction between the gluteal folds with each running stride.
- The hyperpigmentation will spontaneously resolve with rest.

ENVIRONMENTAL INJURY

Sun and Heat

Sunburn

- Prolonged exposure to ultraviolet B (UVB) (290–320 nm) may burn skin, producing symptoms ranging from mild erythema to intense blistering, edema, and pain.
- Ultraviolet A (UVA) (320–400 nm) is 1000-fold less burning to the skin than UVB but is more penetrating and produces chronic damage.
- Ultraviolet exposure increases with altitude and with reflection off snow or water (1).
- Preventive measures include avoiding exercise between 10 a.m. and 2 p.m., applying sun protective factor (SPF) with para-aminobenzoic acid (PABA) at least 20 minutes prior to sun exposure, and recoating after water exposure or sweating (1,24).

Miliaria

- Miliaria rubra, or prickly heat, occurs in hot, humid summer environments.
- Fine, pruritic, erythematous, vesiculopapular rash develops over eccrine sweat glands occluded by clothing (spares the palms and soles) (25).
- Cooling and drying the skin to stop further sweating and application of hydrophilic ointments (Eucerin) and mild topical corticosteroids can open the occluded ducts (11,26).

Solar Urticaria

- Solar urticaria is an uncommon cause of urticaria in athletes.
- Manifested by itching and burning of the skin within minutes after exposure to UVA, UVB, or both wavelengths (27).
- Erythema and wheal formation will follow and clear within 2 hours after exposure (4,19).
- Normally unexposed skin areas of the trunk will be more prone to develop an urticarial reaction than the regularly exposed face or distal extremities.
- Phototesting is recommended to determine the type and treatment of solar urticaria.
- Desensitization by sunlight and a combination of oral psoralen and long-wave ultraviolet light (PUVA) has been shown to decrease symptoms (27).
- Treatment includes sunlight avoidance, sunscreen or zinc lotion, high-dose antihistamines, cyclosporine, chloroquine, and intravenous immunoglobulin (27).

Cholinergic Urticaria

- Pruritic dermatosis occurring during exercise, heat, emotional stress, or eating spicy foods is believed to be mediated by increased sympathetic tone and acetylcholine activity (28).
- Most commonly affects the trunk and extremities, sparing face and neck.
- The condition is characterized by the eruption of pinpoint papular wheals with a surrounding subcutaneous erythematous flare during and after heat exposure or exercise.
- Provocative testing with exercise under controlled circumstances is the safest and surest means to reproduce symptoms. Full resuscitative measures should be available because exercise-induced anaphylaxis may be included in the differential diagnosis (28).
- Treatment with H_1 antihistamines (hydroxyzine and cetirizine) and danazol has been found to be effective if taken 1 hour prior to exercise (29).
- Danazol should be avoided or used with caution in females because it is a strong androgenizing agent (28).
- Propranolol may be effective in refractory cases (28).

Cold

Chilblain

- Chilblain or pernio is the result of repeated or prolonged exposure to cold, but not freezing, temperatures in moist conditions (30).
- Athletes may initially be asymptomatic, but later complain of reddish-blue patches that are pruritic, painful, and tender and then lead to blisters or ulcerations (31).

- Injury is due to hypoxia from local vasoconstriction occurring primarily on the feet, hands, and face, particularly in young, white females (32).
- The area should be rewarmed and protected from further environmental exposure; rubbing or massaging is contraindicated as this may further damage the injured tissue (33).
- Topical corticosteroids or a short burst of oral corticosteroids may be used to minimize the painful, inflammatory skin lesions.
- Insulated and water-resistant outer clothing, moisture-wicking socks and gloves, frequent sock and glove changes, and protective covering over the face aid in preventing this injury.

Frostnip

- Frostnip is the most common of cold injuries and involves only the superficial skin.
- The skin and superficial subcutaneous tissue of the fingertips, toes, nose, cheeks, and ears become pallid and painful, develop paresthesias, and finally lose sensation.
- Penile frostnip has been reported in joggers wearing polyester trousers and cotton undershorts (30).
- Frostnip is completely reversed with rewarming of the affected area, but it is possible for paresthesia to persist for several weeks after the injury (30).
- Prevention includes insulation and skin protection from both wind and cold, not shaving prior to participation to preserve the natural skin oils, and application of a sunscreen or petrolatum-based emollient (30).

Frostbite

- Frostbite occurs when tissue temperature falls below 28 °F (−2 °C) and intra- and extracellular fluid sludges and then crystallizes, mechanically disrupting cell membranes (31).
- The tissue appears cold, white, and hard and will not exhibit pain or sensation to tactile stimulation until thawing occurs.
- Initial management is immobilization and evacuation. Rewarming should not be attempted until the risk of refreezing is eliminated because further freeze-thaw cycles greatly increase tissue damage.
- Once hypothermia has been ruled out or treated, affected areas should be rapidly warmed in a circulating water bath at 104–108 °F (40–42 °C) avoiding rubbing, which increases tissue damage and loss (33).
- Thawing is often intensely painful, and narcotic pain medication may be employed. Consideration should also be given to administration of tetanus toxoid and antibiotic therapy (31).
- Surgical therapy is often delayed up to 2–3 months until dry gangrene or mummification clearly demarcates nonviable tissue (33).

Cold Urticaria

- Cold urticaria is characterized by pruritic wheals or hives in response to exposure to cold weather or objects and will flare after the area is rewarmed (30).
- Urticarial plaques are usually confined to the exposed area, but may be generalized.
- Provocative testing of the forearm with ice cubes for 5 minutes will produce wheals on warming the skin and confirm the diagnosis (4).
- Symptoms will likely recur, so exposure avoidance is recommended.
- The prophylactic use of nonsedating antihistamines such as cyproheptadine (Periactin), 2 mg once or twice a day, or doxepin (Sinequan), 10 mg two or three times daily, has been useful in preventing recurrence (34).

INFECTIOUS INJURY

- Skin infections account for up to 21% of time loss from wrestling practice or competition (2).
- Prevention is important and is possible through athlete self-reporting, preparticipation examinations, personal and equipment hygiene, hand sanitization, avoidance of sharing toiletries or towels, and prompt treatment and isolation of infected individuals.
- NCAA requires infectious skin conditions to be deemed noninfectious and adequately medicated per treatment guidelines and properly covered with a secured impermeable bandage or dressing (2).

Bacterial

Impetigo

- Serosanguinous, honey-crusted pustules on an erythematous base.
- β-*Hemolytic streptococci* more commonly produce impetigo, but staphylococcal species have been isolated from cultured wounds (35).
- Very contagious and common among contact sports, although cases and outbreaks are documented among weightlifters, fencers, and cross-country runners (35).
- Recommended treatment includes both topical antibiotic (mupirocin twice daily) and a second-generation cephalosporin or penicillinase-resistant penicillin derivative for 10 days (36).
- The NCAA requires all wrestlers to be without new lesions for 48 hours before a meet, have completed 72 hours of antibiotic therapy, and have no moist or draining lesions prior to competition (2).
- Active, purulent lesions shall not be covered to allow for participation (2).

Furunculosis

- Erythematous, nodular abscesses found most commonly in the hairy areas of the axillae, buttocks, and groin (37).
- Highly contagious, so routine screening, prompt treatment, and event disqualification of infected players can prevent outbreaks (36).
- Staphylococci are the most frequent bacteria isolated, but all wounds should be cultured to guide therapy because methicillin-resistant *Staphylococcus aureus* (MRSA) is common.

- Acute treatment consists of warm compresses and a 10-day course of a cephalosporin, erythromycin, or penicillinase-resistant penicillin derivative (36).
- Topical mupirocin may be used to eradicate nasal carriage of *Staphylococcus* species among team members if an outbreak occurs (36).
- Incision and drainage are necessary because of the poor hematogenous antibiotic penetration.
- The NCAA guidelines for participation of wrestlers with bacterial infections are described in the previous section on impetigo (2).

Pitted Keratolysis

- A scalloped-bordered plaque with sculpted pits of variable depth forms on the weight-bearing plantar surfaces (heel and toes) and is often misdiagnosed as tinea pedis.
- Hyperhidrosis and gram-positive bacteria, most commonly *Corynebacterium* and *Micrococcus* species, found in the stratum corneum have been implicated in producing the pungent foot odor (36).
- Application of topical antibiotics 2–4 weeks (5% erythromycin or 1% clindamycin in 10% benzoyl peroxide) reduces the bacterial inflammatory component and result in clearing (38).
- Prophylactic therapy includes washing with benzoyl peroxide soap and adding topical foot powders with 20% aluminum chloride (Drysol) to control hyperhidrosis (38).

Erythrasma

- Chronic, bacterial infection affecting the intertriginous areas.
- The causative organism is a gram-positive rod, *Corynebacterium minutissimum*.
- The sharply demarcated reddish-brown plaques are similar in appearance to tinea cruris, but diagnosis can be confirmed by examination with a Wood's lamp, which reveals coral-red fluorescence (39).
- Treatment options include clarithromycin 1 g single dose or 500 mg twice a day for 2 weeks, and erythromycin 250 mg twice to four times a day for 2 weeks or tetracycline 250 mg four times per day for 2 weeks (40).
- The areas should be covered for athletes to participate in practice and competitive contact-related sports.

MRSA

- Community-acquired MRSA (CA-MRSA) is an increasingly common condition affecting athletes.
- MRSA typically presents similar to other bacterial infections as furuncles, carbuncles, and abscesses and is sometimes mistaken as spider bites, and any of these presentations should be evaluated for possible CA-MRSA (35).
- Any suspicious lesion should be cultured to isolate the infective organism and determine susceptibilities.
- Prevention measures are identical to those general principles listed earlier with the addition of showering using antibacterial soap after every practice and game, as well as eliminating cosmetic body shaving because shaving has been demonstrated to increase rates of CA-MRSA (37).
- Definitive treatment of cutaneous lesions is incision and drainage.
- Antibiotic therapy must be guided by culture and sensitivity as well as local susceptibility information.
- Antibiotic regimens most often include oral clindamycin 300–450 mg three times daily or trimethoprim-sulfamethoxazole two double-strength tablets daily.
- MRSA infections can be severe, leading to hospitalization and requiring intravenous antibiotic therapy including vancomycin, clindamycin, or linezolid.

Viral

Verrucae

- The human papilloma virus induces warts, or verrucae vulgaris.
- Plantar warts disrupt the normal dermatoglyphics of the pressure points of the feet and often coalesce to form a gyrate or mosaic pattern.
- Small black dots representing thrombosed capillaries within a hyperkeratotic plaque confirm the diagnosis (7).
- The NCAA requires wrestlers to cover multiple digitate verrucae of the face with a mask, verrucae plana or vulgaris must be adequately covered to compete, and solitary lesions can be curetted prior to the meet but cannot be seeping (2).
- Salicylic acid preparations or topical imiquimod can be applied with an occlusion wrap during the season (41,42).
- Liquid nitrogen cryotherapy can be used concurrently or alone every 2 weeks, but may delay return to training due to pain.

Molluscum Contagiosum

- Characterized by flesh-colored, dome-shaped papules with a central umbilication.
- The pox virus is highly contagious and spreads by direct skin transmission from person to person, autoinoculation, water transmission, and gymnasium equipment (43).
- The papules are typically self-limiting and resolve over weeks to months.
- NCAA wrestling rules require that lesions be removed by sharp curettage or liquid nitrogen and any solitary lesions be covered with a gas-permeable dressing (OpSite, BioClusive) and tape in a manner that can withstand the rigors of competition (2).
- NCAA wrestling rules require trunk and upper thigh lesions to be covered with clothing (2).
- Liquid nitrogen, 0.7% cantharidin, topical tretinoin (Retin-A), electrodesiccation, and the use of imiquimod 5% cream have been successful but may require several treatments (43).

Herpes Gladiatorum

- Herpes gladiatorum or rugbeiorum refers to a herpes simplex virus (HSV-1) outbreak on the face or body of wrestlers or rugby players during "lock-up" or in a scrum. These lesions occur most commonly on the head and neck, followed by the extremities and trunk.
- Classic lesions appear as a cluster of painful vesicles on an erythematous base, and diagnosis is made on clinical appearance, but may be confirmed by Tzanck smear or viral culture (41).
- The virus is passed by direct face-to-face or body-to-body transmission between athletes, and headgear does not decrease the risk of transmission (43).
- Antiviral therapies for acute outbreaks include acyclovir 400 mg three times a day for 5 days, valacyclovir 1 g twice a day for 7–10 days, or famciclovir 250 mg twice or three times a day for 7–10 days (44).
- Athletes with recurrent outbreaks may use suppressive therapy during the season, most commonly with valacyclovir 500–1000 mg daily, acyclovir 400 mg twice a day, or famciclovir 250 mg twice a day (44).
- The NCAA allows a wrestler to participate if free of systemic symptoms, has not developed new lesions during the last 72 hours before the examination, all lesions have a firm adherent crust, and the wrestler has been on antiviral therapy for 120 hours. Active herpetic lesions cannot be covered to allow for participation (2).

Fungal

Tinea Pedis

- A papulosquamous fungal infection producing a pruritic, red, scaly rash on the lateral soles of the feet and between the toes.
- The superficial dermatophytic fungal infection is caused by *Trichophyton rubrum*, *Trichophyton mentagrophytes*, or *Epidermophyton floccosum*.
- The majority of cases respond promptly to topical antifungal creams, such as ketoconazole, clotrimazole, itraconazole, or terbinafine (38).

Tinea Corporis

- A dermatophyte infection produces an annular, ring-like (ringworm) lesion with a sharply demarcated, red scaly border, and central clearing.
- Tinea corporis gladiatorum has been frequently isolated and reported in wrestlers on their head, neck, and upper arms (36).
- In the majority of cases, *Trichophyton tonsurans* is the causative fungus (38).
- Recent studies reveal that oral fluconazole, 100 mg taken once daily for 3 days prior to the season and once again 6 weeks later, decreased the incidence of tinea among wrestlers from 67.4% to 3.5% (45).
- The NCAA requires a minimum of 72 hours of topical therapy for skin lesions, a minimum of 2 weeks of oral therapy for scalp (tinea capitis) lesions, and all lesions must be adequately covered with an impermeable dressing that has been secured with prewrap and stretch tape after evaluation and disposition by a team physician or certified athletic trainer (2).

Tinea Cruris

- An erythematous, pruritic plaque with well-demarcated, scaly borders that extends to the groin, upper thighs, abdomen, and perineum, but typically spares the genitalia (46).
- The appearance of an inflammatory, red rash with satellite lesions involving the scrotum is candidiasis and requires treatment with imidazole creams.
- Diagnosis can be confirmed by the presence of fungal hyphae on a potassium hydroxide slide.
- Topical antifungals are effective, and clotrimazole is the recommended first-line therapy (46).
- Addition of topical corticosteroid with topical antifungal may speed resolution of symptoms (47).
- Oral antifungal agents may be required in recalcitrant cases, if the hair roots are involved.
- Tinea cruris must be differentiated from candida intertrigo (scrotal involvement and satellite lesions), erythrasma (coral-red fluorescence under Wood's lamp), or a chronic irritant dermatitis from elasticized undergarments (46).

Tinea Versicolor

- Also called pityriasis versicolor, overgrowth of the active fungal form of *Malassezia furfur* (also known as *Pityrosporum orbiculare*) causes a chronic, asymptomatic, hyper- or hypopigmented, scaling, macular dermatosis (48).
- Wood's (black) lamp reveals a characteristic yellow-green or coppery orange fluorescence (49).
- Treatment consists of washing the affected area with zinc pyrithione or selenium sulfide shampoo or with topical imidazole treatments such as ketoconazole or clotrimazole (48).
- In extensive or recurrent disease, oral ketoconazole 200 mg daily for 7–15 days or fluconazole 400 mg for one dose may be effective (49).
- The athlete needs to continue exercise and perspire for at least 1 hour after taking ketoconazole to promote absorption into the hair root (11).

Onychomycosis

- Onychomycosis is the most common disease of the nails and represents a fungal infection, with *Trichophyton rubrum*, *Trichophyton mentagrophytes*, or *Epidermophyton floccosum* being the causative organism in 90% of cases (50).
- Risk factors include repeated nail trauma, moist environment, occlusive footwear, genetic predisposition, poor circulation, concurrent diabetes, and immunosuppression.
- Multiple treatment regimens of oral and topical antifungal medications are described, but the mainstay of therapy is

oral agents with terbinafine 250 mg daily for 12 weeks superior to itraconazole (51).

- Oral itraconazole 200 mg daily for 12 weeks with topical amorolfine 5% lacquer applied weekly for 6 months has been shown to have a 94% cure rate (50).
- Prescriber should review medication interactions because these are common among systemic antifungals.
- Baseline liver function tests must be performed, and laboratory monitoring for hepatotoxicity and pancytopenia should be considered during therapy.

MISCELLANEOUS

Contact Dermatitis

- Primary irritant dermatitis is a nonallergic reaction that leads to symptoms within minutes of the exposure. The dermatitis is localized to the contact site and exhibits erythema and a burning sensation. Common irritants are detergents and soaps, adhesive pretape sprays, sunscreens, and fiberglass (36).
- Allergic contact dermatitis is an acquired immune response that develops hours to days after recurrent exposure to an allergen. The dermatitis exhibits patches of erythema, edema, vesicle formation, and extreme pruritus. Equipment with protective rubber coverings (golf clubs), black rubber seals (swim gear), tanned leather straps, latex products, iodine preparations, topical antibiotic ointments, adhesive tape, shoe dyes, and poison ivy or oak have all produced allergic reactions (20).
- Initial treatment includes avoidance and washing with water in an attempt to physically remove the irritant and prevent further systemic progression.
- Alternative equipment has been manufactured using polyurethane, neoprene, and silicone to alleviate allergic reactions.
- Antihistamines, corticosteroids, analgesics, and H_2 antagonists are commonly used for moderate to severe systemic hypersensitivity reactions by either oral or intravenous routes.
- Patch testing can often help identify the allergen triggering the dermatitis.

Envenomation

- Most allergic reactions are from hornets and wasps.
- Hymenoptera venom can be neutralized with meat tenderizer or shaving cream at the site.
- Antihistamines and nonsteroidal anti-inflammatory agents are commonly prescribed for allergic reactions to stings.
- Participants with known allergic reactions to hymenoptera should be advised to use sunscreens with insect repellent formulas.
- Athletic trainers or physicians covering events should always carry an injectable subcutaneous 1:1000 epinephrine syringe (EpiPen kit).
- In the United States, 4000–6000 venomous snake bites occur yearly, and about 70% require antivenom (52).
- Initial treatment of venomous snake bite includes splinting the limb below the level of the heart, removing restrictive clothing from the extremity, and evacuating to a medical facility immediately (52).
- Contraindicated first aid techniques include arterial tourniquet, incision and suction, ice or cryotherapy, venom extractors, electric shock, and application of papain or meat tenderizer (52).
- Antivenom is the primary treatment for envenomations, but should only be given based on the severity of envenomation because antivenom also has a significant risk of causing an allergic reaction.

Swimmer's Itch

- A parasitic dermatitis produced by the cercarial form of freshwater schistosomes commonly found in freshwater lakes of the United States (36).
- 1- or 2-mm macules develop into papules on exposed areas, not under the bathing suit.
- Self-limiting, but symptoms may be reduced with cold packs, antihistamines, and topical steroids (53).

Seabather's Eruption

- Pruritic papules and wheals with onset 2–24 hours after saltwater swimming and occurring in areas covered by a swimming suit, especially under the waistband or shoulder straps (53).
- Free-swimming, larval forms of *Edwardsiella lineata* and *Linuche unguiculata* containing stinging nematocysts are trapped in the swimming suit (54).
- Symptoms typically resolve within 3–7 days, but resolution may take as long as 6 weeks in severe cases (54).
- Oral antihistamines and topical corticosteroid are effective (53).

Green Hair

- Regular swimmers with natural or tinted blonde, gray, or white hair may develop a green tint to their hair from the release of copper from pipes or algicides in swimming pools (55,56).
- Immediately washing the hair and maintaining the pool pH between 7.4 and 7.6 will prevent this condition (4).
- Copper chelating shampoo applied for 30 minutes, hydrogen peroxide soak for 2–3 hours, and ethylenediaminetetraacetic acid (EDTA) conditioner once or twice per season have been effective in returning hair to original color (8).

Exercise-Induced Anaphylaxis

- Exercise-induced anaphylaxis (EIA) is a rare and unpredictable condition that typically occurs with a short duration of submaximal exercise and may occur in sedentary individuals or elite athletes (57).
- Pruritus with large wheals may progress to systemic symptoms of wheezing, nausea, diarrhea, angioedema, hypotension, and shock.
- Running has been found to be the most common exercise predisposed to EIA (36).
- Food-dependent exercise-induced anaphylaxis (FDEIA) is a subtype in which symptoms result only when a particular food is ingested prior to exercise and no symptoms occur with the food or exercise alone.
- FDEIA has been associated with many food allergens, with wheat being the most common (57).
- EIA is a clinical diagnosis, and it is important to differentiate it from more common triggers including foods, ingredients in sports drinks, and latex.
- Plasma histamine levels are elevated in all forms of EIA.
- Preventive measures include not exercising in extremes of either hot or cold weather and the use of nonsedating antihistamines 1 hour prior to exercise (58).
- Athletes who want to continue vigorous exercise should be instructed to exercise with someone (jogging partner) who has knowledge of their condition and can administer an injectable subcutaneous 1:1000 epinephrine syringe (EpiPen kit).

REFERENCES

1. Honsik KA, Romeo MW, Hawley CJ, Romeo SJ, Romeo JP. Sideline skin and wound care for acute injuries. *Curr Sports Med Rep.* 2007;6(3):147–54.
2. Barbee C. *NCAA Wrestling Rules 2023-2024 and 2024-2025.* Indianapolis (IN): The National Collegiate Athletic Association; 2023.
3. Freiman A, Barankin B, Elpern DJ. Sports dermatology part 1: common dermatoses. *CMAJ.* 2004;171(8):851–3.
4. Pharis DB, Teller C, Wolf JE Jr. Cutaneous manifestations of sports participation. *J Am Acad Dermatol.* 1997;36(3 pt 1):448–59.
5. Basler RS. Skin injuries in sports medicine. *J Am Acad Dermatol.* 1989;21(6):1257–62.
6. Urbina F, Leon L, Sudy E. Black heel, talon noir or calcanea petechiae? *Australas J Dermatol.* 2008;49(3):148–51.
7. Mailler-Savage EA, Adams BB. Skin manifestations of running. *J Am Acad Dermatol.* 2006;55(2):290–301.
8. Adams BB, Kindred C. Common and uncommon hair and nail problems in sports. *Cutis.* 2005;75(5):269–75.
9. Yavuz M, Davis BL. Plantar shear stress distribution in athletic individuals with frictional foot blisters. *J Am Podiatr Med Assoc.* 2010;100(2):116–20.
10. Levine N. Dermatologic aspects of sports medicine. *J Am Acad Dermatol.* 1980;3(4):415–24.
11. Bergfeld WF, Elston DM. Diagnosis and treatment of dermatologic problems in athletes. In: Fu FH, Stone DA, editors. *Sports Injuries: Mechanisms, Prevention, Treatment.* Baltimore (MD): Williams & Wilkins; 1994. 781 p.
12. Heymann WR. Dermatologic problems of the endurance athlete. *J Am Acad Dermatol.* 2005;52(2):345–6.
13. Worthing RM, Percy RL, Joslin JD. Prevention of friction blisters in outdoor pururitis: a systematic review. *Wilderness Environ Med.* 2017;28(2):138–49.
14. Stephenson J, Farndon L, Concannon M. Analysis of a trial assessing the long-term effectiveness of salicylic acid plasters compared with scalpel debridement in facilitating corn resolution in patients with multiple corns. *J Dermatol.* 2016;43(6):662–9.
15. Hashmi F, Nester CJ, Wright CRF, Lam S. The evaluation of three treatments for plantar callus: a three-armed randomised, comparative trial using biophysical outcome measures. *Trials.* 2016;17(1):251.
16. Wolfram D, Tzankov A, Pülzl P, Piza-Katzer H. Hypertrophic scars and keloids—a review of their pathophysiology, risk factors, and therapeutic management. *Dermatol Surg.* 2009;35(2):171–81.
17. Daniel CR III, Iorizzo M, Tosti A, Piraccini BM. Ingrown toenails. *Cutis.* 2006;78(6):407–8.
18. Heidelbaugh JJ, Lee H. Management of the ingrown toenail. *Am Fam Physician.* 2009;79(4):303–8.
19. Mayeaux EJ Jr, Carter C, Murphy TE. Ingrown toenail management. *Am Fam Physician.* 2019;100(3):158–64.
20. Kockentiet B, Adams BB. Contact dermatitis in athletes. *J Am Acad Dermatol.* 2007;56(6):1048–55.
21. Rocha BDO, Fernandes JD, Prates FV. Piezogenic pedal papules. *An Bras Dermatol.* 2015;90(6):928–9.
22. Redboard KP, Adams BB. Piezogenic pedal papules in a marathon runner. *Clin J Sport Med.* 2006;16(1):81–3.
23. Tomecki KJ, Mikesell JF. Rower's rump. *J Am Acad Dermatol.* 1987;16(4):890–1.
24. Seité S, Fourtanier A, Moyal D, Young AR. Photodamage to human skin by suberythemal exposure to solar ultraviolet radiation can be attenuated by sunscreens: a review. *Br J Dermatol.* 2010;163(5):903–14.
25. Gauer R, Meyers BK. Heat-related illnesses. *Am Fam Physician.* 2019;99(8):482–9.
26. Seto CK, Way D, O'Connor N. Environmental illness in athletes. *Clin Sports Med.* 2005;24(3):695–718.
27. Gambichler T, Al-Muhammadi R, Boms S. Immunologically mediated photodermatoses diagnosis and treatment. *Am J Clin Dermatol.* 2009;10(3):169–80.
28. Feinberg JH, Toner CB. Successful treatment of disabling cholinergic urticaria. *Mil Med.* 2008;173(2):217–20.
29. Zuberbier T, Aberer W, Asero R, et al. The EAACI/GALEN/EDF/WAO guideline for the definition, classification, diagnosis and management of urticaria. *Allergy.* 2018;73(7):1393–414.
30. Englund SL, Adams BB. Winter sports dermatology: a review. *Cutis.* 2009;83(1):42–8.
31. Golant A, Nord RM, Paksima N, Posner MA. Cold exposure injuries to the extremities. *J Am Acad Orthop Surg.* 2008;16(12):704–15.
32. Yang X, Perez OA, English JC III. Adult perniosis and cryoglobulinemia: a retrospective study and review of the literature. *J Am Acad Dermatol.* 2010;62(6):e21–2.
33. Jurkovich GJ. Environmental cold-induced injury. *Surg Clin North Am.* 2007;87(1):247–67.
34. Krause K, Zuberbier T, Maurer M. Modern approaches to the diagnosis and treatment of cold contact urticaria. *Curr Allergy Asthma Rep.* 2010;10(4):243–9.

35. Kirkland EB, Adams BB. Methicillin-resistant *Staphylococcus aureus* and athletes. *J Am Acad Dermatol.* 2008;59(3):494–502.
36. Adams BB. Dermatologic disorders of the athlete. *Sports Med.* 2002;32(5):309–21.
37. Ibler KS, Kromann CB. Recurrent furunculosis - challenges and management: a review. *Clin Cosmet Investig Dermatol.* 2014;7:59–64.
38. Vlahovic TC, Dunn SP, Kemp KK. The use of a clindamycin 1%-benzoyl peroxide 5% topical gel in the treatment of pitted keratolysis: a novel therapy. *Adv Skin Wound Care.* 2009;22(12):564–6.
39. Miller SD, David-Bajar K. Images in clinical medicine. A brilliant case of erythrasma. *N Engl J Med.* 2004;351(16):1666.
40. Forouzan P, Cohen PR. Erythrasma revisited: diagnosis, differential diagnoses, and comprehensive review of treatment. *Cureus.* 2020;12(9):e10733.
41. Fatahzadeh M, Schwartz RA. Human herpes simplex virus infections: epidemiology, pathogenesis, symptomatology, diagnosis, and management. *J Am Acad Dermatol.* 2007;57(5):737–66.
42. Sterling JC, Gibbs S, Haque Hussain SS, Mohd Mustapa MF, Handfield-Jones SE. British Association of Dermatologists' guidelines for the management of cutaneous warts. *Br J Dermatol.* 2014;171(4):696–712.
43. Pleacher MD, Dexter WW. Cutaneous fungal and viral infections in athletes. *Clin Sports Med.* 2007;26(3):397–411.
44. Gilbert DN, Chambers HF, Saag MS, et al. *The Sanford Guide to Antimicrobial Therapy.* 55th ed. Sperryville (VA): Antimicrobial Therapy Inc.; 2025.
45. Brickman K, Einstein E, Sinha S, Ryno J, Guiness M. Fluconazole as a prophylactic measure for tinea gladiatorum in high school wrestlers. *Clin J Sport Med.* 2009;19(5):412–4.
46. Patel GA, Wiederkehr M, Schwartz RA. Tinea cruris in children. *Cutis.* 2009;84(3):133–7.
47. Onsun N, Pirmit S, Ummetoglu O. Successful therapy of tinea cruris with topical isoconazole in combination with a corticosteroid. *Mycoses.* 2008;51(suppl 4):27–8.
48. Hu SW, Bigby M. Pityriasis versicolor: a systematic review of interventions. *Arch Dermatol.* 2010;146(10):1132–40.
49. Bonifaz A, Gómez–Daza F, Paredes V, Ponce RM. Tinea versicolor, tinea nigra, white piedra, and black piedra. *Clin Dermatol.* 2010;28(2):140–5.
50. Welsh O, Vera-Cabrera L, Welsh E. Onychomycosis. *Clin Dermatol.* 2010;28(2):151–9.
51. Frazier WT, Santiago-Delgado ZM, Stupka KC. Onychomycosis: Rapid evidence review. *Am Fam Physician.* 2021;104(4):359–67.
52. Weinstein SA, Dart RC, Staples A, White J. Envenomations: an overview of clinical toxinology for the primary care physician. *Am Fam Physician.* 2009;80(8):793–802.
53. Basler RS, Basler GC, Palmer AH, Garcia MA. Special skin symptoms seen in swimmers. *J Am Acad Dermatol.* 2000;43(2 pt 1):299–305.
54. Freiman A, Barankin B, Elpern DJ. Sports dermatology part 2: swimming and other aquatic sports. *CMAJ.* 2004;171(11):1339–41.
55. Hinz T, Klingmüller K, Bieber T, Schmid-Wendtner MH. The mystery of green hair. *Eur J Dermatol.* 2009;19(4):409–10.
56. Peterson J, Shook BA, Wells MJ, Rodriguez M. Cupric keratosis: green seborrheic keratoses secondary to external copper exposure. *Cutis.* 2006;77(1):39–41.
57. Robson-Ansley P, Toit GD. Pathophysiology, diagnosis and management of exercise-induced anaphylaxis. *Curr Opin Allergy Clin Immunol.* 2010;10(4):312–7.
58. Fisher AA. Sports-related allergic dermatitis. *Cutis.* 1992;50(2):95–7.

Genitourinary

33

Sean N. Martin and Sean Wise

INTRODUCTION

- Pathology of the genitourinary (GU) system related to sport is either exertional or traumatic in nature.
- Exercise-induced GU pathology presents as post-exercise findings and include hematuria, proteinuria, or acute kidney injury. These conditions are typically benign and self-limiting in nature. Return to play following exertional hematuria, proteinuria, or acute kidney injury can proceed once symptoms have resolved.
- Blunt kidney trauma is classified based on a five-level scale, with escalating degrees of imaging, intervention, risk of surgery, and complication rates.
- Ureter and bladder trauma, often penetrating, requires advanced imaging and urologic specialist consultation.
- Clearance for sport in Athletes with a solitary kidney should be guided by the relative risk of their sport.

EPIDEMIOLOGY

- Hematuria and proteinuria are the most common urinary findings in athletes. It is estimated that between 17% and 22% of marathon runners experience post-race gross or microscopic hematuria (1,2). Similarly, 55% of rowers and football players, 73% of boxers, and 80% of swimmers, lacrosse players, and track athletes experience post-exertional hematuria (3,4). Furthermore, 30%–69% of runners develop proteinuria following the completion of a marathon regardless of gender (1,5). Among 5k runners, 12% developed post-exercise hematuria when a time limit was enforced, whereas 1.3% of participants experienced hematuria when completing the event without a time limit — implying an exertional component (6). Younger runners (less than age 30) appear to have a higher incidence of hematuria than older participants in the 5k event (7). Among ultramarathon runners, approximately 24% experience post-race hematuria (8).
- Acute renal failure in athletes is a rare event and is usually associated with volume depletion, rhabdomyolysis, or the nephrotoxic effects of *nonsteroidal anti-inflammatory drugs* (NSAIDs).
- Although the incidence has not been directly studied, studies have suggested that sports are responsible for up to 30% of renal trauma in the pediatric population (9). Contusion is the most frequent kidney and bladder injury, whereas laceration and rupture may be life-threatening. Athletes in gymnastics, horseback riding, football, ice hockey, rugby, boxing, and soccer have reported cases of renal trauma with bicycle riding consistently identified as the most common sports-related cause of renal injury (10). Overall, individual sports rather than team sports account for the majority renal injuries (2).
- The male genitalia are often subjected to trauma ranging from testicular contusions to penile frostbite. Bikers are at risk for overuse pudendal nerve injury and straddle injuries.
- The prevalence of *sexually transmitted diseases* (STDs) in athletes is similar to that of the general population, although a study of college athletes showed they tend to be at higher risk for certain lifestyle behaviors. These maladaptive behaviors include less safe sex, greater number of sexual partners, and less contraceptive use when compared with their non-athlete peers (5).

PATHOPHYSIOLOGY

Anatomy

- The genitourinary system comprises the kidneys, ureters, bladder, urethra, and genital organs and is located in the lower abdomen and pelvis.
- The kidneys are located high in the retroperitoneum, which provides added protection from blunt trauma. A malpositioned kidney, however, may be prone to injury. In addition, the athlete with a solitary kidney is unable to leverage compensatory circulation from the additional kidney, and is therefore at higher risk for complicated kidney injury.
- The urinary bladder is located in the anterior pelvis and, as a result of its placement within the bony pelvis, is rarely acutely injured.

Physiology

- The kidneys receive more blood flow per unit weight than any other organ in the body. Renal blood travels to the glomerulus via the afferent arteriole and exits via the efferent arteriole. With afferent arteriole constriction, a pressure drop occurs within the glomerulus and filtration fraction decreases, whereas with efferent arteriole vasoconstriction, pressure increases within the glomerulus thereby increasing the filtration fraction.

- Exercise causes acute changes in a variety of organ systems, as exercising muscle requires a significantly larger proportion of cardiac output. Blood flow is shunted away from the kidney to meet the demands of working muscle. Studies have noted a drop in renal blood flow from 1000 mL · min^{-1} to as little as 200 mL · min^{-1} with exercise, a decrease that is proportional to the intensity of exercise (11,12). Interestingly, there is conflicting data correlating intensity and duration of exercise as independent variables causing hematuria (6,13).
- In an attempt to maintain glomerular filtration rate, the efferent arteriole constricts to a greater degree than the afferent arteriole creating a "pressure-head" at the glomerulus. In addition, the nephron becomes partially hypoxic causing increased glomerular permeability. These two mechanisms account for the increased urinary erythrocyte concentration.
- The increase in filtration fraction is attenuated by improving the runner's hydration status. Poorly hydrated individuals have a significantly larger decrease in renal blood flow compared with normally hydrated individuals.
- With moderate exercise (50% VO_{2max}), renal plasma flow decreases by 30%, whereas with heavy exercise (65% VO_{2max}) renal plasma flow decreases by 75%. These changes are temporary as renal blood flow typically returns to preexercise levels within 60 minutes of exercise cessation (14).

HEMATURIA

Clinical Features

- Exercise-induced hematuria is known by a variety of names to include *sports hematuria, stress hematuria, athletic pseudonephritis*, and *10,000-m hematuria* and can be either gross or microscopic in nature. Exercise-induced hematuria can be observed across a variety of contact sports such as boxing, as well as noncontact sports such as rowing, swimming, running, and rarely cycling. This phenomenon typically follows rigorous bouts of effort.
- Hematuria related to exercise typically resolves within 24–72 hours, but may vary by activity. Among 5k runners, 81% of cases resolve within 72 hours, with 12% lasting 3–7 days, and 7% lasting beyond 7 days (15). In ultramarathon runners, hematuria can be seen up to 7 days post event (8).
- That exercise-induced hematuria is a diagnosis of exclusion, other causes of hematuria should be first ruled out. A thorough history should be obtained in athletes who present with gross hematuria, to include the presence of urinary urgency, dysuria, frequency, or clots. Furthermore, a history of trauma, penile discharge, or nephrolithiasis should be ascertained. General historical questions include the presence of bleeding disorders, ongoing menses, recent streptococcal infection, generalized swelling, or risk factors for urologic cancer, such as tobacco use, age greater than 40, and pelvic irradiation. Other important questions include prescription and over-the-counter drug use, dietary supplement use, family history, and diet history. Medications that may result in hematuria include aminoglycosides, oral contraceptives, anticonvulsants, penicillins, diuretics, nonsteroidal anti-inflammatories, and amitriptyline. In addition, the use of anticoagulant medications can result in more visible hematuria. Select products have been implicated through anecdotal experience and case reports, but there is no published list of supplements known to cause hematuria as determining the exact ingredient as the culprit is difficult. Certain foods, such as rhubarb, beets, blackberries, and blueberries can cause the urine to take on a red hue.
- It is important to confirm hematuria on microscopic examination, as hemoglobinuria and myoglobinuria can also manifest as a red to brown urinary stream.
- A complete exercise history should be obtained when microscopic hematuria is discovered incidentally.
- The timing of gross hematuria is an important historical feature. Presence of blood on initiating urination is likely urethral in origin. Hematuria on termination of urination likely originates from the bladder, prostate, or posterior urethra. Continuous hematuria likely originates from the upper urinary tract. The presence of clots suggests the pathology is distal to the nephron and the thickness of the clots increases with more distal pathology.
- A thorough and meticulous physical examination should be completed. Vital signs — especially blood pressure — should always be obtained. The back, flank, abdomen, and genitalia are key components of the examination, particularly seeking signs of trauma or infection.

Differential Diagnosis and Treatment

- Differential diagnosis includes exertional hematuria, urinary tract infection, nephrolithiasis, hydronephrosis, urethritis, prostatitis, glomerulonephritis, cancer of the urologic system, sickle cell disease, polycystic kidney disease, medication effect, kidney/bladder trauma, and myoglobinuria. Furthermore, ingestion of certain foods (beats, berries) is known to cause red-colored urine. Resolution of clinical signs after activity indicates exercises-induced pseudonephritis versus activity-independent nephritis.
- Grossly bloody urine should always be dipstick tested for blood and red blood cells confirmed by microscopy. When myoglobin or hemoglobin is present, urine tests positive for blood but red blood cells are absent on microscopic examination. Medications, dyes, and food coloring often discolor urine. In this case, dipstick testing and microscopy will be negative for blood.
- See Figure 33.1 for evaluation and treatment.

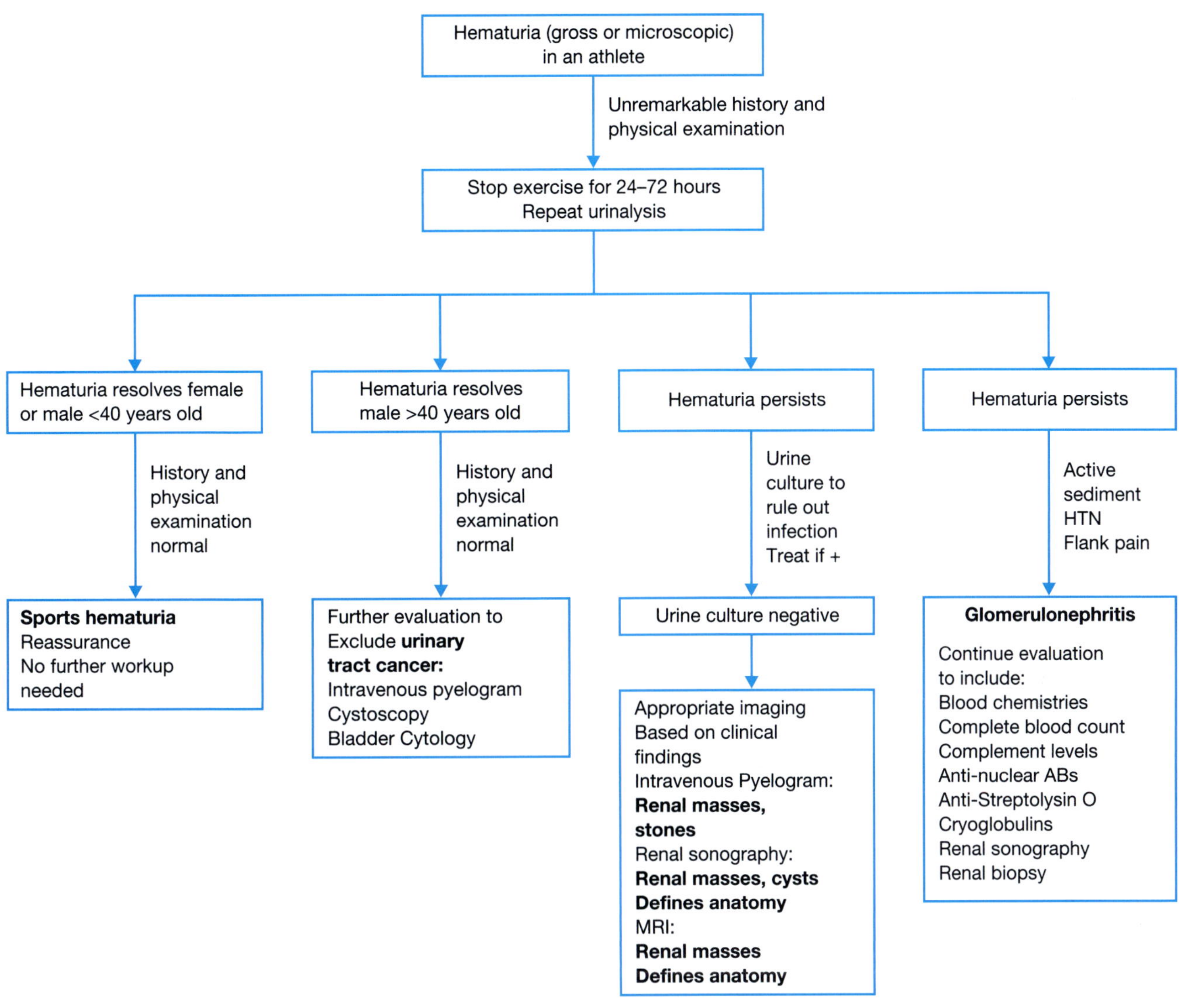

Figure 33.1: Hematuria algorithm. AB, antibody; HTN, hypertension; MRI, magnetic resonance imaging.

Return to Play

- Exercise-induced hematuria has not been shown to result in chronic sequelae. Athletes may return to sport once their symptoms have resolved and it can be concluded that their symptoms are purely related to exertion (16,17).

PROTEINURIA

Clinical Features

- Normal urine protein excretion is composed of 30% albumin, 30% serum globulins, and 40% tissue proteins. Up to 200 mg of protein is excreted in the urine daily. The diagnosis of proteinuria, however, is considered in an athlete with a post-exercise urine protein level above 150 mg. Post-exercise proteinuria is relatively common and has been described for well over 120 years. It occurs in a variety of sports, both contact and noncontact and is associated with strenuous effort more so than duration of exercise (18).
- Although the exact mechanism remains elusive, it is theorized that moderate to strenuous exercise results in an increase in glomerular filtration of albumin. Furthermore, more strenuous degrees of exercise also increase filtration of low molecular weight–proteins to a degree that interstitial tubules cannot adequately resorb resulting in further proteinuria (19).
- Important historical questions include exposure to nephrotoxic medications, IV drug use, and chronic conditions, such as diabetes, systemic lupus erythematosus, or chronic active hepatitis. A family history of hereditary nephritis or polycystic kidney disease is important.

- Often, the proteinuria is an incidental finding and the patient should be questioned about prior exercise, its duration and, more importantly, its intensity.
- Vital signs (especially blood pressure) are essential, followed by a meticulous physical examination. The back, flank, abdomen, skin, and genitalia are examined in routine fashion. The extremities should be evaluated for any signs of edema.
- Like exertional hematuria, proteinuria following exercise usually is transient, with resolution occurring within 1–2 days after cessation of activity (18).

Differential Diagnosis and Treatment

- Differential diagnosis includes exercise-induced proteinuria, orthostatic proteinuria, glomerulonephritis, nephrotic syndrome, and multiple myeloma.
- Proteinuria is usually identified through dipstick testing and, when exercise-induced, is usually 2+ to 3+.
- False positives occur because of very concentrated urine, gross hematuria, alkaline urine, or phenazopyridine.
- Although case reports have reported otherwise, placebo-controlled trials have demonstrated that creatine supplementation, in usual dosing, does not result in increased proteinuria among large groups of participants (20).
- See Figure 33.2 for evaluation and treatment

Return to Play

- Similar to exertional hematuria, post-exercise proteinuria is typically a benign finding. Athletes may return to exercise on follow-up testing that demonstrates resolution of proteinuria.

Preparticipation Screening for Hematuria and Proteinuria

- Routine urine testing for blood or protein is not a recommended component of the preparticipation examination as incidentally positive samples have shown 100% case resolution on follow-up testing with no sequelae (21).

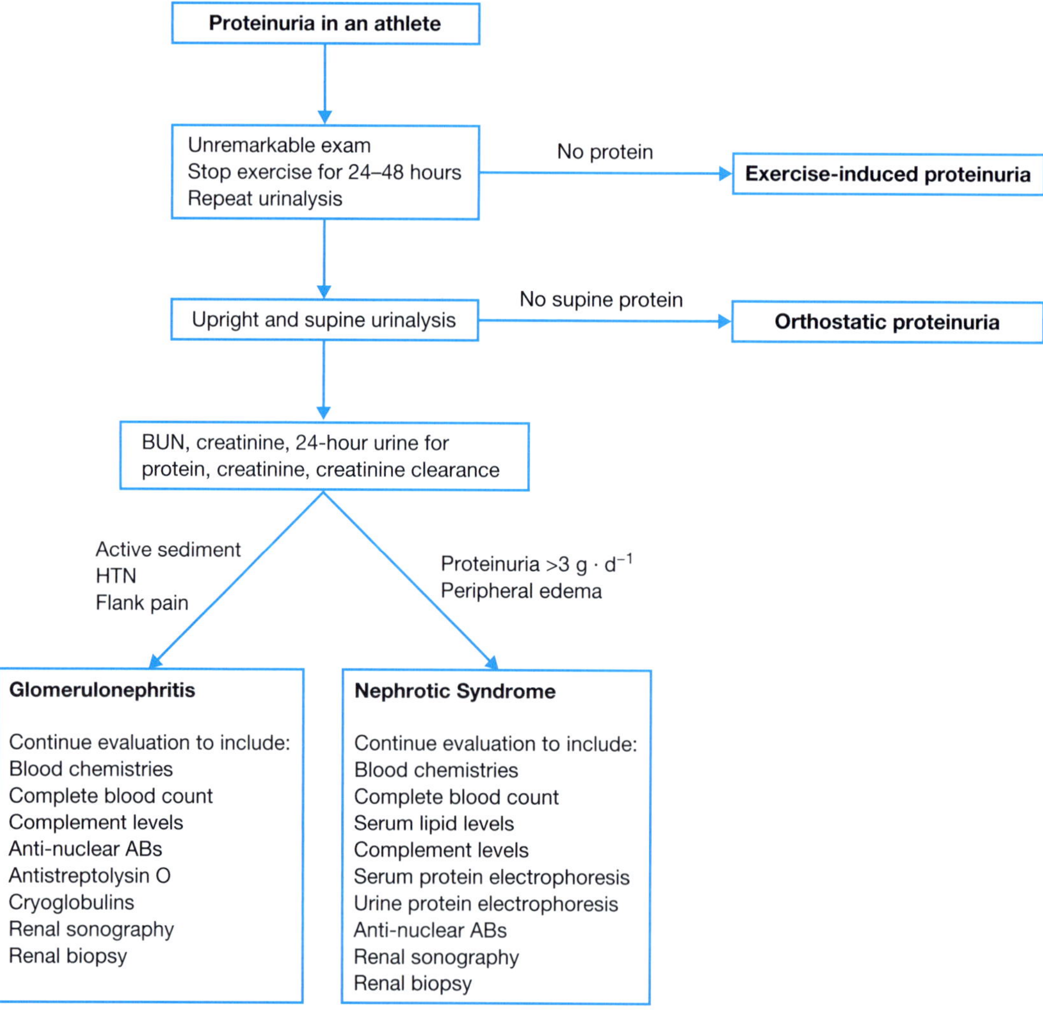

Figure 33.2: Proteinuria algorithm. AB, antibody; BUN, blood urea nitrogen; HTN, hypertension.

ACUTE KIDNEY INJURY

Clinical Features

- Acute kidney injury (AKI) refers to the abrupt decrement in kidney function.
- Acute kidney injury in athletes is typically secondary to acute tubular necrosis caused by complications associated with strenuous exercise such as rhabdomyolysis, dehydration, or hyperpyrexia leading to hemolysis. Hence, risk factors for exertional AKI include prolonged exertion, high ambient temperature, and imbalance of hydration versus fluid losses. More rarely, Obstructive uropathy can lead to acute renal failure.
- Nonsteroidal anti-inflammatory agents inhibit prostaglandins, thereby decreasing renal blood flow and contributing to acute renal failure in athletes. The dose and duration of NSAID usage that results in significantly decreased renal function is not clear, however, and thought to be less contributory than the aforementioned risk factors (22).
- More experienced athletes are at much lower risk to develop acute renal failure than novices.
- The athlete in acute renal failure often presents with nonspecific complaints, such as malaise, weakness, loss of appetite, nausea, anuria or oliguria, and symptoms of dehydration.
- The overall risk of renal failure in athletes is quite low, whereas the multitude of health benefits of exercise, even among patients with chronic kidney disease, is well established.

Diagnosis and Treatment

- Serum laboratory tests include a complete blood count (CBC), blood urea nitrogen (BUN), creatinine, and basic chemistry panel. In addition, osmolality, sodium, and creatinine should be examined in a urine sample. With these data, a fractional excretion of sodium (FE_{Na}) can be calculated to differentiate between prerenal azotemia and acute tubular necrosis as the cause of kidney failure.
- There are multiple definitions and criteria for AKI. The Kidney Disease: Improving Global Outcomes (KDIGO) has become regularly used in clinical practice as a modern and preferred criterium. This KDIGO allows for diagnosis based after correcting for volume status (23).
- The criteria for AKI, per KDIGO, includes: increase in serum creatinine by $\geq$0.3 mg · dL^{-1} ($\geq$26.5 μmol · L^{-1}) within 48 hours, or increase in serum creatinine to $\geq$1.5 times baseline, which is known or presumed to have occurred within the previous 7 days, or urine volume $<$0.5 mL · kg^{-1} · h^{-1} for 6 hours (24).
- Treatment of prerenal azotemia involves rapid and aggressive volume replacement.
- Identification of an endogenous nephrotoxin such as myoglobin in rhabdomyolysis or an exogenous nephrotoxin as in NSAID-induced renal failure is crucial. All reversible causes must be sought and treated.
- Treatment involves appropriate intravenous fluid hydration, electrolyte management, and cardiovascular monitoring. Diuretics are only indicated in fluid overload states. Indications for dialysis include the need for ultrafiltration of a volume-overloaded state or the need for solute clearance, following the same clinical indication guidelines as patients in renal failure who have not exercised recently.
- Creatine supplementation, in usual dosing, does not result in adverse kidney physiology among individuals with normal baseline renal function (24).
- AKI, in general, has been associated with repeat AKI episodes thereafter, cardiovascular events, and progression to chronic kidney disease (24,25). An extensive review of the literature has concluded that exercise-associated AKI as an isolated event, however, does not result in increased risk of progression to chronic kidney disease (26).
- Exertional rhabdomyolysis leading to acute kidney injury is well recognized. A variation of this condition is seen after anaerobic exercise; acute renal failure with severe loin pain after anaerobic exercise (ALPE) has recently been described. Patients with this disorder of AKI present with severe loin pain hours after anaerobic exercise. Rather than myoglobinuria-based disruption of filtration, the proposed mechanism of injury in ALPE is renovascular spasm, in the setting of oxidative stress and muscular damage. This leads to patchy renal vessel vasoconstriction, characteristically appearing as wedge-shaped contrast enhancement of the renal cortex on computed tomography. The resulting vascular spasm is thought to be the cause of the presenting pain (27,28). The resultant clinical presentation is a nonoliguric renal failure in the presence of a mild rhabdomyolysis. The clinical course is generally benign, with athletes at increased risk of recurrence, with subsequent intense exercise. Affected athletes should engage in a graduated return-to-activity program, and be monitored closely for recurrent renal injury.

GENITOURINARY TRAUMA

Renal

- The kidneys are normally well protected by surrounding muscles, ribs, and pericapsular fat in adults. However, these protective factors are not as pronounced in the pediatric population, making them more prone to kidney injury. A blow to the flank or the abdomen can produce a coup-countercoup mechanism of injury. Abnormally located or anomalous kidneys are more prone to injury.
- Flank pain and subsequent hematuria are the most common presenting complaint.
- Kidney injuries are divided into five classes based on severity and type of injury (Table 33.1) (29):
  - Class I: Contusion — most common renal sports injury
  - Class II: Superficial cortical laceration (<1 cm)

Table 33.1 AAST Organ Injury Severity Scale

Grade I	Contusion OR Subcapsular Hematoma, Nonexpanding
Grade II	Cortical renal laceration less than 1 cm without urinary extravasation OR retroperitoneal perirenal hematoma, nonexpanding
Grade III	Laceration extending to medulla, great than 1 cm, without extravasation
Grade IV	Laceration extending through collecting system with extravasation, OR vascular injury or segmental infarction without avulsion of the hilum and contained hematoma
Grade V	Shatter or fractured kidney (multiple grade IV lacerations) OR vascular injury with hilar avulsion and devascularization

Reprinted from Table 1 of Viola TA. Closed kidney injury. *Clin Sports Med.* 2013;32(2):219–27.

- Class III: Deep cortical laceration extending to medulla without extravasation (>1 cm)
- Class IV: Laceration of cortex and collecting system with extravasation, or vascular injury, or segmental infarction
- Class V: Multiple lacerations of grade-IV severity or vascular injury with hilar avulsion and devascularization

- Flank pain or gross hematuria after blunt trauma in an athlete requires consideration of possible renal injury. Physical examination may reveal flank ecchymosis and tenderness.
- Athletes with severe renal injuries (class IV and V) often present in hypovolemic shock. Aggressive intravascular volume replacement, transfusion, and surgical exploration to control life-threatening bleeding are often required for these injuries.
- Computed tomography has become the imaging modality of choice for the evaluation of renal injuries in hemodynamically stable athletes. Hemodynamically unstable athletes should be stabilized prior to imaging. Laboratory examination of blunt trauma should include urinalysis, complete blood count, electrolyte panel, and a pregnancy test in females.
- Treatment of class I–III injuries involve observation, bed rest, and repeat urinalysis to assess for resolution of hematuria. If nonsurgical management is pursued for class IV and V injuries, repeat CT imaging should be accomplished at 48 hours (Table 33.2). The risk of surgical treatment is as follows (Table 33.3) (29):
  - Class I: 0%
  - Class II: 15%
  - Class III: 76%
  - Class IV: 78%
  - Class V: 93%

Ureters

- Ureteral injury is associated with severe trauma, such as pelvic fractures and lower lumbar vertebrae fractures.
- Trauma to the flank or pelvis raises the possibility of ureteral injury. Hematuria is present in 90% of ureteral trauma. The diagnosis is best established utilizing intravenous pyelogram and retrograde pyelogram (30).
- Treatment is accomplished with the placement of a ureteral stent in a partially intact ureter or, as is often the case, open surgical repair.
- Urology consultation is recommended for all ureteral injuries other than those that are very low severity.

Bladder

- Repetitive microtrauma, which may easily remain unknown to the athlete, is a common cause of blunt trauma to the bladder, as demonstrated in a cohort of athletes who received

Table 33.2 Management Based on AAST Grade

AAST Grade	Immediate Treatment	CT Results
I	No gross hematuria: Outpatient management, no routine imaging	N/A
	Gross hematuria: Bed rest until gross hematuria resolves, observation, no routine imaging	N/A
II	Admit for observation, no routine imaging	N/A
III	Admit for observation, no routine imaging	N/A
IV	No urinary extravasation: no routine imaging	N/A
	Urinary extravasation: Repeat CT at 48 h	CT stable: monitor Arterial bleed: consider angiography Urinary extravasation: consider stent vs drain
V	Repeat CT at 48 h	CT stable: monitor Arterial bleed: consider angiography Urinary extravasation: consider stent vs drain

Reprinted from Table 3 of Viola TA. Closed kidney injury. *Clin Sports Med.* 2013;32(2):219–27.

Table 33.3 Risk of Surgical Treatment by AAST Grade

AAST Grade	Surgical Treatment	Nephrectomy
I	0%	0%
II	15%	0%
III	76%	3%
IV	78%	9%
V	93%	86%

Reprinted from Table 2 of Viola TA. Closed kidney injury. *Clin Sports Med.* 2013;32(2):219–27.

cystoscopy following a run greater than 10,000 m (31). That proximity of the bladder walls increases this microtrauma, running with residual urine in the bladder is thought to be protective.

- Patients with bladder contusion present with a history of trauma, suprapubic pain, guarding, hematuria, and possibly dysuria.
- *Biker's bladder is* a complication of aggressive bicycling and presents with abrupt onset of urinary frequency, diminished urinary stream, nocturia, and terminal dribbling.
- Bladder rupture may be intra- or extra-peritoneal and is usually associated with pelvic fracture. Extraperitoneal rupture is often treated with catheter drainage and close observation. Intraperitoneal rupture, however, is often surgically repaired (32).
- Cystography is the definitive study for the diagnosis of bladder rupture. If bladder rupture is present, assessment for pelvic fracture is mandatory. If extraperitoneal rupture is suspected, computed tomography imaging is indicated in the case of pelvic fracture with hematuria or widening of the pubic symphysis more than 1 cm on radiographs (33). If bladder rupture is present, assessment for pelvic fracture is mandatory. Bladder contusions are treated with catheter drainage for a few days.

Genitalia

- Genital trauma may occur in any sport, although it is often seen in gymnastics, cycling, martial arts, and various contact sports.
- Testicular injuries can result from direct trauma and include contusion, torsion, or fracture.
- The extent of testicular trauma and testicular blood flow can be evaluated by ultrasound. Testicular rupture is a urologic emergency requiring surgical management if the testis is to be salvaged. Testicular contusions are treated symptomatically.
- Physical activity does not cause testicular torsion; torsion may occur during or after exercise, or while at rest or sleep. The onset of pain is most often abrupt and can include significant lower abdominal pain with nausea and vomiting. The classic physical examination finding is a high-riding testis; although not required, ultrasound can assist in equivocal cases. Surgical exploration is the standard of care for testicular torsion. Although an attempt at manual detorsion (medial to lateral) may be attempted for patients who cannot be taken to surgery within 2 hours, surgical exploration is still required even after successful manual detorsion (34,35).
- Penile injuries are unusual in athletes. The penis may be injured in straddle-type injuries or by direct blow (36). Irritation of the pudendal nerve in bicycle racers can cause priapism or ischemic neuropathy of the penis. Symptoms usually resolve once the race is over.
- Penile frostbite occurs in runners who wear inadequate clothing in extremely cold conditions.
- Female genitalia may be injured by direct trauma and results in contusion, lacerations, or vulvar hematoma.

Return to Play

- In the case of contusion or minor laceration, athletes may return to sport following resolution of hematuria. They should be withheld from contact sports for a further 6 weeks (16). Extensive injury may necessitate withdrawal from contact sports for 6–12 months.
- Persistence or recurrent hematuria requires imaging evaluation.

SPORT PARTICIPATION AMONG PATIENTS WITH STRUCTURAL GENITORUINARY ABNORMALITIES

- In the presence of a congenital solitary kidney, a search should be undertaken for extrarenal malformations, such as malformation of the genital tract (37).
- Although exercise is known to yield improvement of quality of life in patient with chronic kidney disease, individuals with kidney transplant, ectopic kidney, severe hydronephrosis, or ureteropelvic junction obstruction should refrain from contact sports participation (38).
- Patients with acquired solitary kidney should also avoid excessive salt (>4 $g \cdot d^{-1}$) and protein (>1 $g \cdot kg^{-1} \cdot d^{-1}$) intake. Although postoperative management is not clear, lifestyle measures including regular exercise is recommended after nephrectomy to minimize risk factors for the development of chronic kidney disease (39).
- Patients with solitary kidneys should routinely be followed by a nephrology for the duration of their life (37).
- In patients with a solitary kidney without malformations, sport participation is not restricted, per consensus recommendation of the Italian Society of Pediatric Nephrology, but excessive intake of salt or protein should be avoided (37).
- In 2001, the American Academy of Pediatrics (AAP) opined that a "Qualified yes" be granted to patients with a solitary kidney based on whether that sport was considered Contact/Collision, Limited Contact, or Noncontact (40).

Table 33.4 Proposed Activity Classification System for Pediatric Patients With Solitary Kidneys, Stratified According to Incidence of High-Grade (>3) Renal Injury or Kidney Loss Following Renal Trauma

Highest Risk	High Risk (>1.0%)	Moderate Risk (0.1%–1.0%)	Low Risk (<0.1%)

Reprinted from Table 4 of Papagiannopoulos D, Gong E. Revisiting sports precautions in children with solitary kidneys and congenital anomalies of the kidney and urinary tract. *Urology*. 2017;101:9–14.

- Most recently, after a thorough review of the literature on types of kidney trauma incidence in various sports, a revision to the 2001 AAP Consensus Statement has been proposed based on a sport's unique risk of high-grade renal injury or kidney loss as opposed to the degree of contact (Table 33.4) (41).

SUMMARY

- Exertional hematuria is generally benign and, once more concerning causes are ruled out, athletes may return to sport after resolution, usually within 24–72 hours.
- Exertional proteinuria is often an incidental finding, typically a benign result of high levels of endurance exercise altering filtration of the kidney, and return to sport may occur after resolution, usually occurring without intervention within 24–48 hours.
- Of the variety of definitions of AKI, the KDIGO criteria is currently one of the more universally accepted standards.
- Although AKI are known to result in higher risk for future AKI events, isolated AKI events attributed to exercise have not been shown to lead to chronic kidney disease.
- Exercise is well established as safe and recommended in patients with chronic kidney disease.
- Although well protected in the retroperitoneal space, blunt kidney trauma should be considered in patients presenting with flank pain, hematuria, and/or bruising in the area after trauma.
- The degree of trauma is classified from grade I to V with escalating degrees of imaging requirements, surgical indications, and complications.
- Grade IV and V kidney injuries, often presenting in hypovolemic shock, require immediate stabilization followed by advanced imaging and emergent specialist evaluation.
- Ureteral injury is usually associated with high-grade trauma, with treatment consisting of stent placement and Urologic consultation.
- Pelvic fracture should prompt investigation for bladder rupture and vice versa.
- Testicular trauma should prompt consideration of emergent ultrasound to assess for the disruption of blood flow to the testes.
- Patients with a congenital solitary kidney should undergo a workup for further malformations.
- Patients with chronic kidney disease, individuals with kidney transplant, ectopic kidney, severe hydronephrosis, or ureteropelvic junction obstruction should refrain from contact sports participation.
- Patients with a solitary kidney should avoid excessive salt (>4 $g \cdot d^{-1}$) and protein (>1 $g \cdot kg^{-1} \cdot d^{-1}$) intake.
- Most recent consensus opinion for patients with solitary kidney considers the degree of contact of their chosen sport prior to clearance.

REFERENCES

1. Boileau M, Fuchs E, Barry JM, Hodges CV. Stress hematuria: athletic pseudonephritis in marathoners. *Urology*. 1980;15(5):471–4.
2. McAleer IM, Kaplan GW, Lo Sasso BE. Renal and testis injuries in team sports. *J Urol*. 2002;168(4 pt 2):1805–7.
3. Alyea EP, Parish HH. Renal response to exercise-urinary findings. *J Am Med Assoc*. 1958;167(7):807–13.
4. Amelar RD, Solomon C. Acute renal trauma in boxers. *J Urol*. 1954;72(2):145–8.
5. Nattiv A, Puffer JC, Green GA. Lifestyles and health risks of collegiate athletes: a multi-center study. *Clin J Sport Med*. 1997;7(4):262–72.
6. Ubels FL, van Essen GG, de Jong PE, Stegeman CA. Exercise induced macroscopic haematuria: run for a diagnosis? *Nephrol Dial Transplant*. 1999;14(8):2030–1.
7. Reid RI, Hosking DH, Ramsey EW. Haematuria following a marathon run: source and significance. *Br J Urol*. 1987;59(2):133–6.
8. Kallmeyer JC, Miller NM. Urinary changes in ultra long-distance marathon runners. *Nephron*. 1993;64(1):119–21.
9. Amaral J. Thoracoabdominal injuries in the athlete. *Clin Sports Med*. 1997;16(4):739–53.
10. Gerstenbluth RE, Spirnak JP, Elder JS. Sports participation and high-grade renal injuries in children. *J Urol*. 2002;168(6):2575–8.
11. Jones GR, Newhouse I. Sport-related hematuria: a review. *Clin J Sport Med*. 1997;7(2):119–25.
12. Castenfors J. Renal function during prolonged exercise. *Ann N Y Acad Sci*. 1977;301:151–9.
13. Gerth J, Ott U, Funfstuck R, et al. The effects of prolonged physical exercise on renal function, electrolyte balance and muscle cell breakdown. *Clin Nephrol*. 2002;57(6):425–31.
14. Cianflocco AJ. Renal complications of exercise. *Clin Sports Med*. 1992;11(2):437–51.
15. Varma PP, Sengupta P, Nair RK. Post exertional hematuria. *Ren Fail*. 2014;36(5):701–3.
16. Holmes FC, Hunt JJ, Sevier TL. Renal injury in sport. *Curr Sports Med Rep*. 2003;2:103–9.
17. Lippi G, Sanchis-Gomar F. Exertional hematuria: definition, epidemiology, diagnostic and clinical considerations. *Clin Chem Lab Med*. 2019;57(12):1818–28.
18. Poortmans JR. Exercise and renal function. *Sports Med*. 1984;1(2):125–53.

19. Poortmans JR, Labilloy D. The influence of work intensity on postexercise proteinuria. *Eur J Appl Physiol Occup Physiol.* 1988;57(2):260–3.
20. Groeneveld GJ, Beijer C, Veldink JH, Kalmijn S, Wokke JHJ, van den Berg LH. Few adverse effects of long-term creatine supplementation in a placebo-controlled trial. *Int J Sports Med.* 2005;26(4):307–13.
21. Goldberg B, Saraniti A, Witman P, Gavin M, Nicholas JA. Pre-participation sports assessment-an objective evaluation. *Pediatrics.* 1980;66(5):736–45.
22. McDermott BP, Smith CR, Butts CL, et al. Renal stress and kidney injury biomarkers in response to endurance cycling in the heat with and without ibuprofen. *J Sci Med Sport.* 2018;21(12):1180–4.
23. Khwaja A. KDIGO clinical practice guidelines for acute kidney injury. *Nephron Clin Pract.* 2012;120(4):c179–84.
24. Davani-Davari D, Karimzadeh I, Ezzatzadegan-Jahromi S, Sagheb MM. Potential adverse effects of creatine supplement on the kidney in athletes and bodybuilders. *Iran J Kidney Dis.* 2018;12(5):253–60.
25. Gameiro J, Marques F, Lopes JA. Long-term consequences of acute kidney injury: a narrative review. *Clin Kidney J.* 2021;14(3):789–804.
26. Hodgson LE, Walter E, Venn RM, et al. Acute kidney injury associated with endurance events-is it a cause for concern? A systematic review. *BMJ Open Sport Exerc Med.* 2017;3(1):e000093.
27. Ishikawa I. Acute renal failure with severe loin pain and patchy renal ischemia after anaerobic exercise in patients with or without renal hypouricemia. *Nephron.* 2002;91(4):559–70.
28. Kitahara M, Kurata K, Iwasaki Y. Acute renal failure with severe loin pain and patchy renal vasoconstriction in a patient with march hemoglobinuria. *Clin Nephrol.* 2022;97(4):246–51.
29. Viola TA. Closed kidney injury. *Clin Sports Med.* 2013;32(2):219–27.
30. Hirsch K, Heinz M, Wullich B. Diagnosis and therapeutic management in kidney, ureter, and bladder trauma. *Aktuelle Urol.* 2017;48(1):64–71.
31. Blalock NJ. Bladder trauma in the long-distance runner: "10,000 metres haematuria." *Br J Urol.* 1977;49:129–32.
32. Sagalowsky AI, Peters PC. Genitourinary trauma. In: Walsh PC, Retik AB, Vaughan ED Jr, editors. *Campbell's Urology.* 7th ed. Philadelphia (PA): Saunders; 1998. p. 3085–108.
33. Stern N, Pignanelli M, Welk B. The management of an extraperitoneal bladder injury associated with a pelvic fracture. *Can Urol Assoc J.* 2019;13(6 suppl 4):S56–60.
34. Sessions AE, Rabinowitz R, Hulbert WC, Goldstein MM, Mevorach RA. Testicular torsion: direction, degree, duration and disinformation. *J Urol.* 2003 Feb;169(2):663–5.
35. Eyre R. *Acute Scrotal Pain.* UpToDate. Accessed October 12, 2023.
36. LeRoy JB. Banana-seat hematuria. *N Engl J Med.* 1972;287(6):311.
37. La Scola C, Ammenti A, Bertulli C, et al. Management of the congenital solitary kidney: consensus recommendations of the Italian Society of Pediatric Nephrology. *Pediatr Nephrol.* 2022;37(9):2185–207.
38. Master Sankar Raj V, Patel DR, Ramachandran L. Chronic kidney disease and sports participation by children and adolescents. *Transl Pediatr.* 2017;6(3):207–14.
39. Tantisattamo E, Dafoe DC, Reddy UG, et al. Current management of patients with acquired solitary kidney. *Kidney Int Rep.* 2019;4(9):1205–18.
40. Committee on Sports Medicine and Fitness. American Academy of Pediatrics: medical conditions affecting sports participation. *Pediatrics.* 2001;107(5):1205–9.
41. Papagiannopoulos D, Gong E. Revisiting sports precautions in children with solitary kidneys and congenital anomalies of the kidney and urinary tract. *Urology.* 2017;101:9–14.

34 Ophthalmology

Ronica Martinez

BACKGROUND

- Ocular injuries are relatively uncommon when looking at all types of sports-related injuries.
- Eye injuries often have detrimental effects if not properly treated.
- 90% of ocular injuries in sport can be prevented.
- As with any practice of medicine, more emphasis should be placed on prevention of eye injuries.

EPIDEMIOLOGY

- More than 42,000 eye injuries are brought to the emergency departments every year while participating in sport and recreational activities in the United States (1–6).
- Approximately 30,000 emergency department visits in the United States were due to sports-related ocular injuries (7,8).
- The majority of eye injuries are due to sports-related activity and can lead up to a significant amount of blindness found by a systematic review of 132 studies (9).
- Basketball, baseball, and softball see the most eye injuries in the United States (1,2,6,7).
- Most sports-related eye injuries occur in people under the age of 25 year (1,2).
- Males are likely to have a 4:1 increased risk for sports-related eye injuries compared to females (7,10).
- From 2016 to 2020, the Centers for Disease Control and Prevention reported approximately 5% of emergency departments visits annually in the United States were work-related eye injuries (11).

CLASSIFICATION OF SPORTS FOR OCULAR INJURY

- Four different classifications of sport: high, moderate, low, and eye safe (1,3,12)
- High risk
  - Most activities with hard projectiles, sticks, or close contact:
    - Basketball, baseball/softball, cricket, fencing, hockey, lacrosse (men/women), racquetball, and squash
  - Activities with small, fast projectiles:
    - Air rifle, BB gun, and paintball
  - Activities causing intentional injury:
    - Boxing and full-contact martial arts
- Moderate risk
  - Badminton, fishing, football, gold, soccer, tennis, volleyball, and water polo
- Low risk
  - Bicycling, diving, noncontact martial arts, skiing (snow/water), swimming, and wrestling
- Eye safe
  - Track and field and gymnastics

PREPARTICIPATION EXAM

- Eye exam is a very important element of the preparticipation physical.
- Careful history for prior eye trauma, severe myopia, infections, or retinal detachment should be assessed since these can predispose them for a more visual-threatening injury.
- If the athlete has had a prior ocular history as mentioned above, a referral to an ophthalmologist should be considered if participating in a high-risk sport (12,13).
- Visual acuity should be 20/20 if correction is used; if not, they should be referred to an eye specialist for evaluation (14).
- Athletes with prior history of eye trauma or surgery may be more susceptible to injury due to weakened eye tissue and therefore should be encouraged to wear proper eye protection (12,13).

THE MONOCULAR ATHLETE

- A monocular or functionally one-eyed athlete is defined as having a best-corrected visual acuity of less than 20/40 in the weakest eye. It is strongly recommended that functionally one-eyed athletes wear appropriate eye protection during all sport and recreational activities (1,3,12–14).

- Sports in which you cannot properly protect the eye are contraindicated to the functionally one-eyed athlete (boxing, mixed martial arts, and wrestling).

OCULAR EVALUATION OF THE INJURED ATHLETE

History

- A detailed history of mechanism of injury should be obtained paying close attention to timing of visual loss.
  - Mechanisms can be described as blunt, penetrating, or perforating (15).
- Ask the athlete if there are signs of more serious eye injury such as any diplopia (blowout fracture), blurred vision (hyphema), tearing (foreign body), flashing lights (retinal detachment), floaters (retinal detachment), headache, or pain (corneal abrasion or laceration).

Physical Exam

- Eye exam should be done in an orderly fashion.
- Comparison to uninjured eye should always be done.
- Contact lens should be removed from the affected eye.
- **Visual acuity** of both the uninjured and injured side should be obtained using a Snellen card or other text source. This can be compared with baseline ideally.
  - If an athlete is unable to read, then light perception or finger count should be documented.
- **Visual fields** should be evaluated. Loss of visual fields could be caused by retinal detachment, central nervous system injury, or optic nerve injury (12).
- **Evaluate pupils:** Use a bright light to assess pupillary responses.
  - Pupils should be round, symmetrical, and responsive to light.
  - In a normal exam, pupils will constrict equally and quickly to accommodate light directed to the affected and uninjured eye (consensual light reflex).
  - If light reflex abnormal, a swinging light test can be done to determine if there is an issue with an efferent lesion (pupillary muscle or third nerve) or an afferent lesion (optic nerve or retina).
    - **Swinging light test:** In a dim room, the examiner notes the size of the pupils as the patient gazes at a distance. The examiner swings a penlight from one eye to the other noting pupil size and the pupillary reaction from the penlight. Repeats from eye to eye about five times.
    - **Normal test:** Illuminated pupil should quickly constrict and the opposite pupil also constricts consensually.
    - **Efferent lesion:** Affected eye will dilate regardless where the light is shining and the unaffected eye will respond normally.
    - **Afferent lesion:** Both pupils will dilate when shining on the affected eye and both will constrict when shining on the unaffected eye.
  - Pupillary abnormalities should be evaluated by an ophthalmologist.
- **Anterior chamber:** Use a pen light to evaluate.
  - Check for a hyphema (blood in the anterior chamber). Look closely and compare the unaffected side.
  - Check for foreign bodies, lacerations, or abrasions.
  - If any concern, will need a slit lamp exam for more precise evaluation.
  - Seidel test (to evaluate for global rupture):
    - Prepare a slit lamp and cobalt blue light.
    - Apply a drop of eye anesthetic.
    - Gentle apply moistened, concentrated fluorescein strip to the eye injury site paying close attention to NOT apply pressure to the eye.
    - Visualize injury under cobalt blue light.
    - Positive test:
      - Diluted fluorescein dye seen due to leaking aqueous fluid will be bright green.
- **Extraocular range of motion**
  - Both eyes should have full motility in all positions of gaze.
  - An orbital floor fracture could limit ability to gaze upward.
  - Double vision may suggest entrapment from an orbital floor (blowout) fracture in one or both eyes and should be referred to an ophthalmologist.
- **External examination**
  - Closely exam the adnexal structures (adjacent to eye including eyelids, extraocular muscles, socket, and tear system).
  - Examine for any asymmetry in the bony orbits or eyelids.
  - Palpate the bony orbits checking for crepitus or tenderness.
  - Make note of any bony step-offs of the orbital rim, proptosis, periorbital ecchymosis, or swelling.
  - Pain with opening of the mouth (trismus) usually occurs with fracture of the lateral orbital wall.
  - If there is paresthesia in the trigeminal nerve V2 distribution, this can suggest an inferior orbital wall fracture.
- **Sclera and conjunctiva**
  - Examine for any bleeding under the conjunctiva (subconjunctival hemorrhage) and pay close attention to any signs of a ruptured globe.
  - Signs of a ruptured globe include a 360° subconjunctival hemorrhage, lacerations, or extruding pigment (uveal tissue) or gel (vitreous humor).
  - May need to evert the upper eyelid to fully view the conjunctiva and assess for foreign bodies by using a cotton tip applicator.

- **Cornea**
  - Should be examined for clarity by applying a fluorescein dye to identify any epithelial defects or foreign bodies
  - An ophthalmoscope with a blue light or a pocket Wood's lamp can be used with fluorescein dye to visualize defects.
- **Fundoscopic exam**
  - Use an ophthalmoscope to see red reflex since inability to see a symmetrical red reflex may be one of the only exam findings of a ruptured globe.
  - A small amount of bleeding in the ocular media can obscure the red reflex.
  - Any abnormality requires an ophthalmology referral.
- **Ultrasound** (16)
  - Use of ocular ultrasound is evolving for ocular trauma with some supportive evidence.
  - Can be used to identify retinal detachments, retinal tears, lens dislocations, vitreous hemorrhages, intraocular foreign bodies, and retrobulbar hematomas
  - Most research contraindicates ocular ultrasound to be used for suspected global rupture, but there are several prospective studies showing good sensitivity specificity for penetrating global injury.
  - Ultrasound technique is essential for ocular examinations to minimize any additional pressure to the globe.
- See Table 34.1 for ocular symptoms and signs that require referral to an ophthalmologist (12,13,15).

CLASSIFICATION OF EYE INJURIES (15,17)

- Sports-related eye injuries can be classified using the Birmingham Eye Trauma Terminology, which can be useful when needing to refer to an ophthalmologist to explain the type of injury upon transfer of care.

Table 34.1 Ocular Symptoms and Signs That Require a Referral to an Ophthalmologist (12,13,15)

Diplopia	Vision Loss	Pain With Eye Movement
Hyphema	Visual field loss	Halos around lights
Photophobia with penlight	Irregular pupil size	Proptosis of eye
Suspected global injury	Laceration near medial canthus	Shattered glasses/ broken contact
Floaters/light flashes	Laceration of the lid margin	Asymmetrical pupils
Iris not well visualized	Embedded foreign body	

- Closed globe
  - Contusion
  - Lamellar laceration (partial-thickness injury of the eye wall)
- Open globe
  - Rupture
  - Laceration
    - Penetrating
    - Perforating
    - Intraocular foreign body

COMMON EYE INJURIES SEEN IN SPORT

- Each section will contain symptoms, examination, treatment, and return-to-play (RTP) recommendations.
- RTP guidelines can vary depending on extent of injury and practitioner.

Corneal Abrasions

- Corneal abrasions are the most common eye injury in sport (18).
- They account for about 12% of eye injuries in the National Basketball Association (19,20) and about 33% of eye injuries in Major League Baseball (21). There are more than 20% of eye injuries in young amateur soccer ball–related activities (22).
- They occur when there is damage to the superficial epithelium of the cornea.
- **Symptoms:** sharp pain, tearing, photophobia, and foreign body sensation
- **Exam:** A topical anesthetic drop can be used to resolve the pain.
- Full exam should be done including a lid assessment as to rule out foreign bodies.
- Fluorescein dye can show an epithelial defect when used with a cobalt blue light, which will confirm the diagnosis (Fig. 34.1).
- **Treatment:** Should be with a topical antibiotic to prevent infection (drops or ointment), and if the athlete is a contact wearer, coverage should include *Pseudomonas* (10,15,19,23). No antibiotic appears to be superior than other (24).
- Topical anesthetics should not be given at home because they retard epithelial healing. Caution should be given to topical NSAIDS as well as they can cause local toxicity if used more than 48 hours (15).
- Therapeutic contact lenses and patching can also be used for larger abrasion in conjunction with an ophthalmologist (15). Patching is usually avoided in contact wearers.
- Close daily follow-up is recommended, ideally using a slit lamp.

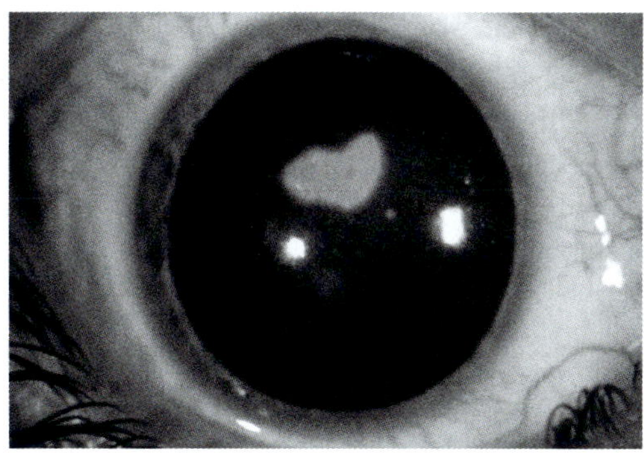

Figure 34.1: Corneal abrasion shown using fluorescein dye and cobalt blue light. *Source:* Figure 3 from Micieli JA, Easterbrook M. Eye and orbital injuries in sport. *Clin Sports Med.* 2017;36(2):299–314.

- Protect from the sunlight during healing.
- **RTP:** Keep athlete out of contact sport until completely healed, which usually takes about 3 days, and use protective eyewear.

Eyelid Injuries

- Usually occurs after blunt or sharp trauma to the eye; like from a pair of broken spectacles.
- **Symptoms:** Localized pain and bleeding around the eye are usually present.
- **Exam:** Check for involvement of the lid margin and assess the depth of laceration to see if orbital fat is exposed.
- If the laceration is medial to the pupil, the lacrimal drainage system needs to be thoroughly examined. A ruptured globe must be ruled out.
- **Treatment if need to refer:** Lid laceration repairs should be based on the team physician's level of comfort, but any laceration involving the lacrimal duct drainage system, full-thickness lacerations, exposure to orbital fat, and lacerations involving the lid margin require an immediate ophthalmology referral.
- **Treatment with no referral needed**
  - Clean the area with betadine and inject lidocaine locally for anesthesia.
  - Explore wound for a foreign body and irrigate with normal saline or lactated Ringer solution.
  - Suturing is done using a 5–0 nylon.
  - Antibiotic ointment is then applied to the area, and a protective shield is placed.
  - Sutures can be removed within 7–10 days.
  - **RTP:** Athletes can usually RTP with sutures but will need to wear proper eye protection until sutures are removed and wound is fully healed.

Subconjunctival Hemorrhage

- Very common in sport after blunt trauma
- Subconjunctival hemorrhages occur when there is bleeding in the subconjunctival space after blood vessel rupture.
- **Symptoms:** Does not cause pain or vision loss but may have a mild discomfort of the eye.
- **Exam:** Assessment is mainly focused on ruling out a ruptured globe or foreign body.
- **Treatment** is reassurance and usually takes about 2–3 weeks to resolve.
- **RTP** is immediate and without restrictions if there are no visual changes (25).

Conjunctival Lacerations

- Often, a subconjunctival hemorrhage is seen with a conjunctival laceration.
- **Symptoms:** Patient presents with mild eye pain, a red eye, and a foreign body sensation.
- **Exam:** A thorough ocular exam should be done.
- Fluorescein exam may show a tear.
- The team physician should pay close attention for a scleral laceration or other evidence for a ruptured globe or subconjunctival foreign body.
- If a conjunctival laceration is suspected, a rigid eye shield should be placed, with immediate referral to an ophthalmologist.
- **Treatment** requires application of a topical broad-spectrum antibiotic and an overnight pressure patch if there is no evidence of a ruptured globe.
- Large lacerations (1–1.5 cm) can require suturing, but this should be reserved for the ophthalmologist.
- **RTP** when released by an ophthalmologist and evidence of epithelium healing has occurred
- Proper eye protection should be worn during sport until patient is fully released by eye specialist.

Corneal Lacerations

- Corneal laceration: Patient usually complains of severe eye pain, tearing, and blurred vision.
- **Exam:** A thorough ocular exam should be done.
- The cornea is best viewed by using a slit lamp but may also be seen with a penlight.

- Any irregularities of the iris, a flattened anterior chamber, or a fold in the cornea are indicative of a corneal tear.
- The team physician should again pay close attention for a scleral laceration or other evidence for a ruptured globe or subconjunctival foreign body.
- **Treatment:** If corneal laceration is suspected, a rigid eye shield should be placed, with immediate referral to an ophthalmologist.
- Corneal lacerations usually include a cycloplegic drop along with a topical antibiotic. Most corneal lacerations will need surgical repair (26).
- **RTP** per ophthalmologist and will need to use the proper eye protection.

Hyphema

- A hyphema is defined as blood in the anterior chamber and can occur with any type of significant blunt trauma.
- The iris is torn either at the pupil margin or the iris root (27).
- **Symptoms** include blurred vision, photophobia, and pain and may be associated with traumatic iritis.
- **Exam:** A complete eye exam must be performed including intraocular pressure and a slit lamp exam. Generally, the blood can layer, but clots or stranding can be seen by slit lamp. Red blood cells floating can be identified, which would suggest a microhyphema.
- There is a traumatic hyphema grading scale that considers severity and outcome. The lesser the injury, the better the outcomes (microhyphema has the best prognosis for 20/50 vision or better). In contrast, grade III and IV hyphema (>50% and 100% blood in the anterior chamber) have the worst prognosis (28).
- **Treatment:** An urgent ophthalmology referral is needed for all hyphemas, and in instances of a large hyphema, the athlete may be admitted for observation, although this remains controversial (26).
- Treatment includes strict bed rest in dim light with elevation of head at 30°.
- A rigid eye shield should be used.
- Ophthalmologist should treat with atropine 1% drops two or three times a day for a microhyphema.
- Athletes should not be on any anti-inflammatory (anticoagulation) medicine and should know sickle cell status as presence of sickle cell trait can lead to increased risk of intraocular pressure increase.
- Daily follow-up by an ophthalmologist is needed to assess intraocular pressure and evidence for rebleed.
- Restrict activity for 4 days because there is risk for rebleed and monitor for resolution.
- **RTP:** When the hyphema is resolved and released by an ophthalmologist. Usually, the athlete is not allowed any strenuous activity for at minimum 1 week from injury or rebleed. Normal activities can resume once hyphema has resolved and out of the rebleed time frame (26).
- American Society for Testing and Materials (ASTM) approved eye protection should be worn after injury.

Traumatic Iritis

- Irritation in the anterior chamber usually occurring 3 days after blunt trauma.
- **Symptoms:** Athletes will complain of a dull ache or throbbing pain, photophobia, and tearing.
- **Exam:** This requires a slit lamp to diagnose, so if suspected, send the athlete for an urgent referral to an ophthalmologist if a slit lamp is not available. A ciliary flush (redness/violet color around the cornea) is seen (29).
- **Treatment** is with cycloplegic drops; steroid drops should not be used if there are any epithelial defects (26,29).
- **RTP:** Athletes can RTP with close ophthalmology follow-up and are asymptomatic with visual fields and acuity have normalized. This can be expected to occur within 7–10 days (29).

Retinal Detachment

- Retinal detachment can occur after any direct trauma to the orbit or from significant head trauma.
- Athletes with myopia are at higher risk.
- **Symptoms:** The athlete complains of floaters or flashing lights (13,15) and may have a blind spot on the edge of a visual field.
- **Exam:** The team physician must check the visual field for defects.
- An afferent pupil defect (see Physical Exam portion of this chapter) may be present if there is a large area of detachment.
- A funduscopic exam should be performed, but a detachment can be hard to identify; they usually begin peripherally.
- **Treatment:** If there is suspicion for a retinal detachment, an urgent referral to an ophthalmologist is warranted for a dilated exam.
- The athlete may need a treatment by the ophthalmologist that will inject an intraocular gas bubble or possibly surgery for a larger detachment.
- **RTP:** The athlete can RTP when released by an ophthalmologist, depending on extent of damage, but 2 weeks is the minimum out of activity (30).

Periorbital Contusions (Black Eye)

- This type of injury can be seen in contact and ball sports.
- **Symptoms:** Appears worse than actually is with periorbital swelling and ecchymosis.
- **Exam:** A thorough eye exam should be done to exclude orbital fracture or other serious eye injury.

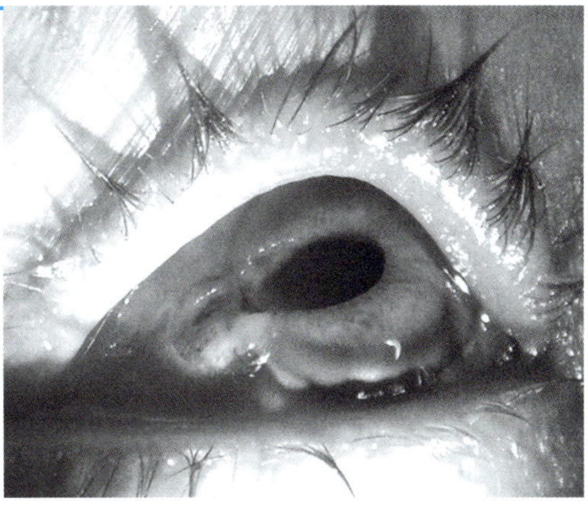

Figure 34.2: Ruptured globe showing a flattened anterior chamber, iris prolapse, and irregular pupil. (*Source:* Fig. 3.14.1 from Bagheri N, Wajda BN, Calvo CM, Durrani AK, Friedberg MA, Rapuano CJ. editors. *The Wills Eye Manuel: Office and Emergency Room Diagnosis and Treatment of Eye Disease*. 7th ed. Philadelphia (PA): Lippincott Williams & Wilkins; 2017. p. 14–44.)

- **Treatment** includes icing. Athletes with significant swelling should undergo follow-up with an ophthalmologist to get full evaluation to rule out a retinal detachment (29).
- **RTP:** Return can occur as tolerated with the athlete and there is full ability to have complete and normal vision.

Globe Injuries/Penetrating Injuries

- These types of injuries occur from direct trauma to the orbit or significant head trauma (Fig. 34.2).
- Athletes with myopia are at higher risk.
- **Symptoms:** The athlete usually presents with a history of trauma, pain, loss of vision, and possibly blepharospasm. (29)
- **Exam:** A thorough exam should be done, but **NO** pressure should be applied to the globe.
- Pay close attention to any dark pigmented tissue exposed (uveal tissue), leaking gel or fluid (vitreous or aqueous humor), or a flattened anterior chamber.
- The presence of a 360° subconjunctival hemorrhage strongly suggests a ruptured globe (26).
- Place a rigid eye shield on the athlete and send the athlete for an immediate ophthalmology consultation.
- **DO NOT** attempt to remove the penetrating object.
- Athlete is to remain NPO (nothing by mouth) due to the high probability for surgical exploration and repair.
- **RTP:** Should be in conjunction with an ophthalmologist. If full vision returns, the athlete can RTP, but if partial vision returns, then the team physician must follow recommendations for the monocular athlete.

Orbital Fractures

- Mostly seen after significant blunt eye trauma.
- Orbital blowout fractures are most commonly seen in baseball after contact with a bat or baseball. It is a fracture involving the inferior floor of the orbit (31).
- **Symptoms:** Athletes present with localized periorbital pain, swelling, or crepitus with nose blowing.
- The athlete may have diplopia, which can suggest extraocular muscle entrapment, most commonly the inferior rectus (Fig. 34.3).
- Numbness on the cheek or upper lip can be indicative of infraorbital nerve involvement.
- **Exam:** A complete eye exam should be done, with focus on extraocular motility, palpitation of the orbits, and facial numbness, which can all be seen in an orbital blowout fracture.

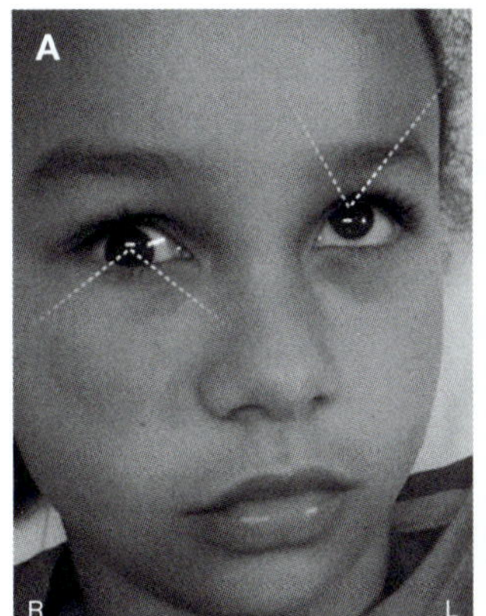

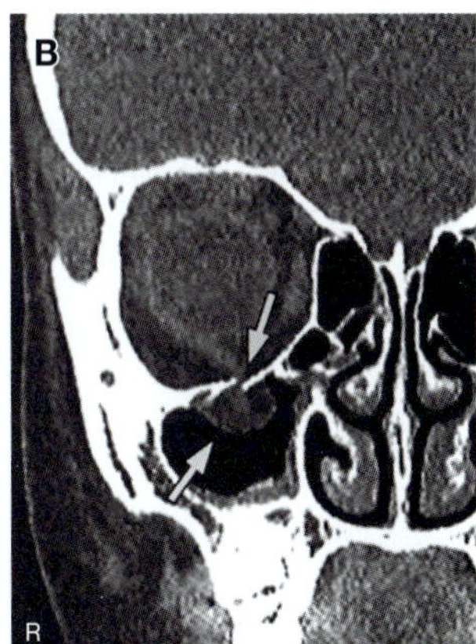

Figure 34.3: Orbital fracture showing nerve entrapment. A, The line of sight of each eye is depicted by the dashed white lines which is caused by the hematoma around the right zygoma; the right eye is unable to elevate. B, The upper arrow shows an orbital floor fracture by CT scan with herniation (lower arrow) of the inferior rectus muscle and orbital soft tissue surrounds the muscle. (*Source:* Figure 1 from Kemps PG, Frank MH. Football causes orbital trapdoor fracture with restricted eye movement. *Lancet*. 2020;395(10221):370.)

- A ruptured globe should be ruled out.
- A CT scan of the orbits should be ordered to further assess orbital wall fracture.
- **Treatment:** Evaluation from ophthalmologist is warranted.
- Treatment by ophthalmologist usually consists of a broad-spectrum antibiotic (cephalexin, amoxicillin/clavulanate, doxycycline, or trimethoprim/sulfamethoxazole) for 7–10 days and oxymetazoline nasal spray twice a day for 3 days should be given to prevent orbital cellulitis.
- Instruct athletes NOT to blow their nose.
- Apply ice for the first 24–48 hours.
- **RTP:** Athlete needs clearance from eye specialist to return to contact play because timing depends on extent of injury. Some orbital wall fractures need immediate repair, while others may need delayed repair 1–2 weeks after initial trauma (26).

Foreign Body

- It is a very common sports-related eye injury.
- It is more common with outdoor sports (dust, debris).
- **Symptoms:** Athletes will complain of eye irritation, tearing, pain, and possibly a "sandy/gravelly sensation" in the affected eye.
- Conjunctival injection can occur due to the constant irritation.
- **Exam:** A thorough eye exam should be done including eversion of the upper eye using a cotton applicator.
  - Fluorescence dye must be done to exclude a corneal abrasion; it may see a vertical dye uptake, which occurs if the foreign body gets lodged under the lid and scratches the cornea with blinking (10).
- **Treatment:** A topical anesthetic in the eye may be used to relieve pain and keep the athlete more comfortable, but the anesthetic should not be administered on a regular basis.
- A superficial foreign body can be removed with a saline-moistened cotton applicator or irrigation with saline.
- If foreign body is unable to be removed or is embedded, removal must be done using a slit lamp by an ophthalmologist.
- If the foreign body was metal, a rust ring may be seen after removal, thus warranting a referral to an ophthalmologist, which is usually easier to remove after 24 hours of foreign body removal (32) (Fig. 34.4).
- Removal of a foreign body may leave an epithelial defect on the cornea, which should be treated as an abrasion.
- **RTP:** Athletes can usually RTP immediately once the foreign body has been removed and visual acuity restored.
- Protective eyewear may be needed for a short time.

SIDELINE KIT RECOMMENDATIONS (29,33)

- Pocket-size Snellen chart
- Ophthalmoscope
- Blue light
- Sterile eye saline
- Fluorescein stain strips
- Topical anesthetic
- Dilating agent
- Eye patch
- Antibiotic ointment
- Cycloplegic drops

COMMON EYE MEDICATIONS

- Antibiotics
  - Erythromycin ointment (34)
    - Coverage includes *Streptococcus*, *Staphylococcus*, and *Mycoplasma pneumoniae*; *Haemophilus influenzae* (not all strains); *Treponema pallidum*; *Corynebacterium diphtheriae*; *Neisseria gonorrhoeae*; and *Chlamydia trachomatis*.
  - Bacitracin ophthalmic ointment (29,35)
    - Most gram-positive coverage such as staphylococci, streptococci, anaerobic cocci, Clostridia, *Corynebacterium*, gonococci, meningococci, and fusobacteria. Can also cover *T. pallidum*, *Treponema vincentii*, and *Actinomyces israelii*.
  - Trimethoprim/polymyxin B solution (29,36)

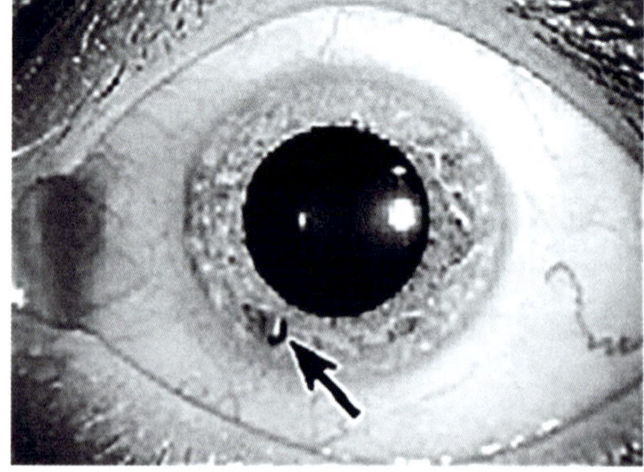

Figure 34.4: Rust ring (arrow) after removal of a metallic foreign body. (*Source:* Figure 4 from Wilson SA, Last A. Management of corneal abrasions. *Am Fam Physician*. 2004;70(1):123–8.)

- Coverage includes *Staphylococcus aureus*, *Staphylococcus epidermidis*, *Streptococcus pneumoniae*, viridans streptococci, and *H. influenzae*
- Ciprofloxacin solution/ointment (29,37)
  - Coverage includes *S. aureus*, *S. epidermidis*, *S. pneumoniae*, viridans group streptococci, *H. influenzae*, *Pseudomonas aeruginosa*, and *Serratia marcescens*
  - Should be used for contact wearer for proper *Pseudomonas* coverage
- Analgesics (29)
  - Tetracaine 0.5%, 1% drops
  - Proparacaine 0.5% drops
  - Analgesic drops should not be prescribed as an outpatient and should only be used for exam purposes.
- Cycloplegic/mydriatic agents (29)
  - Tropicamide 0.5%, 1% drops
    - Causes mydriasis induction (dilates) and cycloplegic refraction (temporarily immobilizes ciliary bodies of the eye)
  - Phenylephrine ophthalmic solution 2.5%
    - Mydriasis induction only

PREVENTION/PROTECTIVE GEAR

- Majority of all eye injuries can be prevented (1,3,5).
- ASTM-approved protective eyewear is mandatory for athletes who are functionally one-eyed (best corrected vision >20/40) or as recommended by an ophthalmologist after ocular trauma or surgery.
- Should be made of polycarbonate lenses (1,3,8,12,13,15,29,33,38–41) or Trivex lenses for racquet sports (8)
- Proper fitting protective eyewear can reduce risk for serious eye injury by 90% (42).
- Contact lenses offer no protection, and prescription glasses offer inadequate protection.
- A protective shield may be integrated if helmet is required for a particular sport.
- Eye protectors should be replaced if they show damage or are yellowed with age.
- Protective eyewear must meet ASTM standards:
  - ASTM F803 for selected sports (basketball, racket sports, women's lacrosse, baseball fielders, soccer (43), and field hockey (1,3))
  - ASTM F910 for youth batter and base runner in youth baseball and softball
  - ASTM 513 facemask on helmet for street hockey and ice hockey
  - ASTM F1587 for ice hockey goaltenders
  - ASTM 659 for skiing
  - ASTM F1776 for paintball
- Ultraviolet protection is needed for skiers, mountain climbers, and water sports.
- Eye protection has been mandated in women's lacrosse since 2005 (33,41,44).
- In 2011, the National Federation of State High School Associations for Field Hockey required protective eyewear (33,44).
- In 2012, the national governing body for U.S. Squash mandated that all hardball and softball players along with coaches wear eye protection during all sanctioned meets (44).

Choosing Eye Protection

- Use eye protection that is up to standard.
- Get professional assistance to properly select eye protection. Professionals can include an ophthalmologist, optometrist, athletic trainer, or optician.
- Know the athlete's eye and vision history.

SUMMARY

- Although eye injuries may be smaller in number compared to total injuries in sport, they can be more severe and detrimental when they occur.
- Physicians, athletic trainers, and coaches should educate people who participate in sports to be more aware of potential hazards if proper eye protection is not worn.
- Professionals need to identify people at high risk for eye injury including the monocular athlete, people with previous eye injury or surgery, or people who wear corrective lenses and participate in a potentially high-risk sport for eye injury.
- Most eye injuries caused by sport can be prevented with proper eye protection that is properly fit and ASTM approved for specific sport (1,3).
- Sports medicine specialists need to have the expertise to know if an athlete needs to be removed from activity after sustaining an eye injury, be allowed to continue participation, be sent for emergent ophthalmic evaluation, or can they be referred to an ophthalmologist (45).

REFERENCES

1. American Academy of Ophthalmology. *Joint Policy Statement: Protective Eyewear for Young Athletes*; 2013. https://www.aao.org/assets/13b282f3-f325-4ea8-bccb-87166ecc5974/635167507795070000/protective-eyewear-for-young-athletes-2013-pdf
2. US Consumer Product Safety Commission. *Sports and Recreational Eye Injuries*; 2000.
3. American Academy of Pediatrics Committee on Sports Medicine and FitnessAmerican Academy of Ophthalmology, Eye Health and Public Information Task Force. Joint policy statement: protective eyewear for young athletes. *Ophthalmology*. 2004;111:600–3.

4. Heimmel MR, Murphy MA. Ocular injuries in basketball and baseball: what are the risks and how can we prevent them? *Curr Sports Med Rep*. 2008;7(5):284–8.
5. Vinger PF. Sports medicine and the eye care professional. *J Am Optom Assoc*. 1998;69(6):395–413.
6. Ohana O, Alabiad C. Ocular related sports injuries. *J Craniofac Surg*. 2021;32(4):1606–11. doi:10.1097/SCS.0000000000007618z
7. Haring RS, Sheffield ID, Canner JK, Schneider EB. Epidemiology of sports-related eye injuries in the United States. *JAMA Ophthalmol*. 2016;134(12):1382–90.
8. Olson DE, Weber T, Allen BF. Eye injuries. In: Madden CC, Putukian M, Young CC, McCarty EC, editors. *Netter's Sports Medicine*. 3rd ed. Philadelphia (PA): Saunders Elsevier; 2023:371–8.
9. Motlagh BF, Zamani N, Ghojazadeh M, et al. Prevalence of sports-related eye injuries: a systematic review and meta-analysis. *Arch Trauma Res*. 2021;10:114–32.
10. Olitsky SE, Marsh JD. Injuries to the Eye, Chapter 653. In: Kliegman RM, editor. *Nelson Textbook of Pediatrics*. 21st ed. Elsevier Inc.; 2020:3393–7.
11. Center for Disease Control and Prevention. Estimated number of nonfatal occupational injuries and illnesses treated in the U.S. hospital emergency departments from NEISS Query Results 2016-2020. Content source: National Institute for Occupational Safety and Health (NIOSH) Division of Safety Research. https://wwwn.cdc.gov/wisards/workrisqs/workrisqs_estimates_results.aspx
12. Rodriguez JO, Lavina AM, Agarwal A. Prevention and treatment of common eye injuries in sports. *Am Fam Physician*. 2003;67(7):1481–8. 1481–8,1494–6.
13. Martinez RA, Ellini KA. Ophthalmology. In: O'Connor FG, Sallis RE, Wilder RP, St Pierre P, editors. *Just the Facts Sports Medicine*. New York: McGraw-Hill; 2005:162–5.
14. Bernhardt DT, Roberts WO. *Preparticipation Physical Evaluation*. 5th ed. Itasca (IL): American Academy of Pediatrics; 2019:103–10.
15. Micieli JA, Easterbrook M. Eye and orbital injuries in sports. *Clin Sports Med*. 2017;36(2):299–314.
16. Ray JW, Gende AM, Hall MM, Coe I, Situ-LaCasse E, Waterbrook A. Ultrasound in trauma and other acute conditions in sports, Part II. *Curr Sports Med Rep*. 2020;19(12):546–51.
17. Website of American Academy of Ophthalmology Eyewiki, Rousselot A, Murchison A, Justin G. *Birmingham Eye Trauma Terminology*. Obtained 29 Dec 2022. https://eyewiki.aao.org/Birmingham_Eye_Trauma_Terminology_(BETT
18. Youn J, Sallis RE, Smith G, Jones K. Ocular injury rates in college sports. *Med Sci Sports Exerc*. 2008;40(3):428–32.
19. Zagelbaum BM. Treating corneal abrasions and lacerations. *Phys Sportsmed*. 1997;25(3):38–44.
20. Zagelbaum BM, Starkey C, Hersh PS, Donnenfeld ED, Perry HD, Jeffers JB. The National Basketball Association eye injury study. *Arch Ophthalmol*. 1995;113(6):749–52.
21. Zagelbaum BM, Hersh PS, Donnenfeld ED, Perry HD, Hochman MA. Ocular trauma in major league baseball players. *N Engl J Med*. 1994;330(14): 1021–3.
22. Burke MJ, Sanitato JJ, Vinger PF, Raymond LA, Kulwin DR. Soccerball-induced eye injuries. *JAMA*. 1983;249(19):2682–5.
23. Ahmed F, House RJ, Feldman BH. Corneal abrasions and corneal foreign bodies. *Prim Care*. 2015;42(3):363–75.
24. Algarni AM, Guyatt GH, Turner A, Alamri S. Antibiotic prophylaxis for corneal abrasion. *Cochrane Database Syst Rev*. 20225(5):Art. No.: CD014617. Accessed 29 Dec 2022. doi:10.1002/14651858.CD014617.pub2
25. Usman S. Management of head and neck injuries by the sideline physician. *Am Fam Physician*. 2022;106(5):543–8.
26. Bagheri N, Wajda BN, Calvo CM, Durrani AK, Friedberg MA, Rapuano CJ, editors. *The Wills Eye Manuel: Office and Emergency Room Diagnosis and Treatment of Eye Disease*. 7th ed. Philadelphia (PA): Lippincott Williams & Wilkins; 2017:14–44.
27. MacEwen CJ, McLatchie GR. Eye injuries in sport. *Scott Med J*. 2010;55(2):22–4.
28. Andreoli CM, Gardiner MF. Traumatic Hyphema: Management. Bachur RG, Trobe J, Moreira ME, editors. *UpToDate*. Walltham (MA): UpToDate Inc. Access on February 16, 2023. http://www.uptodate.com
29. Aerni GA. Blunt visual trauma. *Clin Sports Med*. 2013;32(2):289–301.
30. Patel DR, Greydanus DE, Baker RJ. *Pediatric Practice Sports Medicine*. 1st ed. New York (NY): McGraw-Hill; 2009. 552 p.
31. Hong S, Choi K, Kim J, Lee H, Lee H, Baek S. Analysis of patients with blowout fracture caused by baseball trauma. *J Craniofac Surg*. 2022;33(4):1190–2. doi:10.1097/SCS.0000000000008492
32. Easterbrook M, Johnston RH, Howcroft MJ. Assessment and management of ocular foreign bodies. *Phys Sportsmed*. 1997 Feb;25(2):77–87.
33. Toldi JP, Thomas JL. Evaluation and management of sports-related eye injuries. *Curr Sports Med Rep*. Jan 2020;19(1):29–34. doi:10.1249/JSR.0000000000000677
34. *Baush and Lomb Incorporated package insert*. Retrieved 31 Dec 2022. https://pi.bausch.com/globalassets/pdf/PackageInserts/Pharma/Rx-Generics/Erythromycin-Ophthalmic-Ointment.pdf
35. Lexicomp. *Bacitracin (Ophthalmic): Drug Information*. UpToDate; n.d. 2022. Retrieved December 31, 2022.
36. Lexicomp. *Trimethoprim and Polymyxin B: Drug Information*. UpToDate; n.d. 2022 Retrieved December 31, 2022.
37. Lexicomp. *Ciprofloxacin (Ophthalmic): Drug Information*. UpToDate; n.d. 2022. Retrieved December 31, 2022.
38. Website for American Academy of Ophthalmology. Obtained 28 Dec 2022. https://www.aao.org/eye-health/tips-prevention/injuries-protective-eyewear https://www.aao.org/eye-health/tips-prevention/injuries-protective-eyewear
39. Website for American Academy of Ophthalmology. *Historic Moments in Eyewear*. Obtained 28 Dec 2022. https://www.aao.org/eye-health/tips-prevention/sports-eye-protection-history
40. Vinger PF. A practical guide for sports eye protection. *Phys Sportsmed*. 2000;28(6):49–69.
41. Cass SP. Ocular injuries in sports. *Curr Sports Med Rep* [Internet]. 2022 [cited 2022 Dec 31]; 11(1). pp. 11–15, Jan/Feb 2012. | Available from: https://journals.lww.com/DOI:10.1249/JSR.0b013e318240dc06
42. Jeffers JV. An ongoing tragedy: pediatric sports-related eye injuries. *Semin Ophthalmol*. 1990;5:216–23.
43. Vinger PF, Capão Filipe JA. The mechanism and prevention of soccer eye injuries. *Br J Ophthalmol*. 2004;88(2):167–8.
44. *The American Academy of Ophthalmology Website* [Internet]. Retrieved 31 Dec 2022. Available from: https://www.aao.org/eye-health/tips-prevention/sports-eye-protection-history
45. Moe MC, Özmert E, Baudouin C, et al. International Olympic Committee (IOC) consensus paper on sports-related ophthalmology issues in elite sports. *BMJ Open Sport Exerc Med*. 2023;9(3):e001644. doi:10.1136/bmjsem-2023-001644

Otorhinolaryngology

35

Charles W. Webb and Patrick J. St. Martin

INTRODUCTION

- Facial injuries are among the most common injuries in athletics. They comprise 4%–19% of all sports-related injuries depending on age and gender. Of all facial injuries, 3%–29% are sports related, with the majority (60%–90%) occurring in males aged 10–29 years (1–3). The gender difference increases with age from 1.5:1 male to females during the ages of 1–10 years, to 12:1 in the 16- to 18-year-olds (4,5). With the addition of facemasks and mouth guards in football and hockey (1950s and 1970s respectively), the number of severe facial injuries has declined dramatically (6,7).

ASSESSMENT OF FACIAL INJURIES ON THE SIDELINE

- Sideline management of the athlete with a facial injury begins with the ABCs (airway, breathing, circulation). Blood, avulsed teeth, mouth guards, or other objects are airway hazards. Cervical spine precautions must be observed in all head injuries, especially when the player is unconscious (6).
- The history should include the mechanism of injury, assessment for related injuries, and the presence of any other injuries past or present (3,8).
  - Most facial injuries are the result of direct trauma. Assess the nature of the impact and the presence or absence of protective equipment.
  - Ask about alertness, orientation, headaches, vision symptoms, and neurological deficits to assess for concussion or intracranial injury (8).
  - Ask about neck pain and take appropriate cervical spine precautions.
  - Other questions to ask: Can you breathe through both sides of your nose? Are you having any trouble speaking? Is your hearing normal? Have you had any previous facial injuries or surgeries, including procedures to correct vision (*e.g.*, LASIK)? When you close your mouth, do your teeth line up?
- Physical examination includes observation, palpation, and imaging (if there is any question about the diagnosis).
  - Observation includes evaluation of facial symmetry, bruising, lacerations, and swelling. Asymmetry is especially important to assess on the sideline because it may be a clue to facial fracture and can become obscured by swelling and hematoma quickly (3,8,9).
  - Bruising around the mastoid process is called the Battle sign and is suggestive of a basilar skull fracture.
  - Observation of the nares includes the septum, which can be seen with an otoscope. A bluish tinted bulge represents a septal hematoma and requires prompt treatment (6).
  - Palpation includes the orbital rim, nasal bones, maxillary bones, mandible, temporomandibular joint, mastoid process, and the upper and lower jaws (9–11).
  - The nares should be inspected for any type of fluid drainage. This may be blood or cerebrospinal fluid (CSF). The "ring test" is a method of detecting CSF on the sideline. It is done by placing a drop of blood from the nares on a piece of paper or gauze, CSF will form a halo (clear fluid ring) around the drop of blood. This represents a severe facial fracture and requires immediate transport (5,12,13).
  - Imaging is usually of limited value. X-rays may be helpful in determining the presence of a facial fracture; however, computed tomography (CT) is the gold standard (2,6,9).
  - Return-to-play guidance is based on the history and physical examination. Suspected fractures (except some nasal fractures), airway obstruction or impending obstruction, uncontrolled bleeding, loss of consciousness, and changes in vision are contraindications for return to play.

EAR INJURIES

Ear Laceration

- The more common ear injuries encountered in sports include lacerations, hematomas, otitis externa, and exostosis of the outer ear, and tympanic membrane (TM) rupture (traumatic and barometric) of the inner ear.
- The auricle consists of avascular cartilage, which derives its nutrition from the tightly adhered perichondrium. Overlying that is closely adhered skin with little subcutaneous tissue (14).

- Signs and symptoms: Pain and bleeding around the ear with a history of trauma.
- Examination: Must evaluate for cartilage involvement and for radial extension to the scalp.
- Treatment
  - Cartilage tears must be repaired unless they are very small and can be readily approximated. Absorbable 5-0 suture is preferred.
  - Local anesthesia is best achieved with nerve blocks of the great auricular nerve (along the superficial body of the sternocleidomastoid muscle 6.5 cm inferior to the auditory canal) and V3 nerve (2.5 cm anterior to the tragus in the notch between the condyle and coronoid process of the mandible) to avoid local tissue swelling (15–17).
  - Lacerations should be irrigated thoroughly prior to suturing, being careful to avoid removing the perichondrium.
  - Debridement of cartilage should be kept to a minimum to maintain cosmetic appearance and minimize risk of chondritis.
  - All exposed cartilage must be covered after the repair.
  - After the repair, apply a pressure dressing to prevent formation of auricular hematoma (15–17).
  - Prophylactic antibiotics may be used to prevent chondritis.

Auricular Hematoma

- "Wrestler's ear" or "cauliflower ear" is caused by bleeding between the skin (perichondrium) and the auricular cartilage. This occurs secondary to repetitive contusions to the auricle. This can evolve into a permanent cosmetic deformity with chronic hematomas, secondary to an increased pressure and eventual necrosis of the cartilage.
- Signs and symptoms: Acute throbbing pain, tenderness, and edema.
- Examination: Soft hematoma within the auricle.
- Treatment
  - Definitive treatment is aspiration and complete evacuation of hematoma as soon as possible, followed by compression (14).
  - Compression may be achieved by mattress sutures through the ear with or without cotton bolstering. A circumferential pressure dressing is also acceptable but less desirable.
  - The athlete should not return to play until after the removal of the compression device in 7–10 days and should always wear proper ear protection (head gear).
  - An alternative treatment method is repeated aspiration of the hematoma. This allows the athlete to return to play quickly (same day with headgear); however, this treatment method usually leads to a permanent cauliflower ear. Both the athlete and the parents should be informed of the risk and the permanence of this defect (14,17,18).

Otitis Externa

- Infection of the external auditory canal is most caused by bacteria (90%), primarily *Pseudomonas aeruginosa*, *Staphylococcus aureus*, or occasionally other aerobic and anaerobic species. Fungal infections cause 10% of cases (19).
- Acute otitis externa (OE) is unilateral in 90% of patients.
- Most common in children 7–12 years old, rare after age 50.
- Risk factors include high humidity, warm water, ear trauma, and immune compromise. It is most common in water sports and has an increased incidence in poorly chlorinated pools and fresh water (20,21).
- Evaluation
  - Mild: Erythema of the canal with mild discomfort and pruritus and a watery discharge.
  - Moderate: Developing edema and mucopurulent discharge.
  - Severe: Obstruction of the lumen with surrounding cellulitis, parotitis, or adenopathy.
  - Debris may be seen in the lumen, which should be removed (directly or by lavage) to visualize the TM and facilitate effective treatment.
  - Always ensure TM integrity before irrigation or using ototoxic topical medications.
- Differential diagnosis
  - Other dermatologic conditions may manifest in the ear, such as contact dermatitis, eczema, or psoriasis.
  - Contact dermatitis from ototopicals is not uncommon, occurring in 5%–18% of patients using neomycin.
  - Consider fungal other causes if not responding to antibacterial treatment.
- Treatment
  - Mild cases, including most fungal causes, may be treated with astringents such as 2% acetic acid, 2.75% boric acid, or rubbing alcohol.
  - Moderate to severe cases should be treated with a topical antibiotic with or without topical corticosteroid. Commonly used medications include aminoglycosides, Cortisporin Otic (neomycin/polymyxin B/hydrocortisone), and fluoroquinolones.
  - Fluoroquinolones are the only topical antibiotic approved for ruptured TM.
  - Tolnaftate or clotrimazole can be used for fungal infections.
  - Pain control with nonsteroidal anti-inflammatory drugs (NSAIDs) or mild opiates.
  - Consider oral antibiotics after getting a culture for severe cases or moderate disease in high-risk patients: those who are elderly, are immunocompromised, or have diabetes.
  - If the canal is swollen, a cotton wick may be used to help deliver the antibiotic.
  - Swimmers may use alcohol or acidifying drops to prevent OE (19–21).

TYMPANIC MEMBRANE RUPTURE

- This usually occurs secondary to a diving, water skiing, surfing, or slap injury.
- Signs and symptoms: Acute pain, sudden unilateral hearing loss, nausea, and vertigo.
- Examination: Visualization of the defect with an otoscope.
- Treatment: Observation and reassurance are the treatments of choice, as 90% will heal in 8 weeks.
- Antibiotics are recommended only if an infection develops.
- No water sports until perforation completely healed (20,21).

AUDITORY EXOSTOSES

- Exostoses are benign broad-based osseous lesions typically presenting after a history of cold-water exposure.
- They are usually multiple and bilaterally symmetrical.
- More commonly in male teenagers or young adults.
- Presents with conductive hearing loss, from external auditory canal obstruction.
- Pain with palpation or with cold-water exposure (22).
- Bony outgrowths of the temporal bone into the auditory canal.
- Related to cold-water exposure, primarily in surfers.
- Surgical referral for excision is advised for large growths, or progressive hearing loss.
- Protective equipment such as ear plugs is the treatment as well as preventative for cold-water athletes.
- Treatment is ear plugs, avoidance of cold water, and surgery in severe cases (21).

NASAL INJURIES

Nasal Fractures

- Most common sports-related facial fracture as well as the most common facial structure injured. Direct end-on blows usually result in comminuted fractures of both the bone and the cartilage. Side blows usually result in simple fractures with deviation to the opposite side.
- Signs and symptoms: Acute pain, tearing, epistaxis, facial swelling, and ecchymosis.
- Examination: Crepitus over the nasal bridge and observation of nasal deformity.
- If bleeding is present, a ring test should be performed.
- Careful evaluation for other injuries.
- X-rays: Seldom helpful for treatment decisions in the clinic or emergency room but may be useful in documentation.
- Treatment: Reduction of the displaced nasal fracture may be done on the sideline and is semipainless if done immediately.
  - If unable to reduce, an otorhinolaryngology referral is required in 5–7 days for reduction.
  - Follow up within 48 hours to ensure no septal hematoma.
  - Athletes should not return to play the same day unless there are no other associated injuries, and the nose can be protected. Return to play is typically not advised for at least the first week post reduction. External protective devices are recommended for the first 4 weeks postinjury (6,12).

Septal Hematoma

- Accumulation of blood between the septal cartilage and the overlying perichondrium.
- Septal hematomas are prone to abscess formation and may lead to pressure necrosis of the underlying bone and cartilage (saddle nose deformity) if not treated (3).
- Signs and symptoms: Acute pain, facial swelling, and nasal obstruction.
- Examination: A bluish bulge is seen on the nasal septum.
- Treatment: Prompt aspiration is the key to successful treatment.
  - Aspiration is done using an 18- to 20-gauge needle or scalpel, then packing the nose with bilateral nasal packing for 4–5 days to prevent recurrence.
  - The use of prophylactic broad-spectrum antibiotics for 10–14 days to prevent abscess formation, especially in children, is often recommended although not proven to reduce complications.
  - Complications: Minor: Minor esthetic deformities, and septal alterations with no airway compromise. Major: Nasal deformation causing esthetic impairment, deviation of the septum with naris obstruction, and swelling of the cartilage, or complete erosion of the septal cartilage with saddle deformity of the nose (5,12,13).

Epistaxis

Anterior Epistaxis

- 90%–95% of all nosebleeds are anterior. The most common site for bleeding is from the Kiesselbach plexus in the Little area on the anterior septum (17).
- Causes include blunt trauma, digital trauma, dry mucosa, chemical irritants, mucosal atrophy (topical steroids), and illicit drug (cocaine) use. NSAIDs are a common medication in athletes that may worsen bleeding. Other antiplatelet or anticoagulant medications are important to ask about.
- Signs and symptoms: Dripping blood from the nostril.
- Examination: Every effort should be made to visualize the location of bleeding. Common equipment needed for complete nasal examination include bayonet forceps, nasal speculum, Frazier suction tip, posterior double balloon system and

syringe for inflation, packing materials, including nonadherent gauze impregnated with petroleum jelly and 3% bismuth tribromophenate (Xeroform), Merocel, and Gelfoam.

- Treatment: Ice and compression of the nasal ala are the mainstays of treatment.
  - Topical vasoconstrictors can be used, such as phenylephrine and oxymetazoline (Afrin).
  - Cautery may be considered if pressure fails, and the bleeding site can be identified (silver nitrate or electrocautery pen).
  - Nasal packing is the next option when compressive therapy fails for anterior bleeds. There are multiple commercially available products including polyvinyl acetate polymer sponges, Merocel, and inflatable nasal balloons, Rhino Rocket, and Rapid Rhino. Packing is typically left in place for 48 hours. Oral antibiotics are typically started to prevent staph-induced sinusitis and toxic shock syndrome, despite little supporting evidence.
  - Return to play should not be allowed with nasal packing in place as the potential for airway obstruction exists.
  - If no packing is required and the bleeding is controlled, the athlete may return to play (5,12,13).

Posterior Epistaxis

- 5%–10% of nosebleeds.
- Bleeding occurs from branches of the internal maxillary, sphenopalatine, and descending palatine arteries.
- Signs and symptoms: Bleeding that drains mainly through the posterior pharynx and does not stop with direct pressure.
- Evaluation: The bleeding cannot be directly visualized. Must evaluate for other facial trauma to include orbital fracture and nasal fracture. Most posterior bleeds require more than an on-the-field assessment. These athletes should be evacuated to a hospital for ENT (ear, nose, and throat) surgical consultation.
- Treatment: Emergent hemostasis can be achieved with a small Foley catheter, inserted through the naris, inflated in the posterior pharynx, and then pulled snug against the posterior naris, tamponading the bleeding and protecting the airway. If available a nasal balloon can be inserted. There are several commercially available products (*i.e.*, Rhino Rocket, Rapid Rhino, Epi-Max, T3100 Epistaxis Catheter). These products typically have two balloons: one anterior and one posterior. It is recommended that all posterior bleeds be admitted to the hospital for antibiotics, observation, and ENT evaluation (5,12,13).

FACIAL INJURIES

Lacerations

- Knowledge of facial anatomy is important for assessing damage to underlying structures such as nerves, blood vessels, glands, ducts, and delicate facial musculature.
- Superficial facial lacerations should be thoroughly irrigated, and all foreign bodies removed. Repair can be done with 6-0 or smaller suture, or skin adhesive such as Dermabond. Tissue adhesive works especially well on lacerations less than 4 cm, not under tension, and in children (9,15–17).
- Deeper lacerations may be repaired in the training room using absorbable sutures for subcutaneous approximation and skin closure as mentioned earlier. Care must be taken to assess for damage to underlying structures and cosmetically sensitive areas.
- Lip lacerations should be referred if they cross the vermillion border, or affect the orbicularis oris muscle ("kissing muscle").
- With cheek lacerations, evaluate for damage to the parotid duct.
- Tongue lacerations seldom need repair, but this can be done with absorbable suture or covered with saline-soaked gauze and referred.
- Eyelid lacerations should be closed within 12–36 hours. Packing with iced saline gauze can decrease swelling to allow for better repair. Some simple lacerations may be repaired on site, but referral to a qualified provider is strongly recommended for any involvement of the lid margins, tear ducts, lacrimal sac, or levator palpebrae muscle (9,15–17).
- Tetanus status should be assessed.

Fractures

- Assessment should be done immediately before swelling obscures bony deformity.
- 75% of facial fractures involve the nose, zygoma, and mandible (2).
- With all suspected facial fractures, other than simple nasal fractures (discussed separately), the athlete should be removed from competition and referred for further evaluation.
- CT is the gold standard for imaging facial bones.
- Zygomatic fractures are caused by blunt trauma to the cheek. They can affect vision, jaw function, and the width of the face (2,6).
- Mandibular fractures may present with malocclusion or numbness of the inferior alveolar nerve in addition to pain and swelling. 50% of fractures are multiple. Surgical reduction and fixation is the treatment.
- Orbital fractures are caused by direct blunt trauma to the orbit. They most commonly affect the inferior wall and less commonly the medial wall. Vision and extraocular movement should be assessed. A deficit in either is an indication for emergent transfer due to risk of globe rupture or extraocular muscle entrapment.
- Maxillary fractures are classified according to the Le Fort system. These fractures may create an unstable midface that could complicate the airway. Surgical airway is sometimes needed.

- Return to play for noncombat athletes can begin with light activity at 21 days, noncontact training at 31 days, and full contact at 41 days. Protective masks may speed the return to contact. Combat athletes should wait 3 months before return to activity (2,6,9,10).

TRACHEAL INJURIES

- Blunt trauma to the anterior neck can have devastating effects on the larynx and the trachea, causing serious airway compromise. Hockey, football, softball, baseball, wrestling, soccer, lacrosse, and gymnastics are the sports more commonly associated with tracheal/laryngeal injury. Hockey, baseball, softball, lacrosse, and fencing all require the athlete to wear neck protecting extensions or masks to protect the anterior neck. Blunt trauma to this region can produce both contusions and fractures of the larynx and the trachea.

Laryngeal Fracture

- Typically, a result of high force trauma and is associated with other maxillofacial injuries.
- The signs and symptoms include airway compromise (stridor, shortness of breath), voice changes (hoarseness), subcutaneous emphysema, neck hematoma, and palpable fracture.
- It is of the utmost importance to establish an airway, protect it, and then transport the athlete to the nearest health care facility. If there is an associated facial injury, it may be impossible to place an orotracheal tube or a nasotracheal tube. In these cases, the surgical airway of choice is the cricothyroidotomy (1,3,8,23).

Cricothyroidotomy

- The decision to do a surgical Cricothyroidotomy can be determined by following the simple algorithm provided in Figure 35.1.

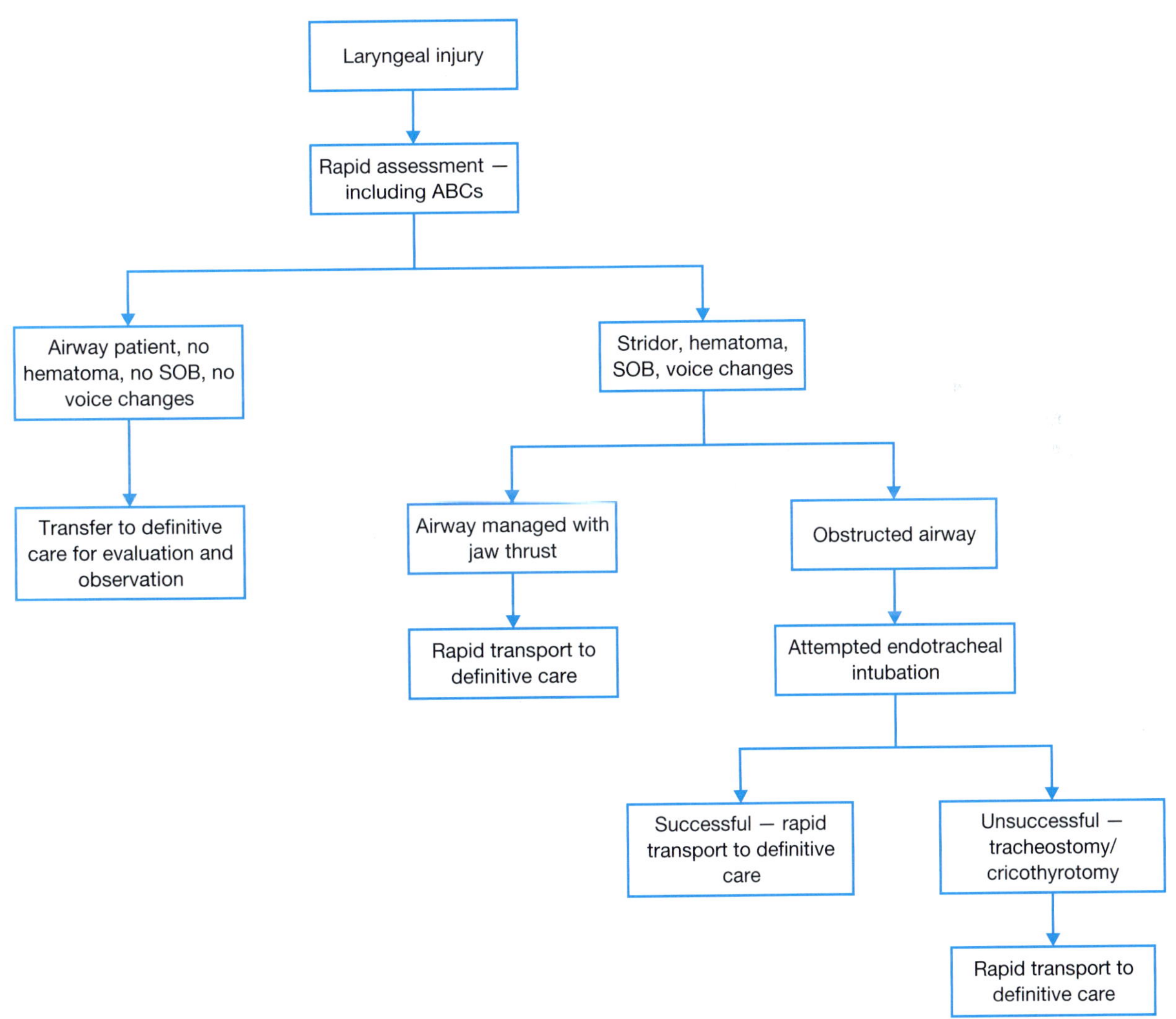

Figure 35.1: Laryngeal fracture management.

- Cricothyroidotomy is placement of a catheter through the cricothyroid membrane to establish an airway. This surgical airway may be used as a temporizing airway when oral and nasal intubation is not possible.
  - This is done by first identifying the anatomy. The cricothyroid membrane is located between the thyroid cartilage and the cricoid cartilage. The first landmark to find is the thyroid cartilage (Adam's apple), and then move inferiorly to the groove below the thyroid cartilage. The cricothyroid membrane is in the space between the thyroid cartilage and the cricoid cartilage located as the next hard ring of tissue inferior to the thyroid cartilage.
  - If time permits, the neck should be prepped with alcohol, chlorhexidine, or povidone-iodine and the skin anesthetized locally before the first incision is made.
  - The initial incision is made vertically through the skin (3–4 cm) over the cricothyroid membrane.
  - The next step is to identify the cricothyroid membrane immediately inferior to the thyroid cartilage. Once it is identified, a 1–2 cm horizontal incision is made.
  - Insert a tracheostomy tube or a 5–6 mm endotracheal tube (3 mm for a child) and secure the tube with tape.
- If there is not enough time to perform the surgical procedure, a needle cricothyroidotomy may be performed by locating the cricothyroid membrane as mentioned earlier and inserting a 12–16 gauge over the needle catheter that is attached to a syringe can be utilized. This allows the syringe to be connected to a pressurized oxygen source or a 3.0 endotracheal tube for ventilation while transport is taking place.
- There are prepackaged cricothyroidotomy kits available commercially. These kits will come prepackaged for either the blind percutaneous method or the insertion through the skin incision. The contents for a sideline cricothyroidotomy kit are outlined in Table 35.1. The complications to this procedure should be weighed against the risk of death in the athlete prior to availability of definitive care. The complications as well as the contraindications are listed in Table 35.2 (1,3,8,23).

Table 35.1 Sideline Cricothyroidotomy Kit

Alcohol pads	Povidone-iodine pads or swabs
# 11 scalpel	3- or 5-mL syringe with needle
25-gauge needle	1% or 2% lidocaine with or without epinephrine
4-in hemostat	5- to 6-mm endotracheal tube or tracheostomy tube
3-mm endotracheal tube	12- to 16-gauge catheter over needle

Table 35.2 Risks and Contraindications for Surgical Airway

	Contraindications	
Risks	**Absolute**	**Relative**
Hemorrhage	Ability to place another type of airway	Coagulopathy
Esophageal perforation		Overlying tumor
Subcutaneous emphysema		Hematoma Infection longer than 3 d
Tracheal stenosis		Age less than 10 yr
Vocal cord damage		Indistinct landmarks
Aspiration		Previous intubation longer than 3 d
Infection		

SUMMARY

- Ear, nose, and throat injuries are common injuries seen on the sidelines and can be quite serious in nature. The team physician must have a thorough knowledge of the anatomy to provide adequate care to the injured athlete. These injuries can range from cosmetic (wrestler's ear), to the severely life-threatening (laryngeal fracture). Essential equipment and training for the team physician can mean the difference between life and death.

REFERENCES

1. Grewal HS, Dangayach NS, Ahmad U, Ghosh S, Gildea T, Mehta AC. Treatment of tracheobronchial injuries: a contemporary review. *Chest.* 2019;155(3):595–604.
2. Meeuwisse WH. Full facial protection reduces injuries in elite young hockey players. *Clin J Sport Med.* 2002;12(6):406.
3. Hsiao J, Pacheco-Fowler V. Videos in clinical medicine. Cricothyroidotomy. *N Engl J Med.* 2008;358(22):e25.
4. Jaworski CA. Advances in emergent airway management. *Curr Sports Med Rep.* 2002;1(3):133–40.
5. Manes RP. Evaluating and managing the patient with nosebleeds. *Med Clin North Am.* 2010;94(5):903–12.
6. Chukwulebe S, Hogrefe C. The diagnosis and management of facial bone fractures. *Emerg Med Clin North Am.* 2019;37(1):137–51.
7. Shaikh ZS, Worrall SF. Epidemiology of facial trauma in a sample of patients aged 1-18 years. *Int J Care Injured.* 2002;33(8):669–71.
8. Liberman M, Mulder DS. Airway injuries in the professional ice hockey player. *Clin J Sport Med.* 2007;17(1):61–7.
9. Reehal P. Facial injury in sport. *Curr Sports Med Rep.* 2010;9(1):27–34.
10. Romeo SJ, Hawley CJ, Romeo MW, Romeo JP, Honsik KA. Sideline management of facial injuries. *Curr Sports Med Rep.* 2007;6(3):155–61.

11. Truman B, Gooch B, Sulemana I, et al. Reviews of evidence on interventions to prevent dental caries, oral and pharyngeal cancers, and sports-related craniofacial injuries. *Am J Prev Med.* 2002;23(1 suppl):21–54.
12. Krulewitz NA, Fix ML. Epistaxis. *Emerg Med Clin North Am.* 2019 Feb;37(1):29–39. doi:10.1016/j.emc.2018.09.005
13. Womack JP, Kropa J, Jimenez Stabile M. Epistaxis: outpatient management. *Am Fam Physician.* 2018;98(4):240–5.
14. Brickman K, Adams DZ, Akpunonu P, Adams SS, Zohn SF, Guinness M. Acute management of auricular hematoma: a novel approach and retrospective review. *Clin J Sport Med.* 2013;23(4):321–3.
15. Brown DJ, Jaffe JE, Henson JK. Advanced laceration management. *Emerg Med Clin North Am.* 2007;25(1):83–99.
16. Forsch RT, Little SH, Williams C. Laceration repair: a practical approach. *Am Fam Physician.* 2017;95(10):628–36.
17. Giles WC, Iverson KC, King JD, Hill FC, Woody EA, Bouknight AL. Incision, and drainage followed by mattress suture repair of auricular hematoma. *Laryngoscope.* 2007;117(12):2097–9.
18. Zimmerman ZA, Sidle DM. Soft tissue injuries including auricular hematoma management. *Facial Plast Surg Clin North Am.* 2022;30(1):15–22.
19. Osguthorpe JD, Nielsen DR. Otitis externa: review and clinical update. *Am Fam Physician.* 2006;74(9):1510–6.
20. Rosenfeld RM, Schwartz SR, Cannon CR, et al. Clinical practice guideline: acute otitis externa. *Otolaryngol Head Neck Surg.* 2014 Feb;150(1 suppl):S1–24.
21. Taylor KS, Zoltan TB, Achar SA. Medical illnesses and injuries encountered during surfing. *Curr Sports Med Rep.* 2006;5:262–7.
22. Climstein M, Simas V, DeBeliso M, Walsh J. A novel method for the determination of exostosis severity in the external auditory canal. *Clin Otolaryngol.* 2021;46(6):1247–50.
23. Verschueren DS, Bell RB, Bagheri SC, Dierks EJ, Potter BE. Management of laryngo-tracheal injuries associated with craniomaxillofacial trauma. *J Oral Maxillofac Surg.* 2006;64(2):203–14.

36 Dental Injuries

Elizabeth M. O'Connor and Kristina M. Ceravolo

INTRODUCTION

- There are many benefits to participating in athletic activities, such as enhanced physical fitness and the enjoyment from competition. However, sports also increase the risk of sustaining an injury, especially injuries to the oral cavity and its counterparts such as gingival tissue and the oral mucosa.
- Sports medicine physicians are in an ideal position to facilitate early intervention to preserve dental health and promote proper preventative strategies.

EPIDEMIOLOGY

- An oral injury can be defined as any of the following: dental avulsions, dental fractures, dental luxations, lacerations or contusions to the gum, cheeks, tongue, and lips, and jaw injuries (fracture, locked open or closed, temporomandibular joint (TMJ) pain, and chewing difficulty). A concussion from a blow under the chin can also be included (1).
- The most prevalent signs and symptoms of TMJ dysfunction in athletes and nonathletes are masticatory muscle pain on palpation (66.8% and 60%, respectively), teeth clenching or grinding in athletes (50%), and clicking in nonathletes (20%) (2).
- Contact sports, such as basketball, hockey, and football, have a great risk of orofacial-related injuries. These injuries are the result of an increased risk of body-to-body or object/surface-to-oral cavity contact and are incrementally compounded by the speed of the sport. According to a study by Tesini and Soporowski (3), based on 159 injuries reported by pediatric dentists during a 1-year period, the sports receiving the most orofacial injuries were baseball and biking, followed by hockey and basketball.
- Noncontact sports, such as golf, billiards, and bowling, have a much lower incidence of orofacial injury. Although not a contact sport, biking, as previously noted, has an increased risk of orofacial injury (3).
- Dental trauma data report that 25% of people of ages 6–50 have sustained an oral injury to their anterior teeth (4).
- The most common mechanism of injury described in athletics was contact with another player, followed by contact with apparatus (5).
- Despite parents being more inclined to have their sons wear a dental mouthguard in sports compared to their daughters, males demonstrate 300% more orofacial sports–related injuries than females (3). In majority of dental injuries, the athlete was not wearing a mouthguard when the dental injury was sustained (5).
- Studies have also demonstrated that by the time a student graduates from secondary school, one out of three boys and one out of four girls will have suffered from a traumatic dental injury (3).
- Injury rates appear to be highest from about 7–14 years of age (6).

ANATOMY

- The tooth is composed of three layers: enamel, dentin, and the pulp chamber (Fig. 36.1).
- The enamel is the most external layer of the three. Enamel protects the crown of the tooth because of its hardness and structure. Enamel is the hardest substance in the human body.
- The next layer is called dentin. Dentin is softer than enamel and has dentinal tubules that contain neurovascular structures. When dentin is exposed, it is very prone to decay and sensitivity.
- The innermost layer is the pulp. This structure contains the blood vessels and nerves that supply each tooth from the jaw.
- The *periodontal ligament* (PDL) connects the alveolar bone to the root and anchors the tooth in the socket.
- The *root* of a tooth is covered in a layer of *cementum*. Most anterior teeth have one root, while most posterior teeth have more than one. Roots contain canals of pulpal tissue.
- The TMJ is a synovial joint composed of the temporal bone and the head of the mandible, a fibrocartilaginous articular disk, articular ligaments, and surrounding muscles.

FIELD-SIDE ASSESSMENT

- It is important not to overlook dental injuries as part of the sideline evaluation (7,8).

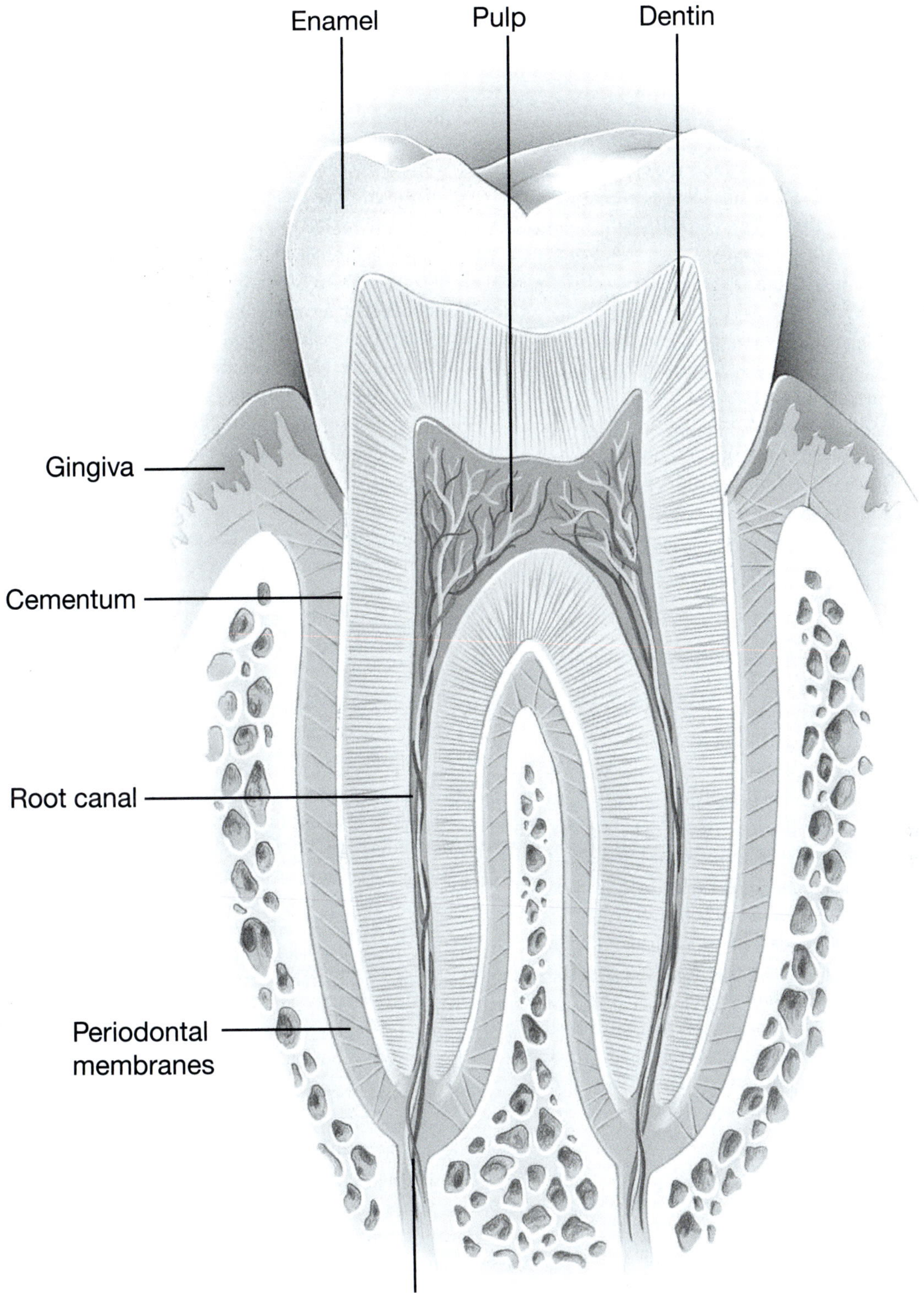

Figure 36.1: Anatomy of the tooth.

- Initial examination should be external, beginning with checking for lacerations of the head or injury to the neck. The TMJ can be externally palpated, while the patient opens and closes the jaw. The opening pattern should be closely evaluated to check for deviation, which could indicate a unilateral mandibular fracture. Palpation of the zygomatic arch, angle, and lower border of the mandible should be checked for tenderness, swelling, and bruising to rule out bone fracture.
- Signs of a mandibular fracture include pain and swelling originating from the jaw, inability to properly align teeth, loose teeth, and inability to open and close as normal.
- Intraoral examination of the lips, tongue, cheek, palate, and floor of the mouth should be completed to check for possible laceration or a dislodged tooth fragment. Gingival trauma needs to be assessed.
- If there is a laceration to the lip or tongue, it must be palpated and, if need be, radiographed to rule out embedded foreign bodies from the sustained trauma.
- Careful daily cleaning and triple antibiotic ointment can be used for lacerations outside the mouth. Prophylactic antibiotics, such as penicillin VK or amoxicillin/clavulanate, usually are indicated for lip and oral injuries (9).
- Difficulty controlling hemorrhage may be contributed to by a damaged artery; dental or otolaryngologist referral would be warranted.

SPECIFIC INJURIES

Trauma

- The most common recorded types of dental and oral injuries were lacerations (37%) followed by fractures (17%), contusions (10%), avulsions (5%), and dislocations (5%) (5).
- Unfavorable maxillomandibular relationships can increase the risk for orofacial injury. A class II molar relationship (a malocclusion where the upper teeth protrude past the lower teeth, also called an *overbite* or *buck teeth*), having an overjet greater than 4 mm, having a short upper lip, having incompetent lips (having to forcefully close lips over teeth at resting position), and being a mouth breather are all biologic factors that increase the risk of dental injury. A referral to an orthodontist to evaluate for orthodontic correction to reduce such risks is very important (8).
- Damage to the TMJ can cause myofascial pain, clicking upon opening, and discomfort to palpation. Treatment includes joint mobilization and soft-tissue work to improve function and reduce pain, ice packs, moist heat, and passive opening exercises are all helpful (2).
- A tooth fracture can be classified based on location and severity. Fractures can occur in both the root of a tooth and the crown of a tooth and can occur vertically or horizontally. A vertical fracture extending down the root of the tooth has a poor prognosis. A small chip in the enamel has an excellent prognosis.
- The most serious complication of the tooth fracture would involve injury to the pulp. Pulpal involvement can be seen by examining the fractured area and looking for a bleeding spot or a red dot. This type of involvement can be painful and prone to infection, so care should be taken not to expose the tooth to cold air, saliva, or substances/food. A patient with such a tooth fracture, involving injury to the pulp, should see their dentist for an examination and treatment on an emergent basis (within 2 hours of injury is ideal). A patient with dentin involvement should also not return to play and seek immediate dental attention. A patient with enamel-only involvement does not need immediate referral and can return to normal play with a protective mouthguard, but must see a dentist for follow-up within 24 hours.
- A tooth with a minor chip and without displacement does not need immediate dental attention, but should be evaluated at a near future date, preferably within 24–48 hours (10). Any tooth fragments that can be saved should be given to the patient to bring to the dental examination. These fragments are ideally stored in Hank balanced salt solution (HBSS).
- Intrusion is the most complicated and controversial types of luxation injury. If the intrusion is >6 mm, then the prognosis is extremely poor. The eventual outcome of an intrusive injury depends on the severity of the injury, concurrent crown fracture, and treatment methods. The permanent tooth loss due to severe intrusion is quite possible. This type of injury needs an immediate referral to a dentist. The tooth should not be attempted to be put back in the correct position (8). If the tooth is salvageable, the intruded tooth will need a root canal.
- A tooth that has had an extrusion (pushed out of its socket) injury will interfere with normal occlusion — the patient will likely contact prematurely on the injured tooth causing discomfort and malocclusion. The displaced tooth will be in front of or behind the normal tooth position. These teeth will be quite painful to return to normal position; therefore, these patients need immediate dental evaluation, treatment, and follow-up. An extruded tooth may be gently attempted to be repositioned in the field if not too painful (8,11).
- An avulsed tooth is a tooth that has completely come out of the socket. The tooth has been separated from the socket, and often, there are vital periodontal ligament cells on the root surface. The prognosis is much higher for successful reimplantation if the tooth is not given a chance to dry out and is stored in the proper environment. The tooth must first be located; it may be in the patient's mouth, on their clothing, or near the injury site. The avulsed tooth should be handled very carefully — only by the crown/enamel, therefore not causing further damage to the root surface. The tooth should be implanted within the first 20 minutes of injury to increase the success of reimplantation. Immediate reimplantation onsite gives the best prognosis but requires onsite knowledge of emergency treatment (10). The tooth should be gently cleansed with saline and repositioned in the socket. Once the tooth has been reimplanted, a splint is needed to maintain

the position and increase stabilization. Temporary splinting can be done with aluminum foil, silly putty, or chewing gum to the surrounding teeth (10). The athlete should then follow-up with a dentist immediately for definitive diagnosis and management (12).

- If reimplantation is not able to be done onsite, then a proper medium for tooth transport is critical.
- Immediate referral to a dentist is necessary because the speed of treatment affects prognosis. A tooth that has been out of the mouth for greater than 30 minutes has a decreased chance of survival.
- If the tooth is reimplanted within 15–30 minutes, there is a 90% chance the tooth will be retained for life (6).
- The most suitable transport medium is HBSS because of its pH-preserving fluid and trauma-reducing suspension. Save-a-Tooth (Biologic Rescue Products, Conshohocken, PA) is one HBSS-type product. HBSS should be readily available at schools, in emergency rooms, in athletic coach trainer kits, and at private medical offices.
- If HBSS is not available, then milk, saliva, and physiologic saline are good alternatives. Tap water is not a good alternative because it can cause periodontal cell death within minutes (10). Cool milk has been shown to work as a better medium than warm milk. Also, getting the tooth into a medium within the first 15 minutes increases cell survival and reimplantation success (11).
- Ankylosis and root resorption can occur if the tooth becomes too dry.
- Primary avulsed teeth should not be reimplanted because this could injure the permanent tooth follicle that has not yet erupted (6).

Infection

- Pulpitis is inflammation of the pulp. The pulp can be reversibly inflamed, irreversibly inflamed, or necrotic (dead). Secondary to this, inflammation around the apex of the tooth can occur. The tooth will then have localized pain and swelling and sensitivity to percussion. Referral to the dentist for either a root canal or extraction is needed. Over-the-counter pain medication may be given, but antibiotics are not necessary (6).
- An apical abscess, characterized by suppuration and pain, is localized. If not treated, cellulitis may follow. Cellulitis is a diffuse painful swelling. This infection may spread into the fascial spaces of the head and neck, possibly causing airway problems. The infection may spread to the periorbital area with complications, such as loss of vision, cavernous sinus thrombosis, and central nervous system involvement. A patient with cellulitis should be placed on antibiotics, and incision and drainage should be performed whether cellulitis is indurated or fluctuant to allow for a pathway of drainage.
- Antibiotics are administered if patients have fever or lymphadenopathy or if the infection has spread to soft tissues. Penicillin VK 500 mg for four times daily and clindamycin 300 mg for four times daily are the first-line antibiotics (9).
- Patients with severe swelling in the head/neck with possible airway compromise often need hospitalization. These patients will need surgical drainage and intravenous broad-spectrum antibiotics immediately.
- Periodontal disease is an inflammatory destructive process resulting in loss of attachment of tooth and bone. The PDL and alveolar bone are destroyed by bacterial plaque. Athletes with evidence of periodontal disease, such as mobile teeth, should be referred to the care of a periodontist.
- Dental decay or caries are caused by oral bacterial demineralizing tooth enamel and dentin. The acid production from the fermentation of dietary carbohydrates by oral bacteria demineralizes the tooth. Dental caries begin with no symptoms, but can be seen as opaque areas on the enamel that progress to brownish cavities (13).
- Antibiotics should be prescribed for most sport-related and through-and-through oral lacerations. They are also recommended when there is an avulsed tooth, root fracture, or fracture of alveolar bone, mandible, or maxilla. Amoxicillin clavulanate or a cephalosporin is recommended (4).

Prevention

- A properly fitted mouthguard should be protective, comfortable, resilient, tear resistant, odorless, tasteless, not bulky, cause minimal interference to speaking and breathing, and have excellent retention, fit, and sufficient thickness in critical areas. Mouthguards are worn in football, and football has been reported to have 0.07% orofacial injuries. On the contrary, in basketball, where mouthguards are not routinely worn, the orofacial injury rate is 34% (5). The American Dental Association (ADA) estimates mouthguards have prevented 200,000 injuries per year. A properly fitting mouthguard will protect the teeth and may reduce the incidence of concussion from a blow to the jaw (13).
- Overall injury reduction from a recent literature review was noted to be between 1.6- and 1.9-fold (14).
- The literature to this point does not support mouthguards preventing concussions (15).
- There are four types of mouthguards: stock, boil and bite, vacuum custom, and pressure-laminated custom.
- Stock mouthguards are available at most sporting goods stores and are the least expensive and least protective. They are ready to use out of the package but considered bulky and have little retention.
- Boil and bite mouthguards are the most common on the market. The mouthguard is immersed in boiling water and formed in the mouth by fingers, tongue, and biting pressure. This mouthguard does not cover all the posterior teeth, decreasing the protective qualities and possibly increasing concussion chance.
- Custom mouthguards are made by a dentist after a complete dental examination and proper questioning. An impression is taken of the athlete's mouth, allowing the dentist to make a stone cast of the mouth. A single-layer thermoplastic

mouthguard material is adapted over the cast. A vacuum custom mouthguard can be made in the office.

- Increased evidence has shown that a multilayer guard or laboratory pressure laminated guard may be preferred to a single-layer guard. These either can be made by the dentist in the office if proper materials are available or need to be sent to a qualified laboratory.
- Thickness is the major factor for sports mouthguard's mechanical performance and shock absorption, with the literature consensus suggesting that the optimal thickness should be approximately 4 mm (16).
- When properly worn, helmets and facemasks will increase safety and decrease morbidity. They protect the skin and bones of the head and face. Full face shields should be worn in hockey because wearing half shields is associated with a 2.31% increased risk of facial laceration and 9.90% increased risk of dental injury (17).
- The ADA recommends mouthguard use for 29 sports: acrobatics, basketball, bicycling, boxing, equestrian, extreme sports, field events, field hockey, football, gymnastics, handball, ice hockey, inline skating, lacrosse, martial arts, racquetball, rugby, shot putting, skateboarding, skiing, skydiving, soccer, softball, squash, surfing, volleyball, water polo, weightlifting, and wrestling (18).
- Injury rates in football have gone from 50% to less than 1% since the onset of mouthguard and face mask use (1).
- In athletes who are undergoing orthodontic treatment (braces are a greater risk for orofacial injuries), a custom mouthguard is indicated (19).
- Compliance can be a problem with mouthguard use — coaches, parents, and athletic trainers are encouraged to explain to the athletes the benefit of mouthguard use (19).

DENTAL MAINTENANCE

- It is important for athletes as well as the general public to have regular dental checkups. An initial comprehensive dental examination should be performed, including chief complaint, health history, intraoral and extraoral examination, and radiographs where applicable; then the dentist will recommend a recall schedule as needed dictated by the evaluation.
- Oral jewelry has become a recent fad with the youth of this country. Dental professionals are advised to give these patients all relevant information about the problems that can occur with the jewelry. Tongue piercing can cause teeth fractures and gingival stripping. Dental professionals should also inform patients that the jewelry should be removed prior to any contact sports participation to minimize risk.
- Dentists can also screen patients who are using smokeless (snuff) tobacco and inform them that it is not a safe substitute for smoking. These patients are at an increased risk for developing oral cancer. Smoking decreases protective saliva function.
- Anorexia and bulimia nervosa can also be picked up during routine dental checkup. The clinical signs are erosion of the lingual enamel of the teeth, bilateral swelling of the parotid gland, and floating amalgam restorations because of quicker erosion of enamel versus metal.
- It is important for patients to follow through with any recommended dental treatment, thereby preventing any future problems.

REFERENCES

1. Kvittem B, Hardie NA, Roettger M, Conry J. Incidence of orofacial injuries in high school sports. *J Public Health Dent*. 1998;58(4):288–93.
2. Starr CL, McGrew C. TMJ disorders in athletes. *Curr Sports Med Rep*. 2023;22(1):10–4. doi:10.1249/JSR.0000000000001026
3. Tesini D, Soporowski N. Epidemiology of orofacial sports-related injuries. In: Holland K, editor. *The Dental Clinic of North America Advances in Sports Dentistry*. Philadelphia: Saunders; 2000. p. 8.
4. Ranalli DN. Dental injuries in sports. *Curr Sports Med Rep*. 2005;4(1):12–7.
5. Azadani EN, Peng J, Townsend JA, Collins CL. Traumatic dental injuries in high school athletes in the United States of America from 2005 to 2020. *Dent Traumatol*. 2023;39(2):109–18. doi:10.1111/edt.12800
6. Douglass AB, Douglass JM. Common dental emergencies. *Am Fam Physician*. 2003;67(3):511–6.
7. Cohen S, Burns RC. Traumatic injuries. In: Cohen S, Burns RC, editors. *Pathways of the Pulp*. 8th ed. St. Louis: Mosby; 2002. p. 605.
8. Roberts WO. Field care of the injured tooth. *Phys Sportsmed*. 2000;28(1):101–2.
9. Inouye J, McGrew C. Dental problems in athletes. *Curr Sports Med Rep*. 2015;14(1):27–33. doi:10.1249/JSR.0000000000000114
10. Kenny DJ, Barrett EJ. Recent developments in dental traumatology. *Pediatr Dent*. 2001;23(6):464–8.
11. Trope M. Clinical management of the avulsed tooth: present strategies and future directions. *Dent Traumatol*. 2002;18(1):1–11.
12. Padilla RR. *Sports dentistry site. Dental communications*; [cited 2010 Nov 1]. Available at: https://www.drraypadilla.com/services/sports-dentistry/
13. Dorn SO. Sports dentistry for endodontists. *J Endod*. 2002;28(9):669.
14. Knapik JJ, Marshall SW, Lee RB, et al. Mouthguards in sport activities: history, physical properties and injury prevention effectiveness. *Sports Med*. 2007;37(2):117–44.
15. Benson BW, Hamilton GM, Meeuwisse WH, McCrory P, Dvorak J. Is protective equipment useful in preventing concussion? A systematic review of the literature. *Br J Sports Med*. 2009;43(suppl 1):i56–i67.
16. Roberts HW. Sports mouthguard overview: materials, fabrication techniques, existing standards, and future research needs. *Dent Traumatol*. 2023;39(2):101–8. doi:10.1111/edt.12809
17. Benson BW, Mohtadi NG, Rose MS, Meeuwisse WH. Head and neck injuries among ice hockey players wearing full face shields vs half face shields. *JAMA*. 1999;282(24):2328–32.
18. American Dental Association. For the dental patient: The importance of using mouthguards. Tips for keeping your smile safe. *J Am Dent Assoc*. 2004;135(7):1061.
19. Ranalli DN. Sports dentistry and dental traumatology. *Dent Traumatol*. 2002;18(5):231–6.

Infectious Disease and the Athlete

37

Mark D. Harris

INTRODUCTION

- Physical activity and sports participation are associated with improved health-related quality of life in children and adults (1).
- Moderate exercise of up to 45–60 minutes in duration improves immunity in athletes, especially in those with poor baseline fitness, underlying chronic medical problems, and older age (2). This effect is represented as a J curve (3).
- High-intensity exercise and prolonged exercise can impair immunity in nonelite athletes. However, it may not impair immunity in elite athletes (2). This effect is represented as an S curve (3).

IMMUNOLOGY AND EXERCISE

- The J hypothesis argues that infection risk declines after moderate exercise (5–60 minutes at 40%–60% of maximum heart rate) and increases continuously after strenuous exercise (70%–80% of maximum heart rate) or after prolonged exercise (more than 60 minutes) (4).
- The S hypothesis argues that infection risk declines after moderate exercise and increases temporarily but then decreases again for elite athletes (3). Proponents suggest that overtraining and genetic factors, rather than strenuous or prolonged exercise per se, cause the increased risk of infection. The impact of exercise on elite athletes is compounded by the fact that in elite competitions, athletes face intense psychological pressure, lack of good sleep, altered diet, and long-duration ground or air travel with circadian disruption (2).
- The Open Window theory suggests that the risk of upper respiratory tract infection increases immediately after vigorous exercise and then closes again after 24 hours (3).
- The innate immune system includes barriers such as skin, hair, turbulent nasal airflow, gastric acidity, and mucous membranes. Pathogen and debris removal systems such as the mucociliary elevator assist.
- The innate immune system also includes natural killer (NK) cells, phagocytes, toll-like receptors, cytokines (such as the tumor necrosis factor), and complement factor (5). The innate immune system provides immediate protection against all pathogens but is not adapted to defend against any single one.
- The adaptive or acquired immune system includes both T lymphocytes (thymus) and B lymphocytes (bone marrow), which produce monoreactive antibodies (immunoglobulins IgM, IgG, IgA, IgD, and IgE), and cytokines (5). The adaptive immune system provides targeted but about 7 days delayed protection against specific pathogens on the first encounter. Protection from the adaptive immune system occurs in only a few days on subsequent encounters. Lymphoid tissue, which facilitates the mingling of pathogens and immune cells, includes the spleen, Peyer patches, tonsils, appendix, and lymph nodes (5). Thymic activity is reduced by strenuous exercise (6).
- The innate and adaptive immune systems overlap notably, cooperating to protect the host. For example, phagocytes engulf pathogens, digest them, and present them to lymphocytes to induce antibody production.
- Secretory IgA, which comprises about 75% of all immunoglobulins in the body, is excreted from mucous membranes, unlike other immunoglobulins which dwell in serum and central organs (7). IgA ensures mutualism with commensal bacteria, defends against toxins, and reduces the burden of viral particles (7).
- Broadly cross-reactive natural antibodies, usually IgM, activate the complement cascade, clear debris, neutralize invaders, and suppress inflammatory and autoimmune responses (8).
- Environmental factors such as sun, wind, temperature, and humidity, and physical trauma can break down physical barriers such as skin and mucous membranes. Nasal breathing allows incoming air to be warmed, filtered, and moisturized prior to entry into the lungs, but the increased air flow required for strenuous activities requires mouth breathing, which bypasses these protections. With thicker and colder mucous, the mucociliary elevator can no longer remove debris as effectively. Air pollution increases lung inflammation (6).
- Exercise in sports can augment the immune system. Moderate exercise lasting 5–60 minutes increases neutrophil counts, NK cell counts, and secretory IgA levels (4). Exercise in sports can also impair the immune system. Strenuous exercise decreases levels of NK cells, T cell proliferation, neutrophil phagocytic function, and IgA. The IgA can decrease up to 65% (4). In one study, decreased IgA levels were shown to be predictive of upper respiratory tract infections (URTIs) in rugby players (9).

INFECTIONS AND EXERCISE

- Fever is a vital part of the body's response to infection. It is traditionally defined as an oral or rectal body temperature greater than 100.4°F (4). Fever of unknown origin, however, can be defined as an oral or rectal body temperature greater than 101°F (10). Higher temperatures enhance the body's immunological response, impair the replication of microorganisms, and decrease blood glucose (4). Such changes deny fuel to bacteria and promote the production of acute-phase reactants. Temperature amplitudes are higher in physically active individuals (4).
- Fever impairs performance, increases insensible fluid loss, and causes temperature dysregulation (4). Speed and coordination fall. Muscle strength declines 5%–15% and endurance falls 13%–18% compared to baseline owing to a cytokine-mediated loss in muscle proteins (4). Fluid losses decrease stroke volume. If the heart rate cannot compensate, cardiac output drops, thus decreasing VO_{2max} (3).
- Fever can be treated with acetaminophen up to 4 g · d^{-1} divided into doses every 4–6 hours. Nonsteroidal anti-inflammatory drugs can also be used.
- Drugs used to treat acute infections can also impact athletes. Antihistamines can cause drowsiness, and antibiotics can result in diarrhea. Many drugs are banned by sports organizations, and taking them will disqualify an athlete from competing.
- Cardiorespiratory, musculoskeletal, and metabolic deconditioning can occur in less than 4 weeks of a lack of exercise (3).

RHINORRHEA AND NASAL CONGESTION

Upper Respiratory Tract Infections

- Healthy adults get up to six URTIs each year, with URTI accounting for half of training room visits (3). Caused by viruses, especially the rhinovirus and coronavirus, transmission is typically via respiratory droplets from hand to nose, eyes, or mouth. Athletes are at highest risk from early autumn to early spring, probably due to crowding and competition in indoor venues. Athletes are more likely to complain of nasal symptoms than sedentary people (11).
- Symptoms include nasal congestion, sore throat, dry cough, malaise, and low-grade fever (12). Signs include rhinorrhea, inflamed nasal mucosa, and oropharyngeal edema. Symptoms usually resolve at 10 days. The median symptom duration in children is 8 days, but symptoms resolve in 90% by 23 days (12).
- Treatments for adults include antipyretics, analgesics, antihistamines, decongestants, zinc, lactobacillus, and ipratropium for cough (12). Nasal saline irrigation may be beneficial. Avoid antibiotics unless clear evidence of bacterial infection (*i.e.*, strep pharyngitis, bacterial sinusitis, bacterial otitis) is present.
- Treatments in children up to age 18 include analgesics, honey, ipratropium, acetylcysteine, and vitamin C. Avoid antitussives, antihistamines, and decongestants (12). Avoid antibiotics unless the infection is clearly bacterial.
- Adequate sleep, good nutrition, stress management, and up-to-date vaccinations are key preventive measures. Athletes should not share water bottles or other personal items. Handwashing and the use of hand sanitizer impair URTI transmission. Isolate ill persons from healthy ones. Coaches and staff must ensure adequate rest between workouts. Athletes can return to their sport when symptoms resolve, but should gradually increase first frequency, then duration, and finally intensity. Expect impaired exercise performance for 2–4 days after recovery from a URTI (6).
- Carbohydrate ingestion, especially during strenuous exercise, may impair exercise-induced inflammation (6). By facilitating iron absorption, vitamin C may benefit immune status. Vitamins D and E and probiotics may reduce the risk of URTI in athletes (6). Additionally, omega-3 polyunsaturated fatty acids may decrease exercise-induced inflammation (6). One meta-analysis discovered that probiotic supplementation decreased total symptom severity score in URTI in athletes (13). Sivamaruthi et al. noted that probiotics had a wide range of beneficial effects, including improvements in URTI and gastrointestinal symptoms (14).
- Repetitive mild hyperthermia, like sitting in a 40°C sauna on a cold day, augments the immune system. Massage boosts the immune response. Breath control can help reduce stress (6).

Sinusitis

- Acute sinusitis is defined as sinonasal symptoms of acute onset and lasting less than 4 weeks' duration. In 2016, there were 8 million US ambulatory visits for acute sinusitis, which is often associated with URTI (15). Acute sinusitis is usually viral but can be of bacterial origin (*Haemophilus influenza, Streptococcus pneumoniae, Moraxella* (*Branhamella*) *catarrhalis*) (16). Only 0.5%–2% of all URTI cases are complicated by acute bacterial paranasal sinusitis (15).
- Presenting complaints include nasal congestion, cough, headache, and fever (16). Bacterial rhinosinusitis, for which antibiotics may be useful, can be differentiated from viral sinusitis, by the presence of C-reactive protein >1.5/dL (15/L), maxillary toothache, tender maxillary sinus, purulent nasal discharge, fetid breath odor, and preceding respiratory tract infection (15). Erythrocyte sedimentation rate greater than 10, fever, and "double sickening" (in which a patient develops a URTI, seems to recover, and within a week develops sinusitis) also suggest a bacterial origin (16). Imaging is not often helpful.
- In acute bacterial sinusitis, antibiotics can decrease the time to resolution in 5–11 patients per 100 (15). Nonetheless, between 70% and 90% of these patients receive antibiotics. Antibiotics of choice include amoxicillin with or without clavulanate,

doxycycline, or azithromycin, each for 5–7 days (16). Nasal saline irrigation, analgesics, and intranasal corticosteroids can help.

- Preventive measures and return-to-play guidelines are similar to those of URTI.

Allergic and Nonallergic Rhinitis

- Allergic rhinitis is an allergen-induced inflammation of the nasal mucous membranes. Release of histamine, mediated by IgE, causes watery eyes, conjunctival erythema, pruritus, and rhinorrhea (17). Plant pollen and animal dander are common allergens, and symptoms can be related to the amount of allergen in the environment. Cigarette smoke and other pollutants worsen symptoms. Persistent allergic rhinitis presents with symptoms for at least 4 $d \cdot wk^{-1}$ for 4 $wk \cdot y^{-1}$ (17).
- Nonallergic rhinitis shares similar clinical features with allergic rhinitis (18). Acute symptoms are related to vasomotor rhinitis, but chronic symptoms derive from atrophic rhinitis, drug-induced rhinitis, geriatric rhinitis, gustatory rhinitis, hormonal rhinitis, nasal eosinophilia syndrome, nonallergic rhinopathy, and occupational rhinitis (18).
- Rhinitis treatment involves nasal steroids, antihistamines, nasal irrigation with saline, and decongestants. Rhinorrhea and sneezing improve with intranasal cromolyn and leukotriene receptor agonists. Dust mite prevention has limited effectiveness (17).
- Outside activities can increase exposure to environmental pollens due to higher concentrations. The increased respiratory rate and tidal volume associated with exercise increases the likelihood of allergic symptoms because more air is moving through the respiratory system during each unit of time.
- Athletes may return to play when their symptoms have resolved or are at least well controlled.

COUGH

Acute Cough

- Cough is the presenting complaint for nearly 7 million outpatient and emergency department visits per year in the United States (19). Athletes presenting with acute cough span the severity spectrum from routine to life threatening. The latter includes severe asthma exacerbation, pulmonary embolism, severe pneumonia, and heart failure, but these are uncommon in the athlete population. More likely causes include infections such as URTI, bronchitis, and less-severe pneumonia. Acute cough lasts less than 3 weeks, and subacute cough lasts 3–8 weeks (20). Endurance athletes in cold environments, such as Nordic skiers, are especially prone to develop cough. Allergens, automobile exhaust, emotional stress, and irritants in sporting venues such as nitrous oxide from arena resurfacing and chlorine from pools can exacerbate cough (20). Dehydration, changes to the osmolality of the respiratory mucous, and cold temperatures stimulate the vagus nerve, resulting in cough, bronchoconstriction, and increased mucous production (20).
- Acute bronchitis is acute inflammation of the large and medium-sized airways without evidence of pneumonia (19). Viruses cause over 90% of cases, but *Mycoplasma pneumoniae*, *Bordetella pertussis*, and *Chlamydia pneumoniae* can be seen (3). Clinical features include dyspnea, cough, nasal congestion, headache, and low-grade fever. The median duration of cough is 18 days (19). Laboratory and radiographic testing are usually not indicated unless the clinical suspicion of pneumonia or some other cause is high.
- Treatment is symptomatic and, since only 10% of acute bronchitis cases are bacterial, antibiotics are rarely indicated (19). Evidence for antihistamines and decongestants is weak. β-Agonists should be used if wheezing is present (19). Pertussis can benefit from antibiotics and is covered later.
- Influenza presents with myalgia, and other symptoms similar to but often more severe than URTI. Patients who are aged, immunocompromised, or pregnant are at higher risk for poor outcomes. Diagnostic testing may not be necessary in a healthy, young athlete with no risk factors, but may be of benefit in preventing a larger outbreak in an athletic program (3). Neuraminidase inhibitors such as oseltamivir and zanamivir decrease symptoms if started in the first 48 hours after symptom onset (3). Athletes should take the annual influenza vaccine. Symptoms should improve between days three and seven. Patients at high risk should receive antiviral treatment regardless of timing of symptoms (21).
- Pneumonia is an infection of the lung parenchyma causing 60,000 deaths annually in the United States (22). The annual incidence is 248 cases per 100,000 adults and is higher in older adults (23). Clinical features include productive cough, dyspnea, hypoxia, fever, and tachypnea (22). Examination, radiograph, and ultrasound can identify lung field consolidation. The CURB-65 score (including confusion of new onset, blood urea nitrogen > 7, respiratory rate 30 or greater, blood pressure < 90/60, and age >65) and the Pneumonia Severity Index (including age, vitals, serious comorbidities, and mental status) are validated tools for pneumonia risk stratification (23). Diagnostic cultures and antigen testing are appropriate for patients with severe symptoms (23).
- Macrolides, doxycycline, β-lactam antibiotics, and fluoroquinolones are appropriate for outpatient therapy for community-acquired pneumonia (23). Corticosteroids reduce the risk of adult respiratory distress syndrome in severely ill patients. Older runners and those at higher risk of disease should get the pneumococcal vaccination.

Chronic Cough

- Lasting greater than 8 weeks, chronic cough can dramatically impair sleep, training, cause incontinence, and contribute to depression. Infections (pertussis, tuberculosis), medications (angiotensin-converting enzyme (ACE) inhibitors), smoking, and other factors (upper airway cough syndrome, chronic bronchitis, chronic obstructive pulmonary disease (COPD), nonasthmatic eosinophilic bronchitis, gastroesophageal reflux disease (GERD), asthma) cause chronic cough (24).

- 7%–10% of the general population in North America has asthma, compared to 25%–50% of endurance athletes (20). Asthma can be asymptomatic, but acute exacerbations present with wheezing, dyspnea, nasal flaring, chest tightness, and intercostal retractions. Spirometry demonstrates reversible bronchoconstriction. Treatment includes inhaled bronchodilators and inhaled steroids, and for severe symptoms: epinephrine, intravenous steroids, supplementary oxygen, and ventilatory support (24).
- Pertussis is caused by aerosol transmission of *B. pertussis*. In the catarrhal phase (1–2 weeks), patients present with mild, intermittent cough, coryza, and low-grade fevers (3). In the paroxysmal phase (1–6 weeks), inspiratory whoop, spasmodic cough, and posttussive emesis develop (3). During the convalescent phase (1 week to several months), symptoms resolve. Polymerase chain reaction (PCR) testing confirms the diagnosis. Macrolides for 14 days are indicated. Trimethoprim/sulfamethoxazole (TMP/SMX) can be used. Isolate patients for the first 5 days of treatment (3). Athletes without medical contraindications should receive booster vaccinations against pertussis.
- Other causes of chronic cough such as infection, COPD, GERD, smoking, and ACE inhibitor use should be treated appropriately.
- Athletes can resume exercise after their symptoms have resolved, but only slowly advance to their normal intensity.

SORE THROAT

- URTI-related viruses, group A β-hemolytic streptococcus (GABHS), *Mycoplasma*, gonococcus, herpes simplex virus, and Epstein-Barr virus (EBV) cause pharyngitis (25). GABHS pharyngitis and infectious mononucleosis deserve discussion.

Pharyngitis

- Patients with GABHS present with painful sore throat, white tonsillar exudates, bright red swollen tonsils, local lymphadenopathy, fever, headache, and abdominal discomfort. URTI-type symptoms such as cough and nasal congestion are typically absent (25).
- The Modified Centor Score can help predict the likelihood of GABHS, and rapid strep tests are 70%–90% sensitive for diagnosing strep throat (26).
- Acute otitis media (AOM), acute sinusitis, and peritonsillar abscess (quinsy) are uncommon suppurative complications. Acute rheumatic fever and acute glomerulonephritis are nonsuppurative complications, and they are rare in the athlete population (25).
- Penicillin (500 mg twice per day for 10 days) remains an effective treatment for GABHS, but watchful waiting can be a better option. Untreated, 40% of patients will be symptom-free in 3 days and 85% will be symptom-free in 7 days (25). Acetaminophen, saltwater gargles, and throat lozenges may decrease pain. Azithromycin and erythromycin can be used in refractory cases. Corticosteroids, acetaminophen, and nonsteroidal anti-inflammatory medications can improve symptoms.
- Athletes should be asymptomatic before resuming their training.

Infectious Mononucleosis

- Caused by the Epstein-Barr virus (EBV), infectious mononucleosis is generally self-limited and is primarily seen in patients 15–24 years old (27). By age 35, 90% of the global population has developed antibodies to EBV.
- Symptoms and signs include lymphadenopathy, exudative pharyngitis, splenomegaly, and maculopapular, urticarial, or petechial rash (28). Older adults are more likely to develop jaundice.
- Heterophile antibody testing (Monospot) is the best available diagnostic tool with a sensitivity of 63%–84% and specificity of 84%–100% (27). False negatives are more likely in the first weeks of symptoms, so repeat negative tests at 4 weeks.
- A later study, however, found that Monospot sensitivity and specificity were 80.0% and 90.6%, and recommended confirmation with EBV antibody testing (29). Liver transaminases were typically elevated (29). Lymphocytosis is common, and a lymphocyte level of less than 4000 mm^3 has a 99% negative predictive value for infectious mononucleosis (IM) (27).
- Treatment is symptomatic. Corticosteroids decrease throat soreness in the first 12 hours, but no more than other analgesics. Neither glucocorticoids nor antivirals decrease the duration or severity of illness (27). Avoid aspirin since patients with IM are more likely to develop Reye syndrome.
- Patients with IM typically develop splenomegaly, but splenic rupture is uncommon, occurring in 0.1%–0.2% of patients with IM (28). The risk is increased in the first 3 weeks of illness. Athletes should not participate in their sport or in any other strenuous activities during this period.
- Airway compromise occurs in up to 5% of patients with EBV, typically in children due to palatal and nasopharyngeal tonsil hypertrophy (27). Other complications include acute interstitial nephritis, cranial nerve palsies, encephalitis, hemolytic anemia, meningitis, mononeuropathies, myocarditis, neurologic abnormalities, retrobulbar neuritis, and thrombocytopenia (27). Patients with immunosuppression or an X-linked lymphoproliferative syndrome are at much higher risk for poor outcomes.

OTHER COMMON HEAD, EAR, AND EYE CONDITIONS

Otitis Media and Externa

- AOM is responsible for 13.6 million office visits per year in children but is less common in adults. Adults typically present with ear pain and URTI symptoms, while children often present with ear pain, fever, irritability, otorrhea, and anorexia (30). Physical exam may reveal a red, bulging, and immobile tympanic membrane. Pneumatic otoscopy is up to 94% sensitive and 90% specific for identifying middle ear effusion (30). Tympanometry is 70%–94% sensitive and 90% specific for identifying middle ear effusion (30). Evidence of middle ear effusion is necessary for a diagnosis of AOM.

- Antibiotics are not indicated in uncomplicated AOM for adults, adolescents, and older children (30). Amoxicillin, with or without clavulanate, and azithromycin are appropriate for patients with mastoiditis, with diabetes, or who are immunocompromised.
- Otitis externa (OE), inflammation of the external ear canal, has a lifetime prevalence of 10% and is common in water sports athletes (31). OE is primarily caused by *Pseudomonas aeruginosa* and *Staphylococcus aureus*, although *Aspergillus* has been identified. OE presents with ear pain, tenderness when pulling on the ipsilateral tragus, canal edema and erythema, and purulent discharge (31).
- Avoid putting foreign objects into the ear canal. Topical corticosteroids with antimicrobials or antibiotics such as acetic acid, aminoglycosides, polymyxin B, and quinolones are the treatment of choice in uncomplicated cases (32).

Conjunctivitis

- Conjunctivitis is inflammation of the conjunctiva of the eye(s) caused by allergies, viruses, bacteria (*Staphylococcus epidermidis*, *Streptococcus*, *Haemophilus*), or other factors (mechanical irritation from rubbing, excessive brightness, foreign bodies, and irritants). Of infectious conjunctivitis, viruses cause up to 75%. Gluing of the eyelids and lack of itching suggest a bacterial cause (33).
- Presenting complaints include red eyes, itching, discharge (clear if allergic, purulent if bacterial), and irritation. Severe symptoms such as a loss of visual acuity or a visual field defect suggest a more serious diagnosis (33). Contact lens wearers are more likely to develop keratitis and gram-negative infections. If symptoms do not resolve spontaneously in 1–2 days, provide an ophthalmic antibiotic preparation (33).
- Athletes with conjunctivitis must be restricted from participation in high contact sports (such as wrestling) and water sports until asymptomatic.

Meningitis

- Meningitis is inflammation of the meninges, tissue layers covering the spinal cord and brain. Aseptic meningitis is usually viral (*i.e.*, *Enterovirus*, coxsackievirus, herpes simplex virus) or involving other organisms (*i.e.*, Rickettsia, fungi, protozoa, tuberculosis). It is self-limited and has an incidence of 7.6 cases per 100,000 per year (34). Septic meningitis is usually bacterial (pneumococcus, *Neisseria meningitidis*, *H. influenza*) and has high rates of permanent disability or death. Meningitis is most common in the summer and spreads by fecal-oral transmission.
- The classic clinical presentation includes fever, neck stiffness headache, and altered mental status. Focal neurological deficits may appear. Typical signs like the Kernig sign and Brudzinski sign are unreliable, and less than half of patients have the classic triad of fever, stiff neck, and headache (34). Therefore, diagnosis requires cerebrospinal fluid (CSF) analysis, typically obtained by a lumbar puncture. Serum C-reactive protein, serum procalcitonin, and CSF lactate levels can help distinguish between aseptic and bacterial meningitis (34).
- Athletes with meningitis should be evaluated and treated rapidly. Ceftriaxone and vancomycin or meropenem and vancomycin are first-line drugs for bacterial meningitis (34).
- Close contacts, which often include teammates, should receive chemoprophylaxis with rifampin, ceftriaxone, ciprofloxacin, penicillin, clindamycin, or vancomycin, depending upon the causative agent, within 24 hours of diagnosis (34).
- All athletes for whom it is not contraindicated should be vaccinated against *N. meningitidis* and *H. influenza*. Fecal-oral transmission can be averted by regular handwashing and not sharing personal items such as water bottles.

MYOCARDITIS

- Myocarditis is one of the leading causes of cardiac dysfunction and death in otherwise young and healthy people. Common viral causes include adenovirus, *Enterovirus* (coxsackie B), COVID-19, parvovirus B19, and herpesviruses (35). Bacteria, fungi, and protozoa can be involved, and as sport venues span the globe, clinicians must consider schistosomiasis, Chagas disease, tuberculosis, hepatitis viridae, and Lyme disease (35). Myocarditis can be related to noninfectious agents, such as inflammatory diseases and many drugs.
- Patients may present with fatigue, palpitations, light-headedness, tachycardia, fever, myalgia, and exercise intolerance. In severe cases, dyspnea on exertion, jugular venous distension, syncope, or even aborted sudden cardiac death may occur. Laboratory studies should include cardiac biomarkers (troponins, CK-MB [creatine kinase-myocardial band]), and electrocardiogram, echocardiography, Holter, and cardiac MRI (35). Refer for endomyocardial biopsy in patients with cardiogenic shock or acute heart failure (36).
- Many athletes recover with only supportive care, but immunotherapies are available for severe or refractory disease. Corticosteroids inhibit inflammation but are not generally needed in uncomplicated myocarditis (36). ACE inhibitors and diuretics decrease cardiac afterload and thereby decrease stress on the myocardium. Complications include permanent myocardial damage, heart failure, and death.
- Athletes with proven or suspected myocarditis and altered left ventricular (LV) function should immediately stop all competitive sports and strenuous exercise training for 6 months from the onset of symptoms (35). Thereafter, athletes may

begin a gradual return to sport if cardiac size, function, and wall motion are normal on echocardiogram. Also, clinically significant arrhythmias must be absent, a 12-lead ECG must be normal, and cardiac enzymes and other markers of inflammation and failure must be normalized. Recent recommendations suggest that athletes with no symptoms and normal LV function may begin a gradual return to sport as early as one to 3 months after symptom onset (35).

GASTROENTERITIS — ACUTE DIARRHEA

- Up to 40% of travelers to developing countries will experience acute diarrhea, commonly from foodborne infection (3). Viruses (esp. norovirus) cause 10% of cases of traveler's diarrhea (3). Bacteria (esp. *Salmonella*, *Shigella*, and *Escherichia coli*, *Campylobacter*, *Clostridioides difficile*, *Vibrio cholera*) cause up to 90% of cases of travelers diarrhea. Protozoa (esp. *Giardia*, *Cyclospora*, cryptosporidium) causes a small minority of cases. Clinical features include three or more loose and watery stools in less than 24 hours (37). Most cases are self-limited, requiring only adequate fluid intake to avoid dehydration. Antimotility agents can improve symptoms.
- Fever, dehydration, bloody stools, and abdominal pain mark severe diarrhea. Depending upon the history, fecal occult blood, stool culture, lactoferrin, ova and parasite testing, endoscopy, and imaging may be required.
- Antibiotics are generally indicated in healthy patients with severe diarrhea, and in patients at higher risk of complications (37). These include advanced HIV, organ transplantation, or severe inflammatory bowel disease. Choices include azithromycin (*Campylobacter*), metronidazole (*Clostridium difficile*, giardiasis, *Entamoeba histolytica*), ciprofloxacin (enterotoxigenic *E. coli*, *Shigella*), doxycycline (*V. cholera*), TMP/SMX DS (*Cyclospora*), and albendazole (microsporidia).
- Prevent acute diarrhea with handwashing, avoiding suspect foods, and vaccination. Rifaximin is effective for prophylaxis. Athletes may return to their sport once they are afebrile, symptom-free, rehydrated, and tolerating solid foods.

BLOODBORNE INFECTIONS

- The human immunodeficiency virus (HIV) and hepatitis viruses B, C, and D (HBV, HCV, and HDV) are bloodborne pathogens (BBPs) in that they are transmitted by blood and other body fluids. Sexual contact, needle sharing, tattooing, and body piercing are high-risk activities (38). Standard precautions including handwashing and glove use when at risk for encountering body fluids minimize the risk of transmission.
- HIV is a double-stranded RNA virus that attacks helper T lymphocytes (CD4). In the United States, 1.1 million people are infected with HIV, half are not being adequately treated, and 38% of transmissions to noninfected individuals are from people who do not know they are infected (39). Patients are usually asymptomatic but may have unusual opportunistic infections. Saliva and sweat do not transmit HIV disease (38). Casual contact does not transmit HIV, and there have been no documented cases of HIV transmission during sports, but HIV has been transmitted during street fights (38). HIV is poorly infectious and not stable in the environment.
- Anti-retroviral therapy suppresses the virus and restores immune function. Properly treated, patients infected with HIV can have near-normal lifespans (39). All people between ages 15 and 65 should be screened for HIV at least once (39). Patients who are HIV positive can receive standard vaccines, but those who have a low CD_4 count should avoid live virus vaccines.
- Serum, semen, and saliva all transmit HBV. There are three case series (584 cases) of HBV transmission resulting from sports participation (38). HBV is highly infectious and can survive on environmental surfaces for over a week (38). High-risk patients, such as men who have sex with men and injectable drug users, should be screened for HBV and HCV. Athletes should take the HBV vaccination unless contraindicated.
- HCV can survive for 16 hours in the environment (38). There are no documented cases of transmission through sports. The USPSTF recommends HCV screening once for adults born between 1945 and 1965. Potentially curative treatments are available.
- HDV requires HBV for assembly, replication, and transmission, and the modes of transmission and clinical features are similar (38).
- Clinicians should consider pre- and postexposure prophylaxis for BBPs. Exercise benefits patients who are chronically infected with BBPs (38). For example, patients with HIV who exercise enjoy more efficient oxygen consumption, higher insulin sensitivity, and fewer depressive symptoms. Strenuous exercise, however, may be detrimental (38).

SEXUALLY TRANSMITTED INFECTIONS

- The US Centers for Disease Control and Prevention (CDC) estimate that one in five Americans currently has a sexually transmitted infection. Forty-two million have human papilloma virus (HPV); 19 million have herpes simplex virus 2 (HSV-2); 2.6 million have trichomonas; 2.4 million have chlamydia; one million have HIV; 210,000 have gonorrhea; 156,000 have syphilis; and 103,000 have HBV (40). These numbers indicate prevalence, and the incidence of new cases of chlamydia and gonorrhea is much higher.
- Chlamydia may present with vaginal or urethral discharge but is usually asymptomatic, especially in women. Gonorrhea

has similar symptoms. HSV and syphilis have cutaneous manifestations such as vesicles and sores, respectively. All females younger than 25 years should be screened for chlamydia and gonorrhea. HIV screening should be offered to all adolescents (41).

- HPV is vaccine preventable, and the CDC recommends that athletes of both sexes receive vaccination. Genital warts can be treated with topicals (*i.e.*, imiquimod, podofilox) or cryotherapy. HSV-2 commonly presents with vesicles and is responsive to acyclovir, valacyclovir, or famciclovir. Chlamydia responds to doxycycline or azithromycin. Gonorrhea is treated with ceftriaxone (41). Penicillin remains the drug of choice for syphilis, as metronidazole does for trichomonas.

URINARY TRACT INFECTIONS

- Half of all women experience at least one urinary tract infection during their lifetime (42). Common causes in women include *Escherichia coli* (86%), *Staphylococcus saprophyticus* (4%), *Klebsiella* species (3%), *Proteus* species (3%), *Enterobacter* species (1.4%), *Citrobacter* species (0.8%), or *Enterococcus* species (0.5%) (42).
- Women with an increased frequency of urination and dysuria have a 90% likelihood of having a UTI and need no further testing before treatment (3). Females with atypical symptoms and males should have a urinalysis and culture. UTI is uncommon in men, so imaging of the genitourinary tract may be necessary. Diagnosis and management by telephone produces short-term outcomes similar to in-person office care (42).
- Uncomplicated infection in females can be treated with TMP/SMX or nitrofurantoin for 3 days. Males and females with complications require 7 days of antibiotic therapy. Drinking cranberry juice decreased the risk of UTI by 26% in one meta-analysis (3). Athletes who are asymptomatic and rehydrated may return to their sport.

CORONAVIRUS (COVID-19)

- COVID-19 is an enveloped, single-stranded RNA coronavirus, which emerged in Wuhan, China, in 2019 and caused the most notable pandemic since the Spanish flu in 1918. Athletes are at lower risk for severe COVID-19 symptoms than the general population (43). Considering global data, approximately 85% of people with COVID-19 have mild illness, whereas 14% require hospitalization (44). Five percent of adults and 2% of children need admission to an intensive care unit (44). The incubation period is 2–14 days, but symptoms usually begin within 5 days of exposure.
- Clinical presentation includes absent or altered taste and smell, fever, fatigue, shortness of breath, dry cough, myalgias, and occasionally diarrhea, nausea, and vomiting (44). Radiographs demonstrate ground glass opacities and inter- or intralobular thickening. All coronavirus-infected patients should be isolated while they are symptomatic. Outpatient management is supportive, and telephone management is appropriate for patients with mild disease who need to maintain isolation (44).
- Acute COVID-19, the first stage, lasts up to four weeks. Ongoing symptomatic COVID-19, the second stage, goes from four to twelve weeks. Post-COVID-19, the final stage, lasts beyond twelve weeks (43). Long COVID-19 refers to signs and symptoms that develop after acute COVID-19.
- Athletes with acute COVID-19 should rest until asymptomatic and slowly resume moderate exercise, including a gradual return to their sport. COVID-19 can cause myocarditis, so athletes with persistent symptoms must be evaluated. Athletes with no symptoms for 7 days and no structural abnormality on echocardiogram can slowly return to their sport (43).
- The incidence of COVID-19 myocarditis in young, healthy adults is 450 cases per million (45). Treatment is noted in the myocarditis section.
- Athletes with COVID-19 myocarditis should completely abstain from exercise for 3–6 months. Athletes can return to play when they (1) have no cardiopulmonary symptoms, (2) have no residual laboratory evidence of infection, (3) have normal LV systolic function, and (4) have no spontaneous or inducible arrhythmias on ECG and exercise testing (45).
- Among COVID-19 patients, 10%–15% will have persistent symptoms over weeks to months (46). Women are more likely to have prolonged symptoms than men. Athletes aged 45–60, those with a normal body mass index, and Caucasians are also more likely to have prolonged symptoms (46). Cardiopulmonary, neuropsychological, and common symptoms such as fatigue should be addressed as they would in any other event.
- Athletes who lack contraindications should get vaccinated against COVID-19 or be checked for antibody titers. Sport medicine personnel should have an emergency action plan to treat athletes with acute myocardial complications from COVID-19 (47).

REPORTABLE DISEASES

- Bloodborne pathogens, sexually transmitted infections, and other diseases of public health importance such as meningitis or active tuberculosis are usually reportable. Clinicians should check their state requirements.
- Every health care facility, including sports medicine personnel supporting high school, college, professional, or other teams, should have a reliable and easy-to-use disease reporting system.

EXERCISE IN UNUSUAL PLACES

- Extreme sports events often occur in jungles, deserts, and mountains, and dangers of waterborne, tick-, and parasite-related diseases are high. Traveler's diarrhea is common.

RETURN TO PLAY AFTER INFECTION

- Asymptomatic athletes with fever greater than 100.4°F and symptomatic athletes with a temperature of 0.5°–1° increase from baseline and elevated pulse by 10 bpm should rest until symptoms resolve (4).
- Athletes with a respiratory infection but having symptoms only above the neck ("neck check") may do 15 minutes of light exercise. If symptoms do not worsen, they may increase their exercise as tolerated. Athletes with worsening symptoms, systemic symptoms, or other symptoms below the neck should rest (3).
- In general, for every day missed from training, the athlete should expect and allow 2–3 days of graded return to play. Athletes should increase frequency, then duration, and finally intensity by 10% at a time until they are fully recovered (3). A slower return-to-sport schedule is generally not necessary.
- Return-to-play recommendations are also noted under the individual sections in this chapter.

CURRENT AND FUTURE PROSPECTS FOR PREVENTION AND TREATMENT

- Athletes can minimize their chances of developing infections that can impair their play. Frequent handwashing reduces viral spread, and medical personnel can wear gloves, masks, and gowns when appropriate. Together these interventions in athletes and medical staff are up to 91% effective in preventing transmission of dropletborne infectious disease (4). Athletes should not share personal items such as water bottles, towels, and razors. Living conditions are often crowded, meals are poor, and sleep is difficult. Beware of excessive alcohol use and sexually transmitted diseases.
- Vaccinations minimize the risk of infectious diseases. All athletes should have all immunizations recommended by the US CDC based on their age and health status. Arm and leg workouts decreased reports of local adverse reactions, including pain, tenderness, and swelling, in female adolescents and young adults. Exercise reduced self-reported systemic adverse reactions such as fever, feeling ill, and reduced appetite (48).
- Health care providers should focus on early detection and treatment of infectious diseases in all athletes. Being available to the athletes, including by telemedicine, enhances diagnosis. Treatment and rehabilitation must be timely. Disease prevention is the ultimate goal.

REFERENCES

1. Moeijes J, van Busschbach JT, Wieringa TH, Kone J, Bosscher RJ, Twisk JWR. Sports participation and health-related quality of life in children: results of a cross-sectional study. *Health Qual Life Outcomes*. 2019;17(1):64. doi:10.1186/s12955-019-1124-y
2. Simpson RJ, Campbell JP, Gleeson M, et al. Can exercise affect immune function to increase susceptibility to infection? *Exerc Immunol Rev*. 2020;26:8–22.
3. Jaworski CA, Rygiel V. Acute illness in the athlete. *Clin Sports Med*. 2019;38(4):577–95. doi:10.1016/j.csm.2019.05.001
4. Dick NA, Diehl JJ. Febrile illness in the athlete. *Sports Health*. 2014;6(3):225–31. doi:10.1177/1941738113508373
5. Yatim KM, Lakkis FG. A brief journey through the immune system. *Clin J Am Soc Nephrol*. 2015;10(7):1274–81. doi:10.2215/CJN.10031014
6. Cicchella A, Stefanelli C, Massaro M. Upper respiratory tract infections in sport and the immune system response: a review. *Biology*. 2021;10(5):362. doi:10.3390/biology10050362
7. Geuking MB, McCoy KD, Macpherson AJ. The function of secretory IgA in the context of the intestinal continuum of adaptive immune responses in host-microbial mutualism. *Semin Immunol*. 2012;24(1):36–42.
8. Maddur MS, Lacroix-Desmazes S, Dimitrov JD, Kazatchkine MD, Bayry J, Kaveri SV. Natural antibodies: from first-line defense against pathogens to perpetual immune homeostasis. *Clin Rev Allergy Immunol*. 2020;58(2):213–28. doi:10.1007/s12016-019-08746-9
9. Tiernan C, Lyons M, Comyns T, Nevill AM, Warrington G. Salivary IgA as a predictor of upper respiratory tract infections and relationship to training load in elite rugby union players. *J Strength Cond Res*. 2020;34(3):782–90. doi:10.1519/jsc.0000000000003019
10. David A, Quinlan J. Fever of unknown origin in adults. *Am Fam Physician*. 2022;105(2):137–43.
11. Walker AC, Surda P, Rossiter M, Little SA. Nasal disease and quality of life in athletes. *J Laryngol Otol*. 2018;132(9):812–5. doi:10.1017/s0022215118001408
12. DeGeorge KC, Ring DJ, Dalrymple SN. Treatment of the common cold. *Am Fam Physician*. 2019;100(5):281–9.
13. Łagowska K, Bajerska J. Probiotic supplementation and respiratory infection and immune function in athletes: systematic review and meta-analysis of randomized controlled trials. *J Athl Train*. 2021 Jan 22;56(11):1213–23. doi:10.4085/592-20
14. Sivamaruthi BS, Kesika P, Chaiyasut C. Effect of probiotics supplementations on health status of athletes. *Int J Environ Res Public Health*. 2019;16(22):4469. doi:10.3390/ijerph16224469
15. Barry A, Fahey T. Clinical diagnosis of acute bacterial rhinosinusitis. *Am Fam Physician*. 2020;101(12):758–9.
16. Aring AM, Chan MM. Current concepts in adult acute rhinosinusitis. *Am Fam Physician*. 2016;94(2):97–105.
17. Sur DKC, Plesa ML. Treatment of allergic rhinitis. *Am Fam Physician*. 2015;92(11):985–92.
18. Sur DKC, Plesa ML. Chronic nonallergic rhinitis. *Am Fam Physician*. 2018;98(3):171–6.
19. Kinkade S, Long N. Acute bronchitis. *Am Fam Physician*. 2016;94(7):560–5.
20. Boulet LP, Turmel J. Cough in exercise and athletes. *Pulm Pharmacol Ther*. 2019;55:67–74. doi:10.1016/j.pupt.2019.02.003

21. Gaitonde D, Moore FC, Morgan MK. Influenza: diagnosis and treatment. *Am Fam Physician.* 2019;100(12):751–8.
22. Kaysin A, Viera AJ. Community-acquired pneumonia in adults: diagnosis and management. *Am Fam Physician.* 2016;94(9):698–706.
23. Womack J, Kropa J. Community-acquired pneumonia in adults: rapid evidence review. *Am Fam Physician.* 2022;105(6):625–30.
24. Michaudet C, Malaty J. Chronic cough: evaluation and management. *Am Fam Physician.* 2017;96(9):575–80.
25. Kenealy T. Sore throat. *Am Fam Physician.* 2015;91(10):689–90.
26. Mantzourani E, Evans A, Cannings-John R, et al. Impact of a pilot NHS-funded sore throat test and treat service in community pharmacies on provision and quality of patient care. *BMJ Open Qual.* 2020;9(1):e000833. doi:10.1136/bmjoq-2019-000833
27. Womack J, Jimenez M. Common questions about infectious mononucleosis. *Am Fam Physician.* 2015;91(6):372–6.
28. Putukian M, O'Connor FG, Stricker P, et al. Mononucleosis and athletic participation: an evidence-based subject review. *Clin J Sport Med.* 2008;18(4):309–15.
29. Wang EX, Kussman A, Hwang CE. Use of monospot testing in the diagnosis of infectious mononucleosis in the collegiate student–athlete population. *Clin J Sport Med* 2022;32(5):467–70, doi:10.1097/jsm.0000000000000996
30. Gaddey HL, Wright MT, Nelson TN. Otitis media: rapid evidence review. *Am Fam Physician.* 2019;100(6):350–6.
31. Schaefer P, Baugh RF. Acute otitis externa: an update. *Am Fam Physician.* 2012;86(11):1055–61.
32. Rosenfeld RM, Schwartz SR, Cannon CR, American Academy of Otolaryngology-Head and Neck, Surgery Foundation, et al. Clinical practice guideline: acute otitis externa executive summary. *Otolaryngol Head Neck Surg.* 2014;150(2):161–8. doi:10.1177/0194599813517659
33. Epling J. Bacterial conjunctivitis. *Am Fam Physician.* 2010;82(6):665–6.
34. Mount HR, Boyle SD. Aseptic and bacterial meningitis: evaluation, treatment, and prevention. *Am Fam Physician.* 2017;96(5):314–22.
35. Halle M, Binzenhöfer L, Mahrholdt H, Johannes Schindler M, Esefeld K, Tschöpe C. Myocarditis in athletes: a clinical perspective. *Eur J Prev Cardiol.* 2021;28(10):1050–7. doi:10.1177/2047487320909670
36. Ammirati E, Frigerio M, Adler ED, et al. Management of acute myocarditis and chronic inflammatory cardiomyopathy. *Circ Heart Fail.* 2020;3(11):e007405. doi:10.1161/circheartfailure.120.007405
37. Meisenheimer ES, Epstein C, Thiel D. Acute diarrhea in adults. *Am Fam Physician.* 2022;106(1):72–80.
38. McGrew C, MacCallum DS, Narducci D, et al. AMSSM position statement update: blood-borne pathogens in the context of sports participation. *Br J Sports Med.* 2020;54(4):200–7. doi:10.1136/bjsports-2019-100650
39. Goldschmidt R, Chu C. HIV infection in adults: initial management. *Am Fam Physician.* 2021;103(7):407–16.
40. US Centers for Disease Control and Prevention. *STI Prevalence, Incidence, and Cost Estimates Infographic.* Atlanta, GA: Centers for Disease Control and Prevention; 2021. https://www.cdc.gov/sti-statistics/annual/summary.html
41. Klein DA, Valerio CR, Cofield ZN. Sexually transmitted infections: updated guideline from the CDC. *Am Fam Physician.* 2022;105(5):553–7.
42. Colgan R, Williams M. Diagnosis and treatment of acute uncomplicated cystitis. *Am Fam Physician.* 2011;84(7):771–6.
43. Lindsay RK, Wilson JJ, Trott M, et al. What are the recommendations for returning athletes who have experienced long term COVID-19 symptoms? *Ann Med.* 2021;53(1):1935–44. doi:10.1080/07853890.2021.1992496
44. Cheng A, Caruso D, McDougall C. Outpatient management of COVID-19: rapid evidence review. *Am Fam Physician.* 2020;102(8):478–86.
45. Gluckman TJ, Bhave NM, Allen LA, et al. 2022 ACC expert consensus decision pathway on cardiovascular sequelae of COVID-19 in adults: myocarditis and other myocardial involvement, post-acute sequelae of SARS-CoV-2 infection, and return to play. A report of the American College of Cardiology Solution Set Oversight Committee. *J Am Coll Cardiol.* 2022;79(17):1717–56.
46. Giusto E, Asplund CA. Persistent COVID and a return to sport. *Curr Sports Med Rep.* 2022;21(3):100–4. doi:10.1249/jsr.0000000000000943
47. Drezner JA, Heinz WM, Asif IM, et al. Cardiopulmonary considerations for high school student-athletes during the COVID-19 pandemic: update to the NFHS-AMSSM guidance statement. *Sports Health.* 2022;14(3):369–71. doi:10.1177/19417381221077138
48. Lee VY, Booy R, Skinner SR, Fong J, Edwards KM. The effect of exercise on local and systemic adverse reactions after vaccinations: outcomes of two randomized controlled trials. *Vaccine.* 2018;36(46):6995–7002. doi:10.1016/j.vaccine.2018.09.067

38 Endocrinology and Sports

Alena Comella and Adriana Isacke

INTRODUCTION

- The endocrine system is a complex framework of glands and hormones that receives input and provides feedback through the hypothalamic-pituitary axis. The hormones are often ubiquitous and ultimately govern many key physiologic functions, such as metabolism, growth, and muscle function.
- Hormones are responsible for the machinery that allows us to exercise, and when deficient, provides a management challenge to both the athlete and the sports medicine physician.
- This chapter will review some of the key components of the endocrine system and the implications of disease of this system in sports.

PANCREATIC HORMONES

- Insulin and glucagon are secreted by the islet cells in the pancreas. *Glucagon* is a catabolic hormone and it stimulates gluconeogenesis, thereby acting as a counterbalance to insulin through its stimulation of gluconeogenesis.
- *Insulin* is an anabolic hormone that regulates glucose channels and insulin receptors, stimulates protein and glycogen synthesis, and generally inhibits catabolism. When it is absent, lipolysis produces fatty acids and ketones as the primary fuel source, resulting in a metabolic acidosis. Insulin is also involved in growth and development through its numerous interactions with other mediators of growth such as growth hormone (GH) and insulin-like growth factor-1 (IGF-1) (1).
- During exercise, insulin levels decrease while glucagon and catecholamines drive hepatic glycogenolysis and free fatty acid production to provide glucose to stressed cells. In this state, active muscles use glucose through insulin-independent means and potentiate the action of residual insulin through adaptations in the affinity for and quantity of insulin receptors.
- After exercise, insulin production and sensitivity are increased in response to elevated blood glucose. Insulin drives replenishment of glycogen and protein stores and downregulates counterregulatory hormones.

DIABETES AND EXERCISE

- Because insulin is administered exogenously in people with diabetes, this cascade relies heavily on proper management. Excess insulin prior to exercise inhibits catecholamines, suppressing the liver's ability to mobilize fuel while muscles continue to use circulating glucose. This results in hypoglycemia, with blood sugar <70 mg $\cdot$ dL^{-1}.
- **Hypoglycemic emergencies** arise as exogenous insulin inhibits counterregulatory hormones. Following exercise, enhanced glucose uptake and insulin sensitivity predisposes the athlete with insulin-dependent diabetes to hypoglycemia for as long as 12–24 hours.
  - Pallor, diaphoresis, confusion, headache, shakiness, irritability, and a change in mental status are common presentations and may progress to syncope, seizure, or coma if left untreated.
  - Athletes with long-standing diabetes have a blunted stress response and may not exhibit these warning signs, which are the result of sympathetic activation. Fatigue, hunger, and irritability may be the only clues (2).
  - **Treatment,** if alert, is oral replacement with 15 g of glucose.
    - Repeat blood sugar every 15 minutes until euglycemic.
    - If obtunded, administer glucagon 1 mg intramuscularly (IM)/subcutaneously (SC) if >100 lb or 0.5 mg if <100 lb.
    - Glucagon has a short half-life and should be continuously supplemented with additional carbohydrates on awakening, until glucose normalizes (3).
- **Hyperglycemia** can also be problematic for athletes when insufficient insulin is present during exercise. When blood glucose control is poor prior to exercise, athletes may have high blood glucose and subsequent polyuria resulting in dehydration. Without insulin's inhibitory effect on lipolysis, ketogenesis contributes to the deteriorating metabolic state.
  - Counterregulatory hormones are normally active in the stressed state but in this setting, they will contribute detrimentally to the hyperglycemia. Diabetic ketoacidosis may be the end result. These athletes need urgent supplemental insulin and hydration.

Therapeutic Use Exemption

- Insulin is listed as a prohibited substance under S4 — Hormone and Metabolic Modulators of the World Antidoping Agency (WADA) Prohibited List. All individuals with insulin-dependent diabetes require a therapeutic use exemption (TUE).
- Documentation from a specialist in the management of diabetes is recommended.
- For type 1 diabetes, a TUE may be granted for insulin for up to 10 years, with a documented review every few years.
- For type 2 diabetes, a TUE may be granted for 12 months, then undergo review for an additional 10 years (4).

Return to Play

- Athletes with routine hypoglycemia can return to play when repeat blood glucose measurements have stabilized. Blood glucose in excess of 250 mg · dL^{-1} or ketonuria is a relative contraindication to play. Athletes with blood glucose between 150 and 249 mg · dL^{-1} should be monitored closely but can continue to play (5).

PARTICIPATION GUIDELINES

Preseason

- Assess athlete's disease literacy.
  - Nutrition, carbohydrate counting
  - Ability to monitor blood sugars with appropriate frequency
  - Recognizes the symptoms of hypoglycemia and hyperglycemia
  - Knows how to treat diabetic emergencies, sick day plan
  - Medical alert bracelet
- Screen for long-term complications of diabetes.
  - Recent hemoglobin A1c, blood pressure, lipid profile, creatinine, microalbumin
  - Screen for peripheral neuropathy, foot care education
  - Screen for retinopathy, and if present, avoid activities that could increase intraocular pressure (*e.g.*, vigorous intensity aerobic or resistance training, high-impact training) (6)
  - Consider screening for coronary artery disease
  - Graded exercise testing if older than 35 or 25 with >15 years of diabetes
- Create a plan with sports medicine staff for diabetic emergencies.
- The athlete should experiment in preseason with insulin regimens.
  - Start season conditioning to minimize changes in insulin needs that develop with fitness.
  - Experiment with injection site and effects of exercise and climate on absorption, although the abdomen is the recommended injection site for consistent absorption (5).

Before Exercise

- Estimate intensity, duration, and energy demand of the event.
- Reduce SC insulin based on intensity and duration of exercise.
  - For exercise lasting <1 hour, decrease insulin by 30%
  - Exercise lasting 1–2 hours, decrease insulin by 40%
  - Exercise lasting >2 hours, decrease insulin by 50%
  - If exercise is scheduled in the evening, also reduce mealtime insulin by 50% to avoid post-exercise hypoglycemia (5)
- Insulin pump users should reduce basal rate by 50% at least 1 hour prior to sport.
  - May remove pump for up to 2 hours for sport, especially water or contact sports
  - Frequent glucose checks
  - Contingency plan for extended events (5)
- Check blood sugars prior to exercise.
  - If blood glucose < 100 mg · dL^{-1}, ingest 15 g of carbohydrate. Wait for 15 minutes, and recheck blood sugar. Repeat as needed.
  - If blood glucose is between 180 and 249 mg · dL^{-1}, increase frequency of blood sugar checks. Hold carbohydrate intake pending clinical course.
  - If blood glucose > 250 mg · dL^{-1}, postpone exercise, measure urine ketone, and administer insulin.

During Exercise

- Add 15 g of carbohydrate for the first 30–60 minutes of exercise.
  - During events of longer duration, 30–60 g · h^{-1} carbohydrate should be ingested every 15–30 minutes.
- Attention to adequate hydration.
- Monitor glucose levels at least hourly.

Post-exercise

- Meal within 30 minutes of activity and increased caloric intake for 12–24 hours after activity
- Continued blood glucose surveillance, especially overnight
  - Watch for late-onset hypoglycemia.
  - Adjust insulin as needed.
- Proper foot care
- Attention to adequate hydration.

ADRENAL GLAND

Adrenal Cortex

- Adrenocorticotropin (ACTH), synthesized in the anterior pituitary, is secreted under the control of corticotropin-releasing hormone (CRH) and vasopressin. ACTH stimulates the adrenal glands to secrete glucocorticoids, mineralocorticoids, and androgens.

- Superficially, the *zona glomerulosa* produces mineralocorticoids; primarily aldosterone. Aldosterone helps maintain blood volume by binding to receptors in the kidney under direction of the renin-angiotensin-aldosterone system. Aldosterone increases reabsorption of sodium and excretion of potassium and hydrogen ions in the kidney, colon, and salivary glands (7).
- In the *zona fasciculata*, glucocorticoids (*e.g.*, cortisol) are produced diurnally, with the highest concentrations secreted in the morning. The key function of cortisol is to increase blood glucose through gluconeogenesis and glycolysis. Cortisol is a potent anti-inflammatory hormone, decreases bone formation, strengthens cardiac muscle contractions, and causes water retention (8). Glucocorticoids are secreted in response to stress, hypotension, fever, and hypoglycemia under the direction of ACTH and catecholamines (7). Glucocorticoids provide negative feedback to the hypothalamus when steroid levels are adequate, downregulating the Hypothalamus-Pituitary-Adrenal (HPA) axis.
- The deepest layer is the *zona reticularis* where weak androgens are produced. They are secreted with cortisol in response to stress and in a diurnal fashion. Please refer to the section on androgens for more details (8).

Primary Hyperaldosteronism

- Primary aldosteronism (PA) is estimated to account for 10% of all cases of hypertension (9).
- Early identification is important, as PA can cause severe hypertension and the treatment differs from other types of hypertension.
- The etiology is excessive, autonomous production of aldosterone in the adrenal gland, either by bilateral hyperplasia or aldosterone-producing adenomas.
- Renin is secreted by the kidney and converts angiotensin into angiotensin I and launches the RAAS system to produce aldosterone. Renin is suppressed by a negative feedback loop when aldosterone is high (9).
- Symptoms include hypokalemia (only 9%–37% of patients), blood pressure >150/100 mm Hg taken on three different days, hypertension in patients less than 30 year old, drug-resistant hypertension, hypertension with adrenal incidentaloma, hypertension with a family history of cerebrovascular events at a young age.
- **Diagnosis** can be made by checking a complete metabolic panel and renin and aldosterone in the morning after the patient has been out of bed for 2 hours (10).
  - Low serum renin (<1.0 ng · mL^{-1} · h^{-1}) and high aldosterone levels (>10 ng · dL^{-1}) are suggestive of PA.
  - Calculating an aldosterone to renin ratio (ARR) is more sensitive, as early stages of PA can have episodes of normal renin and aldosterone. ARRs between 20 and 40 ng · dL^{-1} are suggestive of PA.
  - If these tests come back positive, nephrology consult is recommended for confirmatory testing (11).
- **Treatment** is determined by the cause of PA, and can include medication management or adrenalectomy

Adrenal Insufficiency

- Insufficiency can present at any age and can be a result of either primary (adrenal), secondary (pituitary), or tertiary (hypothalamic) dysfunction.
- *Autoimmune primary adrenal insufficiency* most commonly presents between 20 and 50 years old, with a higher prevalence in women. It can present in combination with autoimmune thyroid disease, type 1 diabetes, and premature ovarian insufficiency (12).
- *Secondary adrenal insufficiency* is often caused by a pituitary gland tumor and can be seen in combination with other pituitary hormone deficiencies. Drugs, such as chronic steroids or opiates, can cause secondary adrenal insufficiency. Chronic steroid treatment is combined with Cushingoid features as a consequence of the drug (12).
- Patients present with fatigue, lethargy, nausea, abdominal pain, unintentional weight loss, abdominal pain, arthralgias, myalgias, hypoglycemia, and hypovolemia with orthostatic hypotension due to urinary salt losses. Hyperpigmentation of high friction areas of the skin can occur due to high concentrations of ACTH, which stimulates dermal melanocortin receptors (12).

Diagnosis

- Adrenal insufficiency is suggested by hypoglycemia, hyponatremia, hypothyroidism, and hyperkalemia.
- Cortisol and ACTH levels should be ordered to confirm the diagnosis.
- A fasting morning basal cortisol level <100 nmol · L^{-1} and ACTH double the upper limit of normal is diagnostic.
- Once the diagnosis of adrenal insufficiency is confirmed, consultation with an endocrinologist is recommended to help determine the cause.

Treatment

- Hydrocortisone 15–25 mg orally in divided doses thrice a day (or fludrocortisone 0.1–0.2 mg every day for primary adrenal insufficiency with aldosterone deficiency).
- In primary adrenal insufficiency, salt substitution is required, with special attention paid to athletes to determine the accurate dosages based on symptoms during and after exercise.
- Some athletes report requiring higher doses during prolonged exercise. Athletes may require a 2.5–5 mg dose of hydrocortisone before exercise, with a repeat dose every 2–4 hours during exertion (12).

Acute Adrenal Crisis

- In those with adrenal insufficiency, an *acute adrenal crisis* may be precipitated by extreme stresses (surgery, infection, dehydration, gastroenteritis, dental procedures) or rapid withdrawal of long-term glucocorticoid therapy.

- These individuals may present with shock, an "acute" abdomen, headache, nausea, vomiting, myalgias, pyrexia, or be comatose.
- Normal exercise does not require stress doses of corticosteroids, but a fracture, moderate blood loss, or vomiting may precipitate an emergency.

- **Treatment** includes 100 mg of injectable hydrocortisone or 4 mg of dexamethasone.
  - Medication should be available at all times.
  - The athlete and sports medicine staff should be educated about how and when to use these rescue medications (*i.e.*, during acute illness or during high-stress medical procedures).
  - Hydrocortisone needs to be dosed every 6 hours or given continuously through IV infusion, along with fluid resuscitation. Thus, patients in adrenal crisis should be admitted to the hospital for close monitoring and treatment (12).
- **Therapeutic use exemption**
  - Glucocorticoids are banned for use in competition under the World Antidoping Agency guidelines.
  - For adrenal insufficiency, a TUE can be granted if the medical professional confirms the diagnosis and can prove that using glucocorticoids is reasonable and acceptable medical treatment.
  - The TUE is valid for 10 years after completion.
  - There should be an annual review of the condition by an endocrinologist.
  - A plan for adrenal crisis in times of high stress should be integrated into the TUE.
  - The athlete should report the use of stress doses on the doping control form at the time of testing.
  - The TUE requires affirmation that the treatment is not performance enhancing beyond a return to the athlete's previous state of health (13).
  - A TUE for functional adrenal insufficiency resulting from glucocorticoid withdrawal can be granted for a period of 4–12 weeks.
  - Given the controversy surrounding the efficacy of and need for dehydroepiandrosterone (DHEA) supplementation, an independent expert should be consulted (13).
- **Return to play**
  - With adequate therapy and a TUE, there are no restrictions.

Adrenal Medulla

- The adrenal medulla is a collection of postganglionic neurons under the direct control of the central nervous system through autonomic preganglionic fibers. The medulla secretes catecholamines into the blood under direct stimulation of the autonomic nervous system in response to stress and exercise.
- Catecholamines, which include norepinephrine and epinephrine, act at adrenergic receptors located throughout the body, activating the sympathetic division of the nervous system. They increase heart rate, cardiac output, and arterial pressure through the α-adrenergic receptors. Catecholamines also cause bronchodilation, vasodilatation, and mydriasis.
- Ephedra alkaloids are weak sympathomimetic agents with actions similar to epinephrine. Some studies have shown that ephedrine supplementation can enhance athletic performance by promoting weight loss, increasing aerobic capacity, reducing fatigue, and increasing alertness and reaction time during exercise. These studies, however, were flawed, so the actual ergogenic effects of ephedrine are still under debate (14).
- High doses of the compound can cause insomnia, anxiety, headache, delirium, irritability, aggression, hypertension, loss of appetite, urinary retention, and tachyarrhythmia (14).
- **Therapeutic Use Exemption**
  - Ephedrine and stimulants, in general, are banned during competition. There is no TUE available.
  - There are several other agents acting on the adrenergic axis that are prohibited by WADA; please refer to a current prohibited substances list for details.

THYROID HORMONE

- Thyroid hormone (TH), produced by the thyroid gland under direction of the hypothalamic-pituitary axis, is secreted in response to elevated thyroid-stimulating hormone (TSH) when TH levels are low. When there is adequate hormone, negative feedback decreases production.
- TH actually represents the combination of the two main hormones that your thyroid gland releases: thyroxine (T4) and triiodothyronine (T3). T3 is the active form of TH; T4 is converted in the periphery to T3.
- TH plays an important role in development through cell differentiation and organogenesis, as well as maintaining thermogenic and metabolic homeostasis in adults (15).
- TH upregulates β-adrenergic receptors, resulting in an enhanced response to circulating catecholamines. During exercise, TH helps maintain ventilation in response to hypoxia and hypercapnia, and it improves oxygen consumption in metabolically active tissues. TH also increases the rate of carbohydrate absorption and stimulates breakdown of fatty acids for energy (16).

Hypothyroidism

- Manifestations are that of a slowed metabolic state that includes fatigue, slowed movement, cold intolerance, constipation, weight gain, delayed relaxation of deep tendon reflexes, and bradycardia.

- In athletes, however, the complaint may be as simple as a decrease in performance or fatigue.
- Patients with hypothyroidism often present with muscular complaints, including cramps, weakness, stiffness, and poor exercise tolerance.
- The lack of TH likely affects the metabolism and production of energy within muscle cells, leading to suboptimal contractile function. Rhabdomyolysis is a rarer consequence of hypothyroidism (17).
- Function of the cardiovascular system is greatly affected by hypothyroidism. Both systolic function and diastolic function are reduced, and the relaxation of vascular smooth muscles is impaired, increasing systemic vascular resistance (18).
- In children, TH is a key component in bone and muscle development, brain maturation, and onset of puberty. Thus, a young athlete with hypothyroidism may present with stunted growth, delayed onset of puberty, or cognitive impairment (19).

Diagnosis

- An elevated TSH and a low free T_4 are suggestive of primary hypothyroidism.

Treatment

- Replacement starts with levothyroxine at 1.6 μg · kg^{-1} · d^{-1}, typically 50–100 μg · d^{-1}, with subsequent increases every 6–8 weeks by 12.5–25 μg until the patient responds (20).

Therapeutic Use Exemption

- A TUE is not required for thyroid replacement (4).

Return to Play

- Return to play is largely based on symptoms; there are no particular restrictions.

Hyperthyroidism

- Hyperthyroidism is often the result of autoimmune disease, which results in excess TH and leads to a hypermetabolic condition (21).
- Symptoms may include unexplained weight loss despite an increased appetite, anxiety, sweating, hyperactivity, and palpitations, all signs of sympathetic activation. Like hypothyroid individuals, however, their only complaint may be a decrease in performance.
  - Thyrotoxicosis should be included in the differential diagnosis of any well-trained athlete with resting tachycardia.
  - Female athletes may have oligomenorrhea or secondary amenorrhea and increased bone turnover leading to lower bone mineral density, thereby increasing the risk of fracture (22).
- Exogenous thyroid use has historically been a tool of many weight loss clinics in an effort to produce a hypermetabolic state in hopes of enhancing weight loss.
  - Although thyroid hormone can stimulate both lipogenesis and lipolysis, hyperthyroidism ultimately leads to a reduction in adipose tissue (23).
  - Factitious TH use is linked to myocardial infarction and other overt characteristics of thyrotoxicosis (24).

Diagnosis

- TSH is the best initial test and is low or undetectable in true thyrotoxicosis.
- Elevated free T_4 and total triiodothyronine (T_3) support the diagnosis (25).

Treatment

- Antithyroid medications, which include methimazole and propylthiouracil, are often first line and may be used in combination with β-blockers (21).

Therapeutic Use Exemption

- β-blockers are banned during competition for a number of sports requiring concentration. There are a select number of sports where they are also banned outside of competition. Please refer to WADA guidelines (26).

Return to Play

- As with hypothyroidism, there are no restrictions on return to play. However, any athlete with ongoing thyrotoxicosis is at risk for tachyarrhythmia and should be encouraged to avoid exercise until the disease is stabilized.

GROWTH HORMONE

- Growth hormone (GH) is produced in the anterior pituitary, under the direction of GH-releasing hormone in a very complex interaction with many peripheral inputs. GH secretion occurs in response to hypoglycemia, androgens, sleep, stress, protein ingestion, and exercise.
- GH inhibitors include glucocorticoids, hyperglycemia, and fatty meals (27).
- GH is produced in a pulsatile manner throughout the day but peaks an hour after sleep begins. GH's primary function is to increase height by promoting chondrocyte proliferation. It also promotes lipolysis, glucose availability, calcium homeostasis, and regulation of lean body mass (27). However, it seems to exert most of its effect through IGF-1.
- IGF-1 is produced in the liver and promotes cell proliferation. It inhibits apoptosis, causing skeletal muscle hypertrophy and activation of chondrocytes and osteocytes (28).

GH Deficiency

- GH deficiency (GHD) most often presents in childhood, at a prevalence between 1:4000 and 1:10,000. It typically presents with growth failure, decreased bone age, and other signs of pituitary dysfunction.
- Adult onset idiopathic GHD is rare and may not be an obvious syndrome. It is commonly diagnosed in the setting of multiple anterior pituitary deficiencies and other hormone deficiencies in the setting of central nervous system disease,

infection, cranial irradiation, pituitary disease, or head trauma.

- Symptoms of GHD are short stature (more than 2 SD below the mean), increased intra-abdominal visceral fat, insulin resistance, decreased lean muscle mass, maintenance of prepubertal voice, hypertension, hyperlipidemia, and systolic dysfunction.
  - Bone mineralization is reduced, and an athlete may present with osteopenia or a pathologic fracture (28).

Diagnosis

- GH levels are often not helpful.
- A low serum IGF-1 concentration is suggestive of GHD. The diagnosis should be confirmed with a GH secretion provocation test.
- An endocrinologist should be consulted prior to initiating treatment.

Treatment

- In adults, human GH is given at a starting dose of 0.1–0.3 mg · d^{-1} SC every night, with higher starting doses given to pediatric patients, which mimics natural age-related decline in GH (27).
- The dose is titrated based on serial IGF-1 levels.

Therapeutic Use Exemption

- In adults, treatment of partial GH deficiency remains debatable, and for WADA purposes, only documented severe GH deficiency is eligible for TUE.
- An endocrinologist should independently review each case, a log book should be kept by the athlete of each self-administration of the medication, and the diligent medical records of each prescription given by the physician need to be kept.
- Treatment monitoring includes documenting BMI, IGF-1 levels, blood glucose and hemoglobin A1C levels, bone density, and quality of life measures. The results of regular monitoring should be reviewed yearly.
- A TUE is granted for 8 years if there is genetic, congenital, irradiation, or HPA structural abnormalities.
- The TUE is granted to 2 years (adult) or 4 years (children/adolescent) if GHD is due to brain trauma or is idiopathic (29,30).

Return to Play

- There are no restrictions on return to play with GHD.

Doping and GH

- Historically, athletes and trainers have felt that GH increases lean body mass and strength in highly trained athletes. It has been an intriguing substance to athletes given its ability to augment lean muscle mass and strength and because there have been limited methods to detect GH abuse.
- Although administration of GH has been shown to improve muscle mass, VO2max, and decreased total body fat in GHD individuals, this has not been proven to occur in healthy individuals supplementing with GH. In fact, exercise capacity, strength, and VO2max may actually worsen with the chronic use of exogenous GH in healthy adults (31).
- IGF-1 can be used by athletes to enhance the anabolic effects of GH, but it is difficult to obtain and prepare so is not as commonly abused.
- The health risks associated with excess GH use includes acromegaly, gynecomastia, vision changes, headaches, macroglossia, sleep apnea, water retention, diabetes mellitus, hypertension, cardiomyopathies, valve disorders, arrhythmias, and higher risk of some cancers.

Detection

- Due to its short half-life, pulsatile excretion, and low urinary excretion, direct GH testing is challenging to interpret.
- IGF-1 and N-terminal extension peptide of procollagen type III, which are markers of GH activity, are being studied for validity at this time and are not being routinely used.
- GH isoforms are also being used to detect GH abuse. Normal GH secretion from the pituitary includes a variety of isoforms, including varies configurations of both 22- and 20-kd forms.
  - Exogenous GH has only a 22-kd monomer, which downregulates the production of natural forms through negative feedback. A positive test is flagged when the ratio of 22-kDA isoform to other isoforms is increased compared to normal levels (27,31).

PARATHYROID HORMONE

- The parathyroid gland is located on the poles of the thyroid gland and secretes parathyroid hormone (PTH), which plays a role in governing serum calcium and phosphorus. Calcium and phosphorus are key mediators of bone health, blood coagulation, muscle contraction, and nerve function. PTH is stimulated by low serum calcium and mobilizes calcium from bone, increasing renal reabsorption and intestinal absorption of calcium.
- Hypercalcemia inhibits the secretion of PTH. *Calcitonin*, produced in the thyroid gland, opposes PTH, and is secreted in response to hypercalcemia ($Ca^+ > 9.5$ mg · dL^{-1}). It subsequently inhibits bone resorption and encourages calciuria (32). A hyperactive gland results in hypercalcemia, causing bone pain, weakness, myalgias, cognitive impairment, and osteoporosis.

Primary Hyperparathyroidism

- Primary hyperparathyroidism is common with an estimated prevalence of 66 cases per 100,000 person-years in women and 25 per 100,000 person-years in men (33).
- In this disorder, PTH is autonomously produced from one or more abnormal parathyroid glands and presents with hypercalcemia and either normal or high PTH levels.

- Symptoms include nephrolithiasis, fragility fractures (due to osteopenia), fatigue, depression, or impaired memory. In severe hypercalcemia, patients can present with neuromuscular weakness, or altered mental status (33).

Diagnosis

- High serum calcium concentrations with normal or high serum PTH concentrations, showing an inappropriate PTH level given the degree of hypercalcemia.
- Once the diagnosis is made, renal ultrasound, 24-hours urine calcium, and a bone density test should be performed.

Treatment

- Primary hyperparathyroidism requires surgical removal of the abnormal parathyroid tissue.

VITAMIN D

- Vitamin D is produced in the skin from cholesterol, a process stimulated by sunlight exposure, forming vitamin D_3 (cholecalciferol). Vitamin D_3 is 25-hydroxylated in the liver to 25-hydroxycholecalciferol [25(OH)D] and then is 1α-hydroxylated in the kidney, creating the more active metabolite, 1,25-dihydroxycholecalciferol.
- PTH also stimulates the induction of bioactive 1,25-dihydroxycholecalciferol from 25-hydroxycholecalciferol in the kidney in response to hypocalcemia.
- Vitamin D is responsible for the absorption and transport of Ca^{2+} and PO_4^{3-} from the intestine and inhibits calciuria by decreasing renal excretion. It also stimulates osteoblasts and plays a role in appropriate bone mineralization. Vitamin D is loosely regulated but appears to be inhibited by hypercalcemia (34).

Vitamin D Deficiency

- Deficiency results in defective calcification of the bone matrix and is implicated in a number of disease states.
  - Miller et al. (35) measured vitamin D levels in 53 patients who had confirmed stress fractures, and 83% had vitamin D deficiency or insufficiency.
  - Vitamin D likely plays a role in protein synthesis, mitochondrial metabolism, and energy production, although more research is needed to further clarify the cellular mechanisms (36).
  - Athletes who participate in indoor sports have a greater risk of developing vitamin D deficiency compared to those who play outdoors (37).
  - Osteomalacia is seen in adults with inadequate amounts of vitamin D and is characterized by softening of the bones due to defective bone mineralization.
    - The disease is the result of inadequate calcium absorption and common in malabsorptive states and those with eating disorders (38).
    - Patients present with bone pain, lumbar back pain, and occasionally have pathologic fractures and proximal muscle weakness (39).

Diagnosis

- Vitamin D insufficiency is defined by 25(OH)D levels less than 12–20 ng · mL^{-1}, and deficiency is defined as 25(OH)D levels less than 12 ng · mL^{-1} (40).
- The U.S. Preventive Services Task Force (USPSTF) has insufficient evidence to advise on screening, but supplementation is generally considered low risk.

Treatment

- The recommended daily intakes of vitamin D 600–800 IU for most adults.
- Those with deficiency can be treated with 50,000 units of vitamin D_3 every week for 6–8 weeks initially, then 800 IU daily.
- Currently, the treatment for those with vitamin D insufficiency is more controversial. It is reasonable to treat these individuals with 800–1000 IU of vitamin D_3 daily, then check serum levels in 3 months (40).

Return to Play

- There are currently no WADA restrictions on therapy and no rules governing return to play (26).

POSTERIOR PITUITARY HORMONES

- The posterior pituitary is a collection of axons that extend from the hypothalamus producing, among other hormones, antidiuretic hormone (ADH).
- ADH plays an important role in maintaining the body's osmotic balance, blood pressure regulation, sodium homeostasis, and kidney function (41).
- ADH maintains serum osmolality between 280 and 295 mOsm · kg^{-1} H_2O by adjusting the kidney's ability to reabsorb water. Secretion of ADH is initiated by small changes in serum osmolality.
- ADH secretion is also stimulated by hypovolemia — low blood pressure is sensed by baroreceptors in the aortic arch, left atrium, and carotid arteries, which stimulates the vagus nerve and promotes the secretion of ADH. This response to hypovolemia will occur even in hypoosmotic states.
- Other factors, such as nausea, stress, pain, hypoxia, angiotensin II, hypoglycemia, and many medications, including nonsteroidal anti-inflammatory drugs (NSAIDs), sensitize the kidneys to ADH and are also commonly implicated in stimulation of ADH secretion (41).
- ADH acts on antidiuretic receptors in the collecting duct of the kidney, causing an increase in permeability of the plasma membrane and reabsorption of water in the kidney, creating concentrated urine to conserve water. ADH also acts on vascular smooth muscle, increasing total peripheral vascular resistance, and increasing blood pressure.

- A number of clinical conditions result in a condition of vasopressin excess, otherwise known as the syndrome of inappropriate antidiuretic hormone (SIADH). With this excess, a surplus of free water results, leading to hyponatremia and subsequent neurologic and metabolic disturbances.

Exercise-Associated Hyponatremia

- Exercise-Associated Hyponatremia (EAH) is diagnosed when a serum sodium level below 135 mmol · L^{-1} develops during or up to 24 hours after physical activity (42,43).
- The current practice of aggressive fluid replacement with water or hypotonic sports drinks in excess of typical and insensible fluid loss seems to play a role.
- Sweat sodium is hypotonic to serum sodium, thus fluid needs during exercise are likely overestimated by athletes who develop EAH.
- The majority of hypervolemic EAH cases results from overdrinking associated with abnormal fluid retention from exercise-induced inappropriate ADH secretion (43).
- Hypovolemic EAH is, in part, caused by sustained sweat sodium losses stimulated by ADH secretion, although the amount of sodium lost is minor.
- Sweat becomes the primary source of water and electrolyte loss during exercise above 50% VO2max. This is due to exercise-induced increases in renin and ADH. This increases the potential for electrolyte abnormalities during prolonged exercise.
- Euvolemic EAH is mediated by SIADH, where nonosmotic ADH is secreted in response to nausea/vomiting, serum volume contraction, high temperatures, hypoglycemia, inflammatory mediators, or other endocrine mediators. This decreases urinary excretion to improve plasma volume.
- Many athletes with hyponatremia are asymptomatic, whereas others look pale and have weakness, dizziness, headache, nausea, muscle cramps, fatigue, puffiness, irritability, and subtle changes in mental status. Symptoms can progress in severity to agitation, dyspnea, altered mental status, phantom running, seizures, coma, and decorticate posturing.
- When sodium is rapidly lowered, water crosses the blood-brain barrier seeking to equilibrate tonicity across the membrane. The resulting influx of water causes swelling and an increased cerebral pressure, which explains many of the neurologic symptoms accompanying hyponatremia. Given enough time, typically 24 hours, the brain can shunt water and electrolytes to the cerebrospinal fluid, restoring balance (43).

Risk Factors

- History of overdrinking, prolonged endurance exercise, event inexperience, high fluid availability, warmer ambient conditions, high or low BMI, and slower event times.

Diagnosis

- Hypervolemic/euvolemic EAH: Body weight gain, serum sodium level below 135 mmol · L^{-1}, low BUN, urine sodium above 30 mmol · L^{-1}.
- Hypovolemic EAH: Body weight loss, elevated BUN, urinary sodium below 30 mmol · L^{-1}.

Treatment

- Asymptomatic and mild EAH: fluid restriction and observation or oral administration of hypertonic saline solution (4 bouillon cubes in 125 mL of water or 100 mL of 3% saline with flavoring) until the onset of urination.
- Moderate EAH: favor treating with oral administration of hypertonic saline solution rather than observation and fluid restriction.
- Severe EAH is a medical emergency, and these patients should be transferred to the nearest medical facility. These individuals often need 3% saline to rapidly correct a portion of the sodium deficit in the setting of life-threatening neurologic disorders. Central pontine myelinolysis (osmotic demyelination) is not observed with rapid correction of EAH, as this is an acute hyponatremia and the brain has not adapted to the changes in serum sodium.
- Unless clearly hypovolemic EAH, normal saline should be avoided as it is isotonic.
- Currently, there is insufficient evidence to support the suggestion that ingestion of sodium prevents or decreases the risk for EAH.
- Sodium consumption during exercise does not prevent EAH. There is a large variation between individuals and the rate at which they lose sodium and water during exercise (44).
- Armstrong (44) advised that the aim of rehydration should be to consume a volume of fluid that avoids dehydration (weight loss of >4%). A goal of 400–800 mL · h^{-1} of fluid intake has been recommended as a baseline but must be individualized.

Return to Play

- There are no strict rules governing return to play following EAH. Clearly, a more appropriate fluid management strategy and close monitoring should be employed in subsequent events.

SEX HORMONES

Estrogen

- Estrogens are a group of steroid hormones that are manufactured in the ovaries and, in small amounts, in the male testes plus the adrenal glands, brain, and fat.
- Luteinizing hormone (LH) stimulates the production of androstenedione from cholesterol, which is then converted to estradiol. In fat, liver, muscle, and brain cells, estrogen is also created through aromatization, under the direction of follicle-stimulating hormone (FSH), converting androgens

to estrogens (45). Estrogen is a regulatory factor in the female menstrual cycle, contributes to the development of secondary sexual characteristics, reduces bone resorption, increases clotting of blood, and decreases both LDL cholesterol and fat deposits (46). Please refer to Chapter 131, The Female Athlete for more details.

Testosterone

- Testosterone is the predominant male sex hormone that is primarily produced in Leydig cells of the testicle and its production is regulated by LH.
- DHEA and androstenedione are precursors to testosterone and have a weak androgenic effect. Testosterone is anabolic and leads to muscle growth by increasing synthesis and limiting breakdown of protein. It also contributes to the development of male secondary sex characteristics (47).
- Hypogonadism refers to a decrease in one or both of the major functions of the testes: sperm production or testosterone production. Testosterone deficiency prior to puberty results in underdeveloped genitals and failure to complete puberty. In adults, symptoms may include low energy, decreased libido, and depressed mood. Manifestations such as muscle weakness and hair loss typically do not develop for a few years (48).

Diagnosis

- Total testosterone (drawn between 8 and 10 a.m.), LH and FSH, and TSH are reasonable first steps in making the diagnosis. For the purpose of WADA and a TUE, interpretation and evaluation by an endocrinologist is preferred.

Treatment

- Testosterone can be given as an injection 50–100 mg IM every week or 100–200 mg IM every 2 weeks, applied daily to skin in gel form (50–100 mg of 1% concentration), or applied as a 2- to 6-mg daily patch. Serial total testosterone levels are needed to monitor efficacy (49).

Therapeutic Use Exemption

- A TUE for testosterone replacement is required in the setting of appropriately diagnosed hypogonadism and requires an organic etiology as opposed to a functional disorder.
- TUE is subject to yearly review.
- Given the potential controversy associated with the use of testosterone, management by an endocrinologist and the opinion of an independent expert are strongly recommended (26).

Return to Play

- There are no restrictions on return to play.

Testosterone Misuse

- A large Centers for Disease Control and Prevention survey found that 2.9% of adolescents in high school reported taking androgenic steroids without a doctor's prescription; the prevalence was higher among male (3.3%) students compared to female (2.4%) (50). It can be challenging to determine which athletes are using these drugs.
- With testosterone, especially at supratherapeutic doses, there is an increase in lean body mass through hypertrophy of existing muscle fibers and through growth of new fibers. This is accomplished through enhanced protein synthesis, interactions with GH, and inhibition of cortisol's catabolic actions.
- Studies have demonstrated associations with a number of different adverse effects including, but not limited to, dyslipidemia and increased coronary atherosclerotic burden, increased thrombosis, increased likelihood of ventricular arrhythmias, impaired insulin sensitivity, aggressive behavior, and increased practice of other high-risk behaviors (51).
- Androstenedione and DHEA are precursors to testosterone and have been utilized by athletes for performance, although there is little evidence to support any clinical significance. Androstenedione does not have an anabolic effect like testosterone, and it does not increase testosterone levels. DHEA is available over the counter as a supplement; it does not have any androgenic effects itself, and has been shown to increase testosterone levels in women but not men (52).

Side Effects of Androgen Misuse

- Gynecomastia, virilization, acne, and deepening of the voice are some of the cosmetic complications of testosterone.
- Testicular atrophy is a result of the inhibition of natural testosterone production by high exogenous concentrations through negative feedback. Some will try to combat this by using human chorionic gonadotropin (52).
- Hepatotoxicity, cardiomyopathies, and mood disorders have also been described as complications from exogenous androgenic steroid use (52).
- In young athletes, testosterone may stimulate premature epiphyseal fusion, resulting in short stature.

Drug Testing

- Androgens other than testosterone can be detected by gas chromatography and mass spectrometry.
- It is not currently possible to distinguish between exogenous and endogenous testosterone. The conventional method is to determine the urinary ratio of testosterone to epitestosterone glucuronide (T/E ratio), which ranges from 1:1 to 3:1 (52).
  - Supplemented testosterone will increase the ratio to 6:1 or higher, although WADA considers misuse when the ratio is greater than 4:1 (52).
  - However, this test is limited by genetic differences in testosterone metabolism (52).
- Measuring the ratio of carbon 13 to carbon 12 in urinary metabolites of testosterone is considered the most accurate method, and a low 13 C:12 C ratio is suspicious for exogenous use (52).

REFERENCES

1. Mantzoros C, Serdy S. Insulin action. In: Post, TW, editor. *UpToDate*. Waltham (MA): UpToDate; 2022.
2. Cryer P. Hypoglycemia in adults with diabetes mellitus. In: Post, TW, editor. *UpToDate*. Waltham (MA): UpToDate; 2022.
3. Levitsky L, Madhusmita M. Hypoglycemia in children and adolescents with type 1 diabetes mellitus. In: Post TW, editor. *UpToDate*. Waltham (MA): UpToDate; 2022.
4. Therapeutic Use Exemptions [Internet]. *World Anti Doping Agency*. WADA; 2022 [cited 2022 Nov 17]. Available from: https://www.wada-ama.org/en/what-we-do/science-medicine/therapeutic-use-exemptions
5. Yurkewicz M, Cordas M Jr, Zellers A, Sweger M. Diabetes and sports: managing your athlete with type 1 diabetes. *Am J Lifestyle Med*. 2017;11(1):58–63. doi:10.1177/1559827615583648
6. Mendes R, Sousa N, Reis VM, Themudo-Barata JL. Prevention of exercise-related injuries and adverse events in patients with type 2 diabetes. *Postgrad Med J*. 2013 Dec;89(1058):715–21. doi:10.1136/postgradmedj-2013-132222
7. Lotfi CFP, Kremer JL, Dos Santos Passaia B, Cavalcante IP. The human adrenal cortex: growth control and disorders. *Clinics (Sao Paulo)*. 2018 Sep 6;73(suppl 1):e473s.
8. Hannibal KE, Bishop MD. Chronic stress, cortisol dysfunction, and pain: a psychoneuroendocrine rationale for stress management in pain rehabilitation. *Phys Ther*. 2014 Dec;94(12):1816–25.
9. Schilbach K, Junnila RK, Bidlingmaier M. Aldosterone to renin ratio as screening tool in primary aldosteronism. *Exp Clin Endocrinol Diabetes*. 2019 Feb;127(2-03):84–92.
10. Funder JW, Carey RM, Mantero F, et al. The management of primary aldosteronism: case detection, diagnosis, and treatment—an endocrine society clinical practice guideline. *J Clin Endocrinol Metab*. 2016 May;101(5):1889–916.
11. Nieman LK, Lacroix A, Martin KA. *Diagnosis of Adrenal Insufficiency in Adults*. UpToDate [Internet]. 2022. Available from: https://pubmed.ncbi.nlm.nih.gov/?term=the+diganosis+of+adrenal+insufficiency+in+adults&filter=datesearch.y_5
12. Husebye ES, Pearce SH, Krone NP, Kämpe O. Adrenal insufficiency. *Lancet*. 2021 Feb 13;397(10274):613–29.
13. World Antidoping Agency [Internet]. *TUE Physician Guidelines - Adrenal Insufficiency. Version 7.0*. February 2022. [cited 2023 Jan 1]. Available from: https://www.wada-ama.org/sites/default/files/2022-02/02.%20TUE%20Physician%20Guidelines_Adrenal%20Insufficiency_Final%20%28February%202022%29.pdf
14. Sellami M, Slimeni O, Pokrywka A, et al. Herbal medicine for sports: a review. *J Int Soc Sports Nutr*. 2018 Mar 15;15:14.
15. Jameson JL, Mandel SJ, Weetman AP. Thyroid gland physiology and testing. In: Loscalzo J, Fauci A, Kasper D, Hauser S, Longo D, Jameson JL, editors. *Harrison's Principles of Internal Medicine*. 21st ed. New York (NY): McGraw-Hill Education; 2022.
16. Esfandiari NH, McPhee SJ. Thyroid disease. In: Hammer GD, McPhee SJ, editors. *Pathophysiology of Disease: An Introduction to Clinical Medicine*. 8th ed. New York (NY): McGraw-Hill Education; 2019.
17. Sindoni A, Rodolico C, Pappalardo MA, Portaro S, Benvenga S. Hypothyroid myopathy: a peculiar clinical presentation of thyroid failure. Review of the literature. *Rev Endocr Metab Disord*. 2016;17(4):499–519. doi:10.1007/s11154-016-9357-0
18. Klein I. Cardiovascular effects of hypothyroidism. In: Post TW, editor. *UpToDate*. Waltham (MA): UpToDate; 2022.
19. Bartz S, Chan CM, Cree-Green M, Davis S, Hsu S. Endocrine disorders. In: Bunik M, Hay WW, Levin MJ, Abzug MJ, editors. *Current Diagnosis & Treatment: Pediatrics*. 26th ed. New York (NY): McGraw-Hill Education; 2022.
20. Jameson JL, Mandel SJ, Weetman AP. Hypothyroidism. In: Loscalzo J, Fauci A, Kasper D, Hauser S, Longo D, Jameson JL, editors. *Harrison's Principles of Internal Medicine*. 21st ed. New York (NY): McGraw-Hill Education; 2022.
21. Jameson JL, Mandel SJ, Weetman AP. Hyperthyroidism and other causes of thyrotoxicosis. In: Loscalzo J, Fauci A, Kasper D, Hauser S, Longo D, Jameson JL, editors. *Harrison's Principles of Internal Medicine*. 21st ed. New York (NY): McGraw-Hill Education; 2022.
22. Luksch JR, Collins PB. Thyroid disorders in athletes. *Curr Sports Med Rep*. 2018;17(2):59–64. doi:10.1249/jsr.0000000000000452
23. Baranowska-Bik A, Bik W. The association of obesity with autoimmune thyroiditis and thyroid function-possible mechanisms of bilateral interaction. *Int J Endocrinol*. 2020 Dec 14;2020:8894792. doi:10.1155/2020/8894792
24. Ross DS. Exogenous hyperthyroidism. In: Post TW, editor. *UpToDate*. Waltham (MA): UpToDate; 2022.
25. Ross DS. Diagnosis of hyperthyroidism. In: Post TW, editor. *UpToDate*. Waltham (MA): UpToDate; 2022.
26. The Prohibited List [Internet]. *World Anti Doping Agency*. WADA; 2022 [cited 2022 Nov 17]. Available from: https://www.wada-ama.org/en/prohibited-list
27. Siebert DM, Rao AL. The use and abuse of human growth hormone in sports. *Sports Health*. 2018 Sep/Oct;10(5):419–26.
28. Aguiar-Oliveira MH, Bartke A. Growth hormone deficiency: health and longevity. *Endocr Rev*. 2019 Apr 1;40(2):575–601.
29. World Antidoping Agency [Internet]. *TUE Physician Guidelines—Growth Hormone Deficiency and Other Indications for Growth Hormone Therapy. Version 2.1*. October 2022. [cited 2023 Jan 1]. Available from: https://www.wada-ama.org/sites/default/files/2022-11/tue_physician_guidelines_growth_hormone_deficiency_children_and_adolescent_final_november_20221.pdf
30. World Antidoping Agency [Internet]. *TUE Physician Guidelines—Growth Hormone Deficiency. Version 2.2*. 2020 Jul. [cited 2023 Jan 1]. Available from: https://www.wada-ama.org/sites/default/files/resources/files/tue_physician_guideline_ghadult_version2.1_july2020.pdf
31. Anderson LJ, Tamayose JM, Garcia JM. Use of growth hormone, IGF-I, and insulin for anabolic purpose: pharmacological basis, methods of detection, and adverse effects. *Mol Cell Endocrinol*. 2018 Mar 15;464:65–74.
32. Goltzman D. Physiology of parathyroid hormone. *Endocrinol Metab Clin North Am*. 2018 Dec;47(4):743–58.
33. Yun Leung EK. Parathyroid hormone. In: Makowski GS, editor. *Advances in Clinical Chemistry*. Vol. 101. 1st ed. Cambridge (MA): Academic Press; 2021. p. 42–73.
34. Pazirandeh S, Burns DL. Overview of vitamin D. In: Post TD, editor. *UpToDate*. Waltham (MA): UpToDate; 2022.
35. Miller JR, Dunn KW, Ciliberti LJ Jr, Patel RD, Swanson BA. Association of vitamin D with stress fractures: a retrospective cohort study. *J Foot Ankle Surg*. 2016 Jan-Feb;55(1):117–20. doi:10.1053/j.jfas.2015.08.002
36. Montenegro KR, Cruzat V, Carlessi R, Newsholme P. Mechanisms of vitamin D action in skeletal muscle. *Nutr Res Rev*. 2019 Dec;32(2):192–204. doi:10.1017/S0954422419000064
37. Millward D, Root AD, Dubois J, et al. Association of serum vitamin D levels and stress fractures in collegiate athletes. *Orthop J Sports Med*. 2020 Dec 9;8(12):2325967120966967. doi:10.1177/2325967120966967

38. Cohen A, Drake MT. Epidemiology and etiology of osteomalacia. In: Post TD, editor. *UpToDate*. Waltham (MA): UpToDate; 2022.
39. Cohen A, Drake MT. Clinical manifestations, diagnosis, and treatment of osteomalacia. In: Post TD, editor. *UpToDate*. Waltham (MA): UpToDate; 2022.
40. Dawson-Hughes B. Vitamin D deficiency in adults: definition, clinical manifestations, and treatment. In: Post TD, editor. *UpToDate*. Waltham (MA): UpToDate; 2022.
41. Cuzzo B, Padala SA, Lappin SL. Physiology, vasopressin. [2022 Aug 22]. In: *StatPearls* [Internet]. Treasure Island (FL): StatPearls Publishing; 2022 Jan.
42. Buck E, Miles R, Schroeder JD. Exercise-associated hyponatremia. [2022 Aug 9]. In: *StatPearls* [Internet]. Treasure Island (FL): StatPearls Publishing; 2022 Jan.
43. Hew-Butler T. Exercise-associated hyponatremia. *Front Horm Res.* 2019;52:178–89.
44. Armstrong LE. Rehydration during endurance exercise: challenges, research, options, methods. *Nutrients.* 2021 Mar 9;13(3):887.
45. Barrett KE, Barman SM, Brooks HL, Yuan JXJ. Reproductive development & function of the female reproductive system. In: *Ganong's Review of Medical Physiology*. 26th ed. New York (NY): McGraw-Hill Education; 2019.
46. Bubier C. The reproductive system. In: Janson LW, Tischler ME, editors. *The Big Picture: Medical Biochemistry*. New York (NY): McGraw-Hill Education; 2018.
47. Barrett KE, Barman SM, Brooks HL, Yuan JXJ. Function of the male reproductive system. In: *Ganong's Review of Medical Physiology*. 26th ed. New York (NY): McGraw-Hill Education; 2019.
48. Snyder PJ. Clinical features and diagnosis of male hypogonadism. In: Post TD, editor. *UpToDate*. Waltham (MA): UpToDate; 2022.
49. Snyder PJ. Testosterone treatment of male hypogonadism. In: Post TD, editor. *UpToDate*. Waltham, MA: UpToDate; 2022.
50. Kann L, McManus T, Harris WA, et al. Youth risk behavior surveillance—United States, 2017. *MMWR Surveill Summ.* 2018; 67(8):1–114.
51. Bhasin S. Men's health. In: Loscalzo J, Fauci A, Kasper D, Hauser S, Longo D, Jameson JL, editors. *Harrison's Principles of Internal Medicine*. 21st ed. New York (NY): McGraw-Hill Education; 2022.
52. Snyder PJ. Use of androgens and other hormones by athletes. In: Post TD, editor. *UpToDate*. Waltham (MA): UpToDate; 2022.

Hematology in the Athlete

39

William B. Adams and Preston DeHan

INTRODUCTION

- Athletes as a group tend to be healthier, but they are still susceptible to the same hematologic diseases as nonathletes. However, symptoms from hematologic disturbances may manifest earlier and at lower severity, often presenting as impaired physical performance (1,2).
- Maximal or prolonged exertion efforts typically cause transient changes in several hematologic indices. Regular endurance and altitude training generally results in more sustained alterations of hematologic parameters. Dietary inadequacies, not uncommon in athletes, may cause hematologic problems because of a deficit of calories or critical nutrients (1–5).

ANEMIA

- Anemia is a deficiency of total red blood cell (RBC) mass that manifests as RBC volume (hematocrit [Hct] or hemoglobin [Hb]) concentration below normal values. Symptoms and physical manifestations depend on reduction in RBC volume, the decrement in oxygen delivery to tissues, the rate at which these changes occur, and compensatory capacity of the cardiopulmonary system (1,6).
  - Prevalence in US males: 3.5% overall, 0.8% in those ages 15–29, and highest of 26.3% in adults 80–85 (6).
  - Prevalence in US nonpregnant women of all ages is 7.5%. Black women have anemia at rates 4–7 times that of white women and Hispanics noted to have anemia at rates 2–3 times that of whites, with a higher proportion (24%) of black women having anemia. Prevalence in all women ages 19–40 is 8% (6).
  - Anemia arises from either excessive loss or inadequate production of RBCs or a combination of both (6–8).
  - Athletes trying to restrict weight or follow special diets that are deficient in iron, vitamins, or calories may have a higher prevalence of anemia (3,5).

ATHLETIC PSEUDOANEMIA

- Regular consistent aerobic or endurance-level training causes an increase in both RBC production and plasma volume; however, plasma volume expansion typically exceeds the increase in RBC mass, causing a slight reduction in Hb and Hct in the resting state. This condition, common in athletes, is not a true anemia but rather a physiologic adaptation that promotes increased cardiac output and enhanced oxygen delivery to tissues and protects against hyperviscosity (1).
  - Plasma volume can decrease 5%–20% with endurance exercise (sweat losses and intravascular fluid shifts) (9).
  - Conditioned endurance athletes tend to have greater transient reductions in plasma volume as a result of greater sweat losses.
  - Hb values typically run 0.5 $g \cdot dL^{-1}$ lower for athletes regularly pursuing moderate-intensity training and 1.0 $g \cdot dL^{-1}$ lower for elite-level athletes (9,10).
  - Diagnosis may be confirmed by the following:
    - Retesting the athlete after several days of rest from training as the hemodilution of conditioning reverses within days of terminating endurance-level training (10,11).
    - The following laboratory findings are consistent with pseudoanemia:
      - Normal RBC indices and reticulocyte distribution width (RDW) on complete blood count (CBC)
      - Normal reticulocyte count
      - Normal serum ferritin level

IRON DEFICIENCY ANEMIA

- In the United States, iron deficiency affects 3%–5% of premenopausal women, and iron deficiency without anemia affects 16% of women (12). Compared to their sedentary counterparts, active women are twice as susceptible to iron deficiency without anemia (13,14). This is important because iron deficiency has been demonstrated to impact oxidative metabolism and physical performance (15). In addition to menstrual bleeding in the female athlete, iron deficiency may be secondary to gastrointestinal (GI) losses, poor dietary intake, and altered intestinal absorption (16).
- Laboratory testing reveals a low Hb and Hct with low mean corpuscular volume (MCV) and mean corpuscular hemoglobin.
- RDW is increased, unless iron deficiency is longstanding.

- Peripheral smear reveals hypochromic microcytic cells with a low-to-normal reticulocyte count.
- Serum ferritin levels are low, typically <12 μg · L^{-1} (note, however, that ferritin levels of 12–35 μg · L^{-1} may reflect inadequate iron stores with associated decrement in athletic performance without anemia manifesting) (3).
- Total iron-binding capacity (TIBC) tends to be elevated.
- Transferrin saturation (serum iron × 100/TIBC) tends to be low (particularly <16%) (16).

ANEMIA FROM BLOOD LOSS

- Anemia may arise from acute bleeding or massive hemolysis, as well as chronic cumulative losses from insidious bleeding or persistent accelerated destruction of RBCs (1,17,18). Acute hemorrhage is typically obvious from history or examination findings of gross blood, melena, or manifestations of hypovolemia. Bleeding contained within tissues or the body cavity may be less obvious, particularly in the retroperitoneal space. Characteristics of rapid blood loss include the following:
  - Hb and Hct (both concentration values) are initially normal in the absence of any fluid administration (19).
  - Platelet counts initially drop with hemorrhage but become elevated within 1 hour if hemorrhage stops (19).
  - Hb and Hct values decline over the ensuing days with plasma volume expansion.
  - RBC indices are initially normal. After 3–5 days, MCV and RDW start to increase because of reticulocyte response (20).
  - Bilirubin levels are normal unless bleeding is internal. Similar to hemolysis, internal bleeding causes a rise in unconjugated bilirubin and lactate dehydrogenase (LDH) but without evidence of hemolysis on peripheral smear.
- If blood loss is slow and insidious, as in chronic low-grade GI bleeding or menstrual blood loss in women, anemia may not manifest until iron stores are depleted. This situation may be revealed by a reticulocytosis with concomitant increase in RDW well before iron stores are depleted and MCV becomes low.
- **GI blood loss:** GI bleeding is a very common and often serious cause of anemia. It may arise from peptic ulcer disease, vascular anomalies, inflammatory bowel diseases, ischemic bowel syndromes, infection, diverticula, or tumors. Thus, stool occult blood testing is indicated in any anemia evaluation (21). Note that it is not uncommon for athletes to manifest mild transient GI bleeding from marathons and similar endurance events (exercise-associated GI bleeding — see Chapter 41, Gastroenterology).
- Features of exercise-associated GI bleeding include the following:
  - Occurs exclusively with prolonged endurance events and is low grade (22,23).
  - Source of bleeding is seldom detectable; it is theorized to arise from acute transient ischemia or mechanical contusion (*e.g.*, cecal slap syndrome) (22,23).
  - In the absence of this or other pathology, bleeding is seldom significant enough to cause anemia (23).
- Note that regular use of nonsteroidal anti-inflammatory drugs (NSAIDs) is common among athletes. In addition to NSAID-induced acute GI bleeding, chronic use may cause enough insidious blood loss over time to impact RBC mass (24,25). All GI bleeding warrants thorough investigation to rule out serious causes.
- **Menstrual blood loss:** Menstrual bleeding with concomitant loss of iron coupled with inadequate iron replacement is a common cause of anemia in women. When evaluating any woman for anemia, the provider should estimate the volume of menstrual blood loss and adequacy of iron replacement. Treatment is focused on reduction of menstrual flow if excessive and enhancing iron replacement. Clues for significant iron losses through menstruation include the following:
  - Heavy and/or frequent menses
  - Twelve or more soaked pads throughout menses
  - Passage of clots beyond the first day
  - Flow greater than 7 days
  - More than one episode of menstrual flow per month
  - Diet inadequate to compensate for cumulative menstrual losses (*e.g.*, low intake of dietary iron sources) (17)
- **Exertional hemolysis (i.e., foot-strike hemolysis):** Intravascular destruction of RBCs may occur in association with various exertional activities. Originally described as "march hemoglobinuria" in foot soldiers in the late 1800s, it was thought to arise from the foot strike causing compression of capillaries and rupturing RBCs; however, it is also seen in swimmers, rowers, and weightlifters, although usually to a much lesser degree. It is now hypothesized that intravascular turbulence, acidosis, and elevated temperature in muscle tissues may be causative factors as well (1,18,26).
  - Typically, hemolysis is not significant enough to affect CBC parameters (26).
  - Reticulocyte count, RDW, and MCV may be elevated (26,27).
  - Haptoglobin levels may be reduced if there is enough cumulative hemolysis (26,27).
  - Transient hemoglobinuria may occur if hemolysis exceeds the binding capacity of serum haptoglobin (approximately 20 mL of blood) (27).
- Generally, no treatment is necessary; reducing impact forces to the feet (*e.g.*, improved shoe cushioning, softer running terrain) may benefit some, particularly distance runners (18).

SICKLE CELL TRAIT

- Sickle cell trait (SCT), the heterozygous state where Hb S is present with Hb A in RBCs, is a common condition. It typically does not cause anemia and causes little impairment of athletic performance (28). In symptomatic cases, collapse from exertional sickling can often be confused with sudden collapse from heatstroke, exercise-associated muscle cramping, or cardiac dysrhythmias. It is important to note that exertional sickling may be typified as soft or flaccid muscles, weakness, and pain (28–30). See Table 39.1.

- Present in 7%–9% of blacks in the United States (31).
- May confer heightened risk of complications with exercise at altitude: Sickling may be provoked in hypoxic environments, particularly altitudes above 10,000 ft, and cause a clinical picture similar to sickle cell anemia. Vigorous exertion at altitudes of 5000 ft or more may result in enough hypoxic and metabolic stress to induce sickling and its sequelae (30).
- Epidemiologic data suggest an increased risk of sudden death in heat stress environments and settings of rapid accelerated conditioning and sustained maximal exertion efforts (30,32).
- Sickle cell trait and exertional collapse (ECAST) is further discussed in Chapter 17, Catastrophic Sports Injury.

ERYTHROCYTHEMIA (POLYCYTHEMIA)

- RBC mass may be increased as a physiologic response to hypoxic stress, disease processes, or drug use. Smoking, carbon monoxide exposure (*e.g.*, ice rinks), and training at altitude may also increase RBC mass in athletes. A spurious erythrocytosis may also arise from transient plasma volume contraction (*e.g.*, exercise, dehydrated status) (28). True polycythemia arises from conditions of excess RBC production, either as part of a hyperplastic marrow response (polycythemia vera) or secondary response to excess erythropoietin production (secondary polycythemia).

ETIOLOGIES OF ERYTHROCYTOSIS

- **Pseudoerythrocytosis:** Patient in a dehydrated state when phlebotomy is performed.
- **Polycythemia vera:** A myeloproliferative disorder involving trilineage marrow hyperplasia. RBC mass increase is associated with leukocytosis and thrombocytosis. Erythropoietin levels are low, with markedly elevated Hct. These patients require regular phlebotomy to prevent a hyperviscosity state (33).
- **Secondary erythrocytosis:** Results from intrinsic elevated erythropoietin or excess erythrocyte production (34).
  - Hypoxic stress
  - Endogenous conditions of excessive erythropoietin production
  - Endogenous conditions of isolated excess erythrocyte production
- **Blood doping**
  - Transfusion (phlebotomy later followed with autologous blood transfusion).
  - Exogenous erythropoietin characterized by elevated RBC and erythropoietin levels with normal white blood cell (WBC) and platelet counts (35,36). Erythropoietin produced by recombinant DNA techniques is identical to endogenous human erythropoietin, making detection difficult (37,38).

WBC LINE ABNORMALITIES

- Strenuous or prolonged vigorous exercise may acutely produce profound transient perturbations of WBC populations. This effect, however, resolves with rest and is not typically associated with persistent abnormalities of WBC lines. Various drugs may either elevate or depress WBC production, as may infection. Persistent leukopenia may be indicative of human immunodeficiency virus infection or marrow disorders. Some populations (*e.g.*, black males) may manifest a mild neutropenia that is nonpathologic (39).
- If blood work indicates a pathologic alteration of the WBC population, examination should include a thorough assessment of lymphatic and hematologic systems with investigation for infectious, toxic, or oncologic causes.
- Readily treatable etiologies, such as infection, are addressed as indicated. Otherwise, referral to a hematologist for bone marrow assessment may be necessary, particularly if there is profound leukopenia, leukocytosis, or disturbances of other cell lines suggestive of malignancy (40).

Table 39.1 Differentiating Features of Common Causes of Exertional Collapse

ECAST	Muscle Cramping	Exertional Heatstroke	Cardiac Collapse
Slumps to the Ground	Hobbles to a Halt	Variable from Bizarre Behavior to Collapse	Falls like a Rock
Weakness > Pain	Pain > Weakness	Fuzzy Thinking	No Cramping
Can talk at First	Yelling in Pain	Variable Cognitive Dysfunction	Unconscious
Muscles Normal	Muscles Locked Up	Variable	Flaccid or Seizing
Temp <103 F	Temp <103	Temp >104	Temp Nonspecific
Can Occur Early in Exercise	Usually Occurs Later in Exercise	Usually Occurs Later in Exercise	Limited to No Warning

Source: Eichner ER, Anderson S. Exertional sickling. In: Casa DJ, editor. *Preventing Sudden Death in Sport and Physical Activity*. Sudbury (MA): Jones & Bartlett Learning; 2012. p. 131–41.

ABNORMALITIES OF PLATELETS AND COAGULATION

- The effects of exercise, particularly endurance activities, seem to have a net neutral effect on platelets and coagulation. Athletes manifesting petechiae, unusual bruising, or bleeding problems should undergo prompt investigation for causes of these disorders. Longstanding history of mild prolonged bleeding, slow clotting, or bruising problems may indicate von Willebrand disease or mild factor VIII or IX deficiency (41). Some medications such as aspirin-containing compounds, often a component in analgesics, directly or indirectly impair platelet or clotting activity. Disseminated intravascular coagulation (DIC) may be induced by autoimmune disorders, infections, certain drugs, toxins, malignancies, and other conditions, resulting in thrombocytopenia ranging from mild to severe (42). Diets deficient in green vegetables may manifest coagulopathy because of impairment of vitamin K–dependent factors (43).
- Evaluation of platelet and coagulation disorders focuses on assessment for causative conditions as listed earlier. Laboratory assessment should start with a CBC with peripheral smear looking for abnormalities in all hematologic cell lines. Coagulation studies (prothrombin time [PT], partial thromboplastin time [PTT], and international normalized ratio) should be conducted as well. If the clinical picture suggests DIC (low platelets, fragmented RBCs, and prolonged coagulation times), confirmatory testing to include fibrinogen, fibrin split products, and D-dimer should be added (42).
- Thrombocytosis is often a transient condition, typically a manifestation of an acute response to physiologic stress. Transient isolated thrombocytosis is rarely of significance. Persistent thrombocytosis should prompt investigation for infection, inflammatory disorders, malignancies, or other hyperproliferative disorders (*e.g.*, polycythemia vera, myeloproliferative diseases) (44,45).

OTHER DISORDERS CAUSING ANEMIA/ CELL LINE ABNORMALITIES

- Anemia and other cell line abnormalities may result from several other conditions, such as inherited disorders (*e.g.*, thalassemia), or as a consequence of various disease processes. These may manifest in the form of accelerated cell destruction or hemolysis or through impaired erythropoiesis. Details regarding diagnosis and evaluation of these conditions may be found in hematology reference books (46).

EXERTIONAL RHABDOMYOLYSIS

- Rhabdomyolysis is a condition of skeletal muscle breakdown with release of myocyte contents into the circulation. Exertional rhabdomyolysis is the term applied to rhabdomyolysis precipitated by exercise or exertion. It is most frequently seen in running or prolonged exertional activity, particularly in settings of accelerated physical training. Often, it occurs with exertional heat illness (47–49). Biochemically, muscle injury causes a release of myoglobin and muscle enzymes — creatine phosphokinase (CPK), LDH, and transaminases. Severe states with a large volume of muscle damage typically cause electrolyte disturbances (potassium, phosphate, and calcium) plus extracellular fluid shifts into injured tissues. Various extrinsic and intrinsic factors may enhance susceptibility to rhabdomyolysis (47–49). These include the following:
  - Drug or toxin exposure (*e.g.*, stimulants, antihistamines, alcohol, ephedra, and statin drugs)
  - Infection
  - Heatstroke
  - Dehydration
  - Excessive muscle overload activities (especially eccentric loading)
  - Genetic muscle diseases/enzyme deficiencies
  - Metabolic diseases or disorders (diabetes, thyroid disease, chronic electrolyte disorders, or acidosis)
  - SCT
  - Autoimmune disorders (*e.g.*, polymyositis)
  - Deconditioned state (especially with rapidly accelerated physical training)
- Exertional rhabdomyolysis is a spectrum condition. Manifestations range from mild muscle injury with negligible symptoms or systemic effects to fulminate cases with large muscle mass injury, severe metabolic derangements, DIC, and death (47–50). Myoglobin release may cause nephrotoxicity, but occurrence may not directly correlate with the degree of muscle enzyme elevation or severity of metabolic disturbance. Severity of rhabdomyolysis is gauged initially by magnitude of symptoms and early perturbations of blood chemistries. Collapse short of a finish line, severe pain with inability to walk, and early sustained acidosis are ominous indicators. Alternately, symptoms may start off relatively mild but progressively worsen in subsequent hours or days. Muscle enzyme levels following insult may be deceptively low early on but subsequently rise and peak 1–3 days after the injury (if there is no persistent or recurrent muscle insult).
- Management of rhabdomyolysis requires a high index of suspicion to allow for early recognition, initiation of interventions appropriate to degree of injury, and monitoring for progression. Initial laboratory studies should include basic electrolyte panel including creatinine (Cr), CPK, transaminases, LDH, uric acid, CBC, and urinalysis with microscopy. In more severe cases, calcium, phosphate, PT, PTT, fibrinogen, and fibrin split products should be added (50).
- Urinalysis demonstrating positive Hb with no RBCs is used to infer the presence of myoglobinuria because results of myoglobin tests in most settings are not available quickly enough to be of value in acute management (47–50). Muddy casts indicate heavy myoglobin load and likely renal toxicity (51).

MILD RHABDOMYOLYSIS

- Mild muscle soreness that typically resolves within 1–2 days; otherwise, no complaints.
- On examination, the patient has mild soreness to palpation and minimal to no soreness with passive muscle stretch.
- Laboratory studies reveal isolated CPK elevation (generally <3000 mg · L^{-1} but may be up to 5000 mg · L^{-1}); transaminases may peak slightly above normal in 1–2 days (generally less than 3 times normal values).
- Treat with oral hydration and avoidance of strenuous exertion for 1–2 days.
- Monitor for escalation or recurrence of symptoms; educate patients regarding preventive measures.
- Patients may return to activity the next day after becoming asymptomatic and after laboratory studies improved.

MODERATE RHABDOMYOLYSIS

- Symptoms of moderate muscle soreness or stiffness.
- On examination, the patient has moderate muscle soreness to palpation with pain toward extremes of passive stretch.
- Moderate elevation of CPK in first few hours with mild increase in Cr (1.5–2 mg · L^{-1}), LDH, aspartate aminotransferase (AST), and alanine aminotransferase (ALT) (3 times normal or more) several hours to 1 day after injury, with CPK peak typically <30,000 mg · L^{-1}; uric acid and electrolyte studies remain normal.
- Initial treatment is 2 L of intravenous (IV) isotonic fluids and assessment of response (symptoms and studies):
  - No worsening of symptoms and laboratory studies improved: Oral hydration and reevaluate in 12–24 hours.
  - Symptoms improved but laboratory studies little changed: Assess the need for further hydration; reassess every 4–6 hours until laboratory studies improve or refer for hospitalization if studies worsen or do not improve.
  - Symptoms not improving and laboratory studies rising: Refer to hospital for continued IV hydration and monitoring (watch for progression to severe or fulminant state).
  - If urine is positive for myoglobin or strongly positive for hemoglobin on urine dipstick testing, and not improving, continuous IV fluid therapy is needed (typically in hospital) for treatment of myoglobinuria.

SEVERE RHABDOMYOLYSIS

- Severe rhabdomyolysis has marked muscle soreness and pain with any muscle activity.
- Examination reveals tight muscles that are painful to palpation and limited passive stretch.
- Laboratory studies reveal transient acidosis, elevated uric acid, and minor electrolyte alterations that resolve with hydration; Cr is elevated typically >2 mg · L^{-1}; and CPK progressively rises well above 30,000 mg · L^{-1}; LDH, AST, and ALT progressively rise, peaking above 3 times normal at 2–3 days after insult.
- Treatment is IV fluids (2 L bolus); arrange for continued IV fluid therapy (150–200 mL · h^{-1}). Repeat laboratory studies after fluid bolus and then again after the next 3–4 hours of IV fluid therapy.
  - Symptoms and laboratory studies improved: Oral hydration and evaluate response over the next 12–24 hours.
  - Symptoms improved but laboratory studies little changed: Assess the adequacy of hydration and need for additional measures (*e.g.*, compartment pressure testing); reassess every 4–6 hours.
  - Symptoms not improving and laboratory studies rising: Transfer to the intensive care unit (ICU) addressing comorbid issues of electrolyte disturbances, myoglobinuria, and compartment syndrome.
  - If urine is positive for myoglobin or strongly positive for hemoglobin on urine dipstick testing, and not improving, continuous IV fluid therapy is needed at 150–200 mL · h^{-1} for treatment of myoglobinuria.
- In a subacute setting (presenting days after injury), if symptoms and labs are stable or improving, condition may be managed as moderate rhabdomyolysis with assessment for renal injury and exclusion of myoglobinuria.

FULMINANT RHABDOMYOLYSIS

- Patients often present with an initial conscious collapse with early to delayed obtundation. Extreme muscle tightness and pain with weakness and extreme difficulty moving involved muscle(s).
- Often associated with findings typical of heatstroke, shock, and dehydration (50). Fulminant rhabdomyolysis is thought to be the mechanism associated with ECAST (52).
- May manifest as progressively escalating symptoms refractory to less-aggressive interventions.
- On examination, involved muscles are tense, very tender, and extremely painful to any passive stretch.
- Initial laboratory studies collected near the time of collapse typically manifest acidosis, hypokalemia, hypocalcemia, elevated uric acid, and/or decreased phosphate. Initial CPK levels may be deceptively low. In subsequent hours, serum chemistries manifest persistent acidosis with a shift to hyperkalemia, hypercalcemia, and hyperphosphatemia with rapidly rising CPK, LDH, AST, and ALT (51).
- Treatment necessitates the early provision of oxygen, cardiac monitoring for dysrhythmias in this setting with advanced life support capability, aggressive IV fluid hydration, and transfer to the ICU for management of the metabolic derangements (53).

- Consult an orthopedic surgeon for potential fasciotomy evaluation. Mild to moderate increased compartment pressures perpetuate muscle necrosis and the condition improves with early fasciotomy of the involved muscle areas (54).

RHABDOMYOLYSIS OF AN ISOLATED MUSCLE OR MUSCLE GROUP

- Typically occurs with excessive overload in weightlifting or excessive repetition of a calisthenic exercise.
- CPK levels may become elevated into the tens of thousands.
- Typically, this is self-limited, rarely manifesting systemic effects beyond the involved muscle, although sometimes myoglobinuria may be significant enough to require treatment.

RHABDOMYOLYSIS FOLLOW-UP

- Healthy individuals with **uncomplicated** mild to moderate rhabdomyolysis may return to activity in a graduated manner after resolution of symptoms and 3 consecutive days of decline in muscle enzymes (particularly transaminases) below 50% of peak value or level back to near normal. Graduation of activity should be limited by fatigue or provocation of soreness or tightness in affected muscles. Recurrent bouts of rhabdomyolysis and any severe or fulminant episodes warrant investigation for an underlying disease process, muscle enzyme deficiencies, or underlying myopathy (52,55,56).

SUMMARY

- With the exception of athletic pseudoanemia, it is uncommon to encounter significant persistent hematologic alterations from exercise. Although high-intensity and prolonged endurance training may result in alterations of several hematologic parameters and occasional lysis of RBCs, rarely are these of pathologic significance. However, signs and symptoms of hematologic disease may manifest at an earlier state in the athlete because of physiologic demands that require maximal hematologic system performance.
- The condition of exertional rhabdomyolysis may occasionally manifest in athletes advancing training too rapidly but may also appear in a conditioned athlete in association with underlying disease states or as a consequence of severe overexertion or exertional heat illness. Identification and early treatment of those with myoglobin release or severe myocyte injury are crucial to preclude serious complications.

REFERENCES

1. Damian MT, Vulturar R, Login CC, Damian L, Chis A, Bojan A. Anemia in sports: a narrative review. *Life (Basel)*. 2021 Sep 20;11(9):987. doi:10.3390/life11090987
2. Akabas SR, Dolins KR. Micronutrient requirements of physically active women: what can we learn from iron? *Am J Clin Nutr*. 2005;81(5):1246S–51S.
3. Lukaski HC. Vitamin and mineral status: effects on physical performance. *Nutrition*. 2004;20(7-8):632–44.
4. Rodriguez NR, Dimarco NM, Langley S. American Dietetic Association position statement: nutrition and athletic performance—vitamins and minerals [Internet]. [cited 2010]. Available from: http://www.medscape.com/viewarticle/717046
5. Sim M, Garvican-Lewis LA, Cox GR, et al. Iron considerations for the athlete: a narrative review. *Eur J Appl Physiol*. 2019 Jul;119(7):1463–78. doi:10.1007/s00421-019-04157-y
6. Le CH. The prevalence of anemia and moderate-severe anemia in the US population (NHANES 2003-2012). *PLoS One*. 2016 Nov 15;11(11):e0166635. doi:10.1371/journal.pone.0166635
7. Hinton PS. Iron and the endurance athlete. *Appl Physiol Nutr Metab*. 2014 Sep;39(9):1012–8. doi:10.1139/apnm-2014-0147
8. Elghetany MT, Banki K. Erythrocytic disorders. In: McPherson RA, Pincus MR, editors. *Henry's Clinical Diagnosis and Management by Laboratory Methods*. 21st ed. St. Louis (MO): Saunders; 2007. p. 504–44.
9. Varamenti E, Nikolovski Z, Elgingo MI, Jamurtas AZ, Cardinale, M. Training-induced variations in haematological and biochemical variables in adolescent athletes of Arab origin throughout an entire athletic season. *J Hum Kinet*. 2018 Oct 15;64:123–35. doi:10.1515/hukin-2017-0187
10. Schumacher YO, Garvican LA, Christian R, et al. High altitude, prolonged exercise, and the athlete biological passport. *Drug Test Anal*. 2015 Jan;7(1):48–55. doi:10.1002/dta.1717
11. Silva ASR, Santhiago V, Papoti M, Gobatto C. Hematological parameters and anaerobic threshold in Brazilian soccer players throughout a training program. *Int J Lab Hematol*. 2008;30(2):158–66. doi:10.1111/j.1751-553X.2007.00919.x
12. Cogswell ME, Looker AC, Pfeiffer CM, et al. Assessment of iron deficiency in US preschool children and nonpregnant females of childbearing age: National Health and Nutrition Examination Survey 2003-2006. *Am J Clin Nutr*. 2009;89(5):1334–42.
13. Della Valle DM, Haas JD. Iron status is associated with endurance performance and training in female rowers. *Med Sci Sports Exerc*. 2012;44(8):1552–9.
14. Sinclair L, Hinton, P. Prevalence of iron deficiency with and without anemia in recreationally active men and women. *J Am Diet Assoc*. 2005;105(6):975–8.
15. DellaValle DM. Iron supplementation for female athletes: effects on iron status and performance outcomes. *Curr Sports Med Rep*. 2013 Jul-Aug;12(4):234–9. Erratum in: *Curr Sports Med Rep*. 2013 Sep-Oct;12(5):349. doi:10.1249/JSR.0b013e31829a6f6b
16. Gaffney-Stomberg E, McClung JP. Inflammation and diminished iron status: mechanisms and functional outcomes. *Curr Opin Clin Nutr Metab Care*. 2012;15(6):605–13.
17. Bruinvels G, Burden R, Brown N, Richards T, Pedlar C. The prevalence and impact of heavy menstrual bleeding (menorrhagia) in elite and non-elite athletes. *PLoS One*. 2016 Feb 22;11(2):e0149881. doi:10.1371/journal.pone.0149881

18. Lippi G, Sanchis-Gomar F. Epidemiological, biological and clinical update on exercise-induced hemolysis. *Ann Transl Med.* 2019 Jun;7(12):270. doi:10.21037/atm.2019.05.41
19. Killeen RB, Tambe A. Acute anemia. [Updated 2023 Aug 17]. In: *StatPearls* [Internet]. Treasure Island (FL): StatPearls Publishing; 2023 Jan. Available from: https://www.ncbi.nlm.nih.gov/books/NBK537232/
20. Salvagno GL, Sanchis-Gomar F, Picanza A, Lippi G. Red blood cell distribution width: a simple parameter with multiple clinical applications. *Crit Rev Clin Lab Sci.* 2015;52(2):86–105. doi:10.3109/10408363.2014.992064
21. Milovanovic T, Dragasevic S, Nikolic AN, et al. Anemia as a problem: GP approach. *Dig Dis.* 2022;40(3):370–5. doi:10.1159/000517579
22. Packer N, Hoffman-Goetz L, Ward G. Does physical activity affect quality of life, disease symptoms and immune measures in patients with inflammatory bowel disease? A systematic review. *J Sports Med Phys Fitness.* 2010 Mar;50(1):1–18.
23. Costa RJS, Snipe RMJ, Kitic CM, Gibson PR. Systematic review: exercise-induced gastrointestinal syndrome—implications for health and intestinal disease. *Aliment Pharmacol Ther.* 2017;46(3):246–65. doi:10.1111/apt.14157
24. Van Wijck K, Lenaerts K, Van Bijnen AA, et al. Aggravation of exercise-induced intestinal injury by Ibuprofen in athletes. *Med Sci Sports Exerc.* 2012 Dec;44(12):2257–62. doi:10.1249/MSS.0b013e318265dd3d
25. Lambert GP, Boylan M, Laventure JP, Bull A, Lanspa S. Effect of aspirin and ibuprofen on GI permeability during exercise. *Int J Sports Med.* 2007 Sep;28(9):722–6. doi:10.1055/s-2007-964891
26. Lippi G, Schena F, Salvagno GL, Aloe R, Banfi G, Guidi GC. Foot-strike haemolysis after a 60-km ultramarathon. *Blood Transfus.* 2012 Jul;10(3):377–83. doi:10.2450/2012.0167-11
27. Hoffman MD, Stuempfle KJ, Fogard K, Hew-Butler T, Winger J, Weiss RH. Urine dipstick analysis for identification of runners susceptible to acute kidney injury following an ultramarathon. *J Sports Sci.* 2013;31(1):20–31. doi:10.1080/02640414.2012.720705
28. Naik RP, Haywood C Jr. Sickle cell trait diagnosis: clinical and social implications. *Hematology Am Soc Hematol Educ Program.* 2015;2015(1):160–7. doi:10.1182/asheducation-2015.1.160
29. Eichner ER. Sickle cell considerations in athletes. *Clin Sports Med.* 2011 Jul;30(3):537–49. doi:10.1016/j.csm.2011.03.004
30. O'Connor FG, Bergeron MF, Cantrell J, et al. ACSM and CHAMP summit on sickle cell trait: mitigating risks for warfighters and athletes. *Med Sci Sports Exerc.* 2012 Nov;44(11):2045–56. doi:10.1249/MSS.0b013e31826851c2
31. Pecker LH, Naik RP. The current state of sickle cell trait: implications for reproductive and genetic counseling. *Blood.* 2018 Nov 29;132(22): 2331–8. doi:10.1182/blood-2018-06-848705
32. Mitchell BL. Sickle cell trait and sudden death. *Sports Med Open.* 2018 May 23;4(1):19. doi:10.1186/s40798-018-0131-6
33. Tefferi A, Vannucchi AM, Barbui T. Polycythemia vera: historical oversights, diagnostic details, and therapeutic views. *Leukemia.* 2021 Dec;35(12):3339–51. doi:10.1038/s41375-021-01401-3
34. Babakhanlou R, Verstovsek S, Pemmaraju N, Rojas-Hernandez CM. Secondary erythrocytosis. *Expert Rev Hematol.* 2023 Apr;16(4):245–51. doi:10.1080/17474086.2023.2192475
35. Means RT. Polycythemia: erythrocytosis. In: Greer JP, Foerester J, Rogers GM, editors. *Wintrobe's Clinical Hematology.* 10th ed. Baltimore: Lippincott Williams & Wilkins; 1999.
36. Simon TL. Induced erythrocythemia and athletic performance. *Semin Hematol.* 1994;31(2):128–33.
37. World Anti-Doping Agency. *World Anti-doping Code: Athlete Biological Passport Operating Guidelines and Compilation of Required Elements (Version 2.1)* [Internet]. 2010 [cited 2011 Mar 31]. Available from: http://www.uci.ch/Modules/BUILTIN/getObject.asp?MenuId=&ObjTypeCode=FILE&type=FILE&id=NjA2NzM&LangId=142
38. Jelkmann W, Lundby C. Blood doping and its detection. *Blood.* 2011 Sep 1;118(9):2395–404. doi:10.1182/blood-2011-02-303271
39. Eichner ER. Sports medicine pearls and pitfalls: benign neutropenia in athletes. *Curr Sports Med Rep.* 2009 Jul-Aug;8(4):162–3. doi:10.1249/JSR.0b013e3181ae00f0
40. Chabot-Richards DS, George TI. Leukocytosis. *Int J Lab Hematol.* 2014 Jun;36(3):279–88. doi:10.1111/ijlh.12212
41. Weyand AC, Flood VH. Von Willebrand disease: current status of diagnosis and management. *Hematol Oncol Clin North Am.* 2021 Dec;35(6):1085–101. doi:10.1016/j.hoc.2021.07.004
42. Levi M, Sivapalaratnam S. Disseminated intravascular coagulation: an update on pathogenesis and diagnosis. *Expert Rev Hematol.* 2018 Aug;11(8):663–72. doi:10.1080/17474086.2018.1500173
43. Mladěnka P, Macáková K, Kujovská Krčmová L, et al. Vitamin K - sources, physiological role, kinetics, deficiency, detection, therapeutic use, and toxicity. *Nutr Rev.* 2022 Mar 10;80(4):677–98. doi:10.1093/nutrit/nuab061
44. Parnes A, Ravi A. Polycythemia and thrombocytosis. *Prim Care.* 2016 Dec;43(4):589–605. doi:10.1016/j.pop.2016.07.011
45. Vannucchi AM, Barbui T. Thrombocytosis and thrombosis. *Hematology Am Soc Hematol Educ Program.* 2007:363–70. doi:10.1182/asheducation-2007.1.363
46. Viprakasit V, Ekwattanakit S. Clinical classification, screening and diagnosis for thalassemia. *Hematol Oncol Clin North Am.* 2018 Apr;32(2):193–211. doi:10.1016/j.hoc.2017.11.006
47. Rawson ES, Clarkson PM, Tarnopolsky MA. Perspectives on exertional rhabdomyolysis. *Sports Med.* 2017 Mar;47(suppl 1):33–49. doi:10.1007/s40279-017-0689-z
48. Huerta-Alardín AL, Varon J, Marik PE. Bench-to-bedside review: rhabdomyolysis—an overview for clinicians. *Crit Care.* 2005 Apr;9(2): 158–69. doi:10.1186/cc2978
49. Landau ME, Kenney K, Deuster P, Campbell W. Exertional rhabdomyolysis: a clinical review with a focus on genetic influences. *J Clin Neuromuscul Dis.* 2012 Mar;13(3):122–36. doi:10.1097/CND.0b013e31822721ca
50. Tietze DC, Borchers J. Exertional rhabdomyolysis in the athlete: a clinical review. *Sports Health.* 2014 Jul;6(4):336–9. doi:10.1177/1941738114523544
51. Varghese V, Rivera MS, Alalwan A, et al. Concomitant identification of muddy brown granular casts and low fractional excretion of urinary sodium in AKI. *Kidney360.* 2022 Jan 19;3(4):627–35. doi:10.34067/KID.0005692021
52. O'Connor FG, Franzos MA, Nye NS, et al. Summit on exercise collapse associated with sickle cell trait: finding the "Way Ahead." *Curr Sports Med Rep.* 2021 Jan 1;20(1):47–56.
53. Long B, Koyfman A, Gottlieb, M. An evidence-based narrative review of the emergency department evaluation and management of rhabdomyolysis. *Am J Emerg Med.* 2019 Mar;37(3):518–23. doi:10.1016/j.ajem.2018.12.061
54. Schmidt AH. Acute compartment syndrome. *Orthop Clin North Am.* 2016 Jul;47(3):517–25. doi:10.1016/j.ocl.2016.02.001
55. O'Connor FG, Brennan FH Jr, Campbell W, Heled Y, Deuster P. Return to physical activity after exertional rhabdomyolysis. *Curr Sports Med Rep.* 2008 Nov-Dec;7(6):328–31. doi:10.1249/JSR.0b013e31818f0317
56. Nye NS, Kasper K, Madsen CM, et al. Clinical practice guidelines for exertional rhabdomyolysis: a Military medicine perspective. *Curr Sports Med Rep.* 2021 Mar 1;20(3):169–78.

40 Neurology

Joel Shaw

INTRODUCTION

- Concussion is a common injury seen by sports medicine physicians and is often a difficult scenario due to the athlete's desire to return to play, coaches' desire to have their athletes available, and the social pressure of parents and media. Due to the potential sequelae of injury, it is important to understand how to evaluate the patient initially looking for potentially dangerous symptoms and to be comfortable in how to safely return an athlete to sports.
- Due to the frequency of headaches in athletes and the general population and the potential to limit activity, it is important to understand how to diagnose the type of headache and how to treat each type to enable an athlete to return to activity.
- The history of limiting athletes with epilepsy from participation has led to many unwanted effects including obesity and its health effects, social isolation, depression, and anxiety. It is important for their long-term health to increase their ability to participate in sports.

CONCUSSIONS

Definition

- Concussion is defined as "a traumatic brain injury induced by biomechanical forces" (1). Concussion can be caused either by a direct blow to the head and face or by transmitted forces from contact to another part of the body. This results in a rapid onset of impairment that resolves spontaneously. The symptoms are primarily caused by a functional disturbance in the brain without structural damage, although sometimes with related neuropathological changes. In most patients the symptoms resolve in a sequential pattern, although in rare cases the post-concussion symptoms may be prolonged. Concussions do not result in changes on typical neuroimaging studies. As originally discussed in the Prague guidelines, the majority of concussions (80%–90%) resolve quickly (10–14 days), with a possible extended resolution period in children and adolescents (2,3).

CONCUSSION EVALUATION

Signs and Symptoms

- In evaluating a patient with presumed concussion, the medical evaluation should include an extensive injury history, clinical symptoms, physical signs, behavior, balance, and cognition.
- Symptoms may include but are not limited to headache, a sensation of fogginess, drowsiness, and lability.
- Physical signs include amnesia and possible loss of consciousness.
- Cognitive impairment may include slowed reaction times, irritability, anxiety, or depressed mood.
- It is important to remember that in some cases the symptoms may not appear until several hours after the injury.

Sideline Evaluation

- When a patient shows any potential features of a concussion, the athlete should initially be evaluated by emergency procedures including the ABCs of emergency care, with a special emphasis on evaluating for a possible cervical spine injury. The disposition based on emergency protocol should be determined by the treating healthcare provider.
- A stable patient should next be evaluated by a sideline tool designed for concussion evaluation, such as the Sports Concussion Assessment Tool (SCAT5) or smart phone applications such as Concussion Assessment and Response: Sport Version (CARE). The SCAT5 includes essential evaluations including: red flags, memory assessment (Maddocks Questions), Glasgow Coma Scale, cervical spine assessment, symptom evaluation, cognitive screening, neurological screening, balance examination, and delayed recall.
- It is important to understand the SCAT tool is useful immediately after injury, but effectiveness wanes 3–5 days after injury. Additional information can come from evaluating reaction time, balance assessment, and oculomotor screening.
- After diagnosis of a concussion, a player should not be left alone with serial monitoring for several hours after the injury. Based on the Zurich (2008) and Berlin (2016) consensus conference statements, reinforced by the AMSSM Position Statement on Concussion in Sport (2019) and the ACSM Team Physician

Consensus Conference (TPCC) on Sport Related Concussion (2021) guidance, an athlete should not be allowed to return to competition on the same day as the injury (4–6).

- The Amsterdam Concussion guidelines were published in October 2022 with new methodologies including anonymous voting by consensus members, summaries of alternate viewpoints, and inclusion of athlete voice, parasport athletes, and ethical viewpoints. Some prevention recommendations of this guideline include some recommended rule changes to reduce collisions, recommended neuromuscular training in warm-ups, and recommended mouthguard use in ice hockey.
- The SCAT tool was updated (SCAT6) along with a new office tool to better guide evaluation and management in the office 72 or more hours after injury — the Sports Concussion Office Assessment Tool-6 (SCOAT6). Other important updates include new return-to-learn and return-to-sport strategies, increased evidence supporting early intervention with physical activity and aerobic exercise treatment, and recommendation of cervicovestibular rehabilitation for athletes with neck pain, headaches, dizziness, and/or balance problems as part of their symptom complex (7).
- One essential part of sideline evaluation is testing of cognitive function.
  - Standard orientation questions (*e.g.*, time, place, and person) have been shown to be ineffective in sideline evaluations compared to memory assessment (8).
  - Brief tests for memory, recall, and concentration have been shown to be effective, including the Maddocks questions (8) and the Standardized Assessment of Concussion (SAC) (9).
  - These tests are effective for rapid sideline evaluation, but in questions of more subtle, persistent changes they are not able to replace the effectiveness of comprehensive neuropsychological testing.
- Follow-up evaluation may occur in the emergency room or preferably in the doctor's office. Follow-up examination should include a comprehensive history of the event and persistent symptoms.
  - Neurologic exams should include cognitive function, oculovestibular function, gait, and balance assessment. The decision to move to advanced or emergent imaging may be needed for severer symptoms concerning for brain injury related to structural abnormalities.

Advanced Outpatient Testing

- The use of neuroimaging studies is still not effective for the standard evaluation of concussions.
- Brain CT and MRI are normal in concussive injuries, but should still continue to be used when there are symptoms suspicious for possible intracerebral structural lesions. These situations include prolonged disturbance in consciousness, focal neurologic deficits, or worsening symptoms.
- Newer studies, including perfusion and diffusion MRI's, functional MRI, positron emission tomography, and magnetic resonance spectroscopy show some future promise. There is also significant research underway regarding fluid biomarkers and genetic testing, but in current state these are important research tools, but further validation is needed before they provide benefit in initial clinical evaluation and treatment planning.
- Objective balance assessment can provide additional information in concussed patients. Studies consistently show, whether by sophisticated force plate testing or clinical balance tests, that postural stability deficits persist for about 72 hours. These tests are useful tools to evaluate the motor portion of neurologic function.
- Neuropsychological testing (NP) gives critical information that can be valuable in concussion evaluation and recovery.
  - In some cases, cognitive recovery and symptom recovery follow the same pattern, but studies have demonstrated that frequently cognitive recovery lags behind symptom recovery. In these cases, NP testing would be beneficial in determining the patients who are not fully recovered functionally.
  - It is important to recognize that NP assessment should not be used singularly to make return-to-play decisions, but it is effective as an addition to clinical decision making.
  - Based on the data from several studies, NP testing is best used in return-to-play decisions after the patient is asymptomatic (10). See Chapter 30 for further discussion on Neuropsychometric Testing.

Concussion Management

- The current evidence no longer supports that complete physical and cognitive rest will result in symptom resolution. Although the current guidelines (7) recommend a brief 24–48-hour period of rest, there does appear to be a benefit to gradual and progressive increase in activity after that period. The activity progression should not advance to a level that causes increased cognitive or physical symptoms and initially should not involve vigorous exertion.
- A graduated return to play protocol is listed in Table 40.1. The athlete needs to remain asymptomatic to continue along the stepwise progression. Each stage should last for 24 hours. If any post-concussion symptoms develop, the patient should return to the previous asymptomatic stage.
- Previous consensus statements suggested elite athletes may be able to return on the day of injury or earlier than adolescent athletes, but an update in the Berlin guidelines states "all athletes, regardless of level of participation, should be managed using the same management principles" (1).
- Based on this recommendation, any athlete should be led through some version of a return-to-play protocol similar to Table 40.1 that allows for progression of activity and no same day return to play.

Table 40.1 Return-to-Play Protocol

Stage/Aim	Activity	Goal of Step
1. Symptom-limited activity	Complete physical and cognitive rest	Gradual reintroduction
2. Light aerobic exercise	Walking, swimming, or stationary cycling keeping intensity <70% MPHR; no resistance training	Increase heart rate
3. Sport-specific exercise	Skating drills in ice hockey, running drills in soccer; no head impact activities	Add movement
4. Noncontact training	Progression to more complex drills: training drills, eg, passing drills in football and ice hockey; start progressive resistance training	Exercise Coordination Thinking
5. Full contact practice	Following medical clearance, participate in normal training activities	Confidence Assess
6. Return to play	Normal game play	

- Several studies have shown high–school- and college-age athletes often continue to show NP deficits despite being asymptomatic on the sidelines and are more likely to have delayed onset of symptoms (11,12). The evidence of persistent neuropsychologic changes despite clinical resolution has led to more caution around rapid return to play.
- There are several factors that should cause the physician to consider a more deliberate approach to return to play.
  - One controversial factor is loss of consciousness (LOC). Although prior guidelines that were primarily based on the presence or absence of LOC have been shown to be less helpful, LOC is still an important indicator of severity. If LOC lasts greater than a minute, it is an indicator of a more severe concussion that will likely require longer recovery time.
  - Presence of amnesia is still difficult to interpret but may correlate with prolonged recovery (13). Athletes with multiple concussions should be given more time to recover.
  - Athletes with repeated concussions occurring with progressively less impact are likely to require a longer period of recovery.
- Several factors appear to predict a prolonged course of symptoms and limitations.
  - Increased severity of initial symptoms continues to be the best predictor of slower recovery, and conversely a lower level of symptoms in the first day typically indicates a better prognosis.
  - The development of migraine headaches or depressive symptoms often correlates with symptoms lasting longer than a month.
  - Athletes from children to young adults with preinjury history of mental health disorders and migraine headaches are more likely to have prolonged symptoms greater than a month.
  - Although more coordination and planning are needed to support athletes with attention deficit disorder and learning disabilities while recovering, most recent evidence does not correlate with a higher risk of prolonged symptoms (14).
- Second impact syndrome (SIS) is one reason for the graduated return to play, although there is some controversy on whether SIS exists. The controversy relates to several factors include the rarity of cases, lack of reports in Australian football compared to American football, and no similar reports from European literature (15). This occurs in an athlete who returns to contact before resolution of the symptoms and physiologic changes associated with concussion. A second traumatic event results in loss of cerebral vasomotor control. This results in uncontrollable cerebral edema and increasing intracranial volume and pressure. This often leads to neurologic collapse and death.

Post-Concussion Syndrome

- Post-concussion syndrome is a poorly defined entity. It can be defined as persistence of cognitive, physical, or emotional symptoms of concussion lasting longer than what are normally expected. The time frame is not well defined but usually refers to symptoms lasting more than a couple of weeks. The cause of persistent symptoms is controversial, but appears to be a combination of psychogenic and physiologic changes. The condition is a clinical diagnosis made by an intensive history with minimal changes on physical exam and normal imaging techniques.
- There are several symptoms and historical factors that correlate with increased likelihood of persistent symptoms. Amnesia is connected with the risk of symptoms lasting more than 5 days but not necessarily for longer periods (16). Migraine symptoms (17) and noise sensitivity (18) are connected with increased risk of prolonged symptoms. Several studies show that athletes with several previous concussions are more likely to develop post-concussion syndrome (12,19). The preexistence of psychiatric issues also appears to correlate with prolonged symptoms.
- The effect of previous concussions has been well documented. One study confirmed a significant increase in

cognitive deficits in professional football players with a history of at least three concussions (20). Other studies have shown similar results in younger athletes with cumulative effects from less violent hits. Athletes with prior concussions require longer recovery time and are at increased risk for future head injuries.

- The symptoms include the typical cognitive and physical symptoms of concussion, but especially headache, distractibility, and poor concentration. Other common symptoms include depression, anxiety, personality changes, irritability, and apathy.
- Treatment of post-concussion syndrome is controversial. There are several options to try for the cognitive deficits (21).
  - Dopaminergic agents including amantadine, levodopa, and bromocriptine have some evidence supporting their beneficial effect on cognitive deficits.
  - Due to the similarities with Alzheimer's, there has been an effort to treat cholinergic dysfunction with physostigmine and donepezil with some effect.
  - The mood disorders associated with this syndrome are best treated with psychiatric counseling (22). Selective serotonin reuptake inhibitors and buspirone are effective in the treatment of mood disorders, including anxiety and depression.
  - Topiramate and tricyclic antidepressants have been shown to be effective for migraines, including migraines related to post-concussion injury.
  - Trazodone or Melatonin or beneficial for the associated sleep disturbances (23).
  - Benzodiazepines and antipsychotics should be avoided as they may exacerbate cognitive changes.
- Regarding long-term consequences of recurrent head trauma and the potential to develop chronic traumatic encephalopathy (CTE), there is still significant research required to confirm the true cause-and-effect relationship. There also is not enough evidence yet to confirm a direct relationship between exposure to contact sports and CTE. But the risk for long-term sequelae of CTE, cognitive impairment, and/or depression should lead to a more thoughtful and cautious approach to managing athletes with traumatic brain injuries.

HEADACHES

Classification

- Primary exercise headache (previously termed exertional headache) was defined by the International Classification of Headache Disorders, 3rd edition (ICHD-3), published in 2018 (24).
- It is important to correctly diagnose an exertional headache as opposed to other causes of potentially more significant headaches.
  - Exercise headache requires the presence of the following criteria: at least two headache episodes, brought on by and occurring only during or after strenuous exercise, and lasting less than 48 hours while not better accounted for by another ICHD-3 diagnosis.
  - The headache is often described as pulsatile head pain and would only be brought on by exercise.
  - The headaches are typically bilateral and throbbing in quality and are unlikely to involve nausea and vomiting.
  - Theories of the pathophysiology vary, but likely involve some type of increased intracranial pressure from either vascular congestion or distention impacting the pain-sensitive vascular or meningeal tissues (25).
  - Underlying abnormalities may include previous traumatic injury, supratentorial and posterior fossa space-occupying lesions, vascular abnormalities such as aneurysm or arteriovenous malformation, and intracranial hemorrhage (26).
- The first responsibility is to determine the severity of the headache. Severe headaches require immediate in-depth evaluation and treatment. Neurologic symptoms require a more intensive initial evaluation.
  - An athlete who describes a "thunderclap headache" should be taken seriously as it could be a sign of a subarachnoid hemorrhage or brain aneurysm.
  - An athlete with a traumatic headache that is rapidly increasing in severity or associated with neurologic symptoms should be evaluated with further imaging to look for cerebral hemorrhage or infarct.
  - Neurologic symptoms that should be evaluated further include mental status changes, nausea, vomiting, increased neck stiffness, or focal neurologic findings. It is important to look for these abnormalities as one study found that 10% of patients with exertional headache had an organic lesion as the cause of headache.
- Exercise headaches are the most common type of headache in athletes. These headaches are often preceded by prodromal migraine symptoms. These symptoms may include scotomata, photopsia, vertigo, aphasia, ataxia, or paresthesias. The aura usually occurs 10–20 minutes prior to the headache and ceases prior to the headache.
  - Generally, the headache is bilateral and throbbing in nature. It will last between 5 minutes and 48 hours. It usually occurs with high-intensity exertion. The associated increased intracranial pressure appears to be the cause.
  - According to one study, patients who suffer from recurrent headaches are more likely to have myofascial trigger points and postural abnormalities associated with cervical and thoracic dysfunction (27). It is important to remember to treat the associated musculoskeletal abnormalities that may lead to recurrent headaches.
- Weightlifter's headache is one type of exertional headache (28). It most commonly occurs during power lifting or maximal lifts. The presumed mechanism is breath holding during lifting associated with the Valsalva maneuver. The increase

in intracranial pressure leads to headache in the posterior occipital region.

- The headache begins sharp and intense, often incapacitating. Symptoms often last at least several days, lasting longer than the other benign headaches.
- If these headaches become more severe or recurrent then further evaluation should be completed with MRI looking for Arnold-Chiari malformation or aneurysm.

- Effort headaches occur in endurance activities such as long-distance running or triathlons.
  - The headaches tend to be similar to migraines, often unilateral with associated nausea, vomiting, and visual aura.
  - Besides endurance, these headaches appear to occur in relation to heat, humidity, altitude, dehydration, or poor nutrition.
  - The best treatment for this type is preventative, including hydration, proper conditioning, and avoidance of altitude changes.

Treatment

- Treatment of migraines should be multifactorial. To treat migraines most effectively, it is important to have an accurate diagnosis. There are three main stages of treatment to include prevention, acute treatment, and in some cases prevention.
- Prevention is the most effective form of treatment. A healthy lifestyle is essential to limit headaches, including a healthy, well-balanced diet, adequate sleep (8 hours a day), and good hydration. According to several studies, the use of riboflavin 200 mg twice a day (29) and magnesium citrate 200 mg has shown questionable benefit. The riboflavin improves mitochondrial energy and the magnesium decreases neurologic hyperexcitability. Proper warm-up and breathing techniques will help limit the effects of breath holding and Valsalva maneuver.
- Acute treatment of headaches is most commonly treated with typical nonsteroidal anti-inflammatory drugs (NSAIDs), including Ibuprofen and Naproxen.
  - When the pattern is more typical of migraines, 5-hydroxytryptamine blockers such as sumatriptan or ergotamine is effective.
  - Prophylactic treatment may include medications such as indomethacin or other NSAIDs, amitriptyline, and selective serotonin reuptake inhibitors (SSRIs).
  - β-blockers would be a less common choice for athletes due to potential side effects of fatigue and bradycardia. For difficult-to-manage patients several alternative treatments have been shown to be effective.
  - Botulinum toxin type A is effective and safe as prophylaxis for chronic headaches (30).
  - A randomized controlled trial showed that acupuncture improves quality of life and decreases headache pain (31).

EPILEPSY

Introduction

- There is a long history of controversy involving epileptic patients and their safety to participate in athletics and exercise. For the past several decades, the concerns of parents, administrators, and coaches have led to restrictions on athletic involvement for epileptic patients. Medical recommendations for a long period supported the exclusion of these patients and have only recently made some progress in allowing participation.
- Until 1974, organizations such as the American Medical Association (AMA) and the American Academy of Pediatrics (AAP) recommended significant restrictions in activity due to fear of injury and induction of seizure activity. Articles published in 1973 argued both for and against participation for epileptic patients (32,33). This discussion led to a change in the recommendations of the AMA in 1974 allowing participation in contact sports in some cases to assist in adjustment to school, social interactions, and the diagnosis of seizure disorder (34).
- In 1983 the AAP adjusted their recommendation to allow participation in most sports, including contact sports, as long as seizures were adequately controlled and supervision was available.
- Epilepsy is present in 1%–2% of the population. About 75% of these patients have their first seizure by the age of 20 (35). About 30%–40% of patients who have an initial seizure will have a recurrent episode and then are likely to have repetitive episodes in the future. Despite this frequency, based on a study in 1997, 80% of patients are well controlled on two or fewer antiepileptic medications (36). This should reassure patients and physicians that these patients would benefit from exercise.
- Multiple studies confirm the connection of decreased exercise and activity in epileptic patients with decreased self-esteem, increased anxiety and depression, and diseases associated with poor physical fitness, such as obesity, heart disease, and diabetes. For this reason, the psychosocial and psychologic benefits of physical activity should be used to encourage patients with well controlled epilepsy to be involved frequently in physical activity, athletics, and exercise.

Classification

- Partial seizures are localized to 1 area of the brain with activation of a smaller number of neurons. Partial seizures are further classified as simple or complex in reference to the effect on consciousness. Seizures with no LOC are termed partial seizures but may include motor, sensory, or autonomic symptoms. Seizures associated with altered consciousness, which may include diminished responsiveness, staring, lip smacking, and repetitive swallowing, are termed complex seizures.

- Generalized seizures are seizures associated with bilateral discharges on electroencephalography (EEG) and involve the entire cortex. Generalized seizures can be either convulsive or nonconvulsive. Nonconvulsive generalized seizures include absence and myoclonic seizures.

Risks of Participation

- It is important for patients and physicians to understand the things that may make participation in sports dangerous or unsafe.
- We need to understand factors that may precipitate seizures. These may include fatigue, emotional stress, fever, hormonal changes of the menstrual cycle, alcohol, caffeine, heat, humidity, and sleep deprivation.
  - These factors vary depending on the patient and should be individualized.
  - There are rare cases when exercise may be a trigger for a specific patient.
  - In two separate studies only 1%–2% of patients had identified exercise as a trigger for seizure activity (37,38).
  - Hypoglycemia and hyponatremia are also common abnormalities that may lower the seizure threshold.
- The concern for an increased risk of injury with sports participation is unfounded in most sports (39), although there are certain activities that are connected with higher risk and will be discussed in a later section.

Benefits of Exercise

- As stated before, epileptic patients have a higher rate of obesity, body mass index, and body fat ratio (40).
- To counteract this medical risk, according to a study by Eriksen et al. (41), an active exercise program decreased cholesterol levels and increased aerobic performance. This same study showed that a regular exercise program reduces sleep problems and fatigue, improves psychosocial functioning, and increases sense of well-being.
- There are multiple studies, including the study by Eriksen et al., which show decreased seizure risk in patients who follow a regular exercise program. Two studies showed improved EEG results, including a decrease in occurrence of epileptiform discharge, normalization of EEG changes, and raising of the seizure threshold (42–44).

Sports Participation

- Based on these benefits of athletic participation, it is important to support epileptic patient participation whenever possible and safe. Because of the potential risk, it is important to do everything possible to make participation safe, including controlling risk when possible and using protective equipment when available.
- The International League Against Epilepsy Task Force on Sports and Epilepsy published a consensus paper regarding physical exercise and sports participation for patients with seizure disorder or epilepsy in 2015 (45). The group of experts used numerous studies and articles to develop standards for participation.
  - Sports were divided into three categories: Group 1 sports with no significant additional risk, Group 2 sports with moderate risk to athletes but not bystanders, and Group 3 sports with high risk for athletes and potential risk to bystanders (see Table 40.2).

Table 40.2 Epilepsy Participation Categories

Group 1 Sports
Ground sports including baseball, basketball, football, rugby, field hockey, volleyball
Cross-country skiing
Dancing
Golf
Bowling
Group 2 Sports
Alpine skiing
Archery
Biathlon, triathlon, cycling
Boxing, karate
Fencing
Gymnastics
Horse riding
Pole vault
Skating
Snowboarding
Swimming
Water skiing
Weightlifting
Group 3 Sports
Aviation
Climbing
Diving
Horse racing
Motor sports parachuting
Rodeo
Scuba diving
Ski jumping
Solitary sailing
Surfing

Source: Adapted from Table 1 from Capovilla, G, Kaufman, KR, Perucca, E, Moshé, SL, Arida, RM. Epilepsy, seizures, physical exercise, and sports: a report from the ILAE Task Force on Sports and Epilepsy. *Epilepsia.* 2015;57(1):6–12.

  - Participation recommendations were determined based on these categories. General standards in all categories included: if an athlete is seizure free for 12 months or longer, they can participate in any sports; if an athlete has had no seizure for 10 or more years and no seizure medications for 5 or more years, their epilepsy was considered resolved with no further restrictions or follow-up required, and the only restrictions for category I sports (which includes football, rugby, judo, and wrestling) are the requirement for treating neurologist input if there were recent seizures with impaired awareness or a recent change or withdrawal of seizure medication.
  - Other recommendations for risk reduction include adequate rest, proper hydration, and a well-balanced diet to decrease the risk of hypoglycemia or other abnormalities that may lower the seizure threshold.

Sports Specific Participation

Contact and Collision Sports

- Per the ILAE categories, most collision and contact sports fit in group 1, except for boxing and karate. This supports and aligns with the recommendations of the AMA and AAP, that there should be no restrictions for well-controlled epileptics to participate in football, hockey, rugby, soccer, basketball, or baseball.
  - The only reason for pause in contact and collision sports, such as football, rugby, and wrestling, is if the athlete has had a seizure in the recent past associated with impaired awareness that has a question of possible seizure precipitating factors related to the actual sport activity, or has had a recent change in medication.
  - In those cases, involving their neurologist in athletic participation decisions would be recommended.
- With boxing and karate as group 2 sports, there should be no restrictions if the athlete has been seizure free for 12 months or more. If the athlete has had seizures more recently associated with impaired awareness, we would recommend participation based on recommendations from the treating neurologist; only allowing participation after this discussion, informed consent on risks, and when there is appropriate medical surveillance and supervision during the athletic activity.

Swimming and Water Sports

- Obviously, the main concern with swimming is the risk of drowning if a seizure occurs while in the water. One study showed a four-fold increase in the risk of drowning or near drowning from submersion in epileptic patients.
- Swimming also fits in the group 2 sports category. The consensus is that epileptic patients with no seizures for 12 or more months may participate in water competition and swimming, although we would recommend direct visual supervision by someone adequately trained in rescue and resuscitation techniques. This should only be done in events with clear water.
  - Patients with poor control and frequent seizures should be restricted from swimming.
- Scuba diving (a group 3 sport) is much more restricted due to the risk of dislodging the regulator, the poor airway protection during an emergency rapid ascent increasing the risk of aspiration or "the bends," and the potential for injury to the rescue partner.
  - Any patient with poor control of seizures should not be allowed to dive, and even allowing the well-controlled epileptic to scuba dive should only happen after significant deliberation and consideration including input from the treating neurologist.

Sports from Heights

- Sports in which a fall could cause serious injury require more serious consideration of seizure control and the benefit or participation for the athlete.
- Gymnastics (group 2 sport) requires appropriate planning and preparation for each individual. When seizures are well controlled, close observation and assistance by coaches and trainers is essential. In some cases, the use of safety harnesses may be beneficial.
- Horseback riding and harnessed rock climbing may be possible with good seizure control and the assistance of a partner who can provide first aid and can contact emergency personnel, as long as the patient has full understanding of the risks.

Motor Sports

- The risk of injury to the driver, other drivers, or spectators in motor sports due to the high speed and force of collision is severe. For this reason, any effort to reduce the frequency of accidents and the risk of severe injury is essential.
- The general recommendation is that all epileptic patients should avoid participation in motor sports.

Medical Treatment of Epilepsy

- Medical treatment of epilepsy is difficult in the athletic population due to the frequent side effects from these medications that may affect the performance of athletes. We will discuss side effects of several medications that may impact athletic performance, but the main point is that each patient must be treated individually for better seizure control with reduction of side effects.
- **Gabapentin** is well tolerated compared to most antiepileptic medications with minimal side effects or drug interactions.
- **Lamotrigine** has the potential to cause dizziness, movement disorders, sedation, and headaches.
- **Valproate** is known to cause increased appetite resulting in weight gain and tremors. Sedation and cognitive impairment are much less common.
- **Carbamazepine** may cause sedation, ataxia, nausea, and dizziness.
- **Phenytoin** is known to result in sedation, depressed cognitive function, and depressed activity.

REFERENCES

1. McCrory P, Meeuwisse W, Dvorak J, et al. Consensus statement on concussion in sport-the 5th international conference on concussion in sport held in Berlin, October 2016. *Br J Sports Med.* 2017;51(11):838–47.
2. McCrory P, Johnston K, Meeuwisse W, et al. Summary and agreement statement of the second international conference on concussion in sport, Prague 2004. *Br J Sports Med.* 2005;29:196–204.
3. Zimmerman SD, Vernau BT, Meehan WP III, Master CL. Sports-related concussions and the pediatric patient. *Clin Sports Med.* 2021 Jan;40(1):147–58.
4. McCrory P, Meeuwisse W, Johnston K, et al. Consensus statement on Concussion in Sports 3rd International Conference on Concussion in Sport, Zurich 2008. *Clin J Sport Med.* 2009;19(3):185–200.
5. Herring S, Kibler WB, Putukian M, et al. Selected issues in sport-related concussion (SRC| Mild Traumatic Brain Injury) for the Team Physician: A consensus statement. *Curr Sports Med Rep.* 2021 Aug;20(8):420–31.
6. Harmon KG, Clugston JR, Dec K, et al. American medical society for sports medicine position statement on concussion in sport. *Clin J Sport Med.* 2019 Mar;29(2):87–100.
7. Patricios JS, Schneider KJ, Dvorak J, et al. Consensus statement on concussion in sport: the 6th International Conference on Concussion in Sport-Amsterdam, October 2022. *Br J Sports Med.* 2023;57(11):695–711.
8. Maddocks DL, Dicker GD, Saling MM. The assessment of orientation following concussion in athletes. *Clin J Sport Med.* 1995;5(1):32–5.
9. McCrea M. Standardized mental status assessment of sports concussion. *Clin J Sport Med.* 2001;11(3):176–81.
10. Lovell MR. The relevance of neuropsychologic testing for sports-related head injuries. *Curr Sports Med Rep.* 2002;1:7–11.
11. Collins M, Field M, Lovell M, et al. Relationship between post-concussion headache and neuropsychological test performance in high school athletes. *Am J Sports Med.* 2003;31(2):168–73.
12. Collins M, Grindel S, Lovell M, et al. Relationship between concussion and neuropsychological performance in college football players. *JAMA.* 1999;282(10):964–70.
13. Meehan W, Stracciolоni A, Elbin R, Collins M. Symptom severity predicts prolonged recovery from sports-related concussion, but age and amnesia do not. *J Pediatrics.* 2013 Sep;163(3):721–5.
14. Manley G, Gardner AJ, Schneider KJ, et al. A systematic review of potential long-term effects of sport-related concussion. *Br J Sports Med.* 2017 Jun;51(12):969–77.
15. McCrory P. Does second impact syndrome exist? *Clin J Sport Med.* 2001;11(3):144–9.
16. Collins M, Iverson GL, Lovell MR, McKeag DB, Norwig J, Maroon J. On-field predictors of neuropsychological and symptom deficit following sports-related concussion. *Clin J Sport Med.* 2003;13(4):222–9.
17. Lau B, Lovell MR, Collins MW, Pardini J. Neurocognitive and symptom predictors of recovery in high school athletes. *Clin J Sport Med.* 2009;19(3):216–21.
18. Dischinger PC, Ryb GE, Kufera JA, Auman KM. Early predictors of postconcussive syndrome in a population of trauma patients with mild traumatic brain injury. *J Trauma.* 2009;66(2):289–97.
19. Moser RS, Schatz P, Jordan BD. Prolonged effects of concussion in high school athletes. *Neurosurgery.* 2005;57(2):300–6.
20. Guskiewicz KM, Marshall SW, Bailes J, et al. Recurrent concussion and risk of depression in retired professional football players. *Med Sci Sports Exerc.* 2007;39(6):903–9.
21. Jones JC, O'Brien MJ. Medical therapies for concussion. *Clin Sports Med.* 2021 Jan;40(1):123–31.
22. Chen CL, Lin MY, Huda MH, Tsai PS. Effects of cognitive behavioral therapy for adults with post-concussion syndrome: a systematic review and meta-analysis of randomized controlled trials. *J Psychosom Res.* 2020 Sep;136:110190.
23. Barlow KM, Brooks BL, Esser MJ, et al. Efficacy of melatonin in children with postconcussive symptoms: a randomized clinical trial. *Pediatrics.* 2020 Apr;145(4):e20192812.
24. Arnold M. Headache Classification Committee of the International Headache Society (IHS) The International Classification of Headache Disorders, 3rd edition. *Cephalalgia.* 2018;38(1):1.
25. Doepp F, Valdueza JM, Schreiber SJ. Incompetence of internal jugular valve in patients with primary exertional headache: a risk factor? *Cephalalgia.* 2008;28(2):182–5.
26. Sands GH, Newman L, Lipton R. Cough, exertional, and other miscellaneous headaches. *Med Clin North Am.* 1991;75(3):733–47.
27. Esterov D, Thomas A, Weiss K. Osteopathic manipulative medicine in the management of headaches associated with postconcussion syndrome. *J Osteopath Med.* 2021 Apr;121(7):651–6.
28. Simpson M. Weightlifter's headache. *Pract Neurol.* 2016;16(3):215–16.
29. Schoenen J, Jacquy J, Lenaerts M. Effectiveness of high-dose riboflavin in migraine prophylaxis. A randomized controlled trial. *Neurology.* 1998;50(2):466–70.
30. Blumenfeld A. Botulinum toxin type A as an effective prophylactic treatment in primary headache disorders. *Headache.* 2003;43(8):853–60.
31. Coeytaux RR, Kaufman JS, Kaptchuk T, et al. A randomized controlled trial of acupuncture for chronic daily headache. *Headache.* 2005;45(9):1113–23.
32. Livingston S, Berman W. Participation of epileptic patients in sports. *JAMA.* 1973;224(2):236–38.
33. McLaurin RL. Epilepsy and contact sports: factors contraindicating participation. *JAMA.* 1973;225(3):285–87.
34. Corbitt RW, Cooper DL, Erickson DJ, Kriss FC, Thornton ML, Craig TT. Editorial: epileptics and contact sports. *JAMA.* 1974;229(7):820–21.
35. Daniel JC, Nassiri JD, Wilckens J, Land BC. The implementation and use of the standardized assessment of concussion at the U.S. Naval Academy. *Mil Med.* 2002;167(10):873–6.
36. Baker GA, Jacoby A, Buck D, Stalgis C, Monnet D. Quality of life of people with epilepsy: a European study. *Epilepsia.* 1997;38(3):353–62.
37. Frucht MM, Quigg M, Schwaner C, Fountain NB. Distribution of seizure precipitants among epilepsy syndromes. *Epilepsia.* 2000;41(12):1534–39.
38. Nakken KO. Physical exercise in outpatients with epilepsy. *Epilepsia.* 1999;40(5):643–51.
39. Aisenson MR. Accidental injuries in epileptic children. *Pediatrics.* 1948;2(1):85–8.
40. Steinhoff BJ, Neususs K, Thegeder H, Reimers CD. Leisure time activity and physical fitness in patients with epilepsy. *Epilepsia.* 1996;37(12):1221–27.
41. Eriksen HR, Ellertsen B, Gronningsaeter H, Nakken KO, Løyning Y, Ursin H. Physical exercise in women with intractable epilepsy. *Epilepsia.* 1994;35(6):1256–64.
42. Gotze W, Kubicki S, Munter M, Teichmann J. Effect of physical exercise on seizure threshold (investigated by electroencephalographic telemetry). *Dis Nerv Syst.* 1967;28(10):664–7.
43. Nakken KO, Loyning A, Loyning T, Gløersen G, Larsson PG. Does physical exercise influence the occurrence of epileptiform EEG discharges in children? *Epilepsia.* 1997;38(3):279–84.
44. Capovilla G, Kaufman KR, Perucca E, Moshé SL, Arida RM. Epilepsy, seizures, physical exercise, and sports: a report from the ILAE Task Force on Sports and Epilepsy. *Epilepsia.* 2016;57(1):6–12.
45. Carter JM, McGrew C. Seizure disorders and exercise/sports participation. *Curr Sports Med Rep.* 2021 Jan 1;20(1):26–30.

41 Gastroenterology

David L. Brown and Thea J. Dennis-Arends

INTRODUCTION AND EPIDEMIOLOGY

- From a gastrointestinal (GI) perspective, long-distance runners have been the most scrutinized group, but studies have also looked at the GI symptoms of long-distance walkers, cyclists, triathletes, and weightlifters. Lower GI symptoms predominate nearly two to one over upper GI symptoms in endurance runners. Upper and lower GI tract symptoms occur with equal prevalence in cyclists. Whether running or riding, these same patterns also hold true in triathletes (1). In low-intensity long-distance walking, the overall occurrence of GI symptoms is much lower than that in other sports studied. The most common symptoms are flatulence and nausea, which occur at similar rates to those of the baseline population (only 5% of walkers) (2).
- Symptomatic gastroesophageal reflux is extremely common in athletes. GI symptoms increase with duration of activity, intensity of activity, and dehydration (3). Weightlifters have the highest rates of reflux, followed by runners and cyclists, who may experience less agitation during activity. All groups have increased reflux when exercising postprandially. Whereas cyclists have been demonstrated to have a modest increase in reflux after eating, weightlifters nearly double and runners triple their reflux (4).
- The prevalence of peptic ulcer disease (PUD) in the United States is 8.4%, with two-third of patients reporting no symptoms (5). PUD is associated with the primary risk factors of *Helicobacter pylori* infection and nonsteroidal anti-inflammatory drug (NSAID) use. The most common symptom is epigastric pain. *H. pylori* is associated with 65%–95% of gastric ulcers and 75% of duodenal ulcers. The estimated risk of a clinically significant NSAID-induced event, including bleeding and perforation, is 1%–4% per year for nonselective NSAID. Either of these factors alone increases ulcer risk 20-fold. When both risk factors are present, an individual is 61 times more likely to develop ulcer disease (6).
- The primary lower GI condition of athletes is runner's diarrhea, affecting up to 26% of marathon runners (7). One study on triathletes showed GI distress in 93% of participants (8). Runner's diarrhea is not typically associated with bleeding; however, studies in marathon runners showed that 20% of runners completing a marathon had occult blood in their stools, another 6% had bloody diarrhea, and 17% had frank hematochezia while in training (9).

UPPER GI DISEASES

Gastroesophageal Reflux Disease

- The most common presenting complaints for gastroesophageal reflux disease (GERD) are heartburn and acid regurgitation. The classic presentation is retrosternal burning, exacerbated by meals, intense workouts, and recumbency with resolution on antacids. Symptoms are typically more common during initial training periods with improvement as the athlete becomes more conditioned (10). Atypical symptoms include nausea, excessive salivation (water brash), bloating, and belching (11). Extraintestinal complaints include sore throat, exertional dyspnea, cough, or wheezing (Table 41.1).
- GERD pathophysiology involves retrograde movement of gastric acid and the proteolytic enzyme pepsin, which causes irritation of the esophageal epithelium. Reflux alone is insufficient to explain why individuals become symptomatic because affected patients have reflux rates similar to those of healthy individuals (12). The critical factor in symptom development appears to be that the contact time between refluxed material and the epithelium is so excessive that the normal gastric contents overwhelm the epithelial protective mechanisms. Alternatively, symptoms may develop when normal contact time occurs in the face of insufficient protective mechanisms.
- Symptomatic reflux episodes during exercise are likely multifactorial but correlate best with transient lower esophageal sphincter relaxations (TLESRs) (13). This vagally mediated reflex facilitates lower esophageal sphincter (LES) relaxation and gas venting in response to gaseous stomach distention. The decrease in LES tone and reflux associated with TLESRs last longer and are not accompanied by a swallow-induced peristaltic sweep, leading to prolonged acid exposure. Supine or forward-flexed posture during particular modes of exercise increases intra-abdominal pressure, overcoming the mechanical protection of the LES and negating bolus acid clearance achieved by gravity. Increasing exercise intensity is associated with increased reflux episodes and duration of acid exposure (14). This is particularly pronounced when maximum oxygen consumption, VO2, was greater than or equal to 70% (15). As exercise intensity increases, the frequency, duration, and amplitude of esophageal contractions progressively decrease. High-intensity exercise also reduces

Table 41.1 GERD Symptom Patterns

Classic Symptoms	Atypical Symptoms/Signs	Red Flag Symptoms
Heartburn	**Pulmonary**	Chronic untreated symptoms
Acid regurgitation	Asthma	Dysphagia
Nonspecific Symptoms	Chronic cough	Weight loss
Nausea	**ENT**	Hematemesis
Dyspepsia	Dental erosions	Melena
Bloating	Halitosis	Odynophagia
Belching	Lingual sensitivity	Vomiting
Indigestion	Chronic pharyngitis	Early satiety
Hypersalivation/water brash	Hoarseness Rhinitis/sinusitis Globus **Cardiac** Atypical chest pain	

ENT, ear, nose, and throat; GERD, gastroesophageal reflux disease.

splanchnic blood flow, which may inhibit restoration of acid-base balance and deprive the epithelium of the oxygen and nutrients needed for damage repair.

- If the history and physical examination raise red flags, symptoms are particularly severe, or the diagnosis is unclear, the athlete should be referred for gastroenterology evaluation (Fig. 41.1). In patients with extraintestinal manifestations or atypical GERD symptoms, providers can consider an initial therapeutic trial. If empiric therapy fails, it is important not only to consult gastroenterology, but also the specialty that would evaluate for extraintestinal complications (Fig. 41.2).
- Behavioral and training interventions may improve symptoms such as decreasing the intensity of training briefly, then gradually increasing it as tolerated. Other interventions include avoiding postprandial exercise or waiting to exercise for at least 3 hours after a meal. Avoiding high-calorie meals and fatty foods prior to exercise may also help symptoms (10). Physical manipulation may also provide some relief from symptoms. Cervical traction and trunk stabilization maneuvers decrease pressure in the upper and lower esophageal sphincters, leading to relief from symptoms (16).

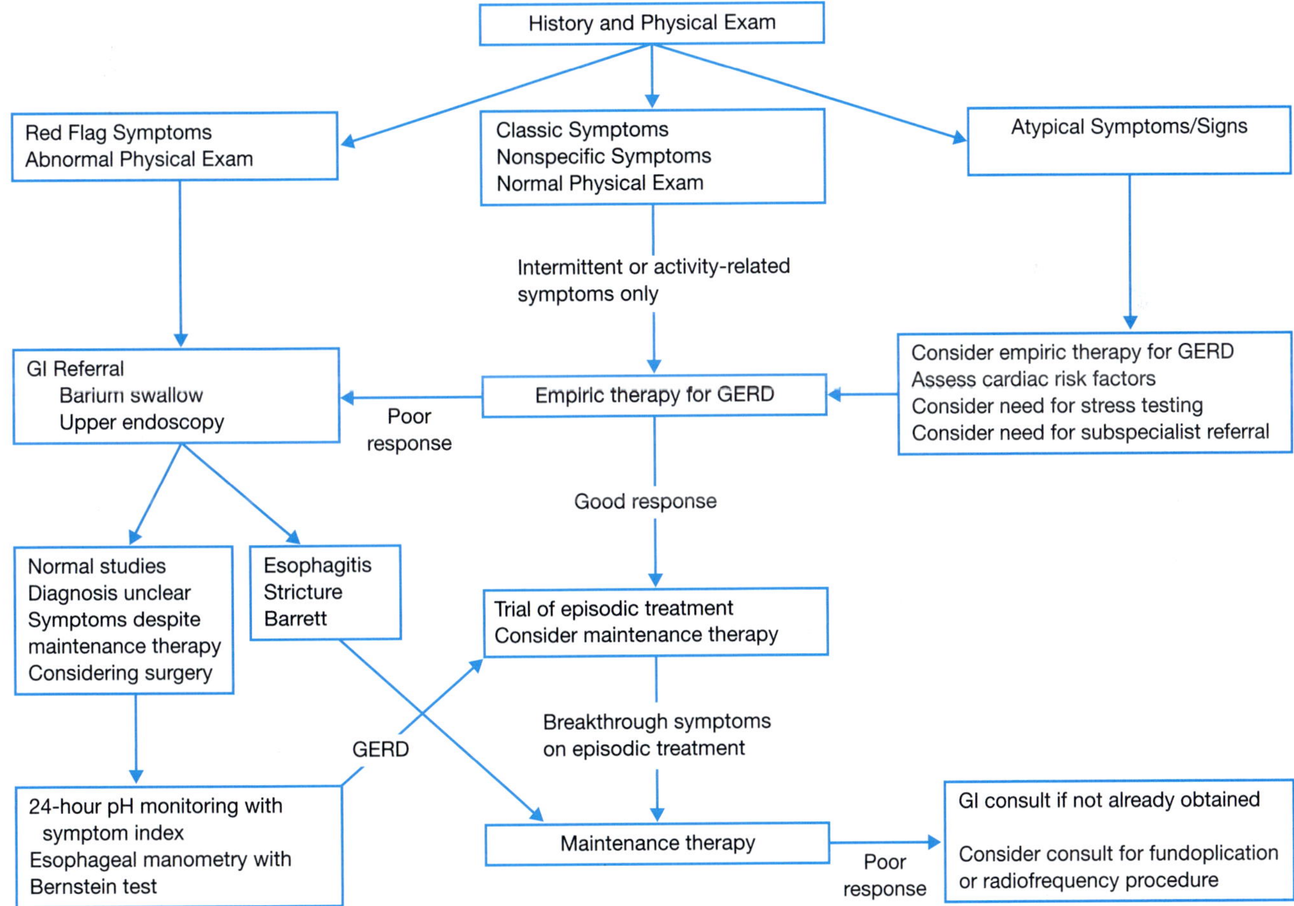

Figure 41.1: Evaluation of gastroesophageal reflux disease (GERD). GI, gastrointestinal. (Adapted with permission from O'Connor, FG. Gastrointestinal problems in runners. In: O'Connor, FG, Wilder, R, editors. *Textbook of Running Medicine*. 1st ed. New York: McGraw-Hill; 2001. pp. 307–14.)

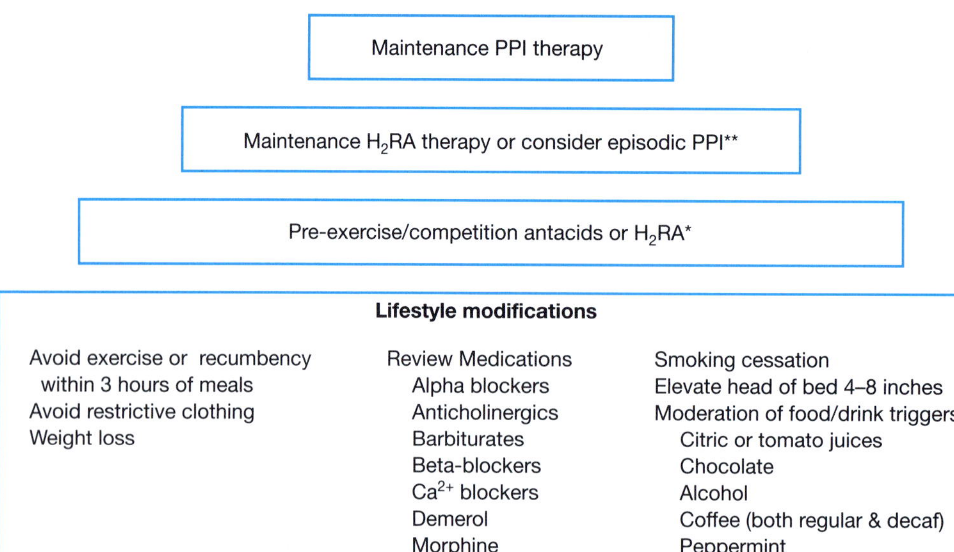

Figure 41.2: Therapeutic pyramid for exercise-related gastroesophageal reflux disease. (Adapted with permission from O'Connor, FG. Gastrointestinal problems in runners. In: O'Connor, FG, Wilder, R, editors. *Textbook of Running Medicine*. 1st ed. New York: McGraw-Hill; 2001. p. 307–14.)

- Persistent symptoms despite behavioral interventions warrant medical therapy. Episodic complaints are treated with over-the-counter (OTC) antacids, as needed, or antireflux medication, such as histamine 2 receptor antagonists (H_2RAs) or standard-dose proton pump inhibitors (PPIs) (10). This can be advanced to prescription-strength antireflux (H_2RA or PPI) therapy if control is insufficient. PPIs provide more rapid relief of symptoms (17) and are more likely than H_2RAs to heal and prevent recurrence of erosive esophagitis (18). PPIs are considered first line due to better symptom control and improved healing when compared to H_2RAs (19). Different PPI agents are equally efficacious in controlling heartburn and have similar healing and relapse rates (20). Because reported differences in initial bioavailability and antisecretory potency are not clinically significant with longstanding use, one PPI cannot be recommended over another (21). If the response to episodic treatment is generally favorable but symptoms are occurring on a more chronic basis, maintenance therapy may be beneficial. Because their efficacy is dose-dependent, PPI therapy can be stepped up to control symptoms. Should symptoms continue after 8 weeks of medication therapy, neither continuing the therapy nor increasing the dose is likely to achieve control (19,22). Recent data from nested case-control studies and meta-analyses suggest that long-term/high-dose PPIs utilization may be associated with an increased risk of hip fragility fractures. Impairment of calcium, magnesium, and vitamin B absorbance, hypergastrinemia, an increased secretion of histamine, play an important role in determining the increased fracture risk. Sports physicians should carefully evaluate the risk of fractures in long-term high-dose PPIs users and suggest adequate calcium/vitamin D supplementation (23).
- It was previously common practice to consider add-on therapy with a prokinetic agent to improve LES tone, gastric emptying, and peristalsis. These agents all have side effects that make them undesirable for use in athletes. Bethanechol has generalized cholinergic effects. Metoclopramide has a high incidence of fatigue, restlessness, tremor, and tardive dyskinesia, making it a poor choice for anything more than sporadic use. Cisapride, formerly the prokinetic agent of choice, was found to be associated with arrhythmia development, especially with concomitant use of macrolides, imidazoles, or protease inhibitors (3). This discovery led to severe prescribing restrictions in the United States. Current guidelines do not recommend adding a medication in PPI nonresponders (19).
- Failure to respond to high-dose PPI therapy requires gastroenterologist evaluation to rule out complications of GERD. In the absence of findings consistent with reflux disease, further GI testing will be necessary to confirm GERD and assess for other esophageal disorders.
- More invasive treatments are available for patients with an established diagnosis of GERD who respond poorly to PPIs, who are intolerant of medical therapy, or who desire a permanent solution to potentially eliminate their need for medication. Laparoscopic antireflux surgery has a range of efficacy from 10% to 93% for symptom reduction (24). A recent retrospective study showed significant symptom improvement

in surgery patients when compared to medication use alone (25). Other endoscopic therapies, including suturing, radiofrequency ablation, injection therapy, and bulking therapy, are performed in certain patient populations and are still being looked at in terms of long-term efficacy.

Peptic Ulcer Disease

- Epigastric pain is the hallmark of PUD. Both gastric and duodenal ulcers typically present with deep burning or gnawing pain, sometimes with radiation to the back. Duodenal ulcer symptoms usually develop 2–3 hours after meals and are relieved with food or antacids. Gastric ulcer symptoms develop sooner after meals but are less consistently relieved with food or antacids. Food ingestion can actually precipitate gastric ulcer pain in some individuals. Most PUD patients have associated anorexia and weight loss. Some patients, particularly with duodenal ulcers, experience hyperphagia and weight gain, presumably because of the mitigating effects of food. Commonly, the initial presentation of PUD can be life-threatening upper GI hemorrhage or perforation (26).
- Peptic ulcers are erosions in the surface of the stomach or duodenum that extend down to the muscularis mucosa. *H. pylori* induces ulcers by both direct and indirect mechanisms. Bacterial phospholipases weaken the protective mucus barrier, allowing the toxic compounds created from its breakdown of urea to directly damage the epithelium. The same urease enzyme that promotes this direct cell damage acts as a potent antigenic stimulator of immune cells. By inciting an exuberant host inflammatory response, *H. pylori* produces indirect epithelial damage as well (27).
- NSAID inhibition of prostaglandins affects multiple layers of the GI tract's protective barrier. With increasing concentration, NSAIDs diminish mucosal blood flow and penetrate the epithelial cells, eventually leading to mitochondrial oxidative uncoupling and cell death (28). There are no studies directly relating NSAID use to upper GI symptoms or bleeding specifically in athletes. Nevertheless, the increased mucosal permeability and decreased splanchnic blood flow that occurs with prolonged exercise may magnify the effects of *H. pylori* and the NSAIDs.
- Athletes should be questioned regarding any relationship of symptom onset with NSAID use. Laboratory analysis should assess for occult GI bleeding and anemia. If any alarm signs or symptoms are present or if an individual has new-onset dyspepsia after the age of 45 or has a family history of gastric cancer, early gastroenterology referral is recommended.
- If NSAID use is discovered, it should be discontinued if possible. If analgesic therapy is crucial, replacing a nonselective NSAID with acetaminophen or a cyclooxygenase-2 (COX-2) inhibitor would be prudent. Among individual NSAIDs, ibuprofen, celecoxib, and diclofenac have the lowest relative risk of upper GI complications whereas ketorolac has one of the highest (29). Upper GI safety and tolerability studies have shown that COX-2 inhibitors have a 46% lower rate of medication withdrawal for adverse events, a 71% lower risk of ulcers on endoscopy, and a 39% lower incidence of symptoms because of ulcers, perforations, bleeding, or obstruction compared to nonselective NSAIDs (30). COX-2 inhibitors are also recommended over the use of combined NSAID with proton-pump inhibitors (PPI). Combining NSAIDs with PPIs can have some protective effect, but this is limited to the upper GI tract. A systematic review comparing the effectiveness of these two regimens showed that COX-2 inhibitors are protective throughout the GI tract and have lower rates of GI complications (31).
- If symptoms are not predominantly GERD related, there are no markers for severe disease, and medication-induced disease is eliminated, consensus recommendations support stepwise therapy. *H. pylori* infection and testing should be considered in adults less than 60 years of age without alarm symptoms (32). Urea breath analysis is the favored test, with the stool antigen assay and whole blood or serum serology as alternatives. Symptomatic individuals who test positive for *H. pylori* require eradication therapy. Treatment regimen depends on local antibiotic resistant rates as well as patient tolerance. Options include clarithromycin with amoxicillin and a PPI, clarithromycin with metronidazole and a PPI, and Bismuth quadruple therapy (Table 41.2).
- Those who are *H. pylori*–negative can be managed with lifestyle and dietary modifications, along with medication. Mild symptoms can be managed with OTC antacids, or prescription H_2RA twice a day. Patients who fail this regimen or have severe symptoms should start PPI therapy daily. If symptoms are refractory to PPI use, diagnostic endoscopy should be performed as well as ambulatory esophageal pH-metry study. Referral to gastroenterology for further evaluation should also be considered.

Table 41.2 Regimens for the Treatment of *Helicobacter Pylori* Infection

Regimen	Duration	Eradication Rate[a]
Bismuth Quadruple	10–14 d	77.6%
Bismuth subcitrate (300 mg or 524 mg) qid		
Metronidazole 500 mg tid		
Tetracycline 500 mg qid		
PPI bid		
Clarithromycin Triple	14 d	68.9%
Clarithromycin 500 mg bid		
Amoxicillin 1 g bid OR Metronidazole 500 mg tid		
PPI bid		

bid, twice a day; PPI, proton pump inhibitor; qid, four times a day.
Source: O'Connor, FG. Gastrointestinal problems in runners. In: O'Connor, FG, Wilder, R, editors. *Textbook of Running Medicine*. 1st ed. New York: McGraw-Hill; 2001, p. 307–14; with permission.
[a]All eradication rates are based on a 7-day regimen. Although European data suggest 7 days are adequate, this has not been confirmed by U.S. studies. Thus, a full 14-day treatment course is recommended.

LOWER GI DISEASES

Runner's Diarrhea

- Lower GI symptoms occur more frequently in endurance athletes and more frequently affect women than men (33). Runner's diarrhea is a spectrum of exertional or immediately postexertional lower GI symptoms. Complaints range from abdominal cramping and fecal urgency to diarrhea and frank incontinence. Often, runner's diarrhea occurs in association with increases in training mileage or with particularly strenuous training sessions and competitions. An individual may be able to endure an episode by transiently reducing their pace. When symptoms are severer, it may be necessary to suspend their workout and quickly seek relief.
- Although the true etiology of runner's diarrhea remains unknown, several physiologic mechanisms have been proposed. Increased parasympathetic output during moderate exercise may intensify peristalsis, leading to cramping and rapid bowel transit. The mechanical effect of running, such as abdominal vibration, has been proposed as a cause (34). Strenuous exercise may lead to rapid shifts in intestinal fluid and electrolytes, causing colonic irritability (35). Another hypothesis is that the 70%–80% reduction in splanchnic blood flow with vigorous exercise may lead to ischemic enteropathy. Poor tissue perfusion maintained over the length of the exercise session could cause mucosal ischemia, leading to fluid shifts and diarrhea. This theory could explain the high prevalence of GI bleeding in marathon runners (36). Gut dysbiosis has also been proposed as a mechanism. Gut dysbiosis refers to an abnormal composition of gut microbiota, which can lead to GI disorders including diarrhea. A recent study found that female endurance runners had gut microbiota that differed from control subjects, specifically more inflammatory-type bacteria. This could indicate a link between dysbiosis and prevalence of GI symptoms in athletes (37).
- In addition to the basics, the history should document any recent travel, unusual food ingestion, or exposure to sick contacts to determine a potential infectious etiology. Diarrhea not associated with training should prompt a more intensive investigation. A focused lab assessment includes fecal occult blood testing and a complete blood count to look for anemia. In the presence of severe diarrhea, serum electrolytes should be drawn. Liver enzymes and pancreatic enzymes can be considered. If the history is suggestive of an infectious process, the stool should be examined for leukocytes, ova, parasites, and stool cultures.
- Treatment starts with a temporary reduction in training intensity and duration for 1–2 weeks. In most cases, this alone is enough to abolish symptoms (38). During this time, cross-training with low-impact or nonimpact activities at a level that does not trigger symptoms can be used to maintain the athlete's aerobic capacity. Any dietary or fluid replacement triggers should be eliminated. If a specific trigger is not identified, individuals with ongoing symptoms may benefit from dietary manipulation. A diet low in fiber can be helpful. Although not an adequate regimen for the control of chronic symptoms, some individuals may benefit from a complete liquid diet on the day prior to competition or scheduled intense exercise session. Once the diarrhea is under control, a full return to high-intensity exercise can be achieved by gradually increasing training as symptoms tolerate. Antidiarrheal medication should be used sparingly and with great caution. Antispasmodics, such as loperamide, are generally safe; however, anticholinergic medications, such as diphenoxylate with atropine (Lomotil), are to be avoided because of the increased heat injury risk secondary to their effect on sweating. Consult GI for unresolved symptoms despite conservative therapy or for red flag symptoms.

Abdominal Pain — "Side Stitch"

- In the young, active population, abdominal pain with exertion is common. The conditions previously discussed notwithstanding, the "side stitch," or exercise-related transient abdominal pain (ETAP), is the most common cause of this in athletes. Most often seen in swimmers, runners, and equestrians, it presents as a somewhat pleuritic aching sensation, usually in the right upper abdominal quadrant (39). Of the athletes who report experiencing ETAP, 90% complain of pain described as sharp, stabbing, cramping, aching, or pulling (6,21). It is often seen in deconditioned individuals starting an exercise program but can also be observed in athletes intensifying their training. Exercise in the postprandial period is a frequent exacerbating factor. Side stitches usually stop immediately on ceasing exercise. As an individual gains aerobic fitness, the frequency and severity of attacks tend to subside.
- Although their true etiology remains elusive, there are many theories including hypoxia-induced diaphragmatic muscle spasm (40). Other potential etiologies include pleural irritation, hepatic capsule irritation, symptomatic abdominal adhesions, and right colonic gas pain (41). Stress and anxiety are also thought to play a role (42).
- The management involves using the history to rule out not only the other GI diseases discussed in this chapter but also other exertional pain syndromes, especially angina. Fortunately, other serious causes of abdominal pain with exercise, such as mesenteric ischemia, bowel infarction, omental infarction, and hepatic vein thrombosis, are rare; however, in the setting of unremitting pain, especially with signs of systemic illness or shock, these conditions need to be considered in the differential and patients referred for potential surgical evaluation.
- Athletes with the typical features of a side stitch should be reassured that this is a benign process and will get better as their conditioning improves. They should be advised against exercise immediately after eating. If an episode of pain does occur, temporarily stopping exercise, stretching the right arm over their head, and exhaling through pursed lips can help abort it quickly (26).

Elevated Liver Enzymes

- Liver enzyme elevations observed in otherwise asymptomatic long-distance runners and other athletes are usually incidental findings. The suspected etiology is an ischemic insult secondary to reduced splanchnic blood flow and oxygen tension during vigorous exercise (43). Observed increases in alanine aminotransferase (ALT), aspartate aminotransferase (AST), alkaline phosphatase, creatinine phosphatase, and lactate dehydrogenase are confounded by the fact that these enzymes can be elevated in response to musculoskeletal injury. Hepatocellular injury can be confirmed by measuring glutamate dehydrogenase and γ-glutamyltransferase (GGT), enzymes more specific to the liver (44).
- Because these asymptomatic enzyme abnormalities are often discovered in the convalescent setting, the history and physical examination should focus on recent training sessions and environmental exposure, evaluating for evidence of a missed heat injury or episode of exertional rhabdomyolysis. The athlete should be questioned regarding any history of chronic liver disease or alcohol dependence and their medication list reviewed for any potentially hepatotoxic agents. With the nearly ubiquitous use of nutritional supplements, it is crucial to investigate this often-overlooked area.
- The majority of athletes can be reassured that this is a benign process and the enzyme abnormalities usually revert to normal within just 1 week after abstaining from exercise. The first step in the laboratory evaluation is to obtain a repeat liver enzyme panel after abstaining from acetaminophen, alcohol, and exercise for 1 week. If the liver enzymes are elevated at that time, they can be rechecked in 1 month. If the liver enzyme abnormalities persist on serial examinations, further evaluation should start with an iron panel, total iron-binding capacity, and hepatitis serologies to look for viral hepatitis or hemochromatosis. Second-tier tests include antinuclear antibody titer, anti-smooth muscle antibody, ceruloplasmin, α_1-antitrypsin, and serum protein electrophoresis, which would look for other causes for elevated aminotransferases, such as muscle disorders, Wilson disease, or thyroid disease. A right upper quadrant ultrasound is useful to evaluate for fatty liver, cholelithiasis, or other obstruction.
- GI referral should occur for abnormal lab testing, mildly elevated liver enzymes for over 6 months despite a negative evaluation, significantly elevated AST or ALT (>150) without improvement for 2 months, or signs of evolving hepatic insufficiency (44).

REFERENCES

1. Peters HP, Zweers M, Backx FJ, et al. Gastrointestinal symptoms during long-distance walking. *Med Sci Sports Exerc.* 1999;31(6):767–73.
2. Rehrer N, Janssen GM, Brouns F, Saris WH. Fluid intake and gastrointestinal problems in runners competing in a 25-km race and a marathon. *Int J Sports Med.* 1989;10(suppl 1):S22–5.
3. Waterman JJ, Kapur R. Upper gastrointestinal issues in athletes. *Curr Sports Med Rep.* 2012;11(2):99–104.
4. Collings KL, Pierce Pratt F, Rodriguez-Stanley S, Bemben M, Miner PB. Esophageal reflux in conditioned runners, cyclists, and weightlifters. *Med Sci Sports Exerc.* 2003;35(5):730–5.
5. Kavitt RT, Lipowska AM, Anyane-Yeboa A, Gralnek IM. Diagnosis and treatment of peptic ulcer disease. *Am J Med.* 2019;132(4):447–56.
6. Viola T. Evaluation of the athlete with exertional abdominal pain. *Curr Sports Med Rep.* 2010;9(2):106–10.
7. Keeffe EB, Lowe DK, Goss JR, Wayne R. Gastrointestinal symptoms of marathon runners. *West J Med.* 1984;141(4):481–4.
8. Jeukendrup AE, Vet-Joop K, Sturk A, et al. Relationship between gastro-intestinal complaints and endotoxaemia, cytokine release and the acute-phase reaction during and after a long-distance triathlon in highly trained men. *Clin Sci.* 2000;98(1):47–55.
9. Nilius M, Malfertheiner P. *Helicobacter pylori* enzymes. *Aliment Pharmacol Ther.* 1996;10(suppl 1):65–71.
10. Pate R. Principles of training. In: Kulund D, editor. *The Injured Athlete.* Philadelphia (PA): JB Lippincott; 1988.
11. Soffer EE, Merchant RK, Duethman G, Launspach J, Gisolfi C, Adrian TE. Effect of graded exercise on esophageal motility and gastroesophageal reflux in trained athletes. *Dig Dis Sci.* 1993;38(2):220–4.
12. Hirschowitz BI. A critical analysis, with appropriate controls of gastric acid and pepsin secretion in clinical esophagitis. *Gastroenterology.* 1991;101(5):1149–58.
13. Herregods TVK, van Hoeij FB, Oors JM, Bredenoord AJ, Smout AJPM. Effect of running on gastroesophageal reflux and reflux mechanisms. *Am J Gastroenterol.* 2016;111(7):940–6.
14. Spechler JS. Peptic ulcer disease and its complications. In: Feldman M, Friedman LS, Sleisinger MH, editors. *Sleisenger and Fordtran's Gastrointestinal and Liver Disease.* 7th ed. Philadelphia (PA): Saunders; 2002.
15. Mendes-Filho AM, Moraes-Filho JP, Nasi A, et al. Influence of exercise testing in gastroesophageal reflux in patients with gastroesophageal reflux disease. *Arq Bras Cir Dig.* 2014;27(1):3–8.
16. Bitnar P, Stovicek J, Hlava S, et al. Manual cervical traction and trunk stabilization cause significant changes in upper and lower esophageal sphincter: a randomized trial. *J Manip Physiol Ther.* 2021;44(4):344–51.
17. Bardhan KD, Müller-Lissner S, Bigard MA, et al. Symptomatic gastro-oesophageal reflux disease: double-blind controlled study of intermittent treatment with omeprazole or ranitidine. The European Study Group. *BMJ.* 1999;318(7182):502–7.
18. Chiba N, De Gara CJ, Wilkinson JM, Hunt RH. Speed of healing and symptom relief in grade II to IV gastroesophageal reflux disease: a meta-analysis. *Gastroenterology.* 1997;112(6):1798–810.
19. Katz PO, Dunbar KB, Schnoll-Sussman FH, Greer KB, Yadlapati R, Spechler SJ. ACG clinical guideline for the diagnosis and management of gastroesophageal reflux disease. *Am J Gastroenterol.* 2022;117(1):27–56.
20. Caro JJ, Salas M, Ward A. Healing and relapse rates in gastroesophageal reflux disease treated with the newer proton-pump inhibitors lansoprazole, rabeprazole, and pantoprazole compared with omeprazole, ranitidine, and placebo: evidence from randomized clinical trials. *Clin Ther.* 2001;23(7):998–1017.
21. Wysowski DK, Bacsanyi J. Cisapride and fatal arrhythmia. *N Engl J Med.* 1996;335(4):290–1.
22. Kahrilas PJ, Fennerty MB, Joelsson B. High- versus standard-dose ranitidine for control of heartburn in poorly responsive acid reflux disease: a prospective, controlled trial. *Am J Gastroenterol.* 1999;94(1):92–7.
23. Briganti SI, Naciu AM, Tabacco G, et al. Proton pump inhibitors and fractures in adults: a critical appraisal and review of the literature. *Int J Endocrinol.* 2021 Jan 15;2021:8902367.

24. Sidwa F, Moore AL, Alligood E, Fisichella PM. Surgical treatment of extraesophageal manifestations of gastroesophageal reflux disease. *World J Surg*. 2017 Oct;41(10):2566–71.
25. Johannessen R, Petersen H, Olberg P, Johnsen G, Fjøsne U, Kleveland PM. Airway symptoms and sleeping difficulties in operated and non-operated patients with gastroesophageal reflux disease. *Scand J Gastroenterol*. 2012;47(7):762–9.
26. Stamford B. Sports medicine adviser. *Phys Sportsmed*. 1985;13(5):187.
27. Parmelee-Peters K, Moeller JL. Gastroesophageal reflux in athletes. *Curr Sports Med Rep*. 2004;3(2):107–11.
28. Lichtenstein DR, Syngal S, Wolfe MM. Nonsteroidal anti-inflammatory drugs and the gastrointestinal tract. The double-edged sword. *Arthritis Rheum*. 1995;38(1):5–18.
29. Castellsague J, Riera-Guardia N, Calingaert B, et al. Individual NSAIDs and upper gastrointestinal complications: a systematic review and meta-analysis of observational studies (the SOS project). *Drug Saf*. 2012;35(12):1127–46.
30. Deeks JJ, Smith LA, Bradley MD. Efficacy, tolerability, and upper gastrointestinal safety of celecoxib for treatment of osteoarthritis and rheumatoid arthritis: systematic review of randomised controlled trials. *BMJ*. 2002;325(7365):619–23.
31. Jarupongprapa S, Ussavasodhi P, Katchamart W. Comparison of gastrointestinal adverse effects between cyclooxygenase-2 inhibitors and non-selective, non-steroidal anti-inflammatory drugs plus proton pump inhibitors: a systematic review and meta-analysis. *J Gastroenterol*. 2013 Jul;48(7):830–8.
32. Moayyedi PM, Lacy BE, Andrews CN, Enns RA, Howden CW, Vakil N. ACG and CAG clinical guideline: management of dyspepsia. *Am J Gastroenterol*. 2017;112(7):988–1013.
33. Ho GW. Lower gastrointestinal distress in endurance athletes. *Curr Sports Med Rep*. 2009;8(2):85–91.
34. Rehrer NJ, Meijer GA. Biomechanical vibration of the abdominal region during running and bicycling. *J Sports Med Phys Fitness*. 1991 Jun;31(2):231–4.
35. Richter JE. Typical and atypical presentations of gastroesophageal reflux disease. The role of esophageal testing in diagnosis and management. *Gastroenterol Clin North Am*. 1996;25(1):75–102.
36. Bounous G, McArdle AH. Marathon runners: the intestinal handicap. *Med Hypotheses*. 1990;33(4):261–4.
37. Morishima S, Aoi W, Kawamura A, et al. Intensive, prolonged exercise seemingly causes gut dysbiosis in female endurance runners. *J Clin Biochem Nutr*. 2021;68(3):253–8.
38. Fogoros RN. Runner's trots. Gastrointestinal disturbances in runners. *JAMA*. 1980;243(17):1743–4.
39. Morton DP, Callister R. Characteristics and etiology of exercise-related transient abdominal pain. *Med Sci Sports Exerc*. 2000;32(2):432–8.
40. Peters HP, Bos M, Seebregts L, et al. Gastrointestinal symptoms in long-distance runners, cyclists, and triathletes: prevalence, medication, and etiology. *Am J Gastroenterol*. 1999;94(6):1570–81.
41. Lauder TD, Moses FM. Recurrent abdominal pain from abdominal adhesions in an endurance triathlete. *Med Sci Sports Exerc*. 1995;27(5):623–5.
42. Wilson PB. Perceived life stress and anxiety correlate with chronic gastrointestinal symptoms in runners. *J Sports Sci*. 2018;36(15):1713–9.
43. Lijnen P, Hespel P, Fagard R, et al. Indicators of cell breakdown in plasma of men during and after a marathon race. *Int J Sports Med*. 1988;9(2):108–13.
44. *Liver enzyme elevation referral guideline* [Internet]. [cited 1999]. Available from: http://www.mamc.amedd.army.mil/referral/guidelines

Pulmonary

42

Carrie A. Jaworski and Jacqueline Leemputte

INTRODUCTION

- Patients with pulmonary disorders can benefit greatly from exercise when their disease process is under proper control.
- Awareness of when and when not to participate and the ability to use pharmacologic agents and environmental controls greatly enhance one's ability to participate safely.

ASTHMA

- Asthma is a chronic pulmonary disorder characterized by varying degrees of airflow obstruction, bronchial hyperresponsiveness, and underlying chronic inflammation (1).
- Approximately, 25 million adults and 5.5 million children in the United States have chronic asthma (1).
- The National Heart, Lung, and Blood Institute (NHLBI) has set forth guidelines on the diagnosis and management of asthma in an effort known as the National Asthma Education and Prevention Program. This program is evidence based and routinely updates its recommendations based on the newest research. The third edition was completed in 2007, and in 2020, there was a revision of selected topics; the latest recommendations can be found at the NHLBI Web site: http://www.nhlbi.nih.gov/ (2).
- While in the past, patients with asthma were discouraged from exercise, today it is recognized that regular exercise can reduce airway reactivity and decrease medication use (3). Current data support this trend, with decreased numbers of patients with asthma reporting limitations in their activity (1,4).

Diagnosis of Asthma

- History or presence of episodic symptoms of airflow obstruction, such as wheezing, chest tightness, shortness of breath, or cough. Absence of symptoms at the time of examination does not exclude diagnosis.
- Airflow obstruction needs to be at least partially reversible, as demonstrated through the use of spirometry. First, establish airflow obstruction: forced expiratory volume in 1 second (FEV_1) <80% predicted and FEV_1/forced vital capacity (FVC) ratio <70% or below the lower limit of normal. Then establish reversibility by an FEV_1 increase of ≥12% from baseline or ≥10% of predicted FEV_1 after using a short-acting inhaled β_2-agonist (5).
- It must exclude other diagnoses, such as exercise-induced laryngeal obstruction (EILO) (previously referred to as vocal cord dysfunction), vascular rings, and reflux disease, if spirometry is normal.
- Classification of asthma severity is based on history and spirometry (Table 42.1).
- Management should focus on patient education, environmental control, and objective monitoring.
- **Patient education:** Patients and their families should understand signs and symptoms of an asthma exacerbation, the chronicity of the disease, and potential triggers of an attack. A written plan should be reviewed, and instruction on proper use of inhaled medications and peak flow monitoring should be provided.
- **Environmental control:** Avoidance of exposure to precipitating factors is paramount. Potential triggers include pollen, mold, ozone, exercise, and cold air. Athletes should exercise indoors on bad weather days or use measures, such as masks, to decrease the chance of attack. Indoor swimming is considered an excellent option secondary to the warm, moist environment at the pool. Some patients with asthma are susceptible to aspirin and nonsteroidal anti-inflammatory drugs, so judicious use must be exercised (6).
- **Monitoring:** Athletes need to be monitoring their peak flows daily to recognize decline in function, as well as response to treatment. Formal spirometry is recommended for initial diagnosis, after treatment and peak flows have stabilized, and then every 1–2 years when asthma is stable, or more often when unstable (1).
- Pharmacologic therapy should be instituted to control inflammation and treat episodes of bronchoconstriction. Use a stepwise approach to treatment as outlined in Table 42.2.

Medication Classes

- The two main classes of asthma medications are long-term control medications that are used to treat and control the persistent symptoms of asthma and short-acting agents that provide quick relief of symptom exacerbations.

Table 42.1 Severity Classification

	Components of Control	Classification of Asthma Control (Youth ≥12 Y of Age and Adults)		
		Well Controlled	**Not Well Controlled**	**Very Poorly Controlled**
Impairment	Symptoms	≤2 d a week	>2 d a week	Throughout the day
	Nighttime awakening	≤2 × a month	1–3 × a week	≥4 × a week
	Interference with normal activity	None	Some limitation	Extremely limited
	Short-acting β_2-agonist use for symptom control (not prevention of EIB)	≤2 d a week	>2 d a week	Several times per day
	FEV_1 or peak flow	>80% predicted/personal best	60%–80% predicted/personal best	<60% predicted/personal best
	Validated questionnaires			
	ATAQ	0	1–2	3–4
	ACQ	≤0.75[a]	≥1.5	N/A
	ACT	≥20	16–19	≤15
Risk	Exacerbations	0–1 a year	≥2 a year (see note)	
		Consider severity and interval since last exacerbation		
	Progressive loss of lung function	Evaluation requires long-term follow-up care		
	Treatment-related adverse effects	Medication side effects can vary in intensity from none to very troublesome and worrisome. The level of intensity does not correlate to specific levels of control but should be considered in the overall assessment of risk.		

ACQ, Asthma Control Questionnaire; ACT, Asthma Control Test; ATAQ, Asthma Therapy Assessment Questionnaire; EIB, exercise-induced bronchospasm; FEV_1, forced expiratory volume in 1 second.
[a]ACQ values of 0.76–1.4 are indeterminate regarding well-controlled asthma.

LONG-TERM CONTROLLERS

- **Corticosteroids:** Mechanism is to block late-phase reaction to allergens, decrease airway hyperresponsiveness, and inhibit inflammatory cell actions. Inhaled corticosteroids (ICSs) are the mainstay of treatment in the long-term control of asthma. ICSs are considered to be the most potent and consistently effective anti-inflammatory asthma medication (1,7–10). ICSs must be taken on a regular basis. Side effects can include local irritation, dysphonia, and oral candidiasis. Systemic forms may be needed in asthma flares and cases recalcitrant to inhaled glucocorticoids.
- **Khellin derivatives:** Cromolyn sodium (Intal) and nedocromil sodium (Tilade) act to stabilize mast cells, thus preventing the release of inflammatory mediators. Both are inhaled medications with a strong safety profile and can be considered as an alternative to ICSs but are not a preferred therapy. Cromolyn is approved for children of all ages, whereas nedocromil is approved in children older than age 6. Both take about 2 weeks to demonstrate a therapeutic response.
- **Leukotriene modifiers:** Zileuton (Zyflo), a 5-lipoxygenase inhibitor, blocks the synthesis of leukotrienes, whereas zafirlukast (Accolate) and montelukast (Singulair), leukotriene receptor antagonists (LTRAs), block the effects of leukotrienes after they are formed. All three medications decrease airway inflammation and offer another alternative to ICSs. Montelukast and zafirlukast are approved in children, have a favorable safety profile, and are taken orally every day or twice a day. Less desirable is zileuton, which is not approved in children <12 years old and requires dosing 4 times a day and monitoring of hepatic function.
- **Long-acting β_2-agonists (LABAs)** are bronchodilators that last up to 12 hours after 1 dose. Examples include salmeterol (Serevent) and formoterol (Foradil). LABAs are the recommended medication to be used in combination with ICSs for management of moderate to severe asthma (11–13). Based on most recent guidelines, ICS-formoterol may also be taken as needed in the management of persistent asthma (1). Concern regarding the use of LABA as monotherapy and an increased risk of asthma exacerbations and asthma-related deaths has caused a black box warning to be placed on all preparations containing a LABA (14,15). An expert panel recommends weighing the benefit of LABA use in uncontrolled patients with asthma versus the small increased risk (1).
- **Long-acting muscarinic antagonists (LAMAs)** are a class of long-acting bronchodilators that can be considered in individuals older than 12 with uncontrolled persistent asthma that is not controlled by an ICS-LABA combination, or if the individual cannot tolerate the addition of a LABA to ICS therapy. Currently, the only FDA-approved LAMA for asthma is tiotropium bromide (Respimat) (1).

Table 42.2 Treatment: Stepwise Approach

Intermittent Asthma	Management of Persistent Asthma in Individuals Ages 12+ Years				
Step 1	**Step 2**	**Step 3**	**Step 4**	**Step 5**	**Step 6**
Preferred: SABA PRN	***Preferred:*** Daily low-dose ICS and PRN SABA or PRN concomitant ICS and SABA*	***Preferred:*** Daily and PRN combination low-dose ICS-formoterol	***Preferred:*** Daily and PRN combination medium-dose ICS-formoterol	***Preferred:*** Daily medium-high dose ICS-LABA + LAMA and PRN SABA*	***Preferred:*** Daily high-dose ICS-LABA + oral systemic corticosteroids + PRN SABA
	Alternative: *Daily LTRA and PRN SABA* or Cromolyn, or nedocromil, or zileuton or theophylline, and PRN SABA	***Alternative:*** Daily medium-dose ICS and PRN SABA or Daily low-dose ICS-LABA, or daily low-dose ICS + LAMA, or daily low-dose ICS + LTRA, and PRN SABA or Daily low-dose ICS + theophylline or zileuton and PRN SABA	***Alternative:*** *Daily medium-dose ICS-LABA or daily medium-dose ICS + LAMA and PRN SABA* or Daily medium-dose ICS + LTRA, or daily medium-dose ICS + theophylline, or daily medium-dose ICS + zileuton and PRN SABA	***Alternative:*** Daily medium-high dose ICS-LABA or daily high-dose ICS + LTRA, and PRN SABA	
	Steps 2–4: Conditionally recommend the use of subcutaneous immunotherapy as an adjunct treatment to standard pharmacotherapy in individuals ≥5 years of age whose asthma is controlled at the initiation, buildup, and maintenance phases of immunotherapy			Consider adding asthma biologics (*e.g.*, anti-IgE, anti-IL5, anti-IL5R, anti-IL4/IL13)	

ICS, inhaled corticosteroid; LABA, long-acting beta$_2$-agonist; LAMA, long-acting muscarinic antagonist; LTRA, leukotriene receptor antagonist; SABA, inhaled short-acting beta$_2$-agonist.

- **Immune modulators:** Omalizumab (Xolair) is a monoclonal antibody that prevents binding of immunoglobulin E to mast cells and basophils. It can be used as adjunctive therapy in patients older than 12 years with allergies and severe asthma. It is for those with severe persistent asthma not controlled with a combination of high-dose ICS and LABA (16,17). It has been shown to decrease severe allergic asthma attacks irrespective of blood eosinophil levels (17). Other immune modulators target interleukin 5 (IL-5), the IL-5 receptor, or the IL-4 receptor α-unit. These are indicated in severe eosinophilic asthma and repetitive exacerbations irrespective of blood eosinophil levels (17).
- **Methylxanthines:** Sustained-release theophylline is a bronchodilator with mild anti-inflammatory effects that is an alternative, but not preferred, adjunctive therapy with ICS. It requires monitoring of blood levels, which makes it less ideal.

SHORT-ACTING AGENTS

- **Short-acting β_2-agonists (SABAs):** Inhaled albuterol is the main rescue medication for acute bronchoconstriction and prevention of exercise-induced asthma (EIA). Inhaled forms have a good safety profile with primarily mild central nervous system side effects. Medication has an immediate effect and is, therefore, subject to overuse. Chronic use can also lead to decreases in efficacy and increased bronchial hyperreactivity. Oral forms are not approved for use by the International Olympic Committee or National Collegiate Athletic Association.
- **Anticholinergics:** Ipratropium bromide (Atrovent) is a bronchodilator used more often in patients with chronic obstructive pulmonary disease (COPD). It can be an adjunct for patients who have an inadequate response to β_2-agonists. The duration of action is 3–4 hours with an onset of 30–90 minutes.

ASTHMA MANAGEMENT

- The goal of therapy is to maintain control of asthma with the least amount of medication necessary. Use a stepwise approach while minimizing impairment and risk (1). See Table 42.2.
- Use caution when prescribing medications to collegiate, professional, and elite athletes. Always check with the sport's governing body regarding banned substances. The U.S. Olympic Committee has an up-to-date list available through their Web site (http://www.usantidoping.org), or you can call their drug control hotline at 1-800-233-0393.

- Once asthma is well controlled, exercise should be encouraged. Studies have demonstrated decreased numbers of exacerbations, less medication use, and fewer missed days of work or school in patients with asthma who exercised (1,18).
- The exercise prescription should include a pre-exercise assessment to document control. FEV_1 should be ≥80% of expected levels (8). The exercise goal should be consistent with the American College of Sports Medicine's recommendation to exercise on most days of the week for 20–30 minutes (19). The type of exercise can be anything that the patient enjoys but should provide aerobic benefit, as well as strength and flexibility conditioning.
- Advise caution on risky activities, such as exercising outside on a cold day, when wheezing or when peak flows suggest a decline in lung function because exercise can trigger symptoms of bronchoconstriction. (See next section.)

EXERCISE-INDUCED ASTHMA/ BRONCHOSPASM

- EIA is defined as the transitory increase in airway resistance that typically occurs following vigorous exercise in a patient with chronic asthma. Exercise-induced bronchospasm (EIB) refers to those individuals with no symptoms outside of exercise. EIB is the preferred term, but it is important to understand that some patients with asthma will only mount symptoms with exercise, so ensuring that no symptoms or reductions in pulmonary function exist at rest is paramount in guiding treatment (5).
- Ninety percent of patients with chronic asthma will have EIB, and 40% of patients with allergic rhinitis or atopic dermatitis will have EIB (20).
- The prevalence of EIB in athletes varies by sport with ranges between 12% and 55% (21), and EIB occurs in amateur to elite-level athletes. Higher risk sports include those with high-minute ventilation, such as basketball, track, and soccer, as well as those done in cool, dry air, such as cross-country skiing, ice skating, and hockey. Environmental exposures such as allergens or chloramines from pools may also affect athletes (22,23).
- The pathophysiology of EIB remains debatable. Two main theories exist.
  - The *water loss theory* attributes EIB to the loss of water through the bronchial mucosa as the body tries to warm rapidly inhaled air during exercise. This dries the mucosa and causes local changes in pH, osmolarity, and the temperature of the airway, which may trigger bronchoconstriction (24).
  - The *thermal expenditure theory* holds that EIB is the result of respiratory heat loss that occurs during exercise. The increased ventilation of exercise causes a cooling of the airways. Once exercise ceases, the blood vessels dilate and engorge to rewarm the epithelium, which may lead to rebound hyperemia and bronchoconstriction (24).
- Some studies demonstrate that the presence of inflammatory mediators are also involved in EIB (25–28).

Presentation

- Clinical symptoms may include coughing, wheezing, chest tightness, or shortness of breath during or minutes after intense exercise. Symptoms usually peak 5–10 minutes after exercise and last for 20–30 minutes. Atypical symptoms can include stomach cramps, chest pain, nausea, headache, or feeling out of shape. Examination during an attack may demonstrate increased respiratory rate, prolonged expiration, decreased breath sounds, and wheezing. Some athletes may describe a late response 6–8 hours after the onset of exercise.

Diagnosis

- The diagnosis of EIB is often based on history and self-reported symptoms. Numerous studies have demonstrated that this approach is unreliable and can both underdiagnose and overdiagnose the condition (29–31). Parsons et al. (29) found that 36% of athletes with a positive eucapnic voluntary hyperventilation (EVH) test did not report any symptoms and that only 35% of athletes with symptoms were found to have positive tests. More reliable diagnosis is based on pulmonary function testing after a thorough history and physical examination have ruled out any other explanation of the symptoms.
- Office spirometry should be done at rest to rule out underlying chronic asthma in anyone suspected of having EIB. A normal resting test with suspicion of EIB warrants a bronchoprovocation test. Many physicians will give a trial of a prophylactic bronchodilator if classic history and mild symptoms exist.
- Normal testing with no response to medication should prompt consideration of EILO as the diagnosis. Gastroesophageal reflux and cardiac disorders need to be considered as well.
- Options for confirming EIB include indirect and direct challenge tests. (See Chapter 28 Exercise-Induced Bronchoconstriction Testing, for detailed discussion.)

INDIRECT CHALLENGE TESTS (SEE CHAPTER 27 EXERCISE-INDUCED BRONCHOCONSTRICTION TESTING)

Exercise Challenge Test

- Performed either in a laboratory or in the field, this test seeks to simulate the athlete's sport in order to provoke EIB. Formal pulmonary function tests are done, with FEV_1 being the index most often measured in the lab versus peak expiratory flow rate (PEFR) in the field. Solitary EIB will have a pre-exercise baseline FEV_1 or PEFR between 80% and 100% of normal predicted values. The exercise is most commonly free or treadmill running for 5–8 minutes at a high intensity (≥85%–90% maximum predicted heart rate). FEV_1 or PEFR is measured at 1-, 3-, 5-, 10-, and 15-minute intervals. Positive test = a decrease in FEV_1 or PEFR of 15%. Mild EIB = 15%–25% decrease. Moderate EIB = 25%–40% decrease. Severe EIB = a decrease of >40% (32).

- Field testing offers the advantage of more closely mimicking actual sport, but it can be difficult to control environmental factors and hard to control/monitor rate of exertion.
- Laboratory testing is more costly and eliminates possible contributing environmental triggers. It offers the advantages of controlled cardiovascular workload and ability to monitor pulmonary and cardiovascular function during exercise (33).
- Other indirect challenge tests include the EVH challenge test, the hyperosmolar saline challenge test, and the mannitol challenge test. EVH testing is considered the "gold standard" by many; however, it is not readily available other than at research centers (34).

DIRECT CHALLENGE TESTS

- Direct challenge testing involves administration of increasing doses of a pharmacologic agent, such as methacholine, to cause bronchoconstriction. These tests are highly sensitive but have a poor specificity for EIB.

Treatment

- Good long-term control of chronic asthma should allow participation in athletics without any EIB symptoms. If symptoms are occurring, adjustment to the treatment needs to be made (Table 42.2). A variety of agents are available to treat EIB. Treatment should be tailored to the individual athlete and their sport.

PHARMACOLOGIC TREATMENTS (ALSO SEE LONG-TERM CONTROLLERS SECTION)

- SABAs: First-line therapy is usually with an inhaled SABA, such as albuterol, two to four puffs taken 15–30 minutes prior to activity. Albuterol's onset of action is ≤5 minutes and duration of effect is ~2–6 hours. It will prevent EIB in >80% of patients (1). All athletes with EIB should carry a SABA inhaler with them during exercise to relieve acute exacerbations that occur despite prophylaxis.
- LABAs can be protective for up to 12 hours and should be considered in athletes involved in endurance/all-day events, as well as in children where activity is unpredictable. When used daily, shortening of duration of action occurs (35). Frequent use of LABAs for EIB is not recommended because it may disguise poorly controlled persistent asthma (1).
- Cromolyn or nedocromil can be used as an alternative to SABAs, but they are not as effective. Both should be administered as two to four puffs 20 minutes prior to exercise. The duration of action is ~2 hours. They are not to be used to treat acute symptoms but are useful for repeated bouts of exercise because they have minimal/no side effects. Combining cromolyn with SABA can be helpful (36).
- LTRAs offer the advantage of oral administration and long duration of action. Attenuation of EIB symptoms occurs in up to 50% of patients (1). Montelukast is administered at 10 mg daily in adults and 5 mg in 6- to 14-year-old children. It has a 3- to 4-hour onset of action and a duration of 24 hours. Zafirlukast is administered at 20 mg twice a day in adults and 10 mg twice a day in children 5–11 years old. It has an onset of action of 30 minutes and duration of 12 hours.
- ICSs are not effective as prophylaxis prior to exercise but need to be considered in patients refractory to the aforementioned medications; patients should also be reevaluated for chronic asthma.

NONPHARMACOLOGIC TREATMENTS

- The use of masks or scarves to decrease the amount of heat and water lost with exercise in cold weather may diminish EIB.
- Aerobic conditioning may reduce severity of EIB by improving rate of ventilation during exercise, but there is no proof it prevents EIB (34).
- Appropriate cooldowns help decrease EIB. Cooling down helps by allowing gradual rewarming of the airways, which decreases vascular dilation and edema.
- **Refractory period:** Defined as the time after spontaneous recovery from an episode of EIB where >50% of athletes will not experience another episode of bronchoconstriction with exercise. Effect is usually 1–2 hours in duration. It can benefit athletes who experience this effect in that they can induce a refractory period prior to their actual competition to lessen the severity of EIB during their event. Various methods exist to induce the effect, including 20–30 minutes of low-intensity exercise or seven 30-second sprints separated by short intervals (3,34,37,38). Studies demonstrate that the most consistent decrease in EIB symptoms was seen with a warm-up comprised of either high-intensity intervals or a variable intensity warm-up that goes from low to very high intensity (39). Studies also demonstrate that this effect is inhibited with the use of nonsteroidal anti-inflammatories (40). Athletes should be counseled to still use their prescribed EIB medications because effect is partial for most people (41).

CHRONIC OBSTRUCTIVE PULMONARY DISEASE

- COPD is a progressive disease that primarily refers to emphysema and chronic bronchitis. It is a condition of slowly deteriorating pulmonary function whereby expiratory airflow obstruction leads to dyspnea and deconditioning. While exercise cannot reverse the process, it can provide improvements in quality of life and decreased disability (42).
- Estimated worldwide prevalence is 7%–19%, but COPD is largely underdiagnosed (43). Death rates from COPD continue to rise, and it is the sixth leading cause of death in the United States (43).
- The primary cause is chronic tobacco use, but other etiologies, such as α_1-antitrypsin deficiency and environmental exposures, do play a role.
- The pathophysiology of COPD is multifactorial. Airway hyperreactivity and/or increased respiratory secretions lead to chronic obstruction. This results in air trapping and respiratory muscle dysfunction, which, over time, causes generalized deconditioning. Additionally, the emphysematous component causes destruction of alveolar capillary membranes, which leads to hypoxemia. Chronic hypoxemia results in pulmonary hypertension and right ventricular failure (32).
- Severe limitations in respiratory function and chronic hypoxemia cause great fear and anxiety in patients with COPD, including a fear of exercise and thus further deconditioning (44).
- Our role as sports medicine physicians is to enable patients with COPD to exercise comfortably and safely.
- **Evaluation:** Prior to providing an exercise prescription, patients must have an assessment of their current status through a physical examination and pulmonary function testing. One can expect reductions in FEV_1 and increased ventilatory muscle effort.
  - A careful assessment of cardiac risk and exercise capacity, including exercise testing, is recommended for all patients. Many protocols exist for both treadmill and stationary cycle testing. Exercise testing can help to determine safe levels of exercise to prevent arrhythmias and hypoxemia, the amount of supplemental oxygen needed during exercise, and any need for bronchodilators.
- **Management:** The care of the patient with COPD is aimed at maintaining, or improving, the functional capacity through a multidisciplinary approach.
- **Exercise:** Studies demonstrate that exercise improves dyspnea, provides an aerobic training response, reduces ventilation, and improves overall exercise tolerance (45). No evidence exists that exercise lengthens life expectancy in the patient with COPD, but it provides immense physical and psychological benefits.
  - Supervised exercise through a pulmonary rehabilitation program is warranted if patient has significant disease. Most can graduate to independent exercise within 6 weeks (42).
  - Independent exercise goal should be to exercise 3 days a week at 60%–80% of maximal heart rate for 20–30 minutes. Type of exercise will vary based on patient's ability and comorbidities. Stationary cycling is useful initially because many patients are unsteady on their feet, and arm ergometry can be used for those with lower extremity limitations. These goals may take months to reach, if at all. Start with several minutes of exercise and progress at a rate appropriate for the individual (45,46).
  - Exercise aids can include supplemental oxygen and medications. Bronchodilators and anticholinergics are the mainstay of pharmacologic therapy in COPD and should be used aggressively. Mucolytics can assist with excessive secretions. ICS can also assist in decreasing airway inflammation. Oral corticosteroids are reserved for more severe cases, and theophylline remains a controversial therapy.
  - Bronchopulmonary toilet and pursed-lip breathing are two other mechanical techniques that can aid patients with COPD in achieving activity goals.
- Careful attention to preventive health care, such as influenza, COVID-19, and polyvalent pneumococcal immunizations, can help patients with COPD avoid setbacks in their exercise programs and enhance overall well-being.

CYSTIC FIBROSIS

- Cystic fibrosis (CF) is an autosomal recessive disorder that affects multiple organ systems, including the pulmonary, gastrointestinal, reproductive, and skeletal systems, as well as the sweat glands. Chronic pulmonary disease is the leading cause of morbidity and mortality because the thick mucus found with CF leads to infection and inhibits pulmonary function. Aerobic exercise has been shown to aid in the clearance of secretions and improve quality of life in patients with CF (47). Standardized exercise testing has recently been endorsed as a routine part of the regular assessment of patients with CF (48).
- Diagnosis of CF is made by an abnormal sweat chloride test. Prenatal screening is now available and should be offered to couples at higher risk, particularly those of Northern European descent. Pulmonary function tests are similar to a patient with asthma but also demonstrate a decreased FVC.
- Management of CF is dependent on the extent of disease. A goal of preventing recurrent respiratory infections is attempted through chest physiotherapy, bronchodilators, and antibiotics. Corticosteroids, oxygen, recombinant deoxyribonuclease I, and possibly lung transplantation in advanced cases may also be warranted.

- Exercise can augment mobilization of secretions when combined with chest physiotherapy (49,50). A study also demonstrated less loss of FVC compared to controls (51). In mild forms of CF, athletes should be allowed to participate as their pulmonary function allows. Moderate to severe cases of CF benefit from more formal rehabilitation programs where the need for supplemental oxygen can be tracked.
- All athletes with CF need to be counseled on safe exercise in the heat because they are subject to increased sodium and chloride losses in their sweat when compared to those without CF. This is particularly important when athletes with CF partake in more intense endurance exercise as this places them at an increased risk of exercise-associated hyponatremia. These athletes should be educated on proper steps to mitigate this risk through proper hydration/electrolyte replacement techniques.

RESPIRATORY INFECTIONS

- Respiratory tract infections are one of the most common medical problems encountered in the care of athletes. Upper respiratory tract infections (URIs) comprise the majority of these infections (52).
- Immune function affects avoidance and occurrence of URIs. Studies demonstrate that moderate exercise can protect against URIs, whereas intense exercise can decrease immunity and increase the risk of URIs (53).
- Prevention of URIs can be augmented through avoidance of overtraining, adequate sleep, proper nutrition, and limiting stress. Influenza vaccination of athletes in winter sports should be considered. Vaccination against COVID-19 should also be considered for all athletes.
- Treatment of URIs is primarily symptomatic. Nasal ipratropium bromide and oral/topical decongestants can be helpful in the short term. Caution must be exercised with antihistamines in athletes because they can impair temperature regulation and cause sedation. Inhaled β-agonists can help with URI-associated coughs. Antibiotics are only indicated if progression to a secondary bacterial infection occurs. Zinc and vitamin C may reduce the duration of URI symptoms (54,55).
- Athletes with a common cold can continue to participate to a lesser degree provided no fever is present. Care should be taken to increase hydration and cease activity if constitutional symptoms occur, such as fever, myalgias, productive cough, vomiting, or diarrhea.
- Progression to diseases, such as pneumonia and complicated bronchitis, warrants up to 10–14 days of rest before resuming full activity. Return to play after a COVID-19 infection should be based on the severity of symptoms experienced (see Chapter 38 on Infectious Diseases).

EXERCISE-INDUCED LARYNGEAL OBSTRUCTION

- EILO is a type of inducible laryngeal obstruction that occurs due to narrowing at the glottic or supraglottic level during exercise. It is important to identify and treat EILO appropriately as it may lead to exercise avoidance if left untreated.
- EILO is a common condition in young individuals, particularly in athletes, and occurs due to a failure in the abduction of the glottic and aryepiglottic folds that should normally occur during exercise. This may be due to anatomic mechanisms including airway size and compliance or neurologic factors. Other contributors may include asthma, reflux, rhinosinusitis, behavioral or genetic components, and differences in anatomic structure (56).
- Athletes with EILO commonly present with inspiratory stridor and shortness of breath during exercise with full resolution of symptoms within a couple minutes of stopping exercise. Symptoms may vary among athletes but may also include cough, stridor, globus sensation, hoarseness, choking sensation, and chest tightness.
- Evaluation should include a thorough history to determine the timing of symptoms in relation to onset of exercise, resolution of symptoms with exercise cessation, history of comorbid conditions, and other known exposures/triggers.
- Patients reporting stridor at rest should be further evaluated for other forms of inducible laryngeal obstruction. Other conditions including asthma and exercise-induced bronchoconstriction should be included in the differential diagnosis.
- Continuous laryngoscopy during exercise (CLE) is the gold standard for diagnosis of EILO. CLE utilizes flexible nasolaryngoscopy with an exercise challenge that is sport-specific when possible (eg, treadmill test or cycle ergometry) to evaluate adduction of supraglottic structures and glottic folds during exercise with abrupt resolution after discontinuing stress testing (57). Evaluation for EILO should include spirometry to assess flow volume loops at rest to identify coexisting conditions including asthma, vocal fold paralysis, or subglottic stenosis. Methacholine or mannitol bronchoprovocation is useful to evaluate for asthma and exercise-induced bronchoconstriction (58).
- First-line treatment for EILO is speech-behavioral therapy focusing on relaxation and retraining of laryngeal muscles and coordinating breathing patterns (59). Therapeutic laryngoscopy can be used during exercise to provide biofeedback to teach specific exercises and techniques for muscle relaxation. The majority of patients improve with these measures alone, but for patients with refractory symptoms, a supraglottoplasty that involves incision into portions of aryepiglottic folds and arytenoids may be necessary (60,61).

REFERENCES

1. U.S. Department of Health and Human Services. *2020 Focused Updates to the Asthma Management Guidelines* [Internet]. [cited2020]. Available from: https://www.nhlbi.nih.gov/health-topics/asthma-management-guidelines-2020-updates
2. National Institute of Health. *Highlights of the Expert Panel Report 3: Guidelines for the Diagnosis and Management of Asthma*. Bethesda (MD): National Institutes of Health Publication; 2007. National Institutes of Health, National Heart, Lung, and Blood Institute.
3. Disabella V, Sherman C. Exercise for asthma patients: little risk, big rewards. *Phys Sportsmed*. 1998;26(6):75–84.
4. Bundgaard A. Exercise and the asthmatic. *Sports Med*. 1985;2(4):254–266.
5. U.S. Department of Health and Human Services. *EPR-2. Expert Panel Report 2: Guidelines for the Diagnosis and Management of Asthma (EPR-2 1997)*. Bethesda (MD): U.S. Department of Health and Human Services, National Institutes of Health, National Heart, Lung, and Blood Institute, National Asthma Education and Prevention Program. NIH Publication No. 97-4051; 1997.
6. Stevenson DD, Szczeklik A. Clinical and pathologic perspectives on aspirin sensitivity and asthma. *J Allergy Clin Immunol*. 2006;118(4):773–88. quiz 787–8.
7. Garcia Garcia ML, Wahn U, Gilles L, Swern A, Tozzi CA, Polos P. Montelukast, compared with fluticasone, for control of asthma among 6- to 14-year-old patients with mild asthma: the MOSAIC study. *Pediatrics*. 2005;116(2):360–9.
8. Ostrom NK, Decotiis BA, Lincourt WR, et al. Comparative efficacy and safety of low-dose fluticasone propionate and montelukast in children with persistent asthma. *J Pediatr*. 2005;147(2):213–20.
9. Szefler SJ, Phillips BR, Martinez FD, et al. Characterization of within-subject responses to fluticasone and montelukast in childhood asthma. *J Allergy Clin Immunol*. 2005;115(2):233–42.
10. Zeiger RS, Szefler SJ, Phillips BR, et al. Response profiles to fluticasone and montelukast in mild-to-moderate persistent childhood asthma. *J Allergy Clin Immunol*. 2006;117(1):45–52.
11. Bateman ED, Bantje TA, João Gomes M, et al. Combination therapy with single inhaler budesonide/formoterol compared with high dose of fluticasone propionate alone in patients with moderate persistent asthma. *Am J Respir Med*. 2003;2(3):275–81.
12. Bateman ED, Boushey HA, Bousquet J, et al. Can guideline-defined asthma control be achieved? The Gaining Optimal Asthma Control study. *Am J Respir Crit Care Med*. 2004;170(8):836–44.
13. U.S. Department of Health and Human Services. *EPR-Update 2002. Expert Panel Report: Guidelines for the Diagnosis and Management of Asthma. Update on Selected Topics 2002*. NIH Publication No. 02-5074. Bethesda (MD): U.S. Department of Health and Human Services, National Institutes of Health, National Heart, Lung, and Blood Institute, National Asthma Education and Prevention Program; 2002.
14. Mann M, Chowdhury B, Sullivan E, Nicklas R, Anthracite R, Meyer RJ. Serious asthma exacerbations in asthmatics treated with high-dose formoterol. *Chest*. 2003;124(1):70–4.
15. Nelson HS, Weiss ST, Bleecker ER, Yancey SW, Dorinsky PM, SMART Study Group. The Salmeterol Multicenter Asthma Research Trial: a comparison of usual pharmacotherapy for asthma or usual pharmacotherapy plus salmeterol. *Chest*. 2006;129(1):15–26. [published correction appears in *Chest*. 2006;*129*(5):1393].
16. Humbert M, Beasley R, Ayres J, et al. Benefits of omalizumab as add-on therapy in patients with severe persistent asthma who are inadequately controlled despite best available therapy (GINA 2002 step 4 treatment): INNOVATE. *Allergy*. 2005;60(3):309–16.
17. Katsaounou P, Buhl R, Brusselle G, et al. Omalizumab as alternative to chronic use of oral corticosteroids in severe asthma. *Respir Med*. 2019 Apr;150:51–62.
18. Eichenberger PA, Diener SN, Kofmehl R, Spengler CM. Effects of exercise training on airway hyperreactivity in asthma: a systematic review and meta-analysis. *Sports Med*. 2013;43(11):1157–70. doi:10.1007/s40279-013-0077-2
19. Physical Activity Guidelines for Americans. 2nd ed. Accessed 12 Jan 2022. https://health.gov/sites/default/files/2019-09/Physical_Activity_Guidelines_2nd_edition.pdf
20. Feinstein RA, LaRussa J, Wang-Dohlman A, Bartolucci AA. Screening adolescent athletes for exercise-induced asthma. *Clin J Sport Med*. 1996;6(2):119–23.
21. Langdeau JB, Boulet LP. Prevalence and mechanisms of development of asthma and airway hyperresponsiveness in athletes. *Sports Med*. 2001;31(8):601–616.
22. Boulet LP, O'Byrne PM. Asthma and exercise-induced bronchoconstriction in athletes. *N Engl J Med*. 2015;372(7):641–8.
23. Bougault V, Loubaki L, Joubert P, et al. Airway remodeling and inflammation in competitive swimmers training in indoor chlorinated swimming pools. *J Allergy Clin Immunol*. 2012;129(2):351–8.e1.
24. Anderson SD, Kippelen P. Exercise-induced bronchoconstriction: pathogenesis. *Curr Allergy Asthma Rep*. 2005;5(2):116–22.
25. Duong M, Subbarao P, Adelroth E, et al. Sputum eosinophils and the response of exercise-induced bronchoconstriction to corticosteroid in asthma. *Chest*. 2008;133(2):404–11.
26. Anderson SD. Single-dose agents in the prevention of exercise-induced asthma: a descriptive review. *Treat Respir Med*. 2004;3(6):365–379.
27. Anderson SD, Brannan JD. Long-acting beta 2-adrenoceptor agonists and exercise-induced asthma: lessons to guide us in the future. *Paediatr Drugs*. 2004;6(3):161–175.
28. Carlsen KH, Carlsen KC. Exercise-induced asthma. *Paediatr Respir Rev*. 2002;3(2):154–60.
29. Parsons JP, Kaeding C, Phillips G, Jarjoura D, Wadley G, Mastronarde JG. Prevalence of exercise-induced bronchospasm in a cohort of varsity college athletes. *Med Sci Sports Exerc*. 2007;39(9):1487–92.
30. Thole RT, Sallis RE, Rubin AL, Smith GN. Exercise-induced bronchospasm prevalence in collegiate cross-country runners. *Med Sci Sports Exerc*. 2001;33(10):1641–46.
31. Tikkanen HO, Peltonen JE. Asthma-cross-country skiing. *Med Sci Sports Exerc*. 1999;31(5 suppl):S99.
32. Smith BW, MacKnight JM. Pulmonary. In: Safran MR, McKeag DB, VanCamp SP, editors. *Manual of Sports Medicine*. Philadelphia: Lippincott-Raven; 1998. p. 244–54.
33. Rundell KW, Wilber RL, Szmedra L, Jenkinson DM, Mayers LB, Im J. Exercise-induced asthma screening of elite athletes: field versus laboratory exercise challenge. *Med Sci Sports Exerc*. 2000;32(2):309–16.
34. Holzer K, Brukner P, Douglass J. Evidence-based management of exercise-induced asthma. *Curr Sports Med Rep*. 2002;1(2):86–92.
35. Simons FE, Gerstner TV, Cheang MS. Tolerance to the bronchoprotective effect of salmeterol in adolescents with exercise-induced asthma using concurrent inhaled glucocorticoid treatment. *Pediatrics*. 1997;99(5):655–9.
36. Spooner CH, Spooner GR, Rowe BH. Mast-cell stabilising agents to prevent exercise-induced bronchoconstriction. *Cochrane Database Syst Rev*. 2003;2003:CD002307.
37. Elkins MR, Brannan JD. Warm-up exercise can reduce exercise-induced bronchoconstriction. *Br J Sports Med*. 2013;47(10):657–8.
38. Kippelen P, Fitch KD, Anderson SD, et al. Respiratory health of elite athletes — preventing airway injury: a critical review. *Br J Sports Med*. 2012;46(7):471–6.

39. Stickland MK, Rowe BH, Spooner CH, Vandermeer B, Dryden DM. Effect of warm-up exercise on exercise-induced bronchoconstriction. *Med Sci Sports Exerc.* 2012;44(3):383–91.
40. O'Byrne PM, Jones GL. The effect of indomethacin on exercise-induced bronchoconstriction and refractoriness after exercise. *Am Rev Respir Dis.* 1986;134(1):69–72.
41. Storms WW, Joyner DM. Update on exercise-induced asthma: a report of the olympic exercise asthma summit conference. *Phys Sportsmed.* 1997;25(3):45–55.
42. Mink BD. Exercise and chronic obstructive pulmonary disease: modest fitness gains pay big dividends. *Phys Sportsmed.* 1997;25(11):43–52.
43. Murphy SL, Kochanek KD, Xu JQ, Arias E. *Mortality in the United States, 2020.* Hyattsville (MD): National Center for Health Statistics; 2021. NCHS Data Brief No. 427. doi:10.15620/cdc:112079
44. Casaburi R. Exercise training in chronic obstructive lung disease. In: Casaburi R, Petty TL, editors. *Principles and Practice of Pulmonary Rehabilitation.* Philadelphia: Saunders; 1993:204–224.
45. Ries AL, Bauldoff GS, Carlin BW, et al. Pulmonary rehabilitation: joint ACCP/AACVPR evidence-based clinical practice guidelines. *Chest.* 2007;131(5 suppl l):4S–42S.
46. Storer TW. Exercise in chronic pulmonary disease: resistance exercise prescription. *Med Sci Sports Exerc.* 2001;33(7 suppl l):S680–S692.
47. Wilkes DL, Schneiderman JE, Nguyen T, et al. Exercise and physical activity in children with cystic fibrosis. *Paediatr Respir Rev.* 2009;10(3):105–9.
48. Hebestreit H, Arets HG, Aurora P, European Cystic Fibrosis Exercise Working Group, et al. Statement on exercise testing in cystic fibrosis. *Respiration.* 2015;90(4):332–351.
49. Rand S, Prasad SA. Exercise as part of a cystic fibrosis therapeutic routine. *Expert Rev Respir Med.* 2012;6(3):341–52.
50. Thomas J, Cook DJ, Brooks D. Chest physical therapy management of patients with cystic fibrosis: a meta-analysis. *Am J Respir Crit Care Med.* 1995;151(3 pt. 1):846–850.
51. Schneiderman-Walker J, Pollock SL, Corey M, et al. A randomized controlled trial of a 3-year home exercise program in cystic fibrosis. *J Pediatr.* 2000;136(3):304–310.
52. Jaworski C, Rygiel V. Acute illness in the athlete. *Clin Sports Med.* 2019 Oct;38(4):577–95.
53. Nieman DC. Is infection risk linked to exercise workload?. *Med Sci Sports Exerc.* 2000;32(7 suppl l):S406–S411.
54. Hemilä H. Does vitamin C alleviate the symptoms of the common cold?—A review of current evidence. *Scand J Infect Dis.* 1994;26(1):1–6.
55. Mossad SB, Macknin ML, Medendorp SV, Mason P. Zinc gluconate lozenges for treating the common cold. A randomized, double-blind, placebo-controlled study. *Ann Intern Med.* 1996;125(2):81–88.
56. Clemm HH, Olin JT, McIntosh C, et al. Exercise-induced laryngeal obstruction (EILO) in athletes: a narrative review by a subgroup of the IOC Consensus on 'acute respiratory illness in the athlete'. *Br J Sports Med.* 2022;56(11):622–9.
57. Olin JT, Deardorff EH, Fan EM, et al. Therapeutic laryngoscopy during exercise: a novel non-surgical therapy for refractory EILO. *Pediatr Pulmonol.* 2017;52(6):813–19.
58. Røksund OD, Olin JT, Halvorsen T. Working towards a common transatlantic approach for evaluation of exercise-induced laryngeal obstruction. *Immunol Allergy Clin North Am.* 2018;38(2):281–92.
59. Chiang T, Marcinow AM, deSilva BW, Ence BN, Lindsey SE, Forrest LA. Exercise-induced paradoxical vocal fold motion disorder: diagnosis and management. *Laryngoscope.* 2013;123(3):727–31.
60. Maat RC, Roksund OD, Olofsson J, Halvorsen T, Skadberg BT, Heimdal JH. Surgical treatment of exercise-induced laryngeal dysfunction. *Eur Arch Otorhinolaryngol.* 2007;264(4):401–7.
61. Mehlum CS, Walsted ES, Godballe C, Backer V. Supraglottoplasty as treatment of exercise induced laryngeal obstruction (EILO). *Eur Arch Otorhinolaryngol.* 2016;273(4):945–51.

43 Rheumatology

Daniel Diaz

INTRODUCTION

- Individuals with rheumatologic and autoimmune conditions experience musculoskeletal pathology caused by overload, repetitive movements, and poor posture.
- These diseases may also be aggravated following sports participation or recreational activities that involve high physical demands.
- Both healthy individuals and those with a medical history linked to the musculoskeletal system (i.e., previous trauma, autoimmune diseases, inflammations, degenerative, or genetic diseases) are subject to the same risks (1).
- The most frequent rheumatologic conditions encountered in sports medicine are represented by periarticular conditions of the shoulder, hip, knee, ankle, and foot.
- In most cases, diagnosis is clinical, and treatment is conservative. Diagnostic investigations are only required in cases where there is suspicion of system disease.
- Patients typically require ongoing management including activity modification, rehabilitation to correct biomechanical deficits, appropriate use of braces and assistive devices, and medical therapy to decrease inflammation and slow joint destruction (2).

CHALLENGES OF RHEUMATOLOGIC TESTS IN CLINICAL MEDICINE

- The utilization of clinical testing in diagnosing autoimmune and connective tissue disorders in clinical medicine can be complex and confusing.
- There is no single definitive laboratory test that can diagnose all connective tissue disorders and rheumatologic conditions. Diagnosis often relies on a combination of clinical assessment, patient history, imaging, and multiple lab tests.
- Rheumatoid factor (RF), anticyclic citrullinated peptide antibodies (CCP Ab), and antinuclear antibodies (ANA) are common serological markers, but their presence or absence alone does not confirm or rule out specific conditions.
- Specificity versus Sensitivity: Many lab tests used for these conditions have varying specificity and sensitivity levels, leading to false positives and negatives. Clinicians must interpret results cautiously.
- Overlap Syndromes: Some patients present with overlap syndromes, where features of multiple rheumatologic conditions coexist, making diagnosis and treatment decisions more challenging.
- Lab results should always be interpreted in the context of the patient's clinical presentation and history, as variations in lab values are common.
- Table 43.1 summarizes common tests to consider when diagnosing connective tissue disorders and was adapted from the American Academy of Family Physicians article on "*Rheumatoid Arthritis: Common Questions About Diagnosis and Management.*"

RHEUMATOID ARTHRITIS

- Rheumatoid arthritis (RA) is the most common chronic form of inflammatory arthritis, affecting approximately 1% of the population (3,4).
- The pathogenesis of RA is complex, with multiple genetic, environmental, immunologic, and other factors contributing to the development and expression of disease (4–6).
- Susceptibility to RA depends on a pattern of inherited genes, most importantly those in the human leukocyte antigen (HLA) major histocompatibility complex (MHC) (7).
- RA expression usually involves environmental triggers at mucosal surfaces (*i.e.*, exposure to cigarette smoke in the airway) (7).

Early Recognition

- Should be suspected in any adult patient who presents with inflammatory polyarthritis or unexplained synovitis in a single joint in the absence of inflammatory bowel disease (IBD) or systemic rheumatic disease such as systemic lupus erythematous (SLE).
- Those complaining of morning stiffness for greater than 30 minutes
- Physical Findings:
  - Joints boggy and tender/joint effusion
  - Joints of wrist and hand classically involved
    - RA: MCP and PIP; <10% of cases involve DIP

Table 43.1 Tests for Suspected Connective Tissue Disorders

Connective Tissue Disorder	Screening Test	Follow-up Test
Mixed connective tissue disease	Antinuclear antibody (ANA)	Anticardiolipin antibodies, anticyclic citrullinated peptide antibodies, anti-Jo-1antibodies, antiribonucleoprotein anti-bodies, anti-Scl 70 antibodies, rheumatoid factor
Dermatomyositis/polymyositis	ANA, creatine kinase	Myositis-specific antibodies, including anti-Jo-1 antibodies
Rheumatoid arthritis	Rheumatoid factor	Anticyclic citrullinated peptide antibodies
Sjögren syndrome	ANA	Sjögren antibodies
Systemic lupus erythematosus	ANA	Anticardiolipin antibodies, anti–double-stranded DNA antibodies, Sjögren antibodies, anti-Smith antibodies, antiribonucleoprotein U1 antibodies, lupus anticoagulant
Vasculitis	Antineutrophil cyto-plasmic antibodies	Antiproteinase 3 antibodies, antimyeloperoxidase antibodies

Source: Ali Y. Rheumatologic tests: A primer for family physicians. *Am Fam Physician.* 2018;98(3):164–70.

Diagnosis

Lab Evaluation

- **RA specific:** Rheumatoid factor (RF) and anticitrullinated peptide antibodies (ACPA): Both positive increases sensitivity for RA.
  - Both can be negative on presentation in up to 50% of patients.
  - **Nonspecific:** Erythrocyte sedimentation rate (ESR) and serum C-reactive protein (CRP)
  - **Differential Diagnosis:** ANA testing, Complete blood count (CBC) with differential and platelet count, Complete Metabolic Panel (CMP), serum uric acid, and urinalysis
  - **Synovial fluid analysis:** include a cell count and differential, crystal search, and Gram stain and culture
    - Exclusion of gout, pseudogout, or an infectious arthritis
  - **Specialty Lab Evaluation: Assessing for chronic infection**
    - In those with very short duration of symptoms and seronegative for RF and ACPA
    - Human parvovirus B19, hepatitis B virus (HBV), and hepatitis C virus (HCV). In areas endemic for Lyme disease consider Lyme titers.
- **Classification System:** based on the 2010 American College of Rheumatology (ACR)/European Alliance of Associations for Rheumatology (EULAR) guidelines (Table 43.2).
- **Imaging:** X-ray can be helpful in grading severity of disease and driving treatment. Magnetic resonance imaging (MRI) and ultrasound do not have an established role in diagnosing RA, but can be useful in identifying synovitis and ruling out other diagnosis on the differential.

Treatment

- Physical therapy, exercise, and activity modification:
  - Customized therapy Rx based on symptom severity, presence of erosive disease, and serological testing
  - Low-impact exercises
  - Avoid combative, collision, or contact sports if there is any atlantoaxial instability (2)
- Disease-modifying antirheumatic drug (DMARD) therapy
  - DMARD therapy should be initiated early in all patients diagnosed with RA. Early initiation has been associated with slowing the progression of disease (5,6,8).
  - Methotrexate is first-line therapy in most cases
  - Biologic agents should be added if there is inadequate response to first-line treatment (2,8):
    - TNF Alpha antagonist, B-Cell targeting/Anti-CD20 therapies, and Interleukin-6 inhibitors
- Other pharmacological agents include oral or intra-articular glucocorticoids and/or NSAIDs
- Nonpharmacological therapies
  - Joint replacement surgery or arthrodesis
  - Fatty acid supplementation
  - Regular exercise and activity
- **Sports-Specific Considerations:** Same as those for osteoarthritis.

OSTEOARTHRITIS

- Osteoarthritis (OA) is the most common form of arthritis and possesses marked variability of disease expression (9).
- The hallmarks of this disease are joint pain and functional impairment (9).
- The age of disease onset, sequence of joint involvement, and disease progression vary from person to person.
- OA ranges from an asymptomatic, incidental finding on clinical or radiologic examination to a progressive disabling disorder eventually culminating in "joint failure" (9).

Signs and Symptoms

- Commonly pain is worse with activity and improved with rest.
- Patients can experience joint tenderness, limitation of motion, bony swelling, and recurrent joint effusions.
- Joint deformity — sign of advanced joint damage

Table 43.2 Scoring Criteria for Rheumatoid Arthritis Diagnosis

Target population: Patients who (i) have at least 1 joint with clinical synovitis and (ii) with the synovitis not better explained by another disease.

	Score
A. Joint involvement (tender/swollen)	
1 large joint	0
2–10 large joints	1
1–3 small joints (± involvement of large joints)	2
4–10 small joints (± involvement of large joints)	3
>10 joints (at least 1 small joint)	5
B. Serology	
Negative RF & ACPA	0
Low-positive RF/low-positive ACPA	2
High-positive RF/high-positive ACPA	3
C. Acute-phase reactants	
Normal CRP & ESR	0
Abnormal CRP & ESR	1
D. Duration of symptoms	
<6 wk	0
≥6 wk	1

Add score of categories A–D:
≥6/10 = definite RA

ACPA, anticitrullinated protein antibodies; CRP, C-reactive protein; ESR, erythrocyte sedimentation rate; RA, rheumatoid arthritis; RF, rheumatoid factor.
Source: Aletaha D, Neogi T, Silman AJ, et al. 2010 Rheumatoid arthritis classification criteria: an American College of Rheumatology/European League Against Rheumatism collaborative initiative. *Arthritis Rheum.* 2010;62(9):2569–81.

- Instability — Often a "pseudo-laxity" due to joint degeneration and altered patellar tracking (with lateral patellar subluxation). However, true joint instability may also be present.
- Joint distribution in OA can be variable and isolated to a single joint or present in multiple joints
- There is no correlation between patient symptoms and severity of osteoarthritic disease (10).

Diagnosis

- Diagnosis can be made clinically without imaging
  - Persistent usage-related joint pain in one or a few joints
  - Age ≥45 years
  - Morning stiffness ≤30 minutes
- Conventional radiography is the most widely used imaging modality in OA and allows for detection of characteristic features of OA, including marginal osteophytes, localized joint space narrowing, subchondral sclerosis, and cysts (11,12).
- Radiography is considered an appropriate initial imaging modality for evaluating patients with chronic atraumatic joint pain such as OA (13,14).
- MRI is not necessary but can help identify OA at earlier stages of the disease before radiographic changes become apparent.
- Ultrasound (US) is not necessary for diagnosing but can be helpful in detecting specific pathologic features such as synovial inflammation, effusion, and osteophytosis. US can also be useful in diagnosing OA in smaller superficial joints but has limited benefit with deeper and larger joints.

Treatment

- Primary treatment is through activity modification, exercise, and weight loss.
  - Loss of at least 10% of body weight through a combination of diet and exercises has been associated with a 50% reduction in pain scores in patients who are overweight or have obesity with knee OA after 18 months (15).
  - Depending on OA severity, low-impact exercise and water-based therapy may be beneficial and yield better results.
  - Exercise and sport participation recommendations should be based on disease severity, symptoms (*i.e.*, presence of pseudo-laxity and/or instability), and joint alignment.
  - Walking aids and knee braces for patients with malalignment (tibiofemoral or patellofemoral OA) may improve pain and should be considered as adjunctive treatments (16).
- Pharmacological management include:
  - NSAIDs
    - Trial of topical prior to oral
    - Recommend lowest dose required to control the patient's symptoms on an as-needed basis.
  - Opioids are not indicated for long-term treatment of OA.
  - Intra-articular corticosteroids
    - Pain relief short-lived (~4 weeks) and usually requires repeat injections.
  - Intra-articular hyaluronic acid (HA) injections:
    - Most evidence demonstrates only a small superiority over intra-articular placebo.
    - Given low risk and side-effect profile HA is still a reasonable option and commonly used.
  - Platelet-rich plasma
    - Research thus far has not demonstrated benefit both in terms of pain and structural changes (17).

- Supplements
    - No clear evidence demonstrating a clinically important benefit with glucosamine, chondroitin, vitamin D, diacerein, avocado soybean unsaponifiables (ASU), and fish oil use.
- Surgical management for OA includes joint replacement surgery or arthrodesis.
    - Surgical intervention recommended, once trial of nonoperative treatment has failed

Sports-Specific Considerations

- Encourage low-impact sports and activities such as swimming, cycling, and elliptical training to reduce joint stress while maintaining cardiovascular fitness.
- Emphasize the importance of joint protection techniques, including proper warm-up, cool-down, and stretching routines, to minimize the risk of exacerbating osteoarthritis symptoms.
- Provide sport-specific advice on technique and form to minimize joint strain and reduce the risk of injury during activities such as golf, tennis, or running.
- Develop individualized exercise plans that focus on strengthening the muscles around affected joints. Physical therapy and targeted exercises can help improve joint stability.
- Cross-Training: Encourage cross-training to diversify physical activities and reduce the risk of overuse injuries. Suggest complementary exercises that maintain fitness while reducing joint stress.
- Monitor patients' progress and symptoms during sports participation. Regular follow-up appointments can help identify issues early and adjust exercise plans accordingly.
- Recommend appropriate assistive devices such as braces, orthotics, or canes to provide support and reduce joint stress during sports activities.
- Educate patients about the importance of self-care, including weight management, nutrition, and hydration, to promote overall joint health.

SPONDYLOARTHROPATHIES

- Spondyloarthritis (SpA) is used for a family of disorders, including ankylosing spondylitis, nonradiographic axial spondyloarthritis (nr-axSpA), forms of arthritis associated with psoriasis and with inflammatory bowel diseases, and other conditions (18).
- The different forms of SpA share a group of clinical features; the most distinguishing features are inflammation of axial joints (especially the sacroiliac [SI] joints), asymmetric oligoarthritis (especially of the lower extremities), dactylitis (sausage fingers), and enthesitis (inflammation at sites of ligamentous or tendon attachment to bone) (18).
- Additional features include skin and genital lesions, eye and bowel inflammation, an association with preceding or ongoing infectious disorders, positive family history, and elevated acute phase reactants (18).
- Patients with SpA have higher frequencies of the HLA B27, and of sacroiliitis by radiography or MRI (19).
- Patients with axSpA are classified one of two subgroups, termed radiographic axSpA (*i.e.*, Ankylosing spondylitis [AS]) or nonradiographic axSpA.
- Peripheral SpA include those with predominantly peripheral involvement whose symptoms consist mainly of peripheral arthritis, peripheral enthesitis, and/or dactylitis and who do not meet criteria for axSPA.
- Symmetry of sacroiliac involvement distinguishes two groups of SpA (2):
    - Bilateral involvement is consistent with AS or Enteropathic arthritis.
    - Unilateral involvement is consistent with reactive arthritis and psoriatic arthritis.

Ankylosing Spondylitis

Symptoms

- Back pain: Chronic with onset before the age of 40 years
    - Insidious onset, morning stiffness >30 minutes
    - Improvement with exercise, No improvement with rest.
- Enthesitis: Most commonly at the Achilles tendon insertion
- Dactylitis
- Extra-articular manifestations:
    - Acute anterior uveitis (Frequency of uveitis in patients with SpA is approximately 25%–35%) (20)
- Associated conditions: inflammatory bowel disease (IBD) and psoriasis
- Family history of SpA or other rheumatologic conditions, history of IBD

Physical Exam Findings

- **Positive Schober Test**
    - Assesses flexibility of the lumbar spine.
    - Patient stands upright with back straight and feet shoulder-width apart.
    - Two points marked on the skin (one at dimples of Venus, one 10 cm above).
    - Patient bends forward maximally while keeping knees straight.
    - Normal increase in distance between points: at least 5 cm (2 in).
    - Less than 5 cm increase suggests limited lumbar flexion, possibly ankylosing spondylitis.
- **Lateral Spinal Flexion Test**
    - Assesses side-to-side bending of the spine.
    - Patient stands with feet together and arms relaxed at sides.
    - Examiner stabilizes pelvis from behind.
    - Patient laterally bends as far as possible without rotating trunk or raising heels.

- Symmetric distances on both sides are normal.
- Significant difference may indicate limited range of motion or spinal abnormality.

Diagnosis

- Laboratory findings are generally nonspecific
- Positive HLA-B27
  - Present in 85%–95% of white patients with AS (21)
  - However positive test is not diagnostic, and a negative test does not rule out AS
- CRP, ESR may or may not be elevated
- Imaging studies: extremely important in the diagnosis of axSpA
- X-ray: X-ray pelvis recommended to assess for sacroiliitis.
- MRI SI Joint: Can be beneficial if suspicion of axSpA is high, x-rays are negative, and HLA-B27 is positive.
- Ultrasound: Can be helpful in evaluation of enthesitis
- Colonoscopy: To assess for IBD and rule out enteropathic arthritis

Treatment

- Physical therapy and symptom-based activity modification
- NSAIDs — First-line treatment
- Tumor necrosis factor (TNF) inhibitor — second-line treatment
  - If inadequate response to initial therapy with two different NSAIDs
  - Can also trial sulfasalazine (SSZ)
- Intra-articular corticosteroid injections
- Surgical treatment: Joint replacement surgery, spine surgery.
- Counsel on risk of return to contact sport and higher risk of fracture (2)

REACTIVE ARTHRITIS

- Reactive arthritis is conventionally defined as an arthritis that arises following an infection, although the pathogens cannot be cultured from the affected joints (22).

Symptoms

- Occur 1–4 weeks after inciting infection. Interval between infection and the onset of arthritis considered by expert consensus is a minimum of several days and a maximum of several weeks (23).
- In at least half of the patients, all symptoms resolve in less than 6 months (24)
- Three main clinical manifestations:
  - Preceding infection
    - GI
      - Salmonella
      - *Shigella*
      - *Yersinia*
      - *Campylobacter*, especially *Campylobacter jejuni*
      - *C. difficile*
    - GU: *Chlamydia*
- Axial and/or peripheral musculoskeletal signs and symptoms
  - Peripheral arthritis
  - Inflammatory low back pain
  - Dactylitis and enthesitis
- Extra-articular signs and symptoms
  - Ocular symptoms, such as conjunctivitis, and less frequently, anterior uveitis.
  - Gastrointestinal and genitourinary symptoms
  - Oral and skin lesions
  - Psoriatic like nail changes

Diagnosis

- The diagnosis of reactive arthritis is a clinical diagnosis based on the pattern of findings and exclusion of other diseases. There is no single definitive diagnostic test, nor are there validated diagnostic criteria (25).

Treatment

- Treat underlying infection
  - However, antibiotic treatment did not significantly reduce the likelihood of failing to achieve remission of the reactive arthritis (26)
- NSAIDs first-line treatment
- Consider Intra-articular or systemic glucocorticoids.
- DMARDs can be used for cases not responding to NSAID treatment

PSORIATIC ARTHRITIS

- Psoriatic arthritis (PsA) is an inflammatory musculoskeletal disease associated with psoriasis, which was initially considered a variant of rheumatoid arthritis, but subsequently emerged as a distinct clinical entity (27,28).

Symptoms

- Psoriatic skin lesions
- Pain and stiffness in joints associated with fatigue and morning stiffness lasting >30 minutes.
  - Fatigue was found to occur in 22% of patients with PsA (29)
- Arthritis
  - Distal arthritis, *i.e.*, DIP joints
  - Asymmetric oligoarthritis, less than five small and/or large joints are affected in an asymmetric distribution
  - Symmetric polyarthritis, similar to RA
  - Arthritis mutilans
  - SpA, including both sacroiliitis and spondylitis

- Nail lesions to include nail pits, onycholysis, nail bed hyperkeratosis, and splinter hemorrhages
- Dactylitis, enthesopathy, tenosynovitis
- Ocular symptoms similar to other SpAs

Diagnosis

- Mostly based on history and clinical features, and should be the leading diagnostic consideration in a patient who has both psoriasis and an inflammatory arthritis in a pattern typical of PsA (30)

Treatment

- Treatment dependent on whether patient has active or severe psoriasis as well as arthritis.
- Treatment when psoriasis present and active may include Methotrexate, Tumor necrosis factor (TNF), and Interleukin (IL) 17 inhibitors.
- Arthritic treatment is similar to the treatment for Osteoarthritis (OA) except that DMARDs can be utilized if patient is not responding to initial arthritic treatment.
- Exercise recommendations same as those for patients with OA

ENTEROPATHIC ARTHRITIS

- Inflammatory bowel disease (IBD)-associated arthritis should be suspected whenever an IBD patient develops joint pain, stiffness, or symptoms of inflammatory back pain (31).
- In SpA patients who develop abdominal pain, diarrhea, or weight loss, or who manifest an unexplained anemia, a referral to a gastroenterologist should be considered (31).

Symptoms

- Peripheral arthropathy
  - Type 1: Acute, self-limiting, affecting less than 6 joints, occurs early in the course of the bowel disease, and is nonerosive.
  - Type 2: chronic and recurrent polyarticular disease, with metacarpophalangeal joints being particularly involved (32). One half of the patients will experience migratory arthritis.
- Enthesitis, and less often, dactylitis
- Spondylitis and sacroiliitis

Diagnosis

- There are no labs that are diagnostic of EA and diagnosis is made based on clinic findings and symptoms
- HLA-B27 is found in 50%–75% of the patients with IBD-associated axial arthritis (33)
- Synovial fluid demonstrates predominantly polymorphonuclear leukocytes.
- Imaging demonstrates findings consistent with arthritis and SpA

Treatment

- Treatment of EA associated with inflammatory bowel disease (IBD) is similar to the treatment of other forms of SpA. NSAIDs being first-line treatment; selected conventional DMARDs for peripheral arthritis resistant to initial therapy, if biologics are not already required for axial or gastrointestinal disease manifestations (34).
- TNF inhibitors can be beneficial for peripheral arthritis resistant to conventional nonbiologic DMARDs and for axial disease resistant to NSAIDs (34).

Sports Specific Considerations in Spondyloarthropathies

- Conduct a thorough assessment of the patient's spondyloarthropathy, considering factors such as disease activity, joint involvement, and any related comorbidities.
- Encourage low-impact sports and exercises, such as swimming, stationary cycling, and yoga, to minimize the risk of exacerbating joint symptoms and spinal inflammation.
- Core strengthening: Emphasize the importance of core muscle strengthening exercises to help stabilize the spine and reduce the risk of injury or deformity progression.
- Promote regular stretching and flexibility exercises to maintain joint mobility, especially in the spine, hips, and shoulders.
- Pain management: Work closely with patients to manage pain effectively, using a combination of medications, physical therapy, and other modalities as appropriate.
- Regularly monitor disease activity using clinical assessments and lab tests to gauge inflammation levels and adjust treatment plans accordingly.
- Discuss the use of DMARDs with patients to control inflammation and improve joint function.
- Educate patients about the increased risk of fractures, particularly in patients with ankylosing spondylitis, and advise on fall prevention strategies.
- Recommend adaptive sports equipment and techniques, such as ergonomic backpacks and proper footwear, to reduce strain on the spine and joints.
- Encourage patients to adapt their chosen sports to their individual capabilities and limitations, focusing on techniques and modifications that reduce stress on affected joints.

SYSTEMIC LUPUS ERYTHEMATOSUS

- SLE is a chronic autoimmune disease, of unknown cause, that can affect any joint or organ in the body. Immunologic abnormalities, especially the production of several antinuclear antibodies (ANA), are a prominent feature of the disease (35).
- Symptoms can vary in severity and range from mild joint and skin involvement to life-threatening kidney, hematologic, or central nervous system involvement. The clinical

heterogeneity of SLE and the lack of pathognomonic features or tests pose a diagnostic challenge for the clinician (35).

- There are no pathognomonic features or test and diagnosis of SLE is generally based on clinical and laboratory findings after excluding alternative diagnoses.
- Should be considered in any patient with recurrent fever of unknown etiology, unexplained symptoms in two or more organ systems, and arthritis and arthralgias.

Clinical Manifestations

- Constitutional symptoms
  - Fatigue, present in 80%–100% of patients and not associate with disease severity (35)
  - Fever and myalgias
  - Weight change, decrease due to disease or medications, increase usually due to salt retention, increase appetite when on glucocorticoids, depression
- Arthritis and arthralgias
  - Occurs in over 90% of patients with SLE and is often the earliest manifestation (36)
  - Tends to be moderately painful, migratory, polyarticular, and symmetrical. It usually does not cause erosion, and is rarely deforming.
- Mucocutaneous symptoms
  - Patients develop skin and mucous lesions, there is high variability in symptoms with the most common presentation being a malar rash or "butterfly rash."
- Cardiac involvement and vascular manifestations
  - Pericarditis, with or without an effusion, is the most common cardiac manifestation of SLE, occurring in approximately 25% of patients at some point during their disease course (37)
  - Raynaud phenomenon
  - Vasculitis
  - Thromboembolic disease — Can affect both venous and arterial circulations
- Hematologic abnormalities
  - Common symptom of SLE than can affect all three blood lines.
  - Anemia of chronic disease is the most common type of anemia among patients with SLE. Leukopenia is also common occurring in approximately 50% of SLE patients (38)
- Renal involvement
  - Renal involvement is clinically apparent in approximately 50% of SLE patients and is a significant cause of morbidity and mortality (39)
  - Patients should undergo periodic screening for the presence of lupus nephritis
    - Urinalysis: key indicator of kidney damage and is often one of the first signs of lupus nephritis.
    - Serum Creatinine
    - Blood Urea Nitrogen (BUN)
    - Complete Blood Count (CBC): Anemia and a decrease in platelet count may be seen in lupus nephritis.
    - Protein-to-Creatinine Ratio (PCR) or albumin-to-creatinine ratio: can assess proteinuria over time.
- Pulmonary involvement
  - Common manifestation of SLE to include pleuritis (with or without effusion), pneumonitis, interstitial lung disease, pulmonary hypertension, shrinking lung syndrome, and alveolar hemorrhage.
- Neurologic and neuropsychiatric involvement
  - Manifestations include a broad range of neurologic and psychiatric manifestations, most commonly, stroke, seizures, cognitive dysfunction, delirium, psychosis, and/or peripheral neuropathies.
- Ophthalmologic involvement
  - Any structure in the eye can be involved, with keratoconjunctivitis sicca being the most common manifestation as a result of secondary Sjögren syndrome (40)
  - Retinal vasculopathy in the form of cotton wool spots
  - Photosensitivity

Diagnosis

- Given the broad range of clinical manifestations of SLE, a thorough history and physical exam is necessary
- Basic laboratory evaluation includes a complete blood count, serum creatinine, urinalysis with urine sediment, ESR, C-reactive protein levels, urine PCR, and serum protein electrophoresis.
- Specialized laboratory testing includes ANA, Anti-double-stranded DNA (anti-dsDNA), Antiphospholipid antibodies, Anti-Smith (Sm) antibody, Anti-Ro/SSA, and anti-La/SSB antibodies
- If the ANA is positive, one should test for other specific antibodies. Positive ANA must be interpreted in the setting of other clinical and laboratory findings. Nearly 15% of the U.S. population has a positive ANA, but only 10% of those with positive ANA have a true autoimmune disorder (41)
- Diagnostic Criteria: **2019 EULAR/ACR criteria** (The European League Against Rheumatism/American College of Rheumatology)
  - The classification for SLE requires the presence of positive antinuclear antibodies (ANA) as an entry criterion. Additive criteria consist of seven clinical (*i.e.*, constitutional, hematologic, neuropsychiatric, mucocutaneous, serosal, musculoskeletal, renal), and three immunologic (*i.e.*, antiphospholipid antibodies, complement proteins, SLE-specific antibodies) categories, each of which are weighted from 2 to 10. Patients are classified as having SLE with a score of 10 or more points.

Treatment

- Treatment of SLE must be individualized mostly on clinical manifestations, disease activity and severity.
- General measures include, diet and exercise, smoking cessation, assuring immunizations are up to date, and photoprotection.
    - Exposure to ultraviolet (UV) light may exacerbate or induce systemic manifestations of SLE (42).

Medication Management

- Hydroxychloroquine is recommended for all patients with SLE with any degree and type of disease activity (43).
    - The benefits of hydroxychloroquine or chloroquine in SLE are broad and include relief of constitutional symptoms, musculoskeletal manifestations, and mucocutaneous manifestations (43).
- Escalation in medication management based on disease activity, severity, and organs involved.
- For mild to moderate disease, prednisone is used in addition to hydroxychloroquine until hydroxychloroquine becomes effective and prednisone is then subsequently tapered.
- In moderate disease a glucocorticoid-sparing immunosuppressive agent (*e.g.*, azathioprine) is often required to control symptoms (43).
- With severe disease when organ-threatening manifestations are present, initial period of intensive immunosuppressive therapy (induction therapy) many times in addition to high-dose glucocorticoids are required to control the disease and halt tissue injury (43).
    - Initial therapy is subsequently followed by a longer period of less-intensive, and ideally less-toxic, maintenance immunosuppressive therapy to consolidate remission and prevent flares (43).

Prognosis

- Course is variable ranging from a relatively benign illness to a rapidly progressive disease resulting in organ failure and death.
- Although 5-year survival has improved dramatically to greater than 90% in recent years (44), mortality remains two to five times higher than that of the general population (45,46).
- Complete remission is difficult to achieve and usually short lasting (1–2 years).

Sports-Specific Considerations in SLE

- Protection against sun exposure
- Evaluate and monitor renal function in athletes. Consider screening before high-intensity, long-distance, and endurance activities. Special consideration should be taken when activity is in high-temperature environments. Monitor hydration status during activity.
- Discourage exercise during flares when fever present due to increased risk of endocarditis, vasculitis, and worsening synovitis (2).
- Recommend baseline echocardiogram to rule out pericarditis and follow-up echocardiogram prior to clearance for moderate- to high-intensity exercise (2).
- Consider screening for coronary artery disease in older athletes with long-standing SLE when starting a new exercise regime (47).
    - Carotid US and stress echo are noninvasive and low-risk screening modalities
- Counseling should be given to athletes exercising perioperatively, under times of stress, and peripregnancy as there is higher risk of SLE flare.

MANAGEMENT CONSIDERATIONS IN THE ELITE ATHLETE WITH INFLAMMATORY ARTHROPATHY (48)

- Joint effects of inflammatory arthritis
    - Diagnosing inflammatory arthritis in elite athletes is challenging due to potential differentials such as overuse injuries or muscular strains.
    - Overuse tendinopathy shares similarities in pathophysiology with inflammatory autoimmune enthesitis. An inflammatory response driven by proinflammatory cytokines (IL1, IL6, TNFα) occurs at the entheses, leading to tendon swelling, pain, and reduced tensile strength.
    - Both overuse injuries and inflammatory conditions exhibit a prolonged low-grade inflammatory state that inhibits tendon healing, making them more susceptible to injury.
    - Histological analysis shows commonalities in collagen structure loss, noncollagenous components increase, and increased vascularity in both overuse tendinopathy and enthesitis from inflammatory arthritis.
    - Overuse injuries are prevalent in elite athletes, with a significant number diagnosed during events such as the Olympics. These injuries, often attributed to overuse, could potentially serve as the initial presentation of an underlying inflammatory arthropathy.
    - Systemic inflammatory arthritides involve more than just joint destruction; they affect entheses and other body systems, impacting high-performing athletes.
    - Distinguishing sports-related injuries from early inflammatory arthritis in elite athletes presents challenges due to overlapping symptoms and clinical nuances.
    - Early diagnosis is crucial for prompt medical treatment and improved prognosis, with better outcomes in radiological joint damage if treatment starts within 3 months of symptom onset.

- Pain in the axial skeleton in elite athletes
  - Back pain is prevalent in both the general population and elite athletes, with up to 30% experiencing it. Trauma from contact sports or overuse injuries can result in spinal pain, resembling inflammatory arthropathies.
  - Repetitive trauma can lead to degenerative conditions such as spondylolysis and disc degeneration.
  - Imaging, including radiographs, CT, and MRI scans, helps diagnose degenerative conditions and soft-tissue injuries. AxSpA may present with bone marrow edema in sacroiliac joints on MRI scans.
  - Athletes, especially in contact sports, may experience cervical spine discomfort, with some presenting symptoms resembling RA. RA involving the cervical spine can lead to atlantoaxial instability, potentially causing spinal cord injury.
  - Early diagnosis of cervical involvement in axSpA is vital to prevent complications.
- Drug management in the elite athlete
  - Treating inflammatory arthritis in elite athletes is challenging due to strict regulations on prescribed medications.
  - When deciding on medical management, it is important to reference the banned medication list provided by the World Anti-Doping Agency (WADA). Noncompliance with WADA rules can result in fines and bans from competitive sports.
  - Athletes requiring medications prohibited by WADA must obtain a therapeutic use exemption.
  - DMARDs are not on the prohibited list and have reduced the need for corticosteroids and anti-inflammatories.
  - DMARDs have potential side effects, including gastrointestinal issues, rashes, pulmonary fibrosis, neuropathies, and increased infection risk.
  - Regular monitoring with blood tests is required due to the risk of myelosuppression and anemia.
  - Short-term use of over-the-counter analgesics may raise pain thresholds and potentially enhance performance.
  - Analgesics may modulate pain feedback in the nervous system and play a role in neuromuscular fatigue development.
- Fatigue and exercise in elite athletes
  - Intensive exercise leads to muscle fatigue, requiring rest and recovery to regain maximal contraction ability. Inflammatory arthropathies can cause systemic symptoms such as fatigue, related to a reduction in muscle strength.
  - Fatigue in RA patients is partially attributed to cachexia and sarcopenia, resulting from factors such as increased metabolic rate, poor nutrition, and lack of exercise.
  - High-intensity exercise may reduce cachexia and sarcopenia by maintaining joint and muscle health.
  - Anemia of chronic disease, present in up to 60% of RA patients, can contribute to fatigue.
  - Exercise has been shown to reduce joint pain and inflammation, improve mental health and self-esteem, and decrease bone loss in inflammatory arthropathies.
  - Intensive exercise has led to improvements in blood markers, fatigue levels, and cognitive function in RA and axSpA patients.
  - In animal studies, high-intensity exercise suppressed inflammatory cytokine production and joint destruction.
  - Neuromuscular changes in inflammatory arthritis can lead to peripheral fatigue, whereas psychological factors such as motivation and depression play a role in fatigue perception.
  - Elite athletes typically possess high mental toughness, but injuries and overtraining can lead to anxiety and depression.
  - Mental health risks in athletes are highest during their competitive peak, especially when sidelined due to injury, requiring appropriate support and management.

SUMMARY

- In conclusion, this chapter has explored the intricate realm of rheumatologic conditions, highlighting their complexities and the multifaceted challenges they present in the field of orthopedic and sports medicine, and emphasizing the paramount importance of early recognition. As orthopedic and sports medicine physicians, a firm grasp of the high-yield diagnostic testing points outlined here is invaluable.
- Timely identification and intervention not only enhance patient outcomes but also contribute to the overall well-being and quality of life of those affected by these conditions.
- By integrating the knowledge shared in this chapter into their practice, physicians are poised to make a significant impact, offering the best possible care to individuals facing rheumatologic challenges while enabling them to pursue their active lifestyles with confidence and comfort.

REFERENCES

1. Alexescu T, Szolga B. *Implications of Rheumatology in Sports Medicine*. Saarbrücken, Germany: Lambert Academic Publishing; 2018.
2. Harrast MA, Finnoff JT. *Sports Medicine: Study Guide and Review for Boards*. New York: Demos Medical Publishing; 2017.
3. Smolen JS, Aletaha D, Barton A, et al. Rheumatoid arthritis. *Nat Rev Dis Primers*. 2018;4:18001.
4. Firestein GS, McInnes IB. Immunopathogenesis of rheumatoid arthritis. *Immunity*. 2017;46(2):183–96.
5. Singh JA, Saag KG, Bridges SL Jr, et al. 2015 American College of Rheumatology guideline for the treatment of rheumatoid arthritis. *Arthritis Care Res (Hoboken)*. 2016;68:1–26.
6. Knevel R, Schoels M, Huizinga TW, et al. Current evidence for a strategic approach to the management of rheumatoid arthritis with disease-modifying antirheumatic drugs: a systematic literature review

informing the EULAR recommendations for the management of rheumatoid arthritis. *Ann Rheum Dis.* 2010;69(6):987–94.
7. Firestein G, Guma M. Pathogenesis of rheumatoid arthritis. In: Seo P, editor. UpToDate; 2021. Retrieved 2023 March 02. Available from: https://www.uptodate.com/contents/pathogenesis-of-rheumatoid-arthritis
8. Fraenkel L, Bathon JM, England BR, et al. 2021 American College of Rheumatology guideline for the treatment of rheumatoid arthritis. *Arthritis Rheumatol.* 2021 Jul;73(7):1108–23. doi:10.1002/art.41752
9. Doherty M, Abhishek A. Clinical Manifestations and diagnosis of osteoarthritis. In: Seo P, editor. UpToDate; 2022. Retrieved 2023 March 3. Available from: https://www.uptodate.com/contents/clinical-manifestations-and-diagnosis-of-osteoarthritis
10. Steenkamp W, Rachuene PA, Dey R, Mzayiya NL, Ramasuvha BE. The correlation between clinical and radiological severity of osteoarthritis of the knee. *SICOT J.* 2022;8:14. doi:10.1051/sicotj/2022014
11. Hayashi D, Roemer FW, Guermazi A. Imaging for osteoarthritis. *Ann Phys Rehabil Med.* 2016;59(3):161–9.
12. Roemer FW, Eckstein F, Hayashi D, Guermazi A. The role of imaging in osteoarthritis. *Best Pract Res Clin Rheumatol.* 2014;28(1):31–60.
13. American College of Radiology — ACR Appropriateness Criteria: Chronic Knee Pain; 2018. https://acsearch.acr.org/docs/69432/Narrative/
14. American College of Radiology — ACR Appropriateness Criteria: Chronic Hip Pain; 2018. https://acsearch.acr.org/docs/69425/Narrative
15. Messier SP, Mihalko SL, Legault C, et al. Effects of intensive diet and exercise on knee joint loads, inflammation, and clinical outcomes among overweight and obese adults with knee osteoarthritis: the IDEA randomized clinical trial. *JAMA.* 2013;310(12):1263–73.
16. McAlindon TE, Bannuru RR, Sullivan MC, et al. OARSI guidelines for the non-surgical management of knee osteoarthritis. *Osteoarthr Cartil.* 2014;22(3):363–88.
17. Bennell KL, Paterson KL, Metcalf BR, et al. Effect of intra-articular platelet-rich Plasma vs placebo injection on pain and medial tibial cartilage volume in patients with knee osteoarthritis: the RESTORE randomized clinical trial. *JAMA.* 2021;326(20):2021–30.
18. Yu D, Tubergen A. Overview of the clinical manifestations and classification of spondyloarthitis. In: Seo P, editor. UpToDate; 2022. Retrieved 2023 March 10. Available from: https://www.uptodate.com/contents/overview-of-the-clinical-manifestations-and-classification-of-spondyloarthritis
19. Sepriano A, Ramiro S, van der Heijde D, et al. What is axial spondyloarthritis? A latent class and transition analysis in the SPACE and DESIR cohorts. *Ann Rheum Dis.* 2020;79(3):324–31.
20. Yu D, Tubergen A. Clinical manifestations of axial spondyloarthritis (ankylosing spondylitis and nonradiographic axial spondyloarthritis) in adults. In: Seo P, editor. UpToDate; 2023. Retrieved 2023 March 10. Available from: https://www.uptodate.com/contents/clinical-manifestations-of-axial-spondyloarthritis-ankylosing-spondylitis-and-nonradiographic-axial-spondyloarthritis-in-adults
21. Bakland G, Nossent HC. Epidemiology of spondyloarthritis: a review. *Curr Rheumatol Rep.* 2013 Sep;15(9):351. doi:10.1007/s11926-013-0351-1
22. Ahvonen P, Sievers K, Aho K. Arthritis associated with Yersinia enterocolitica infection. *Acta Rheumatol Scand.* 1969;15(3):232–53.
23. Braun J, Kingsley G, van der Heijde D, Sieper J. On the difficulties of establishing a consensus on the definition of and diagnostic investigations for reactive arthritis. Results and discussion of a questionnaire prepared for the 4th International Workshop on Reactive Arthritis, Berlin, Germany, July 3-6, 1999. *J Rheumatol.* 2000;27(9):2185–92.
24. Garcia Ferrer HR, Azan A, Iraheta I, et al. Potential risk factors for reactive arthritis and persistence of symptoms at 2 years: a case-control study with longitudinal follow-up. *Clin Rheumatol.* 2018;37:415–22.
25. Yu D, Tubergen A. Reactive arthritis. In: Seo P, editor. UpToDate; 2023. Retrieved 2023 March 10. Available from: https://www.uptodate.com/contents/reactive-arthritis
26. Barber CE, Kim J, Inman RD, Esdaile JM, James MT. Antibiotics for treatment of reactive arthritis: a systematic review and metaanalysis. *J Rheumatol.* 2013;40(6):916–28.
27. Brockbank J, Gladman D. Diagnosis and management of psoriatic arthritis. *Drugs.* 2002;62(17):2447–57.
28. Wright V, Moll JM. Psoriatic arthritis. *Bull Rheum Dis.* 1971;21(5):627–32.
29. Eder L, Haddad A, Rosen CF, et al. The incidence and risk factors for psoriatic arthritis in patients with psoriasis: a prospective cohort study. *Arthritis Rheumatol.* 2016;68(4):915–23.
30. Gladman D, Ritchlin C. Clinical manifestations and diagnosis of psoriatic arthritis. In: Seo P, editor. UpToDate; 2022. Retrieved 2023 March 15. Available from: https://www.uptodate.com/contents/clinical-manifestations-and-diagnosis-of-psoriatic-arthritis
31. Inman R. Clinical manifestations and diagnosis of arthritis associated with inflammatory bowel disease and other gastrointestinal diseases. In: Seo P, editor. UpToDate; 2022. Retrieved 2023 March 15. Available from: https://www.uptodate.com/contents/clinical-manifestations-and-diagnosis-of-arthritis-associated-with-inflammatory-bowel-disease-and-other-gastrointestinal-diseases
32. Wordsworth P. Arthritis and inflammatory bowel disease. *Curr Rheumatol Rep.* 2000;2:87–8.
33. Weiner SR, Clarke J, Taggart N, Utsinger PD. Rheumatic manifestations of inflammatory bowel disease. *Semin Arthritis Rheum.* 1991;20:353.
34. Inman R. Treatment of arthritis associated with inflammatory bowel disease. In: Seo P, editor. UpToDate; 2022. Retrieved 2023 March 15. Available from: https://www.uptodate.com/contents/treatment-of-arthritis-associated-with-inflammatory-bowel-disease
35. Wallace DJ, Gladman DD. Clinical manifestations and diagnosis of systemic lupus erythematosus in adults. In: Seo P, editor. UpToDate; 2022. Retrieved 2023 March 15. Available from: https://www.uptodate.com/contents/clinical-manifestations-and-diagnosis-of-systemic-lupus-erythematosus-in-adults
36. Greco CM, Rudy TE, Manzi S. Adaptation to chronic pain in systemic lupus erythematosus: applicability of the multidimensional pain inventory. *Pain Med.* 2003;4(1):39–50.
37. Miner JJ, Kim AH. Cardiac manifestations of systemic lupus erythematosus. *Rheum Dis Clin N Am.* 2014;40(1):51–60.
38. Newman K, Owlia MB, El-Hemaidi I, Akhtari M. Management of immune cytopenias in patients with systemic lupus erythematosus - old and new. *Autoimmun Rev.* 2013;12(7):784–91.
39. Danila MI, Pons-Estel GJ, Zhang J, Vilá LM, Reveille JD, Alarcón GS. Renal damage is the most important predictor of mortality within the damage index: data from LUMINA LXIV, a multiethnic US cohort. *Rheumatology.* 2009;48(5):542–5.
40. Silpa-archa S, Lee JJ, Foster CS. Ocular manifestations in systemic lupus erythematosus. *Br J Ophthalmol.* 2016;100(1):135–41.
41. Satoh M, Chan EK, Ho LA, et al. Prevalence and sociodemographic correlates of antinuclear antibodies in the United States. *Arthritis Rheum.* 2012;64(7):2319–27.
42. Lehmann P, Homey B. Clinic and pathophysiology of photosensitivity in lupus erythematosus. *Autoimmun Rev.* 2009;8(6):456–61.
43. Wallace DJ. Overview of the management and prognosis of systemic lupus erythematosus in adults. In: Seo P, editor. UpToDate; 2022. Retrieved 2023 March 16. Available from: https://www.uptodate.com/contents/overview-of-the-management-and-prognosis-of-systemic-lupus-erythematosus-in-adults
44. Trager J, Ward MM. Mortality and causes of death in systemic lupus erythematosus. *Curr Opin Rheumatol.* 2001;13(5):345–51.

45. Borchers AT, Keen CL, Shoenfeld Y, Gershwin ME. Surviving the butterfly and the wolf: mortality trends in systemic lupus erythematosus. *Autoimmun Rev*. 2004;3(6):423–53.
46. Singh RR, Yen EY. SLE mortality remains disproportionately high, despite improvements over the last decade. *Lupus*. 2018;27(10):1577–81.
47. Croca SC, Rahman A. Imaging assessment of cardiovascular disease in systemic lupus erythematosus. *Clin Dev Immunol*. 2012;2012:694143. doi:10.1155/2012/694143
48. Kin-Hoo Koo K, Chinoy H, Creaney L, Hayton M. Inflammatory arthropathy in the elite sports athlete. *Curr Sports Med Rep*. 2021 Nov 1;20(11):577–83. doi:10.1249/JSR.0000000000000903

Allergic Diseases in Athletes

44

David L. Brown, Nathan P. Falk, and Linda L. Brown

INTRODUCTION

- Allergic rhinitis alone affects over 60 million Americans (1). It is the fifth most common chronic disease and the most prevalent in patients under 18 years of age, affecting up to 40% of children (1–3). Allergic rhinitis coexists in 75%–80% of asthma patients (2).
- Urticaria and angioedema affect 20%–30% of the population during their lifetime (4).
- Approximately 20,000–50,000 patients with anaphylaxis present for medical care in the United States each year. Annual mortality figures are difficult to quantify, but available estimates indicate anaphylaxis causes up to 1000 deaths each year (5).

ALLERGIC RHINITIS

- Allergic rhinitis occurs when an individual develops immunoglobulin (Ig) E sensitization to aeroallergens. Inhalation of the aeroallergens leads to mast cell activation and release of histamine and other chemical mediators of inflammation.
- Common symptoms include rhinorrhea, postnasal drip, congestion, sneezing, cough, and pruritus of the nose and soft palate. Patients may complain of generalized irritability and fatigue. Eye pruritus, injection, irritation, and watery discharge may indicate coexisting allergic conjunctivitis.
- Symptoms recur on exposure to any aeroallergen to which a patient is sensitized.
- Spring and early summer exacerbations occur with tree and grass pollination. Late summer and fall symptoms are usually related to weeds and mold. Indoor flares suggest sensitivity to cockroach, dust mites, pet dander, or molds. Perennial symptoms may be sensitive to a combination of these allergens or indicate nonallergic rhinitis.

NONALLERGIC RHINITIS

- The occurrence of nonallergic rhinitis is independent of an IgE-mediated mechanism.
- Excluding infectious causes, this category includes exercise-related rhinitis as well as vasomotor, drug-induced, food-induced, hormonal, nonallergic occupational, atrophic, NARES (nonallergic rhinitis with eosinophilia syndrome), and rhinitis of the elderly (2).
- Prominent complaints can include nasal congestion and/or clear nasal secretions. Nasal, eye, and soft-palate pruritus are usually absent.
- With vasomotor rhinitis, symptoms are often perennial and triggered by strong odors or smoke. Seasonal air temperature, humidity, and barometric pressure changes may lead to exacerbations, making it difficult to distinguish from allergic rhinitis.

Evaluation

- The history should focus on isolating an allergen exposure. A personal or family history of asthma, allergies, and eczema leads to a higher suspicion for allergic rhinitis.
- Physical examination will not distinguish allergic from nonallergic rhinitis.
  - The nasal mucosa in allergic rhinitis is classically pale or bluish, but can be red or edematous or appear normal. Postnasal drip of any etiology causes posterior pharyngeal cobblestoning. "Allergic shiners" from infraorbital venous congestion are also nonspecific.
  - Findings suggestive of allergic rhinitis include an accentuated transverse nasal crease (seen in children who repeatedly rub their nose because of pruritus), atopic stigmata, such as eczema, and wheezing on auscultation.

Management

- Allergen avoidance is essential in managing allergic rhinitis.
  - Avoidance of animal dander is always best. Exclusion of the pet from the bedroom and high-efficiency particulate air (HEPA) filter use may provide some benefit.
  - For dust mite allergy, use occlusive covers on the pillows, mattress, and box springs. Frequent washing of bed linens and blankets in hot water is helpful. Dehumidifiers and removing carpet may help. HEPA filters are ineffective because dust mite products are not airborne for an extended period of time.
  - Mold allergen can be difficult to control, but dehumidifiers and scrupulous cleaning can be beneficial.

Medical Therapy

- Medical therapy is initiated in a stepwise fashion (Fig. 44.1). Available medications include nasal corticosteroids, antihistamines, decongestants, cromolyn, leukotriene receptor blockers, and nasal ipratropium bromide.
- Nasal corticosteroids are the most effective therapy for persistent or severe symptoms (6). Several days of treatment are usually necessary for maximal effectiveness. They can be used periodically for an athlete's allergy season, but once initiated, the steroid needs regular administration for optimal efficacy (Table 44.1). Side effects are low and include irritation, burning, sneezing, and bloody nasal discharge.
- Chronic nasal steroids, when used properly, are not associated with significant adrenal suppression, nasal or pharyngeal candidiasis, cataracts, or glaucoma (7–9). Studies using mometasone furoate and fluticasone in children showed no difference in growth compared to placebo (10–12).
- Nasal antihistamines can be beneficial in both allergic and nonallergic rhinitis (Table 44.2). Side effects include drowsiness and an unpleasant aftertaste. Whereas nasal steroids provide greater relief of nasal symptoms, nasal antihistamines are also considered first-line therapy. Combination therapy with nasal steroid and nasal antihistamine should be considered for athletes with moderate to severe rhinitis when monotherapy is ineffective (2,13).
- Oral antihistamines relieve sneezing, itching, and rhinorrhea in allergic rhinitis. Their efficacy is roughly equivalent to nasal cromolyn but less than nasal steroids. They provide little relief of nasal obstruction and are generally ineffective in the treatment of nonallergic rhinitis. First-generation antihistamines can cause significant sedation, decreased alertness, and performance impairment and are not recommended for chronic management, especially in competitive athletes (2). These effects can exist without an individual's awareness and can be present even with nighttime-only dosing. Second-generation antihistamines are at least as effective as first-generation antihistamines and possess much lower rates of sedation (Table 44.3). Antihistamines can decrease heat dissipation by their anticholinergic effects on sweat glands and should be used with caution in athletes.
- Oral decongestants relieve congestion in allergic and nonallergic rhinitis. In allergic rhinitis, they are most effective when combined with an oral antihistamine (14). Side effects include insomnia, irritability, tachycardia, and palpitations. Because they decrease heat dissipation via peripheral

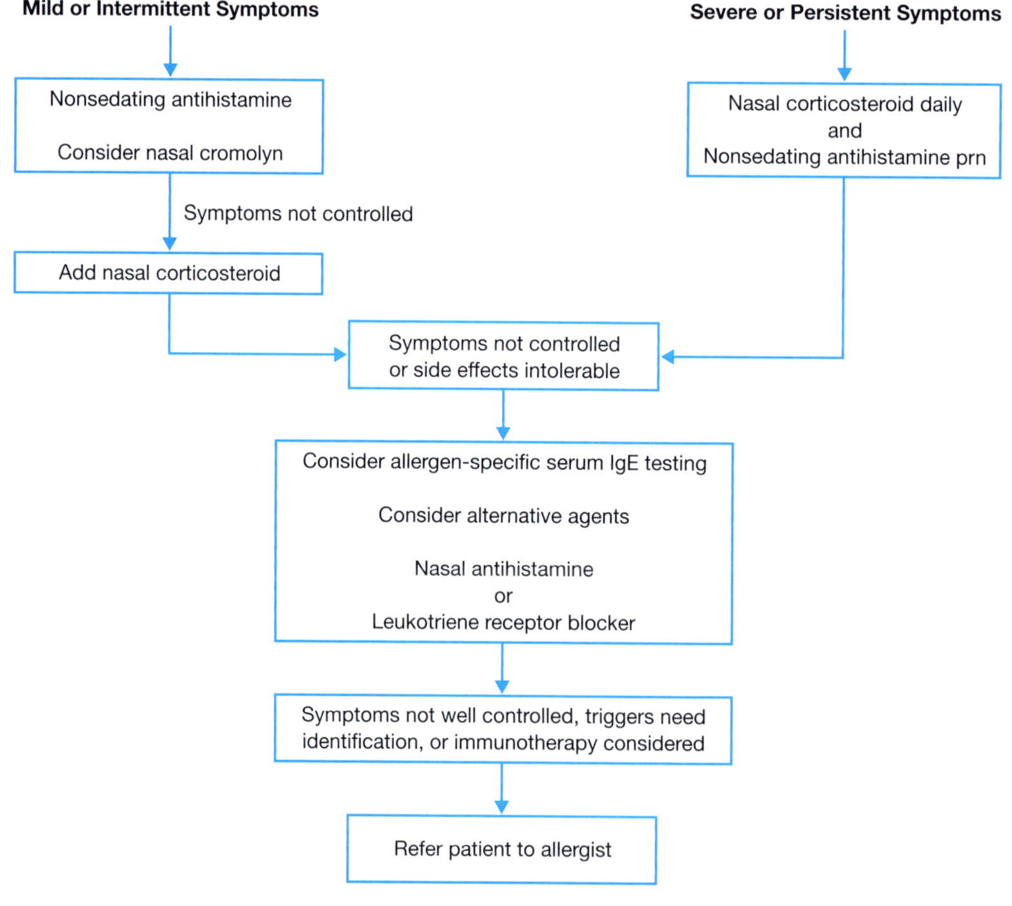

Figure 44.1: Suggested therapeutic strategy for allergic rhinitis in athletes. IgE, immunoglobulin E; prn, as needed.

Table 44.1 Nasal Corticosteroids

Nasal Corticosteroid	Dose: Sprays per Nostril
Flonase, Sensimist (fluticasone)	Age ≥12: 2 daily Age 4–11: Same but start at 1 daily
Nasonex (mometasone furoate)	Age ≥12: 2 daily Age 2–11: 1 daily
Rhinocort Aqua (budesonide)	Age ≥12: 1–4 daily Age 6–11: 1–2 daily
Omnaris (ciclesonide)	Age ≥6: 2 daily
Nasarel (flunisolide)	Age ≥15: 2 bid to tid Age 6–14: 1 tid or 2 bid
Nasacort AQ (triamcinolone)	Age ≥12: 2 daily Age 6–11: 1–2 daily
Beconase and Vancenase AQ (beclomethasone)	Age ≥12: 1–2 bid Age 6–11: 1 bid

bid, twice a day; tid, three times a day.

vasoconstriction, they should be avoided during training or competition in the heat. Athletes must be aware of the rules of their particular sport. Governing bodies for competitive sports have individual guidelines that may ban certain decongestants (see later section, Athlete-Specific Medication Issues).

- Topical nasal decongestants are for short-term control of severe congestion. Their use should not exceed 5 days. If used for more than 5–7 days, they can cause severe rebound congestion and rhinorrhea.
- Cromolyn, a topical mast cell stabilizer, provides modest improvement in the sneezing, itching, and rhinorrhea associated with allergic rhinitis and has a low potential for toxicity. It is useful when given prior to allergen exposure but often requires dosing up to 4–6 times daily to be effective.
- Leukotriene receptor antagonists (LRAs) provide mild improvement in allergic rhinitis with some studies showing efficacy similar to second-generation antihistamines (15). However, there have been reports of serious neuropsychiatric events including suicidal thoughts and actions in patients taking montelukast. The FDA has advised that montelukast only be considered when other alternative therapies are ineffective or have intolerable side effects (2).
- Ipratropium bromide 0.03% nasal spray is effective for treating rhinorrhea, particularly rhinorrhea triggered by exercise, cold air, and food. It has no effect on pruritus or congestion. Side effects include occasional epistaxis and nasal dryness but no systemic anticholinergic or rebound effects. It is effective when dosed 30 minutes prior to exercise or exposure.
- When treatments fail, consider medication inadequacy and noncompliance, as well as the possibility of other diagnoses, such as anatomic or physical obstruction and/or chronic sinusitis.

Table 44.2 Nasal Antihistamines

Topical Agent	Mechanism of Action	Dose per Nostril
Patanase (olopatadine)	Mast cell blocker/ antihistamine	Age 6–11: 1 spray bid Age ≥12: 2 sprays bid
AstePro (Azelastine)	Antihistamine	Age 6 mo–6 y 0.1% 1 spray bid Age 6–12 0.1% or 0.15% 1 spray bid Age >12 0.1% or 0.15% up to 2 sprays bid

Athlete-Specific Medication Issues

- Because restrictions on over-the-counter and prescription medications can change, an athlete should discuss a medication's status with the governing body for their particular sport or level of competition prior to its use. This would include the National Collegiate Athletic Association (NCAA) and the World Anti-Doping Agency (WADA).

Table 44.3 Second-Generation Oral Antihistamines

Second-Generation Oral Antihistamine	Dose	Sedation
Fexofenadine (Allegra)	Age ≥12: 180 mg daily or 60 mg bid Age 2–11: 30 mg bid	No different from placebo
Cetirizine (Zyrtec)	Age ≥6: 5–10 mg daily Age 2–5: 2.5–5 mg daily (syrup)	Slightly higher than placebo but less than first generation
Levocetirizine (Xyzal)	Age ≥12: 5 mg daily Age 6–11: 2.5 mg daily Age 2–5: 1.25 mg daily (syrup)	Slightly higher than placebo but less than first generation
Loratadine (Claritin)	Age ≥6: 10 mg daily Age 2–5: 5 mg daily	No different from placebo at 10 mg; sedating at higher doses
Desloratadine (Clarinex)	Age ≥12: 5 mg daily Age 6–11: 2.5 mg daily Age 2–5: 1.25 mg daily	No different from placebo[a]

bid, twice a day.
[a]Seven percent of population may have sedation because of decreased metabolism of the drug.

- The NCAA has no restrictions on any allergy-related products with the exception that any products containing ephedrine are banned.
- The WADA standards are more stringent. Ephedrine and pseudoephedrine are both banned. However, the urinary concentration of pseudoephedrine associated with normal therapeutic use typically falls below the WADA limit of 150 $\mu g \cdot mL^{-1}$. Oral glucocorticoids are also banned. Injected epinephrine (EpiPen) for emergency use requires a therapeutic use exemption (TUE). Antihistamines, cromolyn, and leukotriene receptor blockers, as well as topical and nasal steroids, are not banned and do not require a TUE. The WADA releases a new list of banned substances each year and requires review by participants and medical staff to ensure compliance (16).

ALLERGY TESTING

- In patients with a history suggestive of allergic rhinitis, indications for referral for skin testing include targeting allergens for avoidance, as well as institution of immunotherapy when medical therapy is failing. Allergy consultation is recommended prior to drastic environmental interventions, such as pet elimination, taking up carpets, or purchasing new mattresses, bedding, dust mite covers, and the like.
- Antihistamines should be stopped 1 week prior to testing, so as not to blunt the cutaneous response to skin testing.
- Allergy testing is contraindicated in the setting of severe lung disease or poorly controlled asthma.
- Skin testing is preferred by most allergists because it is felt to be more sensitive than in vitro allergen-specific serum IgE testing with radioallergosorbent testing (RAST) or ImmunoCAP. Serum testing is a reasonable alternative when skin testing cannot be performed and is helpful for validating the diagnosis and supporting environmental controls.

ALLERGEN IMMUNOTHERAPY

- Allergen immunotherapy (AIT) is effective for allergic rhinitis and allergic asthma. Advantages include long-lasting symptom remission and a reduction in the risk of developing new allergies and asthma in children (3). Notable symptom relief usually takes several months of treatment. Three to five years of AIT are required to sustain symptom remission. Any individual who cannot fully commit to treatment, has poorly controlled asthma, or is on a β-blocker should not receive AIT. It should be prescribed and administered by a board-certified allergist to ensure a thorough discussion of the benefits and potential risks of therapy and to provide ongoing follow-up.

ALLERGIC CONJUNCTIVITIS

- Etiology is the same as for allergic rhinitis. Symptoms occur on inoculation of the allergen onto the mucosa of the eyes.
- Symptom control can be achieved with the same measures as discussed for allergic rhinitis. Persistent eye symptoms may require targeted ocular medications (Table 44.4). Using a combination of mast cell blocker and antihistamine topical therapy is very effective. Other options include topical mast cell blockers or antihistamine alone, topical decongestants, and topical mast cell stabilizers. Topical decongestants should be reserved for short-term use because rebound hyperemia occurs with chronic application. Topical corticosteroids are associated with significant complications and should only be used after consultation with an ophthalmologist.

Table 44.4 Allergic Conjunctivitis Topical Medications

Topical Agent	Mechanism of Action	Dose
Patanol (olopatadine)	Mast cell blocker/antihistamine	Age ≥3: 1 drop bid
Zaditor (ketotifen)	Mast cell blocker/antihistamine	Age ≥3: 1 drop 2–3 times daily
Alomide (lodoxamide)	Mast cell blocker	Age >2: 1–2 drops qid
Alamast (pemirolast)	Mast cell blocker	Age ≥3: 2 drops qid
Livostin (levocabastine)	Antihistamine	Age ≥12: 1 drop qid
Alocril (nedocromil)	Inhibits activation and mediator release from inflammatory cells	Age >3: 1–2 drops bid
Emadine (emedastine)	Antihistamine	Age ≥3: 1 drop qid
Optivar (azelastine)	Antihistamine	Age ≥3: 1 drop bid
Crolom (cromolyn)	Mast cell blocker	Age >4: 1–2 drops qid
Naphcon-A, Opcon-A, Visine-A	Antihistamine/decongestant	Age ≥6: 1 drop up to 4 times daily

bid, twice a day; qid, four times a day.

URTICARIA AND ANGIOEDEMA

Pathophysiology

- Urticaria is caused by mast cell degranulation in the superficial dermis and is characterized by pruritic, erythematous, cutaneous elevations that blanch with pressure. Hives may appear anywhere on the body but occur primarily on the trunk and extremities. Mast cell mediators involved include histamine, prostaglandins, leukotrienes, platelet-activating factor, anaphylatoxins, bradykinin, and Hageman factor. All cause blood vessel dilation and tissue edema.
- Angioedema is similar to urticaria but occurs in the deeper dermis and subcutaneous tissues. It is more painful and burning than pruritic and often involves the face.
- Acute urticaria is defined as new-onset symptoms of less than 6 weeks in duration. If symptoms persist more than 6 weeks, it is considered chronic urticaria.
- In chronic urticaria, 75% have symptoms for over 1 year, 50% have symptoms for over 5 years, and 20% have symptoms for decades. Urticaria occurs at any age but is most common in children and young adults. Approximately 50% of patients at presentation have both urticaria and angioedema, 40% have urticaria only, and 10% have angioedema only (17).
- Most cases are considered autoimmune, but potential triggers are medications, insect stings, and infections as well as foods and food additives. Table 44.5 lists the most common known triggers.
- Physical stimuli can also cause urticaria. Physical urticarias represent 20% of chronic urticaria cases and are important to consider in athletes because they are triggered by conditions occurring during practice and competition (18). (See Table 44.6 for their evaluation and management) (19).
    - Cholinergic urticaria, from elevation in core body temperature, is precipitated by exercise or use of hot tubs. Classically, patients develop small, punctate wheals with prominent erythematous flare. Symptoms usually occur within 2–30 minutes of exposure and last up to 90 minutes.
    - Cold urticaria is precipitated by contact with cold air or objects. Within 2–5 minutes, the exposed area develops swelling and pruritus. Symptoms generally worsen as the area rewarms and last up to 2 hours. Patients with cold urticaria should avoid swimming and diving because this condition carries a risk of anaphylaxis during rewarming if patients have a significant drop in core body temperature.
    - Aquagenic urticaria, which is extremely rare, is caused by contact with water itself. For athletes in water sports, this condition could be confused with cholinergic or cold urticaria. Aquagenic urticaria differs from cholinergic urticaria because it occurs even in cool water and even if the athlete is not exercising while in the water. Unlike cold urticaria, aquagenic urticaria will not be precipitated by application of a cold object that is not water-based.
    - Solar urticaria occurs with exposure to ultraviolet light. Anaphylaxis could occur if large body areas are exposed.
    - Pressure urticaria (angioedema) is precipitated by direct pressure on the skin. Skin pressure is followed 3–12 hours later by localized hives, fever, malaise, and leukocytosis. It can be precipitated by running, clapping, sitting, or using hand equipment. Symptoms can last up to 24 hours.
    - Symptomatic dermatographism is another type of physical urticaria. Patients develop linear, pruritic wheals 2–5 minutes after an area of skin is stroked.

Table 44.5 Common Triggers for Urticaria

Medications
Antibiotics
β-Lactams
Sulfa compounds
NSAIDs
Progesterone
Local anesthetics
Opioid analgesics
Physical Contacts
Latex
Nickel
Plants and plant resins
Fruits/vegetables
Raw fish
Animal saliva
Insect Stings
Foods and Food Additives
Milk
Egg
Peanut
Nuts
Soy
Wheat
Fish/shellfish
Sulfites
Infections
Coxsackie A and B
Hepatitis A, B, and C
HIV
Ebstein-Barr virus
Herpes simplex
Intestinal parasites
Dermatophyte infections

HIV, human immunodeficiency virus; NSAIDs, nonsteroidal anti-inflammatory drugs.

Evaluation

- In the acute setting, providers should assess for symptoms indicating anaphylaxis rather than isolated urticaria or angioedema (20). (See later section, Anaphylactic and Anaphylactoid Reactions.)

Table 44.6 Physical Urticarias

Type	Precipitant	Evaluation	Treatment
Cholinergic urticaria	Elevation in core temperature; exercise, hot tubs, etc.	History and classic pencil eraser-sized punctate wheals	Premedicate with nonsedating antihistamine prior to exercise
Cold urticaria	Contact with cold object	Place cold object on skin for 15 min	Nonsedating antihistamines as needed; avoidance of swimming and diving sports because of risk of anaphylaxis
Aquagenic urticaria	Water contact	History; expose skin to water	Nonsedating antihistamines
Solar urticaria	Ultraviolet light exposure	Expose small, unprotected patch of skin to sunlight	Limit sun exposure; protective clothing and sunscreen use
Pressure urticaria/ angioedema	Direct pressure on skin. Running, prolonged sitting, clapping, etc.	Place 15-lb weight on patient for 20 min and look for skin changes; test for fever and leukocytosis 3–12 h later	Avoidance of precipitants; nonsedating antihistamines and NSAIDs; consider steroid burst/taper if symptoms severe
Symptomatic dermatographism	Stroking or rubbing skin; areas where clothing or equipment abrades skin	Look for linear, pruritic wheal 2–5 min after rubbing the skin	Loose-fitting clothing; treatment usually not necessary; nonsedating antihistamines only for severe symptoms

NSAIDs, nonsteroidal anti-inflammatory drugs.

- Although in most cases the precipitant remains unknown, a detailed history may isolate the cause. Searching for a trigger is more beneficial in acute urticaria as compared to chronic urticaria where the cause is found in less than 10% of cases. For known causes, drug hypersensitivity is most common. Individuals should be asked about any recent prescription medication, over-the-counter medication, or supplement use. Food and food additives rarely cause isolated urticaria, but the relationship to food inhalation, contact, and consumption should be documented. It is important to document physical triggers, occupational exposures, insect envenomations, and any recent illnesses. A thorough review of systems will help rule out any disease associations, such as an acute bacterial or viral illness, parasitic infection, autoimmune/collagen vascular disease, serum sickness, endocrine disease, or malignancy (21).
- The physical examination is especially helpful in the acute setting when skin manifestations are present. It can help document whether urticaria and angioedema are occurring together or in isolation and whether there are any signs of anaphylaxis. The examination should also look for evidence of other diseases that are rarely associated with urticaria and angioedema.
- The use of laboratory and imaging studies should be targeted by the history and physical.
- Consider the following tests: Monospot or Epstein-Barr virus antibody titers if acute mononucleosis is suspected; hepatitis A, B, and C panel; and human immunodeficiency virus (HIV) testing given the right clinical setting. The association of urticaria with other viral infections remains unclear, and routine testing for other viral pathogens is not recommended.
- If a significant travel history is discovered and the complete blood count shows eosinophilia, stool studies should be obtained looking for intestinal parasites. Progressive weight loss and/or the presence of lymphadenopathy or hepatosplenomegaly on examination would warrant an evaluation for an underlying lymphoreticular malignancy.
- If enlargement or nodularity of the thyroid is present, a thyroid function panel, thyroid autoantibodies, thyroid ultrasound, and nuclear medicine thyroid studies should be considered.
- Testing for C1 esterase inhibitor deficiency should be considered for any athlete presenting with recurrent isolated angioedema.
- A skin biopsy for vasculitis is indicated when individual urticarial lesions last longer than 24 hours or are associated with purpura, pain, hyperpigmentation, or systemic symptoms (4).
- If the history and physical examination are unrevealing, a limited laboratory evaluation consisting of a complete blood count with differential, urinalysis, erythrocyte sedimentation rate, thyroid-stimulating hormone, and liver panel is reasonable to screen for occult conditions.

Management

- After the initial evaluation, the management of urticaria and angioedema becomes primarily symptomatic (22,23). Known triggers should be avoided if possible. Mild symptoms can be controlled with a second-generation antihistamine (Table 44.2). Athletes with exercise-induced symptoms only, such as cholinergic urticaria, can take the antihistamine 1–2 hours prior to exercise to maximize effect. Those who exercise regularly and those with chronic symptoms often require daily medication to prevent exacerbations. For moderate or poorly controlled symptoms, the antihistamine should be increased to twice daily dosing prior to considering add-on therapy. Although there is limited data on their effectiveness, additive therapies such as H_2 blockers and leukotriene antagonists are options. Nighttime hydroxyzine or doxepin can be employed but the potential for sedation and adverse effects on cognition and performance must be considered. For periods of moderate to severe symptoms, prednisone therapy can be helpful, but chronic use should be avoided because of the risk of long-term side effects. Omalizumab (XOLAIR) is an FDA-approved anti-IgE therapy for patients whose symptoms remain uncontrolled; it is well tolerated and has shown good efficacy. It is administered as an injection, 150–300 mg once a month (24,25).

- Because food and food additives are a rare cause of chronic urticaria and angioedema, elimination diets are unnecessary unless the history pinpoints a specific food.
- Referral to an allergist is recommended when there is suspicion of an allergic component precipitating symptoms, when there is a history of respiratory distress and hypotension suggesting anaphylaxis, when there is severe angioedema, and when symptoms are not well controlled with standard treatment and XOLAIR therapy is being considered. The athlete should be referred to dermatology for skin biopsy if urticarial vasculitis is suspected.

ANAPHYLACTIC AND ANAPHYLACTOID REACTIONS

Pathophysiology

- Anaphylaxis is an acute, life-threatening, systemic reaction mediated through IgE antibodies and their receptors. It requires previous sensitization and subsequent reexposure to an allergen.
- Anaphylactoid reactions are clinically indistinguishable from true anaphylaxis. Both are caused by massive release of potent chemical mediators from mast cells and basophils. The differences are that IgE antibodies do not mediate anaphylactoid reactions, they do not require prior sensitization, and they are less commonly associated with severe hypotension and cardiovascular collapse. Both are managed with the same treatment measures discussed here.
- Anaphylaxis includes cutaneous signs or symptoms accompanied by obstructive respiratory symptoms and/or hemodynamic changes. Additional features include gastrointestinal complaints and experiencing a "sense of impending doom" (Table 44.7). The onset of symptoms typically begins seconds to minutes after the inciting cause. More rarely, symptoms may be delayed for up to 2 hours.
- Approximately 80% of anaphylaxis cases have a uniphasic course with abrupt onset of symptoms. In the most fulminant cases, symptoms can be followed by death within minutes despite treatment. Up to 20% of patients have a biphasic presentation with a 1- to 8-hour asymptomatic period following the acute phase. After the symptom-free period, a late-phase reaction ensues with recurrence of severe symptoms. The late phase can be protracted, persisting for several hours in 28% of individuals (15).

Table 44.7 Symptoms and Signs of Anaphylaxis

Psychological
"Sense of impending doom"
Cutaneous
Tingling/pruritus
Generalized erythema
Urticaria
Angioedema
Upper Airway
Nasal congestion
Rhinorrhea
Sneezing
Globus sensation
Throat tightness
Dysphonia
Dysphagia
Lower Airway
Dyspnea
Wheezing
Cough
Cardiovascular
Lightheadedness
Syncope
Palpitations
Shock
Gastrointestinal
Abdominal cramps
Bloating
Nausea/vomiting

Evaluation

- The diagnosis of anaphylaxis is affected by variability in the standard case definition. Obtaining as much information from the affected athlete and any witnesses will define the time course, severity of the reaction, and potential cause.
- Anaphylaxis triggers include food, medications, and insect stings (Table 44.8). Any food exposure prior to the onset of symptoms should be documented. Of special concern would be exposure to the most common food allergens, which include eggs, peanut, cow's milk, nuts, fish, soy, shellfish, and wheat. Several medications have been known to cause anaphylaxis, with the most common being β-lactam antibiotics. Documenting exposure to prescription medications, as well as over-the-counter medications and supplements, is important. Bee-sting sensitivity should be suspected in any athlete with a reaction that occurs outdoors, even if the patient does not recall being stung.
- Exercise-induced anaphylaxis is a rare condition associated with exercising within 2–4 hours after food ingestion. It is characterized by the usual manifestations of anaphylaxis beginning

Table 44.8 Causes of Anaphylaxis

Idiopathic
Medications
Antibiotics
Intravenous and local anesthetics
Aspirin/NSAIDs
Chemotherapeutic agents
Opiates
Vaccines
Allergy immunotherapy sera
Radiographic contrast media
Blood products
Latex
Hymenoptera envenomation
Foods
Eggs
Peanut
Cow's milk
Nuts
Seafood
Soy
Wheat
Exercise

NSAIDs, nonsteroidal anti-inflammatory drugs.

within 5–30 minutes of exercise and lasting up to 3 hours. The medical history should explore the relationship of symptom onset to physical exercise to assess for this rare trigger.

- The physical manifestations of anaphylaxis involve multiple sites, including the skin, upper airway, lower airway, and cardiovascular system. The physical examination should start by evaluating upper airway patency by listening for inspiratory stridor and looking for oral or pharyngeal edema. The athlete's work of breathing and accessory muscle use can be used to assess their respiratory status. Auscultation may reveal wheezing, indicating acute bronchospasm. A set of vital signs is critical to patient management, looking for any evidence of cardiovascular or respiratory compromise. Once the ABCs (airway, breathing, and circulation) are assessed and secured, the skin can be examined for the presence of generalized erythema, urticaria, and angioedema.

Acute Management

- Initial management of anaphylaxis should always start with prompt administration of 0.01 mg · kg^{-1} of epinephrine 1:1000 (maximum of 0.5 mL in adults and 0.3 mL in children) even when symptoms are mild. It can be given intramuscular (IM) or subcutaneous (SC). The IM route is preferred, especially in children, due to quicker onset of action. Doses may be repeated every 10–15 minutes if symptoms persist. Intravenous (IV) epinephrine at 1 μg · min^{-1} of 1:10,000 (10 μg · mL^{-1}) can be considered for symptoms resistant to repeated IM or SC administration. The IV dosage can be increased to 2–10 μg · min^{-1} for severe reactions. Patients on β-blockers may not respond to epinephrine. In these cases, glucagon 2–5 mg IM/SC is beneficial. Supportive therapy includes oxygen for hypoxemia, recumbent positioning and IV fluids for hypotension, and inhaled β-agonists or racemic epinephrine for bronchospasm. Antihistamines (diphenhydramine 1–2 mg · kg^{-1} or 25–50 mg IV or orally) may provide additional benefit for pruritus and hives. Although evidence is lacking, corticosteroids (prednisone 0.5–2.0 mg · kg^{-1} up to 125 mg) are frequently given in an effort to help prevent late-phase reactions. Neither antihistamines nor steroids should be used as substitutes for epinephrine. Their onset of action is much slower, and they are insufficient to prevent or treat severer anaphylaxis with respiratory or cardiovascular involvement (26).
- Athletes who have had anaphylaxis should be observed until symptom free. Current evidence does not clearly define the required length of observation. Patients with a mild episode and known trigger can be released after 1 hour of asymptomatic observation. Extended observation should be considered for patients with an unknown trigger as well as for patients with severe symptoms and/or those requiring more than one dose of epinephrine. If an athlete is considered high risk for a late-phase reaction, does not have ready access to emergency services, does not have access to epinephrine, or has poor self-management skills, extended observation of 6 hours or longer or hospitalization may be the best course of action (26).

Long-Term Management

- All patients with anaphylaxis need an action plan to include allergen identification, symptom recognition, and appropriate treatment. A provider knowledgeable in allergic disease should provide education on allergen avoidance, hidden allergens, and cross-reacting substances. All individuals should have an epinephrine autoinjector with them at all times and be educated on the indications and proper technique for its use. The trainer and coach should be familiar with anaphylaxis recognition and epinephrine use as well. The athlete should wear a medical alert bracelet at all times, indicating their condition and allergy if known.
- Because there are no measures proven to prevent exercise-induced anaphylaxis, affected athletes should never exercise alone. Pretreatment with antihistamines is not effective. The primary preventative strategy is to avoid eating for 4 hours prior to exercise. Other measures that may limit attacks are to avoid nonsteroidal anti-inflammatory drugs and aspirin prior to exercise and to avoid outdoor exercise during periods of high humidity, temperature extremes, and the individual's allergy season (27). Occasionally, skin testing can identify a

specific food that the patient can avoid, but often the results are inconclusive. Athletes should carry an epinephrine auto-injector on their person when they do not have immediate access to their gear bag. They should discontinue exercise at the first sign of symptoms and self-administer epinephrine.

- Indications for allergy referral include when further testing is necessary for an unclear diagnosis or an unknown inciting agent, when reactions are recurrent and difficult to control, or when desensitization is required, such as for stinging insects or antibiotic administration. Allergists also serve as an important resource for athletes, parents, and coaches needing education on allergen avoidance, as well as institution or reinforcement of an individual's action plan.

REFERENCES

1. American Academy of Allergy. *Asthma and Immunology. The Allergy Report*; 2010 [cited 2010 Oct 8]. Available from: http://www.aaaai.org/
2. Dykewicz MS, Wallace DV, Amrol DJ, et al. Rhinitis 2020: a practice parameter update. *J Allergy Clin Immunol.* 2020;146(4):721–67.
3. Ledford DK. Efficacy of immunotherapy. *Immunol Allergy Clin North Am.* 2000;20(3):503–25.
4. Kaplan AP. Urticaria and angioedema. In: Middleton E, Reed CE, Ellis EF, et al., editors. *Allergy: Principles and Practice.* St. Louis: Mosby; 1993. p. 1553–80.
5. Neugut AI, Ghatak AT, Miller RL. Anaphylaxis in the United States: an investigation into its epidemiology. *Arch Intern Med.* 2001;161(1):15–21.
6. Benninger M, Farrar JR, Blaiss M, et al. Evaluating approved medications to treat allergic rhinitis in the United States: an evidence-based review of efficacy for nasal symptoms by class. *Ann Allergy Asthma Immunol.* 2010;104(1):13–29.
7. Boner AL. Effects of intranasal corticosteroids on the hypothalamic-pituitary-adrenal axis in children. *J Allergy Clin Immunol.* 2001;108(suppl l):S32–9.
8. Bruni FM, De Luca G, Venturoli V, Boner AL. Intranasal corticosteroids and adrenal suppression. *Neuroimmunomodulation.* 2009;16(5):353–62.
9. Krahnke J, Skoner D. Benefit and risk management for steroid treatment in upper airway diseases. *Curr Allergy Asthma Rep.* 2002;2(6):507–12.
10. Allen DB, Meltzer EO, Lemanske RF Jr, et al. No growth suppression in children treated with the maximum recommended dose of fluticasone propionate aqueous nasal spray for one year. *Allergy Asthma Proc.* 2002;23(6):407–13.
11. Schenkel EJ, Skoner DP, Bronsky EA, et al. Absence of growth retardation in children with perennial allergic rhinitis after one year of treatment with mometasone furoate aqueous nasal spray. *Pediatrics.* 2000;105(2):E22.
12. Skoner DP, Rachelefsky GS, Meltzer EO, et al. Detection of growth suppression in children during treatment with intranasal beclomethasone dipropionate. *Pediatrics.* 2000;105(2):E23.
13. Yáñez A, Rodrigo GJ. Intranasal corticosteroids versus topical H1 receptor antagonists for the treatment of allergic rhinitis: a systematic review with meta-analysis. *Ann Allergy Asthma Immunol.* 2002;89(5):479–84.
14. Sussman GL, Mason J, Compton D, Stewart J, Ricard N. The efficacy and safety of fexofenadine HCL and pseudoephedrine alone and in combination in seasonal allergic rhinitis. *J Allergy Clin Immunol.* 1999;104(1):100–6.
15. Kemp SF. Current concepts in the pathophysiology, diagnosis, and management of anaphylaxis. *Immunol Allergy Clin North Am.* 2001;21(4):611–34.
16. World Anti-Doping Agency. *World Anti-Doping Code International Standard Prohibited List 2023* [Internet]. 2023. Available from: https://www.wada-ama.org/sites/default/files/2022-09/2023list_en_final_9_september_2022.pdf
17. Tharp MD. Chronic urticaria: pathophysiology and treatment approaches. *J Allergy Clin Immunol.* 1996;98(6 pt. 3):S325–30.
18. Fernando S, Broadfoot A. Chronic urticaria—assessment and treatment. *Aust Fam Physician.* 2010;39(3):135–8.
19. Casale TB, Sampson HA, Hanifin J, et al. Guide to physical urticarias. *J Allergy Clin Immunol.* 1988;82(5 pt. 1):758–63.
20. Frigas E, Park MA. Acute urticaria and angioedema: diagnostic and treatment considerations. *Am J Clin Dermatol.* 2009;10(4):239–50.
21. Stafford CT. Urticaria as a sign of systemic disease. *Ann Allergy.* 1990;64(3):264–70.
22. Bernstein JA, Lang DM, Khan DA, et al. The diagnosis and management of acute and chronic urticaria: 2014 update. *J Allergy Clin Immunol.* 2014;133(5):1270–7.
23. Kaplan AP. Clinical practice. Chronic urticaria and angioedema. *N Engl J Med.* 2002;346(3):175–9.
24. Kaplan AP, Popov TA. Biologic agents and the therapy of chronic spontaneous urticaria. *Curr Opin Allergy Clin Immunol.* 2014 Aug;14(4):347–53.
25. McCormack PL. Omalizumab: a review of its use in patients with chronic spontaneous urticaria. *Drugs.* 2014 Sep;74(14):1693–9.
26. Shaker MS, Wallace DV, Golden DBK, et al. Anaphylaxis – A 2020 practice parameter update, systematic review, and Grading of Recommendations, Assessment, Development and Evaluation (GRADE) analysis. *J Allergy Clin Immunol.* 2020;145(4):1082–123.
27. Shadick NA, Liang MH, Partridge AJ, et al. The natural history of exercise-induced anaphylaxis: survey results from a 10-year follow-up study. *J Allergy Clin Immunol.* 1999;104(1):123–7.

45 Overtraining Syndrome

Elizabeth Gannon and Thomas M. Howard

INTRODUCTION

- Overtraining has been described and has been well known to athletes and trainers for decades. In 1923, Dr. Parmenter described overtraining as "a condition difficult to detect and still more difficult to describe. Evaluation should focus on training load, nutrition, sleep, rest, competition stress, and psychological state" (1).
- There are multiple hypotheses on the cause of overtraining. There continues to be research on overtraining to further define the condition and pathophysiology and identify markers for diagnosis, treatment, and prevention (2).
- Overtraining, if left unrecognized or untreated, can result in injury, poor performance, and early retirement.
- Overtraining syndrome (OTS) is a condition that arises along a continuum of fatigue.
- The diagnosis of overtraining syndrome is one of exclusion and often requires an extensive workup of the athlete. As the precise etiology of overtraining syndrome remains elusive, the ideal battery of laboratory testing does not exist (3,4).
- Treatment of overtraining syndrome is rest; however, it often requires a multidisciplinary approach involving the physician, trainers, nutritionist, and often, a sports psychologist.

DEFINITIONS

- **Training:** A series of stimuli or displacement of homeostasis to provide stimulation for adaptation. A progressive overload in an effort to improve performance.
- **Adaptation:** A physiologic response to stress that results in an adjustment in function.
- **Recovery:** Period of time following a training stimulus when adaptation occurs, resulting in supercompensation to allow better performance in the future (*i.e.*, the training effect). Recovery includes hydration, nutritional replenishment, sleep/rest, stretching, relaxation, and emotional recovery.
- **Periodization:** Planned sequencing of increased training loads and recovery periods within a training program.
- **Overreaching:** A short-term decrease in performance after a period of overload (intensity or volume). This acute phase is thought to last 1–2 weeks. Some authors even consider overreaching to represent normal physiologic fatigue to overload training (5).
- **Overtraining syndrome:** This syndrome is defined as prolonged decrease in sport-specific performance, usually >2 weeks. It is manifested by premature fatigability, emotional and mood changes, lack of motivation, sleep disorders, pronounced vegetative somatic complaints, overuse injuries, and immune dysfunction (5–7). It is the result of prolonged heavy exercise over an extended period of time with inadequate recovery time between training sessions.

PHYSIOLOGIC CHANGES WITH TRAINING

Immunologicals

- Decreased salivary immunoglobulin A (IgA)
- Increased white blood cells (WBCs), lymphocytes, natural killer cells, and polymorphonuclear cell (PMN) activity
- Transient decrease in T helper/T suppressor (Th/Ts) ratio
- Decreased serum glutamine

Endocrine

- Increased testosterone proportional to exercise intensity.
- Increased muscle mass stimulating glycogen regeneration and protein synthesis (anabolism).
- Transient increase in cortisol relative to the duration and intensity of exercise. The stress response (catabolism).
- The ratio of free testosterone to cortisol (FTCR) represents the balance of anabolism and catabolism. A 30% decrease in this ratio may suggest inadequate recovery or overreaching (8).
- Norepinephrine increases before exercise (anticipation) and early in exercise, stimulating lipolysis.
- Epinephrine increases proportional to exercise intensity.
- Decreased sex hormone binding globulin (SHBG) production with intense exercise.
- Suppression of pulsatile secretion of gonadotropin-releasing factor (GnRH), probably affected by stress and poor nutrition.
- Growth hormone peak secretion at night; blunted response with intense exercise.

EPIDEMIOLOGY

- Overtraining has a lifetime prevalence of 30% for nonelite athletes and 60% in elite athletes (9).
- More commonly seen in endurance events, such as swimming, cycling, or running. Overtraining in powerlifters is probably different.
- Susceptible athletes include highly motivated, goal-oriented individuals; athletes who design exercise programs by themselves; and athletes who tend to be focused, conventional, and conservative.

HYPOTHESES

- **Glycogen depletion:** Chronic nutritional deficiency and extensive periods of heavy training lead to glycogen depletion in muscles, resulting in peripheral fatigue (5). Central fatigue is interrelated to changes in branched-chain amino acids (BCAAs); see central fatigue hypothesis (10).
- **Central fatigue hypothesis/BCAA hypothesis:** Peripheral fatigue and nutrient depletion lead to the consumption of BCAAs with subsequent change in the BCAA to free tryptophan ratio in plasma. This favors transport of tryptophan into the central nervous system. Tryptophan is a precursor for serotonin 5-hydroxytryptamine, which causes central fatigue (11,12).
- **Autonomic imbalance:** An increase in sympathetic activity from stress and overloaded target organs and increased catabolism leading to decreased sympathetic intrinsic activity. Chronically increased catecholamine levels cause downregulation of receptors and fatigue (13).
- **Glutamine hypothesis/immune dysfunction:** Overload training leads to decreased glutamine production from stressed muscle tissue. Glutamine deficiency, as well as acute exercise stress on the immune system, creates an immunologic open window leading to repeated minor infections and systemic stress (14).
- **Cytokine hypothesis:** Incomplete recovery of locally damaged tissue causes a local inflammatory response that becomes systemic with elevated proinflammatory cytokines interleukin (IL)-1β, tumor necrosis factor-α, and IL-6. These cytokines cause central nervous system fatigue (6). Cheng et al. recently published an excellent review of the literature in their discussion of the intramuscular mechanisms of overtraining (7).

CATEGORIES OF OVERTRAINING

- **Sympathetic overtraining:** Probably represents early overtraining. It is manifested by increased resting heart rate (HR) and blood pressure, loss of appetite, loss of lean body mass (LBM), irritability, sleep disturbances, and fatigue (8).
- **Parasympathetic overtraining:** Probably represents more chronic state, prolonged overtraining. It is manifested by low resting HR and blood pressure, sleep disturbances, depressed mood, and fatigue (8).

Physical Findings

- Elevated resting HR (usually >10 beats per minute [bpm] over baseline)
- Decreased LBM
- Depressed mood on various evaluation tools
- Otherwise, normal physical exam

Differential Diagnosis

Common Causes

- Caffeine withdrawal, environmental allergies, exercise-induced bronchospasm, infectious mononucleosis, insufficient sleep, iron deficiency with or without anemia, overtraining, performance anxiety, mood disorder (anxiety, depression, adjustment reaction), psychosocial stress, and upper respiratory infection

Less-Common Causes

- Dehydration, diabetes mellitus, eating disorder, hepatitis (A, B, or C), hypothyroidism, inadequate carbohydrate or protein intake, lower respiratory infection, medication side effect (antidepressants, antihistamines, anxiolytics, β-blockers), post-concussive syndrome, pregnancy, and substance abuse

Relatively Rare Causes, but Important

- Adrenocortical insufficiency or excess, congenital or acquired heart disease, arrhythmia, bacterial endocarditis, congestive heart failure, coronary heart disease, human immunodeficiency virus, malabsorption, lung disease, Lyme disease, malaria, malignancy, neuromuscular disorder, renal disease, and syphilis

Evaluation (Fig. 45.1)

First Visit

- A thorough history focusing on the chief complaints, training program, diet, medications, nutrition, illness, review of systems (ROS), and an assessment of the goals of the athlete's training program.
- Initial lab studies to consider: complete blood count (CBC), erythrocyte sedimentation rate (ESR), metabolic panel, thyroid-stimulating hormone (TSH), ferritin, serum β-human chorionic gonadotropin (β-hCG), monospot, and other specifically indicated tests based on history, ROS, and examination.
- Prescribe decrease in intensity or even absolute rest for 2 weeks. During that time, consider cross-training for enjoyment and evaluation of other confounding stressors.

Second Visit

- Review lab results, training over the past 2 weeks, and symptoms.

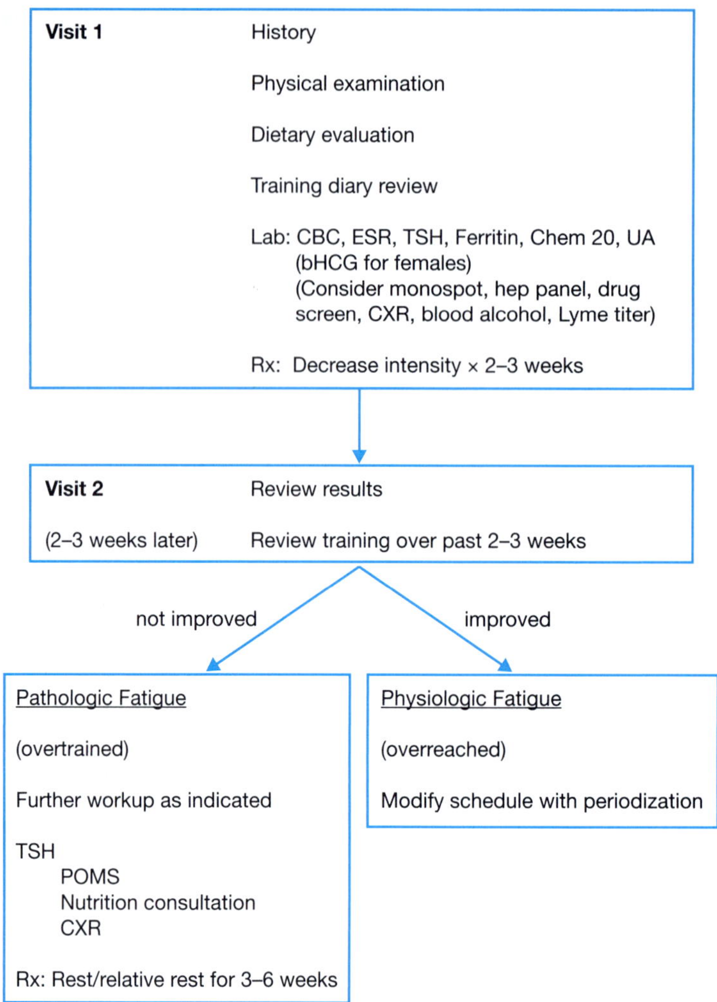

Figure 45.1: Algorithm for evaluation of fatigue in the athlete. bHCG, β-human chorionic gonadotropin; CBC, complete blood count; CXR, chest x-ray; ESR, erythrocyte sedimentation rate; Hep, hepatitis; POMS, Profile of Mood States; TSH, thyroid-stimulating hormone; UA, urinalysis.

- If improved, consider the diagnosis of physiologic fatigue (overreaching) and focus on adjustments to the training schedule with periodization, cross-training, and addressing the other stressors identified.
- If no improvement, consider the diagnosis of pathologic fatigue or overtraining. Patients will require prolonged relative rest from intense training and further workup. Consider consulting with a sports psychologist and dietician and further evaluation to work through the differential diagnosis.
- Recent publications from the Endocrine and Metabolic Response to Overtraining (EROS) have outlined combinations of clinical and biochemical markers that can more reliably diagnose OTS. One of the many publications from this study identified nine clinical (anger, fatigue, tension and vigor on Profile of Mood States [POMS], dietary consumption of protein, carbohydrates and total calories, % body fat, and muscle mass) and nine biochemical markers (growth hormone, prolactin, total testosterone, TE ratio and Insulin tolerance test to measure cortisol, ACTH, growth hormone, and prolactin) to be nearly 100% accurate in confirming the diagnosis of overtraining syndrome (15–17).

TREATMENT

- The first line of treatment should be prevention. To try to prevent overtraining syndrome, review the athlete's training schedule and concepts of cross-training and emphasize adequate rest and minimization of coexisting life stressors.
- When prevention fails, the treatment is rest. There is no quick fix. An initial rest period of 2–4 weeks should be considered.
- Life stressors should be reviewed in depth, as well as a review of the athlete's diet, sleep schedule, and training and competition schedules.
- A multidisciplinary approach is recommended. Consultation with a nutritionist and sports psychologist can be beneficial.
- Close monitoring of the athlete is recommended. On return to practice and competition, the athlete should pay careful attention to sleep, nutrition, social stress, and competition stress with slow advancement of training. The sequence of advancing activity should focus on frequency, then duration, and finally the intensity of the sessions.

MONITORING

- Poor markers for overtraining include body mass, hemoglobin, ferritin, and creatine phosphokinase and are not recommended for monitoring.
- Indicators of inadequate recovery, but not necessarily overtraining, include FTCR ratio decrease >30%, a decrease in SHBG, and a glutamine-to-glutamate level <3.58 (18,19).
- Psychiatric indicators generally change before biologic markers.
- **Good markers for monitoring:** Athletes, trainers, and coaches often use baseline HR. An increase of >10 bpm from baseline is considered abnormal. This rise represents an imbalance between sympathetic and parasympathetic systems with heightened sympathetic tone (5,20). Resting HR can easily be obtained, but can be affected by illness, consumption of stimulants.
- Decrease in HR variability also indicates inadequate recovery (5,21). With new wearable HR monitors it is much easier to obtain the HR variability and track it daily and over time. Similar to resting HR, it represents the HR response to sympathetic and parasympathetic tone. It rises with training and will decrease with heavy overload. Sudden decreases in this value should alert the athlete or coach to inadequate recovery.
- Monitor performance in time trials and standard exercise challenges.
- Foster (22) described a "session RPE," or rating of perceived exertion, as the athlete's self-described intensity of the training session multiplied by the duration of the session. Daily mean load and standard deviation (SD) can be calculated to quantitative monotony (daily mean/SD) and strain (weekly load × monotony) (22).
- **Psychological tools:** POMS — 65 questions assessing 5 negative mood states (tension, depression, anger, fatigue, and confusion) and 1 positive mood state (vigor) (23). Concerning trends indicated by increased negative mood symptoms and decrease in the positive.
- Total Quality Recovery (TQR) action and RPE scales (15). An athlete or coach assesses the various aspects of quality recovery and assigns a score to track trends.
  - Action: A total score in four major areas of recovery
    - Nutrition/hydration: 10 points
    - Sleep/rest: 4 points
    - Relaxation/emotional support: 3 points
    - Stretching/active rest: 3 points
  - Perceived: A reverse Borg RPE scale of perceived recovery (Table 45.1)
- Recovery-Stress Questionnaire for Athletes (RESTQ-Sport) (24): 90-question survey tool answered on a Likert-type scale to assess training stress and recovery.

Table 45.1 Total Quality Recovery Action

Rating of Perceived Exertion	Total Quality Recovery
6	6
7 Very, very light	7 Very, very poor recovery
8	8
9 Very light	9 Very poor recovery
10	10
11 Faintly light	11 Poor recovery
12	12
13 Somewhat hard	13 Reasonable recovery
14	14
15 Hard	15 Good recovery
16	16
17 Very hard	17 Very good recovery
18	18
19 Very, very hard	19 Very, very good recovery
20	20

PREVENTION

- Individualized and variable training programs
- Coaching and supervised training
- Periods of "time out"
- Cross-training
- Reasonable goal setting (short- and long-term)
- Relaxation and visualization techniques or use of a sports psychologist

REFERENCES

1. Parmenter DC. Some medical aspects of the training of college athletes. *Boston Med Surg J*. 1923;189:45–50.
2. Weakley J, Halson SL, Mujika I. Overtraining syndrome symptoms and diagnosis in athletes: where is the research? A systematic review. *Int J Sports Physiol Perform*. 2022 May 1;17(5):675–81.
3. Meeusen R, Duclos M, Foster C, et al. Prevention, diagnosis, and treatment of the overtraining syndrome: joint consensus statement of the European College of Sport Science and the American College of Sports Medicine. *Med Sci Sports Exerc*. 2013 Jan;45(1):186–205.
4. Carfagno DG, Hendrix JC III. Overtraining syndrome in the athlete: current clinical practice. *Curr Sports Med Rep*. 2014 Jan-Feb;13(1):45–51.
5. Snyder AC. Overtraining and glycogen depletion hypothesis. *Med Sci Sports Exerc*. 1998;30(7):1146–50.
6. Smith DJ, Norris SR. Changes in glutamine and glutamate concentrations for tracking training tolerance. *Med Sci Sports Exerc*. 2000;32(3):684–9.
7. Cheng AJ, Jude B, Lanner JT. Intramuscular mechanisms of overtraining. *Redox Biol*. 2020;35:101480. doi:10.1016/j.recdox.2020.101480

8. Fry AC, Kraemer WJ. Resistance exercise overtraining and overreaching. Neuroendocrine responses. *Sports Med.* 1997;23(2):106–29.
9. Cardoos N. CAQ review. *Curr Sports Med Rep.* 2015;14(3):157–8.
10. Load, overload, and recovery in the athlete: select issues for the team physician—a consensus statement. *Med Sci Sports Exerc.* 2019;51(4):821.
11. Davis JM, Bailey SP. Possible mechanisms of central nervous system fatigue during exercise. *Med Sci Sports Exerc.* 1997;29(1):45–57.
12. Gastmann UA, Lehmann MJ. Overtraining and the BCAA hypothesis. *Med Sci Sports Exerc.* 1998;30(7):1173–8.
13. Lehmann M, Foster C, Dickhuth HH, Gastmann U. Autonomic imbalance hypothesis and overtraining syndrome. *Med Sci Sports Exerc.* 1998;30(7):1140–5.
14. Walsh NP, Blannin AK, Robson PJ, Gleeson M. Glutamine, exercise and immune function. Links and possible mechanisms. *Sports Med.* 1998;26(3):177–91.
15. Cadegiani FA, Kater CE. Hormonal aspects of overtraining syndrome: a systematic review. *BMC Sports Sci Med Rehabil.* 2017;9:14. doi:10.1186/s13102-017-0079-8
16. Cadegiani FA, da Silva PH, Abraro TC, Kater CE. Diagnosis of overtraining syndrome: results of the endocrine and metabolic responses on overtraining syndrome study—EROS-diagnosis. *J Sports Med.* 2020;2020:3937819. doi:10.1155/2020/3937
17. Cadegiani FA, Kater CE. Novel insights of overtraining syndrome discovered from the EROS study. *BMJ Open Sport Exerc Med.* 2019;5(1):e000542. doi:10.1136/bmjsem-2019-000542
18. Halson SL, Lancaster GI, Jeukendrup AE, Gleeson M. Immunological responses to overreaching in cyclists. *Med Sci Sports Exerc.* 2003;35(5):854–61.
19. Smith LL. Cytokine hypothesis of overtraining: a physiological adaptation to excessive stress? *Med Sci Sports Exerc.* 2000;32(2):317–31.
20. Dressendorfer RH, Hauser AM, Timmis GC. Reversal of runner's bradycardia with training overstress. *Clin J Sport Med.* 2000;10(4):279–85.
21. Pichot V, Busso T, Roche F, et al. Autonomic adaptations to intensive and overload training periods: a laboratory study. *Med Sci Sports Exerc.* 2002;34(10):1660–6.
22. Foster C. Monitoring training in athletes with reference to overtraining syndrome. *Med Sci Sports Exerc.* 1998;30(7):1164–8.
23. McNair DM, Lorr M, Dropplemen L. *EdITS for the Profile of Mood States (POMS).* San Diego (CA): Educational & Industrial Testing Service; 1971.
24. Kellmann M, Günther KD. Changes in stress and recovery in elite rowers during preparation for the Olympic Games. *Med Sci Sports Exerc.* 2000;32(3):676–83.

Exercise and Chronic Disease

46

Shane Hudnall, Karl B. Fields, Catherine R. Rainbow, Kenneth P. Barnes, and Wes Bailey

- Chronic diseases such as diabetes, hypertension, and coronary artery disease directly cause or are risk factors in over 70% of deaths each year.
- Approximately 60% of Americans have at least one chronic disease whereas 40% have two or more chronic diseases.
- Evidence shows a healthy diet, avoiding tobacco and excessive alcohol, and being physically active can prevent and decrease the risk of many chronic diseases.
- In this chapter, we review the effects of exercise on chronic diseases and current recommendations for physical activity participation with these conditions.

OBESITY

- Obesity in adults is defined as a BMI > 30 and severe obesity as a BMI > 40.
- In children and adolescents, obesity is defined as a BMI-for-age in the 95th percentile or greater. Severe obesity is BMI-for-age at 120% of the 95th percentile or greater; A BMI-for-age >35 kg/m^2 also constitutes severe obesity in children and adolescents.
- According to data collected from the National Health and Nutrition Examination Survey (NHANES) from 2017 to March 2020, the prevalence of obesity in adults 20 and older was 41.9%, an 11.4% increase from 1999 to 2000. 9.2% of adults were severely obese.
- The prevalence of obesity in children and adolescents aged 2–19 was 19.7%, increased from 13.9% in 1999–2000 data.
- Overall morbidity and mortality related to obesity has been well documented.
- Obesity correlates with increased death from coronary artery disease, cerebrovascular disease, and several different types of cancer (especially liver, endometrial, and kidney).
- Obesity is associated with type 2 diabetes, dyslipidemia, hypertension, heart failure (HF), venous thromboembolism, gallbladder disease, sleep apnea, osteoarthritis, and other chronic diseases.
- Abdominal obesity in which the waist-to-hip ratio is high indicates a subset of individuals at much higher risk of cardiovascular diseases, mortality from cardiovascular diseases, and cancer mortality. A waist circumference of 35 in in women and 40 in in men is considered high risk.
- Observational studies have demonstrated a decreased risk of chronic diseases in those who exercise regularly (1).
- High BMI is associated with a greater risk of injury in youth sports, especially in the lower extremities (2).
- The odds of sustaining a musculoskeletal injury increase with BMI. Overweight individuals are 15% more likely. Those with class III Obesity (BMI > 40) are 48% more likely to have an exercise-related injury (3).
- Obesity also poses a much greater risk of heat illness during competition in sports.
- Despite the health risks of obesity, several overweight athletes have achieved high levels of sports success. In some sports, including football, weight throws in track and field, heavyweight wrestling, and powerlifting, excessive weight has generally been considered advantageous.
- Highly competitive athletes may need to consume 1500–2000 excess calories per day to account for the calorie expenditure of intense training. Dietary calorie consumption appears to be a learned behavior and appetite often does not decline with a reduction in activity levels in the off-season or after retirement. This can lead to weight gain and obesity.
- Regular exercise reduces the risk of developing obesity. In a cohort study of nonobese adults averaging 6 years of follow-up, participants who met physical activity guidelines for resistance or aerobic exercise (resistance exercise 2 or more times a week, aerobic exercise over 500 MET-minutes per week) had a lower risk of developing obesity. Those who met both guidelines had the lowest risk (4).
- All forms of muscular activity burn calories but aerobic activity generally serves as the backbone of a weight loss program. There is a dose-dependent relationship between aerobic exercise and weight loss. Although less than 150 min · wk^{-1} of aerobic exercise results in little change in body weight, this type of activity performed between 225 and 420 min · wk^{-1} results in 5–7.5 kg weight loss (5).
- Combining a moderately reduced calorie diet with increased physical activity results in greater initial weight loss and sustained weight loss at 1 year. However, when caloric intake is

more severely limited, the addition of physical activity does not seem to confer additional benefit for weight loss.

- Resistance exercise may provide benefits in lean muscle mass but does not appear to promote weight loss or prevent weight regain after weight loss. Sustained aerobic exercise, however, is important in helping prevent weight regain (5).
- Medications to assist in the treatment of obesity are not recommended in athletes although continued research with GLP-1 inhibitors in individuals with severe obesity could change future guidelines (6).

TYPE 2 DIABETES

- As of 2022, over 37 million Americans have diabetes; more than 90% of those have type 2 diabetes. Approximately 20% of Americans are unaware they have diabetes.

Improved Glycemic Control

- Exercise improves insulin sensitivity in liver, muscle, and fat cells.
- The insulin sensitizing effect of exercise disappears after about 48 hours. Repeated exercise causes a persistent increase in insulin action in insulin-resistant individuals.
- Multiple studies have demonstrated a decrease in HbA1c with regular exercise (7–9).
- All types of exercise lead to statistically significant reductions in A1c levels but a combination of aerobic and resistance exercise may confer the best benefit.
- A dose-response relationship has been demonstrated for aerobic and combined exercise programs with greater reductions in those who exercise more than 150 min · wk^{-1} compared to those who exercised 150 minutes or less.
- In a meta-analysis of supervised aerobic exercise programs lasting more than 12 weeks, it was demonstrated HbA1c is reduced by 0.22% for every 30 min · wk^{-1} of supervised moderate-vigorous aerobic exercise (10).
- High-intensity resistance exercise has greater effects on A1c and insulin levels than low-moderate resistance exercise.
- High-intensity aerobic and resistance exercise is contraindicated in diabetics with proliferative retinopathy (11).
- High-intensity interval training (HIIT) improves HbA1c with a reduction similar to that seen in moderate continuous training.

Lower Mortality Risk

- Regular physical activity is associated with a lower mortality risk in diabetics.
- Each increase of 10 metabolic equivalent task hours of physical activity per week lowers mortality by 4% in those with type 2 diabetes (12).

Cardiovascular Benefits

- Diabetes mellitus is considered a cardiac equivalent because of the strong association of this disease with cardiovascular problems. Maintaining a good fitness level lowers the risk of cardiac death and is associated with longevity.
- Regular physical activity has beneficial effects on cardiac risk factors, autonomic tone, and myocardial ischemia.
- Diabetics beginning a gradual exercise program only need stress testing if they are symptomatic or higher risk (11).
- In a large group of diabetics, walking at least 2 hours a week lowered cardiovascular mortality rates. This level of walking prevented 1 death · y^{-1} for every 61 patients (13). A similar study demonstrated patients who performed moderate-to-vigorous exercise had a 40% lower risk of cardiovascular disease than those who did not exercise (14).
- Several studies and meta-analyses have shown regular exercise helps lower blood pressure in type 2 diabetes (8,9). Aerobic exercise may also delay or prevent the development of hypertension. Good control of blood pressure lessens the risk of complications in diabetic patients.
- Aerobic exercise improves lipid profiles in type 2 diabetics. In a meta-analysis of patients undergoing a supervised aerobic training program, improvements were shown in total cholesterol, triacylglycerol levels, and low-density lipoprotein (LDL) cholesterol (15).

Decreased Risk of Developing Type 2

- Exercise may help individuals with impaired glucose tolerance and lead to prevention of type 2 diabetes especially when combined with weight reduction and dietary changes (16).
- Structured programs combining physical activity and modest weight loss have been shown to reduce the risk of developing type 2 diabetes by up to 58% in high-risk populations (17).

OTHER BENEFITS OF EXERCISE IN TYPE 2 DIABETES

Improved Balance/Decreased Falls

- Exercise may improve balance in type 2 diabetics.
- Combined resistance and balance training for older type 2 diabetics (age 50–75) over 6+ weeks was associated with decreased risk of falls (18).

Body Composition

- Aerobic, resistance, and combined training lead to abdominal fat reduction with aerobic exercise being the most effective.
- Other studies have demonstrated decrease in BMI, waist circumference, and body fat with improvements in muscle strength (7,9).

VO_{2max}

- Aerobic exercise improves maximum oxygen consumption and aerobic capacity (9).
- High-intensity interval training also improves VO_{2max}.

Mental Health

- Aerobic exercise training has positive effects on mental health, anxiety, insomnia, and subscales of physical symptoms (19).

Improved Cognition

- Exercise may improve cognition in those with type 2 diabetes but more trials are needed.

Decreased Bone Loss

- Combined resistance and weight-bearing aerobic exercise helps prevent excessive bone loss.

Improved Nerve Function and Decreased Neuropathic Pain

- Aerobic exercise training may positively affect nerve function in type 2 diabetes (20).

Recommended Physical Activity and Exercise

- High levels of sedentary behavior are associated with a greater risk of type 2 diabetes (21).
- The American College of Sports Medicine (ACSM) and the American Diabetes Association have concurred that physical activity has major benefits for individuals with type 2 diabetes.
- Similar to recommendations for all adults, diabetics are encouraged to perform over 150 min · wk^{-1} of moderate-intensity aerobic exercise or 75–150 min · wk^{-1} of vigorous-intensity aerobic exercise.
- Given the insulin-sensitizing effects of exercise disappear after about 48 hours, there should not be more than 2 consecutive days between bouts of physical activity.
- Muscle-strengthening activities should be performed 2–3 d · wk^{-1} but not on consecutive days.
- Specific recommendations should be tailored to the individual patient based on their baseline activity level, health status, and fitness goals (11).

TYPE 1 DIABETES

- Exercise in type 1 diabetes has not been studied as rigorously as type 2 diabetes.
- Individuals with type 1 diabetes exercise less than the general population. These patients report hypoglycemia and fear of hypoglycemia as the two greatest barriers preventing them from exercising.
- In general, physical activity has not been shown to have a statistically significant difference in HbA1c in type 1 diabetics, but more studies are needed.
- Resistance training may be beneficial for glycemic control in those with type 1 diabetes. Blood glucose is reduced for a more prolonged period following resistance exercise compared to aerobic exercise that may account for reduced A1c seen in some studies of resistance exercise (22).
- Physical activity is associated with decreased glycemic variability in type 1 diabetics. Furthermore, resistance exercise before aerobic exercise improved glycemic stability throughout exercise, reducing severity of post-exercise hypoglycemia in type 1 diabetes (23).
- Exercise training in type 1 diabetics improves body mass index, strength, VO_{2max}, and LDL in adults; exercise improves insulin dose, waist circumference, LDL, triglycerides, quality of life, and physical fitness in children.
- An epidemiologic study following males with type I diabetes for 20 years showed those who participated in high school or college sports had lower mortality and lower incidence of macrovascular disease than sedentary counterparts.
- Continuous glucose monitoring allows type 1 diabetics to exercise more consistently within a safe glucose range. Preliminary data suggests that this increases exercise activity (24).

HYPERTENSION

- For children and adolescents, The National High Blood Pressure Education Program recommends the evaluation of blood pressure using percentiles based on age, height, and gender.
- For children aged 1–12 years, normal blood pressure is less than the 90th percentile; elevated blood pressure is ≥90th percentile to <95th percentile **OR** 120/80 mm Hg to <95th percentile (whichever is lower); stage 1 hypertension is ≥95th percentile to <95th percentile + 12 mm Hg **OR** 130/80 to 139/89 mm Hg (whichever is lower); and stage 2 hypertension is ≥95th percentile + 12 mm Hg **OR** ≥ 140/90 mm Hg (whichever is lower).
- For adolescents aged 13–17 years, normal blood pressure is <120/80 mm Hg; elevated blood pressure is 120/<80–129/<80 mm Hg; stage 1 hypertension is 130/80–139/89 mm Hg; and stage 2 hypertension is ≥140/90 mm Hg.
- In adults, the International Society of Hypertension defines normal blood pressure as <120/80 mm Hg; elevated blood pressure is ≥120/80; grade 1 hypertension depends on the location of measurement — in the office 140/90–159/99 mm Hg, at home measurement 135/85–159/99 mm Hg; grade 2 hypertension is ≥160/100 mm Hg irrespective of location of measurement (25).

- Blood pressure is a product of cardiac output multiplied by peripheral resistance. Peripheral resistance must fall dramatically during exercise or else blood pressure rises excessively as increasing physical activity requires a higher cardiac output than rest.
- In patients whose blood pressure rises too dramatically during dynamic exercise, the relative risk of subsequent hypertension is higher.
- A meta-analysis of 54 clinical trials of aerobic exercise showed reductions of systolic and diastolic blood pressure in both hypertensive and normotensive individuals (26).
- The Osaka Health Survey demonstrated that a daily walk of 20 minutes or more reduced the risk of hypertension in men. In fact, for every 26 men who walked, one case of hypertension was prevented. Vigorous exercise for as little as 30 minutes, just once weekly, also reduced risk.
- Endurance exercise lowers blood pressures of hypertensives by 5–7 mm Hg after an exercise session or following a period of exercise training. Blood pressure can remain reduced for up to 22 hours following a bout of endurance exercise. The greatest decreases occur in those with severe hypertension (27).
- Increased risk of myocardial infarction and stroke are well established with hypertension. Moreover, there is a higher risk of developing aneurysms in comparison to normotensive patients (28).
- Exercise can reduce future cardiovascular events and mortality.
- Most resistance exercise seems to benefit hypertensive athletes, although maximal resistance efforts pose theoretical risks. Resistance exercise can supplement endurance activities (27).
- Hypertensive individuals sustain higher blood pressure increases in comparison to normotensive patients with exercise. They also have slower recovery of blood pressure during exercise intervals (28).
- Heavy resistance exercise, particularly weightlifting, can cause dramatic rises in blood pressure that are transient. One major barrier to confident exercise prescription is the concern regarding this rapid and potentially large rise in systolic blood pressure during resistance exercise. This rise can possibly be mitigated by adjusting the training protocol: For example, combining more sets with less repetitions and shorter rest intervals (28).
- To further elucidate the optimal exercise recommendations for hypertensives, more studies are needed with particular focus on hypertensives and with consideration of the following variables: demographics, comorbidities (*e.g.*, pulmonary hypertension, HF, etc.), and medications (*i.e.*, diuretics, ace-inhibitors, angiotensin receptor blockers, calcium channel blockers, beta blockers, antiarrhythmics).
- A mix of aerobic exercises and resistance exercises is generally advised (27,28).
- The ACSM recommends performance of low-to-moderate exercise (*e.g.*, walking); at 40%–59% of oxygen reuptake reserve (VO_2R), 5–7 $d \cdot wk^{-1}$, for a total of at least 30 minutes daily (27). The ACSM also recommends resistance training for 2–3 sessions per week.
- Patients on alpha blockers, calcium channel blockers, or vasodilators are at risk of hypotension in the immediate post-exercise period. Risk can be mitigated by avoidance of sudden exercise cessation and by undertaking an extended cool down period of light activity.
- β-blockers and diuretics can impair thermoregulation. This can be mitigated by limiting exercise intensity in hot or humid weather, ensuring adequate hydration, and by wearing clothing that promotes cooling.

CORONARY ARTERY DISEASE

- Patients with known coronary artery disease can reduce their risk of coronary events by maintaining high fitness levels.
- Exercise has been shown to decrease cardiovascular mortality and all-cause mortality (29).
- Patients with CAD who develop fitness to achieve a 10.7 MET level workload have a normal age-adjusted mortality rate.
- Exercise increases myocardial oxygen demand (thereby stimulating increased coronary flow), improves endothelial and coronary smooth muscle function, improves coronary vasodilation, stimulates collateralization (vital for ischemic myocardium), and slows progression of atherosclerosis and restenosis (30).
- High-intensity activities result in higher contractility and reduced diastolic filling times (31). More studies are needed to elucidate the benefit and risk profiles of high-intensity exercise activities for CAD patients, particularly with respect to the degree of CAD and the existence of other comorbidities.
- Research suggests that exercise lowers C-reactive protein (CRP) levels. Athletes such as swimmers and runners have significantly lower CRP levels than the average individual. The more intensely they train, the greater the decline in their CRP level. Speculation centers as to whether this may be one of the mechanisms by which exercise lowers the risk of cardiovascular disease.
- Ideal exercise routines achieve the following: avoidance of high afterload, favorable effects on heart rate variability (HRV), improved endurance, and involvement of multiple muscle groups. Aerobic exercise and resistance training generally favor HRV (31).
- High repetition, low load resistance (HRLL) regimens can mitigate risk of high afterload, promote favorable effects on heart rate (HR) and HRV, and promote significant increases in muscle strength and endurance. HRLL type regimens are those typically advised for CAD patients (31). There is an unclear role of low repetition, low-load regimens. The type of resistance training (*e.g.*, high intensity, eccentric, etc.) might be a factor (30).

- Exercise prescriptions are under-utilized in CAD patients. It is estimated that only 20%–30% of eligible patients receive referrals for cardiac rehabilitation (30).
- The individual's exercise capacity should be measured by exercise tolerance testing (32).
- A mix of aerobic exercises and resistance exercises is generally advised (29). The American Heart Association and the American College of Cardiology recommend 30 minutes of moderate-intensity aerobic exercise per day, 5–7 d · wk^{-1}. Resistance training can supplement these exercises 2 d · wk^{-1} (32).
- CAD-related absolute contraindications to exercise and exercise tolerance testing include acute myocardial infarction (within 2 days) and ongoing unstable angina. Obstructive left main coronary artery stenosis is a relative contraindication (33).
- As CAD becomes more advanced (*e.g.*, 70% or greater stenosis) chronic compensatory coronary vasodilation sets in. This causes functional impairments in coronary blood flow (30). More studies of this patient population are needed to foster consensus on exercise prescription recommendations for advanced CAD.
- High-risk patients (*e.g.*, those with recent acute coronary syndrome or revascularization, or HF) should be medically supervised during exercise (32).
- See Chapter 31 Coronary Artery Disease and Table 31.5 for the latest recommendations from the American Heart Association and American College of Cardiology for athletes with coronary artery disease.

EXERCISE POST-CEREBROVASCULAR ACCIDENT

- Post-stroke patients often suffer from weakness, paralysis, sensory loss, and decreased overall exercise capacity. Less than 1 month after stroke, patients develop a significant compromise in exercise capacity.
- The oxygen cost of exercise in hemiplegic patients is up to 2 times that of controls. This can lead to inactivity and secondary deconditioning, atrophy, osteoporosis, and impaired leg circulation.
- Exercise trainability may be comparable to that of age-matched controls (34,35).
- The role and timing of exercise stress testing post stroke is controversial.
- During the immediate post-stroke period the role of exercise is limited by increased risk of recurrent stroke and secondary cardiac complications.
- A supervised exercise program for stroke survivors with multiple comorbidities is effective at improving fitness while potentially decreasing the risk of further disease and disability.
- Exercise becomes increasingly important beyond the first several months to increase aerobic capacity and sensorimotor function (35).
- Fewer than 50% of post-CVA patients reliably have their risk factors assessed, treated, or controlled. This can pose natural challenges to safe exercise prescription.
- Exercise is important in primary and secondary prevention of cardiovascular and stroke risk. A study of over 16,000 men found an inverse relationship between cardiovascular fitness and stroke mortality (36).
- Post-stroke patients who increased activities of daily living showed a significant increase in peak oxygen intake. In addition, post-stroke patients' training on treadmills showed significant improvements of VO_2max; gait; and overall functional mobility, balance, and muscular activity (37,38).
- A randomized controlled trial of 42 hemiparetic stroke survivors demonstrated that they could increase their fitness by a magnitude similar to healthy controls in similar programs. Aerobic training 3 times weekly for 10 weeks improved peak oxygen consumption, workload, submaximal blood pressure response, exercise time, and sensorimotor function (35).
- Another randomized controlled trial of 88 men with CAD and disability (2/3 were stroke victims) who completed a 6-month home exercise training program showed significant increases in peak left ventricular ejection fraction and HDL cholesterol and decreases in resting heart rate and total serum cholesterol (34).
- Aerobic conditioning can enhance glucose regulation, mobilization of fat stores, blood pressure, CRP, triacylglycerol (TG), total cholesterol (TC), low-density lipoprotein (LDL), and HDL.
- Six months of treadmill aerobic exercise allowed patients to perform activities of daily living at sub-maximal energy expenditure.
- Strength training can safely be used in most post-stroke rehabilitation to improve muscle strength and overall balance. Caution should be used in patients with uncontrolled hypertension as well as avoidance of lifting excessive weight and Valsalva.
- More data are needed regarding consensus exercise prescription after CVAs (29). A mix of aerobic exercises and resistance exercises is generally advised (37).
- Flexibility stretches 2–3 d · wk^{-1} can help prevent contractures and improve range of motion.
- Coordination and balance activities 2–3 days weekly can improve safety during performance of ADLs.
- Current recommendations regarding exercise are primarily based on individuals with mild to moderate stroke and at sub-acute to chronic phases of recovery (37):
    1. Aerobic Exercise — 3–5 days weekly; 20- to 40-minute session duration; moderate intensity; 12–13 on 20-point Rate of Perceived Exertion (RPE) scale; 40%–59% of heart rate reserve; can split sessions. Gradual progression with initial focus on duration or frequency before finally progressing intensity as tolerated.

2. Resistance Exercise — 2–3 days weekly. Start with major muscle groups and include 8–10 exercises of 1–3 sets with 10–15 repetitions per set, performed at 30%–50% of one-repetition maximum (1-RM) as tolerated.
3. Exercises can be performed seated if there are balance or fall concerns.
4. It is important to screen for cardiovascular risk factors. Vitals signs should be monitored.
5. Assess for psychological barriers (*e.g.*, low motivation, depression).

HEART FAILURE

- HF is a complex syndrome of cardiac (particularly left ventricular) dysfunction, which can be asymptomatic in its early stages. Previously associated primarily with decreased left ventricular ejection fraction (LVEF), diagnosis and management of HF has become more complex over the years amid increasing cognizance of HF with preserved ejection fraction (HFpEF), which commonly involves asymptomatic diastolic dysfunction (39).
- HF is a leading cause of morbidity and mortality associated with hospital admissions and high healthcare costs (39).
- Prevalence data are conflicting given evolving definitions of HF subtypes, lack of worldwide consensus echocardiogram criteria for diastolic dysfunction, and worldwide differences in data collection among healthcare and public health systems. Generally accepted prevalence is 2% for at-large adult population, with an increase to 5%–9% in adults aged 65 years or more (39).
- Consistent performance of physical activity is conducive to reducing symptoms, improving quality of life, reducing the risk of hospitalization due to HF, and reducing morbidity and mortality (40).
- Exercise antagonizes peripheral skeletal muscle wasting and promotes left ventricular reverse remodeling with cardiomegaly reduction and ejection fraction improvement in patients with heart failure with reduced ejection fraction (HFrEF) (29).
- Prospective randomized studies have shown aerobic endurance training interventions to be safe and effective in HFrEF (29).
- Endurance training reverses cardiac remodeling with reduced end-diastolic volume (EDV), improved systolic function, and improved diastolic function.
- Meta-analyses show significant improvement in exercise capacity, quality of life, and HF-related hospitalization.
- It is unclear whether this decreases all-cause mortality and cardiovascular mortality.
- HIIT can promote greater improvements in exercise capacity and quality of life without undesirable left ventricular (LV) remodeling effects (29).
- Exercise training exerts a lusitropic effect on left ventricular diastolic function in patients with preserved ejection fraction (HFpEF) (29).
- Evidence is greatest for aerobic exercise training in HF although a mix of aerobic and resistance exercise is generally advised for most patients.
- HF patients typically have impaired exercise capacity due to central and peripheral pathology. Hence, exercise regimens typically emphasize peripheral muscles while mitigating central cardiac stress.
- Physical frailty is considered an ominous prognostic indicator (40):
  1. This is characterized by reduced skeletal muscle mass, capillary density, oxidative capacity, and strength presumably mediated by multiple factors such as inflammation, reduced tissue perfusion, mitochondrial dysfunction, autonomic dysfunction, and deconditioning. Frailty is also associated with lower levels of testosterone and overexpression of negative growth factors such as myostatin.
  2. Data are lacking regarding the ideal exercise regimen for the frail and/or elderly.
- Patients with more advanced HF might be intolerant of longer exercise sessions. Multiple short sessions throughout the day, as opposed to one continuous session, are a viable alternative.
- More data are needed regarding consensus exercise prescriptions for certain cases of HF (*e.g.*, advanced HF) (29).

CHRONIC KIDNEY DISEASE

- Dehydration, hyperpyrexia, hyperkalemia, and rhabdomyolysis may all occur as a result of exercise. This may lead to renal damage, which can be permanent.
- Rhabdomyolysis, especially in untrained athletes, can lead to renal ischemia and nephrotoxins. This may result in permanent renal damage. Subsets of athletes such as those with sickle cell trait may have a higher risk of rhabdomyolysis and renal failure.
- Adequate hydration is important in minimizing muscle damage, promoting myoglobin elimination, and maintaining renal blood flow.
- Athletes reduce the risk of rhabdomyolysis and secondary renal failure through adequate fluid intake, avoidance of excessive heat stress, not exercising at the time of febrile illness, appropriate carbohydrate intake to avoid glycogen depletion, and exercising within the limits of their muscular tolerance.
- Chronic Kidney Disease (CKD) negatively affects skeletal muscle function including atrophy, weakness, fatigue, and abnormal mitochondria (41). Sarcopenia is common. Exercise in those with CKD has been shown to increase muscle mass and muscle endurance (42,43).

- Cardiovascular disease accounts for most deaths in patients with end-stage renal disease (ESRD).
- Exercise is generally safe for hemodialysis (HD) and predialysis patients. Limited data exist regarding the effects of exercise on the progression of CKD. Established benefits are linked to beneficial effects on comorbidities (*e.g.*, CAD, hypertension) (42).
- VO_2 peak (peak oxygen uptake) has been purported to strongly predict survival in ESRD patients. Patients with CKD have significantly reduced VO_2 peaks in comparison to age and gender matched controls. Moderate exercise (~60% VO_2 peak) for 10–20 minutes can produce modest improvements although CKD patients do not reach predicted VO_2 peak.
- Resistance training can increase muscle size and strength on a low-protein diet in patients with chronic renal insufficiency.
- Combined cardiovascular and resistance training helps improve cardiovascular function, strength, endurance, and muscle size. This exercise regimen produced greater increases in VO_2 peak likely via effects of resistance training on skeletal muscle function, which thereby improved VO_2 peak.
- Exercise has also been tied to favorable vascular effects and increased exercise capacity (43).
- Exercise can have positive effects on VO_2 peak, systolic blood pressure, diastolic blood pressure, muscle mass, muscle endurance, and exercise capacity (42,43).
- Physical activity has been tied to improvements in eGFR and to improved management of comorbidities such as hypertension and hyperlipidemia (44).
- Studies of exercise in CKD patients have heavily focused on ESRD. More studies are needed of the predialysis population.
- A mix of aerobic exercises and resistance exercises is generally advised (42).
- It is important to assess other cardiovascular risk factors when devising an exercise regimen for CKD patients.
- Most studies support performance of moderate-intensity exercise for at least 30 minutes, at least 3 days weekly (42). More studies are needed to refine recommended modes, frequency, and intensity of aerobic and resistance activities for CKD patients.
- Contraindications to exercise in CKD include systolic blood pressure of 200 mm Hg or more, diastolic pressure of 110 mm Hg or more, electrolyte abnormalities, recent myocardial infarction, or recent change in the electrocardiogram.

THYROID DISEASE

Hypothyroidism

- Hypothyroidism and subclinical hypothyroidism are associated with decreased exercise tolerance (45,46).
- Patients with autoimmune thyroiditis have worse perceived exercise tolerance than all other types of hypothyroidism (46).
- Patients often develop muscle weakness, cramps, and fatigue, which is worse in elderly patients (47).
- This exercise intolerance is due to increased systemic vascular resistance, which decreases blood flow to exercising muscles. This leads to reduced oxygen delivery and blood-borne substrate availability (47).
- Exercise appears to decrease vascular resistance and serum TSH levels during acute bouts of exercise (48).
- Aerobic exercise training programs can help improve health-related quality of life indicators for patients with subclinical hypothyroidism.
- Overtraining of nonelite female athletes does not appear to cause hypothyroidism.
- Replacement of thyroxin is the mainstay of treatment.
- Exercise is safe when adequate replacement is maintained.

Hyperthyroidism

- Hyperthyroidism is associated with decreased exercise tolerance.
- Higher blood lactate, depletion of glycogen, and relative hyperthermia may all contribute to decreased performance that is due to mitochondrial dysfunction (47).
- Patients with hyperthyroidism have an increased heart rate, blood volume, left ventricular stroke volume, ejection fraction, and cardiac output as well as decreased systemic vascular resistance at rest. They also have an overall increased preload and decreased afterload (47).
- When patients with hyperthyroidism exercise, they have an impaired inotropic and chronotropic response to incremental exercise leading to a plateau in exercise capacity (47).
- Patients with hyperthyroidism reach anaerobic threshold faster than controls. Although their heart rate is elevated at baseline, hyperthyroid individuals have a lower increase in heart rate from baseline to the anaerobic threshold compared to controls as well as an increased respiratory rate (49).
- β-blockers can be helpful in the treatment of hyperthyroidism but may have a negative effect on performance and are banned for specific sports under Olympic regulations.
- Exercise is safe after appropriate treatment and close supervision.

Osteoporosis

- Data from the NHANES survey from 2017 to 2018 indicated 19.6% of women and 4.4% of men over the age of 50 in the United States have osteoporosis. An additional 51.5% of women and 33.5% of men over age 50 have low bone mass.
- It is estimated that half of women and one in five men over age 50 will sustain an osteoporosis-related fracture (50).
- Exercise at an early age is important to develop adequate bone density. Multiple studies on young men and women have shown that both resistance and endurance exercise programs can lead to site-specific increases in bone mineral

density (BMD) (51). BMD is reported to be higher in athletic young adults than in their sedentary peers.

- A Cochrane review of exercise in postmenopausal women demonstrated exercise slightly improves BMD and reduces the risk of fracture.
  - Strength training decreases bone loss by 1.03% at the hip, whereas combinations of exercise types reduce bone loss in the lumbar spine by 3.2% compared to no exercise.
  - The risk of fracture was decreased by 4% in those who exercise (52).
- It is recommended that women with osteoporosis exercise 3–5 times a week at moderate to high intensity for 30–60 minutes a day. Exercise should comprise weight-bearing activities 3–5 times a week and resistance exercise 2–3 times a week (53).
- Performing different exercises leads to improvements in strength, flexibility, quality of life, balance, physical fitness, and a reduced risk of falls (54).
- Exercise goals for individuals with osteoporosis should include reducing pain, increasing mobility, improving muscle endurance, balance, and stability to improve quality of life and reduce the risk of falling.
- Exercise should not take the place of other treatments for osteoporosis if medically necessary. It should instead be a component of osteoporotic therapy.

EPILEPSY

- Patients with epilepsy exercise less than those without epilepsy. Reasons cited by patients include fear of having a seizure during exercise, fear of injury should they have a seizure, lack of interest, fatigue from medication, and, in some cases, having been told by a medical provider to avoid physical activity due to their seizure disorder. Education and improved medical control allow more patients with epilepsy to exercise and participate in sports.
- Studies have demonstrated either decreased or unchanged seizure frequency in patients who undergo an aerobic exercise program (55), but there is a lack of high-quality prospective research on the subject. Epileptic patients undergoing intense exercise have fewer epileptic discharges on electroencephalography during and after exercise (56).
- The mechanism through which exercise decreases seizures is incompletely understood but is likely multifactorial. Exercise has been shown to modulate brain metabolism, neurotrophins, and neurotransmitters (GABA, noradrenaline), which help mediate the inhibitory/excitatory balance of neurons. The increased mental alertness and attention during exercise has also been proposed to play a role in the reduction of seizure activity (57).
- Exercise helps reduce anxiety and depression and lead to improvements in quality of life (55). It also improves self-esteem and the overall sense of well-being in epileptics. In a population where isolation and depression are common, participation in exercise may improve self-worth and social integration.
- In a large cohort study of Swedish cross-country skiers, there was a 40%–50% decreased incidence of focal and unspecified epilepsy compared to the general population suggesting physical activity may prevent or delay the development of epilepsy (58).
- Regarding sports participation in patients with known epilepsy, a patient with uncontrolled epilepsy (seizure within the past year) should avoid the following activities: scuba diving, hang gliding, parachuting, skydiving, aviation, motor sports, riflery, and archery (59).
- Athletes with controlled epilepsy can generally participate in all sports (including contact and collision sports) when appropriate safety equipment is used (60).
- Water sports and swimming should be undertaken with supervision owing to the increased risk of submersion and drowning in people with epilepsy. Life vests should be worn when participating in water sports (61).
- Consensus does not exist for participation in many high-risk sports including boxing. The recommendation on whether to participate should be individualized based on several factors: type of seizure, timing of seizure occurrence, probability of seizure, athlete's willingness to accept risk, and the sport involved (60).

CEREBRAL PALSY

- In patients with cerebral palsy and other chronic neuromuscular syndromes, physical therapy has become a mainstay in treatment. The purpose of therapy is to enhance motor development and minimize the development of contractures. Emphasis is generally placed on range of motion, both passive and active. Neuromuscular electric stimulation has been added to improve mobility, control muscular movements, increase strength, and to decrease spasticity. Although there is some evidence for effectiveness of upper extremity training, more well-designed studies are needed on overall efficacy of physical therapy in this population (62).
- Several chronic health conditions are more prevalent in those with cerebral palsy including diabetes, hypertension, stroke, and arthritis.
- Physical activity counseling should be prioritized by healthcare professionals with the hopes of improving physical fitness safely and decreasing chronic disease risk factors (63).
- Concurrent with recommendations for all individuals, health professionals should encourage all patients with cerebral palsy to decrease sedentary behavior.
- There are no consensus guidelines on strength training and aerobic exercise for individuals with cerebral palsy.

- Strength training has been avoided in cerebral palsy owing to a theory that it can lead to increased spasticity in antagonist muscles; however, multiple studies have shown that strength training can improve motor skills and strength without decreased range of motion or increased spasticity. In addition, strength training may lessen the amount of bone loss that frequently occurs in less mobile patients with cerebral palsy (64).
- Many patients with cerebral palsy do not participate in aerobic activities. Several studies have demonstrated improvements in cardiorespiratory endurance through short-term aerobic training appropriate for the individual's motor function classification (65). This has also been shown to improve patients' social skills, behavioral and emotional problems, and overall sense of well-being.
- Caution must be used in planning an exercise program for patients with cerebral palsy. Patients must have sufficient motor skills to safely participate in an exercise program. Scoliosis, contractures, chronic arthritis, and risk of hip subluxation can limit a patient's physical ability. Likewise, patients often suffer from sensory defects, such as poor vision. Last, behavioral and emotional maladjustments can be present, so special accommodations may need to be made.

EXERCISE-INDUCED ASTHMA/ EXERCISE-INDUCED BRONCHOCONSTRICTION

- Exercise-induced asthma (EIA) describes those with persistent or chronic asthma who also get episodic bronchospasm with exercise.
- EIA is a misleading term, as exercise is not an independent risk factor for asthma, but a trigger of bronchoconstriction in patients with underlying asthma. Therefore exercise-induced bronchoconstriction (EIB) is a more accurate reflection of the underlying pathophysiology.
- EIB refers to the phenomenon of transient airway narrowing that occurs during or after physical exertion in patients who have bronchospasm with exercise with no history of asthma.
- EIB is defined as a decrease in lung function, usually greater than a 10% fall in forced expiratory volume in one second (FEV_1), occurring within 30 minutes after vigorous exercise, at a power output that elicits 85% or more of maximal O_2 consumption for 4–10-minute periods (66).
- The estimated prevalence of EIB varies from 5% to 20% in the general population. In comparison, up to 90% of patients with symptomatic asthma have some degree of EIB. EIB occurs in 10% of patients without known asthma or atopy.
- The prevalence of EIB appears to be higher among elite athletes and has been evaluated in a number of studies (66,67).
- In a study of athletes participating in the summer Beijing and Athens Olympic Games, the sports most frequently associated with a Therapeutic Use Exemption (TUE) for asthma were swimming, cycling, triathlon, pentathlon, and rowing, with prevalences of approximately 18%, 16%, 12%, 13%, 7%, respectively (67).
- In contrast, the prevalence of asthma among athletes in disciplines without endurance demands, such as gymnastics, fencing, and sailing, was less than 5% (67).
- In a separate study, positive eucapnic hyperventilation was noted in 39% of swimmers and 24% of winter sport athletes (68).
- Patients with EIB typically have initial bronchodilation during the first 6–8 minutes of exercise, followed by bronchoconstriction that peaks within 10–15 minutes and resolves within 60 minutes (69).
- In most patients with EIB, bronchoconstriction is followed by a refractory period, during which repeated exertion causes less bronchoconstriction. This refractory period is generally less than 4 hours. Inhibitory prostaglandins (particularly prostaglandin E2) released during the refractory period probably protect against repeated episodes of EIB.
- The diagnosis and management of EIA and EIB are detailed in Chapters 27 Exercise Induced Asthma Testing, and 42 Pulmonary.
- Exercise should be encouraged in patients with EIB with a focus on appropriate prevention and management. Be more aware in environments that put an athlete at greater risk (cold weather, chlorinated swimming pools for example). And recognize the potential need for TUEs and medications that may be banned for elite athletes.
- Systematic reviews have reached different opinions about the effect of vitamin C in reducing EIB possibly due to the small number of subjects and differing choices of outcome measurements (70). Overall, the data appear inconclusive.
- Lycopene supplements have not been shown to reduce EIB (69).
- All medications should be initiated, and their use monitored under the supervision of a physician.
- World Anti-doping Agency (WADA) has published guidelines for the diagnosis and management of asthma in athletes and a list of medications that require a TUE (71).
- The WADA lists β2-agonists on its prohibited medication list due to concerns about performance enhancement (71).
- However, inhaled albuterol (salbutamol), maximum dose 1600 μg/24 hours and 800 μg/12 hours, inhaled formoterol, maximum delivered dose 54 μg/24 hours, and inhaled salmeterol, maximum dose 200 μg/24 hours, are acceptable and do not need a TUE (71). Nebulized β2-agonists may reach levels above those permitted. Urinary levels of albuterol over 1000 ng/mL or formoterol over 40 ng/mL are in excess of therapeutic use to prevent EIB (71).
- In terms of potential effects on performance, a study of 16 athletes found that high-dose salbutamol (albuterol) 1600 $\mu g \cdot d^{-1}$ for 6 weeks did not increase strength, power, or endurance relative to placebo (72).

- Inhaled glucocorticoids are permitted by the WADA and do not need a TUE (WADA). Systemic glucocorticoids are prohibited in competition, and a TUE may need to be filed for use outside of competition (71).

CHRONIC LUNG DISEASE IN CHILDREN

Cystic Fibrosis

- Patients with cystic fibrosis often refrain from physical activity due to fatigue and shortness of breath, which are believed to be caused by deficits in skeletal muscle aerobic and anaerobic capacity, muscle strength deficits, and decreased pulmonary function (73).
- Short- and long-term studies suggest both aerobic and anaerobic training have a positive effect on exercise capacity, strength, and lung function (74).
- Strength and aerobic training both increase physical work capacity and patient strength.
- Decreased breathlessness allows greater mobility and participation with peers in social and sporting activities, improves confidence and self-esteem, and creates a greater pleasure in life for the individual patient.
- Limitations in exercise performance appear related to the extent of lung disease and compromised nutritional status.
- Exercise testing is recommended in those with cystic fibrosis to guide exercise prescription. Cycle ergometry with pulse oximetry and gas exchange measures utilizing the Godfrey protocol is the preferred method of testing (75).
- Oxygen therapy during exercise improves oxygenation but causes a mild hypercapnia, which may not be clinically significant. Patients can exercise longer while using oxygen (76).
- Exercise and physiotherapy programs have limited evidence suggesting that they may decrease intravenous antibiotic requirements and lower the risk for hospitalizations (77).
- A consensus of pediatric pulmonary specialists feels that exercise should be encouraged as part of the treatment of cystic fibrosis (77).
- Measurable changes in pulmonary function secondary to an exercise program are difficult to demonstrate (77).

Bronchopulmonary Dysplasia

- There is limited information suggesting that exercise programs may be able to improve exercise tolerance, exercise capacity, and flexibility in preterm children with bronchopulmonary dysplasia.
- Children with moderate to severe bronchopulmonary dysplasia born extremely premature tend to have expiratory flow limitation and an exaggerated ventilatory response limiting their exercise (78).

Bronchiectasis

- There is limited evidence of the benefits of inspiratory muscle training, which improved endurance exercise capacity and quality of life measured on chronic respiratory questionnaires.
- Therapeutic exercise programs have low to moderate evidence for stabilizing pulmonary function, improving quality of life, functional exercise capacity, cough-related quality of life, and psychological symptoms (79).
- Ventricular function is affected in bronchiectasis although the myocardial performance of patients is dependent on their pulmonary status (80).

CHRONIC OBSTRUCTIVE PULMONARY DISEASE IN ADULTS

- Exercise training and pulmonary rehabilitation should be considered for all patients with chronic obstructive pulmonary disease (COPD) who experience exercise intolerance despite optimal medical therapy (81).
- Before prescribing an exercise program, patients with COPD require careful evaluation to assess cardiac risk and exercise capacity.
- A combination of strength and endurance exercise probably reduces dyspnea most effectively (81–83).
- The three medical determinations that would preclude patients with COPD from exercising include cor pulmonale, resting hypercapnia and dyspnea at rest.
- Studies consistently demonstrate that peripheral muscles are weak in patients with COPD exhibiting effort-dependent strength scores that are 70%–80% of these measures in age-matched healthy subjects (84).
- In COPD patients, up to 40% of total oxygen intake during low-level exercise is devoted to the respiratory muscles, compared to 10%–15% in healthy persons.
- Exercise tolerance may improve following exercise training because of gains in aerobic fitness, peripheral muscle strength, enhanced mechanical skill, efficiency of exercise, improvements in respiratory muscle function, breathing pattern, and lung hyperinflation while decreasing anxiety, fear, and dyspnea associated with exercise (81,82).
- Pulmonary rehabilitation improves symptoms of dyspnea and health-related quality of life while decreasing the number of hospital days, hospital admissions, and other health care utilization (83).
- Increasing physical activity or maintaining a moderate to high level of regular physical activity at a low level of intensity can reduce the rate of hospitalizations for acute COPD exacerbations.
- Exercise training of the muscles of ambulation is highly recommended as a component of pulmonary rehabilitation.

- Both low- and high-intensity exercise training leads to clinical benefits for patients with COPD. Strength training also increases muscle strength and mass (85).
- Unsupported endurance training of the upper extremities is beneficial for patients with COPD although this type of exercise leads to faster fatigue (86).
- There is some evidence that fully active patients with COPD can see some reduction in their mortality risks, improve their heart rate responses, and increase their life expectancy (87).
- Endothelial function can improve in patients who have severe and very severe COPD with increased steps taken per day (88).
- Oxygen should be used during exercise in patients who develop severe exercise-induced hypoxemia but can also be used in patients without exercise-induced hypoxemia to improve endurance (89).
- Oxygen desaturation during exercise in patients with COPD conveys a higher risk of mortality (90).
- Exercise training has low evidence for improving fatigue symptoms in patients with COPD.
- Short-acting bronchodilators have little effect on exercise capacity whereas long-acting bronchodilators reduce dyspnea associated with moderate exercise intensity.

OSTEOARTHRITIS

- Patients with arthritis have substantially worse health-related quality of life than those without arthritis.
- The Centers for Disease Control and Prevention advocate physical activity for patients with arthritis recommending 150 minutes of moderate-intensity aerobic activity or 75 minutes of vigorous activity in addition to muscle-strengthening activities at least 2 $d \cdot wk^{-1}$ in all adults.
- A study has shown that those patients who do not meet the 150 minutes of moderate- to vigorous-intensity physical activity tend to have the following characteristics: women, older age, higher body mass index, nonwhites, depressive symptoms, not working who have frequent knee symptoms (91).
- There are limited high-quality studies that have reviewed long-term outcomes on exercise therapy and osteoarthritis.
- Systematic reviews of exercise for hip osteoarthritis are limited but suggest that exercise programs may reduce pain slightly but may not improve physical function.
- There is high-quality level of evidence that land-based exercise has short-term benefits for patients with osteoarthritis of the knee by reducing pain and improved physical function (92).
- Running and walking regularly, including at the elite and recreational levels up to the marathon distance, do not increase a patient's risk for developing knee osteoarthritis or risk of knee replacement surgery (93). However, obese males may hit a threshold of higher-level physical activity, which can lead to a possible increase in osteoarthritis.
- Running appears to reduce the risk for hip replacement surgery in part because runners, as opposed to walkers, tend to have a lower body mass index.
- More walking has been associated with fewer functional limitations, decreased stiffness, and less-reported pain in patients with knee osteoarthritis.
- There are some older studies that suggest intense, high-level physical activity could lead to an increased risk of knee and hip osteoarthritis. However, more recent studies suggest that strenuous exercise and high-level physical activity do not increase the risk of knee osteoarthritis (91,92).
- Patients with osteoarthritis of the knee benefit from both high- and low-intensity aerobic exercise training, which significantly improves their functional status, gait, pain, and aerobic capacity.
- A combination of aerobic and resistance training improved pain and function scores for patients with knee osteoarthritis (94).
- Both high- and low-resistance training improves muscle strength as well as self-reported measures of pain and physical function for knee osteoarthritis (95). Messier et al, however, reported in 2021 although that both high- and low-intensity strength training did not significantly reduce knee pain or knee joint compressive forces in his study (96).
- Concentric and eccentric resistance training improve activity-related osteoarthritis knee pain, but concentric resistance training more effectively decreased the severity of pain during ambulation and pain after walking.
- Strength training of the whole body appears to be more beneficial than limiting work to the muscles around the affected joint.
- Studies testing biomarkers associated with inflammation and cartilage turnover have low-level evidence suggesting that these biomarkers are not increased post exercise (97).
- Increased physical activity does not appear to increase knee cartilage loss and may even be protective for women based on MRI imaging studies.
- Moderate daily recreational or sport activities of any kind are not a consistent risk factor for clinical or radiological changes associated with knee or hip osteoarthritis (98).
- Aquatic exercises may have some beneficial short-term effects for patients with hip and/or knee osteoarthritis. Aquatic resistance training is beneficial for preventing stiffness although this was not found to be true in the long term (99).
- Swimmers do appear to have less knee osteoarthritis although compared to controls especially if the swimming exercise was started before 35 years of age (100). Regular swimming can decrease pain and stiffness, increase muscle strength, and improve functional capacity.

- The benefits of exercise therapy do not appear to be sustained in the long term (greater than 6 months) for knee and hip osteoarthritis unless the patient continues to exercise.
- Data from the Fitness Arthritis and Seniors Trial suggested that beneficial effects of exercise on functional capacity in osteoarthritis patients are independent of exercise type.
- High-impact activities that include running and jumping may be detrimental for established osteoarthritis of lower extremity joints if the osteoarthritis is more severe.

REFERENCES

1. Lee I, Shiroma E, Lobelo F, et al. Effect of physical inactivity on major non-communicable diseases worldwide: an analysis of burden of disease and life expectancy. *Lancet*. 2012;380(9838):219–29.
2. Toomey C, Whittaker J, Richmond S, Owoeye OB, Patton DA, Emery CA. Adiposity as a risk factor for sport injury in youth: a systematic review. *Clin J Sport Med*. 2022;32(4):418–26.
3. Finkelstein EA, Chen H, Prabhu M, Trogdon JG, Corso PS. The relationship between obesity and injuries among U.S. adults. *Am J Health Promot*. 2007;21(5):460–8.
4. Brellenthin AG, Lee DC, Bennie JA, Sui X, Blair SN. Resistance exercise, alone and in combination with aerobic exercise, and obesity in Dallas, Texas, US: a prospective cohort study. *PLoS Med*. 2021;18(6):e1003687.
5. Donnelly JE, Blair SN, Jakicic JM, et al. American College of Sports Medicine Position Stand. Appropriate physical activity intervention strategies for weight loss and prevention of weight regain for adults. *Med Sci Sports Exerc*. 2009;41(2):459–71.
6. Wilding JPH, Batterham RL, Calanna S, et al. Once-weekly semaglutide in adults with overweight or obesity. *N Engl J Med*. 2021 Mar 18;384(11):989–1002.
7. Shah SZA, Karam JA, Zeb A, et al. Movement is improvement: the therapeutic effects of exercise and general physical activity on glycemic control in patients with type 2 diabetes mellitus. A systematic review and meta-analysis of randomized controlled trials. *Diabetes Ther*. 2021;12(3):707–32.
8. Mannucci E, Bonifazi A, Monami M. Comparison between different types of exercise training in patients with type 2 diabetes mellitus: a systematic review and network metanalysis of randomized controlled trials. *Nutr Metab Cardiovasc Dis*. 2021;31(7):1985–92.
9. Lora-Pozo I, Lucena-Anton D, Salazar A, Galan-Mercant A, Moral-Munoz JA. Anthropometric, cardiopulmonary and metabolic benefits of the high-intensity interval training versus moderate, low-intensity or control for type 2 diabetes: systematic review and meta-analysis. *Int J Environ Res Public Health*. 2019;16(22):4524.
10. Jayedi A, Emadi A, Shab-Bidar S. Dose-dependent effect of supervised aerobic exercise on HbA1c in patients with type 2 diabetes: a meta-analysis of randomized controlled trials. *Sports Med*. 2022;52(8):1919–38.
11. Kanaley JA, Colberg SR, Corcoran MH, et al. Exercise/physical activity in individuals with type 2 diabetes: a consensus statement from the American College of Sports Medicine. *Med Sci Sports Exerc*. 2022 Feb 1;54(2):353–68.
12. Geidl W, Schlesinger S, Mino E, Miranda L, Pfeifer K. Dose-response relationship between physical activity and mortality in adults with noncommunicable diseases: a systematic review and meta-analysis of prospective observational studies. *Int J Behav Nutr Phys Act*. 2020; 17(1):109.
13. Gregg EW, Gerzoff RB, Caspersen CJ, Williamson DF, Narayan KM. Relationship of walking to mortality among US adults with diabetes. *Arch Intern Med*. 2003;163(12):1440–7.
14. Hu FB, Stampfer MJ, Solomon C, et al. Physical activity and risk for cardiovascular events in diabetic women. *Ann Intern Med*. 2001;134(2): 96–105.
15. Pan B, Ge L, Xun YQ, et al. Exercise training modalities in patients with type 2 diabetes mellitus: a systematic review and network meta-analysis. *Int J Behav Nutr Phys Act*. 2018 Jul 25;15(1):72.
16. Uusitupa M, Khan TA, Viguiliouk E, et al. Prevention of type 2 diabetes by lifestyle changes: a systematic review and meta-analysis. *Nutrients*. 2019;11(11):2611.
17. Colberg SR, Sigal RJ, Fernhall B, et al. Exercise and type 2 diabetes: the American college of Sports Medicine and the American Diabetes Association. Joint position statement. *Diabetes Care*. 2010 Dec;33(12): e147–67.
18. Morrison S, Colberg SR, Mariano M, Parson HK, Vinik AI. Balance training reduces falls risk in older individuals with type 2 diabetes. *Diabetes Care*. 2010 April 1;33(4):748–50.
19. Sardar MA, Boghrabadi V, Sohrabi M, Aminzadeh R, Jalalian M. The effects of aerobic exercise training on psychosocial aspects of men with type 2 diabetes mellitus. *Glob J Health Sci*. 2014 Jan 20;6(2):196–202.
20. Gu Y, Dennis SM, Kiernan MC, Harmer AR. Aerobic exercise training may improve nerve function in type 2 diabetes and pre-diabetes: a systematic review. *Diabetes Metab Res Rev*. 2019;35(2):e3099.
21. Katzmarzyk PT, Powell KE, Jakicic JM, et al. Sedentary behavior and health: update from the 2018 Physical Activity Guidelines Advisory Committee. *Med Sci Sports Exerc*. 2019;51(6):1227–41.
22. Yardley JE, Kenny GP, Perkins BA, et al. Resistance versus aerobic exercise: acute effects on glycemia in type 1 diabetes. *Diabetes Care*. 2013 March 1;36(3):537–42.
23. Yardley JE, Kenny GP, Perkins BA, et al. Effects of performing resistance exercise before versus after aerobic exercise on glycemia in type 1 diabetes. *Diabetes Care*. 1 April 2012;35(4):669–75.
24. Abdulrahman A, Manhas J, Linane H, et al. Use of continuous glucose monitoring for sport in type 1 diabetes. *BMJ Open Sport Exerc Med*. 2018;4(1):e000432.
25. Clarke SL. Hypertension in adults: initial evaluation and management. *Am Fam Physician*. 2023 Oct;108(4):352–9.
26. Whelton SP, Chin A, Xin X, He J. Effect of aerobic exercise on blood pressure: a meta-analysis of randomized, controlled trials. *Ann Intern Med*. 2002;136(7):493–503.
27. Pescatello L, Franklin B, Fagard R, et al. American College of Sports Medicine position stand. Exercise and hypertension. *Med Sci Sports Exer*. 2004;36(3):533–53.
28. Paulo AC, Forjaz CLM, Mion D Jr, Silva GV, Barros S, Tricoli V. Blood pressure increase in hypertensive individuals during resistance training protocols with equated work to rest ratio. *Front Physiol*. 2020;11:481.
29. Gielen S, Laughlin MH, O'Conner C, Duncker DJ. Exercise training in patients with heart disease: review of beneficial effects and clinical recommendations. *Prog Cardiovasc Dis*. 2015;57(4):347–55.
30. Bruning RS, Sturek M. Benefits of exercise training on coronary blood flow in coronary artery disease patients. *Prog Cardiovasc Dis*. 2015;57(5):443–53.
31. Caruso FR, Arena R, Phillips SA, et al. Resistance exercise training improves heart rate variability and muscle performance: a randomized controlled trial in coronary artery disease patients. *Eur J Phys Rehabil Med*. 2015;51(3):281–9.
32. Smith SC Jr, Benjamin EJ, Bonow RO, et al. AHA/ACCF secondary prevention and risk reduction therapy for patients with coronary and

other atherosclerotic vascular disease. 2011 update: a guideline from the American Heart Association and American College of Cardiology Foundation. *Circulation*. 2011;124(22):2458–73.

33. Fletcher GF, Ades PA, Kligfield P, et al. Exercise standards for testing and training: a scientific statement from the American Heart Association. *Circulation*. 2013;128(8):873–934.
34. Fletcher BJ, Dunbar SB, Felner JM, et al. Exercise testing and training in physically disabled men with clinical evidence of coronary artery disease. *Am J Cardiol*. 1994;73(2):170–4.
35. Potempa K, Lopez M, Braun LT, Szidon JP, Fogg L, Tincknell T. Physiological outcomes of aerobic exercise training in hemiparetic stroke patients. *Stroke*. 1995;26(1):101–5.
36. Lee CD, Blair SN. Cardiorespiratory fitness and stroke mortality in men. *Med Sci Sports Exerc*. 2002;34(4):592–5.
37. Kim Y, Lai B, Mehta T, et al. Exercise training guidelines for multiple sclerosis, stroke, and Parkinson disease: rapid review and synthesis. *Am J Phys Med Rehabil*. 2019;98(7):613–21.
38. Ali A, Tabassum D, Baig SS, et al. Effect of exercise interventions on health-related quality of life after stroke and transient ischemic attack: a systematic review and meta-analysis. *Stroke*. 2021;52(7): 2445–55.
39. Van Riet EE, Hoes AW, Wagenaar KP, Limburg A, Landman MAJ, Rutten FH. Epidemiology of heart failure. The prevalence of heart failure and ventricular dysfunction in older adults over time: a systematic review. *Eur J Heart Fail*. 2016;18(3):242–52.
40. Laddu DR, Ozemek C, Sabbahi A, Severin R, Phillips SA, Arena R. Prioritizing movement to address the frailty phenotype in heart failure. *Prog Cardiovasc Dis*. 2021;67:26–32.
41. Thome T, Kumar RA, Burke SK, et al. Impaired muscle mitochondrial energetics is associated with uremic metabolite accumulation in chronic kidney disease. *JCI Insight*. 2020 Dec 8;6(1):e139826.
42. Gould DW, Graham-Brown MP, Watson EL, Viana JL, Smith AC. Physiological benefits of exercise in pre-dialysis chronic kidney disease. *Nephrology*. 2014;19(9):519–27.
43. Van Craenenbroeck AH, Van Craenenbroeck EM, Kouidi E, Vrints CJ, Couttenye MM, Conraads VM. Vascular effects of exercise training in CKD: current evidence and pathophysiological mechanisms. *Clin J Am Soc Nephrol*. 2014;9(7):1305–18.
44. Zhang L, Wang Y, Xiong L, Luo Y, Huang Z, Yi B. Exercise therapy improves eGFR, and reduces blood pressure and BMI in non-dialysis CKD patients: evidence from a meta-analysis. *BMC Nephrol*. 2019;20(1):398.
45. Lankhaar JAC, de Vries WR, Jansen JA, Zelissen PMJ, Backx FJG. Impact of overt and subclinical hypothyroidism on exercise tolerance: a systematic review. *Res Q Exerc Sport*. 2014;85(3):365–89.
46. Lankhaar JAC, Kemler E, Hofstetter H, et al. Physical activity, sports participation and exercise-related constraints in adult women with primary hypothyroidism treated with thyroid hormone replacement therapy. *J Sports Sci*. 2021;39(21):2493–502.
47. Kahaly G, Kampmann C, Mohr-Kahaly S. Cardiovascular hemodynamics and exercise tolerance in thyroid disease. *Thyroid*. 2002;12(6): 473–81.
48. Masaki M, Koide K, Goda A, Miyazaki A, Masuyama T, Koshiba M. Effect of acute aerobic exercise on arterial stiffness and thyroid-stimulating hormone in subclinical hypothyroidism. *Heart Vessels*. 2019;34(8):1309–16.
49. Kahaly G, Hellermann J, Mohr-Kahaly S, Treese N. Impaired cardiopulmonary exercise capacity in patients with hyperthyroidism. *Chest*. 1996;109(1):57–61.
50. Coughlan T, Dockery F. Osteoporosis and fracture risk in older people. *Clin Med*. 2014 Apr;14(2):187–91.
51. Friedlander AL, Genant HK, Sadowsky S, Byl NN, Glüer CC. A two-year program of aerobics and weight training enhances bone mineral density of young women. *J Bone Miner Res*. 1995;10(4):574–85.
52. Howe TE, Shea B, Dawson LJ, et al. Exercise for preventing and treating osteoporosis in postmenopausal women. *Cochrane Database Syst Rev*. 2011;7:CD000333.
53. Kohrt WM, Bloomfield SA, Little KD, Nelson ME, Yingling VR, American College of Sports Medicine. American college of sports medicine position stand: physical activity and bone health. *Med Sci Sports Exerc*. 2004;36(11):1985–96.
54. Linhares DG, Borba-Pinheiro CJ, Castro JBP, et al. Effects of multicomponent exercise training on the health of older women with osteoporosis: a systematic review and meta-analysis. *Int J Environ Res Public Health*. 2022;19(21):14195.
55. Arida RM, Scorza FA, Gomes S, et al. The potential role of physical exercise in the treatment of Epilepsy. *Epilepsy Behav*. 2010;17(4):432–5.
56. Vancini RL, de Lira CAB, Scorza FA, et al. Cardiorespiratory and electroencephalographic responses to exhaustive acute physical exercise in people with temporal lobe epilepsy. *Epilepsy Behav*. 2010;19(3):504–8.
57. Arida RM. Physical Exercise and seizure activity. *Biochim Biophys Acta Mol Basis Dis*. 2021 Jan 1;1867(1):165979.
58. Ahl M, Avdic U, Strandberg MC, et al. Physical activity reduces epilepsy incidence: a retrospective cohort study in Swedish cross-country skiers and an experimental study in seizure-prone synapsin II knockout mice. *Sports Med Open*. 2019 Dec 16;5(1):52.
59. Pimentel J, Tojal R, Morgado J. Epilepsy and physical exercise. *Seizure*. 2015;25:87–94.
60. Capovilla G, Kaufman KR, Perucca E, Moshe SL, Arida RM. Epilepsy, seizures, physical exercise, and sports: a report from the ILAE Task Force on Sports and Epilepsy. *Epilepsia*. 2016;57(1):6–12.
61. Arida RM, Cavalheiro EA, da Silva AC, Scorza FA. Physical activity and epilepsy: proven and predicted benefits. *Sports Med*. 2008;38(7):607–15.
62. Anttila H, Autti-Rämö I, Suoranta J, Mäkelä M, Malmivaara A. Effectiveness of physical therapy interventions for children with cerebral palsy: a systematic review. *BMC Pediatr*. 2008 Apr 24;8:14.
63. Verschuren O, Peterson MD, Balemans ACJ, Hurvitz EA. Exercise and physical activity recommendations for people with cerebral palsy. *Dev Med Child Neurol*. 2016;58(8):798–808.
64. Dodd KJ, Taylor NF, Damiano DL. A systematic review of the effectiveness of strength-training programs for people with cerebral palsy. *Arch Phys Med Rehabil*. 2002;83(8):1157–64.
65. Slaman J, Roebroeck M, van der Slot W, et al. Can a lifestyle intervention improve physical fitness in adolescents and young adults with spastic cerebral palsy? A randomized controlled trial. *Arch Phys Med Rehabil*. 2014;95(9):1646–55.
66. Pope JS, Koenig SM. Pulmonary disorders in the training room. *Clin Sports Med*. 2005;24(3):541–64.
67. Mountjoy M, Fitch K, Boulet LP, Bougault V, van Mechelen W, Verhagen E. Prevalence and characteristics of asthma in the aquatic disciplines. *J Allergy Clin Immunol*. 2015;136(3):588–94.
68. Bougault V, Turmel J, Boulet LP. Bronchial challenges and respiratory symptoms in elite swimmers and winter sport athletes. Airway hyperresponsiveness in asthma: its measurement and clinical significance. *Chest*. 2010;138(2 suppl l):31S–7S.
69. Parsons JP, Hallstrand TS, Mastronarde JG, et al. An official American Thoracic Society clinical practice guideline: exercise-induced bronchoconstriction. *Am J Respir Crit Care Med*. 2013;187(9):1016–27.
70. Milan SJ, Hart A, Wilkinson M. Vitamin C for asthma and exercise-induced bronchoconstriction. *Cochrane Database Syst Rev*. 2013 Oct 23;2013(10):CD010391.

71. World Anti-Doping Agency. *Therapeutic Use Exemption Physician Guidelines: Asthma* [Internet]. [cited 2022 Dec 10]. Available from: https://www.wada-ama.org/sites/default/files/resources/files/tuec_asthma_version6.1.pdf
72. Dickinson J, Molphy J, Chester N, Loosemore M, Whyte G. The ergogenic effect of long-term use of high dose salbutamol. *Clin J Sport Med.* 2014;24(6):474–81.
73. Shoemaker MJ, Hurt H, Arndt L. The evidence regarding exercise training in the management of cystic fibrosis: a systematic review. *Cardiopulm Phys Ther J.* 2008;19(3):75–83.
74. Radtke T, Smith S, Nevitt SJ, Hebestreit H, Kriemler S. Physical activity and exercise training in cystic fibrosis. *Cochrane Database Syst Rev.* 2022;8(8):CD002768.
75. Hebestreit H, Arets HG, Aurora P, et al. Statement on exercise testing in cystic fibrosis. *Respiration.* 2015;90(4):332–351.
76. Elphick HE, Mallory G. Oxygen therapy for cystic fibrosis. *Cochrane Database Syst Rev.* 2009;1:CD003884.
77. Pérez M, Groeneveld IF, Santana-Sosa E, et al. Aerobic fitness is associated with lower risk of hospitalization in children with cystic fibrosis. *Pediatr Pulmonol.* 2014;49(7):641–9.
78. MacLean JE, DeHaan K, Fuhr D, et al. Altered breathing mechanics and ventilatory response during exercise in children born extremely preterm. *Thorax.* 2016;71(11):1012–19.
79. Lee AL, Gordon CS, Osadnik CR. Exercise training for bronchiectasis. *Cochrane Database Syst Rev.* 2021;4(4):CD013110.
80. Gencer M, Ceylan E, Yilmaz R, Gur M. Impact of bronchiectasis on right and left ventricular functions. *Respir Med.* 2006 Nov;100(11):1933–43.
81. Bourjeily G, Rochester CL. Exercise training in chronic obstructive pulmonary disease. *Clin Chest Med.* 2000;21(4):763–81.
82. Li N, Li P, Lu Y, et al. Effects of resistance training on exercise capacity in elderly patients with chronic obstructive pulmonary disease: a meta-analysis and systematic review. *Aging Clin Exp Res.* 2020;32(10):1911–22.
83. Puhan MA, Gimeno-Santos E, Scharplatz M, et al. Pulmonary rehabilitation following exacerbations of chronic obstructive pulmonary disease. *Cochrane Database Syst Rev.* 2010;11:CD005305.
84. Frazão M, Santos ADC, Araújo AA, et al. Neuromuscular efficiency is impaired during exercise in COPD patients. *Respir Physiol Neurobiol.* 2021;290:103673.
85. Liao WH, Chen JW, Chen X, et al. Impact of resistance training in subjects with COPD: a systematic review and meta-analysis. *Respir Care.* 2015;60(8):1130–45.
86. Yekefallah L, Zohal MA, Keshavarzsarkar O, Barikani A, Gheraati M. Comparing the effects of upper limb and breathing exercises on six-minute walking distance among patients with chronic obstructive pulmonary disease: a three-group randomized controlled clinical trial. *Adv Respir Med.* 2019;87(2):77–82.
87. Shu CC, Lee JH, Tsai MK, Su TC, Wen CP. The ability of physical activity in reducing mortality risks and cardiovascular loading and in extending life expectancy in patients with COPD. *Sci Rep.* 2021;11(1):21674.
88. Kohlbrenner D, Clarenbach CF, Thiel S, Roeder M, Kohler M, Sievi NA. A few more steps lead to improvements in endothelial function in severe and very severe COPD. *Respir Med.* 2021;176:106246.
89. Vitacca M, Paneroni M, Zampogna E, et al. High-flow oxygen therapy during exercise training in patients with chronic obstructive pulmonary disease and chronic hypoxemia: a multicenter randomized controlled trial. *Phys Ther.* 2020;100(8):1249–59.
90. Kim C, Ko Y, Lee JS, et al. Predicting long-term mortality with two different criteria of exercise-induced desaturation in COPD. *Respir Med.* 2021;182:106393.
91. Chang AH, Song J, Lee J, Chang RW, Semanik PA, Dunlop DD. Proportion and associated factors of meeting the 2018 Physical Activity Guidelines for Americans in adults with or at risk for knee osteoarthritis. *Osteoarthr Cartil.* 2020;28(6):774–81.
92. Skou ST, Bricca A, Roos EM. The impact of physical activity level on the short- and long-term pain relief from supervised exercise therapy and education: a study of 12,796 Danish patients with knee osteoarthritis. *Osteoarthr Cartil.* 2018;26(11):1474–8.
93. Lo GH, Musa SM, Driban JB, et al. Running does not increase symptoms or structural progression in people with knee osteoarthritis: data from the osteoarthritis initiative. *Clin Rheumatol.* 2018;37(9):2497–504.
94. Kabiri S, Halabchi F, Angoorani H, Yekaninejad S. Comparison of three modes of aerobic exercise combined with resistance training on the pain and function of patients with knee osteoarthritis: a randomized controlled trial. *Phys Ther Sport.* 2018;32:22–8.
95. Peeler J, Leiter J, MacDonald P. Effect of body weight-supported exercise on symptoms of knee osteoarthritis: a follow-up investigation. *Clin J Sport Med.* 2020;30(6):e178–85.
96. Messier SP, Mihalko SL, Beavers DP, et al. Effect of high-intensity strength training on knee pain and knee joint compressive forces among adults with knee osteoarthritis: the START randomized clinical trial. *JAMA.* 2021;325(7):646–57.
97. Bricca A, Struglics A, Larsson S, Steultjens M, Juhl CB, Roos EM. Impact of exercise therapy on molecular biomarkers related to cartilage and inflammation in individuals at risk of, or with established, knee osteoarthritis: a systematic review and meta-analysis of randomized controlled trials. *Arthritis Care Res.* 2019;71(11):1504–15.
98. Lefèvre-Colau MM, Nguyen C, Haddad R, et al. Is physical activity, practiced as recommended for health benefit, a risk factor for osteoarthritis? *Ann Phys Rehabil Med.* 2016;59(3):196–206.
99. Munukka M, Waller B, Häkkinen A, et al. Effects of progressive aquatic resistance training on symptoms and quality of life in women with knee osteoarthritis: a secondary analysis. *Scand J Med Sci Sports.* 2020;30(6):1064–72.
100. Lo GH, Ikpeama UE, Driban JB, et al. Evidence that swimming may be protective of knee osteoarthritis: data from the osteoarthritis initiative. *PM R.* 2020;12(6):529–37.

Environmental Injuries: Hypothermia, Frostbite, Heat Illness, and Altitude Illness

47

Blair B. Rhodehouse and Micah K. Watson

INTRODUCTION

- Participation in sporting activities can expose athletes to a wide range of environmental conditions during training or competitive events. Health care providers need to promptly identify and respond to medical conditions associated with environmental exposures as injuries can be severe, even catastrophic. Early recognition and treatment of environmental injuries can be lifesaving; however, proper preparation and prevention is equally, if not more, important. In this chapter we address four of the most common environmental injuries including hypothermia, frostbite, heat illness, and altitude illness. The focus of each topic will address the basics of pathophysiology, clinical presentation, treatment, and prevention.

HYPOTHERMIA

Definition

- Hypothermia occurs when an individual's core body temperature decreases below 35 °C (95 °F) and can be further divided into mild (32–35 °C [90–95 °F]), moderate (28–32 °C [82–90 °F]), and severe (<28 °F [<82 °F]) (1,2).

Epidemiology

- Populations and individuals at increased risk include:
  - Prolonged exposure to inclement environments (homeless, hikers, hunters, adventure sport enthusiasts).
  - Individuals younger than 2 years of age because of their increased surface-to-volume ratio.
  - Adults older than 60 years of age due to blunted thermoregulatory responses secondary to underlying medical conditions, medications, and decreasing muscle and subcutaneous fat mass.
  - History of psychiatric illnesses (*i.e.*, schizophrenia, epilepsy and seizure disorders, psychosis), use of intoxicants (alcohol, opioids, sedative hypnotics, barbiturates, etc.), medical illnesses, sleep deprivation, dehydration, malnutrition, and trauma. Impaired judgment resulting from psychiatric illness, or the use of ethanol, is the most common predisposing factor (1).

Pathophysiology

- The human body tightly regulates core body control in the "thermoneutral zone" (36.5 °C/97.7 °F to 37.5 °C/99.5 °F) by balancing heat-producing and heat-reducing mechanisms.
- The body combats the fall in core temperature through several mechanisms including increased metabolic rate, blood pressure, and preshivering muscle tone with maximum shivering at 95 °F.
  - When the core temperature drops below 35 °C (95.0 °F), individuals become poikilothermic and cool to the ambient temperature as the body can no longer maintain thermal homeostasis.
- Central nervous system (CNS) function is directly depressed by the cold. The electroencephalogram becomes abnormal below at temperatures of 33.5 °C (92.5 °F) and silent at 19 °C (66 °F) (2).
- Initial reflex tachypnea continues until core temperature falls below 30 °C (86 °F). Failure of brainstem control of respiratory drive and the freezing of the thoracic musculature eventually lead to a cessation of breathing.
- Cold triggers peripheral vasoconstriction and tachycardia.
- Below 34 °C (93 °F), bradycardia, hypotension, decreased cardiac output, and a lengthening of cardiac electrical conduction ensue. A J-wave (Osborn hypothermic hump) may be noted at the QRS-ST junction. The myocardium becomes increasingly irritable, and spontaneous atrial and ventricular dysrhythmias can occur (2).
- Below 28 °C (82 °F), ventricular fibrillation can develop with minor stimuli, such as removing a patient's wet clothing or ambulance transport.

Clinical Features

- Nonspecific symptoms and signs predominate and mimic the effects of mild dementia, ethanol intoxication, hypoglycemia, and diabetic ketoacidosis/hyperosmolar hyperglycemic state.
  - The CNS effects of hypothermia lead to progressive cerebral impairments beginning with executive dysfunctions (*i.e.*, planning, organizing, emotional regulation, memory, perception, and speech) and ending with global cessation of neural activity.
  - Initial hypertension, tachycardia, and tachypnea diminish with increasing hypothermia leading to decreased perfusion and oxygenation compounding CNS impairments. Moderate to severe hypothermia increases myocardium irritability and predisposition for dysrhythmias, specifically ventricular fibrillation.
  - A cold-induced ileus, abdominal spasm, and rigidity can mimic an acute abdomen.

Diagnosis

- An accurate core temperature is crucial and is ideally obtained with a rectal thermistor probe. At a minimum, a rectal temperature obtained with a thermometer scaled for hypothermia is required. Oral and ear temperatures are grossly inaccurate. A core temperature above 35 °C (95.0 °F) can rapidly exclude hypothermia.
- Hypothermia is classified as mild, moderate, or severe based on the core temperature (Table 47.1).
- Common laboratory findings include a falsely elevated hematocrit caused by dehydration, a low leukocyte count caused by sequestration, hyperamylasemia resulting from pancreatic injury, an aberrant coagulation profile, hypokalemia, and hypoglycemia caused by glycogen depletion. Below 30 °C (86.0 °F), insulin is rendered inactive, and a paradoxical hyperglycemia can ensue.

Table 47.1 Hypothermia Severity and Treatment

Temperature	Clinical Features	Treatment
Mild		
35 °C/95 °F	Maximum shivering	Passive external rewarming
33 °C/91 °F	Ataxia, apathy, tachypnea	Passive external rewarming
Moderate		
32 °C/90 °F	Stupor, shivering stops	Active core rewarming (± active external rewarming)
Severe		
28 °C/82 °F	Decreased ventricular fibrillation threshold, hypoventilation	Active core rewarming
14 °C/57 °F	Lowest adult accidental hypothermia survival	Active core rewarming
9 °C/48 °F	Lowest therapeutic survival	Active core rewarming

Treatment

- Field treatment should focus on *gentle handling* of the victim, to prevent cardiac dysrhythmias. Wet clothing should be removed and dry clothing or a blanket applied. Massage of cold-injured limbs should be avoided; it can damage fragile, frozen parts and trigger dysrhythmias. Traumatic injuries to the spine or limbs should be stabilized (2).
- An airway should be maintained, and cardiac monitoring begun, **if available.** When assessing pulse, check a carotid pulse for at least 1 min as patients will be bradycardic and hypotensive. When assessing for respiration, watch for chest movement and listen for breath sounds for at least 30 seconds as patients will have bradypnea. When attaching electrode pads for cardiac monitoring, note if the skin is frozen as this can impair adhesive properties of pads. If this occurs, needle electrodes should be used or can be fashioned by passing a 20-gauge needle through an electrode pad into the frozen skin. If the patient is alert and warm, noncaffeinated beverages can be provided. Fluid resuscitation with intravenous (IV) 5% dextrose in normal saline (D5NS) should be started. Avoid use of lactated ringers in hypothermic patients due cold-induced stress or injury of the liver, which impairs its ability to metabolize lactate. Emergency room treatment should focus on rewarming the patient. Follow basic life support (BLS) and advanced life support (ALS) guidelines apart from prolonged checking of pulses (carotid recommended) and respiration as stated earlier.
  - In patients identified to have absence of a nonperfusing rhythm, follow traditional BLS and ALS management. The hypothermic heart may be unresponsive to cardiovascular drugs, pacemaker stimulation, and defibrillation; however, the data to support this are essentially theoretical. If shockable rhythm persists after a single shock, the value of deferring subsequent defibrillations until a target temperature is achieved is uncertain. There is no evidence to suggest a benefit from deviating from standard BLS protocol for defibrillation (Class IIB, level of evidence [LOE] C, Emergency Cardiovascular Care Guidelines of the American Heart Association [AHA], 2020) (3).
- Medications may be less effective with severe hypothermia, but it is not unreasonable to consider use of vasopressors according to standard ACLS algorithms (Class IIb, LOE C, AHA ACLS guidelines, 2020) (3).
- Passive external rewarming by covering the victim with a blanket or wrap is ideal in an alert patient whose core temperature is greater than 32 °C (90 °F).
- Below 90 °F, rewarming should proceed with active core rewarming (ACR) concurrent with active external rewarming (AER). ACR can be accomplished with IV D5NS warmed to 40–42 °C (104–108 °F) or the inhalation of humidified

oxygen warmed to 104–108 °F. More invasive techniques include peritoneal lavage with dialysate warmed to 104–108 °F, thoracic lavage with normal saline at 104–108 °F, or warming of the gastrointestinal tract with gastric/colonic lavage (LOE C).

- AER (fires, hot water bottles, and heating pads) should be employed when ACR has already begun to avoid the life-threatening risk of core temperature afterdrop. This devastating process occurs when sudden exposure of vasoconstricted cool extremities to AER causes peripheral vasodilatation, a drop in central blood pressure, and a sudden influx of cool blood from the periphery to the core that can trigger dysrhythmias and shock (2). Table 47.1 provides an overview of hypothermia severity and ideal treatment modalities (2).

Prevention

- Good conditioning, proper nutrition, experienced leadership in backcountry environments, normal hydration, avoidance of ethanol or tobacco, and habituation to the cold environment (both physiologic and behavioral), along with the use of proper clothing help prevent hypothermia (4).
- Clothing choice centers on the 3 Ls: layered, loose, and lightweight. A waterproof outer layer is key. If exercise is occurring in a temperature of <0 °F, three-layered hand and footwear are optimal for the prevention of frostbite.

FROSTBITE

Definition

- Frostbite is a cold-related injury that leads to cellular ischemia due to vasospasms and small vessel thromboses as a result of tissue freezing. Frostnip is a reversible cold-related injury with no permanent *tissue damage*. Chilblains is an *autoimmune* lymphocytic vasculitis, common in women, which leads to localized nodules or ulcers on the extremities 12 hours after cold exposure (5).

Epidemiology

- Frostbite is most common in active individuals from 30–49 years of age. High-risk outdoor activities in inclement environments account for a large percentage of injuries.
- Risk factors for frostbite are shown in Table 47.2. Ethanol and psychiatric problems underlie up to 70% of frostbite cases. The need for amputation correlates more with the *duration* of cold exposure rather than how low the temperature. This explains why impaired judgment from ethanol use and psychiatric illness account for such a large percentage of injuries (5,6).
- Anatomic sites of injury include the following, in order of most common occurrence: feet and hands (90% of all frostbite), ears, nose, cheeks, and the penis (a particular concern for runners).

Table 47.2 Risk Factors for Frostbite

Predisposing Factors	
Behavioral	**Organic**
Ethanol use	Prior cold injury
Psychiatric illness	Wound infection
Motor vehicle problems	Atherosclerosis
Homelessness	Diabetes mellitus
Smoking	Fatigue
Improper clothing	
High-risk outdoor activities (back-country skiing/ mountaineering)	

Pathophysiology

- There are three synchronous pathways that lead to tissue damage in frostbite: tissue freezing, hypoxia, and the release of inflammatory mediators. Each pathway multiplies and catalyzes the damage caused by the other pathways. Freezing leads to denaturation of the membrane lipid-protein matrix and cellular disruption. Hypoxia occurs from cold-induced vasoconstriction that triggers acidosis, increased viscosity, microthrombosis, and vessel endothelial damage. Inflammatory mediators (prostaglandin $F_2\alpha$, thromboxane A_2) are released from damaged endothelium, which triggers more vasoconstriction, platelet aggregation, thrombosis, hypoxia, and cell death. The same prostaglandins are found in the blister fluid of heat- and frostbite-damaged skin (7–9).
- The release of these prostaglandins peaks during rewarming; *therefore, cycles of recurrent freezing and rewarming must be avoided to lessen the extent of injury* (7–9).

Clinical Features

- Symptoms include numbness, clumsiness, tingling, and throbbing pain after rewarming.
- The signs of frostbite were classically divided into first through fourth degrees; however, this scheme can be simplified into superficial (first and second degree) and deep (third and fourth degree). Superficial injury is characterized by normal skin color, large blisters filled with clear or milky fluid, intact pinprick sensation, and skin that will indent with pressure. Deep frostbite shows small blood-filled dark blisters, nonblanching cyanosis, and skin that is wooden to the touch and will not indent with pressure.

Diagnosis

- Tissue viability is not ultimately determined until 22–45 days after injury. The primary utility of diagnostic tests is to help define tissue viability at an earlier time.

- Doppler flow studies and angiography can determine tissue viability and predict the need for surgical intervention as early as 7 days after injury. Technetium-99m scintigraphy can be employed as soon as 72 hours from injury to assess tissue viability with a positive predictive value (PPV) of 0.84 for viable tissue. A scan on day 7 raises the PPV to 0.92 (LOE A, randomized clinical trial) (10).
- Magnetic resonance imaging/magnetic resonance angiography (MRI/MRA): Case reports suggest MRA is superior to ^{99}Tc due to ability to direct visualization of occluded vessels and surrounding tissue helping to demarcate the areas of ischemic tissue; however, no large prospective studies have been performed (7).

Treatment

- Field warming should not be instituted until refreezing can be prevented. Wet or constrictive clothing should be removed, and the injured tissue should be protected with a loose bulky splint during transport for definitive care. Hypothermia should be treated first. Smoking, ethanol, direct exposure to heating systems, open fire, and massage of the frozen part should be avoided. Definitive emergency department care is outlined in Table 47.3. It is based on the work of Heggers et al. (14) and McCauley et al. (9). Adjuvant therapies with heparin, warfarin, steroids, dextran, vitamin C, and hyperbaric oxygen have not been universally accepted (13). Pentoxifylline (Trental) has been shown to be useful in pedal frostbite (9).

Table 47.3 Stepwise Treatment of Frostbite
Treat hypothermia and any concomitant injuries.
Rapidly rewarm the affected parts in water at 40–42 °C (104–108 °F) until thawing is complete and the skin is pliable in texture (typically 15–30 min of rewarming).
Debride blisters filled with clear or milky fluid. Apply aloe vera (at least 70%; Dermaide aloe). Cover with a bulky dressing.
Leave hemorrhagic blisters intact.
Splint and elevate the extremity.
Administer ibuprofen 400 mg every 12 h orally. (Avoid aspirin or steroids, but consider use of pentoxifylline 400 mg orally twice a day.)
Give tetanus toxoid and tetanus immune globulin if >10 yr since the last booster.
Consider starting broad-spectrum antibiotics to cover for staph, strep, and pseudomonal species if concern for secondary infection (11–13).
Clindamycin is the recommended alternative for penicillin-allergic patients.
Treat pain with parenteral narcotics as needed. Can consider local anesthetic injections for pain control (11,12).
Begin daily hydrotherapy with hexachlorophene at 40 °C for 30–60 min daily.
No smoking.

HEAT ILLNESS

Definitions

- Exertional heat injuries can be seen as a spectrum of disease and severity from heat cramps and heat syncope, to exertional heat exhaustion (EHE), exertional heat injury (EHI), and ultimately to life-threatening exertional heatstroke (EHS).
- Heat cramps are involuntary, painful contractions of skeletal muscle typically occurring during or after prolonged exercise.
- Heat syncope is a brief loss of consciousness associated with vasodilation and blood pooling of the extremities during heat exposure without elevation of core temperature. Can be associated with EHE and is quickly reversible with removal from heat and rehydration.
- EHE is a syndrome of hyperthermia with a core temperature <40 °C (104 °F) at time of collapse or debilitation following activity. Individuals have minimal (headache and/or dizziness) to no neurological symptoms. Heat exhaustion is a signal of significant systemic vascular strain as the body's attempt to maintain normothermia; *if untreated, it may progress to heat injury or heatstroke.*
- EHI: Occurs when individuals have evidence of heat exhaustion and signs of end-organ damage (*e.g.*, liver and/or kidney injuries) and/or muscle damage (*e.g.*, rhabdomyolysis) without any neurological symptoms. The level of end-organ damage can range from mild to severe.
- EHS is a potentially life-threatening syndrome of hyperthermia defined by having a core temperature usually >40 °C (104 °F) with associated signs and symptoms of CNS dysfunction (confusion, delirium, stupor, and/or coma), which can begin prior to cessation of activity or present as collapse. Failure to recognize and initiate prompt treatment may lead to severe end-organ dysfunction and even death (15).

Epidemiology

- Risk of heat illness correlates with the wet bulb globe temperature (WBGT). WBGT uses humidity, dry air temperature, wind, and solar radiation to measure environmental conditions during exercise. Exercise modification based on region and WBGT can reduce the risk of EHI. Work rest cycles and heat safety tables using WBGT are recommended.
- Other risk factors for EHS include obesity, low physical fitness, dehydration, fatigue, recent episode of heat illness, concomitant febrile illness, sleep deprivation, wear of impermeable garments, lack of acclimatization, and use of medicines or supplements that decrease sweating and increase thermogenesis (antihistamines, ephedra, caffeine, diuretics) (15).

Pathophysiology

- The etiology of heat cramps is not fully understood; however, dehydration, electrolyte disturbances, and fatigue are contributing factors. EHI occurs when heat storage outpaces heat loss that leads to deleterious changes at the cellular level. Core temperature >41 °C leads to a release of many inflammatory mediators to include interleukin 1, interleukin 6, and tumor necrosis factor. These cytokines amplify cellular and endothelial damage that triggers systemic vascular collapse and multiorgan failure (15,16).

Clinical Features

- Symptoms of heat exhaustion, heat injury, and heatstroke overlap making the differentiation between them challenging.
  - Individuals with EHE generally have nondescript symptoms such as headache, dizziness, fatigue, irritability, anxiety, chills, nausea, vomiting, and heat cramps.
  - Individuals with EHI can have all the above symptoms along with a core temperature greater than 40 °C, tachycardia, hyperventilation, hypotension, and associated laboratory changes (see diagnosis), A lack of spontaneous cooling with cessation of exertion and profuse sweating that *ceases* despite an elevated core temperature are both ominous signs of EHI and EHS.
  - Individuals with EHS will have mental status changes that can be progressive with rapid decline to a comatose state or be complicated by a febrile seizure.
    - Signs include a core temperature greater than 40 °C, tachycardia, hyperventilation, and hypotension. A lack of spontaneous cooling with cessation of exertion and profuse sweating that *ceases* despite an elevated core temperature are both ominous signs that point toward heatstroke (15,16).

Diagnosis

- The diagnosis hinges on an elevated core temperature *combined* with the presence of the symptoms and signs noted earlier. This temperature should be rectal in the clinical setting. Any collapse during exertion should include exertional heat-related illnesses in the differential, with early core temperature measurement being crucial for diagnosis. Other etiologies such as exercise collapse associated with sickle-cell trait and arrhythmias must also be included.
  - Of note, healthy athletes can raise their core temperature to 39 °C simply from exertion alone and be asymptomatic.
- Laboratory tests are generally normal in EHE; however, they can become abnormal in EHIs and EHS. Lab evaluation can be very important in guiding treatment and return to activity. Some laboratory studies of note are:
  - Complete blood count and coagulation studies: Low platelets can indicate severe liver injury.
  - Serum liver function tests (LFTs): LFTs may not peak until days after initial injury are essential to evaluate for signs of liver injury and assess severity of injury.
  - Serum electrolytes, blood urea nitrogen (BUN), and creatinine: Abnormal sodium and potassium levels along with increases in BUN/creatinine can be seen with renal injury.
  - Creatine kinase and blood and urine myoglobin elevations are seen in rhabdomyolysis along with other cases of EHI.

Treatment

- When an individual is suspected to have a heat-related injury, it is imperative that treatment not be delayed. Immediate treatment increases the likelihood of the body's return to normal thermoregulation and prevents progression to heatstroke.
- Field treatment should focus on:
  - Cessation of activity and movement to/creation of a shaded, cool environment.
  - Heat cramps can be treated with passive stretching of the affected muscles (8).
  - Fluid replacement: With normal mentation, oral fluids are an appropriate first option. If there are concerns for EHI or EHS, obtain IV access and give IV fluids (preferably NS).
- In case of altered mental status, seizures, or a core temperature greater than 104 °F, heatstroke should be presumed; **immediate whole body (active) cooling with available resource (*e.g.*, cold water immersion or ice sheets) is the key to a successful outcome, and an attempt to cool the patient should be done prior to being evacuated** (15). Active cooling can be done using:
  - Cold water immersion: (Consider gold standard) Produces fastest whole-body cooling with best outcomes. The individual is placed in a tub/tank with cold water up to the nipple line with active temperature monitoring while water is agitated frequently to speed cooling. The individual should be directly supervised to prevent drowning if they become unconscious.
  - Ice sheets/fans: Use of sheets/blankets submerged in ice water and then placed over junctional areas. This is the most resource concise and easier to do in an austere environment.
  - Endovascular cooling in the emergency department for recalcitrant cases (17).
  - Stop active cooling recommended once core temp reaches 38 °C (101 °F) or the athlete begins to shiver to prevent hypothermic overshoot (15).
- Heatstroke treatment recommendations are outlined in Table 47.4 (18,19). Concerns that ice water immersion would increase seizures or trigger shivering thermogenesis have been allayed by recent studies (LOE A, ACSM 2023 Consensus Statement: Exertional Heat Illness) (15). If the patient responds to field treatment, they should avoid exertion for at least 7 days to avoid a transient, but increased risk of recurrent heat illness and follow graduated return to activity. Return to activity varies but is typically achieved within 2–4 weeks. Consider referral and consider heat tolerance testing if return to activity is not achieved by 4–6 weeks (15).

Table 47.4 Treatment of Heatstroke

Immediate cooling with available resources. Ice water immersion is best. If not, use available resources to aggressively cool before transport. Cool until rectal temperature reaches 38 °C (101 °F).
Avoid antipyretics. The hypothalamic set point is normal! Antipyretics can aggravate hepatic or renal injury.
Avoid alcohol baths. Vasodilated skin can lead to systemic absorption.
Monitor core temperature until it is <38 °C (101 °F).
Consider diazepam (5 mg) or lorazepam (2 mg) to control shivering and as prophylaxis against seizures.
Monitor renal function closely. Early dialysis is indicated.
Correct *persistent* electrolyte abnormalities.
Check coagulation profile at admission and serially until 72 h have passed.
Use fresh frozen plasma and/or platelets as needed.
Rehydrate vigorously; monitor for fluid overload and hyponatremia.
Consider N-Acetyle Cysteine in setting of shock liver or pending liver failure.

Five Keys to Prevention

- *Acclimatization* to high heat and humidity for 10–14 days prior to competition is ideal. The first 4–5 days are when 2 key physiologic changes occur: changes in sweat composition and an increase in the ability of the body to rapidly dissipate heat.
- *Clothing* should be light colored, lightweight, and offer sun protection.
- *Medications* that impair heat loss should be stopped or changed, for example, change antihistamines to nasal steroids to treat allergic rhinitis and stop ephedra compounds.
- *Activity planning or reduction* should be based on the WBGT scale: <65, low risk for heat illness; 65–72, high-risk individuals should be monitored or told not to compete; 72–78, risk rises for all; 78–82, high-risk individuals should not exercise; 82–86, unacclimated or unfit athletes should stop; 86–90, exercise should be limited for even fit and acclimated individuals; and >90, all activities should stop (15).
- *Prehydration and hydration per ACSM recommendations.* These can be summarized for patients as follows: Prehydrate by slowly drinking fluids 5–7 $mL \cdot kg^{-1}$ body weight 4 hours before activity. The goal of drinking is to prevent a greater than 2% body weight loss and should be customized to the activity and the athlete. Pre- and postexercise body weight is ideal to estimate sweat rate, total fluid losses, and fluid replacement volume. After exercise, replace each kilogram of weight lost with approximately 1.5 L of fluids. Prolonged exercise or exercise causing large fluid losses (>2%) should include fluid replacement with beverages containing electrolytes and carbohydrates to support fluid-electrolyte balance (20).

ALTITUDE ILLNESS

Definitions and Clinical Syndromes

- Rapid ascent past 6500 ft leads to the onset of the physiologic effects of decreased oxygen concentration at altitude. These effects are most pronounced for those attempting exercise at altitude. Several clinical syndromes exist.
- High-altitude headache (HAH) is the first symptom of altitude exposure. It may or may not progress to acute mountain sickness (AMS).
- AMS is a syndrome that includes HAH and at least one of four symptoms: nausea/vomiting, fatigue/lassitude, dizziness, or insomnia. The Lake Louise Acute Mountain Sickness Scoring System can be used as a tool to screen for AMS. High-altitude cerebral edema (HACE) is the clinical progression of AMS, so that severe CNS symptoms develop, such as ataxia, altered consciousness, confusion, drowsiness, stupor, or coma.
- High-altitude pulmonary edema (HAPE) is the most common cause of altitude-related death. It is characterized by classic signs of pulmonary edema: wet cough, dyspnea at rest, weakness, and orthopnea.

Epidemiology

- Altitude illness is most common in the unacclimatized, regardless of fitness level, who ascend rapidly past 8000 ft but can occur as low as 6500 ft. The severity is linked to the rate of ascent, altitude attained, sleeping altitude, length of altitude exposure, level of exertion, and an individual's inherent physiologic susceptibility that remains static despite reexposure (21).

Pathophysiology

- A rapid rate of ascent, an inappropriately slowed hypoxic ventilatory response to ambient hypoxia and hypercarbia, fluid retention, and vasogenic edema are the initial pathologic changes. Days later, cerebral edema, pulmonary hypertension, and alveolar leakage lead to death if untreated (22,23).
- Maximal oxygen uptake (O_{2max}) falls 10% for each 3281 ft of altitude gained over 5000 ft. O_{2max} at sea level is *not* predictive of performance at altitude. Many of the world's elite mountaineers have average sea level O_{2max} values. Past performance and personal problems with altitude illness are the best predictors of future performance and the need for aggressive preventive interventions (23).

Differential Diagnosis

- Any of the symptoms of AMS on ascent past 6500 ft should trigger suspicion for altitude illness. Key differential diagnostic considerations include dehydration, hypothermia, and a viral infection. Dehydration can be differentiated by response to a fluid challenge. Hypothermia can be distinguished by a low core temperature and improvement with exertion/increased body temperature. Altitude illness worsens with exertion. Although viral syndromes have similar symptoms, they are typically accompanied by fever, myalgia, or diarrhea and are more subacute in onset than AMS. Dyspnea at rest, worsening of symptoms after sleeping, and gait disturbance point toward altitude illness. Abnormal tandem gait is a sensitive examination finding for severe AMS progressing to HACE. Improvement with descent confirms the diagnosis.

Treatment

- Initial field treatment involves stopping the ascent and rest. A lack of improvement in 12 hours should lead to a descent in altitude. Typically, descending 1000–3000 ft is sufficient. Acetazolamide (250 mg twice a day) should be given. Doses of 125 mg twice a day can be given 48 hours before ascent to help prevent AMS (21). If available, low-flow oxygen (maintain SPO2 > 90%) and portable hyperbaric bags are helpful. Additional useful medications are ibuprofen or aspirin for headache and promethazine (25–50 mg) or prochlorperazine (5–10 mg) for nausea and vomiting but should not delay definitive treatment/descent (21).
- Treatment of HACE or HAPE should include *immediate* descent and evacuation. Dexamethasone (8 mg initial dose then 4 mg oral/intramuscular every 6 hours) for HACE and nifedipine (30 mg of the extended-release tablet twice a day) should be instituted for HAPE (LOE 1B) (21,24).
- Hospital treatment will also include high-flow oxygen or hyperbaric oxygen and loop diuretics for pulmonary edema. Mechanical ventilation is only required in cases of coma.

Prevention

- Altitude illness can be prevented by proper acclimatization. Physiologic changes of hyperventilation, tachycardia, erythropoiesis, and a variety of cellular changes take from minutes to months to reach their peak. Recommendations for the prevention of altitude illness are provided in Table 47.5 (21).

Table 47.5 Prevention of Altitude Illness

Begin exertion below 8000 ft. Spend 2–3 nights sleeping between 8000 and 10,000 ft before ascending above 10,000 ft.
Sleep no more than 1500 ft higher each day above 10,000 ft.
Avoid alcohol or sedatives.
Avoid dehydration or hypothermia.
Consider acetazolamide 125 mg orally twice a day beginning 1–2 d before ascent: for any individual with a prior history of acute mountain sickness (AMS), when climbing above 11,400 ft, or when acclimatization is not possible. (Continue until after 48 h at maximum altitude.) Tadalafil (10 mg every 12 h) and Sildenafil (50 mg every 8 h) can also be considered for prevention of high-altitude pulmonary edema.
If Lake Louise AMS score of 3 or higher, do not ascend. Descend if symptoms do not improve in 12 h.
Reserve dexamethasone (4 mg every 6 h) for the treatment of severe AMS or high-altitude cerebral edema.

REFERENCES

1. Danzl DF, Pozos RS. Accidental hypothermia. *N Engl J Med.* 1994;331(26):1756–60.
2. Dow J, Giesbrecht GG, Danzl DF, et al. Wilderness medical society clinical practice guidelines for the out-of-hospital evaluation and treatment of accidental hypothermia: 2019 update. *Wilderness Environ Med.* 2019 Dec;30(4 suppl):S47–69. doi:10.1016/j.wem.2019.10.002
3. Panchal AR, Bartos JA, Cabañas JG, et al. Part 3: adult basic and advanced life support — 2020 American Heart Association guidelines for cardiopulmonary resuscitation and emergency cardiovascular care. *Circulation.* 2020;142(16_suppl_2):S366–468.
4. Castellani JW, Young AJ, Ducharme MB, et al. American College of Sports Medicine position stand: prevention of cold injuries during exercise. *Med Sci Sports Exerc.* 2006;38(11):2012–29.
5. Sheridan RL, Goverman JM, Walker TG. Diagnosis and treatment of frostbite. *N Engl J Med.* 2022;386(23):2213–20. doi:10.1056/NEJMra1800868
6. Reamy BV. Frostbite: review and current concepts. *J Am Board Fam Pract.* 1998;11(1):34–40.
7. Lorentzen AK, Davis C, Penninga L. Interventions for frostbite injuries. *Cochrane Database Syst Rev.* 2020 Dec 20;12(12):CD012980. doi:10.1002/14651858.CD012980.pub2
8. Markenson D, Ferguson JD, Chameides L, et al. Part 17: first aid—2010 American Heart Association and American Red Cross guidelines for first aid. *Circulation.* 2010;122(18 suppl 3):S934–46.
9. McCauley RL, Hing DN, Robson MC, Heggers JP. Frostbite injuries: a rational approach based on the pathophysiology. *J Trauma.* 1983;23(2):143–7.
10. Cauchy E, Marsigny B, Allamel G, Verhellen R, Chetaille E. The value of technetium 99 scintigraphy in the prognosis of amputation in severe frostbite injuries of the extremities: a retrospective study of 92 severe frostbite injuries. *J Hand Surg Am.* 2000;25(5):969–78.
11. Herring SA, Bernhardt DT, Boyajian-O'Neil L, et al. Selected issues in injury and illness prevention and the team physician: a consensus statement. *Med Sci Sports Exerc.* 2007;39(11):2058–68.
12. Persitz J, Essa A, Ner EB, Assaraf E, Avisar E. Frostbite of the extremities — recognition, evaluation and treatment. *Injury.* 2022;53(10):3088–93.
13. Murphy JV, Banwell PE, Roberts AH, McGrouther DA. Frostbite: pathogenesis and treatment. *J Trauma.* 2000;48(1):171–8.
14. Heggers JP, Robson MC, Manavalen K, et al. Experimental and clinical observations on frostbite. *Ann Emerg Med.* 1987;16(9):1056–62.
15. Roberts WO, Armstrong LE, Sawka MN, Yeargin SW, Heled Y, O'Connor FG. ACSM expert consensus statement on exertional heat illness: recognition, management, and return to activity. *Curr Sports Med Rep.* 2023 Apr 22;22(4):134–49.
16. Casa DJ, DeMartini JK, Bergeron MF, et al. National athletic trainers' association position statement: exertional heat illnesses. *J Athl Train.* 2015 Sep;50(9):986–1000.
17. Bursey MM, Galer M, Oh RC, Weathers BK. Successful management of severe exertional heat stroke with endovascular cooling after failure of standard cooling measures. *J Emerg Med.* 2019 Aug;57(2):e53–6. doi:10.1016/j.jemermed.2019.03.025
18. O'Connor FG, Nye NS, DeGroot D, Deuster PA. *Clinical Practice Guideline for the Prevention, Diagnosis, and Management of Exertional Heat Illness.* Consortium for Health and Military Performance (CHAMP). Maryland: Bethesda; 2024.
19. Will JS, Snyder CJ, Westerfield KL. N-Acetylcysteine (NAC) for the prevention of liver failure in heat injury-mediated Ischemic Hepatitis. *Mil Med.* 2019 Oct;184(9–10):565–7.
20. American College of Sports Medicine, Sawka MN, Burke LM, et al. American College of Sports Medicine position stand. Exercise and fluid replacement. *Med Sci Sports Exerc.* 2007;39(2):377–90.

21. Luks AM, Auerbach PS, Freer L, et al. Wilderness medical society clinical practice guidelines for the prevention and treatment of acute altitude illness: 2019 update. *Wilderness Environ Med.* 2019;30(4 suppl):S3–18.
22. Fiore DC, Hall S, Shoja P. Altitude illness: risk factors, prevention, presentation and treatment. *Am Fam Physician.* 2010;82(9):1103–10.
23. Hackett PH, Roach RC. High-altitude illness. *N Engl J Med.* 2001;345(2):107–14.
24. Bärtsch P, Maggiorini M, Ritter M, Noti C, Vock P, Oelz O. Prevention of high-altitude pulmonary edema by nifedipine. *N Engl J Med.* 1991;325(18):1284–9.

SECTION IV

Musculoskeletal Problems in the Athlete

Head Injuries

Dennis A. Cardone, Naina Rao, and Eric J. Strauss

48

BACKGROUND

- There are an estimated 1.6–3.8 million sports-related head injuries that occur annually in the United States, with many not seeking prompt medical care (1). Almost 70% of these visits are in patients 20 years or younger (2).
- Pediatric and adolescent athletes make up the majority of these visits with approximately 1.1–1.9 million concussions or head injuries annually (3).
- Head injuries trigger neurometabolic disruptions that contribute to long-term neuronal impairment. The brain is capable of neither regeneration nor, unlike many other body parts and organs, transplantation. Every effort must be made to protect the athlete's head during competition because even minor injuries have been demonstrated to have lifelong cognitive effects (4).
- Head injuries include acute subdural hemorrhage (ASDH), acute epidural hematoma, cerebral contusion, traumatic cerebrovascular accidents, diffuse brain swelling, diffuse axonal injury, skull fractures, and sports-related concussion (SRC).
- American football, cycling, and baseball had the highest total number of head injuries treated at U.S. emergency rooms, whereas rugby, ice hockey, and American football had the highest incidence rates per 1000 athlete exposures of all organized sports (5,6).
- Concussion rates for American football are 33.2–39.1 per 10,000 athletes at the high school level and account for the most amount of concussions across all sports at the collegiate level (7,8).
- From 2012 to 2014, the incidence of concussions in the National Football League (NFL) was found to be 27.8 per 1000 athletes (9).
- ASDH is the leading cause of catastrophic death in high school and collegiate football players, making up 90% of all catastrophic head injuries in the sport (10,11).
- Almost all patients who sustain an ASDH are senior high school students or younger (12).
- From 1990 to 2011, there were 243 American football fatalities in high school and college football players. Brain injury was the second most common cause of fatalities (sudden cardiac death was the most common cause). Subdural hematoma (SDH) was responsible for 79% of deaths in the brain injury group (13).
- While there is no difference in head injury risk among different football positions for high school students, in the NFL (14), defensive secondary and offensive line positions incurred the most number of head injuries, whereas tight ends/wide receivers had the highest rates of concussion (15).
- Most brain injury–related fatalities are sustained by high school football players while making tackles or being tackled (10,16).
- Per 100,000 participants, American football is less likely to result in a fatal head injury when compared to horseback riding, skydiving, or car or motorcycle racing and has about the same risk of a fatal head injury as gymnastics and ice hockey (17).
- Other sports historically have been shown to have a high rate of head injury, including wrestling, cheerleading, martial arts, boxing, automobile racing, skiing, and snowboarding (18–20).

CEREBRAL CONCUSSION

- Concussion comes from the Latin word *concutere*, which means to shake violently.
- According to the Consensus Statement on Concussion in Sport from 2016, SRC is a traumatic brain injury (TBI) caused by biomechanical forces. Some common features that can be used in a clinically relevant manner to define the condition include (21):
    - May be caused by direct blow to head or indirect blow with impulsive force transmitted to head.
    - Typically, rapid (seconds to minutes) onset of short-lived impairment of neurologic function with spontaneous resolution.
    - Acute clinical symptoms largely reflect functional disturbance rather than a structural injury and may not be visible on standard imaging.
    - Concussion results in a graded set of clinical symptoms that may or may not involve loss of consciousness and the subsequent resolution of clinical and cognitive symptoms typically follows a sequential course.

- Rates of concussion in several popular sports are listed in Table 48.1 (22).
- Rates of adolescent concussions may be grossly underestimated because approximately 50% of concussions sustained by high school athletes go unreported, making accurate determination of incidence difficult (3).
- The risk of sustaining a subsequent concussion is 3–5 times greater in an athlete who sustained a concussion within the year than those without a history of concussion in the same time period (14,23).
- In 2021, the American College of Sports Medicine's Team Physician Consensus Conference (TPCC) initiative published guidance on SRC. The TPCC is an annual project-based alliance of six major professional associations. The goal of this TPCC statement is to assist the team physician in providing optimal medical care for the athlete with SRC (24).
- Diagnosis of acute concussion involves an assessment of clinical symptoms, physical signs, behavior, balance, sleep, and cognition.
- List of signs and symptoms are included in Table 48.2.
- Most adult patients recover spontaneously within 7–14 days, but adolescents may take up to 4 weeks or longer (24).
- Strict bed rest after SRC has been shown to slow recovery and prolong symptoms (24).
- After a brief period of relative rest (24–48 hours), athletes may gradually and progressively resume cognitive and physical activity at a level that does not produce new symptoms or exacerbate existing symptoms (subthreshold) (24).

Table 48.1 Concussion Rates per 10,000 AE and Rate Ratios Comparing Competitions Versus Practices in High School and College Sports (22)

		High School				College			
		Overall Rate	**Competition Rate**	**Practice Rate**	**Rate Ratio: Competition vs. Practice (95% CI)**	**Overall Rate**	**Competition Rate**	**Practice Rate**	**Rate Ratio: Competition vs. Practice (95% CI)**
Men's sports	American football	7.28	25.73	3.54	7.27 (6.78, 7.79)	6.31	30.09	3.99	7.53 (6.89, 8.24)
	Baseball	0.69	1.33	0.34	3.87 (2.59, 5.79)	1.13	2.25	0.53	4.22 (2.70, 6.58)
	Basketball	1.53	3.27	0.79	4.14 (3.27, 5.23)	6.18	12.62	4.52	2.79 (2.35, 3.32)
	Ice hockey	6.83	17.66	1.5	11.74 (8.24, 16.72)	6.95	22.88	2.06	11.12 (8.76, 14.12)
	Lacrosse	4.87	12.18	1.63	7.46 (5.76, 9.66)	4.51	16.98	2.19	7.75 (5.74, 10.47)
	Soccer	2.78	7.68	0.68	11.28 (8.81, 14.45)	4.02	12.36	1.73	7.16 (5.58, 9.19)
	Wrestling	3.13	5.85	2.17	2.70 (2.24, 3.25)	6.72	27.95	4.1	6.81 (5.05, 9.18)
Women's sports	Basketball	2.98	7.39	1.08	6.82 (5.55, 8.38)	4.99	9.99	3.54	2.82 (2.31, 3.44)
	Field hockey	2.67	5.94	1.16	5.14 (3.63, 7.29)	4.19	11.29	1.86	6.08 (3.80, 9.73)
	Lacrosse	3.67	8.34	1.57	5.33 (3.85, 7.36)	5.07	14.23	2.88	4.94 (3.56, 6.83)
	Soccer	4.5	12.84	0.92	13.92 (11.13, 17.40)	6.44	19.11	2.33	8.19 (6.73, 9.98)
	Softball	1.4	2.2	0.97	2.26 (1.66, 3.07)	2.61	4.19	1.5	2.80 (2, 3.92)
	Volleyball	1.18	1.9	0.8	2.39 (1.77, 3.23)	2.29	3.26	1.88	1.73 (1.22, 2.46)

Abbreviations: AE, athlete exposure, one athlete participating in one practice or competition; CI, confidence interval; HS RIO, High School Reporting Information Online database; NCAA-ISP, NCAA Injury Surveillance Program.

High School Reporting Information Online (2005/06–2013/14) and the National Collegiate Athletic Association Injury Surveillance Program (2004/05–2013/14).

HS RIO and the NCAA-ISP collect injury and exposure data from national samples of high school and collegiate sports programs, respectively. Data presented in this table were collected from each surveillance system during the same time periods. HS RIO began data collection of lacrosse, ice hockey, and field hockey in 2008/09.

Source: Pierpoint LA, Collins C. Epidemiology of sport-related concussion. *Clin Sports Med.* 2021;40(1):1–18.

Table 48.2 Signs and Symptoms That May Suggest Concussion (25)

Somatic	Vestibular and/or Oculomotor	Cognitive	Emotional	Sleep
Headache	Vision problems	Confusion	Irritable	Drowsiness and/or fatigue
Nausea and/or vomiting	Hearing problems and/or tinnitus	Feeling mentally "foggy"	More emotional than usual	Feeling slowed down
Neck pain	Balance problems	Difficulty concentrating	Sadness	Trouble falling asleep
Light sensitivity	Dizziness	Difficulty remembering	Nervous and/or anxious	Sleeping too much
Noise sensitivity		Answers questions slowly		Sleeping too little
		Repeats questions		
		Loss of consciousness		

Source: Halstead ME, Walter KD, Moffatt Ket al. Sport-related concussion in children and adolescents. *Pediatrics.* 2018;142(6):e20183074.

- Recent studies have shown that progressive moderate aerobic exercise within the first week after SRC helps safely speed recovery. Cognitive activities should be modified or limited to that which does not produce or exacerbate symptoms (24).
- After successful completion of a graduated program of exertion, most athletes can be medically cleared for return to competition.
- Concussion diagnosis and management, to include the Amsterdam Guidelines published in October 2022, are further discussed in Chapter 30, Neuropsychological Testing in Concussion and Chapter 40, Neurology (26).

POSTCONCUSSION SYNDROME

- A second late effect of concussion is the postconcussion syndrome (PCS), which refers to the persistence of concussion symptoms for an extended period (months to years). This syndrome can consist of fatigue, sleep disturbance, headache, dizziness/vertigo, irritability/aggression, affective disturbance, personality change, and apathy (25,27).
- The persistence of these symptoms reflecting altered neurotransmitter function can have a delayed presentation after the initial injury (28).
- The precise definition and diagnostic criteria lack consensus among physicians. However, the most common time to diagnose PCS clinically was 1–3 months with a minimum of at least one symptom (29).
- The most important factor that is associated with the development of PCS is the severity of the early concussion symptoms following the head injury. Comorbidities such as preexisting migraine or psychiatric disorders may also increase the risk (30,31).
- When these symptoms persist, patients should be treated with the goal of minimizing symptom severity through health education and pharmacologic and/or nonpharmacological interventions.

LONG-TERM RISKS AFTER CONCUSSION

- Mental health issues
  - Retired professional football players with a history of concussions develop moderate to severe depression at 2.4 times the rate than those who had no concussion in their career (32–34).
  - Caregivers and family members should be vigilant of this increased risk of depression.
- Chronic traumatic encephalopathy (CTE)
  - There is concern for delayed development of CTE, a progressive neurodegenerative tauopathy that evolves into dementia, in athletes who have sustained multiple mild (unreported) TBIs (35,36).
  - In a postmortem study of 202 former American football players who competed at different levels of play, overall 87% were neuropathologically diagnosed with CTE, with 99% of former NFL players having the condition (35).
  - The neuropathological severity of CTE was distributed according to the level of play with high school players having mild pathology and professional players having severe pathology (35).
  - Current evidence does not show an increased risk of CTE in young athletes who sustain multiple SRCs (24).
  - Clinical manifestations of CTE include dysarthria, tremors, attention difficulty, memory deficits, executive function dysfunction, and pyramidal signs (37).
  - The incidence, prevalence, and pathophysiology of CTE are unknown (24).
  - The diagnosis of CTE is made only via examination of the brain at autopsy.
  - In most cases, the symptoms of CTE will not be clinically apparent until decades after exposure to trauma (24).

INTRACRANIAL HEMORRHAGE

- The leading cause of death from athletic head injury is intracranial hemorrhage. There are four types of hemorrhage: epidural, subdural, subarachnoid, and intracerebral, to which the examining trainer or physician must be alert in every instance of head injury.

Neuroimaging in Head Injury

- Computed tomography (CT) and magnetic resonance imaging (MRI) are rarely necessary in concussion management except when there is suspicion of intracranial hemorrhage, cervical spine injury, or skull fracture (38,39).
- CT is the test of choice for detecting skull fractures and intracranial bleeding within the first 48 hours.
- MRI is superior to CT for diagnosis of cerebral contusion, petechial hemorrhage, and white matter injury (40).
- Box 48.1 includes a list of signs and symptoms indicative of further neuroimaging.
- There are several guidelines that help assess the need for neuroimaging, of which two are frequently used:
  1. Canadian CT Head Rule: CT should be used if the patient has a Glasgow Coma Scale (GCS) <15, a suspected open skull or basal skull fracture, 2+ episodes of vomiting, retrograde amnesia, or dangerous mechanism of injury or is older than 65 years (41).
  2. New Orleans Criteria: CT should be used if the patient presents with severe headache, vomiting, age above 60 years, drug or alcohol intoxication, short-term memory loss, trauma above the clavicles, or seizure (42).
- Any patient with worsening symptoms should undergo neuroimaging.
- Patients with loss of consciousness for 30 seconds or more are at higher risk for intracranial bleeding and should undergo neuroimaging (43).

48.1 Concussion Danger Signs

- Convulsions or seizures (shaking or twitching)
- Not able to recognize people or places
- Repeated nausea or vomiting
- Unusual behavior, increased confusion, restlessness, or agitation
- Loss of consciousness with increasing drowsiness, inability to wake up, or inability to stay awake
- Slurred speech, weakness, numbness, or decreased coordination
- A headache that gets worse and does not go away
- One pupil larger than the other or double vision

Source: Centers for Disease Control and Prevention. Available at: https://www.cdc.gov/heads-up/signs-symptoms/index.html

- A normal imaging study acutely after injury does not rule out a chronic SDH or future neurobehavioral abnormalities, so continued observation and management may still be required (43).

Epidural Hematoma

- Most patients with an epidural hematoma will also have a concurrent skull fracture that damages the middle meningeal artery or vein (44).
- The "lucid interval" is the period of time after loss of consciousness/altered mental state where the athlete appears asymptomatic for minutes to hours.
- On a noncontrast head CT an epidural hematoma typically appears as a biconvex (lens-shaped) hyperdense area. Treatment is surgical decompression. Early treatment is correlated with improved survival. (45).
- Frequent serial monitoring is required to identify deterioration.

Subdural Hemorrhage

- Subdural hemorrhage is the most common type of traumatic brain lesion that occurs in 20%–40% of catastrophic head injuries. It results when the bridging veins between brain and dura are torn (46).
- Athletes with acute SDH (within 24 hours) are usually not conscious. However, presentation can vary and the injured athlete can even be asymptomatic.
- It often presents with concomitant brain parenchyma contusions, which suggests worse clinical outcomes (47).
- Diagnosis requires noncontrast head CT imaging to identify crescent-shaped, hyperdense mass along the skull (48).
- Prompt surgical evacuation is crucial to reduce mortality as a delay of more than 4 hours can increase the mortality to 90% (49).
- It has been suggested that recent prior head injury can increase the risk of ASDH in an athlete (47).

Intraventricular Hemorrhage (50,51)

- Intraventricular hemorrhage occurs from a torn artery with direct bleeding into the brain parenchyma after a tensile or shearing force.
- Typically, presentation does not have a lucid interval but does vary greatly depending on the location.
- Initially symptoms can include headache, confusion, retrograde amnesia, and focal deficits and can quickly deteriorate to coma.
- Clinical monitoring with serial exams is required due to the high likelihood of mass effect caused by delayed edema.
- Because all four types of intracranial hemorrhage may be fatal, a rapid and accurate initial assessment, as well as an appropriate follow-up, is mandatory after an athletic head injury.

POSTTRAUMATIC SEIZURE

- Posttraumatic seizures (PTS) are classified as "early" if they occur within 7 days and "late" if it is later.
- Risk factors for early PTS include GCS of ≤10; amnesia lasting longer than 30 min; skull fracture; a penetrating head injury; subdural, epidural, or intracerebral hematoma; and cortical contusion (43).
- One trial has shown that phenytoin can decrease the incidence of early PTS but not late PTS. While levetiracetam has been gaining popularity, it has no benefit compared to phenytoin (52,53).
- If a seizure occurs in an athlete with a head injury, it is important to logroll the patient onto their side. By this maneuver, any blood or saliva will roll out of the mouth or nose and the tongue cannot fall back and obstruct the airway.
- These events are usually dramatic, last several minutes, and then cease. Majority of cases return to play (RTP) within 2 weeks and only a fraction develops long-term sequelae (54).

MALIGNANT BRAIN EDEMA

- Pathology studies cellular or cytotoxic edema that results within minutes of the head injury and affects multiple types of cells in the brain.
- Prompt recognition is extremely important because there is little initial brain injury, and the seriousness of fatal neurologic outcome is secondary to raised intracranial pressure with herniation (55).
- Key signs that suggest cerebral insult are altered mental status and development of fixed and dilated pupils. Those who have these symptoms should undergo CT to reveal the edema.
- Prompt treatment with positioning, intubation, hyperosmolar therapy, antipyretics, sedative, hyperventilation, and osmotic agents has helped to reduce the mortality. Decompressive craniectomy should be considered as a last resort if other intracranial pressure-lowering methods have failed (56,57).

SECOND IMPACT SYNDROME

- This syndrome, while rare and not well known, is most commonly defined as catastrophic brain injury in a person who suffers from head trauma while still recovering from the effects of a recent concussion (58,59).
- Validated cases have indicated that second impact syndrome (SIS) occurs nearly exclusively in male athletes, those who play American football, and athletes below the age of 20 years (59).
- The mechanism of injury is thought to originate from axonal shearing, causing rapid depolarization, neurotransmitter release, and extracellular leakage of potassium. The subsequent dysfunctional cerebral blood flow autoregulation leads to an increase in intracranial pressure and ultimately brain herniation and brain stem injury (60).
- The second blow may be remarkably minor, perhaps only involving a blow to the chest that jerks the athlete's head and indirectly imparts accelerative forces to the brain (61).
- Usually within seconds to minutes of the second impact, the athlete — quite precipitously collapses to the ground, entering a semicomatose state, with rapidly dilating pupils, loss of eye movement, and evidence of respiratory failure (62).
- Radiologically, there is evidence of cerebral swelling that is often associated with ASDH.
- Prevention is accomplished by strict adherence to RTP guidelines outlined previously.
- Overall incidence is unknown because it is very rare, with 36 documented cases among American football players from 1946 to 2015 (61).
- Mortality rate approaches 100%; prevention is key.

DIFFUSE AXONAL INJURY

- This condition results when severe shearing forces are imparted to the brain and cause extensive damage to the white matter tracts by severing the axonal connections, in the absence of intracranial hematoma (43).
- The patient is usually deeply comatose with a low GCS score and a negative head CT, and immediate neurologic triage for treatment of increased intracranial pressure is indicated (63).
- It is seen radiographically most often on T2 MRI and gradient echo sequences as subtle hemorrhagic foci in places such as corona radiata, corpus callosum, internal capsule, brain stem, and thalamus (64).

TRAUMATIC CEREBROVASCULAR DISEASE (11)

- Cerebral infarction caused by sports is very rare and mostly occurs due to arterial dissection.
- This is observed in a variety of sports such as soccer, rugby, judo, winter sports, bowling, wrestling, and scuba diving.
- The most common cause is internal carotid artery dissection from blunt trauma.
- Symptoms include amaurosis, anterior neck pain, transient ischemic attack, and Horner syndrome.
- CT, magnetic resonance angiography, and ultrasound are best for diagnosing this condition.
- Those who have a history of dissection are recommended to not participate in any sport that requires neck rotation or hyperextension

48.2 Canadian CT Head Rule Guidelines

Under the Canadian CT Head Rule patients with minor head injuries should only receive CT scans if one or more of the following criteria are met:

- Glasgow Coma Scale score lower than 15 at 2 hours after injury.
- Suspected open or depressed skull fracture.
- Any sign of basal skull fracture.
- Two or more episodes of vomiting.
- Age 65 or older.
- Amnesia before impact of 30 or more minutes.
- Dangerous mechanism (this is defined by Stiell et al. (2005) as "a pedestrian struck by a motor vehicle, an occupant ejected from a motor vehicle, or a fall from an elevation of 3 or more feet or 5 stairs."

The first five criteria are considered "high-risk", whereas criteria 6 and 7 are considered "medium-risk".

Source: Stiell IG, Wells GA, Vandemheen K, et al. The Canadian CT Head Rule for patients with minor head injury. *Lancet.* 2001;357(9266):1391–6.

MANAGEMENT GUIDELINES (21,65)

- **Immediate treatment:** With a head injury, the ABCs of first aid must be followed. Before a neurologic examination is undertaken, the treating physician must determine if the airway is adequate and the circulation is being maintained. Thereafter, attention may be directed to the neurologic examination. It is important to understand that all players who have had a concussion must be removed from competition.
- **Definitive treatment:** Definitive treatment of severe concussions as well as of the SIS and intracranial hematoma should take place at a medical facility where neurosurgical and neuroradiologic capabilities are present (65).
- **What tests to order and when:** After a concussion, observation alone may be all that is indicated. In instances of a more severe concussion, however, a CT scan or MRI of the brain is recommended. Please see the Canadian CT Head Rule (Box 48.2) guidelines for a list of red flags that would be an indication for further imaging studies.
- **When to refer:** More severe head injuries should be referred for neurologic or neurosurgical evaluation following removal of the athlete from the contest.
- **Appropriate time course for resolution:** In cases of head injury, the RTP guidelines outlined in this chapter may be used as a reference. Each case needs to be considered on an individual basis.

SUMMARY

- While head injuries may always be a part of athletic competition, we must continue to strive to decrease their effect on athletes and their incidence overall.
- Great strides have been made, including increased recognition and appropriate treatment at athletic competitions and strict regulations regarding RTP criteria at all levels of sport.
- We must continue to move in this direction by installment of rules that continue to respect the nature of competition while protecting athletes from harm.

REFERENCES

1. Harmon KG, Clugston JR, Dec K, et al. American Medical Society for Sports Medicine position statement on concussion in sport. *Br J Sports Med.* 2019;53(4):213–25.
2. Coronado VG, Haileyesus T, Cheng TA, et al. Trends in sports- and recreation-related traumatic brain injuries treated in US emergency departments: the national electronic injury surveillance system-all injury Program (NEISS-AIP) 2001-2012. *J Head Trauma Rehabil.* 2015;30(3):185–97.
3. Bryan MA, Rowhani-Rahbar A, Comstock RD, Rivara F, Seattle Sports Concussion Research Collaborative. Sports- and recreation-related concussions in US youth. *Pediatrics.* 2016;138(1):e20154635.
4. Brett BL, Gardner RC, Godbout J, Dams-O'Connor K, Keene CD. Traumatic brain injury and risk of neurodegenerative disorder. *Biol Psychiatry.* 2022;91(5):498–507.
5. Agarwal N. *Sports-related Head Injury.* American Association of Neurological Surgeons; 2018.
6. Pfister T, Pfister K, Hagel B, Ghali WA, Ronksley PE. The incidence of concussion in youth sports: a systematic review and meta-analysis. *Br J Sports Med.* 2016;50(5):292–7.
7. Kerr ZY, Wilkerson GB, Caswell SV, et al. The first decade of web-based sports injury surveillance: descriptive epidemiology of injuries in United States high school football (2005-2006 through 2013-2014) and national collegiate athletic association football (2004–2005 through 2013-2014). *J Athl Train.* 2018;53(8):738–51.
8. Zuckerman SL, Kerr ZY, Yengo-Kahn A, Wasserman E, Covassin T, Solomon GS. Epidemiology of sports-related concussion in NCAA athletes from 2009-2010 to 2013-2014: incidence, recurrence, and mechanisms. *Am J Sports Med.* 2015;43(11):2654–62.
9. Lawrence D, Hutchison M, Comper P. Descriptive epidemiology of musculoskeletal injuries and concussions in the national football League, 2012-2014. *Orthop J Sports Med.* 2015;3(5):2325967115583653.
10. Kucera KL, Yau RK, Register-Mihalik J, et al. Traumatic brain and spinal cord fatalities among high school and college football players—United States, 2005-2014. *MMWR Morb Mortal Wkly Rep.* 2017;65(52):1465–9.
11. Mizobuchi Y, Nagahiro S. A review of sport-related head injuries. *Korean J Nutr.* 2016;12(1):1–5.
12. Mueller FO. Catastrophic head injuries in high school and collegiate sports. *J Athl Train.* 2001;36(3):312–5.
13. Boden BP, Breit I, Beachler JA, Williams A, Mueller FO. Fatalities in high school and college football players. *Am J Sports Med.* 2013;41(5):1108–16.
14. Tsushima WT, Siu AM, Ahn HJ, Chang BL, Murata NM. Incidence and risk of concussions in youth athletes: comparisons of age, sex, concussion history, sport, and football position. *Arch Clin Neuropsychol.* 2019;34(1):60–9.

15. Mack CD, Solomon G, Covassin T, Theodore N, Cárdenas J, Sills A. Epidemiology of concussion in the national football League, 2015-2019. *Sports Health*. 2021;13(5):423–30.
16. Bailes JE, Patel V, Farhat H, Sindelar B, Stone J. Football fatalities: the first-impact syndrome. *J Neurosurg Pediatr*. 2017;19(1):116–21.
17. Kappelhof JP, Vrensen GF. The pathology of after-cataract. A minireview. *Acta Ophthalmol Suppl (1985)*. 1992;1992(205):13–24.
18. *D.R. C. National High School Sports-Related Injury Surveillance Study: Summary Report,* 2015-2016 *School Year*. Colorado School of Public Health, Pediatric Injury Prevention E, and Research (PIPER) program; 2017.
19. Stewart TC, Gilliland J, Fraser DD. An epidemiologic profile of pediatric concussions: identifying urban and rural differences. *J Trauma Acute Care Surg*. 2014;76(3):736–42.
20. Fernandes FA, de Sousa RJA. Head injury predictors in sports trauma – a state-of-the-art review. *Proc Inst Mech Eng H*. 2015;229(8):592–608.
21. McCrory P, Meeuwisse W, Dvorak J, et al. Consensus statement on concussion in sport—the 5th international conference on concussion in sport held in Berlin, October 2016. *Br J Sports Med*. 2017. bjsports-2017-0.
22. Pierpoint LA, Collins C. Epidemiology of sport-related concussion. *Clin Sports Med*. 2021;40(1):1–18.
23. Reneker JC, Babl R, Flowers MM. History of concussion and risk of subsequent injury in athletes and service members: a systematic review and meta-analysis. *Musculoskelet Sci Pract*. 2019;42:173–85.
24. Herring S, Kibler WB, Putukian M, et al. Selected issues in sport-related concussion (SRC|mild traumatic brain injury) for the team physician: a consensus statement. *Br J Sports Med*. 2021;55(22):1251–61.
25. Ahmed BZ, Benton AH, Serra-Jovenich M, Toldi JP. Postconcussion symptoms and neuropsychological performance in athletes: a literature review. *Curr Sports Med Rep*. 2023;22(1):19–23.
26. Patricios JS, Schneider KJ, Dvorak J, et al. Consensus statement on concussion in sport: the 6th International conference on concussion in sport-Amsterdam, October 2022. *Br J Sports Med*. 2023;57(11):695–711.
27. Morgan CD, Zuckerman SL, Lee YM, et al. Predictors of postconcussion syndrome after sports-related concussion in young athletes: a matched case-control study. *J Neurosurg Pediatr*. 2015;15(6):589–98.
28. Kim K, Priefer R. Evaluation of current post-concussion protocols. *Biomed Pharmacother*. 2020;129:110406.
29. Rose SC, Fischer AN, Heyer GL. How long is too long? The lack of consensus regarding the post-concussion syndrome diagnosis. *Brain Inj*. 2015;29(7–8):798–803.
30. Hubertus V, Marklund N, Vajkoczy P. Management of concussion in soccer. *Acta Neurochir*. 2019;161(3):425–33.
31. Quinn DK, Mayer AR, Master CL, Fann JR. Prolonged postconcussive symptoms. *Am J Psychiatry*. 2018;175(2):103–11.
32. Kerr ZY, Evenson KR, Rosamond WD, Mihalik JP, Guskiewicz KM, Marshall SW. Association between concussion and mental health in former collegiate athletes. *Inj Epidemiol*. 2014;1(1):28.
33. Kerr ZY, Thomas LC, Simon JE, McCrea M, Guskiewicz KM. Association between history of multiple concussions and health outcomes among former college football players: 15-year follow-up from the NCAA concussion study (1999–2001). *Am J Sports Med*. 2018;46(7):1733–41.
34. Montenigro PH, Alosco ML, Martin BM, et al. Cumulative head impact exposure predicts later-life depression, apathy, executive dysfunction, and cognitive impairment in former high school and college football players. *J Neurotrauma*. 2017;34(2):328–40.
35. Mez J, Daneshvar DH, Kiernan PT, et al. Clinicopathological evaluation of chronic traumatic encephalopathy in players of American football. *JAMA*. 2017;318(4):360–70.
36. Mez J, Daneshvar DH, Abdolmohammadi B, et al. Duration of American football play and chronic traumatic encephalopathy. *Ann Neurol*. 2020;87(1):116–31.
37. Galgano M, Toshkezi G, Qiu X, Russell T, Chin L, Zhao LR. Traumatic brain injury: current treatment strategies and future endeavors. *Cell Transplant*. 2017;26(7):1118–30.
38. Pulsipher DT, Campbell RA, Thoma R, King JH. A critical review of neuroimaging applications in sports concussion. *Curr Sports Med Rep*. 2011;10(1):14–20.
39. Master CL, Mayer AR, Quinn D, Grady MF. Concussion. *Ann Intern Med*. 2018;169(1):ITC1–16.
40. Mutch CA, Talbott JF, Gean A. Imaging evaluation of acute traumatic brain injury. *Neurosurg Clin N Am*. 2016;27(4):409–39.
41. Stiell IG, Wells GA, Vandemheen K, et al. The Canadian CT Head Rule for patients with minor head injury. *Lancet*. 2001;357(9266):1391–6.
42. Haydel MJ, Preston CA, Mills TJ, Luber S, Blaudeau E, DeBlieux PM. Indications for computed tomography in patients with minor head injury. *N Engl J Med*. 2000;343(2):100–5.
43. Azim A, Joseph B. *Traumatic Brain Injury*. Springer International Publishing; 2018:1–10.
44. Talbott JF, Gean A, Yuh EL, Stiver SI. Calvarial fracture patterns on CT imaging predict risk of a delayed epidural hematoma following decompressive craniectomy for traumatic brain injury. *AJNR Am J Neuroradiol*. 2014;35(10):1930–5.
45. Clement MO. Imaging of brain trauma. *Radiol Clin North Am*. 2019;57(4):733–44.
46. Carek SM, Clugston JR. Acute sports-related head injuries. *Prim Care*. 2020;47(1):177–88.
47. Yengo-Kahn AM, Gardner RM, Kuhn AW, Solomon GS, Bonfield CM, Zuckerman SL. Sport-related structural brain injury: 3 cases of subdural hemorrhage in American high school football. *World Neurosurg*. 2017;106:1055.e5–1055.e11.
48. Bates TJ, Lee P, Ellison TM, Ahuero JS, Schmitz MR. Acute subdural hematoma in an elite-level rugby union player. *Trauma Case Rep*. 2020;26:100295.
49. Sindelar B, Bailes JE. Neurosurgical emergencies in sport. *Neurol Clin*. 2017;35(3):451–72.
50. Schweitzer AD, Niogi SN, Whitlow CT, Tsiouris AJ. Traumatic brain injury: imaging patterns and complications. *Radiographics*. 2019;39(6): 1571–95.
51. Mata-Mbemba D, Mugikura S, Nakagawa A, et al. Intraventricular hemorrhage on initial computed tomography as marker of diffuse axonal injury after traumatic brain injury. *J Neurotrauma*. 2015;32(5): 359–65.
52. Temkin NR, Dikmen SS, Wilensky AJ, Keihm J, Chabal S, Winn HR. A randomized, double-blind study of phenytoin for the prevention of post-traumatic seizures. *N Engl J Med*. 1990;323(8):497–502.
53. Yang Y, Zheng F, Xu X, Wang X. Levetiracetam versus phenytoin for seizure prophylaxis following traumatic brain injury: a systematic review and meta-analysis. *CNS Drugs*. 2016;30(8):677–88.
54. Kuhl NO, Yengo-Kahn AM, Burnette H, Solomon GS, Zuckerman SL. Sport-related concussive convulsions: a systematic review. *Phys Sportsmed*. 2018;46(1):1–7.
55. Hawryluk GWJ, Rubiano AM, Totten AM, et al. Guidelines for the management of severe traumatic brain injury: 2020 update of the decompressive craniectomy recommendations. *Neurosurgery*. 2020;87(3):427–34.
56. Nehring SM, Tadi P, Tenny S. *Cerebral Edema*. StatPearls; 2023.
57. Pinto VL, Tadi P, Adeyinka A. Increased intracranial pressure. In: *StatPearls*. Treasure Island (FL): StatPearls Publishing; 2022.
58. Stovitz SD, Weseman JD, Hooks MC, Schmidt RJ, Koffel JB, Patricios JS. What definition is used to describe second impact syndrome in sports? A systematic and critical review. *Curr Sports Med Rep*. 2017;16(1):50–5.
59. Engelhardt J, Brauge D, Loiseau H. Second impact syndrome. Myth or reality? *Neurochirurgie*. 2021;67(3):265–75.

60. May T, Foris LA, Donnally CJ. *Second Impact Syndrome.* StatPearls; 2025.
61. McLendon LA, Kralik SF, Grayson PA, Golomb MR. The controversial second impact syndrome: a review of the literature. *Pediatr Neurol.* 2016;62:9–17.
62. Cantu RC. Second-impact syndrome. *Clin Sports Med.* 1998;17(1):37–44.
63. Georges A, Das JM. Traumatic brain injury. In: *StatPearls.* Treasure Island (FL): StatPearls Publishing; 2022.
64. Benson C. Diffuse axonal injury. In: Aminoff MJ, Daroff RB, eds. *Encyclopedia of the Neurological Sciences* 2nd ed. Oxford: Academic Press; 2014:998–9.
65. Silverberg ND, Iaccarino MA, Panenka WJ; American Congress of Rehabilitation Medicine Brain Injury Interdisciplinary Special Interest Group Mild TBI Task Force, et al. Management of concussion and mild traumatic brain injury: a synthesis of practice guidelines. *Arch Phys Med Rehabil.* 2020;101(2):382–93.

Cervical Spine

49

Aaron Bolds and Bryan Murtaugh

BACKGROUND

- Sports-related cervical spine injuries, while relatively uncommon, can be season ending, career ending, life altering, or even fatal.
- While the spectrum of cervical injuries includes more serious, permanently disabling injuries, most are ligament sprains, muscle strains, or contusions (1).
- The sports medicine physician can take steps to help prevent catastrophic neck injuries in athletes. The training of physicians who wish to care for athletes, therefore, should impart an understanding of the mechanisms and management of cervical spine injuries.
- The percentage of cervical spine injuries associated with certain sports varies by region. For example, those occurring in ice hockey are higher in Canada, whereas rugby injuries are more common in Europe, South Africa, and Australia (2).
- Regardless of the sport, the principles for management of athletic cervical spine injuries remain constant.

EPIDEMIOLOGY

- There are approximately 17,000 spinal cord injuries yearly in the United States, with 10% sustained by athletes (3).
- Sports with a greater risk of cervical spine injuries include diving, football, rugby, surfing, skiing, boxing, ice hockey, wrestling, and gymnastics (4).
- A five-year epidemiology study in the National Collegiate Athletic Association looked at data across 22 different varsity collegiate sports, which showed an estimated 11,510 neck and cervical spine injuries over this 5-year period.
- In sex-comparable sports, there was a 1.36 times increase in cervical spine injuries in men versus women (5).
- While the prevalence of sports-related cervical spine injuries has not been adequately researched, it is estimated that 10%–15% of football players may experience a soft-tissue or neurologic injury of the cervical spine that results in time loss from sport (6).
- A 10-year epidemiology study collected data on cervical spine injuries in high school athletes in the United States, which showed a cervical spine injury rate of 3.04 per 100,000 exposures.
- Overall, the most common mechanisms of injury were player-to-player contact (70.7%) and contact with the playing surface (16.1%) (7).
- In football, those most at risk play defensive positions, that is defensive backs, linemen, and linebackers (8,9).
- The prevalence of the stinger or burner (*i.e.*, neurapraxic injury to the nerve root or brachial plexus) is reported to be ≥50% in football players (10).
- Helmets have decreased fatalities but may have increased the risk of nonfatal cervical spine injury due to the emergence of spear tackling and by imparting a sense of invincibility to the athlete in their "armor" (11).

FUNCTIONAL ANATOMY

- There are seven cervical vertebrae and eight exiting nerve roots.
- The cranium articulates with C1 at the atlanto-occipital joint, where approximately 50% of all flexion and extension occur (the "yes" joint). The first and second cervical vertebrae form the atlantoaxial joint and are uniquely designed to allow for 50% of all cervical rotatory motion (the "no" joint).
- Lateral bending occurs coupled with rotation via motion from C3 to C7.
- Intervertebral discs between C2 and C7 serve to dissipate and transmit compressive or axial loads.
- The discs are thicker anteriorly and this design contributes to the normal cervical lordosis.
- Normal sagittal diameter of the cervical spinal canal between C3 and C7 is ≥15 mm, and spinal stenosis is suggested and may be present below 13 mm. Functional spinal stenosis refers to the loss of protective cushioning from cerebrospinal fluid around the spinal cord as documented on magnetic resonance imaging (MRI), computed tomography (CT), or myelography (12).
- Each nerve root occupies between 25% and 33% of the neural foramen, which is bordered by the uncovertebral joints anteromedially, the intervertebral disc medially, the zygapophyseal or facet joints posterolaterally, and superiorly/inferiorly by the

pedicles of adjoining vertebrae. Degenerative arthritic changes of any of the structures that form or border the foramina may contribute to nerve root compression.

- From C2 to C7, the nerve roots exit above their corresponding numbered vertebral body, whereas C1 exits between the occiput and atlas, and C8 exits between the C7 and T1 vertebrae (13).
- There is a 45° facet angle in lower cervical segments (C3–C7), which allow for cervical flexion and extension and limit axial rotation (2).
- The cervical spine depends on both static (*i.e.*, osseocartilaginous and ligamentous) and dynamic (*i.e.*, musculotendinous) stabilizing factors to absorb and/or dissipate forces.
- Pain in the cervical spine is mediated by free nerve endings in the outer one-third of the annulus fibrosus of each intervertebral disc, in the zygapophyseal (facet) joints, in the ligaments (*i.e.*, posterior longitudinal ligament, ligamentum flavum, interspinous and supraspinous ligaments), and in the supporting musculature.

SPORT-SPECIFIC BIOMECHANICS

- The cervical spine is normally able to absorb significant multidirectional external forces by virtue of several supportive mechanisms.
- The cervical lordosis aids in dissipating axial loads through the intervertebral discs, facet joints, interspinous ligaments, and paraspinal muscles.
- Once cervical flexion occurs past 30°, the lordosis is lost, which is synonymous to tucking chin during a tackle or prior to impact. Forces applied in this position are no longer dissipated through the surrounding cervical anatomy, and instead straight down the spinal column (2).
- Axial loading has been shown to be the mechanism of catastrophic cervical spine injury in all National Football League (NFL) cases that were documented well enough to allow detailed analysis (14).
- Hyperflexion or hyperextension of the cervical spine in an athlete with a congenitally or developmentally narrowed canal may cause neurologic injury by a *pincer* mechanism (15).
- External forces that cause a combination of lateral bending and extension may lead to neuroforaminal compression and the neurologic injury commonly called a stinger or burner.
- A second proposed mechanism for the stinger or burner is flexion or extension combined with lateral bending and ipsilateral shoulder depression resulting in a traction injury to the cervical nerve roots.
- Acceleration/deceleration forces, such as those that occur in whiplash injuries, occur commonly in contact/collision sports and commonly cause injury to the muscular or ligamentous supports (cervical strain/sprain) or the cervical facet joints.

CLINICAL FEATURES

Differential Diagnosis of Neck Pain in the Athlete

- Cervical muscle strain or ligament sprain
- Herniated nucleus pulposus
- Burner/stinger (*i.e.*, cervical nerve root, brachial plexus, or peripheral nerve neurapraxia)
- Cervical radiculopathy
- Brachial plexopathy
- Fracture or dislocation
- Facet arthropathy
- Medical causes of neck pain, such as cardiovascular (myocardial infarction), endocrine (thyroid), pulmonary (pneumomediastinum), or infection (osteomyelitis or diskitis)

History

- Sideline physicians at an athletic event should keep in mind that most cervical spine injuries in athletes are cervical sprains or strains, followed by the stinger or burner. Fortunately, fracture-dislocation injuries are rare (16).
- That said, the sports medicine physician must err on the side of caution. Neck pain in any downed athlete is treated as an unstable cervical spine injury until proven otherwise.
- The stinger or burner (cervical nerve root, brachial plexus, or peripheral nerve neurapraxia) typically involves the C5 and C6 innervated muscles (*i.e.*, deltoid, biceps, and rotator cuff), and so the athlete may complain of an inability to raise the arm (17).
- Head injuries frequently occur concomitantly with spinal injuries. An athlete with both a suspected concussion and neck pain should be considered to have a cervical spine injury until proven otherwise.
- The examiner should always inquire about the following:
  - Neck, shoulder, arm, and leg pain
  - Arm or leg numbness, tingling, or weakness
- Rule of thumb (simple guidelines):
  - Symptoms in one arm → peripheral nerve injury
  - Symptoms in two arms or in one or both legs → spinal cord injury
  - Signs of head injury such as headache, blurred vision, dizziness, and disorientation
  - Previous head or neck injuries
  - Bowel or bladder dysfunction
  - Prior treatments and functional status (if not seen acutely)
- It is important to know your athletes and inquire about any history of cervical spine injuries or congenital canal stenosis.
- Athletes with Down syndrome (trisomy 21) and rheumatoid arthritis may be at increased risk for rupture of the transverse and/or alar ligaments and atlantoaxial instability.

Minor trauma in such persons may cause complete atlanto-axial dissociation.

Physical Examination

- Physical exam should begin with a primary survey and quickly evaluating CAB (circulation, airway, and breathing).
- After primary survey, be sure to use history and clinical judgment to rule out cervical instability prior to moving the athlete. If cervical spine instability is suspected, immobilize the spine-injured athlete immediately to prevent further neurologic deterioration (18).
  - Inspection for the normal spinal curvature, ecchymosis, laceration, and obvious deformity
  - Palpation for deformity or step-off and bony or soft-tissue tenderness
  - Range of motion (ROM), including flexion, extension, lateral bending, and rotation
  - Strength examination via manual muscle testing
  - Sensation testing in all cervical dermatomes
  - Reflex assessment of the C5 (biceps), C6 (brachioradialis), C6/7 (pronator), and C7 (triceps), as well as the L4 (patellar), L5 (medial hamstring), and S1 (Achilles) myotomes
  - Pathologic reflex testing (Hoffman and Babinski)
  - Special tests such as the Spurling and Lhermitte signs

DIAGNOSTIC STUDIES

Imaging

- Plain radiographs are appropriate if osseoligamentous disruption is a concern or in cases of recurrent stingers or burners or cervical cord neurapraxia. Anterior-posterior, lateral, and open-mouth views should always be obtained. Flexion and extension views may be indicated to rule out abnormal segmental motion.
- Studies of intact cadaver cervical spine segments have shown that horizontal movement of one vertebra on the next does not normally exceed 3.5 mm, and the angular displacement of one vertebral body on another is always ≤11°. These measurements may be made with lateral neutral or flexion/extension radiographs. One caveat, however, is that younger athletes are more likely to demonstrate ligamentous laxity, and these criteria may not always be applicable (1,17,19,20).
- The Torg-Pavlov ratio compares the diameter of the spinal canal to that of the vertebral body. A ratio of less than 0.8 is used to predict cervical stenosis and has been found commonly in persons with an episode of transient cervical cord neurapraxia. The ratio has been found, however, to have low positive predictive value for determining future injury. It is not, therefore, a recommended screening tool.
- However, MRI signal changes (T2 signal hyperintensity) after cervical cord injury should be used in conjunction with Torg-Pavlov ratio when considering return-to-play (RTP) decision and an athlete's risk for further injury (21).
- Advanced imaging modalities have also provided improved screening parameters. The mean subaxial cervical space available for the spinal cord is more accurate and has a higher positive predictive ratio than Torg-Pavlov ratio. This could have application in regard to chronic stingers and deciding on RTP (22).
- A diagnosis of "spear tackler's spine" constitutes an absolute contraindication to participation in collision sports. It is identified as follows:
  - Developmental cervical canal stenosis
  - Reversal of the normal cervical lordosis on lateral radiographs
  - Preexisting posttraumatic radiographic abnormalities of the cervical spine
  - Documentation of the athlete having used spear tackling techniques
- Advanced imaging such as a CT scan is recommended to investigate a clinically suspected fracture when plain radiographs are unrevealing or equivocal. CT scan with myelography is a sensitive measure of spinal stenosis.
- MRI is used to evaluate soft tissues for ligamentous disruption or herniated nucleus pulposus and can also demonstrate spinal cord contusions. T2-weighted images may be used to determine the extent of *functional* reserve, the protective cushioning of cerebrospinal fluid around the spinal cord.

Electrodiagnostics

- Electromyography and nerve conduction studies (EMG/NCS) may be useful in evaluating an athlete after neurologic insult with persistent motor or sensory abnormalities. Such testing can help delineate whether the lesion is at the level of the nerve root, brachial plexus, or peripheral nerve.
- EMG and NCS are typically utilized at least 2–3 weeks after an injury. This is secondary to Wallerian degeneration, which is retrograde degeneration of an axon's distal end after a nerve lesion (23) (see Chapter 24 for a further discussion of Electrodiagnostic Testing).

TREATMENT

- The sideline physician should ensure that an emergency action plan (EAP) is in place and that all equipment, including an automated external defibrillator, is available. The EAP should be reviewed and rehearsed at least yearly with medical staff (see Chapter 15, Sideline Emergencies).
- There should also be awareness of where the ambulance entrance to the field is and which hospital athletes will be transported to in case of emergency.
- Sideline management of any athlete with neck pain or tenderness and neurologic symptoms, excluding those with a

clear diagnosis of a stinger or burner, includes immobilizing the athlete on a spine board and emergent transport to a trauma center for evaluation by a spine specialist.

- Cervical injury red flags to be aware of include:
  - Bilateral symptoms
  - Unconscious athlete
  - Focal C-spine tenderness to palpation
  - Paralysis
  - Apprehension to or restriction to ROM
- In these events, the helmet should not be removed. However, in the event of altered mental status or loss of airway, the face mask can be removed. If helmet or pads must be removed, they should be removed together and only if trainers and physicians are trained in equipment removal (24).
- Fractures should be referred to an orthopedic spine specialist for definitive treatment.
- Cervical sprains or strains are generally self-limited injuries managed with relative rest, icing, nonsteroidal anti-inflammatory medications for pain and inflammation, and early mobilization and strengthening in a pain-free ROM.
- There is no benefit to using a soft cervical collar for cervical sprains or strains other than perhaps providing a sense of security and local warmth. In fact, the use of a collar can delay recovery by causing a decrease in cervical spine ROM.
- Stingers or burners are generally self-limited, with symptom resolution in minutes to hours. Once an athlete's neurologic examination has normalized, a tailored rehabilitation program should be instituted to prevent recurrence.
- Unresolved neurologic symptoms should be observed closely for progression and further assessment.

REHABILITATION

- Rehabilitation is the cornerstone of ensuring prompt return of an athlete to competition and for preventing recurrent injury. Alternative methods of conditioning should be used while the athlete is kept out of play.
- Cervical spine and concussion can occur concurrently. In this case, rehabilitation should include concussion protocol as well, such as balance and vestibular-ocular training.
- The sports rehabilitation paradigm is as follows:
  - Decrease pain and inflammation.
  - Restore pain-free, full cervical spine ROM.
  - Optimize head and neck posture.
  - Strengthen the cervical spine musculature (dynamic stabilizers), scapular stabilizers, upper extremities, and trunk.
  - Maintain cardiovascular endurance according to the demands of the sport.
  - Direct sport-specific training.
  - Review and refine specific techniques such as tackling skills. Determine, if possible, the issues surrounding the initial injury.
  - Restore muscular imbalances, which can be risk factors for cervical injuries.
  - Optimize use of well-fitted protective gear (*e.g.*, pads, collars).

RTP GUIDELINES

- RTP decisions should be determined on a case-by-case basis, given the variety in mechanisms, severity, and complexity of injuries.
- Several authors have published guidelines to assist clinicians in determining when an athlete should be allowed to return to collision sports following a cervical spine injury (1,16,19). All of these guidelines are based on expert opinion (Table 49.1).
- In general, RTP may be contemplated when the athlete:
  - Demonstrates full and pain-free ROM.
- Displays a normal neurologic examination including strength, sensation, and reflexes.
- Does not have an osseous or unstable ligamentous injury.
- Controversy exists over returning an athlete to sport after sustaining an episode of cervical cord neurapraxia (transient quadriparesis).
- Burners or stingers are common cervical injuries and approximately 85% of collision athletes who experience them are not kept from subsequent practices or games (22).
  - After sustaining one stinger in a game, the player can RTP with complete symptom resolution and baseline exam. Consensus is that a player should not return to a game if multiple stingers occur in that game.
  - If there are three or more stingers in a season, the athlete should sit out the remainder of the season, or at least until potential congenital anomalies, foramina cervical stenosis, or further cord compromise is ruled out (22).
- Intervertebral disc pathology requiring nonsurgical management is safe for RTP if there is normal strength, pain-free ROM, and neurological exam is intact.
  - If surgery such as anterior cervical discectomy and fusion is performed at one level, there can be RTP once fusion is solid, there is full strength and painless ROM, and no MRI T2 signal changes. However, 2- and 3-level procedures are relative (granted no MRI T2 signal changes) and absolute contraindications, respectively, for RTP (21).
  - In 2011, a research group examined NFL athletes who underwent single-level operative treatment for cervical disk herniations. They found that those undergoing single-level spine surgery returned to play at a higher rate compared to nonsurgical (72% and 46%, respectively) (25).
    - The operative group returned to play for 29 games over a 2.8-year span and the nonoperative group returned to play for 15 games over a 1.5-year span. This was statistically significant, given the average NFL career is 3.5 years (25).

Table 49.1 Torg and Ramsey-Emrhein Collision Sport Participation Guidelines

No Contraindication
Congenital
Spina bifida occulta
Type II Klippel-Feil at C3 and below, if no signs or symptoms of cervical spine pathology
Developmental
Torg-Pavlov ratio <0.8 if asymptomatic
Nondisplaced stable healed fracture at compression or endplate, no posterior involvement, or clay shoveler's fracture
Healed herniated nucleus pulposus
One-level fusion
Relative Contraindication
Developmental
Torg-Pavlov ratio <0.8, with motor and/or sensory neurapraxia
Previous episodes of neurapraxia
Two-level fusions
Healed but displaced stable fracture C3–C7 at posterior ring or compression fracture
Healed, nondisplaced stable fracture C1–C2
Instability <3.5 mm or 11°
Healed herniated nucleus pulposus with residual facet instability
Absolute Contraindication
Congenital
Odontoid (C2) abnormalities such as odontoid agenesis, odontoid hypoplasia, or os odontoideum
Atlantooccipital fusion
C1–C2 anomaly or fusion
Klippel-Feil anomaly with congenital fusion of one or more vertebral segments and a loss of segmental motion, instability, disc disease, degenerative changes, or occipitocervical anomalies
Developmental
Spear tackler's spine
Residual pain or limited range of motion
Acute fracture or central herniated nucleus pulposus
Recurrent cervical cord neurapraxia
Fracture or ligamentous laxity at C1–C2
Acute or chronic hard disc
C1–C2 fusion
Instability >3.5 mm or 11°
Body fracture with sagittal compression, arch fracture, ligament injury, and fragmentation at canal
Lateral mass fracture with facet incongruity
≥Three-level fusion

Source: Malanga GA. The diagnosis and treatment of cervical radiculopathy. *Med Sci Sports Exerc.* 1997;29(7 suppl):S236–45; Torg JS, Guille JT, Jaffe S. Current concepts review — injuries to the cervical spine in American football players. *J Bone Joint Surg Am.* 2002;84–A(1):112–22; Hsu WK. Outcomes Following nonoperative and operative treatment for cervical disc herniations in National Football League athletes. *Spine.* 2011;36(10):800–5.

- Guidelines for deciding RTP for episodes of cervical cord neuropraxia:
  - Canal/vertebral body ratio of 0.8 or less is not a contraindication for RTP in an asymptomatic athlete.
  - Canal/vertebral body ratio of 0.8 or less and one episode of cervical cord neuropraxia is a relative contraindication for RTP.
  - >1 episode of cervical cord neuropraxia with intervertebral disc disease and/or degenerative changes is a relative contraindication for RTP.
  - Episode of cervical cord neuropraxia with MRI evidence of cord defect or cord edema is controversial and viewed as either relative or absolute contraindication.
  - Episode of cervical cord neurapraxia with ligamentous instability or neurological symptoms that persists >36 hours is an absolute contraindication (16).
- Most cervical fractures have no contraindications for RTP if it is healed, stable, and the athlete has no residual symptoms (neurological or strength deficits, pain, ROM restrictions). However, the following fractures are exceptions.
- Fractures absolutely contraindicated for RTP include:
  - Acute cervical fractures
  - Cervical vertebral body fractures with sagittal component or involving posterior elements
  - Fracture leading to retropulsion and canal compromise (16)
- Fractures that have relative contraindications include:
  - Healed, stable displaced vertebral body
  - Healed, stable fractures involving posterior elements (16)
- Congenital anomalies seen as absolute contraindications to contact sports include:
  - Odontoid genesis, odontoid hypoplasia, and os odontoidium are absolute contraindications to collision activities because of the associated C1–C2 instability (16).
  - Atlantooccipital fusion in isolation or in conjunction with other abnormalities
  - Klippel-Feil anomaly is characterized by congenital fusion of two or more cervical vertebrae.
  - All lesion types of Klippel-Feil anomalies are absolute contraindications to collision activities except type II, given the athlete has full cervical ROM and no occipitocervical anomalies, instability, disc disease, or degenerative changes (16).

PREVENTION

- Programs are being implemented to teach proper safety protocols at an early age. The goal is to educate youth football athletes so that they can utilize these techniques as they age and continue to play.
- Heads Up Football instructs coaches on health and safety protocols as well as on-field fundamentals, which include proper equipment fitting and shoulder tackling and blocking.

- Reductions in the numbers of cervical spine injuries in sport can be made by the following:
  - Rule changes: In the NFL, for instance, rule changes in 1976 eliminated the head as an initial contact area for blocking and tackling. Coaches are encouraged to instruct players to block and tackle with their head up. Spearing with the head has been banned.
  - Conditioning exercises to strengthen the neck and sports-specific training
  - Prohibiting spearing or tackling using the head as a battering ram or grabbing the face mask
  - Strict enforcement of the rules by officials and intolerance of illegal play
  - Understand that football players playing defensive positions are more likely to sustain a catastrophic injury, so safe blocking and tackling techniques should be reinforced and stressed.
  - Ensuring that equipment properly fits
  - Expert on-site medical care: A certified athletic trainer and, if possible, a sports medicine physician should be available at the playing field. A plan for managing a catastrophic neck injury must be rehearsed and be in place.
  - Any athlete with a suspected head or neck injury should be managed as if they have an unstable cervical spine fracture until proven otherwise. The player should be instructed not to move, the head and neck should be immobilized, and trained professionals should coordinate safe transfer onto a spine board and referral to a trauma center.
  - When possible, identifying congenital anomalies of the spine through a thorough preparticipation history and physical examination

REFERENCES

1. Cantu RC. Cervical spine injuries in the athlete. *Semin Neurol.* 2000;20(2):173–8.
2. Oshlag B, Ray T, Boswell B. Neck injuries. *Prim Care.* 2020 Mar;47(1):165–76.
3. National Spinal Cord Injury Statistical Center. *Facts and Figures at a Glance.* Birmingham, (AL): University of Alabama at Birmingham; 2019.
4. Vaccaro AR, Watkins B, Albert TJ, Pfaff WL, Klein GR, Silber JS. Cervical spine injuries in athletes: current return-to-play criteria. *Orthopedics.* 2001;24(7):699–705.
5. Deckey D, Makovicka J, Chung A, et al. Neck and cervical spine injuries in National College Athletic Association athletes. A 5-year epidemiologic study. *Spine.* 2020;45(1):55–64.
6. Meyer SA, Schulte KR, Callaghan JJ, et al. Cervical spinal stenosis and stingers in collegiate football players. *Am J Sports Med.* 1994;22(2):158–66.
7. Meron A, McMullen C, Laker S, Currie D, Comstock D. Epidemiology of cervical spine injuries in high school athletes over a ten-year period. *PM&R J.* 2018;10(4):365–72.
8. Cantu RC, Mueller FO. Catastrophic football injuries: 1977–1998. *Neurosurgery.* 2000;47(3):673–7.
9. Castro FP Jr, Ricciardi J, Brunet ME, Busch MT, Whitecloud TS III, Whitecloud TS III. Stingers, the Torg ratio, and the cervical spine. *Am J Sports Med.* 1997;25(5):603–8.
10. Levitz CL, Reilly PJ, Torg JS. The pathomechanics of chronic, recurrent cervical nerve root neurapraxia. The chronic burner syndrome. *Am J Sports Med.* 1997;25(1):73–6.
11. Torg JS, Vegso JJ, Sennett B, Das M. The National football head and neck injury registry. 14-Year report on cervical quadriplegia, 1971 through 1984. *JAMA.* 1985;254(24):3439–43.
12. Cantu RC, Bailes JE, Wilberger JE Jr. Guidelines for return to contact or collision sport after a cervical spine injury. *Clin Sports Med.* 1998;17(1):137–46.
13. Malanga GA. The diagnosis and treatment of cervical radiculopathy. *Med Sci Sports Exerc.* 1997;29(7 Suppl):S236–45.
14. Torg JS, Guille JT, Jaffe S. Current concepts review — injuries to the cervical spine in American football players. *J Bone Joint Surg Am.* 2002;84-A(1):112–22.
15. Penning L. Some aspects of plain radiography of the cervical spine in chronic myelopathy. *Neurology.* 1962;12:513–9.
16. Torg JS, Ramsey-Emrhein JA. Management guidelines for participation in collision activities with congenital, developmental, or post-injury lesions involving the cervical spine. *Clin J Sport Med.* 1997;7(4):273–91.
17. Feinberg JH. Burners and stingers. *Phys Med Rehabil Clin N Am.* 2000;11(4):771–84.
18. McAlindon RJ. On field evaluation and management of head and neck injured athletes. *Clin Sports Med.* 2002;21(1):1–14.
19. Morganti C, Sweeney CA, Albanese SA, Burak C, Hosea T, Connolly PJ. Return to play after cervical spine injury. *Spine.* 2001;26(10):1131–6.
20. White AA III, Johnson RM, Panjabi MM, Southwick WO. Biomechanical analysis of clinical stability in the cervical spine. *Clin Orthop Relat Res.* 1975;109:85–96.
21. Schroeder G, Vaccaro A. Cervical spine injuries in the athlete. *J Am Acad Orthop Surg.* 2016;24:122–33.
22. Bowles D, Canseco J, Alexander T, Schroeder G, Hecht A, Vaccaro A. The prevalence and management of stingers in college and professional collision athletes. *Curr Rev Musculoskelet Med.* 2020;13(6):651–62.
23. Preston D, Shapiro B. *Electromyography and Neuromuscular Disorders: Clinical-Electrophysiologic-Ultrasound Correlations.* 4th ed. Elsevier Health Sciences; 2020. 720 p.
24. Usman S. Management of head and neck injuries by the sideline physician. *Am Fam Physician.* 2022;106(5):543–8.
25. Hsu WK. Outcomes Following nonoperative and operative treatment for cervical disc herniations in National Football League athletes. *Spine.* 2011;36(10):800–5.

Thoracic and Lumbar Spine

50

Luke Mugge, Reginald S. Fayssoux, and John Hamilton

INTRODUCTION

- Nonspecific low back pain is a commonly encountered pathology that contributes to significant disease burden worldwide (1). It is a frequent complaint and source of morbidity among athletes in all sports and accounts for as much as 5%–8% of all injuries (2).
- While the treatments available are numerous, the diverse etiologies that contribute to low back pain make appropriate application unclear and challenging (3).
- Sports are common contributors to low back pain and spine injuries in general. Nearly 15% of all spinal cord injuries, including cervical, thoracic, and lumbar in the United States, are related in some way to sports or other recreational activities. The distribution across sports is not homogeneous, as certain mechanics involved in sports predispose to injury more frequently than others. Despite the relative prevalence of spinal injuries in various sports, little has been done in the way of prevention; winter sports stand as an example (4).

EPIDEMIOLOGY

- Musculoligamentous injury is common in sports that require truncal or axial rotation including golf, tennis, and basketball. This is commonly contrasted with contact sports such as basketball, football, and soccer or sports that resulted in injury due to repetition such as gymnastics, swimming, diving, or volleyball. Specifically, American football, ice hockey, and rugby, full contact sports, are notorious for causing spinal cord injury. This is particularly true of the cervical spine (see Chapter 49, Cervical Spine). And while the thoracic and lumbar spine are less commonly involved, injuries to other segments of the spine are possible. This is because the sports listed above involve axial loading or forward flexing of the neck, making it prone to injury (5). Conversely, spondylolisthesis and malalignment can result from lumbar hyperextension.
- The conditions and high-speed nature of some winter sports, specifically downhill skiing and snowboarding, are frequently associated with spinal cord injury. Risk factors with the sports include poorly groomed slopes, equipment failure, unfavorable weather conditions, overcrowded skiing slopes, and loss of control (6). Jumping associated with freestyle versions of winter sports is also a common contributor to injuries being responsible for approximately 80% of spinal injuries and typically affecting the thoracolumbar region (7). Further, snowboarders are much more likely to suffer injury compared to skiers because snowboarders have their feet fastened to the board where skiers do not (8).
- As patients age, low back pain and spinal cord injury in general become more prevalent. Degenerative changes, which occur with aging throughout the spine, contribute to stenosis and decrease the physiological reserve of the spine while increasing its rigidity. This process challenges both prevention and diagnosis and treatment. Decisions regarding return to play (RTP) and recommendations for appropriate activities in elderly patient populations are complicated, especially if patients have had prior surgery or known stenosis, which may predispose them to further injury.

ANATOMY

- The spine is a complex neuromuscular structure with osseous components and needs to be understood in all of its intricacies in order to appreciate the full spectrum of possible injury, permit accurate diagnosis, and assign the most appropriate treatment.
- The purpose of the spine is to provide support to the rest of the appendicular skeleton while simultaneously providing protection for the enclosed neural structures. Every aspect of the spine from the osseous anatomy, the articulating structures, the intervertebral discs, the muscular ligamentous complex, and nerve structures is subject to injury during any number of activities.

Osseous Anatomy

- The spinal column is the foundation of the axial skeleton and extends from the pelvis to the cranial base. It articulates directly with the skull at the occipital condyles most cranially and with the pelvis via the sacrum most caudally. The midsection articulates with the rib cage. The spinal column can be subdivided into five different segments. There are 7 cervical, 12 thoracic, 5 lumbar, 5 sacral, and 5 coccygeal vertebrae.

Each subdivision of the spine has unique anatomical features that render it susceptible to various kinds of injury and fractures.

- In the normal anatomical position, the head is situated directly over the pelvis. The spine is not straight in the sagittal plane. The cervical spine is lordotic, the thoracic spine is kyphotic, and the lumbar spine is lordotic again. Appropriate amounts of kyphosis and lordosis are needed to maintain normal posture. The relative degree of kyphosis and lordosis is in part due to the anatomical shape of the vertebral bodies in each corresponding segment of the spine. An additional component is the intervertebral disc. The combination of the intervertebral discs and proper spine alignment provides resiliency to axial loading as well as flexing and extending. In contrast to the sagittal plane with the lordosis and kyphosis, the spine should be completely straight in the coronal plane. In the absence of congenital deformity or trauma, the head will be centered over the pelvis in both the coronal and sagittal planes. When this occurs, the spine is considered "balanced."
- In the cervical spine, the most anterior portion of the vertebrae is the vertebral body itself. This is a round-shaped bone. Directly lateral to this are the lateral masses. These are connected by pedicles. More posteriorly, the lamina projects from each lateral mass. These join and form the posterior spinous process. The facets, in the cervical spine, are along the superior and inferior portions of the lateral masses. Most laterally, there are transverse processes extending laterally from the lateral masses. See Chapter 49, Cervical Spine, for further discussion.
- For the thoracic spine, the vertebral body is larger. In this case, there are no lateral masses and the pedicles terminate in the pars. The pars is the confluence of the lamina, the pedicle, the transverse process, and the facet. The transverse process, in the thoracic spine, articulates with ribs directly. Like the cervical spine, the laminae conjoin posteriorly to form the spinous process, which projects inferiorly in thoracic spine. The vertebral bodies in this segment are often wedge-shaped, which aids in normal kyphosis over this area. However, if there is greater than 5° of anterior wedging in the thoracic spine over more than three contiguous vertebrae, a diagnosis of Scheuermann's kyphosis should be applied (9). This diagnosis should be considered when patients have abnormal posture, despite efforts to stand up straight. The thoracic spine is inherently more stable than the other segments, secondary to the rib cage and sternum, which provide anterior support and serve to limit overall segmental mobility.
- The lumbar spine has the largest vertebral bodies. Like the thoracic spine, the pedicles extend from the vertebral body and continue to the pars, a confluence of the superior and inferior articulating facets, the lamina, and the pars. The transverse processes extend laterally from the pars. Posteriorly, the lamina forms the spinous process. The transition zone between the thoracic and lumbar spine (T12 and L1) is a significant site of injury (10). The reason for the high concentration of injuries in this segment of the spine is a subject of debate. It is speculated that the transition between a semirigid thoracic spine to a highly mobile lumbar spine stresses the region beyond capacity. Even under normal conditions, this area has a high degree of physiologic mobility.
- The sacral spine under normal circumstances is a nonmobile segment. These five vertebrae are fused together and join laterally with the sacral ala. The sacrum is important in two ways. First, it functions to join the spine with the pelvis. And second, it forms the most posterior portion of the pelvic ring. From a biomechanical perspective, it transitions the weight of the upper body into the lower appendicular skeleton.
- Regardless of the level of the spine or the vertebrae considered, each vertebra is composed of a thin cortical bone that surrounds a soft or trabecular cancellous bone. This is analogous to many other long bones in the body. This anatomical consideration is most important in the context of elderly patients where osteoporosis may play a role. Softening of the outer cortical bone as a result of this disease process increases frequency of compression fractures (11). These fractures are more commonly seen in the lower segments of the spine where axial loading forces increase in an upright posture and as the segments are more involved in weight bearing.

Articular Anatomy

- Not only is the bony anatomy unique throughout the spinal column, but the joint anatomy, or more accurately, the facet, is also unique. The facets are different among the cervical, thoracic, and lumbar spine. Each has implications for associated pathology. The facets are crucial for posterior linkage of the vertebral bodies and distinctly important in facilitating normal spine motion. The facets are superior and posteriorly oriented within the cervical spine. In the thoracic spine, they are posteriorly oriented. Facets in the lumbar spine lie medial to lateral and superior in orientation. The orientation of the facets is central to the motion that it permits. For example, in the cervical spine, the more superior orientation of the facets permits flexion, extension, and rotational movement. The more sagittal plain facets of the thoracic spine predominantly support extension and flexion. The medial to lateral orientation of the lumbar spine facets allow for rotational movement in addition to extension and flexion.
- Apart from their structure, facets can also contribute to spinal pathology. An essential component to degenerative spine disease is facet hypertrophy and degeneration. Instability of the joint and compensatory hypertrophy of the capsule can cause compression of neural elements. This causes direct compression because of the facet's posterior orientation in relation to the exiting nerve root. A more detailed description of the nerve anatomy is provided below. As the facet hypertrophies, it will cause compression both on the exiting nerve root and on the thecal sac, which is located medially and ventrally. Degenerative pain and spondylolisthesis, described more completely below, can result from facet joint dysfunction

where the joint instability causes one vertebral body to slip on the other, resulting in pain directly from its disassociation. In isolation, facet disease can cause mechanical back pain.

- Beyond the facet joints between the vertebral bodies, the costovertebral joints, located between the ribs and the vertebral bodies of the thoracic spine, are an additional location of pathology. These, like the facet joints, or synovial joints permit articulation between the rib head in the transverse process of the associated thoracic spine vertebral body. The final joints of significance in this region are the costochondral joints, which form the articulations between the distal rib in the sternum ventrally. These potentially can be involved in costochondritis.

Intervertebral Disc Anatomy

- Intervertebral discs are another critical portion to the spinal column. Discs contribute to the spine's overall mobility and alignment. Anatomically, intervertebral discs are present in the thoracic and lumbar spine. There are no discs between the lateral masses in the cervical spine, and the sacral spine is fused. Discs are also subject to significant degradation with age, a source of major pathology, and often responsible for low back pain.
- The disc itself is composed of two layers in the outer fibrous annulus and an inner nucleus pulposus. The outer fibrous annulus is a thick ring composed of fibrocartilaginous material situated in concentric rings. The inner nucleus pulposus is the remnant of the embryonic notochord. It is a loose, gelatinous, and randomly oriented collagen matrix, composed mostly of glycosaminoglycans and water.
- As patients age, the water content in the disc decreases, lowering overall disc volume, which results in a decreased disc height. This has implications for spinal alignment particularly in the thoracic spine. With age, decreased disc height secondary to loss of water in the disc itself increases the thoracic kyphosis. More globally, it decreases the patient's height. Additionally, the outer annulus weakens with age or with trauma. When there is a violation of the outer annulus, the inner nucleus can herniate causing compression on neural elements.
- The disks themselves are situated against the hyaline cartilage, which lies between the disc and the vertebral end plate. The blood supply to the disc itself is obliterated in the first 3 decades of life. With this cessation of blood flow, a rapid decrease in dispersion of nutrients occurs. Afterward, the disc must rely on diffusion to get nutrients from the end plate. Together, this results in an overall decline in disc health with age that further contributes to the loss in height and discogenic disease seen in later decades.

Musculoligamentous Anatomy

- The ligamentous anatomy of the spine is a complicated network involving all columns of the spine. Starting at the cranial base and extending all the way down to the pelvis, multiple sets of ligaments contribute to its stability. Starting at the cranium, the atlas and the axis, the first two cervical vertebrae, are anchored to the skull by strong alar ligaments and the tectorial membrane. The transverse ligament runs between the lateral masses of C1 and keeps the odontoid process in place. The apical ligament runs from the tip of the odontoid process to the base of the skull. A strong anterior longitudinal ligament (ALL) runs along the ventral portion of the cervical vertebral bodies. There is a weaker posterior longitudinal ligament (PLL), which runs along the dorsal aspect of the cervical vertebral bodies. Between the spinous processes runs the posterior ligamentous complex.
- The ALL and PLL run the full length of the spine and are seen in the thoracic and lumbar spine. Other components of the posterior ligamentous complex include the supraspinous ligament, the inner spinous ligament or nuchal ligament, and the ligamentum flavum, which is over the dorsal surface of the dura in the fibrous capsule of the facet joint. The posterior ligamentous complex plays a critical role in stabilizing the posterior elements of the spine and preventing hyperflexion. Disruption of this ligament, as can occur during significant trauma, results in instability of the spine and kyphosis of that segment. This can occur in the cervical, thoracic, or lumbar segments of the spine.
- As it relates to discogenic disease, the PLL is a thin ligamentous complex in the lumbar spine compared to the ALL. When combined with the relatively weak annulus, as is seen in elderly patients, violation of both layers by a disc can cause direct compression of neural elements, as suggested above. The ligamentum flavum lies just dorsal to the dura. It forms throughout the spinal column as an incomplete, discontinuous layer between two adjacent laminae. With degenerative spinal disease, this ligament hypertrophies, causes direct spinal cord or nerve root compression, and can greatly contribute to central stenosis. This commonly results in a condition known as neurogenic claudication.
- The musculature of the spinal column is a complex network that connects the vertebrate and other components of the appendicular skeleton. Multiple sets of muscles exist in the cervical, thoracic, and lumbar spine and are unique to each area. In the more cephalad region, innervation occurs via the dorsal scapular nerve to the rhomboids and, via the spinal accessory nerve, to the trapezius. All other nerves are innervated by the dorsal rami.
- Anatomically, the musculature can be divided into layers. The most superficial layers, starting cranially and going caudally, are the trapezius, latissimus dorsi, and the dorsal lumbar fascia. Deep to this, in the cervical spine, lies the levator scapulae in the rhomboid major and minor. The deepest layer in the cervical spine includes the semispinalis capitis. The middle layers in the thoracic and lumbar regions include the erector spinal muscle groups consisting of the spinalis, longissimus, and the iliocostalis. Finally, the deepest layer in the thoracolumbar region includes the multifidi, rotatores, and intertransversarii muscles.

Nervous System Anatomy

- Just as the osteocyte anatomy is unique in the different segments of the spine, so is the nervous anatomy. True spinal cord resides in both the cervical and thoracic region. The spinal cord terminates in the conus medullaris, which is typically situated between L1 and L2 of the lumbar spine. If the cord terminates lower than this level, cord tethering via the filum terminale should be considered. Nerve roots come off laterally at both the cervical and thoracic levels. There are eight levels of cervical nerve roots and 12 levels of thoracic nerve roots. The nerve roots in the lumbar spine emerge from the conus medullaris and travel down in a bundle known as the cauda equina. These nerve roots exit the spinal canal in both the lumbar and sacral portions. Laterally, the nerve exits between the vertebral bodies through an opening called the foramen, which is composed of the pedicles and facets of the vertebral bodies positioned superior and inferiorly. The nerve root then divides into ventral and dorsal rami after it has exited the framing.
- After exiting the foramen and contributing to the ventral rami, the nerve roots from the cervical spine, beginning at C5 and extending down to T1, coalesce to form the brachial plexus. As they exit, they are situated in the center of the foramen. These nerve roots then serve to innervate the musculature of the upper appendages. Throughout the thoracic spine region, nerve roots exit through the foramen and innervate the spinal erector muscles. Similar to the cervical spine, the nerve root is positioned in the center of the foramen. Nerve roots in the lumbar spine and upper portion of the sacral spine merge together to form the lumbosacral plexus after they leave the spinal canal. These nerve roots are then responsible for the innervation of the musculature of the lower extremities. The sinuvertebral nerve is a sensory nerve that originates in the periphery and coalesces to contribute to the dorsal root ganglia prior to entering the spinal column. It supplies sensation to the PLL, the posterior annulus of the disc, and the posterior vertebral body. It is one of the nerves thought to be responsible for causing low back pain.
- The orientation of the nerve root in the frame and found in the lumbar spine differs significantly compared to the orientation in the cervical and thoracic spine. Here, the nerve root hugs the inferior border of the pedicle as it exits via the lateral recess and finally through the framing. Because of this orientation, it is subject to compression by disc herniation. As the nerve traverses the level above, it is susceptible to compression by a paracentral disc herniation. In the foreman, it is susceptible to compression by the disc at the same level. This herniation must occur laterally in order to produce compression. For example, an L4-L5 paracentral disc herniation will injure the traversing L5 nerve root. Conversely, a foraminal or lateral disc herniation will injure the exiting nerve root at that level. Very large disc herniations that occur centrally in the lumbar spine will cause significant compression of the cauda equina. This results in cauda equina syndrome where patients present with urinary retention, fecal incontinence, satellite esthesia, and significant lower extremity weakness and the inability to walk.

INITIAL EVALUATION

- While certain sports carry a more elevated risk of spinal column and spinal cord injury compared to others, physicians should always have an awareness that such injuries can occur with all sports. The on-field management algorithm for injured athletes with suspected spinal cord trauma is discussed more comprehensively elsewhere in this text. In brief, the main goals of on field treatment in a patient with a suspected spinal cord injury revolve around prevention of secondary injury (12,13). There needs to be a high index of suspicion when evaluating patients who have sustained an injury that involves hyperextension, flexion, or axial loading, which results in significant pain.
- Given the risk of secondary injury, an unknown stable spine injury should be suspected as each of the above scenarios represents a potential mechanism of injury. Patients with acute onset of severe neck or back pain with any degree of neurological symptoms or dysfunction should be suspected of a spinal cord injury. Further, unconscious patients should be treated as if they have significant spinal cord injury until it is proven otherwise. Early recognition of an initial spinal cord injury is essential to prevent secondary injury. Upon recognition, initiation of the appropriate management and protocols in conjunction with engagement of emergency medical services can result in improved outcomes in the context of spinal cord injury. Indeed, evidence suggests that protocols that enhance efficiency and engage subspecialized medical services early in a way that permits early surgical intervention, when needed, promote better neurological outcomes (14). The same can be applied to all athletes and their injuries.
- During the evaluation of athletes at follow-up, which most frequently occurs in the office, assessing a patient whose complaints are concerning for spinal cord or spinal column injury can be challenging. Implications of a specific spinal cord trauma can be complex and diverse; therefore, a thorough investigation should take place. Understanding the spinal column from an anatomical and biomechanical perspective is necessary to realize the implications of a trauma on the anatomy. There are also several sports where specific attention is required. For example, volleyball frequently involves flexion and extension injuries, whereas sports that involve impact, such as football and rugby, require axial loading. A further complicating aspect of spinal cord injury is the time of injury to the onset of symptoms does not necessarily presume causality. Indeed, the development of symptoms may in fact represent secondary injury, which results in the wake of a prior, more significant, primary spinal cord injury. This requires the physician to keep a broad differential in mind and to consider all aspects of the involved anatomy.

- Significant symptoms to consider involve any neurological deficit, hyperreflexia, difficulty with balance, or any dysfunction in bowel or bladder function, including urinary retention or fecal incontinence. While these symptoms in themselves are not pathognomonic for spinal cord injury, the presence of such symptoms should indicate the possibility of their presence, necessitating further investigation to rule them out. Box 50.1 presents a summary of the historical information that should be obtained from each athlete who presents with low back pain.
- Low-level injury to the spinal column frequently presents with isolated back pain. While back pain or neck pain are the most frequent presenting symptoms, they are not the most concerning. Box 50.2 is a summary of the most significant red flag symptoms for which more urgent workup is necessary to include acquisition of advanced imaging; a more detailed explanation is provided below.

In addition to a detailed history of the patient athlete, the physical exam is just as central in determining the nature and severity of the injury, initial or delayed. Any neurological deficits of abnormal reflexes need to be taken seriously and indicate the possibility of more significant injury being present. A summary of crucial exam findings is provided in Box 50.3.

- When spinal column injury is suspected, either because of physical exam findings or red flags on history, the relative benefits of intervention should be weighed against the cost of further diagnostic investigation. A crucial consideration related to this is the patient's comorbidities. A physician should have an accurate understanding of the patient's overall health and determine if the patient is able to undertake any necessary diagnostic workup safely and then to participate and comply with any recommended treatments. This is most essential in the context of injury to the spinal column if either bracing or surgical intervention is deemed necessary.

IMAGING

- Once it is determined that further investigation is needed based off the physical exam and interview, selection of the best imaging modality is the next clinical decision that must be made. For injuries that involve any portion of the spine, plane film x-rays are useful as the initial evaluation modality. Several guidelines site their utility (15). Generally, plain x-rays are useful in the identification of fractures, dislocations, degenerative spondylosis, spondylolisthesis, spondylolysis, and scoliosis. If instability is suspected because of the noted symptoms and in the absence of any gross deformity on plane x-rays, acquisition of flexion and extension views can be useful to evaluate for the development of listhesis

50.1 Historical Information to Obtain When Evaluating a Patient With Low Back Pain

General health of the patient aids risk-benefit analysis of treatment options

- Age
- Comorbidities

Sport activity level of the patient aids return-to-play decision-making

- Recreational vs. competitive vs. professional athlete

Mechanism of injury suggests diagnosis and treatment options (activity modification)

- Repetitive injury vs. acute injury
- Blunt trauma
- Axial load
- Hyperflexion
- Hyperextension
- Rotation

Location of symptoms can aid in diagnosis

- Back — spinal vs. musculoligamentous
- Buttocks — spinal vs. sacroiliac vs. tendinitis/bursitis (*e.g.*, at the ischial tuberosity)
- Groin — hip joint vs. spinal
- Hips — spinal vs. trochanteric pain syndromes
- Radiating leg pain that does not go past the knee — spinal vs. sacroiliac
- Radiating leg pain past the knee — radicular pain

Severity of symptoms aids selection of treatment options

Neurologic symptoms narrow differential to spinal, plexus, or peripheral nerve involvement

- Anesthesia
- Paresthesia
- Dysesthesia
- Weakness

Character of symptoms can suggest neurologic etiology

- Burning, stabbing

Aggravating and alleviating factors suggest possible diagnoses

- Pain worse with certain motions — mechanical pain
- Pain improves with recumbency — mechanical pain
- Night pain, rest pain — fracture, infection, tumor
- Groin or buttock pain worse with hip motion (putting on socks) — hip pathology
- Radiating chest or leg pain worse with Valsalva maneuver — radicular pain
- Chest pain worse with inspiration and expiration — costochondritis, rib fracture
- Back pain worse when sitting (lumbar spine flexed) — disc herniation
- Buttock or leg pain worse when sitting — disc herniation, ischial bursitis, proximal hamstring injury
- Back or leg pain worse when standing (lumbar spine extended) — spinal stenosis, facet joint pathology

Knowledge of complicating factors aids risk-benefit analysis of treatment options

- Prior spinal surgery
- Secondary gain

50.2 Red Flags

Age >50, significant trauma, rest pain, night pain, history of cancer, unexplained weight loss, steroid usage, fever, intravenous drug use, failure to improve with appropriate treatment, bowel, or bladder dysfunction

in the sagittal plane. Specifically, a change in orientation of the vertebral bodies in relation to each other will be seen in flexion compared to extension and vice versa. While useful, inexpensive, and generally well tolerated, plain x-rays have many shortcomings in terms of their diagnostic utility. Indeed, plane x-rays have been noted to miss fractures in the cervical spine (16). If the pretest probability is high, more advanced imaging is necessary.

- If plain x-rays are inconclusive or the clinical scenario suggests the injury is more severe, computed tomography (CT) is the next imaging modality of choice. This modality, over all other imaging, is best for visualization of bony anatomy because of its propensity to visualize density. Accordingly, CT scans are the most useful for evaluating fractures. Pars defects are commonly seen in the lumbar spine and are a frequent source of back pain in young athletes and are well visualized on CT. Beyond trauma, CT scans are useful for evaluating osteophytes and other bony abnormalities that can cause cord impingement and result in pain. Other features of bony anatomy including facet joint arthrosis, alignment, and dislocation can be evaluated using CT scans. Patients with neurologic deficits who are unable to undergo magnetic resonance imaging (MRI) because of any kind of metal implant can be evaluated using a CT myelogram, which involves the acquisition of a CT after contrast is introduced to the spinal canal via a lumbar puncture. In this way, an assessment can be made of neural compression.
- Soft-tissue assessment is best accomplished with an MRI. This modality is ideal for outlining normal neural elements, intervertebral discs, and ligaments. Pathology, which is compressive in nature but does not involve bone, is best visualized on MRI. Additionally, many aspects of degenerative disc disease are best assessed using MRI images with a relatively high degree of interpreter reliability (17). However, changes throughout the spine are prevalent with age. Yet, the presence of abnormal findings on MRI often does not correlate with symptoms, and a large portion of patients with abnormalities are asymptomatic. Therefore, one should interpret these results with care (18). Numerically, 20% of asymptomatic patients younger than 60 years of age will have radiographic evidence of disc herniation. This number rises to 40% in patients older than 60 years of age. Twenty percent of patients in this cohort will also have evidence of spinal stenosis. Cauda equina is a pathology where MRI is particularly adept at rendering a diagnosis.
- Beyond MRI, bone scans and single-photon emission computed tomography (SPECT) are useful. The centerpiece of this imaging relies on radiolabeled isotopes attached to the

50.3 Physical Examination Findings to Elicit When Evaluating a Patient With Low Back Pain

General health of the patient aids risk-benefit analysis of treatment options

- General appearance
- Body mass index

Neurologic signs can narrow differential to spinal, plexus, or peripheral nerve involvement

- Sensory deficits (dermatomal vs. peripheral nerve distribution)
- Motor weakness (myotomal vs. peripheral nerve distribution)
- Reflex testing
- Presence of pathologic reflexes (*e.g.*, Babinski) suggests upper motor neuron (*e.g.*, myelopathy).

Range of motion (ROM)

- Decreased ROM in the back can predispose the patient to back injury.
- Decreased flexibility in the lower extremities (*i.e.*, hips, knees, ankles) may result in increased load transfer to the lumbar spine with the potential for injury (*e.g.*, increased lumbar torsional strains during the golf swing in a patient with inflexible hips).

Provocative maneuvers can aid in diagnosis.

- Straight leg raise test, Lasègue maneuver (worsening of pain with ankle dorsiflexion), and the femoral nerve stretch test, when positive, suggest radiculopathy.
- Fortin finger test (points to pain within 1 inch of posterior superior iliac spine), flexion-abduction-external rotation (FABER) of the hip, Gaenslen maneuver (hip extension with contralateral hip flexion), and sacroiliac joint thrust/compression, when positive, suggest sacroiliac joint dysfunction.
- Flexion-adduction-internal rotation of the hip suggests intra-articular labral pathology.
- Hip pain with a single leg squat may result from trochanteric pain syndrome.

Gait can suggest diagnosis

- Sciatic list, foot drop, foot slap, and steppage gait suggest neurologic involvement.
- Trendelenburg gait may be evident in patients with hip pathology.

Waddell signs can suggest a nonorganic component to pain. Three or more signs suggest symptom magnification, *not* malingering.

- Superficial or nonanatomic tenderness
- Pain with axial loading or simulated rotation
- Distracted straight leg raise
- Nonanatomic sensory change or breakaway weakness
- Overreaction

ligand of interest. This is useful predominantly in the context of cancer where metabolites are used to localize neoplastic tissue. Occasionally, it can be used to identify reactive areas of bone and specifically the facet, which will appear as a "hot" facet, secondary to the high uptake of the radiolabeled isotope. This is not typically used secondary to the radiation exposure and the high associated cost of operation.

LABORATORY

- After a patient presents with signs and symptoms concerning spine-related pathology, either traumatic or degenerative in nature, a full comprehensive medical workup is necessary. This is true even if the patient does not require surgery. Initial laboratory tests should be comprehensive and include a complete blood count with differential, urethra site sedimentation rate, C-reactive protein, and a basic metabolic panel. In addition to the basic tests, specific tests are indicated depending on the etiology. If infection is possible, obtain full viral and bacterial panels. Additionally, it must be determined whether a lumbar puncture is indicated or not. If osteomyelitis and/or discitis is being considered, a CT guided biopsy would be the initial invasive lab of choice. If a lumbar puncture is obtained, full cerebral spinal fluid testing should follow. If malignancy is possible, and particularly if multiple myeloma is indicated, a biopsy should be the next step. For predominantly inflammatory processes, basic laboratory evaluation is all that is necessary.
- For patients who present with monoradiculopathies, either in the lumbar or cervical spine, acquisition of further electrodiagnostic testing can be useful. Electromyography (EMG) is useful for the assessment and diagnosis of a myriad of neurological conditions. It is helpful in distinguishing neuropathies from radiculopathies. It can further help to localize the pathology, delineating whether the cause is peripheral or central in the context of compressive etiologies. EMG is even helpful in the context of trauma or with various degrees of nerve injury, as it can detect nerve avulsion in injuries. Clinicians should have a low threshold for obtaining this test in any context, and regardless of the etiology, when a mononeuropathy is being considered.

CLINICAL SYNDROMES

Musculoligamentous Injuries

- A common cause of low back pain is thoracolumbar muscular ligamentous injury. This can take the form of either myofascial muscular injury or ligamentous injury or "a back strain." The etiologies for this type of injury are diverse and include any sports-related activity that requires significant rotational or bending force of the trunk. Additionally, such injuries can also occur in high-speed events as in contact sports or motor vehicle accidents. The pain related to this kind of injury is typically delayed on outset and is typically not noticed until much later, most likely secondary to the inflammatory cascade in the time associated with its development.
- Examination of patients with this kind of injury is often unremarkable. There may be tenderness in the surrounding musculature of the affected area or paravertebral muscle spasm. There will not be any focal neurological deficit. Pain may be associated with specific motions or in resisting certain movements when the injured muscle is isolated. Tenderness to the region surrounding the facet may indicate capsular injury. If this is the case, an extensive musculoskeletal exam is needed for localization. Range of motion (ROM) is often limited secondary to pain and when the patient is attempting to guard from potentially painful movement. The presence of any other symptoms or neurological deficits should indicate the need for further diagnostic testing with the imaging.
- Radiographs or other advanced imaging of the thoracolumbar spine is often unremarkable for muscular ligamentous injuries. Occasionally, x-rays can demonstrate a loss of normal lordosis or hyperkyphosis of the thoracic spine. It is more important, however, to avoid missing other critical pathology, including fractures and dislocations, when obtaining radiographs in this context. The diagnosis will often be one of exclusion as radiographs are frequently unremarkable. CT and MRI scans, while having increased sensitivity and specificity for all pathologies in this region, come at great expense. The clinician needs to consider the relative pretest probability prior to ordering more advanced imaging given the high rate of negative findings. This can permit avoidance of unnecessary imaging while still caring for the patient.
- Avoidance of secondary injury is the mainstay of treatment for all muscular ligamentous injury of the thoracolumbar spine. This is achieved first through anti-inflammatories followed by physical therapy. It is important to have adequate pain management throughout the process as well. Initial pain treatment can involve icing with intermittent heat to promote muscle relaxation. When adequate pain levels are achieved, full ROM and strength exercises should be encouraged to restore full flexibility and strength. This should be done in a formalized setting with a trained physical therapist.
- A primary focus of physical therapy should center on the improvement of biomechanics and posture. This will not only decrease the risk of secondary injury in the acute phase but decrease the risk of subsequent injury in the future. Exercises should focus on increasing core strength as improvement in core muscles is associated with alterations in low back pain (19). Further, the abdominal and paraspinal musculature needs to be improved to stabilize the axial skeleton and decrease the risk of injury. These different muscle groups coalesce together to stabilize the spinal and pelvic anatomy, an essential aspect of many sports (20,21) (see Chapter 75, Core Strengthening).
- If nonpharmaceutical interventions are insufficient at providing the pain control necessary for adequate physical

therapy, several pharmaceutical interventions can be considered (see Chapter 73, Pain Management).

- Beyond medications, bracing can occasionally be beneficial. In the acute situation, bracing can allow for the transition of mechanical weight to the brace itself, alleviate stress, and promote healing. Bracing should only be used for a relatively short period as long-term use can be associated with muscle degradation and the inability to support weight with axial loading. Bracing should always be engaged in and with additional stretching in physical therapy, which promotes adequate muscle building. A notable exception to this is when ligamentous injury occurs in the cervical spine. Here, ligamentous injury can lead to significant instability, which could have catastrophic consequences (22). Here, bracing is necessary to avoid more serious injury. Similarly, injury to the posterior ligamentous complex occurring in the thoracolumbar spine often indicates more significant injury and routinely requires surgical intervention (23).
- A crucial distinction to make when evaluating patients for muscular ligamentous injury is in the elderly patient population. Here, arthritic facets or facet arthropathy can mimic muscular ligamentous back pain. This is often seen in the setting of trauma. In this context, trigger point injections are frequently successful at treating pain. Similar for other injuries numerated above, these injections should be done in context with physical therapy and adequate application of pharmaceuticals. Regardless of age, the prognosis is good for patients who suffer myofascial or musculoligamentous injury related to sports. While prognosis is generally contingent on the extent of injury, successful completion of physical therapy often accompanies a good recovery provided there is full restoration, normal ROM, and adequate strength. Patients can generally RTP within one or 2 weeks, but only if they have returned to their baseline neurological status and function and can participate in all aspects of the sport in question without experiencing any pain (24).

Disc Herniations

- Disc herniation and discogenic origin of pain are common after a myriad of sports-related injuries. It is a significant contributor to morbidity after sports-related injury and symptomatically can present with isolated back pain, radiculopathy, either bilateral or unilateral, and even in rare circumstances when the disc causes significant central stenosis, it can cause nerve root compression or cauda equina in the lumbar spine or spinal cord compression in the cervical or thoracic spine. Mechanistically in the lumbar spine, disc herniation occurs when there is injury to the outer annulus. This commonly occurs in sports which involve significant rotational force or axial loading of the spine, which places unusual strain on the ligaments and annulus. Once there is injury to the annulus, it is possible for the inner nucleus pulposus to herniate out and cause compression of nerves or the thecal sac. Disc herniations often occur in patients who have weak ligaments to begin with. As such, these injuries are more common in obese athletes with potentially underdeveloped ligamentous complex.
- The symptoms produced by an acute disc herniation are easily distinguished from other pathologies. The pain is acute with onset. It will occur suddenly with certain hyperflexion of the spine. Herniation will produce a radiating and neuropathic pain which is in the isolated nerve root distribution when the disk is paracentral or foraminal. A singular disc herniation can cause bilateral radiculopathies if it is broad enough to affect both traversing nerve roots. This is in contrast to a muscular ligamentous injury, which has a slower onset and is indolent in nature. Here, the radiculopathy is caused by an acute irritation of the nerve root and can be exacerbated in the subsequent days as the inflammation increases.
- Cauda equina syndrome occurs when there is more profound central compression and the compression involves multiple nerve roots in the lumbar and sacral spine (25). While the exact diagnostic criteria are still a matter of debate, red flag symptoms generally include neurological dysfunction of the lower extremities, urinary retention, bowel incontinence, saddle anesthesia, hyperreflexia, inability to walk, and a lack of rectal tone. When the syndrome is seen, emergent neurosurgical evaluation is warranted for urgent surgical decompression. Conus medullaris syndrome is the result of compression of the most distal aspect of the spinal cord between L1 and L2. These syndromes can have multiple overlapping symptoms, and the presentation can be highly variable (26). As such, urgent evaluation is necessary and clinicians should have a low threshold for obtaining subspecialty consultation in this context.
- Radiographically, plane film x-rays are often insufficient in diagnosing discogenic disease. An MRI without contrast is the gold standard diagnostic imaging modality. This is true regardless of the etiology. Such imaging will reveal a hypointensity in the central canal, lateral recess, or in the framing. In these locations, it should be noted on imaging whether there is compression of the traversing or exiting nerve roots. The definition of discriminations is highly specific and categorized into normal, focal, or broad protrusion, and extrusion (27,28). It is critical to correlate findings on MRI with the patient symptomatically. Changes in disc height and morphology are common with aging (29). Because of this, abnormalities on an MRI scan do not by themselves indicate the presence of pathology. Indeed, these changes can be present in patients who are asymptomatic (18).
- Management of acute disc herniations centers on a multifactorial, conservative approach. Analgesics with nonsteroidal anti-inflammatory drugs (NSAIDs) or a minimal narcotic regimen are reasonable for acute presentations. Medication should be administered concomitantly with formal physical therapy. For patients who have continued pain, administration of epidural steroid injections is the next step in management (30). For those patients who are refractory to medical management, surgical intervention can be considered. It is important to understand, however, that a significant portion of patients who do not undergo surgical intervention will

still experience significant improvement in their symptoms. Intention to treat trials, such as the SPORT trial, suggests that medical and surgical intervention produce equal clinical outcomes (31). When examining the duration of symptoms, surgical and conservative approaches are not equal over the short term with surgery providing faster initial pain relief. However, over an extended period, approaches have equivalent outcomes (32). For many patients, conservative measures are all that is required for symptom resolution, and patients can even demonstrate normal imaging after several years. Because of this, conservative management is always preferred over surgical intervention as the initial step in treating herniations of all kinds.

- As it relates to RTP guidelines, there is no demonstrative difference between patients who undergo surgical intervention versus those who undergo conservative management either in terms of functionality or duration till RTP (33). In general, the duration to RTP for patients who undergo conservative management is approximately 5 months (34). When surgical intervention is necessary, either due to the severity of symptoms or because conservative management failed, there does not appear to be any significant implications for surgical management on athletic performance (35). However, as stated above, given the relative equal outcomes for patients who undergo conservative therapy compared to surgery, conservative measures should be considered as the initial intervention of choice, with surgery reserved for refractory cases.

Fracture, Subluxation, and Dislocation

- The most significant spinal pathologies encountered in sports medicine are fractures, subluxations, and dislocations. Usually caused by trauma, this pathology is often significant and accompanied by neurological injury. The morphology and management of fractures differ significantly throughout the cervical, thoracic, and lumbar spine.
- Indications for bracing and nonoperative management are considerably different depending on the level of the spine involved. Operative intervention is often required given the extent of neurological compromise that accompanies these sorts of injuries. The complexity of these pathologies and the diverse nature of the morphology and presentation make both surgical and nonsurgical management complex, and as such, beyond the scope of this chapter. Clinicians should have a low threshold for engagement of subspecialties when fractures are encountered given their complex presentation and significant associated morbidity.

Osteoporotic Thoracic Vertebral Compression Fractures in the Elderly

- Specific fractures that are within the scope of this chapter include osteoporotic compression fractures within the thoracic spine of the elderly. Given that osteoporosis typically occurs within the aging population, it is not surprising that these types of fractures are seen within this demographic (36). These fractures are particularly common for elderly patients who are playing sports. Considering the patient's age is essential when determining the acuity of a fracture from a morphological standpoint. Two fractures seen in the elderly, particularly in the context of osteoporosis, are often benign and require mere bracing for treatment. Conversely, an equivalent fracture, seen in a relatively young patient, as defined as age less than 60, often indicates the presence of more extensive injury, which would classify the fracture as a burst fracture and possibly indicate an underlying, more extensive disease such as cancer or infection.
- The transition point between the thoracic and lumbar spine is the most common location of involvement for these types of fractures. In general, most fractures in the thoracolumbar spine occur at this junction (37). The main reason is these levels, T11 to L2, represent the transition point between a highly flexible lumbar spine and a relatively rigid thoracic spine. As such, significant biomechanical forces are placed on these vertebral levels at baseline. Consequently, sports involving hyperflexion or axial loading have a propensity to cause such injuries. Patients will present with tenderness at the injured vertebral level, and it will have an acute onset. There will not be a delayed onset. This pain will also be reproducible with palpation over the spinous process at the affected level.
- If osteoporosis is a known condition for the patient in question, diagnosis of a compression fracture is best made by CT scan. Consideration of Hounsfield units on the CT is also helpful in assessing fractures in the context of osteoporosis (38). For conditions where chronicity is in question, an MRI scan without contrast can be helpful as CT scans are relatively insensitive (39). Specifically, hyperintensity on flare signal sequence can indicate edema which is commonly seen in acute fractures. Once a diagnosis is established, treatment focuses on immobilization and pain amelioration. Bracing of the thoracolumbar spine is best achieved with external orthosis. Treatment of pain can either be with NSAIDs or a light narcotic regimen. Pain regimens should be accompanied by physical therapy. If bracing fails, treatment of the fracture with either a vertebroplasty or kyphoplasty can be considered, although this is controversial (40).
- Treatment of such fractures must be combined with the treatment of osteoporosis itself. This can be with either intranasal calcitonin or bisphosphonate therapy. More modern drug regimens including teriparatide, abaloparatide, and romosozumab are now available for the treatment of osteoporosis in adult patients (41). Referral to an endocrinologist to manage these drugs is essential. Indeed, general practitioners should have a low threshold for endocrinology referral in patients who are susceptible to osteoporosis given the high prevalence of concomitant fractures that occur when these individuals engage in athletic activities. This will help identify secondary causes and prevent recurrence. Specifically, young female athletes with osteoporosis, amenorrhea, and anorexia should be evaluated for compression fractures as the presence of this triad increases their relative risk of recurrent fractures (42).

Spondylolysis and Spondylolisthesis

- When there is an acquired defect of the bone in the pars interarticularis, which is the anatomical bone bridge between the inferior and superior articulating facet and the lamina, lumbar spondylolysis occurs. This can be unilateral or bilateral. Spondylolisthesis is the slipping of one vertebral body on another and results in abnormal alignment. In the context of degenerative spine disease, spondylolisthesis is measured by the Meyerding grading system, but others exist as well (43,44).
- Specifically, spondylolysis is a defect in the pars interarticularis, which results from repetitive microtrauma during growth or by repetitive lumbar hyperextension (45). This causes a nonunion of the pars interarticularis and instability, leading to slipping of one vertebra upon another. The most common form of spondylolysis is isthmic spondylolisthesis, which typically occurs between L5-S1 and more rarely at other levels (46).
- Common etiologies include certain high-risk sports that traditionally involve repetitive lumbar hyperextensions and axial loading such as blocks in football, military press in weightlifting, serving in tennis, pitching in baseball, back walkovers in gymnastics, and the butterfly stroke in swimming to name a few. All of these are considered high-risk sports and activities. Athletes who participate in high-risk sports are estimated to be as much as five times likely to have a poor outcome compared to those who participate in low-risk sports (47). While the majority of such injuries are unilateral in nature, rare cases can involve bilateral spondylolysis. Bilateral cases can lead to anterior slippage of the superior vertebral body on the caudal vertebral body. This can result in significant foraminal and central stenosis, creating a myriad of neurological symptoms. This is typical with traumatic etiologies, which are the minority of cases. The more common presentation for isthmic spondylolisthesis is in children with back pain due to alternative causes where this finding is incidental. In these cases, the finding represents a preexisting developmental condition that is often not the cause of the presenting symptom in children or adolescence. Therefore, alternative causes of back pain need to be considered prior to initiating therapy.
- A focused history and physical exam are often helpful in diagnosing and isolating spondylolisthesis as the cause of low back pain. Patients typically present with either focal low back pain or bilateral radiculopathies. The back pain will be mechanical in nature and often exacerbated with axial loading. The radiculopathy is the result of bilateral foraminal stenosis usually caused by the spondylolisthesis itself. This results from nerve compression directly and is a concerning finding. When nerve root involvement is absent, often the area is tender to palpation, which can reproduce the pain. On lateral view, a loss of normal lordosis can occasionally be appreciated on physical exam. Compensatory tightening of the hamstrings is common. In adolescents, this low back pain is frequently refractory to conservative management and does not respond to physical therapy or even appropriate levels of pain management.
- From a diagnostic perspective, while any of the imaging modalities above is appropriate for assessment of this pathology, each has its own strength in terms of rendering diagnostic information. Lateral and oblique lumbar spine x-rays are good for delineating pars defects if the fractures are significant or if the spondylolisthesis is large. Given that L5 is the most affected, plain x-rays are a reasonable initial imaging modality. However, depending on the quality of the image and the extent of the pathology, plane film x-rays have limited utility and even oblique views are often not diagnostic and therefore have significant limitations (44). If the x-ray is not diagnostic for any reason, CT scans are best for outlining bony anatomy. If there is any doubt on plane film x-rays, obtaining a CT scan is the best next step. While CTs do have the limitation of not being able to establish chronicity along with the drawback of involving radiation, CT scans completely define bony anatomy, making it a good option as an early, if not initial imaging modality of choice. Indeed, CT is the gold standard for evaluation of osseous anatomy (44). For very young children, an MRI is more reasonable given its lack of radiation. An MRI has further benefits, as it will show the extent to which there is nerve impingement by the fracture itself. Hyperintensity on short tau inversion recovery (STIR) sequencing can also help physicians identify the acuity of the fracture if the chronicity is uncertain. Finally, SPECT and bone scans should be reserved as the last imaging modality of choice given its associated radiation and cost.
- A similar treatment is used for both spondylolysis and spondylolisthesis. Initial therapy is centered on avoidance of activities that exacerbate the condition and in physical therapy on back strengthening (48). In general, rest, administration of anti-inflammatory medications, and restricted activity are the recommendation. It has been shown that the combination of sport cessation, thoracolumbar external orthosis, and bone stimulator use leads to excellent outcomes in adolescents (49). Occasionally, injections directly into the pars defects can alleviate symptoms and have the added benefit of being diagnostic. Recently shown, a positive response to a steroid injection is associated with better surgical outcomes for isthmic spondylolisthesis in adults (50).
- Operative intervention for both spondylolysis and spondylolisthesis is reserved for patients refractory to conservative management. It is important to note however that the presence of significant spondylolisthesis radiographically does not necessitate operative intervention when the patient is minimally or completely asymptomatic. Indeed, watchful waiting is appropriate and associated with good outcomes in children (51).
- For refractory cases, surgical intervention is necessary, and referral to neurosurgery or orthopedic surgery is crucial. A myriad of surgical interventions exist for these conditions (52). However, some studies suggest that the long-term clinical outcomes among various methods of interbody fusion

may be equivalent (53). Regardless, referral to a subspecialist is necessary.

Facet Joint Syndrome

- The presentation of facet joint syndrome is usually pain, generally localized to the spine and occasionally radiating to the upper buttocks and thigh. However, the exact diagnosis and treatment of this syndrome are still a subject of debate (54).
- Facet joint osteoarthritis is the most common form of facet joint syndrome. Facet joint syndrome in the lumbar spine is a common cause of low back pain (55). It is a mechanical and postural disease. Pain is typically generated and exacerbated by movements which involve extension and increase the load on the facets. It is typically improved with activity. Initial treatment centers on enrolling the patient in physical therapy as this, in combination with an exercise routine, is often sufficient in treating this condition. Particular attention should be paid toward improvement of spine biomechanics and posture.
- For patients who require additional interventions, other therapeutic options include rest, weight control, analgesics, NSAIDs, an exercise aimed at improving lumbosacral support and lumbar flexion. For further refractory cases and particularly when facet osteoarthritis is the cause, facet injections or radiofrequency neuroablation can be considered (56). However, these are never a first line of treatment.

Sacroiliac Joint Dysfunction

- While typically the result of repetitive trauma, sacroiliac (SI) joint dysfunction can also result from direct impact. This joint is the anatomical junction between the iliac crest portion of the pelvis and the sacral ala. At baseline, and under normal physiological conditions, this is a nonmobile joint. However, SI joint dysfunction is an underrecognized cause of low back pain and is estimated to account for up to one-third of all low back pain (57). This is due in part to the presenting symptoms of SI joint dysfunction being similar to other presenting syndromes (58).
- While the presenting pain of the syndrome typically localizes well to the sacral iliac joint, there is often concomitant pain that radiates down the posterior aspect of the leg and knee, mimicking an L5 radiculopathy. Diagnosis requires reproduction of pain with several provocative maneuvers, which is suggestive of the diagnosis (59). In addition to physical exam maneuvers, significant improvement in symptoms with injection into the SI joint is confirmatory of the diagnosis.
- From a treatment perspective, braces can help a subset of patients, providing that body habitus does not prevent adequate accommodation of this brace. For patients who failed conservative management, SI joint fusion is a promising alternative and gaining traction in the surgical community. The adaptation of navigation that permits achievement of fusion of this otherwise immobile joint has decreased the relative surgical risk and morbidity. Currently, a myriad of implants are available to aid surgical fixation of this joint (55).

Costochondritis (Tietze Syndrome)

- Costochondritis is an inflammatory pathology affecting the costal cartilage at the intersection point of the ribs and the sternum. This can result from several sports-related injuries that require repetitive upper extremity motion. These symptoms can often be misinterpreted as acute coronary syndrome as the symptoms present in the same location. The second ribs are the most commonly affected (60).
- Diagnosis is made by palpation of the chest, and particularly, the areas adjacent to the sternum. Palpation will cause reproduction of the symptoms. This reproducibility is crucial in distinguishing the pathology from acute coronary syndrome and other underlying cardiac disease. Additionally, cardiac symptoms will be accompanied by arm and jaw pain as well as shortness of breath. Costochondritis will be isolated sternal pain, which can sometimes be associated with breathing or movement of the upper extremities.
- From a diagnostic perspective, bone scans can occasionally be helpful in confirming the diagnosis as the costal cartilage will show "hot spots" indicating increased inflammatory action.
- Treatment is centered on reducing inflammation principally achieved by the administration of anti-inflammatory medications or, in more refractory conditions, with the injection of corticosteroids over the affected area.

Costovertebral Joint Pain

- Costovertebral joint pain should be contrasted with costochondritis. Whereas costochondritis principally affects the anterior portion of the rib cage, costovertebral joint pain principally affects the posterior aspect and can often present as mid and upper back pain. The pathology of this disease process involves osteoarthritic changes to the joint and articulations between the rib head and the thoracic vertebral body and transverse process. The most involved ribs are those which have singular articulations with the vertebral body including the 1, 11, and 12 ribs. Ribs six through eight are also commonly affected as these are the longest ribs which have the greatest biomechanical strain on the joint and thus are most prone to degradation and arthritic changes.
- Symptomatically, the pain is often unilateral and described as achy, burning, or radiating. The radiating nature of this can often cause it to mimic thoracic disc herniations or other pathologies which cause nerve impingement. On exam, the diagnosis is confirmed clinically when the pain is reproduced with palpation of the costovertebral junction posteriorly. It is further confirmed when the pain is reproduced with rib manipulation such as with deep inhalation or exhalation. More specifically, relief of the symptoms with a local, trigger point injection is confirmatory of the diagnosis.

- Treatment involves injection of the symptomatic joint with cortical steroids and symptomatic treatment with anti-inflammatories and pain medication. For refractory cases, surgical excision of the affected joint can be considered, although this is not common and not a first-line treatment.

Lower Rib Pain Syndrome (Rib-Tip Syndrome)

- Lower rib pain syndromes can result from a myriad of etiologies and typically involve the lowest four ribs. Symptomatically, pain generally radiates from anterior to posterior and hence the alternative name of rib-tip syndrome. Pain is typically reproducible with palpation.
- Similar to the above pathologies, treatment centers on administration of anti-inflammatory medications. For refractory cases, corticosteroid injections can be considered (60).

RTP GUIDELINES

- The decision to allow an athlete to RTP after a spine injury, either a fracture or more serious neurological injury, is complicated and multifactorial. While the desire to RTP often increases young athletes' compliance with physical therapy, the same desire often increases risk-taking and can lead to premature engagement in physical contact sports. In general, there is a wide variation in opinion regarding the most appropriate RTP criteria. Studies in best practice for RTP are few, leaving clinicians limited guidelines of recommendations for patients. Most consensus guidelines recommend that physicians evaluate the neurological status of the patient, the level of pain experienced with normal ROM or with the activity associated with the sport, the average RTP for a given injury, the potential risk for recurrent injury, and the position of a particular sport played (61–63). In the cervical spine, there is consensus that athletes should be allowed to RTP if they are asymptomatic and have stable signal change on MRI or have resolved signal change and a relatively larger canal diameter (64). However, there is no consensus about the timing of RTP. And players are generally discouraged from resuming sports that involve significant physical contact (65). Ultimately, there are several factors, in addition to those listed above, which the physician should consider. These include, but are not limited to, typical healing time and patient's overall health. Of equal importance would be the involved anatomy of the injury and the presence of any congenital predisposition or alteration in anatomy that could put the patient at significant risk of recurrent injury. An example of this is congenitally short pedicles.
- The type of sport in question should be a major consideration as well. Athletes in sports which require frequent or repetitive bending and twisting, such as golf, should generally wait longer prior to returning to play. The skill level of the athlete in question is also important. More skilled athletes potentially have better form which in some instances may be protective against recurrent injury. However, professional athletes can also exert significantly more force depending on the sport in question. Again, golf is an example where players need to wait longer before returning to play as they exert significantly more torsional movements on their spine compared to recreational golfers. Professional football players are also much more likely to sustain substantial recurrent injury from collision due to the harder, direct hits endemic to the sport.
- The timing of RTP also has significant social implications. If the athlete in question is a professional, they may be receiving significant external and secondary pressures from the team or fans to RTP before the optimal time has passed. There may also be economic forces wherein completion of a contract is contingent on the ability to RTP. While all these factors are not universally applicable, all should be considered when evaluating injury to the spinal column, rendering an opinion about the most appropriate time to resume a sport, and determining the most appropriate level of activity following an injury.

REFERENCES

1. Maher C, Underwood M, Buchbinder R. Non-specific low back pain. *Lancet.* 2017 Feb 18;389(10070):736–47. doi:10.1016/S0140-6736(16)30970-9
2. Stanish W. Low back pain in athletes: an overuse syndrome. *Clin Sports Med.* 1987;6(2):321–44.
3. Thornton JS, Caneiro JP, Hartvigsen J, et al. Treating low back pain in athletes: a systematic review with meta-analysis. *Br J Sports Med.* 2021 Jun;55(12):656–62. doi:10.1136/bjsports-2020-102723
4. Bigdon SF, Gewiess J, Hoppe S, et al. Spinal injury in alpine winter sports: a review. *Scand J Trauma Resusc Emerg Med.* 2019 Jul 19;27(1):69. doi:10.1186/s13049-019-0645-z
5. Oshlag B, Ray T, Boswell B. Neck injuries. *Prim Care.* 2020 Mar;47(1):165–76. doi:10.1016/j.pop.2019.10.009
6. Boden BP, Jarvis CG. Spinal injuries in sports. *Neurol Clin.* 2008;26(1):63–78, viii.
7. Levy AS, Smith RH. Neurologic injuries in skiers and snowboarders. *Semin Neurol.* 2000;20(2):233–45.
8. Siu TL, Chandran KN, Newcombe RL, Fuller JW, Pik JH. Snow sports related head and spinal injuries: an eight-year survey from the neurotrauma centre for the Snowy Mountains, Australia. *J Clin Neurosci.* 2004 Apr;11(3):236–42. doi:10.1016/j.jocn.2003.08.003
9. Sardar ZM, Ames RJ, Lenke L. Scheuermann's kyphosis: diagnosis, management, and selecting fusion levels. *J Am Acad Orthop Surg.* 2019 May 15;27(10):e462–72. doi:10.5435/JAAOS-D-17-00748
10. Wood KB, Li W, Lebl DR, Ploumis A. Management of thoracolumbar spine fractures. *Spine J.* 2014 Jan;14(1):145–64. Erratum in: *Spine J.* 2014 Aug 1;14(8):A18. Lebl, Darren S [corrected to Lebl, Darren R]. doi:10.1016/j.spinee.2012.10.041
11. Imamudeen N, Basheer A, Iqbal AM, Manjila N, Haroon NN, Manjila S. Management of osteoporosis and spinal fractures: contemporary guidelines and evolving paradigms. *Clin Med Res.* 2022 Jun;20(2):95–106. doi:10.3121/cmr.2021.1612
12. Swartz EE, Boden BP, Courson RW, et al. National athletic trainers' association position statement: acute management of the cervical spine-injured athlete. *J Athl Train.* 2009;44(3):306–31.

13. Coen SD. Spinal cord injury: preventing secondary injury. *AACN Clin Issues Crit Care Nurs*. 1992 Feb;3(1):44–54. Erratum in: *AACN Clin Issues Crit Care Nurs*. 1992 Aug;3(3):652. doi:10.4037/15597768-1992-1005
14. Badhiwala JH, Ahuja CS, Fehlings MG. Time is spine: a review of translational advances in spinal cord injury. *J Neurosurg Spine*. 2019;30(1):1–18. doi:10.3171/2018.9.SPINE18682
15. Parreira PCS, Maher CG, Megale RZ, March L, Ferreira ML. An overview of clinical guidelines for the management of vertebral compression fracture: a systematic review. *Spine J*. 2017 Dec;17(12):1932–8. doi:10.1016/j.spinee.2017.07.174
16. Besman A, Kaban J, Jacobs L, Jacobs LM. False-negative plain cervical spine x-rays in blunt trauma. *Am Surg*. 2003 Nov;69(11):1010–4.
17. Zook J, Djurasovic M, Crawford C 3rd, Bratcher K, Glassman S, Carreon L. Inter- and intraobserver reliability in radiographic assessment of degenerative disk disease. *Orthopedics*. 2011 Apr 11;34(4). doi:10.3928/01477447-20110228-07
18. Boden SD, Davis DO, Dina TS, Patronas NJ, Wiesel SW. Abnormal magnetic-resonance scans of the lumbar spine in asymptomatic subjects. A prospective investigation. *J Bone Joint Surg Am*. 1990;72(3):403–8.
19. Huxel Bliven KC, Anderson BE. Core stability training for injury prevention. *Sports Health*. 2013 Nov;5(6):514–22. doi:10.1177/1941738113481200
20. Jeng S. Lumbar spine stabilization exercise. *Hong Kong J Sport Med Sports Sci*. 1999;8:59–64.
21. Pollock ML, Leggett SH, Graves JE, Jones A, Fulton M, Cirulli J. Effect of resistance training on lumbar extension strength. *Am J Sports Med*. 1989;17(5):624–9.
22. Vij N, Tolson H, Kiernan H, Agusala V, Viswanath O, Urits I. Pathoanatomy, biomechanics, and treatment of upper cervical ligamentous instability: a literature review. *Orthop Rev*. 2022 Aug 5;14(3):37099. doi:10.52965/001c.37099
23. Bizdikian AJ, El Rachkidi R. Posterior ligamentous complex injuries of the thoracolumbar spine: importance and surgical implications. *Cureus*. 2021 Oct 14;13(10):e18774. doi:10.7759/cureus.18774
24. Ball JR, Harris CB, Lee J, Vives MJ. Lumbar spine injuries in sports: review of the literature and current treatment recommendations. *Sports Med Open*. 2019;5(1):26. doi:10.1186/s40798-019-0199-7
25. Bulloch L, Thompson K, Spector L. Cauda equina syndrome. *Orthop Clin North Am*. 2022 Apr;53(2):247–54. doi:10.1016/j.ocl.2021.11.010
26. Harrop JS, Hunt GE Jr, Vaccaro AR. Conus medullaris and cauda equina syndrome as a result of traumatic injuries: management principles. *Neurosurg Focus*. 2004 Jun 15;16(6):e4. doi:10.3171/foc.2004.16.6.4
27. Fardon DF. Nomenclature and classification of lumbar disc pathology. *Spine*. 2001 Mar 1;26(5):461–2. doi:10.1097/00007632-200103010-00007
28. Li Y, Fredrickson V, Resnick DK. How should we grade lumbar disc herniation and nerve root compression? A systematic review. *Clin Orthop Relat Res*. 2015 Jun;473(6):1896–902. doi:10.1007/s11999-014-3674-y
29. Shao Z, Rompe G, Schiltenwolf M. Radiographic changes in the lumbar intervertebral discs and lumbar vertebrae with age. *Spine*. 2002 Feb 1;27(3):263–8. doi:10.1097/00007632-200202010-00013
30. Akşan Ö. 309 patients treated with fluoroscopy-guided caudal epidural injection for lumbar disc herniation. *J Int Med Res*. 2022 Oct;50(10):3000605221129031. doi:10.1177/03000605221129031
31. Weinstein JN, Tosteson TD, Lurie JD, et al. Surgical vs. nonoperative treatment for lumbar disk herniation: the Spine Patient Outcomes Research Trial (SPORT). A randomized trial. *JAMA*. 2006 Nov 22;296(20):2441–50. doi:10.1001/jama.296.20.2441
32. Hahne AJ, Ford JJ, McMeeken JM. Conservative management of lumbar disc herniation with associated radiculopathy: a systematic review. *Spine*. 2010 May 15;35(11):E488–504. doi:10.1097/BRS.0b013e3181cc3f56
33. Sedrak P, Shahbaz M, Gohal C, Madden K, Aleem I, Khan M. Return to play after symptomatic lumbar disc herniation in elite athletes: a systematic review and meta-analysis of operative versus non-operative treatment. *Sports Health*. 2021 Sep-Oct;13(5):446–53. doi:10.1177/1941738121991782
34. Iwamoto J, Takeda T, Sato Y, Wakano K. Short-term outcome of conservative treatment in athletes with symptomatic lumbar disc herniation. *Am J Phys Med Rehabil*. 2006;85(8):667–77.
35. Watkins RG IV, Williams LA, Watkins RG III. Microscopic lumbar discectomy results for 60 cases in professional and Olympic athletes. *Spine J*. 2003;3(2):100–5.
36. Rajasekaran S, Kanna RM, Schnake KJ, et al. Osteoporotic thoracolumbar fractures-how are they different?-classification and treatment algorithm. *J Orthop Trauma*. 2017 Sep;31(suppl 4):S49–56. doi:10.1097/BOT.0000000000000949
37. Magerl F, Aebi M, Gertzbein SD, Harms J, Nazarian S. A comprehensive classification of thoracic and lumbar injuries. *Eur Spine J*. 1994;3(4):184–201. doi:10.1007/BF02221591
38. Chen HJ, Xiao ZG, Yu RH, Wang Y, Xu RJ, Zhu XD. CT measurement and analysis of the target vertebral body in elderly patients with uncompressed osteoporotic thoracolumbar fractures. *Eur Rev Med Pharmacol Sci*. 2018 Jul;22(1 suppl l):36–44. doi:10.26355/eurrev_201807_15357
39. Strickland CD, DeWitt PE, Jesse MK, Durst MJ, Korf JA. Radiographic assessment of acute vs. chronic vertebral compression fractures. *Emerg Radiol*. 2023 Feb;30(1):11–8. doi:10.1007/s10140-022-02092-8
40. McCarthy J, Davis A. Diagnosis and management of vertebral compression fractures. *Am Fam Physician*. 2016 Jul 1;94(1):44–50.
41. Reid IR, Billington EO. Drug therapy for osteoporosis in older adults. *Lancet*. 2022 Mar 12;399(10329):1080–92. Erratum in: *Lancet*. 2022 Sep 3;400(10354):732. doi:10.1016/S0140-6736(21)02646-5
42. Hobart JA, Smucker DR. The female athlete triad. *Am Fam Physician*. 2000 Jun 1;61(11):3357–67. [
43. Koslosky E, Gendelberg D. Classification in brief: the Meyerding classification system of spondylolisthesis. *Clin Orthop Relat Res*. 2020 May;478(5):1125–30. doi:10.1097/CORR.0000000000001153
44. Chung CC, Shimer AL. Lumbosacral spondylolysis and spondylolisthesis. *Clin Sports Med*. 2021 Jul;40(3):471–90.
45. Morita T, Ikata T, Katoh S, Miyake R. Lumbar spondylolysis in children and adolescents. *J Bone Joint Surg Br*. 1995;77(4):620–5.
46. Ganju A. Isthmic spondylolisthesis. *Neurosurg Focus*. 2002 Jul 15;13(1):E1. doi:10.3171/foc.2002.13.1.2
47. d'Hemecourt PA, Zurakowski D, Kriemler S, Micheli LJ. Spondylolysis: returning the athlete to sports participation with brace treatment. *Orthopedics*. 2002;25(6):653–7.
48. Mohile NV, Kuczmarski AS, Lee D, Warburton C, Rakoczy K, Butler AJ. Spondylolysis and isthmic spondylolisthesis: a guide to diagnosis and management. *J Am Board Fam Med*. 2022 Dec 23;35(6):1204–16. doi:10.3122/jabfm.2022.220130R1
49. Choi JH, Ochoa JK, Lubinus A, Timon S, Lee YP, Bhatia NN. Management of lumbar spondylolysis in the adolescent athlete: a review of over 200 cases. *Spine J*. 2022 Oct;22(10):1628–33. doi:10.1016/j.spinee.2022.04.011
50. Turtle J, Randell Z, Karamian B, et al. Response to preoperative steroid injections predicts surgical outcomes in patients undergoing fusion for isthmic spondylolisthesis. *Spine*. 2023 Jul 1;48(13):914–19. doi:10.1097/BRS.0000000000004687
51. Lundine KM, Lewis SJ, Al-Aubaidi Z, Alman B, Howard AW. Patient outcomes in the operative and nonoperative management of high-grade spondylolisthesis in children. *J Pediatr Orthop*. 2014 Jul-Aug;34(5):483–9. doi:10.1097/BPO.0000000000000133
52. Alomari S, Judy B, Sacino AN, Porras JL, Tang A, Sciubba D, Witham T, Theodore N, Bydon A. Isthmic spondylolisthesis in adults… A review of the current literature. *J Clin Neurosci*. 2022 Jul;101:124–30. doi:10.1016/j.jocn.2022.04.042

53. Prost S, Giorgi H, Ould-Slimane M, French Spine Surgery Society SFCR, et al. Surgical management of isthmic spondylolisthesis: a comparative study of postoperative outcomes between ALIF and TLIF. *Orthop Traumatol Surg Res*. 2023 Jan;109(6):103560. doi:10.1016/j.otsr.2023.103560
54. Du R, Xu G, Bai X, Li Z. Facet joint syndrome: pathophysiology, diagnosis, and treatment. *J Pain Res*. 2022 Nov 30;15:3689–710. doi:10.2147/JPR.S389602
55. Himstead AS, Brown NJ, Shahrestani S, Tran K, Davies JL, Oh M. Trends in diagnosis and treatment of sacroiliac joint pathology over the past 10 years: review of scientific evidence for new devices for sacroiliac joint fusion. *Cureus*. 2021 Jun 3;13(6):e15415. doi:10.7759/cureus.15415.
56. Baroncini A, Maffulli N, Eschweiler J, Knobe M, Tingart M, Migliorini F. Management of facet joints osteoarthritis associated with chronic low back pain: a systematic review. *Surgeon*. 2021 Dec;19(6):e512–18. doi:10.1016/j.surge.2020.12.004
57. Rashbaum RF, Ohnmeiss DD, Lindley EM, Kitchel SH, Patel VV. Sacroiliac joint pain and its treatment. *Clin Spine Surg*. 2016 Mar;29(2):42–8. doi:10.1097/BSD.0000000000000359
58. Barros G, McGrath L, Gelfenbeyn M. Sacroiliac joint dysfunction in patients with low back pain. *Fed Pract*. 2019 Aug;36(8):370–5.
59. Falowski S, Sayed D, Pope J, et al. A review and algorithm in the diagnosis and treatment of sacroiliac joint pain. *J Pain Res*. 2020 Dec 8;13:3337–48. doi:10.2147/JPR.S279390
60. Errico TJ, Stecker S, Kostuik JP. Thoracic pain syndromes. In: Frymoyer JW, editor. *The Adult Spine: Principles and Practice*. 2nd ed. Philadelphia: Lippincott-Raven; 1997. p. 1623–37.
61. Swiatek PR, Nandurkar TS, Maroon JC, et al. Return to play guidelines after cervical spine injuries in American football athletes: a literature-based review. *Spine*. 2021 Jul 1;46(13):886–92. doi:10.1097/BRS.0000000000003931
62. Huang P, Anissipour A, McGee W, Lemak L. Return-to-play recommendations after cervical, thoracic, and lumbar spine injuries: a comprehensive review. *Sports Health*. 2016 Jan–Feb;8(1):19–25. doi:10.1177/1941738115610753
63. Morganti C. Recommendations for return to sports following cervical spine injuries. *Sports Med*. 2003;33(8):563–73. doi:10.2165/00007256-200333080-00002
64. Schroeder GD, Canseco JA, Patel PD, et al. Updated return-to-play recommendations for collision athletes after cervical spine injury: a modified Delphi consensus study with the Cervical Spine Research Society. *Neurosurgery*. 2020 Sep 15;87(4):647–54. doi:10.1093/neuros/nyaa308
65. Alsobrook J, Clugston JR. Return to play after surgery of the lumbar spine. *Curr Sports Med Rep*. 2008 Feb;7(1):45–8. doi:10.1097/01.CSMR.0000308666.15064.48

Shoulder Instability

Katherine J. Coyner, Samuel R. Engel, and Robert A. Arciero

51

INTRODUCTION

- The glenohumeral joint is the most commonly dislocated joint in the body, with an overall incidence of 17 per 100,000 per year (1–4) with higher incidences in more active patients such as military personnel reported by Owens et al. (5) 1.69 per to be 1000 person-years. The incidence of anterior shoulder dislocation requiring closed reduction is approximately 23 out of 100,000 person-years (6). Recurrence after the initial dislocation is common, and young age and activity level are the strongest risk factors (7–10). After 25 years of follow-up, Hovelius et al. (8) reported in a prospective study of 229 primary dislocations that were treated nonoperatively, 72% of patients originally younger than 22 years had at least 1 recurrent episode of instability, as compared with 27% of patients older than 30 years at the time of initial dislocation. Level I evidence suggests that surgical stabilization may be indicated for young first-time dislocators (11–15).

CLASSIFICATION

- There are three basic categories of instability. Instability should be considered as a spectrum of pathology. Unidirectional traumatic instability is on one end of the spectrum, and acquired instability and atraumatic multidirectional instability (MDI) are at the other end (16).

Traumatic

- Traumatic instability is further classified by the direction the humerus subluxates or dislocates in relationship to the glenoid.
- **Anterior:** Fall with the arm in an abducted and externally rotated position or an anterior force with the arm in abduction and external rotation (arm tackling in football, falling while snow skiing).
- **Posterior:** Posterior directed force with the arm forward elevated and adducted (motor vehicle accident or pass blocking in football). Grand mal seizure or electrical shock can also produce a traumatic posterior dislocation.

Acquired

- **Microinstability:** Subtle instability associated with pain in a throwing athlete or associated with rotator cuff tendinosis/dysfunction. This instability can occur from repetitive stretching of shoulder ligaments from daily activity or sports participation. These patients will present with anterior shoulder pain and sensation of transient instability combined with pertinent clinical exam findings consistent with instability.

Atraumatic

- **Multidirectional:** These patients have symptomatic glenohumeral subluxation or dislocations in more than one direction. Many patients present with severe pain as an initial complaint and not overt instability. For treatment planning, it is essential to identify the *primary direction* of instability based on patient history and physical examination.
  - Primary anterior: Pain associated with the arm in an abducted, externally rotated position
  - Primary posterior: Pain with pushing open a heavy door
  - Primary inferior: Pain associated with carrying heavy objects at the side
- Shoulder instability can be further classified via:
  - *Degree of instability:* Dislocation, subluxation, apprehension
  - *Chronology of instability:* Congenital, acute, chronic, recurrent
  - *Direction of instability:* Anterior, posterior, inferior, superior
  - Laxity is not instability: Laxity refers to translation of the humerus within the glenoid fossa. Many individuals are extremely lax but are asymptomatic. Instability refers to the symptomatic complaint of instability and dysfunction.

PATHOLOGY OF INSTABILITY

- The primary pathologic entity for traumatic instability is disruption of the anterior inferior labrum from the glenoid (Bankart lesion) combined with concomitant but variable damage to the capsule.

- The primary pathology for MDI is a loose, redundant capsule. Most patients with MDI can be treated successfully by conservative methods, such as patient education, a shoulder girdle strengthening program, or modification of the patient's routine activity.

Dynamic Restraints (see Fig. 51.1)

- This is a term that refers to the stability provided by contraction of the rotator cuff (supraspinatus, infraspinatus, subscapularis, and teres minor) and scapular stabilizers (serratus anterior, trapezius, and levator scapulae). The long head of the biceps can stabilize when contracting as well as the acromial arch (coracoacromial ligament and conjoined tendon).

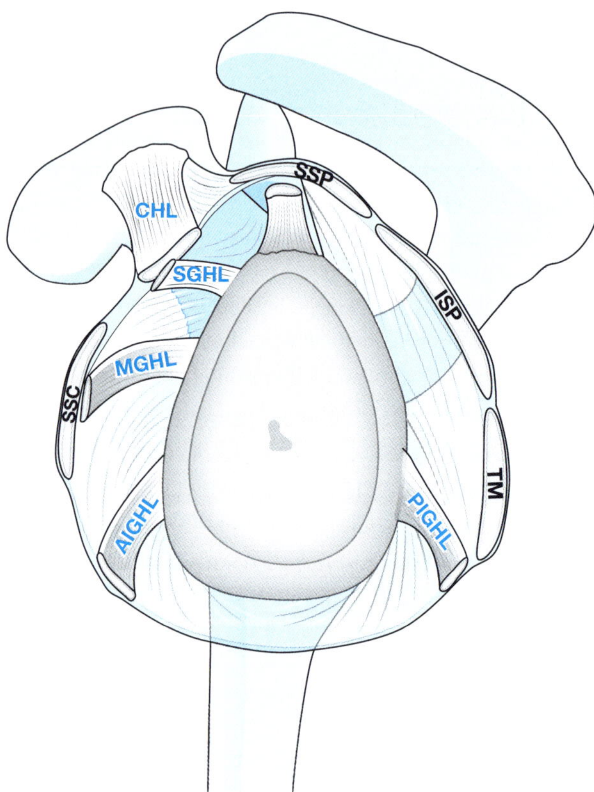

Figure 51.1: Dynamic stabilizers (red) of the glenohumeral joint are the rotator cuff muscles (17). (SSc, subscapularis; SSp, supraspinatus; ISp, infraspinatus; TM, teres minor), and the static stabilizers (blue) are the capsule, labrum, and the glenohumeral ligaments (AIGHL, anterior band of the inferior glenohumeral ligament; CHL, coracohumeral ligament; MGHL, middle glenohumeral ligament; PIGHL, posterior band of the inferior glenohumeral ligament; SGHL, superior glenohumeral ligament). (Adapted with permission from Provencher MT, Midtgaard KS, Owens BD, Tokish JM. Diagnosis and management of traumatic anterior shoulder instability. *J Am Acad Orthop Surg*. 2021:29(2):e51–61.)

Static Restraints (see Fig. 51.1)

- These restraints comprise bony, ligamentous, and labral anatomy that restrains translation statically and is independent of muscle contraction. The static stabilizers have the greatest contribution to shoulder stability at the end range of motion (ROM).
  - The humeral head is large compared with the shallow glenoid fossa, and the inherent stability of the glenohumeral joint relies heavily on glenoid version and soft-tissue stabilizers.
  - The labrum provides stability to the humeral head like a chockablock for a tire. It is a fibrocartilaginous structure attached to both the capsule and the glenoid. It surrounds the entire glenoid and is tightly attached in the anterior inferior quadrant, has a variable attachment in the superior quadrant, and is generally less prominent posteriorly.
  - The glenohumeral ligaments represent thickenings of the shoulder capsule. These are checkreins for stability. They are best visualized arthroscopically on the inside of the capsule but are difficult to distinguish on the outside as with open surgery. The anterior band of the IGHL (inferior glenohumeral ligament) is the main stabilizer. The MGHL (middle glenohumeral ligament) provides restraint with the arm in 45° of abduction and external rotation. The SHGL (superior glenohumeral ligament) provides restraint with the arm at the side.
  - Negative pressure, adhesion/cohesion
  - Finite joint volume limits end ranges of motion.
  - Joint conformity is increased with an intact capsulolabral complex that provides concavity to an otherwise flat glenoid and provides 50% additional glenoid depth.

Congenital Factors

- Individual collagen laxity
- Bone configuration (small glenoid, retroverted glenoid)
- Age

Associated Pathologies

- In addition to the Bankart lesion, several additional pathologies are described; preoperative appreciation of these unique labral and capsuloligamentous is critical for successful surgical management (see Fig. 51.2):
  - An osseous Bankart is defined as a detachment of the anteroinferior labrum associated with a glenoid rim fracture.
  - A reverse Bankart lesion is defined as the detachment of posteroinferior labrum with avulsion of posterior capsular periosteum.
  - A Perthes lesion is a variant of Bankart lesion when the labrum is avulsed from the glenoid, but remains partially attached to the scapula by intact periosteum.

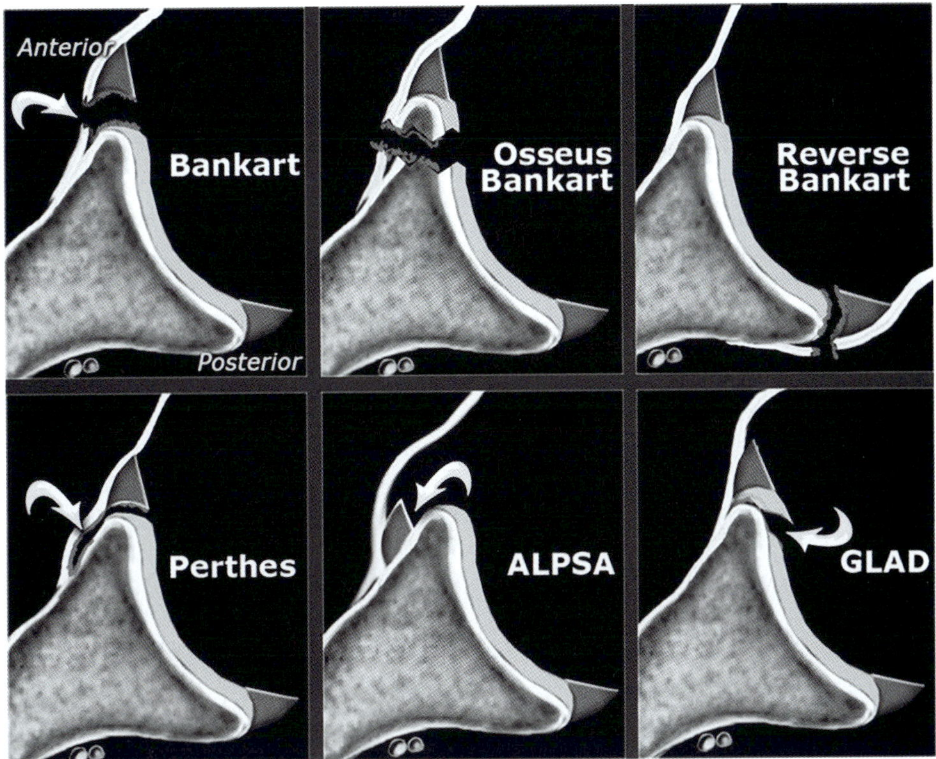

Figure 51.2: Bankart lesions and variants. (*Source:* Smithuis R, van der Woude HJ. Radiology Assistant: Shoulder instability – MRI. Available from: https://radiologyassistant.nl/musculoskeletal/shoulder/instability)

- A glenolabral articular disruption (GLAD) lesion is defined as a superficial anterior inferior labral tear associated with an anterior inferior glenoid articular cartilage injury.
- An anterior labral periosteal sleeve avulsion (APLSA) lesion is defined as a labral detachment, which remains attached to the glenoid periosteum (the sleeve); however, the anterior labroligamentous complex rolls up in a sleeve -like fashion and becomes displaced medially and inferiorly, "the medialized Bankart lesion."
- A humeral avulsion of the glenohumeral ligaments (HAGL) lesion is an avulsion of the inferior glenohumeral ligament (IGHL) from its humeral insertion.
- A Hill-Sachs lesion is defined as a bony defect of the postero-supero-lateral humeral head that occurs in association with anterior shoulder instability.
- A reverse Hill-Sachs lesion is a fracture of the anteromedial portion of the humeral head as a result of a posterior dislocation.

CLINICAL PRESENTATION

- **Physical Examination:** A careful and complete vascular and neurologic examination is essential. The frequency of axillary nerve injuries increases with age, with incidence of 5%–35% (18). Table 51.1 demonstrates a summary of the physical examination.

Traumatic Dislocation

- **Anterior:** This patient is in acute distress. Arm is held in slight abduction and internal rotation. There is a loss of deltoid contour, and there will be a prominence of the acromion (19).
- **Posterior:** Posterior dislocation of the shoulder is a rare injury (<4% of all shoulder dislocations). The diagnosis of this injury is often missed (60%–79%) on initial examination (20). Associated either with a high-energy event with a posterior directed force or a subluxation. Arm is held in significant internal rotation. A hallmark physical examination feature is inability to externally rotate the arm with the humerus lodged behind the posterior edge of the glenoid. Seizure disorders and electrocution are among the medical conditions that can lead to posterior shoulder dislocations.

Atraumatic Multidirectional

- These patients present with complaints of pain and multiple subluxation events. A hallmark physical examination feature is generalized ligamentous laxity and a sulcus sign. These patients may or may not have global joint laxity and, due to pain and spasm, sometimes do not have significant glenohumeral translation (21).

Table 51.1 Clinical Exam Findings Relevant to Assessing Shoulder Instability (17)

Sulcus sign	A test for shoulder laxity. The patient is in a relaxed standing position with their arms at their side. A force is applied to the affected arm. If a sulcus appears at the superior aspect of the humeral head, then the arm is put into external rotation. The test is then repeated, and the test is positive if the sign persists.
Apprehension test	The patient is positioned supine The shoulder is abducted 90° and externally rotated fully. Pain indicates a positive test.
Relocation test	If a posterior directed force is applied at the anterior margin of the glenoid reduces the pain in the apprehension test, the relocation test is considered positive.
Surprise test	The patient is seated with the arm in forward flexion at the shoulder to 90° and internally rotated to 90°. An axial load is quickly applied without warning to the humerus, pushing posteriorly. The test is possible if there is a "clunk" or pain.
Load-and-shift test	The patient is positioned supine with the shoulder at 40°–60° of abduction and 90° of forward flexion. An axial load is applied to the humerus while anterior and posterior translational forces are applied.
Anterior drawer test	The scapula is stabilized with one of the examiner's hands and a force is applied anteriorly at the humeral head with the other hand of the examiner. The test is positive if the patient feels a sense of instability when compared with the contralateral side.
Posterior drawer test	The same method is used as in the anterior drawer test, but the force is applied posteriorly at the humeral head.

Adapted with permission from Provencher MT, Midtgaard KS, Owens BD, Tokish JM. Diagnosis and management of traumatic anterior shoulder instability. *J Am Acad Orthop Surg*. 29(2):e51–61.

IMAGING

Radiographic Examination

- It is essential to obtain at least three views of the shoulder to determine direction of dislocation and also to ascertain the involvement of other bony pathology. It is important to obtain at least two orthogonal views to avoid missing a dislocation.
  - **Anteroposterior (AP):** The arm is held in slight internal rotation. This view will assist in the identification of greater tuberosity fractures. The glenoid in profile or an AP with the beam angled perpendicular to the glenohumeral joint allows more accurate identification of glenoid rim fractures.
  - **West point:** This is a special view taken with the patient prone and the beam directed inferiorly. It is a view that allows visualization of the anterior glenoid with no other overlying bone involvement. A traditional axillary view is also very useful for evaluating the direction of dislocation and fractures of the glenoid.
  - **Supraspinatus outlet view, scapular lateral view, or Y view:** This is a lateral view of the shoulder that can provide information on direction of dislocation as well as angulation of proximal humerus fractures.
  - **Stryker notch:** This is a view taken to evaluate the humeral head. A Hill-Sachs lesion is an impression fracture of the humeral head and, if large enough, can impact the clinical outcome. The patient is supine with the shoulder and elbow flexed and the beam directed through the axilla.
- Various imaging technologies are used to quantify the amount of capsular labral damage as well as evaluate the articular surface, rotator cuff, and bony architecture.
- **Magnetic resonance imaging (MRI):** The MRI allows visualization of the articular cartilage and rotator cuff. It also allows visualization of the glenolabral structures and capsule and can indicate whether there is a HAGL, or other aforementioned pathologies, which would predict a much different operative course. MRI has been validated as an imaging modality through which to assess bone loss.
- **Magnetic resonance arthrography (intra-articular gadolinium):** Shown to have the best sensitivity, specificity, and accuracy when compared to computed tomography (CT) arthrography and MRI for documenting glenolabral pathology (22).
- **CT arthrography:** This study allows axial cuts to evaluate glenoid morphology (amount of excess retroversion or anteversion). CTs are also used for the evaluation of bony injuries and calculation of glenoid bone loss or characterizing size and shape of glenoid fracture fragments.
- Historically "critical" bone loss has been defined as glenoid bone loss >25% (with a range from 20% to 27%) (23–25) and is biomechanically highly unstable. Shoulder stability cannot be restored with soft-tissue stabilization alone and glenoid defect >25% requires bony procedure to restore bone loss (Latarjet-Bristow, other sources of autograft or allograft).
- Increasing attention in recurrent anterior shoulder instability is being focused on bony defects and redefining "critical" bone loss. Yamamoto et al. in 2007 introduced the concept of the "glenoid track," which highlights that the position and orientation of the lesion have been shown to be important (26). A Hill-Sachs lesion that is "on track" cannot engage with the glenoid, whereas an "off track" lesion has a risk of engagement and dislocation and can be preoperatively determined by 3D CT (Fig. 51.3).

METHODS OF REDUCTION

- After a complete history, physical examination, and radiographic evaluation, reduction should be completed as quickly as possible.

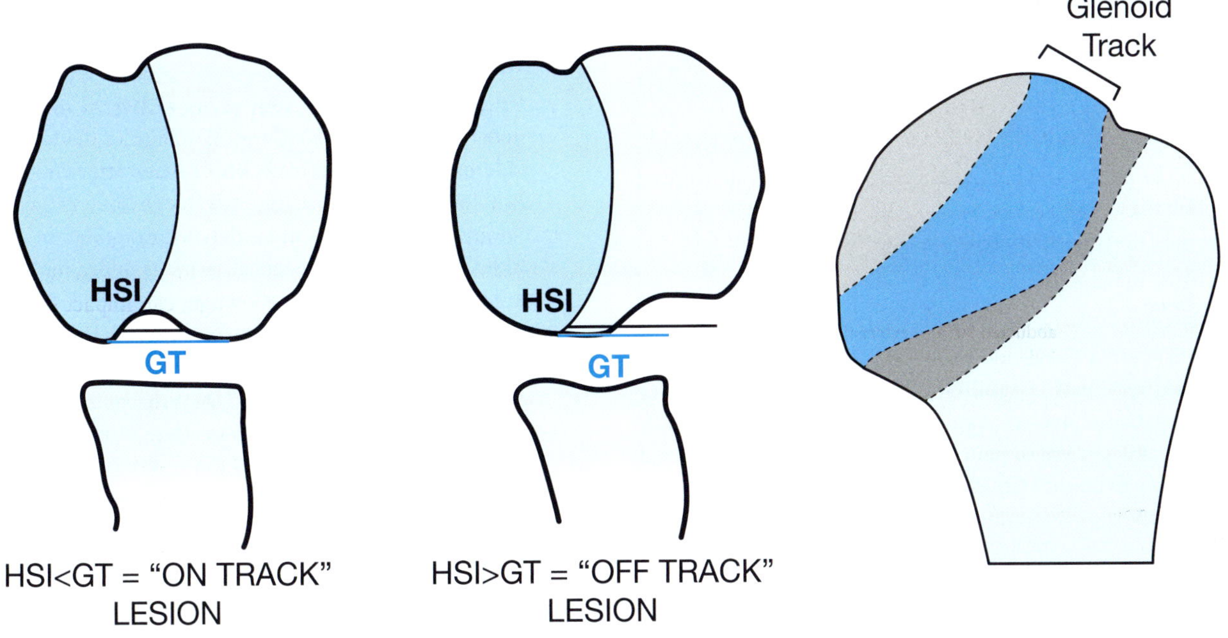

Figure 51.3: Visualization of the glenoid track (27). GT, glenoid track; HSI, hill sachs index. (Adapted with permission from Ventura A, Smiraglio C, Viscomi A, De Salvatore S, Bertucci B. The glenoid track concept: on-track and off-track—a narrative review. *Osteology*. 2022;2(3):129–36.)

- **Rockwood (traction/counter-traction) method:** Most commonly used. An assistant provides counter-traction with a sheet draped around the torso stabilizing the chest. The caregiver then applies counter-traction of the dislocated extremity distally. Slight internal and external rotation may be used to "free" up the engaged humeral head (28).
- **Stimson method:** The patient is placed in a prone position with the thorax supported by the table. Five to 10 lbs of weight are applied to the wrist with the arm straight. In time, the muscle will relax and the shoulder will be reduced (29).
- **Milch technique:** The patient is supine, and the arm is elevated slowly to 90°. It is then abducted with external rotation, and thumb pressure is used to gently reduce the shoulder (30).
- **Kocher technique:** The arm is flexed to 90°, and traction is applied in the line of the humerus. The arm is then fully externally rotated and then adducted across the chest. The arm is then internally rotated until the hand is placed on the opposite shoulder. This has been associated with proximal humerus fractures in the elderly (28).

POSTREDUCTION CARE

- It is paramount to examine and document neurovascular status before and after reduction. A sling can be provided for comfort, and pendulum exercises should be taught to the patient. Studies have not shown any benefit of immobilization >1 week for decreasing recurrence rates (31). Some studies show that immobilization in external rotation decreases recurrence rates in patients <40 by reducing the anterior labrum to the glenoid leading to more anatomic healing (32). However, subsequent studies have refuted this finding and the initially published results have not been reproducible (33).
- Follow-up evaluation should be in 10–14 days when spasm and pain have subsided. Rehabilitation can then be employed to establish full strength and ROM (19).
- goal is to return to sport within 7–21 days once the patient has full ROM and rotator cuff strength.
- **Rotator cuff injury:** In patients over 40 years, tears of the rotator cuff can occur with an incidence of 15% (34). In patients over 50, there is a 63% incidence of rotator cuff pathology or proximal humerus fractures (35).
- **Axillary nerve injury:** This complication has been reported to be between 1% and 7%. At 4 weeks postreduction, if active abduction cannot be established, an electromyogram (EMG) may be necessary to diagnose and follow an axillary nerve injury. Full functional and EMG recovery is typically documented 3–6 months after this complication (19).
- **Proximal humerus fractures:** Fractures of the greater tuberosity have been observed in up to 40% of patients older than the age of 50. Displacement of 1 cm may require surgical treatment.
- *Note:* Associated injuries involving the rotator cuff, proximal humerus fractures, and axillary nerve injuries increase with age at the time of dislocation.

NATURAL HISTORY AND NONOPERATIVE TREATMENT

- **Traumatic anterior:** Recurrence rates after primary dislocation:
  - 65%–95% in patients younger than 20 years depending on the author
  - 60% in patients 20–40 years old
  - 10% in patients older than 40 years old
- **Posterior:** Posterior subluxation patients responded better to nonoperative treatment than anterior subluxation patients (36).
- **Multidirectional instability (MDI):** The natural history of MDI patients involves a much larger spectrum of pathology. Eighty percent of patients diagnosed with MDI respond favorably to nonoperative treatment (36).

REHABILITATION

- Rehabilitation for instability involves activation of the dynamic stabilizers of the shoulder to aid in the overall stabilization. There are three main components — ROM, strengthening, and brace wear.
- **ROM:** Full external, internal, abduction, and forward elevation should be established. This is obtained by passive, active assisted, and finally active ROM. A trained therapist is critical for accuracy of movement, safety, and motivation.
- **Strengthening:** This begins with isometric contractions within a ROM that is comfortable for the patient. Once this is established, dynamic exercise band exercises can begin. Finally, isokinetic and isotonic strengthening with a complete arc of motion complete the program. Strengthening of the rotator cuff and scapular stabilizers is critical. Scapular dyskinesis is often a byproduct of instability and must be corrected to maintain shoulder stability.
- **Brace:** Braces are used to limit the "at-risk" position for return to sports.
  - Shoulder Subluxation Inhibitor (SSI) brace (Boston Brace International): Limits motion and protects against blows.
  - The SAWA Shoulder Orthosis (Brace International) provides anterior support and adds a checkrein.
  - The Duke–wire harness–lace up corset
  - The SSI brace was the most effective in limiting anterior shoulder subluxation, whereas the SAWA was considered to be the most comfortable (37).

OPERATIVE TREATMENT OPTIONS

- **Instability Severity Score:** Balg and Boileau (38) developed the Instability Severity Index Score (ISIS) evaluating six preoperative factors to determine patients appropriate for arthroscopic repair (Table 51.2). A score over six was felt to contraindicate arthroscopic repair.
- **Recurrent traumatic anterior:** Recurrence rates in the young athletic population after nonoperative treatment are unpredictable (65%–95%). Surgical stabilization should be considered in a young athlete who desires return to sport. Arthroscopic surgery has the advantage of creating less morbidity and allowing a more detailed examination of the shoulder. Although controversial, acute stabilization in the high-demand patient has been very successful and should be considered in the correct setting (39–42).
  - **Arthroscopic results:** Arthroscopic techniques have evolved over the last 35 years. Arthroscopic techniques have evolved to the level where they mimic the open technique. This involves plication of redundant inferior capsule, reattachment of the anterior inferior labrum directly to bone with suture anchors, and closure of the rotator interval. Recurrent instability rates following arthroscopic Bankart repair have been reported to be 8.5% (43), whereas in contact athletes the recurrence rate increases to 17.8% (44). Given the most common complication following isolated anterior labral repair is recurrent instability, it is imperative that risk factors for

Table 51.2 Instability Severity Score (38)

Prognostic Factors	Points
Age at Surgery (y)	
≤20	2
>20	0
Degree of Sport Participation (preoperative)	
Competitive	2
Recreational or none	0
Type of Sport (preoperative)	
Contact or forced overhead	1
Other	0
Shoulder Hyperlaxity	
Shoulder hyperlaxity (anterior or inferior)	1
Normal laxity	0
Hill-Sachs on AP Radiograph	
Visible in external rotation	2
Not visible in external rotation	0
Glenoid Loss of Contour on AP Radiograph	
Loss of contour	2
No lesion	0
Total (points)	10

Adapted with permission from Balg F, Boileau P. The instability severity index score. A simple pre-operative score to select patients for arthroscopic or open shoulder stabilisation. *J Bone Joint Surg Br*. 2007;89(11):1470–7.

recurrent shoulder instability such as glenoid or humeral head bone loss are identified and addressed.

- Assessment of the glenoid bone loss is most commonly done preoperatively by looking at the en face view of a CT and using a best-fit circle to determine the percent bone loss and confirming this by arthroscopic measurement (Fig. 51.4). Multiple studies have shown higher failure rates with arthroscopic labral repair in the presence of substantial glenoid bone loss, typically defined as great than 25% (45,46).
- The concept of what is the critical amount of glenoid bone loss has been challenged lately, with several studies that show inferior outcomes of arthroscopic Bankart procedures with bone loss as low as 13.5% (23,47,48). It is also important to assess the amount of bone loss on both the glenoid and humeral side, often referred to as "bipolar bone loss." More recently there has been more debate about managing glenoid bone loss when it is 10%–30% and when there are bipolar lesions on both the glenoid and humeral head. A recent cadaver-based study concluded that combined, bipolar lesions with as little as 8%–15% of the glenoid, with a medium-sized Hill-Sachs lesion, could compromise a Bankart repair (49).

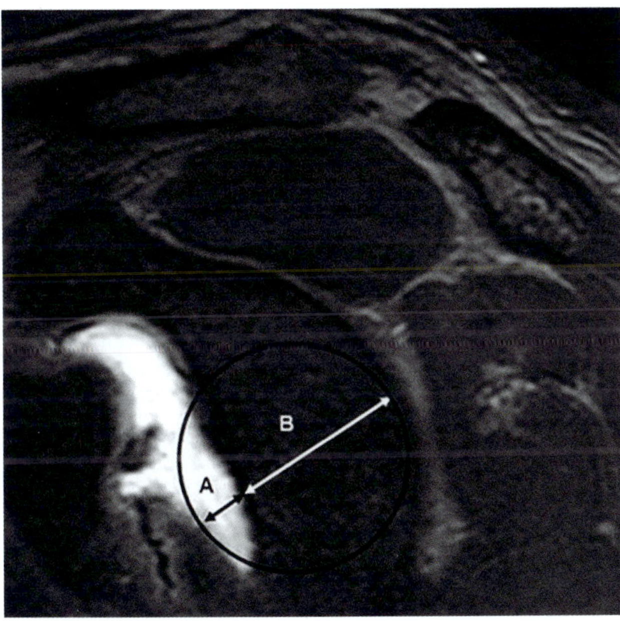

Figure 51.4: Measurement of glenoid bone loss by the best fit circle method (49). Maximum transverse width of the bony glenoid *(B)* is compared with a diameter of best-fit circle *(A + B)*. Glenoid bone loss is percentage reduction in maximum transverse glenoid width relative to diameter of best-fit circle, that is, $A/(A + B) \times 100\%$. Glenoid bone loss in this case was 23%. (Adapted with permission from Arciero RA, Parrino A, Bernhardson AS, et al. The effect of a combined glenoid and Hill-Sachs defect on glenohumeral stability: a biomechanical cadaveric study using 3-dimensional modeling of 142 patients. *Am J Sports Med.* 2015;43(6):1422–9.)

- **Hill-Sachs lesion:** If the humeral head lesion is large (>33%) or "off-track" Hill-Sachs lesions with <20 to 25% glenoid bone loss then various procedures can be considered (40).
- Lesser tuberosity transfer with subscapularis tendon (remplissage) in which the posterior capsule and infraspinatus tendon sutured into the Hill-Sachs lesion. Often performed with concomitant Bankart repair. The goal of the remplissage is to restore the articular surface of the glenoid while eliminating an engaging Hill-Sachs lesion. Hughes and colleagues compared Bankart repair with or without remplissage in the high-risk adolescent population with Hill-Sachs lesions and found that the addition of remplissage significantly decreased recurrence rates (13% vs. 47%), while maintaining similar ROM and patient outcome scores (50).
- Open capsular shift
- Humeral head allograft

- **Open results:** Historically, many procedures have been described for glenohumeral instability. Many of these did not repair the labral lesion, and high rates of instability were still found. Only the open Bankart suture repair and coracoid process transfers (Bristow and Laterjet) are currently being performed.
  - Bankart — suture repair of labrum
  - Laterjet transfer of the coracoid process
- **Open versus arthroscopic results:** A recent systematic review identified over 60 studies reporting results of arthroscopic procedures for chronic anterior shoulder instability or comparisons between arthroscopic and open surgery. The failure rates of older arthroscopic techniques using staples or transglenoid suture techniques were significantly higher than the failure rates for open or arthroscopic stabilization using suture anchors or bioabsorbable tacks. The meta-analysis concluded that arthroscopic stabilization using newer techniques had a similar rate of failure compared to open stabilization after 2 years (51).
- Another recent systematic review comparing arthroscopic with open stabilization procedures concluded that further research is needed. Randomized controlled trials that are sufficiently powered, use validated outcome measures, and have long-term follow-up are required (52).

- Bankart lesions (tears of the anterior inferior labrum) were found in 84% of patients with continued instability after surgery. Stability was restored in 92% with the repair of labrum. Uncorrected capsular redundancy was also a reason for failure in over 80% of patients (53).
  - **Bone reconstruction:** There are instances where the anterior inferior glenoid has a large fracture or is deficient secondary to impaction or chronic instability. In these instances soft-tissue procedures are not adequate, and bone graft may be required.

- **Glenoid deficiency:** For large defects, three procedures exist:
- **Laterjet/Bristow:** Coracoid bone transferred to the glenoid (45).
- **Autograft (tricortical iliac crest or distal clavicle) or allograft (iliac crest or distal tibia).** Indications include bony deficiencies with >20–25% glenoid deficiency (inverted pear deformity to glenoid). These can be performed open or arthroscopic.

- **Recurrent traumatic posterior:** This is a less frequent multifactorial condition with several modes of presentation.
  - **Open capsular posterior shift:** Associated with a posterior Bankart lesion and good success. Posterior capsule is shifted superiorly and laterally through a posterior approach (54).
  - **Arthroscopic:** Suture anchor or bioabsorbable tack fixation arthroscopically of the posterior Bankart lesion; associated with an 8% reoperation rate for failure (55).
  - **Acquired microinstability:** This is a condition that exists in the throwing or overhead athlete. Subtle anterior instability may lead to an impingement of the articular supraspinatus/infraspinatus tendons against the posterior superior labrum termed internal impingement.
- **Multidirectional:** Open inferior shift: This procedure, first reported by Neer and Foster (1980) (21), has been successful. Reports of 2%–8% failure rates in MDI patients (21,56).

REFERENCES

1. Bankart AS. Recurrent or habitual dislocation of the shoulder-joint. *Br Med J.* 1923;2(3285):1132–3.
2. Bigliani LU, Kelkar R, Flatow EL, Pollock RG, Mow VC. Glenohumeral stability. Biomechanical properties of passive and active stabilizers. *Clin Orthop Relat Res.* 1996;330:13–30.
3. Krøner K, Lind T, Jensen J. The epidemiology of shoulder dislocations. *Arch Orthop Trauma Surg.* 1989;108(5):288–90.
4. Romeo AA, Cohen BS, Carreira DS. Traumatic anterior shoulder instability. *Orthop Clin North Am.* 2001;32(3):399–409.
5. Owens BD, Dawson L, Burks R, Cameron KL. Incidence of shoulder dislocation in the United States military: demographic considerations from a high-risk population. *J Bone Joint Surg Am.* 2009;91(4):791–6.
6. Leroux T, Wasserstein D, Veillette C, et al. Epidemiology of primary anterior shoulder dislocation requiring closed reduction in Ontario, Canada. *Am J Sports Med.* 2014;42(2):442–50.
7. Hovelius L. The natural history of primary anterior dislocation of the shoulder in the young. *J Orthop Sci.* 1999;4(4):307–17.
8. Hovelius L, Olofsson A, Sandström B, et al. Nonoperative treatment of primary anterior shoulder dislocation in patients forty years of age and younger. a prospective twenty-five-year follow-up. *J Bone Joint Surg Am.* 2008;90(5):945–52.
9. Rowe CR, Sakellarides HT. Factors related to recurrences of anterior dislocations of the shoulder. *Clin Orthop.* 1961;20:40–8.
10. Simonet WT, Cofield RH. Prognosis in anterior shoulder dislocation. *Am J Sports Med.* 1984;12(1):19–24.
11. te Slaa RL, Wijffels MP, Brand R, Marti RK. The prognosis following acute primary glenohumeral dislocation. *J Bone Joint Surg Br.* 2004;86(1):58–64.
12. Bottoni CR, Wilckens JH, DeBerardino TM, et al. A prospective, randomized evaluation of arthroscopic stabilization versus nonoperative treatment in patients with acute, traumatic, first-time shoulder dislocations. *Am J Sports Med.* 2002;30(4):576–80.
13. Handoll HH, Almaiyah MA, Rangan A. Surgical versus non-surgical treatment for acute anterior shoulder dislocation. *Cochrane Database Syst Rev.* 2004;2004(1):CD004325.
14. Jakobsen BW, Johannsen HV, Suder P, Søjbjerg JO. Primary repair versus conservative treatment of first-time traumatic anterior dislocation of the shoulder: a randomized study with 10-year follow-up. *Arthroscopy.* 2007;23(2):118–23.
15. Kirkley A, Werstine R, Ratjek A, Griffin S. Prospective randomized clinical trial comparing the effectiveness of immediate arthroscopic stabilization versus immobilization and rehabilitation in first traumatic anterior dislocations of the shoulder: long-term evaluation. *Arthroscopy.* 2005;21(1):55–63.
16. Thomas SC, Matsen FA III. An approach to the repair of avulsion of the glenohumeral ligaments in the management of traumatic anterior glenohumeral instability. *J Bone Joint Surg Am.* 1989;71(4):506–13.
17. Provencher MT, Midtgaard KS, Owens BD, Tokish JM. Diagnosis and management of traumatic anterior shoulder instability. *J Am Acad Orthop Surg.* 2021:29(2):e51–61.
18. Blom S, Dahlbäck LO. Nerve injuries in dislocations of the shoulder joint and fractures of the neck of the humerus. A clinical and electromyographical study. *Acta Chir Scand.* 1970;136(6):461–6.
19. Arciero RA. Acute anterior dislocations. In: Warren RF, Craig EV, Altchek DW, eds. *The Unstable Shoulder.* Philadelphia: Lippincott-Raven; 1999. p. 159–75.
20. Hawkins RJ, Neer CS 2nd, Pianta RM, Mendoza FX. Locked posterior dislocation of the shoulder. *J Bone Joint Surg Am.* 1987 Jan;69(1):9–18.
21. Neer CS II, Foster CR. Inferior capsular shift for involuntary inferior and multidirectional instability of the shoulder. A preliminary report. *J Bone Joint Surg Am.* 1980;62(6):879–908.
22. Chandnani VP, Yeager TD, DeBerardino TM, et al. Glenoid labral tears: prospective evaluation with MRI imaging, MR arthrography, and CT arthrography. *AJR Am J Roentgenol.* 1993;161(6):1229–35.
23. Shaha JS, Cook JB, Song DJ, et al. Redefining"critical" bone loss in shoulder instability: functional outcomes worsen with "subcritical" bone loss. *Am J Sports Med.* 2015;43(7):1719–25.
24. Beran MC, Donaldson CT, Bishop JY. Treatment of chronic glenoid defects in the setting of recurrent anterior shoulder instability: a systematic review. *J Shoulder Elbow Surg.* 2010;19(5):769–80.
25. Bigliani LU, Newton PM, Steinmann SP, Connor PM, Mcllveen SJ. Glenoid rim lesions associated with recurrent anterior dislocation of the shoulder. *Am J Sports Med.* 1998;26(1):41–5.
26. Yamamoto N, Itoi E, Abe H, et al. Contact between the glenoid and the humeral head in abduction, external rotation, and horizontal extension: a new concept of glenoid track. *J Shoulder Elbow Surg.* 2007;16(5):649–56.
27. Ventura A, Smiraglio C, Viscomi A, De Salvatore S, Bertucci B. The glenoid track concept: on-track and off-track — a narrative review. *Osteology.* 2022;2(3):129–36.
28. Neer CS, Rockwood CA Jr. Fractures and dislocations of the shoulder. In: Rockwood CA Jr, Green DP, editors. *Fractures in Adults.* 4th ed. Philadelphia: JB Lippincott; 1996.
29. Matsen FA, Thomas SC, Rockwood CA Jr. Anterior glenohumeral instability. In: Rockwood CA Jr, Matsen FA, editors. *The Shoulder.* 2nd ed, Vol. 2. Philadelphia: Saunders; 1998:669–72.

30. Milch H. Treatment of dislocation of the shoulder. *Surg.* 1938;3:732–40.
31. Paterson WH, Throckmorton TW, Koester M, Azar FM, Kuhn JE. Position and duration of immobilization after primary anterior shoulder dislocation: a systematic review and meta-analysis of the literature. *J Bone Joint Surg Am.* 2010;92(18):2924–33.
32. Shinagawa K, Sugawara Y, Hatta T, Yamamoto N, Tsuji I, Itoi E. Immobilization in external rotation reduces the risk of recurrence after primary anterior shoulder dislocation: a meta-analysis. *Orthop J Sports Med.* 2020 Jun;8(6):2325967120925694.
33. Liavaag S, Brox JI, Pripp AH, Enger M, Soldal LA, Svenningsen S. Immobilization in external rotation after primary shoulder dislocation did not reduce the risk of recurrence: a randomized controlled trial. *J Bone Joint Surg Am.* 2011;93(10):897–904.
34. Neviaser RJ, Neviaser TJ, Neviaser JS. Concurrent rupture of the rotator cuff and anterior dislocation of the shoulder in the older patient. *J Bone Joint Surg Am.* 1988;70(9):1308–11.
35. Ribbans WJ, Mitchell R, Taylor GJ. Computerised arthrotomography of primary anterior dislocation of the shoulder. *J Bone Joint Surg Br.* 1990;72(2):181–5.
36. Burkhead WZ Jr, Rockwood CA Jr. Treatment of instability of the shoulder with an exercise program. *J Bone Joint Surg Am.* 1992;74(6):890–6.
37. DeCarlo M, Malone K, Geric J, Hucker M. Evaluation of shoulder instability braces. *J Sports Rehabil.* 1996;5:143–50.
38. Balg F, Boileau P. The instability severity index score. A simple pre-operative score to select patients for arthroscopic or open shoulder stabilisation. *J Bone Joint Surg Br.* 2007;89(11):1470–7.
39. Arciero RA, Wheeler JH, Ryan JB, McBride JT. Arthroscopic Bankart repair versus nonoperative treatment for acute, initial anterior shoulder dislocations. *Am J Sports Med.* 1994;22(5):589–94.
40. Bottoni CR, Smith EL, Berkowitz MJ, Towle RB, Moore JH. Arthroscopic versus open shoulder stabilization for recurrent anterior instability: a prospective randomized clinical trial. *Am J Sports Med.* 2006;34(11):1730–7.
41. Fabbriciani C, Milano G, Demontis A, Fadda S, Ziranu F, Mulas PD. Arthroscopic versus open treatment of Bankart lesion of the shoulder: a prospective randomized study. *Arthroscopy.* 2004;20(5):456–62.
42. Kirkley A, Griffin S, Richards C, Miniaci A, Mohtadi N. Prospective randomized clinical trial comparing the effectiveness of immediate arthroscopic stabilization versus immobilization and rehabilitation in first traumatic anterior dislocations of the shoulder. *Arthroscopy.* 1999;15(5):507–14.
43. Harris JD, Gupta AK, Mall NA, et al. Long-term outcomes after Bankart shoulder stabilization. *Arthroscopy.* 2013;29(5):920–33. doi:10.1016/j.arthro.2012.11.010
44. Leroux TS, Saltzman BM, Meyer M, et al. The influence of evidence-based surgical indications and techniques on failure rates after arthroscopic shoulder stabilization in the contact or collision athlete with anterior shoulder instability. *Am J Sports Med.* 2017;45(5):1218–25.
45. Burkhart SS, De Beer JF. Traumatic glenohumeral bone defects and their relationship to failure of arthroscopic Bankart repairs: significance of the inverted-pear glenoid and the humeral engaging Hill-Sachs lesion. *Arthroscopy.* 2000;16(7):677–94.
46. Boileau P, Villalba M, Héry JY, Balg F, Ahrens P, Neyton L. Risk factors for recurrence of shoulder instability after arthroscopic Bankart repair. *J Bone Joint Surg Am.* 2006;88(8):1755–63.
47. Dickens JF, Owens BD, Cameron KL, et al. The effect of subcritical bone loss and exposure on recurrent instability after arthroscopic Bankart repair in intercollegiate American football. *Am J Sports Med.* 2017;45(8):1769–75.
48. Shin SJ, Kim RG, Jeon YS, Kwon TH. Critical value of anterior glenoid bone loss that leads to recurrent glenohumeral instability after arthroscopic Bankart repair. *Am J Sports Med.* 2017;45(9):1975–81.
49. Arciero RA, Parrino A, Bernhardson AS, et al. The effect of a combined glenoid and Hill-Sachs defect on glenohumeral stability: a biomechanical cadaveric study using 3-dimensional modeling of 142 patients. *Am J Sports Med.* 2015;43(6):1422–9.
50. Hughes JL, Bastrom T, Pennock AT, Edmonds EW. Arthroscopic Bankart repairs with and without remplissage in recurrent adolescent anterior shoulder instability with hill-sachs deformity. *Orthop J Sports Med.* 2018;6(12):2325967118813981.
51. Hobby J, Griffin D, Dunbar M, Boileau P. Is arthroscopic surgery for stabilisation of chronic shoulder instability as effective as open surgery? A systematic review and meta-analysis of 62 studies including 3044 arthroscopic operations. *J Bone Joint Surg Br.* 2007;89(9):1188–96.
52. Pulavarti RS, Symes TH, Rangan A. Surgical interventions for anterior shoulder instability in adults. *Cochrane Database Syst Rev.* 2009;7(4):CD005077.
53. Rowe CR, Zarins B, Ciullo JV. Recurrent anterior dislocation of the shoulder after surgical repair. Apparent causes of failure and treatment. *J Bone Joint Surg Am.* 1984;66(2):159–68.
54. Bigliani LU, Pollock RG, McIlveen SJ, Endrizzi DP, Flatow EL. Shift of the posteroinferior aspect of the capsule for recurrent posterior glenohumeral instability. *J Bone Joint Surg Am.* 1995;77(7):1011–20.
55. Williams RJ III, Strickland S, Cohen M, Altchek DW, Warren RF. Arthroscopic repair for traumatic posterior shoulder instability. *Am J Sports Med.* 2003;31(2):203–9.
56. Cooper RA, Brems JJ. The inferior capsular shift procedure for multidirectional instability of the shoulder. *J Bone Joint Surg Am.* 1992;74(10):1516–21.

52 Rotator Cuff Pathology

Patrick St. Pierre

HISTORY

- John Gregory Smith published the first detailed series of rotator cuff ruptures, describing seven cases obtained by grave robbing, in a letter to the editor of *The London Medical Gazette* in 1834. Muller and Perthes were the first to perform repairs in the late 1800s. Codman and later McLaughlin were pioneers in the early 1900s, describing their approach to the shoulder and detailing rotator cuff repair (RCR) techniques that have been followed until today (1).
- In 1972, Neer (2) first proposed the phrase "impingement syndrome" for pain involving the subacromial bursa and superior rotator cuff. He described the clinical presentation of the painful shoulder and proposed a mechanism for how the pathology developed. He noted that many of these patients had a hooked acromion, and his hypothesis was that the bursa and rotator cuff were impinged between the humeral head and acromion with elevation of the arm. This would usually start as mild inflammation of the tendon, would progress to fibrosis and tendonitis, and eventually could lead to full-thickness rotator cuff tear.

IMPINGEMENT OR ROTATOR CUFF SYNDROME (2,3)

- Stage I, as described by Neer, included edema and hemorrhage in the tendon. Tendinosis of the supraspinatus and, less frequently, the infraspinatus or subscapularis is involved.
- Stage II consisted of fibrosis and tendonitis in the subacromial space. This is a secondary process resulting from the underlying etiology.
- Stage III resulted in the development of spurs and eventually tendon rupture.
- The long head of the biceps tendon may also be involved with pathology ranging from inflammation to rupture (4). Dislocation of the biceps tendon from the bicipital groove is pathognomonic for a tear of the upper border of the subscapularis muscle from its humeral insertion (5,6).
- Pain will often occur along the anterior-lateral acromion, in the infraspinatus fossa, or distally at the deltoid insertion on the humerus. This pain is likely to be referred pain from the inflamed bursa, which irritates the deep deltoid. Pain referring proximally to the neck usually originates from the acromioclavicular (AC) joint (7–10).
- There have been several other etiologies proposed for shoulder pain emanating from the subacromial space following Dr. Neer's initial description (10–12). These different etiologies may or may not lead to actual impingement of the cuff by the acromion. Because multiple pathologies are often factors in this condition, including tendinosis and bursitis, the best global term to describe this condition is rotator cuff syndrome, reserving impingement syndrome for cases of true external impingement caused by AC arthritis or from the development of a coracoacromial (CA) ligament spur. Specific etiologies, as discussed later, may also be used.

PATHOPHYSIOLOGY

Rotator Cuff Syndrome

- Historically, patients will occasionally remember a direct blow or some other form of trauma. There may be a history of a traction injury or a fall directly on a patient's shoulder.
- Overuse injury is also a frequent cause of this syndrome. Patients will often not recall a specific injury but may have carried luggage all weekend, cleaned out their attic, or worked on their car. Frequently, repetitive overhead activity such as tennis, softball, or swimming is the causative factor.
- These conditions occur primarily because of injury to the rotator cuff causing tendinosis and rotator cuff dysfunction. The subacromial impingement occurs chronically with the development of subacromial spurs and superior humeral head migration due to lower rotator cuff inhibition or fatigue.

Secondary Impingement

- Subtle shoulder instability can lead to rotator cuff dysfunction and thus to rotator cuff syndrome. Jobe and colleagues described this as secondary or internal impingement syndrome (11,12). This condition was originally noted in overhead-throwing athletes, but should be suspected in all younger athletes who complain of "impingement"-type pain. Treatment of this condition must address the underlying instability and not just the secondary pathology in the subacromial space.

Posterosuperior Glenoid Impingement

- This condition, as described by Walch et al. (13), has also been proposed as an etiology occurring in patients who play repetitive overhead sports such as baseball, tennis, and swimming. Walch did not find the anterior instability described by Jobe in his patients, but rather noted an impingement of the supraspinatus and infraspinatus tendons between the posterosuperior glenoid labrum and the humeral head.
- These internal impingement syndromes are characterized by partial tears of the articular surface of the rotator cuff, in distinction to the external compression described by Neer (14).
- Whatever the etiology, weakness of the rotator cuff results, especially the lower cuff, and superior humeral head migration occurs. The humeral head then compresses the bursa and tendon into the acromion, leading to impingement. This causes more bursitis, more tendinosis, and eventually more weakness. Often with chronic injury, shoulder mechanics will change, leading to abnormal scapulothoracic motion. Physical therapy will need to include rehabilitation of the scapular stabilizing musculature as well as the lower rotator cuff muscles (15).
- Any subacromial changes, such as lateral hooking, CA ligament calcification, or AC joint arthritis (inferior spurs), will cause the condition to get worse and will more likely need operative intervention than when the acromion is flat.
- Calcific tendinitis
  - The etiology of calcific tendinitis remains unknown. Degenerative changes and relative hypoxia have been suggested as possible explanations. Conservative treatment similar to that for rotator cuff syndrome is reported as successful in 60%–90% of patients (16–18). Repetitive needling and injection of local anesthetic have also been successful in relieving symptoms and often result in disappearance of the calcified mass. Infrequently, the patient's symptoms will persist, and the patient will require operative intervention. The mass is localized within the substance of the tendon while viewing in the subacromial space. The calcified substance is then evacuated and debrided. Some argue that a repair of the tendon is not necessary, but the surgeon should evaluate the cuff after debridement in each case to determine if repair is necessary.

EXAMINATION (19)

- Inspection should focus on normal alignment of chest wall, shoulders, and clavicle. Have the patient perform active range of motion (ROM) in forward flexion, abduction, adduction, external rotation, and internal rotation. Look from the back and front for asymmetric motion or atrophy. Often patients will have a painful arc of motion over 120° of elevation.
- Palpate the AC and sternoclavicular joints, the anterior and lateral acromion edges, and the infraspinatus fossa. Tenderness at the AC joint should lead you to further evaluation and treatment of AC joint arthrosis. Cross-arm adduction is often painful with AC arthrosis. However, this test is not very specific and is often positive with rotator cuff syndrome.
- Palpation of the long head of the biceps tendon within the bicipital groove is helpful to determine biceps involvement. O'Brien active compression test, Speed test, and Yergason test are also used to determine biceps involvement and are covered in Chapter 50.
- Strength testing should involve the deltoid, biceps, and triceps muscles. Although there is no way to totally isolate each of the rotator cuff muscles, the tests that have shown to be most specific are the following (20):
  - Supraspinatus: Active elevation against resistance with the elbow in extension and the arm elevated to 90° and externally rotated to 45°. The hand should be supinated to neutral as if holding a full can of soda.
  - Infraspinatus/teres minor: Active external rotation with arm at the side and elbow flexed to 90°.
  - Subscapularis: Active internal rotation with elbow flexed to 90° and hand placed behind the back. This is often referred to as the Gerber lift-off test (5,6,21). In patients who are unable to internally rotate their hand behind their back, a belly press test or "Napoleon test" is performed. The patient places their hand on their belly and presses hard into their abdomen while bringing their elbow forward in the sagittal plane. Subscapularis tear or dysfunction is indicated if they are unable to do this maneuver and the elbow stays close to the side (22).
- Lag tests are also often used to detect rotator cuff tears. The hornblower sign, external rotation lag, and internal rotation lag tests were described by Gerber and Hertel and are helpful to determine subtle weakness (6,23).
- Special tests include the Neer impingement sign and test and Hawkins sign.
  - The Neer impingement sign is similar to the supraspinatus testing described earlier, except the arm is held in maximal internal rotation as if pouring out a can of soda. This rotates the greater tuberosity under the acromion to elicit a painful response if the bursa or tendons are injured. A positive Neer test is when a subacromial injection of local anesthetic relieves the pain elicited prior to the injection (2,3).
  - The Hawkins test forward flexes the arm to 90° and applies maximum internal rotation to the flexed elbow. If one supplies downward pressure at the elbow while the patient resists, the sensitivity of the exam increases (8,24).
  - The accuracy of these and many other tests in the shoulder has been called into question; however, they remain the standard as the initial baseline test. Clinical history, examination, and diagnostic testing must all be used together to make an accurate diagnosis (25).

- A cervical spine examination should be performed if there is any concern of radicular symptoms as a factor in diagnosis. This is particularly useful in patients older than 50 years of age and if painful symptoms radiate distal to the elbow.

RADIOGRAPHIC EXAMINATION

- Standard radiographs include anteroposterior (AP), axillary, and supraspinatus outlet views. These views will allow you to determine if there is degenerative joint disease in the AC or glenohumeral joints, spurring from the acromion or calcification within the tendon (calcific tendonitis). Chronic rotator cuff tears will often result in superior humeral head migration secondary to atrophy of the lower rotator cuff. A true scapular AP view will allow better examination of the glenoid, and internal and external rotation view will allow better assessment of the humeral head for defects or impression fractures.
- Special radiographs are indicated in certain conditions. A supraspinatus outlet view is often obtained to evaluate the morphology of the acromion in rotator cuff or impingement syndrome. A West Point view is helpful in evaluating the anterior glenoid for bony deficiency in cases of instability.
- Magnetic resonance imaging (MRI) is an excellent tool for determining rotator cuff pathology and should be used if a full rotator cuff tear is suspected.
- Certain signal characteristics are indicative of full tears versus partial tears or tendinitis. An MRI can determine labral pathology (Bankart lesions or superior labral anterior to posterior tears), bursitis, acromial morphology, and articular cartilage condition to include glenohumeral and AC joint arthritis. More details about MRI for upper extremity injuries can be found in Chapter 46.
- An MRI does not need to be obtained immediately if the patient has full ROM and only complains of pain and weakness. These patients can be started on the nonoperative treatment described in the next section, and the vast majority will improve. An MRI can be obtained after the next visit if the patient's symptoms have not resolved with therapy.
- The MRI is useful in determining the extent of the tear and for preoperative planning. In larger, chronic tears, the MRI is useful for determining atrophy of the muscles and efficacy of repair. In older patients, this is also useful to help determine surgical treatment of RCR versus reverse shoulder arthroplasty (26).

NONOPERATIVE TREATMENT (PAIN CONTROL — INJECTIONS)

- Nonsteroidal anti-inflammatory drugs (NSAIDs) are usually helpful to decrease the bursitis and reduce the pain. They are not curative in themselves, but decrease pain so the patient can do therapy. Tylenol can be added to the NSAID regimen to help with pain.
- A subacromial injection can be performed as a diagnostic test or as part of the treatment plan. When the Neer sign is positive, an injection is made into the subacromial space using a local anesthetic. The patient is retested after 3–5 minutes, and the Neer test is positive if the pain is relieved. Many physicians who are certain of their diagnosis will proceed with a therapeutic injection of 2–3 mL of an injectable corticosteroid at the same time. Others will inject a second time if the initial injection relieves the patient's symptoms.
- If there is a diagnostic dilemma between whether the AC joint is the cause of pain or the bursa, injections can be performed in one location and then the second to determine the source. The subacromial injection should be done first because with AC pathology, the capsule is often disrupted and an AC injection is likely to go into the bursa as well. The reader is referred to Chapter 79 on injections for more information.
- Many practitioners are concerned about the effects of corticosteroids on the damaged tendon and several studies have documented an increased risk of infection following corticosteroid injections (27). Many physicians will either forego this step or limit the number of injections. Patients who have developed subacromial spurs and AC arthritis are less likely to improve due to fixed impingement and may require surgery. However, the number of injections and length of nonoperative treatment should be individualized to the patient.
- If an acute, traumatic tear is suspected in an active patient who may require surgery, a corticosteroid injection should be delayed until after an MRI is obtained so as not to delay surgery.
- Platelet-rich plasma (PRP) injections have been used for treatment of partial-thickness rotator cuff tears. A systematic review of PRP compared with corticosteroid revealed short- and long-term relief with both modalities, but significantly more effectiveness in both functional and pain control in the long term (28,29) (see Chapter 78, Orthobiologics).

NONOPERATIVE TREATMENT (REHABILITATION)

- Rotator cuff strengthening is essential for recovery, and many patients improve after surgical intervention because they finally commit themselves to rehabilitation.
- The focus of rehabilitation should be to reduce inflammation (usually bursal), restore motion, and strengthen muscles to help stabilize the scapula and humerus. Therapists will start with anti-inflammatory modalities, work on ROM, and begin periscapular strengthening to stabilize the scapula (15,30).
- Once the pain is reduced and the ROM restored, more aggressive strengthening exercises are instituted. Internal and external rotation exercises using rubber tubing or resistance

bands are very useful, and the patient progresses to heavier tubing as they get stronger. Supine or lateral decubitus exercises with small weights are also started at this time.

- Core strengthening exercises to help stabilize the scapula are also instituted. These exercises are very important and often neglected. Simple exercises such as squeezing the shoulder blades together or scapular rows are often effective. Progress is monitored by observing normal scapulothoracic motion with elevation. If scapular winging is severe or fails to improve with treatment, further workup for other etiologies such as trapezius or long thoracic nerve palsy should occur.
- Deltoid strengthening should include isolated training of all three parts of the deltoid.
- Strengthening of the supraspinatus is not instituted immediately because it will aggravate symptoms. Supraspinatus strengthening should be started when ROM is restored and lower cuff strength is sufficient to allow overhead motion without pain.
- Most patients' symptoms resolve with this program.

SURGICAL INTERVENTION

Subacromial Decompression

- Subacromial decompression was originally described by Neer as an open operation to remove anterior and lateral spurs on the acromion, to remove the inflamed bursa, and for resection or release of the CA ligament (2).
- Many believe the development of spurs is a secondary process and is not causative in nature as once thought by Neer (31). The spurs are usually anterior and medial and due to calcification of the CA ligament. Inspection of the acromion and CA ligament should be performed, with the removal of bone only if abnormal ossification has occurred. Frequently an acromioplasty and CA ligament resection are not necessary. This is especially true for articular-sided tears caused by intrinsic pathology.
- Arthroscopy has led to a less invasive approach to decompression, and the operative goal is usually to convert the acromion to a so-called type I acromion. A bursectomy and inspection of the cuff are included.
- Pathology of the long head of the biceps tendon is often a part of this syndrome. A thorough inspection of the biceps tendon intra-articularly and into the bicipital groove is necessary. Treatment of these conditions is described in Chapter 50.

AC Joint Surgery (see Chapter 49)

- AC joint surgery was originally described as an open operation by Mumford, and 1.5–2.0 cm of the distal clavicle is removed for treatment of AC joint arthritis (7).
- This surgery relies on the coracoclavicular ligaments providing stabilization of the clavicle. The AC ligaments are repaired at closure.
- Arthroscopic surgeons have found that resection of 8–10 mm is all that is necessary for adequate decompression and pain relief.
- Often neglected is medial spurring on the acromion at the AC joint. This should also be resected with either an open or arthroscopic procedure.

Rotator Cuff Repair

- The indications and necessity of RCR remains controversial and often determined by individual characteristics of the patient or the tear. The fact that many patients with a full-thickness rotator cuff tear are asymptomatic indicates that the mere presence of a hole in the supraspinatus tendon does not necessitate surgical repair. Many patients may do well with a simple lower rotator cuff and periscapular rehabilitation program to strengthen and balance the anterior and posterior forces providing humeral head depression (32). This is especially true of chronic tears that present with insidious onset as opposed to those that are traumatic in nature (32).
- However, Yamaguchi et al. (33) have shown that many tears will progress, leading to a dysfunctional shoulder. Once these tears are large, the muscles will atrophy and undergo fatty degeneration, making a functional repair impossible. A recent study following nonoperative treatment of rotator cuff tears by MRI (34) revealed that progression of the tear was predicted by age >60 years, presence of a full-thickness tear, and fatty infiltration of the rotator cuff muscles. Another study in Europe (35) revealed that if initial nonoperative treatment of massive rotator cuff tears was effective, progression of degenerative joint changes occurred over 4 years and often led to reparable tears becoming irreparable.
- The decision for RCR is an individual one made between the surgeon and the patient. Age, activity level, chronicity of the tear, and failure of initial nonoperative treatment all play a factor. The younger and more active patient is likely to require repair. However, an older patient, still active in sports such as pickleball, tennis, and golf may also require repair.
- Smaller, one or two tendon tears, without retraction or atrophy, can be repaired anatomically using arthroscopic techniques. These repairs usually heal and allow the patient to return to all activities (36).
- Larger, massive tears may be retracted and atrophic. Burkhart has shown us that balancing the forces of the infraspinatus and subscapularis, without necessarily a "watertight closure," is often sufficient for a successful repair (37–41). However, for large, massive tears, many advocate decompression alone or tendon transfers to restore some function of the lower rotator cuff (42).
    - Open RCR: Open repair of the rotator cuff to the tuberosities of the humerus had been the gold standard for many years (43,44). The fear of deltoid failure or detachment, and the overall invasiveness of the technique, has led to it being abandoned for less invasive techniques (45).

- Mini-open repair (45): Development of shoulder arthroscopy methods has allowed surgeons to perform arthroscopic evaluation and surgical treatment. Initially, subacromial decompression was performed arthroscopically and then converted to an open repair. This allows visualization of the rotator cuff and the ability to address subacromial bursitis, AC joint pathology, and acromial changes such as the development of spurs or ossification of the CA ligament. The mini-open repair takes advantage of this preparation and utilizes a deltoid split to access the rotator cuff tear and perform an open repair (45). This approach was used during the initial development of arthroscopic techniques and now has been replaced by most surgeons by a completely arthroscopic technique (36).
- Arthroscopic RCR: Further development of arthroscopic suture management, arthroscopic knot tying, and the use of arthroscopically delivered suture anchors have led to the ability to perform RCRs arthroscopically. The procedure is minimally invasive and the ability to preserve cortical bone enhances the strength of fixation while allowing the tendon to heal to bone (46). Arthroscopic RCR is now done as effectively as open repair (19,47–50) and is taught in all residency programs throughout the United States and Europe.

- PRP used at the time of surgery has not been shown to improve re-tear rates or clinical outcome scores compared with surgery alone, but has shown promise with certain types of tears (51). Studies to date have been equivocal, with some studies showing effectiveness (52) and others equivalence (28,51). Further investigations are pending for the use of PRP as well as stem cells to enhance the biologic milieu and influence healing. However, details of PRP processing and characteristics have been reported inconsistently and often studies are not comparable or conclusive (53,54).
- The use of both bone marrow–derived mesenchymal stem cells and adipose-derived mesenchymal stem cells has been studied and a recent systematic review has suggested a possible increased strength and quality of repair in preclinical studies. However, adequate studies to prove effectiveness over conventional repair do not exist at this time (55).

MASSIVE RCR

- A recent Delphi study conducted by the American Shoulder and Elbow Surgeons Neer Circle Committee obtained consensus on possible surgical options for treatment of massive rotator cuff tears. Clinical scenarios were presented and acceptable or preferred treatment selected. As the patient's age, activity level, degree of atrophy, examination, and the degree of subscapularis involvement all contribute to the decision of surgery and what type of surgery, the reader is referred to the study for more details (56). Depending on the clinical scenario, all of the following were recommended for treatment of irreparable rotator cuff tears:
  - Subacromial decompression alone without repair of the rotator cuff (7)
  - Partial RCR (39,57)
  - Graft augmentation of RCR (55,58)
  - Superior capsular reconstruction (59–61)
  - Tendon transfer (59,60,62)
  - Reverse shoulder arthroplasty (63,64)

POSTOPERATIVE REHABILITATION

Subacromial Decompression/Distal Clavicle Resection

- Following surgery, a good rehabilitation program should be instituted to ensure optimal recovery (30). This may be done with formal physical therapy or with a physician-directed program.
- Following arthroscopic subacromial decompression, a sling is used for a few days for comfort, and active motion may be resumed immediately. Once motion is achieved, strengthening exercises are started.
- Strengthening should focus on lower rotator cuff strength and scapular stabilization.
- Pool therapy is often very effective for shoulder rehabilitation for regaining proper motion and allowing protected use of the shoulder muscles in the recovery period.
- Return to sports is recommended when full painless motion is recovered following surgery.

Rotator Cuff Repair

- Following RCR, the recovery is structured to allow the cuff to heal to the bone, while maintaining motion. Histologic studies have shown that this can take up to 12–16 weeks (46).
- The surgeon will direct postoperative ROM based on the size of the tear and the stability of the repair at the time of surgery.
- Many surgeons are following a much more conservative rehabilitation program to allow the rotator cuff to start healing before starting motion.
- Passive motion may be started early, with active motion being delayed for 4–6 weeks.
- Forward elevation should be delayed as the motion will cause stress on the repair.
- Formal rehabilitation is often not started for 6 weeks, and some surgeons are using a home-directed rehabilitation program for independent and motivated patients.
- Full recovery will differ for each patient; however, 6–8 weeks are usually sufficient for decompression alone, and 4–6 months required for RCR.

SUMMARY

- Rotator cuff pathology is a frequent cause of pain in active patients in all stages of life. It is seen in younger patients participating in throwing or racquet sports, in the weekend athlete developing overuse injuries, and in the older patient still active in tennis, golf, and pickleball; the proper diagnosis and treatment of this condition can lead to resolution of symptoms and return the patient to a more functional and usually normal use of their arm.

REFERENCES

1. Burkhead WZ, Habermeyer P. The rotator cuff: a historical review of our understanding. In: Burkhead WZ Jr, editor. *Rotator Cuff Disorders*. Baltimore (MD): Williams & Wilkins; 1996. p. 3–18.
2. Neer CS II. Anterior acromioplasty for the chronic impingement syndrome in the shoulder: a preliminary report. *J Bone Joint Surg Am*. 1972;54(1):41–50.
3. Neer CS II. Impingement lesions. *Clin Orthop Relat Res*. 1983;173:70–7.
4. Crenshaw AH, Kilgore WE. Surgical treatment of bicipital tenosynovitis. *J Bone Joint Surg Am*. 1966;48(8):1496–502.
5. Gerber C, Hersche O, Farron A. Isolated rupture of the subscapularis tendon. *J Bone Joint Surg Am*. 1996;78(7):1015–23.
6. Gerber C, Krushell RJ. Isolated rupture of the tendon of the subscapularis muscle. Clinical features in 16 cases. *J Bone Joint Surg Br*. 1991;73(3):389–94.
7. Chen AL, Rokito AS, Zuckerman JD. The role of the acromioclavicular joint in impingement syndrome. *Clin Sports Med*. 2003;22(2):343–57.
8. Valadie AL III, Jobe CM, Pink MM, Ekman EF, Jobe FW. Anatomy of provocative tests for impingement syndrome of the shoulder. *J Shoulder Elbow Surg*. 2000;9(1):36–46.
9. Warner JJ, Higgins L, Parsons IMIV, Dowdy P. Diagnosis and treatment of anterosuperior rotator cuff tears. *J Shoulder Elbow Surg*. 2001;10(1):37–46.
10. Yocum LA. Assessing the shoulder. History, physical examination, differential diagnosis, and special tests used. *Clin Sports Med*. 1983;2(2):281–9.
11. Jobe FW, Jobe CM. Painful athletic injuries of the shoulder. *Clin Orthop Relat Res*. 1983;173:117–24.
12. Jobe FW, Kvitne RS, Giangarra CE. Shoulder pain in the overhand or throwing athlete. The relationship of anterior instability and rotator cuff impingement. *Orthop Rev*. 1989;18(9):963–75.
13. Walch G, Boileau P, Noel E, Donell ST. Impingement of the deep surface of the supraspinatus tendon on the posterosuperior glenoid rim: an arthroscopic study. *J Shoulder Elbow Surg*. 1992;1(5):238–45.
14. McFarland EG, Hsu CY, Neira C, O'Neil O. Internal impingement of the shoulder: a clinical and arthroscopic analysis. *J Shoulder Elbow Surg*. 1999;8(5):458–60.
15. Jobe FW, Moynes DR. Delineation of diagnostic criteria and a rehabilitation program for rotator cuff injuries. *Am J Sports Med*. 1982;10(6):336–9.
16. DePalma AF, Kruper JS. Long-term study of shoulder joints afflicted with and treated for calcific tendinitis. *Clin Orthop*. 1961;20:61–72.
17. Harmon PH. Methods and results in the treatment of 2,580 painful shoulders, with special reference to calcific tendinitis and the frozen shoulder. *Am J Surg*. 1958;95(4):527–44.
18. Moseley HF. The results of nonoperative and operative treatment of calcified deposits. *Surg Clin North Am*. 1963;43:1505–6.
19. Wilson F, Hinov V, Adams G. Arthroscopic repair of full-thickness tears of the rotator cuff: 2- to 14-year follow-up. *Arthroscopy*. 2002;18(2):136–44.
20. Kelly BT, Kadrmas WR, Kirkendall DT, Speer KP. Optimal normalization tests for shoulder muscle activation: an electromyographic study. *J Orthop Res*. 1996;14(4):647–53.
21. Greis PE, Kuhn JE, Schultheis J, Hintermeister R, Hawkins R. Validation of the lift-off test and analysis of subscapularis activity during maximal internal rotation. *Am J Sports Med*. 1996;24(5):589–93.
22. Warner JJP, Allen AA, Gerber C. Diagnosis and management of subscapularis tendon tears. *Techn Orthop*. 1994;9(2):116–25.
23. Hertel R, Ballmer FT, Lombert SM, Gerber C. Lag signs in the diagnosis of rotator cuff rupture. *J Shoulder Elbow Surg*. 1996;5(4):307–13.
24. Hawkins RJ, Kennedy JC. Impingement syndrome in athletes. *Am J Sports Med*. 1980;8(3):151–8.
25. MacDonald PB, Clark P, Sutherland K. An analysis of the diagnostic accuracy of the Hawkins and Neer subacromial impingement signs. *J Shoulder Elbow Surg*. 2000;9(4):299–301.
26. Allert JW, Sellers TR, Simon P, Christmas KN, Patel S, Frankle MA. Massive rotator cuff tears in patients older than sixty-five: indications for cuff repair versus reverse total shoulder arthroplasty. *Am J Orthop (Belle Mead NJ)*. 2018 Dec;47(12). doi:10.12788/ajo.2018.0109
27. Kompel AJ, Roemer FW, Murakami AM, Diaz LE, Crema MD, Guermazi A. Intra-articular corticosteroid injections in the hip and knee: perhaps not as safe as we thought? *Radiology*. 2019 Dec;293(3):656–63.
28. Barber FA, Hrnack SA, Snyder SJ, Hapa O. Rotator cuff repair healing influenced by platelet-rich plasma construct augmentation. *Arthroscopy*. 2011;27(8):1029–35.
29. Giovannetti de Sanctis E, Franceschetti E, De Dona F, Palumbo A, Paciotti M, Franceschi F. The efficacy of injections for partial rotator cuff tears: a systematic review. *J Clin Med*. 2020 Dec 25;10(1):51.
30. Wilk KE, Arrigo C. Current concepts in the rehabilitation of the athletic shoulder. *J Orthop Sports Phys Ther*. 1993;18(1):365–78.
31. Nirschl RP. Rotator cuff tendinitis: basic concepts of pathoetiology. *Instr Course Lect*. 1989;38:439–45.
32. Burkhart SS, Esch JC, Jolson RS. The rotator crescent and rotator cable: an anatomic description of the shoulder's "suspension bridge". *Arthroscopy*. 1993;9(6):611–6.
33. Yamaguchi K, Tetro AM, Blam O, Evanoff BA, Teefey SA, Middleton WD. Natural history of asymptomatic rotator cuff tears: a longitudinal analysis of asymptomatic tears detected sonographically. *J Shoulder Elbow Surg*. 2001;10(3):199–203.
34. Maman E, Harris C, White L, Tomlinson G, Shashank M, Boynton E. Outcome of nonoperative treatment of symptomatic rotator cuff tears monitored by magnetic resonance imaging. *J Bone Joint Surg Am*. 2009;91(8):1898–906.
35. Zingg PO, Jost B, Sukthankar A, Buhler M, Pfirrmann CW, Gerber C. Clinical and structural outcomes of nonoperative management of massive rotator cuff tears. *J Bone Joint Surg Am*. 2007;89(9):1928–34.
36. MacDermid JC, Bryant D, Holtby R, et al. Arthroscopic versus mini-open rotator cuff repair: a randomized trial and meta-analysis. *Am J Sports Med*. 2021 Oct;49(12):3184–95.
37. Burkhart SS. Arthroscopic repair of massive rotator cuff tears: concept of margin convergence. *Tech Shoulder Elbow Surg*. 2000;1:232–9.
38. Burkhart SS. Arthroscopic treatment of massive rotator cuff tears. *Clin Orthop Relat Res*. 2001;390:107–18.
39. Burkhart SS. Partial repair of massive rotator cuff tears: the evolution of a concept. *Orthop Clin North Am*. 1997;28(1):125–32.

40. Burkhart SS, Nottage WM, Ogilvie-Harris DJ, Kohn HS, Pachelli A. Partial repair of irreparable rotator cuff tears. *Arthroscopy.* 1994;10(4):363–70.
41. Yoo JC, Ahn JH, Koh KH, Lim KS. Rotator cuff integrity after arthroscopic repair for large tears with less-than-optimal footprint coverage. *Arthroscopy.* 2009;25(10):1093–100.
42. Gartsman GM. Massive, irreparable tears of the rotator cuff. Results of operative debridement and subacromial decompression. *J Bone Joint Surg Am.* 1997;79(5):715–21.
43. Cordasco FA, Bigliani LU. The rotator cuff. Large and massive tears. Technique of open repair. *Orthop Clin North Am.* 1997;28(2):179–93.
44. McLaughlin, HL. Lesions of the musculotendinous cuff of the shoulder. The exposure and treatment of tears with retraction. *Clin Orthop Relat Res.* 1994;304:3–9.
45. Blevins FT, Warren RF, Cavo C, et al. Arthroscopic assisted rotator cuff repair: results using a mini-open deltoid splitting approach. *Arthroscopy.* 1996;12(1):50–9.
46. St Pierre P, Olson EJ, Elliott JJ, O'Hair KC, McKinney LA, Ryan J. Tendon-healing to cortical bone compared with healing to a cancellous trough. A biomechanical and histological evaluation in goats. *J Bone Joint Surg Am.* 1995;77(12):1858–66.
47. Ellman H, Kay SP, Wirth M. Arthroscopic treatment of full-thickness rotator cuff tears: 2- to 7-year follow-up study. *Arthroscopy.* 1993;9(2):195–200.
48. Gartsman GM, Khan M, Hammerman SM. Arthroscopic repair of full-thickness tears of the rotator cuff. *J Bone Joint Surg Am.* 1998;80(6):832–40.
49. Murray TF Jr, Lajtai G, Mileski RM, Snyder SJ. Arthroscopic repair of medium to large full-thickness rotator cuff tears: outcome at 2- to 6-year follow-up. *J Shoulder Elbow Surg.* 2002;11(1):19–24.
50. Tauro JC. Arthroscopic rotator cuff repair: analysis of technique and results at 2- and 3-year follow-up. *Arthroscopy.* 1998;14(1):45–51.
51. Saltzman BM, Jain A, Campbell KA, et al. Does the use of platelet-rich plasma at the time of surgery improve clinical outcomes in arthroscopic rotator cuff repair when compared with control cohorts? A systematic review of meta-analyses. *Arthroscopy.* 2016 May;32(5):906–18.
52. Randelli P, Arrigoni P, Ragone V, Aliprandi A, Cabitza P. Platelet rich plasma in arthroscopic rotator cuff repair: a prospective RCT study, 2-year follow-up. *J Shoulder Elbow Surg.* 2011;20(4):518–28.
53. DeClercq MG, Fiorentino AM, Lengel HA, et al. Systematic review of platelet-rich plasma for rotator cuff repair: are we adhering to the minimum information for studies evaluating biologics in orthopaedics? *Orthop J Sports Med.* 2021 Dec 7;9(12):23259671211041971.
54. Bono OJ, Jenkin B, Forlizzi J, et al. Evidence for utilization of injectable biologic augmentation in primary rotator cuff repair: a systematic review of data from 2010 to 2022. *Orthop J Sports Med.* 2023 Feb 3;11(2):23259671221150037.
55. Morgan CN, Bonner KF, Griffin JW. Augmentation of arthroscopic rotator cuff repair: biologics and grafts. *Clin Sports Med.* 2023 Jan;42(1):95–107.
56. St Pierre P, Millett PJ, Abboud JA, et al. Consensus statement on the treatment of massive irreparable rotator cuff tears: a Delphi approach by the Neer Circle of the American Shoulder and Elbow Surgeons. *J Shoulder Elbow Surg.* 2021 Sep;30(9):1977–89.
57. Cuff DJ, Pupello DR, Santoni BG. Partial rotator cuff repair and biceps tenotomy for the treatment of patients with massive cuff tears and retained overhead elevation: midterm outcomes with a minimum 5 years of follow-up. *J Shoulder Elbow Surg.* 2016 Nov;25(11):1803–9.
58. Lee GW, Kim JY, Lee HW, Yoon JH, Noh KC. Clinical and anatomical outcomes of arthroscopic repair of large rotator cuff tears with allograft patch augmentation: a prospective, single-blinded, randomized controlled trial with a long-term follow-up. *Clin Orthop Surg.* 2022 Jun;14(2):263–71.
59. Mercurio M, Castricini R, Castioni D, et al. Better functional outcomes and a lower infection rate can be expected after superior capsular reconstruction in comparison with latissimus dorsi tendon transfer for massive, irreparable posterosuperior rotator cuff tears: a systematic review. *J Shoulder Elbow Surg.* 2022 Dec;14:S1058–2746.
60. Wagner ER, Woodmass JM, Welp KM, Chang MJ, Higgins L, Warner JJP. Early postoperative recovery comparisons of superior capsule reconstruction to tendon transfers. *J Shoulder Elbow Surg.* 2023 Feb;32(2):276–85.
61. Gbejuade H, Patel MS, Singh H, Modi A. Reconstruction of irreparable rotator cuff tears with an acellular dermal matrix in elderly patients without joint arthritis. *Shoulder Elbow.* 2022 Jul;14(1 suppl):83–9.
62. Wagner ER, Elhassan BT. Surgical management of massive irreparable posterosuperior rotator cuff tears: arthroscopic-assisted lower trapezius transfer. *Curr Rev Musculoskelet Med.* 2020 Oct;13(5):592–604.
63. Kobayashi EF, Oak SR, Miller BS, Bedi A. Treatment of massive rotator cuff tears with reverse shoulder arthroplasty. *Clin Sports Med.* 2023 Jan;42(1):157–73.
64. Sevivas N, Ferreira N, Andrade R, et al. Reverse shoulder arthroplasty for irreparable massive rotator cuff tears: a systematic review with meta-analysis and meta-regression. *J Shoulder Elbow Surg.* 2017 Sep;26(9):265–77.

Sternoclavicular, Clavicular, and Acromioclavicular Injuries

53

Michael R. Mancini, Colin L. Uyeki, and Augustus D. Mazzocca

INTRODUCTION

- Injuries to the clavicle and its articulations are very common.
- High-energy injuries have been seen in increasing frequency as more people participate in higher risk sports such as mountain biking and rollerblading.
- Because man is an upper extremity–dependent animal, these injuries can lead to significant disabilities and limitations.

STERNOCLAVICULAR JOINT

- Injury to the sternoclavicular (SC) joint is rare. In one large study conducted by Rowe and Marble, out of 1603 shoulder girdle injuries, there was only a 3% incidence of SC joint injuries (1). In a separate analysis of shoulder girdle injuries at a level I trauma center over 19 years, SC joint injuries had an incidence of only 0.9% (2). This is in comparison to an 85% incidence of glenohumeral injuries and 12% incidence of acromioclavicular (AC) dislocations. That being said, it has also been commented that SC joint dislocations are not as rare as posterior glenohumeral dislocations.
- The SC joint is the only true joint connecting the axial skeleton to the shoulder girdle.
- Despite having such an important role, the SC joint lacks inherent bony stability and relies solely on ligamentous and capsular attachments.

Anatomy and Biomechanics

- The SC joint represents the articulation of the proximal end of the clavicle with the sternum and is a diarthrodial joint.
- Although the clavicle is the first long bone in the body to ossify during the fifth intrauterine week, the medial clavicular epiphysis is the last epiphysis to close. Closure of the medial clavicular epiphysis typically begins at age 18 and is usually fused to the clavicular shaft by age 25. It has even been documented in autopsy studies that complete union of the medial clavicular epiphysis may not occur until age 31 (3).
- Similar to the AC joint, the SC joint has an intra-articular disc, or meniscal homologue. Unlike the AC joint, however, the articular surface of the medial clavicle of the SC joint is covered with fibrocartilage.
- The SC joint is incongruous as the medial clavicle is enlarged, bulbous, and saddle-shaped, whereas the clavicular notch of the sternum is smaller and concave. Because there is such a large discrepancy in shape and size of the clavicle with the sternum, there is relatively little to no bony stability of the joint. In fact, less than half of the medial clavicle actually articulates with the sternum. It has been shown that in 2.5% of patients, the inferior aspect of the medial clavicle actually articulates with the superior aspect of the first rib (4).
- The SC joint articulation is held in place by the SC capsular ligaments, the costoclavicular ligaments, and the infraclavicular ligaments (Fig. 53.1).
- There are two parts of the capsular ligament: the anterior and posterior portions. The capsular ligaments help to support and reinforce the anterosuperior and posterior SC joint. Of the ligaments surrounding the SC joint, the capsular

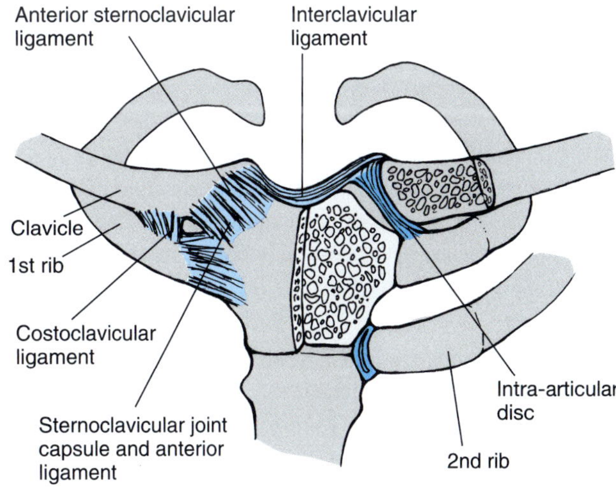

Figure 53.1: Sternoclavicular joint.

ligament is the strongest and most important structure preventing upward displacement of the medial clavicle (5).

- The intra-articular disc ligament arises from the junction of the sternum and first rib and attaches on the superior and posterior aspects of the medial clavicle, after passing directly through the SC joint. The fibers of the intra-articular disc ligament blend into the fibers of the capsular ligaments and help to separate the SC joint into medial and lateral compartments. It prevents medial displacement of the clavicle with compression.
- The costoclavicular ligament shows anatomic variance and can be found as a singular band or two independent fascicles. The costoclavicular ligament is on average 2 cm in width and extends from the inferior surface of the medial clavicle to the first costal cartilage and the medial portion of the first rib. The costoclavicular ligament provides rotational stability during elevation and retraction of the shoulder girdle (6).
- Connecting the two clavicles is the interclavicular ligament, which connects the superomedial aspect of the clavicles and the capsular ligaments. The purpose of this ligament is to maintain "shoulder poise," by holding the clavicle and shoulder up (7).
- Despite the presence of the ligaments and capsule stabilizing the SC joint, a relatively large amount of motion is still seen. There is approximately 30°–35°of upward elevation, 35° of translation in the anterior to posterior plane, and 50° of rotation around the longitudinal axis of the clavicle (8,9).

Classification

- The SC joint can be dislocated anteriorly or posteriorly and be the result of traumatic or atraumatic injury. Anterior and posterior dislocations are described based on the location of the medial clavicle with respect to the sternum. Of the two types of dislocations, anterior dislocations are far more common.
- Atraumatic instability of the SC joint can either be acquired or congenital in etiology. The SC joint may subluxate or dislocate with overhead motion in patients who have systemic ligamentous laxity. Typically, atraumatic instability is not associated with pain.
- Traumatic injury to the SC joint is the most common etiology. Motor vehicle collisions and sports participation are the top two causes of traumatic SC joint injury (10–12). Traumatic SC joint injuries have been classified into three types.
  - Type 1: mild sprain, SC joint is stable and ligaments are intact
  - Type 2: moderate sprain, SC joint subluxates and there is partial disruption of ligaments and capsule
  - Type 3: severe sprain, SC joint is dislocated and ligaments and capsule are completely disrupted

Mechanism of Injury

- Posterior dislocations of the SC joint typically occur as the result of a direct force to the anteromedial clavicle, as can happen during a motor vehicle collision, as a result of the steering wheel hitting the clavicle, or a direct kick to the chest.
- Posterior sprains and dislocations can also occur with a posterolateral force applied to the clavicle. Such an injury has been reported multiple times in the literature, each instance involving a football player who fell onto the posterolateral aspect of their shoulder (13,14).
- Anterior dislocations, on the other hand, rarely occur as a result of direct trauma. Instead, anterior dislocations can occur when an anterolateral force is applied to the clavicle and the shoulder is rolled backward. In three separate studies looking at SC joint dislocations, an indirect force was the most common mechanism of injury (15,16).
- Rockwood describes a common mechanism of indirect SC joint dislocation — a pileup during a football game (15). One player usually falls to the ground with the ball. Other players begin to jump and fall on top of the first player.

Physical Examination

- Often with an acute dislocation, either anterior or posterior, palpable step-off at the SC junction can be appreciated.
- Posterior dislocations, although rare, have more significant symptoms and implications.
  - Posterior dislocations can be associated with venous congestion present in the neck or ipsilateral upper extremity from compression on the subclavian vessels (Fig. 53.2).
  - The posteriorly displaced clavicle can also compress the trachea or esophagus.
  - As such, patients may complain of dyspnea, a choking sensation, difficulty swallowing, or a tight feeling in the throat.
  - In the most severe cases, the posterior dislocation can result in complete shock or a pneumothorax.
- For patients with a type 1 injury (mild sprain), there is usually mild to moderate pain associated with movement of the upper extremity. Instability is usually absent, but the SC joint may be tender to palpation and slightly swollen. With this injury, the ligaments remain intact so the joint should not be unstable.
- Type 2 injuries (moderate sprain) are associated with partial disruption of the ligaments. There may be some instability or subluxation when the joint is manually stressed, but it is not grossly dislocated or dislocatable. These patients usually have more swelling and pain than patients with type 1 injuries, and the SC joint is more tender to palpation.
- Type 3 (severe sprain) injury results in complete dislocation, either anterior or posterior, of the SC joint. Patients with this injury present with severe pain that is exacerbated by any movement of the upper extremity. The ipsilateral shoulder may appear protracted in comparison to the contralateral uninjured shoulder. Patients will often hold the affected arm across the chest in an adducted position and support it with the contralateral arm. The head may be tilted toward the side

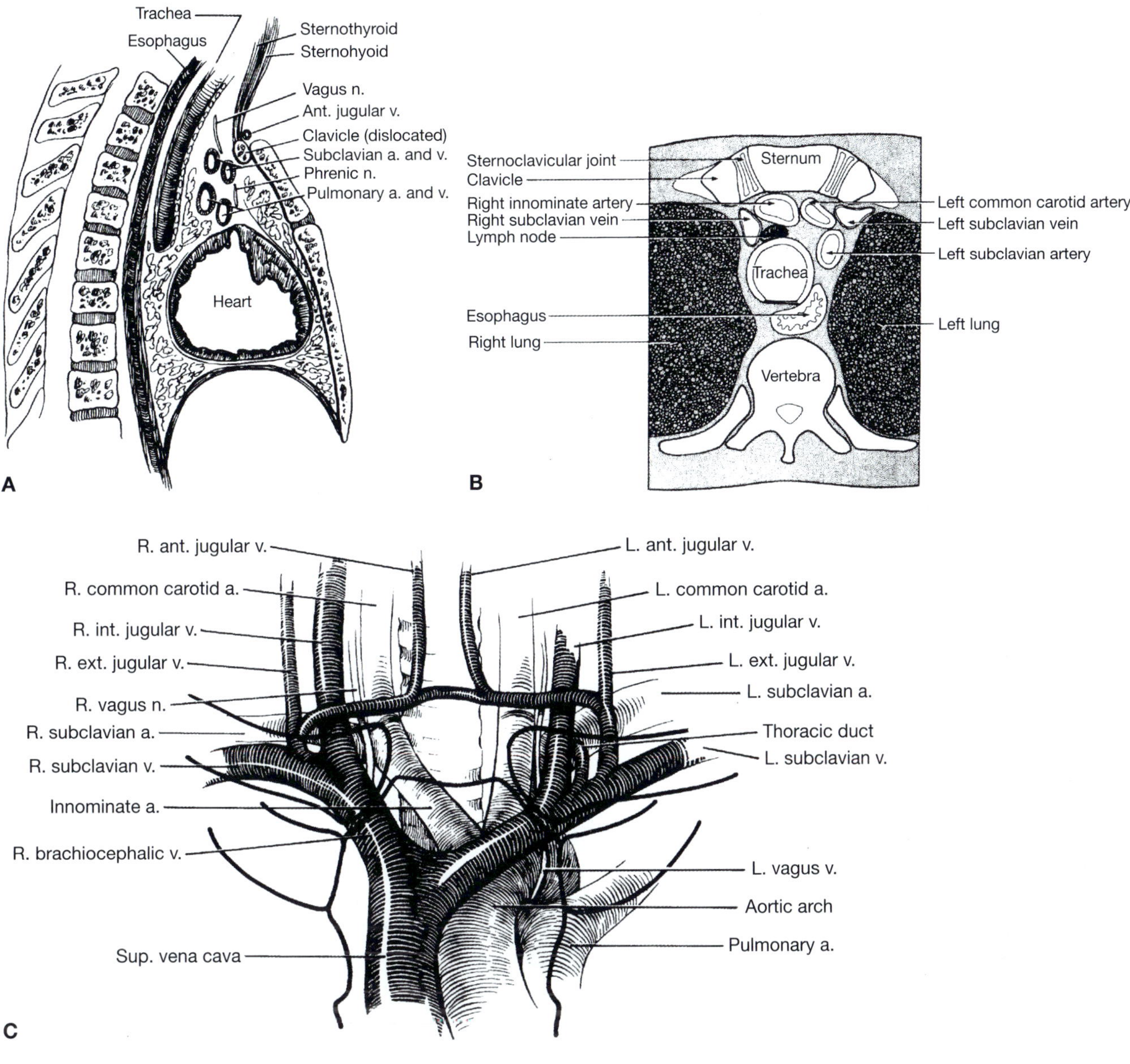

Figure 53.2: Applied anatomy of the vital structures posterior to the sternoclavicular (SC) joint. A and B: Sagittal views in cross-section demonstrating the structures posterior to the SC joint. C: A diagram demonstrating the close proximity of the major vessels posterior to the SC joint.

of the injured clavicle. Examination of the patient lying supine on the examining table will lead to a worsening of symptoms, and the involved shoulder will not lie flat on the table.

Radiologic Evaluation

- A standard anteroposterior (AP) x-ray of the chest or SC joint may suggest an injury to the SC joint; however, this is not the best view for visualizing the joint.
- The serendipity view is the best view to visualize the SC joint. It is taken by tilting the x-ray tube 40° cephalad and centered on the sternum.
- In adolescents and young adults, serendipity views can help to exclude the possibility of a physeal fracture, which may present similarly to an SC joint injury, and in a case series of 48 adolescents with suspected SC joint injuries, the eventual diagnosis was a physeal fracture in 50% of the cases (17).
- Although less commonly obtained, a Hobbs and/or a Heinig radiograph can also help to visualize the SC joint. The Hobbs view requires the patient to sit and lean over the x-ray with the beam directly superior to their neck and centered on the manubrium. The Heinig view produces an image that is perpendicular to the SC joint (13).

- Computed tomography (CT) scan of the chest should include a special note to the radiology technician to do views of the bilateral SC joint for comparison. With a CT scan, axial sections can be viewed of both the injured and uninjured sides on one image. Subtle differences from side to side can be picked up more easily by the physician looking at the axial views.

Nonoperative Treatment

- Type 1 and 2 injuries are often treated nonoperatively. Nonoperative treatment consists of a short period of immobilization in a sling, anti-inflammatory medication, and ice.
- After a short period of immobilization, the patient can gradually return back to activities based on their own level of comfort.
- As in type 2 injuries where the clavicle is subluxated, the joint can be reduced by retracting the shoulders in a figure-of-eight brace. This treatment modality can be incorporated whether the subluxation is anterior or posterior.
- When the SC joint is completely dislocated, as seen in a type 3 injury, an attempt can be made at closed reduction.
- For an anterior dislocation, the patient should be placed supine with a roll in the center of the back between the shoulder blades (Fig. 53.3).

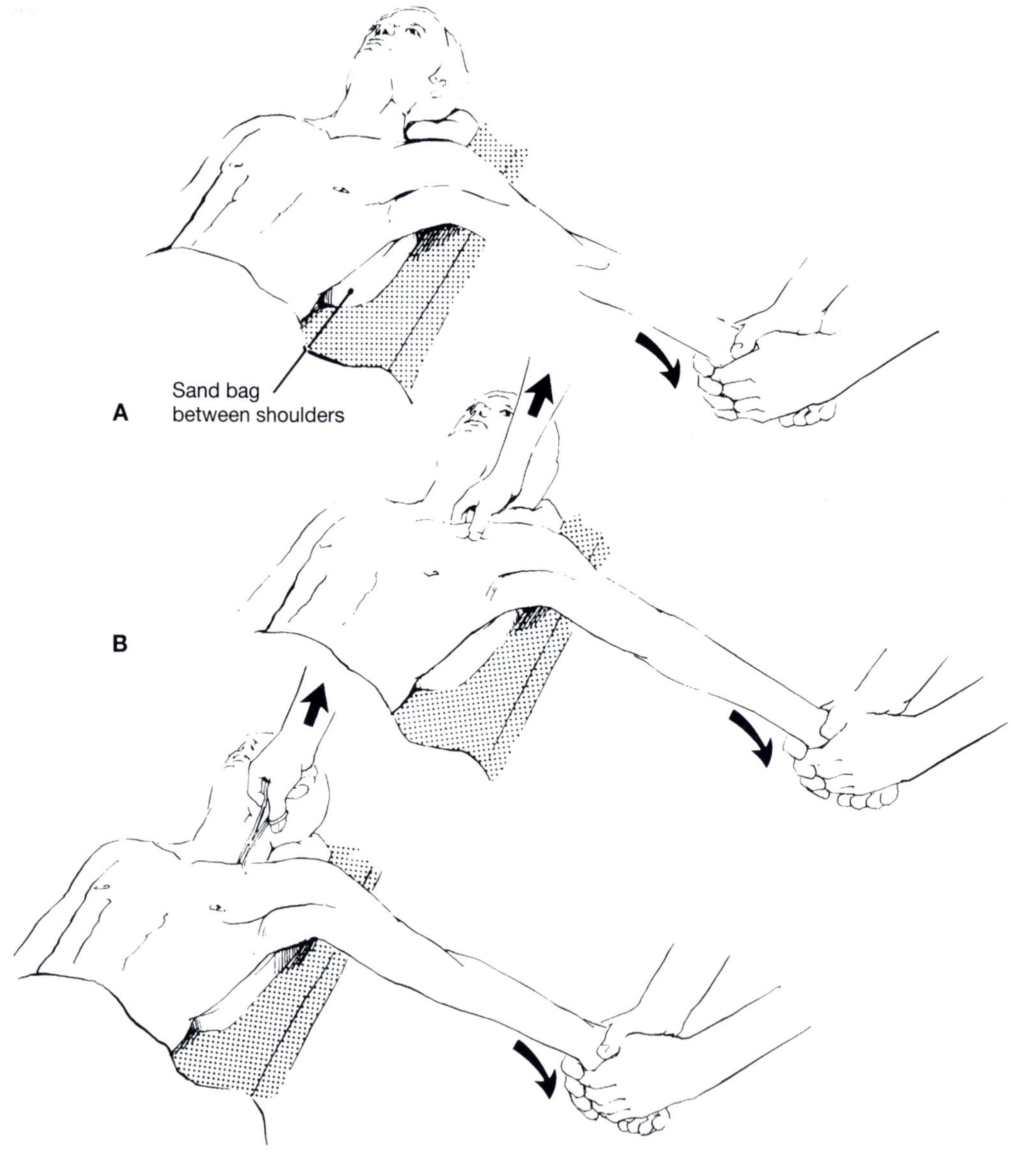

Figure 53.3: Technique for closed reduction of the sternoclavicular joint. A: The patient is positioned supine with a sandbag placed between the two shoulders. Traction is then applied to the arm against countertraction in an abducted and slightly extended position. In anterior dislocations, direct pressure over the medial end of the clavicle may reduce the joint. B: In posterior dislocations, in addition to the traction, it may be necessary to manipulate the medial end of the clavicle with the fingers to dislodge the clavicle from behind the manubrium. C: In stubborn posterior dislocations, it may be necessary to sterilely prepare the medial end of the clavicle and use a towel clip to grasp around the medial clavicle to lift it back into position.

  - This positioning allows the scapula to assume a retracted position and pull the clavicle laterally.
  - A gentle pressure can then be applied to the anteromedial clavicle in order to reduce.
  - Anterior dislocations are often easy to reduce; however, they are usually unstable and will dislocate once the pressure is released.
  - If, however, the SC joint maintains reduction after closed means, the patient should be immobilized in a soft figure-of-eight brace for a period of 6 weeks.
- Prior to any attempt at closed reduction of posteriorly displaced clavicle, injury to local vessels, heart, and lung needs to be ruled out.
- Closed reduction of a posterior dislocation should be done in the operating room with the patient under general anesthesia (Fig. 53.4).
  - Similar to an anterior dislocation, the patient should lay supine with a roll between the scapula.
  - Traction should then be applied to the abducted arm while it is slowly extended. Often the joint will reduce with this maneuver; if not, the clavicle can be manipulated with fingers or a towel clip.
  - The towel clip can be used to grasp the medial clavicle under sterile conditions and pull it anteriorly in order to achieve reduction.
  - Posterior dislocations are usually stable once reduced.
  - It is important to have a vascular surgeon available if the patient is taken to the operating room for an attempted closed reduction because of the potential complications that may arise as a result of the injury or the attempt at reduction.
- The patient with a reduced SC joint should then be placed in a figure-of-eight brace for 4–6 weeks while the ligaments heal.

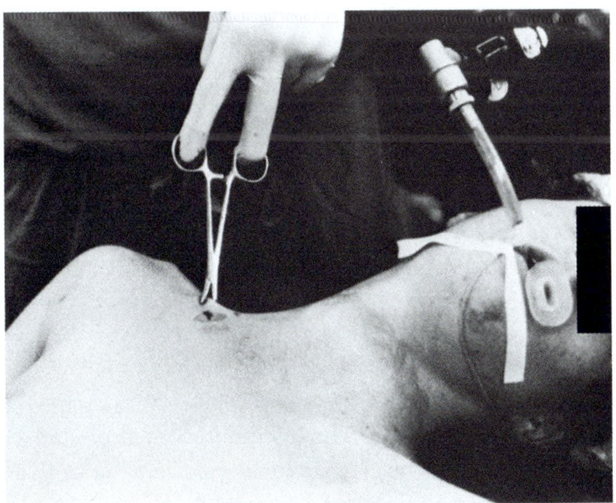

Figure 53.4: Posterior dislocation of the right sternoclavicular joint can be reduced in the operating room under general anesthesia. A rolled towel should be applied between the patient's shoulder blades. A towel clip can be applied to the medial aspect of the clavicle and the clavicle can be pulled anteriorly.

Operative Treatment

- Most SC joint dislocations are best managed nonoperatively and either left unreduced or attempted to be closed reduced.
- Surgical stabilization of the clavicle is not recommended by most authors (18,19). In most cases, the benefits of surgery are outweighed by the risks.
- Numerous complications have been reported in the literature, including infection, recurrence, poor cosmesis, and hardware migration.
- If patients develop symptomatic SC joint instability, then several surgical options exist.
- Good long-term outcomes have been reported in patients who have medial clavicle excision or SC joint reconstruction for SC joint instability (20).
- In a biomechanical analysis of reconstructions for SC joint instability, Spencer and Kuhn tested three SC joint fixation methods in a cadaveric study (21). They concluded that figure-of-eight semitendinosus reconstruction provided superior biomechanical properties to subclavius tendon reconstruction and intramedullary ligament reconstruction.
- Cautiously recommended in the recent literature is a two-stage approach for SC joint instability (22).
  - The first stage involves fixation of the medial clavicle to the sternum with a concomitant midclavicular osteotomy to offload the fixation at the SC joint.
  - The second stage, usually performed 4 months after the first, involves removal of the hardware at the SC joint and plate osteosynthesis at the osteotomy site.
- Any surgery being performed for a posterior SC joint dislocation should be done with a cardiothoracic surgeon present due to risk of injury to surrounding structures.

CLAVICLE

- The clavicle grows through intramembranous ossification like the skull and scapula.
- Ossification begins at the fifth week of gestation, and it is the first bone to ossify.
- It is also the last bone to finish growing as the medial physis closes at age 23–25 years.

Anatomy and Biomechanics

- The clavicle is a subcutaneous double S-shaped bone that articulates with the sternum and the scapula via the SC and AC joints, respectively.
- The acromial end of the clavicle is more broad and flat than the sternal end.
- The undersurface of the acromial end has bony projections called the conoid tubercle and trapezoid line. These projections mark the attachment sites of the conoid and trapezoid ligaments, respectively, of the coracoclavicular ligament complex.

- The trapezius, sternocleidomastoid, and sternohyoid muscles insert on the posterior-superior border of the clavicle.
- The deltoid, clavicular head of the pectoralis major, and subclavius muscles originate from the anterior inferior surface of the clavicle.
- The clavicle acts as a strut that connects the upper limb to the trunk and allows the arm to hang freely.
- The clavicle also functions to protect the neurovascular structures running from the neck to the arm.

Clavicle Fractures

- Clavicle fractures are very common fractures, accounting for nearly 5%–15% of all fractures.
- Classification
  - Allman (23) created the classification system that is still used today.
    - Type I — middle third clavicle fractures
    - Type II — lateral third clavicle fractures
    - Type III — medial third clavicle fractures
  - In 1968, Neer (24) further divided lateral clavicle fractures into three types.
    - Type I — lateral clavicle fracture with intact coracoclavicular ligaments
    - Type II — lateral clavicle fracture with torn coracoclavicular ligaments
    - Type III — intra-articular lateral clavicle fracture involving the AC joint, but coracoclavicular ligaments remain intact
- Of all clavicle fractures, 80% involve the middle third of the clavicle, and 10%–15% involve the lateral third of the clavicle.
- Clavicle fractures most commonly result from a fall on the lateral aspect of the shoulder, but can also result from a direct blow.
- Traditionally, clavicle fractures have been treated nonoperatively with a reported healing rate of 99% (25,26). More recent studies have shown that the clavicle fracture nonunion rate is actually higher than previously reported, at around 15%–25% (27–30).
- With midshaft clavicle fractures, the medial fragment is displaced superomedially due to the pull of the sternocleidomastoid and sternohyoid muscles. The lateral fragment is displaced inferolaterally due to gravity and the pull of the deltoid, trapezius, and pectoralis major muscles.

Physical Examination

- Typically, patients present with a clear history of falling on the lateral aspect of their shoulder or having a direct blow to the clavicle.
- It is important to assess the quality of the skin over the clavicle to make sure that the skin is not ischemic, open, or compromised in any way.
- A complete neurovascular exam is important in order to ensure that there has been no injury to the subclavian vessels or brachial plexus.
- Fractures of the clavicle may occur in isolation, but be sure to assess the scapula, humerus, and ribs for other fractures that may be concomitantly present.

Radiologic Evaluation

- Like other fractures, in order to understand the displacement and angulation of the fracture, views in two different planes are needed. Obtaining an AP of the clavicle and a 45° cephalic tilt AP usually suffices (8). Also a bilateral Zanca view can be helpful for side-to-side comparison.
- If there is any confusion regarding the fracture pattern and displacement, a CT scan can be ordered.
- An axillary view is often helpful in lateral third clavicle fractures to assess posterior displacement of the medial fragment.

Treatment

- Traditionally clavicle fractures have been treated nonoperatively, regardless of the amount of shortening or displacement.
- Surgical treatment of clavicle fractures of all types has been increasing given recent literature findings supporting better functional outcomes (31).
- Certain cases where surgery is indicated include:
  - Open fractures
  - Tenting of the skin, when the skin integrity is compromised
  - Neurovascular injury that is present or is getting progressively worse
  - Floating shoulder injuries where there is an unstable scapula fracture including the glenoid along with a fracture of the clavicle
  - Polytrauma patient where traditional methods of immobilization are difficult
- A relative indication for midshaft clavicle fractures is >100% displacement and ≥2 cm of shortening (31).
- Other relative indications are for patients who are unhappy with the cosmetic appearance of their deformity or patients who cannot tolerate immobilization due to underlying medical issues such as neurologic conditions, parkinsonism, and seizure disorders.

Nonoperative Treatment

- Nonoperative care still remains the treatment of choice for most fractures of the clavicle shaft, especially those that are minimally displaced or nondisplaced.
- Other instances where these fractures should be treated nonoperatively are in the elderly, patients with significant medical comorbidities, or noncompliant patients.
- There is no technique available to successfully close reduce and maintain position of a clavicle fracture.

- Options for immobilization for clavicle fractures include sling, sling and swathe, or figure-of-eight brace.
- Studies have shown that there is no difference in terms of functional outcomes of fractures with any of the previously mentioned forms of immobilization. Overall patients are more satisfied with a sling compared with the other options (32).
- Patients treated with a sling should wear the sling only as needed for comfort and begin shoulder motion as soon as it is comfortable for them.
- The nonunion rate with nonoperative treatment has been reported to be from 15%–30%, with many of the nonunions being symptomatic (33).
- Patients treated nonoperatively often complain of a short, sagging, asymmetric shoulder with functional and cosmetic issues (28,33,34).

Operative Treatment

- Operative treatment is usually of one or two types: plate and screw fixation or intramedullary pin fixation.
- Intramedullary pin fixation has been described and promoted because of less soft-tissue disruption. Disadvantages include difficulty inserting a straight intramedullary pin in a curved bone, inability to control rotation, and the potential of migration of the pin in the lung or surrounding neurovascular structures (35–38).
- In a multicenter prospective clinical trial, 132 patients with a displaced midshaft fracture of the clavicle were randomized to either operative treatment with plate fixation or nonoperative treatment with a sling. Patients treated with surgery had improved functional and subjective outcomes at 1 year compared to patients treated nonoperatively.
- Patients treated with surgical plate fixation also have a reported lower rate of malunion and nonunion (31,39–41).
- Potential problems with surgery include prominent hardware, soft-tissue complications, neurovascular injuries, and often need for a second procedure for hardware removal.
- Lateral third clavicle fractures are often difficult to treat given the location of the fracture. Distal clavicle locking plates have become an option for fixation as have hook plates that hook underneath the acromion. Most surgeons prefer fixation of the clavicle to the coracoid with either a screw or cerclage technique, with excision or saving the lateral clavicle fragment at the surgeon's discretion.
- Lateral third clavicle nonunions often require, in addition to distal clavicle excision, reconstruction of the coracoclavicular ligaments with an autograft or allograft.

AC JOINT

- Injuries of the AC joint represent 9% of all shoulder girdle injuries. It has been previously reported that 43.5% of AC joint injuries occur in patients in their 20s.
- AC joint injuries are five times more common in men and are twice as likely to be incomplete versus complete (42).
- AC joint separations have been found to be the third most common injury in Division I college hockey teams and account for as many as 40% of the shoulder injuries seen in National Football League quarterbacks (3,4).

Anatomy and Biomechanics

- The articulation of the acromion and the distal clavicle represents a diarthrodial joint.
- There are four planes of motion at this articulation: anterior/posterior and superior/inferior.
- Similar to most joints, the AC joint is surrounded by a capsule, has intra-articular synovium, and has an articular cartilage interface.
- There is a meniscal homologue present within the joint that has a large variation in both shape and size.
- The average size of the adult AC joint is 9 mm by 19 mm, but tremendous variation has been documented (8).
- The true articular portion of the distal clavicle varies in both location and size. Articular cartilage can cover the entire distal clavicle or it can cover a smaller percentage, which can complicate the fixation and treatment of AC joint injuries.
- In the frontal plane, the AC joint line can have 20°–50° of lateral inclination (9).
- Motion at the AC joint is facilitated by the clavicle, which allows up to 20°–30° of motion in the vertical, horizontal, and frontal planes (10,12).
- Rockwood et al. (42) have reported that, with full overhead elevation, the clavicle can rotate up to 40°–50°. Most of this motion, however, is achieved with scapular rotation rather than at the AC joint itself.
- Only about 5°–8° of motion have been found to occur at the AC joint with forward elevation and abduction to 180° (42).
- Motion at the AC joint is necessary for full shoulder range of motion (ROM) due to the coupling of clavicle rotation with scapular motion and arm elevation.
- Stability at the AC joint is achieved through a combination of both static and dynamic stabilizers.
- The coracoclavicular, AC, and coracoacromial ligaments comprise the static stabilizers. The dynamic stabilizers include the deltoid and trapezius muscles.
- The fibers of the superior AC ligament coalesce with the dynamic AC joint stabilizers (deltoid and trapezius).
- There are four AC ligaments: superior, inferior, anterior, and posterior.
- The AC joint capsule and the AC ligaments resist movement of the distal clavicle primarily in the horizontal plane (anterior to posterior direction) with respect to the scapula (15).
- Resistance to posterior translation is important because instability of the distal clavicle in the posterior direction can lead to abutment with the spine of the scapula (11).

In sectioning studies where the AC ligaments were serially sectioned, the superior ligament was found to contribute to 56% resistance of posterior clavicle displacement, whereas the posterior ligament contributed to 25%.

- The coracoclavicular ligament complex is the primary restraint to vertical (superior to inferior) translation at the AC joint, but it has significant influence in the horizontal plane as well. This complex is comprised of the conoid and trapezoid ligaments.
  - In addition to stabilizing the AC joint in the vertical plane, the coracoclavicular ligaments also strengthen the AC articulation and mediate scapulohumeral motion by attaching the clavicle to the scapula.
  - The conoid ligament is cone shaped, with the apex attaching at the posteromedial side of the base of the coracoid. The base of the conoid ligament attaches posterior to the conoid tubercle on the undersurface of the clavicle.
  - The trapezoid ligament arises anterior to the conoid ligament at the base of the coracoids and inserts laterally to the conoid ligament on the undersurface of the clavicle.
- For added stability at the AC joint, the superior fibers from the AC ligament blend with the fascia of the deltoid and trapezius muscles (43).
  - Hawthorne et al. demonstrated that injury to the deltotrapezial fascia significantly reduced both anterior and posterior rotational stability of the AC joint (44,45).
- The deltoid origin and trapezius insertion both attach to 37% of the entire clavicular length.
- The deltoid is confluent with greater than 90% of the anterior AC joint and has deep attachments that extend 4.0 mm beneath the anteroinferior clavicular ridge.
- The trapezius has a robust insertion onto the posterosuperior AC joint capsule.
  - Trudeau et al. demonstrated that injury to the trapezius destabilized internal rotation of the AC joint during scapular protraction (46).
- The radiographic anatomic distance between the coracoid and the clavicle has been found to range between 1.1 and 1.3 cm (16). This anatomic distance is important when reviewing radiographs of a suspected AC joint injury and when trying to restore normal functional anatomy during repair or reconstruction of the coracoclavicular ligaments.
- The bilateral Zanca view is used to compare the coracoclavicular distance of the injured side to the contralateral uninjured side.

Classification

- The Rockwood classification is a radiographic classification of AC joint injuries, which represents a continuum of increased soft-tissue injury (Fig. 53.5).
  - Type I: AC ligament sprain with the AC joint intact
  - Type II: AC ligament tear with coracoclavicular ligament intact and AC joint subluxed
  - Type III: AC and coracoclavicular ligaments torn and 100% dislocation in joint
  - Type IV: complete dislocation with posterior displacement of distal clavicle into or through the trapezius muscle
  - Type V: exaggerated superior dislocation of between 100% and 300% dislocation of the joint increasing the coracoclavicular ligament distance two to three times including disruption of the deltotrapezial fascia
  - Type VI: complete dislocation with inferior displacement of distal clavicle into a subacromial or subcoracoid position
- The International Society of Arthroscopy, Knee Surgery and Orthopaedic Sports Medicine (ISAKOS) Upper Extremity Committee modified the Rockwood classification to incorporate functional status and patient outcomes following nonoperative management (47):
  - Type IIIA: stable without evidence of scapular dysfunction
  - Type IIIB: unstable with evidence of scapular dysfunction despite physical therapy

Mechanism of Injury

- Two common mechanisms account for AC joint injury: direct and indirect.
  - The most common mechanism is a result of a direct force to the AC joint. A direct injury occurs when a person falls onto the AC joint with their arm at their side in an adducted position. This is commonly seen in collision sports such as hockey, football, rugby, and karate.
  - An indirect injury to the AC joint can also occur as the result of a fall on an outstretched hand. The fall typically drives the humeral head superiorly into the acromion. In this mechanism of injury, energy is only referred to the AC ligaments, as the coracoclavicular interspace is decreased during loading.

Radiologic Evaluation

- One of the most important things to remember when obtaining an x-ray for evaluation of an AC joint injury is to reduce the penetration by one-third to one-half of that used for a standard glenohumeral x-ray. Failure to do so will result in an over-penetrated (dark) film, which prevents the ability to see small or subtle fractures.
- AP, supraspinatus outlet, and axillary views are the standard views necessary for examining the shoulder.
- As previously mentioned, the axillary view is particularly helpful in visualizing a type IV AC joint injury with a posteriorly displaced distal clavicle.
- When there is a normal coracoclavicular interspace but a complete dislocation of the AC joint, a coracoid fracture should be suspected.
- The best view to visualize a coracoid fracture is the Stryker notch view, which is taken with the patient supine and the

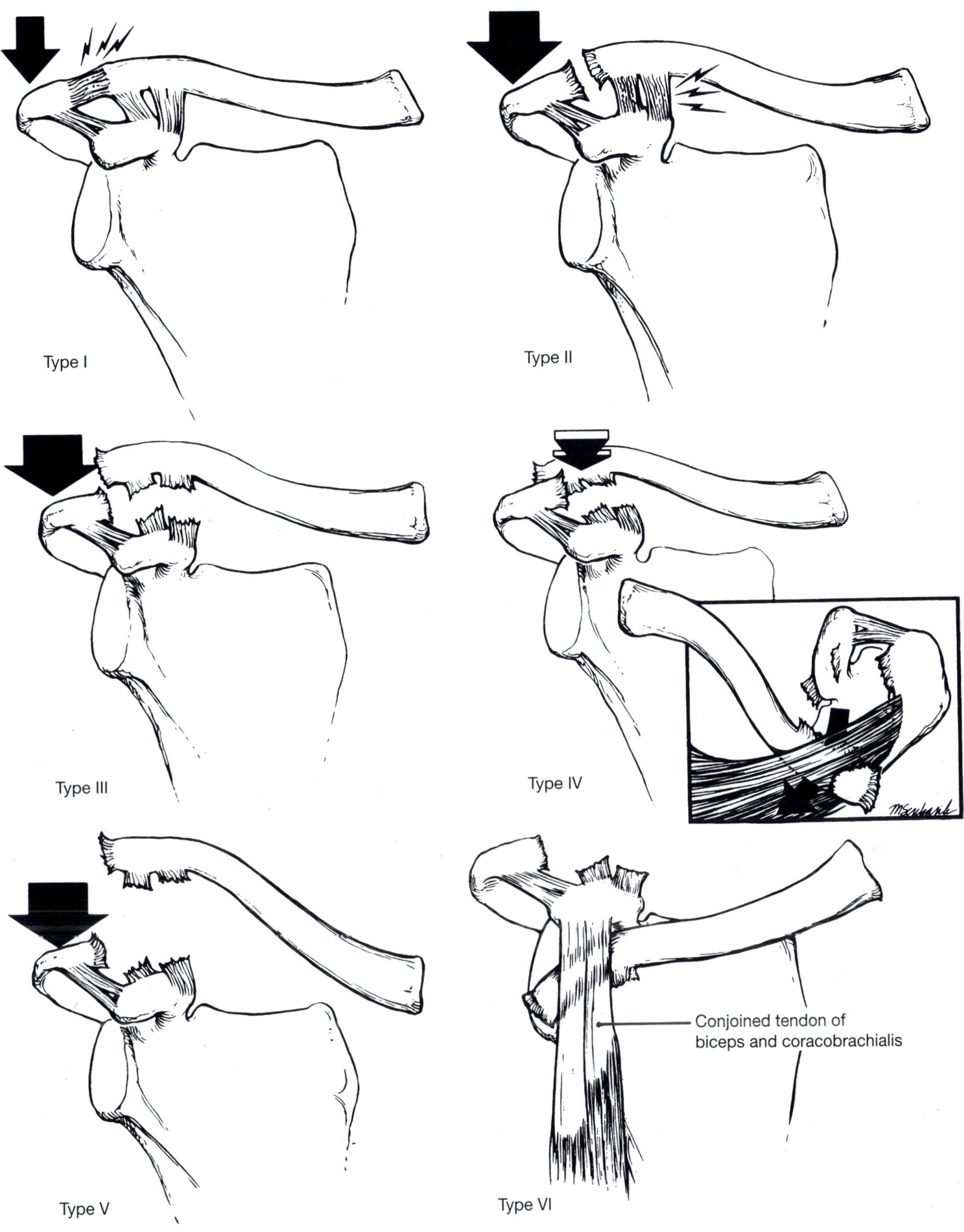

Figure 53.5: Schematic drawings of the classification of ligamentous injuries to the acromioclavicular (AC) joint. Top left: In the type I injury, a mild force applied to the point of the shoulder does not disrupt either the AC or the coracoclavicular ligaments. Top right: A moderate to heavy force applied to the point of the shoulder will disrupt the AC ligaments, but the coracoclavicular ligaments remain intact (type II). Center left: When a severe force is applied to the point of the shoulder, both the AC and the coracoclavicular ligaments are disrupted (type III). Center right: In a type IV injury, not only are the ligaments disrupted, but the distal end of the clavicle is also displaced posteriorly into or through the trapezius muscle. Bottom left: A violent force applied to the point of the shoulder not only ruptures the AC and coracoclavicular ligaments but also disrupts the muscle attachments and creates a major separation between the clavicle and the acromion (type V). Bottom right: This is an inferior dislocation of the distal clavicle in which the clavicle is inferior to the coracoid process and posterior to the biceps and coracobrachialis tendons. The AC and coracoclavicular ligaments are also disrupted (type VI).

palm on their affected side placed on their head. The x-ray beam is then tilted 10° cephalad.

- The Zanca view is the most accurate view to visualize the AC joint.
  - This view is achieved by tilting the x-ray beam 10°–15° cephalad and using one-half of the standard penetrance.
  - Because of the significant variation in AC joint anatomy from one side to another, a bilateral Zanca view is recommended to visualize both AC joints on a single x-ray cassette while maintaining the same orientation of the x-ray beam.
  - By visualizing both AC joints on the same cassette, the coracoclavicular distance can be compared from side to side.
- Barnes et al. (48) has described a cross-arm adduction view of the AC joint. This view is taken with the arm forward elevated to 90° and adducted across the body. If the clavicle overrides the acromion on this view, the injury is considered unstable.
- AP stress views are obtained by hanging 5–10 lb of weight from both of the patient's wrists with wrist straps. The use of wrist straps, as opposed to having the patient hold the weight, encourages full muscle relaxation.
  - Coracoclavicular distance is measured and compared between the injured and uninjured sides.
  - Stress x-rays are most useful to differentiate between type II and type III injuries.
  - Literature has shown that the added cost, time, and patient discomfort associated with stress views are not outweighed by their utility.
  - Patients who have complete dislocations (type II, IV, V, or VI) most often have evidence of coracoclavicular widening on standard AP x-rays.
- On standard x-rays, it has been reported by Zanca that the AC joint space is between 1.0 and 3.0 mm (49). This width decreases with age and has been found to be as small as 0.5 mm by age 60 (50). As previously mentioned, the coracoclavicular interspace has been found to be between 1.1 and 1.3 cm. Bearden et al. (16) reported that an increase in this interspace by 25%–50%, when compared to the uninjured side, indicates complete disruption of the coracoclavicular ligament.

History and Physical Examination

- Pathology of the AC joint is identified by a reproducible triad of point tenderness at the AC joint, pain with cross-arm adduction, and relief of symptoms by injection of a local anesthetic.
- The cross-arm adduction test creates pain at the AC joint because compression forces at the joint are generated with this maneuver. This test is performed with the arm elevated and internally rotated to 90° and the elbow flexed to 90°. The arm is then slowly adducted across the body.
- In addition, patients with AC joint pathology will complain of pain in the superior anterior aspect of the shoulder. This can be explained, in part, by the innervations of the AC joint and superior glenohumeral joint.
  - Gerber et al. (51) studied the patterns of pain produced by irritation of the AC joint and the subacromial space.
  - They found that irritation of the AC joint was referred to the anterolateral neck in the region of the anterolateral deltoid.
  - Conversely, irritation of the subacromial space resulted in pain referred to the lateral acromion and lateral deltoid; no pain was referred to the neck or trapezius.
  - Impingement of the lateral pectoral nerve is referred anteriorly, and impingement of the suprascapular nerve is referred posteriorly.
- Patients with a type V injury, however, may have pain in the neck or trapezius due to the disruption of the deltotrapezial fascia.
- Examination of the patient with a suspected AC injury should be done with the patient standing or sitting, which allows the weight of the arm to stress the AC joint and exaggerate any deformity.
- The O'Brien test results in active compression across the AC joint.
  - The test is performed by having the patient extend the elbow, fully pronate the forearm (resulting in obligate internal rotation of the humerus), elevate the arm to 90°, and adduct it approximately 10°–15°. The patient is then asked to resist a downward force applied by the examiner.
  - AC joint pathology is localized to the superior aspect of the shoulder and confirmed by palpation of the examiner over the AC joint.
  - If, however, pain is referred to the anterior glenohumeral joint, then labral or biceps pathology should be suspected.
  - The O'Brien test is helpful in differentiating AC joint pathology from intra-articular labral pathology.
- Other conditions that have been associated with AC joint pain are pseudogout and synovial chondromatosis.
- In patients with Crohn disease, an aseptic inflammation has been described.
- Patients who have glenohumeral arthritis have been found to have AC joint cysts.
- Distal clavicle osteolysis is a pathologic process resulting in resorption of subchondral bone in the distal clavicle. The condition results from repetitive microtrauma and is commonly seen in weightlifters from bench pressing.

Physical Examination and Radiographic Correlation

- Type I injuries result in minimal to moderate tenderness and swelling over the AC joint.
  - There is no palpable displacement of the joint itself.
  - Patients typically only have minimal pain with movement of the arm.

- Both the AC and coracoclavicular ligaments are intact, and x-ray examination is normal.
- There may be mild soft-tissue swelling on x-ray, but there is no widening, separation, or deformity at the AC joint.

- Type II injuries are characterized by moderate to severe pain at the AC joint.
  - The distal end of the clavicle may be palpated to be slightly superior to the acromion, and shoulder motion produces more pain at the AC joint.
  - The distal clavicle is also found to be unstable in the horizontal plane if grasped and moved anteriorly to posteriorly.
  - The AC ligaments are disrupted, but the coracoclavicular ligaments are not.
  - X-rays may demonstrate that the distal clavicle is slightly elevated, but stress x-rays do not show 100% displacement of the clavicle from the acromion.
  - Stress x-rays also demonstrate that the coracoclavicular interspace is the same in both the injured and uninjured shoulders.
- Type III injuries present with the upper extremity in a supported adducted and elevated position to help relieve pain. The distal clavicle may be prominent enough to tent the skin.
  - These patients have a severe amount of pain with tenderness to palpation at the AC joint.
  - Any movement of the arm, especially abduction, creates pain and discomfort, especially for the first 1–3 weeks.
  - The distal clavicle can be unstable in both the vertical and horizontal planes because both the AC and coracoclavicular ligaments are disrupted, but the deltoid and trapezial fascia are intact.
  - In type IIIA injuries, the AC joint is stable and without evidence of an overriding clavicle on cross-body adduction radiographs.
  - In type IIIB injuries, the AC joint is unstable and demonstrates an overriding clavicle on cross-body adduction radiographs secondary to therapy-resistant scapular dysfunction.
  - Both plain and stress x-rays reveal that the distal clavicle is 100% displaced superiorly in relation to the acromion. In actuality, the position of the clavicle is not altered by the injury. The weight of the upper extremity causes the acromion to displace inferiorly in relation to the horizontal plane of the lateral clavicle.
  - A shrug test has been described to differentiate a type III injury from a type V injury. If when the patient shrugs their shoulders the joint reduces, then the deltotrapezial fascia is intact and a type V injury can be ruled out.
- Type IV injuries are characterized by complete dislocation with posterior displacement of the distal clavicle into or through the fascia of the trapezius.
  - Physical examination of these patients is very similar to patients with type III, but examination of the seated patient from above will reveal that the distal clavicle is inclined posteriorly when compared to the contralateral shoulder.
  - It is possible for the distal clavicle to become "buttonholed" in the trapezius and tent the skin posteriorly.
  - With a type IV injury, it is also important to examine the SC joint for a concomitant anterior dislocation.
  - The posteriorly displaced clavicle is best appreciated on an axillary x-ray of the shoulder.
- Type V injuries represent a greater degree of soft-tissue damage, with the deltoid and trapezial fascia being stripped off the acromion and the clavicle.
  - These injuries present as a more severe type III injury with more pain and a greater amount of displacement at the AC joint.
  - The distal end of the clavicle appears to be grossly displaced superiorly toward the neck.
  - The scapula gets translated anteriorly and inferiorly as it migrates around the thorax.
  - On x-ray, there is 100%–300% increase in the coracoclavicular interspace.
- Type VI injuries are inferior AC joint dislocations. Three cases have been described by Gerber and Rockwood, and other cases have been described by Patterson, McPhee, and Schwarz (18–21).
  - None of the cases described in the literature had accompanying vascular injuries.
  - Type VI injuries are usually seen in high-energy polytrauma patients.
  - The mechanism of injury is extreme hyperabduction and external rotation of the arm combined with retraction of the scapula.
  - The distal end of the clavicle can displace either subcoracoid or subacromial. In a subcoracoid dislocation, the clavicle gets stuck behind the conjoined tendon. As such, the acromion is very prominent with a palpable inferior step-off to the superior surface of the coracoids.
  - Associated injuries include clavicle and upper rib fractures and upper root brachial plexus injuries.
  - It is not uncommon for these patients to have transient paresthesias that subside after reduction.

Treatment

- The goal of treatment for AC joint injuries is pain-free shoulder movement with full ROM and stability.
- Most type I and type II injuries are successfully treated nonoperatively with sling, ice, and a 3- to 7-day period of immobilization, although some can become painful later on.
- Type IV, V, and VI AC joint injuries are usually treated operatively due to the morbidity associated with a chronically dislocated joint and soft-tissue disruption.

- Controversy exists over the appropriate treatment of type III injuries. There has been a trend to treat these injuries nonoperatively, and if nonoperative management fails, then an operative intervention could be pursued.
- Rockwood has previously reported that in patients who participate in contact sports (football, hockey, soccer, and lacrosse) where the risk of reinjury is high, nonoperative treatment is recommended. In the small group of patients who have persistent pain and are unable to return to work or sports after nonoperative treatment, surgical stabilization is encouraged.
- A meta-analysis report supports nonoperative treatment of type III dislocations (52). This analysis included 1172 patients; 88% of those who underwent surgery and 87% of those treated nonoperatively had satisfactory outcomes. Complications included the need for further surgery (59% operative vs. 6% nonoperative), infection (6% vs. 1%), and deformity (3% vs. 37%). Pain and ROM were not significantly affected. The authors did not recommend surgery for type III AC joint injuries in young patients.
- A survey of Major League Baseball team physicians regarding treatment modalities for a type III injury in a pitcher was conducted by McFarland et al. (53) in 1997. Of the physicians surveyed, 69% reported that they would recommend nonoperative treatment for their players. Within the study, 32 pitchers with type III injuries were evaluated. Twenty pitchers were treated nonoperatively and 12 were treated operatively. Eighty percent of the pitchers treated nonoperatively and 91% of those treated operatively had achieved pain relief and normal function.

Nonoperative Treatment

- Nonoperative treatment is typically indicated in type I and type II injuries. Type III injuries are evaluated on a case-by-case basis with regard to treatment. By definition, type IIIA injuries can successfully be managed nonoperatively.
- The goal of treatment, whether operative or not, is to restore the patient back to their preinjury activity level with a painless shoulder.
- Most nonoperative treatment is centered around a brief period of immobilization in a sling accompanied by ice and oral anti-inflammatory medication if tolerated.
- Particularly in patients with type III injuries, surgery may be indicated if pain persists for 6–8 weeks. However, it is important to remember that at the 2-year follow-up, nonoperatively versus operatively treated type III injuries show no difference in strength (54).
- A specific rehabilitation protocol for athletes has been previously described by Gladstone et al. (55). Their rehabilitation protocol consists of four phases:
    - Pain control, immediate protective ROM, and isometric exercises
    - Strengthening exercises using isotonic contractions
    - Unrestricted functional participation to increase strength, power, endurance, and neuromuscular control
    - Return to activity with sports-specific functional drills
- Rehabilitation protocols in the current literature are limited by their standardization and arbitrary timelines, which neglect individual patient characteristics.
- Rehabilitation should be goal-oriented and allow therapists freedom to critically think in order to address individual patient needs.
- The goal of rehabilitation after AC injury is to regain scapular control.
- LeVasseur et al. coined the term "PASS" to characterize common barriers of effective AC injury rehabilitation: Pain, Apprehension, and Stiffness (anterior chest wall) in order to achieve Scapular control (56).
    - Pain — overaggressive rehabilitation can cause regression and persistent pain. Cryotherapy, anti-inflammatory medications, gentle therapist-directed ROM, and closed-chain exercises are practical aids for patients struggling with pain.
    - Apprehension — patients may be hindered by shoulder clicking, subjective weakness, or visual asymmetries of their shoulder girdle (known as an "upper extremity limp"). Counseling and emphasis of goal-directed therapies are beneficial to progress patients beyond their apprehension.
    - Stiffness — prolonged immobilization can cause anterior chest wall stiffness due to pectoralis minor tightness. With the patient supine and a longitudinal bump placed along the thoracic spine, soft-tissue massage and therapist-driven stretching of the anterior chest wall are useful to release the contracted tissues.

Operative Treatment

- There are four basic types of surgical procedures that have been described for treatment of these injuries. These include:
    - Primary repair of the AC joint with pins, screws, or rods
    - Distal clavicle excision with soft-tissue reconstruction (Weaver-Dunn)
    - Anatomic coracoclavicular reconstruction (ACCR)
    - Arthroscopic suture fixation

Primary AC Joint Repair

- AC ligament repair was first advocated by Sage and Salvatore (57) in 1963, who also recommended reinforcement of the superior AC ligament with joint meniscus. Supplementation of this repair with transarticular smooth or threaded pins was subsequently advocated by many surgeons (16,50,58–68).
- Eskola et al. (69) then did a comparative study of smooth pins, threaded pins, and a cortical screw. Of the 86 patients available for follow-up, 13 had osteolysis, and 8 of the 13

patients were among the 25 patients who were initially treated with a Bosworth screw.

- Treatment with a plate or pins across the AC joint has been described by several other authors, with good to excellent results ranging from 60% to 94% (70–73).
- Broos et al. (73) compared the Wolter plate to the Bosworth screw and found no significant difference in outcome.

Distal Clavicle Excision With Soft-Tissue Reconstruction

- Distal clavicle excision with soft-tissue reconstruction was initially described in 1972 as the Weaver-Dunn technique (74). The original description of the procedure involved resection of the distal clavicle followed by release of the coracoacromial ligament from its attachment on the acromion. The detached end of the ligament was then attached to the distal clavicle to help hold it in a reduced position. Although the original description involved a distal clavicle excision, the procedure has also been described without one.
- Arguments have been made that the aforementioned technique for the Weaver-Dunn leads to an obligate anterior displacement of the clavicle based on the location of the coracoid.
- Various other techniques have since been described that include detaching the coracoacromial ligament with a piece of bone attached for transfer. Transfer of the conjoined tendon has most recently been described in 2007, where the lateral half of the tendon is transferred to the distal clavicle (75). After transfer of the conjoined tendon, additional coracoclavicular fixation is achieved through the use of a double-loaded Ethibond suture anchor.
- It has been proposed that transfer of the conjoined tendon is superior to the original Weaver-Dunn technique because the functioning coracoacromial ligament is left intact.

Anatomic Coracoclavicular Ligament Reconstruction

- Coracoclavicular ligament repair was first introduced by Bosworth in 1941 through the placement of a percutaneous screw suspension procedure (76). Bearden et al. and Albrecht et al. described reconstruction of the coracoclavicular ligaments through the use of wire loops around the clavicle and coracoids (16,77). Various other materials have also been reported in the literature for use as a loop around the clavicle and coracoids (49,78–80).
- Based on these data, the ACCR was developed with the use of free grafts (81).
  - The ACCR procedure begins with a diagnostic shoulder arthroscopy.
  - Two drill holes are made in the clavicle at the origins of the conoid and trapezoid ligaments.
  - A gracilis or semitendinosus autograft or allograft is then looped underneath the coracoid and through two drill holes in the clavicle.
  - The graft is then tied to itself in a figure-of-eight fashion or fixed to the clavicle with interference screws.
- Several biomechanical studies that illustrate that ACCR more closely approximates the stiffness of the coracoclavicular ligament complex and produces less anterior to posterior translation at the AC joint compared to the Weaver-Dunn procedure have been completed (82–85).

Arthroscopic Suture Fixation

- Recently, in the literature, two techniques for restoring the coracoclavicular ligaments without a graft have been described.
  - The first technique involves using two suture anchors through four drill holes in the clavicle for fixation (86). The suture anchors are fixed in the coracoid and tied over a bone bridge in the clavicle. As part of this procedure, the coracoacromial ligament is transferred as well.
  - Previously a technique was described using a single suture anchor (87). In a controlled laboratory study on cadaveric shoulders, two tightrope devices were used to reconstruct the coracoclavicular ligaments through two single tunnels in the clavicle and coracoid. Both studies report anatomic restoration of the AC joint with favorable biomechanical results (86,88).

Postoperative Care

- During the first 6–8 weeks, the patients wear a brace that provides support and protects the surgical repair against the force of gravity such as the Lerman Shoulder Brace (DJO Inc., Vista, CA) or a Gunslinger Shoulder Orthosis (Hanger Prosthetics & Orthotics, Inc., Bethesda, MD).
- At 8 weeks, the repair has achieved enough stability that upright ROM exercises may be started.
- By 12 weeks, pain-free ROM and strengthening exercises can be started.
- Weight training may begin at 3–5 months postoperatively, and full-contact sports may be resumed at 6 months.

REFERENCES

1. Fractures and other injuries. By the members of the fracture clinic of the Massachusetts general hospital and the faculty of the Harvard Medical School. Edited by Edwin F. Cave, M.D. 10 × 7 in. Pp. 863 + xviii, with 612 illustrations. 1958. Chicago: The Year Book Publishers Inc. 210s. *Br J Surg.* 2005;46(197):298–9. doi:10.1002/bjs.18004619731.
2. Boesmueller S, Wech M, Tiefenboeck TM, et al. Incidence, characteristics, and long-term follow-up of sternoclavicular injuries: an epidemiologic analysis of 92 cases. *J Trauma Acute Care Surg.* 2016;80(2):289–95. doi:10.1097/TA.0000000000000888

3. Flik K, Lyman S, Marx RG. American collegiate men's ice hockey: an analysis of injuries. *Am J Sports Med.* 2005;33(2):183–7. doi:10.1177/0363546504267349
4. Kelly BT, Barnes RP, Powell JW, Warren RF. Shoulder injuries to quarterbacks in the national football league. *Am J Sports Med.* 2004;32(2):328–31. doi:10.1177/0363546503261737
5. Petersson CJ. Degeneration of the acromioclavicular joint. A morphological study. *Acta Orthop Scand.* 1983;54(3):434–8. doi:10.3109/17453678308996597
6. Tubbs RS, Shah NA, Sullivan BP, et al. The costoclavicular ligament revisited: a functional and anatomical study. *Rom J Morphol Embryol.* 2009;50(3):475–9.
7. Salter EG Jr, Nasca RJ, Shelley BS. Anatomical observations on the acromioclavicular joint and supporting ligaments. *Am J Sports Med.* 1987;15(3):199–206. doi:10.1177/036354658701500301
8. Bosworth BM. Complete acromioclavicular dislocation. *N Engl J Med.* 1949;241(6):221–5. doi:10.1056/nejm194908112410601
9. Palma D, Anthony F. Surgery of the shoulder. *Ind Med Gaz.* 1951;86:282.
10. Lucas DB. Biomechanics of the shoulder joint. *Arch Surg.* 1973;107(3):425–32. doi:10.1001/archsurg.1973.01350210061018
11. Klimkiewicz JJ, Williams GR, Sher JS, Karduna A, Des Jardins J, Iannotti JP. The acromioclavicular capsule as a restraint to posterior translation of the clavicle: a biomechanical analysis. *J Shoulder Elbow Surg.* 1999;8(2):119–24. doi:10.1016/s1058-2746(99)90003-4
12. Kent BE. Functional anatomy of the shoulder complex. A review. *Phys Ther.* 1971;51(8):947.
13. Yang JS, Bogunovic L, Brophy RH, Wright RW, Scott R, Matava M. A case of posterior sternoclavicular dislocation in a professional American football player. *Sports Health.* 2015;7(4):318–25. doi:10.1177/1941738113502153
14. Cruz MF, Erdeljac J, Williams R, Brown M, Bolgla L. Posterior sternoclavicular joint dislocation in a division I football player: a case report. *Int J Sports Phys Ther.* 2015;10(5):700–11.
15. Fukuda K, Craig EV, An KN, Cofield RH, Chao EY. Biomechanical study of the ligamentous system of the acromioclavicular joint. *J Bone Joint Surg Am.* 1986;68(3):434–40.
16. Bearden JM, Hughston JC, Whatley GS. Acromioclavicular dislocation: method of treatment. *J Sports Med.* 1973;1(4):5–17. doi:10.1177/036354657300100401
17. Lee JT, Nasreddine AY, Black EM, Bae DS, Kocher MS. Posterior sternoclavicular joint injuries in skeletally immature patients. *J Pediatr Orthop.* 2014;34(4):369–75. doi:10.1097/BPO.0000000000000114
18. Patterson WR. Inferior dislocation of the distal end of the clavicle. A case report. *J Bone Joint Surg Am.* 1967;49(6):1184–6.
19. Gerber C, Rockwood CA Jr. Subcoracoid dislocation of the lateral end of the clavicle. A report of three cases. *J Bone Joint Surg Am.* 1987;69(6):924–7.
20. McPhee IB. Inferior dislocation of the outer end of the clavicle. *J Trauma.* 1980;20(8):709–10. doi:10.1097/00005373-198008000-00015
21. Schwarz N, Kuderna H. Inferior acromioclavicular separation. Report of an unusual case. *Clin Orthop Relat Res.* 1988;234:28–30.
22. Zanca P. Shoulder pain: involvement of the acromioclavicular joint. (Analysis of 1,000 cases). *Am J Roentgenol Radium Ther Nucl Med.* 1971;112(3):493–506. doi:10.2214/ajr.112.3.493
23. Allman FL Jr. Fractures and ligamentous injuries of the clavicle and its articulation. *J Bone Joint Surg Am.* 1967;49(4):774–84.
24. Neer CS II. Fractures of the distal third of the clavicle. *Clin Orthop Relat Res.* 1968;58:43–50.
25. Stanley D, Trowbridge EA, Norris SH. The mechanism of clavicular fracture. A clinical and biomechanical analysis. *J Bone Joint Surg Br.* 1988;70(3):461–4. doi:10.1302/0301-620X.70B3.3372571
26. Neer CS II. Nonunion of the clavicle. *J Am Med Assoc.* 1960;172:1006–11. doi:10.1001/jama.1960.03020100014003
27. Nowak J, Mallmin H, Larsson S. The aetiology and epidemiology of clavicular fractures. A prospective study during a two-year period in Uppsala, Sweden. *Injury.* 2000;31(5):353–8. doi:10.1016/s0020-1383(99)00312-5
28. Nowak J, Holgersson M, Larsson S. Can we predict long-term sequelae after fractures of the clavicle based on initial findings? A prospective study with nine to ten years of follow-up. *J Shoulder Elbow Surg.* 2004;13(5):479–86. doi:10.1016/j.jse.2004.01.026
29. Harris RI, Wallace AL, Harper GD, Goldberg JA, Sonnabend DH, Walsh WR. Structural properties of the intact and the reconstructed coracoclavicular ligament complex. *Am J Sports Med.* 2000;28(1):103–8. doi:10.1177/03635465000280010201
30. Eskola A, Vainionpää S, Pätiälä H, Rokkanen P. Outcome of operative treatment in fresh lateral clavicular fracture. *Ann Chir Gynaecol.* 1987;76(3):167–9.
31. Canadian Orthopaedic Trauma Society. Nonoperative treatment compared with plate fixation of displaced midshaft clavicular fractures. A multicenter, randomized clinical trial. *J Bone Joint Surg Am.* 2007;89(1):1–10. doi:10.2106/JBJS.F.00020
32. Andersen K, Jensen PO, Lauritzen J. Treatment of clavicular fractures. Figure-of-eight bandage versus a simple sling. *Acta Orthop Scand.* 1987;58(1):71–4. doi:10.3109/17453678709146346
33. Hill JM, McGuire MH, Crosby LA. Closed treatment of displaced middle-third fractures of the clavicle gives poor results. *J Bone Joint Surg Br.* 1997;79(4):537–9. doi:10.1302/0301-620x.79b4.7529
34. Brinker MR, Edwards TB, O'Connor DP. Estimating the risk of nonunion following nonoperative treatment of a clavicular fracture. *J Bone Joint Surg Am.* 2005;87(3):676–7. doi:10.2106/00004623-200503000-00034
35. Jubel A, Andermahr J, Schiffer G, Tsironis K, Rehm KE. Elastic stable intramedullary nailing of midclavicular fractures with a titanium nail. *Clin Orthop Relat Res.* 2003;408:279–85. doi:10.1097/00003086-200303000-00037
36. Grassi FA, Tajana MS, D'Angelo F. Management of midclavicular fractures: comparison between nonoperative treatment and open intramedullary fixation in 80 patients. *J Trauma.* 2001;50(6):1096–100. doi:10.1097/00005373-200106000-00019
37. Chuang TY, Ho WP, Hsieh PH, Lee PC, Chen CH, Chen YJ. Closed reduction and internal fixation for acute midshaft clavicular fractures using cannulated screws. *J Trauma.* 2006;60(6):1315–21. doi:10.1097/01.ta.0000195991.80809.a6
38. Boehme D, Curtis RJ Jr, DeHaan JT, Kay SP, Young DC, Rockwood CA Jr. Non-union of fractures of the mid-shaft of the clavicle. Treatment with a modified Hagie intramedullary pin and autogenous bone-grafting. *J Bone Joint Surg Am.* 1991;73(8):1219–26.
39. Zlowodzki M, Zelle BA, Cole PA, Jeray K, McKee MD, Evidence-Based Orthopaedic Trauma Working Group. Treatment of acute midshaft clavicle fractures: systematic review of 2144 fractures—on behalf of the Evidence-Based Orthopaedic Trauma Working Group. *J Orthop Trauma.* 2005;19(7):504–7. doi:10.1097/01.bot.0000172287.44278.ef
40. Poigenfürst J, Rappold G, Fischer W. Plating of fresh clavicular fractures: results of 122 operations. *Injury.* 1992;23(4):237–41. doi:10.1016/s0020-1383(05)80006-3
41. McKee MD, Seiler JG, Jupiter JB. The application of the limited contact dynamic compression plate in the upper extremity: an analysis of 114 consecutive cases. *Injury.* 1995;26(10):661–6. doi:10.1016/0020-1383(95)00148-4
42. Rockwood CA Jr, Williams GR Jr, Young DC. Disorders of the acromioclavicular joint. In: Rockwood CA Jr, Matsen FA III, editors. *The Shoulder.* Philadelphia (PA): WB Saunders; 1998. p. 483–553.

43. Czerwonatis S, Dehghani F, Steinke H, Hepp P, Bechmann I. Nameless in anatomy, but famous among surgeons: the so called "deltotrapezoid fascia". *Ann Anat.* 2020;231:151488. doi:10.1016/j.aanat.2020.151488
44. Hawthorne BC, Mancini MR, Wellington IJ, et al. Deltotrapezial stabilization of acromioclavicular joint rotational stability: a biomechanical evaluation. *Orthop J Sports Med.* 2023;11(1):23259671221119542. doi:10.1177/23259671221119542
45. LeVasseur MR, Mancini MR, Kakazu R, et al. Three-dimensional footprint mapping of the deltoid and trapezius: anatomic pearls for acromioclavicular joint reconstruction. *Arthroscopy.* 2022;38(3):701–8. doi:10.1016/j.arthro.2021.07.016
46. Trudeau MT, Peters JJ, Hawthorne BC, et al. The role of the trapezius in stabilization of the acromioclavicular joint: a biomechanical evaluation. *Orthop J Sports Med.* 2022;10(9):23259671221118943. doi:10.1177/23259671221118943
47. Beitzel K, Mazzocca AD, Bak K, et al. ISAKOS upper extremity committee consensus statement on the need for diversification of the Rockwood classification for acromioclavicular joint injuries. *Arthroscopy.* 2014;30(2):271–8. doi:10.1016/j.arthro.2013.11.005
48. Barnes CJ, Higgins LD, Major NM, Basamania CJ. Magnetic resonance imaging of the coracoclavicular ligaments: its role in defining pathoanatomy at the acromioclavicular joint. *J Surg Orthop Adv.* 2004;13:69–75.
49. Zanca P, Shoulder pain: involvement of the acromioclavicular joint. (Analysis of 1,000 cases). *Am J Roentgenol Radium Ther Nucl Med.* 1971;112(3):493–506. doi:10.2214/ajr.112.3.493
50. Bundens WD Jr, Cook JI. Repair of acromioclavicular separations by deltoid-trapezius imbrication. *Clin Orthop.* 1961;20:109–15.
51. Gerber C, Galantay RV, Hersche O. The pattern of pain produced by irritation of the acromioclavicular joint and the subacromial space. *J Shoulder Elbow Surg.* 1998;7(4):352–5. doi:10.1016/s1058-2746(98)90022-2
52. Phillips AM, Smart C, Groom AF. Acromioclavicular dislocation. Conservative or surgical therapy. *Clin Orthop Relat Res.* 1998;353:10–7.
53. McFarland EG, Blivin SJ, Doehring CB, Curl LA, Silberstein C. Treatment of grade III acromioclavicular separations in professional throwing athletes: results of a survey. *Am J Orthop (Belle Mead NJ).* 1997;26(11):771–4.
54. Tibone J, Sellers R, Tonino P. Strength testing after third-degree acromioclavicular dislocations. *Am J Sports Med.* 1992;20(3):328–31. doi:10.1177/036354659202000316
55. Gladstone JN, Wilk KE, Andrews JR. Nonoperative treatment ofacromioclavicular joint injuries. *Oper Tech Sports Med.* 1997;5(2):78–87. doi:10.1016/S1060-1872(97)80018-4
56. LeVasseur MR, Mancini MR, Berthold DP, et al. Acromioclavicular joint injuries: effective rehabilitation. *Open Access J Sports Med.* 2021;12:73–85. doi:10.2147/OAJSM.S244283
57. Sage FP, Salvatore JE. Injuries of the acromioclavicular joint: a study of results in 96 patients. *South Med J.* 1963;56:486–95. doi:10.1097/00007611-196305000-00009
58. Zaricznyj B. Late reconstruction of the ligaments following acromioclavicular separation. *J Bone Joint Surg Am.* 1976;58(6):792–5.
59. O'Donoghue DH. Treatment of injuries to athletes. *Northwest Med.* 1958;57(11):1433–8.
60. Neviaser JS. Acromioclavicular dislocation treated by transference of the coraco-acromial ligament. A long-term follow-up in a series of 112 cases. *Clin Orthop Relat Res.* 1968;58:57–68.
61. Mikusev IE, Zainullin RV, Skvortsov AP. Treatment of dislocations of the acromial end of the clavicle. *Vestn Khir Im I I Grek.* 1987;139(8):69–71.
62. Fama G, Bonaga S. Safety pin synthesis in the cure of acromio-clavicular luxation. *Chir Organi Mov.* 1988;73(3):227–35.
63. Dannöhl C. Angulation osteotomy of the clavicle in old luxations of the acromioclavicular joint. *Aktuelle Traumatol.* 1984;14(6):282–4.
64. Bartonícek J, Jehlicka D, Bezvoda Z. Surgical treatment of acromioclavicular luxation. *Acta Chir Orthop Traumatol Cech.* 1988;55(4):289–309.
65. Augereau B, Robert H, Apoil A. Treatment of severe acromio-clavicular dislocations. A coraco-clavicular ligamentoplasty technique derived from Cadenat's procedure (author's transl). *Ann Chir.* 1981;35(9 pt 1):720–2.
66. Ahstrom JP Jr. Surgical repair of complete acromioclavicular separation. *JAMA.* 1971;217(6):785–9.
67. Inman VTMH, Neviaser JS, Rowe C. Treatment of complete acromioclavicular dislocation. *J Bone Joint Surg Am.* 1962;44:1008–11.
68. Moshein J, Elconin KB. Repair of acute acromioclavicular dislocation utilizing the coracoacromial ligament. *J Bone Joint Surg Am.* 1969;51(4):812.
69. Eskola A, Vainionpää S, Korkala O, Rokkanen P. Acute complete acromioclavicular dislocation. A prospective randomized trial of fixation with smooth or threaded Kirschner wires or cortical screw. *Ann Chir Gynaecol.* 1987;76(6):323–6.
70. Voigt C, Enes-Gaiao F, Fahimi S. Treatment of acromioclavicular joint dislocation with the Rahmanzadeh joint plate. *Aktuelle Traumatol.* 1994;24(4):128–32.
71. Henkel T, Oetiker R, Hackenbruch W. Treatment of fresh Tossy III acromioclavicular joint dislocation by ligament suture and temporary fixation with the clavicular hooked plate. *Swiss Surg.* 1997;3(4):160–6.
72. Habernek H, Weinstabl R, Schmid L, Fialka C. A crook plate for treatment of acromioclavicular joint separation: indication, technique, and results after one year. *J Trauma.* 1993;35(6):893–901. doi:10.1097/00005373-199312000-00016
73. Broos P, Stoffelen D, Van de Sijpe K, Fourneau I. Surgical management of complete Tossy III acromioclavicular joint dislocation with the Bosworth screw or the Wolter plate. A critical evaluation. *Unfallchirurgie.* 1997;23(4):153–9. doi:10.1007/BF02630221
74. Weaver JK, Dunn HK. Treatment of acromioclavicular injuries, especially complete acromioclavicular separation. *J Bone Joint Surg Am.* 1972;54(6):1187–94.
75. Jiang C, Wang M, Rong G. Proximally based conjoined tendon transfer for coracoclavicular reconstruction in the treatment of acromioclavicular dislocation. *J Bone Joint Surg Am.* 2007;89(11):2408–12. doi:10.2106/JBJS.F.01586
76. Bosworth BM. Acromioclavicular separation: new method of repair. *Surg Gynecol Obstet.* 1941;73:866–71.
77. Albrecht F, Kohaus H, Stedtfeld HW. The Balser plate for acromioclavicular fixation. *Chirurg.* 1982;53(11):732–4.
78. Kappakas GS, McMaster JH. Repair of acromioclavicular separation using a dacron prosthesis graft. *Clin Orthop Relat Res.* 1978;131:247–51.
79. Goldberg JA, Viglione W, Cumming WJ, Waddell FS, Ruz PA. Review of coracoclavicular ligament reconstruction using Dacron graft material. *Aust N Z J Surg.* 1987;57(7):441–5. doi:10.1111/j.1445-2197.1987.tb01394.x
80. Fleming RE, Tornberg DN, Kiernan H. An operative repair of acromioclavicular separation. *J Trauma.* 1978;18(10):709–12. doi:10.1097/00005373-197810000-00005
81. Mazzocca AD, Arciero RA, Bicos J. Evaluation and treatment of acromioclavicular joint injuries. *Am J Sports Med.* 2007;35(2):316–29. doi:10.1177/0363546506298022
82. Tauber M, Gordon K, Koller H, Fox M, Resch H. Semitendinosus tendon graft versus a modified Weaver-Dunn procedure for acromioclavicular joint reconstruction in chronic cases: a prospective comparative study. *Am J Sports Med.* 2009;37(1):181–90. doi:10.1177/0363546508323255
83. Mazzocca AD, Santangelo SA, Johnson ST, Rios CG, Dumonski ML, Arciero RA. A biomechanical evaluation of an anatomical coracoclavicular ligament reconstruction. *Am J Sports Med.* 2006;34(2):236–46. doi:10.1177/0363546505281795

84. Grutter PW, Petersen SA. Anatomical acromioclavicular ligament reconstruction: a biomechanical comparison of reconstructive techniques of the acromioclavicular joint. *Am J Sports Med.* 2005;33(11):1723–8. doi:10.1177/0363546505275646
85. Costic RS, Labriola JE, Rodosky MW, Debski RE. Biomechanical rationale for development of anatomical reconstructions of coracoclavicular ligaments after complete acromioclavicular joint dislocations. *Am J Sports Med.* 2004;32(8):1929–36. doi:10.1177/0363546504264637
86. Shin SJ, Yun YH, Yoo JD. Coracoclavicular ligament reconstruction for acromioclavicular dislocation using 2 suture anchors and coracoacromial ligament transfer. *Am J Sports Med.* 2009;37(2):346–51. doi:10.1177/0363546508324968
87. Jerosch J, Filler T, Peuker E, Greig M, Siewering U. Which stabilization technique corrects anatomy best in patients with AC-separation? An experimental study. *Knee Surg Sports Traumatol Arthrosc.* 1999;7(6):365–72. doi:10.1007/s001670050182
88. Walz L, Salzmann GM, Fabbro T, Eichhorn S, Imhoff AB. The anatomic reconstruction of acromioclavicular joint dislocations using 2 TightRope devices: a biomechanical study. *Am J Sports Med.* 2008;36(12):2398–406. doi:10.1177/0363546508322524

54

Shoulder Superior Labrum Anterior and Posterior Tears and Biceps Tears

Jeffrey S. Abrams and Robert McCunney

INTRODUCTION

- Superior labrum anterior to posterior (SLAP) lesions are defined as tears or the detachment of the labrum in the superior quadrant of the glenoid and can occur with or without the involvement of the long head of the biceps tendon.
- SLAP lesions are a common shoulder injury in overhead athletes (1).
- SLAP tears can be a cause of shoulder pain following chronic repetitive overhead activities or acute traumatic injuries.
- SLAP injuries can be treated nonoperatively or operatively. Surgery is generally indicated when conservative treatments fail or if there is presence of instability.
- The increased number of postoperative complications following surgical repair have raised questions about patient selection and treatment.
- Successful return to activities of daily living and sport participation is increasing; however, overhead baseball pitchers continue to be problematic and return to preinjury level of play may be successful in only half of the athletes (2,3).

EPIDEMIOLOGY

- SLAP injuries occur in a bimodal distribution most commonly in people 20–29 and 40–49 years of age (4).
- SLAP lesions in overhead athletes are most commonly asymptomatic and are recognized to be related to adaptive anatomical changes from the repetitive throwing motion (5).
- SLAP tears can be present in 72% of middle-aged asymptomatic patients (6).
- Reliable data for SLAP injuries are difficult to obtain due to the increasing reported incidence from improvements in magnetic resonance imaging (MRI) technology, the recent development of a formal Current Procedural Terminology code in 2001, and inconsistent value of reliable physical examination tests (4).

SUPERIOR LABRUM

- The superior labrum is identified as the superior quadrant of the glenoid extending anterior to and posterior from the biceps insertion.
- The superior labrum, biceps tendon, and attached ligaments contribute to humeral head stability.
- SLAP tears can be a source of deep shoulder pain and disability either in isolation or coexistent with other shoulder pathology (7,8).
- The etiology of SLAP tears in overhead athletes, as in baseball pitchers, differs from SLAP injuries following acute trauma in that tears in overhead athletes are related to repetitive microtrauma, gradual labral attrition, and biomechanical strain in the early acceleration phase of throwing (4). This can combine with posterior superior articular rotator cuff tearing termed internal impingement.

Superior Labrum Anatomy

- The labrum is a cartilaginous ring surrounding the perimeter of a shallow glenoid, contributing to depth and humeral head contact (9). Superior labrum lesions can occur alone or can extend to anterior or posterior labral avulsions.
- The labrum consists of dense fibrocartilage and elastin that connects the superior and middle capsular ligaments and long head of the biceps to the glenoid.
- The superior labrum is identified as the superior quadrant of the glenoid extending anterior to and posterior from the biceps insertion. Disruption of the superior labrum affects the attached ligaments and can alter the insertion of the long head of the biceps (10,11).
- Normal variants include a fovea, a Buford complex, and a peel-back labrum. The fovea is an incomplete anterior superior labral attachment to the glenoid with a hole or thin fibrous tissue between the labrum and the glenoid (12). A Buford complex is a thickened middle glenohumeral ligament band that inserts at the biceps labral junction with

an absent anterior superior labrum (13). A large fovea or superior labral absence may mistakenly resemble an avulsion injury. The posterior superior labrum may be attached to the glenoid neck rather than to the articular margin (14). Variations of labral attachment can be normal embryonic variants or repetitive activity adaptations. Anatomic variants and developmental changes with age can resemble tissue failure (15). The greatest success with surgical treatment is following traumatic instability events.

- Arthroscopic evaluation along the undersurface of the labrum and adjacent articular cartilage should demonstrate abnormal wear, suggesting instability of the superior labrum in pathologic settings (16).
- Superior labral tears can allow extra-articular collection of synovial fluids encapsulating as paralabral cysts. These cysts, often recognized on MRI or ultrasound exam, can create pressure on adjacent structures (17).
- The anatomy can be visualized arthroscopically in a static and dynamic exam. The peel-back labrum can be seen arthroscopically as loss of posterior superior, glenoid contact when the shoulder is placed in abduction and external rotation (14). An otherwise normal finding may increase with repetitive stresses, potentially leading to a painful condition.

Superior Labrum Function

- Superior labrum contributes to superior, anteroinferior, inferior, and posterior glenohumeral stability. Superior humeral head translation can be reduced with secure attachment of the superior labrum and its biceps and capsular attachments. Surgeons have noted SLAP tears associated with some patients with posterior and multidirectional shoulder instability (18).
- The rotator cuff interval plays a role in stabilizing the adducted shoulder (19). This interval consists of the superior labrum, superior glenohumeral ligament, middle glenohumeral ligament, and coracohumeral ligament. Reduction of an enlarged interval has decreased inferior translation or sulcus, reduced anterior translation, and external rotation and can be used to augment anterior stabilization.
- Superior translation of the humeral head can be limited with an intact superior labrum and biceps anchor with the humerus in external rotation (20). The long head of the biceps attaches to the superior labrum and glenoid tubercle. When the shoulder is in the cocked throwing position (abduction, external rotation, and extension), the head is translated posteriorly (21). Capsular changes and tears in the superior labrum may alter these relationships.
- The superior labrum may contribute to articular lesions on the undersurface of the rotator cuff. Internal impingement is a common pathologic finding in overhead throwers with shoulder pain and is related to the posterior undersurface of the supraspinatus against the superior labrum during the late cocking phase of throwing. Excessive contact of the posterosuperior labrum with the supraspinatus and infraspinatus during early acceleration can create articular-sided partial-thickness rotator cuff tears. The subscapularis tendon can abrade on the anterosuperior labrum with flexion and internal rotation.

Superior Labral Pathologic Conditions

- SLAP tears have been associated with instability, rotator cuff pathology, and ganglion cysts.
- Etiologies of SLAP tears are divided among acute traumatic injuries and attritional injuries.
- Traumatic SLAP injuries can be divided based on mechanism — compression-type injuries and traction-type injuries (22).
- Compression-type traumatic SLAP injuries commonly result from a fall on an outstretched arm in varying degrees of shoulder abduction, which can translate the humeral head superiorly, causing an injury to the superior labrum.
- Traction-type traumatic SLAP injuries generally involve shoulder hyperextension, as in an arm tackle, seat belt restraint, or during weight lifting. This can place a traction force through the biceps and capsular attachments avulsing the superior labrum. SLAP avulsion can increase inferior translation of the shoulder contributing to shoulder instability and can be related to the development of large Bankart lesions.
- Attritional SLAP injuries can be divided into those arising from a peel-back mechanism and those that are purely degenerative. Attritional SLAP injuries are more likely to be present in the overhead athlete.
- Peel-back SLAP injuries occur with the arm in abduction and external rotation during the late cocking phase of throwing. In this position, forces from both the biceps tendon and the posteriorly directed humerus can result in the posterior labrum to peel off of the posterosuperior quadrant of the glenoid (23).
- Degenerative SLAP lesions develop secondary to chronic overuse with age and may affect overhead laborers.
- SLAP tears often coexist with other shoulder pathology as a result of overuse. Baseball pitchers develop upper extremity velocity by placing the arm in maximum extension as they externally rotate and abduct. Torso forward projection places additional contact forces on the undersurface of the rotator cuff against the superior labrum. Attrition can occur with a single episode or breakdown of throwing biomechanics and fatigue. Internal impingement occurs when excessive compressive forces occur and may be associated with rotator cuff tears, superior labral tears, posterior capsular changes, and scapular dyskinesia.
- SLAP injuries can also be due to a failure of overall athlete conditioning. Overhead throwers can compromise their throwing mechanics when fatigued, resulting in increased shoulder extension and increased wear at the superior labrum.
- Ganglion cysts can develop in the setting of superior labrum injuries, which can lead to weakness of the rotator cuff.

Common locations of ganglion cysts include the suprascapular notch and the spinoglenoid notch. A cyst in the suprascapular notch can cause nerve compression, resulting in weakness in both the supraspinatus and infraspinatus, whereas a cyst in the spinoglenoid notch generally causes weakness to only the infraspinatus.

Superior Labral Diagnosis

- Patients most often complain of pain in provocative positions. A painful click may occasionally be reproducible, especially when associated with instability.
- Physical examination has had variable results (7,8,24). Examination of the biceps with provocative testing has been helpful in anterior tears (Speed, Yergason tests). Translation test (load and shift, jerk tests) and provocative position (relocation test) testing can produce pain but can have similar pain patterns with common complaints exterior to the shoulder (*i.e.*, the acromioclavicular joint). Some SLAP lesions are not diagnosed preoperatively, but rather at the time of arthroscopic surgery (25).
- SLAP tears frequently present in association with other shoulder pathologies and a comprehensive history and physical if imperative.
- Important components to consider when obtaining a patient history include the description of deep shoulder pain, mechanical symptoms such as locking, popping, or catching, shoulder instability, and pain-provoking activities.
- Cervical spine exam should be performed to rule out cervical radiculopathy and other nonshoulder conditions (25,26).
- Provocative testing for biceps tendon lesions include Speed test, uppercut test, Yergason test, belly press test, O'Brien test, anterior slide test, and crank test, among many others.
- The O'Brien test and the crank test have been reported to be the most sensitive, whereas the Yergason and anterior slide test have been reported to be the most specific (27).
- Speed test is positive when the patient experiences pain in the bicipital groove with resisted shoulder flexion while the arm is supinated. The reported sensitivity and specificity are 32% and 75%, respectively (2).
- Anterior slide test involves the patient placing their hand on their ipsilateral hip with the thumb pointing posteriorly. The examiner applies axial compression in the anterosuperior direction from the elbow through the shoulder. The test is positive when pain is elicited or a painful click is felt. The reported sensitivity and specificity is 10% and 82%, respectively (28).
- The O'Brien test is performed when a downward directed force is applied to an arm that is forward flexed, adducted, and internally rotated with the thumb facing downward, reproducing pain and weakness.
- Imaging tests can be helpful. MRI without contrast can identify ganglion cysts adjacent to the shoulder. MRI with articular contrast may illustrate superior labral tear. Anatomic variants may contribute to abnormal imaging findings.
- Juxta-articular ganglions adjacent to the glenohumeral joint have been diagnosed with increasing frequency since MRI of the shoulder has been used. Ganglions often originate from the joint space and communicate with the ganglion with a defect or tear in the superior or posterosuperior labrum (29). Ganglions may be asymptomatic or cause neurologic dysfunction due to peripheral pressure on the suprascapular nerve prior to the supraspinatus innervation at the scapular notch or adjacent to the scapular spine prior to the infraspinatus innervation.

Superior Labral Tear Treatment

- An initial period of rest is indicated in all patients with either acute or acute-on-chronic SLAP injuries.
- Nonoperative treatment is generally pursued for at least 3 months and can include anti-inflammatory medications, corticosteroid injections, and a supervised rehabilitation program (30).
- Operative intervention can be indicated if nonoperative treatment fails to regain pain-free range of motion, near-normal rotator cuff strength, and return to preinjury level of activity or if instability is present (30).
- Three broad categories of instability related to SLAP injuries include those with a bony component, inferior instability seen commonly in gymnasts and wrestlers, and anterior instability seen commonly in overhead throwers.
- Superior labral tears (SLAP tears) have been classified by Snyder as type I degenerative, type II avulsion, type III bucket-handle tears, and type IV combined labral tear and biceps insertion split (31). Expanded classification includes extension of Bankart lesions (32,33).
- Treatment of symptomatic SLAP tears should be individualized (34). Options include debridement (35), SLAP repair (36), or biceps tenotomy or tenodesis. Due to a higher complication rate of shoulder stiffness following a SLAP suture anchor repair, biceps tenodesis has been popularized (37,38).
- The best indications for a suture anchor repair are shoulder instability, shoulder hyperlaxity, overhead throwers with hypermobility of the biceps labral complex, and ganglion resection. Many patients with stable shoulders can achieve satisfactory pain relief with biceps tenodesis or tenotomy.
- One of the most common treatments for type I SLAP lesions is debridement and type III/IV SLAP lesions is biceps tenotomy versus tenodesis. Variability exists in the treatment of type II SLAP lesions between fixation of the superior labrum and biceps tenodesis versus tenotomy (39).
- There has been increasing success in treating younger recreational overhead athletes with biceps tenodesis over SLAP repair (32).
- These repairs may be done in combination with capsulorrhaphies, rotator cuff repairs, ganglion decompression, and subacromial decompressions.
- Superior labral repairs are most commonly performed with suture anchors (40). An anchor is inserted along the articular

margin of an abraded glenoid neck. Sutures are advanced through the labrum and tied as mattress or simple sutures. Anterior labral repairs should not close naturally occurring fovea. Posterosuperior SLAP repairs may require accessory portals to properly place anchors along the glenoid to secure the labrum (41). Knotless anchor technology has been helpful to reduce internal impingement of knots.

- Postoperative management should include immobilization (3–4 weeks) and regulated movement, followed by strengthening. Return to demanding activities takes 3–6 months.
- Focus of rehabilitation should be scapular stabilization and rotator cuff strengthening.
- Shoulder girdle proprioceptive training has been shown to decrease the rate of reinjury (42).
- Risk factors for revision surgery following SLAP repair include age greater than 40, female sex, obesity, smoking, and the presence of concomitant biceps pathology (43,44).

BICEPS (SHOULDER)

- The long head of the biceps is susceptible to injury in multiple locations in the shoulder. The articular portion of the biceps has a twisted pathway before attaching to the superior labrum and glenoid. As the shoulder is positioned in abduction and external rotation, additional stresses are placed on its proximal attachment site (14).
- The articular portion of the tendon exits the shoulder and enters the tuber groove between the humeral tuberosities. Tendinosis may develop due to repetitive humeral movements, friction between the tuberosities with humeral elevation and rotation, impingement below the subacromial arch, and compromised blood supply.
- Instability of the long head of the biceps may occur when pulley ligaments or rotator cuff tendons are disrupted. Patients perceive clicking as the humerus is rotated, which may reproduce these findings in a painful shoulder.
- Tendinopathies and instability of the biceps are most often associated with additional injuries of the shoulder. Rotator cuff pathology and impingement syndromes are common coexistent pathologies.

Biceps Anatomy

- The biceps has two proximal origins and inserts below the elbow on the tubercle of the proximal radius. It traverses both the shoulder and the elbow and plays a role in shoulder flexion, elbow flexion, and forearm supination. From a shoulder perspective, the long head of the biceps is the most susceptible to injury. The short head originates from the coracoid process.
- The musculocutaneous nerve (C5, C6, and C7) innervates the biceps. The nerve can be seen to enter the short head inferior to the coracoid. The second portion is innervated more distally, prior to this nerve becoming a cutaneous nerve along the anterolateral aspect of the forearm. Injury to this nerve can result from anterior surgical approaches from surgical retractors.
- The long head of the biceps originates from the glenoid tubercle and superior labrum (45). This tendon changes direction as it exits the shoulder. Capsular ligaments act as a pulley as the tendon exits the articular space and traverses under the transverse ligament (29). Extra-articularly, it runs within a groove between the greater and lesser tuberosities. The muscle tendon junction is adjacent to the inferior border of the pectoralis major tendon. Anatomic variations, including attachments to the rotator cuff and absence of glenoid attachment, may be rarely found and are nonproblematic.
- Anatomic variability in the anatomy of the biceps origin leads to changes in strain on the superior labrum. The four types of variable biceps origins include posterior complete (28%), posterior dominant (56%), equal posterior anterior (16%), and anterior complete (0%) (46).
- Biceps pathology involving the elbow will be discussed in the appropriate section.

Biceps Function

- The role of the normal biceps in the shoulder includes arm elevation and humeral head stabilization when the arm is positioned in external rotation (23).
- Due to two proximal attachment sites, the long head may rupture and not severely impact shoulder functions if the rotator cuff or short head attachments can compensate for this tear (28).
- During the throwing motion, the biceps is positioned with the arm in abduction, extended, and externally rotated. A complex change in pull occurs as the shoulder changes from cocking to acceleration (32). In addition to shoulder stresses, elbow extension occurs simultaneously, placing additional eccentric tension on the proximal anatomy (20,47).

Biceps Pathologic Conditions

- Shoulder biceps tears can be located adjacent to the superior labrum, along the articular portion, beneath the transverse ligament, within the groove, or at the muscle tendon junction.
- Biceps tendinosis is most commonly located adjacent to the location where the tendon has a directional change as it exits the shoulder. Because the shoulder abducts and adducts, these tears extend proximally and distally and can be seen arthroscopically during the articular and bursal exams as it exits above the bicipital groove (48).
- Biceps tendon subluxation can occur when the supporting capsular ligaments are disrupted (49). This can occur when the superior portion of the subscapularis is detached from

the lesser tuberosity (10). Capsular pulley and coracohumeral ligament injury can allow medial subluxation without significant tendon tear (29). Lateral subluxation can occur if the supraspinatus tears and dorsal interval ligaments are disrupted (50).

- Tears at the muscle tendon junction can result from traumatic events. Abrupt eccentric contraction may create a tear (51).
- Biceps long head tendinosis can be coexistent with rotator cuff pathology in the impingement syndrome (52). The tendon is aligned along the leading edge of the supraspinatus. During forward flexion, these structures can be impinged by the acromion and the coracoacromial ligament.

Proximal Biceps Tendon Injury Diagnosis

- The most common complaint is pain along the anteromedial aspect of the shoulder at the bicipital groove. Some patients can demonstrate a click with rotation of the humerus.
- The impingement test is not specific but can be sensitive to biceps pathology. Localized tenderness along the groove can help distinguish this from supraspinatus tendinosis.
- A Speed test is performed by an examiner applying resistance to arm flexion while the arm is supinated. A Yergason sign reproduces pain while palpating the tendon while applying resistance against supinating a flexed forearm. Pain and weakness caused by pain can be reproduced with these maneuvers (23,48).
- Muscular biceps examination is done with elbow flexion and the arm in neutral and supination. Additional testing can be performed with resistive elbow flexion or supination while the shoulder is in the overhead throwing position (53).
- Disruptions of the long head of the biceps may produce a "biceps Popeye muscle" if the tendon retracts distally beyond the transverse ligament. A tear at the muscle tendon junction can create a similar deformity. This appears as a bulging muscle located distal to the contralateral side. There is often ecchymosis initially, and it is commonly associated with a rotator cuff tear (52).
- Biceps imaging can be best accomplished with MRI without enhancement. The sagittal views can demonstrate the articular portion, and the axial cuts demonstrate the extra-articular portions and may demonstrate the biceps medial to the bicipital groove, signifying a disruption of the subscapularis tendon. Rotator cuff tears in the coronal view may raise suspicion of associated pathology.

Biceps Tendon Tear Treatment

- Biceps pathology is often coexistent with rotator cuff injuries. Tendinosis and impingement can coexist with supraspinatus tears. Biceps instability following trauma can be associated with a subscapularis tear. Diagnosing rotator cuff tears is important in determining treatment options.
- Traditionally, treatment has been divided into biceps tears involving up to 50% of the tendon or greater than 50% of the tendon (48). More mild tears are debrided, and larger tears are considered for tenotomy or tenodesis. This concept is controversial, and sports physicians have individualized treatment rather than relying on degree of tendon involvement (54,55).
- Biceps tendon debridement can be done arthroscopically or through an open approach. The articular part of the tendon can be easily debrided arthroscopically. To visualize the extra-articular portion, the tendon needs to be drawn into the articular viewing area or has to be visualized on the bursal side after the supporting capsule has been divided.
- Current controversy exists between cutting the damaged biceps tendon (tenotomy) (54) versus reattachment of the biceps tendon in a different location (tenodesis) (42,48). Generally, older individuals who are less active are comfortable with tenotomy supported by a minimal postoperative recovery. Younger and high-demand individuals may wish to avoid a possible biceps muscle deformity that may be created by completing the tear of the biceps and prefer a tenodesis. Functional deficits from a long-head rupture or iatrogenic division of the long head of the biceps are usually temporary (28). Patients' concerns and options should be discussed preoperatively.
- Biceps tenodesis can be performed after dividing the tendon adjacent to the superior labrum. The biceps can be fastened to the proximal humerus or to adjacent soft tissue. Tenodesis to bone can be performed with suture anchors, bone tunnels, or interference screw fixation. Soft-tissue repairs can be created with sutures, tendon to tendon, or tendon to capsule.
- Patients can be categorized as rotator cuff intact with biceps tear or coexistent cuff and biceps tears. In the latter, the arthroscopic or open suture anchor repair can be used to create a secure tendon-to-bone repair of both the cuff and the biceps. Patients with an intact cuff may have tenodesis performed but will need postoperative activity restriction during the initial healing period to protect the biceps attachment. Resistive exercises are generally delayed to 8 weeks postoperatively.
- Subpectoral open tenodesis repairs have been popularized when extensive tendon involvement includes the extra-articular portion. This allows for excision of the diseased portion prior to tendon-to-humerus reattachment. The muscle tendon junction is aligned along the inferior border of the pectoralis major tendon.
- In surgically treated SLAP injuries among the general population, there has been an increasing trend of performing a biceps tenodesis over SLAP repair (56).
- In overhead athletes under 35 years of age, recent studies demonstrate comparable outcomes between biceps tenodesis and SLAP repair; however, there is a reported higher possibility of patients modifying their sport or activity postoperatively after undergoing a biceps tenodesis (57).

REFERENCES

1. Fortier LM, Menendez ME, Kerzner B, Verma N, Verma NN. Slap tears: treatment algorithm. *Arthroscopy*. 2022 Dec;38(12):3103–5.
2. Brockmeyer M, Tompkins M, Kohn DM, Lorbach O. SLAP lesions: a treatment algorithm. *Knee Surg Sports Traumatol Arthrosc*. 2016 Feb;24(2):447–55.
3. Fedoriw WW, Ramkumar P, McCulloch PC, Lintner DM. Return to play after treatment of superior labral tears in professional baseball players. *Am J Sports Med*. 2014 May;42(5):1155–60.
4. Varacallo M, Tapscott DC, Mair SD. Superior labrum anterior posterior lesions. In: *StatPearls*. Treasure Island (FL): StatPearls Publishing; 2022 Sep 4.
5. Jost B, Zumstein M, Pfirrmann CW, Zanetti M, Gerber C. MRI findings in throwing shoulders: abnormalities in professional handball players. *Clin Orthop Relat Res*. 2005 May;434:130–7.
6. Schwartzberg R, Reuss BL, Burkhart BG, Butterfield M, Wu JY, McLean KW. High prevalence of superior labral tears diagnosed by MRI in middle-aged patients with asymptomatic shoulders. *Orthop J Sports Med*. 2016 Jan;4(1):2325967115623212.
7. Lafosse L, Reiland Y, Baier GP, Toussaint B, Jost B. Anterior and posterior instability of the long head of the biceps tendon in rotator cuff tears: a new classification based on arthroscopic observations. *Arthroscopy*. 2007;23(1):73–80.
8. Neer CS II, Bigliani LU, Hawkins RJ. Rupture of the long head of the biceps related to the subacromial impingement. *Orthop Trans*. 1977;1:114.
9. Howell SM, Galinat BJ. The glenoid labral socket. A constrained articular surface. *Clin Orthop Relat Res*. 1989;243:122–5.
10. Powell SE, Nord KD, Ryu RKN. The diagnosis, classification, and treatment of SLAP lesions. *Oper Tech Sports Med*. 2004;12(2):99–110.
11. Cooper DE, Arnoczky SP, O'Brien SJ, Warren RF, DiCarlo E, Allen AA. Anatomy, histology, and vascularity of the glenoid labrum. An anatomical study. *J Bone Joint Surg Am*. 1992;74(1):46–52.
12. Cordasco FA, Steinmann S, Flatow EL, Bigliani LU. Arthroscopic treatment of glenoid labral tears. *Am J Sports Med*. 1993;21(3):425–31. discussion 430–1.
13. Petersson CJ. Spontaneous medial dislocation of the tendon of the long biceps brachii. An anatomic study of prevalence and pathomechanics. *Clin Orthop Relat Res*. 1986;211:224–7.
14. Burkhart SS, Morgan CD. The peel-back mechanism: its role in producing and extending posterior type II SLAP lesions and its effect on SLAP repair rehabilitation. *Arthroscopy*. 1998;14(6):637–40.
15. Davidson PA, Rivenburgh DW. Mobile superior glenoid labrum: a normal variant or pathologic condition? *Am J Sports Med*. 2004;32(4):962–6.
16. Rodosky MW, Harner CD, Fu FH. The role of the long head of the biceps muscle and superior glenoid labrum in anterior stability of the shoulder. *Am J Sports Med*. 1994;22(1):121–30.
17. Kim TK, Quele WS, Cosgarea AJ, McFarland EG. Clinical features of different types of SLAP lesions: an analysis of one hundred and thirty-nine cases. *J Bone Joint Surg Am*. 2003;85(1):66–71.
18. Abrams JS. Arthroscopic treatment of posterior instability. In: Tibone JE, Savoie FH III, Shaffer BS, editors. *Shoulder Arthroscopy*. New York (NY): Springer-Verlag; 2003. p. 97–103.
19. Harryman DT II, Sidles JA, Harris SL, Matsen FA III. The role of the rotator interval capsule in passive motion and stability of the shoulder. *J Bone Joint Surg Am*. 1992;74(1):53–66.
20. Abrams JS. Special shoulder problems in the throwing athlete: pathology, diagnosis, and nonoperative management. *Clin Sports Med*. 1991;10(4):839–61.
21. Howell SM, Galinat BJ, Renzi AJ, Marone PJ. Normal and abnormal mechanics of the glenohumeral joint in the horizontal plane. *J Bone Joint Surg Am*. 1988;70(2):227–32.
22. Snyder SJ, Karzel RP, Del Pizzo W, Ferkel RD, Friedman MJ. SLAP lesions of the shoulder. *Arthroscopy*. 1990;6(4):274–9.
23. Burkhead WZ Jr, Arcand MA, Zeman C, et al. The biceps tendon. In: Rockwood CA Jr, Matsen FA, editors. *The Shoulder*. 2nd ed. Philadelphia (PA): W.B. Saunders; 1998. p. 1009–63.
24. Morgan CD, Burkhart SS, Palmeri M, Gillespie M. Type II SLAP lesions: three subtypes and their relationships to superior instability and rotator cuff tears. *Arthroscopy*. 1998;14(6):553–65.
25. Meserve BB, Cleland JA, Boucher TR. A meta-analysis examining clinical test utility for assessing superior labral anterior posterior lesions. *Am J Sports Med*. 2009 Nov;37(11):2252–8.
26. Dean RS, Onsen L, Lima J, Hutchinson MR. Physical examination maneuvers for SLAP lesions: a systematic review and meta-analysis of individual and combinations of maneuvers. *Am J Sports Med*. 2023;51(11):3042–52.
27. Friel NA, Karas V, Slabaugh MA, Cole BJ. Outcomes of type II superior labrum, anterior to posterior (SLAP) repair: prospective evaluation at a minimum two-year follow-up. *J Shoulder Elbow Surg*. 2010;19(6):859–67.
28. McFarland EG, Kim TK, Savino RM. Clinical assessment of three common tests for superior labral anterior-posterior lesions. *Am J Sports Med*. 2002;30(6):810–5.
29. Panossian VR, Mihata T, Tibone JE, Fitzpatrick MJ, McGarry MH, Lee TQ. Biomechanical analysis of isolated type II SLAP lesions and repair. *J Shoulder Elbow Surg*. 2005;14(5):529–34.
30. Michener LA, Abrams JS, Bliven KCH, et al. National athletic trainers' association position statement: evaluation, management, and outcomes of and return-to- play criteria for overhead athletes with superior labral anterior-posterior injuries. *J Athl Train*. 2018 Mar;53(3):209–29.
31. Walch G, Nové-Josserand L, Boileau P, Levigne C. Subluxations and dislocations of the tendon of the long head of the biceps. *J Shoulder Elbow Surg*. 1998;7(2):100–8.
32. Glousman R, Jobe F, Tibone J, Moynes D, Antonelli D, Perry J. Dynamic electromyographic analysis of the throwing shoulder with glenohumeral instability. *J Bone Joint Surg Am*. 1988;70(2):220–6.
33. Snyder SJ, Banas MP, Karzel RP. An analysis of 140 injuries to the superior glenoid labrum. *J Shoulder Elbow Surg*. 1995;4(4):243–8.
34. Alpert JM, Wuerz TH, O'Donnell TF, Carroll KM, Brucker NN, Gill TJ. The effect of age on the outcomes of arthroscopic repair of type II superior labral anterior and posterior lesions. *Am J Sports Med*. 2010;38(11):2299–303.
35. Altchek DW, Warren RF, Wickiewicz TL, Ortiz G. Arthroscopic labral debridement: a three-year follow-up study. *Am J Sports Med*. 1992;20(6):702–6.
36. Brockmeier SF, Voos JE, Williams RJ III, et al. Outcomes after arthroscopic repair of type-II SLAP lesions. *J Bone Joint Surg Am*. 2009;91(7):1595–603.
37. Boileau P, Parratte S, Chuinard C, Roussanne Y, Shia D, Bicknell R. Arthroscopic treatment of isolated type II SLAP lesions: biceps tenodesis as an alternative to reinsertion. *Am J Sports Med*. 2009;37(5):929–36.
38. Frantz TL, Shacklett AG, Martin AS, et al. Biceps tenodesis for superior labrum anterior-posterior tear in the overhead athlete: a systematic review. *Am J Sports Med*. 2021 Feb;49(2):522–8.

39. Stathellis A, Brilakis E, Georgoulis JD, Antonogiannakis E, Georgoulis A. Treatment of SLAP lesions. *Open Orthop J*. 2018 Jul 31;12:288–94.
40. Pfahler M, Haraida S, Schulz C, et al. Age-related changes of the glenoid labrum in normal shoulders. *J Shoulder Elbow Surg*. 2003;12(1):40–52.
41. Westerheide KJ, Karzel RP. Ganglion cysts of the shoulder: technique of arthroscopic decompression and fixation of associated type II superior labral anterior to posterior lesions. *Orthop Clin North Am*. 2003;34(4):521–8.
42. Frost A, Zafar MS, Maffulli N. Tenotomy versus tenodesis in the management of pathologic lesions of the tendon of the long head of the biceps brachii. *Am J Sports Med*. 2009;37(4):828–33.
43. Taylor SA, Degen RM, White AE, et al. Risk factors for revision surgery after superior labral anterior-posterior repair: a national perspective. *Am J Sports Med*. 2017 Jun;45(7):1640–4.
44. Franceschi F, Longo UG, Ruzzini L, Rizzello G, Maffulli N, Denaro V. No advantages in repairing a type II superior labrum anterior and posterior (SLAP) lesion when associated with rotator cuff repair in patients over age 50: a randomized controlled trial. *Am J Sports Med*. 2008;36(2):247–53.
45. Habermeyer P, Walch G. The biceps tendon and rotator cuff disease. In: Burkhead WZ Jr, editor. *Rotator Cuff Disorders*. Baltimore (MD): Williams & Wilkins; 1996. p. 142–59.
46. Tuoheti Y, Itoi E, Minagawa H, et al. Attachment types of the long head of the biceps tendon to the glenoid labrum and their relationships with the glenohumeral ligaments. *Arthroscopy*. 2005 Oct;21(10):1242–9.
47. Andrews JR, Carson WG Jr, McLeod WD. Glenoid labrum tears related to the long head of the biceps. *Am J Sports Med*. 1985;13(5):337–41.
48. Curtis AS, Snyder SJ. Evaluation and treatment of biceps tendon pathology. *Orthop Clin North Am*. 1993;24(1):33–43.
49. Williams MM, Snyder SJ, Buford D Jr. The Buford complex—the "cord-like" middle glenohumeral ligament and absent anterosuperior labrum complex: a normal anatomic capsulolabral variant. *Arthroscopy*. 1994;10(3):241–7.
50. Maffet MW, Gartsman GM, Moseley B. Superior labrum biceps tendon complex lesions of the shoulder. *Am J Sports Med*. 1995;23(1):93–8.
51. Garrett WE Jr, Safran MR, Seaber AV, Glisson RR, Ribbeck BM. Biomechanical comparison of stimulated and nonstimulated skeletal muscle pulled to failure. *Am J Sports Med*. 1987;15(5):448–54.
52. Pagnani MJ, Deng XH, Warren RF, Torzilli PA, Altchek DW. Effect of lesions of the superior portion of the glenoid labrum on glenohumeral translation. *J Bone Joint Surg Am*. 1995;77(7):1003–10.
53. Bell RH, Noble JS. Biceps disorders. In: Hawkins RJ, Misamore GW, editors. *Shoulder Injuries in the Athlete*. New York (NY): Churchill Livingstone; 1996. p. 267–82.
54. Gill TJ, McIrvin E, Mair SD, Hawkins RJ. Results of biceps tenotomy for treatment of pathology of the long head of the biceps brachii. *J Shoulder Elbow Surg*. 2001;10(3):247–9.
55. Mariani EM, Cofield RH, Askew LJ, Li GP, Chao EY. Rupture of the tendon of the long head of the biceps brachii. Surgical versus nonsurgical treatment. *Clin Orthop Relat Res*. 1988;228:233–9.
56. Hong IS, Meade JD, Young BL, et al. Trends in repair vs. Biceps tenodesis for superior labrum from anterior to posterior (SLAP) tear: an epidemiological study. *Cureus*. 2022;14(7):e27096.
57. Lacheta L, Horan MP, Nolte PC, Goldenberg BT, Dekker TJ, Millett PJ. SLAP repair versus subpectoral biceps tenodesis for isolated SLAP type 2 lesions in overhead athletes younger than 35 years: comparison of minimum 2-year outcomes. *Orthop J Sports Med*. 2022;10(6):23259671221105239.

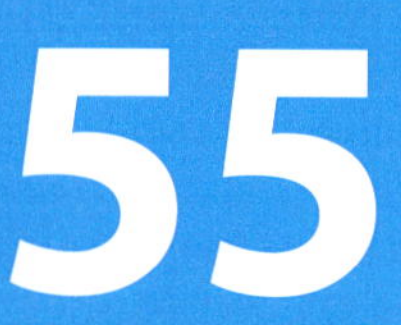

55 The Throwing Shoulder

Gavin Santini Hautala, J. Logan Reynolds, and Mary Lloyd Ireland

INTRODUCTION

- Sports-related throwing injuries represent one of more common injury presentations encountered by the sports medicine physician, with baseball having the highest shoulder injury rates among overhead athletes (1).
- An understanding of throwing biomechanics, adaptive changes, and underlying pathophysiology can assist in establishing an accurate diagnosis and creating an effective treatment plan.
- Injury prevention strategies for the overhead throwing athlete can help athletes to continue to participate.
- Sports-specific recommendations for throwers are further discussed in Chapter 88, Baseball, and Chapter 118, Softball.

THROWING MOTION

- Internal rotation of the shoulder during a baseball pitch is the fastest human movement recorded with angular velocities exceeding $7000° \cdot s^{-1}$. The repetitive nature and high torques associated with the throwing motion lead to increased risk of shoulder injury for these athletes (2). The analysis of the baseball throw is the best understood and most studied; however, the associated biomechanics are often extrapolated to other overhead sports (3).
- Throwing in overhead athletes has been analyzed extensively, especially in baseball, with the specific maneuvers being broken down into six phases (4). The phases of overhead throwing are summarized as follows (Fig. 55.1) (5):
  - Wind up
    - Readying phase
    - Minimal shoulder stress
    - Ground, legs, and trunk are force generators
    - Starts with both feet on ground and finishes when ball separated from glove and knee of stride leg is at max height
  - Early cocking
    - Occurs from the moment stride knee reaches the maximum height to moment when stride foot touches ground
    - Shoulder elevates and begins external rotation.
  - Late cocking
    - Occurs from the moment stride foot touches the ground to the moment of maximal shoulder external rotation
    - Posterior translation of the humeral head as a result of abduction/external rotation (ABER)
    - Shear force across anterior shoulder of 400 N
    - Compressive force of 650 N generated by cuff
    - Medial collateral ligament at the elbow is subject to increased forces during this phase
    - Other associated injuries during this phase of throwing include internal impingement, GIRD (glenohumeral internal rotation defect), SLAP (superior labrum anterior and posterior) tears ("Peel-back" mechanism)
  - Acceleration
    - Phase from maximal shoulder external rotation to ball release
    - Transition from eccentric to concentric forces anteriorly (vice versa posteriorly)
    - Rotation occurs at $7000°–9000° \cdot s^{-1}$
    - Only one-third of the kinetic energy leaves with the ball (the remainder is dissipated through the extremity)
  - Deceleration
    - Begins with ball release and ends with maximum internal rotation of shoulder
    - Most violent phase (responsible for dissipation of energy not imparted to ball)
    - Distractive forces generated by the acceleration phase are countered by contraction of posterior rotator cuff and scapular stabilizers
    - Associated injuries include superior labrum tear (SLAP lesion) and muscle tendon injuries (biceps brachii, brachialis, and teres minor)
    - Largest joint loads
      - Posterior shear force of 400 N

The current authors acknowledge James P. Sostak II and Carlos A Gaunche for their contribution to an earlier version of this chapter in the first edition of this text.

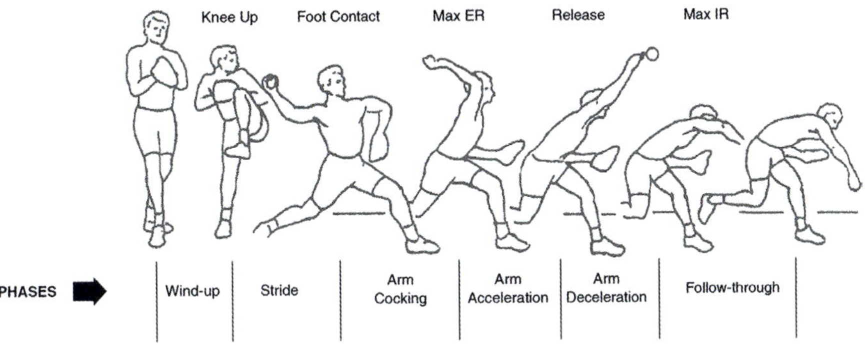

Figure 55.1: Phases of overhead throwing motion. (From Escamilla RF, Barrentine SW, Fleisig GS, et al. Pitching biomechanics as a pitcher approaches muscular fatigue during a simulated baseball game. *Am J Sports Med.* 2007;35 (1):23–33, with permission.)

- Inferior shear forces of >300 N
- Compressive forces of >1000 N
- Adduction torque >80 N·m; horizontal abduction torque of 100 N·m

- Follow-through
  - Rebalancing phase
  - Compressive forces of 400 N
  - Inferior shear of 200 N
- The entire motion takes less than 2 seconds with most of the time (1.5 seconds) taken up by the early phases (wind up and cocking).
  - Three critical points in the motion:
    - Cocking: Point in process where full external rotation/abduction is achieved, shear force on labrum is maximum, biceps vector shifts posteriorly, and the energy generated by trunk/legs is transferred to shoulder; leads to potential injury situation for the shoulder at risk (6,7).
    - Acceleration: The body falls ahead of the shoulder while the internal rotators are maximally contracting and the angular velocity exceeds $7000° \cdot s^{-1}$.
    - Deceleration: Scapular stabilizers and posterior rotator cuff contract violently to counter the distractive force of acceleration and lessen the load on the posterior inferior glenohumeral ligament (PIGHL).

KINETIC CHAIN OF THROWING

- The forces needed to propel the ball and generate the velocity of the throw require contributions from all body segments (6). These contributions help minimize joint stress and allow for the forces to be passed to distal segments as the motion progresses.
- The kinetic chain includes
  - Force generators – ground, legs, trunk
  - Force regulator — shoulder (scapula, clavicle, and humerus) — results in scapulohumeral rhythm (SHR) (8)
  - Force delivery — humerus, forearm, wrist, hand

TERMINOLOGY

- **Dead Arm Syndrome**
  - Any pathologic shoulder condition in which the thrower is unable to throw with preinjury velocity and control because of a combination of pain and subjective unease in the shoulder (7).
- **Glenohumeral Internal Rotation Deficit**
  - Basic definition: defined as the loss in degrees of glenohumeral internal rotation of the throwing shoulder compared with the nonthrowing shoulder (7).
  - Acceptable level of GIRD, as defined by Burkhart et al. (6,7,9) is less than 20° or less than 10% of the total rotation measured in the nonthrowing shoulder.
  - GIRD can also be seen in asymptomatic throwers and, in this case, may be related to increased humeral retroversion (10).
- **Internal Impingement**
  - Rotator cuff compression between the greater tuberosity and posterosuperior glenoid and labrum rim in ABER position. This can result in pain and apprehension and relocation maneuvers.
- **Peel Back Mechanism**
  - A torsional force that is transmitted to the posterior labrum as a result of the long head of the biceps force vector shifting from anterior and horizontal to posterior and vertical in an abduction and external rotation (ABER) extremity. This force "peels back" the labrum and may cause tearing of the fibers.
- **SICK Scapula**
  - **S**capular malposition, **I**nferior medial border prominence, **C**oracoid pain and malposition, and dys**K**inesis of scapular movement. In essence, this is describing scapular dyskinesia.

PATHOPHYSIOLOGY

Current Theory

- Centers around a thickened/contracted PIGHL as the essential problem in pathology of the thrower's shoulder.
- Historically, anterior capsular laxity due to repetitive microtrauma of the throwing motion had been suggested as the essential problem (11).
- However, treatment with anterior capsular plication surgeries had inferior outcomes, suggesting that anterior laxity was not the issue (12,13).
- Cadaveric biomechanical studies show that contracture of the PIGHL causes posterior and superior humeral head translation and increased external rotation, which results in increased throw velocity (14). As increased external rotation is associated with GIRD (6,7), increased labral shear forces (15), and internal impingement (11,16–18), these place a shoulder at risk for injury.

The Pathologic Cascade

- Primary event — Distraction forces during follow-through phase of throw can reach 750 N, and these forces are resisted by posteroinferior capsule/PIGHL and posterior muscles (19,20). Repeated loading results in chronic tearing, which recruits fibroblasts that deposit collagen (21,22). Ultimately, this leads to hypertrophy and thickening of posteroinferior capsule (7,23,24).
  - Posterior superior shift of humeral head on the glenoid occurs in the ABER position (late cocking phase) due to posterior ligament contracture. This can lead to excessive internal impingement beyond the physiologic level, excessive labral shear forces, and excessive posterior biceps vector, thus leading to painful shoulder.
  - Tertiary event of the cascade is anterior capsular failure with resultant instability. This is often limited to veteran throwers, who despite proceeding through the previous points in the cascade over many years have been able to compensate, continuing to throw at an elite level, and only present once the instability tips them over the edge.

LABRAL TEARS (SLAP)

Traction Mechanism

- During deceleration, biceps muscle contraction is strong as both elbow extension and glenohumeral distractions occur. The biceps muscle has been shown to be essential to limiting torsional forces to the shoulder in the ABER position (25). By this mechanism, the effect on the superior labrum would be one of failure either by tension or direct compression.

Peel-Back Mechanism

- Long head biceps tendon force vector shifts from anterior/horizontal to vertical and posterior with ABER extremity. This creates torsional force that is transmitted to posterior labrum (5,26).
- Torsional force "peels back" labrum and possibly causes tearing of fibers. If tearing of fibers occurs, mechanism will repeat with each throw, progressively worsening lesion (5).

ROTATOR CUFF

- Supraspinatus and infraspinatus tear in late cocking to move to maximal external rotation, followed by eccentric firing in deceleration.
- Tensile and torsional stress develops in cuff muscles as external rotation becomes excessive with posterior IGHL tightness.
- These stresses may speed normal degeneration.
- Factors of stressful loading, distraction, and excessive internal and external rotation can cause acute inflammatory responses early (internal impingement) or tendon failure in the later stages (rotator cuff tears).
- Stresses on cuff can also be increased with scapular dyskinesis and a protracted scapula (secondary impingement).

CAPSULAR

External Rotation Excess

Instability Theory

- Excessive external rotation, from repetitive throwing, leads to soft-tissue adaptive changes (anterior capsular stretching) and subsequent instability (27).
- Physical examination should document the full arc of motion on the dominant and nondominant side. Even with increased external rotation, if the arc is symmetrical, the shoulder is at less risk. Associated soft-tissue problems are internal impingement and posterior capsular tightness.

Hyper-External Rotation Theory

- When the anterior capsule is stretched, due to hyper-external rotation and hyper-horizontal abduction, this is a laxity, not instability pattern. The loss of internal rotation and abduction exceeds the increased external rotation, resulting in shoulder injury (28).

Internal Impingement

- Rotator cuff compressed between greater tuberosity and posterosuperior glenoid and labrum rim in ABER position (11,16–18).

- Causes pain in ABER position and correlates with positive apprehension (posterior pain) and relocation maneuvers (17).
- Etiology: two theories
  - Physiologic phenomenon occurring in all individuals that can cause labral and cuff tearing with overuse type/repetitive activity.
  - Secondary internal impingement occurs as a result of the excessive external rotation that developed from repetitive throwing.
- Analysis of rotator cuff contact in throwing and nonthrowing extremities has revealed contact in both arms when in ABER position, lending credence to the theory of physiologic impingement, which develops problems as a result of repetitive trauma (29).

BONY CHANGES

- Bennett lesion: bony reactive changes at the posterior glenoid margin (30,31)
  - Arises from repetitive traction on PIGHL at glenoid rim during deceleration/follow-through phases of throw
  - Leads to an osseous reaction and exostosis typically at the posterior inferior glenoid margin.
- Usually asymptomatic, but when present, symptom complex includes pain in posterior deltoid in follow-through phase.
  - The size of the lesion is not correlated with symptoms.
  - Symptoms may occur gradually or acutely.
- It remains unknown if the Bennett lesion itself is source of pain or if it is concomitant lesions (5).
- Symptomatic exostoses usually respond to rest and occasional steroid injections.
- Surgical options for patients who fail nonoperative treatment include open/arthroscopic excision or addressing associated pathologies (32–36).

MANAGEMENT OF SPECIFIC INJURIES

GIRD

- Mainstay of treatment is nonoperative with posterior capsular stretching and strengthening (37,38).
- Sleeper stretch (Fig. 55.2) and cross body stretch (Fig. 55.3) are common maneuvers, which have shown benefit in symptomatic and asymptomatic GIRD (7,39–42).
- In symptomatic throwers who fail extensive nonoperative management, arthroscopy can be performed (37).

SLAP Lesions

- Variable amounts of detachment encountered. The established classification system defines the clinically unstable lesions as those that involve the biceps anchor (43).
- Type II SLAP lesions in the throwing athlete tend to be located from the biceps anchor extending posterior and less often involve the anterior superior labrum.
- Attempts at rehabilitation center around stretching out the PIGHL to correct GIRD, management of scapulothoracic dyskinesia, and strengthening of the rotator cuff.
- Surgical management is arthroscopic repair. Other capsular surgery, such as posterior capsule release for GIRD greater than 20° is performed based on physical exam and arthroscopic findings (7,9).
- Return to throwing after surgery is approximately 6 months. Rehabilitation programs with scapular stabilization and proper biomechanics are emphasized in the rehabilitation protocol.
- Overhead baseball pitchers continue to be problematic and return to preinjury level of play may be successful in only half of the athletes (44).

Rotator Cuff Tears

- Complete rotator cuff tears are uncommon. Partial tears result from the excessive tension/torsion developed within fibers, as well as internal impingement that occurs in the hyperexternally rotated position.
  - Intra-articular partial tears are most common.
  - Diagnosis is done via magnetic resonance imaging with intra-articular gadolinium.
    - Assess arm in ABER position.
    - Clinical suspicion of diagnosis increases in high-level throwers.
  - Surgical indications:
    - Continued symptoms with exhaustion of conservative management modalities.
    - Debridement is considered with lesions less than 50% thickness and in those with normal preoperative strength.
    - Repair is considered in those lesions greater than 50% of tendon thickness.
    - Consider acromioplasty and/or coracoacromial ligament release if there are signs of primary impingement on exam. Usually, this is not needed because impingement in throwers is often secondary due to scapular protraction and will improve with rehabilitation.

IMPINGEMENT

Primary

- Rare as an isolated entity.
- High incidence of intra-articular pathology.
- A complete diagnostic arthroscopy is indicated in majority of patients to assess for additional pathology. An isolated subacromial decompression is seldom the answer in a thrower with shoulder pain.

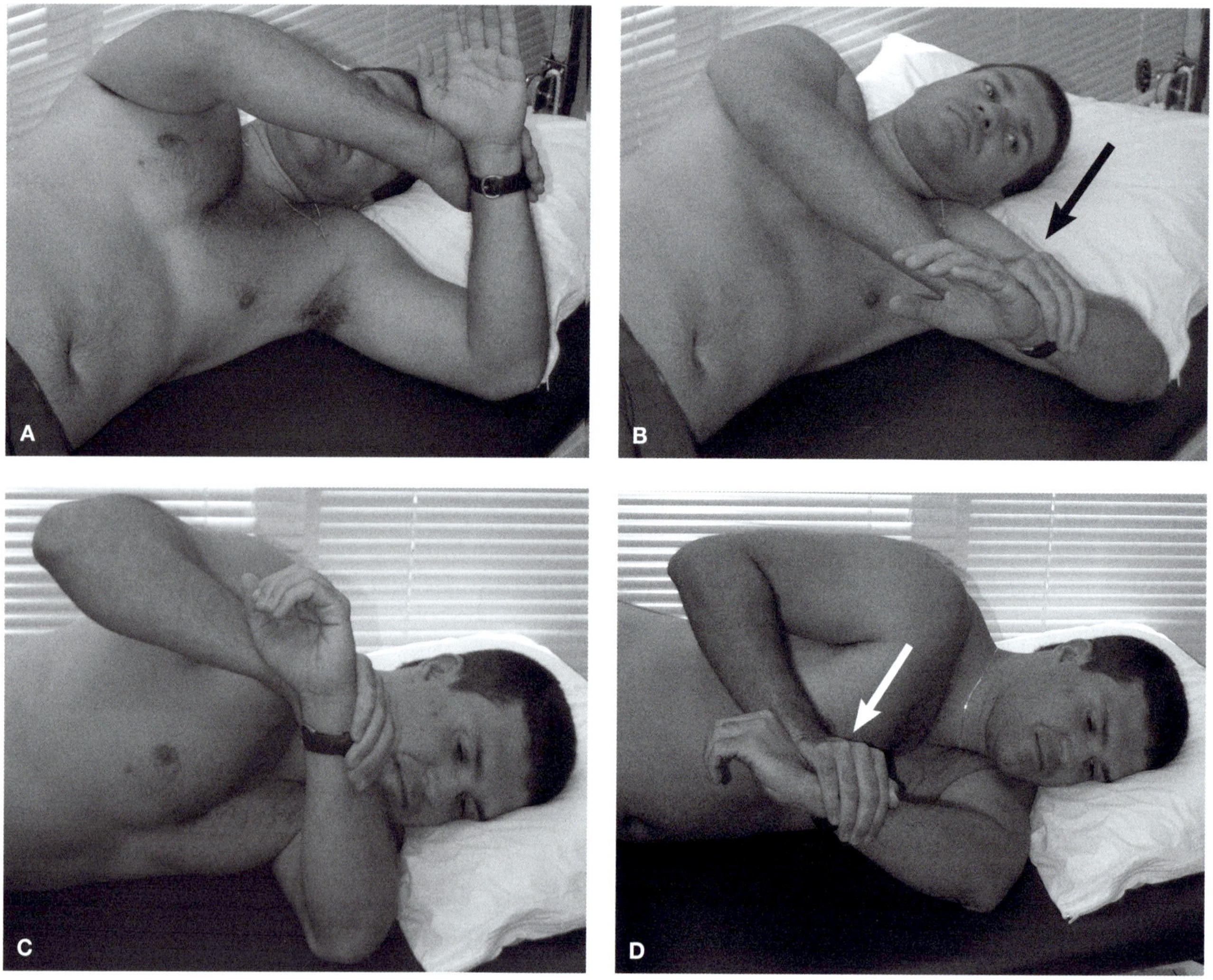

Figure 55.2: A: Sleeper stretch (start). B: Sleeper stretch (finish). C: Rollover sleeper stretch (start). D: Rollover sleeper stretch (finish). (Reprinted with permission from Burkhart SS, Lo IKY, Brady PC. *Burkhart's View of the Shoulder*. Philadelphia (PA): Lippincott Williams & Wilkins; 2000.)

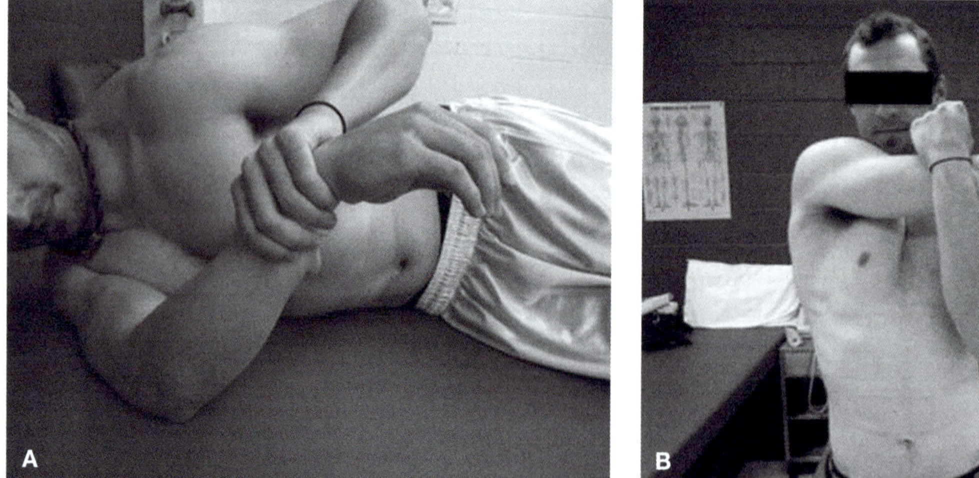

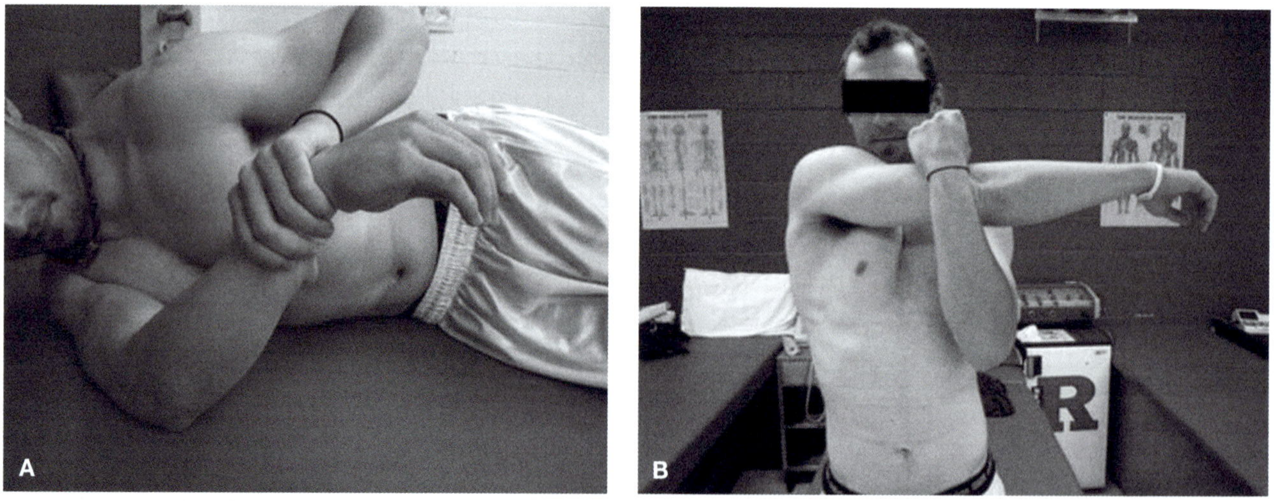

Figure 55.3: A: Sleeper Stretches and (B) Cross-body Stretching as part of a focused posterior-capsule and posterior-cuff stretching program have been shown to prevent and ameliorate symptomatic glenohumeral internal rotation deficit (GIRD). (Reprinted with permission from Miniaci A. *Disorders of the Shoulder: Sports Injuries*. Philadelphia (PA): Lippincott Williams & Wilkins; 2000.)

- In one study, only 43% of patients with surgical decompression returned to preinjury level of competition (45).
- If performing decompression, it should be a conservative resection.

Secondary

- Scapular dyskinesia results because of weak scapular stabilizers. This leads to protracted scapula and impingement in ABER position.
- With a specialized scapular rehabilitation program, this pain generator will resolve.
- This problem needs to be corrected, in addition to intra-articular pathology, or the pathology will recur.

REHABILITATION ISSUES

Scapulothoracic Articulation

- Often the cause of secondary impingement.
- The scapula has five specific functions that have implications in throwers (46).
  - Stable part of the glenohumeral articulation, where rotation of the glenohumeral joint allows maximal concavity and compression
  - Retracts and protracts the shoulder complex along the thoracic wall
  - Acromial elevation to avoid impingement with arm elevation
  - Base for muscular attachments
  - Energy transfer from the legs, back, and trunk

Scapulothoracic Dyskinesia

- Abnormal set of motions and positions affecting the relative position of the scapula and the proximal humerus.
  - Etiologies include nerve or muscle injury, muscle inhibition, and glenohumeral stiffness or laxity.
  - Mechanical dysfunction may result in impingement and insufficient translation of energy from the lower body.
    - Excessive stress results in overuse injuries.
    - Clinical picture is confusing as a result of secondary impingement and capsular changes that may occur as a result of the adaptations to scapular malalignment.

Proprioception

- Excessive joint laxity associated with capsuloligamentous injury and resulting microtrauma cause damage to the neural receptors and lead to deafferentation (47).
- Neuromuscular deficits impair reflexive muscular stabilization, predisposing the shoulder to episodes of functional instability.
  - Diminished joint position sense, kinesthetic awareness, and abnormal humeroscapular firing patterns (48).
  - Abnormal firing patterns documented on electromyography studies in throwers with glenohumeral instability (49).
  - After surgical reconstruction, joint position sense and reproduction of passive positioning improve to baseline levels (48).
- Restoration of functional stability.
  - Traditional strengthening exercises do not address neuromuscular deficits.
  - Four elements are necessary to restore functional stability (48):
    - Peripheral somatosensory: including visual and vestibular
    - Spinal reflexes: sudden alteration in joint position that requires reflex muscular stabilization
    - Cognitive programming: appreciation of joint position
    - Brainstem
  - All four elements need to be addressed to fulfill the objective of stimulating all subsystems:
    - Dynamic stabilization:
      - Promotes coactivation of force couples
      - Centers humeral head.
    - Joint position sensibility:
      - Restore through conscious and unconscious pathways.
    - Reactive neuromuscular control:
      - Reflexive muscular stabilization induced by sudden alterations in joint position.
      - Eccentric activities useful.
    - Functional motor patterns:
      - Progression to the actual throwing activity.
      - Analyze the direction of force, amount of loading, and resultant muscle action to incorporate functional progression.

PREVENTION

- There is a significant overlap of prevention with treatment of throwers shoulder in overhead athletes.
- Increased pitch counts as well as breaking pitches (curveballs, sliders) in adolescents correlate with increased shoulder pain and injury, thus limiting pitch counts and avoiding breaking pitches is recommended for prevention of injury in skeletally immature patients (50,51).
- Preventing injury in the adult thrower begins with rest, followed by a rehabilitation program that addresses global functional deficits (*e.g.*, core stability, lower extremity strength, flexibility) (51).
- The USA Baseball Medical and Safety Advisory Committee has published recommended pitch counts and rest between

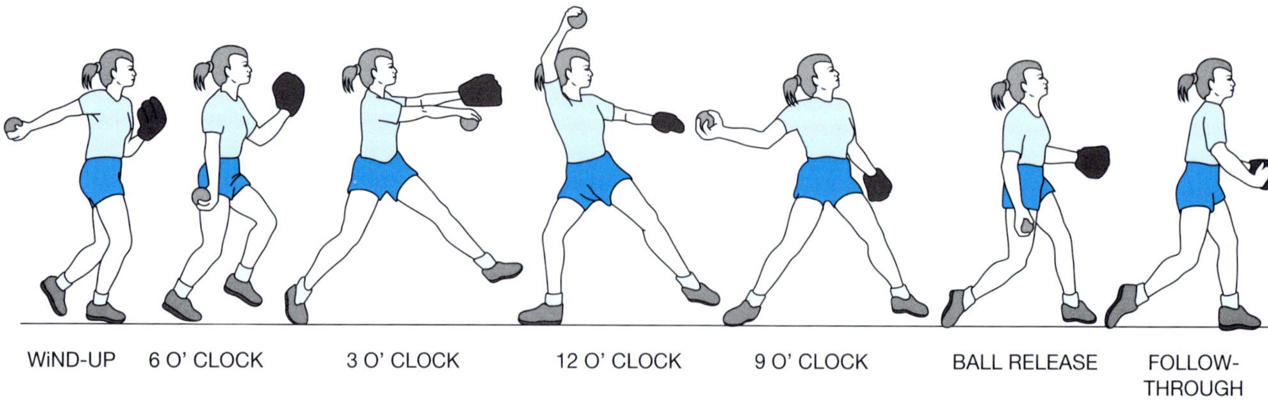

Figure 55.4: Phases of softball (windmill) throwing include the wind-up and circumferential motion labeled above until ball release at the same location as the start point, ending with follow-through. (Maffet MW, Jobe FW, Pink MM, Brault J, Mathiyakom W. Shoulder muscle firing patterns during the windmill softball pitch. *Am J Sports Med.* 1997;25(3):369-374.)

pitching starts at all ages, called the *Pitch Smart Guidelines* (https://www.mlb.com/pitch-smart/pitching-guidelines), which aim to help prevent shoulder injury in throwers (52).

- American Orthopedic Society for Sports Medicine (AOSSM) and the National Council of Youth Sports (NCYS) have collaborated to come up with the *STOP Program* (Sports Trauma and Overuse Prevention), which also has recommended pitch counts and rest duration between starts, as well as warm up and cool down recommendations for baseball athletes (https://ncys.org/safety/sport-specific-resources/) (53).

SOFTBALL PITCHING (WINDMILL THROWING)

- Throwing in softball has more recently been analyzed in the same regard as overhead baseball throwing.
- Softball phases of throwing are back swing, arm rotation, final down swing, release, and follow-through (Fig. 55.4).
- Softball pitchers can have similar overuse injuries as baseball pitchers on the shoulder, but with a different mechanism and kinematic stress on the shoulder.
- The high rate of shoulder injury is theorized to result from overuse attributed to the dynamic and repetitive nature of softball pitching and the high shoulder stresses exhibited throughout the pitching motion (54).
- Injury reports have shown that softball pitchers regularly experience anterior shoulder pain as well as biceps and labral pathology, which might suggest that the biceps-labral complex is under great stress during the windmill pitch (55–57).
- Shoulder distraction stress averaged 80%–94% of body weight (58,59).
- There has not been literature to support an exact pitch count in adolescent or high school softball pitchers to prevent injury, but there have been reports of increased injury with high pitching volume (60,61).

SUMMARY

- Understanding of the biomechanics, adaptations, and pathophysiology of the throwing shoulder continue to evolve.
- As future nonoperative and surgical interventions continue to emerge in the management of the thrower's shoulder, attention should continue to focus on both the prevention and prediction of these injuries in athletes.

REFERENCES

1. Zaremski JL, Wasser JG, Vincent HK. Mechanisms and treatments for shoulder injuries in overhead throwing athletes. *Curr Sports Med Rep.* 2017 May/Jun;16(3):179–88.
2. Wilk KE, Macrina LC, Fleisig GS, et al. Deficits in glenohumeral passive range of motion increase risk of shoulder injury in professional baseball pitchers: a prospective study. *Am J Sports Med.* 2015 Oct;43(10):2379–85.
3. Fleisig GS, Andrews JR, Dillman CJ, Escamilla RF. Kinetics of baseball pitching with implications about injury mechanisms. *Am J Sports Med.* 1995;23(2):233–9.
4. Gowan ID, Jobe FW, Tibone JE, Perry J, Moynes DR. A comparative electromyographic analysis of the shoulder during pitching. Professional versus amateur pitchers. *Am J Sports Med.* 1987;15(6):586–90.
5. Medina G, Bartolozzi AR III, Spencer JA, Morgan C. The thrower's shoulder. *JBJS Rev.* 2022 Mar 18;10(3):e21.
6. Burkhart SS, Morgan CD, Kibler WB. The disabled throwing shoulder: spectrum of pathology. Part III—the SICK scapula, scapular dyskinesis, the kinetic chain, and rehabilitation. *Arthroscopy.* 2003;19(6):641–61.
7. Burkhart SS, Morgan CD, Kibler WB. The disabled throwing shoulder: spectrum of pathology. Part I—pathoanatomy and biomechanics. *Arthroscopy.* 2003;19(4):404–20.
8. Kibler WB, Sciascia AD, Grantham WJ. The shoulder joint complex in the throwing motion. *J Shoulder Elbow Surg.* 2024;33(2):443–9.
9. Burkhart SS, Morgan CD, Kibler WB. The disabled throwing shoulder: spectrum of pathology. Part II—evaluation and treatment of SLAP lesions in throwers. *Arthroscopy.* 2003;19(5):531–9.

10. Tokish JM, Curtin MS, Kim YK, Hawkins RJ, Torry MR. Glenohumeral internal rotation deficit in the asymptomatic professional pitcher and its relationship to humeral retroversion. *J Sports Sci Med*. 2008;7(1):78–83.
11. Jobe CM. Posterior superior glenoid impingement: expanded spectrum. *Arthroscopy*. 1995 Oct;11(5):530–6.
12. Jobe FW, Giangarra CE, Kvitne RS, Glousman RE. Anterior capsulolabral reconstruction of the shoulder in athletes in overhand sports. *Am J Sports Med*. 1991 Sep–Oct;19(5):428–34.
13. Tibone JE, Elrod B, Jobe FW, et al. Surgical treatment of tears of the rotator cuff in athletes. *J Bone Joint Surg Am*. 1986 Jul;68(6):887–91.
14. Grossman MG, Tibone JE, McGarry MH, Schneider DJ, Veneziani S, Lee TQ. A cadaveric model of the throwing shoulder: a possible etiology of superior labrum anterior-to-posterior lesions. *J Bone Joint Surg Am*. 2005;87(4):824–31.
15. Burkhart SS, Morgan CD. The peel-back mechanism: its role in producing and extending posterior type II SLAP lesions and its effect on SLAP repair rehabilitation. *Arthroscopy*. 1998 Sep;14(6):637–40.
16. Bennett GE. Shoulder and elbow lesions distinctive of baseball players. *Ann Surg*. 1947 Jul;126(1):107–10.
17. Walch G, Boileau P, Noel E, Donell ST. Impingement of the deep surface of the supraspinatus tendon on the posterosuperior glenoid rim: an arthroscopic study. *J Shoulder Elbow Surg*. 1992;1(5):238–45.
18. Walch G, Liotard JP, Boileau P, Noël E. Postero-superior glenoid impingement. Another shoulder impingement. *Rev Chir Orthop Reparatrice Appar Mot*. 1991;77(8):571–4.
19. Levitz CL, Dugas J, Andrews JR. The use of arthroscopic thermal capsulorrhaphy to treat internal impingement in baseball players. *Arthroscopy*. 2001 Jul;17(6):573–7.
20. Seroyer ST, Nho SJ, Bach BR Jr, Bush-Joseph CA, Nicholson GP, Romeo AA. Shoulder pain in the overhead throwing athlete. *Sports Health*. 2009 Mar;1(2):108–20.
21. Khan KM, Scott A. Mechanotherapy: how physical therapists' prescription of exercise promotes tissue repair. *Br J Sports Med*. 2009 Apr;43(4):247–52.
22. Yang G, Crawford RC, Wang JHC. Proliferation and collagen production of human patellar tendon fibroblasts in response to cyclic uniaxial stretching in serum-free conditions. *J Biomech*. 2004 Oct;37(10):1543–50.
23. Harryman DT II, Sidles JA, Clark JM, McQuade KJ, Gibb TD, Matsen FA III. Translation of the humeral head on the glenoid with passive glenohumeral motion. *J Bone Joint Surg Am*. 1990 Oct;72(9):1334–43.
24. Thomas SJ, Swanik CB, Higginson JS, et al. Neuromuscular and stiffness adaptations in Division I collegiate baseball players. *J Electromyogr Kinesiol*. 2013 Feb;23(1):102–9.
25. Rodosky MW, Harner CD, Fu FH. The role of the long head of the biceps muscle and superior glenoid labrum in anterior stability of the shoulder. *Am J Sports Med*. 1994;22(1):121–30.
26. Morgan CD, Burkhart SS, Palmeri M, Gillespie M. Type II SLAP lesions: three subtypes and their relationships to superior instability and rotator cuff tears. *Arthroscopy*. 1998;14(6):553–65.
27. Kvitne RS, Jobe FW. The diagnosis and treatment of anterior instability in the throwing athlete. *Clin Orthop Relat Res*. 1993;291:107–23.
28. Rubenstein DL, Jobe FW, Glousman RE, Kvitne RS, Pink M, Giangarra CE. Anterior capsulolabral reconstruction of the shoulder in athletes. *J Shoulder Elbow Surg*. 1992;1(5):229–37.
29. Halbrecht JL, Tirman P, Atkin D. Internal impingement of the shoulder: comparison of findings between the throwing and nonthrowing shoulders of college baseball players. *Arthroscopy*. 1999;15(3):253–8.
30. Bennett GE. Elbow and shoulder lesions of baseball players. *Am J Surg*. 1959;98:484–92.
31. Braun S, Kokmeyer D, Millett PJ. Shoulder injuries in the throwing athlete. *J Bone Joint Surg Am*. 2009 Apr;91(4):966–78.
32. Ferrari JD, Ferrari DA, Coumas J, Pappas AM. Posterior ossification of the shoulder: the Bennett lesion. Etiology, diagnosis, and treatment. *Am J Sports Med*. 1994 Mar–Apr;22(2):171–6. discussion 175–6.
33. Lombardo SJ, Jobe FW, Kerlan RK, Carter VS, Shields CL Jr. Posterior shoulder lesions in throwing athletes. *Am J Sports Med*. 1977;5(3):106–10.
34. Meister K, Andrews JR, Batts J, Wilk K, Baumgarten T. Symptomatic thrower's exostosis. Arthroscopic evaluation and treatment. *Am J Sports Med*. 1999;27(2):133–6.
35. Vo AM, Rogers KM, Bonner KF. Arthroscopic resection of symptomatic Bennett lesions. *Arthrosc Tech*. 2019 Nov 13;8(12):e1463–7.
36. Yoneda M, Nakagawa S, Hayashida K, Fukushima S, Wakitani S. Arthroscopic removal of symptomatic Bennett lesions in the shoulders of baseball players: arthroscopic Bennett-plasty. *Am J Sports Med*. 2002 Sep-Oct;30(5):728–36.
37. Rose MB, Noonan T. Glenohumeral internal rotation deficit in throwing athletes: current perspectives. *Open Access J Sports Med*. 2018 Mar 19;9:69–78.
38. Wilk KE, Macrina LC. Nonoperative and postoperative rehabilitation for injuries of the throwing shoulder. *Sports Med Arthrosc Rev*. 2014;22(2):137–50.
39. Cools AM, Johansson FR, Cagnie B, Cambier DC, Witvrouw EE. Stretching the posterior shoulder structures in subjects with internal rotation deficit: comparison of two stretching techniques. *Shoulder Elbow*. 2012;4(1):56–63.
40. Escamilla RF, Yamashiro K, Mikla T, Collins J, Lieppman K, Andrews JR. Effects of a short-duration stretching drill after pitching on elbow and shoulder range of motion in professional baseball pitchers. *Am J Sports Med*. 2017;45(3):692–700.
41. Mine K, Nakayama T, Milanese S, Grimmer K. Effectiveness of stretching on posterior shoulder tightness and glenohumeral internal-rotation deficit: a systematic review of randomized controlled trials. *J Sport Rehabil*. 2017;26(4):294–305.
42. Tyler TF, Nicholas SJ, Lee SJ, Mullaney M, McHugh MP. Correction of posterior shoulder tightness is associated with symptom resolution in patients with internal impingement. *Am J Sports Med*. 2010;38(1):114–19.
43. Snyder SJ, Karzel RP, Del Pizzo W, Ferkel RD, Friedman MJ. SLAP lesions of the shoulder. *Arthroscopy*. 1990;6(4):274–9.
44. Brockmeyer M, Tompkins M, Kohn DM, Lorbach O. SLAP lesions: a treatment algorithm. *Knee Surg Sports Traumatol Arthrosc*. 2016 Feb;24(2):447–55.
45. Tibone JE, Jobe FW, Kerlan RK, et al. Shoulder impingement syndrome in athletes treated by an anterior acromioplasty. *Clin Orthop Relat Res*. 1985;198:134–40.
46. Kibler WB. The role of the scapula in athletic shoulder function. *Am J Sports Med*. 1998;26(2):325–37.
47. Lephart SM, Henry TJ. Restoration of proprioception and neuromuscular control of the unstable shoulder. In: Lephart SM, Fu FH, editors. *Proprioception and Neuromuscular Control in Joint Stability*. New York (NY): Human Kinetics; 2000. p. 405–13.
48. Lephart SM, Henry TJ. The physiological basis for open and closed kinetic chain rehabilitation for the upper extremity. *J Sport Rehab*. 1996;5(1):71–87.
49. Glousman R, Jobe FW, Tibone J, Moynes D, Antonelli D, Perry J. Dynamic electromyographic analysis of the throwing shoulder with glenohumeral instability. *J Bone Joint Surg Am*. 1988;70(2):220–6.
50. Lyman S, Fleisig GS, Andrews JR, Osinski ED. Effect of pitch type, pitch count, and pitching mechanics on risk of elbow and shoulder pain in youth baseball pitchers. *Am J Sports Med*. 2002;30(4):463–8.
51. Limpisvasti O, ElAttrache NS, Jobe FW. Understanding shoulder and elbow injuries in baseball. *J Am Acad Orthop Surg*. 2007 Mar;15(3):139–47.

52. Pitch Smart | Pitching Guidelines, MLB.com. 2019. Available from: https://www.mlb.com/pitch-smart/pitching-guidelines
53. Sport Specific Resources | National Council of Youth Sports. Ncys.org; n.d. Available from: https://ncys.org/safety/sport-specific-resources/
54. Werner SL, Suri M, Guido JA, Meister K, Jones DG. Relationships between ball velocity and throwing mechanics in collegiate baseball pitchers. *J Shoulder Elbow Surg*. 2008;17(6):905–8.
55. Paul J, Brown SM, Mulcahey MK. Injury prevention programs for throwing injuries in softball players: a systematic review. *Sports Health*. 2021;13(4):390–5.
56. Shanley E, Thigpen C. Throwing injuries in the adolescent athlete. *Int J Sports Phys Ther*. 2013;8(5):630–40.
57. Rojas IL, Provencher MT, Bhatia S, et al. Biceps activity during windmill softball pitching: injury implications and comparison with overhand throwing. *Am J Sports Med*. 2009 Mar;37(3):558–65.
58. Werner SL, Jones DG, Guido JA, Brunet ME. Kinematics and kinetics of elite windmill softball pitching. *Am J Sports Med*. 2006;34(4):597–603.
59. Werner SL, Guido JA, McNeice RP, Richardson JL, Delude NA, Stewart GW. Biomechanics of youth windmill softball pitching. *Am J Sports Med*. 2005 Apr;33(4):552–60.
60. Shanley E, Michener L, Ellenbecker T, Rauh M. Shoulder range of motion, pitch count, and injuries among interscholastic female softball pitchers: a descriptive study. *Int J Sports Phys Ther*. 2012;7(5):548–57.
61. Gooch B, Lambert BS, Goble H, McCulloch PC, Hedt C. Relationship between pitch volume and subjective report of injury in high school female fast-pitch softball pitchers. *Sports Health*. 2022 Sep–Oct;14(5):702–9.

56

Elbow Instability

Mark R. Hutchinson, Michael P. Foy, and Navya Dandu

INTRODUCTION

- The elbow is a compound hinge, trochleoginglymoid, synovial joint, and is a critical element of the kinetic chain of the upper extremity that allows positioning of the hand in space as well as transfer of forces from the hand to the axial skeleton.
- Elbow instability may present as gross instability related to an acute trauma or as functional instability related to chronic repetitive use or failure of healing of an acute injury. Either may lead to dysfunction related to sports participation, especially throwing.
- Acute elbow injury is very common. The elbow is the second most common dislocated major joint in adults with an incidence of 5.2/100,000 persons per year (1). In addition, soft-tissue injuries including LCL and UCL injuries are also quite common, particularly in throwing athletes. There are data from Major League Baseball that approximately 24% of all elbow injuries were UCL related, and in collegiate baseball the incidence is as high as 4.4 per 100 player seasons for pitchers (2,3).
- Injury patterns related to specific mechanisms of injury will directly impact treatment options and prognosis. Posterolateral rotatory forces are associated with injuries of the lateral ulnar collateral ligament and stability of the radiocapitellar joint. Valgus extension overload forces are associated with injuries of the medial collateral ligament with associated compression of the capitellum with impingement of the olecranon in the posterior fossa. Complete elbow dislocations are described based on the location of the distal bones relative to the humerus (posterior, anterior, posterior-lateral, or posterior-medial) and each injury pattern is associated with unique patterns of associated ligament, capsule, and bony injuries that impact prognosis.

FUNCTIONAL ANATOMY

- The elbow joint comprises three bones (humerus, radius, and ulna); their articulations (radiocapitellar, ulnohumeral, and proximal radioulnar); seven primary muscles that act on the elbow (biceps brachii, brachioradialis, brachialis, pronator teres, supinator, triceps brachii, anconeus); nine secondary muscles that anchor on the epicondyles but act on the wrist and hand (flexor carpi radialis, flexor carpi ulnaris, palmaris longus, flexor digitorum superficialis, extensor carpi radialis longus, extensor carpi radialis brevis, and extensor digitorum); as well as a complex capsuloligamentous complex (medial ulnar collateral ligament [MCL], the lateral ulnar collateral ligament, the annular ligament [LCL], radiocollateral ligament), which conjointly contribute to elbow stability.
- The lateral portion of the distal humerus, the capitellum, articulates with the radial head. The medial portion of the humerus, the trochlea, articulates with the trochlear notch or "greater sigmoid notch" of the ulna. The radial notch of the ulna articulates with the radial head (4).
- The ulnohumeral joint affords flexion and extension of the elbow with the medial distal humeral articular surface articulating in the sigmoid notch of the ulna and the lateral distal humeral articulating surface (the capitellum) articulating with the radial head. Indeed, the convex articulating hemisphere of the capitellum also allows a rotational degree of freedom with the concave proximal radial head. The proximal radioulnar joint affords pronation and supination of the radial head within the radial notch of the ulna.
- Bony architecture provides primary stability at the extremes of elbow flexion and extension.
- The capsule-ligamentous complex with associated dynamic muscle tendon function provides primary stability in the mid-range of motion (5).
- The MCL is the main constraint to valgus instability. It originates on the antero-inferior medial epicondyle and consists of an anterior band inserting on the sublime tubercle of the coronoid process and provides most stability at all arcs of flexion. The posterior band inserting on the medial margin of the semilunar notch of the ulna and provides stability at 90° of flexion. The MCL can be injured off the humerus, the sublime tubercle, or mid-substance, and the specifics may guide treatment options.
- The LCL complex originates from the lateral epicondyle and consists of four parts: (a) the radial collateral ligament; (b) the lateral ulnar collateral ligament (LUCL), which provides most lateral stability; (c) the annular ligament, which encircles the radial head; and (d) the accessory LCL. Injury patterns can include avulsions of the complex from the humeral origin or mid-substance injuries with the specific findings guiding treatment and impacting prognosis.

HISTORY

Dislocations

- Elbow dislocations are high-energy injuries more commonly associated with contact and collision sports, but are also associated with falls from heights that occur with gymnastics, cheerleading, and equestrian.
- The most common injury mechanism is a fall on an outstretched arm. Judo is a unique sport in which a competitor may be subjected to an elbow lock by his opponent forcing his elbow into hyperextension, leading to a dislocation if the athlete does not concede defeat.

Medial Ulnar Collateral Ligament

- Symptomatic MCL injuries are most commonly seen in overhead-throwing athletes such as baseball pitchers, and javelin throwers but may be seen in overhead racquet sports such as tennis or in upper extremity dominant sports such as gymnastics (6). The underhand windmill pitch in softball players does not appear to be predisposed to MCL injuries, but other position players in softball can sustain symptomatic MCL injuries. Athletes in sports with less loading and throwing demands may be more tolerant of mild to moderate MCL instability.
- The most common complaint is pain over the medial aspect of the elbow typically felt during late cocking and early acceleration phase of the throwing motion. Throwing velocity and accuracy may also be diminished.
- The onset is usually gradual; however, some athletes are able to identify a single episode of throw where they felt a pop and acute onset of pain. In those cases, most have a prodrome of milder pain complaints.
- Athletes do not usually complain of symptoms of gross elbow instability; however, associated abnormalities such as synovitis, plica, or loose bodies, may present with locking, snapping, or catching symptoms. Classic valgus-extension-overload includes the presentation of both medial elbow pain but also posterior elbow pain as the olecranon impinges in the olecranon fossa.
- Patients may also present with neuritis symptoms of the ulnar nerve with numbness and tingling in the ulnar digits as well as loss of strength in the finger intrinsic muscles. This may occur due to inflammatory changes along the medial side of the elbow or traction of the ulnar nerve within the cubital tunnel.

Lateral Ulnar Collateral Ligament

- Injuries to the LUCL are less common than MCL injuries and are more commonly the result of elbow trauma such as dislocation or fracture-dislocation compared to chronic overuse. The "terrible triad" of radial head fracture, coronoid fracture, and elbow dislocation is commonly associated with lateral ligament instability.
- The most common mechanism of injury is a fall on the outstretched hand.
- Insufficiency of the LUCL is the essential lesion leading to lateral elbow instability.
- Clinicians need to have a high index of suspicion for LCL injuries because the diagnosis of LCL injury is commonly delayed compared to MCL injuries.
- The main complaints of athletes with LCL instability are popping and clicking over the lateral elbow with a sensation of giving way. Push-ups or pushing oneself up from a chair may be painful or bring on symptoms of instability or giving way.
- The LUCL is stressed in activities of daily living (*e.g.*, lifting milk out of the refrigerator or shifting a manual transmission in a car), so unlike an MCL tear, patients will complain of pain and/or instability during normal activities, not just sports (7).

PHYSICAL EXAMINATION

Medial Ulnar Collateral Ligament

- Direct tenderness over the MCL and pain with tension along the MCL are the most common clinical findings. Pain with palpation is 80%–90% sensitive but only 22% specific for MCL tears (4).
- An astute clinician will carefully palpate over the medial epicondyle, flexor-pronator muscle mass, and cubital tunnel to separate out the differential diagnoses of medial epicondyle avulsions in skeletally immature, flexor-pronator muscle strains such as "golfer's elbow," and or ulnar neuritis/cubital tunnel syndrome/instability.
- Tenderness to the posteromedial olecranon may also be associated with valgus extension overload or "pitcher's elbow," which presents as pain in extension. This occurs secondary to repetitive stress of pitching and tension at the MCL.
- An assessment of valgus stability should be performed near full extension to assess bony stability and with slight flexion to assess ligamentous stability. Comparison with the contralateral elbow is helpful and the goal is to assess both the amount of gapping and quality of endpoint. The ability to assess the endpoint is accentuated by asking the patient to lie down and fully externally rotating the shoulder. This technique removes the upper extremity rotation, which allows the examiner to more clearly feel the endpoint (8). Valgus stress test is considered to be 66% sensitive and 60% specific (4).
- The milking maneuver is performed with the ipsilateral elbow locked near the patient's torso with the elbow flexed about 90° while the examiner (or patient) pulls on the ipsilateral thumb creating a valgus load at the elbow. Reproduction of symptoms suggests MCL injury (8).

- The moving valgus stress test is similar to the milking maneuver but includes placing the elbow through a range of motion while the valgus stress is being placed across the elbow. According to O'Driscoll, the test was 100% sensitive and 75% specific (7).

Lateral Ulnar Collateral Ligament

- Pain over the posterior lateral aspect of the elbow is common; however, the key is to palpate instability or recreate the symptoms of instability.
- A useful test in the clinic setting is to gently hold the patient's elbow at 90° while the patient is relaxed in the sitting position. With the examiner's thumb over the radiocapitellar joint, the forearm is passively rotated into full supination. Subtle increased displacement of the radial head represents lateral ligament laxity. This can be compared to the contralateral side. Indeed, accentuating the instability by performing a drawer maneuver of the radial head can help recreate symptoms (8).
- The athlete may also recreate symptoms as they assist themselves to rise from a chair with arm rests by placing both hands on the armrests and then using their arms to rise. If this recreates their symptoms, it is highly suspicious of posterolateral instability of the elbow. Prone push-ups plus seated chair push-ups have been noted to be 87% sensitive as individual tests and 100% sensitive when used in combination (4).
- The lateral pivot shift test can be used for diagnosis. As originally described by O'Driscoll et al. (8), the patient is supine with the shoulder at 90° of flexion with the elbow flexed 90° overhead. The examiner gently supinates the forearm, and a valgus moment is applied. The arm is brought from near extension to flexion. The athlete should have apprehension during the beginning of the test, with further flexion causing a reduction of subluxation and diminution of the apprehension. The test can also be performed from flexion to extension as the elbow moves from reduced to subluxed.
- The lateral pivot shift test is rarely positive in an awake patient unless there is gross instability. Frank palpable subluxation and reduction is rare, unless the patient is under general anesthesia. Under anesthesia, the test is considered to be 100% sensitive compared to only 38% in awake patients (4).

IMAGING STUDIES

- Plain radiographs may reveal associated intra-articular loose bodies, osteophytes, or calcifications associated with chronic MCL or LCL instability (9).
- Comparison views should be obtained in the skeletally immature.
- Point of service ultrasonography can be used to rapidly assess ligamentous injury with a high degree of sensitivity 77% and specificity of 94%. Dynamic stressing can further enhance the sensitivity of diagnostic ultrasonography (10).
- Manual or instrumented radiographic stress views with a valgus or varus force can show a side-to-side difference confirming MCL or LUCL insufficiency. Caution should be taken when assessing asymptomatic patients as subtle side-to-side differences have been noted in elite-level throwers that may simply represent chronic/developmental changes and may not be pathologic (9).
- Computed tomography (CT) carries significant advantages over other imaging modalities when assessing complex elbow fracture dislocations or subtle bony injuries such as coronoid fractures. CT arthrograms are considered 71%–86% sensitive and 91% specific for MCL injuries (4).
- MRI carries significant advantages to evaluate soft-tissue injuries. Nonenhanced MRI scans have been reported to be 57%–79% sensitive and 100% specific for MCL injuries with improved accuracy with MR arthrography up to 97% sensitive and 100% specific. The sensitivity and specificity for lateral injuries has been debated but is certainly less (4).
- It is important to remember that in an active overhead athlete who has been competing for several years, the MRI is almost never "normal," and results should be interpreted in light of the physical examination.

TREATMENT

Elbow Dislocations

- Document the neurovascular examination before and after any interventions.
- Elbow dislocations should be reduced urgently by a clinician comfortable with the procedure.
- Post-reduction x-rays should be obtained to look for associated fractures (coronoid, radial head, olecranon) should be performed.
- Reduction can be accomplished acutely on the sideline or in the emergency room with sedation. After assessing prereduction neurovascular status, any medial-lateral translation should be corrected followed by a gradual movement from extension to flexion with the examiner's thumbs pushing the tip of the olecranon distally into the olecranon fossa. Traction is applied simultaneously along the axis of the forearm to translate the coronoid over the trochlea and gently reduce the joint.
- Once the joint is reduced, it is placed through a gentle range of motion to assess how stable the articulation is. In most simple dislocations, the elbow should be stable from full flexion to extension. This assessment will help guide restrictions in postoperative rehabilitation. Applying a varus or valgus force to test the ligaments is not helpful because they are almost always torn and will show increased laxity, which does not warrant operative treatment.

- If the elbow dislocates as the elbow approaches extension, then options include immobilization at 90° or more for 7–10 days or bracing that prevents full extension.
- Follow-up radiographs should be obtained in several days to confirm continued reduction.
- Early motion is beneficial due to the propensity of the elbow to get stiff.
- Significant bony injuries will likely require surgical interventions.
- For simple dislocations, most patients do NOT require surgical intervention.
- In chronic cases with recurrent instability ligamentous reconstruction may be required.

MCL and LUCL Injuries

- When considering treatment options for ligament injuries about the elbow, the clinician must consider not only anatomic pathology and severity of injury (partial or complete) but also functional demands, specific sport, and what activities reproduce symptoms. For most patients, nonoperative treatment will provide satisfactory return to daily activities.
- Steroid injections should be avoided for fear or weakening ligaments.
- Platelet-rich plasma (PRP) injections have allowed some young athletes to return to play and avoid surgery. Mills et al. demonstrated a 52% return to baseline performance with a combined treatment protocol of PRP, physical therapy, and a rehabilitation program, in a retrospective study of 61 throwing athletes ranging from high school to professional level of play. Success rates were significantly lower in patients with type IV UCL injuries (tear/pathology in more than one location) (11).
- A meta-analysis of return to sport (RTS) after nonoperative management of UCL injury identified an overall rate of 79.7% return to play (RTP) and 77.9% RTLP, with excellent outcomes in lower-grade injuries. RTS rates were significantly higher for proximal tears (12).
- For MCL injuries, the indications for surgery are a failure of a quality rehabilitation regimen and the athlete's desire to return to previous level of activity. The surgical treatment consists of either primary repair or tendon graft augmentation of the MCL (13).
- Primary repair is limited to soft-tissue or bony avulsions from the medial epicondyle or sublime tubercle. Mean RTS rate after repair is estimated to be around 87%, with approximately 95% of patients achieving excellent/good outcomes by the Andrews-Carson Score. This study included patients who underwent repair with suture anchors, direct repair, or repair via drill holes (14).
- A separate case series of nonthrowing athletes by Rothermich et al. demonstrated a 93% RTP rate at a mean of 7.4 months, mean American Shoulder and Elbow Surgeons score of 94, and low complication rates at minimum 2 years follow-up after UCL repair (15).
- Reconstruction techniques can use either allograft or autograph tissue (13). The original MCL reconstruction described by Jobe et al. used bone tunnels with a tendon weave. Newer techniques have worked to optimize the outcomes and limiting complications taking advantage of safer surgical approaches, limiting tunnels, and modernizing fixation devices. In a study of over 900 athletes undergoing UCL reconstruction at minimum 2-year follow-up, 83% returned to previous level of competition or higher, with return to competition at 11.6 months postoperatively (16).
- For LUCL injuries, avoidance of varus stress with use of a splint or brace can be helpful. Range-of-motion exercises in the supine position with the arm overhead allow avoidance of varus stress. In a study by Anakwe et al., after simple elbow dislocation treated conservatively with closed reduction and a short period of immobilization, the most frequent complications included residual pain (62%) and stiffness (56%), as well as 8% reporting residual instability (17). No clinical outcomes studies have been published, to the authors' knowledge, on nonsurgical management of persistent instability associated with LUCL injury.
- For LUCL injuries, indications for surgical reconstruction are pain and dysfunction, either with activities of daily living or secondary to athletic demands. Surgical treatment consists of either repair of the LUCL to the humeral origin or surgical reconstruction of the LUCL with a tendon graft (9). In a systematic review of LUCL reconstruction in 168 patients, 93% regained functional range of motion. However, recurrent instability was a frequent complication (15%) (18).

REFERENCES

1. Pipicelli JG, King GJW. Rehabilitation of elbow instability. *Hand Clin.* 2020;36(4):511–22.
2. Ciccotti MG, Pollack KM, Ciccotti MC, et al. Elbow injuries in professional baseball: epidemiological findings from the Major League Baseball injury surveillance system. *Am J Sports Med.* 2017;45(10):2319–28.
3. Rothermich MA, Conte SA, Aune KT, Fleisig GS, Cain EL Jr, Dugas JR. Incidence of elbow ulnar collateral ligament surgery in collegiate baseball players. *Orthop J Sports Med.* 2018;6(4):2325967118764657.
4. Karbach LE, Elfar J. Elbow instability: anatomy, biomechanics, diagnostic maneuvers, and testing. *J Hand Surg Am.* 2017;42(2):118–26.
5. Ahmed I, Mistry J. The management of acute and chronic elbow instability. *Orthop Clin North Am.* 2015;46(2):271–80.
6. Hariri S, Safran MR. Ulnar collateral ligament injury in the overhead athlete. *Clin Sports Med.* 2010;29(4):619–44.
7. Rodriguez MJ, Kusnezov NA, Dunn JC, Waterman BR, Kilcoyne KG. Functional outcomes following lateral ulnar collateral ligament reconstruction for symptomatic posterolateral rotatory instability of the elbow in an athletic population. *J Shoulder Elbow Surg.* 2018;27(1):112–17.
8. O'Driscoll SW, Lawton RL, Smith AM. The "moving valgus stress test" for medial collateral ligament tears of the elbow. *Am J Sports Med.* 2005;33(2):231–9.

9. Giannicola G, Sacchetti FM, Greco A, Cinotti G, Postacchini F. Management of complex elbow instability. *Musculoskelet Surg.* 2010; 94(suppl):25–36.
10. Sutterer BJ, Boettcher BJ, Payne JM, Camp CL, Sellon JL. The role of ultrasound in the evaluation of elbow medial ulnar collateral ligament injuries in throwing athletes. *Curr Rev Musculoskelet Med.* 2022;15(6):535–46.
11. Mills FB IV, Misra AK, Goyeneche N, Hackel JG, Andrews JR, Joyner PW. Return to play after platelet-rich plasma injection for elbow UCL injury: outcomes based on injury severity. *Orthop J Sports Med.* 2021 Mar 17;9(3):2325967121991135. doi:10.1177/2325967121991135
12. Gopinatth V, Batra AK, Khan ZA, et al. Return to sport after nonoperative management of elbow ulnar collateral ligament injuries: a systematic review and meta-analysis. *Am J Sports Med.* 2023;51(14):3858–69. doi:10.1177/03635465221150507
13. Giannicola G, Calella P, Piccioli A, Scacchi M, Gumina S. Terrible triad of the elbow: is it still a troublesome injury? *Injury.* 2015;46(suppl 8):S68–76.
14. Erickson BJ, Bach BR Jr, Verma NN, Bush-Joseph CA, Romeo AA. Treatment of ulnar collateral ligament tears of the elbow: is repair a viable option? *Orthop J Sports Med.* 2017;5(1):2325967116682211. doi:10.1177/2325967116682211
15. Rothermich MA, Pharr ZK, Mundy AC, et al. Clinical outcomes of ulnar collateral ligament surgery in nonthrowing athletes. *Am J Sports Med.* 2022;50(12):3368–73. doi:10.1177/03635465221120654
16. Cain EL, Andrews JR, Dugas JR, et al. Outcome of ulnar collateral ligament reconstruction of the elbow in 1281 athletes: results in 743 athletes with minimum 2-year follow-up. *Am J Sports Med.* 2010;38(12):2426–34.
17. Anakwe RE, Middleton SD, Jenkins PJ, McQueen MM, Court-Brown CM. Patient-reported outcomes after simple dislocation of the elbow. *J Bone Joint Surg Am.* 2011 Jul 6;93(13):1220–6. doi:10.2106/JBJS.J.00860
18. Badhrinarayanan S, Desai A, Watson JJ, White CHR, Phadnis J. Indications, outcomes, and complications of lateral ulnar collateral ligament reconstruction of the elbow for chronic posterolateral rotatory instability: a systematic review. *Am J Sports Med.* 2021;49(3):830–7.

57 Elbow Articular Lesions and Fractures

Matthew Eads and Benjamin Wilson

INTRODUCTION

- Elbow articular lesions and fractures are common in the athlete. Approximately 7% of all fractures that an athlete will sustain occur in the elbow (1). Because of their prevalence, it is important for the sports physician to become familiar with patterns of injury and treatment options for athletic injuries of the elbow.
- Athletes involved in sports who require throwing (*i.e.*, baseball), upper extremity weight bearing (*i.e.*, gymnastics), or using the upper extremity to brace a fall (*i.e.*, wrestling) are at high risk for sustaining elbow trauma.
- The elbow's high degree of bony congruity, soft-tissue restraints, and high potential for stiffness make the elbow uniquely challenging to treat after athletic injury. A common theme of elbow injuries is that early protected motion is important to minimize stiffness and to nourish the joint. Range of motion (ROM) required for activities of daily living is defined as 30°–130° of flexion/extension and 50° of supination/pronation (2). However, athletic activities often require more motion than this.
- Not only does the athlete have their own considerations, but pediatric and adult elbow fractures differ considerably and will be discussed separately.

PEDIATRIC FRACTURES

Radiographic Evaluation

- Physicians evaluating pediatric elbow fractures must be familiar with normal developmental anatomy. Due to the presence of multiple secondary ossification centers about the elbow, imaging findings that are normal developmentally can be often confused for injuries.
- When obtaining radiographs, it can be helpful to obtain a contralateral comparison view for comparison to differentiate between normal ossification centers and fractures.
- Multiple radiographic relationships have been described to assist in the interpretation of the pediatric elbow radiograph.
  - The proximal radius should point to the capitellum in all views.
  - The long axis of the ulna should line up with or be slightly medial to the long axis of the humerus on a true anteroposterior (AP) view.
  - The anterior humeral line should bisect the capitellum on the lateral view for children older than five, for younger than five it should be within the anterior one third of the capitellum.
  - The humeral-capitellar (Baumann) angle should be within the range of 9°–26° of valgus (3).
- A posterior fat pad sign is always considered to be an abnormal radiographic finding and represents an elbow fracture 76% of the time (4).
- An anterior fat pad sign represents a superficial part of anterior fat pad and should be in front of the coronoid fossa. In normal elbow, the anterior fat pad should be barely visualized. With joint effusion, there will be anterior and superior displacement of anterior fat pad (4).

Ossification Centers of the Elbow

- The secondary ossification centers of the developing elbow reliably appear and close in a predictable order (Fig. 57.1). By knowing what is normal for each age group, one can differentiate between a fracture and a normal radiograph. There are many mnemonics to remember this order such as "you *Can't Resist My Team Of Lawyers*."
  - Capitellum (appears at age 1–2 years)
  - Radial head (appears at age 2–4 years)
  - Medial epicondyle (appears at age 4–6 years)
  - Trochlea (appears at age 8–11 years)
  - Olecranon (appears at age 9–11 years)
  - Lateral epicondyle (appears at age 10–11 years) (3)

Supracondylar Humerus Fractures

- Supracondylar humerus fractures are the most common elbow fracture in the pediatric population and represent 10% of all pediatric fractures.
- Most occur due to a fall on the hand or elbow. Extension pattern is far more common (98%) (3).

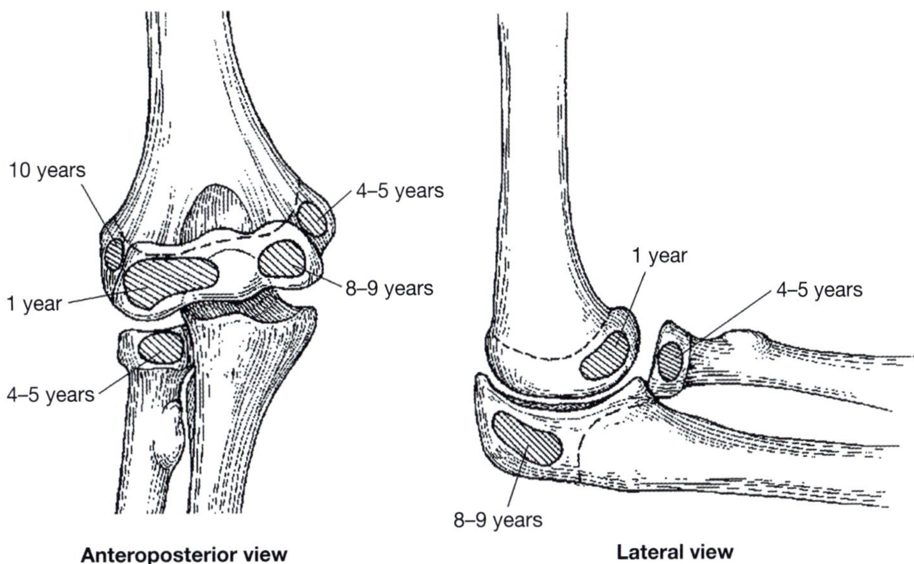

Figure 57.1: Secondary ossification centers of the distal humerus. The average ages for appearance are shown for both males and females. (Reproduced with permission from Skaggs DL. Elbow fractures in children: diagnosis and management. *J Am Acad Orthop Surg*. 1997;5:303–12.)

- Performance of a careful neurovascular examination is crucial. Any of the neurovascular structures crossing the elbow joint may be at risk.
- The pulseless, poorly perfused hand is a true emergency, therefore it is important to rule out vascular injury. Vascular injuries are more commonly associated with posterolateral displacement and higher-grade injuries in which the medial fracture spike may tether the brachial artery.
- One must perform frequent rechecks of the radial pulse to document its presence, as well as its quality. An intimal arterial injury may not be initially apparent but may develop over hours.
- Compartment syndromes must be treated emergently, and a high degree of clinical suspicion for this complication must be maintained, as a missed compartment syndrome may lead to catastrophic results (5). Children pose an increased challenge in assessing compartment syndrome, therefore the three A's are helpful: increased anxiety, agitation, analgesia requirement.
- Nerve injuries may also occur. The anterior interosseous (AI) nerve is the most frequently injured nerve, but most recover spontaneously within 6 months. With posteromedial displacement, the lateral spike of the proximal fragment may tether the radial nerve (6). A simple nerve exam is to have the child perform the following three hand signs that correlate with the motor nerves listed as follows:
  - A-OK — Anterior Interosseous Nerve
  - Thumb's Up — Radial Nerve
  - Crossed Fingers — Ulnar Nerve
- Other concerning clinical signs include the "dimple sign" that occurs when the fracture ends are caught in the brachialis and subcutaneous soft tissues.
- The olecranon and the two epicondyles should form a straight line in the extended position and a triangle when the elbow is flexed to 90°. This relationship is unchanged in a supracondylar fracture but is altered by an elbow dislocation (7).
- Treatment is defined by stability of fracture pattern as defined by Gartland classification.
  - Type I is nondisplaced
  - Type II exhibits anterior gapping, without rotational malalignment, due to an intact posterior hinge.
  - Type III fractures have no cortical continuity and are completely unstable.
- Type I fractures may be treated with immobilization; types II and III require reduction and most require operative intervention to maintain stability while in a 90° position of flexion (7).
- Following reduction, it is crucial to perform a repeat neurovascular examination and again check radiographs.
- Potential long-term sequelae of the supracondylar fracture include the following:

Cubitus varus is the most common complication following supracondylar humerus fracture. It is primarily a cosmetic deformity and does not usually create a loss of function. Earlier, cubitus varus was thought to be created by growth disturbance, but it is now believed to be due to imperfect fracture reduction, especially if medial comminution is present. It is extremely important to have perfect fracture rotation.

Volkmann contracture can be caused by brachial artery injury leading to a severe compartment syndrome, muscle necrosis, and degeneration. This was often a result of maintaining the arm in maximum flexion to maintain a reduction. A closed reduction should be maintained with the arm in 90° of flexion. If more flexion is needed to maintain the reduction, percutaneous pinning should be considered. Treatment options are focused on restoring vascular flow and reducing compartment pressure. It is usually too late to avoid severe morbidity. It is imperative to avoid this complication with proper fracture care and neurovascular monitoring.

Arterial injury occurs in approximately 5% of children with supracondylar fractures. If no pulse is present before and after reduction, emergent surgery is required.

Nerve injuries are usually AI or radial nerve injuries and can be quite common (up to 50% AI injury with type III fractures). Most nerve palsies resulting from supracondylar fractures are neurapraxias and will resolve spontaneously within 3–6 months.

Lateral Condyle Fractures

- Lateral condyle fractures are the second most common type of pediatric elbow fracture, second only to the previously discussed supracondylar humerus fracture.
- These fractures can be intra-articular, and therefore must be considered as potentially unstable.
- An internal oblique radiograph can help show the true amount of displacement and further evaluate the fracture; therefore, it should be obtained in addition to the typical anteroposterior and lateral radiographs.
- Advanced imaging with magnetic resonance imaging (MRI) or computed tomography (CT), or an arthrogram may be needed to appreciate a questionable intra-articular component of fracture.
- If there is less than 2 mm of displacement at the lateral cortex, the fracture may be treated with cast immobilization but must be followed closely with serial radiographs.
- Fracture displacement greater than 2 mm must be surgically reduced and fixed (8,9).
- Even benign-appearing injuries may develop displacement and high complication rates. Potential complications include nonunion, delayed union, and tardy ulnar nerve palsy secondary to progressive cubitus valgus (9).

Medial Epicondyle Fractures

- Medial epicondyle fractures occur later into adolescents than supracondylar or lateral condyle fractures, and are often sport-related injuries.
- Must test for signs of instability, as it is possible that the elbow is dislocated and spontaneously reduced because youths have less inherent stability than adults (10).
- It is very important to evaluate for a fragment entrapped in the joint as this necessitates removal either by closed or operative means.
- Careful neurologic examination at the time of injury must be performed, as the ulnar nerve may be involved (9).
- Even minimally displaced fractures may be well tolerated in the nonathlete (9). However, in the young athlete who is expected to have valgus stress on the elbow (throwers), operative intervention is more likely necessary. Surgical indications include the following (9):
    - Displacement greater than 10 mm may cause loss of strength of the flexor mass and should be fixed.
    - Ulnar neuropathy with displaced fracture
    - Valgus instability, as determined earlier
    - Entrapped fragment in the joint
    - Displaced fracture that blocks joint motion

Olecranon Fracture

- Fractures of the olecranon process occur with other elbow fractures 20% of time.
- Displacement of 5 mm and articular step-off of 2 mm are operative indications.
- Hardware used depends on stability of fracture pattern, with plates used for less-stable injury.
- Treat nonoperatively in 20° of flexion to minimize triceps pull (3).
- Something to consider is an olecranon avulsion fracture, which can be concerning for osteogenesis imperfecta.

Proximal Radius Fracture

- Radial neck fractures are more common in 8- to 12-year-olds.
- Treatment is determined by angulation. Less than 30° of angulation of the neck is accepted. Greater than 30° requires reduction, and greater than 60° may require operative intervention to improve reduction (3).

ADULT ELBOW TRAUMA

Distal Humerus Fractures

- These fractures are rare in the athlete. High energy is required to cause this injury in the young adult population.
- In the general population, these fractures represent one-third of elbow fractures or 2% of all fractures (2).
- All these injuries have a high propensity for stiffness. It is important to maintain a functional ROM for activities of daily living.
- Nonoperative treatment is used only for nondisplaced fractures.
- Operative treatment for displaced articular fractures aims for anatomic reduction and early motion to minimize stiffness.
- Intra-articular distal humerus fractures tend to be extremely complicated to treat operatively, and discussion of operative techniques is beyond the scope of this book.

Capitellar Fracture

- These fractures are rare (<1% of all elbow fractures) (2). They are often associated with radial head fractures.
- Diagnosis may be difficult, and the lateral plain film must be carefully checked. A CT scan may be necessary to better delineate the fracture type.
- Nonoperative treatment is used for nondisplaced fractures.

- There are three basic types of capitellar fractures:
  - Hahn-Steinthal fracture includes a large portion of bone with the capitellar articular surface and usually is able to be primarily reduced and fixed operatively.
  - The Kocher-Lorenz fragment involves a small amount of articular surface of the capitellum only and must often be excised.
  - A third type of fracture is comminuted and is also difficult to fix.
- Early motion is mandatory after these injuries.

Radial Head Fractures

- These fractures are common: 20%–30% of elbow fractures (2).
- Adults tend to sustain radial head fractures, as opposed to neck fractures, which are seen in children.
- May be isolated or associated with elbow dislocation, ulnar shaft fractures, distal radial joint injury (Essex-Lopresti lesion), or carpal fractures, as well as additional fracture patterns.
- Must rule out associated medial collateral ligament (MCL) injury, interosseous membrane injury, and distal radioulnar joint injury.
- Operative indications include displacement greater than 2 mm, mechanical block to motion (pain may be ruled out as cause with intra-articular lidocaine injection), >20%–30% articular depression, or open fracture (11)
- Surgical options depend on fracture type as well as associated lesions and include excision, open reduction internal fixation (ORIF), or hemiarthroplasty.
- The radial head should never be excised with an interosseous ligament or MCL injury.

Olecranon Fracture

- Nondisplaced fractures <2 mm are treated nonoperatively with long arm casting. Care must be taken to avoid prolonged immobilization and stiffness (2).
- Displaced fracture requires ORIF, with technique dependent on fracture pattern stability.
- Although excision of up to 50% of olecranon has been described (6), this should only be used in very low-demand patients and not in the athletic population.

OSTEOCHONDRITIS DISSECANS

- Osteochondritis dissecans (OCD) of the capitellum occurs in adolescent and young adult athletes who are involved in repetitive exercises that load the upper extremity exercise such as: throwers, gymnasts, and weightlifters.
- OCD is a focal disease of the bone that can affect the overlying cartilage and can lead to the development of loose bodies, or osteoarthritis if left untreated.
- Etiology involves repetitive microtrauma in a hypovascular area of bone, but the exact cause is uncertain.
- It is believed to be due to valgus high-stress forces cause during the acceleration phase of throwing, when the capitellum becomes loaded.
- An area of lucency on the capitellum seen on the AP and lateral radiographs are usually sufficient for diagnosis, but early changes can be subtle
- MRI or CT may be helpful to further delineate the extent and stage of lesion (12).
- Symptoms include poorly defined lateral elbow pain, with later stages of disease showing catching and locking.
- Patients should be strictly restricted from throwing for 8–12 weeks or until full, pain-free motion is restored for nondisplaced lesions with intact articular cartilage (11).
- Indications for surgery include partially or completely detached fragments that are painful or cause mechanical symptoms.
- Treatment options are dependent on lesion type and chronicity and include removal and debridement, reattachment, drilling, or osteochondral autograft transfer. Operative techniques continue to evolve (11).
- Osteochondrosis of the capitellum or Panner disease is a similar condition that occurs in children aged 4–8 years and involves the *entire* ossific nucleus. It is self-limiting with conservative treatment (11).

REFERENCES

1. Regan WD. Acute traumatic injuries of the elbow in the athlete. In: Griffin LY, editor. *Orthopaedic Knowledge Update Sports Medicine*. Rosemont (IL): American Academy of Orthopedic Surgeons; 1994. p. 191–204.
2. Scheling GJ. Elbow and forearm: adult trauma. In: Koval KJ, editor. *Orthopaedic Knowledge Update 7*. Rosemont (IL): American Academy of Orthopedic Surgeons; 2002. p. 307–16.
3. Vitale MG, Skaggs DL. Elbow. Pediatric aspects. In: Koval KJ, editor. *Orthopaedic Knowledge Update 7*. Rosemont (IL): American Academy of Orthopedic Surgeons; 2002. p. 299–306.
4. Skaggs DL, Mirzayan R. The posterior fat pad sign in association with occult fracture of the elbow in children. *J Bone Joint Surg Am*. 1999;81(10):1429–33.
5. Shaw BA, Kasser JR, Emans JB, Rand FF. Management of vascular injuries in displaced supracondylar humerus fractures without arteriography. *J Orthop Trauma*. 1990;4(1):25–9.
6. Ippolito E, Caterini R, Scola E. Supracondylar fractures of the humerus in children. Analysis at maturity of fifty-three patients treated conservatively. *J Bone Joint Surg Am*. 1986;68(3):333–44.
7. Harris IE. Supracondylar fractures of the humerus in children. *Orthopedics*. 1992;15(7):811–7.

8. Tejwani N, Phillips D, Goldstein RY. Management of lateral humeral condylar fracture in children. *J Am Acad Orthop Surg.* 2011;19(6):350–8.
9. Wilson NI, Ingram R, Rymaszewski L, Miller JH. Treatment of fractures of the medial epicondyle of the humerus. *Injury.* 1988;19(5):342–4.
10. Fowles JV, Slimane N, Kassab MT. Elbow dislocation with avulsion of the medial humeral epicondyle. *J Bone Joint Surg Br.* 1990;72(1):102–4.
11. Schenck RC Jr, Goodnight JM. Osteochondritis dissecans. *J Bone Joint Surg Am.* 1996;78(3):439–56.
12. Chen FS, Diaz VA, Loebenberg M, Rosen JE. Shoulder and elbow injuries in the skeletally immature athlete. *J Am Acad Orthop Surg.* 2005;13(3):172–85.

Elbow Tendinopathies

58

David Savin and Patrick St. Pierre

INTRODUCTION

- Elbow tendinosis is a result of tendon overuse and a failure of tendon healing.
- Elbow tendinosis can affect the elbow laterally (extensor carpi radialis brevis [ECRB], extensor digitorum communis), medially (pronator teres, flexor carpi radialis), or posteriorly (triceps) (1,2).
- Medial epicondylitis often referred to as golfer's elbow, lateral epicondylitis often referred to as tennis elbow. Both conditions can occur with either etiology.
- Incidence in the working population varies between 0.9 and 4.9 per 100 worker years (3).
- General population incidence is around 3.3–3.5 per 1000 (4).

SYMPTOMS/SIGNS

- Initial symptoms are activity-related pain followed by pain at rest as the condition becomes more chronic.
- Repetitive activities, such as golf, tennis, pickleball, and typing are often the inciting activities for this condition.
- Some loss of extension is common in medial elbow tendinosis, but often the patients maintain full range of motion.
- Tenderness is common over the extensor mass or flexor pronator mass origins.
- Pain is increased over the medial or lateral elbow with provocative examination maneuvers. For lateral epicondylitis this includes wrist and middle finger extension, and gripping. For medial epicondylitis this includes wrist and middle finger flexion, resisted pronation, and finger press to cheeks (1,5).
- Because medial and lateral affected tendon units cross the elbow joint, pain is more severe with provocative testing with the elbow in extension. Therefore, pain with provocative testing with the elbow flexed indicates severer involvement.
- Functional strength loss is common.
- Over 80% of patients will have resolution of symptoms by 6 months. Often self-limiting but early treatment can improve symptoms and shorten the duration of pain (4).
- For those who have pain >6 months, median duration of pain is >2 years (4).

HISTOPATHOLOGY

- Histology of surgically resected tissue fails to reveal inflammatory cells. Thus, the term "tendinosis" is preferable to "tendonitis."
- The epicondyle (bone) itself is not affected in the disease process. Therefore, epicondylitis is a misnomer. However, a bony exostosis may be noted as a companion problem in 20% of lateral elbow tendinosis cases.
- Chronic injury to the tendon leads to tendon disrepair thus creating disorganized collagen (3).
- Pathologic tendinosis shows disruption of normal collagen matrix by the characteristic invasion of fibroblasts and vascular granulation tissue termed "angiofibroblastic proliferation" or angiofibroblastic hyperplasia (6).

DIFFERENTIAL DIAGNOSIS/ ASSOCIATED LESIONS

- Lateral tendinosis can be confused with the rare entity of posterior interosseous nerve (PIN) entrapment, also termed radial tunnel, which would cause diffuse pain along the radial nerve in the extensor mass of the proximal forearm, approximately 3–5 cm distal to lateral epicondyle. Pain will be reproduced with resisted forearm supination in extension that is reduced in flexion. Electrodiagnostic studies are usually inconclusive and a diagnostic injection with a positive wrist drop with reduction of pain can confirm diagnosis (7,8).
- Lateral tendinosis can be seen in combination or association with intra-articular abnormalities, such as synovitis, plica, chondromalacia, and osteochondritis dissecans (OCD) (3).
- Posterior lateral rotatory instability (PLRI) can also be seen with severe lateral epicondylitis, repeated cortisone injections, or trauma. Exam findings include pain and subtle subluxation of the radial head with testing for PLRI including extension, supination, and varus loading (9).
- Medial elbow–associated abnormalities may include degeneration/rupture of medial collateral ligament, entrapment of the ulnar nerve, and congenital or traumatic subluxation of the ulnar nerve (1,8).

- Posterior elbow–associated abnormalities may include extra-articular olecranon bursitis and intra-articular olecranon fossa issues (synovitis, chondromalacia, and loose fragments).
- The mesenchymal syndrome, coined by Nirschl, has been used to describe a subset of patients with apparent decreased tissue durability who present with multiple affected areas. These are often bilateral, including rotator syndrome or tear, medial and lateral elbow tendinosis, carpal tunnel syndrome, trigger finger, de Quervain disease, plantar fasciitis, Achilles insertional tendinosis, and hip trochanteric bursitis (6).

TREATMENT CONCEPTS

- Anti-inflammatory medications can be helpful in controlling pain and can be a first-line therapy, allowing patients to comfortably proceed with curative rehabilitative exercises (3).
- Promotion of a tendon-healing response (neovascularization and fibroblastic infiltration with collagen deposition and maturation) can be accomplished by:
  - Rehabilitative exercise
  - High-voltage electrical stimulation
  - General conditioning/aerobic conditioning, which provides increased regional blood perfusion and minimization of loss of strength of adjacent tissue
  - Rest from inciting trauma, do not push through pain
- Eccentric exercises have been shown to be useful in the rehabilitative exercise program with either medial or lateral disease. A recent review suggests eccentric loading can significantly reduce pain scores when compared to other exercise regimens (10). Eccentric exercises for other tendinopathies have been effective as well and should be included in the first course of treatment for tendinopathy around the elbow (10).
- Cortisone injections, when done under the origin of the ECRB or flexor-pronator mass, can also be effective in acutely relieving pain. However, cortisone injections have risks and some studies suggest worse clinical outcomes and tissue degradation (11). Multiple injections can significantly affect tendon quality and may lead to failure of surgical treatment (12).
- Physical modalities such as high-voltage electrical stimulation, ultrasound, heat/cold, and dexamethasone iontophoresis also are useful in relieving pain (13).
- Control of force loads
  - Counterforce strap bracing to constrain key muscle groups while maintaining muscle balance (14)
  - Improved sports technique, such as improved backhand stroke in tennis (lateral tendinosis) and less trailing arm activity in the golf swing (medial tendinosis)
  - Equipment changes in sports, such as low string tension on tennis racquets and perimeter weighting in golf clubs

BIOLOGIC TREATMENTS

- Platelet rich plasma (PRP) has become a popular option for management of epicondylitis. In comparison to CSI, PRP shows more favorable long-term results (15).
- Autologous blood injection (ABI) and platelet-rich plasma (PRP) have been increasingly used and studied over the past 10 years (16–19). Using ABI and PRP has been shown to demonstrate effectiveness in several studies, with PRP having better results than ABI in one study (16,19).
- Studies suggest leukocyte-rich PRP may be superior to leukocyte poor PRP (20).
- Dry needling is an effective treatment and may be a viable treatment option when PRP is not available (21).
- Although multiple studies support its use due to statistically significant improvements in pain and function, there is a lack of heterogeneity in clinical studies and further research is needed (22,23).

INDICATIONS FOR SURGERY

- Chronic symptoms usually of at least 6 months and often exceeding 1 year in duration (1–3,6).
- Failure of response to a good-quality rehabilitation program.
- Resolution of pain with diagnostic injection.
- Unacceptable quality of life as determined by the patient.

Surgical Principles

- Historically, elbow tendinosis was treated by the total release of the origin of the combined tendon groups from the epicondyle.
- Currently, surgical treatment is directed at resecting only the pathologic tissue and protecting or repairing all normal tissues and attachments, followed by quality postoperative rehabilitation.
- Surgical goals can be accomplished through a small incision (≤3 cm).
- Associated lesions including OCD, loose bodies, and synovitis, can be addressed with a mini-arthrotomy at the time of the tendinosis resection (24).
- Arthroscopic treatment of lateral elbow tendinosis has been shown to be very effective, with satisfactory results of over 90% in several studies (25–27). Associated intra-articular lesions can also be managed arthroscopically (27). For skilled elbow arthroscopists, this is an effective treatment; although the mini-open technique is recommended for most surgeons.
- Ulnar nerve entrapment is associated with medial elbow tendinosis and should be evaluated by exam and possible nerve conduction study (7).

TREATMENT RESULTS

- The vast majority of patients with elbow tendinosis respond to nonoperative intervention (3).
- Of those who do require surgery, up to 97% will experience significant or total pain relief and return of strength with minimal complications (2,25,27).

REFERENCES

1. Nirschl RP. Elbow tendinosis/tennis elbow. *Clin Sports Med*. 1992; 11(4):851–70.
2. Nirschl RP, Ashman ES. Tennis elbow tendinosis (epicondylitis). *Instr Course Lect*. 2004;53:587–98.
3. Keijsers R, de Vos RJ, Kuijer PPF, van den Bekerom MP, van der Woude HJ, Eygendaal D. Tennis elbow. *Shoulder Elbow*. 2019;11(5):384–92. doi:10.1177/1758573218797973
4. Sanders TL, Maradit Kremers H, Bryan AJ, Ransom JE, Smith J, Morrey BF. The epidemiology and health care burden of tennis elbow: a population-based study. *Am J Sports Med*. 2015;43(5):1066–71. doi:10.1177/0363546514568087
5. Amin NH, Kumar NS, Schickendantz MS. Medial epicondylitis: evaluation and management. *J Am Acad Orthop Surg*. 2015;23(6):348–55. doi:10.5435/JAAOS-D-14-00145
6. Nirschl RP, Pettrone FA. Tennis elbow. The surgical treatment of lateral epicondylitis. *J Bone Joint Surg Am*. 1979;61(6A):832–9.
7. Lubahn JD, Cermak MB. Uncommon nerve compression syndromes of the upper extremity. *J Am Acad Orthop Surg*. 1998;6(6):378–86. doi:10.5435/00124635-199811000-00006
8. Strohl AB, Zelouf DS. Ulnar tunnel syndrome, radial tunnel syndrome, anterior interosseous nerve syndrome, and pronator syndrome. *J Am Acad Orthop Surg*. 2017;25(1):e1–10. doi:10.5435/JAAOS-D-16-00010
9. Kholinne E, Liu H, Kim H, Kwak JM, Koh KH, Jeon IH. Systematic review of elbow instability in association with refractory lateral epicondylitis: myth or fact? *Am J Sports Med*. 2021;49(9):2542–50. doi:10.1177/0363546520980133
10. Yoon SY, Kim YW, Shin IS, Kang S, Moon HI, Lee SC. The beneficial effects of eccentric exercise in the management of lateral elbow tendinopathy: a systematic review and meta-analysis. *J Clin Med*. 2021;10(17):3968. doi:10.3390/jcm10173968
11. Coombes BK, Bisset L, Brooks P, Khan A, Vicenzino B. Effect of corticosteroid injection, physiotherapy, or both on clinical outcomes in patients with unilateral lateral epicondylalgia: a randomized controlled trial. *JAMA*. 2013;309(5):461–9. doi:10.1001/jama.2013.129
12. Dean BJF, Lostis E, Oakley T, Rombach I, Morrey ME, Carr AJ. The risks and benefits of glucocorticoid treatment for tendinopathy: a systematic review of the effects of local glucocorticoid on tendon. *Semin Arthritis Rheum*. 2014;43(4):570–6. doi:10.1016/j.semarthrit.2013.08.006
13. Nirschl RP, Rodin DM, Ochiai DH, Maartmann-Moe C, DEX-AHE-01-99 Study Group. Iontophoretic administration of dexamethasone sodium phosphate for acute epicondylitis. A randomized, double-blinded, placebo-controlled study. *Am J Sports Med*. 2003; 31(2):189–95. doi:10.1177/03635465030310020601
14. Kroslak M, Pirapakaran K, Murrell GAC. Counterforce bracing of lateral epicondylitis: a prospective, randomized, double-blinded, placebo-controlled clinical trial. *J Shoulder Elbow Surg*. 2019;28(2):288–95. doi:10.1016/j.jse.2018.10.002
15. Li A, Wang H, Yu Z, et al. Platelet-rich plasma vs corticosteroids for elbow epicondylitis: a systematic review and meta-analysis. *Medicine (Baltimore)*. 2019;98(51):e18358. doi:10.1097/MD.0000000000018358
16. Creaney L, Wallace A, Curtis M, Connell D. Growth factor-based therapies provide additional benefit beyond physical therapy in resistant elbow tendinopathy: a prospective, single-blind, randomised trial of autologous blood injections versus platelet-rich plasma injections. *Br J Sports Med*. 2011;45(12):966–71. doi:10.1136/bjsm.2010.082503
17. Edwards SG, Calandruccio JH. Autologous blood injections for refractory lateral epicondylitis. *J Hand Surg Am*. 2003;28(2):272–8. doi:10.1053/jhsu.2003.50041
18. Peerbooms JC, Sluimer J, Bruijn DJ, Gosens T. Positive effect of an autologous platelet concentrate in lateral epicondylitis in a double-blind randomized controlled trial: platelet-rich plasma versus corticosteroid injection with a 1-year follow-up. *Am J Sports Med*. 2010;38(2):255–62. doi:10.1177/0363546509355445
19. Thanasas C, Papadimitriou G, Charalambidis C, Paraskevopoulos I, Papanikolaou A. Platelet-rich plasma versus autologous whole blood for the treatment of chronic lateral elbow epicondylitis: a randomized controlled clinical trial. *Am J Sports Med*. 2011;39(10):2130–4. doi:10.1177/0363546511417113
20. Shim JW, Lee JS, Park YB, Cho HC, Jung HS. The effect of leucocyte concentration of platelet-rich plasma on outcomes in patients with lateral epicondylitis: a systematic review and meta-analysis. *J Shoulder Elbow Surg*. 2022;31(3):634–45. doi:10.1016/j.jse.2021.10.036
21. Uygur E, Aktaş B, Yilmazoglu EG. The use of dry needling vs. corticosteroid injection to treat lateral epicondylitis: a prospective, randomized, controlled study. *J Shoulder Elbow Surg*. 2021;30(1):134–9. doi:10.1016/j.jse.2020.08.044
22. Chen XT, Fang W, Jones IA, Heckmann ND, Park C, Vangsness CT. The efficacy of platelet-rich plasma for improving pain and function in lateral epicondylitis: a systematic review and meta-analysis with risk-of-bias assessment. *Arthroscopy*. 2021;37(9):2937–52. doi:10.1016/j.arthro.2021.04.061
23. Wong JRY, Toth E, Rajesparan K, Rashid A. The use of platelet-rich plasma therapy in treating tennis elbow: a critical review of randomised control trials. *J Clin Orthop Trauma*. 2022;32:101965. doi:10.1016/j.jcot.2022.101965
24. Kraushaar BS, Nirschl RP, Cox W. A modified lateral approach for release of posttraumatic elbow flexion contracture. *J Shoulder Elbow Surg*. 1999;8(5):476–80. doi:10.1016/s1058-2746(99)90080-0
25. Lattermann C, Romeo AA, Anbari A, et al. Arthroscopic debridement of the extensor carpi radialis brevis for recalcitrant lateral epicondylitis. *J Shoulder Elbow Surg*. 2010;19(5):651–6. doi:10.1016/j.jse.2010.02.008
26. Owens BD, Murphy KP, Kuklo TR. Arthroscopic release for lateral epicondylitis. *Arthroscopy*. 2001;17(6):582–7. doi:10.1053/jars.2001.20098
27. Savoie FH, VanSice W, O'Brien MJ. Arthroscopic tennis elbow release. *J Shoulder Elbow Surg*. 2010;19(2 suppl):31–6. doi:10.1016/j.jse.2009.12.016

59 Soft-Tissue Injuries of the Wrist and Hand

Denver Kraft, Curtis Henn, and Landon Mueller

INTRODUCTION

- Injuries to the wrist and hand are common in all sports. In the past, soft-tissue injuries were frequently designated as "sprains." However, the "waste basket" terms *wrist sprain* and *jammed finger* have been refined with specific diagnoses and defined treatment plans. An understanding of wrist and hand anatomy, biomechanics, and function allows the physician to identify specific pathology and treatment, allowing quicker return to sport for the athlete with a wrist or hand injury. Missed, misdiagnosed, and under-treated injuries can result in permanent deformity and loss of function. Radiographs are indicated in nearly all cases to evaluate for fracture, dislocation, and joint incongruity.

EPIDEMIOLOGY

- The incidence of injuries to the wrist varies according to sport. In the general population, 47% of sports injuries occur in the hand or wrist; of these, 22% are soft-tissue injuries (1). Hand and wrist injuries occur more frequently in younger athletes than adults. A study performed at the Cleveland clinic found that 9% of all athletic participants under the age of 16 sustained injuries involving the wrist (2). In another study, 35% of all injuries in adolescent football players involved the wrist(3). Joint hypermobility and ligamentous laxity can lead to partial or complete ligament tears following a loading of the wrist or may predispose athletes to repetitive stress injury. Overuse syndromes of the wrist are also common in athletes as a result of tension failure or shear stresses (4).

We thank D. Nicole Deal and A. Bobby Chhabra for their contribution on this chapter, as authors of the chapter in the previous edition.

DORSAL WRIST SYNDROMES

- Chronic wrist pain on the dorsal aspect of the wrist can be a result of dorsal ganglion cysts, dorsal impaction/dorsal impingement syndromes, dorsal carpal capsulitis, or distal posterior interosseous nerve syndrome (5).
- Ganglion cysts are the most common soft-tissue masses of the wrist. About 60%–70% originate from the dorsal scapholunate ligament and are extra-articular connections to the scapholunate joint. A history of wrist trauma is present in 15% of patients with a dorsal ganglion (6). Although larger cysts are easily diagnosed with palpation of a firm, mobile mass that transilluminates, an occult dorsal ganglion is difficult to be detected on clinical examination and may only be palpable with extreme flexion (6). Patients with occult ganglion cysts present with pain with weight-bearing on the extended wrist, localized tenderness, limitation of motion, and/or grip weakness.
- Ultrasound and magnetic resonance imaging (MRI) are equally effective in detecting occult cysts (7). Initial treatment should include anti-inflammatory medications, aspiration with or without steroid injections, and at least 6 weeks of immobilization with a forearm-based palmar wrist support splint (8). When conservative treatment has failed to relieve the symptoms, excision of the capsule and ganglion from the scapholunate ligament is performed. Results are generally favorable, with return to full activities in most cases.
- Dorsal impaction syndromes occur from repetitive loading of the wrist in maximum extension, as frequently seen in weightlifters and gymnasts. The shear forces from loading can lead to localized synovitis or osteocartilaginous fractures (9). The athlete will often complain of pain and point tenderness on the middorsal aspect of the wrist, particularly with extension, at the projection of the capitolunate joint or over the dorsal scaphoid (10). Radiographic changes may be seen with disease progression, including development of a hypertrophic ridge on the dorsal rim of the scaphoid or the dorsal border of the lunate as a result of impingement with the capitate during hyperextension. Treatment includes restriction of

wrist hyperextension, strengthening of the wrist flexors, local steroid injection, and cessation from sport for 4–6 weeks. If symptoms persist, the patient may either abandon the activity or undergo surgical treatment with limited synovectomy and cheilectomy of hypertrophic margins that impinge during hyperextension.

- Distal posterior interosseous nerve (PIN) syndrome results from repetitive hyperextension. On examination, the patient will be tender over the fourth extensor compartment, where the PIN resides, and the pain is reproduced with hyperextension. Treatment begins with anti-inflammatories and rest, with PIN exploration, neurolysis, and often excision, indicated in refractory cases (11).

CARPAL INSTABILITY

- Carpal instability may be seen in contact athletes following a traumatic injury or noncontact athletes as a result of repetitive loading of the hand and wrist. Carpal instability includes a wide spectrum of injury and dysfunction. Injury to the scapholunate interosseous ligament is the most common cause of carpal instability. Initial presentation may demonstrate minimal changes and little functional deficit, but can progress to dynamic instability, then static instability, and ultimately to scapholunate advanced collapse (SLAC) (12). Dynamic instability is only apparent on stress radiographs obtained with pronated clenched fist views. Static instability can be seen on routine radiographs with widening of the scapholunate interval (13) (Fig. 59.1). This instability will progress to radiocarpal arthritis and can lead to pancarpal collapse if not diagnosed and treated (14).

Scapholunate Dissociation

- Scapholunate instability occurs with injury to the scapholunate ligament, which allows the scaphoid to settle into flexion, the lunate into extension, and increased space between these two bones (15). The mechanism is most commonly a sudden impact force with the wrist in extension, ulnar deviation, and carpal supination.
- The carpal instability associated with this injury is a dorsal intercalated segmental instability (DISI) deformity. This can be reproduced clinically during physical examination by performing the Watson shift test, which is positive for scapholunate instability when there is a clunk or pain as the wrist moves from ulnar to radial deviation while pressure is applied to the palmar aspect of the scaphoid tubercle.
- Radiographs may show widening of the scapholunate interval (compared to the uninjured wrist, normally less than 2 mm), an increase in the scapholunate angle (>70°; normal, 30°–60°), and a cortical *ring* sign in which the distal pole of the perpendicular scaphoid is seen end-on on the anteroposterior view of the wrist (14).
- Treatment consists of anti-inflammatory medications, splinting, and possible steroid injections in mild cases of ligament strain without radiographic changes. If widening is noted on radiographs, treatment may consist of closed reduction and percutaneous pinning if initiated within the first 3–4 weeks after injury. In most cases, open reduction, ligamentous repair or reconstruction, and internal fixation with Kirschner wires

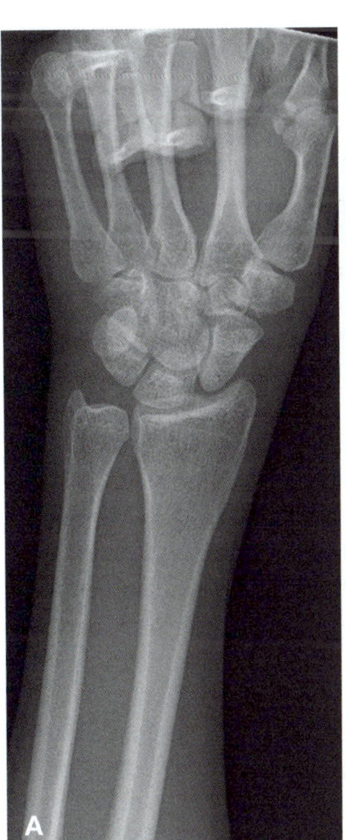

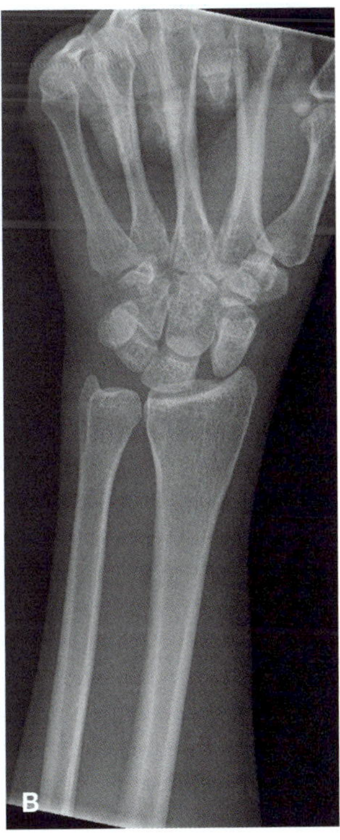

Figure 59.1: PA (A) and PA clenched fist (B) radiographs, demonstrating dynamic scapholunate widening.

is required. For chronic scapholunate dissociation without arthritic changes, a dorsal capsulodesis and ligament reconstruction may be performed (16,17). If ligament reconstruction is not possible, a scaphotrapezial-trapezoidal fusion may be used to correct scaphoid flexion and attempt to prevent radioscaphoid arthritis (18). Prompt identification and referral of these injuries is necessary, as early intervention yields the best return to play. Return to play is significantly limited if salvage procedures (*i.e.*, fusion procedures) are needed (19).

Lunotriquetral Instability

- Injuries to the lunotriquetral ligaments range from sprain to partial tear to complete tear with or without carpal malalignment. The associated carpal instability is a volar intercalated segmental instability (VISI) deformity. A complete tear rarely occurs in athletes.
- Symptoms consist of pain on the dorso-ulnar side of the carpus with a positive lunotriquetral ballottement test (20). Injection of local anesthetic to the lunotriquetral joint usually relieves symptoms and restores grip strength.
- Routine radiographic evaluation may show static instability by volar flexion of the lunate on the lateral radiograph. MRI may demonstrate incomplete or complete tears of the lunotriquetral ligaments. MRI may also detect simultaneous injury to the triangular fibrocartilage, particularly in an ulnar positive patient where the ulna abuts the triquetrum.
- Treatment of acute or chronic injuries with no evidence of a tear consists of injection of a corticosteroid preparation followed by immobilization. If pain is disabling and the patient does not want to cease the pain-provoking activity or sport, surgical repair of the ligament may be possible. Arthroscopy is used to confirm the diagnosis and assist in reduction and pinning of the lunotriquetral joint in the absence of advanced collapse and arthritis (21). In patients with an ulnar positive variance, ulna shortening with ligament debridement may be necessary. Lunotriquetral arthrodesis may be used in chronic cases of instability but is rarely performed in athletes hoping to return to full activity (21).

ULNAR TRANSLOCATION

- Ulnar translocation is an extremely rare injury that is usually a result of a severe violent impact, as may be seen in motor sports. For complete translocation of the carpus to occur, complete disruption of both the volar and dorsal radiocarpal ligaments must occur. The mechanism is typically hyperextension, pronation, and ulnar deviation on a fixed hand (22). As a result, the carpus is free to translate ulnarly along the incline of the radius. Physical examination includes severe swelling, loss of motion, and deformity. Radiographic evaluation will demonstrate carpal translation, rotation of the proximal carpal row into palmar flexion, and scapholunate diastasis due to ulnar displacement of the lunate.
- This is a highly unstable injury and surgery is required in all cases. Radiolunate arthrodesis may be required to maintain reduction that can result in a stable, pain-free wrist with preservation of some motion through the midcarpal joint. Return to strenuous activity is possible if full wrist range of motion is not mandatory (14).

TRIANGULAR FIBROCARTILAGE COMPLEX INJURY

- The triangular fibrocartilage complex (TFCC) is made up of the triangular fibrocartilage, a cartilaginous disc that lies on the ulnar head and several supporting ligaments and acts as a stabilizer of the distal radioulnar joint (DRUJ). Injury to this structure may result in perforation of the disc (traumatic or degenerative) or avulsion (traumatic) of the disc with or without avulsion of the supporting ligaments. Avulsion of the TFCC occurs following acute dislocation or subluxation of the distal ulna at the DRUJ. Degenerative tears usually occur after the third decade (23). Ulnar variance may play a role in degenerative changes of the TFCC, with increased risk in ulnar positive patients (24). Young athletes who are ulnar positive and participate in repetitive loading of the wrist are susceptible to degenerative changes of the TFC similar to older patients (10). Lunotriquetral tears may occur following degenerative perforation of the TFCC leading to carpal instability.
- Patients with injury to the TFCC frequently complain of ulnar-sided wrist pain exacerbated by forearm rotation. It is important to discern injury to TFCC from injury to the DRUJ. TFCC injury is suspected when tenderness is present between the ulna and triquetrum. Relief of pain during manual stabilization of the DRUJ during forearm rotation may indicate DRUJ instability. Diagnostic evaluation includes plain radiographs to evaluate for ulnar variance, MRI to evaluate for ulnolunate "kissing" lesions, arthrography to evaluate for communication between the radiocarpal joint and the DRUJ, and/or arthroscopy. An injection into the ulnocarpal space with steroid may be helpful diagnostically and therapeutically.
- Treatment of acute injury of the TFCC starts with immobilization of the wrist in neutral rotation for 4–6 weeks. Gradual progression of activities may begin with supportive splinting. If the athlete is unable to return to sport and symptoms persist, a steroid injection into the ulnocarpal joint may be performed. If symptoms recur or persist following the injection, surgical debridement and/or repair of the TFCC should be performed (25). If the patient has ulnar positive variance contributing to the TFCC pathology, then ulnar shortening (26) osteotomy or distal ulnar wafer procedure may be performed at the time of TFCC surgery. If advanced DRUJ arthritis has developed DRUJ excisional hemiarthroplasty (27), or the Kapandji procedure (28) may be required. If a peripheral tear in the outer 15%–20% of the TFCC is present,

repair may be needed. For patients with ulnar negative variance, debridement of the TFCC defect may relieve pain and will not increase load transmission if only the central third is removed. For acute avulsions of the TFCC causing DRUJ instability, immobilization of both the wrist and elbow with the DRUJ reduced is usually successful. If instability persists, reattachment of the TFCC is performed, usually at the fovea of the ulnar styloid using suture and drill holes (29).

FINGERTIP INJURIES

- Fingertip injuries are the most common hand injuries seen in the emergency department, and are frequently encountered in athletes. Most injuries require a digital block prior to thorough evaluation and treatment.

Subungual Hematoma

- Crush injuries to the fingertips often damage the nail and underlying matrix, leading to a hematoma beneath the nail and throbbing pain. These injuries may be associated with tuft fractures of the distal phalanx, which can be open fractures if they disrupt the nail matrix (30).
- Hematoma involving less than 50% of the nail matrix may be drained for pain control. An 18-gauge needle or cautery may be used to create one or multiple holes in the nail. Soaking the finger in sterile water with peroxide will facilitate drainage. A sterile dressing should then be applied, with a stack splint in cases involving fracture.
- Hematoma involving more than 50% of the underlying nail bed may be treated by surgical removal of the nail, thorough irrigation and debridement of the wound, repair of the nail matrix, and replacement of the nail with splinting (30). The nail bed may be repaired with either absorbable suture or 2-Octyl cyanoacrylate (31).

Nail Avulsion

- If nail avulsion occurs without damage to the underlying sterile matrix, the wound should be thoroughly cleansed and dressed with a nonadherent dressing. If the proximal portion of the nail has also been avulsed from the nail fold and germinal matrix, the patient's cleansed nail or a piece of sterile gauze or foil may be slid under the eponychial fold to prevent adherence (30).
- If any part of the sterile or germinal matrix has been torn or lacerated, removal of any remaining nail fragments, and repair of the nail bed injury are required with the eponychial fold splinted open (30).

Finger Pulp Injuries

- Simple lacerations may be cleansed and sutured using nonabsorbable monofilament in adults or absorbable suture in children. Grossly contaminated wounds may be cleansed and left open.
- Partial amputations with soft-tissue loss measuring less than 1 cm will heal by secondary intention and may be treated with cleansing and serial dressing changes, and even larger defects will heal well in children (6). Larger wounds involving exposed bone or tendon, nail bed injury, or more proximal amputation should be cleansed and a nonadherent sterile dressing applied. Depending on the degree of injury, emergency department referral and/or operative treatment by a hand surgeon may be required (30).

JOINT INJURIES OF THE FINGERS

- Dislocations are characterized by pain, limited movement, and digit deformity and should be radiographed (ideally pre- and post-reduction) to assess for associated fracture. Dislocations should be reduced and splinted expeditiously. Any irreducible dislocation or dislocation associated with an open wound requires evaluation by a hand surgeon (32).

Distal Interphalangeal Joint

- Distal interphalangeal (DIP) joint dislocations are uncommon, almost always dorsal, and often open. These injuries are frequently associated with tendon disruption or interposition (see sections on mallet and jersey finger).
- After closed reduction, stability may be assessed. Most injuries are immediately stable and thus require only a few days of splinting to control swelling followed by early range of motion.

Proximal Interphalangeal Joint

- Proximal interphalangeal (PIP) joint injuries are the most common joint injuries in sports, primarily occurring in athletes who participate in contact sports and ball handling (33,34).

DORSAL DISLOCATIONS

- Dorsal PIP dislocations are frequently seen in football and basketball. Hyperextension with axial load leads to this injury pattern with distal volar plate rupture with or without bony avulsion. A true lateral x-ray should be obtained to rule out a fracture (34).
- Reduction should be performed acutely. Dynamic and static stability should be assessed after reduction, including collateral ligament stability (34).
- If there is no associated fracture and the joint is stable, splinting should be limited to a few days followed by buddy taping for sports for 4–6 weeks. Recurrent dislocation is rare, but stiffness is frequent and can be permanent. Swelling and

tenderness can persist for several months. Motion exercises as soon as comfort permits are critical to minimize stiffness (34).

VOLAR DISLOCATIONS

- Volar dislocations of the PIP joint are less common, more difficult to reduce, and associated with more complications than their dorsal counterparts. They are caused by axial load and rotation with PIP joint flexion and may be associated with extensor tendon central slip avulsion, volar plate disruption, or collateral ligament tears (34).
- If closed reduction is successful, the PIP joint should be splinted in full extension for 3–4 weeks if a central slip disruption is detected. Early range of motion may also be attempted if the central slip is felt to be intact. If a boutonniere deformity develops, then one must assume the central slip is disrupted and full-time extension splinting of the PIP initiated. The DIP joint should remain free; an active and passive DIP flexion should be encouraged. Night splinting for an additional 3–4 weeks then follows. If closed reduction is not possible, urgent open reduction and pinning are necessary (34). Patients should be warned of the possibility of late boutonnière deformity development.

ROTARY PROXIMAL INTERPHALANGEAL JOINT SUBLUXATION

- Rotatory PIP subluxation typically presents as an irreducible dislocation of the PIP joint with buttonholing of 1 condyle of the proximal phalanx through a longitudinal rent in the extensor hood between the central slip and the lateral band. A lateral radiograph will show a lateral profile of the proximal phalanx with an oblique profile of the middle phalanx (34), but radiographs may also show only subtle persistent PIP subluxation (Fig. 59.2).

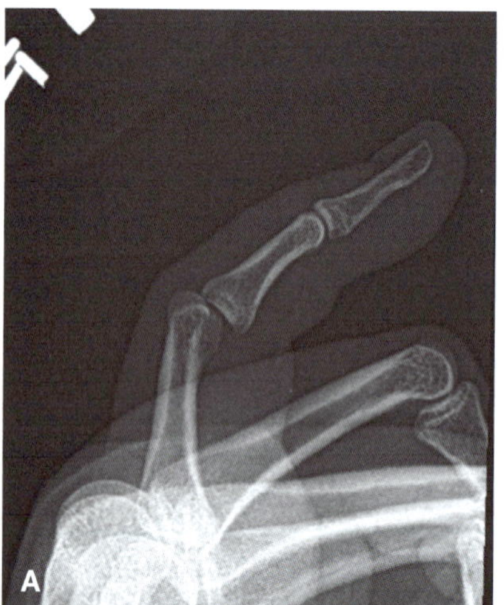

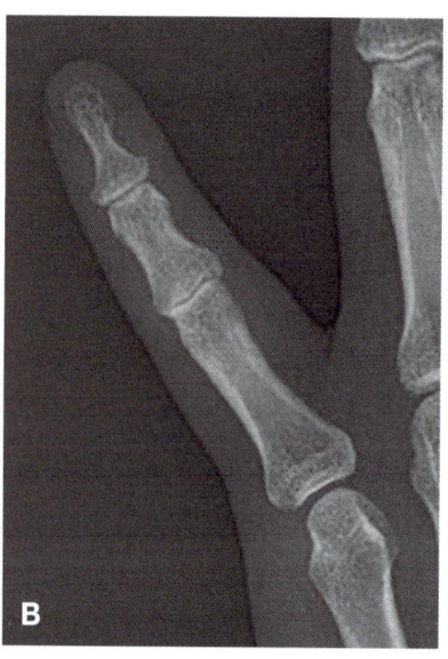

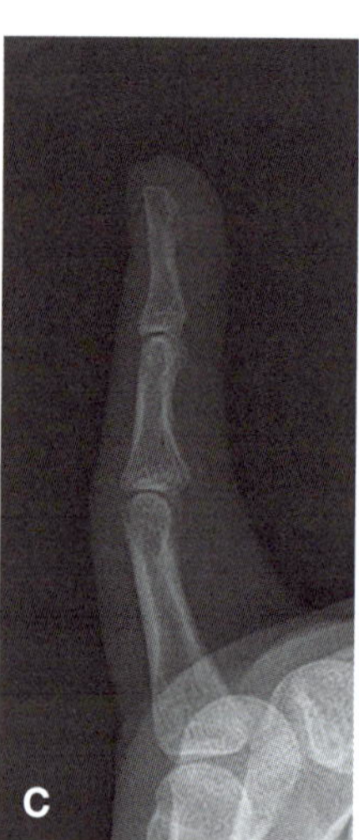

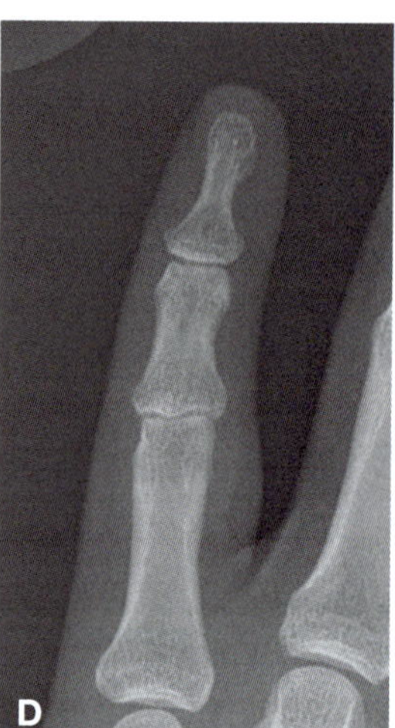

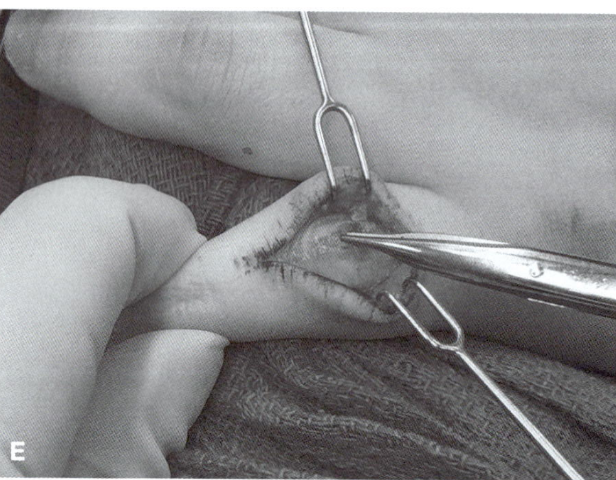

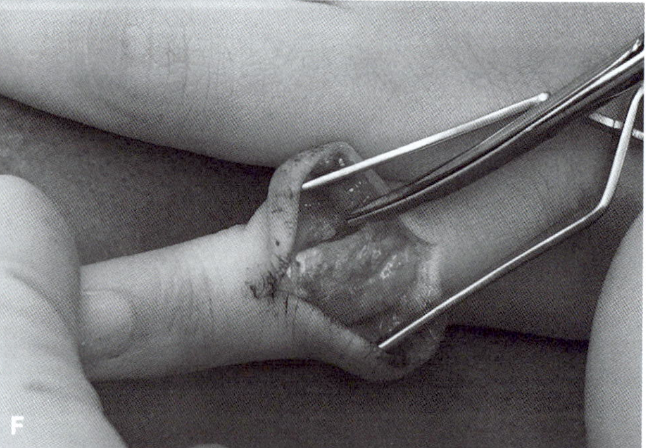

Figure 59.2: Lateral (A) and PA (B) radiographs demonstrating subtle volar rotatory subluxation of the PIP joint. Lateral (C) and PA (D) radiographs following open reduction. Intraoperative photographs demonstrating the buttonhole in the extensor tendon and radial collateral ligament interposed between the central slip and lateral band (E) and normal extensor tendon course following reduction of the collateral ligament (F).

- Open reduction is typically necessary to disengage the proximal phalanx condyle and collateral ligament from its buttonholed position.

COLLATERAL LIGAMENT INJURIES

- "Jammed" fingers are frequently injuries to the collateral ligaments, which are crucial for pinch strength. Diagnosis is made based on swelling and tenderness localized to a collateral ligament, or with instability or pain varus or valgus stress. Collateral ligament injuries result from radial or ulnar stress on the joint, commonly seen in football, wrestling, and basketball. Disruption usually occurs at the proximal attachment, with radial collateral injury more common than ulnar collateral injury (35).
- Radiographs should be obtained to rule out fracture. MRI is rarely used, but it can be helpful if examination is equivocal.
- Most collateral ligament injuries are treated with buddy taping to an adjacent finger for 3–6 weeks with continued participation in athletic activity. Index finger radial collateral ligament injury may require surgical repair to restore pinch strength.

Metacarpophalangeal Joint

- Metacarpophalangeal (MCP) dislocations are rare and usually involve dorsal dislocation of the proximal phalanx. The index finger is the most common, followed by the thumb (36).
- Dorsal dislocations are reduced with the wrist in flexion to take tension on the flexors, with direct pressure over the dorsal aspect of the proximal phalanx. It is important to not pull longitudinal traction, as this may pull the volar plate into the joint and create an irreducible situation. After the reduction, early active range of motion with a dorsal blocking splint is needed. Volar dislocations are reduced with direct pressure over the volar proximal phalanx and should be immobilized in 30° of flexion after reduction (36). Complex dislocations involve buttonholing of the metacarpal head between the flexor tendon and the lumbrical with volar plate interposition into the dislocated joint. These usually require open reduction.
- Collateral ligament injuries are relatively common and can be purely ligamentous injuries or avulsion fractures.
- Examination will exhibit tenderness over the collateral ligament and pain or instability when the collateral ligament is stressed with the MCP passively flexed 90°.
- Treatment largely consists of buddy strapping until pain and/or instability resolves.
- Radial collateral ligament injuries to the index finger, although, often require repair to restore stability.

INJURIES OF THE THUMB

Interphalangeal Joint

- Thumb interphalangeal (IP) dislocations are uncommon injuries and are managed similarly to finger DIP dislocations.

Metacarpophalangeal Joint

- Dislocations of the thumb MCP joint are usually dorsal dislocations, resulting from hyperextension at the MCP joint with volar plate rupture. The metacarpal head may protrude through the volar plate, where it becomes buttonholed between the flexor pollicis longus and flexor pollicis brevis tendons (37).
- The volar plate, flexor pollicis longus, or sesamoids may be interposed, preventing reduction, but closed reduction is usually possible, with splinting recommended for 3–4 weeks after reduction.

Thumb Collateral Ligament Injury

- Ulnar collateral ligament (UCL) injuries of the thumb MCP joint are also known as *skier's thumb* in acute injuries or *gamekeepers thumb* in cases of chronic attenuation. The UCL is necessary for effective pinch and grasping with the thumb. Patients present with tenderness and swelling over the ulnar aspect of the thumb MCP joint with instability of the UCL on radial stress. Stability should be assessed with the MCP in 30° of flexion and at full extension to evaluate both the proper and accessory UCL, respectively (33,38).
- A palpable or visible mass over the ulnar metacarpal head suggests a Stener lesion, which occurs when the UCL displaces superficial to the aponeurosis of adductor pollicis (Fig. 59.3). This prevents nonoperative healing of the ligament. It may be directly visualized with ultrasound or MRI, and is present in up to 70% of acute UCL tears (33).
- In the absence of clinical instability with less than 15° of variation from the uninjured side, patients are treated with immobilization for 4–6 weeks. Surgical intervention with reattachment of the UCL is indicated if there is greater than 15° of variation, a Stener lesion, or large, displaced bony avulsion (33,38).

Radial Collateral Ligament Injury

- Radial collateral ligament injuries occur 10× less frequently than ulnar injuries and present with radial MCP pain, tenderness, and/or instability.
- Nonoperative and surgical management is similar to UCL injuries; however, there is no analogous Stener lesion on the radial side. The abductor pollicis brevis aponeurosis extends proximal enough to completely cover the RCL, making a radial Stener lesion not possible. Complete RCL injuries may

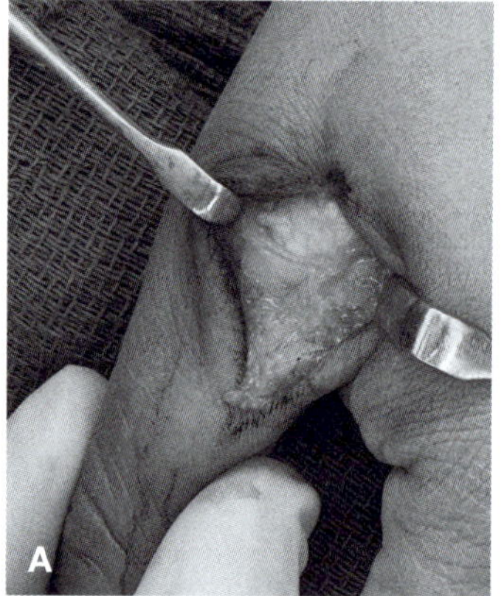

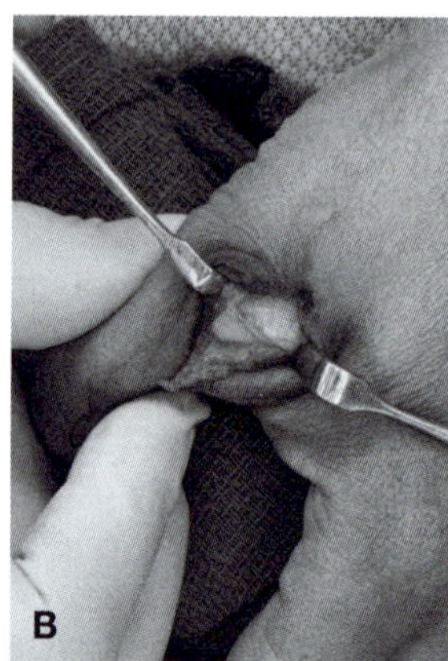

Figure 59.3: Intraoperative photographs of a Stener lesion with the thumb MCP reduced (A) and radially deviated (B). In both positions the entirety of the UCL (on the right of the wound) is superficial to the transverse fibers of the adductor aponeurosis (on the left half of the wound).

also be associated with volar subluxation of the joint and may require surgical stabilization (39).

TENDON INJURIES

Mallet Finger

- Mallet fingers may be seen in any contact or noncontact sport, but are most common in football receivers, baseball players, and basketball players. Mallet finger refers to a disruption of the extensor mechanism insertion into the distal phalanx, resulting from forced flexion of an actively extended DIP joint. A variably sized piece of bone may be avulsed with tendon (40).
- The patient characteristically exhibits a flexed DIP joint at rest and is unable to actively extend the joint (40).
- Treatment is continuous extension splinting of the DIP joint for 6–8 weeks while allowing PIP motion, then up to 4 weeks of nighttime splinting. It is important to stress that patients cannot allow the DIP to flex during their treatment course, as they risk disruption of the extensor mechanism healing. Surgical treatment may be necessary for chronic presentations, in cases with associated fracture involving over 50% of the articular surface, volar subluxation of the DIP, or in the presence of arthritis (40).
- Patients often attain an excellent functional result despite an average of 10° of extensor lag (40).

Boutonnière Deformity

- Boutonnière deformities result from extensor tendon central slip injuries over the PIP, and occur from lacerations, dislocations, traumatic avulsions, or capsular distension in rheumatoid patients. The ruptured central slip leads to reliance on the lateral bands to act as the extensors of both the DIP and PIPs. Initially active extension at the PIP and DIP will be possible. Over time, the lateral bands then subluxate volarly to the center of rotation of the PIP joint and become flexors at the PIP and extensors at the DIP (41).
- The Elson test is a reliable diagnostic tool prior to full deformity progression. The examiner should bend the PIP 90° over a surface and ask the patient to extend the middle phalanx against resistance. A rigid DIP is evidence of central slip injury (Fig. 59.4).
- Treatment of acute cases involves extension splinting or pinning of the PIP for 6 weeks, allowing DIP motion, followed by gradual PIP motion. Cases associated with large bony

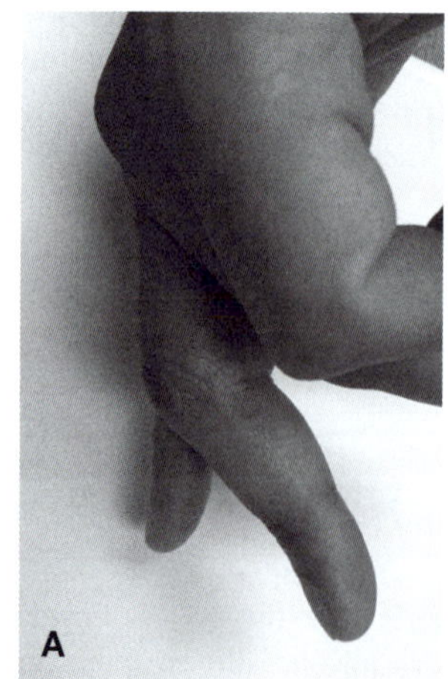

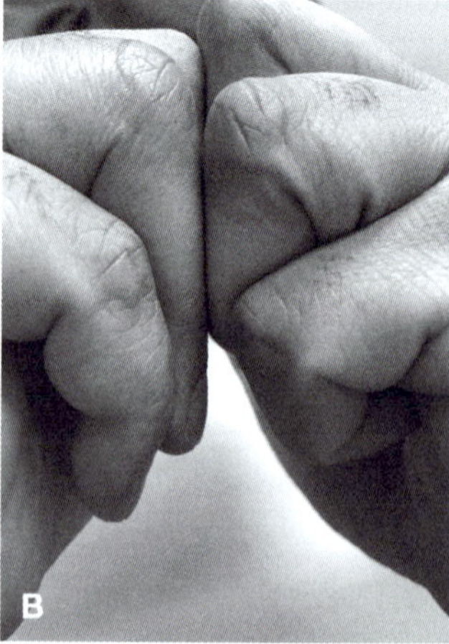

Figure 59.4: Clinical photographs demonstrating boutonniere deformity of the ring finger (A) and positive Elson test on the right ring finger, as evidenced by the full, rigid extension of the ring finger DIP joint on the right ring finger when the PIP is actively extended against resistance at 90° of flexion (B). Note the DIP flexion of all the other digits.

fragments and chronic cases are typically treated surgically. Maintenance of passive range of motion in the chronic deformities is necessary to facilitate later surgical reconstruction.

Pseudo-Boutonnière Deformity

- This injury is caused by a hyperextension injury to the PIP joint, disrupting the volar plate and either the radial collateral ligament or UCL. Tissue contraction causes a progressive PIP flexion deformity. Patients with a pseudo-boutonnière exhibit equivalent active and passive ranges of motion at the PIP joint, whereas patients with true central slip injuries may maintain full passive extension. Pseudo-boutonnières also do not exhibit the classic DIP hyperextension deformity seen in true boutonnière deformities (42).
- Static progressive and dynamic splinting under the direction of a hand therapist is recommended if the PIP deformity is less than 45°. Surgical intervention is reserved for deformities that fail to improve with 3–6 months of dedicated hand therapy (42).

Sagittal Band Injuries

- Sagittal band injury to the extensor tendons at the level of the MCP joint may lead to EDC subluxation or dislocation. Radial sagittal band injury and ulnar EDC subluxation usually result from a direct blow to the digit forcing sudden flexion and ulnar deviation. Ulnar sagittal band injury and radial subluxation are rare. The middle finger is most commonly affected. Patients present with swelling and tenderness over the MCP joint, pain with resisted extension, inability to initiate extension or fully extend the MCP joint from a flexed position, but maintenance of extension power once the MCP is passively extended. There is often palpable or visible tendon subluxation or dislocation (43).
- Acute injuries (4–6 weeks) often respond to relative extension splinting of the MCP joint with a yoke splint. Chronic or recalcitrant cases may require surgical repair or reconstruction of the sagittal band (44).
- Repetitive direct trauma to the dorsal MCP joint may lead to EDC, sagittal band, or dorsal capsule injury, commonly called "Boxer knuckle." It most commonly involves the index and middle digits in professional athletes, and ring and little digits in amateurs. The injury manifests as pain and localized swelling over involved joints (44). Range of motion and strength is typically preserved.
- Rest, cessation of boxing, splinting, and glove alterations often lead to improvement in pain and may resolve the swelling. Exploration with surgical repair of the injured structures may be undertaken in chronic cases in patients who wish to return to boxing (44).

Jersey Finger

- Jersey finger is an avulsion of the flexor digitorum profundus (FDP) tendon from its insertion on the distal phalanx, commonly occurring in football and rugby players. Greater than 75% of cases involve the ring finger because during grip, the ring finger is 5 mm more proximal than the others (42,44).
- Injury is caused by forced DIP extension during maximal FDP contraction, as in grabbing someone's jersey while attempting to tackle. Clinical findings include the inability to actively flex the DIP joint with normal passive range of motion. The resting posture of the hand may demonstrate relative extension of the injured digit (Fig. 59.5). There may also be a painful mass in the palm, a result of the retracted tendon. Radiographs are usually negative unless a bony fragment is avulsed with the tendon (43).
- Injuries are graded based on the degree of tendon retraction. In type I injuries, the tendon retracts into the palm. In type II injuries, the tendon retracts to the level of the PIP joint. In type III injuries, the tendon retracts only to the A4 pulley, limited by a large avulsed bony fragment (42,44). Type 4 injuries include both fracture and tendon avulsion from the fractured segment. Type 5 involves bony comminution with tendon avulsion.
- All require surgical reinsertion of the tendon into the distal phalanx (Fig. 59.5). The greater the degree of retraction, the more quickly surgical intervention is required. Type I injuries should be addressed within 7–10 days, whereas type III injuries may be successfully treated up to 2–3 months after the injury, but should be attempted by 3 weeks for optimal outcomes (44).

VASCULAR INJURY

Hypothenar Hammer Syndrome

- This syndrome is caused by repetitive impact to the hypothenar region of the hand, causing trauma to the ulnar artery in the region of Guyon canal resulting in arterial constriction, thickening, thrombosis, and possible aneurysm formation. It is most commonly seen in judo, karate, cycling, and lacrosse (45).
- Symptoms are caused by distal ischemia and include cold intolerance, pain in the palm or ulnar digits, and an abnormal Allen test. Ulnar nerve compression and the corresponding symptoms may occur secondary to aneurysm formation.
- Treatment includes rest from inciting activities, increased padding of the hypothenar area, vagolytic agents, or surgical intervention with excision of the thrombosed segment and artery ligation or reconstruction (45).

Chronic Digital Ischemia

- Chronic compression or microtrauma to the hand and digital vasculature may cause distal ischemia. This is occasionally seen in baseball pitchers and catchers and handball players. Typical symptoms include cold intolerance, pallor, and pain in the involved digits (46).

Figure 59.5: Clinical photographs (A) demonstrating loss of resting flexion of the DIP of the small finger following FDP avulsion. Fluoroscopic AP (B) and lateral (C) images demonstrating micro suture anchors used to repair the avulsed tendon to the distal phalanx.

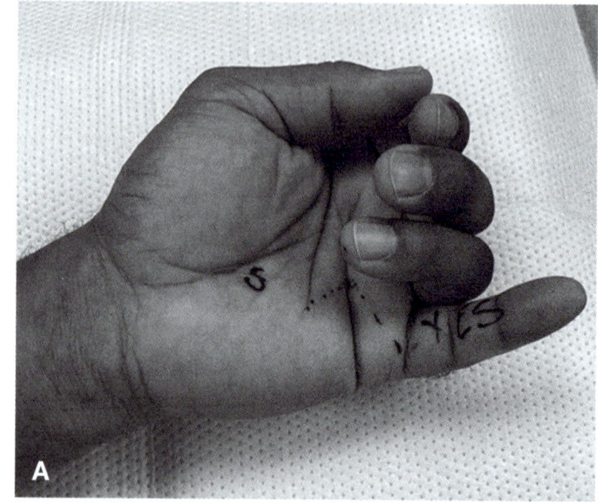

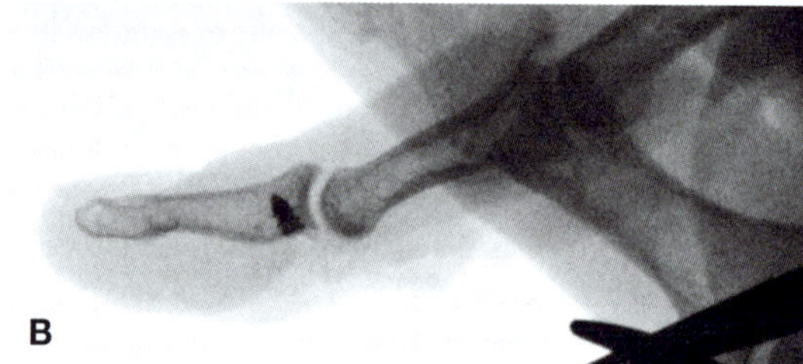

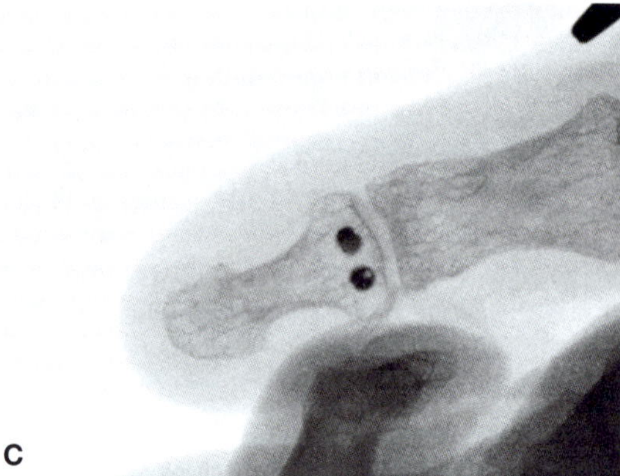

- Increased padding during causative activities, use of pharmacologic agents, or surgical exploration may be needed.

Frostbite

- Ischemic cold injury depends on the duration and severity of exposure, as well as the presence of constrictive clothes, vasospasm, and wetness. Early symptoms include erythema, burning, and itching, followed by numbness, then the formation of vesicles and ulcers (47).
- First-degree frostbite is a superficial injury from which full recovery is expected. Second-degree injury involves partial-thickness dermal loss. In third-degree injury, full-thickness dermal loss occurs. Fourth-degree injury involves deeper structures, including tendon and bone (48). Third- and fourth-degree injuries are considered deep and have a poor prognosis.
- Treatment involves gradual rewarming of involved digits in 40–42 °C water. Advanced injuries and gangrenous areas require surgical debridement, amputation, or skin grafting once gangrene is fully demarcated.

OVERUSE INJURIES

- Wrist syndromes account for the most common upper extremity overuse injuries (49). Repetitive activities, such as gymnastics, racquet sports, rowing, and throwing sports, result in a high number of overuse injuries.

De Quervain Tenosynovitis

- De Quervain tenosynovitis is a stenosing inflammation of the abductor pollicis long (APL) and extensor pollicis brevis

(EPB) in the first dorsal compartment. It occurs in athletes who perform forceful grasp with repetitive use of the thumb and radial-ulnar deviation such as those who play racquet sports, golf (particularly the left thumb in right-handed golfers), fly-fishing, javelin, and discus throwing. Athletes endorse radial-sided wrist pain worsened by gripping and raising objects with the wrist in neutral rotation. On exam, there is localized tenderness over the first dorsal compartment at the level of the radial styloid, occasionally with visible swelling. The Finkelstein test is performed by passively ulnarly deviating the patient's wrist with the thumb adducted. Reproduction of the patient's pain is positive and indicative of de Quervain (49).

- Initial treatment includes anti-inflammatory medication, thumb spica splinting, and corticosteroid injection into the first dorsal compartment. Poor response from injection may be due to a longitudinal septum, which separates the APL and EPB in 20%–30% of cases (10). If conservative measures do not permanently alleviate the symptoms, surgical treatment involves the release of the APL and EPB tendons at the first dorsal compartment. Complications of surgery include persistence of symptoms (possibly due to inadequate release), injury to the superficial radial nerve, and tendon subluxation. Most athletes return to full participation following surgical decompression in 3–4 weeks.

Intersection Syndrome

- Intersection syndrome is tenosynovitis of the second dorsal compartment tendons (extensor carpi radialis longus [ECRL] and extensor carpi radialis brevis [ECRB]) in the dorsoradial distal forearm where the first dorsal compartment muscles cross over the second dorsal compartment. It occurs in athletes exposed to repetitive wrist motions, such as rowers, racquet sports participants, weightlifters, and canoeists (50). Athletes endorse dorsoradial forearm pain and tenderness 5 cm proximal to the wrist that is worse with resisted wrist and thumb extension. Patients may also have obvious crepitus over the intersection. Initial treatment consists of rest, splinting, anti-inflammatory medication, corticosteroid injections, and activity modification and is successful 95% of the time (50). If conservative treatment fails, release of the second dorsal compartment, exploration, and debridement of the intersection zone and bursal tissue, and release of the fascial sheaths of the tendons in the first dorsal compartment is usually effective. Postoperatively, the wrist is splinted for 7–10 days followed by a stretching and strengthening program and return to sport is allowed when the patient is symptom free.

Extensor Carpi Ulnaris Tendinitis/Subluxation

- Extensor carpi ulnaris (ECU) tendonitis is the second most common stenosing tenosynovitis of the hand after de Quervain (49). It occurs in athletes involved in repetitive wrist motion, such as racquet sports, baseball, golf, and rowing. It may also happen after traumatic ECU subluxation with rupture of the fibrous sheath overlying the ECU during forced supination, flexion, and ulnar deviation of the wrist (similar to a baseball swing) (20). Athletes endorse pain and swelling distal to the ulnar head, worsened by resisted wrist extension. A painful snap may be elicited as subluxation of the ECU occurs with supination and ulnar deviation of the wrist (50).
- Initial treatment includes rest, splinting, anti-inflammatory medication, corticosteroid injection, and activity modification. Patients who fail to respond to nonoperative treatment require surgical decompression of the sixth dorsal compartment with radial release of the fibro-osseous tunnel and repair of the extensor retinaculum to prevent postoperative subluxation. After surgery, the wrist is immobilized in 20° of extension for 3 weeks prior to starting activity. Patients with acute ECU subluxation may be treated with long-arm casting with the wrist in full pronation and slight dorsiflexion, but often requires stabilization of the ECU (50).

Flexor Compartment Tendinopathies

- Inflammation of the flexor tendons most commonly occurs in the FCR and flexor carpi ulnaris (FCU) as a result of repetitive wrist motions, such as in golf and racquet sports (51). FCR tendonitis usually presents with pain over the volar aspect of the wrist, proximal to the wrist crease over the FCR tendon, or at the FCR insertion near the scaphoid tubercle. Pain may be elicited with abrupt wrist extension or resisted wrist flexion and radial deviation. Athletes with FCU tendonitis may complain of pain and swelling distal or proximal to the pisiform. Pain may be exacerbated with passive wrist extension or resisted wrist flexion and ulnar deviation.
- Initial treatment includes rest, anti-inflammatory medication, splinting, and corticosteroid injection. If symptoms persist, surgical decompression of the fibro-osseous tunnel containing the FCR is performed in the case of FCR tendonitis. Surgical treatment of FCU tendonitis includes FCU lengthening with or without pisiform excision (51).

Trigger Finger

- Trigger fingers result from inflammation of the flexor tendons at the leading edge of the flexor tendon sheath over the volar MCP, leading to pain, catching, and locking of the finger. Most occur secondary to chronic degenerative changes of the involved flexor tendon and/or the A1 pulley, but direct pressure from racquets, baseball bats, or golf clubs can also cause acute inflammation of the pulley and tendons.
- Initial treatment is splinting, anti-inflammatory medications, and steroid injections into the tendon sheath at the A1 pulley. This provides definitive relief in 60%–90% of patients. If nonoperative treatment fails, surgical release of the Al pulley is effective in over 90% of patients (49).

PEDIATRIC INJURIES

Distal Radial Physeal Stress Syndrome (Gymnast's Wrist)

- There has been a rise in the frequency of wrist pain in skeletally immature athletes, particularly as sports such as gymnastics have grown in popularity. Up to 75% of all male and 50% of all female competitive gymnasts endorse some degree of wrist pain. This is most likely due to repetitive axial loading across a hyperextended wrist. Injuries result from either acute, high-energy trauma or chronic and repetitive stress (52).
- X-rays may reveal stress-related changes of the distal radial epiphysis, including widening of the growth plate, epiphyseal cystic changes with beaking of the distal epiphysis, and metaphyseal irregularity. These changes may lead to premature physeal closure and a higher incidence of ulnar positive variance. As a result, following skeletal maturity, gymnasts may present with ulnar abutment syndrome or Madelung-like deformity. MRI may be useful in determining the presence or extent of physeal injury and assist in determining return to sports participation, especially in the face of normal plain radiographs (52).
- It is rare that the treatment of wrist pain in a skeletally immature athlete is other than rest and withdrawal from the offending activity. Prevention may be the best form of treatment by using protective gear, spotters, proper warm-up, and preclusion of sudden changes in activity intensity. If a physeal injury is diagnosed, monitoring for growth disturbance is crucial to prevent late-onset deformity. It may also be possible to remove the gymnast from the specific event causing symptoms and allow continued competition in other events that do not exacerbate symptoms.

REFERENCES

1. Simpson D, McQueen MM. Acute sporting injuries to the hand and wrist in the general population. *Scott Med J.* 2006;51(2):25–6. doi:10.1258/rsmsmj.51.2.25
2. Bergfeld JA, Weiker GG, Andrish JT, Hall R. Soft playing splint for protection of significant hand and wrist injuries in sports. *Am J Sports Med.* 1982;10(5):293–6. doi:10.1177/036354658201000506
3. Roser LA, Clawson DK. Football injuries in the very young athlete. *Clin Orthop Relat Res.* 1970;69:219–23.
4. Pitner MA. Pathophysiology of overuse injuries in the hand and wrist. *Hand Clin.* 1990;6(3):355–64.
5. Steinberg BD, Kleinman WB. Occult scapholunate ganglion: a cause of dorsal radial wrist pain. *J Hand Surg Am.* 1999;24(2):225–31. doi:10.1053/jhsu.1999.0225
6. Angelides AC, Wallace PF. The dorsal ganglion of the wrist: its pathogenesis, gross and microscopic anatomy, and surgical treatment. *J Hand Surg Am.* 1976;1(3):228–35. doi:10.1016/s0363-5023(76)80042-1
7. Cardinal E, Buckwalter KA, Braunstein EM, Mih AD. Occult dorsal carpal ganglion: comparison of US and MR imaging. *Radiology.* 1994;193(1):259–62. doi:10.1148/radiology.193.1.8090903
8. Richman JA, Gelberman RH, Engber WD, Salamon PB, Bean DJ. Ganglions of the wrist and digits: results of treatment by aspiration and cyst wall puncture. *J Hand Surg Am.* 1987;12(6):1041–3. doi:10.1016/s0363-5023(87)80108-9
9. Linscheid RL, Dobyns JH. Athletic injuries of the wrist. *Clin Orthop Relat Res.* 1985(198):141–51.
10. Halikis MN, Taleisnik J. Soft-tissue injuries of the wrist. *Clin Sports Med.* 1996;15(2):235–59.
11. Carr D, Davis P. Distal posterior interosseous nerve syndrome. *J Hand Surg Am.* 1985;10(6 pt 1):873–8. doi:10.1016/s0363-5023(85)80165-9
12. Lewis DM, Osterman AL. Scapholunate instability in athletes. *Clin Sports Med.* 2001;20(1):131–40. doi:10.1016/s0278-5919(05)70251-9
13. Taleisnik J. Post-traumatic carpal instability. *Clin Orthop Relat Res.* 1980;149:73–82.
14. Slade JF III, Milewski MD. Management of carpal instability in athletes. *Hand Clin.* 2009;25(3):395–408. doi:10.1016/j.hcl.2009.05.002
15. Ramponi D, McSwigan T. Scapholunate dissociation. *Adv Emerg Nurs J.* 2016;38(1):10–4. doi:10.1097/tme.0000000000000094
16. Blatt G. Capsulodesis in reconstructive hand surgery. Dorsal capsulodesis for the unstable scaphoid and volar capsulodesis following excision of the distal ulna. *Hand Clin.* 1987;3(1):81–102.
17. Brunelli GA, Brunelli GR. A new surgical technique for carpal instability with scapholunate dissociation. *Surg Technol Int.* 1996;5:370–4.
18. Watson HK, Hempton RF. Limited wrist arthrodeses. I. The triscaphoid joint. *J Hand Surg Am.* 1980;5(4):320–7. doi:10.1016/s0363-5023(80)80169-9
19. Morrell NT, Moyer A, Quinlan N, Shafritz AB. Scapholunate and perilunate injuries in the athlete. *Curr Rev Musculoskelet Med.* 2017;10(1):45–52.
20. Reagan DS, Linscheid RL, Dobyns JH. Lunotriquetral sprains. *J Hand Surg Am.* 1984;9(4):502–14. doi:10.1016/s0363-5023(84)80101-x
21. Weiss LE, Taras JS, Sweet S, Osterman AL. Lunotriquetral injuries in the athlete. *Hand Clin.* 2000;16(3):433–8.
22. Rettig AC, Rettig LA, Jelinek JA. Ulnar translocation of the wrist in a professional quarterback: a case report. *Am J Sports Med.* 2010;38(3):608–12. doi:10.1177/0363546509350744
23. Mikić ZD. Age changes in the triangular fibrocartilage of the wrist joint. *J Anat.* 1978;126(pt 2):367–84.
24. Palmer AK, Glisson RR, Werner FW. Relationship between ulnar variance and triangular fibrocartilage complex thickness. *J Hand Surg Am.* 1984;9(5):681–2. doi:10.1016/s0363-5023(84)80013-1
25. McAdams TR, Swan J, Yao J. Arthroscopic treatment of triangular fibrocartilage wrist injuries in the athlete. *Am J Sports Med.* 2009;37(2):291–7. doi:10.1177/0363546508325921
26. Linscheid RL. Ulnar lengthening and shortening. *Hand Clin.* 1987;3(1):69–79.
27. Bowers WH. Distal radioulnar joint arthroplasty: the hemiresection-interposition technique. *J Hnd Surg Am.* 1985;10(2):169–78. doi:10.1016/s0363-5023(85)80100-3
28. Gonçalves D. Correction of disorders of the distal radio-ulnar joint by artificial pseudarthrosis of the ulna. *J Bone Joint Surg Br.* 1974;56B(3):462–4.
29. Hermansdorfer JD, Kleinman WB. Management of chronic peripheral tears of the triangular fibrocartilage complex. *J Hand Surg Am.* 1991;16(2):340–6. doi:10.1016/s0363-5023(10)80123-6
30. Fassler PR. Fingertip injuries: evaluation and treatment. *J Am Acad Orthop Surg.* 1996;4(1):84–92. doi:10.5435/00124635-199603000-00003
31. Hallock GG. Expanded applications for octyl-2-cyanoacrylate as a tissue adhesive. *Ann Plast Surg.* 2001;46(2):185–9. doi:10.1097/00000637-200102000-00020

32. Peterson JJ, Bancroft LW. Injuries of the fingers and thumb in the athlete. *Clin Sports Med.* 2006;25(3):527–42, vii–viii. doi:10.1016/j.csm.2006.02.001
33. Morgan WJ, Slowman LS. Acute hand and wrist injuries in athletes: evaluation and management. *J Am Acad Orthop Surg.* 2001;9(6):389–400. doi:10.5435/00124635-200111000-00004
34. Caggiano NM, Harper CM, Rozental TD. Management of proximal interphalangeal joint fracture dislocations. *Hand Clin.* 2018;34(2):149–65. doi:10.1016/j.hcl.2017.12.005
35. Carlo J, Dell PC, Matthias R, Wright TW. Collateral ligament reconstruction of the proximal interphalangeal joint. *J Hand Surg Am.* 2016;41(1):129–32. doi:10.1016/j.jhsa.2015.10.007
36. Kaplan EB. Dorsal dislocation of the metacarpophalangeal joint of the index finger. *J Bone Joint Surg Am.* 1957;39-A(5):1081–6.
37. Kahler DM, McCue FC III. Metacarpophalangeal and proximal interphalangeal joint injuries of the hand, including the thumb. *Clin Sports Med.* 1992;11(1):57–76.
38. Abrahamsson SO, Sollerman C, Lundborg G, Larsson J, Egund N. Diagnosis of displaced ulnar collateral ligament of the metacarpophalangeal joint of the thumb. *J Hand Surg Am.* 1990;15(3):457–60. doi:10.1016/0363-5023(90)90059-z
39. Daley D, Geary M, Gaston RG. Thumb metacarpophalangeal ulnar and radial collateral ligament injuries. *Clin Sports Med.* 2020;39(2):443–55. doi:10.1016/j.csm.2019.12.003
40. Lin JS, Samora JB. Surgical and nonsurgical management of mallet finger: a systematic review. *J Hand Surg Am.* 2018;43(2):146–63.e2. doi:10.1016/j.jhsa.2017.10.004
41. McKeon KE, Lee DH. Posttraumatic boutonnière and swan neck deformities. *J Am Acad Orthop Surg.* 2015;23(10):623–32. doi:10.5435/jaaos-d-14-00272
42. Leddy JP. Soft-tissue injuries of the hand in the athlete. *Instr Course Lect.* 1998;47:181–6.
43. Aronowitz ER, Leddy JP. Closed tendon injuries of the hand and wrist in athletes. *Clin Sports Med.* 1998;17(3):449–67. doi:10.1016/s0278-5919(05)70096-x
44. Rettig AC. Closed tendon injuries of the hand and wrist in the athlete. *Clin Sports Med.* 1992;11(1):77–99.
45. Trommeter RA, Freeman CL, Shah KS, McKinzie JP, Smith AT. Hypothenar hammer syndrome. *J Emerg Med.* 2019;56(1):105–6. doi:10.1016/j.jemermed.2018.09.042
46. Sugawara M, Ogino T, Minami A, Ishii S. Digital ischemia in baseball players. *Am J Sports Med.* 1986;14(4):329–34. doi:10.1177/036354658601400417
47. McAdams TR, Swenson DR, Miller RA. Frostbite: an orthopedic perspective. *Am J Orthop (Belle Mead NJ).* 1999;28(1):21–6.
48. Hutchison RL. Frostbite of the hand. *J Hand Surg Am.* 2014;39(9):1863–8. doi:10.1016/j.jhsa.2014.01.035
49. Rettig AC. Wrist and hand overuse syndromes. *Clin Sports Med.* 2001;20(3):591–611. doi:10.1016/s0278-5919(05)70271-4
50. Patrick NC, Hammert WC. Hand and wrist tendinopathies. *Clin Sports Med.* 2020;39(2):247–58. doi:10.1016/j.csm.2019.10.004
51. Wood MB, Dobyns JH. Sports-related extraarticular wrist syndromes. *Clin Orthop Relat Res.* 1986;202:93–102.
52. Mauck B, Kelly D, Sheffer B, Rambo A, Calandruccio JH. Gymnast's wrist (distal radial physeal stress syndrome). *Orthop Clin North Am.* 2020;51(4):493–7. doi:10.1016/j.ocl.2020.06.012

60 Wrist and Hand Fractures

Denver Kraft, Landon Mueller, and Curtis Henn

EPIDEMIOLOGY

- Wrist and hand injuries account for 47% of sporting injuries in the general population. Of these, 76% were fractures (1).
- Gymnasts have the highest level of wrist and hand injuries among athletes, with up to 43% suffering chronic injuries. In one series, 88% of elite male gymnasts complained of wrist pain and 58% required nonsteroidal anti-inflammatory drug (NSAID) therapy to continue competing (2).

GENERAL PRINCIPLES

- Diagnosis of hand and wrist fractures in the athlete is often straightforward following a thorough physical exam and orthogonal radiographs.
- Clinical deformity is often present and point tenderness is often quite specific.
- Rotational deformity may be assessed by asking the athlete to attempt to make a fist or by passively extending the wrist and allowing the digits to flex via tenodesis (Fig. 60.1).
- When initial radiographs are negative and a high index of suspicion of fracture remains, the treating physician may obtain an MRI to confirm or rule out an occult fracture. The physician may also elect to initiate treatment of a presumed fracture and repeat the radiographs at weekly intervals until tenderness resolves or evidence of a healing nondisplaced fracture is detected radiographically.
- Initial treatment of hand and wrist fractures is dictated by the severity of the injury. Neurovascular compromise, significant soft-tissue injury, or open fractures require emergent treatment.
- Significantly displaced fractures with clinical deformity require urgent reduction and splinting, while closed fractures without clinical deformity may be splinted and evaluated semi-urgently (ideally the same day).
- Surgical versus nonsurgical treatment is often dictated primarily by the location, displacement, and stability of the fracture. Operative fixation may also be undertaken to facilitate earlier and safer return to play.
- Fractures that are treated conservatively following closed reduction require close radiographic follow up to ensure maintenance of acceptable alignment.
- Return to play is always a case-specific decision that depends on many factors, including fracture and fixation characteristics, clinical and radiographic evidence of healing, patient characteristics and goals, risk tolerance of the physician and the patient, the patient's sport and position, the athlete's level and career path, and where the team is during the season.

DISTAL RADIUS FRACTURES

- Distal radius fractures account for 10% of all bony injuries, up to 75% of all fractures to the forearm, and 16% of all fractures treated in the emergency room (3,4).
- Injury often occurs during running or contact sports when the hand is planted on the ground and the wrist hyperextends and the forearm rotates.
- Patients with distal radius fractures will have swelling, pain, and limited range of motion (ROM). In the case of displaced fractures, clinical deformity may also be present and is often obvious.
- It is often not possible to evaluate the stability of the distal radioulnar joint (DRUJ) in the setting of an acute distal radius fracture without adequate anesthesia, but DRUJ instability has been found in 2%–37% of patients after the distal radius fracture has healed. Two-thirds of these patients are symptomatic with ulnar-sided wrist pain and decreased pronation/supination (5,6).
- Carpal tunnel symptoms (numbness, paresthesias, and/or pain in the median nerve distribution) may be present in up to 15% of patients. Median nerve injury from the initial trauma will present as immediate median neuropathy and will improve following reduction. These cases are often observed following closed reduction and may undergo concurrent carpal tunnel release at the time of definitive fixation in a nonurgent manner. Median nerve injury from the initial trauma must be distinguished from acute carpal tunnel syndrome, which will present as progressive, worsening median nerve dysfunction and pain in the fingers. Acute carpal

We thank D. Nicole Deal and A. Bobby Chhabra for their contribution on this chapter, as authors of the prior edition.

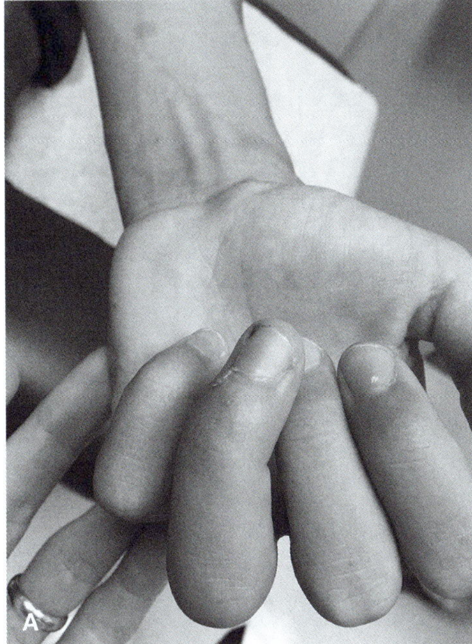

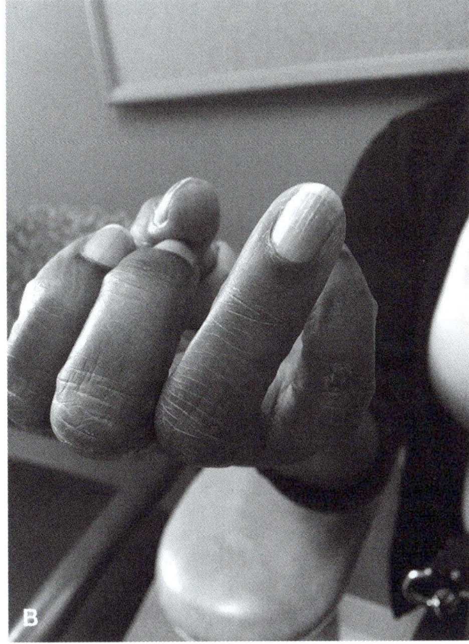

Figure 60.1: Rotational deformity is assessed by asking the athlete to make a fist. Clinical photographs demonstrate obvious rotational deformity from a middle phalangeal fracture (A) and a metacarpal fracture (B).

tunnel syndrome requires emergent carpal tunnel release to prevent permanent nerve damage (7).

- Soft-tissue injuries are reported in 70% of distal radius fractures. The triangular fibrocartilage complex (TFCC) is injured in 40%, scapholunate ligament in 30%, and lunotriquetral ligament in 15% (8). The TFCC is a major stabilizer of the DRUJ. There is an increased likelihood of TFCC disruption if there is 2 mm of coronal displacement at the DRUJ, with greater than 10° of dorsal or volar angulation (5). The clinical significance of these concomitant ligament injuries found during routine arthroscopy at the time of distal radius fixation is not known. Concurrent ligament repair at the time of distal radius fixation is typically undertaken only in the setting of obvious, complete ligament disruption.

Radiographic Evaluation

- Posteroanterior (PA), oblique, and lateral views are useful to assess radial inclination, length, and volar tilt (8). Computed tomography (CT) scan may provide useful information regarding the nature of the fracture and associated injuries when planning for fracture management (8). CT may demonstrate comminution, fracture extension into the DRUJ, and the extent of articular displacement.

Management of Distal Radius Fractures

- Treatment depends on fracture stability and displacement, as well as patient age and activity demands. Most stable fractures can be treated nonsurgically with bracing or casting for nondisplaced fractures or closed reduction and casting for displaced fractures.
- Two millimeters of articular displacement increases the risk for subsequent degenerative arthritis (9). Surgical treatment of fractures is often performed in cases of post-reduction shortening over 3 mm, dorsal tilt over 10°, or intra-articular displacement or step-off over 2 mm (10). Other predictors of fracture instability may lead to surgical treatment, including volar comminution, excessive prereduction displacement, or concurrent distal ulnar metaphyseal fracture (Fig. 60.2).
- **Extra-articular fractures:** Stable, minimally displaced, or nondisplaced fracture treatment consists of placement of a well-fitted short arm splint or cast. Displaced fractures are treated with closed reduction followed by application of a sugar-tong splint, clam-shell short arm splint, or short arm cast with a three-point mold (8). Splints may then be converted to well-molded short arm casts after acute swelling has subsided and fractures have begun to heal, typically at 2 or 3 weeks following reduction. Weekly radiographic follow-up for the first 3 weeks is recommended to assess for loss of reduction and potential need for surgical management. Unstable extra-articular fractures may require surgical management if satisfactory alignment is unable to be attained or maintained.
- **Noncomminuted intra-articular fractures:** Barton fractures are the result of shear forces across the volar or dorsal lip of the distal radius, resulting in one large dorsal or volar articular fragment. Closed reduction is rarely effective and often not attempted except in cases of significant initial displacement or deformity. Due to the inherent instability of

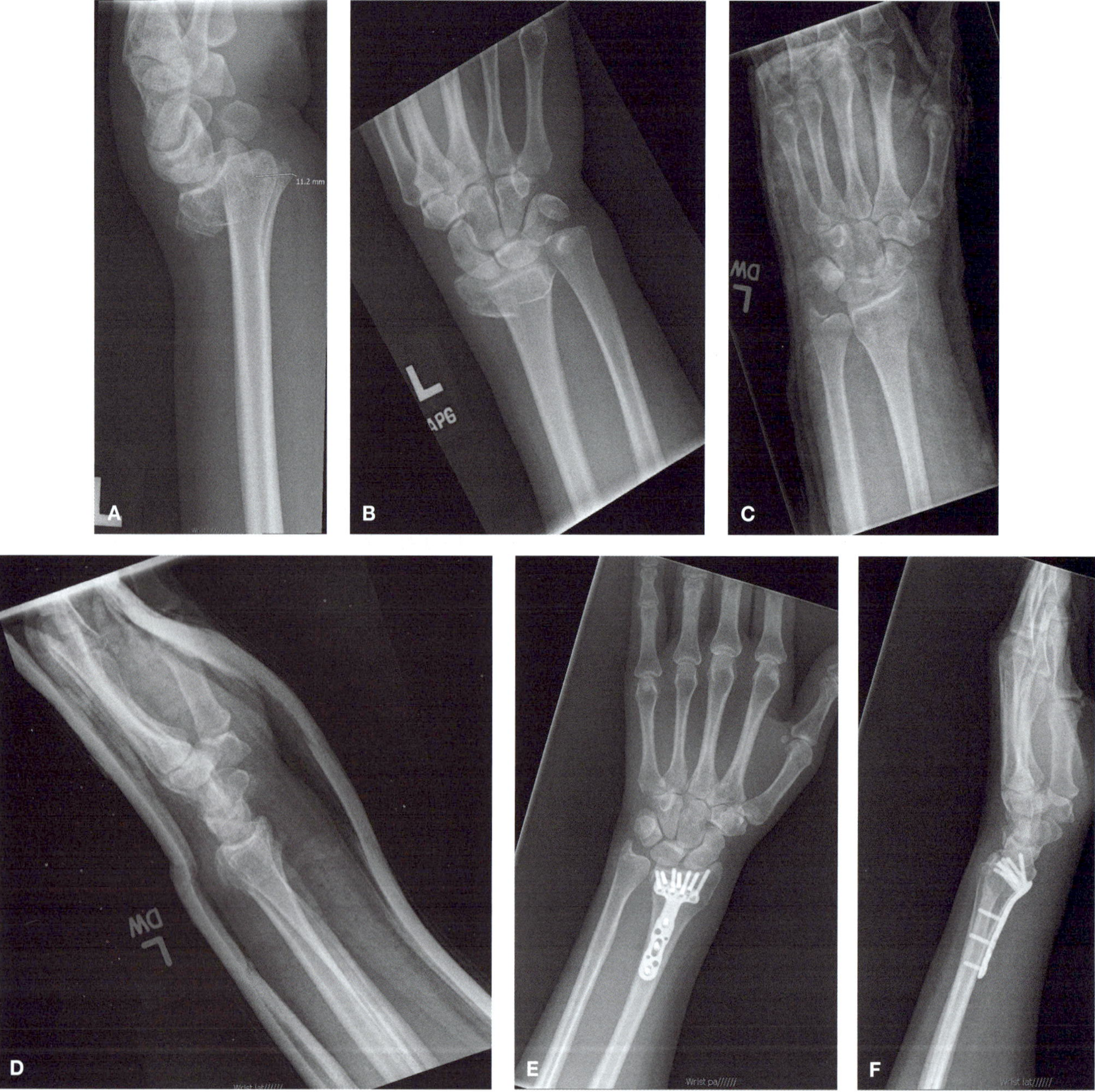

Figure 60.2: Prereduction (A and B), postreduction (B and C), and final (D–F) radiographs of an operatively treated distal radius fracture. Surgical indications include significant prereduction displacement (A), persistent dorsal translation postreduction (D), and volar comminution (A and D).

these fractures and articular displacement, surgical stabilization is nearly always required (11).

- **Comminuted or complex intra-articular fractures:** Distal radius fractures with significant dorsal comminution or articular comminution frequently collapse and shorten without surgical fixation (12,13).

Complications

- Nonunion following distal radius fracture is a rare occurrence, whereas malunion — most commonly shortening and loss of volar tilt — is a common complication (14). Correction of malunion should be considered when there is persistent pain, loss of function, or significant shortening or dorsal tilt. Adaptive carpal instability may indicate unacceptable dorsal angulation and prompt malunion correction (Fig. 60.3).
- Carpal tunnel syndrome can be a late complication of distal radius fractures, seen in 30% of high-energy fractures. The incidence of this complication can be reduced by not immobilizing the patient in flexion or ulnar deviation (14).

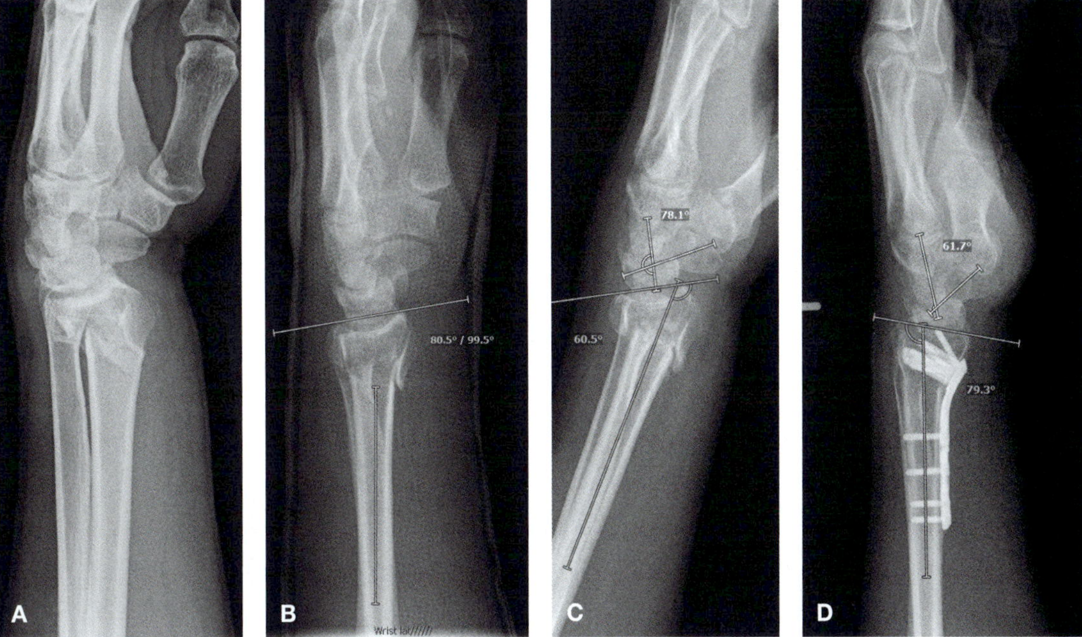

Figure 60.3: Lateral radiographs of a displaced intra-articular distal radius fracture that underwent closed reduction and conservative treatment at an outside hospital. A: Prereduction and (B) postreduction radiographs demonstrate overall satisfactory restoration of alignment. Lateral radiograph at 6 weeks post injury (C) demonstrate worsening dorsal tilt (yellow measurement) and adaptive carpal instability evidence by the >60° scapholunate angle (white measurement). Corrective osteotomy restored distal radial alignment (D, yellow measurement) and scapholunate alignment (D, white measurement).

- Symptomatic hardware, tenosynovitis, and tendon rupture are also possible complications. Modern techniques and implants can minimize these complications.

Return to Sports

- Patients treated nonoperatively with a splint or cast should be immobilized for 4–8 weeks. The athlete may then begin to rehabilitate the wrist using a removable thermoplastic splint. Return to sport is variable, but a general guideline is pain-free ROM and strength equal to 80% of the contralateral side (15). Return to sports without protection is usually not allowed until 3 months from the time of injury. Fractures treated with rigid internal fixation can be protected by a thermoplastic splint with early ROM exercises. Once radiographic evidence of healing is present, progressive strengthening exercises may commence. Full unprotected return to sport is not permitted before 3 months and typically discouraged until full motion and strength have been restored.

SCAPHOID FRACTURES

- Scaphoid fractures are the most common carpal bone fracture (1 in 100 college football players per year) and often a result of a fall on an outstretched hand (16).
- The most common mechanism of injury is axial load across a hyper-dorsiflexed, pronated, and ulnarly deviated wrist.
- The proximal 80% of the scaphoid relies on retrograde blood flow and is susceptible to avascular necrosis and nonunion when a displaced scaphoid waist fracture disrupts the interosseous blood supply.
- On examination, the patient will have tenderness in the anatomic snuff box, dorsally over the proximal pole, and/or volarly over the scaphoid tubercle. The scaphoid compression test is performed by creating an axial load across the scaphoid by loading the thumb metacarpal.
- Radiographs include PA, lateral, semipronated (45°) oblique, and a scaphoid view. The scaphoid view is taken with the wrist in 30° of extension and 20° ulnar deviation.
- If radiographs are negative but suspicion is high, treatment of a presumed nondisplaced fracture should be initiated. Interval radiographs at weekly intervals then may demonstrate a nondisplaced fracture 2–3 weeks after the injury.
- MRI may also be obtained acutely to identify occult fractures with negative initial radiographs.
- CT may be useful for further characterizing fracture displacement to determine if surgical intervention is necessary and for surgical planning.
- Proximal pole fractures are nearly universally treated operatively to minimize the risk of nonunion and/or avascular necrosis.
- Distal pole fractures are treated nonoperatively and reliably heal with immobilization.

- Optimal management of scaphoid waist fractures depends on fracture stability, displacement, and return-to-play goals.
- Nondisplaced fractures (<1 mm of displacement) may be treated nonoperatively with immobilization and a high rate of union can be expected (17,18).
- Immobilization is generally with a short arm cast with or without the thumb included for 6–10 weeks or until healing is evident clinically and radiographically, usually within 3 months (19).
- If there is no evidence of healing by 2–3 months or if there is evidence of avascular necrosis, surgical management is considered.
- Early operative intervention for nondisplaced fractures with percutaneous compression screw fixation is controversial but may allow the athlete to return earlier to sports, decrease the risk of fracture displacement, and reduce total rehabilitation time (20,21).
- Displaced fractures are treated with open reduction internal fixation (ORIF) with headless compression screws to restore anatomic alignment, optimize union rate, and decrease the risk of avascular necrosis.

Return to Sports

- Return to sport is controversial, and must be individualized based on the fracture location, fracture stability, fixation confidence and nature of the sport, and the athlete's position. A survey of professional team physicians noted 51% allowed full return 4–6 weeks after ORIF of nondisplaced fractures, whereas 32% allowed return with protected play (22). Once 50% of cortical bridging has occurred on CT and the athlete has full ROM, return to play is safe (23) (Fig. 60.4).

HAMATE FRACTURES

- Hook or body of the hamate fractures constitute 2%–4% of carpal fractures (24).

Hook of the Hamate Fractures

- The injury commonly occurs from the direct force of a bat, club, or racket to the volar ulnar palm (25).
- Athletes will have sudden pain and difficulty with wrist ROM, digital ROM, and/or gripping. They may localize pain to the hypothenar eminence.
- Exam may initially be difficult to localize, but tenderness over the hook of the hamate is nearly always present.
- The pull test is a sensitive, provocative maneuver where resisted small finger flexion with the wrist ulnarly deviated reproduces significant pain.
- The fracture is often nonvisualized on standard wrist radiographs, and thus the diagnosis is often missed or delayed.
- Carpal tunnel view X-rays or CT scans with 1 mm cuts are often needed for diagnosis. MRI, although, is the most sensitive test if suspicion is high and imaging is negative, given its ability to identify even nondisplaced hamate fractures (25) (Fig. 60.5).
- The natural history of conservatively treated or even untreated hook of hamate fractures is not known, but nonunion of the hook of hamate is common.
- Direct repair of hook of hamate fractures is technically challenging and results in high nonunion rates. Therefore, excision of the hook of hamate is the standard surgical treatment of choice. Indications for surgery include high-level athletes with acute fractures, patients with concomitant ulnar nerve pathology, or patients with symptomatic nonunions (24,25).

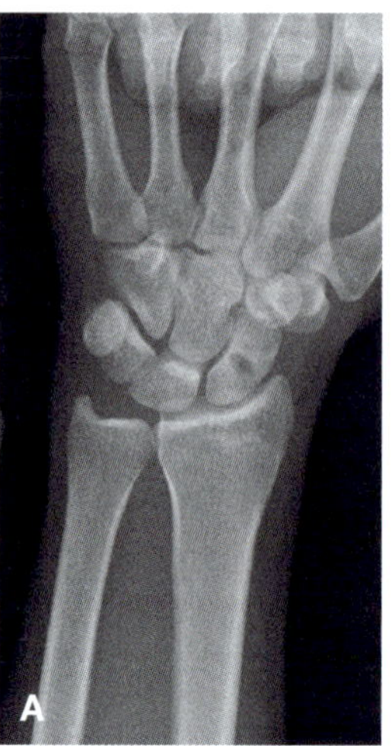

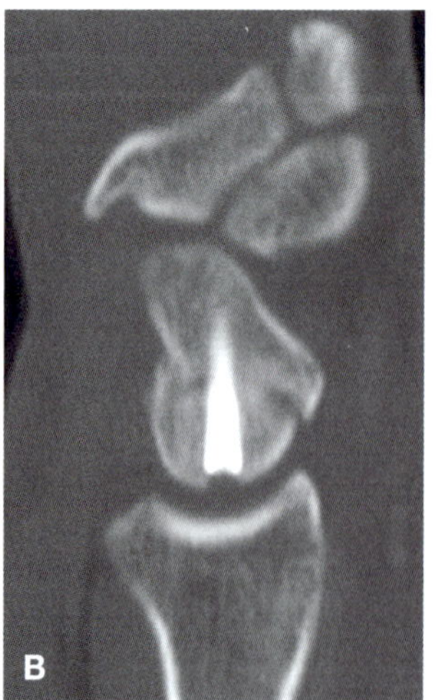

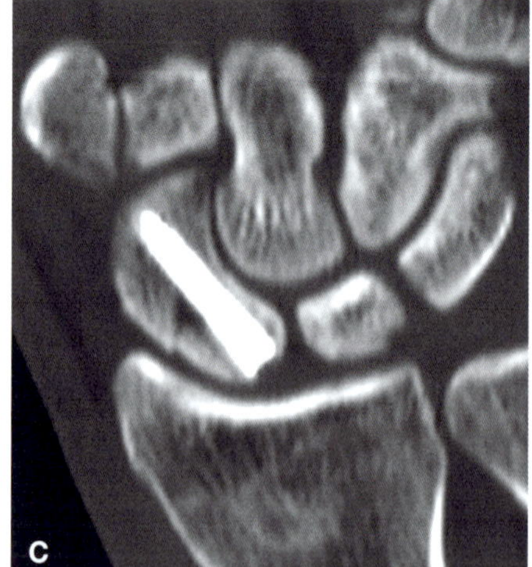

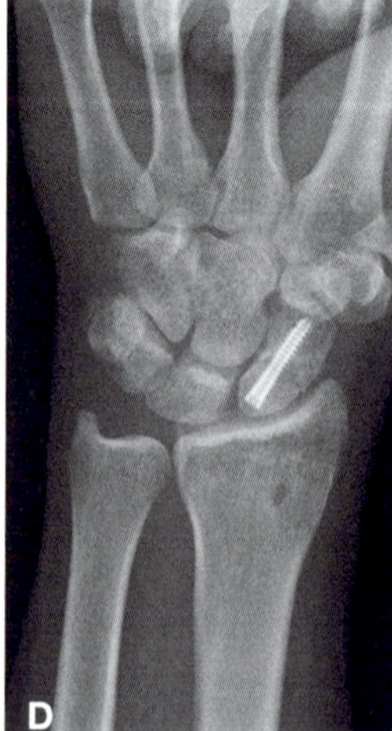

Figure 60.4: Professional ice hockey player with a nondisplaced scaphoid waist fracture found 6 weeks after injury (A). The patient underwent screw fixation with distal radial autograft. CT scan at 5 weeks postop demonstrates bridging bone (B and C). The patient returned to full, unrestricted play at 7 weeks when radiographs confirmed continued healing (D) and the patient attained full, painless ROM with resolution of snuffbox tenderness.

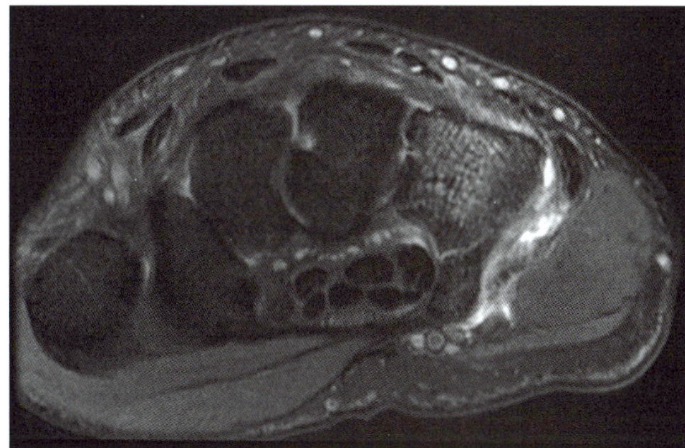

Figure 60.5: Axial T2 MRI image showing acute nondisplaced hook of hamate fracture in a collegiate lacrosse player.

- Excision of the hook of hamate nonunion imparts a higher risk of transient ulnar nerve dysfunction postoperatively than excision of acute hook of hamate fractures. Hook of hamate nonunions is also associated with flexor tendon rupture and ulnar nerve neuropathy. As a result, excision of acute hook of hamate fractures is often the preferred treatment for surgeons and athletes alike.

Body of the Hamate Fractures

- This is a rare (<2%) carpal fracture that frequently occurs due to axial load with clenched fist. It is often associated with fourth and fifth metacarpal fractures or dislocation (26).
- Oblique radiographs of the carpus provide the best visualization. CT scans with 1 mm cuts can assist in diagnosing the fracture and determining optimal treatment.
- Nondisplaced extra-articular fractures are treated with cast immobilization for 4–6 weeks.
- Displaced or intra-articular fractures are treated with closed versus open reduction, Kirschner wire (K wire) or screw fixation, and immobilization for 4–6 weeks (26).

Return to Sports

- Athletes with stable fractures treated by conservative measures may return to sport immediately with protection until pain-free.
- Athletes treated with excision of the hook of hamate may return to sport as tolerated once the wound is healed; hypothenar tenderness may last for several months and may require the use of well-padded gloves for return to sport (20).
- Athletes with surgically treated fractures are restricted from sport until healing is evident on radiographs and the K wires (if used) have been removed (typically 4–6 weeks). Participation may resume with splint or cast protection until normal strength and ROM return (20).

CAPITATE FRACTURES

- Fractures of the capitate account for only 1%–2% of all carpal fractures (27), likely because the capitate is well protected in the center of the carpus.
- Fractures often occur from either a direct blow to the dorsum of the wrist or from forced dorsiflexion or volar flexion. Capitate fractures are often associated with scaphoid fractures and perilunate dislocations (27), which are high-energy injuries that require urgent reduction and often urgent surgical intervention.
- Radiographic assessment is performed with PA, oblique, and lateral views, CT scan, or MRI.
- Nondisplaced fractures are treated with immobilization in short arm cast for 6–8 weeks.
- Displaced capitate fractures are associated with poor outcomes because the fractures are inherently unstable, and delayed union, nonunion, and avascular necrosis are common complications (28).
- Displaced fractures (2 mm of displacement) are treated with ORIF with K wires or screw fixation and immobilized in a short-arm cast for 6 weeks.

Return to Sports

- Athletes with stable, nonoperative fractures may return to sport immediately with protective casting. Close follow-up must be maintained to assure that fracture displacement does not occur, which would necessitate operative intervention (20).
- Athletes with surgically treated fractures are restricted from sport until healing is evident (4–6 weeks). Participation may resume with splint or cast protection for an additional 3 months or until normal strength and ROM return (20).

PISIFORM FRACTURES

- Pisiform fractures are rare and usually occur from direct blow to the palm or fall on the outstretched hand and account for 1%–3% of all carpal fractures (28). Half of pisiform fractures are associated with other carpal injuries (27).
- Patients have tenderness over the hypothenar region or ulnar aspect of the wrist (27).
- Fractures are best visualized on 30° supinated oblique radiographs but often require CT for diagnosis or confirmation.

- Acute, nondisplaced fractures are managed conservatively in a short arm cast for 3–6 weeks.
- Severely comminuted and displaced fractures, symptomatic nonunions, and those associated with persistent ulnar nerve symptoms are managed with pisiform excision, with care to preserve the flexor carpi ulnaris tendon (29).

Return to Sports

- Athletes return to sports as soon as acute pain subsides with taping, padded gloves, or casting as needed. Symptomatic nonunions may be excised subacutely after the season (20,30).

TRIQUETRUM FRACTURES

- Triquetrum fractures are the most common nonscaphoid carpal bone fractures in sports, accounting for 4%–29% of all carpal bone injuries (27).
- Fractures commonly consist of avulsion of the dorsal cortex following hyperextension injury causing impingement with the distal ulna (Fig. 60.6A). The patient will have point tenderness over the fracture, and often pain with flexion and extension of the wrist (27). Other fracture locations include the body or palmar cortex, and are more often associated with other carpal or ligamentous injuries (27). Isolated fractures through the body of the triquetrum are rare injuries and are often associated with scapholunate ligamentous disruption (31).
- PA, lateral, and 45° pronated radiographs are used to identify the fracture.
- Treatment of dorsal cortical fractures is immobilization in short arm cast or brace for 3–4 weeks (27). Treatment of body or palmar cortical fractures is determined by the associated injuries.
- Nonunion of dorsal triquetral fractures occur but are rarely symptomatic and thus rarely, if ever, require further treatment (Fig. 60.6B).

Return to Sports

- Athletes may return to sport wearing a semirigid cast as soon as acute pain resolves or without immobilization when pain does not interfere with sporting activity (32).

LUNATE FRACTURES

- Fractures of the lunate are rare (1% of carpal fractures), in large part to the congruence of the lunate and the lunate facet of the distal radius (27).
- Athletes present with pain and swelling over the dorsum of the wrist.
- Lunate fractures occur through either a compressive force between the capitate and the distal radius or through avulsion-type fractures of the scapholunate or lunotriquetral ligaments (20).
- CT or MRI is often needed for diagnosis.
- Prompt diagnosis, immobilization, and protection from further injury until union are critical to prevent avascular necrosis, carpal instability, or midcarpal arthritis (33).
- Nondisplaced fractures are immobilized in a short arm cast for 6 weeks.
- Displaced fractures require ORIF versus percutaneous fixation to restore radiocarpal and midcarpal stability and alignment, as well as lunate vascularity. Immobilization is continued until fracture healing is evident on radiographs or CT.

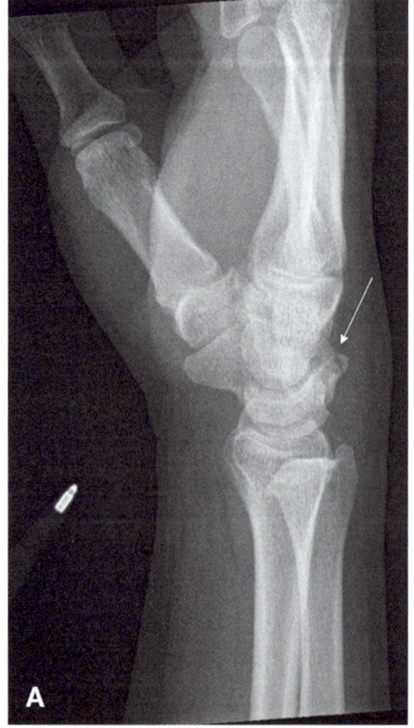

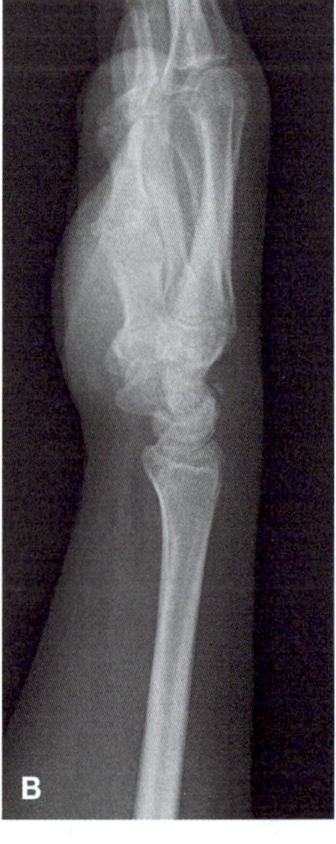

Figure 60.6: Lateral radiographs demonstrating a dorsal triquetral avulsion fracture (A) and subsequent asymptomatic nonunion (B).

Return to Sports

- Athletes may return to sport once fracture healing is evident. Protective splinting is recommended when athletes return to competition until full strength and pain-free ROM is achieved.

TRAPEZIUM FRACTURES

- Fractures of the trapezium constitute 1%–5% of all carpal fractures (20,34). They involve either the longitudinal ridge (the attachment site for the transverse carpal ligament) or the body. They are frequently associated with first metacarpal or distal radius fractures (27).
- Ridge fractures are usually the result of direct trauma such as fall on outstretched hand or being struck by a ball. Body fractures are more common and result from falling on outstretched thumb with resultant splitting of the trapezium body and displacement of the thumb carpometacarpal joint.
- The patient will present with pain distal to the distal pole of the scaphoid, pain with thumb motion, and sometimes weakness with pinch (27).
- Fractures of the trapezium body can be seen on AP and lateral views. A pronated PA view can help visualize the articular surface to detect displacement. The carpal tunnel view is useful to visualize trapezial ridge fractures. A CT scan may be necessary to identify minimally displaced or horizontal fractures.
- Nondisplaced fractures of the trapezium are treated with thumb spica immobilization for 4–6 weeks. ROM and strengthening are then initiated with continued use of a removable thumb spica splint for an additional 2–4 weeks (20).
- Body fractures can be unstable and subject to displacement, requiring close follow-up and vigilance until fracture union is evident (20).
- Displaced body fractures are managed with ORIF with compression screws, K wires, or a combination of both and repair of the capsular structures. Stable internal fixation allows early mobilization (30,35).
- Trapezial ridge fractures with minimal displacement have high rates of nonunion, and surgical excision of the fragment allows for an uncomplicated recovery and early return to sport (36).

Return to Sports

- Patients with nondisplaced fractures treated nonoperatively may return to sport with full activity at 6–8 weeks after treatment initiation (27).
- Trapezial body fractures treated operatively should be protected with immobilization until complete healing and strength and motion have been restored.
- Patients with trapezial ridge fractures treated with excision may return to sport once soft-tissue healing occurs; padded gloves are often required to minimize wound sensitivity that may last for several months (20,30).

TRAPEZOID FRACTURES

- The trapezoid is well-protected position anatomically by the surrounding bones and is the least commonly fractured carpal bone, involved in less than 1% of carpal fractures (20).
- Fracture of the trapezoid is the result of high-energy axially directed trauma along the index metacarpal.
- Trapezoid fractures are visualized on standard AP, lateral, and oblique views, and will show the commonly associated index metacarpal fracture or dislocation as well (27).
- Nondisplaced fractures are treated with immobilization. Displaced fractures or residual joint incongruity are treated with closed reduction and pinning or ORIF with pinning of the index metacarpal in a reduced position (27). The K wires can be removed at 6 weeks, followed by the initiation of hand therapy to restore motion and strength (20).

Return to Sports

- Athletes may return to sport wearing a protective splint once the K wires are removed (20).

METACARPAL FRACTURES

- Metacarpal and phalangeal fractures are the most common fractures in the skeletal system, accounting for greater than 14% of all emergency room visits and greater than 36% of all hand fractures (37,38). The metacarpal neck is the most common site of injury, and the fifth metacarpal is the most commonly injured bone.
- They are often the result of a direct blow or crush injury to the hand or secondary to a fall onto the hand with axial load and rotation.
- Metacarpal fractures typically present with apex dorsal angulation secondary to deforming forces of intrinsic muscles.
- Rotational alignment must be assessed clinically in all metacarpal fractures.
- Fractures are best visualized with standard AP, lateral, and internal and external oblique radiographs of the hand.
- Metacarpal fractures may be classified as transverse, oblique, spiral, and comminuted.

TRANSVERSE FRACTURES

- Apex dorsal fracture angulation is secondary to forces applied by intrinsic muscles. These forces are neutralized by metacarpophalangeal joints (MCP) joint flexion.

- Reduction is typically indicated for angulation in the second and third metacarpals over 10°–20°, for the fourth metacarpal over 30°, and for the fifth metacarpal over 40° (38). For any digit, over 2–5 mm of shortening is often not accepted.

Treatment

- Most stable fractures within the acceptable reduction parameters without any rotational deformity can be treated with cast or brace immobilization for 4 weeks (38). The MCP joints should be immobilized in 90° of flexion and the PIP joints should be left free.
- Treatment for unstable fractures or fractures that fail closed treatment involves closed reduction and percutaneous pinning, cross pinning to an adjacent metacarpal, or open reduction and internal fixation with an intramedullary screw or a dorsal plate and screws (38,39).
- Stable fixation requires no protection postoperatively except for sport, with light active use permitted at 5 days postoperatively (38).

OBLIQUE AND SPIRAL FRACTURES

- Oblique and spiral fractures result from torsional forces to the metacarpal. This is an unstable pattern and often leads to shortening and rotational deformity.
- Any rotational deformity is unacceptable because 5° of malrotation can lead to 1.5–2.0 cm of digit overlap.
- Up to 5 mm of shortening can be accepted without functional deficit (11).

Treatment

- Isolated, minimally displaced fractures may be treated by closed methods similar to the treatment of transverse fractures.
- Fractures that cannot be maintained with closed methods require either percutaneous pinning or ORIF.
- Interfragmentary lag screw fixation may be used if fracture length is twice the bone diameter and provides the most biomechanically stable construct. For fractures with a shorter obliquity, a lag screw and dorsal neutralization plate can provide stable fixation, permitting early return to sport (40).

COMMINUTED FRACTURES

- Comminuted fractures are usually the result of high-energy trauma and may be associated with soft-tissue loss.
- The treatment often requires ORIF or external fixation to maintain metacarpal length and may require delayed or primary bone grafting.
- Return to play following these injuries requires significantly more time to restore satisfactory stability, typically 4–6 weeks, or occasionally longer.

METACARPAL HEAD FRACTURES

- These are rare fractures that occur from axial loading or direct trauma and must be examined closely to ensure there is not an open wound. Any wound over the dorsum of the MCP joint should be considered an open "fight bite" until proven otherwise.
- Nondisplaced fractures may be treated nonoperatively with splint immobilization followed by buddy taping and early ROM (41).
- Any amount of displacement requires ORIF to restore anatomic alignment and articular congruity. If early motion cannot be started, then immobilization in the intrinsic plus position should be maintained until motion can be initiated (41).
- Complications include loss of motion and arthritis. MCP arthroplasty or fusion are salvage surgical options in cases of severe comminution or arthritis.

METACARPAL NECK FRACTURES

- Metacarpal neck fractures most commonly involve the fourth or fifth metacarpals (boxer's fracture).
- Apex dorsal angulation and volar comminution may complicate maintenance of reduction with cast immobilization.
- Angular deformity of 50°–60° is acceptable in the small finger, 30°–40° in the ring finger, and 10°–15° in the index or middle fingers. The difference in acceptability is due to the mobility of the carpometacarpal joints increasing from the index to the small finger (38).
- Initial treatment is closed reduction by the Jahss technique (40) and immobilization in a short arm ulnar gutter splint with the fingers in the intrinsic plus position for 2 weeks, then buddy taping and motion are initiated (42).
- Radiographs should be obtained weekly to assure that reduction is not lost.
- Surgical intervention is indicated for fractures outside the acceptable parameters listed hereinbefore, open fractures, or fractures with any rotational malalignment. Operative intervention may include closed or open reduction with percutaneous pinning or internal fixation with a plate or intramedullary screw (38).
- Bouquet pinning with the insertion of multiple small intramedullary K wires down the metacarpal shaft and across the fracture into the metacarpal head can provide stable fixation and early return of unrestricted hand function in fractures that would otherwise require lengthy immobilization (38).

- The hand is immobilized in a splint for 2 weeks, after which motion is initiated with return to sports at preinjury level within 6 weeks.

METACARPAL BASE FRACTURES

- Metacarpal base fractures are rare. They usually have a stable configuration secondary to a set of four strong interosseous ligaments.
- Second and third carpometacarpal joints have limited motion, whereas the fourth and fifth carpometacarpal joints have 15° and 30° of mobility, respectively (38).
- Nondisplaced or minimally displaced fractures are treated in a short arm cast typically with the MCP joints and the interphalangeal joints free.
- Immobilization is maintained for 6 weeks, followed by buddy taping for 2 weeks to maintain rotational control and allow initiation of motion (41).
- Displaced fractures often require closed or open reduction followed by percutaneous fixation with splint immobilization, then gradual restoration of motion at 6 weeks after injury (38,41).
- Patients with malunited fractures may experience grip weakness or pain with progression of arthritis. These patients may be treated with arthrodesis (41).

Return to Sports After Metacarpal Fractures

- Almost all patients are able to return to sports at preinjury levels of competition, typically within 3–4 weeks. Return to sports may be initiated within 1–2 weeks from injury depending on the requirements of the specific sport and nonoperative versus operative treatment. Fractures treated with rigid internal fixation may allow the athlete earlier return to play than nonoperative treatment (43).
- Athletes may return to contact sports without protection as early as 2 weeks after internal fixation of non-thumb metacarpal fractures treated with internal fixation (44).

THUMB METACARPAL FRACTURES

- Thumb metacarpal fractures are unique due to the thumb's critical role in hand functions, grasp, and power pinch (45).
- Over one-fourth of all metacarpal fractures are to the thumb metacarpal, with 80% of those occurring at the base, resulting from axial load across the partially flexed thumb (45).
- Radiographic imaging of the thumb includes AP (Robert's view) and lateral (hand with 30° pronation and beam directed 15° distally) projections (45).
- The thumb carpometacarpal joint is a reciprocal saddle-shaped surface of the distal trapezium and proximal metacarpal that allows for flexion-extension and abduction-adduction of the thumb (45).
- Intra-articular Bennett (partial articular) and Rolando (complete articular) fractures are commonly displaced dorsally and radially due to the pull of abductor pollicis longus and extensor pollicis longus. Adductor pollicis creates a supination and adduction force on the shaft fragment (46).
- Anatomic joint reduction is necessary to decrease the risk of early arthritis (45).
- Extra-articular fractures with greater than 30° angulation, intra-articular fractures with over 1 mm step-off or comminution require operative treatment with either closed reduction and percutaneous pinning or internal fixation (38).
- Closed reduction and thumb spica casting for nonoperative fractures may be attempted with traction, abduction, and pronation of the thumb (38).
- Severely comminuted intra-articular Rolando fractures may require external fixation followed by limited ORIF with bone grafting (42).
- Immobilization is necessary for a minimum of 6 weeks followed by initiation of ROM and hand therapy for optimal results (45).

Return to Sports

- Athletes may return to sport with immobilization in thumb spica splint or cast as symptoms and sport-specific activity permit. Protection should be maintained until fracture healing is evident on radiographs and strength, stability, and motion are restored.
- Operative intervention with stable fixation may allow for earlier initiation of motion and return to sports than nonoperative management (46) (Fig. 60.7).

PHALANGEAL FRACTURES

Proximal and Middle Phalanx Fractures

- Proximal and middle phalanx fractures are very common in athletes participating in contact sports or ball-catching sports. Phalanx fractures are the most common skeletal injury.
- Fracture displacement depends on the mechanism of injury and subsequent deforming forces of the intrinsic and extrinsic flexors and extensors.
- Proximal phalanx fractures typically have apex volar angulation with the proximal segment flexed by the interossei and the distal segment extended by the central slip portion of the extensor mechanism (38).
- Middle phalanx fractures are deformed by both the central slip and by the flexor digitorum superficialis resulting in either volar or dorsal angulation depending on the location of the fracture relative to these tendon insertions (38).

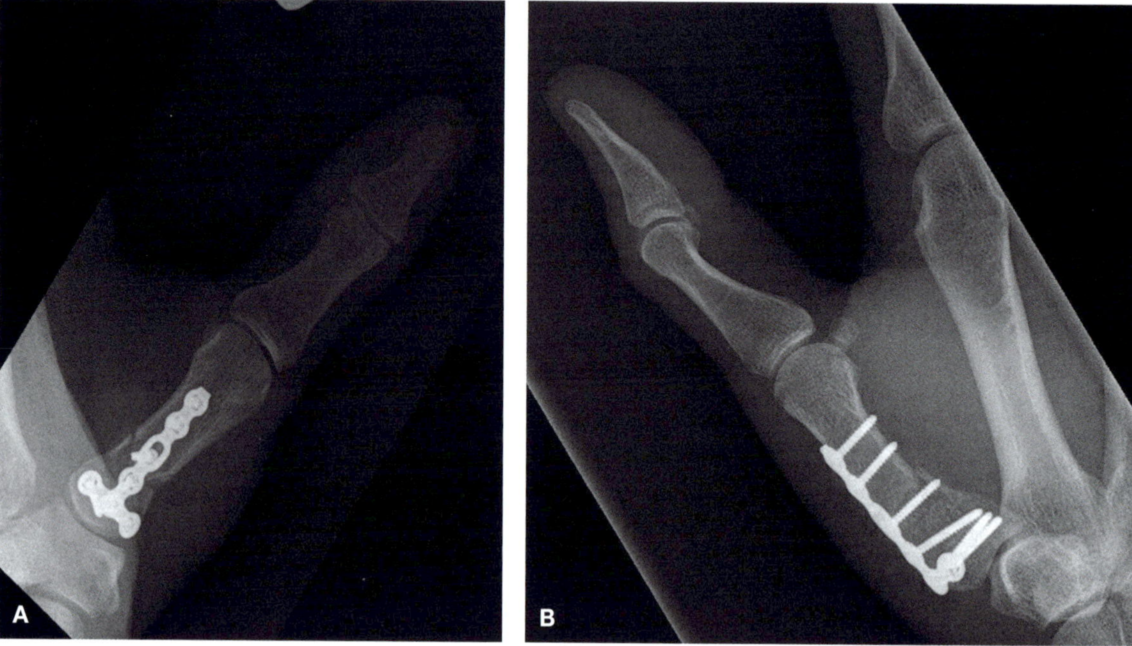

Figure 60.7: AP and lateral (A and B) radiographs of a professional ice hockey player who underwent plate and screw fixation for a displaced, extra-articular thumb metacarpal fracture 3 weeks before. The patient returned to full sport with a protective splint 4 weeks after surgery.

- Treatment depends on the stability of the fracture, rotational deformity, and angulation. Any rotational deformity, shortening greater than 2 mm, articular displacement more than 2 mm, and angular deformity greater than 10° requires correction.
- Nondisplaced and stable fractures can be treated with buddy taping and early ROM (38).
- Displaced fractures require closed reduction and immobilization with cast or splint. (38).
- Fracture immobilization should be limited to 3 weeks, followed by initiation of hand therapy to facilitate maximal restoration of motion, and protective splinting should be continued during sport-specific activities until healing is evident (38).
- Intra-articular, unstable, or rotationally displaced fractures may benefit from open or closed reduction and internal or percutaneous fixation to restore anatomic alignment and rotational control (47).
- If rigid fixation is obtained, mobilization to regain ROM and edema control should begin within the first week, permitting earlier return to sport and a more predictable functional outcome (38).
- Protective splinting should be maintained for 4 weeks or until fracture healing is evident. Buddy taping should be continued until ROM and strength are restored (47).

Distal Phalanx Fractures

- Distal phalanx fractures account for 50% of all hand fractures, most commonly to the thumb and middle finger.
- It is important to examine for associated nail bed injuries.
- Tuft fractures occur at the distal aspect of the distal phalanx and are stable due to the overlying nail plate and underlying volar pulp. They may be associated with nail bed lacerations.
- If a nail bed injury is present and the nail plate has been disrupted, the nail bed must be repaired to prevent nail deformity (48).
- Immobilization is restricted to the distal interphalangeal joint for a period of 3–4 weeks, after which motion is initiated (38).
- Tenderness may persist for over 6 months, requiring a program of desensitization to allow full return of function (18).
- Bony mallet finger injuries result in loss of continuity of extensor mechanism. In the absence of joint subluxation, nonoperative treatment is usually successful, with continuous extension splinting of the distal interphalangeal (DIP) joint for a minimum of 6 weeks followed by the removal of the splint several times a day for active ROM exercises for an additional 2 weeks.

Return to Sports After Phalangeal Fractures

- Athletes with stable fractures treated nonoperatively may return to sports with rigid cast immobilization, thermoplast splint protection, or buddy taping (as sport-specific activities permit) as soon as symptoms allow (49).
- Close follow-up must be maintained to ensure that loss of reduction or malrotation does not occur.

- Protection should be maintained until radiographic evidence of healing is evident and functional recovery of ROM and strength is complete.
- Athletes with surgically treated fractures may return to sports with protective splinting or casting once soft-tissue healing allows.
- Edema control and active motion are typically initiated at 2 weeks, and by 4 weeks, 75% of motion should have been regained and strengthening can be initiated. Protective splinting should be maintained for sport-specific activities until healing is evident (38). Buddy taping should be maintained until strength and motion have been regained.

SUMMARY

- Athletes of all levels frequently sustain hand and wrist fractures that vary greatly in severity and significance.
- These fractures can lead to significant disability and time away from sport, or they may allow expeditious return to play and return to normal function.
- Many factors are considered when the physician and athlete decide to return to sport, and the decision is always made on a case-by-case basis after all these factors have been considered.

REFERENCES

1. Simpson D, McQueen MM. Acute sporting injuries to the hand and wrist in the general population. *Scott Med J.* 2006;51(2):25–6. doi:10.1258/rsmsmj.51.2.25
2. Mandelbaum BR, Bartolozzi AR, Davis CA, Teurlings L, Bragonier B. Wrist pain syndrome in the gymnast. Pathogenetic, diagnostic, and therapeutic considerations. *Am J Sports Med.* 1989;17(3):305–17. doi:10.1177/036354658901700301
3. Owen RA, Melton LJ III, Johnson KA, Ilstrup DM, Riggs BL. Incidence of Colles' fracture in a North American community. *Am J Public Health.* 1982;72(6):605–7. doi:10.2105/ajph.72.6.605
4. Jupiter JB. Fractures of the distal end of the radius. *J Bone Joint Surg Am.* 1991;73(3):461–9.
5. Nypaver C, Bozentka DJ. Distal radius fracture and the distal radioulnar joint. *Hand Clin.* 2021;37(2):293–307. doi:10.1016/j.hcl.2021.02.011
6. Mohanti RC, Kar N. Study of triangular fibrocartilage of the wrist joint in Colles' fracture. *Injury.* 1980;11(4):321–4. doi:10.1016/0020-1383(80)90105-9
7. Pope D, Tang P. Carpal tunnel syndrome and distal radius fractures. *Hand Clin.* 2018;34(1):27–32. doi:10.1016/j.hcl.2017.09.003
8. Koval K, Haidukewych GJ, Service B, Zirgibel BJ. Controversies in the management of distal radius fractures. *J Am Acad Orthop Surg.* 2014;22(9):566–75. doi:10.5435/jaaos-22-09-566
9. Knirk JL, Jupiter JB. Intra-articular fractures of the distal end of the radius in young adults. *J Bone Joint Surg Am.* 1986;68(5):647–59.
10. Lichtman DM, Bindra RR, Boyer MI, et al. Treatment of distal radius fractures. *J Am Acad Orthop Surg.* 2010;18(3):180–9. doi:10.5435/00124635-201003000-00007
11. Jupiter JB, Fernandez DL, Toh CL, Fellman T, Ring D. Operative treatment of volar intra-articular fractures of the distal end of the radius. *J Bone Joint Surg Am.* 1996;78(12):1817–28. doi:10.2106/00004623-199612000-00004
12. Bass RL, Blair WF, Hubbard PP. Results of combined internal and external fixation for the treatment of severe AO-C3 fractures of the distal radius. *J Hand Surg Am.* 1995;20(3):373–81. doi:10.1016/s0363-5023(05)80090-5
13. Geissler WB, Freeland AE, Savoie FH, McIntyre LW, Whipple TL. Intracarpal soft-tissue lesions associated with an intra-articular fracture of the distal end of the radius. *J Bone Joint Surg Am.* 1996;78(3):357–65. doi:10.2106/00004623-199603000-00006
14. Cooney WP III, Dobyns JH, Linscheid RL. Complications of Colles' fractures. *J Bone Joint Surg Am.* 1980;62(4):613–9.
15. Sobel AD, Calfee RP. Distal radius fractures in the athlete. *Clin Sports Med.* 2020;39(2):299–311. doi:10.1016/j.csm.2019.10.005
16. Zemel NP, Stark HH. Fractures and dislocations of the carpal bones. *Clin Sports Med.* 1986;5(4):709–24.
17. Symes TH, Stothard J. A systematic review of the treatment of acute fractures of the scaphoid. *J Hand Surg Eur Vol.* 2011;36(9):802–10. doi:10.1177/1753193411412151
18. Dias JJ, Wildin CJ, Bhowal B, Thompson JR. Should acute scaphoid fractures be fixed? A randomized controlled trial. *J Bone Joint Surg Am.* 2005;87(10):2160–8. doi:10.2106/jbjs.D.02305
19. Gellman H, Caputo RJ, Carter V, Aboulafia A, McKay M. Comparison of short and long thumb-spica casts for non-displaced fractures of the carpal scaphoid. *J Bone Joint Surg Am.* 1989;71(3):354–7.
20. Geissler WB. Carpal fractures in athletes. *Clin Sports Med.* 2001;20(1):167–88. doi:10.1016/s0278-5919(05)70254-4
21. Rizzo M, Shin AY. Treatment of acute scaphoid fractures in the athlete. *Curr Sports Med Rep.* 2006;5(5):242–8. doi:10.1097/01.csmr.0000306422.24038.1f
22. Dy CJ, Khmelnitskaya E, Hearns KA, Carlson MG. Opinions regarding the management of hand and wrist injuries in elite athletes. *Orthopedics.* 2013;36(6):815–9. doi:10.3928/01477447-20130523-30
23. Jernigan EW, Morse KW, Carlson MG. Managing the athlete with a scaphoid fracture. *Hand Clin.* 2019;35(3):365–71. doi:10.1016/j.hcl.2019.03.011
24. Bishop AT, Beckenbaugh RD. Fracture of the hamate hook. *J Hand Surg Am.* 1988;13(1):135–9. doi:10.1016/0363-5023(88)90217-1
25. Parker RD, Berkowitz MS, Brahms MA, Bohl WR. Hook of the hamate fractures in athletes. *Am J Sports Med.* 1986;14(6):517–23. doi:10.1177/036354658601400617
26. Price MB, Vanorny D, Mitchell S, Wu C. Hamate body fractures: a comprehensive review of the literature. *Curr Rev Musculoskelet Med.* 2021;14(6):475–84. doi:10.1007/s12178-021-09731-6
27. Mahmood B, Lee SK. Carpal fractures other than scaphoid in the athlete. *Clin Sports Med.* 2020;39(2):353–71. doi:10.1016/j.csm.2019.12.006
28. Rand JA, Linscheid RL, Dobyns JH. Capitate fractures: a long-term follow-up. *Clin Orthop Relat Res.* 1982;165:209–16.
29. Arner M, Hagberg L. Wrist flexion strength after excision of the pisiform bone. *Scand J Plast Reconstr Surg.* 1984;18(2):241–5. doi:10.3109/02844318409052845
30. Rettig ME, Dassa GL, Raskin KB, Melone CP Jr. Wrist fractures in the athlete. Distal radius and carpal fractures. *Clin Sports Med.* 1998;17(3):469–89. doi:10.1016/s0278-5919(05)70097-1
31. Herzberg G, Comtet JJ, Linscheid RL, Amadio PC, Cooney WP, Stalder J. Perilunate dislocations and fracture-dislocations: a multicenter study. *J Hand Surg Am.* 1993;18(5):768–79. doi:10.1016/0363-5023(93)90041-z
32. Höcker K, Menschik A. Chip fractures of the triquetrum. Mechanism, classification and results. *J Hand Surg Br.* 1994;19(5):584–8. doi:10.1016/0266-7681(94)90120-1

33. Beckenbaugh RD, Shives TC, Dobyns JH, Linscheid RL. Kienböck's disease: the natural history of Kienböck's disease and consideration of lunate fractures. *Clin Orthop Relat Res.* 1980;149:98–106.
34. Botte MJ, Gelberman RH. Fractures of the carpus, excluding the scaphoid. *Hand Clin.* 1987;3(1):149–61.
35. Cordrey LJ, Ferrer-Torells M. Management of fractures of the greater multangular. Report of five cases. *J Bone Joint Surg Am.* 1960;42-A:1111–8.
36. Palmer AK. Trapezial ridge fractures. *J Hand Surg Am.* 1981;6(6):561–4. doi:10.1016/s0363-5023(81)80132-3
37. Packer GJ, Shaheen MA. Patterns of hand fractures and dislocations in a district general hospital. *J Hand Surg Br.* 1993;18(4):511–4. doi:10.1016/0266-7681(93)90161-8
38. Capo JT, Hastings H II. Metacarpal and phalangeal fractures in athletes. *Clin Sports Med.* 1998;17(3):491–511. doi:10.1016/s0278-5919(05)70098-3
39. Taghinia AH, Talbot SG. Phalangeal and metacarpal fractures. *Clin Plast Surg.* 2019;46(3):415–23. doi:10.1016/j.cps.2019.02.011
40. Black D, Mann RJ, Constine R, Daniels AU. Comparison of internal fixation techniques in metacarpal fractures. *J Hand Surg Am.* 1985;10(4):466–72. doi:10.1016/s0363-5023(85)80067-8
41. Palmer RE. Joint injuries of the hand in athletes. *Clin Sports Med.* 1998;17(3):513–31. doi:10.1016/s0278-5919(05)70099-5
42. Buchler U, McCollam SM, Oppikofer C. Comminuted fractures of the basilar joint of the thumb: combined treatment by external fixation, limited internal fixation, and bone grafting. *J Hand Surg Am.* 1991;16(3):556–60. doi:10.1016/0363-5023(91)90032-7
43. Geoghegan L, Scarborough A, Rodrigues JN, Hayton MJ, Horwitz MD. Return to sport after metacarpal and phalangeal fractures: a systematic review and evidence appraisal. *Orthop J Sports Med.* 2021;9(2):2325967120980013. doi:10.1177/2325967120980013
44. Yalizis MA, Ek ETH, Anderson H, Couzens G, Hoy GA. Early unprotected return to contact sport after metacarpal fixation in professional athletes. *Bone Joint J.* 2017;99-B(10):1343–7. doi:10.1302/0301-620x.99b10.Bjj-2016-0686.R3
45. Soyer AD. Fractures of the base of the first metacarpal: current treatment options. *J Am Acad Orthop Surg.* 1999;7(6):403–12. doi:10.5435/00124635-199911000-00006
46. Langford SA, Whitaker JH, Toby EB. Thumb injuries in the athlete. *Clin Sports Med.* 1998;17(3):553–66. doi:10.1016/s0278-5919(05)70101-0
47. Kozin SH, Thoder JJ, Lieberman G. Operative treatment of metacarpal and phalangeal shaft fractures. *J Am Acad Orthop Surg.* 2000;8(2):111–21. doi:10.5435/00124635-200003000-00005
48. Simon RR, Wolgin M. Subungual hematoma: association with occult laceration requiring repair. *Am J Emerg Med.* 1987;5(4):302–4. doi:10.1016/0735-6757(87)90356-1
49. Alexy C, De Carlo M. Rehabilitation and use of protective devices in hand and wrist injuries. *Clin Sports Med.* 1998;17(3):635–55. doi:10.1016/s0278-5919(05)70106-x

Upper Extremity Nerve Entrapment

Justin Tu and Jeffrey Jenkins

61

GENERAL PRINCIPLES OF UPPER EXTREMITY NERVE ENTRAPMENT

Epidemiology

- The most common nerve entrapment is the carpal tunnel syndrome (CTS). Its occurrence is 3.46 cases per 1000 person-years. Female-to-male ratio is about 3.1 (1). The next highest incidence is entrapment of the ulnar nerve at the elbow. Krivickas and Wilbourn (2) studied 180 athletes with sports injuries in the electrodiagnostic (EDX) laboratory, of whom 23% had median nerve injuries, 22% stingers, 10.5% radial nerve lesions, 10.5% ulnar nerve compression syndromes, 12% axillary nerve problems, and 7.8% entrapment of the suprascapular nerve (SSN) only. Per Olivo and Tsao, nerve injuries occurring during a particular sport were responsible for less than 0.5% of all traumatic peripheral nerve injuries, but concede that this rate could be higher in the United States (3).

Pathophysiology

- Nerve entrapment occurs when a nerve passes through a tight space, placing it at risk for mechanical compression as well as ischemia secondary to pressure on the vasa nervorum. Persistent compression results in predictable, progressive degrees of nerve damage, as classified by Seddon: neurapraxia, axonotmesis, and neurotmesis (1). The degree of nerve damage can be further classified based on damage to the endoneurium, perineurium, and/or epineurium, as per the Sunderland classification (see Chapter 9, Nerve Injury, for further discussion).
    - Neurapraxia (conduction block) is reversible. Demyelination may result.
    - Large myelinated fibers are most vulnerable. Duration of compression determines degree of damage (may last minutes to months).
    - Axonotmesis specifies axonal damage, with endoneurium and perineurium variably injured as per the Sunderland classification. Wallerian degeneration ensues. Preservation of endoneurial tubes will provide a guide for regeneration of axons. Recovery can take months.
    - Neurotmesis represents complete disruption of axons, including the endoneurium, perineurium, and epineurium. There is poor functional outcome. Surgery usually indicated.

Risk Factors

- Narrowed space in bony and/or muscular tendinous/fibrous canals/tunnels.
    - Examples: thoracic outlet, quadrilateral space, Struthers ligament, anomalous bone spurs, muscles or fibrous bands, cubital tunnel, radial tunnel, carpal tunnel, Guyon canal, excessive callous formation after (especially malunited) fracture
- Injury
    - Acute: compression, stretch, percussion
    - Chronic: repetitive motion, excessive pressure from equipment
    - Paralysis of cervical/thoracic muscles secondary to myelopathy
- **Medical conditions:** endocrine problems (pregnancy, hypothyroidism, diabetes mellitus), compartment syndrome, peripheral neuropathy

Symptoms and Signs

- Pain, paresthesias, and weakness in distribution of the affected nerve
- Lesions of pure motor nerves (anterior/posterior interosseous, suprascapular, and long thoracic nerves) cause weakness and/or muscle atrophy

Evaluation

- Special tests: Tinel test at the wrist and elbow, Durkan/carpal compression test, Phalen's test, Spurling's maneuver, Adson maneuver, Wright (hyperabduction) test, Roos test, and pectoralis minor and costoclavicular maneuvers that may reproduce symptoms
- Persistent minor pain due to entrapment may cause a regional pain syndrome — type 1 CRPS, previously referred to as reflex sympathetic dystrophy.

Electrodiagnosis (see Chapter 23, Principles of Electrodiagnosis)

- Electromyography (EMG) and nerve conduction studies (NCS) are significant factors in establishing the correct diagnosis of entrapment syndromes. Typical findings include the following:
  - EMG shows decreased motor unit recruitment, increase in polyphasia, action potential durations and amplitudes, and in more severe cases, fibrillations and positive sharp waves. Complex repetitive discharges denote chronicity. EMG demonstrates the severity of the abnormality, especially if there is evidence of denervation, which has considerable impact on treatment decisions.
  - Conduction delay across the site of compression; reduced amplitudes due to blocking or axonal loss (with normal duration) proximal to the site of compression, or secondary to demyelination (with increased duration).

Differential Diagnosis

- Major diagnoses to be ruled out with EMG and NCS are:
  - Radiculopathy
  - Peripheral neuropathy
  - Plexopathy, including neuralgic amyotrophy (Parsonage-Turner syndrome), myopathy, and malingering

Treatment

- Several studies have demonstrated improvement of symptoms seen with mild CTS with 5 percent dextrose in water (D5W) and platelet-rich plasma injectates (4).
- A study from Gill et al. revealed improvement of symptoms attributable to radial tunnel syndrome with ultrasound-guided hydrodissection (5).
- See Chapter 9, Nerve Injury, for a further discussion of additional management considerations.

SPECIFIC NERVE ENTRAPMENTS OF THE UPPER EXTREMITY (SEE TABLE 61.1)

Radiculopathy

- Major differential diagnosis in all entrapment syndromes. However, it also is subject to its own compression and entrapment (C7 > C6 > C8) (6).

Anatomy

- Entrapment is caused by pressure on a spinal nerve as it exits the spine. Primary anterior compression (disc herniation) may selectively affect motor fibers. It may spare the dorsal ramus, sparing sensation. Posterior compression may selectively affect sensory fibers. Compression of the nerve root can occur from any direction within the intervertebral foramen but most commonly occurs due to posterolateral disc herniation or facet degeneration.

Risk Factors

- Cervical spondylosis
- Cervical disc degeneration/herniation
- Facet degeneration
- Space-occupying lesions
- Prior cervical spine trauma or surgery

Symptoms and Signs

- Sensory complaints
- Weakness and reflex changes in root distribution
- Provocative maneuvers including Spurling often positive

Evaluation

- Motor, sensory, and reflex examination
- Provocative maneuver: Spurling — pressure on laterally and posteriorly tilted head reproduces typically sensory symptoms in the affected root distribution
- Shoulder abduction test: Evaluate for relief of symptoms with shoulder abduction as the nerve is taken off tension
- Imaging modalities (cervical spine plain films, magnetic resonance imaging)

Differential Diagnosis

- Peripheral neuropathy
- Brachial plexitis
- Entrapment neuropathies
- Neurologic disease

Treatment

- Indications for immediate surgical referral are as follows:
  - Progressive neurological deficit, bowel or bladder dysfunction, and severe pain refractory to other approaches including physical therapy, modalities, oral and topical analgesics, and epidural steroid injections.
  - Surgery usually includes nerve root decompression, laminectomy, and discectomy if needed, and possible cervical fusion.
- Conservative treatment
  - Pain medications, nonsteroidal anti-inflammatory drugs (NSAIDs)
  - Antispasmodics, antiepileptics, and antidepressants
- Physical therapy modalities:
  - Strengthening exercises, biomechanical mobilization
  - Cervical traction
  - Flexibility
  - Alignment and postural techniques as indicated
  - Transcutaneous electrical nerve stimulation (TENS) and biofeedback
- Epidural steroid injections may help facilitate physical therapy and reduce pain and inflammation.

Table 61.1 Clinical Features of Common Upper Extremity Entrapment Neuropathies

Nerve	Site(s) of Compression	Motor Findings	Sensory Findings	Other Findings
Spinal accessory	Posterior triangle of the neck	Difficulty with shrug of the ipsilateral shoulder; if more proximal lesion, could see weakness with turning head to opposite side	Pain at the neck and upper back, occasionally to the ipsilateral arm	Lateral winging of the scapula
Dorsal scapular	Within the middle scalene muscle	Weakness with pressing the elbow backward against resistance with hand along the hip, or with pushing the palm backward against resistance with arm folded behind the back		Scapular winging with lateral displacement
Long thoracic	Supraclavicular region	Weakness in raising arm above the head		Scapular winging medially with patient pushing arm against wall and with elbow extended
Suprascapular	Suprascapular notch	Weakness with abduction and external rotation of shoulder		Deep scapular pain
	Spinoglenoid notch	Weakness of external rotation of shoulder		Deep scapular pain
Musculocutaneous	At the coracobrachialis	Elbow flexor and forearm supination weakness	Lateral forearm	Proximal forearm pain; decreased biceps reflex
Axillary	Lateral aspect of humerus; quadrilateral space	Weakness of shoulder abduction between 15° and 90°	Lateral shoulder	Deltoid atrophy
Median	Carpal tunnel	Potentially weak hand grip; weakness with thumb flexion, abduction, and opposition with advanced disease	Intermittent, nocturnal paresthesias and numbness in digits 1–3 and radial half of digit 4	Positive Tinel sign at wrist and Phalen sign; positive carpal compression maneuver
	Proximal arch of FDS, pronator teres	Weak handgrip	Numbness of thumb and index finger	Aching pain with resisted flexion to middle finger; pain with active resisted forearm pronation, elbow flexion, and finger flexion; possible Tinel over pronator teres
	Typically forearm within fibrous arch of FDS, less often by Gantzer muscle (accessory FPL)	Weakness with thumb, index, and third finger flexion; forearm pronation	No sensory symptoms	
	Ligament of Struthers	Weakness with all median nerve–innervated muscles	Tingling and numbness in median nerve distribution	Swelling of hand forearm with brachial vein constriction, and blanching with brachial artery compromise
Ulnar nerve	Retro-epicondylar groove	Weakness and possible atrophy in ulnar-innervated hand intrinsic muscles; diminished grip strength	Pain, paresthesias, and numbness in fifth and ulnar half of fourth digits, as well as hypothenar eminence	Positive Tinel sign at elbow; Wartenberg and Froment signs
	Cubital tunnel	Similar to entrapment at retro-epicondylar groove	Similar to entrapment at retro-epicondylar groove	Similar to entrapment at retro-epicondylar groove
	Guyon canal	Potentially weak hand grasp	Numbness and tingling at volar fifth and ulnar half of fourth digits	Positive Wartenberg and Froment signs

(continued)

Table 61.1 Clinical Features of Common Upper Extremity Entrapment Neuropathies (*Continued*)

Nerve	Site(s) of Compression	Motor Findings	Sensory Findings	Other Findings
Radial nerve	Spiral groove	Weak forearm extensors (wrist drop), slight weakness of elbow flexors with brachioradialis involvement; possible triceps involvement	Pain, paresthesias, and numbness in posterior forearm and dorsal hand	
	Supinator syndrome (arcade of Frohse)	Partial wrist drop, weakness in posterior interosseous nerve distribution	No notable sensory deficit	
	Distal radial nerve (Cheiralgia paresthetica, Wartenberg syndrome)	No motor deficits	Sensory deficits in distal superficial radial nerve distribution	

FDS, flexor digitorum superficialis; FPL, flexor pollicis longus.
Adapted from Floranda EE, Jacobs BC. Evaluation and treatment of upper extremity nerve entrapment syndromes. *Prim Care*. 2013 Dec;40(4):925–43, ix.

Spinal Accessory Nerve: Cranial Nerve XI

Anatomy

- The trapezius, the major muscle supplied by the spinal accessory nerve, is a significant scapular stabilizer and thereby critical for the maintenance of efficient shoulder function (7).
- It originates on the occipital protuberance, the ligamentum nuchae, and spinous processes of C7–T12. The upper portion inserts at the lateral clavicle and the acromion (upward rotation of the scapula), the middle portion inserts in the spine of the scapula (retracts the scapula), and the lower portion inserts in the root of the spine of the scapula (depresses and upward rotates the scapula).
- Nerve supply is through the spinal component of cranial nerve (CN) XI. It originates from the anterior horn cells of the cervical spinal cord (C1–C4) (8). Fibers enter the skull through the foramen magnum. The cranial component of the accessory nerve arises from the caudal part of the nucleus ambiguous. It is closely related to the vagus nerve (CN X). The cranial and spinal components, together with CN X, leave the skull through the jugular foramen and then separate again.
- An important fact of the central connections is that the corticobulbar tract from the midbrain eventually terminates in the brainstem, where the fibers to the trapezius muscle are crossed (therefore, central lesions cause contralateral deficit), whereas the corticobulbar fibers to the sternocleidomastoid muscle are either uncrossed or, more likely, double decussate (therefore, lesions are ipsilateral). These deficits help to localize the lesion.
- In the neck, the spinal component of the accessory nerve passes through the posterior triangle (anterior border: sternocleidomastoid; posterior: trapezius; and inferior: clavicle). The roof is the platysma, and the floor is the splenius capitis, levator scapulae, and medial and posterior scalene muscles.
- The triangle is subdivided by the traversing omohyoid. The superior space is the occipital triangle and below is the supraclavicular triangle.
- The contents of the occipital triangle are as follows:
  - Superior trunk of brachial plexus between the anterior and middle scalene muscles
  - Branches of C5, C6, and C7
  - Dorsal scapular nerve (supplies levator scapulae and rhomboids)
  - Long thoracic nerve (innervates serratus anterior)
- The spinal accessory nerve also passes through this space, after giving off a branch to supply the sternocleidomastoid muscle. It then supplies the trapezius muscle. This location is vulnerable for injury and compression. (Also, space for nerve stimulation and conduction studies.)
- The contents of the supraclavicular triangle are as follows:
  - Middle trunk of brachial plexus
  - SSN (supplies the supraspinatus and infraspinatus muscles)
  - Nerve to subclavius muscle
  - Lower trunk of brachial plexus (C8)
  - Subclavian artery
  - External jugular vein descends across sternocleidomastoid muscle to drain into subclavian vein

Risk Factors

- Intracranial: head injuries (especially basal skull fracture)
- Intraspinal cord: posttraumatic syrinx
- Cervical:
  - Percussion or compression of the accessory nerve in the posterior triangle in sports leading to nerve contusion potentially (football, ill-fitting shoulder pads, judo, karate, kickboxing) (9)
  - Blows to the shoulder with a hockey stick
  - Backpack straps and shoulder dislocations
  - Mild to moderate (rarely severe) lesions results in stingers/burners, and occasionally involve nerve roots (10)
  - Traumatic penetrating neck injuries

- Atraumatic, iatrogenic lesions, acute or delayed, mainly after radical neck dissections or lymph node biopsies
- Cannulation of internal jugular vein or after carotid endarterectomies (due to hemorrhages, hematomas, malpositioned suction drainage, infection, or scarring)
- Deep tissue massage
- Spontaneous accessory nerve lesion (trapezius weakness) (11)
- Tumor
- Must rule out neuropathic or myopathic diseases

Symptoms and Signs

- Shoulder syndrome: consists of shoulder drooping, acromion prominence, limited lateral abduction, and impaired forward shoulder flexion
- Lateral winging visualized due to unopposed action of the serratus anterior muscle (8)
- Aberrant scapular rotation, abnormal scapulohumeral rhythm
- Abnormal EDX findings
- Significant pain and tenderness over trapezius, exacerbated by shoulder movement
- Feeling of heaviness in the affected arm may be present
- Difficulty with overhead activities, heavy lifting, prolonged writing, or driving
- Possible impingement pain secondary to inability to rotate scapula, thereby causing the greater tuberosity to abut the acromion (12)
- Late onset of pain is mostly due to adhesive capsulitis, a common sequela of spinal accessory nerve injury
- Proximal lesions of the spinal accessory nerve are less common, but would result in sternocleidomastoid weakness in addition to trapezius weakness

Evaluation

- Test trapezius strength by resistance to lateral abduction of the arm from about 100° to 180° with arm internally rotated and hand pronated (12); check endurance. Isolation of trapezius must be assured since shoulder elevation can also be accomplished with the levator scapula and the rhomboids.
- Test strength of sternocleidomastoid muscles by resisting head turning, opposite to the side of the muscle tested. Also test tilting. Resistance to head flexion tests both sternocleidomastoid muscles at the same time.
- The scapula is laterally translocated with medial rotation of the inferior angle. Shoulder winging caused by trapezius weakness is most pronounced by arm abduction, whereas weakness secondary to long thoracic nerve lesion is most pronounced by arm flexion (pushing upper extremity against a wall).
- EDX testing may be helpful (EMG looking for denervation or other neurogenic changes).
- NCS from posterior triangle to trapezius may be abnormal.
- High-resolution ultrasonography can be used to evaluate the nerve and its surrounding structures (13).

Differential Diagnosis

- Radiculopathy
- Other proximal neuropathy, including dorsal scapular neuropathy resulting in lateral scapular wining (8)
- Posttraumatic focal shoulder elevation dystonia (14)
- Capsulitis
- Plexus lesions
- Neuralgic amyotrophy
- Motor neuron disease
- Meningitis

Treatment

- NSAIDs
- TENS
- Shoulder orthosis
- Physical therapy: Both passive and active range of motion (ROM) exercises to prevent contracture and stiffness; resistive exercises to restore strength. If not successful, surgery may be considered if neurologic deficits are present (EMG confirmed) or dense paralysis (13).
  - Neurolysis
  - Nerve anastomosis
  - Graft procedures
  - Muscle transfers

Brachial Plexus

Anatomy

- The anterior rami (motor) and the posterior rami (sensory) of C5–T1 combine to form the brachial plexus. A prefixed plexus consists of nerve roots C4–C8, and a postfixed plexus consists of nerve roots C6–T2. The C5–C6 roots together become the upper trunk, the C7 alone the middle trunk, and C8–T1 the lower trunk. Under and slightly below the clavicle, the trunks divide into three anterior and three posterior divisions. The anterior, upper, and middle divisions join to become the lateral cord, and the lower division forms the medial cord. All divisions participate to develop the posterior cord (positioned under the pectoralis minor). The cords divide into the major nerves of the upper extremities. (Terminal branches are median, ulnar, radial, axillary, and musculocutaneous nerves.)

Risk Factors

- Compression, stretch, or a combination of both
- Direct trauma

- Excessive pressure on the plexus after prolonged anesthesia, post–median sternotomy, coronary bypass surgery, jugular vein cannulation
- Difficult deliveries (Erb palsy)
- Shoulder dislocation (concern for axillary nerve palsy in particular with anterior dislocation)
- Neoplasm (Pancoast tumor; metastasis from lymphoma, breast cancer, and lung cancer; primary nerve sheath tumors)
- Radiation injury
- Presence of cervical rib with associated fibrous band, resulting in neurogenic thoracic outlet syndrome (TOS) (8)

Symptoms and Signs

- Pain in shoulder and/or arm or hand
- Weakness of upper extremity, in one or multiple muscles
- Numbness, tingling, coldness
- Sensory loss
- Horner syndrome (ptosis, apparent enophthalmos, decreased sweating in affected side of face, miosis) possible with C8–T1 lesions such as tumors, radiculopathy (often root avulsion)

Evaluation

- Test ROM and strength in all muscle groups of the upper extremity
- Sensory examination (pinprick, light touch, temperature, and proprioception)
- Reflex testing
- Nerve conduction tests and EMG
- If necessary, MRI or sonography of the brachial plexus

Differential Diagnosis

- Brachial plexitis
- Rotator cuff lesions
- Tendinitis
- Peripheral neuropathy
- Proximal mononeuropathy
- Lesions secondary to radiation
- Radiculopathy

Treatment

- Rest
- Temporary splinting
- Pain medication: NSAIDs; antiseizure medications (phenytoin, carbamazepine, gabapentin, tricyclic antidepressants) may be helpful to reduce stabbing pains
- ROM exercises
- After reinnervation, strengthening exercises
- If no significant progress after 6 months (mostly if root avulsion is present), surgery should be considered:
  - Neurolysis
  - Nerve grafting
  - Neurotization
- Further surgical options to consider without appropriate recovery or with failure of the first surgical procedure include arthrodesis, tendon transfer, and functioning free muscle transplantation (15).

Upper Trunk Plexopathy

Anatomy

- The upper trunk is formed from the combination of the C5 and C6 nerve roots/spinal nerves. From this region, the SSN and the nerve to the subclavius arise. The fibers to the musculocutaneous, axillary, median, and radial nerves pass through the upper trunk of the brachial plexus. An important landmark is the Erb point. This location is about 2.5 cm above the clavicle, posterolateral to the sternocleidomastoid about the level of the sixth vertebra. This place is vulnerable to injury (compression, entrapment, stretch, or sharp disruption) and, in fact, is the area involved in the stinger/burner injury (16). At this point, the C5 and C6 roots, the SSN, and fibers of the musculocutaneous and axillary nerves can be electrically stimulated simultaneously, which can be helpful in establishing the correct diagnosis.
- The mechanisms of injury considered are (17):
  - Nerve root compression in the neural foramina (lack of protective epineurium and perineurium at that site)
  - Brachial plexus stretch (traction injury)
  - Direct blow to the plexus (percussion, compression)
  - A combination of stretch and percussion/compression

Risk Factors

- Football (highest incidence in defensive backs)
- Wrestlers
- Participants in other collision sports (ice hockey, field hockey, boxing)
- Shoulder laxity (18)
- Rugby
- Ill-fitting shoulder pads, neck rolls, or other equipment (19)
- Faulty techniques (especially during tackling)
- Carrying heavy loads for a long-time including backpacks
- Foraminal stenosis (19,20)
- High-risk childbirth (forceps, breech delivery, shoulder dystocia in large infant) (8)

Symptoms and Signs

- Burning pain and dysesthesia in the affected arm on impact lasting seconds to hours, followed by mostly transient weakness and no sensory symptoms. At times, there is prolonged loss of strength (16).
- Occasionally, the only objective change may be seen as postural abnormality (drooping of the shoulder, especially if the accessory nerve is also involved).
- Weakness of shoulder muscles, especially supraspinatus and infraspinatus, deltoid, biceps.

Evaluation

- Check for the positive Tinel sign at the Erb point
- Spurling test to rule in or out radiculopathy

- More severe injuries may involve the middle and lower trunk. There also may be denervation, which can be identified with EMG (earliest 2 weeks after the injury to allow for Wallerian degeneration to occur).

Differential Diagnosis

- Radiculopathy
- Cervical cord neurapraxia (CCN)
- Shoulder dislocation
- Tendinitis
- Neuralgic amyotrophy
- Rotator cuff injury

Treatment

- Only treatment is prevention of recurrences (improved techniques, appropriate shoulder pads, neck rolls, orthoses).
- With associated weakness and symptoms including tingling, numbness, and burning, these athletes should be followed for at least 2 weeks, as episodes of neurapraxia will typically resolve during this time frame (21).
- In severe lesions, inactivity and slow return to strength and flexibility with gradually increasing collision work and improved tackling techniques are necessary before returning to contact sports.
- Emphasis is placed on postural exercises with cervicothoracic stabilization training and resistive exercises to shoulder muscles (when there is no evidence of denervation).
- The athlete may return to participation in contact sports on reestablishment of pain-free motion, resolution of sensory symptoms, and full recovery of strength and functional status (21).
- Contraindication for return to play is two or more episodes of transient CCN, cervical myelopathy, evidence of neurologic deficit, significantly decreased ROM, and/or neck pain (21,22).
- In the case of severe lesions, with concern for neurotmesis or root avulsion, treatment will likely be surgical.

Lower Trunk Plexopathy

Anatomy

- Positioned between clavicle and first rib. It carries sensory and motor fibers of C8–T1 distribution (median and ulnar nerves). The closeness of median motor and ulnar sensory fiber at this level has EDX significance.
- The best known and most debated compression syndrome is TOS.

Thoracic Outlet Syndrome

Anatomy

- Thoracic outlet clinically refers to the thoracic inlet, the anatomic structure of a bony ring (first thoracic vertebra, first pair of ribs, and the manubrium). The clavicle articulates with the manubrium, which represents the anterior border of the inlet. Several vital structures pass through that opening (brachial plexus, and the subclavian artery and vein). TOS is due to the impingement of the brachial plexus and/or subclavian artery in the region of the scalene muscles (anterior and medial), the first rib, and the clavicle. The subclavian vein lies on top of the anterior scalene but joins the nerve and artery before the tight area between the clavicle and first rib. Compression/entrapment can also occur a bit more inferior (pectoralis minor syndrome).
- TOS is frequently caused by hyperextension injuries of the neck due to accidents, repetitive motion stress at work, and overhead activities like continued reaching for high-placed items. Muscles become tight (scar tissue has been found throughout the muscles by microscopic examination), or ligaments or bands press on the neurovascular structures, mostly just behind the collar bone.
- Several subtypes of TOS are identified by location:
  - Between the anterior and middle scalene muscles
  - The scalenus anticus syndrome: Nerve entrapment between the insertion of the scalenus anticus, the clavicle, and the first rib (especially in the presence of a cervical rib) (23)
  - Costoclavicular syndrome: Nerve entrapment in the narrowed space between clavicle and first rib; prolonged downward and backward shoulder pressure as by heavy loads on the shoulder; worse with abnormal clavicle or malunion or nonunion of clavicle fracture
  - Pectoralis minor syndrome (between chest wall and pectoralis minor)
- Classification by structures involved:
  - Neurogenic thoracic outlet syndrome (NTOS): incidence of 1 in 1,000,000 (24); compression of brachial plexus (lower trunk)
  - Venous thoracic outlet syndrome (VTOS) (Paget-Schrötter syndrome): obstruction of the subclavian vein; presents with arm swelling, pain, and cyanosis, possible thrombosis
  - Arterial thoracic outlet syndrome (ATOS): 1%–2% only (25); emboli arising from subclavian artery stenosis or aneurysm obstruct blood flow and cause ischemia; usually a cervical rib or anomalous first rib is present (26)
  - Clinical TOS without objective findings is very common. Identification as such depends on the diagnostician

Risk Factors

- Cervical rib (with fibrous bands to the first rib) (27)
- Slim, asthenic females (with long "swan neck" and droopy shoulders)
- Accessory nerve lesion (weak trapezius muscle causing droopy shoulders)
- Sternotomy (at risk for pectoralis minor syndrome, especially those with premorbid impaired shoulder motion)

- Neoplasm (*e.g.*, Pancoast tumor, bulky lymphadenopathy in setting of metastases)
- Radiculopathy
- Klippel-Feil anomaly (28)
- Swimmers and other sports using repeated overhead motion
- Scalene hypertrophy (23)
- Heavy backpack

Symptoms and Signs

- Vague pain and fatigue (claudication)
- Color change (pallor and/or cyanosis)
- Distended veins of arm and chest wall
- Cool temperature of upper limb
- Feeling of arm heaviness
- Paresthesias along the medial aspect of the affected hand and forearm
- Pain in neck, shoulder, and arm, especially when elevating the arm
- Thenar wasting and weakness of the abductor pollicis brevis (APB)
- Ulnar hand intrinsics may also be weak and atrophic
- Cervical spine plain films and CT or MRI can help identify bony abnormalities (25)
- Confirmatory tests: arteriography, venography, MR neurography, and EDX studies

Evaluation

- Physical examination: Tenderness over scalene muscles, sometimes causing tingling radiating into arm; possible armpit tenderness (pectoralis minor syndrome); reduced sensation to light touch in involved hand and forearm; weakness and atrophy of APB may be present
- Electrodiagnosis: NCS
- Median antebrachial cutaneous response amplitude decreased
- Median motor response amplitude decreased
- Ulnar sensory response amplitude decreased
- Ulnar motor response amplitude decreased
- Median sensory response amplitude preserved (innervated by middle/upper trunk, lateral cord)
    - EMG may show denervation in lower trunk–innervated musculature (*i.e.*, C8-T1 nerve root distribution).
- Provocative maneuvers: unfortunately, not very reliable
- Adson test: head turned to ipsilateral side, shoulders in military position, taking a deep breath. This decreases the space between clavicle and the first rib. It is positive when the radial pulse can no longer be palpated and/or the symptoms are reproduced. However, there are many false-positive and false-negative results.
- Upper limb tension (Elvey) test: abducting arms to 90° in external rotation, which causes symptoms to appear within 60 seconds (comparable to straight leg raising test) (26)
- Test for costoclavicular compression: Shoulders are placed in military position and clavicles forced downward posteriorly.
- Hyperabduction (Wright) test: tries to reproduce symptoms experienced due to pectoralis minor syndrome
- Roos test (elevate arm stress test, aka EAST): Patient abducts shoulders to 90° in external rotation, opening and closing hands slowly over a 3-minute period.

Differential Diagnosis

- Brachial plexitis
- Radiculopathy
- Cervical myelopathy
- Peripheral neuropathy
- Complex regional pain syndrome
- Fibromyalgia
- Plexopathy after trauma or radiation
- Pancoast tumor
- Glenohumeral instability
- Raynaud syndrome
- Proximal mononeuropathy
- CTS
- Ulnar neuropathy (cubital tunnel syndrome, Guyon canal syndrome)

Treatment

- Physical therapy: physical therapy program including biomechanical retraining and shoulder and ribcage elevation exercises that enlarge the entrapped space. Emphasis on stretching rather than strengthening. Pain should be addressed with specific agents for neuropathic pain (*e.g.*, tricyclics, anticonvulsants, Neurontin, etc.).
- For ATOS and VTOS, urgent thrombolysis is indicated, if not possible surgery.
- Prognosis for surgical results may be assessed by injecting Xylocaine (lidocaine) into the scalene muscles and/or pectoralis muscle.
- After results with anesthetic injection, a simple tenotomy may be performed (especially the pectoralis minor).
- Botulinum toxin type A to the anterior scalene and/or pectoralis muscle demonstrate varying levels of success (29).
- Surgical options: Major procedures include transaxillary versus supraclavicular versus infraclavicular approaches to first rib resection, scalenectomy, and combined rib resection and scalenectomy (30), which may be indicated in cases of vascular etiology or the presence of a cervical rib or other prominent first rib bony abnormality.
- Postsurgical complications are of concern. Recurrence through scarring is a definite possibility. However, following surgical intervention for neurogenic TOS, Urschel and Razzuk discussed that 95% revealed "excellent" results (29).

Long Thoracic Nerve

Anatomy

- C5/C6/C7 anterior primary rami are the origin of the long thoracic nerve. They together pierce the middle scalene muscle forming the long thoracic nerve upper division. Together with the C7 spinal nerve, they travel between the anterior and middle scalene muscles, located in the supraclavicular triangle. It supplies the serratus anterior muscle.

Risk Factors

- Carrying heavy loads, backpacks
- Body building and weightlifting
- Archery, shooting (31)
- Football
- Judo, karate, kickboxing
- Back-stroke swimming
- Volleyball
- Wrestling, gymnastics
- Motor vehicle accidents
- Chiropractic manipulation
- Deep massage
- Heavy labor
- Blow to shoulder or downward traction of the arm (may cause compression of the long thoracic nerve against the second rib)
- Heart surgery
- Trauma to the upper thorax and cervical region
- Infiltrating tumors
- Iatrogenic during radical mastectomy or axillary lymph node dissection
- Idiopathic entrapment

Symptoms and Signs

- Medial scapular winging
- Pain in the shoulder, neck, and arm
- Weakness in the upper extremity, especially with overhead activities
- Frequently found weakness also in deltoid, biceps, supraspinatus, and infraspinatus muscles (additional cervical plexus involvement)
- Shoulder instability
- Severe pain in shoulder lasting several days to weeks followed by shoulder dysfunction and weakness due to neuralgic amyotrophy and the long thoracic nerve being involved in isolation (8)

Evaluation

- Test strength and ROM of shoulder. Forward flexion will be decreased to 90°. Winging will be present when patient presses arms against a wall (compared to winging secondary to trapezius weakness, when abduction produces the greatest amount of winging). Measure angle of scapula plane to chest wall. Strength of the serratus muscle can be determined by distance of scapular angle to chest. More than 5 cm represents severe loss of function.
- NCS not particularly reliable to evaluate the long thoracic nerve; EDX will rely on the EMG portion.

Differential Diagnosis

- Neuralgic amyotrophy (32), also known as brachial plexitis or Parsonage-Turner syndrome (the long thoracic nerve is preferentially affected)
- Trapezius, rhomboid, suprascapular muscle lesions
- Motor neuron disease
- Poliomyelitis
- Radiculopathy
- Fracture
- Neoplasm
- Idiopathic long thoracic nerve palsy

Treatment

- Physical therapy: If denervation is present, ROM exercises are important to prevent contractures of the serratus as well as antagonist muscles (rhomboid and levator scapulae and pectoralis minor). (Stretching denervated muscles is contraindicated because of possible harm.) Muscle-strengthening exercises will begin upon reinnervation, focusing on the scapular stabilizing muscles including the trapezius, rhomboid, and levator scapulae muscles (33).
- Prognosis for spontaneous recovery is good, with cases of atraumatic long thoracic nerve neuropathy resolving by 1 year (34), except in the case of root avulsion.
- A temporary shoulder orthosis is advised.
- If complete denervation persists after 6 months, a nerve graft may be necessary (*i.e.*, intercostal to long thoracic nerve) or neurolysis (33).

Axillary Nerve

Anatomy

- The origin of the axillary nerve stems from roots C5 and C6. Fibers travel through the upper trunk of the brachial plexus. Their path continues through the posterior divisions followed by the posterior cord. The first terminal branch is the axillary nerve. It crosses the anteroinferior aspect of the subscapularis muscle, then through the quadrilateral space. It divides into a posterior trunk that supplies the teres minor and the posterior deltoid and terminates as the lateral brachial cutaneous nerve. The anterior trunk supplies the anterior and middle deltoid. The axillary nerve is the most common nerve affected in shoulder lesions. (Boundaries of the quadrilateral space are teres minor superior, teres major inferior, long head of triceps medial, and surgical neck of the humerus lateral).
- Points of possible compression/entrapment are:
    - At the origin from the posterior cord

- At the anterior and inferior aspect of the subscapularis muscle
- The subfascial surface of the deltoid
- The quadrilateral space

Risk Factors

- Throwing athletes
- Football (accounts for majority of axillary nerve injuries) (Cass), rugby, crew, swimming, backpacking
- Volleyball, wrestling (31)
- Direct blow to the deltoid
- Glenohumeral joint anterior dislocation (35), humerus fractures or surgery
- Muscle hypertrophy and possibly fibrous bands
- Tumors
- Improper use of crutches (leaning on the axilla when standing)
- Inappropriate application of casts or orthoses
- Iatrogenic

Symptoms and Signs

- In quadrilateral space syndrome, there is posterior shoulder pain.
- Paresthesias over a circular location of the lateral arm
- Weakness of deltoid muscle
- Forward flexion and/or abduction and external rotation of the humerus aggravate the symptoms, though patient able to compensate with supraspinatus and infraspinatus for abduction and external rotation, respectively (8)
- Difficulty lifting arm above the head
- Possibly abnormal EDX studies, evaluating for abnormal deltoid compound muscle action potential (CMAP) amplitudes and denervation in the deltoid and/or teres minor muscles (8)

Evaluation

- ROM and strength testing of shoulder muscles; sensory testing of bilateral upper extremities.
- Subclavian arteriography may show compression of the posterior humeral circumflex artery with abduction and external rotation of the arm (36).
- EDX studies may be abnormal.

Differential Diagnosis

- Tendinitis
- Rotator cuff tear
- Frozen shoulder
- Radiculopathy
- Brachial plexopathy
- Parsonage-Turner syndrome
- Cervical radiculopathy

Treatment

- Many patients, especially young patients, recover full shoulder abduction even with continued denervation of the deltoid by substituting the supraspinatus for the deltoid. Throwing athletes experience difficulty. The deltoid provides 50% of the torque about the shoulder.
- With a direct blow to the deltoid, prognosis is poorer than with lesions from other causes.
- Acute injury: Rest, pain control, and treatment of bony or other injuries must be taken care of. ROM and passive exercises to rotator cuff muscles, deltoid, and periscapular muscles, progressing to resistive exercises as muscles are reinnervated. Shoulder contracture must be avoided. There could be an indication for electrical stimulation (37).
- Muscle retraining and/or job changes are recommended. Most patients will recover with the above conservative treatment (33). If there is no evidence of reinnervation after 6 months, surgical exploration must be considered.
- Surgery for quadrilateral space syndrome aims to decompress by release of fascia and fibrous bands around the axillary nerve and posterior humeral circumflex vessels (36).
- For more extensive lesions, neurorrhaphy, neurolysis nerve repair, nerve grafts, nerve transfer, and/or muscle transfer are possibilities (13).
- If there is also root avulsion, grafting and nerve transfers are the optimal procedures to regain function (38).

Suprascapular Nerve

Anatomy

- The C5–C6 spinal nerves are the origin of the SSN. Fibers travel through the upper trunk of the brachial plexus, pass through the supraclavicular fossa, and then through the scapular notch covered by the transverse scapular ligament. Just distal to the notch, the SSN sends branches to the acromioclavicular joint and the subacromial bursa and extends to the shoulder joint. After innervating and passing through the supraspinatus muscle, the SSN bends around the spine of the scapula to innervate the infraspinatus. Per Cass, up to 2% of all shoulder disorders could be related to underlying SSN injury (33).
- Points of possible compression/entrapment:
  - Scapular notch
  - Spinoglenoid notch
  - Fascia between the scapular and the spinoglenoid notches (39)

Risk Factors

- Traumatic:
  - Presence of large retracted rotator cuff tears (40)
  - Shoulder arthrodesis
  - Fracture of the scapula

- Nontraumatic:
  - Repetitive overhead loading activities
  - Volleyball
  - Weightlifting
  - Boxing
  - Basketball
  - Baseball, particular pitchers
  - Painting
  - Backpack straps
  - Ganglion cysts at scapular notch
  - Superior glenoid labrum, spinoglenoid notch cysts
  - Rarely cases of mass lesions, including ganglion cysts, sarcomas, and metastatic carcinoma (8)

Symptoms and Signs

- Vague, deep, dull, and chronic pain shoulder pains with possible radiation in suprascapular or radial nerve distribution (33)
- Vague shoulder and/or acromioclavicular joint pain
- Weakness in supraspinatus and/or infraspinatus muscles with possible atrophy noted

Evaluation

- Test ROM and muscle strength in shoulder muscles.
- Test for the Tinel sign at the scapular notch.
- Overhead activities may worsen symptoms.
- The crossed arm abduction test should exacerbate symptoms on the affected side.
- Advanced imaging including MRI can look for soft tissue masses and indirect signs of denervation (41).
- EDX studies may show abnormality.

Differential Diagnosis

- Cervical radiculopathy
- Discogenic pain
- Shoulder acromioclavicular joint pathology
- Rotator cuff tear
- Musculoskeletal pain syndromes
- Brachial plexitis

Treatment

- Avoidance of exacerbating activities (overhead).
- Physical therapy focuses on maintaining ROM of the scapula and on improving rotator cuff, deltoid, and periscapular stabilizer muscle strength.
- Correct the scapulohumeral rhythm as much as possible.
- Injection of local anesthetic into the suprascapular or spinoglenoid notch may assist in the diagnosis and treatment.
- If no adequate response to conservative measures, consider surgery.
- Surgical decompression arthroscopically (through subacromial space or other portals), particularly in the setting of paralabral cyst or labral injury (33,42).

Musculocutaneous Nerve

Anatomy

- The musculocutaneous nerve is the terminal branch of the lateral cord of the brachial plexus (fibers from C5–C7). The nerve passes through the coracobrachialis, which it innervates, as well as the brachialis and biceps brachii. In many subjects, the brachialis also receives a branch of the radial nerve.
- Just above the elbow, the musculocutaneous motor nerve becomes the sensory nerve, lateral antebrachial cutaneous nerve, which innervates the volar and dorsal forearm along the radial aspect, but not the hand.
- Entrapment is uncommon.

Risk Factors

- Excessive resistive elbow extension (push-ups or arm presses in weightlifters)
- Baseball players
- Strenuous forearm pronation
- Tight biceps aponeurosis (16)
- Shoulder dislocation
- A hypertrophic coracobrachialis muscle; the lateral antebrachial cutaneous nerve may be compressed as it enters the forearm

Symptoms and Signs

- Coracobrachialis entrapment: elbow flexor weakness, lateral arm pain (burning), and/or loss of sensation
- Positive Tinel sign at areas of entrapment
- Decreased biceps reflex possible
- Distal entrapment may present only with lateral forearm pain and/or sensory deficit

Evaluation

- Meticulous history and physical examination.
- Point of maximal tenderness is important for possible surgery.
- Symptoms of pain and/or paresthesias increase with elbow extension and forearm pronation with potential involvement of the distal musculocutaneous sensory nerve (8).
- Electrodiagnosis: Motor and sensory conduction may be slowed and amplitudes reduced. In severe lesions, EMG of biceps may show abnormal neurogenic findings.

Differential Diagnosis

- Shoulder dislocation
- Rotator cuff lesion
- Brachial plexitis
- Tendinitis
- Lateral epicondylitis
- Cervical radiculopathy
- Median or superficial radial nerve entrapment

Treatment

- Rest, ROM, active assistive ROM, gentle stretching, massage
- Anti-inflammatory medication
- Modalities
- Lateral antebrachial cutaneous nerve entrapment near the cubital fossa typically needs surgical decompression (8)

Median Nerve

- Anatomy: The median nerve originates from the C6–T1 spinal roots/nerves. It traverses the upper, middle, and lower trunk; the anterior divisions; and the lateral and medial cord. It is one of the three nerves supplying all muscles of the forearm and hand.

Entrapment Site 1: Ligament of Struthers

Anatomy

- Median and ulnar nerves and brachial artery can be entrapped by a fibrous band from a rare supracondylar process on the anterior humerus to its medial epicondyle or underneath the lacertus fibrosis.

Risk Factors

- Approximately 1%–2% of the population who have the anomaly (8)
- Distal humerus fracture
- Space-occupying lesion

Symptoms and Signs

- Tingling, numbness in the median innervated area
- Weakness in all median nerve–innervated muscles
- Deficits in ulnar nerve distribution, if the ulnar is also entrapped
- Swelling of hand and forearm (brachial vein) and blanching (brachial artery)
- Attenuated radial pulse with supination of the forearm and extension of the elbow (8)
- Ape hand (severe involvement of the whole median nerve)

Evaluation

- Good history and extensive physical examination are paramount.
- Imaging of humerus to confirm the presence of a spur or osteochondroma.
- EDX studies can be helpful. Pronator maybe involved, but not in pronator syndrome.

Differential Diagnosis

- Pronator syndrome
- Humerus fracture
- Humeral osteochondroma (spur oriented away from the joint in opposite to the anomalous supracondylar process, which points toward the joint)
- Radiculopathy

Treatment

- Reduction of aggravating activities
- Anti-inflammatory medications may help some
- Surgery will usually be the treatment of choice (spur excision; in absence of spur, ligament incision and lacertus fibrosis wedge removal) (43)

Entrapment Site 2: Pronator Syndrome

Anatomy

- In the antecubital area the median nerve is located underneath the bicipital aponeurosis (lacertus fibrosis). Then it passes between the superficial and deep heads of the pronator teres, underneath the flexor digitorum superficialis.
- Entrapment by these structures: pronator syndrome. An accessory head of the flexor pollicis longus (FPL), called Gantzer muscle, may contribute to this syndrome as well as the anterior interosseous nerve syndrome. More entrapment syndromes are described by Tubbs et al. (44).

Risk Factors

- Enlarged median artery
- Musicians (pianists, fiddlers, harpists)
- Athletes (baseball players)
- Arm fractures can injure the brachial artery by compression, thereby preventing blood flow and causing ischemia. Resulting scarring of flexor muscles may cause flexion deformity at wrist and fingers (Volkmann contracture)
- Occupational (*e.g.*, machine milkers and dentists)

Symptoms and Signs

- Weak handgrip (weakness of flexor pollicis longus, flexor digitorum profundus to digits 2 and 2, and opponens pollicis) (8)
- Aching pain with resisted flexion to the middle finger, increased activities
- Pain on active resistive forearm pronation, elbow flexion, and finger flexion (6)
- Possible cramping of fingers (writer's cramp)
- Numbness of thumb and index finger
- Possible positive Tinel test over pronator teres muscle
- Negative Phalen test
- Significant loss of median nerve function will cause the "Benediction hand"
- Pronator teres spared

Evaluation

- Precise history and physical
- Strength test, especially pronation against resistance with elbow extended, elbow flexion with forearm supinated, and resistive finger flexion
- Provocative maneuver: Paresthesias in the hand after 30 seconds or less of manual compression of the median nerve over the pronator teres muscle
- EMG and NCS may be helpful

Differential Diagnosis

- Tendinitis
- Entrapment under ligament of Struthers
- CTS
- Entrapment under the sublime bridge
- Brachial plexitis
- Cervical radiculopathy

Treatment

- Avoidance of offending activity, rest, splinting
- Anti-inflammatory drugs
- Possible steroid injections into the area of entrapment
- If there is no improvement in 6 months, surgical exploration is recommended.
- Surgery: Release of pronator teres and offending structure leads to full recovery, unless severe axonotmesis is present (10,45)

Entrapment Site 3: Anterior Interosseous Nerve Syndrome (Kiloh-Nevin Syndrome)

Anatomy

- In the forearm, the median nerve gives off a large deep motor branch, the anterior interosseous nerve, that supplies the FPL, the two lateral heads of the flexor digitorum profundus, and the pronator quadratus. Anterior interosseous lesions are rare.

Risk Factors

- Supracondylar humerus fracture (especially in children)
- Venipuncture
- Anatomic variants
- Tumor
- Neuralgic amyotrophy/Parsonage-Turner syndrome
- Repetitive forearm flexion or pronation

Symptoms and Signs

- No sensory symptoms
- Weakness in thumb flexion, finger flexion, forearm pronation

Evaluation

- Careful examination of forearm and hand.
- ROM and strength evaluation mainly of thumb and finger flexion and pronation.
- Look for the "O" sign: Patients are unable to hold and resist the opening of the index finger to thumb tip-to-tip pinch; the two distal phalanges align flat against each other to hold the pinch.
- EMG is helpful to identify the involved muscles.

Differential Diagnosis

- Neuralgic amyotrophy (Parsonage-Turner syndrome)
- Pronator teres syndrome
- Radiculopathy

Treatment

- Conservative management with avoidance of repetitive elbow flexion, pronation, or forced gripping, and splitting.
- Spontaneous improvement can occur within 6–18 months after onset (46).
- Surgery may become necessary, but literature has described varying results of median nerve decompression (29,46).

Entrapment Site 4: Carpal Tunnel Syndrome

Anatomy

- The carpal tunnel is formed by the arched carpal bones covered by the carpal ligament (retinaculum), which spans from the pisiform and hamate to the trapezium and scaphoid. It contains, in addition to the median nerve, arteries, and veins, tendons of nine flexor muscles: flexor digitorum superficialis (4 tendons), flexor digitorum profundus (4 tendons), and flexor pollicis longus (1 tendon). The flexor carpi radialis tendon has its own synovial sheath to prevent compression when passing through the radial attachment to the retinaculum. It travels with the radial artery and the palmar cutaneous branch superficial to the flexor retinaculum, underneath which the other flexor tendons are located (in the carpal tunnel).
- In the hand, the median nerve supplies the lateral two lumbricals and most of the thenar muscles, except for the deep head of the flexor pollicis brevis (deep motor branch of the ulnar nerve). Sensory fibers, after traveling through the carpal tunnel, supply the lateral three and one-half digits, and the distal one-third of the dorsal aspect of the digits 1–3, one-half of the dorsal distal digit of the ring-finger, and the lateral palm, except for a small area over the thenar eminence (radial nerve supply).

Risk Factors

- Repetitive motion activities (job related, knitting, sewing, etc.)
- Low ratio of depth to width (<0.70) of the wrist (47)
- Hypothyroidism
- Myxedema
- Pregnancy, premenstrual swelling
- Tumor
- Other causes of excessive soft tissue swelling
- Wheelchair athletics
- Tennis
- Baseball, volleyball
- Musicians (violin and piano playing)
- Wheelchair athletes, bikers, bodybuilding/weightlifting
- Archery, wrestlers (48)

Symptoms and Signs

- Nocturnal numbness (Flick sign)
- Tingling and wrist pain, increased with activities
- Patients prone to dropping things
- Sensory impairment in median nerve distribution in the hand, with thenar eminence spared

- Weak hand grip
- When holding a pinch against resistance, patients frequently will use the ulnar innervated deep flexor pollicis to oppose the index, instead of the APB
- In the hand, severe median nerve loss will eventually cause an ape hand deformity because of the loss of thenar muscles and, thereby, loss of opposition and flexion of the thumb

Evaluation

- Meticulous history and examination of muscle strength
- Sensory examination of all modalities (superficial and deep sensation, temperature, position sense, two-point discrimination)
- Neuromuscular ultrasound of the right median nerve particularly at the wrist and forearm
- Electrodiagnosis is extremely helpful in the diagnosis of CTS, especially to rule out radiculopathy and to identify CTS even when peripheral neuropathy is also present. Nerve conduction velocity slowing across the wrist, conduction block, EMG findings in the median nerve–innervated hand intrinsic muscles

Differential Diagnosis

- Cervical radiculopathy
- Brachial plexopathy, particularly NTOS
- Peripheral neuropathy
- Diabetes mellitus
- Tendinitis
- Space-occupying lesion
- Nerve injury or post-surgical complication

Treatment

- Night splints in neutral position
- Splints for activities that produce discomfort (avoiding constant wearing)
- Nonsteroidal pain medication
- TENS effectiveness was objectively confirmed with functional MRI (48)
- Steroid injections into the painful area; if no response, surgery may be considered
- Surgery entails release of confining ligament.
- Endoscopic with minimal invasiveness

Entrapment Site 5: Digital Nerve Entrapment

Anatomy

- The median nerve sensory fibers in the hand are located at the medial and lateral side of digits 1–3 and on the lateral side of digit 4. They may become entrapped.

Risk Factors

- Vibration syndrome
- Athletes (baseball players, bowlers, etc.)
- Musicians
    - Flutists (lateral side of left index finger)
    - Violinists, cellists (right thumb)
    - Percussionists (left middle finger)

Symptoms and Signs

- Numbness and tingling in fingers
- Pain in fingers
- Cramping, dystonia

Evaluation

- Careful history and physical, especially a meticulous sensory examination, all modalities
- Sensory nerve conduction may be of help (finger stimulation and finger recording)

Differential Diagnosis

- Radiculopathy
- Peripheral neuropathy
- Reynaud syndrome
- Dependent arm swelling
- Median neuropathy at the wrist
- Sensory ganglionopathy

Treatment

- NSAIDs
- Splinting
- Steroid injections (last resort)
- Surgical release

Radial Nerve

- Anatomy: The radial nerve originates from fibers of the C5–T1 nerve roots and emerges as the terminal branch of the posterior cord (brachial plexus). It runs between the medial and long heads of the triceps and later along the spiral groove of the humerus, where the posterior antebrachial cutaneous nerve branches off and then supplies the skin of the extensor forearm. The radial nerve pierces the lateral intermuscular septum, travels anterior to the lateral epicondyle, and divides into a superficial sensory and deep motor branch in the cubital fossa. The latter continues in the radial tunnel through the arcade of Frohse, lying between the superficial and deep supinators, and becomes the posterior interosseous nerve (PIN), supplying the extensor forearm muscles (except the extensor carpi radialis longus (ECRL)). The superficial branch courses laterally at the wrist. It supplies sensation to the dorsoradial wrist and the proximal dorsal aspect of the first 3 and one-half digits.

Entrapment Site 1: Radial Nerve Proximal to Elbow — Spiral Groove

Risk Factors

- Humerus fracture: Estimated incidence of radial entrapment is about 11.8% (49). Most lesions are neurapraxic; functional return is seen in 4–5 months (1).
- Saturday night (honeymooner's) palsy: most common, due to prolonged compression of the nerve in or near the spiral groove.

Symptoms and Signs

- Weakness of forearm extensors (wrist drop)
- Slight weakness of elbow flexors if brachioradialis is involved
- Triceps may or may not be involved
- Triceps reflex absent if triceps involved
- Pain and sensory change in posterior antebrachial cutaneous and/or distal superficial radial nerve distribution

Evaluation

- History: trauma to humerus, recent obtundation due to alcohol or other inebriation.
- Physical examination: weakness in extension of wrist, sensory loss to pinprick and/or light touch in distal radial nerve distribution.
- Electrodiagnosis is recommended.
- NCS: Recording radial nerve velocity and amplitude across the point of injury may demonstrate the deficit; evaluate for conduction block and/or amplitude loss.
- Needle exam — Involved muscles may show denervation.

Differential Diagnosis

- Radiculopathy
- Brachial plexitis, particularly posterior cord
- Space-occupying lesion
- Musculocutaneous nerve lesion
- Extensor tenosynovitis

Treatment

- Assure bony stability in the setting of humerus fracture to prevent further nerve injury; start with immobilization followed by functional bracing and pain control.
- Prognosis in lesion above elbow is good (neurapraxia).
- Conservative management with physical therapy, modalities.
- If no recovery in several months or clinical decline, surgical exploration is indicated.

Entrapment 2: Radial Tunnel Syndrome

- This syndrome is controversial. Compression may occur anywhere in the tunnel. The cause of these symptoms often is a treatment resistant chronic tennis elbow. Generally, no definite neurological deficit can be demonstrated clinically or by electrodiagnosis.
- Management would include splinting, activity modification, and NSAIDs (50).

Entrapment 3: Supinator Syndrome — Arcade of Frohse

- This syndrome is a compression at the arcade of Frohse where the radial nerve pierces the supinator and becomes the purely motor PIN. The supinator itself and the extensor carpi radialis brevis are mostly innervated by the PIN before it enters the arcade of Frohse.

Risk Factors

- Repetitive motion
- Fracture of proximal radius
- Fracture/dislocation at elbow (Monteggia fracture)
- Rheumatoid arthritis
- Lacerations, scarring
- Lipomas, other tumors
- Tennis players, body builders, swimmers, gymnasts (48)

Symptoms and Signs

- Pain and/or weakness in radial distributions distal to elbow
- Partial wrist drop, radial deviation on wrist extension (ECRL innervation above elbow)
- Interossei appear weak secondary to loss of wrist stabilization
- No sensory deficit

Evaluation

- Given risk factors, consider advanced imaging such as MRI to identify possible compressive lesions (33).
- Physical examination: Forced supination with arm fully flexed will reproduce pain in lesions proximal to supinator.
- Forced extension of third digit may be weak (not in extensor tenosynovitis).
- Electrodiagnosis: most reliable is the needle examination of the radial-innervated muscles. NCS are not always helpful. The technique would be as the previously described radial nerve study.
- Imaging helps demonstrate the cause.

Differential Diagnosis

- Radiculopathy
- Brachial plexitis, particularly posterior cord
- Tumor (neuroma), rheumatoid arthritis
- Musculocutaneous nerve lesion
- Extensor tenosynovitis
- Lateral epicondylitis, *i.e.*, tennis elbow

Treatment

- Conservative management with activity modification, rest, splinting, NSAIDs, and physical therapy incorporating stretching (33)
- If refractory or rapidly progressive (denervation on EMG study), consider surgical release

Entrapment Site 4: Distal Radial Nerve Lesion ("Handcuff Neuropathy" or Cheiralgia Paresthetica)

- Due to compression at the wrist and is mostly purely sensory

Risk Factors

- Prisoners
- Tight wristwatch
- With more severe injury, multiple nerves may be involved

Symptoms and Signs

- Sensory deficits in distal superficial radial nerve distribution
- No weakness

Treatment

- Conservative management

- Recovery usually complete within 6–8 weeks
- It may predispose patient to complex regional pain syndrome

Ulnar Nerve

- Anatomy: The ulnar nerve (C8–T1) is the terminal branch of the inferior trunk and the medial cord of the brachial plexus. It accompanies the brachial artery and median nerve in a neurovascular bundle. It then travels between the coracobrachialis and triceps. At midpoint of the upper arm, the nerve enters the posterior compartment, piercing the intermuscular septum. The nerve runs along the medial head of the triceps in a tough investing fascia that comprises the arcade of Struthers. At the elbow, the nerve leaves this fascia and passes posterior to the medial epicondyle of the humerus (ulnar sulcus). It enters the cubital tunnel at the humeroulnar aponeurotic arcade (Osborne ligament), pierces the flexor carpi ulnaris (FCU), and lies between its two heads. It exits at the distal end of the cubital tunnel through the deep flexor pronator aponeurosis (DFPA). At the wrist, the nerve passes through the Guyon canal (borders: medially, pisiform bone; laterally, hook of hamate; roof, tendon of FCU; and floor, carpal ligament) into the palm of the hand. In the canal, the ulnar nerve divides into a deep branch accompanied by the ulnar artery, which winds around the hook of the hamate and supplies the interossei, the third and fourth lumbricals, the adductor pollicis, the first dorsal interosseous, and the deep head of the flexor pollicis brevis. The superficial branch supplies the palmaris brevis and terminates as sensory nerve to digits 4 and 5.

Entrapment Site 1: Arcade of Struthers

Risk Factors

- Prior trauma
- Surgery (*e.g.*, ulnar transposition)

Symptoms and Signs

- Decreased sensation in ulnar nerve distribution proximal to wrist
- Severe lesion may involve ulnar motor innervation (FCU, flexor digitorum profundus to digits 4 and 5)
- Weakness of the FCU will reveal radial deviation of wrist with flexion

Evaluation

- Advanced imaging (MRI or diagnostic ultrasound).
- EMG/NCS may be negative until case is advanced; motor fibers are well protected. Motor study of ulnar nerve with stimulation proximal to suspected lesion. May be difficult to discern entrapment here from tardy ulnar palsy, without clinical suspicion.

Differential Diagnosis

- Radiculopathy/myelopathy
- Lower trunk (nTOS) versus medial cord plexopathy
- Pancoast tumor
- Ulnar entrapment further distally
- Double crush

Treatment

- Conservative management is usually not adequate.
- Surgery to release constriction band is often favored.

Entrapment Site 2: Ulnar Sulcus/Retro-Epicondylar Groove (Tardy Ulnar Palsy)

- Second most common nerve entrapment of the upper extremity

Risk Factors

- Leaning on elbows
- Tight casting
- Compressive trauma
- Bony deformity
- Epicondyle fracture (nonunion)
- Wrestling without elbow pads
- Excessive flexion (as in prolonged driving)
- Repetitive motion at elbow
- Chronic subluxation
- High body mass index in women, older age in men
- Rheumatoid arthritis
- Occupational or recreational activities
- Prolonged use of vibrating tools
- Bodybuilding/weightlifting, judo, karate, kickboxing, baseball (48)

Symptoms and Signs

- Pain, paresthesia, and/or numbness in volar aspect of fifth and medial fourth digits and hypothenar eminence, increasing with elbow flexion
- Weakness and/or atrophy in ulnar-innervated hand intrinsic muscles
- Flexion contracture of proximal interphalangeal joint of fifth digit
- Possible claw hand (partial flexion of the proximal and distal interphalangeal joints, with extension of the metacarpophalangeal joints)
- Diminished grip strength

Evaluation

- Dynamic assessment to look for chronic nerve subluxation
- Tinel sign at elbow
- EMG/NCS may assist in the diagnosis (51)
- Consider ulnar inching study (multiple potential sites of entrapment)
- Consider neuromuscular ultrasound of ulnar nerve at elbow compared to forearm

Differential Diagnosis

- Ulnar entrapment distally or proximally
- Systemic disease with high incidence of mononeuropathies (*e.g.*, diabetes, alcoholism, thyroid)

- Compression: extrinsic or intrinsic, postoperative
- Peripheral neuropathy
- Lower trunk (nTOS) versus medial cord brachial plexopathy
- Valgus ligament instability
- Elbow injury and deformities
- Fractures and dislocations
- Cubitus valgus or varus
- Space-occupying lesions: ganglia, tumors, osteophytes, bursae
- Perineural adhesions
- Burns and heterotopic bone
- Osteophytes, synovitis

Treatment

- Conservative management (elbow pad, elbow extension brace, ulnar nerve glides), pain control
- Correct underlying etiology if possible
- Muscle strengthening
- ROM
- Relative rest including avoiding exacerbating activities
- Padding and/or splinting around the elbow
- If neurologic symptoms progress, consider surgery (ulnar nerve release or ulnar nerve transposition)

Entrapment Site 3: Cubital Tunnel Syndrome

- Compression at the entry (Osborne ligament) or exit (DFPA)

Risk Factors

- Lesions mostly nontraumatic
- Repetitive motion injuries
- Anatomic predisposition

Symptoms and Signs

- Findings similar to tardy ulnar palsy
- Tinel sign over the cubital tunnel, not over sulcus
- Wartenberg sign (fifth digit abduction due to weakness of third palmar interosseous muscle)
- Froment sign: Patient pinches a piece of paper between first and second metacarpals. In response to a strong pull, patient contracts the FPL and index long finger flexors to substitute for weak first dorsal interosseous and adductor pollicis

Differential Diagnosis

- Similar to entrapments sites 1–2 discussed earlier

Treatment

- Conservative as with entrapment at retro-epicondylar groove
- Progressive symptoms with motor decline
- Surgery (cubital tunnel release)

Entrapment Sites 4 and 5: Guyon Canal and Palmar Entrapment

- Motor or sensory fibers, or both, may be involved depending on the location of the compression. Entrapment distal to the Guyon canal (deep palmer branch) results in weakness of ulnar-innervated intrinsic muscles. Occasionally, the abductor digiti minimi is spared. In the canal, both may be compressed. The superficial branch causes sensory loss of the ulnar half of the fourth digit and the fifth digit. The dorsal sensory nerve branches off proximal to the canal.

Risk Factors

- Bicycling, snowmobiling (handlebar palsy)
- Wheelchair athletes
- Push-ups
- Flute or violin playing
- Vibrational trauma
- Scars, tumor, ganglion cyst, lipoma
- Ulnar artery aneurysm
- Fracture, especially hook of hamate

Symptoms and Signs

- Wrist/hand pain
- Weakness in grasp
- Numbness and tingling in distal ulnar nerve distribution; often worse at night

Evaluation

- History and physical
- Advanced imaging (MRI, computed tomography, ultrasound)
- Helpful EDX studies on NCS are ulnar and dorsal ulnar cutaneous SNAP (sensory nerve action potential) velocities and amplitudes; CMAP latency across the wrist and amplitude recording from the first dorsal interosseous and abductor digiti minimi muscles
- Tinel's at wrist, Froment's sign

Differential Diagnosis

- See entrapment sites 1–3 discussed earlier
- Wrist flexor tendonitis

Treatment

- Conservative management
- Activity modification
- NSAIDs
- Padding gloves and handlebars
- Possible steroid injections
- If no improvement in 3 months or increased neurological signs, consider surgery particularly for space-occupying lesions

REFERENCES

1. Kimura J. *Electrodiagnosis in Diseases of Nerve and Muscle: Principles and Practice*. 3rd ed. New York (NY): Oxford University Press; 2001. p. 717–8.
2. Krivickas LS, Wilbourn AJ. Peripheral nerve injuries in athletes: a case series of over 200 injuries. *Semin Neurol*. 2000;20(2):225–32.

3. Olivo R, Tsao B. Peripheral nerve injuries in sport. *Neurol Clin.* 2017;35(3):559–72.
4. Buntragulpoontawee M, Chang KV, Vitoonpong T, et al. The effectiveness and safety of commonly used injectates for ultrasound-guided hydrodissection treatment of peripheral nerve entrapment syndromes: a systematic review. *Front Pharmacol.* 2020;11:621150.
5. Gill B, Rahman R, Khadavi M. Ultrasound-guided hydrodissection provides complete symptom resolution in radial tunnel syndrome: a case series and scoping review on hydrodissection for radial nerve pathology. *Curr Sports Med Rep.* 2022;21(9):328–35.
6. Iyer S, Kim HJ. Cervical radiculopathy. *Curr Rev Musculoskelet Med.* 2016;9(3):272–80.
7. Ewing MR, Martin H. Disability following radical neck dissection; an assessment based on the postoperative evaluation of 100 patients. *Cancer.* 1952;5(5):873–83.
8. Preston DC, Shapiro BE. *Electromyography and Neuromuscular Disorders: Clinical-Electrophysiologic-Ultrasound Correlations.* Philadelphia, PA: Elsevier; 2021.
9. Toth C, McNeil S, Feasby T. Peripheral nervous system injuries in sport and recreation: a systematic review recreation. *Sports Med.* 2005;35(8):717–38.
10. Markey KL, Di Benedetto M, Curl WW. Upper trunk brachial plexopathy. The stinger syndrome. *Am J Sports Med.* 1993;21(5):650–5.
11. Eisen A, Bertrand G. Isolated accessory nerve palsy of spontaneous origin. A clinical and electromyographic study. *Arch Neurol.* 1972;27(6):496–502.
12. Bigliani LU, Compito CA, Duralde XA, Wolfe IN. Transfer of the levator scapulae, rhomboid major, and rhomboid minor for paralysis of the trapezius. *J Bone Joint Surg Am.* 1996;78(10):1534–40.
13. Al Shareef S, Newton B. Accessory nerve injury. In: *StatPearls.* Treasure Island (FL): StatPearls Publishing; 2023.
14. Cossu G, Melis M, Melis G, Ferrigno P, Molari A. Persistent abnormal shoulder elevation after accessory nerve injury and differential diagnosis with post-traumatic focal shoulder-elevation dystonia: report of a case and literature review. *Mov Disord.* 2004;19(9):1109–11.
15. Sakellariou VI, Badilas NK, Stavropoulos NA, et al. Treatment options for brachial plexus injuries. *J Bone Joint Surg Am.* 2014;2014(1):314137.
16. Di Benedetto M, Markey K. Electrodiagnostic localization of traumatic upper trunk brachial plexopathy. *Arch Phys Med Rehabil.* 1984;65(1): 15–7.
17. Stracciolini A. Cervical burners in the athlete. *Pediatr Case Rev.* 2003;3(4):181–8.
18. Unlü MC, Kesmezacar H, Akgün I. Brachial plexus neuropathy (stinger syndrome) occurring in a patient with shoulder laxity. *Acta Orthop Traumatol Turc.* 2007;41(1):74–9.
19. Castro FP Jr. Stingers, cervical cord neurapraxia, and stenosis. *Clin Sports Med.* 2003;22(3):483–92.
20. Kelly JDIV, Aliquo D, Sitler MR, Odgers C, Moyer RA. Association of burners with cervical canal and foraminal stenosis. *Am J Sports Med.* 2000;28(2):214–7.
21. Belviso I, Palermi S, Sacco AM, et al. Brachial plexus injuries in sport medicine: clinical evaluation, diagnostic approaches, treatment options, and rehabilitative interventions. *J Funct Morphol Kinesiol.* 2020;5(2):22–19.
22. Weinberg J, Rokito S, Silber JS. Etiology, treatment, and prevention of athletic "stingers". *Clin Sports Med.* 2003;22(3):493–500, viii.
23. Baltopoulos P, Tsintzos C, Prionas G, Tsironi M. Exercise-induced scalenus syndrome. *Am J Sports Med.* 2008;36(2):369–74.
24. Ferrante MA, Ferrante ND. The thoracic outlet syndromes: part 1. Overview of the thoracic outlet syndromes and review of true neurogenic thoracic outlet syndrome. *Muscle Nerve.* 2017;55(6):782–93.
25. Jones M, Prabhakar A, Viswanath O, et al. Thoracic outlet syndrome: a comprehensive review of pathophysiology, diagnosis, and treatment. *Pain Ther.* 2019 Apr 29;8(1):5–18. DOI: 10.1007/s40122-019-0124-2
26. Sanders RJ, Hammond SL, Rao NM. Diagnosis of thoracic outlet syndrome. *J Vasc Surg.* 2007;46(3):601–4.
27. Wilbourn AJ. Thoracic outlet syndromes. *Neurol Clin.* 1999;17(3):477–97, vi.
28. Konstantinou DT, Chroni EM, Constantoyiannis C, Dougenis D. Klippel-Feil syndrome presenting with bilateral thoracic outlet syndrome. *Spine.* 2004;29(9):E189–92.
29. Dang AC, Rodner CM. Unusual compression neuropathies of the forearm, part II: median nerve. *J Hand Surg.* 2009;34(10):1915–20.
30. Chang DC, Rotellini-Coltvet LA, Mukherjee D, De Leon R, Freischlag JA. Surgical intervention for thoracic outlet syndrome improves patient's quality of life. *J Vasc Surg.* 2009;49(3):630–7.
31. Toth C. Peripheral nerve injuries attributable to sport and recreation. *Phys Med Rehabil Clin N Am.* 2009;20(1):77–100.
32. Suarez GA, Giannini C, Bosch EP, et al. Immune brachial plexus neuropathy suggestive evidence for an inflammatory-immune pathogenesis. *Neurology.* 1996;46(2):559–61.
33. Cass S. Upper extremity nerve entrapment syndromes in sports: an update. *Curr Sports Med Rep.* 2014;13(1):16–21.
34. Friedenberg SM, Zimprich T, Harper CM. The natural history of long thoracic and spinal accessory neuropathies. *Muscle Nerve.* 2002;25(4):535–9.
35. Toolanen G, Hildingsson C, Hedlund T, Knibestöl M, Oberg L. Early complications after anterior dislocation of the shoulder in patients over 40 years. An ultrasonographic and electromyographic study. *Acta Orthop Scand.* 1993;64(5):549–52.
36. Cahill BR, Palmer RE. Quadrilateral space syndrome. *J Hand Surg Am.* 1973;8(1):65–9.
37. Safran MR. Nerve injury about the shoulder in athletes, part 1: suprascapular nerve and axillary nerve nerve and axillary nerve. *Am J Sports Med.* 2004;32(3):803–19.
38. Bhandari PS, Sadhotra LP, Bhargava P, et al. Surgical outcomes following nerve transfers in upper brachial plexus injuries. *Indian J Plast Surg.* 2009;42(2):150–60.
39. Duparc F, Coquerel D, Ozeel J, Noyon M, Gerometta A, Michot C. Anatomical basis of the suprascapular nerve entrapment and clinical relevance of the supraspinatus fascia. *Surg Radiol Anat.* 2010;32(3): 277–84.
40. Moen TC, Babatunde OM, Hsu SH, Ahmad CS, Levine WN. Suprascapular neuropathy: what does the literature show? *J Shoulder Elb Res.* 2012;21(6):835–46.
41. Dong Q, Jacobson JA, Jamadar DA, et al. Entrapment neuropathies in the upper and lower limbs: anatomy and MRI features. *Radiol Res Pract.* 2012;2012:230679.
42. Ghodadra N, Nho SJ, Verma NN, et al. Arthroscopic decompression of the suprascapular nerve at the spinoglenoid notch and suprascapular notch through the subacromial space. *Arthroscopy.* 2009;25(4): 439–45.
43. Suranyi L. Median nerve compression by Struthers ligament. *J Neurol Neurosurg Psychiatry.* 1983;46(11):1047–9.
44. Tubbs RS, Marshall T, Loukas M, Shoja MM, Cohen-Gadol AA. The sublime bridge: anatomy and implications in median nerve entrapment. *J Neurosurg.* 2010;113(1):110–2.
45. Eversmann WW. Proximal median nerve compression. *Hand Clin.* 1992;8(2):307–15.
46. Chi Y, Harness NG. Anterior interosseous nerve syndrome. *J Hand Surg.* 2010;35(12):2078–80.

47. Gordon C, Johnson EW, Gatens PF, Ashton JJ. Wrist ratio correlation with carpal tunnel syndrome in industry. *Am J Phys Med Rehabil.* 1988;67(6):270–2.
48. Kara M, Ozçakar L, Gökçay D, et al. Quantification of the effects of transcutaneous electrical nerve stimulation with functional magnetic resonance imaging: a double-blind randomized placebo-controlled study. *Arch Phys Med Rehabil.* 2010;91(8):1160–5.
49. Shao YC, Harwood P, Grotz MR, Limb D, Giannoudis PV. Radial nerve palsy associated with fractures of the shaft of the humerus: a systematic review. *J Bone Jt Surg Br.* 2005;87(12):1647–52.
50. Naam NH, Nemani S. Radial tunnel syndrome. *Orthop Clin N Am.* 2012;43(4):529–36.
51. Dumitru D, Amato AA, Zwarts MJ, editors. *Electrodiagnostic Medicine.* 2nd ed. Philadelphia (PA): Hanley & Belfus; 2002.

62 Pelvis, Hip, and Thigh Injuries

Zackary Birchard, Melissa Martinez, Guy Ball, Nicholas Walla, and Brian Busconi

AVULSION FRACTURES AND APOPHYSEAL INJURIES

History/Findings

- Avulsion fractures about the hip and pelvis are the result of failure of the bone at the tendinous insertion rather than the tendon itself. These injuries are more common in skeletally immature athletes with open apophyses that are more susceptible to failure than the tendinous insertion. These are usually the result of a sudden, forceful concentric or eccentric contracture or rapid, excessive passive lengthening.
- Common sites of these avulsions about the pelvis are the insertion of the sartorius into the anterior-superior iliac spine, the rectus femoris superior head insertion into the anterior-inferior iliac spine, and the insertion of the hamstrings into the ischial tuberosity. These injuries are also seen in the proximal femur with the insertion of the hip abductors into the greater trochanter and the insertion of the iliopsoas into the lesser trochanter.
- In a 2015 review, Schuett showed males represent 76% of apophyseal avulsion fractures. About 49% occur at the anterior inferior iliac spine (AIIS), 30% occur at the anterior superior iliac spine (ASIS), 11% occur at the ischial tuberosity, and only 10% occur along the iliac crest (1).
- Radiographs may show avulsions that involve the bone. Magnetic resonance imaging (MRI) is a more sensitive test and can demonstrate the extent of injury to the muscle.

Treatment

- Nonsurgical management with rest, protected weight-bearing, and nonsteroidal anti-inflammatory drugs has been the mainstay of treatment in most series with good to excellent results reported (2).
- Indications for surgery include complete ruptures of the origin of the hamstring with retraction in active patients with functional disability, chronic ruptures associated with sciatic nerve compression, and large bone avulsion fragments that result in discomfort with sitting, symptomatic nonunion, painful heterotopic bone growth (2–4). Although most authorities do not recommend surgery for these injuries, a 2017 meta-analysis by Eberbach et al. showed a higher successful return to sport rate with surgical fixation (5). However, this idea has been challenged by Schiller and colleagues in their 2017 JAOSS article (3).
- Schiller further highlights the original work of Metzmaker and Pappas (3,6) who described a five-phase rehabilitation treatment protocol for these injuries including (a) rest, using proper positioning to unload the injured apophyses and ice/analgesics; (b) initiation of gentle active and passive range-of-motion (ROM) exercises; (c) progressive resistance beginning when 75% of motion is achieved and ending when 50% of strength is returned; (d) integration of stretching and strengthening exercises with functional activity; and (e) return to competitive sport at 8–10 weeks. Skeletally immature patients are also susceptible to chronic traction injuries at these apophyses, and this is referred to as apophysitis. Apophysitis is treated conservatively with rest followed by functional rehabilitation of the involved muscle group.

STRESS FRACTURES

Pelvis

- Pelvic stress fractures should be suspected in athletes such as long-distance runners and military recruits. The most common site is the junction between the ischium and inferior pubic ramus. Tenderness to palpation directly over the fractured bone can be helpful in locating the lesion. A positive standing sign has been described in which a patient develops discomfort in the groin while standing unsupported on the ipsilateral leg.
- Plain radiographic signs, such as periosteal reaction or fracture line, can lag behind the clinical presentation by as long as 3 weeks. MRI and bone scan can provide an earlier diagnosis. Tumors should at least be considered in the differential diagnosis.
- Treatment consists of rest with emphasis on protected weight-bearing, flexibility, and aerobic nonimpact exercises such as swimming or cycling. Return to sport can be delayed for up to 6 months.

Femoral Neck

- Femoral neck stress fractures also typically occur in military recruits and endurance athletes (7).
- Femoral neck stress fractures account for 3%–5% of all sports-related stress fractures (8).
- Women are at a disproportionate risk for femoral neck fracture (9).
- Although femoral neck stress fractures are not as common as pelvic stress fractures, if treated incorrectly, the results can be disastrous. Similar to pelvic stress fractures, these present with groin pain and an antalgic gait. Pain will be worsened by flexion and internal rotation of the hip. Again, radiographic evidence may lag by 3–4 weeks. Current research has shown that 90% of initial radiographs and 50% of 4–6 week follow-up radiographs are normal. MRI and bone scan may be helpful in earlier diagnosis (8,10).
- Several classification systems exist for femoral neck stress fractures. In 2018, Steele presented a new classification system with three types: Compression-sided, tension-sided, and displaced. Type I is a compression-side femoral neck stress fracture that he further divides into no fracture line, fracture line <50% without effusion, fracture line <50% with effusion, fracture line >50% with or without effusion. Compression-sided fractures occur at the inferior medial aspect of the neck and if <50% of the femoral neck will usually respond to non–weight-bearing status until radiographic evidence of healing has occurred. However, in Steele's classification system if the fracture is <50% of the femoral neck and associated with an effusion, or >50% of the femoral neck, strong consideration should be given to early operative intervention. Type II is a tension-side femoral neck stress fracture. This is a transverse fracture along the superior margin of the neck. Internal fixation is recommended for type II fractures. Type III fractures are displaced fractures, and immediate closed or open reduction and internal fixation is recommended for displaced fractures (10,11). Fracture displacement can lead to avascular necrosis of the femoral head.

SOFT-TISSUE INJURIES

Muscle Strains

- Soft-tissue injuries to the periarticular structures surrounding the hip and pelvis are the most common injuries seen in athletes. In general, the great majority of soft-tissue injuries about the hip and pelvis are musculotendinous strains.
- The type of injury sustained is highly dependent on (a) skeletal age of the athlete, (b) physical condition, and (c) biomechanical forces involved in both the sport and nature of the trauma. The degree of injury can range from repetitive microinjury associated with each performance to a more significant single macroinjury caused by an abnormal biomechanical force. A certain degree of microtrauma occurs with every major exertional performance immediately manifested by swelling, sensitivity, and a recovery interval. If additional moderate or severe microinjury or macroinjury occurs, there may not be a normal healing response, which may lead to more significant changes in tissue structure and a negative effect on future athletic performance (12,13).
- A strain is an injury to a musculotendinous structure caused by an indirectly applied force. The most common mechanism of injury is a result of eccentric contraction or stretching of an activated muscle. The site of injury is influenced by the rate of loading, mechanism of injury, and local anatomic factors. Low rates of loading will result in a failure at the tendon-bone junction by bone avulsion or disruption at its insertion. High rates of loading result in intratendinous or myotendinous juncture injuries.
- These injuries can be graded on a three-scale clinical grading system. Grade 1 injuries involve a simple stretching of soft-tissue fibers. Grade 2 strains involve partial tearing of the musculotendinous unit; and grade 3, which are unusual, are secondary to extreme violent forces causing complete disruptions.

Contusions

- Among the most frequently experienced hip and pelvic injuries sustained by athletes are soft-tissue contusions. Contusions usually result from direct blows to a specific soft-tissue area usually overlying a bony prominence. Contusions are most common in contact sports, especially football, but are also seen in other sports as well. In contact sports, the blow is usually caused by contact with another athlete. In noncontact sports, athletes usually sustain blows from contact with equipment (gymnastics), contact with high-velocity projectiles (lacrosse ball), or contact from the playing surface.
- Contusions are often found over areas of bony prominences of the pelvis including the iliac crest (hip pointer), greater trochanter, ischial tuberosity, and pubic rami. Because of the varied anatomy of the pelvis, contusions can be superficial, especially when they overlie a relatively subcutaneous bone or lie deep within a large muscle mass. It is important to determine possible presence and extent of muscular hemorrhage because an increase in muscular hemorrhage often results in severer symptoms and longer time before returning to sport (13).

HIP POINTER

- Pain and hemorrhage over the iliac crest have been referred to as a hip pointer. These injuries include contusions, avulsion of the iliac apophysis, periostitis, or avulsion of the muscles that insert onto the iliac crest. On physical examination, the patient will have superficial or muscular hemorrhage, which will be painful on palpation. It is important to note

by touch a defect, which would indicate an avulsion injury. Patients will have difficulty with rotation and side bending of the trunk (14).

- Anterior-posterior and oblique x-rays of the pelvis will rule out an avulsion fracture, periostitis, or an acute fracture of the iliac wing.

HAMSTRING SYNDROME

- Hamstring syndrome, described in track athletes, involves severe pain in and around the ischial tuberosity that radiates down the posterior aspect of the thigh to the popliteal area. Any activity that puts the hamstring in stretch can create this radiating pain. Sprinting, hurdling, and even sitting for long periods will cause pain.
- Physical examination elicits exquisite tenderness at the ischial tuberosity and, at times, reproduction of sciatic pain with percussion of the nerve at the ischial tuberosity. Resisted leg extension will reproduce the pain. The sciatic nerve is thought to be entrapped between the semitendinosus and the biceps femoris by a fibrous band that constricts the two muscles (13,15).

THIGH CONTUSIONS/QUADRICEPS INJURY

- Thigh contusions are common athletic injuries, most often encountered in football from direct trauma. These injuries can involve significant muscular damage, hematoma formation, and swelling. Therefore, the athlete can be extremely uncomfortable.
- Initial treatment is rest, ice, and compression to minimize hematoma formation. Immobilization in flexion and initiation of early flexion exercises have been recommended to decrease myositis ossificans formation and improve functional outcome (16).

MOREL-LAVALLEE LESION

- Morel-Lavallee lesions (MLLs) are closed soft-tissue degloving injuries that result in the separation of the dermis from the underlying fascia. These injuries most commonly occur along the proximal lateral thigh, in the peritrochanteric region; they can additionally be identified in the gluteal, lumbosacral, and abdominal areas. These injuries are the result most commonly of a high energy, shearing trauma, in areas where there may be skin hypermobility.
- Treatment of the MLL can be nonoperative or operative based on lesion size, location, and proximity to the site of anticipated surgical procedures. Smaller lesions may be amenable to nonsurgical management or focused aspiration (<50 cm^3). Large or symptomatic MLLs, especially when located in the proximity of intended surgical incisions, should be addressed with débridement and irrigation through a single incision or multiple incisions to reduce the risk of undesired sequelae. Complications can include a high rate of recurrence and pseudocyst formation (17).

SPECIFIC CONDITIONS

Athletic Pubalgia

History/Findings

- The term athletic pubalgia is often used interchangeably with sports hernia. It is a condition of chronic groin pain. The condition is common in soccer and ice hockey athletes. Typically, the patient reports activity-related pain that resolves with rest. Most patients describe a hyperextension injury in association with hyperabduction of the thigh. Usually, the abdominal pain involves the inguinal canal near the insertion of the rectus abdominis muscle at the pubis.
- Maneuvers that increase intra-abdominal pressure, such as a resisted sit-up, can reproduce the symptoms. A gross hernia is not detected. On imaging studies, 12% of patients have derangement of the insertion of the rectus on MRI. Adductor longus inflammation can also be present. Dynamic ultrasound can detect posterior wall defects.

Pathophysiology

- The rectus insertion on the pubis with or without the origin of the adductor longus tendon appears to be the primary site of pathology (18).
- The proposed mechanism of injury involves repetitive hyperextension of the trunk in association with hyperabduction of the thigh pivoting on the anterior pelvis and pubic symphysis. Only a small percentage of patients are found to have occult hernia at the time of surgery (18).

Treatment

- The initial treatment of athletic pubalgia consists of rest, ice, compression, and anti-inflammatory therapy. The role of steroid injections remains controversial and there is a lack of evidence for its widespread use at this time (18). There are medical-grade compression shorts that can help alleviate symptoms. After the symptoms resolve, an overseen slow transition back to sport is employed.
- Athletes with chronic recalcitrant tears that have exhausted conservative management for greater than 6 months may benefit from adductor tenotomy. Acute complete adductor tears can be successfully treated operatively with repair (18).

Outcomes

- With appropriate indications and surgical techniques, return to previous level of performance without pain has been reported at 80%–97% (19).

Osteitis Pubis

- Osteitis pubis is a painful inflammation of the pubis bone, symphysis, and surrounding structures. The pelvic pain can be sharp or aching. It originates over the symphysis and can radiate to the medial thigh along the adductor musculature.
- Physical exam findings include the presence of a positive lateral compression test. With the patient in a lateral decubitus position, force is applied to the iliac crest. This should reproduce the symptoms at the pubis. MRI and computed tomography (CT) findings consist of bone resorption, widening of the symphysis pubis, and periarticular sclerosis.

Pathophysiology

- The condition can be associated with a primary infection or secondary to repetitive microtrauma from the pull of the rectus muscle or gracilis.

Treatment

- Nonoperative management is typically successful. A period of rest, ice, compression, and anti-inflammatory therapy is followed with aggressive rehabilitation protocol to strengthen the pelvic girdle's musculature (18). If there is an infectious component, antibiotics are added.
- Many experts recommend at least 9 months of conservative management before considering operative intervention. If conservative options are exhausted surgical alternatives include debridement of the joint with curette, arthrodesis, and an either partial or complete resection of the joint (18).

Outcomes

- Surgical outcomes of osteitis pubis are variable (20).

Trochanteric Pain Syndrome

History/Findings

- Trochanteric pain syndrome refers to pain at the lateral and posterior aspect of the hip. There are two related conditions that contribute to the symptoms. Trochanteric bursitis is an inflammation of the bursa overlying the trochanter. Patients are typically found to have a tight iliotibial (IT) band. This can be tested with the Ober test; taking the hip from extension and abduction into an adducted position demonstrates tightness and an inability to reach the neutral position.
- Gluteus medius syndrome is recognized as a common cause of posterolateral hip pain. It is an overuse syndrome that can lead to tendinosis and partial and complete tears of the tendon. Single-leg squat or simulated stair step can reproduce the symptoms. Resisted abduction and external rotation from an internally rotated position also produce symptoms.

Pathophysiology

- Bursitis can be secondary to direct injury, overuse of the adjacent musculotendinous structures, or degenerative changes in those structures. The bursa is lined with synovial tissue. Systemic conditions that lead to synovitis can affect the bursa as well.
- Gluteus medius syndrome is an overuse injury to the tendon. It is common in women who participate in running or step aerobics.

Treatment

- In both conditions, the first line of treatment is activity modification, ice, massage, and stretch of the involved muscle. Local anesthetic and steroid injection can be a useful clinical and therapeutic tool. Recalcitrant cases may require surgery to alleviate the symptoms. The posterior aspect of the IT band can be lengthened or released for bursitis. The gluteus medius tendon may be debrided or repaired depending on the type of injury.

Piriformis Syndrome

History/Findings

- Piriformis syndrome involves compression of the sciatic nerve as it exits deep to the piriformis muscle. Patients complain of pain in the sciatic nerve distribution. A history of an acute injury to the buttock is common.
- On physical exam, the low back should be examined to rule out more proximal nerve root impingement. In the case of piriformis syndrome, typically the area of maximal tenderness is over the piriformis muscle in the gluteal area. Provocative tests include Pace sign — pain and weakness on resisted abduction and external rotation of the thigh. Forced internal rotation on an extended thigh can also reproduce the symptoms.
- An MRI can demonstrate sciatic nerve inflammation in the area of the piriformis tendon. Depending on the cause of the syndrome, myopathic and neuropathic changes can be present on electromyographic studies including a prolonged H-reflex.

Pathophysiology

- Piriformis syndrome can be caused by a traumatic injury to the piriformis muscle that leads to hypertrophy and impingement of the sciatic nerve. There can also be anatomic variations that contribute to the development of the syndrome.
- Examination of the relationship between the muscle and nerve in 240 cadavers revealed that, in 90% of the cases, the sciatic nerve emerges from below the piriformis muscle; in 7%, the piriformis and the sciatic nerve are divided, with one branch of the sciatic nerve passing through the split and the other branch passing distal to the muscle; in 2%, only the sciatic nerve is divided; and in 1%, the piriformis is divided by the sciatic nerve (21,22).

Treatment

- Treatment of piriformis syndrome with a history of trauma is directed toward soothing the muscle. Anti-inflammatory medications and muscle relaxants can provide relief. Directed massage, heat, and ultrasound can help break up scar tissue. Physical therapy can assist with these modalities as well as muscle stretch and activity modification. Often muscle imbalance is a contributing factor. Injections of anesthetic and cortisone can help with diagnosis and provide therapeutic benefit.

- If these treatments fail to provide relief, surgery can evaluate the relationship between the piriformis muscle and the sciatic nerve. The nerve can be decompressed, and the muscle can be released to provide relief.

Outcomes

- Benson and Schutzer (21,23) reported the results of 15 cases of traumatic piriformis syndrome. They had 11 excellent and four good results with clinical follow-up at 2 years.

Internal/External Snapping Hip

History/Findings

- A snapping hip, or coxa saltans, refers to the catching of a muscle as it crosses the hip joint. The two most common muscles that can get caught are the IT band as it crosses the greater trochanter and the iliopsoas as it crosses over the anterior hip joint.
- The posterior aspect of the IT band catches at the greater trochanter at the outside of the hip joint and is referred to as an external snapping hip. The patient is often able to make the hip snap. Visually, it can appear dramatic and be confused with a subluxing hip. Over time, the catching can lead to irritation at the trochanteric bursa.
- The internal snapping hip involves the iliopsoas getting caught as it crosses the iliopectineal eminence. The internal snapping hip is often associated with an audible "pop." The bursa around the muscle can be irritated over time and lead to pain. The snap is reproduced when taking the hip from flexion, abduction, and external rotation to a neutral extended position. MRI is useful to rule out other conditions and can demonstrate associated bursitis.

Pathophysiology

- Both snapping hip conditions are associated with tight muscles. In adolescents, a growth spurt can precede the development of muscle tightness. Typically, the snapping muscle does not cause pain, but over time, the compression and shear across the bursa can lead to the development of irritation and bursitis, which is painful.
- In each condition, it is important to rule out additional pathology. The external snapping hip can be associated with tears of the gluteus medius. Both the gluteus medius and the IT band assist in abduction of the hip. If surgical intervention is considered, a tear must be ruled out first.
- The internal snapping hip is common in cases of intra-articular pathology. The iliopsoas or hip flexor crosses directly over the anterior superior labrum. An intra-articular hip derangement can lead to an effusion that exacerbates the symptoms. Conditions such as loose bodies, labral tears, and impingement should be ruled out in a persistent symptomatic internal snapping hip.

Treatment

- Initial management focuses on the treatment of the tight muscle. Physical therapy is an essential adjuvant to selectively stretch the responsible muscle and tendon. Deep massage and ultrasound can assist in alleviating symptoms. An elastic spica wrap or medical-grade compression shorts help control symptoms while stretching the muscles. IT band syndrome and external snapping hip are associated with hill training. Activity modification and cross-training assist in reducing symptoms. When the condition has become painful, steroid injections can decrease the inflammation of the bursa.
- With failed nonoperative management, there are a number of surgical interventions that can lengthen the muscle and address the bursa. More recently, these procedures have been performed endoscopically with encouraging results.

Outcomes

- Ilizaliturri and Camacho-Galindo (7,24) reviewed their results of both endoscopic IT band releases and iliopsoas releases. With at least 2 years of follow-up, 10 patients with endoscopic release of the IT band had resolution of pain. One patient had a painless snapping hip (25). For the hip flexor release, six patients were followed for at least 2 years. All patients had complete relief of symptoms. There was no residual flexion weakness (24,26).

Femoroacetabular Impingement

History/Findings

- Femoroacetabular impingement is an abnormal contact between femur and acetabulum, specifically the anterosuperior femoral head/neck and acetabulum rim. This abnormal contact can lead to damage to the labrum and chondral surface over time.
- Patients typically present in young to middle age with decreased ROM and progressive groin pain exacerbated with physical activity. The abnormal contour of the hip is not by definition painful, but the lesions to the cartilage and labrum result in symptoms.
- On physical exam, pain in the groin and catching with flexion, adduction, and internal rotation are associated with chondral damage and labral injury at the anterolateral rim of the acetabulum. Often patients describe the discomfort as deep within the hip by cupping their hand; this is referred to as the "C" sign. Decreased ROM with flexion, abduction, and external rotation is also indicative of impingement.
- Plain films can demonstrate an abnormal orientation of the acetabulum and contour of the femoral head-neck junction. The crossover sign, also known as the "figure of 8" sign, which evaluates the orientation of the anterior and posterior acetabular walls, can be identified on plain films and indicates acetabular retroversion. CT scans with three-dimensional reconstructions are useful to evaluate the

relationship between the acetabulum and femoral head-neck junction for abnormal cases of impingement. An MRI arthrogram is necessary to evaluate soft-tissue damage to the labrum and articular surface of the acetabulum.

Pathophysiology

- The two components of femoroacetabular impingement are impingement from the acetabulum, or "pincer," and impingement from the femoral head neck junction, or "cam."
- Pincer impingement is the result of a deep acetabulum (coxa profunda) or abnormal orientation of the acetabulum resulting in anterior overcoverage (acetabular retroversion).
- Cam impingement is typically an aspherical contour of the anterolateral head-neck junction. This can be visualized on the frog leg lateral view of the femur and the axial images of a CT scan or MRI.
- Most patients present with a mixture of cam and pincer impingement. The abnormal anatomy can be congenital or acquired (27,28).

Treatment

- Treatment is dependent on the degree of abnormal anatomy and the patient goals. The use of an anti-inflammatory medication to calm down the soft-tissue irritation followed by physical therapy to strengthen the surrounding musculature and adjust pelvic tilt to avoid the abnormal contact is the first line of treatment.
- Often, these patients present after months or years of pain and limitation. In these cases, the nonoperative modalities can exacerbate the symptoms and necessitate surgery. In the past, the impingement was treated with open surgical dislocation of the hip and osteoplasty of the femur and acetabulum. Within the last 15 years, many of the procedures to address the abnormal anatomy and soft-tissue injuries have been performed arthroscopically (27,29).

Outcomes

- The midterm results of both open and arthroscopic procedures are directly related to the degree of osteoarthritis at the time of surgery. Patients with minimal arthritis treated arthroscopically have demonstrated good and excellent results after 3 years of follow-up with significant improvement in pain and function (27,30).

Acetabular Labral Tear

History/Findings

- The labrum is the fibrocartilaginous rim around the articular surface of the acetabulum. Biomechanical studies have shown that it has little function in the distribution of forces or in stability. The labrum functions significantly as a hydraulic seal.
- The clinical findings depend on the location of the labral tear and can be variable. Groin pain and mechanical symptoms with flexion, adduction, and internal rotation are indicative of an anterior-superior lesion.
- An MRI arthrogram with radial reconstructions is the study of choice to evaluate the labrum. Fluid can be seen tracking under the injured labrum.

Pathophysiology

- Labral tears can be the result of abnormal morphology such as femoroacetabular impingement or normal anatomy that is placed in supraphysiologic positions. Isolated labral tears are common in elite athletes and dancers who present with groin pain. These injuries can also be seen in acute trauma, such as a hip dislocation or subluxation. Isolated labral tears are rare in patients who present with an insidious onset of pain. In these cases, it is important to rule out associated conditions such as femoroacetabular impingement. Degenerative tears of the labrum occur with the progression of osteoarthritis.

Treatment

- Initial management of labral tears consists of rest, anti-inflammatory medications, and physical therapy followed by a slow transition back to sport.
- If the symptoms fail to resolve with rest or recur with advancing activity, surgical management is a consideration. The majority of the treatments to address the labrum can now be performed arthroscopically. The choice of a removal of the irritated portion of the labrum versus repair is dependent on a number of factors including the location of the tear, age of the patient, chronicity of the injury, and associated findings.

Outcomes

- A recent study with 10-year follow-up demonstrated 82% continued successful outcomes in patients treated with labral debridement in the absence of osteoarthritis (31,32). Long-term results of arthroscopic repair have not been reported to date. Conceptually, it would make sense that restoration of the anatomy and maintenance of the fluid seal would be beneficial. Regardless of whether the labrum is repaired or removed, it is essential that additional pathology be diagnosed and addressed at the time of surgery.

Loose Bodies

History/Findings

- Loose bodies are common after acute trauma to the hip including subluxations and dislocations. In the setting of dislocation, the incidence has been reported at 92% (33,34). The patient typically reports mechanical symptoms, including locking, catching, or clicking.
- Plain films, CT, and MRI can demonstrate the presence of loose bodies.

Pathophysiology

- The overall stability of the hip joint is related to bony congruence. With a traumatic dislocation, the force at the edge of the acetabulum can lead to a fracture or commonly a shear injury to the cartilage at the edge of the acetabulum. With reduction of the dislocation, those fragments can be caught within the joint. Even without radiographic evidence of loose bodies, arthroscopic evaluation can demonstrate fragments in the joint.

- Other atraumatic conditions that are associated with loose bodies include synovial chondromatosis, dislodged osteophytes, and foreign bodies (33,35).

Treatment

- Mechanical symptoms in the presence of a corresponding clinical history are an indication for arthroscopic evaluation.

Ruptured Ligamentum Teres

History/Findings

- The ligamentum teres is the connection between the cotyloid fossa of the acetabulum and the fovea capitis of the femoral head. It provides blood supply to the developing hip. After adolescence, the function of the structure is not fully known. It is postulated that it provides additional stability and resists dislocation forces at the hip. Injury to the ligamentum teres results in catching, popping, locking, and giving way. These findings are common in intra-articular pathology.
- There is no physical exam test that is pathognomonic for ligamentum teres injury. Imaging findings can be variable as well. In a study by Byrd and Jones (36,37), the diagnosis was made preoperatively in 2 of 23 patients.

Pathophysiology

- Disruption of the ligamentum teres is common after trauma and hip dislocation, but it can occur without dislocation as well. The structure is tight in adduction, flexion, and external rotation. Acute disruptions are believed to occur with exaggerated adduction and external rotation.

Treatment

- The symptoms associated with an injury to the ligamentum teres are believed to be secondary to hyperplasia of the surrounding tissue and soft-tissue impingement. Initial management should consist of modalities to rest the hip and control inflammation.
- Arthroscopic management consists of debridement of the torn fibers of the ligamentum teres.

Outcomes

- Byrd and Jones (36,37) published the results of their experience in 23 cases of traumatic tears. The results demonstrated a significant improvement in pain and function.

REFERENCES

1. Schuett DJ, Bomar JD, Pennock AT. Pelvic apophyseal avulsion fractures: a retrospective review of 228 cases. *J Pediatr Orthop*. 2015;35(6):617–23.
2. Yeager KC, Silva SR, Richter DL. Pelvic avulsion injuries in the adolescent athlete. *Clin Sports Med*. 2021;40(2):375–84.
3. Schiller J, DeFroda S, Blood T. Lower extremity avulsion fractures in the pediatric and adolescent athlete. *J Am Acad Orthop Surg*. 2017;25(4):251–9.
4. Cohen S, Bradley J. Acute proximal hamstring rupture. *J Am Acad Orthop Surg*. 2007;15(6):350–5.
5. Eberbach H, Hohloch L, Feucht MJ, Konstantinidis L, Südkamp NP, Zwingmann J. Operative versus conservative treatment of apophyseal avulsion fractures of the pelvis in the adolescents: a systematical review with meta-analysis of clinical outcome and return to sports. *BMC Musculoskelet Disord*. 2017;18(1):162. doi:10.1186/s12891-017-1527-z
6. Metzmaker JN, Pappas AM. Avulsion fractures of the pelvis. *Am J Sports Med*. 1985;13(5):349–58.
7. Ilizaliturri VM Jr, Camacho-Galindo J. Endoscopic treatment of snapping hips, iliotibial band, and iliopsoas tendon. *Sports Med Arthrosc Rev*. 2010;18(2):120–7.
8. Bernstein E, Kelsey T, Cochran G, Deafenbaugh B, Kuhn K. Femoral neck stress fractures: an updated review. *J Am Acad Orthop Surg*. 2022;30(7):302–11.
9. Kupferer KR, Bush DM, Cornell JE, et al. Femoral neck stress fracture in Air Force basic trainees. *Mil Med*. 2014;179(1):56–61.
10. May LA, Chen DC, Bui-Mansfield LT, O'Brien SD. Rapid magnetic resonance imaging evaluation of femoral neck stress fractures in a US active duty military population. *Mil Med*. 2017;182(1):e1619–25.
11. Steele CE, Cochran G, Renninger C, Deafenbaugh B, Kuhn KM. Femoral neck stress fractures: MRI risk factors for progression. *J Bone Joint Surg Am*. 2018;100(17):1496–502.
12. Hammond KE, Kneer L, Cicinelli P. Rehabilitation of soft tissue injuries of the hip and pelvis. *Clin Sports Med*. 2021;40(2):409–28.
13. Busconi BD, Wixted JJ, Owens BD. Differential diagnosis of the painful hip. In: McCarthy JC, editor. *Early Hip Disease: Advances in Detection and Minimally Invasive Treatment*. New York (NY): Springer-Verlag; 2003. p. 97–103.
14. Hall M, Anderson J. Hip pointers. *Clin Sports Med*. 2013;32(2):325–30.
15. Park JW, Lee YK, Lee YJ, Shin S, Kang Y, Koo KH. Deep gluteal syndrome as a cause of posterior hip pain and sciatica-like pain. *Bone Joint J*. 2020;102-B(5):556–67.
16. Lempainen L, Mechó S, Valle X, et al. Management of anterior thigh injuries in soccer players: practical guide. *BMC Sports Sci Med Rehabil*. 2022;14(1):41.
17. Scolaro JA, Chao T, Zamorano DP. The Morel-Lavallée lesion: diagnosis and management. *J Am Acad Orthop Surg* 2016;24(10):667–72.
18. Elattar O, Choi HR, Dills VD, Busconi B. Groin injuries (athletic pubalgia) and return to play. *Sports Health*. 2016;8(4):313–23.
19. Paajanen H, Brinck T, Hermunen H, Airo I. Laparoscopic surgery for chronic groin pain in athletes is more effective than nonoperative treatment: a randomized clinical trial with magnetic resonance imaging of 60 patients with sportsman's hernia (athletic pubalgia). *Surgery*. 2011;150(1):99–107.
20. Choi H, McCartney M, Best TM. Treatment of osteitis pubis and osteomyelitis of the pubic symphysis in athletes: a systematic review. *Br J Sports Med*. 2011;45(1):57–64.
21. Cass SP. Piriformis syndrome: a cause of nondiscogenic sciatica. *Curr Sports Med Rep*. 2015;14(1):41–4.
22. Beaton LE, Anson BJ. The sciatic nerve and the piriformis muscle: their interrelation a possible cause of coccygodynia. *J Bone Joint Surg Am*. 1938;20(3):686–8.
23. Benson ER, Schutzer SF. Posttraumatic piriformis syndrome: diagnosis and results of operative treatment. *J Bone Joint Surg Am*. 1999;81(7):941–9.

24. Walker P, Ellis E, Scofield J, Kongchum T, Sherman WF, Kaye AD. Snapping hip syndrome: a comprehensive update. *Orthop Rev*. 2021;13(2):25088.
25. Ilizaliturri VM Jr, Martinez-Escalante FA, Chaidez PA, Camacho-Galindo J. Endoscopic iliotibial band release for external snapping hip syndrome. *Arthroscopy*. 2006;22(5):505–10.
26. Ilizaliturri VM Jr, Villalobos FE Jr, Chaidez PA, Valero FS, Aguilera JM. Internal snapping hip syndrome: treatment by endoscopic release of the iliopsoas tendon. *Arthroscopy*. 2005;21(11):1375–80.
27. Egger AC, Frangiamore S, Rosneck J. Femoroacetabular impingement: a review. *Sports Med Arthrosc Rev*. 2016;24(4):e53–8.
28. Safran MR. Hip joint injuries. In: Kibler WB, editor. *Orthopaedic Knowledge Update*. Rosemont (IL): American Academy of Orthopaedic Surgeons; 2009. p. 91–100.
29. Safran MR. Hip arthroscopy: the basics. In: Wiesel SW, editor. *Operative Techniques in Orthopaedic Surgery*. Philadelphia (PA): Lippincott Williams & Wilkins; 2010. p. 191–202.
30. Philippon MJ, Briggs KK, Yen YM, Kuppersmith DA. Outcomes following hip arthroscopy for femoroacetabular impingement with associated chondrolabral dysfunction: minimum two-year follow-up. *J Bone Joint Surg Br*. 2009;91(1):16–23.
31. Hyland SS Jr, Maeso AD, Rogers M, Goforth M, Brolinson PG. Comparative analysis between operative and non-operative acetabular labral tear injuries in division 1 collegiate athletes. *Sci Rep*. 2023;13(1):9461.
32. Byrd JW, Jones KS. Prospective analysis of hip arthroscopy with 10-year followup. *Clin Orthop Relat Res*. 2010;468(3):741–6.
33. Khanna V, Harris A, Farrokhyar F, Choudur HN, Wong IH. Hip arthroscopy: prevalence of intra-articular pathologic findings after traumatic injury of the hip. *Arthroscopy*. 2014;30(3):299–304.
34. Mullis BH, Dahners LE. Hip arthroscopy to remove loose bodies after traumatic dislocation. *J Orthop Trauma*. 2006;20(1):22–6.
35. Djaja YP, Kim S, Lee GY, Ha YC. Acetabular ossicles: epidemiology and correlation with femoroacetabular impingement. *Arthroscopy*. 2020;36(4):1063–73.
36. de SA D, Phillips M, Philippon MJ, Letkemann S, Simunovic N, Ayeni OR. Ligamentum teres injuries of the hip: a systematic review examining surgical indications, treatment options, and outcomes. *Arthroscopy*. 2014;30(12):1634–41.
37. Byrd JW, Jones KS. Traumatic rupture of the ligamentum teres as a source of hip pain. *Arthroscopy*. 2004;20(4):385–91.

63 Knee Meniscal Injuries

James Alexander McIntyre, Matthew J. Salzler, and John C. Richmond

INTRODUCTION

- The meniscus plays an important role in weight distribution, reduction in joint contact stresses, joint stabilization, and energy absorption (1–5). Injury to the meniscus can result in marked physical impairment.
- Once thought to be a vestigial organ, it is now recognized that meniscectomy often leads to a recognizable pattern of joint deterioration including joint space narrowing, osteophyte formation, and squaring of the femoral condyles (2).
- Meniscal preservation is the goal of new surgical procedures.
- Arthroscopy facilitates optimal treatment of meniscal tears with minimally invasive techniques.

ANATOMY AND BASIC SCIENCE

- Each of the medial and lateral compartments of a knee has an intervening meniscus located between the femur and tibia.
- The menisci are peripherally thick and convex and centrally taper to a thin free margin (1).
- The meniscal surfaces conform to the femoral and tibial contours.
- Each meniscus has anterior and posterior bony attachment sites called the meniscal roots.

Medial Meniscus

- The medial meniscus is semicircular and crescent shaped and measures approximately 3.5 cm in length.
- The medial meniscus covers 50%–60% of the medial tibial plateau. The posterior horn is wider than the anterior horn in the anteroposterior dimension (4,5).
- The attachment site for the anterior horn is variable, in the area of the intercondylar fossa in front of the anterior cruciate ligament (ACL), often to the anterior surface of the tibial plateau.
- The posterior fibers of the anterior horn merge with the transverse fibers of the intermeniscal ligament, which connects the anterior horns of the medial and lateral menisci. The intermeniscal ligament is located approximately 8 mm anterior to the ACL (1).
- The posterior horn is firmly attached to the posterior intercondylar fossa of the tibia, anterior and medial to the posterior cruciate ligament (PCL) attachment site (1).
- The peripheral fibers are attached to the capsule throughout its length, and the tibial portion of this attachment is called the coronary ligament. In addition, at its midpoint, the medial meniscus is firmly attached to the femur and tibia through a condensation of the joint capsule known as the deep medial collateral ligament (5).

Lateral Meniscus

- The lateral meniscus is almost circular in gross morphology and covers 70%–80% of the lateral tibial plateau (1,5).
- The lateral meniscus is nearly uniform in width from front to back.
- The bony attachments of the lateral meniscus are much closer to each other than those of the medial meniscus. The anterior root attaches adjacent to the ACL, and the posterior root attaches just posterior to the ACL, which is anterior to the posterior horn of the medial meniscus.
- There is a loose peripheral attachment of the lateral meniscus to the joint capsule that allows over two times as much excursion when compared to the medial meniscus (11.2 vs. 5.2 mm) (1).
- The area of the lateral meniscus with no coronary ligament attachment, anterior to the popliteus tendon, is called the bare area of the lateral meniscus, or popliteal hiatus.

Lateral Meniscus Attachments

- Motion of the lateral meniscus is guided by the capsular attachments, as well as additional ligamentous attachments. These ligaments include the meniscofemoral ligaments (MFLs) and the anterior inferior and posterior superior popliteomeniscal fascicles from the popliteus muscle.
- The posterior horn has variably present attachments to the medial femoral condyle through the MFLs. The MFLs originate from the posterior horn of the lateral meniscus.
- The anterior MFL (of Humphrey) passes anterior to the PCL to insert on the femur between the distal margin of the femoral attachment of the PCL and the edge of the condylar articular cartilage.

- The posterior MFL (of Wrisberg) passes posterior to the PCL to insert at the proximal margin of the femoral attachment of the PCL.
- The overall incidence of at least one MFL is 91%. In the knees demonstrating at least one structure, the incidence of an anterior MFL is 48.2%, and the incidence of posterior MFL is 70.4%. The incidence of both ligaments coexisting in one knee is 31.8% (6).

Meniscal Variants

- Three types exist — incomplete and complete Discoid and Wrisberg.
- Discoid variants occur with an estimated incidence of 0.7%–5.0%, most commonly the incomplete type (7).
- Though usually unilateral, it has been reported to be bilateral in 5%–25% of cases (7).
- Discoid meniscus is almost universally located in the lateral compartment.
- X-rays are most commonly normal, but may sometimes reveal cupping of the lateral tibial plateau and squaring of the lateral femoral condyle.
- Both the incomplete and complete types have firm posterior tibial attachments and are considered stable.
- The Wrisberg variant occurs when the posterior root attachment and posterior meniscocapsular attachments are absent. Thus, the posterior MFL of Wrisberg is the only stabilizing structure (3,7).

Microscopic Anatomy

- The menisci are fibrocartilaginous tissue composed of cells interspersed in a matrix largely composed of collagen bundles, along with noncollagenous proteins including elastin and proteoglycans.
- Two cell types are present — a more fusiform, fibroblastic cell, and a more rounded, chondrocytic cell.
- Water constitutes 72% of the extracellular matrix, and collagen makes up 75% of the dry weight (4).
- Elastin is estimated to be less than 0.6%, and noncollagenous proteins 8%–13%, of the meniscus dry weight in humans (4).
- Type I collagen represents 90% of collagen present, and types II, III, V, and VI are present in varying quantities depending on the location and age (4).
- The principal orientation of collagen fiber bundles is circumferential, with few radially directed "tie" fibers. Tie fibers provide structural rigidity to help resist forces that would split the circumferential fibers with compressive loading (1,4).
- Fiber orientation changes with depth from the surface. Surface fibers are arranged as a network of irregularly oriented bundles. The deeper fibers are primarily circumferential (4).

Neurovascular Anatomy

- Both medial and lateral menisci demonstrate an extensive microvascular network, arising from the respective superior and inferior genicular arteries, which are branches of the popliteal artery (5,8).
- The perimeniscal capillary plexus is oriented circumferentially and branches extensively into smaller vessels to supply the peripheral border of the meniscus through its attachment to the capsule.
- The branches terminate after supplying the peripheral 10%–30% of the meniscus, leaving the remainder avascular (4,8).
- Free nerve endings and specialized end receptors are present within the menisci. The most densely innervated regions are the anterior and posterior horns of both menisci (4).
- Nerve fibers originate in the perimeniscal tissues and radiate into the peripheral 30% of the meniscus, mimicking the vascular anatomy of the meniscus.
- Three receptor types have been identified — Ruffini endings, Golgi tendon organs, and Pacinian corpuscles (9).
- Ruffini endings are unmyelinated, slow adapting fibers that sense changes in joint deformation and pain.
- Golgi tendon organs are myelinated fibers that contribute to neuromuscular inhibition at terminal range of motion.
- Pacinian corpuscles are myelinated fibers that respond to tension and pressure changes.
- It is hypothesized that the nerves play a proprioceptive role in normal joint function. Meniscal-derived signals generated during deformation and loading may be important to joint position sense and for protective neuromuscular reflex control of joint motion and loading (4).

Nutrition of the Menisci

- The bulk of meniscus nutrition is supplied by the synovial fluid, most notably to the avascular regions.
- Nutrients reach the tissue via passive diffusion and mechanical pumping with intermittent compression during loading (4).

BIOMECHANICS AND MENISCAL FUNCTION

- The menisci serve in load transmission, shock absorption, lubrication, prevention of synovial impingement, synovial fluid distribution, stability, and improved gliding motion (5).
- Long-term follow-up demonstrates that virtually all knees after total meniscectomy develop degenerative changes, and this is less frequent after partial meniscectomy (10,11).

Meniscus Motion

- With knee flexion from 0°–120°, the menisci move posteriorly. In the midcondylar, parasagittal plane, the medial meniscus moves approximately 5.1 mm, and the lateral meniscus moves 11.2 mm (1).

- The medial meniscus lacks the controlled mobility of the lateral meniscus.
- Posterior motion of the medial meniscus is guided by the deep medial collateral ligament and semimembranosus, whereas anterior translation is caused by the push of the anterior femoral condyle (12).
- The posterior oblique fibers of the deep medial collateral ligament limit motion in rotation, and therefore, the medial meniscus is at increased risk of tear (1,8).
- The lateral meniscus is stabilized, and motion guided, by the popliteus tendon, popliteomeniscal ligaments, popliteofibular ligament, MFLs, and lateral capsule.
- Meniscal motion allows continued load distribution during changes of position of the joint, during which the radius of curvature of the femoral condyles changes (12).

Knee Stability

- The medial meniscus provides greater restraint to anterior translation than the lateral meniscus by acting as a buttress (13,14).
- ACL-deficient knees demonstrate increased anterior translation when subjected to an anteriorly directed force, and this translation increases significantly with combined meniscectomy at all angles of flexion. This confirms the role of the ACL as a primary restraint to anterior translation and demonstrates that the medial meniscus acts as a secondary stabilizer to resist anterior translation (14).
- With sufficient anterior translation (in the ACL-deficient knee), the posterior horn of the medial meniscus is wedged between the tibial plateau and the femoral condyle and is the mechanism suggested for the resistance provided by the meniscus.
- In contrast, the soft-tissue attachments of the lateral meniscus do not affix the lateral meniscus as firmly to the tibia. Combined lateral meniscectomy and ACL sectioning do not increase anterior translation significantly over ACL sectioning alone. This implies that the greater mobility of the lateral meniscus prevents it from contributing as efficiently as a posterior wedge to resist anterior translation of the tibia on the femur (13).

Load Sharing

- The menisci serve additional functional roles, including load bearing and shock absorption (5). The menisci transmit large loads across the joint, and their contact areas change with different degrees of knee flexion and rotation.
- An intact meniscus expands to resist a compressive load. It decreases this load on the articular cartilage via hoop stress, defined as a tensile stress that transmits compressive force in the axial along the intact circumferential fibers of the meniscus in the transverse plane (15).
- Up to 50%–70% of compressive load is transmitted through the menisci in extension, and 85% at 90° of flexion (1,3,5,8).
- Removal of a portion of the meniscus results in a decreased contact area and subsequently increased peak contact pressure between the femur and tibia. Medial meniscectomy decreases the contact area by up to 70%.
- Resection of as little as 15%–34% of the meniscus results in increased contact pressure by up to 350% (12).

EPIDEMIOLOGY

- The annual incidence of meniscal injury is 60–70 per 100,000 persons (3).
- Meniscus injury is more common in males, with a male-to-female ratio between 2.5:1 and 4:1 (3).
- Approximately one-third of all tears are associated with ACL injury, and approximately 80% of repairable meniscal tears occur during ACL injury (8).
- Meniscal tears are also commonly associated with tibia plateau fractures and femoral shaft fractures.
- Degenerative tears peak in the fourth through sixth decade in men and remain relatively constant after the second decade in women (3).
- Medial meniscus tears are more common than lateral tears, and tears are most frequently located in the midportion and posterior horns of the meniscus.
- Medial meniscal tears are more commonly longitudinal type, whereas laterally, a radial component is more frequent (8).

DIAGNOSIS OF MENISCAL INJURY

History

- Meniscal injury during sport occurs most frequently during noncontact cutting, deceleration, hyperflexion, or landing from a jump.
- Degenerative meniscal injury with aging (>40 years) often occurs after trivial insult. The tear may not be noticed at the time of injury. The mechanical symptoms that follow often trigger the patient to seek attention.
- Mechanical symptoms of popping, catching, locking, or buckling, along with joint line pain, are suggestive of meniscal tear. These are nonspecific symptoms and may be secondary to chondral injury or patellofemoral chondrosis (3).
- Mild synovitis often results from the injury, with swelling present for several days after the event. The synovitis may be recurrent and activity related.
- An audible pop at the time of injury is more characteristic of an ACL tear; however, a meniscus tear is commonly present in this scenario.

- Immediate swelling suggests bleeding and is frequently not present after isolated meniscus tear; however, it may be present with a more peripherally based tear.
- A delayed effusion is more characteristic of meniscus injury, with the production of reactive joint fluid.
- The reporting of loss of motion with a sensation of a mechanical block to extension is suggestive of a displaced meniscus tear (3).
- A history of a snapping or popping knee may suggest a discoid variant. Mechanical symptoms present in childhood or adolescence, without a history of trauma, should raise the suspicion of the presence of a discoid meniscus (5).
- The complete history should include assessment of the patient's lifestyle, activity level, occupation, and medical history. Younger, more active individuals often require more aggressive management.

Physical Examination

- Examination begins with evaluation of gait. A limp is common after meniscus tear, and pain after an acute injury may result in the inability to bear weight.
- Inspection of the knee includes evaluation for an effusion, as well as thigh asymmetry in the setting of a chronic tear.
- Range of motion is assessed in comparison to the opposite extremity. A displaced tear may block the knee from achieving full extension, as well as impair flexion. A mechanical block to motion is termed the locked knee.
- Palpation of the joint lines is performed in an effort to elicit tenderness and may be the best clinical sign of a tear, with 74% sensitivity and 50% positive predictive value (3).
- Pain at terminal flexion or extension may be present, depending on the location of the tear.
- The McMurray test is performed with the patient supine. The hip and knee are flexed, and the foot is alternately internally and externally rotated during application of a circumduction maneuver to the knee. Concurrently, the examiner palpates the posterolateral and posteromedial joint lines.
- Medial meniscal injury is tested by extending the knee with the foot externally rotated. Lateral meniscal injury is assessed with the foot internally rotated.
- A palpable and audible clunk is considered a positive McMurray test. A true positive test is uncommon, even in the presence of a tear, but is nearly 100% specific. The sensitivity of the test is as low as 15% (3). More commonly, the test elicits pain (16).
- Cysts at or below the joint line may be palpable and are highly correlated with meniscal tears, most commonly lateral (3).
- No clinical examination finding is consistently predictive of meniscus tear; however, the combination of several positive tests from the following list is highly predictive of meniscus tear: joint line tenderness, pain on forced flexion, positive McMurray test, and a block to extension.
- Sensitivity of thorough examination reaches 95% and specificity 72% (3).
- Confounding diagnoses include fibrotic plica, fat pad impingement, chondral lesions, and synovitis.

Imaging

- Diagnostic studies should begin with plain radiography. Radiographs are assessed for associated skeletal injury, loose bodies, and presence of degenerative changes.
- Radiographs should include a 45° flexed knee posteroanterior weight-bearing view for individuals who may have knee arthrosis. Flexion weight-bearing views allow evaluation of the posterior tibiofemoral contact region, which is most frequently involved in early degenerative arthritis. Identification of arthrosis may have significant influence on treatment planning.
- Arthrograms are generally reserved for individuals for whom magnetic resonance imaging (MRI) is not possible. This includes individuals with metal implants (pacemaker, aneurysm clips, foreign body, and the like), individuals too large for the MRI equipment, or individuals with severe claustrophobia.
- MRI is the diagnostic modality of choice to evaluate the menisci.
- Accuracy of modern MRI scans in detection of meniscus tears approaches 95% (3).
- MRI studies have shown that the meniscal substance is not always homogeneous.
- Abnormal signal has been found in up to 30% of asymptomatic patients without any history of knee injury (5).
- Normal anatomic structures adjacent to the meniscus, such as the intermeniscal ligament and hiatus for the popliteus tendon, can be a source of confusion in interpretation of MRI scans (17).
- False-positive results occur more frequently than false-negative results, which emphasize the need for clinical correlation.
- Routine preoperative MRI scan does not significantly improve diagnostic accuracy over clinical examination alone (18). Each has accuracy in competitive athletes of approximately 90% (19).
- MRI does provide information regarding the extent of the tear and identification of occult chondral and osseous injuries.
- Judicious use of MRI is recommended, particularly in patients in whom arthroscopic surgery is anticipated.

MRI Interpretation

- Meniscal signals as shown by MRI have been classified into four grades:
  - Grade 0 signal: Uniformly low signal intensity (normal meniscus)
  - Grade I signal: Irregular increases in intrameniscal signal

- Grade II signal: Linear increases in intrameniscal signal, not communicating with the superior or inferior meniscal surface
- Grade III signal: Abnormal increased signal extends to one meniscal surface
- Grades I and II have no surgical significance. Grade III signal is visible arthroscopically and represents a meniscus tear.

MENISCAL PATHOLOGY

Meniscus Tears and Tear Patterns

- Meniscus injuries are commonly classified by the description of the pattern and location of tear.
- Locations within the meniscus include anterior root, anterior horn, body, posterior horn, and posterior root.
- Location can also be described as red-red, red-white, and white-white.
  - Tear classification based on location is as follows: red-red tear, located at the meniscal periphery within the vascular zone; red-white, no blood supply from the inner surface of the lesion; and white-white, located in the avascular zone.
  - It is important to classify the location of the tear relative to the blood supply of the meniscus in order to predict repair potential.
  - Red-red tears have the greatest potential for healing, and white-white tears the least (8).
- Patterns of tear include vertical longitudinal, oblique (flap, parrot beak), horizontal, radial (transverse), and complex.
- Vertical and oblique patterns constitute approximately 80% of tears (3).
- Complex, degenerative tears increase in frequency with age.
- A complete, displaced vertical tear is termed a bucket-handle tear and is the pattern often associated with mechanical block to motion.
- Radial tears disrupt the circumferential fibers of the meniscus and, when they extend to the periphery, result in loss of the load-bearing function of the meniscus.

MENISCAL ROOT PATHOLOGY

- Complete radial tears within 1 cm of the posterior attachment or avulsion off the insertion is considered to be meniscal root injuries.
- Lack of meniscal root integrity leads to significantly increased contact pressure at the tibiofemoral joint, comparable to those recorded after total meniscectomy (20).
- Posterior medial meniscus root tears are thought to lead to the most deleterious tibiofemoral contact pressure changes due to its inherently more rigid fixation to the tibia via capsulomeniscal connections (15).
- However, complete posterior lateral meniscus root tears can lead to increased contact pressures of up to 50%. This can be an underrecognized pathology in patients with concomitant ACL tears (21).

RAMP LESIONS

- Tear or disruption of the peripheral meniscocapsular attachments of the posterior horn of the medial meniscus (22)
- Important as this attachment contributes significantly as a static stabilizer of the knee and resistance to anterior tibial translation
- Seen in 9%–17% of all ACL tears
- Although the contribution of posterior meniscocapsular junction to knee stability is not as large as that of complete radial tears, posterior root tears, or ACL deficiency, these lesions contribute to external rotation instability and anterior tibial translation (22,23).
- Ramp lesions increase forces seen by the ACL by 33%–50% and are hypothesized to be a contributing factor to ACL reconstruction failure (24).
- Although no definitive recommendations exist to indicate that all ramp lesions should be repaired, the lesion is in the peripheral vascular zone and plays a significant role in knee stability, making it a lesion with good biologic potential for healing while repair reconstitutes a structure that contributes significantly to knee stability and decreases stress on the ACL.

TREATMENT

- Treatment of meniscal injury is influenced by patient factors, as well as the nature of the meniscal pathology. Patient factors include the chronicity of symptoms, tolerance for activity modification following repair versus resection, tolerance for risk of failure, expectations, age, and underlying condition of the joint (8).
- The determinants of successful healing of a torn meniscus include tear location and configuration.
- No more than the peripheral one-third of the meniscus has a vascular supply. Therefore, the central 70%–80% demonstrates inferior conditions for healing.
- Tears in the meniscal roots are more clinically significant from a biomechanical standpoint given their role in knee stability and dissipation of hoop stresses. The posterior medial meniscal root is most clinically significant (15).
- Posterior root tears of the medial meniscus were shown to be biomechanically equivalent to a total meniscectomy (20).

- Contact pressures return to normal when the root is repaired (20). Similar effects were found in the posterior root of the lateral meniscus (15).

Nonoperative Management

- Many meniscus tears can be treated successfully without surgery, including degenerative tears associated with osteoarthritis and atraumatic tears without mechanical symptoms.
- However, surgical treatment is recommended for many meniscal tears, excluding those causing minor symptoms in less active patients.
- If nonoperative management is selected, treatment is directed at minimizing symptoms of pain and swelling.
- A trial of activity modification, rehabilitation, and nonsteroidal anti-inflammatory medications is warranted until symptoms abate. This may be successful; however, symptoms may recur.

Operative Management

- Arthroscopic treatment of meniscal injuries is one of the most common orthopedic surgical procedures in the United States (3).
- Operative treatment of meniscus tears is warranted in patients with high physical demands associated with work or sport, because the activity modification required to reduce symptoms often is not acceptable.
- Surgical indications include bucket-handle meniscus tears, symptoms that affect activities of daily living, work, or sport; failure to respond to nonsurgical management; and absence of other causes of knee pain identified by radiographs or other imaging.
- Results of early treatment of peripheral tears (suspected with development of an effusion over the first 48 hours) are improved with surgical repair performed within the first 4 months from the time of injury (ideally <10 weeks) (25).
- Additional predictors of favorable outcome from repair include peripheral location (within 3 mm of the meniscosynovial junction), patient age less than 30 years, tear length less than 2.5 cm, tear of the lateral meniscus, and simultaneous ACL reconstruction (secondary to intra-articular bleeding and fibrin clot formation) (25,26).
- The goal of meniscal surgery is to maximize meniscal preservation. Tears with the potential to heal should be repaired.
- Tears most likely to heal without treatment include tears less than 10 mm in length, tears with less than 3 mm of displacement on arthroscopic probing, partial-thickness tears (<50% meniscal depth), and radial tears less than 3 mm in length (8).
- Arthroscopic rasping of the tear and synovium, or trephination, of these tears to encourage neovascularization may encourage healing and may be successful in as many as 90% of cases (8,25).
- Displaced tears that result in a block to motion should be treated expeditiously to prevent knee stiffness and scarring.

Meniscus Repair

- Repair techniques include open, arthroscopically assisted (inside-out and outside-in), and all-arthroscopic (all-inside) repair.
- Traditional techniques for repair use suture fixation, passed using a variety of devices that are tied through a posterior counterincision.
- Outside-in technique is useful for anterior horn repairs.
- Meniscus repair implants have continued to evolve since their introduction in the mid-1990s. Current-generation implants incorporate a suture-based repair and allow for an all-arthroscopic technique (27).
- Criteria for meniscus repair include complete vertical longitudinal tear >10 mm in length, location within the peripheral 10%–30% of the meniscus (or within 3–4 mm of the meniscocapsular junction), displaceable more than 3–5 mm on arthroscopic probing, no significant secondary joint degeneration or deformity, and a stable knee (8,25).
- Situations not meeting the above criteria must be individualized. It may be appropriate to extend the indications in younger individuals or in cases where resection would lead to nonfunctional remaining tissue (8).
- Suture repairs should be performed with vertical mattress stitches when possible, because these demonstrate superior repair strength compared to the horizontal pattern (25). This is predominately due to the histologic arrangement of the circumferential fiber bundles within the meniscus (27).
- Meniscal root tears can be repaired using several techniques, though most commonly performed are the transtibial pull-out technique (which uses a drill hole with cortical button suspension fixation) and the suture anchor all-inside direct repair technique (28).
- Meniscal ramp repairs are nearly always performed in conjunction with ACL reconstruction because for a ramp lesion to occur, the tibia has to translate far enough forward that the knee relies on the posterior medial meniscus to act as a secondary restraint to anterior tibial translation. However, there are some reports of isolated ramp lesions and subsequent repair (29).

Partial Meniscectomy

- Meniscal injury leads to partial meniscectomy in the majority of cases, as a result of the anatomy of the tear, underlying degeneration of the substance of the meniscus, or distance from the blood supply.
- Meniscal tears that do not fall into the category of stable (with possible spontaneous healing), or repairable, should be treated with partial meniscectomy to remove unstable fragments, eliminate mechanical symptoms, and reduce pain and associated swelling (3).
- Indications for partial meniscectomy include complete oblique, radial, horizontal, degenerative, or complex tears and tears located in the white-white zone (8).

- The goal during meniscectomy is to remove nonfunctioning tissue, maximize meniscus preservation, maintain hoop stresses, and create a stable configuration of the remaining tissue.

OUTCOMES

- As previously outlined, the meniscus serves a chondroprotective function in the knee.
- Precocious arthropathy may result from partial or total meniscectomy. This is thought to be secondary to the increased contact stresses on the articular surfaces.
- Total meniscectomy in previously normal knees results in significant arthrosis in two-thirds of patients by 15 years from surgery (10).
- Better outcome is noted after successful repair compared to resection, with lower incidence of degenerative change after 5 years (8).
- More rapid degeneration is noted after lateral meniscectomy compared to medial meniscectomy (8,30,31).
- The factor with the greatest impact on long-term outcome is whether articular damage is present at the time of partial meniscectomy (25).
- Other factors that influence risk of future arthritis include amount of resection (more resection, higher risk), type of resection (radial resection destroys the meniscus ability to convert compression forces to hoop stresses), associated instability, overall weight-bearing alignment, body habitus, age, and activity level (8).
- A systematic review (32) concluded that the preoperative and intraoperative predictors of poor clinical and/or radiographic outcomes include the following: total meniscectomy (11), removal of the peripheral meniscal rim (33), lateral meniscectomy (34), degenerative meniscal tears (11), presence of chondral damage (12), genetic predisposition as correlated with the presence of hand osteoarthritis (11), and increased body mass index (35).
- Variables that had poor predictive values of clinical and/or radiographic outcomes include nonvertical meniscal tear pattern, age, mechanical alignment, patient gender, activity level, and meniscal tears associated with ACL reconstruction (32).
- Results of partial meniscectomy remain good or excellent in over 90% of patients not demonstrating articular cartilage damage at the time of meniscectomy, but this declines to approximately 60% if damage is present (25). In general, 80%–90% of patients have documented good to excellent results within the first 5 years after partial meniscectomy (8).
- Functional results do not always correlate with radiographic findings. Up to 50% of patients at 8 years after partial meniscectomy, versus 25% of patients with untreated knees, will demonstrate radiographic changes (3,8,30).
- Meniscus repair is successful in approximately 80% of cases. Healing rates increase to approximately 95% in the setting of concomitant ACL reconstruction (25).
- Meniscal root repair is supported by good biomechanical and clinical data.
- Transtibial root repairs have low failure rates and low revision rates of approximately 6% (36). There are no significant differences in functional outcome between these two repair techniques (37,38).
- Meniscal root repairs have been shown to slow the progression of osteoarthritis, though these studies lack long-term follow-up with most having <5-year follow-up data (39).
- Repair of meniscal ramp lesions in conjunction with ACL reconstruction have been shown to have similar patient-reported outcome scores despite having more unstable knees preoperatively (40,41).
- There are limited reported outcomes on nonsurgical treatment of ramp lesions though missed diagnosis of ramp lesions is thought to be a contributor to ACL reconstruction failure (22).

COMPLICATIONS

- Complications specific to meniscus repair include neurovascular injuries.
- The peroneal nerve is at greatest risk with lateral meniscus repair. The popliteal artery, popliteal vein, and tibial nerve are also at risk.
- The saphenous nerve, particularly the infrapatellar branch, is at greatest risk with medial repair.
- Failure of repair resulting in the need for repeat arthroscopy is possible, and the risk increases as indications for repair are extended.
- Meniscus repair done concurrently with ACL reconstruction increases the risk of motion loss; however, the appropriateness of staged repair remains controversial.

MENISCAL SUBSTITUTES

- Substitutes for meniscus tissue injury, or loss, are in development.
- Current replacements include meniscal allograft transplantation and collagen meniscal implants (CMIs).

Meniscal Allograft Transplantation and Scaffolds

- Meniscal allograft transplantation has been used in humans for over 30 years.
- The general indication has been disabling pain after loss of a meniscus in a skeletally mature individual (42).

- A patient with symptoms referable to a meniscus-deficient tibiofemoral compartment is the most common indication for meniscal transplant (43).
- A patient who has undergone prior meniscectomy should be carefully examined for early onset of joint degeneration, with the physical exam focusing on the presence of effusion, joint-line tenderness, crepitus, stability, and axial alignment (43).
- The allograft tissue is most commonly fresh-frozen or cryopreserved. Fresh allografts have also been used; however, logistical difficulties in the routine use of fresh grafts make them impractical for widespread use (25).
- Four types of meniscus allografts are currently available, including fresh, cryopreserved, fresh-frozen, and lyophilized. Fresh and cryopreserved allografts contain viable cells, whereas fresh-frozen and lyophilized allografts are acellular (43).
- Fresh grafts have the theoretical advantage of harboring viable cells, but the proportion of cells that survive and the duration of cell survival following transplantation are not known (43).
- Immune response against the transplant has been shown; however, frank rejection does not appear to occur (31).
- The technique of allograft transplantation has proved to be reproducible in terms of healing and control of post-meniscectomy pain and swelling. The exact indications for allograft transplantation, however, continue to be developed (31). When properly indicated, transplantation leads to predictable good results in over 90% of patients (8).
- Meniscal allograft transplantation may be considered for patients with symptoms referable to a meniscus-deficient tibiofemoral compartment. These symptoms include pain and swelling, more commonly than mechanical symptoms (8,31).
- It is not possible, at this time, to identify patients who will develop symptomatic arthrosis after meniscectomy, and therefore, prophylactic transplantation in the asymptomatic patient after meniscectomy has not been justified (8).
- Ideally, an objective marker of early pathologic changes to articular surfaces will be identified to allow identification of appropriate patients for early meniscus replacement. Such markers may be found through advanced imaging techniques or synovial fluid analysis for cartilage degradation products.
- Transplantation results are poor in cases of advanced joint degeneration and therefore should only be considered when no more than fibrillation and fissuring of the articular surfaces is present.
- Full-thickness articular cartilage lesions on the flexion weight-bearing zone of the femoral condyle or tibia greater than 10–15 mm in diameter are a contraindication to transplantation (25,31).
- Additionally, in order to be a candidate for transplantation, the knee must be stable, without malalignment. An unstable knee must be stabilized, and malalignment requires correction to avoid direct weight bearing through the involved compartment receiving the meniscus transplant (8,31).
- Several biologics and materials such as autologous tendons, submucosa, collagen matrices, and carbon fiber prostheses were developed, but only CMIs, made from bovine Achilles tendons, have been used clinically with varying success rates (44).
- Despite numerous scaffolds being tested and produced over the past several decades, there have been no clear successes and use of them is not widespread.

FUTURE DIRECTIONS

- Future treatments in both meniscus repair and replacement continue to evolve.
- Several biologic therapies are under investigation as potential adjuncts to potentiate healing, such as notch microfracture, autologous blood clot, platelet-rich plasma, and bone marrow aspirate concentrate (45,46).
- These therapies are being investigated as adjuncts because of literature demonstrating increased healing rates of meniscus repair with concomitant ACL reconstruction compared to meniscus repair alone (47–50).
- Meniscal fibrochondrocytes respond with migration and proliferation to growth factors, including platelet-derived growth factor, hepatocyte growth factor, bone morphogenic protein 2, insulin-like growth factor 1, and transforming growth factor beta (51,52).
- Suggested delivery systems for growth factors include impregnated absorbable scaffolds, impregnated fixation devices, or even virus vectors for gene therapy (53).
- Tissue engineering may be the next step in development of a durable meniscal replacement. This technique combines the technology of cell culture, polymer chemistry, and biology to create tissues that are appropriate for tissue replacement or reconstruction. The implant would incorporate fibrochondrocytes that have been multiplied in cell culture, in appropriate-shaped polymer scaffolds.

REFERENCES

1. Arnoczky S, Mcdevitt C. The meniscus: structure, function, repair, and replacement. In: Buckwalter J, editor. *Orthopaedic Basic Science: Biology and Biomechanics of the Musculoskeletal System*. 2nd ed. Rosemont (IL): American Academy of Orthopedic Surgeons; 2000. p. 531–45.
2. Fairbank T. Knee joint changes after meniscectomy. *J Bone Joint Surg Br*. 1948;30B(4):664–70.
3. Greis PE, Bardana DD, Holmstrom MC, Burks RT. Meniscal injury: I. Basic science and evaluation. *J Am Acad Orthop Surg*. 2002;10(3):168–76.
4. Lo I, Thornton G, Miniaci A, Frank C, Rattner J, Bray R. Structure and function of diarthrodial joints. In: *Operative Arthroscopy*. 3rd ed. Philadelphia (PA): Lippincott, Williams and Wilkins; 2003. p. 41–126.
5. Rath E, Richmond JC. The menisci: basic science and advances in treatment. *Br J Sports Med*. 2000;34(4):252–7.

6. Gupte CM, Bull AMJ, Thomas RDW, Amis AA. A review of the function and biomechanics of the meniscofemoral ligaments. *Arthroscopy.* 2003;19(2):161–71.
7. Niu EL, Lee RJ, Joughin E, Finlayson CJ, Heyworth BE. Discoid meniscus. *Clin Sports Med.* 2022;41(4):729–47.
8. Klimkiewicz JJ, Shaffer B. Meniscal surgery 2002 update: indications and techniques for resection, repair, regeneration, and replacement. *Arthroscopy.* 2002;18(9 suppl 2):14–25.
9. Markes AR, Hodax JD, Ma CB. Meniscus form and function. *Clin Sports Med.* 2020;39:1–12.
10. Andersson-Molina H, Karlsson H, Rockborn P. Arthroscopic partial and total meniscectomy: a long-term follow-up study with matched controls. *Arthroscopy.* 2002;18(2):183–9.
11. Englund M, Lohmander LS. Risk factors for symptomatic knee osteoarthritis fifteen to twenty-two years after meniscectomy. *Arthritis Rheum.* 2004;50(9):2811–19.
12. Simon S, Alaranta H, An K. Kinesiology. In: Buckwalter J, editor. *Orthopaedic Basic Science: Biology and Biomechanics of the Musculoskeletal System.* 2nd ed. Rosemont (IL): American Academy of Orthopaedic Surgeons; 2000. p. 730–827.
13. Levy IM, Torzilli PA, Gould JD, Warren RF. The effect of lateral meniscectomy on motion of the knee. *J Bone Joint Surg Am.* 1989;71(3):401–6.
14. Levy IM, Torzilli PA, Warren RF. The effect of medial meniscectomy on anterior-posterior motion of the knee. *J Bone Joint Surg Am.* 1982;64(6):883–8.
15. Bhatia S, LaPrade CM, Ellman MB, LaPrade RF. Meniscal root tears: significance, diagnosis, and treatment. *Am J Sports Med.* 2014; 42(12):3016–30.
16. Richmond JC. The knee. In: Richmond JC, Shahady E, editors. *Sports Medicine for Primary Care.* Oxford (UK): Blackwell Science; 1996. p. 387–444.
17. Greis AC, Derrington SM, McAuliffe M. Evaluation and nonsurgical management of rotator cuff calcific tendinopathy. *Orthop Clin North Am.* 2015;46(2):293–302.
18. Miller GK. A prospective study comparing the accuracy of the clinical diagnosis of meniscus tear with magnetic resonance imaging and its effect on clinical outcome. *Arthroscopy.* 1996;12(4):406–13.
19. Muellner T, Weinstabl R, Schabus R, Vécsei V, Kainberger F. The diagnosis of meniscal tears in athletes. A comparison of clinical and magnetic resonance imaging investigations. *Am J Sports Med.* 1997;25(1):7–12.
20. Allaire R, Muriuki M, Gilbertson L, Harner CD. Biomechanical consequences of a tear of the posterior root of the medial meniscus. Similar to total meniscectomy. *J Bone Joint Surg Am.* 2008;90(9):1922–31.
21. Feucht MJ, Salzmann GM, Bode G, et al. Posterior root tears of the lateral meniscus. *Knee Surg Sports Traumatol Arthrosc.* 2015;23(1): 119–25.
22. Chahla J, Dean CS, Moatshe G, et al. Meniscal ramp lesions: anatomy, incidence, diagnosis, and treatment. *Orthop J Sports Med.* 2016;4(7):2325967116657815.
23. Peltier A, Lording T, Maubisson L, Ballis R, Neyret P, Lustig S. The role of the meniscotibial ligament in posteromedial rotational knee stability. *Knee Surg Sports Traumatol Arthrosc.* 2015;23(10):2967–73.
24. Papageorgiou CD, Gil JE, Kanamori A, Fenwick JA, Woo SL-Y, Fu FH. The biomechanical interdependence between the anterior cruciate ligament replacement graft and the medial meniscus. *Am J Sports Med.* 2001;29(2):226–31.
25. Greis PE, Holmstrom MC, Bardana DD, Burks RT. Meniscal injury: II. Management. *J Am Acad Orthop Surg.* 2002;10(3):177–87.
26. Eggli S, Wegmüller H, Kosina J, Huckell C, Jakob RP. Long-term results of arthroscopic meniscal repair. An analysis of isolated tears. *Am J Sports Med.* 1995;23(6):715–20.
27. Stärke C, Kopf S, Petersen W, Becker R. Meniscal repair. *Arthroscopy.* 2009;25:1033–44.
28. Banovetz MT, Roethke LC, Rodriguez AN, LaPrade RF. Meniscal root tears: a decade of research on their relevant anatomy, biomechanics, diagnosis, and treatment. *Arch Bone Jt Surg.* 2022;10(5):366–80.
29. Jiang J, Ni L, Chen J. Isolated meniscal ramp lesion without obvious anterior cruicate ligament rupture. *Orthop Surg.* 2021;13(2):402–7.
30. Jaureguito JW, Elliot JS, Lietner T, Dixon LB, Reider B. The effects of arthroscopic partial lateral meniscectomy in an otherwise normal knee: a retrospective review of functional, clinical, and radiographic results. *Arthroscopy.* 1995;11(1):29–36.
31. Rodeo SA. Meniscal allografts—where do we stand? *Am J Sports Med.* 2001;29(2):246–61.
32. Salata MJ, Gibbs AE, Sekiya JK. A systematic review of clinical outcomes in patients undergoing meniscectomy. *Am J Sports Med.* 2010;38(9):1907–16.
33. Higuchi H, Kimura M, Shirakura K, Terauchi M, Takagishi K. Factors affecting long-term results after arthroscopic partial meniscectomy. *Clin Orthop Relat Res.* 2000;377:161–8.
34. Chatain F, Adeleine P, Chambat P, Neyret P, Société Française d'Arthroscopie. A comparative study of medial versus lateral arthroscopic partial meniscectomy on stable knees: 10-year minimum follow-up. *Arthroscopy.* 2003;19(8):842–9.
35. Cicuttini FM, Baker JR, Spector TD. The association of obesity with osteoarthritis of the hand and knee in women: a twin study. *J Rheumatol.* 1996;23(7):1221–6.
36. LaPrade RF, Matheny LM, Moulton SG, James EW, Dean CS. Posterior meniscal root repairs: outcomes of an anatomic transtibial pull-out technique. *Am J Sports Med.* 2017;45(4):884–91.
37. Dzidzishvili L, López-Torres II, Sáez D, Arguello JM, Calvo E. A comparison of the transtibial pullout technique and all-inside meniscal repair in medial meniscus posterior root tear: prognostic factors and midterm clinical outcomes. *J Orthop.* 2021;26:130–4.
38. Kim J-H, Chung J-H, Lee D-H, Lee Y-S, Kim J-R, Ryu K-J. Arthroscopic suture anchor repair versus pullout suture repair in posterior root tear of the medial meniscus: a prospective comparison study. *Arthroscopy.* 2011;27(12):1644–53.
39. Faucett SC, Geisler BP, Chahla J, et al. Meniscus root repair vs meniscectomy or nonoperative management to prevent knee osteoarthritis after medial meniscus root tears: clinical and economic effectiveness. *Am J Sports Med.* 2019;47(3):762–9.
40. Bansal S, Floyd ER, A Kowalski M, et al. Meniscal repair: the current state and recent advances in augmentation. *J Orthop Res.* 2021;39(7):1368–82.
41. DePhillipo NN, Dornan GJ, Dekker TJ, Aman ZS, Engebretsen L, LaPrade RF. Clinical characteristics and outcomes after primary ACL reconstruction and meniscus ramp repair. *Orthop J Sports Med.* 2020;8(4):2325967120912427.
42. Goble EM, Kohn D, Verdonk R, Kane SM. Meniscal substitutes – human experience. *Scand J Med Sci Sports.* 1999;9(3):146–57.
43. Packer JD, Rodeo SA. Meniscal allograft transplantation. *Clin Sports Med.* 2009;28(2):259–83.
44. Sandmann GH, Eichhorn S, Vogt S, et al. Generation and characterization of a human acellular meniscus scaffold for tissue engineering. *J Biomed Mater Res A.* 2009;91(2):567–74.
45. Kwon H, Brown WE, Lee CA, et al. Surgical and tissue engineering strategies for articular cartilage and meniscus repair. *Nat Rev Rheumatol.* 2019;15(9):550–70.
46. Xiao W, Yang Y, Xie W, et al. Effects of platelet-rich plasma and bone marrow mesenchymal stem cells on meniscal repair in the white-white zone of the meniscus. *Orthop Surg.* 2021;13(8):2423–32.
47. Kanto R, Yamaguchi M, Sasaki K, Matsumoto A, Nakayama H, Yoshiya S. Second-look arthroscopic evaluations of meniscal repairs

associated with anterior cruciate ligament reconstruction. *Arthroscopy.* 2019;35(10):2868–77.

48. Lyons LP, Weinberg JB, Wittstein JR, McNulty AL. Blood in the joint: effects of hemarthrosis on meniscus health and repair techniques. *Osteoarthritis Cartilage.* 2021;29(4):471–9.
49. Wasserstein D, Dwyer T, Gandhi R, Austin PC, Mahomed N, Ogilvie-Harris D. A matched-cohort population study of reoperation after meniscal repair with and without concomitant anterior cruciate ligament reconstruction. *Am J Sports Med.* 2013;41(2):349–55.
50. Westermann RW, Wright RW, Spindler KP, et al. Meniscal repair with concurrent anterior cruciate ligament reconstruction: operative success and patient outcomes at 6-year follow-up. *Am J Sports Med.* 2014;42(9):2184–92.
51. Bhargava MM, Attia ET, Murrell GAC, Dolan MM, Warren RF, Hannafin JA. The effect of cytokines on the proliferation and migration of bovine meniscal cells. *Am J Sports Med.* 1999;27(5):636–43.
52. Ochi M, Uchio Y, Okuda K, Shu N, Yamaguchi H, Sakai Y. Expression of cytokines after meniscal rasping to promote meniscal healing. *Arthroscopy.* 2001;17(7):724–31.
53. Martinek V, Usas A, Pelinkovic D, Robbins P, Fu FH, Huard J. Genetic engineering of meniscal allografts. *Tissue Eng.* 2002;8(1):107–17.

64 Knee Instability

Emma L. Klosterman, F. Winston Gwathmey Jr, and Mark D. Miller

INTRODUCTION

- The knee is an encapsulated compound joint consisting of two condyloid joints at the medial and lateral articulations of the tibia and femur and one saddle joint between the patella and femur. Lacking intrinsic bony stability, most of its overall stability is derived from the major ligaments and smaller supporting structures in and around the knee. Disruption of one or more of these ligaments, commonly from injury in athletics or major trauma, results in instability. Injuries to the anterior cruciate ligament (ACL) and medial collateral ligament (MCL) make up the vast majority of ligamentous knee injuries (Figure 64.1A–C).

ANATOMY

Anterior Cruciate Ligament

- The ACL is one of two major intra-articular ligaments of the knee. Its femoral origin is on the posteromedial aspect of the lateral femoral condyle. It inserts on the tibial plateau, just anterior to the area between the intercondylar eminences.
- The ACL comprises two distinct bundles, each identified by their relative insertion on the tibia. The anteromedial bundle tightens in flexion, while the posterolateral bundle tightens in full extension. The overall tension on the ACL is greatest when the knee is in 30° of flexion (1).
- The blood supply to the ACL is from the middle geniculate artery, a branch of the popliteal artery. Innervation from branches of the tibial nerve aids proprioception.
- The primary role of the ACL is to prevent excessive anterior tibial translation in relation to the femur, providing 90% of total anterior translational stability. The anteromedial bundle serves this function, while the posterolateral bundle adds protection against internal rotation (2). The ACL also stabilizes the knee against varus and valgus stress when the knee is in full extension. It contributes to the "screw home" mechanism, by which the femur is internally rotated over the tibia in full extension to "lock" the knee while standing (3).

Posterior Cruciate Ligament

- The intra-articular posterior cruciate ligament (PCL) originates on the anterolateral aspect of the medial femoral condyle and inserts in a depression approximately 1–1.5 cm distal to the articular surface in a fovea between the posterior aspects of the medial and lateral tibial plateaus.
- Like the ACL, the PCL is composed of two bundles, a larger anterolateral bundle that tightens in flexion and a posteromedial bundle that tightens in extension. Overall, the ligament bears the most tension in 90° of knee flexion. These bundles are less distinct than those of the ACL and are described by some as a continuum of one ligament.
- Present in 90% of the population, the meniscofemoral ligaments of Humphry and Wrisberg originate on the posterior horn of the lateral meniscus and straddle the PCL anteriorly and posteriorly before inserting on the medial femoral condyle (4).
- The PCL shares its neurovascular supply with the nearby ACL.
- The primary role of the PCL is to resist posterior tibial translation, providing up to 100% of posterior stability at 90° of flexion (5). It also protects against varus and valgus stress in full extension. With the ACL, it contributes to the "screw-home" mechanism (6).

Medial Collateral Ligament

- The MCL is an extraarticular ligament composed of superficial and deep components. The superficial MCL is 10–12 cm long and originates just proximal and posterior to the medial epicondyle. It courses distally deep to the pes anserinus tendons and inserts on the medial tibial metaphysis approximately 6 cm distal to the joint line. The shorter deep MCL is deep and adherent to the superficial MCL. It is connected to the medial meniscus by its meniscofemoral and meniscotibial components (7).
- Once thought to be a posterior portion of the superficial MCL, the posterior oblique ligament (POL) is a distinct, fan-like ligament spanning from a femoral origin posterior and superior to that of the superficial MCL distally to the joint capsule and distal semimembranosus tendon (8).
- The superficial MCL is the primary restraint to valgus instability of the knee and aids in rotational stability. The POL acts synergistically with the MCL to stabilize the knee against

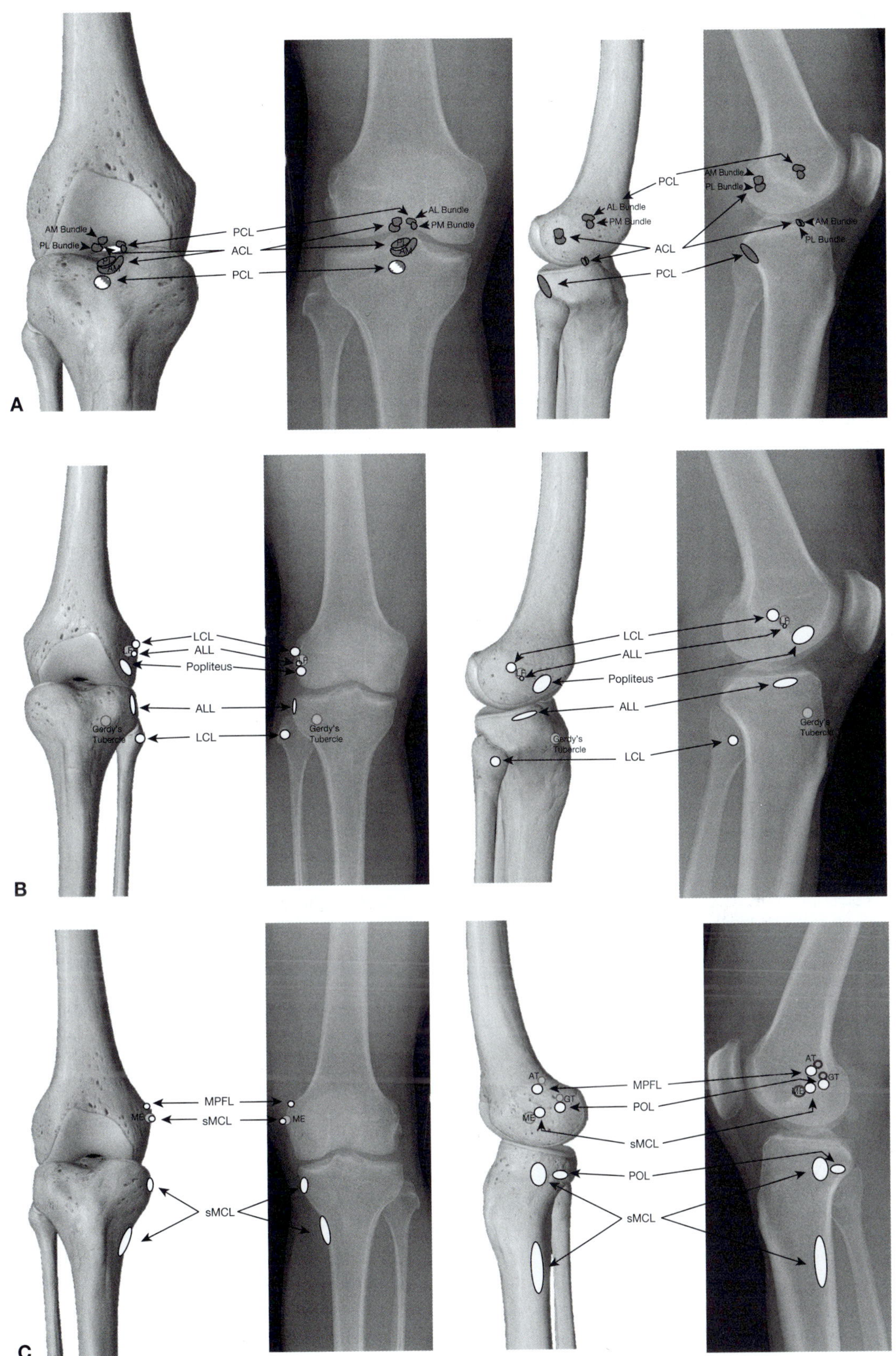

Figure 64.1: A: Central ligaments of the knee anatomy and radiographs. Posterior cruciate ligament with its anterolateral bundle and posteromedial bundle. Anterior cruciate ligament with its anteromedial bundle and posterolateral bundle. ACL, anterior cruciate ligament; AL, anterolateral; AM, anteromedial; PCL, posterior cruciate ligament; PL, posterolateral; PM, posteromedial. B: Lateral ligaments of the knee anatomy and radiographs. ALL,. Anterolateral ligament; LCL, Lateral (fibular) collateral ligament. C: Medial ligaments of the knee anatomy and radiographs. AT, adductor tubercle; GT, gastroc tubercle; ME, medial epicondyle; MPFL, Medial patellofemoral ligament; POL, Posterior oblique ligament; sMCL, Superficial medial collateral ligament.

internal tibial rotation and valgus deformity with the knee in extension (8,9).

- The medial structures of the knee are described in three layers:
  - Layer 1 (superficial): Sartorius, deep fascia
  - Layer 2: Superficial MCL, POL, semimembranosus
  - Layer 3 (deep): Deep MCL, capsule

Posterolateral Corner and Lateral Collateral Ligament

- Multiple static and dynamic stabilizers form a complex, interrelated network to secure the lateral knee against varus deformity, external tibial rotation, and posterior tibial translation. Collectively, these are known as the posterolateral corner (PLC). The lateral collateral ligament (LCL), popliteus muscle, and popliteofibular ligaments are the most important stabilizing structures of the region (10).
- The LCL originates just proximal and posterior to the lateral epicondyle and travels 7 cm distally to insert on the lateral portion of the fibular head. It is the primary restraint to varus instability of the knee and also aids in rotational stability in the extended knee (11).
- From its origin on the posteromedial proximal tibia, the popliteus muscle arcs laterally and proximally. Its tendon becomes intra-articular, coursing through the popliteal hiatus before inserting on the femur deep, distal, and anterior to the LCL. It has interconnections to the fibula, tibia, and meniscus that form the popliteus complex, giving it both static and dynamic stabilizing properties.
- The popliteofibular (arcuate) ligament is a "Y"-shaped structure connecting the popliteus to the fibular head. The popliteus and popliteofibular ligament provide the primary restraint against external tibial rotation (12).
- Other structures involved with the PLC include the fabellofibular ligament, iliotibial band, biceps femoris tendon, lateral head of the gastrocnemius, and the lateral joint capsule. The PLC works in concert with the PCL to prevent excessive posterior tibial translation, contributing more in extension (12,13).
- The lateral structures of the knee can be considered in three layers:
  - Layer 1 (superficial): Fascia, iliotibial band, biceps femoris tendon
  - Layer 2: Patellar retinaculum, patellofemoral ligament
  - Layer 3 (deep): Popliteofibular ligament, popliteus, fabellofibular ligament, LCL, capsule

ANTERIOR CRUCIATE LIGAMENT

Mechanism of Injury

- It is estimated that more than 100,000 ACL injuries occur in the United States each year, many of them during athletic activity. Seventy percent of injuries to the ACL occur by noncontact mechanisms (14). Tension is created primarily by forces in the sagittal plane that cause large anterior tibial sheer forces. A combination of small knee flexion angles, large posterior ground reaction forces, and substantial quadriceps contractions all contribute to anterior sheer stress. This is augmented but not duplicated by rotational and valgus forces acting upon the knee. The posterior sheer forces on the tibia exerted by the hamstrings are protective from ACL injury.
- Common mechanisms of injury include pivoting during acceleration or deceleration and forcefully landing on the heel with a small knee flexion angle (15). Contact-induced injury often involves valgus loading of the fixed and straightened knee (14).
- While males and females sustain an approximately equal number of total ACL injuries, women who participate in athletics are three to eight times more likely than their male counterparts to sustain injury (16,17). Reasons for this discrepancy include smaller ligaments relative to body size, increased joint laxity, higher levels of estrogen, and smaller intercondylar notch dimensions. Females have also been shown to have different neuromuscular mechanics that predispose them to ACL injury. They tend to land from jumps with less knee flexion, have more valgus loading of the knee, and have greater activation of their quadriceps relative to their hamstrings (18).
- Other risk factors for ACL injury include game situations in comparison to practice, an increased coefficient of friction of footwear, and prior ACL injury with or without reconstruction of the ipsilateral or contralateral knee (19).

Evaluation

- A thorough history and physical exam are the most important aspects of the evaluation of a possible ACL injury. Patients often report pain and instability occurring after landing or cutting in a noncontact situation. An audible "pop" is common. Swelling within the joint occurs rapidly, and athletes are typically unable to return to play. It is not uncommon to see ACL, MCL, and lateral meniscal injury from the same event (6).
- The Lachman test is the most accurate physical exam for ACL injuries, performed with the patient supine and the quadriceps relaxed, and the knee is placed in 30° of flexion. The patient's thigh is stabilized, and the examiner grasps the patient's proximal tibia and applies anterior force, noting the amount of anterior translation and the end point. Anterior translation of greater than 3 mm compared to the contralateral knee and a "soft" end point signifies ACL injury. It has a high sensitivity and specificity (81%–85% and 85%–94%, respectively) (20).
- The pivot shift test is an important indicator of rotational instability. With the leg fully extended, the ankle is internally rotated while a valgus force is applied to the proximal tibia. In the ACL-deficient knee, this causes anterior subluxation of the lateral tibial plateau beneath the lateral femoral condyle. As the knee is slowly flexed past 30°, the iliotibial band

induces a sudden reduction of the subluxed lateral tibia, interpreted as a positive pivot shift. Although the test is not very sensitive (24%), it is extremely specific (98%). It is much more sensitive (74%) and comfortable for the patient when performed under anesthesia (20).

- Although not as sensitive or specific as the Lachman test, the anterior drawer test is useful in the evaluation of chronic ACL injury. With a supine patient's knee in 90° of flexion and foot resting on the table, anterior force is applied to the tibia. The difference in anterior translation between the two knees is evaluated (20). All tests have been shown to be highly examiner dependent and are most effectively performed by trained orthopedists (17). Mechanical devices such as the KT-1000 or KT-2000 arthrometers (MEDmetric, San Diego, CA) can evaluate the anterior translation of the tibia in a more standardized fashion but are typically used for research purposes only (3).
- Although radiographs typically do not diagnose ligamentous injury, they are helpful to evaluate for other injuries. Avulsion of the tibial spine and Segond fractures (lateral tibial capsular avulsion fractures) can be seen with ACL injuries, the latter of which is pathognomonic (21). The deep sulcus sign is also associated with ACL injuries (22).
- A magnetic resonance imaging (MRI) is usually not necessary to make the diagnosis of an ACL rupture, but it remains the gold standard and is useful to visualize the ligament, identify characteristic bone bruise on the central lateral femoral condyle and posterior lateral tibial plateau, and to evaluate for other pathology (6,17).

Natural History

- Injury to the ACL rarely occurs in isolation. Approximately half will have meniscal tears, commonly located in the posterior horn of the lateral meniscus in acute injury (23). When meniscal repair is performed concomitantly with ACL reconstruction, there is a greater chance of healing of the meniscus in comparison to delayed treatment.
- Chronic instability of ACL-deficient knees stresses the posterior horn of the medial meniscus, resulting in tears in this region by about 6 months and cartilage lesions by about 1 year (24). Meniscal repairs in the chronically unstable knee typically have poor outcomes (25).
- There is a 50% incidence of clinical and radiographic evidence of osteoarthritis in patients between 10 and 20 years after ACL injury regardless of their treatment. This increased risk of osteoarthritis is especially evident in those who sustain injury to the menisci (26).

Management

- Indications for surgical reconstruction include athletes, patients with associated repairable meniscal injury, patients with complete tears to any of the three other major knee ligaments, and patients experiencing instability that interferes with activities of daily living (27,28).
- Conservative (nonoperative) treatment can be considered for the older patient participating in only linear activities (29). Treatment focuses on regaining normal knee range of motion and strengthening the secondary stabilizers of the knee, in particular the hamstrings. Rotation and lateral movement should be avoided for 6–12 weeks, and competitive situations should be avoided for at least 3 months (30). Bracing may be used for patient comfort but is not necessary. It is important to counsel the patient about episodes of instability and behavioral modifications to protect the joint (31). These patients are typically self-reported to be satisfied with their condition, but suffer from instability issues and a reduction in activity levels (32).
- If surgical treatment is elected, it should be performed after acute hemarthrosis and accompanying synovitis have resolved and knee range of motion has returned to normal, usually 3–4 weeks after injury. Early reconstruction may result in arthrofibrosis, whereas late repair may be associated with additional injury to the joint (31). Restoring range of motion, weight bearing, and closed-chain exercises are key aspects of both preoperative and postoperative management.
- Primary ACL repair has not historically resulted in adequate healing. Though for complete midsubstance ACL rupture, a bridge-enhanced ACL repair technique is currently under clinical investigation (33).
- ACL reconstruction is the accepted surgical treatment for ACL rupture. This involves drilling tunnels through the tibia and femur and placing a graft through these tunnels to serve as scaffolding for new ligament growth. Surgeons commonly use the central third of the patient's patellar tendon with bone plugs from the patella and tibial tubercle (bone-tendon-bone [BTB]), the patient's own semitendinosus and gracilis tendons (hamstring), the patient's quadriceps tendon, or cadaveric (allograft) grafts.
  - BTB autografts have the advantage that they incorporate into the bone tunnels more rapidly and have been shown to have lower static laxity and lower risk of revision surgery than hamstring grafts, making them ideal for active, younger patients. They are associated with increased radiographic osteoarthritis changes as well as anterior knee pain (29,34).
  - Hamstring tendon autografts have lower donor site morbidity and have a greater tensile strength and stiffness when quadrupled, but are slower to incorporate in the tunnels at the bone-tendon interface with increased risk of revision surgery with early rerupture rate (35).
  - Quadriceps tendon with or without a bone block is being increasingly used. It is similar to other graft options in terms of laxity, range of motion, and patient satisfaction (36). It has less donor site morbidity and consistently larger graft cross-sectional area compared to BTB (29).
  - Allografts are associated with no donor site morbidity and decreased operative time. Disease transmission and graft preservation are less of a concern with modern harvesting techniques, but allografts have an increased cost

and delayed graft incorporation. Younger, more active patients have been shown to have significantly higher rates of failure with allografts (37).

- ACL reconstruction augmentation with lateral extra-articular tenodesis to improve rotation stability of the knee is a consideration for patients under 25 years of age, with hyperlaxity and a high-grade pivot shift on exam, participating in a pivoting sport and revision settings (38,39).

Pediatrics

- ACL injuries in skeletally immature patients are increasingly common and now make up 3.3% of all ACL injuries. Children typically suffer from poor outcomes with conservative treatment, but reconstruction is complicated by the proximity of the physeal growth plates to the joint, as the distal tibial and proximal femur contribute to 65% of the growth of the lower extremity. Several different surgical techniques have been shown to be successful in reconstructing the ligament while respecting the physis and thus maintaining normal bone growth (40).

POSTERIOR CRUCIATE LIGAMENT

Mechanism of Injury

- PCL injuries make up approximately 3% of all ligamentous knee injuries, but up to 38% in trauma situations. There are associated injuries in approximately half of all PCL injuries, most notably to the PLC. This proportion rises to 95% in the setting of severe trauma (5,41,42).
- A "dashboard injury" occurs when contact of the tibia with the dashboard during collision exerts a large posterior sheer force on the tibia, often resulting in multiligament damage. In athletics, damage to the PCL is more often isolated and can occur when falling onto a flexed knee with a plantarflexed foot or from a direct blow to the anterior tibia. Severe hyperextension and hyperflexion are other mechanisms of injury (43).
- Unless associated with obvious trauma, the presentation of a PCL injury is subtle, especially if isolated. There is usually no "popping" reported, and athletes are often able to continue competition after injury or may not be able to recall the event at all. Reported symptoms include stiffness, mild swelling, moderate posterior knee pain, and pain with deep knee flexion (43). Acute hemarthrosis due to PCL injury will be mild. Observation of gait may reveal a slight varus deformity in the setting of chronic instability.

Evaluation

- The posterior drawer test is the most important physical examination for evaluation of the PCL, having a sensitivity and specificity of 90% and 99%, respectively. With the patient supine, the knees are flexed to 90° and the hips to 45°, while the feet rest on the table (44). At rest, the tibial plateau should be more than 1 cm anterior to the medial femoral condyle. If it is not, this is detected as a posterior "sag," which is indicative of likely PCL injury. The tibia must be anteriorly reduced to an anatomically neutral position before testing. A posterior force is directed upon the anterior proximal tibia, and the magnitude of displacement and characteristics of the end point are observed. Displacement of 3–5 mm indicates a grade I posterior drawer with the medial tibial plateau remaining anterior to the medial femoral condyle. In grade II displacement, there is 6–10 mm of displacement and the tibial plateau is flush with the femoral condyle. More than 10 mm of displacement, pushing the plateau posterior to the condyle, is a grade III injury (45). In grade III injury, there is likely a concurrent injury to the PCL (46).
- The posterior sag test is done with the patient supine and the hip and knee flexed to 90°. The examiner holds the patient's ankles and observes the knee for a step-off between the tibial plateau and femoral condyles.
- For the quadriceps active test, the supine patient's feet are set flush on the table and the patient is asked to advance the feet away from the body. Anterior shift of the tibial plateau greater than 2 mm is indicative of PCL pathology (43).
- Plain radiographs may show bony avulsions in the acute setting or degenerative changes in the medial and patellofemoral compartments in chronic cases. Stress radiographs are useful to quantify the degree of posterior instability, with greater than 10 mm of displacement compared to the contralateral side indicating injury to the PCL and PLC (46). MRI is excellent for assessment of the PCL and other structures of the knee in acute settings, but lacks adequate sensitivity for detection of chronic PCL injury.

Natural History

- Injuries to the PCL can be subtle and have a varied course. At the time of injury, it is difficult to predict future consequences from instability. One study found that 2% of highly functioning college football players had asymptomatic PCL deficiencies (47).
- MRI studies have shown partial healing ability of the ligament (15). Knee kinematics are altered such that there is persistent anterior subluxation of the medial femoral condyle, leading to increased rates of osteoarthritis in the medial and patellofemoral compartments and higher rates of meniscal tears (48). At 14-year follow-up of nonoperative management, there is about 11% of moderate to severe osteoarthritis (49). Although many do well with conservative treatment, others suffer from continued instability and osteoarthritic changes (50).

Management

- Patients with both acute and chronic isolated grade I, II, or nondisplaced tibial avulsion PCL injuries should undergo nonoperative treatment, because surgical reconstruction has not been shown to be helpful for either. Protected weight bearing in an extension brace is followed by quadriceps rehabilitation and range-of-motion exercises. Return to sports is usually possible within 2–6 weeks (49).

- Surgical intervention is recommended for patients with associated injuries to the ACL, MCL, and PLC (grade III PCL injury), preferably within 1–2 weeks. In the case of chronic injury, a tibial osteotomy may be necessary to correct for varus deformity (51).
- There is no clear superior surgical technique for PCL reconstruction, and results of such procedures are inferior to ACL reconstruction with failure rates from 1% to 25%. Grafts may be single- (anterolateral) or double bundled (42).
- Historically, the graft was fixed to the tibia through a transtibial tunnel. It is forced to make a sharp "killer turn" superiorly over the posterior edge of the tunnel, resulting in loosening of the graft over time. Berg (52) described the tibial inlay technique, using a bony fragment to fix the graft directly to the fovea at the origin of the native PCL, resulting in decreased laxity (53,54). As with ACL reconstruction, exercises are gradually introduced, and full recovery generally takes 9 months.

MEDIAL COLLATERAL LIGAMENT

Mechanism of Injury

- The annual incidence of MCL injuries is 0.24 per 1000 and is twice as common in men (55). They typically occur in isolation and during athletics.
- The mechanism of injury often involves a valgus force on the partially flexed knee, opening the medial compartment of the knee and stressing the medial support structures. Patients often report localized pain and swelling along the medial aspect of the knee. Instability is not a common symptom, but when it does occur, it is described as affecting side-to-side motion (8).

Evaluation

- Physical examination begins with inspection, which may reveal localized swelling or ecchymosis at the site of injury, most often near the femoral origin of the superficial MCL. Areas of tenderness are usually discrete and identifiable.
- Valgus stress testing is done with the knee in 30° of flexion and the patient relaxed. Stabilizing the femur, a valgus load is applied to the tibia. Injury is characterized as grade I for pain and no joint laxity compared to the contralateral knee, grade II for some laxity with a solid end point, and grade III for laxity and a soft or no end point. Grade I and II injuries usually correlate with partial sprains, whereas grade III injuries involve a complete tear. In the case of a grade III tear, careful evaluation should be done for other ligamentous injuries. At 0° of flexion, both the cruciate ligaments and the POL stabilize the knee against valgus deformity; instability in this position should prompt further exam for injury to additional structures (56).
- Radiographic examination can assess for avulsion and for growth plate injury in skeletally immature patients. Valgus stress views are useful to quantify medial compartment opening. A Pellegrini-Stieda lesion, calcification of the MCL at its femoral origin, may be seen with chronic injuries (57).
- Ultrasound is also a useful tool for diagnosis but is highly user dependent (58). MRI is a very sensitive tool for diagnosis and detects bone bruises in almost half of all isolated injuries, mostly in the lateral compartment (59,60).

Natural History

- Although most MCL injuries are isolated, it is important to evaluate for other lesions. Meniscal tears may occur in 5% of presentations. Grade III injuries severe enough to require surgery are associated with POL and ACL injury in 99% and 78% of patients, respectively (61).
- Because of its rich vascular supply, the MCL exhibits excellent healing characteristics. When chronic injury does occur, it exposes other medial knee structures to altered loads that increase the risk of further injury (62).

Treatment

- Most MCL injuries are amenable to nonoperative treatment. For simple grade I and II injuries, a short course of rest, ice, compression, elevation, and possibly bracing may be all that is necessary. Weight-bearing and range-of-motion exercises are initiated as soon as tolerable. Adequate strength and flexibility along with control of pain are the primary goals of treatment (63).
- Nonoperative treatment of grade III injuries and proper rehabilitation have been shown to be just as effective as surgery when the injury is isolated (64). A hinged knee brace is used for 6 weeks after pain and swelling are controlled, and as with lower grade injuries, strength, range of motion, and early weight bearing are key.
- Longer use of bracing is commonly used for comfort in nonoperative patients with grade II or III injuries. Studies of prophylactic bracing by athletes such as football linemen have been shown to be protective of the MCL as well as other knee structures (65).
- Operative treatment is reserved for chronic injuries with instability despite appropriate rehabilitation or MCL injury in combination with other surgically amenable injuries, especially involving the ACL or menisci. Primary repair, imbrications, suture tape augmentation, advancement of insertions, tendon transfers, and reconstruction are all possible techniques, and none has been adequately proven to be superior. Chronic injuries usually require reconstruction of the superficial MCL and POL (66).

- Postoperatively, early range of motion is necessary to prevent adhesions. Closed-chain exercises are started around 6 weeks after surgery, and full weight bearing is permitted shortly thereafter. Wearing a brace throughout rehabilitation will increase the patient's sense of stability and comfort but will not accelerate healing (8,63).

PLC AND LCL

Mechanism of Injury

- Accounting for approximately 16% of knee ligament injuries, damage to the PLC is becoming an increasingly recognized source of instability in the knee. Eighty-seven percent of new presentations have multiple ligament injuries, most often involving the ACL. O'Brien et al. (67) found that chronic PLC deficiency was the most frequently identifiable reason for ACL reconstruction failure.
- The most common mechanism of PLC injury occurs with a blow to the anteromedial tibia. Hyperextension and excessive varus loading can also precipitate injury (68).

Evaluation

- Patients with PLC injury typically report pain along the posterolateral aspect of the knee. Because isolated injury is rare, careful examination of other knee structures is necessary. Peroneal nerve palsy is found in approximately 15% of presentations, and evaluation of foot dorsiflexion, eversion, and sensation is vital (69).
- A patient's gait may be altered, revealing varus thrust, internal rotation with swing, and knee hyperextension in stance. Evaluation of the LCL is completed and graded in the same manner as MCL injury, but with varus stress.
- The external rotation recurvatum test is done by lifting the feet of a supine patient off the table by the greater toes. Hyperextension of the knee, external tibial rotation, and varus deformity are all signs of a PLC lesion.
- The dial test can be done with the patient prone or supine. The patient's feet are externally rotated, and the orientation of the medial sole is compared to that of the femoral shaft. A difference of greater than 10° or 15° with the knee flexed at 30° indicates a PLC injury, and a difference at 90° of knee flexion indicates a combined PLC and PCL injury.
- The posterolateral drawer test is a modification of the posterior drawer test done with the foot externally rotated. Excessive translation indicates PLC injury.
- Plain films may show avulsions of the fibular head in acute presentations or lateral compartment degenerative changes with chronic instability. Varus stress films will show lateral laxity. Although MRI is helpful to identify additional pathology, it may overdiagnose PLC injury due to extensive edema visualized in posterolateral structures. It should be used in combination with physical examination and stress radiographs (70).

Natural History

- Prognosis typically depends on the extent of injury and associated findings. Patients with low-grade injuries typically do quite well in the long run with nonoperative treatment. Complete tears, however, are associated with increased laxity, damage to the ACL, muscle weakness, and osteoarthritis (71,72).

Treatment

- Isolated incomplete injuries are treated nonoperatively. 2–3 weeks of knee immobilization in extension are followed by gradual increases in strength and movement, emphasizing range of motion throughout. A return to full activity is generally seen within 12–14 weeks (73).
- Grade III injuries are treated operatively, ideally between 2 and 3 weeks of an acute injury to avoid excessive scar tissue formation and to allow primary repair. Augmentation of a primary repair with tendon reconstruction is frequently used. Chronic injuries are not amenable to primary repair and require reconstruction. Anatomic and nonanatomic methods have been described (74,75).
- Injuries to other ligaments in the knee should be addressed at the same time or in a staged fashion, because the structures are reliant on one another for stability and proper healing.

KNEE DISLOCATION

Mechanism of Injury

- When an injury leads to disruption of multiple ligaments, there exists the possibility that a femoral-tibial knee dislocation has occurred. In contrast to patellar dislocations, which are common, dislocations between the femur and tibia are much less common and carry a high risk of limb-threatening consequences. Physicians must maintain a high index of suspicion for dislocation because spontaneous reduction may occur prior to examination.
- Dislocations are classified by the direction of tibial displacement in reference to the femur, but because of spontaneous reduction, any injury with three or more damaged ligaments should be considered a dislocation. In most cases, both cruciate ligaments are ruptured, and approximately three-quarters are either anterior or posterior dislocations (76).
- Tethering of the popliteal artery above and below the joint predisposes it to injury in 32%–45% of presentations, with an increased incidence in posterior displacement (77,78). Nerve damage occurs in 16%–40% of patients, more often to the common peroneal nerve, where it is constrained in its path around the proximal fibula (79).
- The mechanism of injury typically involves high-energy impact from motor vehicle accidents, although low-energy injuries do occur in athletes and in the morbidly obese (80).

Evaluation

- After the patient is stabilized, the first step in evaluation is to obtain a brief history, if possible, regarding the mechanism of injury. Reduction is undertaken if the knee is grossly displaced.
- Physical examination starts with palpation for pulses. The ankle-brachial index (ABI) has been shown to be highly sensitive and specific as a screening tool for vascular injury. Any patient with an ABI < 0.9 should undergo further workup and likely has a lesion requiring surgery, whereas the rest can be monitored with serial physical examination (81). Although arteriography has been the gold standard in further evaluation, computed tomography angiography has been shown to be an effective and less invasive alternative (82).
- Sensory and motor exams for tibial or peroneal nerve injury can be difficult in the polytrauma patient, but are important. Anteroposterior and lateral films should be taken before and after manipulation to evaluate for malalignment and for fractures, found in up to 60% of injuries in high-energy trauma (83). Careful evaluation of all ligamentous structures is necessary for proper characterization of the injury (84).

Management

- Emergent surgery is indicated for patients with vascular injury. Other surgical emergencies include compartment syndrome, open injury, and irreducible dislocations (79). Posterolateral dislocations are more likely to be irreducible because of medial femoral condyle entrapment in the medial capsule. Vascular compromise for more than 8 hours has a high association with above-knee amputation (77). Significant instability after reduction may require spanning external fixation.
- In the absence of surgical emergencies and gross instability, the knee should be splinted in extension. Serial vascular examinations are done during a period of observation over the next 24–48 hours. Early surgical intervention within 2–3 weeks is recommended to facilitate primary repair of medial and lateral structures before excessive scar tissue formation. Cruciate reconstruction is concomitant or staged. Nonoperative treatment leads to unacceptable outcomes in terms of stiffness and instability, and thus, surgical treatment is recommended for nearly all knee dislocations (85).
- While most patients are able to return to work after recovery is complete, few are able to return to competitive sports (86,87).

REFERENCES

1. Yu B, Garrett WE. Mechanisms of non-contact ACL injuries. *Br J Sports Med.* 2007;41(suppl 1):i47–51. doi:10.1136/bjsm.2007.037192.
2. Chhabra A, Starman JS, Ferretti M, Vidal AF, Zantop T, Fu FH. Anatomic, radiographic, biomechanical, and kinematic evaluation of the anterior cruciate ligament and its two functional bundles. *J Bone Joint Surg Am.* 2006;88(suppl 4):2–10. doi:10.2106/jbjs.F.00616
3. Miller M. The knee and lower leg. In: Miller MDHJ, MacKnight JM, editors. *Essential Orthopaedics.* Philadelphia: Saunders; 2010.
4. Gupte CM, Smith A, McDermott ID, Bull AM, Thomas RD, Amis AA. Meniscofemoral ligaments revisited. Anatomical study, age correlation and clinical implications. *J Bone Joint Surg Br.* 2002;84(6):846–51. doi:10.1302/0301-620x.84b6.13110
5. Allen CR, Kaplan LD, Fluhme DJ, Harner CD. Posterior cruciate ligament injuries. *Curr Opin Rheumatol.* 2002;14(2):142–9. doi:10.1097/00002281-200203000-00011
6. Baumfeld JAHJ, Miller MD. Sports medicine. In: Miller M, editor. *Review of Orthopaedics.* Philadelphia: Saunders; 2008. p. 245–305.
7. LaPrade RF, Engebretsen AH, Ly TV, Johansen S, Wentorf FA, Engebretsen L. The anatomy of the medial part of the knee. *J Bone Joint Surg Am.* 2007;89(9):2000–10. doi:10.2106/jbjs.F.01176
8. Wijdicks CA, Griffith CJ, Johansen S, Engebretsen L, LaPrade RF. Injuries to the medial collateral ligament and associated medial structures of the knee. *J Bone Joint Surg Am.* 2010;92(5):1266–80. doi:10.2106/jbjs.I.01229
9. Griffith CJ, Wijdicks CA, LaPrade RF, Armitage BM, Johansen S, Engebretsen L. Force measurements on the posterior oblique ligament and superficial medial collateral ligament proximal and distal divisions to applied loads. *Am J Sports Med.* 2009;37(1):140–8. doi:10.1177/0363546508322890
10. LaPrade RF, Bollom TS, Wentorf FA, Wills NJ, Meister K. Mechanical properties of the posterolateral structures of the knee. *Am J Sports Med.* 2005;33(9):1386–91. doi:10.1177/0363546504274143
11. James EW, LaPrade CM, LaPrade RF. Anatomy and biomechanics of the lateral side of the knee and surgical implications. *Sports Med Arthrosc Rev.* 2015;23(1):2–9. doi:10.1097/jsa.0000000000000040
12. LaPrade RF, Ly TV, Wentorf FA, Engebretsen L. The posterolateral attachments of the knee: a qualitative and quantitative morphologic analysis of the fibular collateral ligament, popliteus tendon, popliteofibular ligament, and lateral gastrocnemius tendon. *Am J Sports Med.* 2003;31(6):854–60. doi:10.1177/03635465030310062101
13. Sanchez AR 2nd, Sugalski MT, LaPrade RF. Anatomy and biomechanics of the lateral side of the knee. *Sports Med Arthrosc Rev.* 2006;14(1):2–11. doi:10.1097/00132585-200603000-00002
14. Boden BP, Dean GS, Feagin JA Jr, Garrett WE Jr. Mechanisms of anterior cruciate ligament injury. *Orthopedics.* 2000;23(6):573–8. doi:10.3928/0147-7447-20000601-15
15. Akisue T, Kurosaka M, Yoshiya S, Kuroda R, Mizuno K. Evaluation of healing of the injured posterior cruciate ligament: analysis of instability and magnetic resonance imaging. *Arthroscopy.* 2001;17(3):264–9. doi:10.1053/jars.2001.21540
16. Montalvo AM, Schneider DK, Webster KE, et al. Anterior cruciate ligament injury risk in sport: a systematic review and meta-analysis of injury incidence by sex and sport classification. *J Athl Train.* 2019;54(5):472–82. doi:10.4085/1062-6050-407-16
17. Goldstein J, Bosco JA 3rd. The ACL-deficient knee: natural history and treatment options. *Bull Hosp Jt Dis.* 2001;60(3–4):173–8.
18. Boden BP, Sheehan FT, Torg JS, Hewett TE. Noncontact anterior cruciate ligament injuries: mechanisms and risk factors. *J Am Acad Orthop Surg.* 2010;18(9):520–7. doi:10.5435/00124635-201009000-00003
19. Brophy RH, Silvers HJ, Mandelbaum BR. Anterior cruciate ligament injuries: etiology and prevention. *Sports Med Arthrosc Rev.* 2010;18(1):2–11. doi:10.1097/JSA.0b013e3181cdd195
20. Benjaminse A, Gokeler A, van der Schans CP. Clinical diagnosis of an anterior cruciate ligament rupture: a meta-analysis. *J Orthop Sports Phys Ther.* 2006;36(5):267–88. doi:10.2519/jospt.2006.2011
21. Slagstad I, Parkar AP, Strand T, Inderhaug E. Incidence and prognostic significance of the Segond fracture in patients undergoing anterior cruciate ligament reconstruction. *Am J Sports Med.* 2020;48(5):1063–8. doi:10.1177/0363546520905557

22. Cobby MJ, Schweitzer ME, Resnick D. The deep lateral femoral notch: an indirect sign of a torn anterior cruciate ligament. *Radiology.* 1992;184(3):855–8. doi:10.1148/radiology.184.3.1509079
23. Daniel AV, Krych AJ, Smith PA. The lateral meniscus oblique radial tear (LMORT). *Curr Rev Musculoskelet Med.* 2023;16(7):306–15. doi:10.1007/s12178-023-09835-1
24. Mehl J, Otto A, Baldino JB, et al. The ACL-deficient knee and the prevalence of meniscus and cartilage lesions: a systematic review and meta-analysis (CRD42017076897). *Arch Orthop Trauma Surg.* 2019;139(6):819–41. doi:10.1007/s00402-019-03128-4
25. Bellabarba C, Bush-Joseph CA, Bach BR Jr. Patterns of meniscal injury in the anterior cruciate-deficient knee: a review of the literature. *Am J Orthop.* 1997;26(1):18–23.
26. Lohmander LS, Englund PM, Dahl LL, Roos EM. The long-term consequence of anterior cruciate ligament and meniscus injuries: osteoarthritis. *Am J Sports Med.* 2007;35(10):1756–69. doi:10.1177/0363546507307396
27. Fu FH, Schulte KR. Anterior cruciate ligament surgery 1996. State of the art? *Clin Orthop Relat Res.* 1996(325):19–24. doi:10.1097/00003086-199604000-00004
28. Richmond JC. Anterior cruciate ligament reconstruction. *Sports Med Arthrosc Rev.* 2018;26(4):165–7. doi:10.1097/jsa.0000000000000218
29. Musahl V, Engler ID, Nazzal EM, et al. Current trends in the anterior cruciate ligament part II: evaluation, surgical technique, prevention, and rehabilitation. *Knee Surg Sports Traumatol Arthrosc.* 2022;30(1):34–51. doi:10.1007/s00167-021-06825-z
30. Fithian DC, Paxton EW, Stone ML, et al. Prospective trial of a treatment algorithm for the management of the anterior cruciate ligament-injured knee. *Am J Sports Med.* 2005;33(3):335–46. doi:10.1177/0363546504269590
31. Johnson RJ, Beynnon BD, Nichols CE, Renstrom PA. The treatment of injuries of the anterior cruciate ligament. *J Bone Joint Surg Am.* 1992;74(1):140–51.
32. Muaidi QI, Nicholson LL, Refshauge KM, Herbert RD, Maher CG. Prognosis of conservatively managed anterior cruciate ligament injury: a systematic review. *Sports Med.* 2007;37(8):703–16. doi:10.2165/00007256-200737080-00004
33. Murray MM, Fleming BC, Badger GJ, BEAR Trial Team, et al. Bridge-enhanced anterior cruciate ligament repair is not inferior to autograft anterior cruciate ligament reconstruction at 2 years: results of a prospective randomized clinical trial. *Am J Sports Med.* 2020;48(6):1305–15. doi:10.1177/0363546520913532
34. Hospodar SJ, Miller MD. Controversies in ACL reconstruction: bone-patellar tendon-bone anterior cruciate ligament reconstruction remains the gold standard. *Sports Med Arthrosc Rev.* 2009;17(4):242–6. doi:10.1097/JSA.0b013e3181c14841
35. Foster TE, Wolfe BL, Ryan S, Silvestri L, Kaye EK. Does the graft source really matter in the outcome of patients undergoing anterior cruciate ligament reconstruction? An evaluation of autograft versus allograft reconstruction results: a systematic review. *Am J Sports Med.* 2010;38(1):189–99. doi:10.1177/0363546509356530
36. Mouarbes D, Menetrey J, Marot V, Courtot L, Berard E, Cavaignac E. Anterior cruciate ligament reconstruction: a systematic review and meta-analysis of outcomes for quadriceps tendon autograft versus bone-patellar tendon-bone and hamstring-tendon autografts. *Am J Sports Med.* 2019;47(14):3531–40. doi:10.1177/0363546518825340
37. Borchers JR, Pedroza A, Kaeding C. Activity level and graft type as risk factors for anterior cruciate ligament graft failure: a case-control study. *Am J Sports Med.* 2009;37(12):2362–7. doi:10.1177/0363546509340633
38. Barahona M, Mosquera M, De Padua V, Collaboration, et al. Latin American formal consensus on the appropriate indications of extra-articular lateral procedures in primary anterior cruciate ligament reconstruction. *J isakos.* 2023;8(3):177–83. doi:10.1016/j.jisako.2022.08.007
39. Getgood AMJ, Bryant DM, Litchfield R, STABILITY Study Group, et al. Lateral extra-articular tenodesis reduces failure of hamstring tendon autograft anterior cruciate ligament reconstruction: 2-year outcomes from the STABILITY study randomized clinical trial. *Am J Sports Med.* 2020;48(2):285–97. doi:10.1177/0363546519896333
40. Perkins CA, Willimon SC. Pediatric anterior cruciate ligament reconstruction. *Orthop Clin North Am.* 2020;51(1):55–63. doi:10.1016/j.ocl.2019.08.009
41. Margheritini F, Rihn J, Musahl V, Mariani PP, Harner C. Posterior cruciate ligament injuries in the athlete: an anatomical, biomechanical and clinical review. *Sports Med.* 2002;32(6):393–408. doi:10.2165/00007256-200232060-00004
42. Winkler PW, Zsidai B, Wagala NN, et al. Evolving evidence in the treatment of primary and recurrent posterior cruciate ligament injuries, part 1: anatomy, biomechanics and diagnostics. *Knee Surg Sports Traumatol Arthrosc.* 2021;29(3):672–81. doi:10.1007/s00167-020-06357-y
43. McAllister DR, Petrigliano FA. Diagnosis and treatment of posterior cruciate ligament injuries. *Curr Sports Med Rep.* 2007;6(5):293–9.
44. Feltham GT, Albright JP. The diagnosis of PCL injury: literature review and introduction of two novel tests. *Iowa Orthop J.* 2001;21:36–42.
45. Matava MJ, Ellis E, Gruber B. Surgical treatment of posterior cruciate ligament tears: an evolving technique. *J Am Acad Orthop Surg.* 2009;17(7):435–46. doi:10.5435/00124635-200907000-00004
46. Sekiya JK, Whiddon DR, Zehms CT, Miller MD. A clinically relevant assessment of posterior cruciate ligament and posterolateral corner injuries. Evaluation of isolated and combined deficiency. *J Bone Joint Surg Am.* 2008;90(8):1621–7. doi:10.2106/jbjs.G.01365
47. Parolie JM, Bergfeld JA. Long-term results of nonoperative treatment of isolated posterior cruciate ligament injuries in the athlete. *Am J Sports Med.* 1986;14(1):35–8. doi:10.1177/036354658601400107
48. Logan M, Williams A, Lavelle J, Gedroyc W, Freeman M. The effect of posterior cruciate ligament deficiency on knee kinematics. *Am J Sports Med.* 2004;32(8):1915–22. doi:10.1177/0363546504265005
49. Winkler PW, Zsidai B, Wagala NN, et al. Evolving evidence in the treatment of primary and recurrent posterior cruciate ligament injuries, part 2: surgical techniques, outcomes and rehabilitation. *Knee Surg Sports Traumatol Arthrosc.* 2021;29(3):682–93. doi:10.1007/s00167-020-06337-2
50. Wang D, Graziano J, Williams RJ 3rd, Jones KJ. Nonoperative treatment of PCL injuries: goals of rehabilitation and the natural history of conservative care. *Curr Rev Musculoskelet Med.* 2018;11(2):290–7. doi:10.1007/s12178-018-9487-y
51. Novaretti JV, Sheean AJ, Lian J, De Groot J, Musahl V. The role of osteotomy for the treatment of PCL injuries. *Curr Rev Musculoskelet Med.* 2018;11(2):298–306. doi:10.1007/s12178-018-9488-x
52. Berg EE. Posterior cruciate ligament tibial inlay reconstruction. *Arthroscopy.* 1995;11(1):69–76. doi:10.1016/0749-8063(95)90091-8
53. Kim SJ, Kim SH, Kim SG, Kung YP. Comparison of the clinical results of three posterior cruciate ligament reconstruction techniques: surgical technique. *J Bone Joint Surg Am.* 2010;92(suppl 1):145–57. doi:10.2106/jbjs.J.00185
54. Kim SJ, Kim TE, Jo SB, Kung YP. Comparison of the clinical results of three posterior cruciate ligament reconstruction techniques. *J Bone Joint Surg Am.* 2009;91(11):2543–9. doi:10.2106/jbjs.H.01819
55. Daniel DMPR, O'Connor JJ, Akeson WH. *Daniel's Knee Injuries: Ligament and Cartilage Structure, Function, Injury, and Repair.* 2nd ed. Philadelphia: Lippincott Williams & Wilkins; 2003.
56. Phisitkul P, James SL, Wolf BR, Amendola A. MCL injuries of the knee: current concepts review. *Iowa Orthop J.* 2006;26:77–90.
57. Somford MP, Lorusso L, Porro A, Loon CV, Eygendaal D. The Pellegrini-Stieda lesion dissected historically. *J Knee Surg.* 2018;31(6):562–7. doi:10.1055/s-0037-1604401
58. Lee JI, Song IS, Jung YB, et al. Medial collateral ligament injuries of the knee: ultrasonographic findings. *J Ultrasound Med.* 1996;15(9):621–5. doi:10.7863/jum.1996.15.9.621

59. Meyer P, Reiter A, Akoto R, et al. Imaging of the medial collateral ligament of the knee: a systematic review. *Arch Orthop Trauma Surg*. 2022;142(12):3721–36. doi:10.1007/s00402-021-04200-8
60. Miller MD, Osborne JR, Gordon WT, Hinkin DT, Brinker MR. The natural history of bone bruises. A prospective study of magnetic resonance imaging-detected trabecular microfractures in patients with isolated medial collateral ligament injuries. *Am J Sports Med*. 1998;26(1):15–9. doi:10.1177/03635465980260011001
61. D'Ambrosi R, Corona K, Guerra G, et al. Posterior oblique ligament of the knee: state of the art. *EFORT Open Rev*. 2021;6(5):364–71. doi:10.1302/2058-5241.6.200127
62. Battaglia MJ 2nd, Lenhoff MW, Ehteshami JR, et al. Medial collateral ligament injuries and subsequent load on the anterior cruciate ligament: a biomechanical evaluation in a cadaveric model. *Am J Sports Med*. 2009;37(2):305–11. doi:10.1177/0363546508324969
63. Dold AP, Swensen S, Strauss E, Alaia M. The posteromedial corner of the knee: anatomy, pathology, and management strategies. *J Am Acad Orthop Surg*. 2017;25(11):752–61. doi:10.5435/jaaos-d-16-00020
64. Reider B, Sathy MR, Talkington J, Blyznak N, Kollias S. Treatment of isolated medial collateral ligament injuries in athletes with early functional rehabilitation. A five-year follow-up study. *Am J Sports Med*. 1994;22(4):470–7. doi:10.1177/036354659402200406
65. Albright JP, Powell JW, Smith W, et al. Medial collateral ligament knee sprains in college football. Effectiveness of preventive braces. *Am J Sports Med*. 1994;22(1):12–8. doi:10.1177/036354659402200103
66. LaPrade RF, DePhillipo NN, Dornan GJ, et al. Comparative outcomes occur after superficial medial collateral ligament augmented repair vs reconstruction: a prospective multicenter randomized controlled equivalence trial. *Am J Sports Med*. 2022;50(4):968–76. doi:10.1177/03635465211069373
67. O'Brien SJ, Warren RF, Pavlov H, Panariello R, Wickiewicz TL. Reconstruction of the chronically insufficient anterior cruciate ligament with the central third of the patellar ligament. *J Bone Joint Surg Am*. 1991;73(2):278–86.
68. Quarles JD, Hosey RG. Medial and lateral collateral injuries: prognosis and treatment. *Prim Care*. 2004;31(4):957–75. doi:10.1016/j.pop.2004.07.005
69. LaPrade RF, Terry GC. Injuries to the posterolateral aspect of the knee. Association of anatomic injury patterns with clinical instability. *Am J Sports Med*. 1997;25(4):433–8. doi:10.1177/036354659702500403
70. Chen FS, Rokito AS, Pitman MI. Acute and chronic posterolateral rotatory instability of the knee. *J Am Acad Orthop Surg*. 2000;8(2):97–110. doi:10.5435/00124635-200003000-00004
71. Kannus P. Nonoperative treatment of grade II and III sprains of the lateral ligament compartment of the knee. *Am J Sports Med*. 1989;17(1):83–8. doi:10.1177/036354658901700114
72. Laprade RF, Griffith CJ, Coobs BR, Geeslin AG, Johansen S, Engebretsen L. Improving outcomes for posterolateral knee injuries. *J Orthop Res*. 2014;32(4):485–91. doi:10.1002/jor.22572
73. Chahla J, Murray IR, Robinson J, et al. Posterolateral corner of the knee: an expert consensus statement on diagnosis, classification, treatment, and rehabilitation. *Knee Surg Sports Traumatol Arthrosc*. 2019;27(8):2520–9. doi:10.1007/s00167-018-5260-4
74. Cooper JM, McAndrews PT, LaPrade RF. Posterolateral corner injuries of the knee: anatomy, diagnosis, and treatment. *Sports Med Arthrosc Rev*. 2006;14(4):213–20. doi:10.1097/01.jsa.0000212324.46430.60
75. Levy BA, Stuart MJ, Whelan DB. Posterolateral instability of the knee: evaluation, treatment, results. *Sports Med Arthrosc Rev*. 2010;18(4):254–62. doi:10.1097/JSA.0b013e3181f88527
76. Anazor FC, Baryeh K, Davies NC. Knee joint dislocation: overview and current concepts. *Br J Hosp Med*. 2021;82(12):1–10. doi:10.12968/hmed.2021.0466
77. Green NE, Allen BL. Vascular injuries associated with dislocation of the knee. *J Bone Joint Surg Am*. 1977;59(2):236–9.
78. McDonough EB Jr, Wojtys EM. Multiligamentous injuries of the knee and associated vascular injuries. *Am J Sports Med*. 2009;37(1):156–9. doi:10.1177/0363546508324313
79. Rihn JA, Groff YJ, Harner CD, Cha PS. The acutely dislocated knee: evaluation and management. *J Am Acad Orthop Surg*. 2004;12(5):334–46. doi:10.5435/00124635-200409000-00008
80. Figueras JH, Johnson BM, Thomson C, Dailey SW, Betz BE, Grawe BM. Team approach: treatment of traumatic dislocations of the knee. *JBJS Rev*. 2023;11(4):1–9. doi:10.2106/jbjs.Rvw.22.00188
81. Casey S, Lanting S, Oldmeadow C, Chuter V. The reliability of the ankle brachial index: a systematic review. *J Foot Ankle Res*. 2019;12:39. doi:10.1186/s13047-019-0350-1
82. Redmond JM, Levy BA, Dajani KA, Cass JR, Cole PA. Detecting vascular injury in lower-extremity orthopedic trauma: the role of CT angiography. *Orthopedics*. 2008;31(8):761–7. doi:10.3928/01477447-20080801-27
83. Meyers MH, Moore TM, Harvey JP Jr. Traumatic dislocation of the knee joint. *J Bone Joint Surg Am*. 1975;57(3):430–3. [
84. Fanelli GC, Orcutt DR, Edson CJ. The multiple-ligament injured knee: evaluation, treatment, and results. *Arthroscopy*. 2005;21(4):471–86. doi:10.1016/j.arthro.2005.01.001
85. Ng JWG, Myint Y, Ali FM. Management of multiligament knee injuries. *EFORT Open Rev*. 2020;5(3):145–55. doi:10.1302/2058-5241.5.190012
86. Mortazavi SMJ, Kaseb MH, Maleki RG, Razzaghof M, Noori A, Rezaee R. The functional outcomes of delayed surgical reconstruction in nonsport-induced multiligament knee injuries: a retrospective cohort study. *J Knee Surg*. 2022;35(10):1097–105. doi:10.1055/s-0040-1721788
87. Zhang T, Shasti K, Dubina A, et al. Long-term outcomes of multiligament knee injuries. *J Orthop Trauma*. 2022;36(8):394–9. doi:10.1097/bot.0000000000002348

65 The Patellofemoral Joint

Elizabeth A. Arendt and Raimundo Vial Irarrazal

ANATOMY

- The patella is the largest sesamoid bone in the body. Its blood supply arises mainly from the peripatellar plexus. The patella articulates with the femoral sulcus, otherwise known as the trochlea. It is enveloped by fibers of the quadriceps tendon and blends with the patellar tendon distally. The patella serves as a fulcrum for the quadriceps muscles. The main biomechanical function of the patella is to increase the moment arm of the quadriceps mechanism. With patella alta, the biomechanical action of this lever arm is diminished.
- From a neuromuscular viewpoint, the quadriceps muscle unit encases the patella and crosses two joints (hip and knee). It is responsible for extension of the knee in open kinetic chain function and stabilization and shock absorption of the body in closed chain function.
- The patellar surface is divided into two large facets: medial and lateral, which are separated by a central ridge. The facets are covered by the thickest hyaline cartilage in the body that may measure up to 6.5 mm. The superior three-fourths of the patella are articular, and the inferior one-fourth (the patellar 'nose') is nonarticular, although the percent distribution varies significantly in the population. The contact area between the patella and femur varies with knee flexion angle and with sagittal height of the patella. The patella contacts the femoral trochlea in early flexion; as flexion increases, the contact of the patella moves proximally and medially with the largest area of contact being made at approximately 45°. Contact stresses on the patellofemoral (PF) joint are higher than any other major weight-bearing joint in the body and increases with weight-bearing knee flexion. Compressive forces on the patella can range from 3.3 times body weight with stair climbing up to 7.6 times the body weight with squatting (1).
- Several ossification centers contribute to the patella. Failure of fusion can lead to bipartite patella, with superolateral being most common. The rate of bipartite patellae is approximately 1%; more than 55% are unilateral. A bipartite patella has a firm fibrous union but can become mobile with repeated activity or a single injury. Widening of the fibrous union on repeated imaging, or a bone scan, is helpful is discerning a diagnosis. A bipartite patella may mimic a patellar sleeve fracture in children or an osteochondral fracture after trauma on plain radiographs.
- Patellar soft-tissue stabilizers play a crucial role in patellar joint stabilization. Medial PF complex is the term for the proximal stabilizers (medial patellofemoral ligament [MPFL] and medial quadriceps tendon femoral ligament [MQTFL]), and the distal stabilizers (medial patellotibial and patellomeniscal ligament) (2) (Fig. 65.1).
- The MPFL is the primary static stabilizer of the patella, and accounts for greater than half of the total restraint to lateral patellar displacement (3). The role of the medial distal stabilizers in patellar stabilization continues to evolve (2).
- The lateral retinaculum is composed of a superficial and deep layer and runs from lateral margin of the patella and patellar tendon to the anterior aspect of the iliotibial band.
- The patellar tendon varies in length from 4.0 to 6.9 cm. It connects the apex of the patella to the tibial tuberosity. Sagittal patellar position, or patellar height, can be alta (too superior) or infera (too inferior), in reference to standardized controls. Patellar position is dependent on patellar tendon length and not its tibial insertion, which is more uniform in the population (4). Patellar alta is a major risk factor for lateral patellar dislocations (5), whereas patella infera is commonly a consequence of surgery or trauma.

HISTORY

- It is important to differentiate between acute knee injury and an overuse injury.
- Specific details are listed under the individual categories in the following.
  - If the knee swells within the first 12 hours after knee injury, this signifies blood or a hemarthrosis within the joint. The most common cause of an acute hemarthrosis after a sports-related knee injury is a tear of the anterior cruciate ligament, with the second most common cause being a traumatic lateral patellar dislocation (LPD) with bleeding due to soft-tissue tearing, osteochondral fracture, or both. In the adolescent population (age < 14), the most common cause of an acute hemarthrosis is LPD (6).

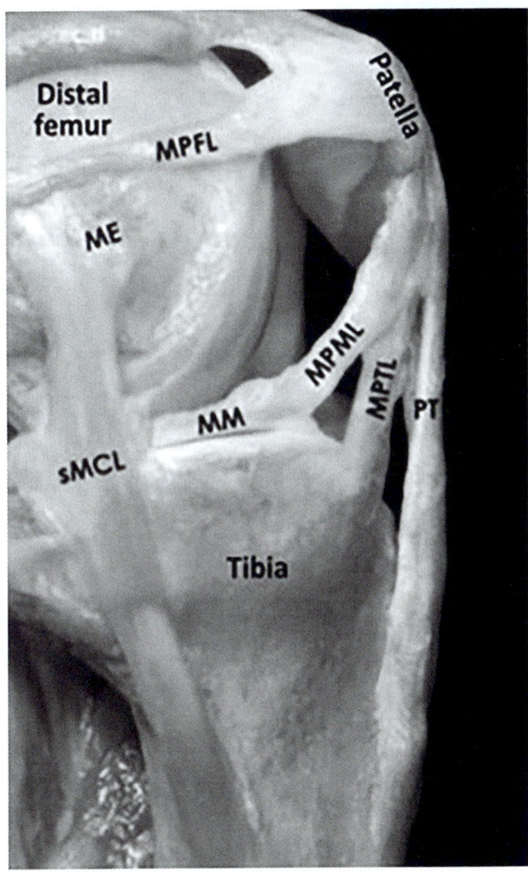

Figure 65.1: Cadaveric dissection of a left knee showing patellar soft-tissue stabilizers. ME, medial epicondyle; MM, medial meniscus; MPFL, medial patellofemoral ligament; MPML, medial patellomeniscal ligament; MPTL, medial patellotibial ligament; PT, patellar tendon; sMCL, superficial medial collateral ligament. (From Kruckeberg BM, Chahla J, Moatshe G, et al. Quantitative and qualitative analysis of the medial patellar ligaments: an anatomic and radiographic study. *Am J Sports Med.* 2018;46(1):153–62. doi:10.1177/0363546517729818)

PHYSICAL EXAMINATION

- One should use a systematic approach to a knee exam including inspection, palpation, testing for tibiofemoral laxity, assessing patellar position, stability, patellar tracking.
- Regarding inspection, the examiner should look for swelling and ecchymosis. Bruising is uncommon in PF disorders excluding an acute injury, so alternative diagnosis should be considered if present. Limb alignment should be assessed both supine and standing and classified as varus (bow-legged), neutral, or valgus (knock-kneed) alignment.
- On palpation, PF crepitus is best elicited by supine or seated active knee range of knee motion. One-finger palpation is important to localize tenderness, especially over the patellar tendon origin and insertion, and quadricep tendon insertion.
- Documentation of the full range of motion (ROM), including knee hyperextension, should be done in the supine position.
- When assessing for patellar instability, measure patellar mobility (patellar glide) (Fig. 65.2). This is based on the maximum amount of passive displacement of the patella (using the quadrant system with the patella divided into four vertical quadrants). Evaluation should include both medial and lateral patellar translation with the knee at 0° and 30° of flexion. This test evaluates the integrity and tightness of the medial and lateral restraints. Any lateral translation greater than two quadrants is considered hypermobile. A side-to-side difference of lateral translation suggests an incompetent MPFL on the more mobile side. Performing lateral translation may cause pain and/or quadricep contraction and is called an "apprehension sign"; this is associated with acute and recurrent lateral patellar dislocation.
- The passive patellar tilt test determines the tension of the lateral restraints. With the knee fully extended, the lateral patellar border is manually elevated. A passive tilt of less than 0° (neutral or below the horizontal plane) may imply lateral retinacular tightness, increased static lateral patellar tilt, and/or a diagnosis of excessive lateral pressure syndrome (ELPS).
- One can also assess patellar tracking; when done with active ROM and open chain, more pathology is elicited. If the patella starts lateral and 'jumps' into the groove in early flexion, or jumps out of the groove in late extension, it is considered a "J sign." (The patella deviates laterally in terminal extension thus mimicking a J.)
- Femoral anteversion (femoral rotation in the axial plane) and tibial torsion (tibial rotation in the axial plane) should be examined with the patient in the prone position. Hip ROM should be included in the nonacute exam. When hip internal rotation is greater than hip external rotation, increased femoral anteversion should be more thoroughly examined (7).

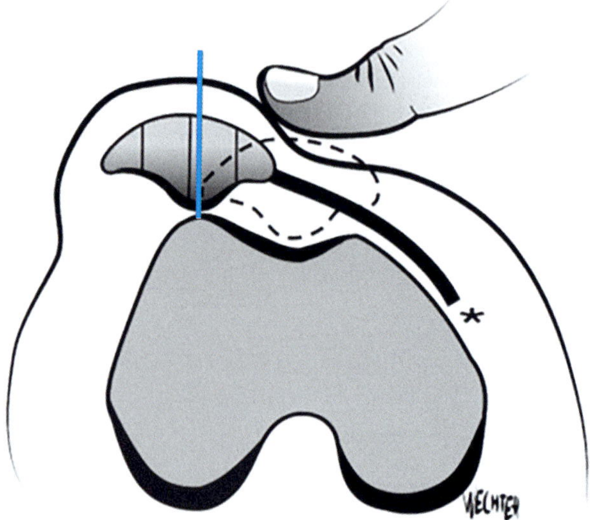

Figure 65.2: The patella has been displaced laterally two quadrants of its width from its original position (dashed line). This is classified as a grade 2 patellar glide.

- Standing alignment as well as double-leg and single-leg squat mechanics are helpful tools to assess for down-the-chain mechanics and alignment. For core strength and stability as well as alignment, these simple maneuvers assess function at the low back, pelvis, hip, knee, ankle, and foot. When observing for both static and dynamic limb alignment, squat mechanics give a snapshot of the forces to which the knee may be subjected while participating in daily activities as well as sport.

RADIOGRAPHS

- Patients who present with PF complaints should undergo standard knee radiographs to rule out associated pathology. Radiographs for ambulatory patients are listed in Table 65.1. The standard patellar radiograph is the axial view or sunrise view. For PF disease and injury, a low flexion angle (Fig. 65.3), which visualize the proximal portion of the femoral groove, is critical for better delineation of joint space narrowing and patella position.

Table 65.1 Radiographs for Ambulatory Patients

Radiographic View	Evaluation
Axial views: Low angle flexion view (20°–30°) (8,9)	Sulcus angle, patella position in the groove (excessive lateral tilt and/or translation), PF joint space narrowing (in older group)
True lateral view (10)	Trochlear dysplasia, patella height, PF joint space narrowing (in older population), etc.
Standing AP	Tibiofemoral joint space narrowing, limb alignment
Standing PA flexion	Tibiofemoral joint space narrowing, particularly lateral compartment

- A computed tomography (CT) scan is most often used to evaluate fractures, healing of fractures, and measurements for limb version (7).
- Knee MRI is most used to detect intra-articular pathology such as meniscal tears, cruciate or collateral ligament injuries, and osteochondral defects. Magnetic resonance imaging (MRI) is most useful for evaluation of the articular surfaces of the PF joint, and for measurement of anatomic (imaging) PF instability risk factors (*e.g.*) tibial tubercle-trochlear groove distance (TT-TG), and the patellar-trochlear index (5,11,12)

GENERAL TREATMENT OF COMMON PATELLOFEMORAL DISORDERS

- PF malalignment is a term that is overused and poorly defined. Confusion arises because malalignment has been used as a clinical diagnosis, a radiographic description of patellar position, and at times a diagnosis. PF malalignment is a concept of imbalance that helps explain PF disorders. Treatment of PF malalignment should include consideration of all contributing factors that includes bony alignment, joint geometry, soft-tissue restraints, neuromuscular control, and functional demands (13). These forces can result in anterior knee pain, PF arthrosis, and/or PF instability, which will be discussed separately.

ANTERIOR KNEE PAIN

- Anterior knee pain (AKP) originates in the anterior knee structures typically in the absence of an identifiable acute injury. AKP is one of the most common conditions presenting to clinicians, particularly those managing an active population.

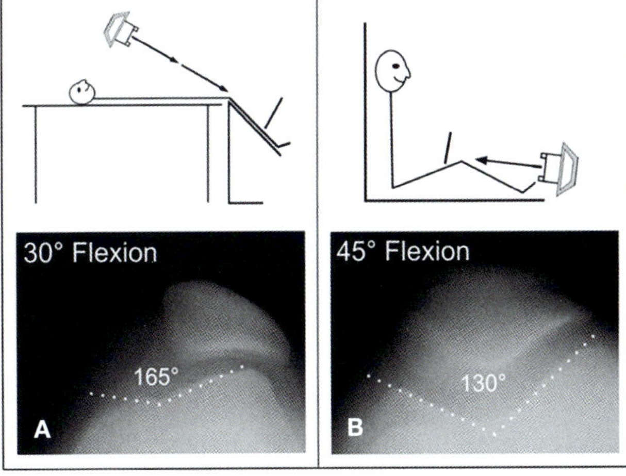

Figure 65.3: Two different ways to obtain an axial patellar x-ray view. A: Laurin view with x-ray beam directed from proximal to distal and a low knee flexion angle. B: Merchant view with the x-ray beam directed from distal to proximal. Note how a lower knee flexion angle allows better appreciation of the proximal trochlea and patellar alignment.

Its primary mechanism lies in overuse injury principles, which can also be useful in directing treatment. This is true although the exact etiology and nature of the pain continues to be poorly understood. An overuse injury is considered repetitive submaximal or subclinical trauma that results in macro- and/or microscopic trauma. The tissue's structural unit is damaged, or at least has overexceeded its clinical responsiveness, and this can lead to pain and/or movement dysfunction. The most common form of an overuse injury is from an endogenous source (*i.e.*, mechanical circumstances) in which the musculoskeletal tissue is subjected to greater tensile force or stress than the tissue can fully absorb.

- The approach to AKP is facilitated by the concept of tissue homeostasis and the envelope effect of function (14). Many patients with AKP have normal imaging. Conversely, many with abnormal findings on imaging have no AKP. No AKP patient should be considered solely from a structural biomechanical perspective; that is, based on imaging alone.
- Increased body mass as well as muscle weakness correlates with increased rates of PF load. This load is felt to be in part a causative factor in AKP. Conversely, a reduction in weight or an increase in strength can diminish the stresses borne by the PF compartment and modulate or reduce pain.
- Faulty body movement patterns can contribute to joint overload in one of two ways: overload at the joint and its surrounding soft-tissue structures through imbalanced or excessive movement within its normal planes of motion; or deviation into abnormal motion planes, which can magnify joint instability and/or malalignment. Both patterns can eventually exceed the joint's capacity to maintain stability and/or exceed the joint structures' tolerance for loading and contribute to pain through tissue overload principles, exceeding the joint's envelope of function (15–17).
- Nonoperative treatment is the mainstay for PF pain (15–17). Load management is advised, and the patient should temporarily avoid activities that consistently reproduce pain. Physical therapy is focused on modifying faulty movement patterns by improving core and lower limb control and increasing load tolerance.
- Simple bracing with a patellar cutout or patellar stabilizing braces may be beneficial to many patients. Differing types of braces act either to help recreate proper tracking or via a lateral buttress effect. Taping techniques, such as those described by Crossley et al. (15,16) to stabilize subluxation or tilt, may also be beneficial to patients.

PF ARTHROSIS

- A patient with isolated PF osteoarthritis (OA) typically describes anterior knee pain in bent knee activities; level ground walking is usually well tolerated. Sometimes there is pseudo-locking and giving way due to the loss of surface gliding at the site of "kissing" bare bone lesions. The patient is often apprehensive doing bent knee activities, especially going down steps.
- Trochlear dysplasia is an anatomic risk factor that is highly correlated to isolated PF arthritis. Although studies are sparse looking at the sex as an independent risk factor for this disease, the available studies show an overwhelmingly female preponderance (18).
- Nonoperative management is similar to medical management of knee arthritis including NSAIDs, injections, and physical therapy aimed at fitness and lower body kinematics. Typically, PFOA is laterally based within the PF compartment, and as such can be 'unloaded' with McConnell taping and bracing, aimed at medial glide and medial tilt.
- Surgical options include:
    - Partial lateral facetectomy with lateral retinacular lengthening/release: ideal in early lateral-sided PF wear associated with lateral tightness and with a positive clinical response to McConnell taping (lateral to medial).
    - Anterio-medialization (AMZ) of the tibial tubercle: ideal in unipolar patellar arthritis based inferior and lateral, with an elevated quadricep vector.
    - Cartilage restoration procedures including osteochondral allografts, and cell-based therapies (*i.e.*) matrix autologous

osteochondral chondrocyte implantation (MACI), are rarely used for PF OA, but reserved for focal unipolar patella or femoral groove lesions.

- PF (uni) arthroplasty is considered when there is radiographic evidence of PF OA, with failed nonoperative management, and no or minimal cartilage wear in the tibiofemoral compartments. Ideal use of PFA is in a patient in whom the implant is expected to last a lifetime. However, the revision of a PFA to a total knee arthroplasty (TKA) is less onerous than a revision TKA. Its use in the younger age group (age 40–55) may acceptably carry with it the expectation of revision to a TKA in their lifetime.

PF INSTABILITY

- Instability is a functional symptom with the patella transiently leaving the femoral groove either partially (subluxation) or completely (dislocation), with LPD being the most common form of PF instability. The patient that has suffered a patellar subluxation or dislocation may describe the feeling of having their kneecap pop out of the knee groove. Dislocation occurs as the knee moves from an extended into a flexed position with valgus and external rotation of the tibia. Usually, the patella will relocate itself. When this does not happen spontaneously, the patella can be relocated by bringing the knee into extension with the quadriceps relaxed if possible. The main soft tissue restraint to lateral subluxation of the patella is the medial PF ligament (3,12); this is usually injured in an acute traumatic patellar dislocation (Fig. 65.4).
- Initial treatment for instability is nonoperative, with the focus on strengthening of the lower extremity musculature including core, and attention to correction of faulty body movement patterns (16).
- Central to the clinical assessment of LPD is knowledge of the anatomic risk factors defined by imaging, initially defined as the four principal factors: trochlear dysplasia, patella alta, excessive quadriceps vector as defined by TT-TG >20 mm, and excessive lateral patellar tilt >20° (5,19).
- Current literature suggests that trochlear dysplasia and patella alta are the dominant anatomic risk factors, along with open physes (20).
- The MPFL has emerged as the major stabilizer against lateral patellar translation in terminal extension. This knowledge has resulted in a paradigm shift in our surgical approach to LPD; reconstruction of the MPFL is currently the cornerstone of surgical solutions for recurrent LPD (19,21).
- Although we have identified anatomic thresholds for the characterization of the patient with a primary LPD, it remains unclear when (at what imaging numerical threshold) and how (what surgical procedure) to reduce each anatomic (imaging) risk factor. We do know, however, that there is a greater chance of redislocation if you have a greater number of anatomic instability risk factors. Recent studies have shown that risk of radiolocation increases as the number of risk factors increases, and range from approx. 20% with no PF instability risk factors to >75% with 3+ risk factors (20).

PATELLAR TENDINOPATHY

- Patellar tendinopathy is an overuse condition of the patellar tendon frequently affecting athletes who play jumping sports (22,23).
- This condition is degenerative rather than inflammatory, so "tendinosis" is the more appropriate term than tendonitis. Repetitive bent knee activity, in particular sports that require

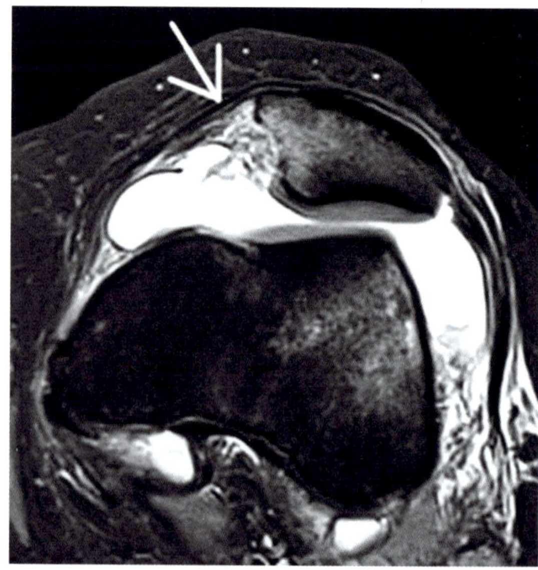

Figure 65.4: PDW FS sequence axial cut of left knee MRI. White arrow shows torn patellar insertion of the medial patellofemoral ligament. Note hyperintense images compatible with "bone bruising" on the medial aspect of the patella and lateral aspect of the femur due to recent patellar dislocation event.

explosive jumping, and inadequate time for healing are risk factors for patellar tendinosis to occur (24).

- Causative risk factors in the development of patellar tendinopathy are largely agreed to be extrinsic factors, including training load and harder training surfaces (25,26). To date intrinsic risk factors, such as patella alta, patellar tilt, coronal plane limb alignment, obesity (BMI) height and weight, have not shown a consistent correlation with patellar tendinopathy (27). However, one prospective study did show that athletes with poor hamstring and quadriceps flexibility were at greater risk to develop patellar tendinopathy (28).
- Treatment of patellar tendinopathy is largely nonoperative, with attention to load management and graduated rehabilitative exercise. The literature is robust with many adjunctive therapies including: platelet-rich plasma (PRP) injections, cryotherapy, patellar strapping, NSAIDs, corticosteroids, aprotinin injections, sclerosing injections with a chemical irritants, glyceryl trinitrate patches, and extracorporeal shockwave therapy (29). The reader is referred to Chapter 76 Medications and Ergogenics, Chapter 78 Orthobiologics, and Chapter 80 Image Guided Procedures, for further discussion.
- Operative treatment should be considered in patients where nonoperative therapy has failed. A recent comprehensive of surgical procedures, including both open and arthroscopic approaches, was conducted with a specific focus on clinical outcomes and return to sports. Both open surgery and arthroscopic surgery for patients with patellar tendinopathy have demonstrated favorable success rates and return-to-sport outcomes, with arthroscopic treatment potentially expediting the recovery process (30).

OSTEOCHONDRAL INJURY

- Osteochondral injuries can occur with blunt knee trauma, but more frequently are encountered following acute traumatic subluxation/dislocation. The patient will commonly give a history of a traumatic event with possible continued instability. They also may have symptoms of a loose body within the knee joint. These injuries are best evaluated with plain x-rays (all four radiographic views), CT scan, and MRI to determine the size and location of the fragment. Osteochondral fractures should be evaluated acutely with arthroscopy. Large articular fragments can and should be fixed acutely, whereas nondisplaced stable fractures can be managed nonsurgically.

FRACTURES

- Fractures of the patella are most commonly from direct trauma to the anterior knee. Patellar fractures are most commonly transverse in orientation and are seen best on a lateral x-ray. Vertical fractures are rare and best seen on the axial view. Nondisplaced fractures with an intact articular surface and preserved extensor mechanism are treated nonoperatively with 6 weeks of bracing/casting in extension followed by progressive ROM exercises. Displaced fractures are those with at least 3 mm of cortical disruption or 2 mm of articular step-off on radiographs. These are treated with open reduction internal fixation (ORIF).
- Patella injury in patients with open growth plates can also occur via indirect mechanisms such as jumping or rapid flexion of the knee with maximal quadriceps contraction and can involve a sleeve injury to the patellar tendon proximal insertion, or an avulsion injury to the apophysis of the tibial tubercle. Most need surgical attention.

REFERENCES

1. Huberti HH, Hayes WC. Contact pressures in chondromalacia patellae and the effects of capsular reconstructive procedures. *J Orthop Res.* 1988;6(4):499–508.
2. Tanaka MJ, Chahla J, Farr J II, et al. Recognition of evolving medial patellofemoral anatomy provides insight for reconstruction. *Knee Surg Sports Traumatol Arthrosc.* 2019;27(8):2537–50.
3. Conlan T, Garth WP Jr, Lemons JE. Evaluation of the medial soft-tissue restraints of the extensor mechanism of the knee. *J Bone Joint Surg Am.* 1993;75(5):682–93.
4. Neyret P, Robinson AH, Le Coultre B, Lapra C, Chambat P. Patellar tendon length--the factor in patellar instability? *Knee.* 2002;9(1):3–6.
5. Arendt EA, England K, Agel J, Tompkins MA. An analysis of knee anatomic imaging factors associated with primary lateral patellar dislocations. *Knee Surg Sports Traumatol Arthrosc.* 2017;25(10):3099–107.
6. Askenberger M, Ekström W, Finnbogason T, Janarv PM. Occult intra-articular knee injuries in children with hemarthrosis. *Am J Sports Med.* 2014;42(7):1600–6.
7. Shih YC, Chau MM, Arendt EA, Novacheck TF. Measuring lower extremity rotational alignment: a review of methods and case studies of clinical applications. *J Bone Joint Surg Am.* 2020;102(4):343–56.
8. Laurin CA, Lévesque HP, Dussault R, Labelle H, Peides JP. The abnormal lateral patellofemoral angle: a diagnostic roentgenographic sign of recurrent patellar subluxation. *J Bone Joint Surg Am.* 1978;60(1):55–60.
9. Merchant AC, Mercer RL, Jacobsen RH, Cool CR. Roentgenographic analysis of patellofemoral congruence. *J Bone Joint Surg Am.* 1974;56(7):1391–6.
10. Dejour H, Walch G, Nove-Josserand L, Guier C. Factors of patellar instability: an anatomic radiographic study. *Knee Surg Sports Traumatol Arthrosc.* 1994;2(1):19–26.
11. Ridley TJ, Hinckel B, Kruckeberg BM, Agel J, Arendt EA. Anatomical patella instability risk factors on MRI show sensitivity without specificity in patients with patellofemoral instability: a systematic review. *J ISAKOS.* 2016;1(3):141–52.
12. Tompkins MA, Rohr SR, Agel J, Arendt EA. Anatomic patellar instability risk factors in primary lateral patellar dislocations do not predict injury patterns: an MRI-based study. *Knee Surg Sports Traumatol Arthrosc.* 2018;26(3):677–84.
13. Post WR, Teitge R, Amis A. Patellofemoral malalignment: looking beyond the view box. *Clin Sports Med.* 2002;21(3):521–46. x.
14. Dye SF. The pathophysiology of patellofemoral pain: a tissue homeostasis perspective. *Clin Orthop Relat Res.* 2005;436:100–10.

15. Crossley K, Bennell K, Green S, Cowan S, McConnell J. Physical therapy for patellofemoral pain: a randomized, double-blinded, placebo-controlled trial. *Am J Sports Med.* 2002;30(6):857–65.
16. Crossley KM, Van Middelkoop M, Callaghan MJ, Collins NJ, Rathleff MS, Barton CJ. 2016 Patellofemoral pain consensus statement from the 4th International Patellofemoral Pain Research Retreat, Manchester. Part 2: recommended physical interventions (exercise, taping, bracing, foot orthoses and combined interventions). *Br J Sports Med.* 2016;50(14):844–52.
17. Hiemstra LA, Kerslake S, Arendt EA. Clinical rehabilitation of anterior knee pain: current concepts. *Am J Orthop (Belle Mead NJ).* 2017;46(2):82–6.
18. Grelsamer RP, Dejour D, Gould J. The pathophysiology of patellofemoral arthritis. *Orthop Clin North Am.* 2008;39(3):269–74. v.
19. Arendt EA, Donell ST, Sillanpää PJ, Feller JA. The management of lateral patellar dislocation: state of the art. *J ISAKOS.* 2017;2:205–12.
20. Huntington LS, Webster KE, Devitt BM, Scanlon JP, Feller JA. Factors associated with an increased risk of recurrence after a first-time patellar dislocation: a systematic review and meta-analysis. *Am J Sports Med.* 2020;48(10):2552–62.
21. Post WR, Fithian DC. Patellofemoral instability: a consensus statement from the AOSSM/PFF patellofemoral instability workshop. *Orthop J Sports Med.* 2018;6(1):2325967117750352.
22. Lian OB, Engebretsen L, Bahr R. Prevalence of jumper's knee among elite athletes from different sports: a cross-sectional study. *Am J Sports Med.* 2005;33(4):561–7.
23. Trojan JD, Treloar JA, Smith CM, Kraeutler MJ, Mulcahey MK. Epidemiological patterns of patellofemoral injuries in collegiate athletes in the United States from 2009 to 2014. *Orthop J Sports Med.* 2019;7(4):2325967119840712.
24. Dan M, Parr W, Broe D, Cross M, Walsh WR. Biomechanics of the knee extensor mechanism and its relationship to patella tendinopathy: a review. *J Orthop Res.* 2018;36(12):3105–12.
25. Sprague AL, Smith AH, Knox P, Pohlig RT, Grävare Silbernagel K. Modifiable risk factors for patellar tendinopathy in athletes: a systematic review and meta-analysis. *Br J Sports Med.* 2018;52(24):1575–85.
26. Visnes H, Bahr R. Training volume and body composition as risk factors for developing jumper's knee among young elite volleyball players. *Scand J Med Sci Sports.* 2013;23(5):607–13.
27. Dan MJ, Mcmahon J, Parr WCH, et al. Evaluation of intrinsic biomechanical risk factors in patellar tendinopathy: a retrospective radiographic case-control series. *Orthop J Sports Med.* 2018;6(12):2325967118816038.
28. Witvrouw E, Lysens R, Bellemans J, Cambier D, Vanderstraeten G. Intrinsic risk factors for the development of anterior knee pain in an athletic population. A two-year prospective study. *Am J Sports Med.* 2000;28(4):480–9.
29. Theodorou A, Komnos G, Hantes M. Patellar tendinopathy: an overview of prevalence, risk factors, screening, diagnosis, treatment and prevention. *Arch Orthop Trauma Surg.* 2023 Nov;143(11):6695–705.
30. Sugrañes J, Jackson GR, Mameri ES, et al. Current concepts in patellar tendinopathy: an overview of imaging, pathogenesis, and nonoperative and operative management. *JBJS Rev.* 2023 Aug 17;11(8):e23.

Soft-Tissue Knee Injuries (Tendon and Bursae)

66

Stephen Rossettie and John J. Klimkiewicz

BIOMECHANICS OF TENDON RUPTURES

Extensor Mechanism Force Ratio

- Position of knee flexion directly affects this ratio. At knee flexion angles <45°, this ratio is >1, whereas at knee flexion angles >45°, this ratio is <1 (1).
- At >45°, the patellar tendon has a mechanical advantage and is less susceptible to injury through tensile failure, whereas at positions <45°, the quadriceps tendon has a mechanical advantage and is less vulnerable to injury.
- Tendon strain in response to tensile load is up to three times greater at the insertion sites than at the tendon midsubstance. Additionally, collagen fiber stiffness is less at the insertion sites. These biomechanical properties contribute to tendon rupture commonly occurring at their insertion sites rather than at their midsubstance (2).
- Failure usually occurs during rapid eccentric muscular contraction when markedly higher forces can be generated compared to concentric muscular contraction (3).
- This most often occurs with trauma causing forced extension of a flexed joint.
- Several metabolic diseases or direct steroid injection can predispose to tendon rupture. These conditions include hyperparathyroidism, calcium pyrophosphate deposition disease, diabetes mellitus, chronic renal disease, gout, systemic lupus erythematosus, and rheumatoid arthritis (4,5).
- Fluoroquinolone antibiotics and isotretinoin treatment have been associated with pathologic tendon alteration and increased incidence of tendon rupture (6,7).

PATELLAR TENDON RUPTURES

- The patellar tendon receives its blood supply from the vessels within the infrapatellar fat pad and retinacular structures (8,9).
- The origin and insertion of the patellar tendon are relatively avascular.
- Ruptures of the patella tendon most typically occur in male patients less than 40 years of age and are frequently associated with sporting activities including football, basketball, and soccer (10).
- Ruptures are most common through the tendon-bone junction at the distal pole of the patella.
- Histologic examination of ruptured tendon often demonstrates an area of degeneration thought to predispose these patients to injury.
- Previous surgeries, including total knee arthroplasty, anterior cruciate ligament (ACL) reconstruction using autograft patellar tendon, and tibial intramedullary nailing, have been associated with postoperative patellar tendon ruptures (11–13).

Clinical Presentation

- At the time of injury, a pop is often heard with an acute onset of pain and swelling. Patient is usually unable to actively extend knee or maintain it in an extended position against gravity. Chronic cases present with an extensor lag (10).
- A palpable defect is commonly present just below the distal pole of the patella.
- Concomitant ACL injuries are not uncommon and should be clinically ruled out (14).
- Plain radiographs often demonstrate a patella alta in comparison to the opposite knee using the Insall-Salvati index (>1.2) (15).
- An osseous fragment is present at times at the distal pole of the patella when an avulsion is part of the injury.
- Magnetic resonance imaging (MRI) is useful in cases where partial injury is suspected.

Treatment

- Partial tendon injuries with an intact extensor mechanism can be treated conservatively by cylinder cast or hinged knee brace with the leg placed in full extension for 4–6 weeks followed by progressive range of motion and strengthening (16).
- Complete ruptures should be directly repaired on an acute basis through suture anchors or transosseous drill holes

through the patella. Suture anchor repair has resulted in less gap formation and decreased rerupture rate compared to transosseous repair (17–19).

- Once secured, the knee should have at least 90 degrees of flexion to avoid overconstraint. Primary repairs are often augmented with wire, Mersilene tape, suture, or autologous hamstring tendon or iliotibial band (20).
- Chronic ruptures can involve proximal patellar migration and can often require quadriceps mobilization or V-Y advancement in order to restore patellar height.
- Semitendinosus/gracilis augmentation is recommended in the chronic scenario. Achilles tendon or patellar tendon allograft has often been found useful to replace/reinforce the reconstruction in chronic situations (21).

Complications

- After surgery, complications include knee stiffness and weakness. Rerupture is rare but more common with transosseous tunnels than suture anchors. Restoration of normal patellofemoral tracking and height at the time of surgery is essential to achieve optimal results. Residual weakness of extensor mechanism is more common in delayed repairs (19).

QUADRICEPS TENDON RUPTURES

- The quadriceps tendon is a coalescence of tendinous portions of the rectus femoris, vastus lateralis, vastus intermedius, and vastus medialis muscles.
- The quadriceps tendon receives its vascular supply from an anastomotic network including the lateral circumflex femoral artery, descending geniculate artery, and medial/lateral geniculate arteries (22).
- There is an avascular region of the deep part of the quadriceps tendon measuring 1.5 × 3.0 cm.
- Ruptures of the quadriceps tendon most typically occur in patients over 40 years of age and are three times more frequent than patella tendon ruptures. Unilateral injuries are up to 20 times more frequent than bilateral injury (23).
- Men are at greater risk with the incidence favoring male-to-female ratio at 8:1 (24).
- The site of rupture usually occurs through a degenerative area within the tendon and seldom occurs in younger individuals. Systemic disease can lead to tendon degeneration and predispose to infrequent bilateral tendon ruptures (25).

Clinical Presentation

- Pain is often present before rupture. At the time of injury, a pop is often heard with an acute onset of pain and swelling.
- In cases of partial injury or complete injuries that do not extend to include the retinacular tissue, the patient may be able to extend and resist gravity with an associated extensor lag, but in complete injuries, this is not possible.
- A palpable defect at the site of rupture is usually felt just superior to the proximal pole of the patella.
- Plain radiographs often demonstrate patellar baja, an avulsion of the superior pole of the patella, spurring of the superior patellar region, or calcification within the quadriceps tendon. Insall-Salvati index is less than 0.8 (15).
- MRI is a useful adjunct study because it can demonstrate partial ruptures or preexisting disease within the quadriceps tendon.

Treatment

- Partial tears are often responsive to conservative treatment when the patient presents primarily with pain and has little loss of strength, retaining the ability to actively extend the knee against gravity.
- Conservative treatment consists of a long leg cylinder cast in full extension for 4–6 weeks, with progressive range of motion and strengthening thereafter for partial injuries.
- Complete ruptures respond best to immediate surgical repair in a direct end-to-end fashion after tendon debridement of necrotic tissue with suture anchors or transosseous tunnels through the patella (26,27).
- Chronic ruptures involving more significant tendon retraction often require quadriceps tendon advancement through a tendon Z-plasty or V-Y tendon lengthening and advancement technique. Interpositional autograft/allograft tendon has been used with success in this scenario (28).
- Success of repair is directly related to the length of time between injury and the time of surgery, with more chronic repairs producing less favorable outcomes. Age is also a factor, with better results in younger patients (29).
- The most common complications after surgery or conservative treatment include decreased quadriceps strength/function with an associated extensor lag and lack of knee flexion.

GASTROCNEMIUS RUPTURE

- Often referred to as *tennis leg*
- Traumatic injury to middle-aged athlete presenting as sudden pain in posterior proximal calf region. Significant pain, swelling, and ecchymosis usually occur within 24 hours.
- Involves tearing of the medial head of the gastrocnemius muscle typically at its musculotendinous junction (30)
- Mechanism of injury combines ankle dorsiflexion in combination with knee hyperextension.

Differential Diagnoses

- Differential diagnoses involve plantaris rupture, thrombophlebitis, and an acute compartment syndrome (31).
- MRI remains the imaging modality of choice. Ultrasound can be employed to rule out thrombophlebitis.
- Can be associated with an acute compartment syndrome secondary to swelling (32)

Treatment

- Treatment of isolated ruptures of the medial gastrocnemius involves compressive wrapping, activity modification including crutches if necessary, ankle range of motion, ice, and anti-inflammatory medications (33).

PATELLAR TENDONITIS

- Caused by activities involving repeated extension of the knee
- Termed *jumper's knee*, because it is most common in sporting activities such as basketball, volleyball, and soccer. Seen most commonly in younger individuals from their adolescent years to 40 years of age (34).
- Predisposing factors include abnormal patellofemoral tracking, patellar alta, chondromalacia, Osgood-Schlatter disease, and leg length discrepancy.
- Can be confused with Sinding-Larsen-Johansson disease, which is a traction apophysitis of the distal pole of the patella that presents with similar complaints in a younger age group (usually under 20 years)
- Involves the most proximal part of the patellar tendon and its attachment to the distal pole of the patella. This area of tendon is thought to impinge under the patella during knee flexion, causing injury to the tendon (35).
- The affected area of tendon resembles tendinosis in the form of tendon degeneration and not inflammation. Histologically, this tissue is characterized as undergoing *angiofibroblastic hyperplasia* with fibroblast proliferation, new blood vessel formation, chondromucoid deposition, and collagen fragmentation (36).

Clinical Presentation

- Pain occurs with palpation in the area of tendon involvement just distal to its insertion on the inferior pole of the patella in full extension (Basset sign) (37).
- Pain is increased with activity requiring knee extension against resistance.
- Tendon may acquire bogginess; however, there is no associated joint effusion.
- Blazina et al. have classified this condition based on the patients' symptoms: (a) pain only after activity; (b) pain is present before activity, and then disappears, only to return near the end of activity with muscular fatigue; (c) pain is constant with both rest and activity; and (d) patellar tendon rupture (38).

Radiographic Evaluation

- Mainly a clinical diagnosis, but plain x-rays, although usually normal, can at times demonstrate an osteopenia at the distal pole of the patella, a traction osteophyte in the area of involvement, and calcification of the tendon.
- Ultrasound may find thickening of the tendon and/or hypoechoic areas.
- MRI is the study of choice in the chronic setting because it can clearly identify the area of tendon involvement. This area usually involves the posterior aspect of the tendon in its proximal third (39).

Treatment

- Conservative treatment is usually successful and includes rest, ice, and anti-inflammatory medication. Therapeutic modalities including ultrasound, iontophoresis, and phonophoresis are helpful in pain relief (40,41).
- Once the pain has subsided, physiotherapy in the form of eccentric quadriceps strengthening and hamstring stretching is begun with gradual return to activity.
- Heavy slow resistance training has good short- and long-term clinical effects as well as pathology improvement and increased collagen turnover (42).
- Corticosteroid injections have good short-term but poor long-term clinical effects, contraindicated due to increased risk of patellar tendon rupture (42).
- An elastic knee sleeve or counterforce brace (Cho-Pat–type brace) has also proved beneficial.
- More chronic cases with pathology demonstrable on MRI scan require surgical debridement and excision of the diseased tendon and adjacent bone through either an open or arthroscopic approach (43–45).
- The use of platelet-rich plasma (PRP) for patellar tendinitis is controversial. Several studies have reported encouraging results, although a recent review affirms that the available evidence is insufficient to guide PRP therapy in patellar tendinopathy (46–53).

QUADRICEPS TENDINITIS

- Quadriceps tendinitis is not as common as patellar tendonitis but has similar risk factors and is most common in male adult athletes.
- Repetitive microtrauma through overuse can lead to localized degeneration of the quadriceps tendon at its insertion into the superior pole of the patella.
- Chronic symptoms in this area appear to be a risk factor for future tendon rupture.

Clinical Presentation

- Pain with exertion and tenderness over the affected area of quadriceps insertion. This most commonly is the lateral aspect of the tendon.
- Radiographs often demonstrate calcification of the tendon at its insertion to the patella or a traction osteophyte at the osseous margin.

Treatment

- Treatment is similar to that of patellar tendonitis. Results of conservative treatment are excellent, although more chronic cases can require open surgical debridement (54).

POPLITEUS TENDINITIS

- Popliteus tendon travels from its origin on the lateral femoral condyle posterolaterally through the popliteal hiatus to insert on the posterior aspect of the proximal tibia (55).
- Injuries to this area are a cause of posterolateral knee pain and can occur both acutely (*i.e.*, ACL rupture or posterolateral corner injuries) or more chronically as an overuse phenomenon. Chronic injuries most often occur with excessive downhill running or walking (*i.e.*, backpacking) (56,57).

Clinical Presentation

- Pain to palpation posterolaterally over the popliteus tendon. This is best appreciated clinically by placing the leg in a figure-of-four position and palpating at the origin of the popliteus just anterior to the lateral femoral epicondyle.
- Can also assess using the Garrick test, which is positive when there is pain in the posterolateral knee occurring with resisted external rotation of the leg while the patient is seated with the hip and knee flexed to 90° (58,59).
- Differential diagnosis includes iliotibial band syndrome, lateral meniscal tear, and biceps femoris tendonitis. Lateral collateral ligament and posterolateral corner ligamentous injuries usually occur with acute trauma as opposed to a chronic injury.

Treatment

- Includes rest and activity modification in the form of eliminating downhill activity. Anti-inflammatory medication and physiotherapeutic modalities are also helpful (56). A generalized knee-strengthening program is instituted following resolution of symptoms.

ILIOTIBIAL BAND SYNDROME

- Most common cause of lateral-sided knee pain in long-distance runners. Also seen in cyclists, weightlifters, football, soccer, and tennis players. Often precipitated by downhill running (60).
- Caused by excessive friction between iliotibial band and lateral epicondyle. Knee flexion angle of 30° maximizes friction between these two structures, causing an ensuing bursitis.
- Anatomic factors predisposing to this condition include limb length discrepancy, genu varum, tibial varum, varus hindfoot, and compensatory foot hyperpronation (61).

Clinical Presentation

- Lateral-sided knee pain that usually is present after initial warm-up that often causes cessation of activity. Pain is generally not present at rest.
- Point of maximal tenderness is approximately 3 cm proximal to lateral joint line over lateral epicondylar region.
- *Ober's* and *Noble's* tests are positive and can confirm diagnosis.
- Ober's test: Patient is placed in lateral decubitus position with the affected extremity upwards. The unaffected knee and hip are flexed. The involved knee is flexed and hip hyperextended and adducted. Tightness or pain along the iliotibial tract will prevent the affected extremity from adducting below the horizontal created by the patient's torso (62).
- Noble's test: Patient is in supine position with the knee flexed 90°. Pain is elicited in the lateral epicondylar region when the patient's knee is extended between 30° and 40°.
- Radiographs are negative in this condition. MRI can confirm more chronic cases unresponsive to conservative treatment.

Treatment

- Conservative treatment focusing on iliotibial tract, hamstring, and hip external rotator stretching combined with strengthening of the hip abductors is usually successful when combined with activity modification and anti-inflammatory treatment. Foot orthotics can also be a useful adjunct in conservative treatment.
- Corticosteroid injections may be used when other conservative measures fail (63).
- Surgical excision of the posterior aspect of the iliotibial tract overlying the lateral epicondyle at 30°–40° of knee flexion is effective in chronic cases not responding to conservative treatment (64).

PREPATELLAR BURSITIS (HOUSEMAID'S KNEE)

- Prepatellar bursa is a potential space of synovial tissue that functions to decrease the friction between the overlying subcutaneous tissue and patella.
- A bursitis can result at any age from an acute injury, infection, systemic disease (*i.e.*, gout), or chronic activity or overuse (65).
- Commonly seen in the sport of wrestling (66)
- Minimum annual incidence of 10/100,000, predominantly affecting male patients (80%) aged 40–60 years (67)

Clinical Presentation

- Patients typically present with swelling superficial to the patella. Knee range of motion may be limited at the extremes of flexion depending on the size of the collection but is painless. There is no associated effusion. Crepitation and thickening of the tissue involving the bursal tissue are often present in more chronic cases.

- Warmth, erythema, and pain to palpation may signify a septic process, but aspiration is necessary to confirm this because not all infected bursae are clinically demonstrable.
- Most common infecting organisms include *Staphylococcus aureus* and streptococcal species (68).
- On synovial fluid analysis, greater than 75% polymorphonuclear cell differential is most accurate in confirming a septic process. Total white blood cell count and glucose levels are less predictable (69).
- Radiographs are usually negative aside from radiolucency in the area of the bursitis. In cases involving gouty deposits, calcific stippling can be seen.

Treatment

- Treatment for aseptic bursitis in this region is activity modification, compressive wrapping, and anti-inflammatory medications. In more chronic situations, aspiration in combination with immobilization in extension can be useful.
- Septic or more chronic aseptic processes are best treated with surgical excision via open or arthroscopic techniques. Cases of septic bursitis should be treated with postoperative antibiotics sensitive to the infecting organism (70).

PES ANSERINE BURSITIS

- Pes anserine bursa is the synovial tissue overlying the attachment of the sartorius, gracilis, and semitendinosus tendons.
- Most commonly seen in overweight middle-aged women, but also common in young athletic adults and older adults with osteoarthritis.
- Risk factors include female sex, diabetes, obesity, and valgus knee deformity (71–73).
- Patients present with pain, swelling, and tenderness over this bursal region (~6–7 cm below the anteromedial joint line of the knee).
- Pain is worse at night and when climbing stairs or arising from a seated position.
- Differential diagnoses include medial collateral ligament injury, medial meniscal tear, medial compartmental arthritis, patellofemoral syndrome, saphenous neuritis, and stress fracture or avascular necrosis of the medial tibial plateau (74).

Treatment

- Treatment comprises activity modification, anti-inflammatory medications, hamstring stretching, and physiotherapy modalities. Recalcitrant cases often respond to a corticosteroid injection (75).

SYNOVIAL PLICAE SYNDROME

- Plicae are defined as synovial folds of tissue within the knee. They are described as suprapatellar, infrapatellar, medial, or lateral based on their position within the knee (76).
- Synovial plicae syndrome affects people of both sexes in their first through third decade, with an average age of 25 (77).
- Ninety percent of cadavers studied on anatomic dissection have the presence of at least one of the synovial plicae described.
- Not all plicae are symptomatic. Differential diagnoses include patellofemoral syndrome and meniscal/chondral pathology. Medial plicae are most associated with symptoms. Its presence noted at the time of arthroscopy in all patients ranges from 19% to 70% (78,79).
- Patients often describe pain over the affected plicae in combination with intermittent snapping or giving way.
- Clinically, this snapping can often be elicited with manipulation of the plicae at varying degrees of flexion between 45° and 60°.
- Radiographic studies, including x-rays and MRI, are usually negative. The latter is often obtained to rule out other intra-articular pathology.

Treatment

- Treatment is usually conservative with nonsteroidal anti-inflammatory drugs and activity modification. Steroid injections, either into the plica or placed into the intra-articular space, have proven to be effective in more unresponsive cases.
- Arthroscopic resection is limited to patients not responding to conservative treatment and has mixed results. Associated chondral injuries and concurrent patellofemoral maltracking have been implicated in arthroscopic failures, which have been reported to be as high as 30% (80).
- Clinical results of arthroscopic plica resection are better in patients without coexisting cartilage lesions (81).

REFERENCES

1. Huberti HH, Hayes WC, Stone JL, Shybut GT. Force ratios in the quadriceps tendon and ligamentum patellae. *J Orthop Res.* 1984;2(1):49–54. doi:10.1002/jor.1100020108
2. Zernicke RF, Garhammer J, Jobe FW. Human patellar-tendon rupture. *J Bone Joint Surg Am.* 1977;59(2):179–83.
3. Garrett WE Jr. Injuries to the muscle-tendon unit. *Instr Course Lect.* 1988;37:275–82.
4. Ford LT, DeBender J. Tendon rupture after local steroid injection. *South Med J.* 1979;72(7):827–30. doi:10.1097/00007611-197907000-00019
5. Rose PS, Frassica FJ. Atraumatic bilateral patellar tendon rupture, A case report and review of the literature. *J Bone Joint Surg Am.* 2001;83(9):1382–6.

6. Scuderi AJ, Datz FL, Valdivia S, Morton KA. Enthesopathy of the patellar tendon insertion associated with isotretinoin therapy. *J Nucl Med.* 1993;34(3):455–7.
7. Williams RJ III, Attia E, Wickiewicz TL, Hannafin JA. The effect of ciprofloxacin on tendon, paratenon, and capsular fibroblast metabolism. *Am J Sports Med.* 2000;28(3):364–9. doi:10.1177/03635465000280031401
8. Arnoczky SP. Blood supply to the anterior cruciate ligament and supporting structures. *Orthop Clin North Am.* 1985;16(1):15–28.
9. Scapinelli R. Studies on the vasculature of the human knee joint. *Acta Anat (Basel).* 1968;70(3):305–31. doi:10.1159/000143133.
10. Matava MJ. Patella tendon ruptures. *J Am Acad Orthop Surg.* 1996;4(6):287–96.
11. Bonamo JJ, Krinick RM, Sporn AA. Rupture of the patellar ligament after use of its central third for anterior cruciate reconstruction. A report of two cases. *J Bone Joint Surg Am* 1984;66(8):1294–7.
12. Crossett LS, Sinha RK, Sechriest VF, Rubash HE. Reconstruction of a ruptured patellar tendon with achilles tendon allograft following total knee arthroplasty. *J Bone Joint Surg Am.* 2002;84(8):1354–61. doi:10.2106/00004623-200208000-00010
13. Keating JF, Orfaly R, O'Brien PJ. Knee pain after tibial nailing. *J Orthop Trauma.* 1997;11(1):10–3. doi:10.1097/00005131-199701000-00004
14. Chow FY, Wun Y-C, Chow Y-Y. Simultaneous rupture of the patellar tendon and the anterior cruciate ligament: a case report and literature review. *Knee Surg Sports Traumatol Arthrosc.* 2006;14(10):1017–20. doi:10.1007/s00167-006-0048-3
15. Aglietti P, Buzzi R, Insall J. Disorders of the patellofemoral joint. In: Insall JN, Scott WN, editors. *Surgery of the Knee.* 3rd ed. New York: Churchill Livingstone; 2001. p. 930–1.
16. Golman M, Wright ML, Wong TT, et al. Rethinking patellar tendinopathy and partial patellar tendon tears: a novel classification system. *Am J Sports Med.* 2020;48(2):359–69. doi:10.1177/0363546519894333
17. Lanzi JT, Felix J, Tucker CJ, et al. Comparison of the suture anchor and transosseous techniques for patellar tendon repair: a biomechanical study. *Am J Sports Med.* 2016;44(8):2076–80. doi:10.1177/0363546516643811
18. O'Donnell R, Lemme NJ, Marcaccio S, et al. Suture anchor versus transosseous tunnel repair for inferior pole patellar fractures treated with partial patellectomy and tendon advancement: a biomechanical study. *Orthop J Sports Med.* 2021;9(8):23259671211022245. doi:10.1177/23259671211022245
19. O'Dowd JA, Lehoang D, Butler RK, De Witt D, Mirzayan R. Transosseous versus anchor repair of acute patellar tendon ruptures. *Orthop J Sports Med.* 2018;6(7_suppl 4):2325967118S00133. doi:10.1177/2325967118s00133
20. Larsen E, Lund PM. Ruptures of the extensor mechanism of the knee joint. Clinical results and patellofemoral articulation. *Clin Orthop Relat Res.* 1986;213:150–3.
21. Hyman J, Rodeo S, Wickiewicz T. Patellofemoral tendinopathy. In: Drez D Jr, DeLee JC, Miller M, editors. *DeLee & Drez's Orthopaedic Sports Medicine: Principles and Practice.* 2nd ed. Philadelphia (PA): Saunders; 2003. p. 1849–54.
22. Petersen W, Stein V, Tillmann B. Blood supply of the quadriceps tendon. *Unfallchirurg.* 1999;102(7):543–7. doi:10.1007/s001130050448
23. Ilan DI, Tejwani N, Keschner M, Leibman M. Quadriceps tendon rupture. *J Am Acad Orthop Surg.* 2003;11(3):192–200. doi:10.5435/00124635-200305000-00006
24. Maffulli N, Wong J. Rupture of the Achilles and patellar tendons. *Clin Sports Med.* 2003;22(4):761–76. doi:10.1016/s0278-5919(03)00009-7
25. Lauerman WC, Smith BG, Kenmore PI. Spontaneous bilateral rupture of the extensor mechanism of the knee in two patients on chronic ambulatory peritoneal dialysis. *Orthopedics.* 1987;10(4):589–91. doi:10.3928/0147-7447-19870401-09
26. Rasul AT Jr, Fischer DA. Primary repair of quadriceps tendon ruptures. Results of treatment. *Clin Orthop Relat Res.* 1993;289:205–7.
27. Petri M, Dratzidis A, Brand S, et al. Suture anchor repair yields better biomechanical properties than transosseous sutures in ruptured quadriceps tendons. *Knee Surg Sports Traumatol Arthrosc.* 2015;23(4):1039–45. doi:10.1007/s00167-014-2854-3
28. Scuderi C. Ruptures of the quadriceps tendon; study of twenty tendon ruptures. *Am J Surg.* 1958;95(4):626–34. doi:10.1016/0002-9610(58)90444-6
29. Konrath GA, Chen D, Lock T, et al. Outcomes following repair of quadriceps tendon ruptures. *J Orthop Trauma.* 1998;12(4):273–9. doi:10.1097/00005131-199805000-00010
30. Miller WA. Rupture of the musculotendinous juncture of the medial head of the gastrocnemius muscle. *Am J Sports Med.* 1977;5(5):191–3. doi:10.1177/036354657700500505
31. Severance HW Jr, Bassett FH III. Rupture of the plantaris--does it exist? *J Bone Joint Surg Am.* 1982;64(9):1387–8.
32. Pai V, Pai V. Acute compartment syndrome after rupture of the medial head of gastrocnemius in a child. *J Foot Ankle Surg.* 2007;46(4):288–90. doi:10.1053/j.jfas.2007.03.007
33. Gecha SR, Torg E. Knee injuries in tennis. *Clin Sports Med.* 1988;7(2):435–52.
34. Ferretti A, Puddu G, Mariani PP, Neri M. The natural history of jumper's knee. Patellar or quadriceps tendonitis. *Int Orthop.* 1985;8(4):239–42. doi:10.1007/BF00266866
35. King JB, Perry DJ, Mourad K, Kumar SJ. Lesions of the patellar ligament. *J Bone Joint Surg Br.* 1990;72(1):46–8. doi:10.1302/0301-620X.72B1.2404986
36. Kannus P, Józsa L. Histopathological changes preceding spontaneous rupture of a tendon. A controlled study of 891 patients. *J Bone Joint Surg Am.* 1991;73(10):1507–25.
37. Rath E, Schwarzkopf R, Richmond JC. Clinical signs and anatomical correlation of patellar tendinitis. *Indian J Orthop.* 2010;44(4):435–7. doi:10.4103/0019-5413.69317
38. Blazina ME, Kerlan RK, Jobe FW, Carter VS, Carlson GJ. Jumper's knee. *Orthop Clin North Am.* 1973;4(3):665–78.
39. Johnson DP, Wakeley CJ, Watt I. Magnetic resonance imaging of patellar tendonitis. *J Bone Joint Surg Br.* 1996;78(3):452–7.
40. Panni AS, Tartarone M, Maffulli N. Patellar tendinopathy in athletes. Outcome of nonoperative and operative management. *Am J Sports Med.* 2000;28(3):392–7. doi:10.1177/03635465000280031901
41. Martens M, Wouters P, Burssens A, Mulier JC. Patellar tendinitis: pathology and results of treatment. *Acta Orthop Scand.* 1982;53(3):445–50. doi:10.3109/17453678208992239
42. Kongsgaard M, Kovanen V, Aagaard P, et al. Corticosteroid injections, eccentric decline squat training and heavy slow resistance training in patellar tendinopathy. *Scand J Med Sci Sports.* 2009;19(6):790–802. doi:10.1111/j.1600-0838.2009.00949.x
43. Coleman BD, Khan KM, Kiss ZS, Bartlett J, Young DA, Wark JD. Open and arthroscopic patellar tenotomy for chronic patellar tendinopathy. A retrospective outcome study. Victorian Institute of Sport Tendon Study Group. *Am J Sports Med.* 2000;28(2):183–90. doi:10.1177/03635465000280020801
44. Griffiths GP, Selesnick FH. Operative treatment and arthroscopic findings in chronic patellar tendinitis. *Arthroscopy.* 1998;14(8):836–9. doi:10.1016/s0749-8063(98)70020-9
45. Romeo AA, Larson RV. Arthroscopic treatment of infrapatellar tendonitis. *Arthroscopy.* 1999;15(3):341–5. doi:10.1016/s0749-8063(99)70048-4
46. Seo WY, Ha JK, Kim JG, Wang BG. Treatment of chronic patellar tendinitis with platelet rich plasma injection. *Korean J Sports Med.* 2012;30(2):110. doi:10.5763/kjsm.2012.30.2.110
47. Andia I, Maffulli N. Use of platelet-rich plasma for patellar tendon and medial collateral ligament injuries: best current clinical practice. *J Knee Surg.* 2015;28(1):11–18. doi:10.1055/s-0034-1384671

48. Baksh N, Hannon CP, Murawski CD, Smyth NA, Kennedy JG. Platelet-rich plasma in tendon models: a systematic review of basic science literature. *Arthroscopy.* 2013;29(3):596–607. doi:10.1016/j.arthro.2012.10.025
49. Zhang J, Wang JH. PRP treatment effects on degenerative tendinopathy—an in vitro model study. *Muscles Ligaments Tendons J.* 2014;4(1):10–7.
50. Dragoo JL, Wasterlain AS, Braun HJ, Nead KT. Platelet-rich plasma as a treatment for patellar tendinopathy: a double-blind, randomized controlled trial. *Am J Sports Med.* 2014;42(3):610–8. doi:10.1177/0363546513518416
51. Charousset C, Zaoui A, Bellaiche L, Bouyer B. Are multiple platelet-rich plasma injections useful for treatment of chronic patellar tendinopathy in athletes? *Am J Sports Med.* 2014;42(4):906–11. doi:10.1177/0363546513519964
52. Vetrano M, Castorina A, Vulpiani MC, Baldini R, Pavan A, Ferretti A. Platelet-rich plasma versus focused shock waves in the treatment of jumper's knee in athletes. *Am J Sports Med.* 2013;41(4):795–803. doi:10.1177/0363546513475345
53. Andriolo L, Altamura SA, Reale D, Candrian C, Zaffagnini S, Filardo G. Nonsurgical treatments of patellar tendinopathy: multiple injections of platelet-rich plasma are a suitable option—a systematic review and meta-analysis. *Am J Sports Med.* 2019;47(4):1001–18. doi:10.1177/0363546518759674
54. James SL. Running injuries to the knee. *J Am Acad Orthop Surg.* 1995;3(6):309–18. doi:10.5435/00124635-199511000-00001
55. Mann RA, Hagy JL. The popliteus muscle. *J Bone Joint Surg Am.* 1977;59(7):924–7.
56. Mayfield GW. Popliteus tendon tenosynovitis. *Am J Sports Med.* 1977;5(1):31–6. doi:10.1177/036354657700500106
57. Naver L, Aalberg JR. Avulsion of the popliteus tendon. A rare cause of chondral fracture and hemarthrosis. *Am J Sports Med.* 1985;13(6):423–4. doi:10.1177/036354658501300611
58. Petsche TS, Selesnick FH. Popliteus tendinitis: tips for diagnosis and management. *Phys Sportsmed.* 2002;30(8):27–31. doi:10.3810/psm.2002.08.401
59. Hyland S, Varacallo M. *Anatomy, Bony Pelvis and Lower Limb, Popliteus Muscle.* Treasure Island (FL): StatPearls; 2022.
60. Orava S. Iliotibial tract friction syndrome in athletes—an uncommon exertion syndrome on the lateral side of the knee. *Br J Sports Med.* 1978;12(2):69–73. doi:10.1136/bjsm.12.2.69
61. Charles D, Rodgers C. A literature review and clinical commentary on the development of iliotibial band syndrome in runners. *Int J Sports Phys Ther.* 2020;15(3):460–70.
62. Renne JW. The iliotibial band friction syndrome. *J Bone Joint Surg Am.* 1975;57(8):1110–1.
63. McKay J, Maffulli N, Aicale R, Taunton J. Iliotibial band syndrome rehabilitation in female runners: a pilot randomized study. *J Orthop Surg Res.* 2020;15(1):188. doi:10.1186/s13018-020-01713-7
64. Martens M, Libbrecht P, Burssens A. Surgical treatment of the iliotibial band friction syndrome. *Am J Sports Med.* 1989;17(5):651–4. doi:10.1177/036354658901700511
65. Dawn B, Williams JK, Walker SE. Prepatellar bursitis: a unique presentation of tophaceous gout in an normouricemic patient. *J Rheumatol.* 1997;24(5):976–8.
66. Mysnyk MC, Wroble RR, Foster DT, Albright JP. Prepatellar bursitis in wrestlers. *Am J Sports Med.* 1986;14(1):46–54. doi:10.1177/036354658601400109
67. Baumbach SF, Lobo CM, Badyine I, Mutschler W, Kanz K-G. Prepatellar and olecranon bursitis: literature review and development of a treatment algorithm. *Arch Orthop Trauma Surg.* 2014;134(3):359–70. doi:10.1007/s00402-013-1882-7
68. Aaron DL, Patel A, Kayiaros S, Calfee R. Four common types of bursitis: diagnosis and management. *J Am Acad Orthop Surg.* 2011;19(6):359–67. doi:10.5435/00124635-201106000-00006
69. Ho G Jr, Tice AD. Comparison of nonseptic and septic bursitis. Further observations on the treatment of septic bursitis. *Arch Intern Med.* 1979;139(11):1269–73.
70. Kaalund S, Breddam M, Kristensen G. Endoscopic resection of the septic prepatellar bursa. *Arthroscopy.* 1998;14(7):757–8. doi:10.1016/s0749-8063(98)70105-7
71. Alvarez-Nemegyei J. Risk factors for pes anserinus tendinitis/bursitis syndrome: a case control study. *J Clin Rheumatol.* 2007;13(2):63–5. doi:10.1097/01.rhu.0000262082.84624.37
72. Uson J, Aguado P, Bernad M, et al. Pes anserinus tendino-bursitis: what are we talking about? *Scand J Rheumatol.* 2000;29(3):184–6. doi:10.1080/030097400750002076
73. Cohen SE, Mahul O, Meir R, Rubinow A. Anserine bursitis and non-insulin dependent diabetes mellitus. *J Rheumatol.* 1997;24(11):2162–5.
74. Larsson LG, Baum J. The syndrome of anserina bursitis: an overlooked diagnosis. *Arthritis Rheum.* 1985;28(9):1062–5. doi:10.1002/art.1780280915
75. Sarifakioglu B, Afsar SI, Yalbuzdag SA, Ustaömer K, Bayramoğlu M. Comparison of the efficacy of physical therapy and corticosteroid injection in the treatment of pes anserine tendino-bursitis. *J Phys Ther Sci.* 2016;28(7):1993–7. doi:10.1589/jpts.28.1993
76. Dandy DJ. Anatomy of the medial suprapatellar plica and medial synovial shelf. *Arthroscopy.* 1990;6(2):79–85. doi:10.1016/0749-8063(90)90002-u
77. Schindler OS. "The Sneaky Plica" revisited: morphology, pathophysiology and treatment of synovial plicae of the knee. *Knee Surg Sports Traumatol Arthrosc.* 2014;22(2):247–62. doi:10.1007/s00167-013-2368-4
78. Joyce JJ, Harty M. Surgery of the synovial fold. In: Cassells W, editor. *Arthroscopy: Diagnosis in Surgical Practice.* Philadelphia (PA): Lea & Febiger; 1984. p. 201–9.
79. Pipkin G. Knee injuries: the role of the suprapatellar plica and suprapatellar bursa in simulating internal derangements. *Clin Orthop Relat Res.* 1971;74:161–76.
80. Dupont JY. Synovial plicae of the knee. Controversies and review. *Clin Sports Med.* 1997;16(1):87–122. doi:10.1016/s0278-5919(05)70009-0
81. Paczesny L, Zabrzynski J, Kentzer R, et al. A 10-year follow-up on arthroscopic medial plica syndrome treatments with special reference to related cartilage injuries. *Cartilage.* 2021;13(1_suppl l):974S–83S. doi:10.1177/1947603519892310

67 Ankle Instability

R. Todd Hockenbury

DEFINITION OF ANKLE SPRAIN

- An ankle sprain is a tear of the ligaments supporting the ankle joint.
- Ankle sprains are common. They constitute 25% of all sports-related injuries (1).
- Ankle sprains make up 21%–53% of basketball injuries and 17%–29% of all soccer injuries (2,3).
- The age group of 10–19 years old is associated with higher rates of ankle sprain. Nearly half of all ankle sprains occur during athletic activity, with basketball (41.1%), football (9.3%), and soccer (7.9%) being associated with the highest percentage of ankle sprains during sports (4).
- A lateral ankle sprain is an injury of the ligaments connecting the fibula to the talus and calcaneus. It is the most common ligament injury of the ankle.
- A high ankle sprain is an injury to the ligaments connecting the fibula to the tibia. Although it is less common than a lateral ankle sprain, greater than 20% of acute ankle sprains in athletes involve the syndesmosis (5). High ankle sprains make up to 25% of ankle sprains in collision sports, such as football, wrestling, rugby, and lacrosse (4,5).
- Combined lateral ankle ligament and syndesmotic ligament injuries have been reported in 17.8% of patients (6).
- Acute isolated deltoid ligament sprains are rare. Deltoid ligament injury almost always occurs in conjunction with fibular fractures and/or syndesmotic injury.

ANATOMY AND PATHOPHYSIOLOGY

Anatomy

- The ankle, or talocrural, joint consists of the talus, tibial plafond, medial malleolus, and lateral malleolus. The distal tibia and lateral malleolus form a mortise, in which the talus sits.
- The talus is wider anteriorly than posterior, thus resulting in a tighter fit and more stable articulation between the talus and mortise during ankle dorsiflexion.
- Ankle joint stability depends on joint congruency and the supporting ligamentous structures.
- The lateral ankle ligaments are the anterior talofibular ligament (ATFL), calcaneofibular ligament (CFL), and posterior talofibular ligament (PTFL). See Figure 67.1.
- The medial ankle ligaments are the deep and superficial portions of the deltoid ligament. The superficial portions of the deltoid ligament are the tibionavicular, tibiospring, and tibiocalcaneal ligaments. The deep portions of the deltoid ligament are the deep anterior tibiotalar and deep posterior tibiotalar ligaments. See Figure 67.2.
- The relative strengths of the ankle ligaments from weakest to strongest are ATFL, PTFL, CFL, and deltoid (7).
- The syndesmotic ligaments connect and stabilize the distal fibula to the distal tibia. The convex medial fibula rests in a concave incisura in the distal lateral tibia. The stabilizing ligaments of the syndesmosis are the anterior inferior tibiofibular ligament, posterior tibiofibular ligament, transverse

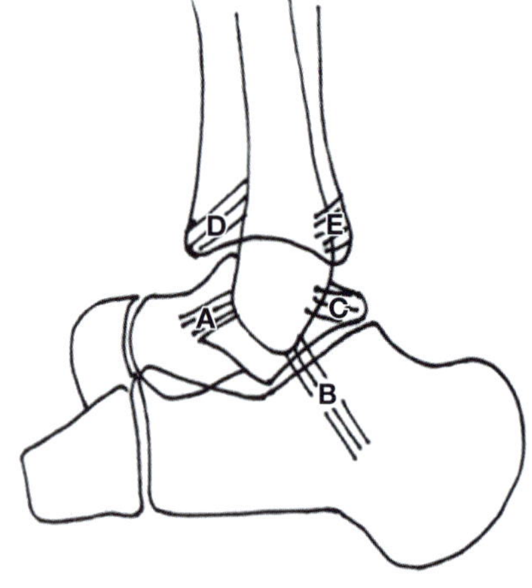

Figure 67.1: Anatomy of lateral ankle ligaments.
A — Anterior talofibular ligament.
B —Calcaneofibular ligament.
C — Posterior talofibular ligament.
D — Anterior inferior tibiofibular ligament.
E — Posterior tibiofibular ligament.

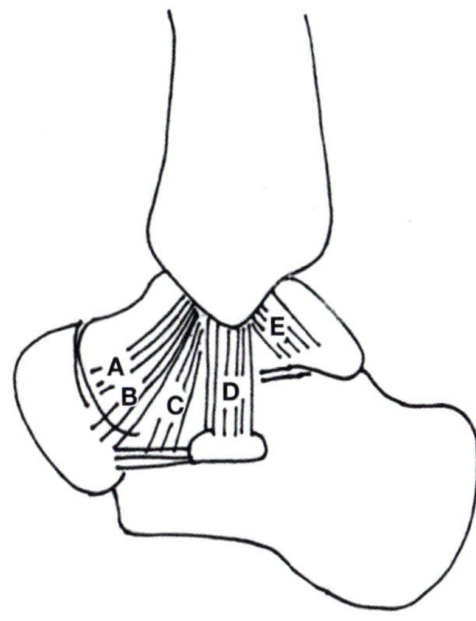

Figure 67.2: Anatomy of medial ankle ligaments.
A — Deep anterior tibiotalar ligament.
B — Tibionavicular ligament.
C — Tibiospring ligament.
D — Tibiocalcaneal ligament.
E — Deep posterior tibiotalar ligament.

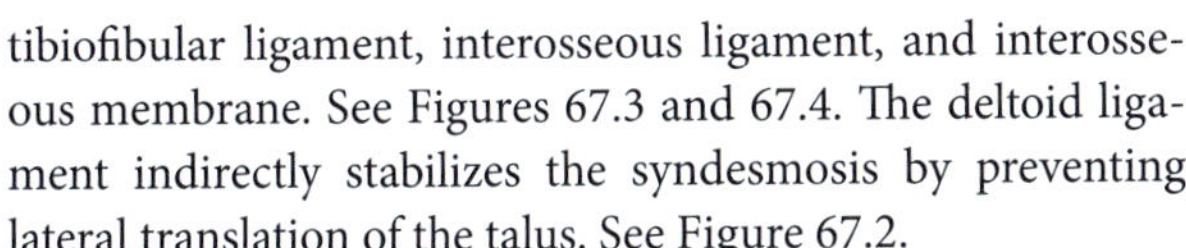

tibiofibular ligament, interosseous ligament, and interosseous membrane. See Figures 67.3 and 67.4. The deltoid ligament indirectly stabilizes the syndesmosis by preventing lateral translation of the talus. See Figure 67.2.

- The subtalar (talocalcaneal) joint lies inferior to the ankle joint and is responsible for hindfoot inversion and eversion. Up to 50% of clinical ankle inversion occurs at the subtalar joint (8).

Joint Mechanics

- The ankle is a hinge joint that permits flexion, extension, and rotation. The talus externally rotates with ankle dorsiflexion and internally rotates during plantarflexion (9).
- The distal fibula externally rotates during ankle dorsiflexion and moves distally during weight bearing, thus deepening and stabilizing the ankle mortise (10).
- The ankle mortise widens with ankle dorsiflexion and weight bearing.
- The ATFL and CFL act synergistically to resist ankle inversion forces. The ATFL resists ankle inversion in plantarflexion, and the CFL resists ankle inversion during ankle dorsiflexion.
- The CFL spans both the lateral ankle joint and the lateral subtalar joint, thus contributing to both ankle and subtalar joint stability (8).
- The PTFL limits posterior talar displacement and external rotation (11).
- The deltoid ligament resists ankle eversion, external rotation, and plantarflexion. In cases of distal fibular fracture and mortise instability, it restrains lateral talar translation (12).

Injury Mechanisms

- The most commonly sprained ankle ligament is the ATFL, followed by the PTFL and then the CFL. An isolated CFL or PTFL tear is rare. A tear of the ATFL almost always precedes a CFL tear. The ATFL is almost always torn, the CFL and

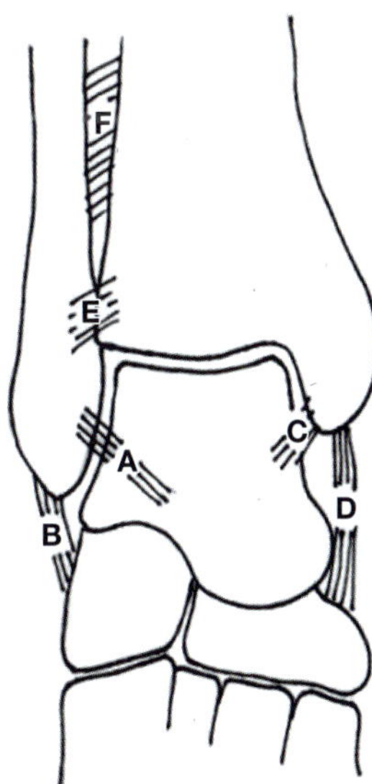

Figure 67.3: Anatomy of syndesmotic ligaments (anterior ankle view).
A — Anterior talofibular ligament.
B — Calcaneofibular ligament.
C — Deep deltoid ligament.
D — Superficial deltoid ligament.
E — Anterior inferior tibiofibular ligament.
F — Interosseous membrane.

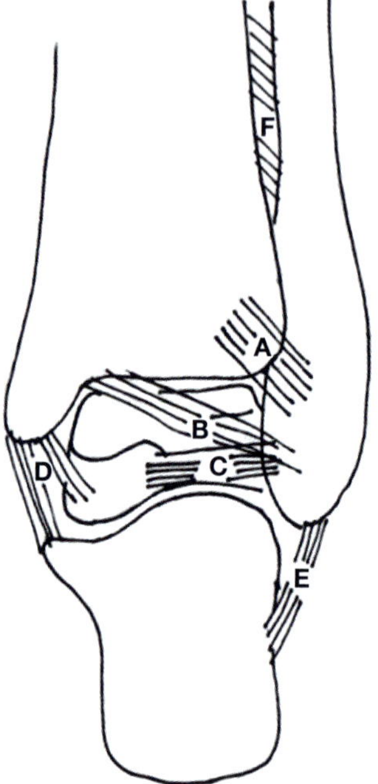

Figure 67.4: Anatomy of syndesmotic ligaments (posterior ankle view).
A — Posterior tibiofibular ligament.
B — Transverse tibiofibular ligament.
C — Posterior talofibular ligament.
D — Deltoid ligament.
E — Calcaneofibular ligament.
F — Interosseous membrane.

PTFL are torn 50%–75% of the time, and the PTFL is torn in <10% of ankle sprains (13).

- Lateral ankle sprains occur as a result of landing on a plantar flexed and inverted foot. These injuries occur while running on uneven terrain, stepping in a hole, stepping on another athlete's foot during play, or landing from a jump in an unbalanced position.
- A syndesmotic ankle sprain, or "high ankle sprain," occurs as a result of forced external rotation of a dorsiflexed foot or during internal rotation of the tibia on a fixed planted foot. A common mechanism is a direct blow to the back of the ankle while the patient is lying prone with the foot externally rotated (14).
- Isolated deltoid ligament sprains are rare and are usually accompanied by a lateral malleolar fracture and/or a syndesmotic injury. The deltoid ligament is injured through a mechanism of external rotation or eversion.

Injury Prevention

- A balance training program has been shown to reduce the rate of ankle sprains in high school soccer and basketball players by one-third to one-half (15,16).
- Studies are mixed regarding the efficacy of prophylactic bracing of athletes. A retrospective study of female college volleyball players who wore bilateral double-upright padded ankle braces showed a 93% reduction in ankle sprain incidence compared to the overall ankle injury rate in the National Collegiate Athletic Association (NCAA) (17). A prospective study of high school volleyball players found that ankle bracing did not overall decrease the incidence of sprains, except in those players who had not had a previous sprain. Players with a previous history of ankle sprain did not benefit from prophylactic bracing to prevent additional sprains. Players who had never had a sprain did show a lower incidence of initial ankle sprains with bracing (18).

Ligament Pathophysiology

- Ligamentous injuries undergo a series of phases during the healing process: hemorrhage and inflammation, fibroblastic proliferation, collagen protein formation, and collagen maturation (19).
- Early mobilization of joints following ligamentous injury actually stimulates collagen bundle orientation and promotes healing, although full ligamentous strength is not reestablished for several months (20–22).
- Early treatment focuses on limiting soft tissue effusion, which speeds up the healing process by lessening the amount of extracellular fluid and hematoma to be reabsorbed (23–25).

PHYSICAL EXAMINATION

- Lateral ankle swelling and ecchymosis are present and are proportional to the degree of ligament damage.
- Careful one-finger palpation is essential to define areas of tenderness and avoid misdiagnosis of associated fractures or tendon ruptures.
- Common fractures that mimic ankle sprains are fractures of the lateral malleolus and medial malleolus, fifth metatarsal base, anterior process of the calcaneus, lateral process of the talus, posterior talar process, talar dome, and navicular.
- Commonly missed tendon injuries are Achilles ruptures, peroneal tendon tears, peroneal tendon subluxation/dislocation,

posterior tibial tendon injuries, anterior tibial tendon tears, and flexor hallucis longus tendon ruptures.

- A careful neurologic examination is essential to rule out loss of sensation or motor weakness, because peroneal nerve and tibial nerve injuries are sometimes seen with severe lateral ankle sprains (26). A traction injury to the superficial peroneal nerve may occur with a plantar flexion inversion injury. This may result in numbness or painful dysesthesia on the dorsum of the foot.

DIAGNOSTIC TESTS

Tests for Lateral Ankle Instability

Anterior Drawer Test

- Tests the integrity of the ATFL.
- Performed by stabilizing the anterior tibia just above the ankle with one hand while grasping the posterior heel with the other hand and applying an anteriorly directed force, and therefore attempting to translate the talus anteriorly.
- The test should be performed on a relaxed leg with the knee bent and the ankle held in slight plantarflexion.
- Normal anterior talar translation is less than 5 mm. The contralateral asymptomatic ankle should also be tested as a baseline.

Inversion Stress Test or Talar Tilt Test

- Tests the integrity of the ATFL and CFL.
- Performed by grasping the heel and inverting the ankle. A clunk may be heard or palpated in unstable ankles, as the medial talar dome impacts the distal tibial medial articular surface, indicating injury to one or both ligaments.
- This test should be performed with the ankle in both dorsiflexion (to test the CFL) and plantarflexion (to test the ATFL).

Suction Sign

- Tests the integrity of the ATFL.
- During performance of the anterior drawer test, an unstable ankle will produce a dimple in the anterolateral ankle as the talus reaches its full anterior excursion. The dimple is formed by negative pressure within the ankle joint (27).

Tests for Syndesmotic Instability

- Although no single test is sufficiently accurate to diagnose syndesmotic injury, the following tests may confirm syndesmotic ligament injury. The most sensitive tests are an inability to hop, syndesmosis ligament tenderness, and the external rotation stress test. The most specific test is the squeeze test (28,29).
- Cadaver studies show that only small displacements of the syndesmosis occur during these stress tests. These findings suggest that pain rather than displacement should be the determinant of positivity for these tests (30).

Squeeze Test

- Tests the integrity of the syndesmotic ligaments.
- The squeeze test is performed by placing the fingers over the proximal half of the fibula and thumb around the tibia and squeezing the two bones together. Pain in the distal ankle may indicate a syndesmotic injury (31).

External Rotation Stress Test

- Tests the integrity of the syndesmotic ligaments.
- The external rotation stress test is performed on the seated patient by externally rotating the foot while stabilizing the tibia with the other hand. Medial ankle pain or lateral talar motion indicates that a syndesmotic injury may be present.
- Confirmatory anteroposterior and lateral external rotation stress radiographs will document widening of the syndesmosis and lateral talar subluxation (32,33).

Cross-Legged Stress Test

- Tests the integrity of the syndesmotic ligaments.
- The seated patient places the injured leg across the knee of the uninjured leg at the junction of the middle and distal two-thirds of the tibia. A gentle force is applied to the medial knee of the injured leg. The presence of ankle pain indicates a positive test.

Fibula Translation Test

- Tests the integrity of the syndesmotic ligaments.
- The tibiotalar joint is stabilized with one hand while the other hand attempts to translate the fibula anteriorly and posteriorly. The presence of pain and increased fibular motion compared to the other side confirms a positive test.

Stabilization or Tape Test

- Tests the integrity of the syndesmotic ligaments.
- The patient's leg is tightly taped just above the ankle joint to stabilize the syndesmosis. The patient is asked to jump on one leg, do toe raises, and walk. If pain decreases after taping the syndesmosis, this is a positive test.

Cotton Test

- Tests the integrity of the syndesmotic ligaments.
- The tibia is stabilized with one hand while the other hand grasps the heel attempting to translate the talus medially and laterally within the ankle mortise.
- Increased pain or translation compared to the uninjured side suggests deltoid ligament disruption associated with syndesmotic injury.

IMAGING

Ottawa Ankle Rules (34)

- Every sprained ankle does not require screening radiographs.
- Anteroposterior, lateral, and oblique radiographs should be obtained if any of the below criteria are present:

- Lateral or medial malleolar bone tenderness.
- Patient is unable to bear weight for four steps, both immediately after injury and in the emergency department.
- The Ottawa ankle rules do NOT apply in the following settings:
  - Age less than 18 years
  - Multiple painful injuries
  - Pregnancy
  - Diminished sensation due to neurologic deficit
- These criteria have been found to be 100% sensitive for detecting fracture while decreasing the incidence of unneeded radiographs (34).

Radiographs

- If radiographs are warranted, they should be examined closely for the following fractures that mimic ankle sprains:
  - Medial or lateral malleolus
  - Talar dome
  - Posterior malleolus (posterior distal tibia)
  - Posterior talar process
  - Lateral talar process
  - Anterior calcaneal process
  - "Flake fracture" off the posterior distal fibular rim, indicating a tear of the superior peroneal retinaculum and peroneal tendon dislocation
  - Navicular fracture
  - Widening of the medial clear space between the medial talar facet and medial malleolus, produced by lateral talar subluxation, indicative of a tear of the deltoid ligament and probable syndesmotic ligament instability

Stress Radiographs

- Not required to make a diagnosis of an acute ankle sprain.
- Used primarily to document mechanical instability as a cause of chronic lateral ankle instability symptoms.
- Can be performed with or without the injection of local anesthetic into the lateral ankle. An injection of 5 mL of 1% Xylocaine (lidocaine) into the anterolateral ankle may yield a more reliable test due to patient comfort.
- Talar tilt test:
  - The talar tilt test is performed by taking an anteroposterior or mortise view of the ankle while performing an inversion stress on the slightly plantarflexed ankle. The tibia is grasped with one hand while the other hand grasps and inverts the calcaneus maximally during the radiograph.
  - The talar tilt angle is obtained by measuring the angle subtended by a line parallel to the distal tibial articular surface and a line drawn along the superior articular surface of the talus.
  - Most authors agree that a difference of 5°–15° in talar tilt between the injured and uninjured side is diagnostic of mechanical ankle instability (35,36).
- Anterior drawer test:
  - Anterior drawer stress radiographs are performed by taking a lateral radiograph of the ankle while attempting to translate the talus anteriorly within the mortise, as in the clinical anterior drawer test.
  - The anterior drawer is measured as the shortest distance between a point on the posterior aspect of the distal tibial articular surface and a point on the posterior aspect of the talar dome.
  - An anterior drawer difference of greater than 5 mm between the injured and uninjured ankle is thought to be diagnostic of ATFL laxity (36).
- Stress radiographs for syndesmotic instability:
  - A mortise stress radiograph of the ankle syndesmosis can be obtained by placing an external rotation force on the ankle while stabilizing the proximal tibia with the knee flexed 90°.
  - Abnormal widening of the mortise and lateral talar shift indicates distal syndesmotic instability.

Magnetic Resonance Imaging

- Magnetic resonance imaging (MRI) is not needed for diagnosis in the acute setting unless an occult fracture or tendon injury is suspected.
- MRI is most useful in diagnosing causes of the "chronically sprained" ankle, and MRI can diagnose talar dome injuries, peroneal tendon tears, bone bruises, or other occult fractures.
- MRI has a sensitivity, specificity, and accuracy of 100%, 93%, and 96%, in diagnosing tears of the anterior inferior tibiofibular ligament (AITFL) and is therefore an excellent imaging modality to diagnose syndesmotic injury (37). Be aware that a positive MRI does not necessarily indicate syndesmotic instability.

Computed Tomography Scan

- Not needed in the acute setting unless an occult fracture is suspected.
- More valuable than MRI in delineating bone or joint pathology (*i.e.*, talar dome fractures, lateral talar process fractures, tarsal coalition, subtalar arthritis, and loose bodies).

GRADING

- Grading of ankle sprains helps to guide treatment, rehabilitation, and prognosis. The grade is based on the number of ligaments injured, degree of ligament tearing (partial vs. complete tear), and amount of swelling and ecchymosis.

Table 67.1 West Point Ankle Sprain Grading System

	Stage 1	Stage 2	Stage 3
Edema/ecchymosis	Localized/slight	Localized/moderate	Diffuse/significant
Weight-bearing ability	Full or partial without significant pain	Difficult without crutches	Impossible
Ligament pathology	Ligament stretch	Partial tear	Complete tear
Instability testing	None	None or slight	Definite
Time to return to sporting activities	11 d	2–6 wk	4–26 wk

- The West Point Ankle Grading System is a useful tool for grading lateral ankle sprains (Table 67.1) (38).
- Grading of syndesmotic ankle sprains (high ankle sprains) is listed in Table 67.2.

INITIAL TREATMENT OF LATERAL ANKLE SPRAINS

PRICE — Protection, Rest, Ice, Compression, Elevation (35)

- Protection — Accomplished with the use of taping, a lace-up splint, a thermoplastic ankle stirrup splint, a functional walking orthosis, or a short leg cast. Early protected range of motion in a flexible or semirigid orthosis is superior to rigid cast immobilization in terms of patient satisfaction, return of motion and strength, and earlier return to function (3,36–42). Protected weight bearing in an orthosis is allowed with weight bearing to tolerance as soon as possible following an injury. Crutches are used until pain-free weight bearing is achieved.
- Rest — Interruption of training in running or jumping sports is essential in limiting swelling and preventing early reinjury. Length of time to return to sports depends on injury grade (see Table 67.1).
- Ice — Cryotherapy is the application of cold to the ankle in the form of ice bags, a cold whirlpool, or a commercially available compressive cuff filled with circulating coolant. Early use of cryotherapy has been shown to enable patients to return to full activity more quickly (43).
- Compression — Compression can be applied to the ankle by means of an elastic bandage, felt doughnut, neoprene or elastic orthosis, or pneumatic device.
- Elevation — This initial treatment attempts to limit the amount of hematoma and extracellular fluid accumulation edema around the ankle in order to speed up ligamentous healing.

Rehabilitation: Five Phases (24,35)

- Acute — PRICE: Goal is to limit effusion, reduce pain, and protect from further injury.
- Subacute — Focus is on eliminating pain, increasing pain-free range of motion, continued protection against reinjury with bracing, limiting loss of strength with isometric exercises, and continued modalities to decrease pain and effusion.
- Rehabilitative — Emphasizes regaining full pain-free motion with joint mobilization and stretching, increasing strength with isotonic and isokinetic exercises, and proprioceptive training.
- Functional — Focuses on sports-specific exercises with a goal to return the patient to sports participation.
- Prophylactic — Seeks to prevent recurrence of injury through preventative strengthening, functional proprioceptive drills, and prophylactic support as needed. An 8-week proprioceptive training program has been shown to reduce the recurrence of ankle sprains and to be cost-effective (44).

Treatment of Syndesmotic Ligament Injury, or "High Ankle Sprain"

- PRICE
- If the mortise is not widened or fractured, protection is in the form of a short leg cast or brace for 4 weeks, followed by physical therapy.

Table 67.2 Grades of Syndesmotic Ligament Injury

	Grade I (Mild)	Grade II (Moderate)	Grade III (Severe)
Ligament injury	Incomplete ligament injury, stable joint	Partial ligament disruption	Complete ligament disruption
Radiographic findings	Normal	Normal	widening of medial clear space, widening of syndesmosis
Stability Tests	Negative	positive external rotation and squeeze tests	All clinical tests positive
Requires surgical stabilization	No	Maybe	Yes

- In the presence of diastasis between the distal fibula and tibia on x-ray, operative stabilization of acute injuries to the syndesmotic ligaments is required. This is accomplished with syndesmotic screws or a suture construct placed through the distal fibula and tibia parallel to the ankle joint.
- For chronic syndesmotic injuries that are more than 6 months old, consideration can also be given to reconstruction of the AITFL or syndesmotic fusion in addition to stabilization of the syndesmosis with screws (45–49).
- The patient should be warned that these injuries result in longer periods of disability than injuries to the lateral collateral ligaments. In one study, only 44% of 16 patients had an acceptable outcome at 6 months (38).
- Heterotopic ossification of the distal syndesmosis has been reported in up to 25% of patients, although no correlation to ossification with functional outcome has been found (50).

Nonsurgical Treatment Results of Lateral Ankle Sprains

- Primary ligamentous repair has not been supported by studies comparing early surgery to functional treatment of ankle sprains (51–53). MRI has documented satisfactory healing of lateral ankle ligaments with the use of a functional ankle brace (54).
- A prospective study of 146 patients with grade 3 ankle sprains, who were randomized into operative and nonoperative groups, found that the group treated with an ankle orthosis returned to work faster. No difference in joint laxity was found on stress radiographs 2 years after injury (55).
- A second controlled prospective study of 51 patients with grade III sprains, randomized into operative and nonoperative groups followed for a mean of 14 years, showed no difference in mean ankle score, ankle stability on stress radiographs, and return to preinjury functional level. Surprisingly, osteoarthritis was more common in the operative group (56).

CHRONIC ANKLE PAIN AND INSTABILITY

Pain Versus Instability

- For residual symptoms following an ankle sprain, initial workup should center on whether the patient's chief complaint is pain or instability. This determination dictates further workup on the different sides of the diagnostic algorithm (Fig. 67.5).

Chronic Ankle Pain

- In a retrospective study of 457 patients treated with immobilization or bracing, 72.6% reported residual symptoms at 6–18 months (57). A study of 96 ankle sprains in West Point cadets found residual symptoms in 40% of ankles at 6 months after injury (38).
- Common causes of chronic ankle pain are occult fractures, tendon tears, nerve injury, ankle soft tissue impingement, or syndesmotic instability.
- An MRI or bone scan (technetium-labeled nuclear medicine study) is an excellent screening test to rule out occult fractures and to guide further treatment. If either test reveals an abnormality, then a spot radiograph or computed tomography scan is useful in further identifying the exact location of fracture.
- Occult or associated injuries to the tendons of the foot and ankle should also be considered. The physical exam is crucial in testing for tendon integrity, strength, or tendon sheath swelling. MRI is the most useful exam to identify and confirm tendon injuries.
- Injury to the lateral ankle ligaments may produce scarring of the ATFL and joint capsule, leading to the formation of "meniscoid tissue" in the anterolateral ankle. This inflamed tissue is pinched between the talus, fibula, and tibia, leading to a condition called anterolateral impingement (58).
- MRI has been shown to have a 78.9% accuracy, 83.3% sensitivity, and 78.6% specificity in the diagnosis of anterolateral soft tissue impingement (59).
- The distal fascicle of the anteroinferior tibiofibular ligament may abrade the anterolateral surface of the talus during ankle dorsiflexion during abnormal anterior translation of the talus (60).
- An anomalous or accessory peroneal tendon may also cause chronic posterolateral ankle pain (61). Its presence is confirmed by an MRI.
- Nerve injury may result due to traction on the nerve during an inversion sprain. Electromyography performed 2 weeks after lateral ankle sprains in 36 patients with grade III injuries showed an 86% incidence of peroneal nerve injury and 83% incidence of tibial nerve injury (26). A cadaver study of a simulated ankle sprain has shown that traction on the superficial peroneal nerve causes nerve strain of enough magnitude to result in nerve injury (62).
- Syndesmotic instability is suggested by pain over the syndesmosis on palpation and by positive clinical tests for syndesmotic instability. MRI is very helpful in diagnosing tears of the AITFL (37,63). Some patients may have painful chronic latent syndesmotic instability but have no frank instability on examination or on stress radiographs (32). The gold standard test for syndesmotic instability is ankle arthroscopy (37,48,63,64). During arthroscopy, the ability to introduce an arthroscopic shaver or probe into the tibiofibular joint from below is indicative of syndesmotic instability. In addition, the shaver can be used to push on the anterior aspect of the distal fibula. Increased posterior translation of the fibula indicates instability of the syndesmosis.

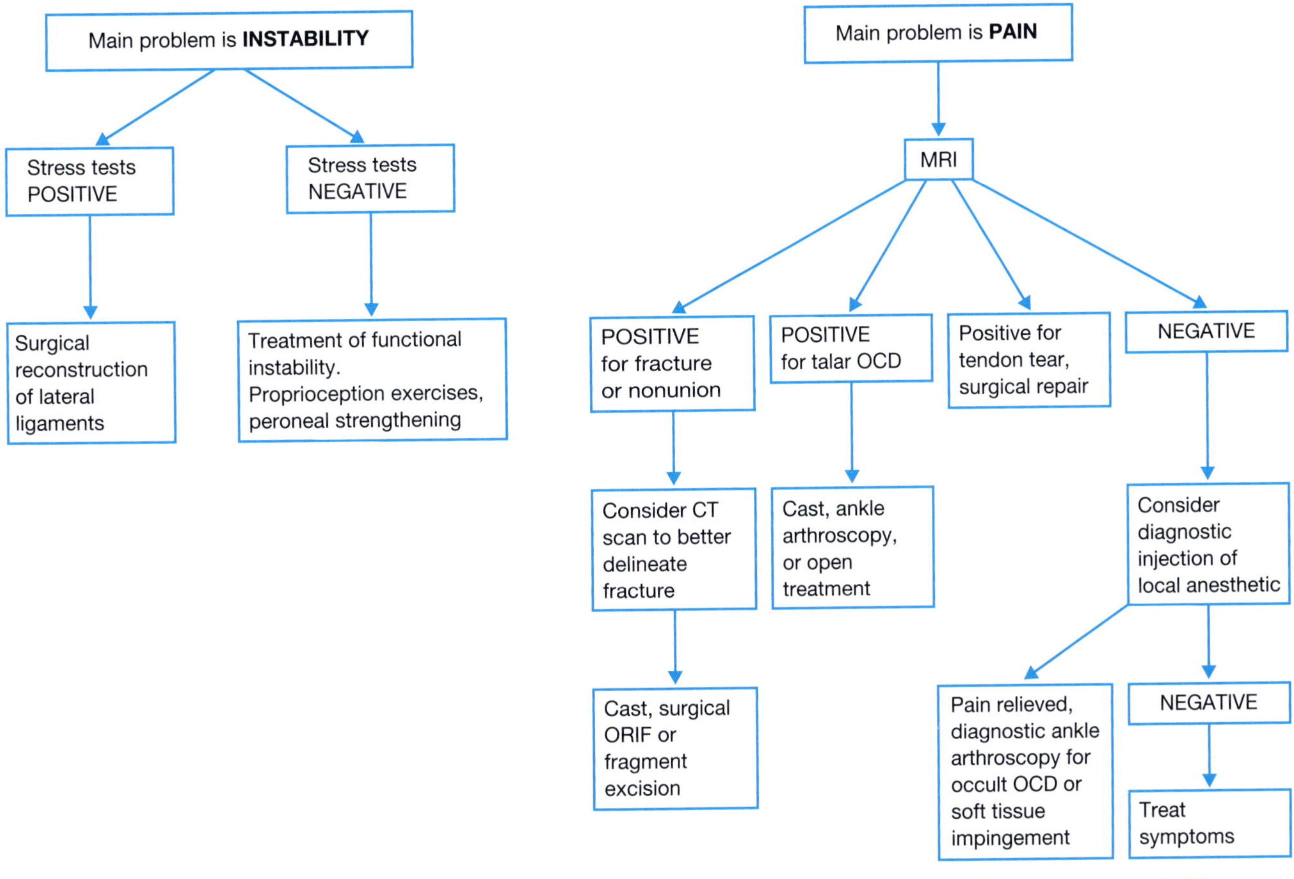

Figure 67.5: Chronic ankle pain algorithm. CT, computed tomography; MRI, magnetic resonance imaging; ORIF, open reduction internal fixation.

Chronic Ankle Instability

- If the primary problem is ankle instability, the patient will experience feelings of "giving way" of the ankle on uneven ground, inability to play cutting or jumping sports, loss of confidence in ankle support, and reliance on braces, and give a history of multiple ankle sprains.
- The ankle should be evaluated with stress radiographs. If the stress radiographs are positive for mechanical lateral ligamentous laxity, then surgery is indicated to reconstruct the deficient ligaments.
- If stress radiographs disprove mechanical laxity of the lateral ankle ligaments, then the patient may have functional ankle instability rather than true mechanical ankle instability. Functional instability is due to deficient neuromuscular control of the ankle, impaired proprioception, and peroneal weakness (65,66). Treatment in this case should be directed toward restoring peroneal tendon strength, restoring ankle motion, and improving ankle proprioception with physical therapy.
- Be aware that the presence of a cavovarus foot deformity with high arch and varus heel position may predispose the patient to lateral ankle ligamentous instability. These patients may benefit from custom orthotic management with a plantar first metatarsal head recess and lateral heel posting. If lateral ankle ligamentous reconstruction is indicated based on symptoms and stress views, the foot position should also be corrected with lateralizing calcaneal osteotomy and possible first metatarsal osteotomy to lower the arch (44,67).
- Chronic recurrent lateral ankle instability is associated with chondral damage. Ankle arthroscopy in 93 patients with chronic ankle instability showed moderate to severe cartilage damage in 41 patients (44%) (68). A retrospective study of 247 patients with ankle arthritis identified 33 patients with ligamentous end-stage ankle osteoarthritis. Eighty-five percent of patients had injured the lateral ligaments, and 15% of patients had injured both medial and lateral ankle ligaments. Mean time from injury to osteoarthritis was 34.3 years (69).
- Other causes for ankle instability not demonstrated by inversion stress radiographs include rotational instability of the talus, subtalar instability, distal syndesmotic (tibiofibular) instability, and hindfoot varus malalignment (44,67).

SURGICAL TREATMENT

Indications for Surgery

- Multiple episodes of mechanical instability, *e.g.*, difficulty walking on uneven ground, inability to play cutting sports, lack of confidence in ankle stability
- Demonstration of mechanical instability on stress radiographs
- Failure of a full course of physical therapy emphasizing peroneal strengthening and proprioceptive training
- Failure of a course of bracing
- Suspected syndesmosis instability based on clinical exam despite normal radiographs and normal external rotation stress radiographs is an indication for arthroscopic evaluation of the syndesmosis. If instability is confirmed at time of arthroscopy, the syndesmosis is stabilized at that time surgically.

Surgical Procedures

- Most procedures are designed to tighten or reconstruct the ATFL and CFL.
- Ankle reconstructive procedures are described either as anatomic or as nonanatomic procedures. Anatomic reconstructions attempt to tighten lateral ligaments or transfer tendons into the exact anatomic locations of the ATFL and CFL. Nonanatomic reconstructions use tendon transfers to act as a tenodesis on the lateral side of the ankle, although they do not attempt to place the transferred tendons to the exact anatomic origins of the ATFL or CFL. Most surgeons agree that anatomic reconstructions are preferable. A retrospective study comparing anatomic to nonanatomic ankle ligament reconstruction in 77 patients showed superior results in the anatomic reconstruction group (70).
- The Brostrom procedure is an anatomic reconstruction in which the ATFL and CFL are divided and imbricated (71). Some authors advance the shortened ligaments into the distal fibula. This procedure is sometimes modified by advancing the extensor retinaculum proximally (the Gould modification) to further tighten the lateral aspects of the ankle and subtalar joints (72).
- The Brostrom procedure can be augmented by placing suture tape over the shortened ATFL and attaching it by suture anchors in the talar neck and distal fibula. This "internal brace" procedure allows for earlier weight-bearing and accelerated rehabilitation protocols (73).
- The arthroscopic Brostrom procedure is now accepted as a safe and effective alternative to open stabilization. A suture anchor is placed arthroscopically into the ATFL footprint of the distal fibula and the attached sutures are used to advance the ATFL and extensor retinaculum proximally to the fibula, thus tightening the lateral ankle ligamentous structures (74).
- Patients with long-standing instability may not have adequate ligamentous tissue for shortening and repair. In these cases, the ligaments are reconstructed. Tendon transfer procedures most commonly employ tendon allografts or one-half of the peroneus brevis tendon. The tendon graft is passed through holes in the talar neck, distal fibula, and lateral calcaneus in order to reconstruct the lateral ligamentous structures. A detailed discussion of all these procedures is beyond the scope of this chapter (75–78).

Postoperative Care

- Following lateral ankle ligamentous reconstructive procedures, most postoperative regimens immobilize the ankle in a cast for 4 weeks, followed by an orthosis for 4 additional weeks.
- Brostrom procedures augmented by suture tape are allowed full weight-bearing in a cast or boot immediately. Range of motion exercises start at postoperative week 2. The Cam boot is discontinued at weeks 4–6, and the patient is transitioned into an ankle brace. High-impact activities are begun at week 6–8.
- Physical therapy is instituted at 6–8 weeks after surgery with an emphasis on peroneal strengthening and proprioceptive training.
- Return to sports occurs at about 3 months after surgery.

REFERENCES

1. Mack RP. Ankle injuries in athletics. *Clin Sports Med.* 1982;1(1):71–84.
2. Ekstrand J, Tropp H. The incidence of ankle sprains in soccer. *Foot Ankle.* 1990;11(1):41–4.
3. Garrick JG, Requa RK. The epidemiology of foot and ankle injuries in sports. *Clin Sports Med.* 1988;7(1):29–36.
4. Waterman BR, Owens BD, Davey S, Zacchilli MA, Belmont PJ Jr. The epidemiology of ankle sprains in the United States. *J Bone Joint Surg.* 2010;92(13):2279–84.
5. Hunt KJ, George E, Harris AH, Dragoo JL. Epidemiology of syndesmosis injuries in intercollegiate football: incidence and risk factors from National Collegiate Athletic Association injury surveillance system data from 2004-2005 to 2008-2009. *Clin J Sport Med.* 2013;23(4):278–82.
6. de César PC, Avila EM, de Abreu MR. Comparison of magnetic resonance imaging to physical examination for syndesmotic injury after lateral ankle sprain. *Foot Ankle Int.* 2011;32(12):1110–14.
7. Attarian DE, McCrackin HJ, DeVito DP, McElhaney JH, Garrett WE Jr. Biomechanical characteristics of human ankle ligaments. *Foot Ankle.* 1985;6(2):54–8.
8. Stephens MM, Sammarco GJ. The stabilizing role of the lateral ligament complex around the ankle and subtalar joints. *Foot Ankle.* 1992;13(3):130–6.
9. Sammarco GJ, Hockenbury RT. Biomechanics of the foot and ankle. In: Nordin M, Frankel VH, editors. *Basic Biomechanics of the Musculoskeletal System.* 3rd ed. Baltimore (MD): Lippincott Williams & Wilkins; 2001. p. 242.
10. Wang Q, Whittle M, Cunningham J, Kenwright J. Fibula and its ligaments in load transmission and ankle joint stability. *Clin Orthop Relat Res.* 1996;330:261–70.

11. Sarrafian SK. *Anatomy of the Foot and Ankle*. 2nd ed. Philadelphia (PA): JB Lippincott; 1993. pp. 159–87, 474–551.
12. Harper MC. Deltoid ligament: an anatomical evaluation of function. *Foot Ankle*. 1987;8(1):19–22.
13. Ferran NA, Maffulli N. Epidemiology of sprains of the lateral ankle ligament complex. *Foot Ankle Clin*. 2006;11(3):659–62.
14. Wuest TK. Injuries to the distal lower extremity syndesmosis. *J Am Acad Orthop Surg*. 1997;5(3):172–81.
15. Emery CA, Meeuwisse WH. The effectiveness of a neuromuscular prevention strategy to reduce injuries in youth soccer: a cluster-randomised controlled trial. *Br J Sports Med*. 2010;44(8):555–62.
16. McGuine TA, Keene JS. The effect of a balance training program on the risk of ankle sprains in high school athletes. *Am J Sports Med*. 2006;34(7):1103–11.
17. Pedowitz DI, Reddy S, Parekh SG, Huffman GR, Sennett BJ. Prophylactic bracing decreases ankle injuries in collegiate female volleyball players. *Am J Sports Med*. 2008;36(2):324–7.
18. Frey C, Feder KS, Sleight J. Prophylactic ankle brace use in high school volleyball players: a prospective study. *Foot Ankle Int*. 2010;31(4):296–300.
19. Chvapil M. *Physiology of Connective Tissue*. London (UK): Butterworth's Scientific Publications; 1967:246–86.
20. Noyes FR, Torvik PJ, Hyde WB, DeLucas JL. Biomechanics of ligament failure: II. An analysis of immobilization, exercise, and reconditioning effects in primates. *J Bone Joint Surg Am*. 1974;56(7):1406–18.
21. Tipton CM, James SL, Mergner W, Tcheng TK. Influence of exercise on strength of medial collateral knee ligaments of dogs. *Am J Physiol*. 1970;218(3):894–902.
22. Vailas AC, Tipton CM, Matthes RD, Gart M. Physical activity and its influence on the repair process of medial collateral ligaments. *Connect Tissue Res*. 1981;9(1):25–31.
23. Hettinga DL. Inflammatory response of synovial joint structures. In: Gould JA, Davies GJ, editors. *Orthopaedic and Sports Physical Therapy*. St. Louis (MO): CV Mosby; 1985. p. 87.
24. Safran MR, Benedetti RS, Bartolozzi AR III, Mandelbaum BR. Lateral ankle sprains: a comprehensive review. Part 1—etiology, pathoanatomy, histopathogenesis, and diagnosis. *Med Sci Sports Exerc*. 1999;31(7 suppl l):S429–37.
25. Thorndike A. *Athletic Injuries: Prevention, Diagnosis, and Treatment*. Philadelphia (PA): Lea & Febinger; 1962. p. 59.
26. Nitz AJ, Dobner JJ, Kersey D. Nerve injury and grades II and III ankle sprains. *Am J Sports Med*. 1985;13(3):177–82.
27. Hockenbury RT, Sammarco GJ. Evaluation and treatment of ankle sprains: clinical recommendations for a positive outcome. *Phy Sportsmed*. 2001;29(2):57–64.
28. Hunt KJ, Phisitkul P, Pirolo J, Amendola A. High ankle sprains and syndesmotic injuries in athletes. *J Am Acad Orthop Surg*. 2015;23(11):661–73.
29. Sman AD, Hiller CE, Rae K, et al. Diagnostic accuracy of clinical tests for ankle syndesmosis injury. *Br J Sports Med*. 2015 Mar;49(5):323–9.
30. Beumer A, van Hemert WLW, Swierstra BA, Jasper LE, Belkoff SM. A biomechanical evaluation of clinical stress tests for syndesmotic ankle instability. *Foot Ankle Int*. 2003;24(4):358–63.
31. Hopkinson WJ, St Pierre P, Ryan JB, Wheeler JH. Syndesmosis sprains of the ankle. *Foot Ankle*. 1990;10(6):325–30.
32. Edwards GS Jr, DeLee JC. Ankle diastasis without fracture. *Foot Ankle*. 1984;4(6):305–12.
33. Xenos JS, Hopkinson WJ, Mulligan ME, Olson EJ, Popovic NA. The tibiofibular syndesmosis: evaluation of the ligamentous structures, methods of fixation, and radiographic assessment. *J Bone Joint Surg*. 1995;77(6):847–56.
34. Stiell IG, Greenberg GH, McKnight RD, et al. Decision rules for the use of radiography in acute ankle injuries: refinement and prospective validation. *JAMA*. 1993;269(9):1127–32.
35. Safran MR, Zachazewski JE, Benedetti RS, Bartolozzi AR III, Mandelbaum R. Lateral ankle sprains: a comprehensive review. Part 2—treatment and rehabilitation with an emphasis on the athlete. *Med Sci Sports Exerc*. 1999;31(7 suppl l):S438–47.
36. Hoffman E, Paller D, Koruprolu S, et al. Accuracy of plain radiographs versus 3D analysis of ankle stress test. *Foot Ankle Int*. 2011;32(10):994–9.
37. Takao M, Ochi M, Oae K, Naito K, Uchio Y. Diagnosis of a tear of the tibiofibular syndesmosis: the role of arthroscopy of the ankle. *J Bone Joint Surg Br*. 2003;85(3):324–9.
38. Gerber JP, Williams GN, Scoville CR, Arciero RA, Taylor DC. Persistent disability associated with ankle sprains: a prospective examination of an athletic population. *Foot Ankle Int*. 1998;19(10):653–60.
39. Ardèvol J, Bolíbar I, Belda V, Argilaga S. Treatment of complete rupture of the lateral ligaments of the ankle: a randomized clinical trial comparing cast immobilization with functional treatment. *Knee Surg Sports Traumatol Arthrosc*. 2002;10(6):371–7.
40. Kerkhoffs GM, Rowe BH, Assendelft WJ, Kelly K, Struijs PA, van Dijk CN. Immobilisation and functional treatment for acute lateral ankle ligament injuries in adults. *Cochrane Database Syst Rev*. 2002;3:CD003762.
41. Klein J, Höher J, Tiling T. Comparative study of therapies for fibular ligament rupture of the lateral ankle joint in competitive basketball players. *Foot Ankle*. 1993;14(6):320–4.
42. Regis D, Montanari M, Magnan B, Spagnol S, Bragantini A. Dynamic orthopaedic brace in the treatment of ankle sprains. *Foot Ankle Int*. 1995;16(7):422–6.
43. Hocutt JE Jr, Jaffe R, Rylander CR, Beebe JK. Cryotherapy in ankle sprains. *Am J Sports Med*. 1982;10(5):316–9.
44. Hintermann B. Biomechanics of the unstable ankle joint and clinical implications. *Med Sci Sports Exerc*. 1999;31(7 suppl l):S459–69.
45. Kwon JY, Stenquist D, Ye M, et al. Anterior syndesmotic augmentation technique using nonabsorbable suture-tape for acute and chronic syndesmotic instability. *Foot Ankle*. 2020;41(10):1307–15.
46. Morris WJ, Rice P, Schneider TE. Distal tibiofibular syndesmosis reconstruction using a free hamstring autograft. *Foot Ankle Int*. 2009;30(6):506–11.
47. Ryan PM, Rodriguez RM. Outcomes and return to activity after operative repair of chronic latent syndesmotic instability. *Foot Ankle Int*. 2016 Feb;37(2):192–7.
48. Wagener ML, Beumer A, Swierstra BA. Chronic instability of the anterior tibiofibular syndesmosis of the ankle. Arthroscopic findings and results of anatomical reconstruction. *BMC Musculoskelet Disord*. 2011 Sep 27;12:212.
49. Olson KM, Dairyko GH Jr, Toolan BC. Salvage of chronic instability of the syndesmosis with distal tibiofibular arthrodesis: functional and radiographic results. *J Bone Joint Surg Am*. 2011;93(1):66–72.
50. Taylor DC, Englehardt DL, Bassett FH III. Syndesmosis sprains of the ankle: influence of heterotopic ossification. *Am J Sports Med*. 1992;20(2):146–50.
51. Sommer HM, Arza D. Functional treatment of recent ruptures of the fibular ligament of the ankle. *Int Orthop*. 1989;13(2):157–60.
52. Weise K, Rupf G, Weinelt J. Die laterale bandverletzung des OSG beim sport. *Aktuelle Traumatol*. 1988;1(18 suppl l):54–66.
53. Zwipp H, Hoffmann R, Wippermann B, Thermann H, Gottschalk F. Fibulare bandruptur am oberen Sprunggelenk. *Orthopä*. 1989;18(4):336–40.
54. De Simoni C, Wetz HH, Zanetti M, Hodler J, Jacob H, Zollinger H. Clinical examination and magnetic resonance imaging in the assessment of ankle sprains treated with an orthosis. *Foot Ankle Int*. 1996;17(3):177–82.

55. Povacz P, Unger SF, Miller WK, Tockner R, Resch H. A randomized, prospective study of operative and non-operative treatment of injuries of the fibular collateral ligaments of the ankle. *J Bone Joint Surg Am.* 1998;80(3):345–51.
56. Pihlajamäki H, Hietaniemi K, Paavola M, Visuri T, Mattila VM. Surgical versus functional treatment for acute ruptures of the lateral ligament complex of the ankle in young men: a randomized controlled trial. *J Bone Joint Surg Am.* 2010;92(14):2367–74.
57. Braun BL. Effects of ankle sprain in a general clinic population 6 to 18 months after medical evaluation. *Arch Fam Med.* 1999;8(2):143–8.
58. Wolin I, Glassman F, Sideman S, Levinthal DH. Internal derangement of the talofibular component of the ankle. *Surg Gynecol Obstet.* 1950;91(2):193–200.
59. Ferkel RD, Tyorkin M, Applegate GR, Heinen GT. MRI evaluation of anterolateral soft tissue impingement of the ankle. *Foot Ankle Int.* 2010;31(8):655–61.
60. Bassett FH III, Gates HS III, Billys JB, Morris HB, Nikolaou PK. Talar impingement by the anteroinferior tibiofibular ligament. A cause of chronic pain in the ankle after inversion sprain. *J Bone Joint Surg Am.* 1990;72(1):55–9.
61. Trono M, Tueche S, Quintart C, Libotte M, Baillon J. Peroneus quartus muscle: a case report and review of the literature. *Foot Ankle Int.* 1999;20(10):659–62.
62. O'Neill PJ, Parks BG, Walsh R, Simmons LM, Miller SD. Excursion and strain of the superficial peroneal nerve during inversion ankle sprain. *J Bone Joint Surg Am.* 2007;89(5):979–86.
63. Han SH, Lee JW, Kim S, Suh JS, Choi YR. Chronic tibiofibular syndesmosis injury: the diagnostic efficiency of magnetic resonance imaging and comparative analysis of operative treatment. *Foot Ankle Int.* 2007;28(3):336–42.
64. Beumer A, Swierstra BA, Mulder PGH. Clinical diagnosis of syndesmotic ankle instability: evaluation of stress tests behind the curtains. *Acta Orthop Scand.* 2002;73(6):667–9.
65. Freeman MA, Dean MR, Hanham IW. The etiology and prevention of functional instability of the foot. *J Bone Joint Surg Br.* 1965;47(4):678–85.
66. Gauffin H, Tropp H, Odenrick P. Effect of ankle disk training on postural control in patients with functional instability of the ankle joint. *Int J Sports Med.* 1988;9(2):141–4.
67. Deben SE, Pomeroy GC. Subtle cavus foot: diagnosis and management. *J Am Acad Orthop Surg.* 2014 Aug;22(8):512–20.
68. Sugimoto K, Takakura Y, Okahashi K, Samoto N, Kawate K, Iwai M. Chondral injuries of the ankle with recurrent lateral instability: an arthroscopic study. *J Bone Joint Surg Am.* 2009;91(1):99–106.
69. Valderrabano V, Hintermann B, Horisberger M, Fung TS. Ligamentous posttraumatic ankle osteoarthritis. *Am J Sports Med.* 2006;34(4): 612–20.
70. Krips R, van Dijk CN, Lehtonen H, Halasi T, Moyen B, Karlsson J. Sports activity level after surgical treatment for chronic anterolateral ankle instability. A multicenter study. *Am J Sports Med.* 2002;30(1):13–9.
71. Broström L. Sprained ankles. VI. Surgical treatment of "chronic" ligament ruptures. *Acta Chir Scand.* 1966;132(5):551–65.
72. Gould N, Seligson D, Gassman J. Early and late repair of lateral ligament of the ankle. *Foot Ankle.* 1980;1(2):84–9.
73. Wittig U, Hohneberger G, Ornig M, et al. Tape augmentation versus Brostrom repair for chronic ankle instability? A systematic review. *Arthroscopy.* 2022 Feb;38(2):597–608.
74. Acevedo JI, Mangone P. Arthroscopic Brostrom technique. *Foot Ankle Int.* 2015;36(4):465–73.
75. Sammarco GJ, DiRaimondo CV. Surgical treatment of lateral ankle instability syndrome. *Am J Sports Med.* 1988;16(5):501–11.
76. Sammarco GJ, Idusuyi OB. Reconstruction of the lateral ankle ligaments using a split peroneus brevis tendon graft. *Foot Ankle Int.* 1999;20(2):97–103.
77. Snook GA, Chrisman OD, Wilson TC. Long-term results of the Chrisman-Snook operation for reconstruction of the lateral ligaments of the ankle. *J Bone Joint Surg Am.* 1985;67(1):1–7.
78. Caprio A, Oliva F, Treia F, Maffulli N. Reconstruction of the lateral ankle ligaments with allograft in patients with chronic ankle instability. *Foot Ankle Clin.* 2006;11(3):597–605.

68

Soft-Tissue Injuries of the Leg, Ankle, and Foot

Arjun Srinath and Tyler Kalbac

- As the number of participants in both recreational and competitive activities increases, soft-tissue injuries to the lower extremity are encountered more frequently by the primary care provider. If left untreated, these injuries could jeopardize participation and quality of life for those affected. The purpose of this chapter is to outline the characteristics and treatment of the more frequently encountered soft-tissue pathologies by region.

SOFT-TISSUE INJURIES OF THE LEG

- The leg extends from the knee to the ankle. Some of the soft-tissue injuries affecting this portion of the extremity include exertional compartment syndrome, posterior tibial tendon injury, and peroneal tendon injury.

Exertional Compartment Syndrome

- Exertional compartment syndrome is activity-related pain caused by an increased intermuscular pressure within an anatomic compartment. In the leg, there are four compartments that contain muscle, blood vessels, and nerves. The compartments are enclosed by fascia, which limit muscular expansion during activity and can cause compression of the contents of the compartment. As pressure within the compartment approaches the mean arterial pressure, the blood flow through the microvasculature is diminished and ischemia ensues.
- Knowledge of the anatomy of the lower leg is vital to the diagnosis of exertional compartment syndrome (Fig. 68.1). The anterior compartment contains the extensor hallucis longus, extensor digitorum longus, peroneus tertius, and tibialis anterior as well as the deep peroneal nerve. The lateral compartment contains the peroneus longus and brevis as well as the superficial peroneal nerve. The superficial posterior compartment contains the gastrocnemius and soleus muscles and the sural nerve. The deep posterior compartment contains the flexor hallucis longus, flexor digitorum longus, and posterior tibialis muscle as well as the posterior tibial nerve.
- The patient is usually asymptomatic upon initiating exercise. The pain will begin at a predictable time during the workout. The pain is described as aching or cramping associated with feelings of swelling, fullness, or tightness. Dysesthesias often accompany the pain along the nerve within the affected compartment. Patients may also complain of altered running style. For example, a runner may state that the foot seems to be slapping the ground when the pain comes on.

Physical Examination

- The physical examination at rest is often normal. In advanced cases, there may be tenderness to deep palpation along the affected compartment or a palpable fascial defect with hernia within the affected compartment.
- Examination immediately after exercise reveals a firm, tender compartment with increased pain on passive stretch of the muscles within the compartment. Fascial defects with resultant herniations are more identifiable at this time.
- Several techniques have been described for measuring compartment pressures: These include needle manometry, wick catheter, and slit catheter. Our preferred method of measuring compartment pressure is with a battery-operated, handheld, digital, fluid pressure monitor. The Stryker Intracompartmental Pressure Monitor (Stryker Corporation, Kalamazoo, MI) is a convenient and easy-to-use measuring device.
- Compartment pressures should be taken before exercise, 1 minute after exercise, and if necessary, 5 minutes after exercise. One or more of the following pressure criteria must be met in addition to a history and physical that is consistent with the diagnosis of exertional compartment syndrome: preexercise pressure >15 mm Hg, 1-minute postexercise pressure >30 mm Hg, or 5-minute postexercise pressure >20 mm Hg (1).

Treatment

- Nonoperative care generally consists of activity modification to levels below symptomatic threshold, ice, nonsteroidal anti-inflammatory medications (NSAIDs), and massage. The patient should be counseled that return to previous level of activity is likely to cause recurrence of symptoms.
- A subcutaneous fasciotomy is the surgical treatment of an exertional compartment syndrome. In this procedure, the

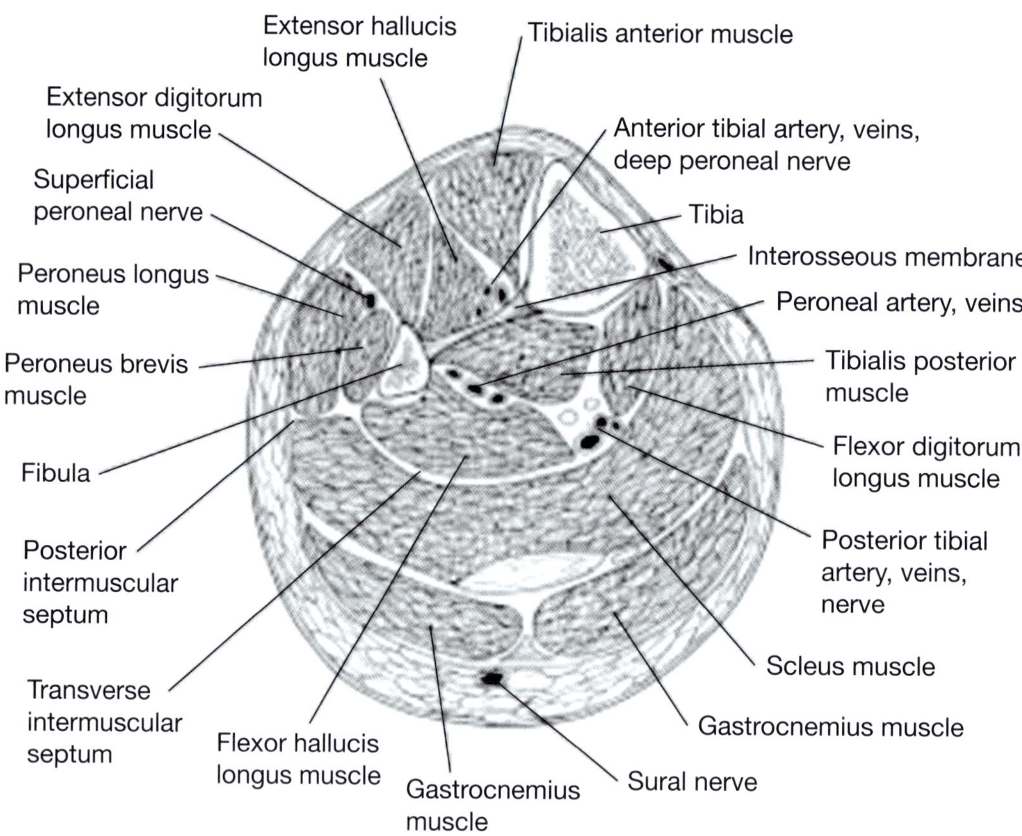

Figure 68.1: Cross-sectional anatomy of the compartments of the leg. (© 2003 American Academy of Orthopedic Surgeons. Reprinted from the *Journal of the American Academy of Orthopedic Surgeons*, 11(4):268–76, with permission.)

fascia is divided longitudinally over the entire length of the involved compartment. Indications for this procedure include an appropriate history for chronic exertional compartment syndrome, a 1-minute postexercise compartment pressure greater than 30 mm Hg, or the presence of a fascial defect.

- Fasciotomy can be successful in relieving pain and allowing for return to full activity in 90% of patients (2).

Popliteal Artery Entrapment Syndrome

- Popliteal artery entrapment syndrome occurs when the popliteal artery, and less commonly the popliteal vein, becomes compressed by the surrounding structures rather than inconsequentially passing between the heads of the gastrocnemius muscles.
- Vascular compression decreases oxygen delivery to muscles in the lower extremity, causing exertional pain, swelling, cramping, and numbness that quickly resolve with rest.
- In patients with popliteal artery entrapment syndrome, a high percentage of concomitant chronic exertional compartment syndrome contributes to diagnostic challenges.

Physical Examination

- Popliteal artery entrapment syndrome presentation consists of intermittent claudication, paresthesia, or lower extremity pain after exercise or with leg elevation.
- Examination findings may include paresthesia in the lower legs and feet along with cramping, blanching, swelling, and cold feet.
- Examination requires close attention to the presence of the popliteal pulse during knee extension with and without ankle dorsiflexion, where active plantarflexion or passive dorsiflexion may cause diminished pedal pulses.

Radiograhic Examination

- Computed tomography angiogram (CTA) is often recommended given its access and availability. It is sufficient to diagnose popliteal artery entrapment syndrome. Evaluation with CTA requires axial imaging performed at rest and with active plantarflexion.
- Magnetic resonance angiography can also be used and its advantages include superior diagnostic imaging quality when performed adequately, anatomical evaluation of the popliteal fossa for surgical planning, and decreased radiation exposure, making it the gold standard for diagnosis (3).

Treatment

- Initial treatment should include relative rest, activity modifications, and analgesics as needed. Avoidance of triggering activities may be achieved via long-term activity modification and observation.
- Botulinum toxin type A has been studied as a treatment, hypothesized to work through paralysis of the muscle occluding the popliteal artery, resultant muscle atrophy, or

arterial smooth muscle relaxation causing arterial dilation; however, this has yet to be validated.

- Surgical intervention focuses on addressing the anatomical abnormality contributing to popliteal artery occlusion, and a posterior or medial approach to the popliteal artery is typically used and remains the gold standard for treatment (3).

Posterior Tibial Tendon Injury

- Injury to the posterior tibial tendon may occur acutely or as a component of chronic overuse syndrome. The posterior tibial tendon helps invert and plantarflex the foot and has an important role in maintaining the longitudinal arch.
- Patients with posterior tibial tendon injury often report pain along the medial aspect of the leg posterior to the medial malleolus. The onset of symptoms is usually gradual with increases in such activities as walking, running, or jumping.

Physical Examination

- There may be loss of the longitudinal arch and a clinical planovalgus deformity. When observing the patient from behind, the affected side will reveal more toes lateral to the heel than the unaffected side, indicating the presence of increased hindfoot valgus.
- With an attempted single-leg heel raise, there is loss of foot supination and heel inversion. In the later stages of posterior tibial dysfunction, patients cannot perform a single-leg heel rise. In earlier stages of dysfunction, patients will perform the single-leg heel rise in a slow deliberated fashion with associated pain.
- There is tenderness and fullness along the course of the tendon.
- Pain and weakness are present with resisted inversion.

Radiographic Examination

- The x-ray evaluation should include standing anteroposterior (AP) and lateral views of the ankle and foot. The AP foot x-ray may show medial talar displacement in relation to the navicular. This is best seen with uncovering of the talar head. The lateral foot x-ray may reveal decreased height of the longitudinal arch and increased overlap of the metatarsals (4).
- Magnetic resonance imaging (MRI) is the test of choice to evaluate the posterior tibial tendon (4). Significant findings on MRI include heterogenous signal along the course of the tendon and possible increase in size.

Treatment

- The initial treatment for posterior tibial tendon deficiency is generally nonoperative and begins with a period of immobilization with the use of a short leg walking boot, short leg walking cast, or posterior tibial tendon brace. Once immobilization is complete, a medial post orthotic should be used to support the arch and relieve stress on the tendon by posting the heel in a neutral position.
- Physical therapy (PT) can be initiated focusing on stretching of the gastrocnemius and posterior tibial tendon.
- Corticosteroid injections are not recommended because of the risk of tendon rupture.
- Surgery should be considered in those who do not respond to nonoperative management after 3–6 months, patients with loss of the arch, or patients with midfoot arthritis (4). Surgical options include synovectomy/debridement, flexor digitorum longus transfer, or calcaneal osteotomy.

Peroneal Tendon Injury

- Peroneal tendon pathology is a commonly missed source of chronic lateral-sided ankle pain. The spectrum of peroneal tendon injury includes tenosynovitis, tendon tear, and peroneal tendon instability.
- The peroneus longus originates from the proximal aspect of the lateral fibula. Its tendinous portion runs posterior to the lateral malleolus before inserting primarily onto the plantar proximal surface of the first metatarsal. Its function is primarily eversion and plantar flexion of the foot. The peroneus brevis originates from the lateral fibula. Its tendinous portion courses anterior and medial to the peroneus longus tendon at the level of the ankle and inserts onto the base of the fifth metatarsal. Its primary function is to evert the foot.
- The patient will often complain of lateral ankle pain that localizes posterior to the lateral malleolus. The patient may also relay a history of pain, "popping," and transient swelling in this area usually after an inversion injury.

Physical Examination

- Pain and swelling over the course of the tendons posterior to the lateral malleolus will be present on examination. The patient may also report pain with resisted eversion of the ankle, passive inversion of the ankle, or resisted plantar flexion of the first metatarsal. In cases of peroneal instability, tendon subluxation or dislocation may be elicited with resisted eversion and dorsiflexion of the ankle.

Radiographic Examination

- Standard radiographic review should include weight-bearing AP, mortise, and lateral x-rays.
- A fleck avulsion of the distal fibula indicates subluxation/dislocation due to injury of the superior peroneal retinaculum.
- Ultrasonography may show areas of heterogeneity within the tendons as well as subluxation.
- MRI may show increased or heterogenous signal within the substance of the tendon. Circumferential fluid within the tendon sheath measuring greater than 3 mm suggests tenosynovitis (5).

Treatment

- The initial treatment of peroneal tendon tenosynovitis begins with rest, ice, and NSAIDs. An ankle brace or lateral heel wedge may also help alleviate symptoms. For more severe cases of tenosynovitis, the patient may be placed in a short leg cast or walking boot for a period of 2–4 weeks. In cases of peroneal tendon instability, nonoperative treatment is associated with a high rate of failure.
- Corticosteroid injections should be used judiciously because of the risk of tendon rupture.
- US-guided platelet-rich plasma has shown promising results (6).

- Operative intervention is indicated if symptoms persist after a trial on nonoperative care. Surgical treatment includes exploration, synovectomy, primary tendon repair, tenodesis, or retinacular repair (7).

SOFT-TISSUE INJURIES OF THE HINDFOOT AND MIDFOOT

- The hindfoot consists of the talus and calcaneus and their articulations, whereas the midfoot consists of the navicular, cuboid, and three cuneiform bones and their related articulations. Foot function hinges on the stability provided by the osseous anatomy and overlying soft-tissue structures. Some of the more frequently encountered soft-tissue pathologies affecting this region include os trigonum, jogger's foot, tarsal tunnel syndrome, plantar heel pain, and posterior heel pain.

Painful Os Trigonum

- The os trigonum is an ossicle present in 7%–11% of the population as a continuation of the posterior talar process. Painful os trigonum syndrome is one cause of posteromedial ankle pain. This syndrome is most prevalent in athletes who perform frequent or forced plantar flexion. The condition may be misdiagnosed as other conditions such as Achilles tendonitis (8).
- Often called posterior ankle impingement syndrome
- Can be associated with flexor hallucis longus tenosynovitis
- Presentation is commonly with pain in the posterior medial ankle that may be worsened with plantar flexion activities (en pointe position in ballet, kicking a soccer ball).

Physical Examination

- On examination, there may be tenderness to palpation over the os or the posteromedial ankle. Passive dorsiflexion/plantar flexion of the great toe may also illicit pain due to the close anatomic relationship of the flexor hallucis longus tendon and the trigonal process.

Radiographic Examination

- Standard radiographs should include weight-bearing AP and oblique and lateral views of the foot. The os trigonum may be appreciated on the lateral view. A plantar flexion lateral may show the os trigonum impinging on the posterior malleolus.
- MRI will demonstrate fluid between the os trigonum and the lateral talar process (9). MRI may also demonstrate associated flexor hallucis longus tenosynovitis.

Treatment

- The initial treatment for symptomatic os trigonum is nonoperative and generally begins with a brief (4–6 weeks) period of immobilization in a short leg cast or controlled ankle movement boot. NSAIDs and activity modification may help alleviate symptoms.
- Diagnostic injection can confirm the diagnosis.
- Surgical excision may be required with failure of nonoperative management and can be performed arthroscopically or open (10).

Compression Neuropathy (Jogger's Foot)

- Entrapment of the medial plantar nerve distal to the tarsal tunnel can cause a neuropathy known as *jogger's foot.* The medial plantar nerve courses plantarward after it exits the tarsal tunnel, where it may be compressed by osteophytes from the talonavicular joint or a fibrotic master knot of Henry.
- Patients often complain of pain or numbness of the medial sole of the foot and medial toes that increases with physical activity.

Physical Examination

- There may be tenderness to palpation along the medial aspect of the longitudinal arch. Numbness and tingling may also be recreated with a Tinel test over this area.

Treatment

- The initial treatment of this condition is generally nonoperative and should consist of rest, NSAIDs, or soft orthoses. Patients with a planovalgus or flatfoot may benefit from a University of California Biomechanics Laboratory orthosis.
- Injection of corticosteroid with local anesthetic can be diagnostic as well as therapeutic.
- Surgical release of the medial plantar nerve may be indicated for cases that fail trials of nonoperative care, with little recurrence seen after release (11).

Tarsal Tunnel Syndrome

- Tarsal tunnel syndrome is the most common compression neuropathy of the foot and ankle. The etiology is entrapment of the posterior tibial nerve in the tarsal tunnel or one of its terminal branches after leaving the tarsal tunnel. Tarsal tunnel syndrome may be posttraumatic, idiopathic, or the result of a space-occupying lesion or accessory muscle (12,13).
- The tarsal tunnel is a fibro-osseous tunnel. The osseous boundaries are the medial surface of the talus, the medial surface of the os calcis, the sustentaculum tali, and inferomedial navicular. The fibrous portion of the canal consists of the flexor retinaculum as the roof and the abductor hallucis with its investing fascia.
- Patients often complain of burning, tingling, or numbness on plantar aspect of foot and may have night pain or discomfort with even light bedcovers.

Physical Examination

- Examination may demonstrate a positive Tinel sign at the tarsal tunnel or reproduction of symptoms with compression for 60 seconds.
- Other causes of peripheral neuropathy should be considered such as diabetes, hypothyroidism, and alcoholism.
- Electrodiagnostic studies are helpful in differentiating tarsal tunnel syndrome from peripheral neuropathy or lumbosacral radiculopathy.

Treatment

- Conservative treatment consists of avoidance of aggravating activities and control of generalized edema, if present, with medications or compressive stockings as indicated. Arch supports or medial heel wedges may help alleviate symptoms. A NSAID or injection of corticosteroid into the tarsal tunnel is often of benefit to patients with tenosynovitis.
- Surgical management consists of complete release of the tibial nerve and all its branches and has been shown to result in improved outcome measures after failure of conservative management (12).

Plantar Fasciitis

- Insertional plantar fasciitis is the most common cause of plantar heel pain. Repetitive or acute trauma leads to microtears at the calcaneal insertion of the plantar fascia. The patient often describes the pain as worse with the "first step in the morning."
- A variation of insertional plantar fasciitis is a posterior fourchette (PF) tear. In this condition, the plantar fascia is acutely torn.
- An infrequent but unique cause of plantar heel pain that can be confused with plantar fasciitis is fat pad insufficiency. This condition is often seen in older athletes or in patients after multiple corticosteroid injections to the heel. Other causes of heel pain should be excluded prior to making the diagnosis of fat pad atrophy. Treatment consists of a viscoelastic heel cup and well-cushioned shoes (6,14).

Physical Examination

- Patients with insertional plantar fasciitis typically present with pain localized to the plantar medial heel. The pain is often worse with the first few steps in the morning or after rest.
- In a PF tear, a palpable defect in the plantar fascia may be appreciated. A loss of arch height may be appreciated in cases of complete tear.

Radiographic Examination

- Standing AP, lateral, and oblique radiographs show a plantar heel spur in 50% of patients with insertional plantar fasciitis and 15% of asymptomatic patients.
- A bone scan can help differentiate plantar fasciitis from calcaneal stress fracture.

Treatment

- The primary treatment of plantar fasciitis is nonoperative, consisting of Achilles and plantar fascia stretching and activity modification.
- Home stretching has been shown to be just as effective as PT (14).
- Hand massage, ice massage, or anti-inflammatories may also be helpful. Cushioned heel cups are often prescribed.
- Injection of corticosteroids with local anesthetic may be considered after failure of other methods. Repeat steroid injections may cause atrophy of the heel fat pad and should be avoided.
- PRP injection may be considered with promising outcomes (15).
- Ninety-five percent of patients with plantar fasciitis will have resolution of their symptoms within 12–18 months.
- For the 5% of patients who fail conservative treatment, surgical release of the plantar fascia may be considered.
- Although surgery generally results in improvement in symptoms, patients should be counseled that recovery can be prolonged and that exercises to maintain Achilles length must be continued.

Insertional Achilles Tendinitis/Tendinosis

- The most common site of posterior heel pain is in the area of the insertion of the Achilles tendon. Factors that predispose this area to pathology include the hypovascular nature of the distal Achilles tendon, the repetitive forces seen at the bone tendon interface, and the prominence of the area becoming irritated with shoe wear.
- Insertional Achilles tendinitis is a common condition in jumping athletes but may also be precipitated by a direct blow or poorly fitting shoes.
- Patients with this condition may complain of pain at the distal portion of the Achilles tendon and note weakness in plantar flexion.
- Acute inflammation is tendinitis, whereas tendinosis refers to the more chronic condition where intratendinous degeneration instead of inflammation counts for the pain.

Physical Examination

- On examination, there is tenderness to palpation directly over the insertion of the Achilles tendon. The patient with this condition may also experience pain with resisted plantar flexion.

Treatment

- Initial treatment is conservative with NSAIDs and activity modification. Felt or Silipos pads placed over the posterior heel may also be beneficial.
- Corticosteroid injections have been associated with tendon rupture and are discouraged.
- The first-line treatment of chronic tendinosis is eccentric stretching; extracorperal shochwave can also be considered (16)
- Operative intervention may be indicated in select cases after a 6-month trial on nonoperative care. Surgical options include Achilles tendon debridement and flexor hallucis longus tendon transfer.

Retrocalcaneal Bursitis

- The retrocalcaneal bursa is a synovial-lined bursa between the posterior calcaneus and the Achilles tendon.
- Patients with this condition frequently present with posterior heel pain and direct tenderness to palpation of the posterior heel.

- Frequently, patients with retrocalcaneal bursitis have an associated pathologic prominence of the posterior superior aspect of the calcaneal tuberosity. This prominence is commonly referred to as a Haglund deformity and is often associated with rigid shoe wear.

Physical Examination

- On examination, there is generally tenderness to palpation just proximal to the insertion of the Achilles tendon. The patient may also demonstrate weakness with plantar flexion of the ankle.
- Patients with an associated Haglund deformity may have a visible prominence at the insertion of the Achilles tendon.

Radiographic Examination

- Standard weight-bearing AP, oblique, and lateral x-rays should be obtained in the initial evaluation. In cases with an associated Haglund deformity, a prominence of the posterior superior portion of the calcaneal tuberosity will be seen on the lateral view.

Treatment

- The initial treatment generally consists of rest, ice, heel cord stretches, and shoe modification.
- In cases that have failed a trial of nonoperative treatment, a bursectomy or surgical excision of the Haglund deformity may be required (17).
- Arthroscopic excision can be performed in select cases.

SOFT-TISSUE INJURIES OF THE FOREFOOT

- The forefoot consists of the metatarsals and phalanges and their corresponding articulations. Injury in this region of the lower extremity is common in both the recreational and competitive athlete.
- During ambulation, the contact forces are equally distributed among the second through fifth metatarsal heads and two sesamoids.
- Because of the higher loads distributed across the first metatarsal phalangeal joint in weight-bearing activities, the great toe is commonly injured.

Hallux Rigidus

- Hallux rigidus is a common disorder, seen in about 1 in 45 individuals over the age of 50. It is characterized by limitation of motion of the first metatarsophalangeal (MTP) joint, particularly in dorsiflexion.
- Patients present complaining of limitation of motion and pain at the MTP joint with ambulation or athletic activity.
- Hallux rigidus has been attributed to many causes, including trauma, inflammatory or metabolic conditions, and congenital disorders.

Physical Examination

- Patients with hallux rigidus will demonstrate pain with both active and passive motion of the first MTP joint. Occasionally, a palpable dorsal exostosis may also be present over the dorsal aspect of the joint.
- Cases with a large exostosis may demonstrate irritation of the overlying skin from improperly fitting shoe wear.

Radiographic Examination

- Weight-bearing AP, oblique, and lateral x-rays obtained during the initial evaluation of hallux rigidus may demonstrate narrowing of the first MTP joint as well as a dorsal osteophyte.

Treatment

- Initial treatment is nonoperative, consisting of NSAIDs and avoidance of high-impact activities.
- A steel or fiberglass shank in the sole of the shoe can relieve symptoms by limiting dorsiflexion. Rocker-bottom shoes and custom insoles may have a similar effect.
- Failure of nonoperative treatment is an indication for surgery. Surgical treatment can consist of cheilectomy for active athletes and arthrodesis for more severe cases.

Hallux Valgus

- Hallux valgus, or bunion deformity, is common in the general population and occurs in athletes as well. Hallux valgus in athletes demands different considerations and treatment than in the general population.
- Hallux valgus occurs with lateral deviation of the great toe and progressive subluxation of the first MTP joint. The medial eminence of the first MTP joint becomes prominent. The overlying soft tissue becomes irritated, swollen, and inflamed, creating the bunion (from the Greek for turnip).
- Several intrinsic and extrinsic factors may contribute to hallux valgus. The most important extrinsic factor is constricting footwear. Shoes with heels and a narrow toe box have been associated with bunions. Athletic activities that increase the lateral stress on the first MTP joint can be another extrinsic cause. Intrinsic factors include a pronated foot, contracted heel cord, hypermobility of the first metatarsocuneiform joint, and metatarsus primus varus. Injury to the first MTP joint, such as turf toe or first MTP dislocation, may weaken the joint capsule and collateral ligament, predisposing to hallux valgus.
- Patients typically present complaining of pain over the medial eminence and irritation with shoe wear. The skin and bursa over the medial eminence may be irritated.

Physical Examination

- The patient's feet should be examined sitting and standing. Standing may accentuate the deformity.
- Range of motion at the first MTP should be noted, as well as any hypermobility at the metatarsocuneiform joint. The foot should be examined for pes planus and pronation.

Radiographic Examination

- Radiographic evaluation consists of AP, lateral, and sesamoid views with the patient standing.
- The angle formed by the proximal phalanx and first metatarsal, or hallux valgus angle, is measured. A normal hallux valgus angle is less than 15°. An angle between 15° and 20° is considered mild hallux valgus. Moderate deformity is characterized by a hallux valgus angle between 20° and 40°, with an angle greater than 40° being severe deformity.
- Other radiographic angles measured include the intermetatarsal angle between the shafts of the first and second metatarsal and the distal metatarsal articular angle, a measurement of joint congruity.

Treatment

- The initial treatment of hallux valgus is nonoperative and consists of shoe wear modification. Irritation of the medial eminence may be relieved with a wider toe box, shoe stretching, or pads around the bunion. Patients with pes planus may benefit from an orthosis.
- Contracture of the Achilles tendon, if present, should be treated appropriately.
- Persistent pain after exhausting nonoperative treatment options is an indication for surgery.
- Surgery can result in not only correction of deformity and pain relief but also postoperative restriction of MTP motion, which should be considered by athletes requiring a great range of MTP motion, such as dancers and sprinters (18).

Turf Toe

- Injury to the first MTP joint has ranked third in collegiate athletes after knee and ankle injuries.
- Turf toe represents an acute injury to the plantar MTP capsuloligamentous structures of the great toe.
- The most common mechanism of injury is when an axial load is delivered to the heel with the ankle plantarflexed and the great toe in dorsiflexion.
- Turf toe is classified into three grades. In grade I, the plantar tissues are stretched but remain intact, and symptoms are minimal. There may be minor swelling but no ecchymosis. Grade II injuries represent a partial tear of the capsule. Symptoms are pain, swelling, ecchymosis, and restricted motion. The patient will be unable to perform at their usual level of sport. Grade III injuries are complete capsuloligamentous tears. There may have been an occult MTP dislocation that spontaneously reduced.

Physical Examination

- On physical examination, there may be swelling or ecchymosis about the MTP joint on inspection. The patient may also demonstrate pain with passive motion and tenderness to palpation. In more severe injuries, there may be instability of the MTP joint.

Radiographic Examination

- X-rays of the affected foot may reveal proximal migration of the sesamoids on the AP view or a lag in sesamoid tracking on the lateral view.
- X-rays of the uninjured foot may be helpful for comparative purposes to evaluate for proximal migration of the sesamoids.
- MRI may reveal increased uptake or frank disruption of the plantar capsuloligamentous structures.

Treatment

- Treatment is generally conservative, consisting of rest, ice, elevation, and possibly anti-inflammatory drugs. Buddy taping or rigid orthoses to limit MTP motion may also provide symptomatic relief.
- Intra-articular steroid injections should be avoided as they mask symptoms.
- Operative treatment may be indicated in patients with sesamoid retraction, joint instability, or symptoms refractory to conservative management.
- Turf toe injuries may predispose toward osteoarthritis of the first MTP joint and hallux rigidus (19,20).

Metatarsalgia

- Metatarsalgia is a descriptive term for pain beneath the metatarsal heads that may have a number of etiologies including stress fracture, synovitis, deformity of the metatarsals, or neuroma.
- Forefoot pain has been associated with tightness of the gastrocnemius-soleus complex. Patients presenting with forefoot or midfoot symptoms have less dorsiflexion on average than asymptomatic controls (21).
- Synovitis of the MTP joint most commonly affects the second metatarsal. It occurs most frequently in middle-aged athletes. Symptoms typically include pain in the forefoot exacerbated by running, walking, or forced dorsiflexion of the MTP joint.
- Interdigital neuroma, or Morton neuroma, is a common cause of forefoot pain that classically presents as neurogenic pain in the ball of the foot between the third and fourth toes. It is thought to be caused by irritation of the interdigital nerve as it passes beneath the deep transverse metatarsal ligament. It occurs in all populations but is most frequently reported in runners and dancers.

Physical Examination

- On examination, there may be swelling dorsally or tenderness to palpation of the MTP joint in cases of MTP synovitis.
- In cases of interdigital neuroma, palpation of the interspace while compressing the forefoot by pressing on the first and fifth metatarsal heads may reproduce the pain.

Radiographic Examination

- Weight-bearing radiographs of the foot should be obtained to rule out joint degeneration, deformity, and metatarsal stress fracture.
- Cases of MTP joint synovitis may demonstrate joint space widening.

Treatment

- Treatment is initially conservative, including activity modification, shock-absorbing insoles, and NSAIDs. Additionally, in cases of interdigital neuroma, avoiding heels or shoes with narrow toe boxes may decrease extrinsic compression on the nerve. In cases where shoe modification has failed, injection of corticosteroid with local anesthetic may give lasting or permanent relief.
- In cases of MTP synovitis, surgical management may be necessary with failure of conservative treatment and development of deformity (22).
- Excision of the neuroma has demonstrated good pain relief in 80% of patients (23).

REFERENCES

1. Pedowitz RA, Hargens AR, Mubarak SJ, Gershuni DH. Modified criteria for the objective diagnosis of chronic compartment syndrome of the leg. *Am J Sports Med.* 1990;18(1):35–40.
2. George CA, Hutchinson MR. Chronic exertional compartment syndrome. *Clin Sports Med.* 2012;31(2):307–19.
3. Neubauer TM, Chin JJ, Hill RD, Hu YE. Popliteal artery entrapment syndrome: updates for evaluation, diagnosis, and treatment. *Curr Sports Med Rep.* 2024 Sep;23(9):310–15.
4. Espinosa N, Maurer MA. Stage I and II posterior tibial tendon dysfunction: return to running? *Clin Sports Med.* 2015;34(4):761–8.
5. Kijowski R, De Smet A, Mukharjee R. Magnetic resonance imaging findings in patients with peroneal tendinopathy and peroneal tenosynovitis. *Skeletal Radiol.* 2007;36(2):105–14.
6. Dallaudière B, Pesquer L, Meyer P, et al. Intratendinous injection of platelet-rich plasma under US guidance to treat tendinopathy: a long-term pilot study. *J Vasc Interv Radiol.* 2014;25(5):717–23.
7. Lugo-Pico JG, Kaiser JT, Sanchez RA, Aiyer AA. Peroneal tendinosis and subluxation. *Clin Sports Med.* 2020;39(4):845–58.
8. Nault ML, Kocher MS, Micheli LJ. Os trigonum syndrome. *J Am Acad Orthop Surg.* 2014;22(9):545–53.
9. Rungprai C, Tennant JN, Phisitkul P. Disorders of the flexor hallucis longus and Os trigonum. *Clin Sports Med.* 2015;34(4):741–59.
10. Sharpe BD, Steginsky BD, Suhling M, Vora A. Posterior ankle impingement and flexor hallucis longus pathology. *Clin Sports Med.* 2020;39(4):911–30.
11. Peck E, Finnoff JT, Smith J. Neuropathies in runners. *Clin Sports Med.* 2010;29(3):437–57.
12. Ferkel E, Davis WH, Ellington JK. Entrapment neuropathies of the foot and ankle. *Clin Sports Med.* 2015;34(4):791–801.
13. Pomeroy G, Wilton J, Anthony S. Entrapment neuropathy about the foot and ankle: an update. *J Am Acad Orthop Surg.* 2015;23(1):58–66.
14. Kaiser PB, Keyser C, Crawford AM, Bluman EM, Smith JT, Chiodo CP. A prospective randomized controlled trial comparing physical therapy with independent home stretching for plantar fasciitis. *J Am Acad Orthop Surg.* 2022;30(14):682–9.
15. Hohmann E, Tetsworth K, Glatt V. Platelet-rich plasma versus corticosteroids for the treatment of plantar fasciitis: a systematic review and meta-analysis. *Am J Sports Med.* 2021;49(5):1381–93.
16. Chen J, Janney CF, Khalid MA, Panchbhavi VK. Management of insertional achilles tendinopathy. *J Am Acad Orthop Surg.* 2022;30(10):e751–9.
17. Okewunmi J, Guzman J, Vulcano E. Achilles tendinosis injuries-tendinosis to rupture (getting the athlete back to play). *Clin Sports Med.* 2020;39(4):877–91.
18. Fournier M, Saxena A, Maffulli N. Hallux valgus surgery in the athlete: current evidence. *J Foot Ankle Surg.* 2019;58(4):641–3.
19. Mason LW, Molloy AP. Turf toe and disorders of the sesamoid complex. *Clin Sports Med.* 2015;34(4):725–39.
20. Nihal A, Trepman E, Nag D. First ray disorders in athletes. *Sports Med Arthrosc Rev.* 2009;17(3):160–6.
21. Digiovani CW, Kuo R, Tejwani N, et al. Isolated gastrocnemius tightness. *J Bone Joint Surg Am.* 2002;84-A(6):962–70.
22. Espinosa N, Brodsky JW, Maceira E. Metatarsalgia. *J Am Acad Orthop Surg.* 2010;18(8):474–85.
23. Kay D, Bennett GL. Morton's neuroma. *Foot Ankle Clin.* 2003;8(1):49–59.

Foot and Ankle Fractures

69

Arjun Srinath and Tyler Kalbac

ANKLE FRACTURES

- The ankle is the most commonly injured weight-bearing joint. The annual incidence is between 71 and 187 per 100,000 people (1).
- A great deal of research has been conducted to determine the incidence of age-related fractures, particularly in the elderly population. Barrett et al. (2) analyzed Medicare data in 1999 and found that ankle fractures were the fourth most common fracture in the elderly population (65–90 years of age). The study also demonstrated that elderly African Americans were less likely than Caucasians to fracture the ankle.

Physical Examination

- The examination of the ankle should begin with a thorough visual inspection noting abnormal swelling, redness, or deformities. The physician should also palpate the ankle to determine the extent of any swelling, identify any abnormal bony prominences or incongruities, determine specific areas of point tenderness or extreme pain, and evaluate the neurovascular status of the patient.
- The neurovascular examination should include an assessment of the dorsalis pedis and posterior tibial pulses. In addition, the physician should evaluate the capillary refill, light touch, and two-point discrimination distal to the ankle.
- Gross deformity of the ankle is a likely indicator of dislocation. Radiographs should be obtained prior to attempted reduction to identify the injury pattern, except in the case of neurovascular compromise. The injury should be reduced and splinted; repeat radiographs should then be obtained to assess the reduction as well as the injury pattern.
- The physician will then evaluate the range of motion of the ankle. The normal range of ankle motion is 30° of dorsiflexion and 45° of plantarflexion. The range of motion necessary for ankle functionality or ambulation is 10° of dorsiflexion and 20° of plantarflexion (3).
- It is important to evaluate the stability of the ankle when suspecting a fracture. The squeeze test is performed to rule out disruption of the tibiofibular syndesmosis. The squeeze test is performed by squeezing the leg, approximating the tibia and fibula, at or slightly above the level of the belly of the gastrocnemius. An indicator of syndesmotic disruption is pain at the distal tibiofibular articulation when the squeeze test is performed (4). The physician should also perform an anterior drawer test and talar tilt test to evaluate the laxity of the complex ligamentous support network of the ankle. Pain with dorsiflexion and external rotation should also be noted because this may represent posterior bony injury or tendinous disruption. In addition, the lateral drawer test has been shown to correlate with findings of ankle instability in isolated Weber B ankle fracture. The maneuver is performed when the examiner uses one hand to stabilize the leg while the other hand grips the hindfoot and performs a direct lateral stress on a neutrally positioned ankle to assess for translational movement (5).

Radiographic Examination

- The *Ottawa ankle rules* are a valuable guideline in determining the need for radiographic examination in a patient suspected to have an ankle fracture. Radiographic examination is required if the patient is unable to bear weight, if the patient has pain with palpation within 6 cm proximal or distal to the talar articulation, or if the patient has bony tenderness at the posterior edge or tip of either malleolus (6).
- The ankle is best examined radiographically with an anteroposterior (AP), lateral, and mortise view. Three-view radiographs demonstrate greater reliability when compared to various combinations of two-view radiographs (7). Abnormal radiographic findings are greater than 2 mm of talar tilt (difference in lateral and medial joint spaces in AP view), misalignment of the talar dome under the tibia in AP or lateral views, widening of the medial clear space greater than 5 mm, and a demonstrated tibiofibular overlap of less than 10 mm on the AP view or the mortise view (1). Stress radiographs may be valuable but are difficult to standardize. Patients are most tolerant of the gravity stress test whereby a mortise view of the ankle is obtained with the patient lying on their injured side and their distal tibia and injured ankle off the table unsupported (8). Although normative data are not adequately reported in the literature, the Telos stress device is being used to standardize the amount of stress about the ankle during routine radiographic stress examinations.
- In addition to dedicated ankle radiographs, full length tibia and fibula radiographs are important to identify potential proximal extension of rotational ankle injuries (1).

- Magnetic resonance imaging (MRI) is best suited for the examination of the integrity of the ankle ligaments, and an MRI is the preferred imaging study to rule out osteochondral lesions in patients with chronic ankle injuries (9).

CLASSIFICATION

- There are three primary classification systems used to define ankle fractures. The Danis-Weber classification is based on the level of an isolated lateral malleolus fracture. The Lauge-Hansen classification describes the ankle fracture according to foot position and movement of the foot in relation to the leg (supination-adduction, supination-external rotation, pronation-abduction, pronation-eversion, and pronation-dorsiflexion). Last, the AO classification is based on the level of the fibula fracture, medial malleolar involvement, and syndesmotic disruption (1). A summary of the aforementioned classifications can be found in Table 69.1.

Treatment

- The goal of treatment of ankle fractures is to restore the anatomic congruity of the ankle joint, promote pain-free restoration of range of motion, and restore and maintain fibular length.
- Nondisplaced, stable ankle fractures with intact deep deltoid and stable mortise on stress examination can be managed nonoperatively with great success. Stable ankle fractures can be treated with weight-bearing as tolerated with immobilization in a controlled ankle motion boot (CAM) or walking cast for approximately 4–6 weeks (10). Diabetics are a special subgroup of patients who may need more time in the short leg cast or CAM boot before adequate bone growth is evident. Diabetes mellitus does increase risks associated with both nonsurgical and surgical treatment of ankle fractures; however, this should not prevent patients from undergoing surgical treatment when necessary. Patients with diabetes mellitus have a higher risk of failed nonsurgical treatment due to their neuropathy and difficulty to maintain weight-bearing

Table 69.1 Classification Systems of Ankle Fractures

Fracture Classification	Type	Location of Fracture	Associated Injuries
Danis-Weber	A	Below ankle mortise and tibiofibular articulation	Syndesmosis likely intact
	B	At level of mortise and tibiofibular articulation	Syndesmosis likely intact
	C	Above level of mortise and tibiofibular articulation	Likely disruption of syndesmosis with positive squeeze test
Lauge-Hansen	Supination-adduction	Transverse fracture of lateral malleolus	Stage 1: Tear of lateral ligaments
			Stage 2: Fracture of medial malleolus
	Supination-external rotation	Avulsion fracture of lateral malleolus	Stage 1: Rupture of anterior tibiofibular ligament
			Stage 2: Spiral or oblique fracture of lateral malleolus
			Stage 3: Posterior tibial fracture
			Stage 4: Fracture of medial malleolus or torn deltoid ligament
	Pronation-abduction	Medial malleolus	Stage 1: Torn deltoid ligament
			Stage 2: Syndesmotic disruption and posterior tibial fracture
			Stage 3: Oblique fracture of fibula above mortise
	Pronation-external rotation	Medial malleolus	Stage 1: Torn deltoid ligament
			Stage 2: Syndesmotic disruption
			Stage 3: Spiral fracture of fibula above mortise
			Stage 4: Posterior tibial fracture
AO	A	Fibula at or below plafond	Intact or possible avulsions medial and posterior
	B	Fibula at plafond extending proximally	Tibiofibular ligaments torn; possible avulsions medially and posteriorly
		Fibula above plafond	Syndesmosis always torn; deltoid ligament torn

restrictions. Surgical indications are the same for patient with or without diabetes mellitus (11).

- Displaced, unstable, open, or unreducible ankle fractures must be treated operatively with reduction and internal or external fixation (10).
- Open fractures require emergent orthopedic consult, and it is very likely that these patients will be taken to the operating room urgently. Recent literature shows that early administration of antibiotics within 3 hours from injury is the most important factor in preventing infection after open fracture (12). Specifically, regarding open ankle fractures, these injuries require operative irrigation and debridement followed by early definitive open reduction and internal fixation (ORIF) versus external fixation with delayed ORIF.
- The most important aspects of ankle fracture management are to perform early reduction of ankle injuries, obtain three-view radiographs of the injured ankle along with full-length tibia films, clean and dress open wounds in a proper sterile fashion, document and evaluate neurovascular status, and apply a posterior splint with a U-shaped component at the ankle when transporting the patient or preparing them for further workup by an orthopedic surgeon.

FOOT FRACTURES

- The foot comprises a total of 26 bones. The hindfoot consists of the talus and calcaneus, whereas the midfoot includes the navicular, cuboid, and cuneiforms, and their articulations with the metatarsal bases. The metatarsals and phalanges make up the forefoot.
- Most foot injuries involve innocuous sprains; however, a small percentage of them involve significant injuries with subtle radiographic findings. Foot injuries involving the talus and tarsometatarsal joints are the most often misdiagnosed. The rarity of these injuries limits physician familiarity and accounts for frequent misdiagnosis (13).

FRACTURES OF THE TALUS

- Fractures of the talus are uncommon injuries only accounting for 3%–6% of all foot fractures (14), and accounting for 0.1%–0.85% of all fractures (15).
- The talus has five articulating surfaces as 60% of the talus is covered with articular cartilage. There are no muscle or tendinous attachments. Blood supply to the talus is tenuous, and fractures can easily disrupt the blood supply, resulting in osteonecrosis (13,16).
- Talus fractures can occur at the talar head, neck, body, or lateral or posterior processes. An os trigonum remains a separate ossicle in 14% of normal feet and can sometimes be mistaken for an acute fracture posterior to the lateral tubercle of the talus (13).

Physical Examination

- Patients with fractures of the talus may present with swelling and ecchymosis of the hindfoot or midfoot. Pain with palpation or with motion of the hindfoot should raise suspicion for the presence of a fracture.

Radiographic Examination

- Physicians evaluating talus fractures should obtain three-view radiographs of both the foot and the ankle. The Canale view can provide an optimal view of the talar neck (13). This is performed with the foot placed flat on the cassette and the ankle in equinus and pronated 15° with the beam directed 15° cephalad from the vertical (Fig. 69.1).
- Computed tomography (CT) is indicated when displacement cannot be ruled out with plain radiographs. A CT will assist with characterization of fracture patterns, displacement, and articular involvement. The role of bone scans or MRI is limited to the evaluation of occult fractures or osteochondral lesions of the talus (OLT).

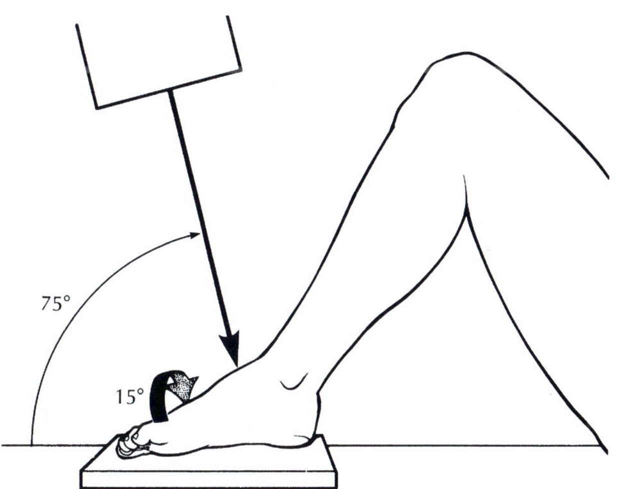

Figure 69.1: Correct position of the foot for x-ray evaluation of the talar neck. (From Bucholz RW, Heckman JD. *Rockwood & Green's Fractures in Adults*. 5th ed. Philadelphia (PA): Lippincott Williams & Wilkins; 2001.)

Talar Neck Fractures

- Most fractures of the talar neck occur from a forced dorsiflexion injury against the anterior margin of the tibia that usually occurs from a motor vehicle accident or fall.
- The Hawkins fracture classification system may be used to guide treatment decisions and predict the risk of osteonecrosis (17). Fracture classification is based on displacement and articular surface involvement (Fig. 69.2). Displaced fractures may injure arteries of the tarsal canal or tarsal sinus, placing the talar body at risk for osteonecrosis.
- Vallier further identified initial fracture displacement and complete joint dislocation as predictors of osteonecrosis (17).
- Nonsurgical treatment is reserved for type I nondisplaced fractures without comminution or articular step-off. Treatment consists of a short leg cast and non–weight-bearing. Nondisplaced fractures must be followed closely with serial radiographs to ensure that the fracture does not displace during nonoperative management (14).
- Operative intervention is indicated for all displaced fractures of the talar neck. Urgent surgical treatment is required when subluxation or dislocation leads to soft-tissue compromise.

Talar Body Fractures

- Talar body fractures are less common than fractures of the talar neck and are usually the result of high-energy injuries during which a rapid deceleration and direct axial load is placed on the injured limb (18).
- Radiographs may underestimate the amount of articular involvement, indicating the need to obtain a CT to identify the fracture pattern and amount of comminution. These fractures can be classified according to their anatomic location.
- ORIF is indicated when there a block to normal motion, there is presence of intra-articular debris, or if the articular surfaces are displaced more than 2 mm (19).

Talar Head Fractures

- Talar head fractures are the least common subtype of talus fractures. These fractures typically result from plantarflexion and compression along the longitudinal axis of the forefoot.
- Radiographic examination should include a careful evaluation of the talonavicular joint for associated navicular injuries or talonavicular joint disruption.
- Nonsurgical treatment consisting of immobilization and non–weight-bearing is indicated for nondisplaced fractures. For displaced fractures, the talonavicular joint should be reduced and the fracture fragments stabilized.

Lateral Process Fractures of the Talus

- Lateral process fractures occur with dorsiflexion and external rotation and most commonly occur during snowboarding. These fractures may be seen on the AP view of the ankle; however, they typically require a CT scan. Physicians should have a high index of suspicion for this injury in patients who

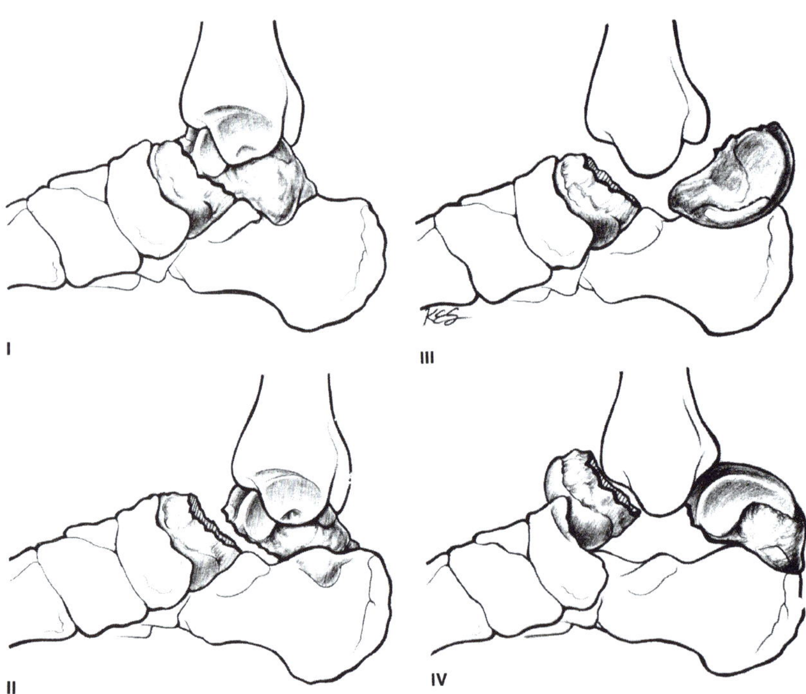

Figure 69.2: Diagrammatic representation of Hawkins classification of talar neck fractures. I nondisplaced; II displaced with associated subtalar joint subluxation; III talar body dislocated from the ankle mortise; IV talonavicular joint subluxated also. (From Hansen ST, Swiontkowski MF. *Orthopaedic Trauma Protocols*. New York (NY): Raven; 1993. 340 p, with permission.)

have anterolateral ankle pain and normal plain radiographs following an ankle injury while snowboarding.

- Nondisplaced lateral process fractures are commonly treated with a period of cast immobilization and non–weight-bearing. ORIF is indicated for fractures displaced more than 2 mm. Comminuted fractures not amenable to ORIF can be treated with casting or excision (20).

Posterior Process Fractures of the Talus

- The posterior process includes the posteromedial and posterolateral tubercles, which are separated by a groove for the flexor hallucis longus tendon. A CT scan is recommended for fractures through this area because they are difficult to visualize on plain radiographs (21).
- Posteromedial tubercle fractures typically occur from an avulsion of the posterior tibiotalar ligament or posterior deltoid ligament. Small avulsion fractures are treated with casting and non–weight-bearing. Large, displaced fragments are treated with ORIF.
- The posterolateral tubercle fractures are usually an avulsion of the posterior talofibular ligament. Clinically, the patient may exhibit pain with flexion and extension of the great toe caused by the flexor hallucis longus rubbing along the fracture fragment.
- Posterolateral tubercle fractures with no subtalar involvement are best treated with nonsurgical management. If there is subtalar involvement, then ORIF is warranted.

FRACTURES OF THE CALCANEUS

- The calcaneus is the most frequently fractured tarsal bone and accounts for 2% of fractures overall. Between 60% and 75% are displaced intra-articular fractures, with open injuries occurring between 7% and 15% of the time. The primary mechanism of injury is an axial load as a result of a fall from a height or motor vehicle accident (3).
- Calcaneus fractures are most common in young, male laborers. These injuries have a profound impact and many patients never return to preinjury employment or activity levels. Short Form (SF)-36 scores for patients with calcaneus fractures at 2 years after injury show similar functional levels to patients who had myocardial infarction or underwent organ transplantation (22).
- The calcaneus has three facets along its superior articular surface with the talus. These include the anterior, middle, and posterior facets. The middle facet lies over the sustentaculum tali and is separated from the posterior facet by the sinus tarsi and its corresponding artery. The posterior facet is the largest of the three facets and is the primary weight-bearing surface (19).

Physical Examination

- Patients with calcaneus fractures typically present with significant swelling and severe heel pain. Ecchymosis around the heel and foot arch is highly suggestive of a fracture of the calcaneus. Fracture blisters are common. To minimize soft-tissue compromise, the foot should be elevated and immediately splinted with the ankle in a neutral position (23).
- Physicians evaluating these injuries should carefully evaluate patients for any neurovascular injury, compartment syndrome, or skin disruption. Wounds associated with open calcaneus fractures typically occur medially (24). Compartment syndrome develops in up to 10% of patients and could lead to a hammer toe deformity (23).
- Associated injuries occur nearly 50% of the time in patients with calcaneus fractures. A thorough exam should be performed on all joints above and below the injury, along with an exam of the lower back. Ten percent of patients with calcaneus fractures also have fractures of the lumbar spine, and 25% have concomitant injuries in the lower extremities (3).

Radiographic Examination

- For patients with a suspected fracture of the calcaneus, appropriate radiographs should include AP, lateral, and oblique views of the foot and ankle, in addition to a Harris axial view. The Harris view helps visualize widening, shortening, or varus position of a tuberosity fragment. This view is obtained with the heel against the plate and the ankle in dorsiflexion. The x-ray beam is aimed approximately 30° cephalad toward the heel of the foot.
- A CT scan is the most complete and reliable means of visualizing and classifying calcaneal fractures. Coronal views are best for evaluating the articular surfaces as well as the position of the peroneal and flexor hallucis tendons. Axial and sagittal views will help evaluate the congruency of the calcaneocuboid joint as well as the posterior facet and calcaneal tuberosity (3,25).
- Other important fracture characteristics include the degree of shortening, widening, and lateral wall displacement, which may cause injury to the peroneal tendons.

Extra-articular Fractures of the Calcaneus

- Extra-articular fractures include the anterior process, tuberosity, medial process, sustentacular, and body fractures. These injuries often occur in patients with osteopenic bone, making secure fixation difficult.
- Tuberosity fractures result from a strong contraction of the gastrocnemius–soleus complex with avulsion at its insertion. This mechanism can create a pattern called the "tongue-type fracture" whereby the posterior tuberosity is displaced superiorly often resulting in skin compromise and necrosis. This pattern if often managed with urgent orthopedic surgery consultation and surgical intervention. Depending on the size of the displaced fragment, surgery may require excision of the fragment versus ORIF (26).
- Anterior process fractures occur with inversion and plantarflexion and result from avulsion of the bifurcate ligament.

Small extra-articular fragments can be treated with casting. Fragments larger than 1 cm may involve the calcaneocuboid joint and require ORIF if joint displacement is present (23).

Intra-articular Fractures of the Calcaneus

- The Sanders classification for calcaneal fractures uses a 30° semicoronal CT to visualize the subtalar joint at its widest point in the coronal plane (Fig. 69.3). Types are based on the number of articular fragments, which may guide treatment options and help predict treatment outcomes (25,27).
- Nonsurgical treatment is reserved for type I nondisplaced fractures. Patients should not bear weight for 10–12 weeks, and range-of-motion exercises are initiated once soft-tissue swelling allows.
- Surgical indications include the following: displaced intra-articular fractures of the posterior facet, fragments with greater than 25% of calcaneocuboid articulation involvement, displaced fractures of the tuberosity, fracture dislocations, and selected open fractures. ORIF generally is delayed for 2–3 weeks to allow for resolution of soft-tissue swelling (23).
- Negative prognostic factors include severity, advanced age, male sex, obesity, bilateral fractures, multiple traumas, tobacco use, and worker's compensation (28).
- A complication rate of up to 40% has been reported. Factors that predict an increased risk of complications include a fall from a height, early surgery, and smoking. Outcomes correlate with the accuracy of the reduction and the number of articular fragments. Type II fractures have better outcomes than type III fractures, whereas type IV fractures have the worst outcomes. Wound-related complications are the most common. Other potential complications include malunion, subtalar arthritis, and lateral impingement with peroneal tendon pathology.

MIDFOOT FRACTURES

- Fractures of the midfoot are relatively uncommon. The bones of the midfoot include the navicular, cuboid, cuneiforms, and bases of the metatarsals. The midfoot has osseous stability due to the recessed articulation of the base of the second metatarsal. The trapezoidal shape of the first three metatarsal bases contributes to stability, as do the plantar ligaments. The calcaneocuboid and talonavicular joints make up the midtarsal joint, whereas the Lisfranc joint complex is between the tarsi and the first two metatarsals (29).
- Most midfoot fractures are a result of high-energy trauma from a motor vehicle collision or the lower energy combination of an axial load and twisting of the foot during an athletic event.

Physical Examination

- When examining a patient with a potential midfoot injury, it is important to recognize there is a wide range of injury severity and patient presentation. Injuries may involve a spectrum of pathology from a simple sprain to a complex midfoot fracture/dislocation.

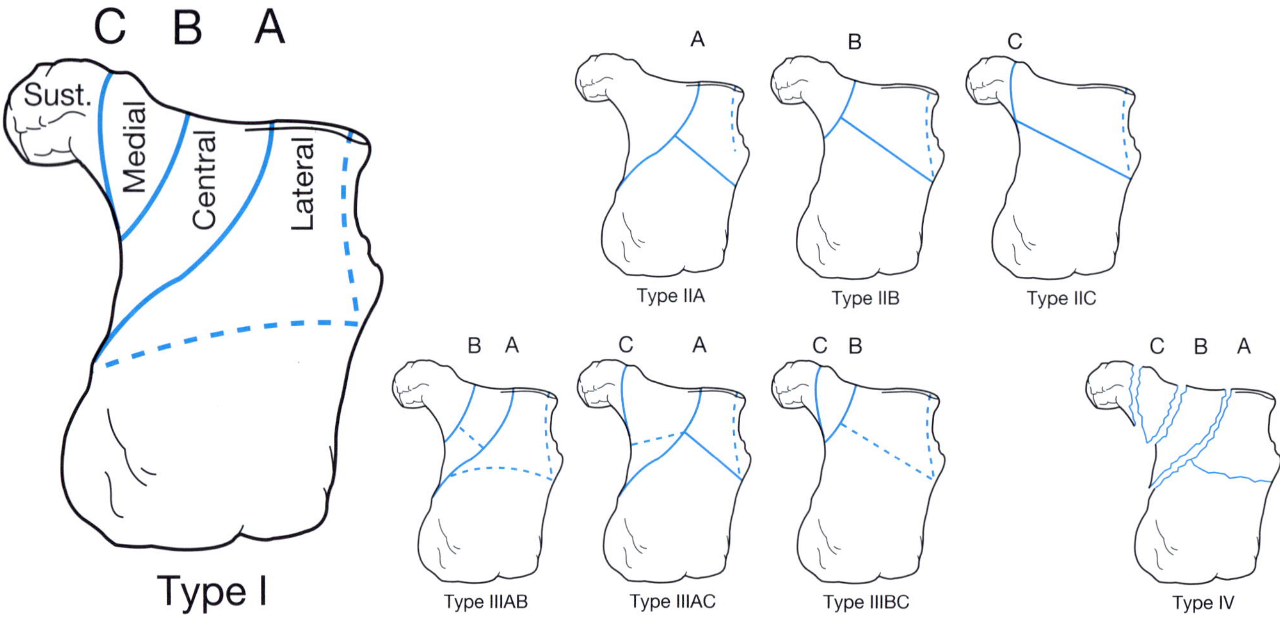

Figure 69.3: Schematic depiction of Sanders classification of intra-articular fractures of the calcaneus. Fracture lines A, B, and C describe the position of the primary fracture line in relation to the posterior facet and the subtalar joint. Types II and III have two or three fragments. Type IV represents severe comminution. (From Bucholz RW, Heckman JD. *Rockwood & Green's Fractures in Adults*. 5th ed. Philadelphia (PA): Lippincott Williams & Wilkins; 2001.)

- Physicians should perform and document a careful neurovascular exam. Serial examinations may be warranted to rule out an impending foot compartment syndrome anytime a patient presents with extreme pain and swelling.

Radiographic Examination

- Three-view radiographs should be obtained including an AP, lateral, and oblique view of the foot as well as an AP, lateral, and mortise view of the ankle. If tolerated, then stress views or weight-bearing films can assist with defining subtle injuries.
- Obtaining a CT can help distinguish any articular incongruities or comminution and can help characterize the fracture pattern. MRI is more beneficial for evaluating a potential ligamentous injury or for the detection of stress fractures.

Navicular Fractures

- The navicular articulates with the cuneiforms, cuboid, calcaneus, and talus. The talonavicular articulation is critical to maintaining inversion and eversion range of motion. The blood supply is limited in the central portion of the navicular, making this area susceptible to fractures.
- Avulsion fractures of the navicular are primarily caused by a plantarflexion injury. Acute treatment consists of immobilization with delayed excision of painful fragments. ORIF is required for fractures involving more than 25% of the articular surface (3).
- Tuberosity fractures commonly result from forced eversion and posterior tibial tendon contraction. An oblique radiograph at 45° of internal rotation can be obtained to appreciate the injury. Most tuberosity avulsions can be managed with cast immobilization. Acute ORIF is indicated with more than 5 mm of diastasis or with large intra-articular fragments (30).
- Fractures of the navicular body are usually caused by axial loading. The Sangeorzan fracture classification is based on the plane of the fracture and degree of comminution. Minimally displaced type I and II fractures are treated nonsurgically, whereas ORIF is used for displaced fractures, disruption of the talonavicular joint, comminution, or type III fractures (30).

Lisfranc Joint Injuries

- Lisfranc injuries can lead to chronic disability if they are not appropriately recognized and treated. The Lisfranc ligament runs from the base of the second metatarsal to the medial cuneiform (Fig. 69.4). This injury can be caused directly from a dorsal force or from an indirect injury by axial loading and twisting on a loaded, plantarflexed foot. Patients may report a history of a fixed foot with rotation of the body around the midfoot (31).
- Physicians evaluating for disruption of the Lisfranc ligament should look for diastasis or a small, avulsed fragment of bone between the base of the first and second metatarsals on an AP radiograph. Anatomic alignment should be maintained on the oblique view, and there should be no dorsal subluxation of the metatarsal bases on the lateral. Weight-bearing or stress radiographs will accentuate the deformity and can be ordered when the results of physical examination and plain radiographs are equivocal.
- Treatment consists of ORIF for displaced midfoot fractures and dislocations. Reduction and screw fixation are indicated to stabilize any intercuneiform instability (29).
- Late posttraumatic osteoarthritis is common, occurring in up to 58% of patients. Anatomic reduction, the presence of an open injury, and comminution will affect long-term outcomes.

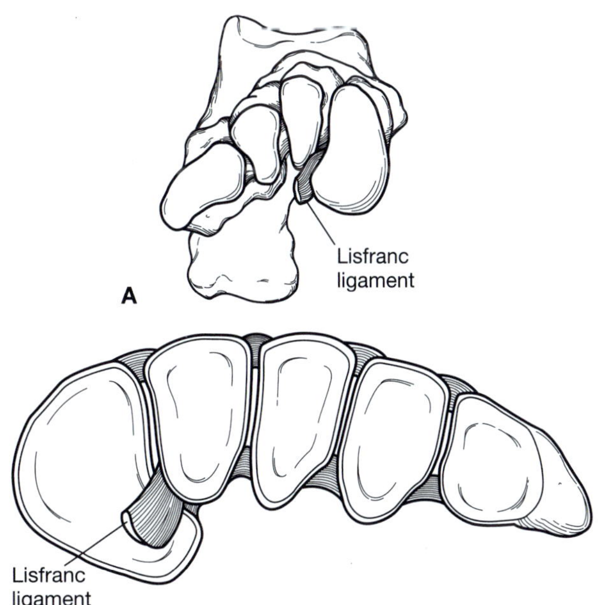

Figure 69.4: Anatomy of the tarsometatarsal joints of the foot. A: Proximal view of the cuneiform and cuboid articular surfaces. B: Distal view of the corresponding articular surfaces of the metatarsals. (From Bucholz RW, Heckman JD. *Rockwood & Green's Fractures in Adults*. 5th ed. Philadelphia (PA): Lippincott Williams & Wilkins; 2001.)

Cuboid Fractures

- Compression fractures of the cuboid can occur as part of a Lisfranc injury, whereas isolated cuboid fractures are uncommon. Cuboid fractures with significant compression can result in collapse of the lateral column requiring the use of an external fixator to restore the length and disimpact the fragments. Avulsion fractures are treated symptomatically (30).

Cuneiform Fractures

- Isolated cuneiform fractures are uncommon. Discovering the mechanism of injury is vital for understanding the severity of the injury as the radiographic appearance does not always demonstrate the inciting displacement.
- Avulsion fractures are treated symptomatically. Displaced fractures and intercuneiform instability can occur as part of a Lisfranc fracture-dislocation and should be treated as such. Displacement should be reduced and stabilized during operative fixation of the tarsometatarsal injuries (30).

METATARSAL AND PHALANGEAL FRACTURES

- Metatarsal and phalangeal fractures are common injuries treated by a variety of physicians. The fifth followed by the first toes are the most frequently injured digits due to their vulnerable positions along the medial and lateral borders of the foot (32).
- Metatarsal fractures can result in a disruption of the major weight-bearing complex of the forefoot leading to other problems such as metatarsalgia or transfer lesions. Injuries to this region should not be overlooked and require a thorough workup and appropriate treatment and referral to avoid further complications and disability. With a careful physical exam, a good history, and appropriate radiographs, the diagnosis of most forefoot injuries is straightforward (29).

Physical Examination

- The physician must always evaluate and document the neurovascular status of the patient with a suspected metatarsal or phalangeal fracture. It is most important to evaluate and document the capillary refill and sensation to each toe.

Radiographic Examination

- Radiographs of a suspected forefoot injury should include AP, oblique, and lateral radiographic views of the foot and ipsilateral ankle.
- CT may aid in determining the precise location, depth, and articular involvement; however, these are not a part of the initial radiologic evaluation for these fractures. MRI may be used to investigate stress fractures, but a bone scan is the radiographic study of choice (32).
- When describing fractures of the metatarsal or phalanx, the reporting physician should include the following: open versus closed, incongruent joints, proximal versus distal, comminution, transverse/spiral/oblique pattern, angulation, and displacement, and shortening or overlap.

Metatarsal Shaft Fractures

- The plantar flexors are the deforming force involved with fractures of the metatarsal shaft. Mechanisms of injury include a direct blow, avulsion, twisting, inversion, or repetitive stress.
- Nonsurgical treatment is appropriate for fractures of the second, third, and fourth metatarsal shafts when there is <3 mm of displacement or <10° of angulation. A prominent plantar fragment can result in callus formation, whereas a dorsiflexion malunion can result in transfer metatarsalgia.
- Indications for surgical treatment include displaced fractures of the first metatarsal. Patients do not tolerate these fractures well because the first ray bears more weight than the lesser metatarsals. Fractures of the second through fourth metatarsals should also undergo operative fixation with >3 mm of displacement, >10° of sagittal displacement, or when there are multiple metatarsal fractures (29).

Metatarsal Neck and Head Fractures

- Metatarsal head and neck fractures are rare and usually occur from a direct blow to the foot involving multiple metatarsals. Failure to recognize and appropriately treat these injuries can disrupt the normal weight-bearing function of the forefoot, causing transfer metatarsalgia (32).
- Most metatarsal head and neck fractures can be treated nonoperatively. Fractures with severe angulation or prominence may require reduction and fixation if closed reduction is unsuccessful (29).

Fifth Metatarsal Base Fractures

- Fifth metatarsal fractures usually result from direct trauma and are generally separated into proximal base and distal spiral fractures. Proximal fractures are further divided into three anatomic fracture zones, which help distinguish treatment options. From proximal to distal, zone 1 includes the tuberosity, zone 2 is from the tuberosity to the metaphyseal-diaphyseal junction, and zone 3 includes the proximal diaphysis (Fig. 69.5).
- Zone 1 fractures are caused by avulsion of the long plantar ligament or the lateral band of the plantar fascia. Treatment consists of weight bearing as tolerated in a stiff-soled shoe. Surgery may be indicated for fractures with large, displaced, intra-articular fragments.
- Zone 2 fractures represent an area of circulatory watershed, resulting in limited blood supply, and are commonly called Jones fractures. Because of the compromised blood supply in this area, the fracture is at risk of nonunion. Therefore,

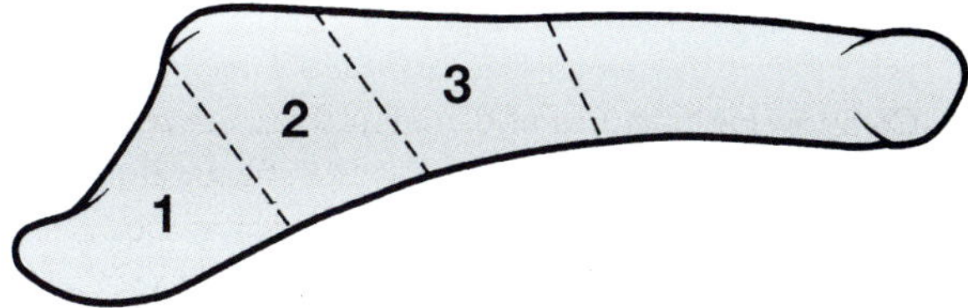

Figure 69.5: Three zones of proximal fifth metatarsal fracture. Zone 1 avulsion fracture. Zone 2 fracture at the metaphyseal-diaphyseal junction. Zone 3 proximal shaft stress fracture. (From Bucholz RW, Heckman JD, Court-Brown C, editors. *Rockwood and Green's Fractures in Adults.* 6th ed. Philadelphia (PA): Lippincott Williams & Wilkins; 2006.)

patients should not bear weight for 6–8 weeks. Acute ORIF using screws is often used in athletes to minimize the possibility of nonunion and prolonged restriction from activity.

- Zone 3 fractures are typically diaphyseal stress fractures. Nonsurgical treatment consisting of non–weight-bearing in a short leg cast is the appropriate treatment for fractures in this zone in the absence of prodromal symptoms (33).

Phalangeal Fractures

- The mechanism of injury is a crush injury or axial loading. Painful subungual hematomas should be evacuated through a hole in the nail.
- Distal phalanx fractures of the hallux are treated nonsurgically, as are lesser toe injuries. Nonsurgical treatment should consist of closed reduction and buddy taping for 4 weeks.
- Surgical treatment is indicated for displaced articular injuries or angulated proximal phalanx fractures of the hallux if closed reduction and percutaneous pinning fail (32).

Sesamoid Fractures

- Sesamoid injuries can occur by either a direct impact with compression, hyperdorsiflexion causing a transverse fracture, or repetitive trauma.
- Plain radiographs can include a sesamoid view to evaluate the articulation of the sesamoid with the plantar aspect of the metatarsal head. MRI is useful in determining the presence of stress reaction or stress fracture; however, a CT is usually not indicated.
- Acute fractures or stress fractures are treated with padding and immobilization in a hard-soled shoe for 4–8 weeks, and patients can be followed up as outpatients. Excision of the sesamoid is used for chronic symptomatic nonunions and not typically for acute fractures (32).

REFERENCES

1. Spiguel A, Jo MJ, Gardner MJ. Ankle and pilon fractures. In: Chou LR, editor. *Orthopaedic Knowledge Update: Foot and Ankle.* 6th ed. Rosemont (IL): American Academy of Orthopaedic Surgeons; 2019. p. 300–16.
2. Barrett JA, Baron JA, Karagas MR, Beach ML. Fracture risk in the U.S. Medicare population. *J Clin Epidemiol.* 1999;52(3):243–49.
3. Koval KJ, Zuckerman JD. *Handbook of Fractures.* 5th ed. Philadelphia (PA): Lippincott Williams & Wilkins; 2014. p. 576–84.
4. Wake J, Martin KD. Syndesmosis injury from diagnosis to repair: physical examination, diagnosis, and arthroscopic-assisted reduction. *J Am Acad Orthop Surg.* 2020;28(13):517–27.
5. Zhao JZ, Ingall EM, Sharma S, et al. The lateral drawer test: a new clinical test to assess mortise instability in Weber B fibula fractures. *Foot Ankle Orthop.* 2022;7(3):24730114221112101.
6. Stiell IG, Greenberg GH, McKnight RD, et al. Decision rules for the use of radiography in acute ankle injuries. Refinement and prospective validation. *JAMA.* 1993;269(9):1127–32.
7. Brandser EA, Berbaum KS, Dorfman DD, et al. Contribution of individual projections alone and in combination for radiographic detection of ankle fractures. *AJR Am J Roentgenol.* 2000;174(6):1691–7.
8. Schock HJ, Pinzur M, Manion L, Stover M. The use of gravity or manual-stress radiographs in the assessment of supination external rotation fractures of the ankle. *J Bone Joint Surg Br.* 2007;89(8):1055–9.
9. Miniaci-Coxhead SL. Osteochondral lesions of the talus. In: Chou LR, editor. *Orthopaedic Knowledge Update: Foot and Ankle.* 6th ed. Rosemont (IL): American Academy of Orthopaedic Surgeons; 2019. p. 408–20.
10. Michelson JD. Ankle fractures resulting from rotational injuries. *J Am Acad Orthop Surg.* 2003;11(6):403–12.
11. Osborne PM. Ankle fractures. In: Ricci WM, Ostrum RF, editors. *Orthopaedic Knowledge Update: Trauma.* 5th ed. Rosemont (IL): American Academy of Orthopaedic Surgeons; 2016. p. 563–74.
12. Atwan Y, Schemitsch EH, Schemitsch EH, Teague D. The top three unanswered questions in the management of open fractures. *OTA Int.* 2020;3(1):e072.
13. Kou JX, Fortin PT. Commonly missed peritalar injuries. *J Am Acad Orthop Surg.* 2009;17(12):775–86.
14. Hak DJ, Martin MP. Talus fractures. In: Chou LR, editor. *Orthopaedic Knowledge Update: Foot and Ankle.* 6th ed. Rosemont (IL): American Academy of Orthopaedic Surgeons; 2019. p. 319–29.
15. Santavirta S, Seitsalo S, Kiviluoto O, Myllynen P. Fractures of the talus. *J Trauma.* 1984;24(11):986–9.
16. Githens M, Tangtiphaiboontana J, Carlock K, Campbell ST. Talus fractures: an update on current concepts in surgical management. *J Am Acad Orthop Surg.* 2022;30(15):e1015–24.
17. Vallier HA, Reichard SG, Boyd AJ, Moore TA. A new look at the Hawkins classification for talar neck fractures: which features of injury and treatment are predictive of osteonecrosis? *J Bone Joint Surg Am.* 2014;96(3):192–7.
18. Daniels TR, Smith JW, Ross TI. Varus malalignment of the talar neck: its effect on the position of the foot and on subtalar motion. *J Bone Joint Surg Am.* 1996;78(10):1559–67.
19. Fortin PT, Balazsy JE. Talus fractures: evaluation and treatment. *J Am Acad Orthop Surg.* 2001;9(2):114–27.
20. Tinner CMD, Sommer CMD. Fractures of the lateral process of the talus. *Foot Ankle Clin.* 2018;23(3):375–95.
21. Berkowitz MJ, Kim DH. Process and tubercle fractures of the hindfoot. *J Am Acad Orthop Surg.* 2005;13(8):492–502.
22. Gotha HEMD, Zide JRMD. Current controversies in management of calcaneus fractures. *Orthop Clin North Am.* 2017;48(1):91–103.

23. Macey LR, Benirschke SK, Sangeorzan BJ, Hansen ST. Acute calcaneal fractures: treatment options and results. *J Am Acad Orthop Surg.* 1994;2(1):36–43.
24. Buckley RE, Tough S. Displaced Intra-articular calcaneal fractures. *J Am Acad Orthop Surg.* 2004;12(3):172–8.
25. Sanders R, Fortin P, DiPasquale T, Walling A. Operative treatment in 120 displaced intra-articular calcaneal fractures. Results using a prognostic computed tomography scan classification. *Clin Orthop Relat Res.* 1993;290:87–95.
26. Hess MMD, Booth BMD, Laughlin RTMD. Calcaneal avulsion fractures: complications from delayed treatment. *Am J Emerg Med.* 2008;26(2):254.e1–254.e2544.
27. Sanders R. Intra-articular fractures of the calcaneus: present state of the art. *J Orthop Trauma.* 1992;6(2):252–65.
28. Potter MQ, Nunley JA. Long-term functional outcomes after operative treatment for intra-articular fractures of the calcaneus. *J Bone Joint Surg Am.* 2009;91(8):1854–60.
29. Schenck RC Jr, Heckman JD. Fractures and dislocations of the forefoot: operative and nonoperative treatment. *J Am Acad Orthop Surg.* 1995;3(2):70–8.
30. Miller CM, Winter WG, Bucknell AL, Jonassen EA. Injuries to the midtarsal joint and lesser tarsal bones. *J Am Acad Orthop Surg.* 1998;6(4):249–58.
31. Solan MC, Moorman CT III, Miyamoto RG, Jasper LE, Belkoff SM. Ligamentous restraints of the second tarsometatarsal joint: a biomechanical evaluation. *Foot Ankle Int.* 2001;22(8):637–41.
32. Early JS. Fractures and dislocations of the midfoot and forefoot. In: Rockwood CA, Green DB, Bucholz RW, , editors. *Fractures in Adults.* 6th ed. Philadelphia (PA): Lippincott Williams & Wilkins; 2006. p. 2337–99.
33. Metzl JA, Bowers MW, Anderson RB. Fifth metatarsal Jones fractures: diagnosis and treatment. *J Am Acad Orthop Surg.* 2022;30(4):e470–9.

Lower Extremity Stress Fractures

70

Michael Fredericson, Julia Arroyo, and Anne M. Kuwabara

INCIDENCE

- Stress fractures account for 0.5%–21% of all injuries in recreational or competitive athletes presenting to sports medicine clinics (1). The highest incidence of stress fractures occurs among track-and-field athletes (6%–20% of total injuries), compared with athletes in other sports such as football, basketball, soccer, or rowing (1–3).
- The site of injury varies by sport. For example, among track athletes, stress fractures of the navicular, tibia, and metatarsals are the most common, whereas in distance runners, the most common locations are the tibia and fibula, and in dancers, the metatarsals (1,4).
- The incidence is postulated to be increasing due to the trend of youth sport specialization (5).

ETIOLOGY

- A stress fracture may best be described as an accelerated bony remodeling in response to repetitive submaximal stress. Histologic studies (6,7) have shown that repetitive response to stress leads to osteoclastic activity that surpasses the rate of osteoblastic new bone formation, resulting in temporary weakening of bone.
- Stress fractures occur due to a combination of increased load after fatigue of supporting structures or to contractile muscular forces acting across and on the bone (7,8).
- If the activity continues, trabecular microfractures result, which are believed to explain the early bone marrow edema seen on magnetic resonance imaging (MRI) scanning (9). The bone responds by forming new periosteal bone for reinforcement. Eventually, if the osteoclastic activity continues to exceed the rate of osteoblastic new bone formation, a full cortical break occurs. It is important to recognize this process as a continuum accumulation of damage that results clinically in a spectrum of injuries, from the early stages called stress reactions, to stress fractures, and ultimately complete bone fractures (4,10). Therefore, these types of injuries are important to identify early to limit an athlete's time out of sport.

RISK FACTORS

- Athletes at great risk include those participating in sports with higher impact and repetitive loads, such as cross-country running, gymnastics, basketball, and outdoor and indoor track (11,12). Most bone stress injuries occur in the lower extremities, particularly the long bones of the leg (tibia and fibula) and foot (metatarsals). However, certain sports are associated with specific bone stress injuries. For example, the spine bone stress injuries are most commonly involved in gymnastics as well as ribs in rowers, humerus in throwing athletes, and distal radius and phalanges in climbers.
- Alteration in the training program is considered one of the most important factors related to the occurrence of stress fractures. Any rapid change in mileage, pace, intensity, or some other factor inserted into the program without adequate time for physiologic adaptation may predispose to stress fractures (13,14). Most commonly this occurs during preseason and transition to competitive season, return from an injury, or moving up to a higher competition level.
- Failure to follow intensive training days with easy ones also can contribute to injury. Hard or cambered training surfaces and training in older shoes are also important precursors to lower extremity overuse injuries (9,15).
- Anatomic variables such as narrow width of the tibia, smaller calf girth, and less muscle mass in the lower limb have been associated with stress fractures. In a study (16) comparing 23 running athletes with a history of tibial stress fractures and 23 healthy runners, the stress fracture group had a significantly smaller tibial cross-sectional area. Bony geometry plays a role in stress fracture development. In runners, repetitive loading in a single plane leads to asymmetric cross-sectional geometry of the tibia in contrast to soccer players who load in multiple directions and are found to have a more robust and symmetric bone geometry (17).
- Statistics suggest that women are at greater risk for sustaining stress fractures than men (1). The female athlete triad (menstrual irregularity, disordered eating, and osteopenia) emphasizes this susceptibility in this group of athletes. Other studies have failed to show a significant gender difference (18).
- Military studies demonstrate that bone stress injury risk varies by race and ethnicity. Compared with black individuals,

non-Hispanic white men and women have 59% and 92% higher risk of bone stress injuries, respectively, while Hispanic and Asian individuals have an intermediate risk (19,20).

- Movement patterns in runners such as greater peak rearfoot eversion and hip adduction and less knee flexion may increase risk. Other variables include altered hip range of motion, leg-length discrepancy, and both pes planus (flat foot) and pes cavus (high arch) (21–28).
- Irrespective of load, runners with a low step rate were found to be at higher risk of bone stress injury (29).
- Exercising on harder surfaces was believed to increase the risk of bone stress injury, but this remains unclear. What is most important is likely a recent and rapid change to an unaccustomed surface (30).
- The role of shoes and inserts on bone stress injury risk also remains unclear (31). Abrupt changes from cushioned shoes to footwear with limited mechanical support may increase the risk of metatarsal injury (32,33).
- Low levels of vitamin D and calcium have been associated with decreased bone strength and increased risk of bone stress injuries. Female distance runners who consumed less than 800 mg of calcium daily had an almost sixfold higher bone stress injury rate than those who consumed more than 1500 mg daily (34–36).
- A family history of bone stress injuries may increase risk (37). Polymorphisms in the purinergic receptor gene *P2X*$_7$ are a potential predisposing factor in the development of bone stress injuries (38). The clinical application of this information remains to be determined.
- Elevated corticosteroid levels (both endogenous and exogenous) are associated with impaired bone health (39,40).
- In a cohort of more than 1 million military recruits, prolonged use of NSAIDs was potentially associated with increased risk of bone stress injuries (41).
- Sleep is suspected to contribute to bone stress injury risk but is not fully understood. A study from the Israeli military found that a lifestyle intervention that included a minimum of 6 hours of sleep resulted in a 62% reduction in bone stress injuries (42).

HISTORY

- The typical history of a stress fracture is that of localized pain that is not present at the start but occurs after or toward the end of physical activity. This pattern is opposite to that of many soft-tissue injuries that cause pain first thing in the morning and with day-to-day activities but reduced pain during physical activity.
- Untreated stress reactions display pain that occurs earlier during the physical activity and lingers longer; with continued training, pain will be present throughout the training and persist into daily ambulation.
- A careful history often reveals some change in the training regimen during the preceding 2–6 weeks, and it is critical that the physician ask detailed questions to identify training changes as a cause. Risk factors described above should be assessed for.

PHYSICAL EXAMINATION

- The physical examination typically reveals local tenderness over the involved bone (8). Other tests for the clinical detection of stress fracture such as the fulcrum test (femur), hop test (tibia), and spinal extension test (pars interarticularis) are helpful but not as reliable as direct palpation (3).
- The fulcrum test is performed by gradually applying a force across the distal femur in the seated position using the edge of the examination table as a fulcrum while fixing the proximal femur (43). In the hop test, patients are asked to repeat single-legged hops over the affected leg. The spinal extension test is performed with the patient standing, balancing on one leg to increase the load over the ipsilateral pars interarticularis. Pain provocation with these maneuvers is a positive finding.
- Assessment of biomechanical factors such as varus alignment of the lower extremity, true leg-length discrepancies, femoral neck anteversion, muscle weakness, excessive Q angles, excessive subtalar pronation, or a pes cavus style is recommended because these may contribute to the mechanical load imparted to the affected site (44).

IMAGING

- Radiographic findings are insensitive in the detection of early-stage stress injuries, and their usefulness is limited to the late phase. The time from onset of pain to positive radiographic evidence of a stress fracture can vary from 2–12 weeks (45). Early radiographic findings of a stress fracture in the long bones may include the visualization of a faint fracture radiolucency in the cortical bone (46). As the bone remodels, the endosteum can become ill defined, thickened, and sclerotic. As the fracture heals and remodels, periosteal reaction follows both on the cortical and endosteal surfaces. Stress fractures present differently in trabecular and cortical bone. The former is characterized by a predictable pattern manifested by a line of sclerosis perpendicular to the trabeculae, whereas the latter demonstrates periosteal reaction or a cortical fracture line.
- Radionuclide scanning is a more sensitive but less specific method for imaging bony stress injuries (45,47). Radionuclide technetium-99 diphosphonate triple-phase scanning can provide the diagnosis as early as 2–8 days after the onset of symptoms (9). In acute stress fractures, all three phases of the bone scan are positive. One must be aware of

the possibility of increased uptake in nonpainful sites, indicating subclinical accelerated remodeling (48).

- MRI is considered as the gold standard for the evaluation of stress injuries (45,48,49). Fat suppression technique allows for early detection of injuries, improving sensitivity and accuracy. A four-stage grading system has been developed: A grade 1 injury simply shows periosteal edema on the fat-suppressed or short tau inversion recovery images. In grade 2 injuries, abnormal increased signal intensity is also seen within the marrow cavity or along the endosteal surface on fat-suppressed T2-weighted images. In grade 3 injuries, signal abnormalities are also present on T1-weighted images. Grade 4 injuries involve an actual fracture line often seen on both T1- and T2-weighted images (9). One study (50) showed that grade 3 and 4 injuries took longer to heal than grade 1 and 2 injuries and demonstrated that the grade of injury has prognostic implications regarding the time of healing. Reported false-negative MRI findings have been because of reader errors, suboptimal choice of imaging planes and sequences, inhomogeneities in fat suppression, and partial volume effects (4).
- Before making therapeutic decisions, it is important to correlate MRI findings with clinical symptoms. Bergman et al. (48) studied 21 asymptomatic runners with MRI of the tibia. Nine (43%) of them showed abnormalities indicating stress injuries. After 12 months, none of the asymptomatic runners developed a bone stress injury. Stress response to exercise may cause bone marrow edema, and interpretation should always be made in conjunction with the patient's clinical history (45).

GENERAL PRINCIPLES OF TREATMENT

- It is important to distinguish stress fractures at higher risk for delayed union, nonunion, displacement, or intra-articular component. These fractures require early diagnosis, aggressive treatment, and occasionally internal fixation. High-risk stress fractures include fractures of the femoral neck (tension side), patella, tibial diaphysis, fifth metatarsal diaphysis (Jones fracture), tarsal navicular, body of the talus, base of second metatarsal, sesamoids, and pars interarticularis.
- Less critical or not-at-risk fractures can be treated with a two-phase protocol. Phase 1 includes pain control with analgesics and physical therapy modalities. Weight bearing is allowed for normal activities within the tolerance of pain.
- A modified activity program such as elliptical, rowing, or cycling can be used to maintain strength and fitness but to reduce impact loading to the skeleton. A program of deep water training or pool running can be indicated. In our experience, we have found it useful to include an antigravity treadmill device as part of the cross-training recovery protocol. This device allows controlled, progressive weight bearing while permitting unrestricted mobility and natural mechanics and enables the athlete to preserve aerobic condition.
- Phase 2, graduated return to sport, generally begins once the athlete has been pain free for 10–14 days. The athlete can return to running only every other day for the first 2 weeks. Then, over a 3- to 6-week period, a gradual increase in distance and frequency is permitted (51).
- Functional foot orthoses may play a role in treatment and prevention of stress fractures (43). Orthoses are useful either for reducing abnormal pronation in patients with a markedly everted rear foot or providing better shock absorption in athletes with a rigid, inverted rear foot (52).
- If there is a positive history of irregular menses or amenorrhea, then consideration should be given to obtaining a bone mineral density test and endocrine workup. Hormonal replacement therapy indication should be cautiously considered only if the athlete is unable to resume normal menses through weight gain and is not indicated as a long-term solution. Calcium and vitamin D supplementation and additional nutritional deficiencies should be assessed and corrected (53).
- The role of calcium and vitamin D supplementation in the prevention of stress fractures is still to be determined. Recent evidence shows that a daily calcium dietary intake of 1500 mg in female adolescent athletes reduced incidence of stress fractures and increased bone mineral density (54).
- There is still no conclusive evidence to prove any beneficial effect of bisphosphonates for the treatment of stress fractures in humans (55,56). Adverse effects should be considered, especially in adolescents with open physis and women of childbearing age. In these patients, the safety of bisphosphonate use has not yet been established (55).
- Electrical stimulation has proven to be effective in enhancing regular fracture healing, but limited experience exists on its benefits for stress fractures (57,58). Electric fields can be useful to accelerate stress fracture healing, but treatment protocol requires compliance with the use of the device for 15 $h \cdot d^{-1}$ in combination with rest and limited weight bearing. Electrical stimulation may be particularly indicated in the more severe cases or in the elite athlete with higher motivation for superior compliance (59).

SPECIFIC SITES OF STRESS FRACTURE

Pelvis

Sacrum

- Stress fractures in the sacrum are most common in women distance runners with low bone density, but can be seen in those with normal bone mineralization. These stress fractures tend to involve the anteroinferior aspect of the sacral wing unilaterally, mimicking a sacroiliitis (60).
- MRI is recommended for diagnosis, with intermediate signal intensity on T1-weighted images and high-signal intensity on T2-weighted images in the anterior aspect of the sacral ala (4).

Pubic Rami

- More commonly, a bony stress reaction may develop in runners at the symphysis pubis (osteitis pubis) or at the inferior pubic ramus adjacent to the symphysis and is believed to be related to overuse of the adductor muscles for pelvis stabilization.
- Treatment for both of the above pelvic stress fractures requires a period of rest and temporary use of crutches if there is any pain during ambulation. Symptoms usually resolve within several weeks, and a gradual return to athletic activity can typically be safely advised between 10 and 12 weeks.

Ischium

- An ischial ramus stress reaction is not considered a true stress fracture, because it is seen in association with proximal hamstring tendinopathy or hamstring bursitis, secondary to chronic traction of the muscle origin (51).

Femoral Neck

- Stress fractures of the femoral neck are high-risk fractures and should be considered in any athlete, especially a distance runner, who presents with hip, thigh, or groin pain. Pain and symptoms are worse with weight bearing, and there is often reduced range of movement in the hip, particularly internal rotation.
- Early detection of femoral neck stress fractures is crucial, because continued stress may lead to a displaced fracture, with associated risk of avascular necrosis and irreversible damages to the joint (61).
- Compression fractures are more common in younger athletic patients and are located at the cortex of the lower medial margin of the femoral neck. The early radiographic appearance of these fractures is subtle endosteal lysis or sclerosis along the inferior cortex of the femoral neck, followed by progressive sclerosis and appearance of a fracture line. If radiographic findings are negative, MRI should be indicated to detect bone marrow edema and the presence or absence of a low signal intensity line that indicates a fracture.
- If there is no fracture line present, treatment is conservative, with a period of non–weight bearing to allow healing (4,62). Athletes are allowed to continue conditioning exercises such as swimming or cycling during the period of rest. The return-to-play criteria are based on asymptomatic full weight bearing, no pain with passive range of motion of the hip, and follow-up imaging studies with signs of a healed fracture. As a rule, 2–3 months are required for complete healing of stress fractures of this type (4).
- Surgical management of this injury is considered under the following circumstances: failure of nonoperative management, prophylactic stabilization of a fracture at high risk for displacement, any displaced femoral stress fracture, and malunion or nonunion (4).

Femoral Diaphysis

- Stress fractures of the femoral diaphysis are relatively common but often misdiagnosed as muscle or tendon injuries. The most common site of injury is the posteromedial cortex of the proximal femur (63).
- Athletes typically complain of an insidious onset of vague poorly localized thigh pain that is activity related. Physical examination may reveal local tenderness, with normal hip range of motion. Hopping on the affected side will typically reproduce pain in the involved bone. The fulcrum test can be helpful in localizing the anatomic site of involvement (3).
- MRI shows periosteal and bone marrow edema involving the medial aspect of the femur approximately at the junction of the proximal and middle thirds of the femoral diaphysis (64).
- If there is no evidence of cortical break or displacement, conservative treatment is indicated. Once the athlete can ambulate without pain, a cross-training program is appropriate and return to athletic activities can be initiated after 8–12 weeks.

Patella

- Stress fracture of the patella is a rare injury that occurs typically in young athletes and jumping sports (65,66).
- The clinical findings are localized tenderness over the patella. Most patellar stress fractures are of the transverse type. These may be confused radiographically with bipartite patella; however, a patella fracture line tends to be more oblique than the bipartite patella.

Tibia

Posterior Medial Tibial Shaft

- Many athletes, particularly runners, commonly experience pain along the medial border of the tibia related to training. Pain in this location from medial tibial stress syndrome (tibial periostitis) and tibial stress fractures accounts for up to 75% of injuries presenting to a sports medicine clinic (67).
- Pain is located along the posteromedial border of the tibia, usually in the middle or distal thirds. It is often difficult to clinically distinguish the more severe tibial stress reaction or fracture from the more common medial tibial stress or shin splint syndrome. It has been suggested that the periostitis (seen as periosteal edema on MRI) may be the initial injury on a spectrum that, if allowed to progress, may evolve into a more serious bone injury (9).
- The physical examination findings such as localized tibial tenderness and pain with direct or indirect (at a distance from the site of tenderness) percussion over the involved bone help distinguish it from the more common medial tibial stress syndrome.
- The pain is occasionally aggravated by testing muscle strength actively, particularly in those muscles that have origins on the posterior medial tibial border including the

soleus (best tested by repetitive toe raises), posterior tibialis, and flexor digitorum longus.

- It is also important to evaluate the lower extremity alignment as well as mechanical gait. Athletes with increased subtalar pronation have shown a tendency toward developing tibial stress injuries (68). It has been found that both the degree of pronation and also the timing of pronation during gait are important discriminators between athletes at higher risk (69).
- The temporary cessation of running is essential to allow for bony remodeling and repair. This can range from a few days to 3 weeks for a minor injury to 12 weeks for a severe injury with frank cortical fracture. If there is pain with daily activities, a pneumatic tibial brace can be used to immobilize distal and midtibial injuries (9).

Anterior Tibial Diaphysis

- Stress fractures of the anterior cortex of the midtibia require a different approach and treatment. They occur most commonly in athletes performing jumping or leaping activities. Located in the tension side of the bone, they are prone to delayed union, nonunion, or even complete fracture (70).
- Radiographs show a radiolucent cortical defect surrounded by sclerosis, known as the dreaded black line for its propensity for nonunion or even progression to complete fracture that may displace (70).
- These patients require treatment in a non–weight bearing brace for 6–8 weeks. Surgical excision and bone grafting or placement of an intramedullary rod are indicated after 3–6 months of failed closed management (71).

Proximal Tibial Metaphysis

- The proximal tibial metaphysis is a less common site of stress fracture. Tenderness is located along the medial aspect of the proximal tibia just below the medial joint line and is often misdiagnosed as pes anserinus tendinitis or bursitis (72).
- Radiographs may show a linear transverse region of sclerosis 2–3 mm wide in the medial plateau close to the level of the epiphyseal scar.
- An MRI examination may demonstrate bone marrow edema of the proximal tibial and medial tibial plateau before radiographic signs appear, with periosteal edema and sometimes a fracture line (64).

Fibula

- Fibular stress fractures are relatively common, accounting for up to 21% of all stress fractures in athletes (15). Although fibular stress fractures can occur more proximally, the majority occur in the lower third of the fibula, just proximal to the tibiofibular ligament attachment.
- The subcutaneous location of the fibula makes it easy to recreate symptoms with direct palpation over the involved bone. These athletes are often found to have a cavus-type foot.
- Radiographs may not be diagnostic at early stages, whereas MRI examination allows for early diagnosis showing periosteal as well as bone marrow edema and often a fracture line (64).
- Fibular stress fractures are noncritical injuries, and a gradual return to running can typically resume when local tenderness resolves.

Medial Malleolus

- The repetitive stress of running and jumping can create a vertical stress fracture starting at the junction of the medial malleolus and the tibial plafond and continuing proximally and slightly medially.
- It is hypothesized that chronic anteromedial impingement of the talus on the medial malleolus during ankle dorsiflexion may result in a medial malleolar stress fracture (73).
- Stress reactions without frank cortical fracture can be treated with temporary immobilization. Unlimited ambulation in a brace is permitted and a gradual return to sport is allowed as symptoms resolve.
- The presence of a radiographically detectable fracture line or displaced fragment, particularly in a high-level or in-season athlete, is considered an indication for surgical intervention (74).

Calcaneus

- Calcaneal stress fractures usually present as heel pain with localized tenderness over the bone, usually in the body of the calcaneus posterior to the talus (75). Initially, these injuries may present similar to plantar fasciitis. A less common stress injury involves the anterior process of the calcaneus (76).
- Pain elicited by squeezing the calcaneus from both sides simultaneously can usually differentiate this condition from retrocalcaneal bursitis, Achilles tendinitis, plantar nerve entrapment, subtalar arthritis, and radiculopathy (51).
- Radiographs generally become positive within the first month after pain presentation and show callus formation perpendicular to the trabecular axis of the calcaneus, usually located between the calcaneal tuberosity and the posterior facet of the subtalar joint.
- This is a noncritical stress fracture with rapid healing, and return to activity is usually possible within 6 weeks following restriction of activity and partial weight bearing.

Navicular Bone

- Tarsal navicular stress fractures are especially important, as they are particularly difficult to diagnose in their early stages and have a high risk of nonunion.
- Patients report an insidious onset of vague foot pain that is worse with certain activities, such as explosive sprinting, rapid changes in direction, jumping, and push-off (77). Tenderness is often located over the dorsal border of the navicular near the talonavicular joint (78).

- Investigation usually requires bone scan or MRI. Computed tomography (CT) is often needed to detect early separation of bone fragments or more clearly define the degree of fracture (64).
- The most common site of stress fracture within the navicular is the central third, which is an area of relative avascularity.
- Treatment of an uncomplicated partial stress fracture should include at least 6 weeks of non–weight-bearing cast immobilization until the navicular is no longer tender. This is followed by a further 6-week program of rehabilitation (51).
- Athletes who have sustained a navicular stress fracture are at high risk of developing a recurrent stress fracture at the same site if they return to their preinjury level of activity. A surgical option should be considered in the athlete to minimize time out of competition and additional risks (77). One study (79) used the CT fracture pattern to classify the lesion and determine the best treatment. Type I shows a cortical break, type II fractures propagate into the navicular body, and type III fractures propagate into the opposite cortex. Early operative intervention was recommended for type II and III injuries, with return to activity of approximately 4 months for all groups.

Talus, Cuboid, and Cuneiform

- Stress fractures of the talus, cuboid, and cuneiform bones are uncommon. In general, joint involvement, displacement, and nonunion do not occur, and treatment can be the same as that for other noncritical stress fractures (78).
- Stress fractures of the talus may have poorer long-term outcomes, and patients may suffer from persistent pain (6). In particular, fractures of the body of the talus can extend into the subtalar joint, which places them into the critical-at-risk category and requires at least 4–6 weeks of immobilization and occasionally open reduction and internal fixation (78,80).

Metatarsals

- Stress fractures of the metatarsal bones were first described in military recruits and referred to as a march fracture. This fracture typically occurs in the neck or distal shaft, with the second and third metatarsals most commonly affected (44,81).
- The stress fracture at the base of the second metatarsals is known as the dancer's fracture. Pain is noted to be greatest when in the full en pointe position. During this maneuver, the foot is maximally plantarflexed, and weight is borne on the plantar aspect and tip of the first and second distal phalanges (82). These injuries can be difficult to differentiate from synovitis of the Lisfranc joint (75). MRI is often necessary for diagnosis. The injury involves the volar and medial aspect of the Lisfranc joint and should be recognized early and treated with at least 4 weeks of non–weight-bearing immobilization (82,83).
- Stress fractures of the proximal fifth metatarsal diaphysis that occur more than approximately 1.5 cm distal to the tuberosity are known as Jones fractures (84). It is important to differentiate this fracture from the acute avulsion fracture of the tuberosity of the fifth metatarsal (80). The avulsion injury is noncritical and is treated with relative rest and then gradual progression. The Jones fracture is notorious for poor healing and requires prolonged immobilization (6–12 weeks) followed by a functional splint for another 4–8 weeks. In the athletic population, open reduction and screw fixation are recommended (83).

Sesamoids

- Stress fracture of a sesamoid of the great toe can be particularly disabling and can result in delayed union or nonunion. Passive distal push of the sesamoid, direct tenderness, and sesamoid area pain with stretch of the flexor hallucis suggest the diagnosis.
- Radiographic changes may be difficult to detect in sesamoid stress fracture, but occasionally, axial views or magnification views can assist in the diagnosis. Separation of the sesamoid fragments and irregular edges suggest a stress fracture rather than a bipartite sesamoid. MRI is often indicated to confirm the diagnosis (64).
- Rest from the offending activity is clearly advised. For nonoperative treatment, it is essential to include a non–weight-bearing 6-week immobilization period with the use of an orthotic designed to off-load the sesamoids and specifically prevent dorsiflexion. Surgical excision is advocated if conservative treatment fails (85).

REFERENCES

1. Snyder RA, Koester MC, Dunn WR. Epidemiology of stress fractures. *Clin Sports Med.* 2006;25(1):37–52. viii.
2. Arendt E, Agel J, Heikes C, Griffiths H. Stress injuries to bone in college athletes: a retrospective review of experience at a single institution. *Am J Sports Med.* 2003;31(6):959–68.
3. Johnson AW, Weiss CB Jr, Wheeler DL. Stress fractures of the femoral shaft in athletes—more common than expected: a new clinical test. *Am J Sports Med.* 1994;22(2):248–56.
4. Fredericson M, Jennings F, Beaulieu C, Matheson GO. Stress fractures in athletes. *Top Magn Reson Imaging.* 2006;17(5):309–25.
5. Patel NM, Mai DH, Ramme AJ, Karamitopoulos MS, Castañeda P, Chu A. Is the incidence of paediatric stress fractures on the rise? Trends in New York State from 2000 to 2015. *J Pediatr Orthop B.* 2020;29(5):499–504.
6. Li GP, Zhang SD, Chen G, Chen H, Wang AM. Radiographic and histologic analyses of stress fracture in rabbit tibias. *Am J Sports Med.* 1985;13(5):285–94.
7. Stanitski CL, McMaster JH, Scranton PE. On the nature of stress fractures. *Am J Sports Med.* 1978;6(6):391–6.
8. Daffner RH, Pavlov H. Stress fractures: current concepts. *AJR Am J Roentgenol.* 1992;159(2):245–52.
9. Fredericson M, Bergman AG, Hoffman KL, Dillingham MS. Tibial stress reaction in runners: correlation of clinical symptoms and scintigraphy with a new magnetic imaging grading system. *Am J Sports Med.* 1995;23(4):472–81.

10. Warden SJ, Creaby MW, Bryant AL, Crossley KM. Stress fracture risk factors in female football players and their clinical implications. *Br J Sports Med.* 2007;41(suppl 1):i38–43.
11. Changstrom BG, Brou L, Khodaee M, Braund C, Comstock RD. Epidemiology of stress fracture injuries among US high school athletes, 2005–2006 through 2012–2013. *Am J Sports Med.* 2015;43(1):26–33.
12. Rizzone KH, Ackerman KE, Roos KG, Dompier TP, Kerr ZY. The epidemiology of stress fractures in collegiate student-athletes, 2004–2005 through 2013–2014 academic years. *J Athl Train.* 2017;52(10):966–75.
13. Hubbard TJ, Carpenter EM, Cordova ML. Contributing factors to medial tibial stress syndrome: a prospective investigation. *Med Sci Sports Exerc.* 2009;41(3):490–6.
14. Macera CA. Lower extremity injuries in runners. Advances in prediction. *Sports Med.* 1992;13(1):50–7.
15. Harrast MA, Colonno D. Stress fractures in runners. *Clin Sports Med.* 2010;29(3):399–416.
16. Crossley K, Bennell KL, Wrigley T, Oakes BW. Ground reaction forces, bone characteristics, and tibial stress fracture in male runners. *Med Sci Sports Exerc.* 1999;31(8):1088–93.
17. Cleek TM, Whalen RT. Effect of activity and age on long bones using a new densitometric technique. *Med Sci Sports Exerc.* 2005;37(10):1806–13.
18. Iwamoto J, Takeda T. Stress fractures in athletes: review of 196 cases. *J Orthop Sci.* 2003;8(3):273–8.
19. Bulathsinhala L, Hughes JM, McKinnon CJ, et al. Risk of stress fracture varies by race/ethnic origin in a cohort study of 1.3 million US Army soldiers. *J Bone Miner Res.* 2017;32(7):1546–53.
20. Knapik J, Montain SJ, McGraw S, Grier T, Ely M, Jones BH. Stress fracture risk factors in basic combat training. *Int J Sports Med.* 2012;33(11):940–6.
21. Bennell KL, Malcolm SA, Thomas SA, et al. Risk factors for stress fractures in track and field athletes: a twelve-month prospective study. *Am J Sports Med.* 1996;24(6):810–18.
22. Dixon SJ, Creaby MW, Allsopp AJ. Comparison of static and dynamic biomechanical measures in military recruits with and without a history of third metatarsal stress fracture. *Clin Biomech.* 2006;21(4):412–19.
23. Milner CE, Hamill J, Davis IS. Distinct hip and rearfoot kinematics in female runners with a history of tibial stress fracture. *J Orthop Sports Phys Ther.* 2010;40(2):59–66.
24. Pohl MB, Mullineaux DR, Milner CE, Hamill J, Davis IS. Biomechanical predictors of retrospective tibial stress fractures in runners. *J Biomech.* 2008;41(6):1160–5.
25. Milner CE, Ferber R, Pollard CD, Hamill J, Davis IS. Biomechanical factors associated with tibial stress fracture in female runners. *Med Sci Sports Exerc.* 2006;38(2):323–8.
26. Finestone A, Shlamkovitch N, Eldad A, et al. Risk factors for stress fractures among Israeli infantry recruits. *Mil Med.* 1991;156(10):528–30.
27. Sullivan D, Warren RF, Pavlov H, Kelman G. Stress fractures in 51 runners. *Clin Orthop Relat Res.* 1984;187:188–92.
28. Simkin A, Leichter I, Giladi M, Stein M, Milgrom C. Combined effect of foot arch structure and an orthotic device on stress fractures. *Foot Ankle.* 1989;10(1):25–9.
29. Kliethermes SA, Stiffler-Joachim MR, Wille CM, Sanfilippo JL, Zavala P, Heiderscheit BC. Lower step rate is associated with a higher risk of bone stress injury: a prospective study of collegiate cross country runners. *Br J Sports Med.* 2021;55(15):851–6.
30. Milgrom C, Finestone AS, Voloshin A. Differences in the principal strain angles during activities performed on natural hilly terrain versus engineered surfaces. *Clin Biomech.* 2020;80:105146.
31. Davis IS, Hollander K, Lieberman DE, Ridge ST, Sacco ICN, Wearing SC. Stepping back to minimal footwear: applications across the lifespan. *Exerc Sport Sci Rev.* 2021;49(4):228–43.
32. Giuliani J, Masini B, Alitz C, Owens BD. Barefoot-simulating footwear associated with metatarsal stress injury in 2 runners. *Orthopedics.* 2011;34(7):e320–3.
33. Lieberman DE, Venkadesan M, Werbel WA, et al. Foot strike patterns and collision forces in habitually barefoot versus shod runners. *Nature.* 2010;463(7280):531–5.
34. Lappe J, Cullen D, Haynatzki G, Recker R, Ahlf R, Thompson K. Calcium and vitamin D supplementation decreases incidence of stress fractures in female Navy recruits. *J Bone Miner Res.* 2008;23(5):741–9.
35. Sonneville KR, Gordon CM, Kocher MS, Pierce LM, Ramappa A, Field AE. Vitamin D, calcium, and dairy intakes and stress fractures among female adolescents. *Arch Pediatr Adolesc Med.* 2012;166(7):595–600.
36. Nieves JW, Melsop K, Curtis M, et al. Nutritional factors that influence change in bone density and stress fracture risk among young female cross-country runners. *PM R.* 2010;2(8):740–94. quiz 794.
37. Field AE, Gordon CM, Pierce LM, Ramappa A, Kocher MS. Prospective study of physical activity and risk of developing a stress fracture among preadolescent and adolescent girls. *Arch Pediatr Adolesc Med.* 2011;165(8):723–8.
38. Varley I, Greeves JP, Sale C, et al. Functional polymorphisms in the P2X7 receptor gene are associated with stress fracture injury. *Purinergic Signal.* 2016;12(1):103–13.
39. Lappe JM, Stegman MR, Recker RR. The impact of lifestyle factors on stress fractures in female Army recruits. *Osteoporos Int.* 2001;12(1):35–42.
40. Poonuru S, Findling JW, Shaker JL. Lower extremity insufficiency fractures: an underappreciated manifestation of endogenous Cushing's syndrome. *Osteoporos Int.* 2016;27(12):3645–9.
41. Hughes JM, McKinnon CJ, Taylor KM, et al. Nonsteroidal anti-inflammatory drug prescriptions are associated with increased stress fracture diagnosis in the US Army population. *J Bone Miner Res.* 2019;34(3):429–36.
42. Finestone A, Milgrom C. How stress fracture incidence was lowered in the Israeli army: a 25-yr struggle. *Med Sci Sports Exerc.* 2008;40(11 suppl):S623–9.
43. Dugan SA, Weber KM. Stress fractures and rehabilitation. *Phys Med Rehabil Clin N Am.* 2007;18(3):401–16. viii.
44. Matheson GO, Clement DB, Mckenzie DC, Taunton JE, Lloyd-Smith DR, MacIntyre JG. Stress fractures in athletes. A study of 320 cases. *Am J Sports Med.* 1987;15(1):46–58.
45. Moran DS, Evans RK, Hadad E. Imaging of lower extremity stress fracture injuries. *Sports Med.* 2008;38(4):345–56.
46. Mulligan ME. The "gray cortex": an early sign of stress fracture. *Skeletal Radiol.* 1995;24(3):201–3.
47. Leffers D, Collins L. An overview of the use of bone scintigraphy in sports medicine. *Sports Med Arthrosc Rev.* 2009;17(1):21–4.
48. Bergman AG, Fredericson M, Ho C, Matheson GO. Asymptomatic tibial stress reactions: MRI detection and clinical follow-up in distance runners. *AJR Am J Roentgenol.* 2004;183(3):635–8.
49. Kiuru MJ, Pihlajamaki HK, Hietanen HJ, Ahovuo JA. MR imaging, bone scintigraphy, and radiography in bone stress injuries of the pelvis and the lower extremity. *Acta Radiol.* 2002;43(2):207–12.
50. Arendt EA, Griffiths HJ. The use of MR imaging in the assessment and clinical management of stress reactions of bone in high-performance athletes. *Clin Sports Med.* 1997;16(2):291–306.
51. Fredericson M, Bergman AG, Matheson GO. Stress fractures in athletes. *Orthopade.* 1997;26(11):961–71.
52. Craig DI. Medial tibial stress syndrome: evidence-based prevention. *J Athl Train.* 2008;43(3):316–8.
53. Fredericson M, Kent K. Normalization of bone density in a previously amenorrheic runner with osteoporosis. *Med Sci Sports Exerc.* 2005;37(9):1481–6.

54. Tenforde AS, Sayres LC, Sainani KL, Fredericson M. Evaluating the relationship of calcium and vitamin D in the prevention of stress fracture injuries in the young athlete: a review of the literature. *PM R.* 2010;2(10):945–9.
55. Shima Y, Engebretsen L, Iwasa J, Kitaoka K, Tomita K. Use of bisphosphonates for the treatment of stress fractures in athletes. *Knee Surg Sports Traumatol Arthrosc.* 2009;17(5):542–50.
56. Sloan AV, Martin JR, Li S, Li J. Parathyroid hormone and bisphosphonate have opposite effects on stress fracture repair. *Bone.* 2010;47(2):235–40.
57. Goldstein C, Sprague S, Petrisor BA. Electrical stimulation for fracture healing: current evidence. *J Orthop Trauma.* 2010;24(suppl 1):S62–5.
58. Mollon B, da Silva V, Busse JW, Einhorn TA, Bhandari M. Electrical stimulation for long-bone fracture-healing: a meta-analysis of randomized controlled trials. *J Bone Joint Surg Am.* 2008;90(11):2322–30.
59. Beck BR, Matheson GO, Bergman G, et al. Do capacitively coupled electric fields accelerate tibial stress fracture healing? A randomized controlled trial. *Am J Sports Med.* 2008;36(3):545–53.
60. Fredericson M, Salamancha L, Beaulieu C. Sacral stress fractures: tracking down nonspecific pain in distance runners. *Phys Sportsmed.* 2003;31(2):31–42.
61. Lombardo SJ, Benson DW. Stress fractures of the femur in runners. *Am J Sports Med.* 1982;10(4):219–27.
62. Volpin G, Hoerer D, Groisman G, Zaltzman S, Stein H. Stress fractures of the femoral neck following strenuous activity. *J Orthop Trauma.* 1990;4(4):394–8.
63. Fredericson M, Jang KU, Bergman G, Gold G. Femoral diaphyseal stress fractures: results of a systematic bone scan and magnetic resonance imaging evaluation in 25 runners. *Phys Ther Sport.* 2004;5:188–93.
64. Bergman AG, Fredericson M. MR imaging of stress reactions, muscle injuries, and other overuse injuries in runners. *Magn Reson Imaging Clin N Am.* 1999;7(1):151–74. ix.
65. Devas MB. Stress fractures of the patella. *J Bone Joint Surg Br.* 1960;42-B:71–4.
66. Drabicki RR, Greer WJ, DeMeo PJ. Stress fractures around the knee. *Clin Sports Med.* 2006;25(1):105–15. ix.
67. Orava S, Puranen J. Athlete's leg pains. *Br J Sports Med.* 1979;13(3):92–7.
68. Moen MH, Tol JL, Weir A, Steunebrink M, De Winter TC. Medial tibial stress syndrome: a critical review. *Sports Med.* 2009;39(7):523–46.
69. Tweed JL, Campbell JA, Avil SJ. Biomechanical risk factors in the development of medial tibial stress syndrome in distance runners. *J Am Podiatr Med Assoc.* 2008;98(6):436–44.
70. Orava S, Hulkko A. Stress fracture of the mid-tibial shaft. *Acta Orthop Scand.* 1984;55(1):35–7.
71. Kaeding CC, Yu JR, Wright R, Amendola A, Spindler KP. Management and return to play of stress fractures. *Clin J Sport Med.* 2005;15(6):442–7.
72. Harolds JA. Fatigue fractures of the medial tibial plateau. *South Med J.* 1981;74(5):578–81.
73. Jowett AJ, Birks CL, Blackney MC. Medial malleolar stress fracture secondary to chronic ankle impingement. *Foot Ankle Int.* 2008;29(7):716–21.
74. Sherbondy PS, Sebastianelli WJ. Stress fractures of the medial malleolus and distal fibula. *Clin Sports Med.* 2006;25(1):129–37. x.
75. Goulart M, O'Malley MJ, Hodgkins CW, Charlton TP. Foot and ankle fractures in dancers. *Clin Sports Med.* 2008;27(2):295–304.
76. Brockwell J, Yeung Y, Griffith JF. Stress fractures of the foot and ankle. *Sports Med Arthrosc Rev.* 2009;17(3):149–59.
77. Mann JA, Pedowitz DI. Evaluation and treatment of navicular stress fractures, including nonunions, revision surgery, and persistent pain after treatment. *Foot Ankle Clin.* 2009;14(2):187–204.
78. Khan KM, Brukner PD, Kearney C, Fuller PJ, Bradshaw CJ, Kiss ZS. Tarsal navicular stress fracture in athletes. *Sports Med.* 1994;17(1):65–76.
79. Saxena A, Fullem B. Navicular stress fractures: a prospective study on athletes. *Foot Ankle Int.* 2006;27(11):917–21.
80. Chuckpaiwong B, Queen RM, Easley ME, Nunley JA. Distinguishing Jones and proximal diaphyseal fractures of the fifth metatarsal. *Clin Orthop Relat Res.* 2008;466(8):1966–70.
81. Heaslet MW, Kanda-Mehtani SL. Return-to-activity levels in 96 athletes with stress fractures of the foot, ankle, and leg: a retrospective analysis. *J Am Podiatr Med Assoc.* 2007;97(1):81–4.
82. Micheli LJ, Sohn RS, Soloman R. Stress fractures of the second metatarsal involving Lisfranc's joint in ballet dancer: a new overuse injury of the foot. *J Bone Joint Surg.* 1985;67(9):1372–5.
83. Khan K, Brown J, Way S, et al. Overuse injuries in classical ballet. *Sports Med.* 1995;19(5):341–57.
84. Jones RI. I. Fracture of the base of the fifth metatarsal bone by indirect violence. *Ann Surg.* 1902;35(6):697–700.2.
85. Cohen BE. Hallux sesamoid disorders. *Foot Ankle Clin.* 2009;14(1):91–104.

Lower Extremity Nerve Entrapments

71

Evan Peck, Jay Smith, and Michael Warwick

INTRODUCTION

- Neurologic conditions account for 10%–15% of all exercise-induced leg pain among runners (1–4). Causes include contusion, compression, stretching, and iatrogenic injury (5–9). The interdigital (interdigital or Morton neuroma), lateral plantar (LPN), medial plantar (MPN), tibial (TN), peroneal (common [CPN], deep [DPN], and/or superficial [SPN]), sural (SN), saphenous, and sciatic (SCN) nerves may be affected (2).
- Figures 71.1–71.7 demonstrate relevant neuroanatomy, including as it pertains to entrapment sites.
- Table 71.1 outlines the anatomic relationship among the lower extremity nerves.

COMMON NERVE ENTRAPMENT SYNDROMES

Interdigital Neuroma (Morton Neuroma)

Definition

- Most commonly affects the third web space, rarely the first or fourth web spaces (Figs. 71.1 and 71.2) (3).
- Typically affects adults age 20 or older; more common in females (2,6,8,10)

Anatomy, Pathophysiology, and Risk Factors

- During push-off, forceful toe dorsiflexion compresses and stretches the interdigital nerve across the dorsal intermetatarsal ligament, resulting in demyelination, scarring, and hypertrophy (6).
- Hyperpronation dorsiflexes the third metatarsal relative to the fourth, exposing the nerve to injury during push-off (2).
- Others suggest that Morton neuromas result from pressure of the metatarsal heads and metatarsophalangeal (MTP) joints (11).
- Idiopathic MTP synovitis may cause local edema and interdigital nerve compression (8).
- Risk factors: prolonged running, squatting, high-heeled or narrow toe-boxed shoes, and demi pointe in ballet (10).

Symptoms and Signs

- Tenderness in affected intermetatarsal space; neuropathic pain, typically between third and fourth toes, increased with running, standing, walking, squatting, and toe dorsiflexion
- Provocative testing: pressure over plantar aspect of the web space between the metatarsal heads, or squeezing metatarsals together during palpation. The squeeze test may also result in a click ("Mulder click") as the neuroma subluxates from between the metatarsals in a plantar direction (2).

Differential Diagnosis and Evaluation

- Differential diagnosis includes proximal and systemic neurologic conditions, stress fractures, MTP joint synovitis or arthritis, and flexor tenosynovitis.
- Diagnostic interdigital nerve block is confirmatory.
- Diagnostic ultrasound (US) can be used for diagnosis or to guide therapeutic injection (12–15).
- Magnetic resonance imaging (MRI) and US have comparable detection rates for Morton neuroma (16).

Treatment

- Activity modification, nonsteroidal anti-inflammatory drugs (NSAIDs), footwear modifications, physical therapy, and biomechanical interventions to reduce toe dorsiflexion, control hyperpronation, and maintain greater metatarsal separation.
- Corticosteroids have been used with good results in some cases (17).
- Sonographically guided neuroma alcohol ablation may be used (13). One study reported pain resolution in 80.3% of cases at a mean follow-up of 36 months (18).

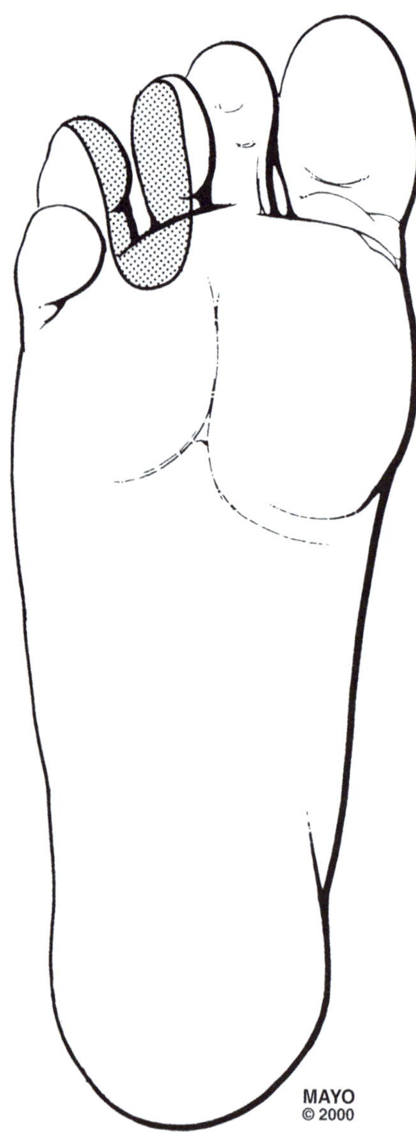

Figure 71.1: Shaded area represents region of sensory loss with an interdigital neuroma in the third intermetatarsal space. (By permission of Mayo Foundation for Medical Education and Research. All rights reserved.)

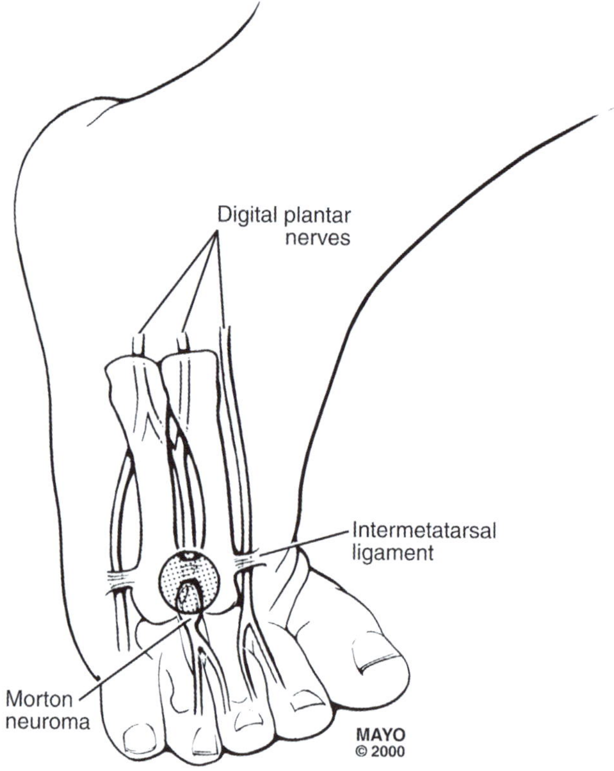

Figure 71.2: Interdigital neuroma in the third intermetatarsal space. (By permission of Mayo Foundation for Medical Education and Research. All rights reserved.)

- Surgery is generally indicated when diagnosis is firm and symptoms refractory. One study noted 76% of cases were asymptomatic at a minimum of 2 years postoperatively after surgical resection (19). Minimally invasive techniques have also been described, with similarly favorable outcomes reported in one small study (20).

TN: TARSAL TUNNEL SYNDROME

Definition

- TN entrapment most commonly occurs at the level of the tarsal tunnel (Fig. 71.3) (3). There is a slight (56%) female predilection (21). TN entrapment may also occur at the level of the medial gastrocnemius (high tarsal tunnel syndrome [TTS]), under the fibromuscular arch of the soleus (soleal sling syndrome), or as a result of popliteus muscle tear (2,6–8,22–24).

Anatomy, Pathophysiology, and Risk Factors

- The TN originates from L4-S3 spinal segments and is the larger terminal branch of the SCN (17). The tarsal tunnel is a fibro-osseous space formed by the flexor retinaculum, medial calcaneus, posterior talus, distal tibia, and medial malleolus and extends from the distal tibia to the navicular. Over 90% of the time, the TN divides into the MPN and LPN within the tarsal tunnel (21). Within 1–2 cm below the medial malleolar-calcaneal line, the MPN and LPN enter separate fibro-osseous canals at the origin of the abductor hallucis muscle (AHM) (2,25). At this point, the LPN may be particularly vulnerable to injury (21).
- Etiologies include trauma, compression by space-occupying lesions (e.g., venous varicosities, ganglion, neurilemmoma, tenosynovitis, os trigonum, bone fragments, tumors, or accessory muscles), systemic disease, and biomechanical factors (25–35). Hyperpronation increases AHM tension and may entrap the TN or

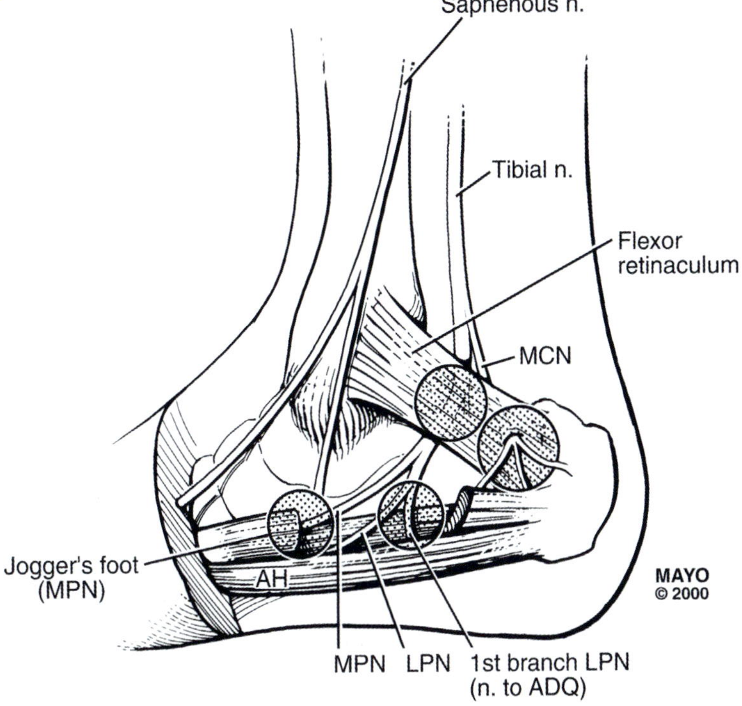

Figure 71.3: Tibial nerve and tarsal tunnel. Shaded areas represent typical sites of nerve entrapment. ADQ, abductor digiti quinti muscle; AH, abductor hallucis muscle; LPN, lateral plantar nerve; MCN, medial calcaneal nerve; MPN, medial plantar nerve. (By permission of Mayo Foundation for Medical Education and Research. All rights reserved.)

plantar nerves (21). Eversion and inversion of the foot and ankle have also been shown to decrease tarsal tunnel compartment volume (36). A specific cause is identified in only 60%–80% of cases (21).

Symptoms and Signs

- Symptoms include cramping, burning, and tingling of the medial ankle and medial and/or plantar foot. The medial heel is usually spared due to the proximal origin of the MCN (21). Symptoms worsen with activity. Running on a banked surface promotes hyperpronation and may aggravate symptoms (17). Resting and night pain may occur in provocative positions, and shaking the foot or walking may provide temporary relief, similar to carpal tunnel syndrome (2,8).
- Examination includes inspection for malalignment, deformity, or muscular atrophy, causing or resulting from TTS, such as forefoot pronation, claw toe, talipes calcaneus, or calcaneovalgus. Percussion testing is performed over the TN and its terminal branches; a Valleix phenomenon (proximal

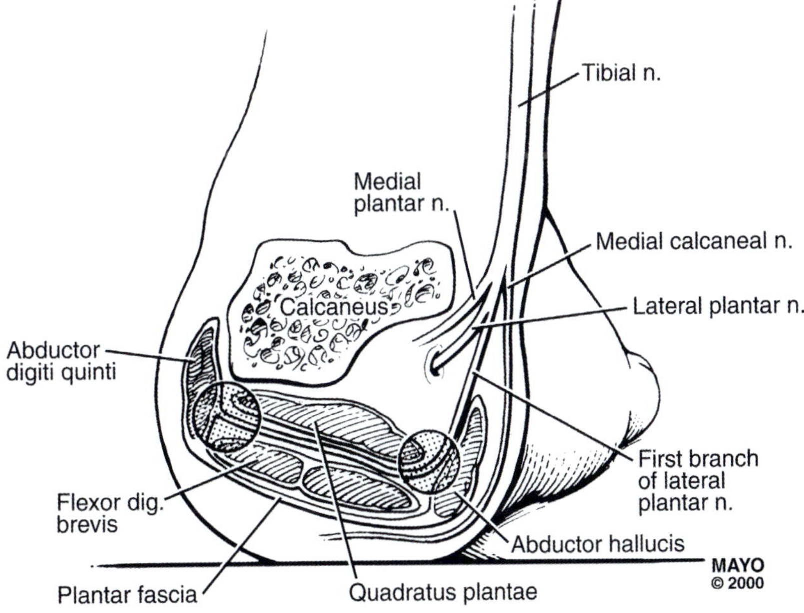

Figure 71.4: First branch of lateral plantar nerve. Shaded areas represent typical sites of entrapment. (By permission of Mayo Foundation for Medical Education and Research. All rights reserved.)

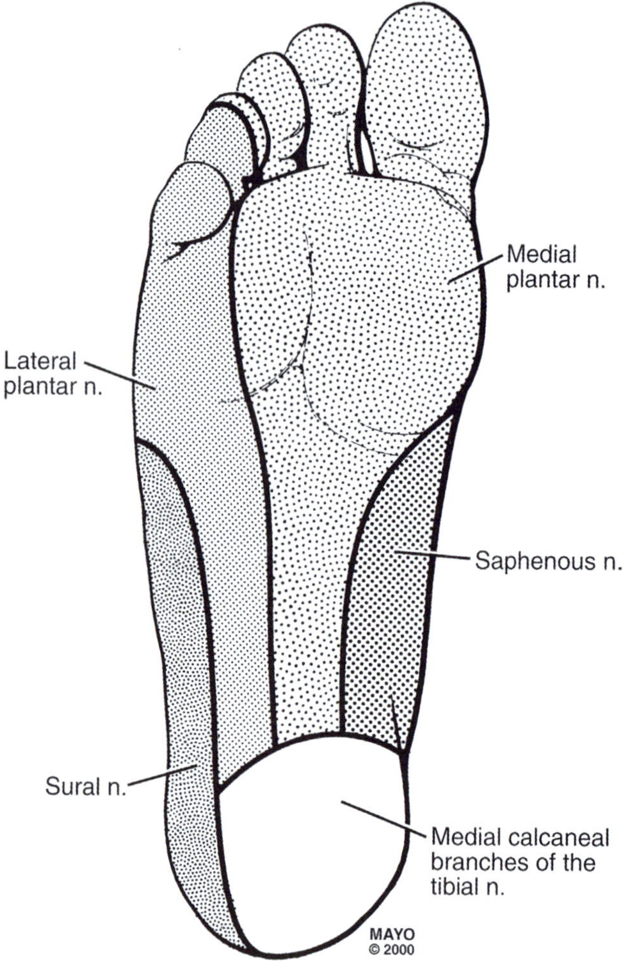

Figure 71.5: Cutaneous innervation of the plantar surface of the foot. (By permission of Mayo Foundation for Medical Education and Research.)

radiation from the site of entrapment) may be elicited (37). Provocative maneuvers include sustained passive eversion, great toe dorsiflexion, and postexercise examination.

- In severe cases, toe plantar flexion weakness manifests with reduced push-off on the affected side (17).

Differential Diagnosis and Evaluation

- Differential diagnosis includes polyneuropathy, proximal or distal mononeuropathy, deep posterior compartment syndrome, popliteal artery entrapment, vascular claudication, venous disease, tenosynovitis, ganglia, plantar fasciitis, tibiotalar or subtalar synovitis, accessory muscle variant, and osseous compression (38,39).
- TN injury just distal to the SN contribution spares gastrocnemius-soleus function and lateral calcaneal and foot sensation. Injury distal to the midportion of the leg affects plantar sensation and results in claw toe deformity due to imbalance between the affected foot intrinsic muscles and the unaffected flexor digitorum longus (FDL) and extensor digitorum brevis (EDB) muscles (17).
- Night pain, proximal radiation, and lack of pain during the first steps in the morning help differentiate TTS from plantar fasciitis (40).
- MRI is effective for examining the tarsal tunnel and reveals an inflammatory lesion or mass in up to 88% of patients with a firm clinical diagnosis of TTS (41). Diagnostic US can also effectively visualize structures within the tarsal tunnel and accurately identify compressive mass lesions and/or focal changes in TN cross-sectional area (29,42,43).
- Electrodiagnostic (EDX) studies may be positive in up to 90% of patients with TTS; whether EDX findings correlate with surgical outcome is controversial (44,45). Of note, increased spontaneous activity can be seen in the AHM in normal subjects (46).

Treatment

- Treatment includes activity modification, NSAIDs, neuromodulatory medications (tricyclic and antiepileptic medications), physical therapy, and biomechanical interventions including pronation control (21). A change in running habits to reduce TN tension may be useful (47).

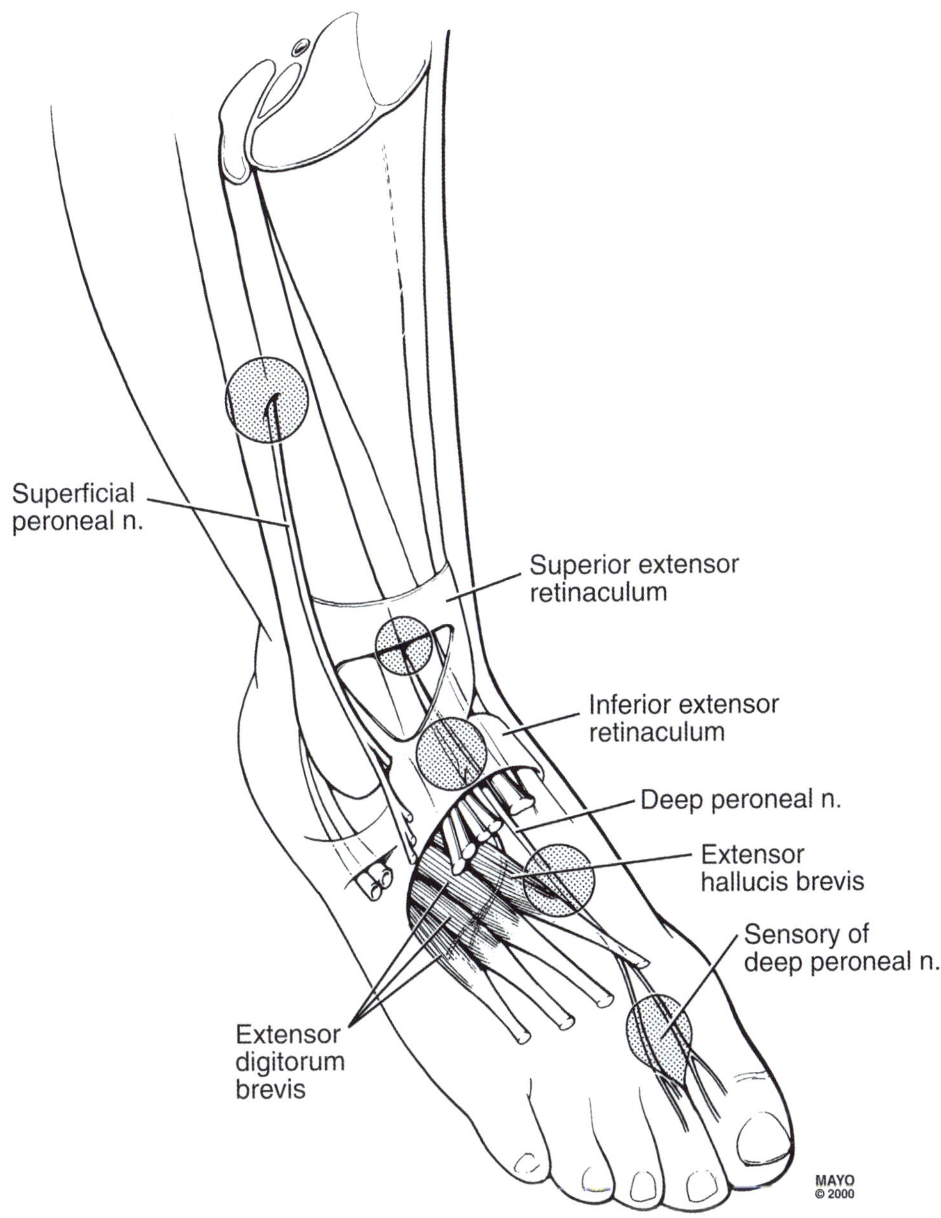

Figure 71.6: Superficial and deep peroneal nerves. Shaded areas represent typical sites of entrapment. (By permission of Mayo Foundation for Medical Education and Research. All rights reserved.)

- Corticosteroid injection may be helpful; a period of postinjection protected weight bearing is recommended (21). Injections around the TN are more accurate with US guidance (48).
- Surgery may be indicated when diagnosis is firm and symptoms refractory (21). Up to 65% of patients required surgical treatment in one study (49).
- Postoperatively, neuropathic symptoms generally improve after 6 weeks, but maximal recovery may take 6 months or more (8). While traditionally good or excellent results were reported in 79%–95% of cases, a more methodologically stringent study indicated only 44% of patients had significant benefit at a minimum 24-month follow-up (21,50). Another investigation found 54% of patients obtained satisfactory benefit following surgical decompression (51). Endoscopic techniques exist, but adequacy of decompression has been questioned (25).

FIRST BRANCH OF THE LATERAL PLANTAR NERVE

Definition

- First branch of the lateral plantar nerve (FB-LPN, also known as inferior calcaneal nerve or Baxter nerve) entrapment is reported to be the most common neurologic cause

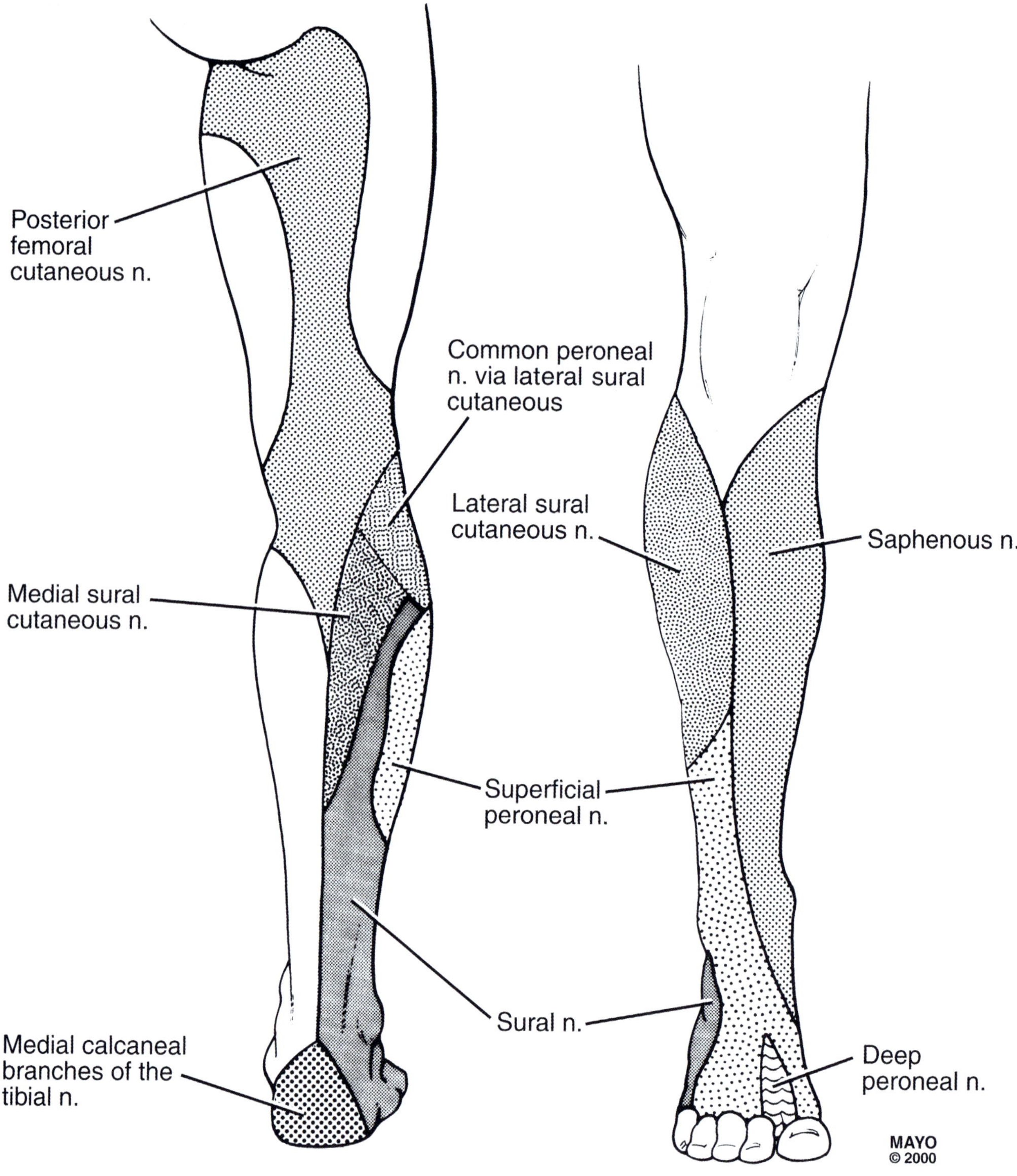

Figure 71.7: Cutaneous innervation of the thigh, leg, and dorsal surface of the foot. (By permission of Mayo Foundation for Medical Education and Research. All rights reserved.)

of heel pain (3,7). Up to 15% of athletes with chronic, recalcitrant heel pain may have FB-LPN entrapment (2). In the largest series to date, the average age was 38 years with 88% being male (7).

Anatomy, Pathophysiology, and Risk Factors

- The FB-LPN usually arises from the LPN in the tarsal tunnel, but in 46% of cases, it may originate directly from the TN (Fig. 71.3) (25). After penetrating the AHM and its fascia,

Table 71.1 Neuroanatomy of the Lower Limb

Sciatic nerve (L4-S3 spinal segments)	Tibial Nerve (TN)	Medial sural cutaneous nerve (MSCN)	Contribution to third interdigital nerve
		Medial calcaneal nerve (MCN)[a]	
		Medial plantar nerve (MPN)	Medial hallucal nerve
		Lateral plantar nerve (LPN)	First branch of LPN (FB-LPN)[b]
	Common peroneal nerve (CPN)	Lateral sural cutaneous nerve (LSCN)	Contribution to third interdigital nerve
		Superficial peroneal nerve (SPN)	
		Deep peroneal nerve (DPN)	
Femoral nerve (FN; L2-4 spinal segments)			Saphenous nerve
Lateral femoral cutaneous nerve (LFCN; L2-3 spinal segments)			
Obturator nerve (ON; L2-4 spinal segments)			

[a]May arise from the LPN or from the bifurcation of the LPN and MPN.
[b]May arise directly from the TN.

the FB-LPN courses inferiorly, passing between the deep fascia of the AHM medially and the medial-caudal margin of the medial head of the quadratus plantae muscle laterally (7). The nerve then courses between the flexor digitorum brevis and quadratus plantae muscles (Fig. 71.4). The FB-LPN ramifies into three terminal branches supplying the flexor digitorum brevis, the medial calcaneal periosteum, and the abductor digiti quinti. The branch to the calcaneal periosteum often supplies branches to the long plantar ligament as well as an inconsistent branch to the quadratus plantae muscle (2).

- FB-LPN entrapment most commonly occurs at the site of inferior to lateral direction change deep to the AHM and less frequently, between the calcaneus and flexor digitorum brevis muscle, or at the plantar aspect of the long plantar ligament (7,52). FB-LPN entrapment has been reported secondary to AHM or quadratus plantae hypertrophy, accessory muscles, abnormal bursae, venous varicosities, calcaneal spurs, and adjacent scar tissue from repetitive injury (6,7,52–54).
- FB-LPN irritation is believed to occur in up to 15%–20% of cases of chronic plantar fasciitis (6–8,17,52). Those with proximal edema of the flexor digitorum brevis or microtears in the plantar fascia may be more susceptible (17). The FB-LPN may be injured by a large calcaneal spur (9).

Symptoms and Signs

- Chronic, neuropathic, and medial heel pain is seen. Symptoms are precipitated by sports in 50% of cases (7). Up to 25% of patients have severe pain in the morning secondary to venous engorgement. Night pain is rare (9).
- A suggested pathognomonic sign of FB-LPN entrapment is maximal pain over the medial heel, superior to the plantar fascia origin along a line drawn parallel to the posterior tibia. In one study, 100% of patients exhibited maximal pain at this site, although 42% also had mild tenderness along the plantar fascia origin (7).

Differential Diagnosis and Evaluation

- Heel pain syndrome, plantar fasciitis, and fat pad disorders are suggested by maximal tenderness in the plantar calcaneal region, anterior medial calcaneus, or mid-medial edge of the plantar fascia, respectively (7). Sensory loss of the medial heel suggests another disorder.
- In 27 patients with 38 symptomatic heels from surgically documented FB-LPN entrapment, only 44% had involvement of the LPN on EDX testing (9).

Treatment

- Most cases of FB-LPN entrapment respond to nonoperative measures (52). Recommended interventions include activity modification, NSAIDs, neuromodulatory medications, physical therapy, biomechanical management for pronation control, and corticosteroid injections (52). One author recommends no more than three injections at 2- to 4-week intervals be attempted (17).
- Most clinicians advocate at least 6–12 months of nonoperative care before considering surgery. Postoperative recovery typically takes 3–6 months, but may be longer if small toe abduction is weak preoperatively (8). With careful patient selection and firm diagnosis, good or excellent results may be seen in approximately 85% of patients (7). A retrospective analysis of outcomes after FB-LPN surgical release found 50% of cases to be asymptomatic and 50% to be mildly symptomatic with activity, at a mean follow-up of 32.8 months (55). Endoscopic techniques have been described (56).

MPN: JOGGER'S FOOT

Definition

- Syndrome of neuropathic pain radiating along the medial heel and longitudinal arch resulting from local entrapment of the MPN (3,47).

Anatomy, Pathophysiology, and Risk Factors

- The MPN enters the sole of the foot, passes superficial to the traversing FDL tendon at the master knot of Henry, and continues distally along the flexor hallucis longus tendon, dividing into terminal medial and lateral branches at the level of the base of the first metatarsal (2). These branches ramify as three terminal common plantar digital nerves within the medial three web spaces. The MPN is a mixed sensorimotor nerve providing sensation to the medial sole and plantar aspect of the first to third and medial fourth toes, as well as motor innervation to the AHM, flexor hallucis brevis, flexor digitorum brevis, and first lumbrical muscles (Figs. 71.3 and 71.5).
- MPN entrapment typically occurs at the AHM fibro-osseous canal or master knot of Henry (6). The MPN may be compressed by AHM hypertrophy, hyperpronation, high-arched orthoses, or in association with hallux rigidus or tibial artery schwannoma (2,6,47,57).

Symptoms and Signs

- Exercise-induced neuropathic pain is reported, radiating along the medial arch toward the plantar aspect of the first and second toes. The most useful palpatory finding is maximal tenderness at the superior aspect of the AHM at the navicular tuberosity, with pain radiating distally (17,47). Provocative testing includes forceful passive heel eversion, percussion over the nerve, and standing on the forefoot. Pre-exercise examination may be normal (6).

Differential Diagnosis and Evaluation

- MPN entrapment typically presents with burning medial heel pain, aching in the longitudinal arch, and medial sole paresthesias (47). Differential diagnosis parallels that of TTS with the addition of local pathologic processes. Resisted great toe plantar flexion or passive dorsiflexion induces pain with flexor hallucis longus tendinopathy but is not typical of nerve entrapment (17).
- EDX studies should be interpreted with caution; asymptomatic runners have been found to have abnormal MPN and SN conduction velocities (58).

Treatment

- Rigid orthoses should be removed to avoid MPN compression. Functional hyperpronation may be addressed by medial arch strengthening, kinetic chain rehabilitation, modifying running mechanics (less valgus) or terrain, or altering footwear (47).
- Surgical release has been successful in refractory cases and is generally a distal extension of TTS surgery.

COMMON PERONEAL NERVE

Definition

- CPN entrapment typically occurs at the fibular head, proximal to the bifurcation into the SPN and DPN, and produces dorsiflexion weakness and neuropathic pain over the anterolateral leg and dorsal foot (3). It is the most prevalent peroneal nerve injury among runners (17,59,60).

Anatomy, Pathophysiology, and Risk Factors

- The CPN contains sensory and motor fibers from L4 to S2 segments and is the smaller terminal branch of the SCN (Figs. 71.5–71.7). The CPN separates from the SCN at the apex of the popliteal fossa, where it supplies innervation to the short head of the biceps femoris muscle and divides into the SPN, DPN, and lateral sural cutaneous nerve at the level of the fibular head.
- The SPN innervates lateral compartment leg muscles and emerges from the lateral compartment by penetrating the crural fascia 10.5–12.5 cm proximal to the tip of the lateral malleolus. It supplies sensation to the anterolateral leg and divides into terminal medial and intermediate cutaneous branches about 6 cm above the lateral malleolus (Figs. 71.6 and 71.7). These branches enter the dorsal foot superficial to the inferior extensor retinaculum and supply sensation to the dorsal foot, with the exception of the first web space.
- The DPN innervates anterior compartment leg muscles, divides into medial and lateral branches 1–2 cm proximal to the ankle, and enters the foot deep to the inferior extensor retinaculum. The medial branch supplies sensation to the first web space; the lateral branch innervates the EDB and local joints. Up to 20% of individuals may have accessory innervation of the EDB from the SPN (17).
- The CPN is vulnerable to compression at the fibular head. Causes include external compression, aneurysms, tumors, tibiofibular joint ganglia, tibiofibular or knee dislocation or instability, Baker cyst, generalized ligamentous laxity, genu varum, genu recurvatum, compartment syndrome, stress fracture, fabella syndrome, fascial compression by the edge of the peroneus longus muscle, direct ice injury, ischemia, and complication of an ankle sprain or after knee surgery (59–69).

Symptoms and Signs

- The DPN is often more severely affected than the SPN. Neuropathic symptoms may affect the anterior or anterolateral leg, extending into the dorsal foot and toe web spaces. The most common complaint is weakness, most often with ankle dorsiflexion (17).
- In one study, postexercise percussion sensitivity or weakness was detected in all seven patients with CPN injury who had normal baseline examinations (59).

Differential Diagnosis and Evaluation

- A focal CPN injury would not involve the TN sensorimotor functions or the cutaneous distribution of the saphenous nerve. Sciatic neuropathy, lumbosacral plexopathy, and L5 radiculopathy may also produce footdrop, but typically produce weakness in nonperoneal innervated muscles, nonperoneal territory sensory loss, and nonperoneal reflex loss. Multiple sclerosis may present as relatively painless, exercise-induced foot drop (Uhthoff phenomenon).
- Diagnostic US can detect intraneural ganglia and other CPN abnormalities (70). EDX abnormalities may only occur postexercise (59).

Treatment

- Treatment may include nerve protection, neuromodulatory medications, transcutaneous electrical nerve stimulation (TENS), biomechanical interventions, dorsiflexion support, knee stabilization, or change in running technique.
- If the clinical diagnosis is firm, operative decompression usually provides satisfactory results. In one small study, 86% of runners returned to normal activities within 6 weeks of surgery (59).

SUPERFICIAL PERONEAL NERVE

Definition

- Typically occurs as the nerve penetrates the crural fascia above the ankle, resulting in neuropathic pain in the SPN distribution (Figs. 71.6 and 71.7). Among athletes, the mean age is 28 years with men and women equally affected (2).

Anatomy, Pathophysiology, and Risk Factors

- May result from sharp fascial edges, chronic ankle sprains, muscle herniation, direct contusion, fibular fracture, edema, varicose veins, wearing tight ski boots or roller blades, biomechanical factors, space-occupying lesions (such as nerve sheath tumors, lipomas, and ganglia), ankle fractures, or a complication of ankle surgery (71–73). Up to 10% of affected individuals may have lateral chronic exertional compartment syndrome (74).

Symptoms and Signs

- Diffuse ache over the sinus tarsi or dorsolateral foot. One third of patients report numbness or tingling (75). Sensation may be an achy distal anterolateral leg discomfort, and proximal radiation has been reported (76). Sensory loss is uncommon (2).
- Examination may reveal percussion tenderness, a fascial defect (60% of patients), or muscular herniation at the exit site approximately 10.5–12.5 cm above the ankle.
- Provocative testing pre- and postexercise is the most useful clinical indicator of SPN entrapment and includes (a) pressure over the exit site during resisted ankle dorsiflexion-eversion, (b) pressure over the same area during passive plantar flexion combined with inversion, and (c) percussion over the SPN course while passive plantar flexion and inversion are maintained. Pain or paresthesias indicate a positive test, and two positive tests strongly supports the diagnosis (74,75).

Differential Diagnosis and Evaluation

- Postexercise nerve conduction testing has been advocated when necessary (74). Diagnostic US can trace the course of the SPN to assess for abnormalities (77).

Treatment

- Parallels that for CPN entrapment, but may also include corticosteroid injection, ankle instability rehabilitation, myofascial release, or lateral heel wedges.
- Though high-quality studies are limited, perineural injection and hydrodissection using normal saline or 5% dextrose water (D5W) has also been increasingly used to successfully treat many entrapment neuropathies including SPN entrapment (78,79) (see Chapter 80: Ultrasound Guided Advanced Procedures for additional details).
- In refractory confirmed cases, surgery typically consists of isolated release at the fascial exit site, reduction of muscular herniation, fat nodule resection, and fasciotomy if compartment syndrome is also documented. One study reported that up to 75% of patients who underwent surgical decompression remained improved at 18-month follow-up; however, only 4 of 17 patients had unlimited activity levels, whereas 10 of 17 patients categorized their activity as improved but still limited (74,75).

DPN: ANTERIOR TARSAL TUNNEL SYNDROME

Definition

- DPN irritation in the vicinity of the extensor retinaculum, resulting in neuropathic pain extending into the dorsomedial foot and first web space (Figs. 71.6 and 71.7) (3).

Anatomy, Pathophysiology, and Risk Factors

- The DPN traverses deep to the extensor retinaculum and between the extensor hallucis longus and extensor digitorum longus tendons, approximately 3–5 cm above the ankle joint. At the level of the oblique superior band of the inferior extensor retinaculum about 1 cm above the ankle joint, the DPN forms its terminal lateral and medial branches. The lateral branch innervates the EDB muscle. The medial branch courses distally with the dorsalis pedis artery, passing deep to the oblique inferior medial band of the inferior extensor retinaculum, where it may be entrapped by processes affecting the talonavicular joint (2).

- DPN entrapment may occur at the inferior aspect of the superior extensor retinaculum where the extensor hallucis longus crosses over the DPN, the inferior extensor retinaculum (most common), or where the EDB crosses the DPN in the first intermetatarsal space. In the latter two cases, an isolated sensory neuropathy of the medial branch occurs. Entrapment may occur due to trauma, shoe contact pressure ("boot top" neuropathy), osteophytic compression, edema, synovitis, or ganglia (80–83).

Symptoms and Signs

- Symptoms include dorsal midfoot pain and neuropathic symptoms extending into the first web space. Symptoms are worse with activity, prolonged standing, and wearing tight fitting or high-top shoes and are relieved by rest. Night pain can occur from pressure or prolonged plantar flexion positioning (25). Depending on entrapment site, symptom provocation may occur with either plantar flexion or dorsiflexion of the ankle (6,25).

Differential Diagnosis and Evaluation

- Parallels that for CPN and SPN entrapments but also includes anterior compartment syndrome. Because CPN entrapments often preferentially affect the DPN fascicles, CPN injury presenting as DPN injury should be excluded (17). Involvement of the EDB localizes injury above the extensor retinaculum.
- Radiographs may reveal dorsal midfoot osteophytes or accessory ossicles that may irritate terminal branches of the DPN (28).

Treatment

- Treatment includes footwear modification to avoid direct pressure, neuromodulatory and anti-inflammatory medications, TENS, edema control, ankle stability rehabilitation, and local corticosteroid injections. Surgery involves partial sectioning of the extensor retinaculum and osteophyte removal. Recovery may take 6–8 weeks.

MISCELLANEOUS NERVE ENTRAPMENT SYNDROMES TN: SOLEAL SLING SYNDROME

Definition, Anatomy, and Pathophysiology

- As previously discussed, TN compression most commonly occurs at the medial ankle within the tarsal tunnel (TTS). More recently, however, the soleal sling, a fibrotendinous arch along the soleus muscle origin, has been recognized as a potential site of proximal TN entrapment (84–87).
- Following SCN bifurcation into CPN and TN branches, the TN courses medially through the proximal leg, deep to the superficial posterior compartment housing the soleus, gastrocnemius, and plantaris. Within the superficial posterior compartment, the soleus, a bipennate muscle originating from the tibia and fibula, is connected by a fascial, "soleal sling," which overlies the TN at the medial junction of superficial and deep posterior compartments, creating an entrapment site as the TN enters the deep posterior compartment to innervate the tibialis posterior, FDL, and flexor hallucis longus (84).

Symptoms and Signs

- Symptoms include proximal, often severe, posterior calf pain with exquisite tenderness and hypersensitivity at the soleal sling, roughly 9 cm distal to the popliteal fossa (86,87). Similar to TTS, pain, numbness, paresthesias, and hypersensitivity may occur along the plantar foot (85,86).
- A positive Tinel sign is frequently described at this level (84,87).
- The motor branch to the flexor hallucis longus is also commonly involved, resulting in great toe flexion weakness (84,86,87).

Differential Diagnosis and Evaluation

- Soleal sling syndrome is traditionally considered a diagnosis of exclusion (85). Differential diagnosis includes lumbosacral radiculopathy, exertional compartment syndrome, popliteal artery entrapment syndrome, medial gastrocnemius tear ("Tennis leg"), popliteus tear, and TTS (84,87). History of failed tarsal tunnel release is often reported (84,86,87).
- EDX studies are of variable utility given TN depth proximally, though are valuable in ruling out lumbosacral radiculopathy, more proximal focal neuropathy, or polyneuropathy (84,86).
- More recently, high-resolution MRI and magnetic resonance (MR) neurography have led to significant advances in diagnosis (84–86). Supportive findings include soleal sling thickening, TN displacement, TN T2 hyperintensity just proximal to the sling, and denervation changes in TN innervated musculature (84,85). Dynamic MRI and US may also be considered to evaluate for TN compression with active plantar flexion or passive dorsiflexion (84,85,88).

Treatment

- Treatment includes activity modification, avoidance of restrictive tights, socks, boots, and other garments, and physical therapy (85). NSAIDs and neuromodulatory agents may be considered.
- For refractory symptoms, proximal TN decompression is warranted. Open release with tibial neurolysis, soleal sling division, and adhesiolysis has demonstrated generally favorable outcomes without any major complications (84,86,87).

SCN: DEEP GLUTEAL SYNDROME

Definition

- Buttock pain and sciatica are common but diagnostically challenging complaints given numerous potential etiologies including intra-abdominal, urogynecological, hip, pelvic, and lumbar spine pathologies (89,90). Buttock, thigh pain, and dysesthesias may also occur from SCN entrapment or injury to any number of structures within the anatomically complex, deep gluteal space (90,91).
- Traditionally, nondiscogenic sciatica has been ascribed to piriformis syndrome, a controversial entity to date. More recently, however, deep gluteal syndrome (DGS) has supplanted this singular model to encompass the multiple pain generators and SCN compression sites within the deep gluteal space (89,90,92).
- Defined as focal and/or radicular pain, paresthesias, or dysesthesias of the posterior buttock, hip, and/or thigh due to SCN irritation from a nonspinal pelvic lesion, DGS includes piriformis syndrome, gemelli-obturator internus syndrome, ischiofemoral impingement syndrome, and proximal hamstring syndrome, overlapping conditions which may present concurrently (89–93).

Anatomy, Pathophysiology, and Risk Factors

- The SCN originates from the ventral rami of L4-S3 nerve roots, forming a single trunk of TN and CPN fascicles before exiting the greater sciatic foramen to the deep gluteal space (90,93). The deep gluteal space is defined anteriorly by the femoral neck and femoroacetabular joint, posteriorly by the gluteus maximus, laterally by the ischial tuberosity, medially by the sacrotuberous ligament, superiorly by the inferior margin of the sciatic notch, and inferiorly by the proximal hamstring origin. From superior to inferior, the deep gluteal space includes the piriformis, superior gemellus, obturator internus, inferior gemellus, and quadratus femoris muscles (89–91,93).
- Exiting the greater sciatic foramen, the SCN courses deep to the piriformis, crosses the obturator internus-gemelli complex just lateral to the ischial tuberosity, and continues superficial to the quadratus femoris through the ischiofemoral space, adjacent to the lesser trochanter (90,91,94). The SCN also maintains a close relationship with the hamstring origin, traveling 1 cm lateral and deep to the proximal insertion (91,94,95).
- Biomechanical studies demonstrate substantial SCN mobility and proximal excursion within the deep gluteal space during routine hip motion. Dynamic narrowing of the deep gluteal space also occurs with hip flexion, abduction, and external rotation (89,90,96). Neural tension and/or impingement at any of these locations may therefore result in SCN dysfunction.

Symptoms and Signs

- Clinical assessment is challenging given overlap with lumbar, SI joint, and intra- and extra-articular hip pathologies, and lumbosacral radiculopathy and hip osteoarthritis should first be ruled out (89,91,93). Presentation is typically insidious, atraumatic, chronic, and unilateral, though acute, traumatic, and bilateral cases have been reported.
- Symptoms include posterior hip or buttock pain and tenderness in the gluteal region with or without radicular, "sciatica-like" pain and paresthesias.
- Increased pain with activity, particularly hip flexion and/or rotation combined with knee extension, gait alterations, sitting intolerance beyond 20 to 30 minutes, sensory disturbances, and worsening nocturnal pain are frequently reported (89,90,92,94). Objective weakness in SCN innervated muscles, including focal deficit such as footdrop, is rare (90,92).
- Examination requires evaluation of the spine, hips, pelvis, and abdomen including pelvic alignment, palpation, active and passive range of motion, gait analysis, provocative maneuvers, and detailed neurovascular testing (90,91,94).
- Tests and signs that may assist in the clinical diagnosis of SCN entrapment, the specifics of which are beyond the scope of this review, include the straight leg raise test and Lasègue sign, Pace sign, Freiberg sign, Beatty test, FADIR test, ischiofemoral impingement test, long stride test, and active and seated piriformis stretch tests (89,92,94,97).

Differential Diagnosis

Piriformis Syndrome

- Piriformis syndrome is a postulated cause of proximal SCN compression either due to a primary cause such as muscle hypertrophy or aberrant SCN anatomy, or more commonly, a secondary process such as overuse (89,92,93). Despite controversy, the piriformis has been most commonly associated with SCN compression in the deep gluteal space, though reported incidence is highly variable (89,91,92,98).
- Traversing the greater sciatic foramen, the piriformis originates along the ventrolateral surface of S2-S4 vertebrae, the gluteal surface of the ileum, and the SI joint capsule, inserting onto the greater trochanter (89).
- The SCN typically runs inferior to the piriformis, rendering it susceptible to compression, though the SCN or one if its divisions, typically the CPN, may course through or above the piriformis, with variants seen in up to 16% of patients (89,91,92,98,99). Despite numerous hypotheses, however, no study has demonstrated a correlation between aberrant piriformis or SCN anatomy and piriformis syndrome (89,91,93,97).
- Provocative factors include sitting, overuse, and repetitive trauma. Exam may demonstrate piriformis contracture, external rotation weakness, and excessive femoral adduction or internal rotation (94,97). When performed together,

active and seated piriformis stretch tests have demonstrated improved sensitivity (0.91) and specificity (0.80) for the clinical diagnosis of SCN entrapment (89,93).

Gemelli-Obturator Internus Syndrome

- Though rare, the gemelli/obturator internus complex should be considered as a cause of SCN irritation in the deep gluteal space. As the SCN passes beneath the piriformis and over the superior gemellus and obturator internus, the SCN may become entrapped between the two muscles, especially with internal hip rotation. A constricting, fibrous band may also be present.
- Similar to piriformis syndrome, dynamic alterations, insertional pathologies including strains and tears, and aberrant anatomical relationships, including SCN penetration of the obturator internus, have been reported as potential causes, though asymmetric hypertrophy of the gemelli or obturator internus is rare (89,92–94).

Ischiofemoral Impingement Syndrome

- The SCN then courses through the ischiofemoral space superficial to the quadratus femoris where impingement may occur between the ischium and lesser trochanter of the femur (89,92,94). Repetitive microtrauma may result in scar tissue formation between the quadratus femoris and SCN, potentiating SCN compression by the lesser trochanter. Less frequently, strains and tears occur at the distal myotendinous junction, resulting in localized edema and SCN irritation (89,92,94).
- Pain is typically lateral to the ischium and notably improved with sitting. Symptoms are reproduced with terminal hip extension and long stride lengths when the femur is approximated to the ischium (91,92,94,96).
- Exam may demonstrate poor pelvic stabilization, increased femoral version, limited hip extension, hip adduction contracture, and gluteal weakness (94).

Hamstring Syndrome

- In the posterior thigh, the SCN runs superficial to the adductor magnus and deep to the hamstring complex (92). As the SCN resides roughly 1 cm from the hamstring origin at the ischial tuberosity, proximal hamstring pathology may result in SCN irritation (91,92).
- Collectively referred to as hamstring syndrome, a wide spectrum of acute and chronic conditions can affect the SCN, including partial and complete muscle or tendon tears, tendinopathy or tendinosis, apophysitis, avulsion fractures, and contusions. Inflammatory changes and adhesions may also lead to fibrosis, resulting in dynamic SCN entrapment with hip or knee motion or static entrapment due to SCN scarring to the hamstrings (89,91,92,94).
- Pain and tenderness at or just lateral to the ischial tuberosity are characteristic with prominent sitting intolerance. Symptoms are exacerbated by hamstring activation, hip flexion, and eccentric lengthening as in heel strike (92,94).
- Exam may demonstrate altered pelvic sagittal alignment, gluteal and hamstring weakness, and in severe cases, tendon retraction (94).

Evaluation

- High-resolution MRI and MR neurography have demonstrated excellent capability in identifying deep gluteal space pathologies. MRI may identify structural causes of SCN entrapment including fibrous bands, muscle hypertrophy or atrophy, partial or complete muscle or tendon tears, anatomic variations, edema, and narrowing of compressible spaces (89,90,93). Pathologic findings on MR neurography include SCN neural enlargement, loss of normal fascicular architecture, increased T2 signal hyperintensity, increased perifascicular fat, and perineural fat stranding (89,92). More recently, high-resolution US has become a reliable diagnostic tool for deep gluteal space visualization, sonopalpation, and dynamic evaluation.
- Diagnostic and potentially therapeutic image-guided injections into the perineural sciatic fat or nerve sheath are also frequently employed to assist in identifying the pain generator (89,90,92,98).
- EDX may demonstrate conduction abnormalities and denervation findings suggestive of sciatic neuropathy. However, no study has found EDX to be of confirmatory value, and primary utility resides in ruling out a radiculopathy or other peripheral cause (90–92,94).

Treatment

- In the absence of a clear surgical indication such as a compressive mass lesion, a graduated therapeutic approach is recommended for all causes of DGS, including rest, activity modification, NSAIDs and neuromodulatory agents, and physical therapy for at least 6 weeks.
- Image-guided local anesthetic and steroid injections can have both diagnostic and therapeutic value, with US-guided piriformis muscle injections most frequently described (89,90,92–94,98). In recalcitrant cases, intramuscular piriformis botulinum toxin injection may be considered, though there is some concern for iatrogenic SCN fibrosis (89,90,96).
- As briefly mentioned, few studies have also investigated US-guided hydrodissection to separate entrapped nerves from surrounding fascia via tissue expansion and adhesiolysis (98,100). SCN perineural hydrodissection involves injection of fluid (typically anesthetic, normal saline, or 5% dextrose in water [D5W]) to dissect the perineural plane and tissue space and may be considered for conditions such as hamstring syndrome in which the SCN is scarred to the hamstrings (90,98,100).
- In refractory cases, surgical treatment is recommended to address any underlying pathology and preserve neural function. Historically, open procedures have been performed. However, endoscopic techniques are gaining more attention

with recent literature supporting the use of SCN endoscopic decompression, neurolysis, and adhesiolysis, with or without muscle resection (89–93,96).

MEDIAL CALCANEAL NERVE

- Medial calcaneal nerve (MCN) entrapment produces neuropathic pain at the medial heel secondary to entrapment in the tarsal tunnel region (3). The purely sensory MCN usually arises from the TN, but may arise from the LPN or at the MPN-LPN bifurcation; thus, the MCN may originate proximal to or within the tarsal tunnel. The MCN pierces the flexor retinaculum to provide cutaneous innervation to the posterior, medial, and plantar surfaces of the heel (Figs. 71.3, 71.5, and 71.7). Entrapment usually occurs as the MCN pierces the flexor retinaculum.
- Contributing factors may include excessive pronation, direct compression, or repetitive heel impact on hard surfaces. Neuropathic pain is limited to the medial heel, and there is no motor or reflex deficit. Symptoms increase with activity. Percussion tenderness may be present, or paresthesias may occur when palpating the MCN as it pierces the retinaculum posterior to the TN (Fig. 71.3). Examination less commonly reveals proximal radiation, or a "lamp cord sign," a hypersensitive, tender thickening of the MCN along its oblique-posterior course (101).
- Differential diagnosis is similar to TTS, but medial heel involvement suggests MCN entrapment.
- Nonoperative management follows general principles previously discussed, including measures to improve pronation control, corticosteroid injections, and cutout pads and footwear alterations to reduce direct pressure on the MCN. A small study showed promising results with extracorporeal shockwave treatment (102). The "lamp cord sign" is often a poor prognostic factor, and surgery is often recommended to remove this "pseudoneuroma" (101).

SURAL NERVE

- The SN is formed by branches of the TN and CPN in the posterior calf, 11–20 cm proximal to the lateral malleolus (3). Two cm proximal to the lateral malleolus, the SN provides a sensory branch to the lateral heel, and then courses subcutaneously inferior to the peroneal tendons to the base of the fifth metatarsal, where it ramifies into distal sensory branches (Figs. 71.5 and 71.7). Causes include recurrent ankle sprains, calcaneal or fifth metatarsal fractures, Achilles tendinopathy, space-occupying lesions such as ganglia, direct contusion, footwear-induced pressure, or iatrogenic (103,104).
- Symptoms consist of achy, posterolateral calf pain, with neuropathic pain in the SN distribution. Examination includes percussion testing along the nerve and provocative testing by passive dorsiflexion and inversion.
- SN conduction studies in asymptomatic runners may be abnormal (58).
- Treatment emphasizes pressure reduction from footwear, Achilles stretching, neuropathic pain treatment, edema control, and ankle stability rehabilitation. When SN block is indicated, US guidance has been shown to improve clinical outcome (105). A retrospective study found good to excellent results in 17 of 18 SN entrapment cases undergoing surgical neurolysis (106).

SAPHENOUS NERVE

- The saphenous nerve is the largest cutaneous branch of the femoral nerve. This purely sensory nerve arises from the femoral nerve in the femoral triangle and courses with the femoral artery to the medial knee, where its infrapatellar branch supplies cutaneous sensation to the medial knee (3). It then courses inferiorly with the saphenous vein to supply cutaneous sensation to the medial calf to the level of the ankle (8). At the ankle, a branch passes anterior to the medial malleolus to innervate the medial foot (Figs. 71.3 and 71.5). The saphenous nerve is most vulnerable at the medial knee, where it pierces the fascia and emerges from the distal subsartorial canal (Hunter adductor canal).
- Causes of saphenous neuropathy include entrapment at the adductor canal, pes anserine bursitis, contusion, patellar dislocation, and iatrogenic injury from knee surgery or injection (107–112).
- Athletes report neuropathic pain and numbness in the area of the medial knee and/or calf, depending on whether there is isolated infrapatellar branch or complete saphenous nerve involvement. Saphenous neuropathy related to pes anserine bursitis may clinically resemble tibial stress fracture (109).
- Examination includes percussion testing along the nerve starting at the adductor canal.
- Differential diagnosis includes all proximal femoral nerve, plexus, and root lesions, as well as musculoskeletal disorders about the knee. Diagnosis and treatment principles resemble those for SN entrapment but focus on different anatomic areas. Surgical release or excision of a neuroma may be necessary.

OBTURATOR NERVE

- Obturator nerve (ON) entrapment is a potential source of groin pain in some athletes (113). The ON arises from the L2–4 spinal segments, exits the pelvis via a fibro-osseous tunnel (obturator canal), and divides into terminal anterior and posterior branches (113). These branches provide the predominant motor innervation to the thigh adductor group and sensory innervations to the distal one-half to two-thirds of the medial thigh (3). ON entrapment most commonly occurs at the exit of the obturator canal due to compressive fibrous bands located in this area (113,114). Rarely, ON entrapment may occur secondary to the local inflammatory changes of osteitis pubis or from an obturator hernia (113,115).

- The athlete will typically complain of activity-related groin pain of a deep, burning, achy quality. Radicular pain, numbness, tingling, and weakness are rare. Examination is largely unremarkable, but assists in excluding more common causes of hip and groin pain among athletes.
- EDX studies may reveal fibrillation potentials in the adductor muscles in some cases but are not uniformly helpful (113,114). Local anesthetic and corticosteroid injections may assist in making the diagnosis and have successfully treated some cases when combined with rehabilitation. Surgical treatment may be necessary (114). A laparoscopic method has been described (116).

LATERAL FEMORAL CUTANEOUS NERVE: MERALGIA PARESTHETICA

- Lateral femoral cutaneous nerve (LFCN) injury has been reported in athletes (117). The purely sensory LFCN arises from the L2–3 spinal segments and typically exits the pelvis by passing underneath or through the lateral aspect of the ilioinguinal ligament, just medial to the anterior superior iliac spine (ASIS) (113). The LFCN then splits into two terminal branches, supplying cutaneous innervation to the anterolateral thigh (3). LFCN injury usually occurs at the level of the ilioinguinal ligament, where the nerve is susceptible to local contusive trauma due to its superficial location and can be injured by repetitive hip flexion-extension.
- Etiologies include rapid weight change, compression from tight clothing or belts, and systemic disease affecting nerves such as thyroid disease and diabetes.
- Athletes report burning, aching discomfort over the anterolateral thigh, with or without clear inciting factors. Examination is often normal but may reveal percussion tenderness or a percussion sign approximately 1 cm anterior and inferior to the ASIS, or a sensory deficit in the cutaneous distribution.
- Differential diagnosis includes focal musculoskeletal pathologies or lesions affecting the lumbosacral plexus or L2–3 nerve roots.
- Treatment involves removal of inciting factors, treatment of neuropathic pain, and injections with local anesthetic and corticosteroid, which may be diagnostic and therapeutic with up to 90% of cases resolving with nonoperative management (118). Successful high-volume perineural injection and hydrodissection with 10–20 mL of D5W has also been described (119,120).
- Surgical release is sometimes necessary (113). One series reported complete symptom resolution in 73% of cases following surgical decompression at a mean follow-up of 4.1 years (121).

MEDIAL HALLUCAL NERVE

- The medial hallucal nerve is a distal terminal branch of the MPN, providing sensation to the medial aspect of the great toe (3). This nerve may be rarely entrapped as it exits the distal end of the AHM, producing medial first MTP joint pain and neuropathic pain extending along the medial great toe. Etiologies include pressure from hallux valgus, prominent tibial sesamoid, abductor hallucis tendinopathy, and poorly fitting footwear.
- Percussion tenderness or a percussion sign over the nerve may be useful on examination. Differential diagnosis includes medial tibial sesamoid disorders, MTP joint disorders, and polyneuropathy. Treatment includes removal of inciting factors and treatment of neuropathic pain as previously described.

SUMMARY

- Lower extremity nerve entrapment represents an uncommon but important cause of exercise and sport-related leg pain and other neurologic symptoms such as numbness, weakness, and paresthesias.
- Successful diagnosis relies heavily on history and neuromuscular examination including recognition of common symptoms and patterns as well as detailed assessment of strength, sensation, and muscle bulk, which may reveal focal abnormalities in a specific peripheral nerve distribution. Exam may additionally be aided by nerve percussion testing, provocative maneuvers, and postexercise examination.
- Diagnostic testing may include plain radiographs, static or dynamic US and MRI, and EDX testing. More recently, high-resolution MR neurography has also greatly improved diagnostic capabilities.
- The majority of peripheral lower extremity nerve conditions can be managed conservatively including relative rest, activity, biomechanical, equipment modifications, NSAIDs, neuromodulatory agents, and physical therapy including modalities.
- Image-guided injections with lidocaine and/or corticosteroid can be both diagnostic and therapeutic. More recently, US-guided peripheral nerve hydrodissection with anesthetic, normal saline, or 5% D5W has also been employed with promising results.
- In the absence of a clear surgical indication such as a compressive mass lesion, most clinicians advocate for at least 6–12 months of nonoperative care. For those cases which remain refractory and have a firm diagnosis, surgical decompression is generally indicated.

REFERENCES

1. Coughlin MJ, Mann RA, Saltzman CL. *Surgery of the Foot and Ankle*. 8th ed. St. Louis (MO): Mosby; 2006. 1511 p.
2. Schon LC, Baxter DE. Neuropathies of the foot and ankle in athletes. *Clin Sports Med*. 1990;9(2):489–509.
3. Smith J, Dahm DL. Nerve entrapments. In: O'Connor FG, Wilder R, Nirschl R, eds. *The Textbook of Running Medicine*. New York: McGraw-Hill; 2001:257–72.
4. Styf J. Chronic exercise induced pain in the anterior aspect of the lower leg. An overview of diagnosis. *Sports Med*. 1989;7(5):331–9.
5. Babcock JL. Cervical spine injuries. Diagnosis and classification. *Arch Surg*. 1976;111(6):646–51.
6. Baxter DE. Functional nerve disorders in the athlete's foot, ankle and leg. *Instr Course Lect*. 1993;42:185–94.
7. Baxter DE, Pfeffer GB. Treatment of chronic heel pain by surgical release of the first branch of the lateral plantar nerve. *Clin Orthop Relat Res*. 1992;279:229–36.
8. Schon LC. Nerve entrapment, neuropathy, and nerve dysfunction in athletes. *Orthop Clin North Am*. 1994;25(1):47–59.
9. Schon LC, Glennon TP, Baxter DE. Heel pain syndrome: electrodiagnostic support for nerve entrapment. *Foot Ankle*. 1993;14(3):129–35.
10. Wu KK. Morton's interdigital neuroma: a clinical review of its etiology, treatment, and results. *J Foot Ankle Surg*. 1996;35(2):112–88.
11. Kim JY, Choi JH, Park J, Wang J, Lee I. An anatomical study of Morton's interdigital neuroma: the relationship between the occurring site and the deep transverse metatarsal ligament (DTML). *Foot Ankle Int*. 2007;28(9):1007–10.
12. Gregg J, Marks P. Metatarsalgia: an ultrasound perspective. *Australas Radiol*. 2007;51(6):493–9.
13. Hughes RJ, Ali K, Jones H, Kendall S, Connell DA. Treatment of Morton's neuroma with alcohol injection under sonographic guidance: follow-up of 101 cases. *AJR Am J Roentgenol*. 2007;188(6):1535–9.
14. Quinn TJ, Jacobson JA, Craig JG, van Holsbeeck MT. Sonography of Morton's neuromas. *Am J Roentgenol*. 2000;174(6):1723–8.
15. Sofka CM, Adler RS. Ultrasound guided interventions in the foot and ankle. *Semin Musculoskelet Radiol*. 2002;6(2):163–8.
16. Lee MJ, Kim S, Huh YM, et al. Morton neuroma: evaluated with ultrasonography and MR imaging. *Korean J Radiol*. 2007;8(2):148–55.
17. McCluskey LF, Webb LB. Compression and entrapment neuropathies of the lower extremity. *Clin Podiatr Med Surg*. 1999;16(1):96–125. vii.
18. Magnan B, Marangon A, Frigo A, Bartolozzi P. Local phenol injection in the treatment of interdigital neuritis of the foot (Morton's neuroma). *Chir Organi Mov*. 2005;90(4):371–7.
19. Espinosa N, Schmitt JW, Saupe N, et al. Morton neuroma: MR imaging after resection—postoperative MR and histologic findings in asymptomatic and symptomatic intermetatarsal spaces. *Radiology*. 2010;255(3):850–6.
20. Zelent ME, Kane RM, Neese DJ, Lockner WB. Minimally invasive Morton's intermetatarsal neuroma decompression. *Foot Ankle Int*. 2007;28(2):263–5.
21. Lau JT, Daniels TR. Tarsal tunnel syndrome: a review of the literature. *Foot Ankle Int*. 1999;20(3):201–9.
22. de Ruiter GC, Torchia ME, Amrami KK, Spinner RJ. Neurovascular compression following isolated popliteus muscle rupture: a case report. *J Surg Orthop Adv*. 2005;14(3):129–32.
23. Feinberg JH, Spielholz NI, eds. *Peripheral Nerve Injuries in the Athlete*. Champaign (IL): Human Kinetics; 2003:106–41.
24. Peri G. The "critical zones" of entrapment of the nerves of the lower limb. *Surg Radiol Anat*. 1991;13(2):139–43.
25. Park TA, Del Toro DR. Electrodiagnostic evaluation of the foot. *Phys Med Rehabil Clin N Am*. 1998;9(4):871–96. vii–viii.
26. Jackson DL, Haglund B. Tarsal tunnel syndrome in athletes. Case reports and literature review. *Am J Sports Med*. 1991;19(1):61–5.
27. Miranpuri S, Snook E, Vang D, Yong RM, Chagares WE. Neurilemoma of the posterior tibial nerve and tarsal tunnel syndrome. *J Am Podiatr Med Assoc*. 2007;97(2):148–50.
28. Murphy PC, Baxter DE. Nerve entrapment of the foot and ankle in runners. *Clin Sports Med*. 1985;4(4):753–63.
29. Nagaoka M, Matsuzaki H. Ultrasonography in tarsal tunnel syndrome. *J Ultrasound Med*. 2005;24(8):1035–40.
30. Park TA, Del Toro DR. The medial calcaneal nerve: anatomy and nerve conduction technique. *Muscle Nerve*. 1995;18(1):32–8.
31. Pasku DS, Karampekios SK, Kontakis GM, Katonis PG. Varicosities as an etiology of tarsal tunnel syndrome and the significance of Tinel's sign: report of two cases in young men and a review of the literature. *J Am Podiatr Med Assoc*. 2009;99(2):144–7.
32. Pla ME, Dillingham TR, Spellman NT, Colon E, Jabbari B. Painful legs and moving toes associates with tarsal tunnel syndrome and accessory soleus muscle. *Mov Disord*. 1996;11(1):82–6.
33. Sammarco GJ, Stephens MM. Tarsal tunnel syndrome caused by the flexor digitorum accessorius longus. A case report. *J Bone Joint Surg Am*. 1990;72(3):453–4.
34. Stefko RM, Lauerman WC, Heckman JD. Tarsal tunnel syndrome caused by an unrecognized fracture of the posterior process of the talus (Cedell fracture). A case report. *J Bone Joint Surg Am*. 1994;76(1):116–8.
35. Yamamoto S, Tominaga Y, Yura S, Tada H. Tarsal tunnel syndrome with double causes (ganglion, tarsal coalition) evoked by ski boots. Case report. *J Sports Med Phys Fitness*. 1995;35(2):143–5.
36. Bracilovic A, Nihal A, Houston VL, Beattie AC, Rosenberg ZS, Trepman E. Effect of foot and ankle position on tarsal tunnel compartment volume. *Foot Ankle Int*. 2006;27(6):431–7.
37. Dumitru D, Amato AA, Zwarts MJ, eds. *Electrodiagnostic Medicine*. 2nd ed. Philadelphia (PA): Hanley & Belfus; 2001. 1103 p.
38. Sammarco GJ, Chalk DE, Feibel JH. Tarsal tunnel syndrome and additional nerve lesions in the same limb. *Foot Ankle*. 1993;14(2):71–7.
39. Turnipseed W, Pozniak M. Popliteal entrapment as a result of neurovascular compression by the soleus and plantaris muscles. *J Vasc Surg*. 1992;15(2):285–94.
40. Jackson DL, Haglund BL. Tarsal tunnel syndrome in runners. *Sports Med*. 1992;13(2):146–9.
41. Frey C, Kerr R. Magnetic resonance imaging and the evaluation of tarsal tunnel syndrome. *Foot Ankle*. 1993;14(3):159–64.
42. Alshami AM, Cairns CW, Wylie BK, Souvlis T, Coppieters MW. Reliability and size of the measurement error when determining the cross-sectional area of the tibial nerve at the tarsal tunnel with ultrasonography. *Ultrasound Med Biol*. 2009;35(7):1098–102.
43. Vijayan J, Therimadasamy AK, Teoh HL, Chan YC, Wilder-Smith EP. Sonography as an aid to neurophysiological studies in diagnosing tarsal tunnel syndrome. *Am J Phys Med Rehabil*. 2009;88(6):500–1.
44. Galardi G, Amadio S, Maderna L, et al. Electrophysiologic studies in tarsal tunnel syndrome. Diagnostic reliability of motor distal latency, mixed nerve and sensory nerve conduction studies. *Am J Phys Med Rehabil*. 1994;73(3):193–8.
45. Gondring WH, Trepman E, Shields B. Tarsal tunnel syndrome: assessment of treatment outcome with an anatomic pain intensity scale. *Foot Ankle Surg*. 2009;15(3):133–8.

46. Boon AJ, Harper CM. Needle EMG of abductor hallucis and peroneus tertius in normal subjects. *Muscle Nerve*. 2003;27(6):752–6.
47. Rask MR. Medial plantar neurapraxia (jogger's foot): report of 3 cases. *Clin Orthop Relat Res*. 1978;134:193–5.
48. Redborg KE, Antonakakis JG, Beach ML, Chinn CD, Sites BD. Ultrasound improves the success rate of a tibial nerve block at the ankle. *Reg Anesth Pain Med*. 2009;34(3):256–60.
49. Cimino WR. Tarsal tunnel syndrome: review of the literature. *Foot Ankle*. 1990;11(1):47–52.
50. Pfeiffer WH, Cracchiolo A III. Clinical results after tarsal tunnel decompression. *J Bone Joint Surg Am*. 1994;76(8):1222–30.
51. Sung KS, Park SJ. Short-term operative outcome of tarsal tunnel syndrome due to benign space-occupying lesions. *Foot Ankle Int*. 2009;30(8):741–5.
52. Johnston MR. Nerve entrapment causing heel pain. *Clin Podiatr Med Surg*. 1994;11(4):617–24.
53. Fredericson M, Standage S, Chou L, Matheson G. Lateral plantar nerve entrapment in a competitive gymnast. *Clin J Sport Med*. 2001;11(2):111–4.
54. Park TA, Del Toro DR. Isolated inferior calcaneal neuropathy. *Muscle Nerve*. 1996;19(1):106–8.
55. Goecker RM, Banks AS. Analysis of release of the first branch of the lateral plantar nerve. *J Am Podiatr Med Assoc*. 2000;90(6):281–6.
56. Lui TH. Endoscopic decompression of the first branch of the lateral plantar nerve. *Arch Orthop Trauma Surg*. 2007;127(9):859–61.
57. Spinner RJ, Scheithauer BW, Amrami KK. Medial plantar nerve compression by a tibial artery schwannoma. Case report. *J Neurosurg*. 2007;106(5):921–3.
58. Colak T, Bamaç B, Gönener A, Ozbek A, Budak F. Comparison of nerve conduction velocities of lower extremities between runners and controls. *J Sci Med Sport*. 2005;8(4):403–10.
59. Leach RE, Purnell MB, Saito A. Peroneal nerve entrapment in runners. *Am J Sports Med*. 1989;17(2):287–91.
60. Møller B, Kadin S. Entrapment of the common peroneal nerve. *Am J Sports Med*. 1987;15(1):90–1.
61. Al-Kashmiri A, Delaney JS. Case report: fatigue fracture of the proximal fibula with secondary common peroneal nerve injury. *Clin Orthop Relat Res*. 2007;463:225–8.
62. Bonnevialle P, Dubrana F, Galau B, et al. Common peroneal nerve palsy complicating knee dislocation and bicruciate ligaments tears. *Orthop Traumatol Surg Res*. 2010;96(1):64–9.
63. Dawson DM, Hallett M, Wilbourn AJ, eds. *Entrapment Neuropathies* 3rd ed. Philadelphia (PA): Lippincott-Raven; 1999:273–8.
64. DiRisio D, Lazaro R, Popp AJ. Nerve entrapment and calf atrophy caused by a Baker's cyst: case report. *Neurosurgery*. 1994;35(2):333–4.
65. Meals RA. Peroneal-nerve palsy complicating ankle sprain. Report of two cases and review of the literature. *J Bone Joint Surg Am*. 1977;59(7):966–8.
66. Moeller JL, Monroe J, McKeag DB. Cryotherapy-induced common peroneal nerve palsy. *Clin J Sport Med*. 1997;7(3):212–6.
67. Nagel A, Greenebaum E, Singson RD, Rosenwasser MP, McCann PD. Foot drop in a long-distance runner. An unusual presentation of neurofibromatosis. *Orthop Rev*. 1994;23(6):526–30.
68. Peicha G, Pascher A, Schwarzl F, Pierer G, Fellinger M, Passler JM. Transsection of the peroneal nerve complicating knee arthroscopy: case report and cadaver study. *Arthroscopy*. 1998;14(2):221–3.
69. Sprowson AP, Rankin K, Shand JE, Ferrier G. Common peroneal and posterior tibial ischemic nerve damage, a rare cause. *Foot Ankle Surg*. 2010;16(2):e16–7.
70. Visser LH. High resolution sonography of the common peroneal nerve: detection of intraneural ganglia. *Neurology*. 2006;67(8):1473–5.
71. Redfern DJ, Sauvé PS, Sakellariou A. Investigation of incidence of superficial peroneal nerve injury following ankle fracture. *Foot Ankle Int*. 2003;24(10):771–4.
72. Stamatis ED, Manidakis NE, Patouras PP. Intraneural ganglion of the superficial peroneal nerve: a case report. *J Foot Ankle Surg*. 2010;49(4):400.e1-400.e4004.
73. Takao M, Ochi M, Shu N, et al. A case of superficial peroneal nerve injury during ankle arthroscopy. *Arthroscopy*. 2001;17(4):403–4.
74. Styf J, Morberg P. The superficial peroneal tunnel syndrome. Results of treatment by decompression. *J Bone Joint Surg Br*. 1997;79(5):801–3.
75. Styf J. Entrapment of the superficial peroneal nerve. Diagnosis and results of decompression. *J Bone Joint Surg Br*. 1989;71(1):131–5.
76. Lowdon IM. Superficial peroneal nerve entrapment. A case report. *J Bone Joint Surg Br*. 1985;67(1):58–9.
77. Canella C, Demondion X, Guillin R, Boutry N, Peltier J, Cotten A. Anatomic study of the superficial peroneal nerve using sonography. *AJR Am J Roentgenol*. 2009;193(1):174–9.
78. Chiang CF, Cheng SH, Wu CH, Özçakar L. Video demonstration of ultrasound-guided hydrodissection for superficial peroneal nerve entrapment. *Pain Med*. 2020;21(7):1509–10.
79. Wu YT, Wu CH, Lin JA, Su DC, Hung CY, Lam SKH. Efficacy of 5% dextrose water injection for peripheral entrapment neuropathy: a narrative review. *Int J Mol Sci*. 2021;22(22):12358.
80. Dallari D, Pellacani A, Marinelli A, Verni E, Giunti A. Deep peroneal nerve paresis in a runner caused by ganglion at capitulum peronei. Case report and review of the literature. *J Sports Med Phys Fitness*. 2004;44(4):436–40.
81. Dellon A. Deep peroneal nerve entrapment on the dorsum of the foot. *Foot Ankle*. 1990;11(2):73–80.
82. Gessini L, Jandolo B, Pietrangeli A. The anterior tarsal syndrome. Report of four cases. *J Bone Joint Surg Am*. 1984;66(5):786–7.
83. Lindenbaum BL. Ski boot compression syndrome. *Clin Orthop Relat Res*. 1979;140:109–10.
84. Chhabra A, Williams EH, Subhawong TK, et al. MR neurography findings of soleal sling entrapment. *AJR*. 2011;196(3):W290–7.
85. Ladak A, Spinner RJ, Amrami KK, Howe BM. MRI findings in patients with tibial nerve compression near the knee. *Skelet Radiol*. 2013;42(4):553–9.
86. Pomeroy G, Wilton J, Anthony S. Entrapment neuropathy about the foot and ankle: an update. *J Am Acad Orthop Surg*. 2015;23(1):58–66.
87. Williams EH, Rosson GD, Hagan RR, Hashemi SS, Dellon AL. Soleal sling syndrome (proximal tibial nerve compression): results of surgical decompression. *Plast Reconstr Surg*. 2012;129(2):454–62.
88. Mastaglia FL. Tibial nerve entrapment in the popliteal fossa. *Muscle Nerve*. 2000;23(12):1883–6.
89. Hernando MF, Cerezal L, Pérez-Carro L, Abascal F, Canga A. Deep gluteal syndrome: anatomy, imaging, and management of sciatic nerve entrapments in the subgluteal space. *Skelet Radiol*. 2015;44(7):919–34.
90. Hu YWE, Ho GWK, Tortland PD. Deep gluteal syndrome: a pain in the buttock. *Curr Sports Med Rep*. 2021;20(6):279–85.
91. Gonzalez-Lomas G. Deep gluteal pain in orthopaedics: a challenging diagnosis. *J Am Acad Orthop Surg*. 2021;29(24):e1282-90.
92. Park JW, Lee YK, Lee YJ, Shin S, Kang Y, Koo KH. Deep gluteal syndrome as a cause of posterior hip pain and sciatica-like pain. *Bone Joint Lett J*. 2020;102-B(5):556–67.
93. Manoharan D, Sudhakaran D, Goyal A, Srivastava DN, Ansari MT. Clinico-radiological review of peripheral entrapment neuropathies – Part 2 lower limb. *Eur J Radiol*. 2021;135:109482.
94. Martin HD, Khoury A, Schröder R, Palmer IJ. Ischiofemoral impingement and hamstring syndrome as causes of posterior hip pain: where do we go next? *Clin Sports Med*. 2016;35(3):469–86.

95. Stępień K, Śmigielski R, Mouton C, Ciszek B, Engelhardt M, Seil R. Anatomy of proximal attachment, course, and innervation of hamstring muscles: a pictorial essay. *Knee Surg Sports Traumatol Arthrosc.* 2019;27(3):673–84.
96. Martin HD, Reddy M, Gómez-Hoyos J. Deep gluteal syndrome. *J Hip Preserv Surg.* 2015;2:99–107.
97. Martin HD, Kivlan BR, Palmer IJ, Martin RL. Diagnostic accuracy of clinical tests for sciatic nerve entrapment in the gluteal region. *Knee Surg Sports Traumatol Arthrosc.* 2014;22(4):882–8.
98. Burke CJ, Walter WR, Adler RS. Targeted ultrasound-guided perineural hydrodissection of the sciatic nerve for the treatment of piriformis syndrome. *Ultrasound Q.* 2019;35(2):125–9.
99. Smoll NR. Variations of the piriformis and sciatic nerve with clinical consequence: a review. *Clin Anat.* 2010;23(1):8–17.
100. Courseault J, Kessler E, Moran A, Labbe A. Fascial hydrodissection for chronic hamstring injury. *Curr Sports Med Rep.* 2019;18(11):416–20.
101. Cohen S. Another consideration in the diagnosis of heel pain: neuroma of the medial calcaneal nerve. *J Foot Ankle Surg.* 1974;13:128.
102. Barrett SL, Reese MM, Tassone J, Buitrago M. The use of low-energy radial shockwave in the treatment of entrapment neuropathy of the medial calcaneal nerve: a pilot study. *Foot Ankle Spec.* 2008;1(4):231–42.
103. Gould N, Trevino S. Sural nerve entrapment by avulsion fracture of the base of the fifth metatarsal bone. *Foot Ankle.* 1981;2(3):153–5.
104. Nakano KK. Entrapment neuropathy from Baker's cyst. *JAMA.* 1978;239(2):135.
105. Redborg KE, Sites BD, Chinn CD, et al. Ultrasound improves the success rate of a sural nerve block at the ankle. *Reg Anesth Pain Med.* 2009;34(1):24–8.
106. Fabre T, Montero C, Gaujard E, Gervais-Dellion F, Durandeau A. Chronic calf pain in athletes due to sural nerve entrapment. A report of 18 cases. *Am J Sports Med.* 2000;28(5):679–82.
107. Ferkel RD, Heath DD, Guhl JF. Neurological complications of ankle arthroscopy. *Arthroscopy.* 1996;12(2):200–8.
108. Gleeson AP, Kerr JG. Patella dislocation neurapraxia — a report of two cases. *Injury.* 1996;27(7):519–20.
109. Hemler DE, Ward WK, Karstetter KW, Bryant PM. Saphenous nerve entrapment caused by pes anserine bursitis mimicking stress fracture of the tibia. *Arch Phys Med Rehabil.* 1991;72(5):336–7.
110. Iizuka M, Yao R, Wainapel S. Saphenous nerve injury following medial knee joint injection: a case report. *Arch Phys Med Rehabil.* 2005;86(10):2062–5.
111. Logue EJ III, Drez D Jr. Dermatitis complicating saphenous nerve injury after arthroscopic debridement of a medial meniscal cyst. *Arthroscopy.* 1996;12(2):228–31.
112. Worth RM, Kettelkamp DB, Defalque RJ, Duane KU. Saphenous nerve entrapment. A cause of medial knee pain. *Am J Sports Med.* 1984;12(1):80–1.
113. McCrory P, Bell S. Nerve entrapment syndromes as a cause of pain in the hip, groin, and buttock. *Sports Med.* 1999;27(4):261–74.
114. Bradshaw C, McCrory P, Bell S, Brukner P. Obturator nerve entrapment. A cause of groin pain in athletes. *Am J Sports Med.* 1997;25(3):402–8.
115. Kopell H, Thompson W. Peripheral nerve entrapments of the lower extremity. *New Engl J Med.* 1962;266:216–9.
116. Rigaud J, Labat JJ, Riant T, Bouchot O, Robert R. Obturator nerve entrapment: diagnosis and laparoscopic treatment—technical case report. *Neurosurgery.* 2007;61(1):E175.
117. Massey EW, Pleet AB. Neuropathy in joggers. *Am J Sports Med.* 1978;6(4):209–11.
118. Williams PH, Trzil KP. Management of meralgia paresthetica. *J Neurosurg.* 1991;74(1):76–80.
119. Becciolini M, Pivec C, Riegler G. Ultrasound of the lateral femoral cutaneous nerve: a review of the literature and pictorial essay. *J Ultrasound Med.* 2022;41(5):1273–84.
120. Nwawka OK, Miller TT. Ultrasound-guided peripheral nerve injection techniques. *Am J Roentgenol.* 2016;207(3):507–16.
121. Siu TL, Chandran KN. Neurolysis for meralgia paresthetica: an operative series of 45 cases. *Surg Neurol.* 2005;63(1):19–23.

SECTION V

Rehabilitation

Principles of Rehabilitation and Return to Sport

72

Joshua E. Lider, Kevin Machino, and Brian A. Davis

INTRODUCTION

- Injury and illness are inherent risks in sports participation (1), which occur when the accumulation of stressors is greater than what the body can tolerate (2).
- When accounting for the multitude of stressors the athlete experiences, it is important to appreciate the varied impact stressors can have on each individual.
- Therefore, the purpose of this chapter is not to create an individualized rehabilitation and return to sport protocol, but to create a framework to guide the clinician through the challenging process of rehabilitation from injury and the return-to-play (RTP) decision. The remaining chapters in this section, 73 through 87, represent adjunctive therapies to assist and augment the recovery process.
- Rehabilitation is a deliberate and multidisciplinary process where the objective is the restoration of optimal form and function. The ultimate goal of the rehabilitation process is to limit the extent of the injury, reduce or reverse the impairment and functional loss, and prevent, correct, or eliminate altogether the disability (3).
- A comprehensive rehabilitation program will expedite the RTP process, reduce future injury risk, and facilitate performance enhancements, allowing the athlete to perform at higher levels upon their return.
- The RTP decision is complex, involving multidimensional circumstances that can be variable throughout the rehabilitation process. Due to the fluidity of circumstances, the RTP decision should not be an isolated conclusion, but should be a part of the continuum throughout the recovery and rehabilitation process.
- In addition, it is important to consider individual factors that may require alteration to the general functional and psychological goals of the rehabilitation program. To further compound this challenge, RTP criteria for many common injuries lack solid scientific evidence and consensus (4).
- Despite the paucity of scientific evidence, there are accepted core principles of a rehabilitation program and RTP decision for the injured or ill athlete. List below was adapted from the American College of Sports Medicine (ACSM) Team Physician Consensus Conference (TPCC) 2012, important to note 2024 ACSM TPCC statement is in press (4–6):
    - Establish an RTP process;
    - Establish a correct diagnosis and identify functional limitations;
    - Apply the most effective interventions to target functional limitations;
    - Aim to return the athlete confidently to sports participation in a timely and safe manner;
    - Clearly document policies and protocols to provide transparency with decisions involved in guiding RTP;
    - Define roles and responsibilities of each member of the RTP team.

PRINCIPLES OF REHABILITATION — THE RTP CONTINUUM

General Considerations

- Treatment and rehabilitation of an injured or ill athlete have important individualized parameters that need to be met prior to progressing to the next phase of treatment. Despite this, the rehabilitation program does not have "defined borders" between phases, but rather is considered a continuum (4,7) (see Figure 72.1).
- To better conceptualize the RTP continuum, we will split up the sections into:
    - Phase 1: acute injury
    - Phase 2: return to participation
    - Phase 3: return to sport
    - Phase 4: return to performance
- Each stage will have a different primary focus, but there will be multiple other overlapping foci that the clinician will have to continue to address across the continuum.

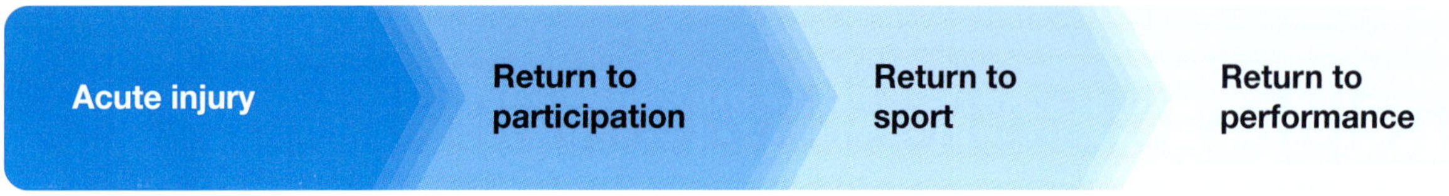

Acute injury → Return to participation → Return to sport → Return to performance

Figure 72.1: The rehabilitation continuum. (Adapted from Ardern CL, Glasgow P, Schneiders A, et al. 2016 consensus statement on return to sport from the First World Congress in Sports Physical Therapy, Bern. *Br J Sports Med*. 2016;50(14):853–64.)

- Important factors to consider when creating and implementing a treatment plan (5,6):
  - Identify the most effective interventions for the individual athlete's diagnosis (pathology, functional limitations, and risk factors) addressing both short- and long-term needs (8).
  - The rehabilitation plan should maintain and restore musculoskeletal, cardiopulmonary, and psychological function as well as the overall health of the injured or ill athlete.
  - When able, the rehabilitation program should be based on evidence and empirical criterion (8).
  - General components addressed in the rehabilitation program:
    - Pain management
    - Range of motion (ROM)
    - Strength: muscle strength and rate of force production
    - Neuromuscular control: balance and proprioception using known recovery patterns
    - Activity tolerance: cardiovascular tolerance, functional capabilities (tolerance of load and confidence in function)
    - Force coupling
    - Psychological well-being
  - Allow for gradual progression in task complexity to facilitate optimal RTP ("crawl → walk → run").
  - Although staffing constraints may limit this, training sessions should be closely monitored (ideally 1 to 1 clinician to athlete ratio) to allow for (8):
    - Application of appropriate timing and dose of interventions to ensure optimal outcomes
    - Timely and logical program progression based on predetermined milestones
    - Evaluate and intervene on potential physiological, psychological, and logistical barriers
    - Monitor for regression: performance deficits, prolonged recovery, pain, swelling, and worsening ROM
  - A documentation system to continue monitoring athlete's progress and to facilitate efficient communication among all stakeholders.
  - Evaluating and intervening on maladaptive physical and psychological responses to injury are important to ensure optimal healing and return to sport.
    - Research has found a negative relationship between psychological distress and wound healing (9).
  - Allow the athlete to collaborate through goal setting for each phase of the rehabilitation process with measurable outcomes to provide confidence in the rehabilitation program.

Phase 1: Acute Injury — Tissue Response

- Duration: 3–6 days
- Characterized by local tissue trauma and resultant inflammation (10–12)
  - Trauma results in local bleeding followed by hemostasis:
    - Hematoma formation
    - Vasoconstriction of damaged blood vessels
    - Clotting cascade initiates inflammatory pathways
  - Inflammation
    - Characteristics: edema, pain, warmth, redness, and neuromusculoskeletal dysfunction
    - Inflammatory process removes damaged tissue and cellular debris through phagocytosis.
  - Muscle dysfunction
    - Secondary to reflexive inhibition (*e.g.*, knee joint effusion inhibiting quadriceps function)
    - Muscle fiber types are affected equally due to muscle inhibition secondary to pain and swelling (13,14).

Phase 1: Acute Injury — Treatment Plan

Interventions

- Protection of injured tissues
  - Minimizing the risk of further injury, while limiting periods of immobilization (15)
  - Rehabilitation tasks should be performed in a controlled environment.
- ROM (16):
  - ROM is often limited by pain and swelling.
- Optimal loading of the injured tissues (12,15):
  - A secondary goal in this stage is to restore muscle function.
  - Progressive functional loading will stimulate connective tissue synthesis, accelerating tissue healing.

- May have some discomfort with tissue loading without detrimental effects to tissue recovery (17,18)
- Overloading will show alterations in movement and muscle activation patterns, indicating loading of the injured tissue should be reduced.

- Interventions for pain and inflammation
  - Analgesia: acetaminophen, nonsteroidal anti-inflammatory drugs (NSAIDs), tramadol, and opioids
    - Avoid analgesics prior and during activity to monitor tissue overload.
    - Research has demonstrated analgesic benefit and attractive benefit-harm ratio with topical NSAIDs, followed by oral NSAIDs, then acetaminophen (19). Opioids should be used sparingly and for short periods if indicated.
      - Avoid opioids whenever possible due to addiction and diversion risk.
    - NSAID:
      - Short course is recommended in treating pain from inflammation (20–22).
      - Controversial use in muscle and bone injury as there is concern that reduced inflammatory response may blunt the normal healing process (12,20,23,24).
    - See Chapter 73, Pain Management in the Athlete, and Chapter 76, Medications, for further discussion.
  - Modalities: ice, compression, and elevation (11,12,16)
    - Commonly recommended interventions in acute injury, despite paucity of clinical studies demonstrating its benefit (25,26)
    - See Chapter 74, Modalities, for more in-depth discussion.
  - Isometric exercise
    - Allows for early neuromuscular training and tissue loading, as this type of muscle activation produces the least amount of force.
    - Isometric exercises have been shown to provide an analgesic effect to the targeted structures (27–29).
- Preoperative rehabilitation
  - For athletes requiring surgical intervention, there is research showing benefits with preoperative rehabilitation programs.
    - Improved outcomes with rehabilitation program to regain full knee extension and regain quadriceps strength prior to anterior cruciate ligament (ACL) reconstruction (30)
    - Reduction of edema for fractures presurgery

Rehabilitation Focus

- Phase goals
  - Primary goal
    - Regain active and passive ROM arc required for sport-specific tasks.
  - Secondary goals
    - Regain motor control and proprioception along the kinetic chain.
    - Regain muscle strength through voluntary contraction.
- Exercise prescription
  - Exercises should be performed in a controlled environment.
  - Exercise progression should focus on increased repetitions, as tissues typically cannot tolerate higher loads used in lower repetition exercises.
  - Include exercises that maintain cardiovascular fitness, while continuing to protect the site of injury or illness
- Restoration of ROM
  - Types of motion
    - Passive range of motion (PROM): individual's joint moved by an external force.
      - Caution: excessive PROM in the acute phase can result in increased pain, inflammation, and further tissue damage.
    - Active-assisted range of motion (AAROM): individual's joint moved with a combination of own force and an external force
    - Active range of motion (AROM): individual's joint moved by own force
    - Resisted range of motion (RROM): individual's joint moved by own force against an opposing force
  - Benefits
    - Decreases pain and edema (31,32)
    - Promotes tissue healing (32)
      - In tendon injuries, fibroblast will produce a collagen scar with collagen fibrils aligned perpendicular to the tendon fibers. With axial tensile loading, the collagen fibrils will realign to a parallel orientation (33).
    - Improved joint ROM and muscle length (31,32,34)
    - Provides neuromuscular training (32)
    - Important for restoration of muscular strength and endurance (32)
    - Mentally gratifying, able to work on function
  - ROM prescription depends on:
    - Healing phase
    - Injury specifics
    - Pain control
  - General sequence: PROM → AAROM → AROM → RROM
    - Directed by the athlete's tolerance and ability
    - PROM and AAROM are most commonly used in the acute phase of injury.
  - Types of stretching to improve ROM:
    - Static: holding the muscle in a lengthened position for a period of time
      - Three to five repetitions of 30–60 seconds

- Proprioceptive neuromuscular facilitation (35)
  - Muscle lengthening that involves muscle contractions
    - Contract-relax of agonist muscle group
    - Contract-relax of antagonist muscle group
    - Contract-relax of agonist-antagonist muscle groups in succession
  - Decreases Golgi tendon organ response/stretch reflex
  - Possibly more efficient acute gains in ROM compared to other forms of stretching; some evidence to suggest better maintenance of ROM gains (36).
  - May require another person to assist
- Ballistic — generally not recommended due to increased risk of injury
  - Through body movements, the muscle is lengthened past its normal ROM.
- Massage and mobilization have been shown to be beneficial in improving ROM (37,38).
  - Massage therapies should be applied by individuals who are professionally trained.
- As ROM improves, it is important to monitor that the joint can tolerate additional motion. Ongoing strengthening should be provided to maintain joint stability (39).
- Common signs of regression
  - Effusion (pain OR pain free), decreased ROM, pain that does not return to baseline in 24–48 hours, performance decrement beyond expected postinjury

Psychological Focus (40)

- Throughout the rehabilitation process, it is important to continue to evaluate the athlete's psychological well-being as it is fluid and has a significant effect on rehabilitation outcomes (41–43).
  - Assess the athlete's readiness to participate in the rehabilitation program (44).
  - Build the athlete's psychological resilience throughout the rehabilitation process (45).
- Factors to help develop confidence during the return-to-sport process:
  - Build a trusting relationship with the treating clinicians.
  - Provide education to the athlete and other stakeholders to set realistic expectations early.
  - Ensure a good social support network.
  - Involve the athlete in goal setting and creation of milestones so they can appreciate objective measures of their improvement.
- Restore self-perceptions
  - Self-confidence
  - Self-esteem
  - Self-identity
- Develop coping strategies
  - The athlete's ability to cope with stress is positively associated with their ability to progress through their rehabilitation program.
  - Coping strategies include:
    - Stress management: shown to decrease the level of negative affective response during the rehabilitation process (46)
    - Problem focus coping: change of perception, viewing the injury as a challenge instead of a threat (47)
    - Reflect on the injury experience as an opportunity for growth.
    - Relaxation techniques (46)
  - There is an association of decreased injury and illness risk in athletes who participate in stress management programs (48).

Phase 2: Return to Participation — Tissue Response

- Duration: 1–3 weeks
- Characterized by tissue growth and repair (10–12)
  - Growth factor release
  - Fibroblast proliferation — type III collagen deposition
  - Formation of granulation tissue
  - Neovascularization
- Collagen deposition may present as tissue adhesions and arthrofibrosis.
  - Presents as joint stiffness and decreased ROM

Phase 2: Return to Participation — Treatment Plan

- Tenuous phase of the rehabilitation course as physical and psychological readiness for progress often do not coincide (49):
  - May have a strong desire to RTP as injured tissue appearance is often better than its function at this point in the healing process
  - May be hesitant to progress in rehabilitation due to the fear of reinjury or lack of confidence in the injured body part.
  - Ongoing education is important to address the physical and psychological disconnects.

Interventions

- Modalities for symptom management — see Chapter 74, Modalities, for further discussion
  - Manual mobilizations to help with tissue restrictions
  - Superficial heat
  - Deep heat: ultrasound (US) (most common), shortwave diathermy
  - Cold therapy
  - Electrotherapy
    - Transcutaneous electrical nerve stimulation

- Medication delivery (iontophoresis)
- Electrical stimulation
  - Direct current electrical stimulation
  - Alternating current electrical stimulation
  - Galvanic electrical stimulation
  - Russian electrical stimulation
- Biofeedback
  - Muscle stimulation in coordination with active muscle contraction has been shown to help combat muscle atrophy (50).

Rehabilitation Focus

- Phase goals
  - Rehabilitation focus: progressively incorporate elements to improve muscle strength, neuromuscular control, and cardiovascular training
  - Exercises should continue to be performed in a controlled environment.
  - Continue to address ROM deficits.
    - Consider not advancing the program if ROM is significantly decreased (*i.e.*, >50% less than expected or preinjury level).
- Exercise prescription
  - Gradually increase loading and complexity of movement patterns, dictated by tissue load tolerance.
  - Program should be focused on allowing the body to adapt to tolerate sport-specific demands.
- Pain control to allow for participation in therapies
  - Medical and manual therapies:
    - If needed, continued use of interventions discussed in phase 1
    - Remaining cognizant of signs of injury recurrence
- Muscle strength
  - Incorporate elements to improve motor control, muscle strength, and endurance.
    - Persistent strength imbalances have been associated with increased reinjury risk.
      - Soccer players with ≥15% hamstring strength asymmetry to the contralateral leg were found to be four times more at risk for hamstring strains if they did not receive intervention (51).
  - Strength gains are specific to the following targeted parameters, although some carryover may exist (*i.e.*, training focused on the phosphagen energy system will also have improvement in other energy systems).
    - ROM and joint position
    - Muscle fiber activation type
    - Speed
    - Energy system
    - Movement pattern
    - External load/resistance
  - Muscle activation types (11)
    - Isometric activation: muscle activation with absence of joint motion or change in muscle length (force against an object or antagonist muscle group coactivating)
      - Indications
        - Often used early in rehabilitation course as it can be done with immobilization
        - Help reduce pain, edema, and atrophy (29)
      - Lowest intensity muscle action
    - Isotonic activation: muscle activation against a constant resistance, resulting in joint motion and a change in muscle length (*e.g.*, standard biceps curl — flexion phase)
      - Concentric: muscle length decreases with activation.
      - Eccentric: muscle length increases with activation.
      - Indication
        - Must have adequate ROM through the joint that the muscles of interest cross
        - Start without counterload, followed by progressing incrementally
    - Isokinetic activation: muscle activation performed at a constant speed with variable resistance resulting in change in joint position and muscle length
      - Slow motion reduces the resistance
      - Faster motion increases the resistance
      - Nonphysiologic (often used in research)
    - Plyometric activation: muscle activation that produces maximum force in short intervals with the goal of increasing power (52)
      - Utilizes the stretch-shortening cycle by utilizing an eccentric movement quickly followed by a concentric movement
      - Phases of plyometric exercise:
        - Eccentric prestretch phase: Stretches the muscle spindle of the muscle-tendon unit and the noncontracting tissue within the muscle
        - Amortization phase (time to rebound): Period of time from the end of the eccentric prestretch phase to beginning of the concentric phase. It is the time delay between overcoming the negative work of the eccentric prestretch phase to generating the force, accelerating muscle contraction, and elastic recoiling in the direction of the plyometric movement pattern.
        - Concentric shortening phase
      - Produces the greatest amount of force
      - Indication:
        - Usually applied at the end of the rehabilitation process and in performance training
- Load progression
  - The balance between applied load and tissue capacity is important to monitor throughout the rehabilitation

process, as well as with sports enhancement and injury prevention training (39).
    - Controlled and gradual load progression is a critical part of the rehabilitation process. Appropriately loading the tissue creates optimal tissue adaptation, resulting in increased load tolerance.
    - Common mistake — inappropriately changing resistance:
        - Increasing resistance in too large of increments resulting in tissue maladaptation
        - Underloading the tissues resulting in inadequate tissue adaptation
    - Optimal loading requires appropriate dosing and timing with ongoing monitoring for adjustments throughout the athlete's training. Factors that can be manipulated include (39):
        - Volume of movements: frequency or repetition of the exercise (per unit time)
        - Velocity of movements: intensity of exercise (rate of energy expenditure [fast/explosive vs slow/controlled movements])
        - External loads: distribution of a load as it is applied to tissue
        - Complexity of movement patterns
    - It is important to recognize different tissues may respond to loading differently (joint vs. ligament vs. tendon/muscle).
    - Monitoring overall training load is especially important for conditions requiring longer rehabilitation programs (*e.g.*, ACL reconstruction):
        - Acute load: training load for the current week
        - Chronic load: training load for the preceding 4 weeks
        - Overloading can be seen in acute, chronic, or both time periods.
- Neuromuscular control
    - Goal to resolve biomechanical deficiencies
    - Progression of activities to train neuromuscular control:
        - Balance training
        - Basic sport-specific technical movements
        - Semicomplex sport-specific movement patterns
        - Complex and dynamic sport-specific movement patterns
- Cardiovascular
    - Cardiovascular endurance training should focus on the energy system of greatest demand in the athlete's sport with continued protection of injured tissues.
    - Goal: Once able to return to sport, the athlete's endurance will allow participation for the duration of the training or competition period.

Psychologic Focus

- As the athlete progresses, it is important to make sure the athlete is psychologically ready to return.
- Fear is the predominant emotion at the time athletes are ready to return to sport (53–56).
    - Usually, the athlete will have low confidence immediately after their injury, with confidence improving gradually through the rehabilitation process (57).
    - Fear of reinjury and underperforming can be a significant reason for athletes not to return after an injury (57,58).
- Emotional integrity (athletes reluctant to discuss their emotions):
    - The athlete may feel alienated or isolated even after RTP (44,59).
    - Provide an environment where the athlete can experience team commodore and/or have social support from friends and family during the rehabilitation process.

Assessing the Athlete's Readiness to Return to Sport (4,57)

- Assessing readiness to RTP should be an integrated process involving all key stakeholders.
- Readiness to train and compete model (1):
    - Health: no injury or illness
        - Medical risk: minimal risk to future health status
        - Performance risk: minimal risk of suboptimal performance
    - Asymptomatic chronic illness or injury:
        - Medical risk: low risk to future health status
        - Performance risk: low risk of suboptimal performance
    - Symptomatic illness or injury — unrestricted training and competition:
        - Medical risk: mild risk to future health status
        - Performance risk: mild risk of suboptimal performance
    - Symptomatic illness/injury with modified training:
        - Medical risk: moderate risk to future health status
        - Performance risk: moderate risk of suboptimal performance
    - Symptomatic illness/injury — removal from training:
        - Medical risk: high risk to future health status
        - Performance risk: high risk of suboptimal performance
- When the athlete has capacity, a shared decision model can be used. Factors that allow for shared decision-making include (60):
    - Choice: discussing reasonable options with the athlete and coach
    - Option: providing more detailed information about different options
    - Decision: guiding the athlete and coach to consider their preference and decide what is best
- The clinician must ensure the following criteria are at a satisfactory level prior to providing clearance for RTP (5,6,61):
    - Functional assessment (45,62)

    - Pain is well controlled.
    - Recovery of joint ROM, strength, and power compared to the contralateral side or preinjury status
    - Neuromuscular readiness (balance, stability, dynamic postural control) to complete sport-specific tasks and skills
    - Functional testing: able to perform functional tests pain free, with normal kinematics and near symmetric performance when compared to preinjury status or contralateral limb (often 85%–90% is the threshold) (8,63)
    - Imaging studies can be used for some conditions to help evaluate interval healing. It is important to appreciate that imaging tends to lag behind functional healing (magnetic resonance imaging and US normalize after an average of 6 months) (64,65).
  - Cardiovascular assessment (45)
    - Ensuring the athlete has appropriate cardiovascular endurance and metabolic capacity that is required for their specific sport demands
  - Psychological assessment (42,45,66,67)
    - Unfortunately, there is not a clear definition of what constitutes psychological readiness nor what is the best way to assess readiness or how to intervene (42).
    - Factors affecting the individual's state of mental preparedness to resume sport-specific activity:
      - Cognitive appraisal: confidence level, expectations, motivations, risk appraisals, internal or external pressures
      - Affective components: anxiety or fears about reinjury or movement
      - Behavioral components: avoidance behaviors (*e.g.*, playing timid)
      - Biopsychosocial factors: Perceived pressure may lead to the athlete returning prematurely (68).
    - Psychological assessment batteries can assist in the evaluation, examples include:
      - Injury-Psychological Readiness to Return to Sport scale (57)
      - ACL-Return to Sport after Injury (69,70).
- Ensure the athlete does not pose undue risk to themselves or other participants; this includes but is not limited to equipment modifications, bracing, and orthoses.
- Compliance with rules and regulations set in place by governing body

Phase 3: Return to Sport — Tissue Response

- Duration: variable, dependent on tissue type; typically, lasting 6 months
  - Bone heals by a regeneration process. Depending on location and fracture type, it usually takes about 6–8 weeks for bone to heal and tolerate loading.
  - Muscle heals by regeneration (new myofibrils) and repair (scar tissue) processes, resulting in tissue never regaining preinjury quality (11).
    - Prior injury is a major risk factor for future injury (71,72).
  - Injured muscle will usually have a mature scar at 21 days that can accept tensile loading (22).
- Characterized by the maturation and remodeling of injured tissues (10–12)
  - During the maturation phase:
    - Type III collagen is replaced by type I collagen.
    - Collagen fibers realign and remodel.
      - This process is dependent on the magnitude and direction of the force applied across injured tissues.
    - Cellularity and vascularity decrease.

Phase 3: Return to Sport — Treatment Plan (Intensive Training)

- Period of progressive reintegration into sport
- Different levels of return to sport that can be considered (73):
  - Return to reduced practice (no contact)
  - Return to normal practice (unrestricted)
  - Return to less competitive games (scrimmages, initially with partial duration of games)
  - Return to competitive games (initially with partial duration of games)
- Most athletes are able to RTP with some increased risk, and the amount depends on the accepted risk tolerance.
  - Many athletes are not clinically "normal" as deficits may still be present:
    - Motion restrictions/imbalances
    - Strength/endurance suboptimal/imbalanced
      - Decreased rate of force development
    - Kinetic chain dysfunction
    - Neuromuscular control deficits
    - Technique alterations
  - Deficits should be measured objectively to provide a basis for progression and RTP decision-making.
    - Best if comparable against the athlete's preinjury status or normative data from similar athletes (normalized to body weight/anthropometric measures)
    - Subjective assessments should be interpreted with caution due to decreased reliability.
  - The number and severity of deficits increase injury risk. Clearance to return to activity should occur when injury risk is low or the consequence of reinjury is minor (74).
  - Rehabilitation progression should be closely monitored; consider video analysis to assist.

- During this phase, it is important to collaborate with the athlete, coaching, and strength staff to help identify:
  - Remaining barriers to RTP
  - Opportunity for gradual return (often affected by competition schedule)
  - Accepted risk tolerance
- Rehabilitation focus
  - Phase goals
    - Return the athlete's function to ≥85%–90% of the pre-injury level (8,63)
    - Neuromuscular control is a primary goal.
      - Speed and agility training
      - Increased movement complexity
    - Muscle strength is a primary goal.
      - Increased strength
      - Improve rate of force development through more explosive movements
    - Address remaining ROM deficits, if applicable.
  - Exercise prescription: sport specific (similar to preseason training)
    - More traditional strength and conditioning training can be incorporated in the rehabilitation program.
      - Continued focus to resolve remaining impairments.
    - Higher rate of force development and on-field sessions facilitate environmental adaptations.
      - Should be able to complete tasks without symptoms during or after training
    - Load monitoring is very important during this phase. Increased loads from training sessions are combined with the continued load from the rehabilitation program.
  - Neuromuscular control
    - Movement patterns require a coordinated interaction between afferent and efferent signals.
      - Afferent: proprioceptive sensory input
      - Efferent: muscle contraction
    - Adequate strength does not guarantee adequate neuromuscular control.
    - Assessment of neuromuscular control through:
      - Balance
      - Movement quality
    - Training progression for neuromuscular control:
      - Gradually increasing the degrees of freedom and speed of task completion while decreasing the amount of environmental control.
        - Acute stage: active ROM, stable ground progressing to unstable ground
        - Return to participation stage: rhythmic stabilization, external perturbation
        - RTP stage: plyometric training, sport-specific training
      - Competitive level can also be adjusted to facilitate smooth return to performance (*e.g.*, playing in minor league baseball games prior to returning to major league baseball competition).
  - If progression fails, evaluate:
    - Content and volume of the rehabilitation program
    - Interventions targeting impairments
    - Ensure proper technique
    - Evaluate total load
      - Can split up rehabilitation program to help reduce load
    - Environmental challenges — family, friends, or athlete's motivation
    - Revisit the diagnosis and functional assessment
- Psychological focus
  - Important to continually assess the athlete's psychological well-being and intervene on any potential deficits
  - Athletes can have an increase in fear and anxiety at this stage of RTP.
  - Athlete may demonstrate signs of fear in different ways (75):
    - Playing timid — especially in similar situations to their mechanism of original injury
    - Heavily taping or padding injured body part

Phase 4: Return to Performance

- Phase goals
  - Motor control
    - Primary goal to ingrain new movement patterns
  - Muscle strength
    - Primary goal to increase power and endurance
  - ROM
    - Focus on maintaining ROM and facilitating recovery
- Exercise prescription: Sport-specific (similar to in-season training)
- At this stage, the athlete should be pain free, have full ROM, and be performing at or above their preinjury level without functional deficits (39).
- It is important to continue working with the athlete, coaching, and strength staff to provide individual injury prevention training after the athlete has returned to competitive level.

RETURN-TO-SPORT GUIDELINES

Stakeholders Composition and Dynamics

- The RTP process is a risk-benefit analysis. It involves a diverse group of individuals who share the mutual goal of returning the athlete to sport in a timely manner, while minimizing the risk of negative future consequences for the athlete (4,5).

- RTP decisions are based on accurate risk and risk tolerance assessments, which can be more complete when there is collaboration among all individuals or stakeholders involved (4,5,8,76,77).
- Stakeholders will have different backgrounds and expertise that influences their values and judgements, which results in prioritizing different factors in the RTP decision (76,78,79). This has been demonstrated in research showing heterogeneity among clinicians within and between different clinical professions (7,62,74,76,80), highlighting the inherent potential for conflict.
    - Athlete: main contributor for subjective information (60)
    - Clinicians: main contributor for objective information (60)
    - Coaching staff: main contributor for contextual information (60)

Team Members and Their Respective Strengths and Weaknesses (1,60,76)

- Athlete
    - Strength
        - Thought to be the best to assess risk tolerance as they have a complete knowledge of the athlete's needs and values (desire to compete, potential financial loss, potential loss of competitive standing)
    - Weakness
        - Limited knowledge of injury and injury sequela
        - Difficult to have an unbiased assessment of risk
        - Potential to be influenced by other team members
    - Potential confounders
        - Internal pressures: strong need to compete for the "love of the game" (56,81)
        - External pressures: sociocultural influences — influences athletes to have higher risk tolerance ("no pain — no gain") (81)
    - Important considerations
        - To be involved in the decision-making process, the athlete must have the ability for informed consent (cognition intact).
        - Consider distracting factors affecting decision-making capacity (time constraints and associated emotions during competition).
- Clinicians
    - Physician
        - Often retains final authority over the decision-making process by default (82)
            - Most jurisdictions place legal liability on the physician.
        - Strength
            - Substantial knowledge of injury risk and injury sequelae as it relates to sport
            - The team physician has privy to information from all members of the team, resulting in a more complete picture of the rehabilitation process.
                - Some notable exceptions for sports psychology/psychiatry
            - Viewed by society and sport associations to be best equipped to evaluate injury risk (short and long term) (76)
        - Weakness
            - Less personal contact with athletes, may not understand the athlete's best interest
            - May work for the team organization, which may represent an inherent conflict of interest (1,83)
        - Specialist: cardiology, neurology, pulmonology, etc.
            - Strength: viewed as the expert on pathology within their specialty
            - Weakness: may have a narrower scope of focus
    - Physical therapists/athletic trainers
        - Strength
            - Substantial knowledge of injury risk and injury sequelae
            - Ability to assess change in risk when protective equipment or activity modification is implemented
            - More interactions with athletes, facilitating increased trust among coaches and athletes
            - Able to modify program rapidly as the athlete improves or declines
        - Weakness
            - Often an employee of the team organization, concern for coercion (perceived or actual)
    - Nutritionist/psychologist
        - Strengths
            - Substantial knowledge of injury risk and sequela within their field of expertise
        - Weakness
            - Often paid consultant to team, concern for coercion (perceived or actual)
            - Less personal contact with athletes
    - Strength and conditioning professionals
        - Strengths
            - Substantial knowledge of strength and conditioning regimen progressions to prepare for specific sport demands
        - Weakness
            - Often an employee of the team organization, concern for coercion (perceived or actual)
            - Limited knowledge of injury risk and injury sequela
- Coaching staff
    - Strength

- Often has a good understanding of the athlete's strengths, desires, and values
- Understands the athlete's performance potential (potential loss of competitive standing)
- Ability to assess the psychological effect on the athlete who is unable to compete
- Weakness
  - Limited experience evaluating injury risk
  - In maximizing performance, the coach may push athletes to their limits (potentially playing while injured).
  - May be biased by emotions associated with competition
  - Financial incentive to RTP
- Front office management
  - Strength
    - Aware of the athlete's career potential and benefits that occur with RTP
  - Weakness
    - May have increased risk tolerance for RTP, even if the athlete would not benefit ("success at all cost")
      - Financial incentive to RTP
- Athlete support (family, friends, agent)
  - Strength
    - Often has a strong knowledge of the athlete's needs and values
  - Weakness
    - Often least knowledgeable with injury risk assessment
    - Potential for bias due to their own personal gain

Intrateam Conflict Management

- Further complicating intrateam dynamics, clinical stakeholders often bias their own profession to have the best skills to assess RTP criteria (76).
- It is important to have a system in place for conflict resolution to help navigate disagreements when they occur. Some recommendations include (4–6,76,79,84,85):
  - Chain of command: Identify, define, and document roles and responsibilities among the team as early as possible. As part of this, it may be beneficial to:
    - Understand the different clinical professions involved (including their training and culture).
    - Identifying professional skill sets best suited for different tasks in the RTP process.
    - Understand values and impact of societal norms in the context of influencing the individual's judgment
  - Document a formal structure of how RTP decisions are made, allowing for transparency of decision reasoning.
  - Formulate a process for clear communication among the RTP team.
  - Create and document a clear dispute resolution system to resolve disagreements and facilitate an unbiased decision.
  - Schedule regular meetings to discuss assessments and review of goals.
    - Acknowledge the challenge of having the entire team involved on decisions that require quick answers.
  - Establish a protocol for the release of information regarding the athlete's ability to RTP.

Establishing an RTP Process

- Prior to being asked to make an RTP decision, it is imperative to have a system in place that provides a structured approach to decide when an athlete can safely return to their sport after an illness or injury.
- RTP decisions are based on accurate risk and risk tolerance assessments in relation to the athlete's well-being. Important elements to guide this assessment include (5,6,84):
  - Need for accurate diagnosis of the athlete's illness or injury
    - Understanding the natural course and sequela of the injury/illness (including future injury risk)
  - Identification and mitigation of risk of illness or injury to other participants from exposure to the affected athlete
    - Injuries resulting from interactions with bracing, casting, or other equipment adaptations that were applied to allow the injured athlete's return to sport
    - Risk of disease transmission (airborne, contact, etc.)
  - Sport-specific evaluation of the athlete in relation to the functional requirements of their sport
    - Ensuring the athlete can meet the functional requirements without placing increased risk of injury to the individual or other participants
    - Functional adaptations to allow the athlete to meet functional requirements:
      - Activity modification: to minimize stress on susceptible tissues
        - Change position on field
        - Alter playing time
        - Alter involvement in different playing situations
      - Equipment modifications: taping, bracing, orthoses, etc.
        - Protect injured tissue: taping, padding, casting, etc.
        - Alter stress on the affected tissue: taping, bracing, orthoses, etc.
        - See Chapters 81–84 for further discussion on orthoses, taping, bracing, and splinting.
      - Medical adaptations: analgesics, inhalers, intravenous fluids, etc.
      - Understand the potential paradoxical increased risk for injury with adaptations, as the athlete may become less cautious with adaptations, negating the intended decreased risk (86).

- Knowledge of the governing body's (international, federal, state, local, institution, and sport association) rules and regulations related to RTP
  - Adaptation allowances (equipment modifications, medical, etc.) (87)
  - Conditions that limit return to sport (skin infections in wrestling, concussion management, etc.) (88)
  - Clearance protocols (involvement of specialists)
    - If a specialist was involved in treating the athlete, they should be involved in clearance decisions.
    - Some conditions require a specialist evaluation prior to return to sport.
- Structured evaluation of risk tolerance for RTP:
  - Contextual considerations (4,84):
    - Injury: acute versus chronic and potential for long-term sequelae
    - Physical demands: contact versus noncontact, cutting, pivoting, landing, and throwing
    - Sport-related factors: point in athlete's season or career, competition level, playing time, and significant future opportunities
    - Social and financial costs: scholarship and endorsements
    - External pressure: family members, friends, and coaches
    - Potential modifiers: fear of litigation, conflict of interest, or other ethical considerations
- Understand the athlete's goals and definition of success (4):
  - Goal focus: return to sustained participation in sport in the shortest time possible
  - Performance focused: returning to a level of prior performance
  - Outcome focused: prevention of new/recurrence or associated injuries
- A process that encourages shared decision-making:
  - Challenging to facilitate athlete autonomy when the physician usually has final decision-making authority (4)
    - In an attempt to retain their autonomy, the athlete may avoid interactions with the clinician (79).
  - Clinicians can optimize the shared RTP decision by considering the biological, psychological, and social factors, including (4,89):
    - Identifying and respecting the athlete's values, goals, and needs, the athlete's support structure can be included as appropriate.
    - Actively involve the athlete in decision-making.
    - Providing access and continuity to coordinated and integrated care throughout the rehabilitation process
    - Sharing information and providing education to the athlete and support structure as appropriate
- Providing education to the athlete and stakeholders on the following:
  - Diagnosis and prognosis of the injury or illness
  - Expectations and goals throughout the rehabilitation course
  - Purpose of treatment interventions to help facilitate buy in
  - Identifying functional improvement milestones that are required prior to advancing to the next phase of the rehabilitation program
  - Future injury risk reduction
- Sports rehabilitation is multidimensional and the clinician will need to manage several parallel foci throughout the athlete's rehabilitation.

RTP Outcomes

- Stakeholders may have different values, which could influence their definition of a successful outcome with RTP (49).
  - The athlete may define success as an expedited return to desired level of performance.
  - The clinician may define success as return to sport without injury or long-term sequela.
- Communicating and agreeing upon the parameters that define a successful outcome should be discussed early, and revisited throughout the rehabilitation process.
- It is important to involve all appropriate stakeholders to assess important elements of the athlete's condition and to set realistic and appropriate goals.
- Potential outcomes for ill-equipped RTP protocols:
  - Miscommunication
  - Loss of trust
  - Potential litigation
  - Declines in participation rates — individual doesn't return to sport
  - Medical complications
  - Injury recurrence

Evaluation: Identifying the Correct Diagnosis and Functional Limitations

Introduction

- Injury or illness occurs when external stressors overcome the load capacity of the body (2,84). May present as:
  - Microtrauma: cumulative trauma over a period of time, commonly seen in overuse injuries
  - Macrotrauma: a specific traumatic event, commonly presenting as an acute injury
  - Acute immune suppression after intense bouts of training or competition (90)

- Risk factors associated with sport participation can positively or negatively affect the body's innate stress tolerance.
- A thorough evaluation, including biological, psychological, and functional status, will allow the clinician to arrive at a complete and accurate diagnosis. In addition, the clinician will be able to account for different risk factors that are associated with poor prognosis (increased duration and/or severity of injury and illness) (91).
    - A proper diagnosis is foundational in guiding management and treatment interventions. In addition, it can help identify future barriers and facilitate a more accurate prognosis for a safe and timely return to sport.
- Please see separate chapters for further discussion on evaluation and diagnosis of individual pathologies for subspecialty organ systems and sports-specific pathologies.

Injury or Illness Evaluation — The Biologic Assessment (5,6,78)

- History should be obtained to better understand the athlete's current health status. Factors to assess include:
    - Mechanism of injury and the acute response of the inciting trauma
    - Athlete's preparation prior to injury (evaluation of previous loading history)
        - Appropriate loading will facilitate subsequent positive tissue adaptation.
        - Pathologic loading:
            - Overloading with inadequate rest will result in subsequent microtrauma and tissue breakdown.
            - Inadequate loading will result in deficient tissue tolerance that is required for performing the functional demands in sport.
    - Athlete's perceived functional limitations in relation to sport demand
    - Response to prior interventions and overall trajectory of injury or illness
    - Evaluate for potential risk factors that contributed to the athlete's current condition or that could affect recovery and rehabilitation prognosis.
- Physical exam should focus on identifying particular pathology and determine if the athlete will require removal from sport to protect against further injury or illness (62).
    - Physical exam should evaluate:
        - Location and severity of pain
        - Identify any inflammation, swelling, angulation/deformity, or joint effusion
        - ROM and strength of affected area in relation to the unaffected contralateral side
        - General definition/tone, muscle defects/atrophy
        - Joint stability
        - Neurological deficits (cognitive, sensation, proprioception)
        - Specific structures affected from illness (*e.g.*, lung sounds — asthma)
        - In-office biomechanics assessment
    - Functional testing: assessing the athlete's ability to perform sport-specific tasks
- Diagnostic workup (imaging, laboratory studies, EKGs)
    - Diagnostic studies are performed to confirm suspected pathologies and severity, guiding therapeutic interventions.
    - Diagnostic studies are also used to assess interval recovery from illness and injury to guide RTP decisions.
- Consider appropriate specialist consultation to assist with management.
    - Formal biomechanics assessment where possible

Evaluation of Potential Risk Factors

- Mechanism of injury is frequently focused on as the causal agent, but frequently there are a multitude of underlying risk factors, both known and unknown, that allow the mechanism of injury to be the causal event (91,92).
- Risk factors are often fluid with variable impact and existence. Hence, it is important to consider risk factor interactions and their potential to be additive, protective, or a confounder (93).
- Routine evaluation of risk factors among all athletes may help form a more comprehensive and effective rehabilitation or injury prevention program, resulting in greater positive outcomes (1).
- Common risk factor categories (2):
    - Modifiable factors: factors that respond to intervention, altering their impact on injury risk
        - Key for injury prevention programs to identify and intervene on these factors
    - Nonmodifiable factors: factors that cannot be changed with intervention
    - Intrinsic risk factors (71,72): factors possessed by the athlete that affects their injury risk (considered the predisposing factor to injury)
        - Biological
            - Cumulative stress (including sport, external responsibilities [school, work, endorsement], life events, and family and friend relationships) (94)
            - Body composition, growth, and maturation
            - Prior injury, health comorbidities, or family history
            - Joint mobility, muscle flexibility, and ligamentous laxity
            - Performance mechanics and skill level
            - Training
                - Biologic tissues preparation for stress tolerance through appropriate loading protocols
                - Energy system preparation through appropriate conditioning

- Recovery
  - Fatigue and recovery status
  - Nutrition and hydration
- Psychological (41)
  - Cognition
    - Goals, motives, and volition
    - Attentional focus
    - Coping and recovery resources
  - Affect
    - Mood state
  - Behaviors
    - Body image and impression management (*e.g.*, toughness)
    - Perfectionism and need to prove
    - Risk behaviors
  - Sociocultural
    - Sports beliefs and attitudes (valor of playing through injury)
    - Life event stress (major and/or accumulation of minor stressors)

- Extrinsic risk factors (71,72): factors the athlete experiences that affect their injury risk (considered the enabling factor that facilitates injury)
  - Physical
    - Sport: playing situation, duration, and interaction with other players — intensity and skill level of play
    - Environment: facility, playing surface, maintenance, weather, safety, security, violence, crowd proximity, and fan behavior
    - Other: medical care, equipment (sport and protective) fit, and usage
  - Sociocultural
    - Sport: rules, etiquette of sport, officiating standards, and sports norms and ethics
    - Organization: coaching quality, organizational stress, and medical interactions
    - Culture: social resources, pressures, cultural context, and media scrutiny

Psychological Assessment

- A comprehensive initial evaluation should include assessment of the athlete's psychological wellness. Injuries may impact athletes differently (68) and can have a significant negative impact on the athlete's psychological state (43,95–97), which can result in poor rehabilitation outcomes (69,96).
  - Positive psychological responses to injury or illness are associated with a faster return, higher rate of return, and increased likelihood of returning to preinjury participation (53).
  - Negative psychological responses to injury or illness are associated with a lower rate of return and a decreased likelihood of returning to preinjury participation (44,47).
  - Typically, as the athlete progresses through the rehabilitation program, there is a decrease in negative emotions and an increase in positive emotions (55,69).
- Factors that influence the athlete's psychological response to injury (41,53,54):
  - Cognition: conscious assessment of injury consequence and serves as the precursor to resultant emotions
    - Sense of loss: missed goals, loss of identity, changed outward impression (toughness), and lost trust in body
    - Pressure: perception of self, letting the team down, and lack of stress outlet
    - Beliefs: optimistic, pessimistic, external locus of control, lower self-esteem, and reduced self-confidence
      - Perception of greater negative injury impact on the athlete's life results in greater risk of not returning to sport (44).
  - Affect: emotional response to injury consequences (44)
    - Emotion (55,69,70): depressed (sadness/grief), anxious/stress (fearful — future implications or movement [kinesiophobia]) (58), anger (often of associated loss), and emotional inhibition (lack of healthy outlet)
    - Feeling:
      - Escape from pressure and relief
      - Burned out, fatigued, guilt, stress, and boredom
      - Socially isolated from team (44)
  - Behavior: resulting action from the athlete's conscious assessment and emotional response to injury
    - Coping: help seeking, social connection (team commodore), psychological interventions, rehabilitation adherence and compliance, and drive to overcome barrier of illness or injury (68)
    - Risky behavior: substance use, suicidal behavior, exercise dependence, and malingering ("faking it")
- Factors affecting the athlete's motivation toward rehabilitation from an injury (54,98,99):
  - Autonomy
    - Ideally, the athlete perceives that they have control in their return to sport (internal locus of control).
    - Alternatively, the athlete may feel that external pressures are what drive the rehabilitation process (external locus of control) (68).
    - Athletes may perceive more autonomy when provided coping strategies aimed at managing the stressful situation (68).
      - Encourage the athlete to work at their own pace and to allow the body to recover fully.
      - Involve the athlete in identifying a realistic date of potential return to sport.

- Work with the athlete with goal setting (100,101):
  - Participation in creating and being aware of the rehabilitation goals resulted in better outcomes (44).
  - Confidence builds as the athlete meets their goals.
- Competence: athlete's perception of their proficiency in their RTP.
  - Aspects that affect competence:
    - Confidence (57,69,70)
    - Risk appraisal (69)
    - Perceived severity of injury (102)
  - Competence can be improved through functional testing — providing a safe environment to allow the athlete to test the injured structure.
- Relatedness
  - Athlete's perception of connectedness or belonging in the social world (feeling they are supported by their team)
    - Providing opportunities for team commodore
  - Athletes may experience a loss of identity and perception of being disconnected from their team.
  - Athletes who are significantly affected by their injury may need support through social interaction (listening and emotional comfort) (68,99).

- Improving autonomy, competence, and relatedness provides the opportunity for the athlete to be intrinsically motivated. Often, this is facilitated by the athlete remaining with the team where possible/appropriate.
- Benefits of intrinsic motivation
  - Improved mental health (103)
  - Positive emotions (104)
  - Greater persistence (104)
  - Improved rehabilitation outcomes (54,98)
- The athlete's emotional response is fluid throughout the rehabilitation process. Routine screening of the athlete's psychological well-being will allow for early identification and intervention against maladaptive responses to injury (53).

Functional Assessment

- Functional assessments should routinely and progressively evaluate the body's ability to tolerate sport-specific stressors.
- The athlete's performance of these assessments allows the clinician to monitor the athlete's response to the rehabilitation program, ensuring the athlete is adequately prepared to safely return to sport (39). The athlete can also see their recovery trajectory, which can help with program adherence.
- Battery of functional tests must be multidimensional to replicate sport-specific stressors in a controlled environment. Sport-specific tasks should be gradually and sequentially increased in difficulty. Factors to replicate in testing include (84):
  - Forces required during muscle contraction
  - Speed required during movement
  - Power expressed during movement
  - Type of movement required (specific or nonspecific to sport)
- In addition, the selected battery of functional tests should be validated to test the structures of interest based on scientific and clinical research (8).
  - Standardized recovery tests are more likely to be known to the athlete.
- When evaluating functional capacity, it should be compared to preinjury values or the contralateral extremity.
- As part of the battery of tests, functional ability can be segmented into three groups to help document and follow rehabilitation trajectory (73,105):
  - Quantitative values: speed, force, and acceleration
  - Qualitative values: movement efficiency
  - Parameter requirements: sport-specific/position-specific load requirements (overall distance covered/contact/energy expenditure)
- Monitoring the athlete's performance on functional tests will show the athlete's recovery trajectory and can identify early signs of injury recurrence.

Removal from Sport

- The goal is to allow the athlete to participate at the highest level without a significant increase in injury risk or long-term injury sequelae.
- When considering level of participation, common designations are listed below:
  - No participation in any activity
  - Strength and conditioning under direction only
  - Practice with modified activity
  - Practice only
  - Compete with a modified role
  - No restrictions
- Absolute removal from sport:
  - Conditions that risk life or extremity
  - Neuromuscular deficits (numbness, strength deficits, altered mental status, etc.)
- Consider removal from sport:
  - The athlete is unable to perform sport-specific functional requirements safely.
  - Unable to tolerate sport-specific load despite adaptations (load reduction, bracing, etc.)
- It is important to comply with governing rules and regulations for removal from sport.
- If the athlete is removed from competition due to injury or illness, it is important to communicate this with the appropriate parties (coaches, medical staff, etc.) (106).

- Any athlete who required treatment during or after the competition should be reevaluated to determine a plan of care, including diagnostic studies, referrals, and plan for follow-up (106).

INJURY PREVENTION

- One of the roles of the team physician is to prevent injury and illness associated with athletic activity (107).
- Preventing injury is crucial for player safety as there is a significant increase in future injury risk after an initial injury (108–110).
- Similar to the evaluation of the injured athlete, multiple factors must be evaluated when setting up an injury prevention program (41,107):
  - Clinicians should understand the pathophysiology of common injury and illness associated with individual sport.
  - Evaluate regional and global biomechanics: ROM, stability, strength, and neuromuscular control
  - Evaluate for known risk factors that influence injury or illness:
    - Internal risk factors:
      - Physiological: neuromuscular control
      - Biomechanical: improper technique
      - Anatomical: extremity alignment
      - Genetic: family history (*e.g.*, hypertrophic cardiomyopathy)
      - Prior injury:
        - Muscle weakness
        - Inflexibility
        - Ligamentous laxity
        - Kinetic chain deficits
      - Medication use
      - Psychologic: burnout, life stressors, and stress coping
    - External risk factors:
      - Inherent demands of the sport: load and recovery
      - Environmental factors
      - Equipment interaction and potential issues (*i.e.*, appropriate cleat for playing surface)
  - Implement interventions to minimize risk factors:
    - Injury prevention programs have been shown to benefit the individual athlete's health and safety and the overall team's performance.
      - Teams with less time loss secondary to injury often have greater league success (111,112).
    - Interventions should be specific for individual factors (sport, injury type, environmental conditions, etc.).
      - Injury prevention programs should be implemented 2 times · wk^{-1}, lasting for 10–15 minutes per episode (39).
    - Education for the player, parents, and coaches is an important intervention to include, as it improves buy-in and program adherence.
    - During the injury prevention program, the athlete's technique should be monitored and corrected to avoid maladaptation.
    - More research is required in this field, but there are injury prevention programs that can be adopted for specific sports (*e.g.*, FIFA 11+ for soccer).
    - Simple interventions such as monitoring loads (*e.g.*, pitch counts) or ensuring hydration can also have a positive effect on injury prevention.
  - After implementing an injury prevention program, it is important to monitor and record outcomes to assess for effectiveness of program:
    - Surveillance data can help identify injury trends and rates (113,114).

SUMMARY

- Rehabilitation is a deliberate, fluid, and multidisciplinary process where the ultimate goal is to limit the extent of the injury, reduce or reverse the impairment and functional loss, and prevent, correct, or eliminate altogether the disability (3).
- The process should be individualized as risk factors inherent to each athlete will result in a varied impact from stressors experienced by the athlete.
- The RTP decision is complex, involving multidimensional circumstances that can be variable throughout the rehabilitation process. Due to the fluidity of circumstances, the RTP decision should not be an isolated conclusion, but should be a part of the continuum throughout the recovery and rehabilitation process.
- The clinician must ensure the athlete's functional, psychological, and cardiorespiratory endurance are at a satisfactory level and the athlete does not pose undue risk to themselves or other participants prior to providing clearance for RTP.

REFERENCES

1. Dijkstra HP, Pollock N, Chakraverty R, Alonso JM. Managing the health of the elite athlete: a new integrated performance health management and coaching model. *Br J Sports Med.* 2014;48(7):523–31. doi:10.1136/bjsports-2013-093222
2. Meeuwisse WH, Tyreman H, Hagel B, Emery C. A dynamic model of etiology in sport injury: the recursive nature of risk and causation. *Clin J Sport Med.* 2007;17(3):215–19. doi:10.1097/JSM.0b013e3180592a48

3. IOC Medical Commission, International Federation of Sports Medicine. In: Frontera WR, editor. *Rehabilitation of Sports Injuries: Scientific Basis*. Blackwell Science; 2003.
4. Ardern CL, Glasgow P, Schneiders A, et al. 2016 consensus statement on return to sport from the First World Congress in Sports Physical Therapy, Bern. *Br J Sports Med*. 2016;50(14):853–64. doi:10.1136/bjsports-2016-096278
5. Herring S, Bergfeld J, Boyd J, et al. The team physician and return-to-play issues: a consensus statement. *Med Sci Sports Exerc*. 2002;34(7):1212–14. doi:10.1097/00005768-200207000-00025
6. Herring S, Kibler W, Putukian M. The team physician and the return-to-play decision: a consensus statement—2012 update. *Med Sci Sports Exerc*. 2012;44(12):2446–8. doi:10.1249/MSS.0b013e3182750534
7. Shultz R, Bido J, Shrier I, Meeuwisse WH, Garza D, Matheson GO. Team clinician variability in return-to-play decisions. *Clin J Sport Med*. 2013;23(6):456–61. doi:10.1097/JSM.0b013e318295bb17
8. Bizzini M, Silvers HJ. Return to competitive football after major knee surgery: more questions than answers? *J Sports Sci*. 2014;32(13):1209–16. doi:10.1080/02640414.2014.909603
9. Gouin JP, Kiecolt-Glaser JK. The impact of psychological stress on wound healing: methods and mechanisms. *Immunol Allergy Clin North Am*. 2011;31(1):81–93. doi:10.1016/j.iac.2010.09.010
10. Rand E, Gellhorn AC. The healing cascade: facilitating and optimizing the system. *Phys Med Rehabil Clin N Am*. 2016;27(4):765–81. doi:10.1016/j.pmr.2016.07.001
11. Järvinen TAH, Järvinen TLN, Kääriäinen M, Kalimo H, Järvinen M. Muscle injuries: biology and treatment. *Am J Sports Med*. 2005;33(5):745–64. doi:10.1177/0363546505274714
12. Baoge L, Van Den Steen E, Rimbaut S, et al. Treatment of skeletal muscle injury: a review. *ISRN Orthop*. 2012;2012:689012. doi:10.5402/2012/689012
13. Hopkins JT, Ingersoll CD. Arthrogenic muscle inhibition: a limiting factor in joint rehabilitation. *J Sport Rehabil*. 2000;9(2):135–59. doi:10.1123/jsr.9.2.135
14. Stockmar C, Lill H, Trapp A, Josten C, Punkt K. Fibre type related changes in the metabolic profile and fibre diameter of human vastus medialis muscle after anterior cruciate ligament rupture. *Acta Histochem*. 2006;108(5):335–42. doi:10.1016/j.acthis.2006.05.005
15. Bleakley CM, Glasgow P, MacAuley DC. PRICE needs updating, should we call the POLICE? *Br J Sports Med*. 2012;46(4):220–1.
16. Orchard JW, Best TM, Mueller-Wohlfahrt HW, et al. The early management of muscle strains in the elite athlete: best practice in a world with a limited evidence basis. *Br J Sports Med*. 2008;42(3):158–9. doi:10.1136/bjsm.2008.046722
17. Smith BE, Hendrick P, Smith TO, et al. Should exercises be painful in the management of chronic musculoskeletal pain? A systematic review and meta-analysis. *Br J Sports Med*. 2017;51(23):1679–87. doi:10.1136/bjsports-2016-097383
18. Hickey JT, Timmins RG, Maniar N, et al. Pain-free versus pain-threshold rehabilitation following acute hamstring strain injury: a randomized controlled trial. *J Orthop Sports Phys Ther*. 2020;50(2):91–103. doi:10.2519/jospt.2020.8895
19. Busse JW, Sadeghirad B, Oparin Y, et al. Management of acute pain from non–low back, musculoskeletal injuries: a systematic review and network meta-analysis of randomized trials. *Ann Intern Med*. 2020;173(9):730–8. doi:10.7326/M19-3601
20. Paoloni JA, Milne C, Orchard J, Hamilton B. Non-steroidal anti-inflammatory drugs in sports medicine: guidelines for practical but sensible use. *Br J Sports Med*. 2009;43(11):863–5. doi:10.1136/bjsm.2009.059980
21. Derry S, Wiffen P, Moore A. Topical nonsteroidal anti-inflammatory drugs for acute musculoskeletal pain. *JAMA*. 2016;315(8):813–14. doi:10.1001/jama.2016.0249
22. Järvinen TAH, Järvinen TLN, Kääriäinen M, et al. Muscle injuries: optimising recovery. *Best Pract Res Clin Rheumatol*. 2007;21(2):317–31. doi:10.1016/j.berh.2006.12.004
23. Dideriksen K. Muscle and tendon connective tissue adaptation to unloading, exercise and NSAID. *Connect Tissue Res*. 2014;55(2):61–70. doi:10.3109/03008207.2013.862527
24. Su B, O'Connor JP. NSAID therapy effects on healing of bone, tendon, and the enthesis. *J Appl Physiol*. 2013;115(6):892–9. doi:10.1152/japplphysiol.00053.2013
25. Bleakley CM, Glasgow P, Webb MJ. Cooling an acute muscle injury: can basic scientific theory translate into the clinical setting? *Br J Sports Med*. 2012;46(4):296–8. doi:10.1136/bjsm.2011.086116
26. Bleakley C, McDonough S, MacAuley D. The use of ice in the treatment of acute soft-tissue injury: a systematic review of randomized controlled trials. *Am J Sports Med*. 2004;32(1):251–61. doi:10.1177/0363546503260757
27. Koltyn KF, Brellenthin AG, Cook DB, Sehgal N, Hillard C. Mechanisms of exercise-induced hypoalgesia. *J Pain*. 2014;15(12):1294–304. doi:10.1016/j.jpain.2014.09.006
28. Vaegter HB, Handberg G, Graven-Nielsen T. Isometric exercises reduce temporal summation of pressure pain in humans. *Eur J Pain*. 2015;19(7):973–83. doi:10.1002/ejp.623
29. Rio E, Kidgell D, Purdam C, et al. Isometric exercise induces analgesia and reduces inhibition in patellar tendinopathy. *Br J Sports Med*. 2015;49(19):1277–83. doi:10.1136/bjsports-2014-094386
30. De Valk EJ, Moen MH, Winters M, Bakker EWP, Tamminga R, Van Der Hoeven H. Preoperative patient and injury factors of successful rehabilitation after anterior cruciate ligament reconstruction with single-bundle techniques. *Arthroscopy*. 2013;29(11):1879–95. doi:10.1016/j.arthro.2013.07.273
31. Rubini EC, Costa ALL, Gomes PSC. The effects of stretching on strength performance. *Sports Med*. 2007;37(3):213–24. doi:10.2165/00007256-200737030-00003
32. Gogate N, Satpute K, Hall T. The effectiveness of mobilization with movement on pain, balance and function following acute and sub acute inversion ankle sprain – a randomized, placebo controlled trial. *Phys Ther Sport*. 2021;48:91–100. doi:10.1016/j.ptsp.2020.12.016
33. Nakamura N, Rodeo S, Alini M, Maher S, Madry H, Erggelet C. Physiology and pathophysiology of musculoskeletal tissues. In: *DeLee & Drez's Orthopaedic Sports Medicine: Principles and Practice*. 4th ed, Vol. 2. Elsevier/Saunders; 2015.
34. Behm DG, Chaouachi A. A review of the acute effects of static and dynamic stretching on performance. *Eur J Appl Physiol*. 2011;111(11):2633–51. doi:10.1007/s00421-011-1879-2
35. Sharman MJ, Cresswell AG, Riek S. Proprioceptive neuromuscular facilitation stretching: mechanisms and clinical implications. *Sports Med*. 2006;36(11):929–39. doi:10.2165/00007256-200636110-00002
36. Amiri-Khorasani M, Kellis E. Acute effects of different agonist and antagonist stretching arrangements on static and dynamic range of motion. *Asian J Sports Med*. 2015;6(4):e26844. doi:10.5812/asjsm.26844
37. Hopper D, Deacon S, Das S, et al. Dynamic soft tissue mobilisation increases hamstring flexibility in healthy male subjects. *Br J Sports Med*. 2005;39(9):594–8. doi:10.1136/bjsm.2004.011981
38. Bradbury-Squires DJ, Noftall JC, Sullivan KM, Behm DG, Power KE, Button DC. Roller-massager application to the quadriceps and knee-joint range of motion and neuromuscular efficiency during a Lunge. *J Athl Train*. 2015;50(2):133–40. doi:10.4085/1062-6050-49.5.03

39. Schwank A, Blazey P, Asker M, et al. 2022 bern consensus statement on shoulder injury prevention, rehabilitation, and return to sport for athletes at all participation levels. *J Orthop Sports Phys Ther.* 2022;52(1):11–28. doi:10.2519/jospt.2022.10952
40. Forsdyke D, Smith A, Jones M, Gledhill A. Psychosocial factors associated with outcomes of sports injury rehabilitation in competitive athletes: a mixed studies systematic review. *Br J Sports Med.* 2016;50(9):537–44. doi:10.1136/bjsports-2015-094850
41. Wiese-Bjornstal DM. Psychology and socioculture affect injury risk, response, and recovery in high-intensity athletes: a consensus statement. *Scand J Med Sci Sports.* 2010;20(suppl 2):103–11. doi:10.1111/j.1600-0838.2010.01195.x
42. Podlog L, Wadey R, Caron J, et al. Psychological readiness to return to sport following injury: a state-of-the-art review. *Int Rev Sport Exerc Psychol.* 2024;17:753–72. doi:10.1080/1750984X.2022.2081929
43. Appaneal RN, Levine BR, Perna FM, Roh JL. Measuring postinjury depression among male and female competitive athletes. *J Sport Exerc Psychol.* 2009;31(1):60–76. doi:10.1123/jsep.31.1.60
44. Johnson U. A three-year follow-up of long-term injured competitive athletes: influence of psychological risk factors on rehabilitation. *J Sport Rehabil.* 1997;6(3):256–71. doi:10.1123/jsr.6.3.256
45. Paster E, Sayeg A, Armistead S, Feldman MD. Rehabilitation using a systematic and holistic approach for the injured athlete returning to sport. *Arthrosc Sports Med Rehabil.* 2022;4(1):e215–19. doi:10.1016/j.asmr.2021.09.036
46. Johnson U. Short-term psychological intervention: a study of long-term-injured competitive athletes. *J Sport Rehabil.* 2000;9(3):207–18. doi:10.1123/jsr.9.3.207
47. Ivarsson A, Tranaeus U, Johnson U, Stenling A. Negative psychological responses of injury and rehabilitation adherence effects on return to play in competitive athletes: a systematic review and meta-analysis. *Open Access J Sports Med.* 2017;8:27–32. doi:10.2147/OAJSM.S112688
48. Perna FM, Antoni MH, Baum A, Gordon P, Schneiderman N. Cognitive behavioral stress management effects on injury and illness among competitive athletes: a randomized clinical trial. *Ann Behav Med.* 2003;25(1):66–73. doi:10.1207/S15324796ABM2501_09
49. Ardern CL, Bizzini M, Bahr R. It is time for consensus on return to play after injury: five key questions. *Br J Sports Med.* 2016;50(9):506–8. doi:10.1136/bjsports-2015-095475
50. Kim KM, Croy T, Hertel J, Saliba S. Effects of neuromuscular electrical stimulation after anterior cruciate ligament reconstruction on quadriceps strength, function, and patient-oriented outcomes: a systematic review. *J Orthop Sports Phys Ther.* 2010;40(7):383–91. doi:10.2519/jospt.2010.3184
51. Croisier JL, Ganteaume S, Binet J, Genty M, Ferret JM. Strength imbalances and prevention of hamstring injury in professional soccer players: a prospective study. *Am J Sports Med.* 2008;36(8):1469–75. doi:10.1177/0363546508316764
52. Davies G, Riemann BL, Manske R. Current concepts of plyometric exercise. *Int J Sports Phys Ther.* 2015;10(6):760–86.
53. Ardern CL, Taylor NF, Feller JA, Webster KE. A systematic review of the psychological factors associated with returning to sport following injury. *Br J Sports Med.* 2013;47(17):1120–6. doi:10.1136/bjsports-2012-091203
54. Podlog L, Eklund RC. The psychosocial aspects of a return to sport following serious injury: a review of the literature from a self-determination perspective. *Psychol Sport Exerc.* 2007;8(4):535–66. doi:10.1016/j.psychsport.2006.07.008
55. Crossman J. Psychological rehabilitation from sports injuries. *Sports Med.* 1997;23(5):333–9. doi:10.2165/00007256-199723050-00005
56. Podlog L, Eklund RC. A longitudinal investigation of competitive athletes' return to sport following serious injury. *J Appl Sport Psychol.* 2006;18(1):44–68. doi:10.1080/10413200500471319
57. Glazer DD. Development and preliminary validation of the injury-psychological readiness to return to sport (I-PRRS) scale. *J Athl Train.* 2009;44(2):185–9.
58. Flanigan DC, Everhart JS, Pedroza A, Smith T, Kaeding CC. Fear of reinjury (kinesiophobia) and persistent knee symptoms are common factors for lack of return to sport after anterior cruciate ligament reconstruction. *Arthroscopy.* 2013;29(8):1322–9. doi:10.1016/j.arthro.2013.05.015
59. Tracey J. The emotional response to the injury and rehabilitation process. *J Appl Sport Psychol.* 2003;15(4):279–93. doi:10.1080/714044197
60. Dijkstra HP, Pollock N, Chakraverty R, Ardern CL. Return to play in elite sport: a shared decision-making process. *Br J Sports Med.* 2017;51(5):419–20. doi:10.1136/bjsports-2016-096209
61. Smith MD, Vicenzino B, Bahr R, et al. Return to sport decisions after an acute lateral ankle sprain injury: introducing the PAASS framework—an international multidisciplinary consensus. *Br J Sports Med.* 2021;55(22):1270–6. doi:10.1136/bjsports-2021-104087
62. Boudier-Revéret M, Mazer B, Feldman DE, Shrier I. Practice management of musculoskeletal injuries in active children. *Br J Sports Med.* 2011;45(14):1137–43. doi:10.1136/bjsm.2009.071233
63. Miller MD, Arciero RA, Cooper DE, Johnson DL, Best TM. Doc, when can he go back in the game? *Instr Course Lect.* 2009;58:437–43.
64. Connell DA, Schneider-Kolsky ME, Hoving JL, et al. Longitudinal study comparing sonographic and MRI assessments of acute and healing hamstring injuries. *AJR Am J Roentgenol.* 2004;183(4):975–84. doi:10.2214/ajr.183.4.1830975
65. Reurink G, Goudswaard GJ, Tol JL, et al. MRI observations at return to play of clinically recovered hamstring injuries. *Br J Sports Med.* 2014;48(18):1370–6. doi:10.1136/bjsports-2013-092450
66. Ardern CL, Webster KE, Taylor NF, Feller JA. Return to sport following anterior cruciate ligament reconstruction surgery: a systematic review and meta-analysis of the state of play. *Br J Sports Med.* 2011;45(7):596–606. doi:10.1136/bjsm.2010.076364
67. Tjong VK, Devitt BM, Murnaghan ML, Ogilvie-Harris DJ, Theodoropoulos JS. A qualitative investigation of return to sport after arthroscopic Bankart repair: beyond stability. *Am J Sports Med.* 2015;43(8):2005–11. doi:10.1177/0363546515590222
68. Bianco T. Social support and recovery from sport injury: elite Skiers share their experiences. *Res Q Exerc Sport.* 2001;72(4):376–88. doi:10.1080/02701367.2001.10608974
69. Langford JL, Webster KE, Feller JA. A prospective longitudinal study to assess psychological changes following anterior cruciate ligament reconstruction surgery. *Br J Sports Med.* 2009;43(5):377–81. doi:10.1136/bjsm.2007.044818
70. Webster KE, Feller JA, Lambros C. Development and preliminary validation of a scale to measure the psychological impact of returning to sport following anterior cruciate ligament reconstruction surgery. *Phys Ther Sport.* 2008;9(1):9–15. doi:10.1016/j.ptsp.2007.09.003
71. Wiese-Bjornstal DM. Sport injury and College athlete health across the Lifespan. *J Intercoll Sport.* 2009;2(1):64–80. doi:10.1123/jis.2.1.64
72. Watson AWS. Sports injuries: incidence, causes, prevention. *Phys Ther Rev.* 1997;2(3):135–51. doi:10.1179/ptr.1997.2.3.135
73. Bizzini M, Hancock D, Impellizzeri F. Suggestions from the field for return to sports participation following anterior cruciate ligament reconstruction: soccer. *J Orthop Sports Phys Ther.* 2012;42(4):304–12. doi:10.2519/jospt.2012.4005
74. Shrier I, Matheson GO, Boudier-Revéret M, Steele RJ. Validating the three-step return-to-play decision model. *Scand J Med Sci Sports.* 2015;25(2):e231–9. doi:10.1111/sms.12306

75. Johnston LH, Carroll D. The context of emotional responses to athletic injury: a qualitative analysis. *J Sport Rehabil.* 1998;7(3):206–20. doi:10.1123/jsr.7.3.206
76. Shrier I, Safai P, Charland L. Return to play following injury: whose decision should it be? *Br J Sports Med.* 2014;48(5):394–401. doi:10.1136/bjsports-2013-092492
77. Barry MJ, Edgman-Levitan S. Shared decision making-pinnacle of patient-centered care. *N Engl J Med.* 2012;366(9):780–1. doi:10.1056/NEJMp1109283
78. Creighton DW, Shrier I, Shultz R, Meeuwisse WH, Matheson GO. Return-to-play in sport: a decision-based model. *Clin J Sport Med.* 2010;20(5):379–85. doi:10.1097/JSM.0b013e3181f3c0fe
79. Shrier I, Charland L, Mohtadi NGH, Meeuwisse WH, Matheson GO. The sociology of return-to-play decision making: a clinical perspective. *Clin J Sport Med.* 2010;20(5):333–5. doi:10.1097/JSM.0b013e3181f465de
80. Mazer B, Shrier I, Feldman DE, et al. Clinical management of musculoskeletal injuries in active children and youth. *Clin J Sport Med.* 2010;20(4):249–55. doi:10.1097/JSM.0b013e3181e0b913
81. Young K, White P, McTeer W. Body talk: male athletes reflect on sport, injury, and pain. *Soc Sport J.* 1994;11:175–94.
82. Stovitz SD, Satin DJ. Professionalism and the ethics of the sideline physician. *Curr Sports Med Rep.* 2006;5(3):120–4. doi:10.1097/01.CSMR.0000306300.03073.d7
83. Testoni D, Hornik CP, Smith PB, Benjamin DK, McKinney RE. Sports medicine and ethics. *Am J Bioeth.* 2013;13(10):4–12. doi:10.1080/15265161.2013.828114
84. Shrier I. Strategic assessment of risk and risk tolerance (StARRT) framework for return-to-play decision-making. *Br J Sports Med.* 2015;49(20):1311–15. doi:10.1136/bjsports-2014-094569
85. Safai P. Healing the body in the "culture of risk": examining the negotiation of treatment between sport medicine clinicians and injured athletes in Canadian intercollegiate sport. *Soc Sport J.* 2003;20:127–46.
86. Hedlund J. Risky business: safety regulations, risk compensation, and individual behavior. *Inj Prev.* 2000;6(2):82–9. doi:10.1136/ip.6.2.82
87. Coppage JM, Carlson MG. Expediting professional athletes' return to competition. *Hand Clin.* 2017;33(1):9–18. doi:10.1016/j.hcl.2016.08.002
88. Barbee C. *2021-2022 and 2022-2023 NCAA Wrestling Rules.* The National Collegiate Athletic Association; 2021.
89. Gerteis M, editor. *Through the Patient's Eyes: Understanding and Promoting Patient-Centered Care.* 1st ed. Jossey-Bass; 1993.
90. Nieman DC. Exercise, upper respiratory tract infection, and the immune system. *Med Sci Sports Exerc.* 1994;26(2):128–39. doi:10.1249/00005768-199402000-00002
91. Bahr R, Holme I. Risk factors for sports injuries—a methodological approach. *Br J Sports Med.* 2003;37(5):384–92. doi:10.1136/bjsm.37.5.384
92. Meeuwisse WH. Assessing causation in sport injury: a multifactorial model. *Clin J Sport Med.* 1994;4(3):166–70. doi:10.1097/00042752-199407000-00004
93. Meeuwisse WH. Athletic injury etiology: distinguishing between interaction and confounding. *Clin J Sport Med.* 1994;4(3):171–5. doi:10.1097/00042752-199407000-00005
94. Guidi J, Lucente M, Sonino N, Fava GA. Allostatic load and its impact on health: a systematic review. *Psychother Psychosom.* 2021;90(1):11–27. doi:10.1159/000510696
95. Park S, Lavallee D, Tod D. Athletes' career transition out of sport: a systematic review. *Int Rev Sport Exerc Psychol.* 2013;6(1):22–53. doi:10.1080/1750984X.2012.687053
96. Hagger MS, Chatzisarantis NLD, Griffin M, Thatcher J. Injury representations, coping, emotions, and functional outcomes in athletes with sports-related injuries: a test of self-regulation theory. *J Appl Soc Psychol.* 2005;35(11):2345–74. doi:10.1111/j.1559-1816.2005.tb02106.x
97. Arvinen-Barrow M, Hemmings B, Weigand D, Becker C, Booth L. Views of chartered physiotherapists on the psychological content of their practice: a follow-up survey in the UK. *J Sport Rehabil.* 2007;16(2):111–21. doi:10.1123/jsr.16.2.111
98. Ryan RM, Deci EL. Self-determination theory and the facilitation of intrinsic motivation, social development, and well-being. *Am Psychol.* 2000;55(1):68–78.
99. Podlog L, Lochbaum M, Stevens T. Need satisfaction, well-being, and perceived return-to-sport outcomes among injured athletes. *J Appl Sport Psychol.* 2010;22(2):167–82. doi:10.1080/10413201003664665
100. Evans L, Hardy L. Sport injury and grief responses: a review. *J Sport Exerc Psychol.* 1995;17(3):227–45. doi:10.1123/jsep.17.3.227
101. Carson F, Polman R. Experiences of professional rugby union players returning to competition following anterior cruciate ligament reconstruction. *Phys Ther Sport.* 2012;13(1):35–40. doi:10.1016/j.ptsp.2010.10.007
102. sÁEZ De Heredia RA, Muñoz AR, Artaza JL. The effect of psychological response on recovery of sport injury. *Res Sports Med.* 2004;12(1):15–31. doi:10.1080/15438620490280567
103. Frederick C, Ryan R. Differences in motivation for sport and exercise and their relations with participation and mental health. *J Sport Behav.* 1993;16:124–46.
104. Vallerand RJ, Losier GF. An integrative analysis of intrinsic and extrinsic motivation in sport. *J Appl Sport Psychol.* 1999;11(1):142–69. doi:10.1080/10413209908402956
105. Bisciotti GN, Volpi P, Alberti G, et al. Italian consensus statement (2020) on return to play after lower limb muscle injury in football (soccer). *BMJ Open Sport Exerc Med.* 2019;5(1):e000505. doi:10.1136/bmjsem-2018-000505
106. Herring SA, Kibler WB, Putukian M. Sideline preparedness for the team physician: a consensus statement—2012 update. *Med Sci Sports Exerc.* 2012;44(12):2442–5. doi:10.1249/MSS.0b013e318275044f
107. Selected issues in injury and illness prevention and the team physician: a consensus statement. *Med Sci Sports Exerc.* 2007;39(11):2058–68. doi:10.1249/mss.0b013e31815a76ea
108. Arnason A, Sigurdsson SB, Gudmundsson A, Holme I, Engebretsen L, Bahr R. Risk factors for injuries in football. *Am J Sports Med.* 2004;32(1 suppl 1):5–16. doi:10.1177/0363546503258912
109. Bahr R, Bahr IA. Incidence of acute volleyball injuries: a prospective cohort study of injury mechanisms and risk factors. *Scand J Med Sci Sports.* 1997;7(3):166–71. doi:10.1111/j.1600-0838.1997.tb00134.x
110. Rebella GS, Edwards JO, Greene JJ, Husen MT, Brousseau DC. A prospective study of injury patterns in high school pole vaulters. *Am J Sports Med.* 2008;36(5):913–20. doi:10.1177/0363546507313571
111. Eirale C, Tol JL, Farooq A, Smiley F, Chalabi H. Low injury rate strongly correlates with team success in Qatari professional football. *Br J Sports Med.* 2013;47(12):807–8. doi:10.1136/bjsports-2012-091040
112. Hägglund M, Waldén M, Magnusson H, Kristenson K, Bengtsson H, Ekstrand J. Injuries affect team performance negatively in professional football: an 11-year follow-up of the UEFA Champions League injury study. *Br J Sports Med.* 2013;47(12):738–42. doi:10.1136/bjsports-2013-092215
113. Fuller CW, Ekstrand J, Junge A, et al. Consensus statement on injury definitions and data collection procedures in studies of football (soccer) injuries. *Scand J Med Sci Sports.* 2006;16(2):83–92. doi:10.1111/j.1600-0838.2006.00528.x
114. Fuller CW, Bahr R, Dick RW, Meeuwisse WH. A framework for recording recurrences, reinjuries, and exacerbations in injury surveillance. *Clin J Sport Med.* 2007;17(3):197–200. doi:10.1097/JSM.0b013e3180471b89

Pain Management in the Athlete

73

Malia Cali and Stanley A. Herring

INTRODUCTION

- Pain, a common complaint in athletes, is influenced by both internal and external factors (1). Accordingly, successful management necessitates an understanding of both the physical demands and training load of the athlete and their unique psychosocial situation.
- The clinical approach to managing pain is dependent on the underlying diagnosis, type of pain, and duration of symptoms.
- Consideration of both nonpharmacologic and pharmacologic treatments is recommended; the treatments implemented for pain management should be clearly documented in the patient's chart.
- A multidisciplinary approach to treatment is often most successful, especially in cases of subacute or chronic pain with associated disability.

TYPES OF PAIN

- Pain is defined as an unpleasant sensory and emotional experience associated with actual or potential tissue damage, or described in terms of such damage (2).
- Pain can be classified as nociceptive, neuropathic, and nociplastic/algopathic/nocipathic (3).
- Nociceptive pain is clearly associated with tissue damage or inflammation. It is generated by activation of nociceptors in peripheral tissue by an actual or potentially tissue-damaging event (2). This is the most common type of pain associated with sports injury.
- Neuropathic pain as defined by the International Association for the Study of Pain (IASP) is the result of a lesion or disease in the somatosensory nervous system. Neuropathic pain can occur acutely due to trauma, toxic substances, or metabolic conditions that affect the neurons centrally or peripherally (4).
- Nociplastic, algopathic, and nocipathic pain are terms that have been proposed for pain in which a specific etiology cannot be identified, but clinical and psychophysical findings suggest altered nociceptive function (5,6). Asking questions about affective and cognitive function is important and often underrepresented.
- It is important for the sports medicine clinician to identify the type of pain in the athlete to better understand the pathophysiology that led to the symptom and ultimately develop an appropriate treatment plan.

TYPES OF INJURY

- Sports injury is defined by the International Olympic Committee as a new or recurring musculoskeletal complaint incurred during competition or training that requires medical attention, regardless of the potential absence from competition or training (7). Types of injury include acute traumatic, subacute recurrent, overuse, and chronic degenerative conditions. Identifying the potential type of injury that occurs is important in addressing an athlete's pain.
- Acute traumatic injury occurs as a result of specific and identifiable events that lead to damage of previously healthy tissue (8).
- Subacute recurrent injuries occur at the same site and of the same type as a previous injury that the athlete had already returned to full function and participation (3).
- Overuse injuries occur due to repetitive submaximal loading of the musculoskeletal system when recovery is not adequate for structural adaptation (9).
- Chronic degenerative conditions can develop independently of a sports injury, but prior acute or overuse injuries may contribute to its development.
- Understanding the occurrence of injury is important in the evaluation of pain in the athlete, although injury can happen without pain and pain without evidence of injury.

ACUTE VERSUS CHRONIC PAIN

- Acute pain is typically self-limited. It can be the result of an acute or overuse injury and is usually classified as nociceptive or neuropathic.
- Pain lasting greater than 6 weeks or the expected time for tissue to heal transitions to subacute pain (4). The risk of transitioning to chronic pain increases with the increased duration of pain. For this reason, the management of acute pain, including proper diagnosis and treatment should be

emphasized. Acute pain that does not resolve should prompt consideration of an alternative diagnosis or further exploration of the individual situation (3).

- Chronic pain is defined by the ISAP as pain lasting greater than 3 months. Pain that transitions from acute to chronic frequently has a nociplastic component and is often best treated with an interdisciplinary, multimodal approach with the goal of improving function (1) (Fig. 73.1).

NONPHARMACOLOGIC PAIN MANAGEMENT

- Nonpharmacologic management is essential in all stages of pain, including acute, subacute, and chronic.
- Pain is modulated by neurobiological, environmental, and cognitive factors, so it is important to consider each individual's situation and experience when determining appropriate treatment modalities (10).
- In the case of acute traumatic injuries, standard treatments such as early relocation of a joint, casting, splinting, or the use of crutches should be practiced to reduce pain and limit injury severity (see Chapters 82, Taping, Chapter 83 Bracing, and Chapter 84 Casting and Splinting).
- In most cases, working with an athletic trainer or physical therapist is important for a variety of reasons. In addition to addressing biomechanical deviations contributing to pain and/or injury and improving strength, range of motion, and endurance, they serve as front-line clinicians who can identify inaccurate conceptualizations of pain as well as psychosocial and contextual influences on pain (3). They can also assist in building confidence in the athlete who may have some fear and anxiety returning to play after experiencing significant pain from injury.
- A wide array of modalities including active and passive techniques may be utilized by the athletic trainer or physical therapist. Manual therapy, such as myofascial release, joint mobilization, or muscle energy techniques may be used in athletes who are unable to tolerate more active techniques early in their rehabilitation (11). Additional physical modalities such as ice, electrical stimulation, or ultrasound may be applied. It is important, however, to recognize that many of these passive techniques are supported by limited evidence and should be considered more for acute treatment (12–16) (see Chapter 74, Modalities).
- Movement and exercise are also important in the treatment of pain, particularly chronic pain, in the athlete. Exercise can help reverse deconditioning and decrease pain. Isometric exercise has been shown to downregulate pain pathways through intracortical inhibition and may result in greater benefit than isotonic and eccentric exercises alone (17–19). Exercise can also activate antinociceptive pathways and endogenous opioid and cannabinoid systems (20–23). Active therapies should serve as the mainstay for longer-term care (see Chapter 75, Core Stability).

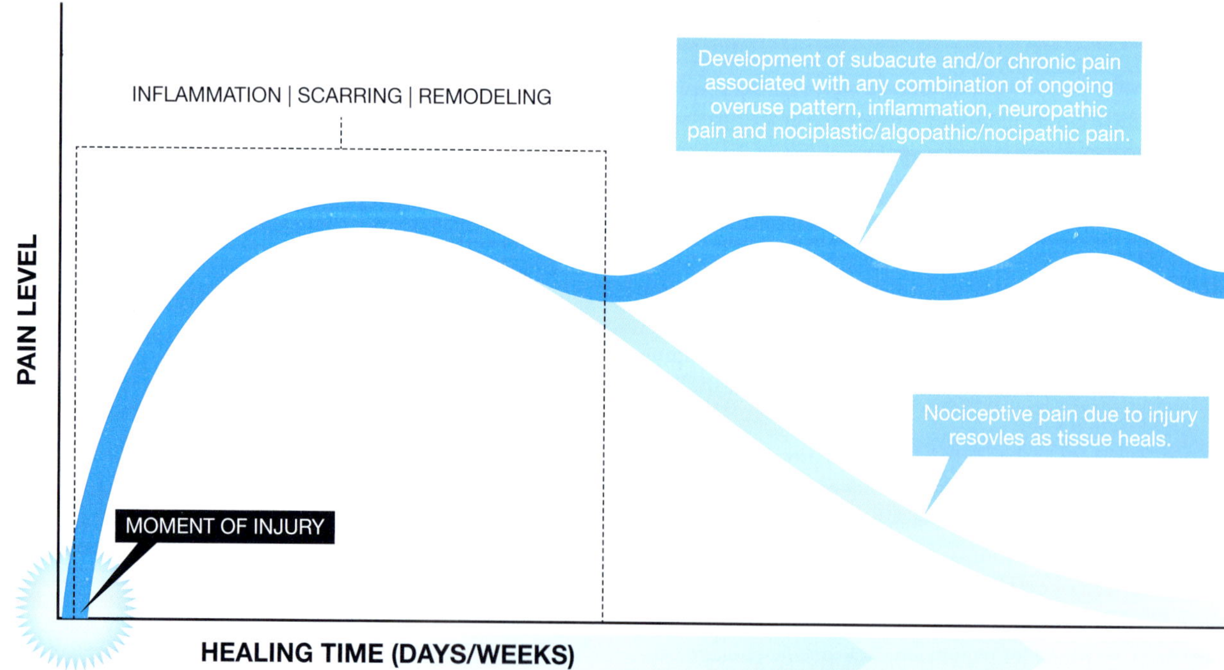

Figure 73.1: Pain variation following injury based on influences of pain. (Adapted with permission from Butler DS, Moseley GL. *Explain Pain Second Edition*. Noigroup Publications; 2013.)

- Sleep and pain are often closely related. Pain can interfere with sleep, and inadequate sleep has been shown to decrease pain thresholds (24–26). In addition to improving pain, the athlete may also experience improvements in performance and overall health with addressing poor-quality sleep (25).
- A proinflammatory load may influence persisting pain in an athlete, suggesting that nutrition may be relevant. Examples of vitamins and supplements that have been studied include vitamin D, vitamin B12, omega-3 fatty acids, turmeric, and curcumin. However, there is no strong evidence demonstrating clear benefit of nutritional supplements for pain management in athletes (27–36). Caution should be exercised with the use of any supplements due to lack of FDA regulation and the potential presence of banned substances (see Chapter 12, Nutrition).
- Psychological interventions can be important in the management of the athlete's pain and wellbeing, especially when time away from their sport is required due to pain in the setting of injury. Techniques such as distraction, relaxation, and imagery may be implemented. Cognitive restructuring and other forms of cognitive behavioral therapy can be helpful for addressing flawed or negative beliefs the athlete may have, developing plans for coping with setbacks, and reducing anxiety (37) (see Chapter 85, Psychology).
- Elective surgery may be considered when there is a structural problem clearly associated with the pain, and, when indicated, all nonoperative interventions have failed (38).

ACUTE PHARMACOLOGICAL PAIN MANAGEMENT

- The use of pharmacologic treatment should be considered as an adjunct to nonpharmacologic strategies and not as the sole treatment of an athlete's pain. See Figure 73.2.
- In general, medications should be prescribed at the lowest effective dose for the shortest period of time. They should be discontinued as pain subsides or if ineffective or not tolerated (1).
- Prior to initiating any medications, a thorough review of the athlete's medical history, including psychological history, should be completed, and potential risks and benefits should be discussed and documented.
- Medications should not be prescribed for injury or pain prevention (3).
- The severity and impact of acute pain on injury and perceived safety should be determined when deciding on appropriate medication management. If same-day return to sport (RTS) is anticipated, first-line medications that are commonly used include acetaminophen, nonsteroidal anti-inflammatory drugs (NSAIDs), and topical analgesics.
- Acetaminophen may be prescribed as a first-line pain medication. When compared to NSAIDs, acetaminophen is metabolized by the liver and does not influence renal function, platelet activity, or gastric mucosa, which should be considered when determining the most appropriate medication. It may be used in combination with NSAIDs.
- Oral NSAIDs are often considered as a mainstay for management. It is important to ensure safety for each individual. There is no high-quality evidence to suggest one NSAID is more beneficial than another. If transitioning from one NSAID to another, the clinician may at least consider one in a different chemical class. Acetaminophen or a cyclooxygenase-2 (Cox-2) selective NSAID may be the medication of choice if the pain is associated with gastrointestinal issues or concern for ongoing hematoma (3).
- Topical medications may also be considered in the treatment of mild to moderate acute pain. Examples of those that affect cutaneous nociception include lidocaine cream or patches, capsaicin, or menthol. Topical NSAIDs, such as diclofenac gel, have a direct anti-inflammatory effect on superficial joints and some systemic absorption. The efficacy of topical medications is variable depending on many factors including the location of pain. Side effects should still be considered, particularly when using in combination with oral medications.
- Rapid onset, temporary relief for moderate to severe pain may also be achieved with injectable medications. Ketorolac is an NSAID that may be judiciously considered. Local anesthetic injections may also be considered for pain localized to a specific location. Injection of anesthetic should be avoided in weight-bearing joints and should not be delivered intratendinously or intraligamentously. Risks include worsening injury or degenerative joint disease, ligament or tendon rupture, pneumothorax, inadvertent major motor nerve block, bleeding, and infection (39). The use of ultrasound guidance may be considered for increased accuracy (see Chapters 79 and 80, Injections and Ultrasound-Guided Procedures).
- Medications that do not allow same day RTP may be administered in the case of acute, severe pain either on the field, sidelines, or in the emergency department.
- For mild to moderate pain that persists beyond the day of injury, oral NSAIDs and acetaminophen as discussed are appropriate for first-line treatment (40). Duration of treatment should not typically exceed 5 days and medication should be reevaluated if pain persists beyond 10 days (41).
- Treatment of persisting moderate to severe pain that is refractory to first-line management with nonopioid alternatives often is facilitated by early mobilization, which is likely to positively impact the athlete's rehabilitation course.
- Opioids are often effective in these cases, but there needs to be an understanding of the potential risks associated with their use (42–45). Guidelines for prescribing opioids that should be followed by the physician include:
  - An assessment of pain and its relationship to the presenting injury should be performed.
  - A review of the athlete's medical history should be completed, particularly with respect to mental health and substance use.

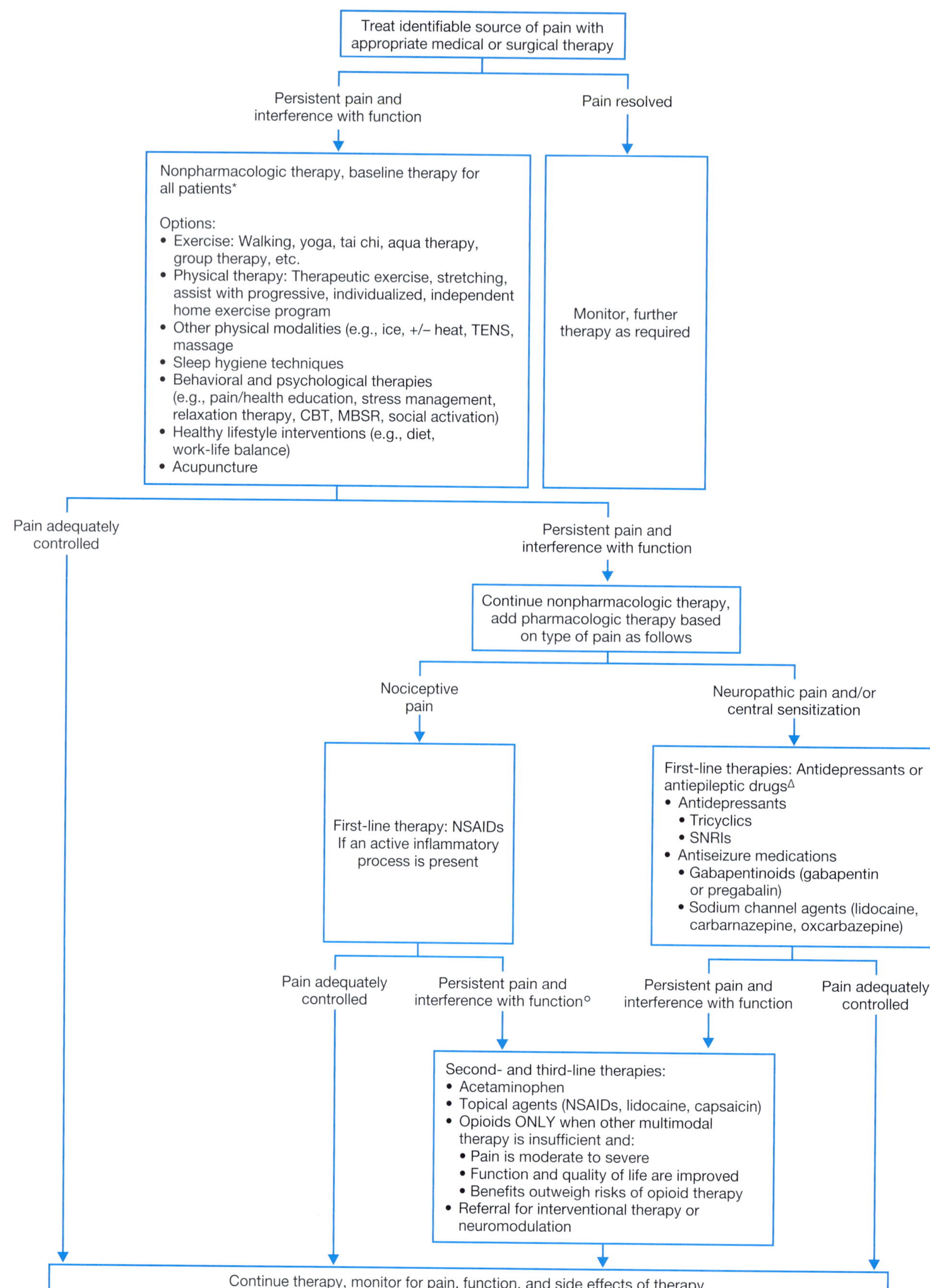

Figure 73.2: Algorithm for pain management. (From Tauben D, Stacey B. Approach to the management of chronic non-cancer pain in adults. *UpToDate*; 2023.)

- If warranted, involvement of additional healthcare professionals should be sought to help mitigate risks of opioid use (44,45).
- Risks including the development of dependence and overdose should be discussed and informed consent obtained.
- Initial prescriptions should not exceed 5 days and need for extension beyond 10 days is rare (3).
- Understanding that opioid use in the treatment of painful musculoskeletal injury for greater than 7 days has been associated with increased odds of disability at 1 year (46).
- For extended opioid use, a plan for limiting risk and discontinuing use should be in place (3).
- Understanding that opioids are on the World Anti-Doping Agency (WADA) prohibited list for in-competition.

- General guidelines for prescribing opioids can be reviewed in Table 73.1.
- Injections including corticosteroids, platelet-rich plasma (PRP), or viscosupplementation have been used for persisting pain depending on the etiology and do not have a role in same day RTS.
  - Corticosteroid injections may be delivered to intra-articular, peritendinous, and epidural structures. Injected steroids reduce inflammation, swelling, and pain through several mechanisms, including suppressing the inflammatory cascade that may impede tissue healing (3,40). A 24-48-hour period of relative rest is often recommended after undergoing a steroid injection. Careful coordination should also be taken with regard to the timing of the injection as corticosteroids are a banned in-competition substance per the WADA. Corticosteroids should not be delivered intratendinously due to the risk of tendon rupture (40).
  - PRP is another injectate that is used for persisting pain. PRP has been used to treat a variety of musculoskeletal conditions, including muscle injury, tendinopathy, and intra-articular pathology. The literature is mixed regarding its effectiveness, and there is a need for more high-quality randomized controlled trials (47–50). Its use should be considered on an individual basis depending on the structural etiology of pain.
  - Viscosupplementation is best studied in the treatment of knee osteoarthritis, but evidence for its use is also mixed (51,52).
- Medications, Injectables, and Orthobiologics are further discussed in Chapters 76 through 79, respectively).

SUBACUTE AND CHRONIC PHARMACOLOGICAL PAIN MANAGEMENT

- The need for pain management in the athlete beyond 6 weeks should prompt reevaluation of the diagnosis and other individual influences on pain and disability. A shift in the treatment approach from relieving pain to improving the function of the athlete is often appropriate as pain transitions from subacute to chronic (3). Nonpharmacological options should be continued as part of a multidisciplinary approach regardless of the use of medications.
- Medications in the treatment of subacute and chronic pain may vary. The continuation of NSAIDs beyond the acute phase has little benefit and is not generally recommended (41).
- Adjuvant medications can be considered depending on the type of pain and are best managed by an experienced clinician (53). Anticonvulsants such as Gabapentin and pregabalin are options, particularly for neuropathic pain management (3).
- Medications in the antidepressant class are also effective adjuvants in the treatment of pain. Serotonin-noradrenaline reuptake inhibitors (*e.g.*, duloxetine, venlafaxine) or tricyclic antidepressants (*e.g.*, amitriptyline or nortriptyline) may be considered.

Table 73.1 Guideline for Prescribing Opioids for Pain Not Related to Sickle Cell, Cancer, Palliative Care, or End-of-Life Care

Opioid Prescribing Guidelines			
Determining Initiation of Opioids	**Selecting Opioid and Dosage**	**Duration of Initial Prescription and Follow-Up**	**Assessing Risk and Addressing Potential Harm of Opioid Use**
• Nonopioid therapies are at least as effective as opioids for **acute** pain. • Non-opioid therapies are preferred for **subacute and chronic** pain • Maximize nonpharmacologic, nonopioid therapies first • Consider for acute pain if benefits outweigh risks • Establish treatment goals for pain and function	• Prescribe immediate release instead of extended-release opioids • Initiate the lowest effective dose • Avoid increasing dosage above levels likely to yield diminishing returns in benefits relative to risks	• Prescribe no greater quantity than needed for the expected duration of pain severe enough to require opioids • Reevaluate within 1–4 wk of starting opioid therapy or escalating dosage and then at regular intervals.	• Evaluate risk for harm before initiation and periodically during treatment • Incorporate strategies to mitigate risk, including offering naloxone • Review patient's prescriptions to help mitigate the risk of overdose • Consider toxicology testing • Use caution when prescribing with CNS depressants • Arrange treatment with evidence-based medications for opioid use disorder

Adapted from the 2022 CDC Guidelines.

PSYCHOLOGY OF PAIN

- When approaching the management of pain in the athlete, it is critical to understand the individual experience. The sensation of pain is modulated by the individual's emotional and cognitive state, which may be influenced by neurobiological, environmental, and cognitive factors (10).
- Pain in the athlete is often associated with uncertainty regarding performance or return to play, which may result in emotional distress (1). The involvement of a licensed mental health provider, such as a sports psychologist, can be helpful in assisting the athlete in developing effective coping strategies. There is always a psychological response to pain, but athletes' resilience and ability to manage the situation may improve when equipped with the proper tools. Those who lack effective coping strategies may rely on self-medication, which may ultimately put them at risk for developing substance use disorder.
- Engaging a mental health provider in the care of the athlete is particularly important in cases where pain is transitioning from acute to persisting pain.
- It is key to identify individuals with coexisting or preexisting mental health disorders as the proper management of underlying conditions will aid in the success of pain management strategies. Psychological factors that may influence pain include but are not limited to individual optimism, self-efficacy, stress, depression, anxiety, coexisting disordered eating, and substance use disorder (1). It is imperative that a psychological history is obtained and a detailed understanding of the athlete's social situation achieved when developing a plan for pain management.

SPECIAL CONSIDERATIONS

Paralympic Athletes

- There is a high incidence of injury and pain within the para-athlete population (54–56). The type of disability and its duration seem to be the major determinants of the prevalence and location of musculoskeletal pain in athletes with disabilities (57).
- Pain and injury in the para-athlete may have severer consequences due to the potentially greater impact on activities of daily living in addition to athletic performance (58).
- There are unique etiologies of pain to consider when treating para-athletes with certain impairments. Patients with amputation may experience pain from the residual limb as well as phantom limb pain. Those with central nervous system disorders, such as stroke, spinal cord injury, and multiple sclerosis, commonly suffer from central neuropathic pain. Spasticity may also be a source of pain in this population and in athletes with cerebral palsy.
- It is not surprising that the use of medications for the management of pain, particularly chronic neuropathic pain, is higher in para-athletes compared to their counterparts without disability (59). Understanding the para-athlete's impairment and disability is key in managing their pain to improve performance and quality of life.

Pediatric Athletes

- The youth and adolescent athlete may have different influences on their experience of pain due to the psychologic and physiologic changes that occur during this time (1). It is important for the practitioner to recognize these factors when assessing and treating the pediatric athlete.
- Awareness of laws regarding privacy and consent in youth and adolescent athletes is especially important (1).
- Caution should be taken in the use and dosing of medications in the pediatric population.

SUMMARY

- Pain is a common complaint in the athlete, and although it may be associated with injury, it is not the same as injury.
- It is important to distinguish the different types of pain to better understand the pathophysiology that led to its occurrence when developing an appropriate treatment plan for the athlete.
- The experience of pain differs among individuals and should consider the athlete's emotional and cognitive state.
- Nonpharmacological treatment should be considered the firstline management of pain with the use of medications only if needed.
- Medications should not be prescribed for the prevention of pain or injury.
- Pain is often best treated with a multidisciplinary approach with the goal of improving function, particularly in the case of subacute and chronic pain.

REFERENCES

1. Herring SA, Kibler WB, Putukian M, et al. Select issues in pain management for the youth and adolescent athlete. *Med Sci Sports Exerc.* 2020;52(9):2037–46.
2. Loeser JD, Treede RD. The Kyoto protocol of IASP basic pain terminology. *Pain.* 2008;137(3):473–7.
3. Hainline B, Derman W, Vernec A, et al. International Olympic Committee consensus statement on pain management in elite athletes [published correction appears in *Br J Sports Med.* 2018 Jan 3]. *Br J Sports Med.* 2017;51(17):1245–58.
4. AlMakadma Y, Eirale C, Chamari K. Neuropathic pain in athletes: basics of diagnosis and monitoring of a hidden threat. *Biol Sport.* 2022;39(4):943–9.
5. Kosek E, Cohen M, Baron R, et al. Do we need a third mechanistic descriptor for chronic pain states? *Pain.* 2016;157(7):1382–6.

6. Hainline B, Turner J, Caneiro J, Stewart M, Lorimer Moseley G. Pain in elite athletes-neurophysiological, biomechanical and psychosocial considerations: a narrative review. *Br J Sports Med*. 2017;51(17):1259–64.
7. Engebretsen L, Soligard T, Steffen K, et al. Sports injuries and illnesses during the London summer Olympic Games 2012. *Br J Sports Med*. 2013;47(7):407–14.
8. Yang J, Tibbetts AS, Covassin T, Cheng G, Nayar S, Heiden E. Epidemiology of overuse and acute injuries among competitive collegiate athletes. *J Athl Train*. 2012;47(2):198–204.
9. DiFiori JP, Benjamin HJ, Brenner J, et al. Overuse injuries and burnout in youth sports: a position statement from the American Medical Society for Sports Medicine. *Clin J Sport Med*. 2014;24(1):3–20.
10. Moseley GL, Vlaeyen JW. Beyond nociception: the imprecision hypothesis of chronic pain. *Pain*. 2015;156(1):35–8.
11. Short S, Tuttle M, Youngman D. A clinically-reasoned approach to manual therapy in sports physical therapy. *Int J Sports Phys Ther*. 2023;18(1):262–71. Published 2023 Feb 1.
12. Brummitt J. The role of massage in sports performance and rehabilitation: current evidence and future direction. *N Am J Sports Phys Ther*. 2008;3(1):7–21.
13. Poppendieck WWM, Ferrauti A, Kellmann M, Pfeiffer M, Meyer T. Massage and performance recovery and injury prevention. *Sports Med*. 2016;46:183–204.
14. Mauntel TC, Clark MA, Padua DA. Effectiveness of myofascial release therapies on physical performance measurements: a systematic review. *Athl Train Sports Health Care*. 2014;6:189–96.
15. Dommerholt J, Bron C, Franssen J. Myofascial trigger Points: an evidence-informed review. *J Man Manip Ther*. 2006;14:203–21.
16. Cox J, Varatharajan S, Côté P, Optima Collaboration. Effectiveness of acupuncture therapies to manage musculoskeletal disorders of the extremities: a systematic review. *J Orthop Sports Phys Ther*. 2016;46(6):409–29.
17. Rio E, Kidgell D, Moseley GL, et al. Tendon neuroplastic training: changing the way we think about tendon rehabilitation—a narrative review. *Br J Sports Med*. 2016;50(4):209–15.
18. Rio E, Moseley L, Purdam C, et al. The pain of tendinopathy: physiological or pathophysiological? *Sports Med*. 2014;44(1):9–23.
19. Rio E, van Ark M, Docking S, et al. Isometric contractions Are more analgesic than isotonic contractions for patellar tendon pain: an in-season randomized clinical trial. *Clin J Sport Med*. 2017;27(3):253–9.
20. Boecker H, Sprenger T, Spilker ME, et al. The runner's high: opioidergic mechanisms in the human brain. *Cereb Cortex*. 2008;18(11):2523–31.
21. Fuss J, Steinle J, Bindila L, et al. A runner's high depends on cannabinoid receptors in mice. *Proc Natl Acad Sci U S A*. 2015;112(42):13105–8.
22. Pagano RL, Fonoff ET, Dale CS, Ballester G, Teixeira MJ, Britto LRG. Motor cortex stimulation inhibits thalamic sensory neurons and enhances activity of PAG neurons: possible pathways for antinociception. *Pain*. 2012;153(12):2359–69.
23. França NRM, Toniolo EF, Franciosi AC, et al. Antinociception induced by motor cortex stimulation: somatotopy of behavioral response and profile of neuronal activation. *Behav Brain Res*. 2013;250:211–21.
24. Kelly GA, Blake C, Power CK, O'keeffe D, Fullen BM. The association between chronic low back pain and sleep: a systematic review. *Clin J Pain*. 2011;27(2):169–81.
25. Tuomilehto H, Vuorinen VP, Penttilä E, et al. Sleep of professional athletes:Underexploited potential to improve health and performance. *J Sports Sci*. 2017;35(7):704–10.
26. Lee YC, Chibnik LB, Lu B, et al. The relationship between disease activity, sleep, psychiatric distress and pain sensitivity in rheumatoid arthritis: a cross-sectional study. *Arthritis Res Ther*. 2009;11(5):R160.
27. Magni G, Caldieron C, Rigatti-Luchini S, Merskey H. Chronic musculoskeletal pain and depressive symptoms in the general population. An analysis of the 1st National Health and Nutrition Examination Survey data. *Pain*. 1990;43(3):299–307.
28. Geusens P, Wouters C, Nijs J, Jiang Y, Dequeker J. Long-term effect of omega-3 fatty acid supplementation in active rheumatoid arthritis. A 12-month, double-blind, controlled study. *Arthritis Rheum*. 1994;37(6):824–9.
29. Gaikwad M, Vanlint S, Mittinity M, Moseley GL, Stocks N. Does vitamin D supplementation alleviate chronic nonspecific musculoskeletal pain? A systematic review and meta-analysis. *Clin Rheumatol*. 2017;36(5):1201–8.
30. Straube S, Derry S, Straube C, Moore RA. Vitamin D for the treatment of chronic painful conditions in adults. *Cochrane Database Syst Rev*. 2015;2015:CD007771.
31. Goldberg RJ, Katz J. A meta-analysis of the analgesic effects of omega-3 polyunsaturated fatty acid supplementation for inflammatory joint pain. *Pain*. 2007;129(1–2):210–23.
32. Mauro GL, Martorana U, Cataldo P, Brancato G, Letizia G. Vitamin B12 in low back pain: a randomised, double-blind, placebo-controlled study. *Eur Rev Med Pharmacol Sci*. 2000;4(3):53–8.
33. Brill S, Sedgwick PM, Hamann W, Di Vadi PP. Efficacy of intravenous magnesium in neuropathic pain. *Br J Anaesth*. 2002;89(5):711–714.
34. Terry R, Posadzki P, Watson LK, Ernst E. The use of ginger (Zingiber officinale) for the treatment of pain: a systematic review of clinical trials. *Pain Med*. 2011;12:1808–18.
35. Agarwal KA, Tripathi CD, Agarwal BB, Saluja S. Efficacy of turmeric (curcumin) in pain and postoperative fatigue after laparoscopic cholecystectomy: a double-blind, randomized placebo-controlled study. *Surg Endosc*. 2011;25(12):3805–10.
36. Henrotin Y, Priem F, Mobasheri A. Curcumin: a new paradigm and therapeutic opportunity for the treatment of osteoarthritis — curcumin for osteoarthritis management. *SpringerPlus*. 2013;2(1):56.
37. De C Williams A, Eccleston C, Morley S. Psychological therapies for the management of chronic pain (excluding headache) in adults. *Cochrane Libr*. 2012;11(11):CD007407.
38. Hainline B. *Back Pain Understood*. Lenoia, NJ: Medicus Press; 2007.
39. Orchard JW. Is it safe to use local anaesthetic painkilling injections in professional football? *Sports Med*. 2004;34(4):209–19.
40. Loveless MS, Fry AL. Pharmacologic therapies in musculoskeletal conditions. *Med Clin North Am*. 2016;100(4):869–90.
41. Mehallo CJ, Drezner JA, Bytomski JR. Practical management: nonsteroidal antiinflammatory drug (NSAID) use in athletic injuries. *Clin J Sport Med*. 2006;16(2):170–4.
42. Aghili RFA, Shiri M. Clinical use of opioids. *J Pharmacoecon Pharm Manage*. 2015;1:1–5.
43. Chou R, Turner JA, Devine EB, et al. The effectiveness and risks of long-term opioid therapy for chronic pain: a systematic review for a National Institutes of Health Pathways to Prevention Workshop. *Ann Intern Med*. 2015;162(4):276–86.
44. Dowell D, Haegerich TM, Chou R. CDC guideline for prescribing opioids for chronic pain – United States, 2016. *JAMA*. 2016;315(15):1624–45.
45. Dowell D, Ragan KR, Jones CM, Baldwin GT, Chou R. CDC clinical practice guideline for prescribing opioids for pain — United States, 2022. *MMWR Recomm Rep (Morb Mortal Wkly Rep)*. 2022;71(3):1–95.
46. Franklin GM, Stover BD, Turner JA, Fulton-Kehoe D, Wickizer TM, Disability Risk Identification Study Cohort. Early opioid prescription and subsequent disability among workers with back injuries: the Disability Risk Identification Study Cohort. *Spine*. 2008;33(2):199–204.
47. Arthur Vithran DT, Xie W, Opoku M, Essien AE, He M, Li Y. The efficacy of platelet-rich plasma injection therapy in the treatment of patients with achilles tendinopathy: a systematic review and meta-analysis. *J Clin Med*. 2023;12(3):995. Published 2023 Jan 28.

48. Idres FA, Samaan M. Intra-articular platelet-rich plasma vs. corticosteroid injections efficacy in knee osteoarthritis treatment: a systematic review. *Ann Med Surg*. 2023;85(2):102–10. Published 2023 Feb 6.
49. Masiello F, Pati I, Veropalumbo E, Pupella S, Cruciani M, De Angelis V. Ultrasound-guided injection of platelet-rich plasma for tendinopathies: a systematic review and meta-analysis. *Blood Transfus*. 2023;21(2):119–36. [published online ahead of print, 2022 Oct 17]. doi:10.2450/2022.0087-22
50. O'Dowd A. Update on the use of platelet-rich plasma injections in the management of musculoskeletal injuries: a systematic review of studies from 2014 to 2021. *Orthop J Sports Med*. 2022;10(12):23259671221140888. Published 2022 Dec 9.
51. Migliore A, Gigliucci G, Alekseeva L, et al. Systematic literature review and expert opinion for the use of viscosupplementation with hyaluronic acid in different localizations of osteoarthritis. *Orthop Res Rev*. 2021;13:255–73. Published 2021 Dec 2.
52. Pereira TV, Jüni P, Saadat P, et al. Viscosupplementation for knee osteoarthritis: systematic review and meta-analysis. *BMJ*. 2022;378:e069722. Published 2022 Jul 6.
53. Flor H, Fydrich T, Turk DC. Efficacy of multidisciplinary pain treatment centers: a meta-analytic review. *Pain*. 1992;49(2):221–30.
54. Derman W, Schwellnus M, Jordaan E, et al. High incidence of injury at the Sochi 2014 Winter Paralympic Games: a prospective cohort study of 6564 athlete days. *Br J Sports Med*. 2016;50(17):1069–74.
55. Derman W, Schwellnus M, Jordaan E, et al. Illness and injury in athletes during the competition period at the London 2012 Paralympic Games: development and implementation of a web-based surveillance system (WEB-IISS) for team medical staff. *Br J Sports Med*. 2013;47(7):420–5.
56. Soligard T, Steffen K, Palmer D, et al. Sports injury and illness incidence in the Rio de Janeiro 2016 Olympic Summer Games: a prospective study of 11274 athletes from 207 countries. *Br J Sports Med*. 2017;51(17):1265–71.
57. Zwierzchowska A, Gaweł E, Rosołek B. Determinants of the prevalence and location of musculoskeletal pain in elite Para athletes. *Medicine (Baltim)*. 2022;101(42):e31268.
58. Fagher K, Lexell J. Sports-related injuries in athletes with disabilities. *Scand J Med Sci Sports*. 2014;24(5):e320–31.
59. Aavikko A, Helenius I, Vasankari T, Alaranta A. Physician-prescribed medication use by the Finnish Paralympic and Olympic athletes. *Clin J Sport Med*. 2013;23(6):478–82.

Physical Modalities in Sports Medicine

74

Joshua E. Lider, Kevin Machino, and Brian A. Davis

INTRODUCTION

- Physical modalities may help reduce pain, decrease swelling or stiffness, and modify the body's inflammatory response to promote healing, which allows the patient to perform rehabilitation exercises more effectively (1).
- These agents are used as part of a comprehensive treatment plan to aid in healing, recovery, and return to play for the athlete. They should not be used in isolation as they are meant to serve as adjuncts to standard exercise and therapy techniques.
- It is imperative for providers to understand the scientific basis of each modality and the principles of implementation for specific injuries to appropriately and effectively prescribe such modalities based on their efficacy during a particular rehabilitation phase (2).

THERAPEUTIC HEAT

- Energy transfer by physical modalities typically occurs by one of three processes: *conduction, convection,* or *conversion.*
- **Conduction:** Heat energy is transferred by contact from the object of highest energy to the object of lowest energy (*e.g.,* hot pack).
- **Convection:** The process of heat energy transfer between a solid object and a moving gas or liquid (*e.g.,* whirlpool).
- **Conversion:** The process of energy transfer that involves converting one form of energy to a different form. Use of high-frequency sound waves or electromagnetic (EM) waves to heat tissue will be discussed (*e.g.,* ultrasound).
- Heating modalities are divided into *superficial* and *deep.*

PHYSIOLOGY OF SUPERFICIAL HEAT

- Predominant mode of heating is conduction; however, some superficial applications use convection or conversion.
- Superficial heat penetration is usually less than 1 cm (3).
- Superficial heat effects include vasodilatation, pain relief, reduction of muscle tone and spasticity, increased cellular metabolic activity, decreased joint stiffness, increased soft-tissue extensibility, and promotion of hyperemia. Elevation of tissue temperature does not generally exceed 40°C and is usually short lived.
- Heat causes local superficial vasodilatation preferentially.
- Changes of 13°C–15°C in the finger joint may change joint viscosity by about 20% (4).
- There is moderate evidence that heat wrap therapy provides short-term pain reduction and disability in patients with acute and subacute low back pain. There is further pain reduction and functional improvement with the addition of exercise (5).

General Indications (3)

- Pain (6)
- Muscle spasm (6)
- Contracture
- Tension myalgia (6)
- Hematoma resolution
- Bursitis
- Tenosynovitis (6)
- Fibromyalgia
- Superficial thrombophlebitis
- Acceleration of metabolic process

General Contraindications and Precautions (3)

- Acute inflammation, trauma, or hemorrhage (7)
- Bleeding dyscrasia
- Ischemia (6)
- Sensation deficits (6)
- Atrophic skin
- Scar tissue
- Inability to communicate
- Poor thermal regulation (systemic applications)
- Malignancy (6)
- Edema

Application Methods

Hot Packs (Hydrocollator)

- Hot pack is applied to a location on the body. Heat energy is transferred by conduction, which results in warming of biologic tissue in the area of application.
- Although this section is focused on hot packs from a hydrocollator, it is important to recognize there are a variety of hot packs that can be used outside the clinical setting (*e.g.*, chemical instant hot packs, electric heating pads, etc.).
- **Application:** Silicate gel in a canvas cover
- When not in use, these packs are kept in thermostatically controlled water baths (hydrocollator) at 70°C–80°C.
- Used in terry cloth insulating covers or used with towels placed between the pack and the patient for periods of 20–30 minutes.
- **Advantages:** Low cost, easy use, long life, and patient acceptance.
- **Disadvantages:** Difficult to apply to curved surfaces, need special equipment.
- **Safety:** One should never have direct contact with the pack, as it is more likely to cause burns. Towels should be applied between the skin and hydrocollator pack.

Heat Lamps

- Heat primarily by the conversion of radiant energy to heat, *i.e.*, the direct application of photons to living tissue leading to heat production.
- **Application:** Simple to use but require some attention to avoid injuries or burns.
- In practice, therapeutic temperatures are usually obtained when the heat sources are about 50 cm from the skin.
- The intensity of heating of point heat sources, such as incandescent bulbs, drops off in accordance with the inverse squared ($1/r^2$) law; the heating effectiveness of linear sources, such as some quartz lamps, may follow a more slowly decreasing $1/r$ relationship (r = distance from light source).
- **Safety:** These agents produce erythema (known as *erythema ab igne* and *erythema calor*). Chronic use may produce a permanent brownish discoloration.

Hydrotherapy

- Heat transfer is primarily by convection.
  - Uses a fluid medium (usually water) to apply heat and cold.
  - Immersion of a large portion of the body in water at neutral temperatures between 36.5°C and 40°C for 20 minutes.
  - Water temperatures are limited to about 39°C if a significant fraction of the body is immersed.
  - Hydrotherapy medium may be stationary or in motion.

Specific Modes

- Whirlpool baths and Hubbard tanks
  - Tanks range in size and construction from small portable units to treat a portion of a limb to fixed Hubbard tanks for the entire body.
  - Hydrotherapy is expensive in terms of labor and resources.

Advantages/Specific Uses

- **Wounds and burns:** Hydrotherapy may lessen pain and speed healing of open wounds (8,9).
- Used for wounds and treatments when gentle mechanical debridement, heat, and solvent actions are desired.
- For larger wounds, a 0.9% NaCl solution improves comfort and lessens the risks of hemolysis and electrolyte imbalance.
- **Musculoskeletal/pain applications:** Hydrotherapy is often used as an adjunct to joint mobilization after cast removal or prolonged immobilization.
- Sitz baths (small warm water bath) for perineal and anal pain.
- Used to treat musculoskeletal pain, spasms, and tension myalgia.
- In clinical institutions where disinfecting procedures are followed and areas of stagnant water are avoided, infection appears to be rare.

Disadvantages

- Should not be used with edematous limbs.
- Treatment systems and infection control are time-consuming.

Contrast Baths

Application

- Contrast baths consist of two baths: a warm bath at 38°C–44°C and a cool reservoir at about 10°C–18°C.
- Treatment begins by soaking the involved limb in the warm reservoir for about 10 minutes and then progressing to about four cycles of 1- to 4-minute cold and 4- to 6-minute warm soaks (10).

Advantages/Disadvantages

- Most commonly used to produce reflex hyperemia and desensitization in patients with complex regional pain syndrome.
- Athletes may find the cold baths uncomfortable.
- May increase superficial blood flow and skin temperature; however, no effect on functional outcome (11).
- Improved blood flow helps remove metabolic waste and thus reduces pain in patients with knee osteoarthritis (12).

Spa Therapy (Balneotherapy)

- Balneotherapy is the use of baths (tubs or pools) containing thermal or mineral water from natural springs or drilled wells.
- Treatment involves immersion in thermal water with a natural temperature of at least 20°C and mineral water with a total mineral content of at least 1 g/L.
- Little research has addressed these modalities for athletes.
- A comparison of the effects of spa therapy and balneotherapy on low-back pain found favorable outcomes in reducing pain and improving function in short and long terms for both modalities; however, the quality of such studies were generally low (13).

Fluidotherapy

Application

- **Heats by convection:** Fine particles fluidized by turbulent, high-velocity hot air, frequently used in hand therapy.
- Despite widespread use, benefits of this high temperature remain poorly established (14,15).
- May be used for analgesia or desensitization.
- There is some evidence to suggest fluidotherapy can help improve pain, hand muscle strength, functional status, and quality of life in the treatment of hand osteoarthritis as well as improve complex regional pain syndrome, hand dexterity, and daily activities in patients with edema who have sustained a stroke (16–18).

Paraffin Baths

Application

- **Heats primarily by conduction:** Liquid mixture of paraffin wax and mineral oil.
- Paraffin bath therapy increases the transduction of tissue fluid, which increases lymphatic flow and local temperature, causing relaxation of muscles and expansion of blood vessels.
- The most common application is the hand. It has been widely used for the treatment of osteoarthritis, systemic sclerosis, eczema, and carpal tunnel syndrome (19).
- Helpful in the treatment of scars and hand contractures. Temperatures (52°C–54°C) are higher than those of hydrotherapy (<40°C–45°C) but are well tolerated due to the low heat capacity of the paraffin-mineral oil mixture and a lack of convection.
- Can be used in combination with exercise for patients with rheumatoid arthritis of the hands with beneficial short-term effects including improved range of motion and function and decreased swelling and pain (20).
- **Treatment:** Dipping, immersion, occasionally brushed onto the area of treatment.
- **Safety:** Burns are the main safety concern with paraffin treatment.
- **Visual inspection is important:** Paraffin baths should have a thin film of white paraffin on its surface or an edging around the reservoir.

DIATHERMY (DEEP HEATING)

- The following differences set diathermy apart from superficial heating:
  - Produces higher temperatures
  - Penetration is about 3–5 cm (3)
  - Heats tissue faster and heat dissipates more slowly
  - Predominantly uses sound waves or EM energy
- Modalities that use diathermy include ultrasound and shortwave diathermy

Deep Heating Modalities

Ultrasound

- *Ultrasound* is defined as sound waves at a frequency above the threshold of human hearing (frequencies above 20 kHz). Therapeutic ultrasound uses a range of 800–2400 kHz (21).

Heats by Conversion

- Ultrasound uses sound waves to heat tissues. A wide range of frequencies are potentially useful, but in the United States, most machines operate between 0.8 and 1 MHz.
- Uses piezoelectric transducers to convert electrical energy into sound.
- Usual doses range from 0.5 to 2.0 W/cm^2 for 5–10 minutes, with 1 or 3 MHz of continuous or pulsed ultrasound applied daily or every other day.
- At depths of 2–5 cm, a 1-MHz continuous mode is used.
- At depths less than 2.5 cm, a 3-MHz frequency is used superficially (22).

Physiology

- The most vigorous and deeply penetrating heating agent can elevate intramuscular temperatures by about 3.5°C–4.0°C (23).
- Penetration is not uniform and depends markedly on tissue properties: Ultrasound beam will selectively heat tissue with high water content (penetrates fat > muscle).
- The ability of ultrasound to heat tissue by the conversion of sound energy into heat is its best-understood capability.
- There are thermal and nonthermal actions.
- Thermal effect is strongest in the border area of heterogeneous tissue structures such as bone and muscle tissue. In practice, therapy is suitable for tissues with high collagen content such as tendons, ligaments, joint capsules as heating increases elasticity without reducing strength.
- Nonthermal effect stimulates the flow of intracellular and extracellular fluids resulting in an anti-inflammatory effect and acceleration of the repair process.
- Nonthermal processes such as *cavitation, shock waves, streaming,* and *mechanical deformation* have been identified.
- Cavitation occurs when small gaseous bubbles are formed in the presence of a high-intensity ultrasound beam and either oscillate stably or grow rapidly in size and collapse (see ECSW section for further discussion) (24).
- No irreversible harmful effects of cavitation have been demonstrated in animal tissue (25).
- Acoustic streaming is described as the movement of objects from one place to another secondary to the force of the wave, as seen with phonophoresis (26).
- Low-intensity ultrasound (15–400 mW/cm^2) may also stimulate cell proliferation, protein synthesis, and cytokine production. Although these findings are limited to the laboratory, they furnish some support for the clinical interest in low-intensity ultrasound in wound healing.

Indications (3)

- Tendonitis and bursitis (6)
- Muscle pain and overuse (6)
- Contractures
- Inflammation and trauma
- Scars and keloids
- The evidence is mixed. In most cases, ultrasound comparisons have been performed against placebo controls; therefore, the relative effectiveness of this agent over that of other conventional approaches is unknown. There is, however, promising evidence of effectiveness in lateral epicondylitis as therapeutic ultrasound have been shown to improve pain (27).

Application

- **Tendinosis:** Apply coupling gel to transducer and move in a circular motion over an injured or painful area. The goal is to warm tendons, muscle, and other tissue to improve blood flow and accelerate healing (28).
- **Fractures:** Low-intensity ultrasound (*e.g.*, 30 mW/cm^2) accelerates bone healing and is approved by the Food and Drug Administration (FDA) for the treatment of some fractures (29).
- Low-intensity pulse ultrasound (LIPUS) has been shown in vivo to enhance collagen synthesis after tendon injury during the granulation phase (2 weeks after injury) but to slow repair during the remodeling phase (4 weeks after injury) (30).
- The results for the use of therapeutic ultrasound in acute and chronic tendinopathy have been poor. Randomized control trials have consistently shown no beneficial effect compared with placebo in pain, functional disability, or range of motion. Therefore, it is difficult to make specific recommendations toward the use of ultrasound therapy in tendinopathies (31).

Precautions

- Ultrasound is typically avoided in the acute stages of an injury due to concerns that it may aggravate bleeding, tissue damage, and swelling (3).
- Due to the local increase in metabolic rate and potential for hematologic spread, ultrasound should be avoided in areas of malignancy (3).
- The subacute situation may be different, because many feel that ultrasound may speed healing and the resolution of symptoms in the later stages of injury.

Phonophoresis

- Ultrasound may be used to deliver medication into tissues. The active substance is mixed into a coupling medium, and ultrasound is used to drive the material through the skin.
- Phonophoresis with corticosteroids or NSAIDs is frequently used in sports medicine.
- Clinical studies are conflicting and current data on the effectiveness of such modalities are mixed and generally consist of small or poorly controlled studies. Therefore, phonophoresis are reasonable second-line alternatives for patients with chronic tendinopathy who have persistent pain despite appropriate rehabilitation exercises (32).
- There is some evidence to suggest that the use of phonophoresis with NSAIDs may be an effective treatment for knee osteoarthritis; however, treatment effect was similar to other topical agents (*e.g.*, Methyl salicylate) (33).
- In a comparison of phonophoresis of 0.05% fluocinonide with ultrasound alone at 1.5 W/cm^2, both treatments were found to be beneficial but were indistinguishable in their effects on superficial musculoskeletal conditions (34).
- Another study did not find lidocaine and corticosteroid phonophoresis to be more effective than the same treatment with an inert coupling agent (35,36).

Contraindications (3)

- Fluid-filled areas (*i.e.*, eye and the pregnant uterus), testicles (6)
- Growth plates, immature or inflamed joints (37–39)
- Malignancy
- Acute hemorrhages, ischemic tissue, tumors, laminectomy sites, infections, and implanted devices such as pacemakers and pumps (6)
- **Caution:** Relatively contraindicated near metal plates or cemented artificial joints because the effects of localized heating (40–42) or mechanical forces on prosthetic-cement interfaces are not well known.

Shortwave Diathermy

Heats by Conversion

- *Shortwave diathermy* (SWD) uses EM energy to interact with tissue and produce heat.
- Both thermal and nonthermal effects are possible.
- Tissue warming is produced by two processes:
  - Resistive heating — tissue resistance to the flow of ions results in tissue heating
  - Degradation of molecular oscillatory motions that EM waves induce when they interact with tissue
- SWD is the dominant EM diathermy in sports medicine, although it is relatively rarely used in comparison to other heating modalities due to cost and equipment requirements.
- Most devices operate at 27.12 MHz. The U.S. Federal Communications Commission also approves frequencies of 13.56 and 40.68 MHz for use.

Mechanism

- An SWD machine is a signal generator that uses either inductive or capacitive electrodes to deliver energy to the body.
- Inductive electrodes act as an antenna, and the body absorbs energy from an EM field produced by the shortwave machine.
- With capacitive electrodes, the portion of the body being treated is placed in series between the electrodes and serves as the dielectric (resistance) between two plates of a capacitor.

- Inductive applicators induce currents that preferentially flow in water-rich tissues such as muscles that are highly conductive.
- Capacitive applicators, however, heat poorly conductive substances, such as fat preferentially (43).
- SWD can increase subcutaneous fat temperatures by 15°C and intramuscular temperatures at depths of 4–5 cm by 4–6°C (44–46).

Technique

- Two common inductive applicators are typically used (pads or drums).
- Pad applicators are moderately flexible mats that contain a coil.
- Drum applicators are characterized by fixed coils and hinges.
- Diathermy with stretching showed improvements in the range of motion compared to stretching alone for the triceps and hamstring muscles. Parameters used were: 150 W/burst, 800 bursts/s, 400 μs burst duration, 800 μs interburst interval with durations of 15–20 minutes (10–15 minutes before stretching and 5 minutes during stretching) (47).

Indications (3)

- Heating in tissues that are either too deep or too extensive to be treated by other modalities, *e.g.*, the low back, the knee.
- Pollet et al performed a recent systemic review and meta-analysis and found SWD is indicated for a variety of acute and chronic musculoskeletal conditions, although research supporting SWD for pain reduction and improved function is poor and lacking evidence (48).

Precautions and Contraindications/Safety (3)

- Jewelry is removed.
- Treatment is performed on nonconductive tables.
- Contraindications include metal implants or electrical devices (*e.g.*, joints, pacemakers, pumps, and metallic intrauterine devices), contact lenses, and a menstruating or pregnant person.
- Treating the immature skeleton is generally not recommended and has not been well studied.

Low-Power and Pulsed EM Field

Heats by Conversion

- Nonthermal effects can be obtained and tissue heating avoided altogether by using low-power fields delivered in either continuous or pulsed modes.
- Pulsed electromagnetic field (PEMF) increases the local cellular activity, provides organization of collagen fibers, increases oxygen use in tissues, and enhances circulation by increasing vasodilation of blood vessels without increasing local temperature.
- A comparison study of the use of PEMF with other physical therapy agents for patients with a rotator cuff tendon tear found that PEMF did not provide additional benefit (49).
- Research offers little to support the specificity or certainty of benefits.

THERAPEUTIC COLD

- The cooling agents are often used for their analgesic, metabolic, and perfusion-limiting effects.
- Cooling therapies are restricted to conductive and convective means.

General Indications (3)

- Acute musculoskeletal trauma (6)
- Pain (6)
- Arthrogenic muscle inhibition
- Muscle spasm: spasticity (6)
- Reduction of metabolic activity

General Contraindication and Precautions (3)

- Ischemia (6)
- Insensitivity (50)
- Cold intolerance (6)
- Raynaud phenomenon and disease (50)
- Severe cold pressor responses (50)
- Cold allergy (6)

Physiology of Cryotherapy

- Superficial cold produces analgesia (51), reduces metabolic activity, slows and may block nerve conduction (52), decreases muscle tone and spasticity (53–55), increases gastrointestinal motility (56), inhibits the release of histamine, and slows chemical reactions (57).
- Relative hyperemia after cold application stimulates tissue repair and healing.
- Ice is the most common cryotherapy agent.
- Skin temperatures initially fall rapidly following the application of ice and then decrease more slowly toward an equilibrium value of 12°C–13°C. The target temperature reduction is 10°C–15°C (58).
- Recent systematic review showed that ice is most effective when applied in repeated applications of 10 minutes, which helps sustain lower muscle temperatures without compromising overlying skin (58).

Technique

- Primary goal of cryotherapy is to maintain a reduced intramuscular temperature for as long as possible in the immediate stages following both injury and exercise to prevent the proliferation of secondary damage (59).
- Ice packs and compression wraps are most common.
- Ice massage is a vigorous approach suitable for limited portions of the body. A piece of ice is rubbed over the painful area for 7–10 minutes.

- Iced whirlpools cool large areas vigorously.
- Vapocoolant and liquid nitrogen sprays produce large (as much as 20°C), rapid drops in skin temperature and are used at times to produce superficial analgesia as well as in *spray and stretch* treatments (60,61).
  - Spray and stretch treatment: Vapocoolant applied to a muscle, followed by a gentle stretch to improve muscle flexibility.
- Chemical ice packs are also common: A mixture of ice water and alcohol was shown to lower skin temperatures significantly more than gels packs or frozen peas (62).
- Postexercise ice water immersion is often used as a method of recovery after intense workouts. It is postulated that ice water immersion will constrict blood vessels, flush waste products and lactic acid out of the affected tissues, slow tissue metabolism, reduce swelling, and prevent further tissue damage (63). Results of several studies on the efficacy of this method in reducing muscle soreness or improving performance and recovery are mixed (63–66).
- Whole-body cryotherapy (WBC) consists of several-minute exposure to very cold air (−110°C to −140°C) in special temperature-controlled cryochambers or cryosaunas. WBC is used to relieve pain and inflammatory symptoms primarily in Europe and is becoming more popular in the United States because of its use in elite athletes. Research is limited; however, recent studies have shown that it does not cause deleterious effects in athletes (67) and provides short-term relief of pain and inflammatory symptoms in rheumatologic patients (68–70).
- Local reflex activity and motor function are impaired for up to 30 minutes after cold application (58).

Trauma Indications

- Cooling applied soon after trauma may decrease edema, lessen metabolic activity, reduce blood flow, lower compartmental pressures, diminish tissue damage, and accelerate healing (71–77).
- *Protect, Rest, Ice, Compression, and Elevation* (PRICE) are the mainstay of treatment (78).
- Opinions regarding the usefulness of cryotherapy for injuries more than 24–48 hours old are divergent.
- Cryotherapy may hasten return to play after ankle sprains (77,79,80).

Precautions and Contraindications

- When sensation is compromised, circulation is impaired, or tissues are compressed (81).
- Rare but possible problems include pressor responses aggravating cardiovascular disease, Raynaud phenomenon, cold hypersensitivity, urticaria, and cold allergy/cryoprecipitation.
- Because reflex activity and motor function are impaired for up to 30 minutes after ice application, return to play should not be immediate to prevent further injury (58).

COMPRESSION THERAPY

- Compression therapy is a widely accepted modality in the PRICE and POLICE (*Protect, Optimal Load, Ice, Compress, Elevate*) acronym for the initial care of acute musculoskeletal injuries (82).
  - Research evaluating compression therapy is lacking and is primarily supported by expert consensus (83).
  - There is evidence to support the use of compression garments as a recovery modality as they have been seen to improve pain scores, perceived soreness for athletes, and may lead to reduced overuse/overload injuries (84).
- Compression therapy for musculoskeletal injuries is typically applied through elastic compression or pneumatic compression.
  - Elastic wraps are applied distal to proximal.
- Compression pressures should be light to moderate (15–35 mm Hg).

General Indications

- Acute injury
  - Reduce edema
  - Reduce tissue damage
  - Faster recovery
- Passive post-exercise recovery
  - Acutely improving muscle pain, soreness, and muscle fatigue (85,86).
  - Research has not shown clinically meaningful improvements for extended subjective or functional benefits (85).

Specific Applications

Cryotherapy

- During acute cryotherapy, compression was found to have an additive cooling effect to the targeted tissues (87–89).

Edema Control

- External compression therapy to acutely injured areas can decrease localized edema response.
  - Compression reduces the amount of fluid leaving local blood vessels, resulting in reduced fluid accumulation at the area of trauma (82).

ELECTROTHERAPY

General Indications

- Today, high-intensity electrical stimulation is used to strengthen muscles and to move paralyzed limbs.
- Less-intense stimulation produces analgesia and delivers medications percutaneously.

- Stimulation at still lower intensities has gained FDA approval for fracture healing.
- Soft-tissue wounds, osteoporosis, and musculoskeletal pain represent additional potentially important, but still investigational, applications (90–92).

Specific Applications

Transcutaneous Electrical Nerve Stimulators

- Small, portable device that delivers electric current to superficial tissues via surface electrodes. Sensation from the current is usually not perceptible.
- It is clear that transcutaneous electrical nerve stimulators (TENS) produce localized analgesia, and research suggests that stimulation at 110 Hz (as well as H-wave therapy at 2 and 60 Hz) results in a hypoalgesia that persists for up to 5 minutes after stimulation is stopped (93).
- Dorsal horn cell activity is reduced following stimulation (94).
- High-frequency, low-intensity TENS (barely or not perceptible, 10–100+ Hz) may work more according to the gate theory than higher-intensity, low-frequency (1–4 Hz) stimulation, which may be more dependent on endorphins.
- Electrodes are usually placed over the painful region, but other locations are common.
- TENS applied close to the site of pain has been shown to reduce the pain intensity during or immediately after treatment with no reported serious adverse effects. TENS may be considered as an adjunct to core treatment to provide short-term symptomatic pain relief via neuromodulation for acute and chronic pain (95).
- Currently, there are inconsistent outcomes and data in the literature regarding the efficacy of TENS in the management of low back pain (96,97). TENS may offer short-term benefit in functional disability but has not been shown to improve symptoms of low back pain (98).
- Acupuncture such as TENS:
  - TENS technique that uses low frequency (2–4 Hz), higher intensity (patient tolerance) with longer pulse width (100/–400 μs) (99).
  - Stimulations create muscle twitches that activate smaller diameter motor afferents creating local analgesia (99).
  - Often used for pain management that has been refractory to conventional TENS (100).

Indications (3)

- Pain reduction

Precautions and Contraindications (3)

- Cardiac pacemakers and implantable cardioverter defibrillator
- Pregnancy
- Epilepsy
- Active malignancy
- Skin irritation or damaged skin

Functional Electrical Stimulation

Neuromuscular Electrical Stimulation/Muscle Stimulation

- Neuromuscular electrical stimulation (NMES) is used interchangeably with electrical stimulation (ES) and often serve a functional purpose. When ES is paired with a functional task, it is referred to as functional electrical stimulation (FES).
- There are many forms of ES that are used to augment muscle action and performance. ES can be used to improve muscle strength, range of motion, edema, atrophy, tissue damage, and pain (101).
- Electrical muscle stimulation is more effective in maintaining muscle mass after an injury than it is in reversing atrophy once it is established (102).
- Review of the literature shows that use of NMES after anterior cruciate ligament reconstruction is associated with increased quadriceps strength compared with exercise alone (103); however, the effect on functional outcome is inconsistent (104).
- The use of NMES after total knee arthroplasty has been shown to attenuate the loss of quadriceps muscle strength and improved functional performance (105).

Galvanic Electrical Stimulation

- Form of NMES that uses interrupted direct current with frequency of 30 Hz and a pulse duration of 1 ms.
- Due to the long pulse duration, this electrical stimulation is ideal for denervated muscle.
- Stimulation results in muscle contraction that mimics voluntary muscle contraction. This results in increased blood flow (increased metabolism and waste product removal).
- Stimulation provides muscle action re-education and minimizes muscle atrophy.
- **Safety:** should not be done over areas of dermatologic conditions (psoriasis, tinea, and eczema), infection, thrombosis, sensation loss, cancer, or cardiac pacemakers.

Iontophoresis

- Iontophoresis uses electrical fields to force charged or polarized substances into tissue (106–108).
- Iontophoretic devices consist basically of a direct-current (possibly pulsed) power source and two electrodes. A dilute solution of the active substance (which must exist in an ionized or polar form) is placed under the electrode of the same polarity, and the device is turned on.
- Medication is not always required as the electric current alone may have therapeutic benefits.
- Iontophoresis with dexamethasone has been shown to be effective in the treatment of bicipital tendonitis, epicondylitis, plantar fasciitis, and tendon sheath inflammation (109–114).
- Direct comparison of iontophoresis with oral medication, transdermal patches, or alternative physical therapy approaches is rare.

- **Safety:** Allergies to the materials (pads, electrodes, and medication) used are always possible, and the passage of electric current into the skin can cause erythema, rashes, and, if the current intensity is high, pain (115).

Interferential and Kilohertz Frequency Currents

- Interferential current (IFC) therapy is a medium frequency alternating current therapy that can reach deeper tissues due to reduced skin impedance.
- Skin impedance (resistance) is inversely proportional to the frequency of an applied current and therefore as frequency increases, the skin impedance decreases.
- As a result, stimuli that are painful at the low <70-Hz frequencies of TENS and many muscle simulators are well tolerated at a few thousand hertz.
- There are at least two ways to take advantage of this fact. One of these arranges two sets of electrodes so that two sine waves in the low-kilohertz range differing by 20–100 Hz cross. The waves thus interfere with each other and produce beneath the skin barrier a *difference* frequency comparable to that of TENS units and muscle stimulators.
- IFC has been shown to have significant analgesic effects in patients with neck pain, low back pain, knee osteoarthritis, and post-operative knee pain (116).
- **Safety:** There is no conclusive and consistent evidence that EM field exposure causes a significant increase in the risk of cancer or neurobehavioral or reproductive dysfunction (117,118).

Russian Electrical Stimulation

- A form of Kilohertz frequency currents that uses alternating currents with medium frequency, typically at 2.5 kHz, with a burst duty cycle less than 50% (119).
- Three major physical parameters:
  - Carrier frequency: number of pulses per second
  - Burst duration
  - Burst duty cycle: ratio between the burst duration and the sum of burst and interburst times.
- Russian scientist Kots created the stimulation regimen: "10/50/10" regimen, 10 second contraction with 2.5 kHz followed by 50 second rest with 50 Hz for 10 repetitions, applied once daily over a period of weeks with reported strength gains (120).
  - Reported strength gains are scrutinized (supporting literature by Knots cannot be accessed and other studies have not been able to recreate strength gains).

COMPLEMENTARY AND ALTERNATIVE THERAPIES

- Athletes and the general population are intrigued by the potential use of complementary and alternative medicine.

Low-Intensity Laser Therapy

- Low level laser therapy (LLLT) is also known as photobiomodulation therapy and is an athermic photochemical modality. Red or near-infrared light is used to stimulate tissue healing and reduce pain and inflammation.
- LLLT is widely used to treat musculoskeletal injuries, speed healing, and lessen pain.
- Lasers have been shown to decrease pain and inflammation in tendinopathies, Achilles tendonitis, and plantar fasciitis (121–123) as well as improve pain and function in osteoarthritis (124).

Static Magnetic Fields (Magnetic Devices)

- Magnetic discs, pads, bandages, and blankets are promoted in sports, veterinary, and general circulation magazines as a cure for a variety of musculoskeletal injuries.
- Various magnetic products have been studied with field strengths generally in the 300–3950 Gs range (125,126).
- Results are generally mixed. In one study, efficacy was demonstrated in patients with painful diabetic neuropathy (127). Another study comparing magnet pad versus control groups suffering from fibromyalgia showed statistical significance for pain relief, but no clear functional improvement in the magnet user group (125). There is also some evidence to suggest that pulsed EM field therapy may provide short-term relief of pain and improvement in function in patients with osteoarthritis (128).
- Many animal studies have shown significant cellular physiologic changes with static magnetic fields, but functional and long-term consequences remain unknown.
- Observed physiologic effects have included increased nerve excitability (129) and circulatory stimulation (130).

Acupuncture

- Treatment consists of using acupuncture needles to pierce the skin to differing depths at designated acupuncture points to bring about pain relief or physiologic change.
- Needles are commonly stimulated by hand, electricity, or heat.
- There are mixed outcomes regarding the efficacy of acupuncture. Some studies have shown that acupuncture provides immediate relief of pain for carpal tunnel syndrome and as an adjunct treatment for low back pain, whereas other studies show inconclusive evidence of the use of acupuncture in shoulder and elbow pathologies (131).
  - Acupuncture has shown mildly greater improvement in the management of carpal tunnel syndrome when compared to oral anti-inflammatory medications (132).
- Research is scarce regarding treatment of athletic injuries; in 1997, the National Institutes of Health sponsored a consensus panel that concluded: "promising results have emerged, for example, showing efficacy of acupuncture in adult

postoperative and chemotherapy associated nausea and vomiting and in postoperative dental pain. There are other situations such as addiction, stroke rehabilitation, headache, menstrual cramps, tennis elbow, fibromyalgia, myofascial pain, osteoarthritis, low back pain, carpal tunnel syndrome, and asthma, in which acupuncture may be useful" (133).

- Dry needling in elite volleyball players during competition provided short-term pain relief and improved function in shoulder injuries (134).
- Acupuncture, in combination with traditional Chinese medicine including massage and herbs, was effective in reducing pain, decreasing edema, and restoring ankle function in acute ankle ligamentous sprains in sports (135).
- Studies have shown increased muscle strength and power, improved performance, and improved hemodynamic parameters in endurance activities after acupuncture. There is also associated decrease in acute muscle soreness with acupuncture (136).
- Single acupuncture treatment improved isometric quadriceps strength in recreational athletes (137).
- Male basketball players treated with acupuncture had decreased maximum heart rate, O_2 max, and blood lactate levels after 30 minutes of exercise compared to controls (138).

BLOOD FLOW RESTRICTION

- Mechanotransduction remains the primary factor for muscle strength and hypertrophy (139,140).
- When compared to type I fibers, type II fibers are more responsive to hypertrophy adaptations and should be preferentially activated (141). Therefore, loading needs to be a significant percentage of the individual's 1-repetition maximum (>65%) (142).
- Blood flow restriction (BFR) is a training augmentation first described in the literature in 1987 (143).
- Strength and hypertrophy gains are obtained through low-weight exercises performed under partial arterial and venous occlusion via external compression applied to the extremity (*i.e.*, inflatable tourniquet).
- Tourniquet pressures should create venous pooling without arterial occlusion. Due to variable cuff and limb sizes, pressures should be adjusted individually to obtain this goal, most accurately via ultrasound. Literature has also suggested arbitrary tourniquet pressures (*e.g.*, 200 mm Hg) or tourniquet pressures based on the brachial systolic blood pressure (bSBP) (*e.g.*, 130% of bSBP), but these have resulted in arterial occlusion (144).
- Similar strength and hypertrophy gains can be obtained with BFR with loads of only 20%–30% of 1-repetition maximum (145). Therefore, strength gains can be obtained in tissues that have reduced loading tolerance.
- In healthy subjects, training benefits (muscular strength, endurance, and hypertrophy) have been observed at the level of the tourniquet (146–149). Research is conflicted for more diffuse benefits (distal, proximal, and contralateral to the tourniquet) (145,150,151).

Physiology

- The mechanism of action for BFR training has not been proven.
- It is theorized that the reduction of blood flow induces a hypoxic environment that enhances the training effect in the exercising muscle (152–155), resulting in the following:
  - Increased plasma growth hormone levels (156)
  - Increased intramuscular stress secondary to the hypoxic environment, resulting in muscle adaptation (157)
  - Increased type II fiber recruitment (157)
  - Greater buildup of anabolic metabolites
  - Increased cellular swelling

General Indications

- BFR training has not been fully evaluated and warrants further research to identify its use in the appropriate populations and determine the most effective treatment protocols.
  - Variable factors to consider include (158,159):
    - Cuff size, pressure, placement, type (static vs dynamic cuff)
    - Duration of occlusion time
    - Load (as % of repetition maximum)
    - Repetition and sets per exercise
    - Frequency of training, rest period
- Consider BFR training to supplement high-load training in elite athletes (160).
- Consider BFR in individuals who cannot tolerate higher load training:
  - Acute and subacute period in postoperative rehabilitation (161–164)
  - Symptomatic osteoarthritis (165)
  - Prevention of sarcopenia in elderly populations (166,167)

General Contraindications and Cautions

- BFR training has been found to be safe, with a similar risk profile to traditional exercise (168).
- There is a need to establish safe and effective protocols.
- Caution in cardiovascular disease (increased heart rate, increased blood pressure, decreased stroke volume) (159).
- Contraindications (159):
  - Bleeding dyscrasias: increased thrombosis risk, easy bruising
  - Hypertension
  - Peripheral vascular disease: poor circulation, varicose veins
  - Inadequate lymphatic system

  - Diabetes
  - Active infection
  - Malignancy
  - Renal compromise
  - Pregnancy

Side Effects (159)

- Common: pain or discomfort during exercise, delayed-onset muscle soreness, and cardiac stress
- Rare: numbness or nerve injury, bruising or ischemic injury, dizziness or fainting, thrombus formation, muscle damage, and rhabdomyolysis.

EXTRACORPOREAL SHOCKWAVE

- Shockwave therapy was originally applied clinically as lithotripsy to treat calcific deposits in the body (*i.e.*, renal calculi). Since the 1990s, shockwave therapy applications have expanded to treat a variety of musculoskeletal conditions.
- Shockwaves are generated from a sudden release of energy within an applicator, which travels through a fluid medium and is transmitted to biologic tissues through coupling gel.

Physiology of Extracorporeal Shockwave

- Shockwaves are a series of single-impulse acoustic waves with certain physical characteristics (169,170):
  - Fast initial rise in pressure (<10 ns)
  - High peak pressure (approximately 50–80 MPa)
  - Low tensile amplitude (up to 10 MPa)
    - Diffraction-induced negative pressure wave that follows the high peak pressure
  - Short cycle life (approximately 10 μs)
  - Broad frequency spectrum (16 Hz–20 MHz)
- Shockwaves emit mechanical forces on targeted tissues through (169):
  - Direct generation of mechanical forces:
    - Low energy release of pressure waves into tissues of similar acoustic impedance to water (fat, muscle, fluid).
    - High energy release of pressure waves into tissues of different acoustic impedance to water (air, bone, lung tissue).
  - Indirect generation of mechanical forces by cavitation bubbles.
- Cavitation bubbles (171)
  - Cavitation bubbles occur from the tensile wave created by the reflected pressure wave off tissues. The tensile wave exceeds the dynamic tensile strength of water, resulting in bubble formation.
  - The bubble diameters oscillate (increasing and decreasing in volume) nonlinearly because the variation in bubble size is not correlated with pressure amplitude.
  - There is a large amount of energy delivered to the bubble as it grows, which is subsequently released in the form of high-energy water jets and high temperature when the bubble collapses.
  - Boundaries of different media (*e.g.*, muscle and calcium deposit) are where the shockwave emits the highest energy and therefore the largest biological effect.

Extracorporeal Shockwave Parameters

- Maximum positive pressure (170)
  - Low energy/impulse: no effect on tissues
  - Midrange energy/impulse: therapeutic effect on tissues
  - High energy/impulse: destructive effect on tissues
- Focal zone
  - Focused shockwaves
    - Generated pressure field converges in an adjustable focus for a selected depth resulting in maximum pressure being reached (170).
    - Shockwaves are generated in water and housed in the applicator through (169,170):
      - Electrohydraulic generator:
        - Found in first generation of orthopedic shockwave machines
        - Spark produced from a charge capacitor vaporizes the surrounding water resulting in a sonic pulse.
        - Shockwave characterized by a fairly large axial diameter of the focal volume and high total energy within that volume.
      - EM generator:
        - Electric current is passed through a coil to produce a strong and variable magnetic field.
        - The strong magnetic field acts on the opposing metal membrane that results in compression of the surrounding fluid medium to produce a shockwave.
        - An acoustic lens is used to focus the shockwaves.
      - Piezoelectric generator:
        - A large number of piezocrystals are mounted in the applicator and receive a rapid electrical discharge resulting in deformation of the crystals that induces a pressure pulse in the surrounding water.
        - The geometric arrangement of the crystals inside the sphere allows for self-focusing of the wave toward the center.
        - Shockwave characterized by a very precise focusing and high energy density within a well-confined focal volume.

  - Radial shockwaves
    - Shockwaves are generated by accelerating a projectile and using compressed air, through a tube on the end of which an applicator is placed. The projectile hits the applicator and the applicator then transmits the generated pressure wave into the body.
    - The divergence of pressure fields from the applicator results in the maximal pressure at the source rather than a selected tissue depth (170).
    - These technically cannot be called shockwaves as they do not have the characteristic shockwave features.
- Energy density: Energy per square area at the focal point (joules per area)
  - Exact cutoffs vary, but general ranges are (172):
    - Low energy shockwaves: <0.08–0.10 mJ/mm^2
      - Beneficial for tendinopathies and spasticity
    - Medium energy shockwaves: 0.08–0.28 mJ/mm^2
      - Beneficial for tendinopathies and spasticity
    - High-energy shockwaves: >0.29 and 0.60 mJ/mm^2
      - Beneficial for calcific tendinopathies and bone disorders
      - For therapy tolerance, may need anesthetic (local or regional)
  - Energy density distinguishing these groupings is not universally accepted, but density above 0.50 mJ/mm^2 should be avoided (173).
- Time: duration of treatment, interval between treatments
- Number of impulses per treatment (accounting for volume of treatment)
- Impulse frequency or number of shockwaves applied per second
  - High frequencies may block the propagation of subsequent waves and reduce the maximum generated pressure (174).
- Localization method (palpation vs. image guidance)
- Anesthesia
  - Use of anesthetics to help with tolerance of therapy
- Concurrent treatments (rest vs. therapeutic exercise)

Proposed Effects of Extracorporeal Shockwave

- Anti-inflammatory
  - Maintaining nitric oxide levels at a physiologic level (175)
  - Decrease in inflammatory cytokines (176)
- Mechanical
  - Pressure waves disrupting calcium deposits and intertissue adhesions.
- Analgesic
  - Hyperstimulation analgesia (177)
- Tissue regeneration (178)
  - Increased tenocyte proliferation
  - Increased release of growth factors (176)
  - Increased collagen synthesis (primarily type 1)
  - Neovascularization (179)

General Indications for Extracorporeal Shockwave

- Overall, evidence supporting extracorporeal shockwave (ECSW) for therapeutic intervention for a variety of musculoskeletal conditions is low to moderate. Likely contributing to this is the paucity of accepted treatment guidelines (174,180,181).
- ECSW therapy has been beneficial in pain and function in:
  - Lower extremity tendinopathies (Achilles, patellar, proximal hamstring, and greater trochanteric pain syndrome) (182,183) and plantar fasciitis (179,184).
    - Achilles tendinopathy responds best with eccentric exercises in combination with extracorporeal shock wave (185)
  - Osteoarthritis (186)
  - Chronic low back pain (187)
  - Calcific tendinopathy of the rotator cuff (180,188)
    - Targeted at the area of calcific deposition
  - Noncalcific tendinopathy of the rotator cuff (180)
    - Targeted at the point of maximum tenderness
  - Lateral and medial epicondylitis (180,189)
  - Adjunct therapy for adhesive capsulitis (190)
  - Adjunct therapy for myofascial pain syndrome (191).
  - Bone healing: bone marrow edema (192), nonunion and delayed healing (193)

General Contraindications and Cautions

- There is not a consensus for general contraindications for ECSW, but most studies exclude individuals with:
  - Malignancy
  - Infection
  - Metal implants
  - Bleeding dyscrasias (including anticoagulation)
  - Cardiac arrhythmias
  - Inflammatory joint disorders
  - Skin wounds over the treatment area
  - Neurologic disorders to the treatment area
  - Pregnancy
  - Skeletal immaturity

SUMMARY

- Physical modalities are a part of a comprehensive treatment plan for healing, recovery, and return to play for the athlete.
- To appropriately and effectively prescribe modalities, the clinician should understand the scientific basis of each

modality and the principles of implementation for specific injuries (i.e., maximize benefit while minimizing risk).

- The clinician should also consider the individual factors that may affect modality application (access, contraindications, compliance, response, etc.).
- Although modalities can augment recovery, they should not be used in isolation, but viewed as adjuncts to facilitate the athlete's ability to participate with standard exercise and therapy techniques.

REFERENCES

1. Statuta S, Pugh K. Training room procedures and use of therapeutic modalities in athletes. *Clin Sports Med.* 2019;38(4):619–38. doi:10.1016/j.csm.2019.06.006
2. Logan C, Asnis P, Provencher M. The role of therapeutic modalities in surgical and nonsurgical management of orthopaedic injuries. *J Am Acad Orthop Surg.* 2017;25(8):556–68. doi:10.5435/JAAOS-D-15-00348
3. Chen W, Annaswammy T, Yang W, et al. Physical agent modalities. In: Cifu DX. editors. *Braddom's Physical Medicine & Rehabilitation.* 5th ed. Elsevier; 2016.
4. Wright V, Johns RJ. Quantitative and qualitative analysis of joint stiffness in normal subjects and in patients with connective tissue diseases. *Ann Rheum Dis.* 1961;20(1):36–46. doi:10.1136/ard.20.1.36
5. Qaseem A, Wilt TJ, McLean RM, , et al. Noninvasive treatments for acute, subacute, and chronic low back pain: a clinical practice guideline from the American College of Physicians. *Ann Intern Med.* 2017;166(7):514–30. doi:10.7326/M16-2367
6. Nadler SF. , Weingand K, Kruse RJ. The physiologic basis and clinical applications of cryotherapyand thermotherapy for the pain practitioner. *Pain Physician.* 2004;3;7(7;3):395–9. doi:10.36076/ppj.2004/7/395
7. Harris ED, McCroskery PA. The influence of temperature and fibril stability on degradation of cartilage collagen by rheumatoid synovial collagenase. *N Engl J Med.* 1974;290(1):1–6. doi:10.1056/NEJM197401032900101
8. Tao H, Butler JP, Luttrell T. The role of whirlpool in wound care. *J Am Coll Clin Wound Spec.* 2012;4(1):7–12. doi:10.1016/j.jccw.2013.01.002
9. Juvè Meeker B. Whirlpool therapy on postoperative pain and surgical wound healing: an exploration. *Patient Educ Couns.* 1998;33(1):39–48. doi:10.1016/S0738-3991(97)00056-6
10. Woodmansey A, Collins DH, Ernst MM. Vascular reactions to the contrast bath in health and in rheumatoid arthritis. *Lancet.* 1938;232(6015):1350–4. doi:10.1016/S0140-6736(00)83051-2
11. Breger Stanton DE, Lazaro R, MacDermid JC. A systematic review of the effectiveness of Contrast baths. *J Hand Ther.* 2009;22(1):57–70. doi:10.1016/j.jht.2008.08.001
12. Fokmare PS, Phansopkar P. A review on osteoarthritis knee management via Contrast bath therapy and physical therapy. *Cureus.* 2022 Jul 27;14(7):e27381. Published online doi:10.7759/cureus.27381
13. Karagülle M, Karagülle MZ. Effectiveness of balneotherapy and spa therapy for the treatment of chronic low back pain: a review on latest evidence. *Clin Rheumatol.* 2015;34(2):207–14. doi:10.1007/s10067-014-2845-2
14. Alcorn R, Bowser B, Henley E, Holloway V. Fluidotherapy and exercise in the management of sickle cell anemia. A clinical report. *Phys Ther.* 1984;64(10):1520–2. doi:10.1093/ptj/64.10.1520
15. Borrell R, Parker R, Henley E, Masley D, Repinecz M. Comparison of in vivo temperatures produced by hydrotherapy, paraffin wax treatment, and fluidotherapy. *Phys Ther.* 1980;60(10):1273–6. doi:10.1093/ptj/60.10.1273
16. Öncel A, Küçükşen S, Ecesoy H, Sodali E, Yalçin Ş. Comparison of efficacy of fluidotherapy and paraffin bath in hand osteoarthritis: a randomized controlled trial. *Arch Rheumatol.* 2021;36(2):201–9. doi:10.46497/ArchRheumatol.2021.8123
17. Sezgin Ozcan D, Tatli HU, Polat CS, Oken O, Koseoglu BF. The effectiveness of fluidotherapy in poststroke complex regional pain syndrome: a randomized controlled study. *J Stroke Cerebrovasc Dis.* 2019;28(6):1578–85. doi:10.1016/j.jstrokecerebrovasdis.2019.03.002
18. Han SW, Lee MS. The effect of fluidotherapy on hand dexterity and activities of daily living in patients with edema on stroke. *J Phys Ther Sci.* 2017;29(12):2180–3. doi:10.1589/jpts.29.2180
19. Kim SG, Kang JW, Boo JH, et al. Effectiveness of paraffin bath therapy for the symptoms and function of hand diseases: a systematic review and meta-analysis of randomized controlled trials. *J Hand Ther.* March 2023;36(3):706–12. Published online doi:10.1016/j.jht.2022.10.005
20. Robinson V, Brosseau L, Casimiro L, Cochrane Musculoskeletal Group, et al. Thermotherapy for treating rheumatoid arthritis. *Cochrane Database Syst Rev.* 2002 Apr 22; 2002(2):CD002826. Published online doi:10.1002/14651858.CD002826
21. Laskowska J, Hadław-Klimaszewska O, Jankowska A, Zdziechowski A, Woldańska-Okońska M. Overview of wellness methods for people practicing sports. *Wiad Lek.* 2021;74(2):355–61. doi:10.36740/WLek202102133
22. Tsai WC, Tang ST, Liang FC. Effect of therapeutic ultrasound on tendons. *Am J Phys Med Rehabil.* 2011;90(12):1068–73. doi:10.1097/PHM.0b013e31821a70be
23. Draper D, Harris ST, Schulthies S, Durrant E, Knight KL, Ricard M. Hot-pack and 1-MHz ultrasound treatments have an additive effect on muscle temperature increase. *J Athl Train.* 1998;33(1):21–4.
24. Flint EB, Suslick KS. The temperature of cavitation. *Science.* 1991;253(5026):1397–9. doi:10.1126/science.253.5026.1397
25. Frizzell L, Dunn F. Biophysics of ultrasound. In: *Therapeutic Heat and Cold.* 4th ed. Williams & Wilkins; 1990. pp. 404–5.
26. Johns LD. Nonthermal effects of therapeutic ultrasound: the frequency resonance hypothesis. *J Athl Train.* 2002;37(3):293–9.
27. Luo D, Liu B, Gao L, Fu S. The effect of ultrasound therapy on lateral epicondylitis: a meta-analysis. *Medicine (Baltim).* 2022;101(8):e28822. doi:10.1097/MD.0000000000028822
28. Miller DL, Smith NB, Bailey MR, et al. Overview of therapeutic ultrasound applications and safety considerations. *J Ultrasound Med.* 2012;31(4):623–34. doi:10.7863/jum.2012.31.4.623
29. Hadjiargyrou M, McLeod K, Ryaby JP, Rubin C. Enhancement of fracture healing by low intensity ultrasound. *Clin Orthop.* 1998;355S(355 suppl):S216–29. doi:10.1097/00003086-199810001-00022
30. Fu SC, Hung LK, Shum WT, et al. In vivo Low-Intensity Pulsed Ultrasound (LIPUS) following tendon injury promotes repair during granulation but suppresses decorin and Biglycan expression during remodeling. *J Orthop Sports Phys Ther.* 2010;40(7):422–9. doi:10.2519/jospt.2010.3254
31. Smallcomb M, Khandare S, Vidt ME, Simon JC. Therapeutic ultrasound and shockwave therapy for tendinopathy: a narrative review. *Am J Phys Med Rehabil.* 2022;101(8):801–7. doi:10.1097/PHM.0000000000001894
32. Childress MA, Beutler A. Management of chronic tendon injuries. *Am Fam Physician.* 2013;87(7):486–90.
33. Martin-Vega FJ, Lucena-Anton D, Galán-Mercant A, et al. Phonophoresis through nonsteroidal anti-inflammatory drugs for knee osteoarthritis treatment: systematic review and meta-analysis. *Biomedicines.* 2022;10(12):3254. doi:10.3390/biomedicines10123254

34. Klaiman MD, Shrader JA, Danoff JV, Hicks JE, Pesce WJ, Ferland J. Phonophoresis versus ultrasound in the treatment of common musculoskeletal conditions. *Med Sci Sports Exerc.* 1998;30(9):1349–55. doi:10.1097/00005768-199809000-00002
35. Antich TJ. Phonophoresis: the principles of the ultrasonic driving force and efficacy in treatment of common orthopaedic diagnoses. *J Orthop Sports Phys Ther.* 1982;4(2):99–102. doi:10.2519/jospt.1982.4.2.99
36. Haney JS. A new look at old principles of ultrasound application. *Phys Therapy Scholarly Projects.* 1993;189.
37. Dussik KT, Fritch DJ, Kyriazidou M, Sear RS. Measurements of articular tissues with ultrasound. *Am J Phys Med.* 1958;37(3):160–5.
38. Weinberger A, Fadilah R, Lev A, Levi A, Pinkhas J. Deep heat in the treatment of inflammatory joint disease. *Med Hypotheses.* 1988;25(4):231–3. doi:10.1016/0306-9877(88)90036-9
39. Weinberger A, Fadilah R, Lev A, Shohami E, Pinkhas J. Treatment of articular effusions with local deep microwave hyperthermia. *Clin Rheumatol.* 1989;8(4):461–6. doi:10.1007/BF02032097
40. Brunner GD, Lehmann JF, McMillan JA, Lane KE, Bell JW. Can ultrasound be used in the presence of surgical metal implants: an experimental approach. *Phys Ther Rev.* 1958;38(12):823–4. doi:10.1093/ptj/38.12.823
41. Gersten JW. Effect of metallic objects on temperature rises produced in tissue by ultrasound. *Am J Phys Med.* 1958;37(2):75–82.
42. Skoubo-Kristensen E, Sommer J. Ultrasound influence on internal fixation with a rigid plate in dogs. *Arch Phys Med Rehabil.* 1982;63(8):371–73.
43. Kantor G. Evaluation and survey of microwave and radiofrequency applicators. *J Microw Power.* 1981;16(2):135–50. doi:10.1080/16070658.1981.11689232
44. Draper DO, Knight K, Fujiwara T, Castel JC. Temperature change in human muscle during and after pulsed short-wave diathermy. *J Orthop Sports Phys Ther.* 1999;29(1):13–22. doi:10.2519/jospt.1999.29.1.13
45. Lehmann JF, de Lateur B. Diathermy and superficial heat and cold therapy. In: *Krusen's Handbook of Physical Medicine and Rehabilitation.* 3rd ed. Saunders; 1982. p. 275.
46. Lehmann JF, DeLateur BJ, Stonebridge JB. Selective muscle heating by shortwave diathermy with a helical coil. *Arch Phys Med Rehabil.* 1969;50(3):117–23.
47. Nakano J, Yamabayashi C, Scott A, Reid WD. The effect of heat applied with stretch to increase range of motion: a systematic review. *Phys Ther Sport.* 2012;13(3):180–8. doi:10.1016/j.ptsp.2011.11.003
48. Pollet J, Ranica G, Pedersini P, Lazzarini SG, Pancera S, Buraschi R. The efficacy of electromagnetic diathermy for the treatment of musculoskeletal disorders: a systematic review with meta-analysis. *J Clin Med.* 2023;12(12):3956. doi:10.3390/jcm12123956
49. Özdemir M, Yaşar MF, Yakşi E. Effect of pulsed electromagnetic field therapy in patients with supraspinatus tendon tear. *Rev Assoc Med Bras.* 2021;67(2):282–6. doi:10.1590/1806-9282.67.02.20200730
50. Paine R. Rehabilitation and therapeutic modalities. Language of exercise and rehabilitation. In: *DeLee and Drez's Orthopaedic Sports Medicine Principles and Practice.* 3rd ed. Elsevier; 2010. pp. 221–331.
51. Malanga GA, Yan N, Stark J. Mechanisms and efficacy of heat and cold therapies for musculoskeletal injury. *Postgrad Med J.* 2015;127(1):57–65. doi:10.1080/00325481.2015.992719
52. Denys EH. AAEM minimonograph #14: the influence of temperature in clinical neurophysiology. *Muscle Nerve.* 1991;14(9):795–811. doi:10.1002/mus.880140902
53. Knight K. *Cryotherapy: Theory, Technique and Physiology.* 1st ed. Chattanooga; 1985.
54. Knutsson E, Mattsson E. Effects of local cooling on monosynaptic reflexes in man. *Scand J Rehabil Med.* 1969;1(3):126–32.
55. Miglietta O. Action of cold on spasticity. *Am J Phys Med.* 1973;52(4):198–205.
56. Bisgard J, Nye D. The influence of hot and cold application upon gastric and intestinal motor activity. *Surg Gynecol Obstet.* 1940;71:172–80.
57. Kunkle BF, Kothandaraman V, Goodloe JB, et al. Orthopaedic application of cryotherapy: a comprehensive review of the history, basic science, methods, and clinical effectiveness. *JBJS Rev.* 2021;9(1):e20.00016. doi:10.2106/JBJS.RVW.20.00016
58. MacAuley DC. Ice therapy: how good is the evidence? *Int J Sports Med.* 2001;22(5):379–84. doi:10.1055/s-2001-15656
59. Kwiecien SY, McHugh MP. The cold truth: the role of cryotherapy in the treatment of injury and recovery from exercise. *Eur J Appl Physiol.* 2021;121(8):2125–42. doi:10.1007/s00421-021-04683-8
60. Oosterveld FGJ, Rasker JJ. Effects of local heat and cold treatment on surface and articular temperature of arthritic knees. *Arthritis Rheum.* 1994;37(11):1578–82. doi:10.1002/art.1780371104
61. Travell J. Ethyl chloride spray for painful muscle spasm. *Arch Phys Med Rehabil.* 1952;33(5):291–8.
62. Kanlayanaphotporn R, Janwantanakul P. Comparison of skin surface temperature during the application of various cryotherapy modalities. *Arch Phys Med Rehabil.* 2005;86(7):1411–15. doi:10.1016/j.apmr.2004.11.034
63. Lateef F. Post exercise ice water immersion: is it a form of active recovery? *J Emerg Trauma Shock.* 2010;3(3):302. doi:10.4103/0974-2700.66570
64. Ingram J, Dawson B, Goodman C, Wallman K, Beilby J. Effect of water immersion methods on post-exercise recovery from simulated team sport exercise. *J Sci Med Sport.* 2009;12(3):417–21. doi:10.1016/j.jsams.2007.12.011
65. Sellwood KL, Brukner P, Williams D, Nicol A, Hinman R. Ice-water immersion and delayed-onset muscle soreness: a randomised controlled trial. *Br J Sports Med.* 2007;41(6):392–7. doi:10.1136/bjsm.2006.033985
66. Wilcock IM, Cronin JB, Hing WA. Physiological response to water immersion: a method for sport recovery? *Sports Med.* 2006;36(9):747–65. doi:10.2165/00007256-200636090-00003
67. Banfi G, Lombardi G, Colombini A, Melegati G. Whole-body cryotherapy in athletes. *Sports Med.* 2010;40(6):509–17. doi:10.2165/11531940-000000000-00000
68. Hirvonen HE, Mikkelsson MK, Kautiainen H, Pohjolainen TH, Leirisalo-Repo M. Effectiveness of different cryotherapy on pain and disease activity in active rheumatoid arthritis. A randomised single blinded controlled trial. *Clin Experim Rheumatol.* 2006;24:295–301.
69. Metzger D, Zwingmann C, Protz W, Jäckel WH. Whole-body cryotherapy in rehabilitation of patients with rheumatoid diseases—pilot study. *Rehabilitation (Stuttg).* 2000;39(2):93–100. doi:10.1055/s-2000-14442
70. Guillot X, Tordi N, Mourot L, et al. Cryotherapy in inflammatory rheumatic diseases: a systematic review. *Expet Rev Clin Immunol.* 2014;10(2):281–94. doi:10.1586/1744666X.2014.870036
71. Basur RL, Shephard E, Mouzas GL. A cooling method in the treatment of ankle sprains. *Practitioner.* 1976;216(1296):708–11.
72. Bert JM, Stark JG, Maschka K, Chock C. The effect of cold therapy on morbidity subsequent to arthroscopic lateral retinacular release. *Orthop Rev.* 1991;20(9):755–8.
73. Hirasé Y. Postoperative cooling enhances composite graft survival in nasal-alar and fingertip reconstruction. *Br J Plast Surg.* 1993;46(8):707–11. doi:10.1016/0007-1226(93)90204-O
74. Ho SSW, Illgen RL, Meyer RW, Torok PJ, Cooper MD, Reider B. Comparison of various icing times in decreasing bone metabolism and blood flow in the knee. *Am J Sports Med.* 1995;23(1):74–6. doi:10.1177/036354659502300112
75. Moore CD, Cardea JA. Vascular changes in leg trauma. *South Med J.* 1977;70(11):1285–6. doi:10.1097/00007611-197711000-00011
76. Schaubel HJ. The local use of ice after orthopedic procedures. *Am J Surg.* 1946;72(5):711–4. doi:10.1016/0002-9610(46)90347-9

77. Sloan JP, Hain R, Pownall R. Clinical benefits of early cold therapy in accident and emergency following ankle sprain. *Emerg Med J.* 1989;6(1):1–6. doi:10.1136/emj.6.1.1
78. Busby C. The PRICE of injury treatment: out with the old and in with the new. *ACSM's Health & Fit J.* 2023;27(1):5–7.
79. Hubbard TJ, Aronson SL, Denegar CR. Does cryotherapy hasten return to participation? A systematic review. *J Athletic Training.* 2004;39(1):88–94.
80. Hocutt JE, Jaffe R, Rylander CR, Beebe JK. Cryotherapy in ankle sprains. *Am J Sports Med.* 1982;10(5):316–9. doi:10.1177/036354658201000512
81. Barlas D, Homan CS, Thode HC. In vivo tissue temperature comparison of cryotherapy with and without external compression. *Ann Emerg Med.* 1996;28(4):436–9. doi:10.1016/s0196-0644(96)70011-2
82. Kellett J. Acute soft tissue injuries--a review of the literature. *Med Sci Sports Exerc.* 1986;18(5):489–500.
83. Bleakley CM. Acute soft tissue injury management: past, present and future. *Phys Ther Sport.* 2013;14(2):73–4. doi:10.1016/j.ptsp.2013.01.002
84. Cullen MFL, Casazza GA, Davis BA. Passive recovery strategies after exercise: a narrative literature review of the current evidence. *Curr Sports Med Rep.* 2021;20(7):351–8. doi:10.1249/JSR.0000000000000859
85. Hoffman MD, Badowski N, Chin J, Stuempfle KJ. A randomized controlled trial of massage and pneumatic compression for ultramarathon recovery. *J Orthop Sports Phys Ther.* 2016;46(5):320–6. doi:10.2519/jospt.2016.6455
86. Heapy AM, Hoffman MD, Verhagen HH, et al. A randomized controlled trial of manual therapy and pneumatic compression for recovery from prolonged running—an extended study. *Res Sports Med.* 2018;26(3):354–64. doi:10.1080/15438627.2018.1447469
87. Gillette CM, Merrick MA. The effect of elevation on intramuscular tissue temperatures. *J Sport Rehabil.* 2018;27(6):526–9. doi:10.1123/jsr.2016-0239
88. Merrick MA, Knight KL, Ingersoll CD, Potteiger JA. The effects of ice and compression wraps on intramuscular temperatures at various depths. *J Athletic Training.* 1993;28(3):236–45.
89. Tomchuk D, Rubley MD, Holcomb WR, Guadagnoli M, Tarno JM. The magnitude of tissue cooling during cryotherapy with varied types of compression. *J Athl Train.* 2010;45(3):230–7. doi:10.4085/1062-6050-45.3.230
90. Banon JJ, Jacobson WE, Tidd G. Treatment of decubitus ulcers. A new approach. *Minn Med.* 1985;68(2):103–6.
91. Wood J, Evans PE III, Schallreuter KU, et al. A multicenter study on the use of pulsed low-intensity direct current for healing chronic stage II and stage III decubitus ulcers. *Arch Dermatol.* 1993;129(8):999–1009.
92. Tiktinsky R, Chen L, Narayan P. Electrotherapy: yesterday, today and tomorrow. *Haemophilia.* 2010;16(suppl 5):126–31. doi:10.1111/j.1365-2516.2010.02310.x
93. McDowell BC, McCormack K, Walsh DM, Baxter DG, Allen JM. Comparative analgesic effects of H-wave therapy and transcutaneous electrical nerve stimulation on pain threshold in humans. *Arch Phys Med Rehabil.* 1999;80(9):1001–4. doi:10.1016/S0003-9993(99)90051-5
94. Garrison DW, Foreman RD. Effects of transcutaneous electrical nerve stimulation (TENS) on spontaneous and noxiously evoked dorsal horn cell activity in cats with transected spinal cords. *Neurosci Lett.* 1996;216(2):125–8. doi:10.1016/0304-3940(96)13023-8
95. Johnson MI, Paley CA, Jones G, Mulvey MR, Wittkopf PG. Efficacy and safety of transcutaneous electrical nerve stimulation (TENS) for acute and chronic pain in adults: a systematic review and meta-analysis of 381 studies (the meta-TENS study). *BMJ Open.* 2022;12(2):e051073. doi:10.1136/bmjopen-2021-051073
96. Leemans L, Elma Ö, Nijs J, et al. Transcutaneous electrical nerve stimulation and heat to reduce pain in a chronic low back pain population: a randomized controlled clinical trial. *Braz J Phys Ther.* 2021;25(1):86–96. doi:10.1016/j.bjpt.2020.04.001
97. Gibson W, Wand BM, Meads C, Catley MJ, O'Connell NE. Transcutaneous electrical nerve stimulation (TENS) for chronic pain - an overview of Cochrane Reviews. *Cochrane Database Syst Rev.* 2019;4(4). Published online April 3. doi:10.1002/14651858.CD011890.pub3
98. Wu LC, Weng PW, Chen CH, Huang YY, Tsuang YH, Chiang CJ. Literature review and meta-analysis of transcutaneous electrical nerve stimulation in treating chronic back pain. *Reg Anesth Pain Med.* 2018;43(4):425–33. doi:10.1097/AAP.0000000000000740
99. Johnson M. Transcutaneous electrical nerve stimulation: mechanisms, clinical application and evidence. *Rev Pain.* 2007;1(1):7–11. doi:10.1177/204946370700100103
100. Dommerholt J, Grieve R, Finnegan M, Hooks T. A critical overview of the current myofascial pain literature – july 2016. *J Bodyw Mov Ther.* 2016;20(3):657–71. doi:10.1016/j.jbmt.2016.07.009
101. Doucet BM, Lam A, Griffin L. Neuromuscular electrical stimulation for skeletal muscle function. *Yale J Biol Med.* 2012;85(2):201–15.
102. Baldi JC, Jackson RD, Moraille R, Mysiw WJ. Muscle atrophy is prevented in patients with acute spinal cord injury using functional electrical stimulation. *Spinal Cord.* 1998;36(7):463–9. doi:10.1038/sj.sc.3100679
103. Toth MJ, Tourville TW, Voigt TB, et al. Utility of neuromuscular electrical stimulation to preserve quadriceps muscle fiber size and contractility after anterior cruciate ligament injuries and reconstruction: a randomized, Sham-controlled, blinded trial. *Am J Sports Med.* 2020;48(10):2429–37. doi:10.1177/0363546520933622
104. Kim KM, Croy T, Hertel J, Saliba S. Effects of neuromuscular electrical stimulation after anterior cruciate ligament reconstruction on quadriceps strength, function, and patient-oriented outcomes: a systematic review. *J Orthop Sports Phys Ther.* 2010;40(7):383–91. doi:10.2519/jospt.2010.3184
105. Stevens-Lapsley JE, Balter JE, Wolfe P, Eckhoff DG, Kohrt WM. Early neuromuscular electrical stimulation to improve quadriceps muscle strength after total knee arthroplasty: a randomized controlled trial. *Phys Ther.* 2012;92(2):210–26. doi:10.2522/ptj.20110124
106. Chantraine A, Ludy JP, Berger D. Is cortisone iontophoresis possible? *Arch Phys Med Rehabil.* 1986;67(1):38–40.
107. Hill AC, Baker GF, Jansen GT. Mechanism of action of iontophoresis in the treatment of palmar hyperhidrosis. *Cutis.* 1981;28(1):69–72.
108. O'malley EP, Oester YT. Influence of some physical chemical factors on iontophoresis using radio-isotopes. *Arch Phys Med Rehabil.* 1955;36(5):310–6.
109. Demirtaş RN, Oner C. The treatment of lateral epicondylitis by iontophoresis of sodium salicylate and sodium diclofenac. *Clin Rehabil.* 1998;12(1):23–9. doi:10.1191/026921598672378032
110. Gudeman SD, Eisele SA, Heidt RS, Colosimo AJ, Stroupe AL. Treatment of plantar fasciitis by lontophoresis of 0.4% dexamethasone: a randomized, double-blind, placebo-controlled study. *Am J Sports Med.* 1997;25(3):312–6. doi:10.1177/036354659702500307
111. Hendricks H, Verbeek A, van de Putte L, Vermeulen R. Effect of dexamethasone-iontophoresis on patients with muscle tendinopathy. *Dutch J Phys Ther.* 1992;102:198–207.
112. Nirschl RP, Rodin DM, Ochiai DH, Maartmann-Moe C, DEX-AHE-01-99 Study Group. Iontophoretic administration of dexamethasone sodium phosphate for acute epicondylitis: a randomized, double-blinded, placebo-controlled study. *Am J Sports Med.* 2003;31(2):189–95. doi:10.1177/03635465030310020601
113. da Luz DC, De Borba Y, Ravanello EM, Daitx RB, Döhnert MB. Iontophoresis in lateral epicondylitis: a randomized, double-blind

clinical trial. *J Shoulder Elb Res.* 2019;28(9):1743–9. doi:10.1016/j.jse.2019.05.020
114. Taskaynatan MA, Ozgul A, Ozdemir A, Tan AK, Kalyon TA. Effects of steroid iontophoresis and electrotherapy on bicipital tendonitis. *J Musculoskelet Pain.* 2007;15(4):47–54. doi:10.1300/J094v15n04_06
115. Berliner MN. Reduced skin hyperemia during tap water iontophoresis after intake of acetylsalicylic acid. *Am J Phys Med Rehabil.* 1997;76(6):482–7. doi:10.1097/00002060-199711000-00010
116. Rampazo ÉP, Liebano RE. Analgesic effects of interferential current therapy: a narrative review. *Medicina (Mex).* 2022;58(1):141. doi:10.3390/medicina58010141
117. Kaiser J. NIH panel revives EMF-cancer link. *Science.* 1998;281(5373):21–2. doi:10.1126/science.281.5373.21b
118. Kaiser J. Panel finds EMFs pose no threat. *Science.* 1996;274(5289):910. doi:10.1126/science.274.5289.910
119. Modesto KAG, Bastos JAI, Vaz MA, Durigan JLQ. Effects of kilohertz frequency, burst duty cycle, and burst duration on evoked torque, perceived discomfort and muscle fatigue: a systematic review. *Am J Phys Med Rehabil.* 2023;102(2):175–83. doi:10.1097/PHM.0000000000001982
120. Kramer JF, Mendryk SW. Electrical stimulation as a strength improvement technique: a review. *J Orthop Sports Phys Ther.* 1982;4(2):91–8. doi:10.2519/jospt.1982.4.2.91
121. Bjordal JM, Lopes-Martins RAB, Iversen VV. A randomised, placebo controlled trial of low level laser therapy for activated Achilles tendinitis with microdialysis measurement of peritendinous prostaglandin E2 concentrations. *Br J Sports Med.* 2006;40(1):76–80. doi:10.1136/bjsm.2005.020842
122. Tumilty S, Munn J, McDonough S, Hurley DA, Basford JR, Baxter GD. Low level laser treatment of tendinopathy: a systematic review with meta-analysis. *Photomed Laser Surg.* 2010;28(1):3–16. doi:10.1089/pho.2008.2470
123. Naterstad IF, Joensen J, Bjordal JM, Couppé C, Lopes-Martins RAB, Stausholm MB. Efficacy of low-level laser therapy in patients with lower extremity tendinopathy or plantar fasciitis: systematic review and meta-analysis of randomised controlled trials. *BMJ Open.* 2022;12(9):e059479. doi:10.1136/bmjopen-2021-059479
124. Ahmad MA, A Hamid MS, Yusof A. Effects of low-level and high-intensity laser therapy as adjunctive to rehabilitation exercise on pain, stiffness and function in knee osteoarthritis: a systematic review and meta-analysis. *Physiotherapy.* 2022;114:85–95. doi:10.1016/j.physio.2021.03.011
125. Alfano AP, Taylor AG, Foresman PA, et al. Static magnetic fields for treatment of fibromyalgia: a randomized controlled trial. *J Altern Complement Med.* 2001;7(1):53–64. doi:10.1089/107555301300004538
126. Vallbona C, Hazlewood CF, Jurida G. Response of pain to static magnetic fields in postpolio patients: a double-blind pilot study. *Arch Phys Med Rehabil.* 1997;78(11):1200–3. doi:10.1016/S0003-9993(97)90332-4
127. Weintraub MI, Wolfe GI, Barohn RA, et al. Static magnetic field therapy for symptomatic diabetic neuropathy: a randomized, double-blind, placebo-controlled trial. *Arch Phys Med Rehabil.* 2003;84(5):736–46. doi:10.1016/S0003-9993(03)00106-0
128. Markovic L, Wagner B, Crevenna R. Effects of pulsed electromagnetic field therapy on outcomes associated with osteoarthritis: a systematic review of systematic reviews. *Wien Klin Wochenschr.* 2022;134(11-12):425–33. doi:10.1007/s00508-022-02020-3
129. Hong CZ. Static magnetic field influence on human nerve function. *Arch Phys Med Rehabil.* 1987;68(3):162–4.
130. Ohkubo C, Xu S. Acute effects of static magnetic fields on cutaneous microcirculation in rabbits. *In Vivo (Athens).* 1997;11(3):221–5.
131. Trofa DP, Obana KK, Herndon CL, et al. The evidence for common nonsurgical modalities in sports medicine, Part 1: Kinesio tape, sports massage therapy, and acupuncture. *JAAOS Glob Res Rev.* 2020;4(1):e1900104. doi:10.5435/JAAOSGlobal-D-19-00104
132. Bahrami-Taghanaki H, Azizi H, Hasanabadi H, et al. Acupuncture for carpal tunnel syndrome: a randomized controlled trial studying changes in clinical symptoms and electrodiagnostic tests. *Alternat Therap.* 2020;26(2):10–6.
133. Acupuncture. *NIH Consens Statement.* 1997;15(5):1–34.
134. Osborne NJ, Gatt IT. Management of shoulder injuries using dry needling in elite volleyball players. *Acupunct Med.* 2010;28(1):42–5. doi:10.1136/aim.2009.001560
135. Fong DT, Chan YY, Mok KM, Yung PS, Chan KM. Understanding acute ankle ligamentous sprain injury in sports. *BMC Sports Sci Med Rehabil.* 2009;1(1):14. doi:10.1186/1758-2555-1-14
136. Ahmedov S. Ergogenic effect of acupuncture in sport and exercise: a brief review. *J Strength Cond Res.* 2010;24(5):1421–7. doi:10.1519/JSC.0b013e3181d156b1
137. Hübscher M, Vogt L, Ziebart T, Banzer W. Immediate effects of acupuncture on strength performance: a randomized, controlled crossover trial. *Eur J Appl Physiol.* 2010;110(2):353–8. doi:10.1007/s00421-010-1510-y
138. Lin ZP, Lan LW, He TY, et al. Effects of acupuncture stimulation on recovery ability of male elite basketball athletes. *Am J Chin Med.* 2009;37(3):471–81. doi:10.1142/S0192415X09006989
139. Schoenfeld BJ. Potential mechanisms for a role of metabolic stress in hypertrophic adaptations to resistance training. *Sports Med.* 2013;43(3):179–94. doi:10.1007/s40279-013-0017-1
140. Khan KM, Scott A. Mechanotherapy: how physical therapists' prescription of exercise promotes tissue repair. *Br J Sports Med.* 2009;43(4):247–52. doi:10.1136/bjsm.2008.054239
141. McCall GE, Byrnes WC, Dickinson A, Pattany PM, Fleck SJ. Muscle fiber hypertrophy, hyperplasia, and capillary density in college men after resistance training. *J Appl Physiol.* 1996;81(5):2004–12. doi:10.1152/jappl.1996.81.5.2004
142. American College of Sports Medicine. American College of Sports Medicine position stand. Progression models in resistance training for healthy adults. *Med Sci Sports Exerc.* 2009;41(3):687–708. doi:10.1249/MSS.0b013e3181915670
143. Eiken O, Bjurstedt H. Dynamic exercise in man as influenced by experimental restriction of blood flow in the working muscles. *Acta Physiol Scand.* 1987;131(3):339–45. doi:10.1111/j.1748-1716.1987.tb08248.x
144. Loenneke JP, Fahs CA, Rossow LM, et al. Blood flow restriction pressure recommendations: a tale of two cuffs. *Front Physiol.* 2013;4:249. doi:10.3389/fphys.2013.00249
145. Bowman EN, Elshaar R, Milligan H, et al. Upper-extremity blood flow restriction: the proximal, distal, and contralateral effects—a randomized controlled trial. *J Shoulder Elb Res.* 2020;29(6):1267–74. doi:10.1016/j.jse.2020.02.003
146. Kang DY, Kim HS, Lee KS, Kim YM. The effects of bodyweight-based exercise with blood flow restriction on isokinetic knee muscular function and thigh circumference in college students. *J Phys Ther Sci.* 2015;27(9):2709–12. doi:10.1589/jpts.27.2709
147. Loenneke JP, Wilson JM, Marín PJ, Zourdos MC, Bemben MG. Low intensity blood flow restriction training: a meta-analysis. *Eur J Appl Physiol.* 2012;112(5):1849–59. doi:10.1007/s00421-011-2167-x
148. Slysz J, Stultz J, Burr JF. The efficacy of blood flow restricted exercise: a systematic review & meta-analysis. *J Sci Med Sport.* 2016;19(8):669–75. doi:10.1016/j.jsams.2015.09.005
149. Sousa J, Neto G, Santos H, Araújo J, Silva H, Cirilo-Sousa M. Effects of strength training with blood flow restriction on torque, muscle activation and local muscular endurance in healthy subjects. *Biol Sport.* 2017;34:83–90. doi:10.5114/biolsport.2017.63738

150. Yasuda T, Ogasawara R, Sakamaki M, Bemben MG, Abe T. Relationship between limb and trunk muscle hypertrophy following high-intensity resistance training and blood flow-restricted low-intensity resistance training. *Clin Physiol Funct Imaging*. 2011;31(5):347–51. doi:10.1111/j.1475-097X.2011.01022.x
151. Bowman EN, Elshaar R, Milligan H, et al. Proximal, distal, and contralateral effects of blood flow restriction training on the lower extremities: a randomized controlled trial. *Sports Health*. 2019;11(2):149–56. doi:10.1177/1941738118821929
152. Takarada Y, Takazawa H, Sato Y, Takebayashi S, Tanaka Y, Ishii N. Effects of resistance exercise combined with moderate vascular occlusion on muscular function in humans. *J Appl Physiol*. 2000;88(6):2097–106. doi:10.1152/jappl.2000.88.6.2097
153. Hoppeler H, Vogt M. Muscle tissue adaptations to hypoxia. *J Exp Biol*. 2001;204(Pt 18):3133–9. doi:10.1242/jeb.204.18.3133
154. Pope ZK, Willardson JM, Schoenfeld BJ. Exercise and blood flow restriction. *J Strength Cond Res*. 2013;27(10):2914–26. doi:10.1519/JSC.0b013e3182874721
155. Scott BR, Loenneke JP, Slattery KM, Dascombe BJ. Exercise with blood flow restriction: an updated evidence-based approach for enhanced muscular development. *Sports Med*. 2015;45(3):313–25. doi:10.1007/s40279-014-0288-1
156. Takarada Y, Tsuruta T, Ishii N. Cooperative effects of exercise and occlusive stimuli on muscular function in low-intensity resistance exercise with moderate vascular occlusion. *Jpn J Physiol*. 2004;54(6):585–92. doi:10.2170/jjphysiol.54.585
157. Takada S, Okita K, Suga T, et al. Low-intensity exercise can increase muscle mass and strength proportionally to enhanced metabolic stress under ischemic conditions. *J Appl Physiol*. 2012;113(2):199–205. doi:10.1152/japplphysiol.00149.2012
158. Wortman RJ, Brown SM, Savage-Elliott I, Finley ZJ, Mulcahey MK. Blood flow restriction training for athletes: a systematic review. *Am J Sports Med*. 2021;49(7):1938–44. doi:10.1177/0363546520964454
159. Lorenz DS, Bailey L, Wilk KE, et al. Blood flow restriction training. *J Athl Train*. 2021;56(9):937–44. doi:10.4085/418-20
160. Luebbers PE, Fry AC, Kriley LM, Butler MS. The effects of a 7-week practical blood flow restriction program on well-trained collegiate athletes. *J Strength Cond Res*. 2014;28(8):2270–80. doi:10.1519/JSC.0000000000000385
161. Wengle L, Migliorini F, Leroux T, Chahal J, Theodoropoulos J, Betsch M. The effects of blood flow restriction in patients undergoing knee surgery: a systematic review and meta-analysis. *Am J Sports Med*. 2022;50(10):2824–33. doi:10.1177/03635465211027296
162. Hughes L, Paton B, Rosenblatt B, Gissane C, Patterson SD. Blood flow restriction training in clinical musculoskeletal rehabilitation: a systematic review and meta-analysis. *Br J Sports Med*. 2017;51(13):1003–11. doi:10.1136/bjsports-2016-097071
163. Ohta H, Kurosawa H, Ikeda H, Iwase Y, Satou N, Nakamura S. Low-load resistance muscular training with moderate restriction of blood flow after anterior cruciate ligament reconstruction. *Acta Orthop Scand*. 2003;74(1):62–8. doi:10.1080/00016470310013680
164. Tennent DJ, Hylden CM, Johnson AE, Burns TC, Wilken JM, Owens JG. Blood flow restriction training after knee arthroscopy: a randomized controlled pilot study. *Clin J Sport Med*. 2017;27(3):245–52.
165. Segal NA, Williams GN, Davis MC, Wallace RB, Mikesky AE. Efficacy of blood flow-restricted, low-load resistance training in women with risk factors for symptomatic knee osteoarthritis. *Pharm Manag PM R*. 2015;7(4):376–84. doi:10.1016/j.pmrj.2014.09.014
166. Abe T, Sakamaki M, Fujita S, et al. Effects of low-intensity walk training with restricted leg blood flow on muscle strength and aerobic capacity in older adults. *Res Rep*. 2010;33(1):34–40.
167. Breen L, Phillips SM. Skeletal muscle protein metabolism in the elderly: interventions to counteract the "anabolic resistance" of ageing. *Nutr Metab*. 2011;8(1):68. doi:10.1186/1743-7075-8-68
168. Loenneke JP, Wilson JM, Wilson GJ, Pujol TJ, Bemben MG. Potential safety issues with blood flow restriction training: safety of blood flow-restricted exercise. *Scand J Med Sci Sports*. 2011;21(4):510–8. doi:10.1111/j.1600-0838.2010.01290.x
169. Ogden JA, Tóth-Kischkat A, Schultheiss R. Principles of shock wave therapy. *Clin Orthop*. 2001;387.
170. McClure S, Dorfmüller C. Extracorporeal shock wave therapy: theory and equipment. *Clin Tech Equine Pract*. 2003;2(4):348–57. doi:10.1053/j.ctep.2004.04.008
171. Delius M. Medical applications and bioeffects of extracorporeal shock waves. *Shock Waves*. 1994;4(2):55–72. doi:10.1007/BF01418569
172. Tenforde AS, Borgstrom HE, DeLuca S, et al. Best practices for extracorporeal shockwave therapy in musculoskeletal medicine: clinical application and training consideration. *PM&R*. 2022;14(5):611–9. doi:10.1002/pmrj.12790
173. Maier M, Tischer T, Milz S, et al. Dose-related effects of extracorporeal shock waves on rabbit quadriceps tendon integrity. *Arch Orthop Trauma Surg*. 2002;122(8):436–41. doi:10.1007/s00402-002-0420-9
174. Van Der Worp H, Van Den Akker-Scheek I, Van Schie H, Zwerver J. ESWT for tendinopathy: technology and clinical implications. *Knee Surg Sports Traumatol Arthrosc*. 2013;21(6):1451–8. doi:10.1007/s00167-012-2009-3
175. Mariotto S, De Prati A, Cavalieri E, Amelio E, Marlinghaus E, Suzuki H. Extracorporeal shock wave therapy in inflammatory diseases: molecular mechanism that triggers anti-inflammatory action. *Curr Med Chem*. 2009;16(19):2366–72. doi:10.2174/092986709788682119
176. Han SH, Lee JW, Guyton GP, Parks BG, Courneya JP, Schon LC. J.Leonard Goldner Award 2008. Effect of extracorporeal shock wave therapy on cultured tenocytes. *Foot Ankle Int*. 2009;30(2):93–8. doi:10.3113/FAI.2009.0093
177. Melzack R. Sensory modulation of pain. *Int Rehabil Med*. 1979;1(3):111–15. doi:10.3109/03790797909163937
178. Vetrano M, d'Alessandro F, Torrisi MR, Ferretti A, Vulpiani MC, Visco V. Extracorporeal shock wave therapy promotes cell proliferation and collagen synthesis of primary cultured human tenocytes. *Knee Surg Sports Traumatol Arthrosc*. 2011;19(12):2159–68. doi:10.1007/s00167-011-1534-9
179. Rhim HC, Kwon J, Park J, Borg-Stein J, Tenforde AS. A systematic review of systematic reviews on the epidemiology, evaluation, and treatment of plantar fasciitis. *Life*. 2021;11(12):1287. doi:10.3390/life11121287
180. Testa G, Vescio A, Perez S, et al. Extracorporeal shockwave therapy treatment in upper limb diseases: a systematic review. *J Clin Med*. 2020;9(2):453. doi:10.3390/jcm9020453
181. Speed C. A systematic review of shockwave therapies in soft tissue conditions: focusing on the evidence. *Br J Sports Med*. 2014;48(21):1538–42. doi:10.1136/bjsports-2012-091961
182. Korakakis V, Whiteley R, Tzavara A, Malliaropoulos N. The effectiveness of extracorporeal shockwave therapy in common lower limb conditions: a systematic review including quantification of patient-rated pain reduction. *Br J Sports Med*. 2018;52(6):387–407. doi:10.1136/bjsports-2016-097347
183. Mani-Babu S, Morrissey D, Waugh C, Screen H, Barton C. The effectiveness of extracorporeal shock wave therapy in lower limb tendinopathy: a systematic review. *Am J Sports Med*. 2015;43(3):752–61. doi:10.1177/0363546514531911
184. Kudo P, Dainty K, Clarfield M, Coughlin L, Lavoie P, Lebrun C. Randomized, placebo-controlled, double-blind clinical trial evaluating

the treatment of plantar fasciitis with an extracoporeal shockwave therapy (ESWT) device: a North American confirmatory study. *J Orthop Res.* 2006;24(2):115–23. doi:10.1002/jor.20008

185. Feeney KM. The effectiveness of extracorporeal shockwave therapy for midportion Achilles tendinopathy: a systematic review. *Cureus.* 2022 Jul 18;14(7):e26960. Published online doi:10.7759/cureus.26960
186. Chen L, Ye L, Liu H, Yang P, Yang B. Extracorporeal shock wave therapy for the treatment of osteoarthritis: a systematic review and meta-analysis. *BioMed Res Int.* 2020;2020. 1907821 p. doi:10.1155/2020/1907821
187. Yue L, Sun M, Chen H, Mu G, Sun H. Extracorporeal shockwave therapy for treating chronic low back pain: a systematic review and meta-analysis of randomized controlled trials. *BioMed Res Int.* In: Song C, editor. 2021;2021:1–7. doi:10.1155/2021/5937250
188. Harniman E, Carette S, Kennedy C, Beaton D. Extracorporeal shock wave therapy for calcific and noncalcific tendonitis of the rotator cuff: a systematic review. *J Hand Ther.* 2004;17(2):132–51. doi:10.1197/j.jht.2004.02.003
189. Yao G, Chen J, Duan Y, Chen X. Efficacy of extracorporeal shock wave therapy for lateral epicondylitis: a systematic review and meta-analysis. *BioMed Res Int.* 2020;2020:2064781–8. doi:10.1155/2020/2064781
190. Zhang R, Wang Z, Liu R, Zhang N, Guo J, Huang Y. Extracorporeal shockwave therapy as an adjunctive therapy for frozen shoulder: a systematic review and meta-analysis. *Orthop J Sports Med.* 2022;10(2):23259671211062222. doi:10.1177/23259671211062222
191. Zhang Q, Fu C, Huang L, et al. Efficacy of extracorporeal shockwave therapy on pain and function in myofascial pain syndrome of the trapezius: a systematic review and meta-analysis. *Arch Phys Med Rehabil.* 2020;101(8):1437–46. doi:10.1016/j.apmr.2020.02.013
192. Häußer J, Wieber J, Catalá-Lehnen P. The use of extracorporeal shock wave therapy for the treatment of bone marrow oedema—a systematic review and meta-analysis. *J Orthop Surg.* 2021;16(1):369. doi:10.1186/s13018-021-02484-5
193. Sansone V, Ravier D, Pascale V, Applefield R, Del Fabbro M, Martinelli N. Extracorporeal shockwave therapy in the treatment of nonunion in long bones: a systematic review and meta-analysis. *J Clin Med.* 2022;11(7):1977. doi:10.3390/jcm11071977

75 Core Strengthening

Joel Press

OVERVIEW

- Core rehabilitation allows the multisegmented spinal column to maintain its center of gravity through multiple ranges of motion, counteracting gravity, and applied forces to decrease torsion and shear on the spinal structures (ligaments, disc, nerve).
- Definition of core
  - The core includes the lumbopelvic hip complex.
  - The core is where the center of gravity is located and where all movement begins (1).
  - An efficient core allows for the maintenance of the normal length-tension relationship of functional agonists and antagonists, which allows for the maintenance of normal force-couple relationships in the lumbopelvic hip complex (1).
- Why is the core important?
  - When a limb is moved, reactive forces are imposed on the spine acting in parallel and opposing those forces producing the movement (2).
  - The spine is particularly prone to the effect of these reactive forces due to its multisegmented nature and the requirement for muscle contractions to provide stability to the spine (3).
  - Without muscular support and contraction, buckling of the spine occurs with compressive forces of as little as 2 kg (4).
  - Significant microtrauma of the lumbar spine will occur with rotation of as little as 2° (5).
  - The musculature of the spine has been shown repeatedly to be most important in maintaining spinal stability during movements (6,7).
  - Function of core muscles: oppose the movements of limbs, hold the spine together, and decrease lumbar shearing.
  - Muscle dysfunction in low back pain is a problem with motor control in the deep muscles related to segmental joint stabilization (8).
  - Back pain can occur as a consequence of deficits in control of the spinal segment when abnormally large segmental motions cause abnormal deformation of ligaments and pain-sensitive structures (9).
    - Loss of joint stiffness.
    - Increase in mobility and abnormal spinal motion.
    - Changes in the ratios of segmental rotations and translations.

WHAT ARE CORE MUSCLES? ANATOMY/ BIOMECHANICS OF THE "CORE"

- Local paravertebral-multifidi.
  - Stabilizing role: Protecting articular structures, discs, and ligaments from excessive bending, strains, and injury.
  - Multisegmented column is unstable and will buckle under compression at individual joints unless locally stabilized.
  - Short muscles provide local support for longer muscles to work (10).
  - Neutral zone control.
  - The neutral zone is a region of intervertebral motion around the neutral posture where little resistance is offered by the passive spinal column (bones and ligaments).
  - Sensitive region for stabilization of joints (9).
  - Multifidi contribute to control of the neutral zone (3,11,12) and contribute more than two-thirds of stiffness increase at L4–L5 (12).
- Polysegmental: Erector spinae
  - Important for posture: Contract intermittently during the swaying movements that take place from an upright position.
  - Contraction of the erector spinae extends the trunk, a movement controlled largely by the opposing activity of the rectus abdominis.
  - In slow trunk flexion movements, the erector spinae lowers the trunk into flexion (eccentrically contract) against the action of gravity during slow movements (13).
  - Role: Balance external loads and minimize forces on the spine (10).
  - Only a very small increase in activation of the multifidi and abdominal muscles is required to stiffen the spinal segments — 5% maximal voluntary contraction (MVC) for activities of daily living and 10% MVC for rigorous activity (14).
  - Endurance of muscles to maintain spinal stability during prolonged activities, not absolute strength, is most important (15).

- Abdominals: transversus abdominis (TrA), internal and external obliques, and rectus abdominis
  - Contraction of abdominals (especially TrA), pelvic floor, and diaphragm correlates closely with increased abdominal pressure in a variety of postural tasks (16–18).
  - TrA: Critical in stabilization of lumbar spine (16).
  - Contracting TrA increases intra-abdominal pressure and tension in the thoracolumbar fascia.
  - Helps create a rigid cylinder, enhancing the stiffness of the lumbar spine (15).
  - Rectus abdominis and oblique abdominals are activated in direction-specific patterns with respect to limb movements, thus providing postural support *before* limb movements (17,19).
  - Contraction increasing intra-abdominal pressure occurs *before* initiation of large segment movement of the upper limbs (17,18,20).
- Quadratus lumborum
  - Fibers cross-link the vertebrae.
  - Extends from transverse processes to the rib cage and iliac crests; can buttress shearing of the spine in all planes.
  - Active during flexion, extension, and lateral bending — not just a frontal plane muscle.
- Diaphragm
  - To minimize the displacement of the abdominal contents within the abdomen and pelvis, it is necessary to elevate the intra-abdominal pressure by simultaneously contracting the diaphragm, the pelvic floor, and the abdominal muscles (14,21).
  - Diaphragm increases intra-abdominal pressure and segmental unloading of the spine, and thus increases trunk stability.
- Pelvic floor
  - Coactivation of the TrA, abdominals, multifidi, and pelvic floor muscles contributes to spine stability (22)
- Lower extremity muscles — gluteus maximus, hamstrings
  - Hip and pelvic muscles: base of support for lumbar spine and upper limbs
  - Thoracolumbar fascia
    - Covers the deep muscles of the back and trunk (including multifidi)
    - Connects the lower limbs to the upper via the latissimus dorsi
    - Internal obliques, TrA, latissimus dorsi, gluteus maximus
    - Enhances stiffness of the lumbar spine
  - Multifidi blend with the superior medial aspect of gluteus maximus
  - Multifidi attach to sacrotuberous ligaments and are mechanically linked to the gluteus maximus

HOW DO WE STRENGTHEN CORE MUSCLES?

- Balance: Control center of gravity (COG) as it moves through various planes of motion and then shifts the COG through various planes
- Goals of core-strengthening exercise:
  - Improve multifidus activity and endurance
  - Restore the control of deep abdominal muscles
  - Restore coordination and position sense
  - Restore mobility, especially in rotational and lateral flexion directions
  - Restore normal gluteal muscle activity and lumbopelvic rhythm
  - Train motor and postural control and balance
  - Make exercises functional

PRACTICAL APPLICATIONS OF CORE STRENGTHENING

- Turn on the light
  - Abdominal bracing: Tightening the abdominal muscles isometrically like you are going to be punched in the stomach
    - May require cueing and instruction
    - Need core stability for global mobility
    - Abdominal bracing is more effective and puts less stress on the spine than hollowing (which is sucking in the abdominal muscles and then holding them tight) (23)
  - Re-education of stabilization muscles — pelvic clocks
    - Learn how to turn on pelvic and hip muscles
- Get the engines going
  - Abdominal bracing in supine > prone, side lying > quadruped
  - Progress to kneeling > sitting > standing
  - Three basic core exercises that put the least load on the spine: plank (Fig. 75.1), side plank (Fig. 75.2), and "bird dog" (Fig. 75.3) (6)

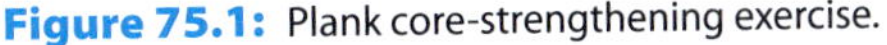

Figure 75.1: Plank core-strengthening exercise.

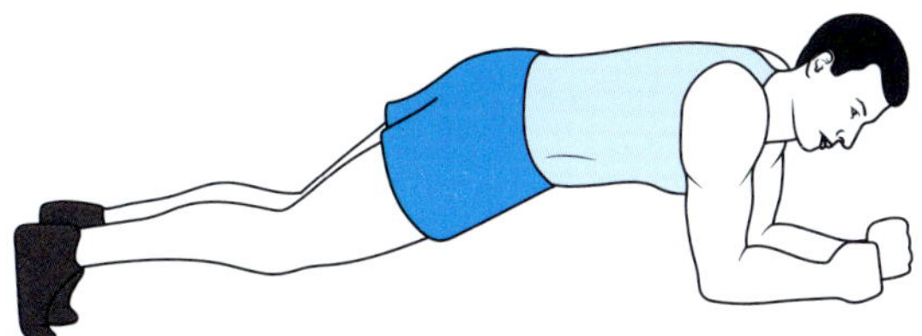

Figure 75.2: Side plank core-strengthening exercise.

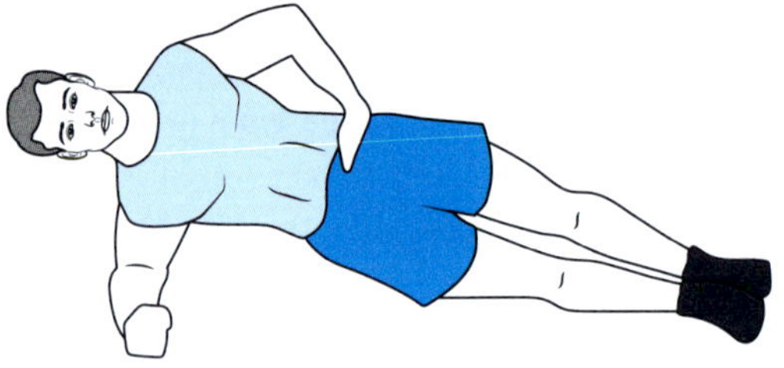

- Make it functional and fun to do
  - Start in pain-free ranges
  - Progress to multiple planes of motion
  - Frontal plane core
  - Sagittal plane core
  - Transverse plane core
  - Dynamic challenges — easy to hard
  - Include balance/proprioception
  - Need to make it subconscious

CORE STABILIZATION: WHAT'S THE EVIDENCE?

Rehabilitation

- Core stability has proven to be an effective rehabilitation strategy for patients with low back pain, decreasing duration of symptoms, decreasing pain, and minimizing disability (24–27).
- Core stability was more effective in improving quality of life, muscular thickness, and lumbar muscle strength compared to minimal or no intervention (28–32).
- Increasing evidence supports core stability exercise in comparison to no intervention, sham intervention, or rest in improving pain and disability. Most current studies observed the superiority of core stability over general exercise protocols with a few studies showing similar effects (33–47).
- Prediction rules indicate that patients most likely to benefit are those in specific subgroups with negative straight leg raise, positive prone instability test, aberrant motion, lumbar hypermobility, or low fear of avoidance (48). If patients are first subgrouped into those responding to specific maneuvers, there is a greater chance of predicting benefit from core exercises.

Performance Enhancement

- Core stability is seen as being pivotal for efficient biomechanical function to maximize force generation and minimize joint loads in all types of activities ranging from running to throwing (49).

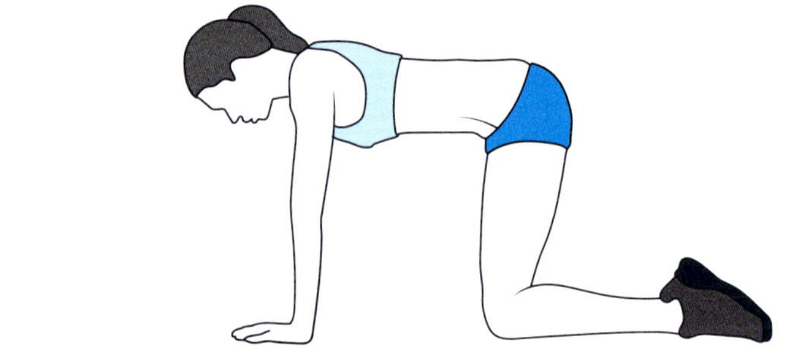

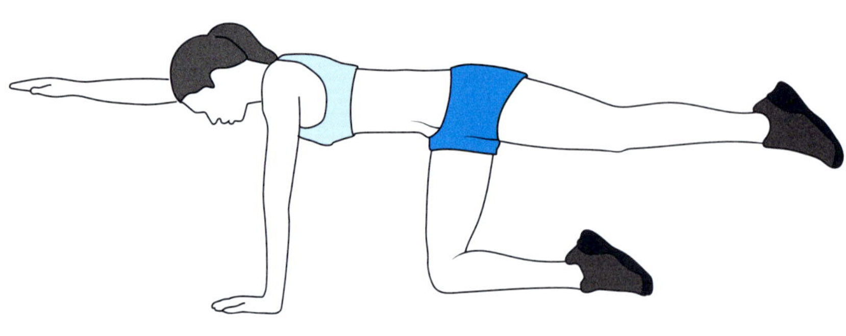

Figure 75.3: "Bird dog" core-strengthening exercise.

- Although the specific effects of core strengthening on performance are evolving, some studies have shown improvements with a functional core stability training program in gymnastics and running (50,51).

SUMMARY

- Core stability can be defined as the ability to control the position and motion of the trunk over the pelvis to allow optimum production, transfer, and control of force and motion to the terminal segment in athletic activities. Core muscle activity is best understood as the preprogrammed integration of local, single-joint muscles and multijoint muscles to provide stability and produce motion.
- The success of the core stability exercise program depends on the patient's compliance and the correct dosage of the exercise program, which should be customized for each patient.

REFERENCES

1. Clark MA, Fater D, Reuteman P. Core (trunk) stabilization and its importance for closed kinetic chain rehabilitation. *Orthop Phys Ther Clin North Am.* 2000;9(2):119–32.
2. Bouisset S, Zattara M. Biomechanical study of the programming of anticipatory postural adjustments associated with voluntary movement. *J Biomech.* 1987;20(8):735–42.
3. Panjabi MM. The stabilizing system of the spine. Part II. Neutral zone and stability hypothesis. *J Spinal Disord.* 1992;5(4):390–6.
4. Morris JM, Lucas DM, Bresler B. Role of the trunk in the stability of the spine. *J Bone Joint Surg Am.* 1961;43:327–51.
5. Gracovetsky S, Farfan H, Helleur C. The abdominal mechanism. *Spine.* 1985;10(4):317–24.
6. Gardner-Morse M, Stokes IA, Laible JP. Role of muscles in lumbar spine stability in maximum extension efforts. *J Orthop Res.* 1995;13(5):802–8.
7. Solomonow M, Zhou BH, Harris M, Lu Y, Baratta RV. The ligamento-muscular stabilizing system of the spine. *Spine.* 1998;23(23):2552–62.
8. Richardson C, Jull G, Hodges PW, Hides JA. *Therapeutic exercise for spinal segmental stabilization in low back pain: scientific basis and clinical approach.* Edinburgh (UK): Churchill Livingstone; 1999:192.
9. Panjabi MM. The stabilizing system of the spine. Part 1. Function, dysfunction, adaptation, and enhancement. *J Spinal Disord.* 1991;5(4):383–9.
10. Bergmark A. Stability of the lumbar spine. A study in mechanical engineering. *Acta Orthop Scand Suppl.* 1989;230:1–54.
11. Steffen R, Nolte LP, Pingel TH. Importance of back muscles in rehabilitation of postoperative lumber instability; a biomechanical analysis. *Rehabilitation.* 1994;33(3):164–70.
12. Wilke HJ, Wolf S, Claes LE, Arand M, Wiesend A. Stability increase of the lumbar spine with different muscle groups. A biomechanical in vitro study. *Spine.* 1995;20(2):192–8.
13. Oddsson LI. Control of voluntary trunk movements in man: mechanisms for postural equilibrium in standing. *Acta Physiol Scan Suppl.* 1990;595:1–60.
14. Cholewicki J, Juluru K, McGill SM. Intra-abdominal pressure mechanism for stabilizing the lumbar spine. *J Biomech.* 1999;32(1):13–7.
15. McGill SM, Norman RW. Reassessment of the role of intra-abdominal pressure in spinal compression. *Ergonomics.* 1987;30(11):1565–88.
16. Cresswell AG, Oddsson L, Thorstensson A. The influence of sudden perturbations on trunk muscle activity and intraabdominal pressure while standing. *Exp Brain Res.* 1994;98(2):336–41.
17. Hodges PW, Butler JE, McKenzie DK, Gandevia SC. Contraction of the human diaphragm during rapid postural adjustments. *J Physiol.* 1997;505(Pt 2):539–48.
18. Hodges PW, Richardson CA. Feedforward contraction of transversus abdominis is not influenced by the direction of arm movement. *Exp Brain Res.* 1997;114(2):362–70.
19. Aruin AS, Latash ML. Directional specificity of postural muscles in feed-forward postural reactions during fast voluntary arm movements. *Exp Brain Res.* 1995;103(2):323–32.
20. Ferreira ML, Ferreira PH, Hodges PW. Changes in postural activity of the trunk muscles following spinal manipulative therapy. *Man Ther.* 2007;12(3):240–8.
21. Daggfeldt K, Thorstensson A. The role of intra-abdominal pressure in spinal unloading. *J Biomech.* 1997;30(11–12):1149–55.
22. Sapsford RR, Hodges PW, Richardson CA, Cooper DH, Markwell SJ, Jull GA. Co-activation of the abdominal and pelvic floor muscles during voluntary exercises. *Neurourol Urodyn.* 2001;20(1):31–42.
23. Grenier SG, McGill SM. Quantification of lumbar stability by using 2 different abdominal activation strategies. *Arch Phys Med Rehabil.* 2007;88(1):54–62.
24. Cairns MC, Foster NE, Wright C. Randomized controlled trial of specific spinal stabilization exercises and conventional physiotherapy for recurrent low back pain. *Spine.* 2006;31(19):E670–81.
25. Goldby LJ, Moore AP, Doust J, Trew ME. A randomized controlled trial investigating the efficiency of musculoskeletal physiotherapy on chronic low back disorder. *Spine.* 2006;31(10):1083–93.
26. McGill SM. *Corrective and therapeutic exercise for the painful lumbar spine: technique matters.* Rochester (MN): American Academy of Neuromuscular and Electrodiagnostic Medicine; 2009.
27. Waseem M, Karimi H, Gilani SA, Hassan D. Treatment of disability associated with chronic non-specific low back pain using core stabilization exercises in Pakistani population. *J Back Musculoskelet Rehabil.* 2019;32(1):149–54. [PubMed].
28. Gong W. The effects of running in place in a limited area with abdominal drawing-in maneuvers on abdominal muscle thickness in chronic low back pain patients. *J Back Musculoskelet Rehabil.* 2016;29(4):757–62.
29. Leonard JH, Paungmali A, Sitilertpisan P, Pirunsan U, Uthaikhup S. Changes in transversus abdominis muscle thickness after llumbo-pelvic core stabilization training among chronic low back pain individuals. *Clin Ter.* 2015;166(5):312–6.
30. Narouei S, Barati AH, Akuzawa H, et al. Effects of core stabilization exercises on thickness and activity of trunk and hip muscles in subjects with nonspecific chronic low back pain. *J Bodyw Mov Ther.* 2020;24(4):138–46.
31. Noormohammadpour P, Kordi M, Mansournia MA, Akbari-Fakhrabadi M, Kordi R. The role of a multi-step core stability exercise program in the treatment of nurses with chronic low back pain: a single-blinded randomized controlled trial. *Asian Spine J.* 2018;12(3):490–502.
32. Paungmali A, Joseph LH, Sitilertpisan P, Pirunsan U, Uthaikhup S. Lumbopelvic core stabilization exercise and pain modulation among individuals with chronic nonspecific low back pain. *Pain Pract.* 2017;17(8):1008–14.
33. Akbari A, Khorashadizadeh S, Abdi G. The effect of motor control exercise versus general exercise on lumbar local stabilizing muscles thickness: randomized controlled trial of patients with chronic low back pain. *J Back Musculoskelet Rehabil.* 2008:105–12.

34. Akhtar MW, Karimi H, Gilani SA. Effectiveness of core stabilization exercises and routine exercise therapy in management of pain in chronic non-specific low back pain: a randomized controlled clinical trial. *Pak J Med Sci.* 2017;33(4):1002–6.
35. Andrusaitis SF, Brech GC, Vitale GF, Greve JMDA. Trunk stabilization among women with chronic lower back pain: a randomized, controlled, and blinded pilot study. *Clinics.* 2011;66(9):1645–50.
36. Bhadauria EA, Gurudut P. Comparative effectiveness of lumbar stabilization, dynamic strengthening, and Pilates on chronic low back pain: randomized clinical trial. *J Exerc Rehabil.* 2017;13(4):477–85.
37. França FR, Burke TN, Hanada ES, Marques AP. Segmental stabilization and muscular strengthening in chronic low back pain: a comparative study. *Clinics.* 2010;65(10):1013–17.
38. Frizziero A, Pellizzon G, Vittadini F, Bigliardi D, Costantino C. Efficacy of core stability in non-specific chronic low back pain. *J Funct Morphol Kinesiol.* 2021;6(2):37. doi:10.3390/jfmk6020037
39. Gatti R, Faccendini S, Tettamanti A, Barbero M, Balestri A, Calori G. Efficacy of trunk balance exercises for individuals with chronic low back pain: a randomized clinical trial. *J Orthop Sports Phys Ther.* 2011;41(8):542–52.
40. Inani SB, Selkar SP. Effect of core stabilization exercises versus conventional exercises on pain and functional status in patients with non-specific low back pain: a randomized clinical trial. *J Back Musculoskelet Rehabil.* 2013;26(1):37–43.
41. Kwon SH, Oh SJ, Kim DH. The effects of lumbar stabilization exercise on transversus abdominis muscle activation capacity and function in low back pain patients. *Isokinet Exerc Sci.* 2020:147–52.
42. Moon HJ, Choi KH, Kim DH, et al. Effect of lumbar stabilization and dynamic lumbar strengthening exercises in patients with chronic low back pain. *Ann Rehabil Med.* 2013;37(1):110–7.
43. Nabavi N, Mohseni Bandpei MA, Mosallanezhad Z, Rahgozar M, Jaberzadeh S. The effect of 2 different exercise programs on pain intensity and muscle dimensions in patients with chronic low back pain: a randomized controlled trial. *J Manip Physiol Ther.* 2018;41:102–10.
44. Shamsi MB, Rezaei M, Zamanlou M, Sadeghi M, Pourahmadi MR. Does core stability exercise improve lumbopelvic stability (through endurance tests) more than general exercise in chronic low back pain? A quasi-randomized controlled trial. *Physiother Theory Pract.* 2016;32(3):171–8. *Funct Morphol Kinesiol.* 2021, 6(37)19:20.
45. Shamsi M, Mirzaei M, HamediRad M. Comparison of muscle activation imbalance following core stability or general exercises in nonspecific low back pain: a quasi-randomized controlled trial. *BMC Sports Sci Med Rehabil.* 2020;12:24.
46. Sipaviciene S, Kliziene I. Effect of different exercise programs on non-specific chronic low back pain and disability in people who perform sedentary work. *Clin Biomech.* 2020;73:17–27.
47. Wang XQ, Zheng JJ, Yu ZW, et al. A meta-analysis of core stability exercise versus general exercise for chronic low back pain. *PLoS One.* 2012;7(12):e52082.
48. Hicks GE, Fritz JM, Delitto A, McGill SM. Preliminary development of a clinical prediction rule for determining which patients with low back pain will respond to a stabilization exercise program. *Arch Phys Med Rehabil.* 2005;86(9):1753–62.
49. Kibler WB, Press J, Sciascia A. The role of core stability in athletic function. *Sports Med.* 2006;36(3):189–98. 0112-1642/06/003-0189.
50. Cabrejas C, Solana-Tramunt M, Morales J, et al. The effects of an eight-week integrated functional core and plyometric training program on young rhythmic gymnasts' explosive strength. *Int J Environ Res Public Health.* 2023 Jan 6;20(2):1041.
51. Sato K, Mokha M. Does core strength training influence running kinetics, lower extremity stability and 5000-M performance in runners? *J Strength Cond Res.* 2009;23(1):133–40.

Medications and Ergogenic Aids

76

Scott D. Flinn and Yao-Wen Eliot Hu

OVERVIEW

- Medications are commonly used by sports medicine providers in the rehabilitative process to alleviate pain and facilitate the rehabilitative process, and potentially augment the healing process. Commonly utilized pharmacologic agents by the team physician include nonsteroidal anti-inflammatories (NSAIDs), anticonvulsants, antidepressants, opioids, cannabinoids, and glucocorticoids. While these agents are commonly employed, their employment and efficacy in athletes have a limited evidence base.
- In addition to prescription pharmaceutical agents, many athletes self-medicate using various pharmacologic or nutritional substances in an effort to improve performance and speed recovery from injury. For example, over-the-counter anti-inflammatory medications are often used to limit pain and inflammation and presumably speed healing from injury. Other substances, which may be legal when given by prescription for U.S. Food and Drug Administration (FDA)-approved indications but are otherwise illegal and/or prohibited by governing authorities, are used specifically in an effort to improve performance.
- This chapter reviews currently employed common ergogenic aids and prescription agents utilized in sports medicine, with a focus on current evidence-based guidance. Injectable agents, to include proliferants, and orthobiologic interventions are reviewed in subsequent chapters (Chapter 77: Prolotherapy, Chapter 78: Orthobiologics, and Chapter 79: Joint Injections). Drug testing is discussed in Chapter 28.
- Strategies for the utilization of medications in the management of acute and chronic pain in the athlete are discussed in Chapter 73: Pain Management in the Athlete.

MEDICATIONS AND ERGOGENIC AIDS BACKGROUND

Definition

- Ergogenic aids are defined as items designed to increase work or improve performance above that of regular training and diet.
- Ergogenic aids are usually classified into five groups: mechanical aids such as running shoes, psychological aids, physiologic aids such as fluids and blood, pharmacologic aids that are thought of as requiring a prescription or used as supplements, and nutritional aids.

History

- Congress passed the Dietary Supplement Health and Education Act in 1994, changing the regulation and marketing of dietary supplements (1). Products labeled and sold as dietary supplements making no claims to be a drug can be sold without FDA approval.
- Because they are not held to the same quality control standards as FDA-approved drugs, they are not evaluated for safety, efficacy, content, or purity and they may contain much more than the amount stated on the label or none at all (2–4).

Evaluating Ergogenic Aids

Efficacy

- Because there is no burden of proof on the manufacturer to prove efficacy or product content like there is for drugs, the amount of the substance listed on the label may vary dramatically from the actual content, which may include substances not listed on the label. These contaminants may have come from previous manufacturing in the same equipment and can cause failed drug tests (5).
- Furthermore, the placebo effect can have an enormous impact on the perceived benefits derived by the user (6).
- Various performance parameters for which ergogenic aids are evaluated include aerobic fitness, anaerobic fitness, strength, body composition, psychological factors, and healing of injuries.
- Aerobic fitness is the ability to produce work using aerobic metabolism, which lasts longer than 1 minute and may last for hours. It is often measured in terms of maximal aerobic power or aerobic capacity.
- Anaerobic fitness is fueled primarily through anaerobic metabolism and is important in activities lasting less than 1 minute.
- Maximum strength is usually measured by the one-repetition maximum and refers to the amount of power that

can be generated in a brief burst. It is fueled by anaerobic metabolism.

- Body composition can affect performance by increasing lean muscle mass. More muscle can perform more work, whereas decreasing body fat decreases the inert weight that must be carried through space to the finish line.
- Psychological factors may affect performance through various mind-body mechanisms including decreased perceptions of fatigue and pain. It is sometimes measured as time to exhaustion.
- Enhancing the healing of injuries and soreness promotes a more rapid return to training and maintenance of fitness.

Safety Considerations

- Ergogenic aids can have side effects like any other substance.
- Heart attacks, seizures, strokes, coma, and death have been attributed to the use of ergogenic products (2).
- Injectable products carry the risk of disease transmission if needles are shared.

Ethical and Legal Considerations

- Athletes will try ergogenic aids to gain a competitive advantage even though the product has not been shown to work, has serious side effects, or is banned by the sport's governing body ruling over the sport in which the athlete is competing.
- Anabolic steroids had become so widespread by the 1964 Olympic Games that drug testing began at the 1968 Olympic Games in Mexico City, with the National Collegiate Athletic Association (NCAA) following in 1986.
- The American College of Sports Medicine and other organizations have taken a position on anabolic steroids stating that they are unethical, they have dangerous side effects, and their use should be deplored (7).
- The Anabolic Steroids Control Act of 1991 made anabolic steroids a Schedule III controlled substance.
- Various amateur and professional sports governing organizations have instituted drug policies targeted toward substances that may be dangerous, be illegal, and/or give an unfair competitive advantage. The U.S. Anti-Doping Agency (USADA) was formed in 2000 as an independent antidoping organization for Olympic sports in the United States.
- The World Anti-Doping Agency (WADA) was created in 2004 to "develop, harmonize and coordinate anti-doping rules and policies across all sports and countries" and provides a list of prohibited substances and methods: https://www.wada-ama.org/en/resources/world-anti-doping-program/prohibited-list (8). This list is updated every January and is freely available on the WADA website. It also provides a process to apply for Therapeutic Use Exemptions (TUEs) to authorize athletes to take needed medications. This is described below.
- The NCAA has their list of prohibited methods and substances at https://www.ncaa.org/sports/2015/6/10/ncaa-banned-substances.aspx (9) and specific drugs and supplements may be researched at https://axis.drugfreesport.com/inquiries (10).
- Because the lists are continually changing, physicians caring for athletes governed by these or other organizations should always consult the governing body prior to writing a prescription or suggesting over-the-counter remedies.
- Testing is usually done by analyzing urine samples through several methods, with most confirmatory tests done using gas chromatography/mass spectrometry. In the future, blood or hair samples may be used to detect banned substances. See Chapter 25: Drug Testing.
- Further discussion of ethical considerations related to supplements, medications, and ergogenic aids can be found in Chapter 2: Ethical Considerations in Sports Medicine.

Therapeutic Use Exemptions

- WADA is the organization that oversees antidoping policies and determines the list of substances (and doping methods) that are banned from sports. This includes hormonal and nonhormonal drugs as well as dietary supplements.
- Some athletes have illnesses or conditions that require them to take medications that may be on the prohibited list. A request for an exception to authorize the athlete to take the needed medication can be granted through a TUE.
- In the United States, the TUE is issued by the USADA (11) and may be found at https://www.usada.org/athletes/testing/tue/.
- The process for obtaining a TUE is defined on the USADA website. The first step is determining if a TUE is needed for that particular drug and sport. A direct link is provided to the Global Drug Reference Online (12), which tells the user if the substance is prohibited in competition and/or out of competition (https://www.globaldro.com/home/index). A reference number for the query is provided by Global Drug Reference Online. Then a TUE Pre-Check form is submitted to USADA to see if a TUE is required. USADA reviews the information and in 3 to 5 business days tells if a TUE is needed and what supporting documentation will be required. A formal TUE with the requested supporting documentation is then submitted online to USADA.
- The TUE is used for prescription therapies and not for supplements; the athlete is taking the supplements at their own risk and is responsible for anything ingested.

MEDICATIONS

Nonsteroidal Anti-Inflammatory Drugs

Efficacy

- NSAIDs are used by millions of people daily both in prescription and over-the-counter form to treat acute and chronic injuries. No one NSAID appears to be more efficacious than others and there is wide individual variation in the response to different NSAIDs (13). Selection of NSAID should be individualized to not only consider efficacy but also limit adverse effects.

- The major pharmacologic effect of NSAIDs is to inhibit the enzyme cyclooxygenase (COX), thus decreasing prostaglandin production. The decreased prostaglandins lead to decreased inflammation and promote analgesia in the injured tissue. There are at least two forms of the COX enzyme, COX-1 and COX-2.
- COX-1 is important in the production of prostaglandins involved in the homeostasis of various tissues including gastric mucosa, platelets, and renal parenchyma.
- COX-2 produces prostaglandins involved in pain and inflammation. Most NSAIDs inhibit both COX-1 and COX-2 at various levels, with some agents developed to be more COX-2 selective to limit adverse effects.
- Both oral and topical NSAIDs have been shown to decrease pain, increase functional ability, and allow for a more rapid return to training in ankle sprains (14,15).
- NSAIDs decrease pain following acute injury (16).

Safety

- The major adverse side effects from use of NSAIDs include gastrointestinal (GI) bleeding, cardiovascular (CV) complications, and kidney damage.
- Although there are published studies of slowed tendon healing in rats, there is no published human data that show delayed tendon healing (17).
- NSAIDs can potentially damage the GI tract mostly through systemic effects including disruption of the mucous layer, decreased bicarbonate secretion, and vasoconstriction, as well as a direct topical effect causing epithelial necrosis (18). GI bleeds can occur with both chronic and acute use, sometimes within days of starting the medication.
- Risk factors for GI bleed with NSAIDs include history of previous bleed, age over 64, and concomitant aspirin use (19).
- Effective measures to reduce GI toxicity in patients who are susceptible to GI adverse events include using alternative therapies like acetaminophen, giving medications for a short duration, using NSAID topical agents to avoid systemic absorption, using a COX-2–selective NSAID, or adding a GI protective agent such as a proton pump inhibitor or misoprostol when using either nonselective or COX-2–selective NSAIDs (20).
- Neither use of H2 blockers (21) nor use of enteric coated aspirin (22) was shown to reduce GI toxicity.
- NSAIDs including the COX-2 inhibitor celecoxib have been shown to increase the risk of both fatal and nonfatal CV events. In one meta-analysis, naproxen did not have an increased risk of CV events (23), but a later study showed that naproxen had the same risk as ibuprofen and celecoxib (24).
- COX-2–selective NSAIDs were introduced in the 1990s to decrease the GI bleed risk, but some had a higher risk of CV side effects including myocardial infarction and had to be withdrawn from the market. One is currently available in the United States — celecoxib — and has no worse risk of adverse CV events than other NSAIDs (24).
- For patients with both high risk of GI bleed and cardiac complications, the use of a COX-2 NSAID plus a proton pump inhibitor may be prudent because the risk of a fatal bleed may be higher than a CV event.
- If the patient will be on NSAIDs for a long duration, consideration should be given to *Helicobacter pylori* eradication (25).
- Both COX-2–selective and nonselective NSAIDs can cause kidney ischemia, decrease in glomerular pressure, and acute kidney injury (26).

Legality

- NSAIDs are allowed by the International Olympic Committee (IOC), NCAA, and WADA (8,9).

Anticonvulsants

Efficacy

- Because of their ability to attenuate hyperactive neuronal states in epilepsy, anticonvulsants such as pregabalin and gabapentin have been studied with respect to chronic pain management (27).
- For low back and chronic neuropathic pain, gabapentin and pregabalin are effective first-line medications for management (27). Specifically, gabapentin was shown to be more effective than placebo in decreasing chronic pain by 50% in patients with neuropathic pain, phantom limb pain, spinal cord injury, and other neuropathies (28).
- Gabapentin has also been shown to provide short-term improvements in symptom burden in patients with concussion, but the long-term outcomes show similar improvement compared to those who were not prescribed medication treatment (29).
- For patients with chronic pain due to fibromyalgia, pregabalin at higher doses has been shown to reduce pain by 30% when compared to amitriptyline and duloxetine, but this was not the case when evaluating for 50% pain reduction (30).
- Carbamazepine has been shown to decrease neuropathic pain associated with diabetic neuropathy and trigeminal neuralgia, but literature support is lacking for its use in controlling musculoskeletal pain (27).

Safety

- Gabapentin may cause peripheral edema, somnolence, dizziness, ataxia, or gait disturbance (31). Pregabalin may cause sedation, dizziness, peripheral edema, and dry mouth but otherwise has limited metabolic, idiosyncratic, and teratogenic effects (32). Thus, caution must be exhibited in the dosing of anticonvulsants.

Legality

- Anticonvulsants are allowed by the IOC, NCAA, and WADA (8,9).

Antidepressants

Efficacy

- Antidepressants increase serotonin, norepinephrine, and dopamine levels, resulting in decreased pain transmission in the body (27). Specific classes of antidepressants including selective serotonin reuptake inhibitors (SSRIs), serotonin and norepinephrine reuptake inhibitors (SNRIs), and tricyclic antidepressants (TCAs) have been studied as treatment for chronic pain syndromes such as fibromyalgia, back pain, and other musculoskeletal pain syndromes with varying degrees of evidence.
- Data are lacking for SSRIs to be used solely for controlling chronic pain although SSRIs have been shown to be efficacious in treating chronic pain with comorbid mood and anxiety disorders (27,33).
- SNRIs such as venlafaxine and duloxetine have shown efficacy in the treatment of neuropathic pain, fibromyalgia, chronic back pain, and postoperative pain (30,33,34). However, the use of SNRIs to treat pain due to osteoarthritis lacks evidence (34).
- Like gabapentin, the TCA amitriptyline has been shown to provide short-term improvements in symptom burden in patients with concussion, but the long-term outcomes show similar improvement compared to those who were not prescribed medication treatment (29).
- Although amitriptyline was shown to be efficacious in the treatment for fibromyalgia where it achieved 50% reduction in pain when compared to duloxetine and pregabalin (30), there was evidence only to support amitriptyline use in neuropathic pain (33). Current literature is inconclusive in supporting amitriptyline treatment for back pain and other musculoskeletal conditions (33,35).

Safety

- SSRIs, SNRIs, and TCAs may cause a variety of autonomic, cardiac, nervous, GI, and urogenital adverse effects including dry mouth, sexual dysfunction, sedation, dizziness, dyspepsia, QT prolongation, and weight gain (36–38). In general, SNRIs are associated with less serious side effects when compared to SSRIs (39), while TCAs are associated with increased cardiac events (38). Thus, caution should be exhibited when prescribing antidepressants due to the potential for medication interactions, serotonin syndrome, and cardiac events.

Legality

- Antidepressants are allowed by the IOC, NCAA, and WADA (8,9).

Opioids

Efficacy

- Opioids block the presynaptic C fibers at the peripheral-spinal junction to decrease transmission of pain (27). Although opioids are the most effective medications for severe acute pain in a dose-dependent manner (39), there is no evidence to support their use in osteoarthritis (40) or in chronic pain syndromes (27).

Safety

- Opioids have high addiction potential, have tendency to develop tolerance, and are associated with various adverse effects such as constipation, nausea, sedation, urinary retention, and dyspepsia (27). The potential for cognitive, behavioral, and reaction time deficits also decreases athletic performance and may place athletes at risk in specific sports (39). Thus, opioids should be prescribed for severe acute pain due to injury with special attention paid to the athlete's mental health and substance use history.

Legality

- Opioids are banned by the NCAA. WADA and the IOC have banned opioids for in-competition athletes and for those anticipating same day return to play (8,9). However, the IOC consensus statement does allow for opioid use as short-term treatment for severe acute pain in injured athletes who are not expected to return to play the same day (39).

Cannabinoids

Efficacy

- Nineteen percent of patients reported cannabidiol (CBD) use to treat joint-related issues in sports medicine (41). With its increasing popularity and more states relaxing their laws, more attention needs to be centered around CBD use for pain control.
- The cannabis plant is composed of more than one hundred cannabinoid products, with the most abundant being delta-9-tetrahydrocannabinol (THC) and CBD (42,43). To modulate pain, THC acts as a partial agonist of the cannabinoid receptors 1 and 2, while CBD acts as an allosteric modulator of various receptor sites.
- Currently, no studies have demonstrated cannabinoid effectiveness in treating severe acute pain (39,43). However, CBD has been shown to provide therapeutic and disease-modifying benefits in osteoarthritis although it has not yet obtained FDA approval (42). With respect to chronic pain syndromes and neuropathic pain, CBD has shown moderate efficacy as treatment (39,42,43).
- Data are extremely limited when studying the efficacy of CBD as treatment for sport-related concussion (42,43). Similarly, the literature is also lacking regarding CBD use for muscle recovery, delayed onset muscle soreness, and sport performance anxiety.

Safety

- Cannabinoids may cause nausea, GI effects, irritability, lethargy, and other cognitive and psychogenic adverse effects (43). They also have high potential for addiction (39), medication interactions, and hepatocellular injuries (42). Given the limited evidence on their therapeutic effects and the potential for adverse effects, caution must be exhibited when prescribing cannabinoid products for pain control.

Legality

- THC, marijuana, and other synthetic cannabinoids are banned by the NCAA (9). WADA prohibits the in-competition use of cannabis and cannabis products, natural and synthetic THC, and synthetic cannabinoids that mimic the effects of THC (8). However, CBD is specifically exempted from the WADA list. The IOC does not support the use of cannabinoids for pain management in elite athletes (39).
- Due to changing federal and state laws, special attention must also be paid to the political landscape regarding cannabinoids.

Glucocorticoids

Efficacy

- Glucocorticoids upregulate the production of anti-inflammatory proteins and downregulate the expression of inflammatory genes in cells, thus decreasing inflammatory cytokines and enzymes.
- Glucocorticoids are commonly used for a variety of acute and chronic injuries, though the literature supporting their use is mostly case series or retrospective studies.
- When used to treat musculoskeletal injuries, they are usually given orally, as a topical agent, or via injection.
- Systemic glucocorticoids help in acute radicular low back pain but not in nonradicular back pain (44,45).
- In patients with acute elbow epicondylitis, a single glucocorticoid injection had a short-term beneficial effect but poorer intermediate and long-term outcomes (46–48), whereas for chronic epicondylitis, outcomes were worse throughout (49).
- Trigger finger responds well to corticosteroid injection with up to 50% of patients getting long-term relief with a single injection (50).
- Subacromial injections for rotator cuff tendinopathy have been shown to improve range of motion in two randomized placebo controlled trials but were no better than lidocaine injection alone in another (51,52). Other studies provide limited support for glucocorticoid injection (53–55).
- When performing corticosteroid injections, there is no evidence-based guideline or consensus on the number, interval, type, or dose of steroid that should be used at a particular site. Various suggestions include mixing anesthetic with the corticosteroid to provide some immediate pain relief, not injecting directly into the tendon or peritendinous area, limiting injections to at least 6 weeks apart, and having no more than three injections at any one site.

Safety

- Corticosteroid injection has a complication rate of 1%–5%, with infection, hypopigmentation, postinjection flare, and fat pad atrophy being the most common adverse effects (56).
- Steroid injection directly into a tendon weakens it and may cause tendon rupture (57).
- Long-term therapy can suppress the hypothalamic-pituitary-adrenal axis and lead to adrenal crisis if steroids are stopped suddenly. Other adverse effects include reduced muscle mass and weakness, osteoporosis, diabetes, hypertension, weight gain and abdominal obesity, cataracts, and various psychiatric symptoms.

Legality

- WADA prohibits all glucocorticoids when administered by oral, intravenous, intramuscular, or rectal routes in competition, but other routes of administration including inhaled, topical, intranasal, ophthalmological, otic, and perianal are not prohibited when used within approved dosage and indication (8). They are not banned by the NCAA (9).

β_2-Adrenergic Receptor Agonists

Efficacy

- β_2-adrenergic agonists, such as albuterol and salmeterol, are sympathomimetics and are used widely as bronchodilators for the treatment of many types of asthma, including exercise-induced asthma. They are effective for treating asthma but have not been found to have any performance enhancement effect on endurance, strength, aerobic, or sprint performance (58,59).
- Clenbuterol is an oral β_2-adrenergic agonists that is used in agriculture in some countries like Mexico and China to increase lean body mass and decreases adipose tissue in animals like cattle and horses. Eating red meat in those countries may result in a positive test (60).
- Clenbuterol was shown to increase lean muscle mass in patients with congestive heart failure but not endurance (61), but no other human studies support its purported ergogenic effect. Athletes use it either as an anabolic steroid substitute or to prevent some of the muscle loss after cessation of anabolic steroids (62).

Safety

- Side effects of β_2-agonists are common and like other sympathomimetics include tachycardia, tremor, palpitations, anxiety, headache, anorexia, and insomnia. Serious rare side effects include dysrhythmias, cardiac muscle hypertrophy, myocardial infarction, or stroke (63).

Legality

- Because of its potential ergogenic effect, clenbuterol in all its forms and all oral β_2-agonists are banned by WADA and NCAA (8,9). Of note, oral clenbuterol and similar substances are classified by WADA as anabolic agents (8). Inhaled salbutamol, salmeterol formoterol, and vilanterol are allowed by WADA when used in accordance with manufacturer's recommendations and specific urinary concentrations are not to be exceeded. The NCAA allows inhaled β_2-adrenergic agonists with a prescription (9).

Table 76.1 Ergogenic Aids, Their Effect on Fitness Components, and Dangerous Side Effects

Product	Aerobic	Anaerobic	Strength	Body Composition	Psychological	Healing	Danger
Anabolic steroids	–	–	+	+	+	?	+
Androstenedione/DHEA	–	–	+	+	+	?	+
β2-agonist (clenbuterol)	?	–	–	?	?	–	?
Blood doping	+	–	–	–	–	–	++
Caffeine	+	+	–	–	?	–	–
Corticosteroids	–	–	–	–	–	?	?
Creatine	–	+	?	+	–	?	–
Ephedrine/amphetamines	+	+	+	+	+		++
Gene therapy	?	?	?	?	?	?	?
Growth hormone	–	–	–	+	–	–	?
NSAIDs	–	–	–	–	–	?	+

–, no effect; ?, unknown effect; +, positive effect; DHEA, dehydroepiandrosterone; NSAIDs, nonsteroidal anti-inflammatory drugs.

ERGOGENIC AIDS

- Specific ergogenic aids will be reviewed here regarding their efficacy, safety, and use in competition. Table 76.1 gives an overview of many ergogenic aids, their efficacy, and their safety.

Anabolic-Androgenic Steroids, Dehydroepiandrosterone, Androstenedione, and Other Testosterone Boosters

Efficacy

- Administration of anabolic-androgenic steroids increases muscle strength, lean body mass, endurance, and power in a dose-dependent fashion (7,64). The performance improvement gained by using steroids is enhanced by a progressive training program and an adequate diet.
- Androstenedione, a testosterone precursor, if taken at extremely high doses can increase both testosterone and estradiol, but studies have failed to demonstrate any significant change in lean body mass or strength (65–67).
- Dehydroepiandrosterone (DHEA) is an adrenal hormone precursor to both androgens and estrogens. DHEA levels peak in young adulthood and gradually fade as aging progresses. A randomized placebo-controlled study of DHEA (100 mg/d), androstenedione, or placebo in 40 trained male athletes showed no differences in fat-free mass and muscle mass between the two drug groups and the placebo group (67).
- DHEA did slightly increase testosterone in older women but not older men (68) Another study showed that DHEA did not appear to affect energy, protein metabolism, or testosterone levels in young males and does not appear to have an ergogenic effect (69)
- Selective androgen receptor modulators (SARMs) are nonsteroidal substances that were developed to bind steroids to androgen receptors in muscle and bone preferentially over receptors in genital tissue. The idea is that these molecules would improve muscle weakness and osteoporosis with less risk of worsening prostate diseases in men or causing virilization in women (70). SARMs have not been approved for use in humans in any country but are available via the internet (4).
- The use of estrogen blockers and aromatase inhibitors may increase testosterone slightly and limit the estrogenic side effects such as gynecomastia from exogenous testosterone use (71).
- Human chorionic gonadotropin (hCG) may increase athletes' testosterone levels while maintaining normal testosterone-to-epitestosterone levels, making it hard to detect (72).

Safety

- Anabolic steroids have an extensive list of reported side effects, mostly in case reports. Of note, steroids have been shown to significantly decrease high-density lipoprotein in both male and female users and increase low-density lipoprotein (73) However, no direct link has been established to increase CV mortality (74).
- Hemoglobin and hematocrit are increased due to testosterone though adverse clinical outcomes are limited to case reports (75)
- Gynecomastia occurs in men taking certain exogenous testosterone products due to the peripheral conversion of testosterone to estrogen. This is mitigated by taking estrogen blockers or aromatase inhibitors or using testosterone products that have certain modifications that prevent peripheral conversion (71).
- Exogenous testosterone use in men suppresses endogenous gonadotropin and testosterone and causes testicular atrophy and infertility. Normal function returns within 4–12 months after discontinuation (76,77).

- Other side effects include acne and female masculinization — alopecia, hirsutism, clitoromegaly, and deepening of the voice. The deepening of the voice is irreversible (78).
- A survey of anabolic steroid users showed increases in the incidence of mood disorders and in aggression (79), though other controlled studies showed little or no variance (80).
- Prolonged use of high doses of androgens (principally the 17-α alkyl-androgens) has been associated with development of hepatic adenomas, hepatocellular carcinoma, and peliosis hepatis — all potentially life-threatening complications.

Legality

- Anabolic steroids are DEA Schedule III controlled substances. Legal indications to prescribe steroids include a confirmed diagnosis of hypogonadism and the presence of associated symptoms.[81]
- Anabolic steroids, DHEA, androstenedione, hCG, estrogen blockers, aromatase inhibitors, SARMs, and masking agents are banned by WADA and the NCAA (8,9). Athletes with certain medical conditions requiring androgen replacement therapy (*e.g.*, bilateral orchiectomy for testicular cancer treatment) may apply for a TUE (8,9,82).

Growth Hormone and Insulin-Like Growth Factor

Efficacy

- Growth hormone (GH) is secreted by the hypothalamus and is important in the growth and development of normal bones and muscle.
- GH has been shown to decrease fat mass, increase lean mass, and, in one randomized trial, improve sprint capacity but no other performance factors (83). This effect was increased with coadministration of testosterone. Other studies have likewise shown increases in lean muscle mass and decrease in fat but no increases in strength or endurance (84,85).
- Insulin-like growth factor (IGF-1) is often administered with short-acting insulin because of purported anabolic effects on muscle and similar effects as GH on increasing lean body mass and decreasing adipose tissue (86). This effect has not yet been proven.
- Although there are myocardial receptors for GH, administration of recombinant human GH did not affect CV performance as measured by left ventricular ejection fraction, heart rate, or blood pressure in seven normal male volunteers (87).
- In summary, GH and IGF-1 appear to increase lean body mass and decrease body fat, but the only performance improvement documented to date is in sprint capacity.

Safety

- Long-term human GH doping will probably result in the symptoms of acromegaly: sodium and fluid retention, hypertension, and an increased risk of insulin resistance and resulting hyperglycemia. Other risks include premature epiphyseal closure, cardiomegaly, and myopathy (86).
- IGF-1 and insulin usage can lead to hypoglycemia, so many athletes ingest copious amounts of sugars to prevent this (88).

Legality

- GH and IGF are banned by WADA and the NCAA, and insulin is banned by WADA. An athlete with a legitimate medical need may obtain a TUE.

Blood Doping and Erythropoietin

Efficacy

- Blood doping refers to the process of artificially increasing red blood cell (RBC) mass to improve exercise performance. RBC mass can be increased by infusion of RBCs by homologous or autologous transfusions or using recombinant erythropoietin (rEPO) to stimulate RBC production (89).
- Increasing the RBC mass improves oxygen-carrying capacity with a resultant increase in maximal aerobic power, aerobic capacity, and exercise tolerance. The increased O_{2max} and time to exhaustion enables improvements in race performance, especially in distance runners and cyclists (90).
- Blood doping also helps performance in the heat, especially in acclimatized individuals (90).

Safety

- Although rare, the major risk from blood transfusions is transfusion reactions. Other complications include infection from the blood or procedure.
- Major risks associated with abnormally high hemoglobin and hematocrit levels include myocardial infarction, stroke, and thromboembolic disease (89). Deaths among cyclists have been attributed to rEPO-induced hyperviscosity, causing vascular sludging and myocardial artery occlusion (90,91).
- Blood pressure may also be increased by rEPO and is contraindicated in uncontrolled hypertension (89).

Legality

- Blood doping, rEPO, and other methods of manipulating blood and blood components are banned by WADA and NCAA (8,9).
- Autologous blood transfusions are exceedingly difficult to detect and other methods like monitoring hemoglobin and hematocrit levels to look for sudden increases can be used. Homologous blood transfusions are easy to detect (90). Erythropoietin isoforms can be measured directly from blood testing and in the urine, but because rEPO currently can only be detected for a few days after administration but has effects that last for weeks, reliable testing is difficult (89).

Caffeine, Guarana, and Energy Drinks

Efficacy

- Caffeine has been shown to enhance muscle endurance, muscle strength, anaerobic power, and aerobic endurance performance (92). Caffeine ingestion improved exercise capacity in short duration, high intensity exercise lasting 1–5 minutes, sustained high intensity training lasting 20 minutes to an hour, and during prolonged submaximal exercise lasting over 90 minutes.

- During resistance exercise, caffeine supplementation increases movement velocity in both the upper and lower body, suggesting that caffeine is beneficial for weightlifting, throwing, and jumping sports, and other activities that rely on powerful movement (93).
- Caffeine's effectiveness as an ergogenic aid has not been shown for single-event high-intensity sports such as discus throwing, weightlifting, sprinting, or jumping (94).
- The dosage of caffeine needed to have an ergogenic effect range from 1 to 6 mg/kg and habitual use does not decrease its effect (95). The response to caffeine varies widely as do the development of side effects, and there may be genetic variation in its effectiveness (96).
- Caffeine is rapidly absorbed and equally effective whether ingested as pill, liquid, or gum, though chewing gum with its oral mucosa absorption may be the quickest (97).
- Guarana's active ingredients include guaranine, which is chemically identical to caffeine, while primary active ingredient in energy drinks is also caffeine, with the amount being highly variable (98). There is currently no data that show guarana or energy drinks have an ergogenic effect above that of the caffeine content.

Safety

- Caffeine does not appear to increase risk for heatstroke or compromise CV activity in endurance performance (99), nor cause dehydration (100,101).
- There is wide variation in side effects from caffeine with some individuals being highly susceptible to irritability, diarrhea, insomnia, restlessness, tremor, and anxiety (102).
- Most observational studies show an inverse relationship between coffee consumption and all-cause mortality as well as CV mortality (103).

Legality

- Caffeine is no longer banned by WADA and the IOC (8). However, the NCAA still has a cutoff for caffeine at 15 μg/mL urine concentration, which is roughly two cups of coffee ingested just prior to testing (9). Caffeine concentrations in urine vary based on amount ingested (in milligrams), body size, metabolic rate, and other factors.

Creatine

Efficacy

- Creatine is a naturally occurring organic acid stored in skeletal muscle predominantly as the phosphocreatine form. Phosphocreatine is a source of phosphate for the rapid resynthesis of adenosine triphosphate, which muscles rely on for energy during short-duration, high-intensity exercise. Creatine supplementation increases the rate of phosphocreatine resynthesis during recovery between high intensity exercise bouts, thereby enhancing recovery and performance (104). In addition, creatine may have direct cellular effects via upregulation of genes and increased activity of enzymes involved in protein synthesis and other activities with anabolic effects (105).
- Creatine has been shown to be effective at improving training and performance of short-duration, high-intensity exercise. In young men and women, it has been shown to increase strength, power, maximum weight anaerobic, and aerobic performance (106–108).
- Creatine has not been shown to be beneficial in endurance events (109).
- Creatine supplementation may increase mass with most weight gain postulated to be from fluid retention. The increased body water appears to aid thermoregulation and creatine may be beneficial when exercising in hot, humid conditions (110).
- As in any supplement, some people do not respond to creatine supplementation.

Safety

- Concerns that increased uptake of water by muscle may hinder heat tolerance and hydration status or that metabolism of creatine by the kidneys may result in kidney damage have not been supported by controlled trials (110,111). Creatine supplementation does not have any proven long-term adverse effects and appears safe (112).

Legality

- The use of creatine by athletes is allowed by WADA and the NCAA. The latter organization did ban the purchase and dispersal of this supplement to athletes by its affiliated universities and university employees (*i.e.*, coaches and athletic trainers) (8,9).

Ephedra, Pseudoephedrine, and Amphetamines

Efficacy

- Ephedra, pseudoephedrine, and amphetamines are stimulants that are used by athletes to try to improve performance by increasing alertness, improving concentration, and promoting weight loss (113). Studies are generally lacking to confirm ergogenic effects.
- *Ephedra sinica*, a.k.a. Ma Huang, is a plant that contains alkaloids that are used as a supplement to promote alertness, endurance, and strength even though no studies have demonstrated a positive performance effect by themselves (114). Ephedra and its derivatives ephedrine, pseudoephedrine, and phenylpropanolamine are sympathomimetic amines and are used as stimulants, appetite suppressants, and decongestants.
- Ephedrine and pseudoephedrine, and phenylalanine when used alone, do not seem to have an ergogenic effect (115–117). However, ephedra in combination with caffeine has been shown to improve time to exhaustion during exercise

tests probably through its central nervous system effects as no changes were seen in VO_{2max} or other physiologic performance parameters (118–120).

- Amphetamines are used by athletes to increase alertness and concentration (121).
- Methylphenidate likewise is used illicitly by athletes to improve alertness (122).
- Amphetamines act as appetite suppressants.

Safety

- Ephedrine was banned as a diet aid due to the increased risk of heart attack and stroke (113).
- Deaths have been associated with the use of these drugs due to myocardial infarctions, arrhythmias, cerebrovascular accidents, and heat stroke (123). Other problems include seizures, arrhythmias, hypertension, and vomiting.
- Amphetamine and its derivatives are DEA Schedule II drugs and are considered potentially addicting with chronic use.

Legality

- Amphetamines are banned by both WADA and NCAA (8,9). Although amphetamines are prohibited, dextroamphetamine and methylphenidate may be granted a TUE for prescription use for treatment of some conditions including attention deficit hyperactivity disorder.
- Ephedrine is illegal as a food supplement in the United States (113). It is banned by the NCAA; WADA allows a small amount and is monitored by urine concentration (8,9).
- Pseudoephedrine is allowed in Olympic competition in small amounts and may be monitored by urine concentration (8). It is allowed by the NCAA (9). Because of their potential to be used in the manufacture of methamphetamine, pseudoephedrine was regulated in the United States by the Combat Methamphetamine Epidemic Act of 2005 and has limits on daily sales, 30-day purchases, and other restrictions regarding their sale (124).
- WADA allows epinephrine (adrenaline) for local administration (e.g., nasal, ophthalmologic, or coadministration with local anesthetic) and is monitored by urine concentration (8). Epinephrine needs a medical exception for the NCAA (10).

Gene Therapy

Efficacy

- The human genetic code is complex and many disease risks as well as performance characteristics are contained in the mitochondrial genome, nuclear genome, and microbial metagenome (125). There are three broad categories of genetic therapies: use of a new exogenous gene for bulk replacement of affected genetic compartments, addition of exogenous genetic material to compensate for genetic errors, and correction of genetic errors using gene editing.
- Genetic therapies have been studied in animal models that can increase blood oxygen carrying capacity of the blood through various means including increased production of erythropoietin, vascular endothelial factor, and other angiogenic factors (126). Additional genetic therapies are being studied, which can increase strength through stimulation of muscle fibers, IGF, and inactivation of myostatin (127–130).
- Cell gene therapies that use viral vectors to infect human somatic cells and transfer genetic material have been developed. These can be cultured ex vivo and rapidly developed to include in vivo applications to produce specific effects (125).
- Clustered regularly interspaced short palindromic repeats (CRISPR)/CRISPR-associated protein 9 gene editing technology is one of the therapies that may be able to treat diseases by permanently correcting deleterious base mutations or disrupting disease-causing genes with great precision and efficiency (131). Similarly, this process could be used to insert specific performance-enhancing genes or adjust performance-limiting genes. However, there are challenges in effectively delivering the CRISPR system to cells in vivo, resulting in slow development and FDA approval for CRISPR therapies, two are on the near-term horizon for sickle cell disease and beta thalassemia.
- Genetic therapies being investigated in animal models for increasing muscle size and strength are primarily designed to inhibit the myostatin gene. Myostatin is a regulator of myocytes limiting the number and growth of myocytes (132). Myostatin inhibitors and antagonists have been encoded into viral DNA and in animal studies results in significantly increased size and strength of hind limb and fore limb skeletal muscles, which persists for more than 2 years. These results held true for both young and middle-aged animals (133). The myostatin inhibitors include myostatin binding proteins like follistatin and myostatin antibodies like domagrozumab.

Safety

- Manipulating the human genome to correct, prevent, or eliminate disease has an enormous potential for genetic therapy. However, there are risks that include damaging the DNA in the wrong place, which could cause tumors or other errors, targeting the wrong cells, vector mutation, which may induce disease, and an unwanted immune reaction from the host.

Legality

- Gene doping is prohibited by WADA and the NCAA (8,9). WADA defines gene doping as “the use of nucleic acids or nucleic acid analogues that may alter genome sequences and/or alter gene expression by any mechanism. This includes but is not limited to gene editing, gene silencing and gene transfer technologies.” It also includes “the use of normal or genetically modified cells.”
- Myostatin inhibitors and related substances are likewise prohibited under the WADA category hormone and metabolic modulators (8).

REFERENCES

1. Glade MJ. The dietary supplement health and education act of 1994—focus on labeling issues. *Nutrition.* 1997;13(11-12):999–1001.
2. Butterfield G. Ergogenic aids: evaluating sport nutrition products. *Int J Sport Nutr.* 1996;6(2):191–7.
3. Cohen PA, Sharfstein J, Kamugisha A, Vanhee C. Analysis of ingredients of supplements in the national institutes of health supplement database marketed as containing a novel alternative to anabolic steroids. *JAMA Netw Open.* 2020;3(4):e202818.
4. Van Wagoner RM, Eichner A, Bhasin S, Deuster PA, Eichner D. Chemical composition and labeling of substances marketed as selective androgen receptor modulators and sold via the internet. *JAMA.* 2017;318(20):2004–10.
5. Newsholme P, Krause M, Newsholme EA, Stear SJ, Burke LM, Castell LM. BJSM reviews: A to Z of nutritional supplements — dietary supplements, sports nutrition foods and ergogenic aids for health and performance — part 18. *Br J Sports Med.* 2011;45(3):230–2.
6. Ortega Á, Salazar J, Galban N, et al. Psycho-neuro-endocrine-immunological basis of the placebo effect: potential applications beyond pain therapy. *Int J Mol Sci.* 2022 Apr 11;23(8):4196. doi:10.3390/ijms23084196
7. Bhasin S, Hatfield DL, Hoffman JR, et al. Anabolic-androgenic steroid use in sports, health, and society. *Med Sci Sports Exerc* 53(8):p 1778–94, Aug 2021. doi: 10.1249/MSS.0000000000002670
8. World Anti-doping Association Banned List 2023. https://www.wada-ama.org/en/resources/world-anti-doping-program/prohibited-list
9. National Collegiate Athletic Association Banned List 2023. https://www.ncaa.org/sports/2015/6/10/ncaa-banned-substances.aspx
10. Axis 2023. https://axis.drugfreesport.com/
11. United States Anti-Doping Agency (USADA). https://www.usada.org/athletes/testing/tue/for2023. https://www.usada.org/athletes/testing/tue/for2023.
12. Global Drug Reference Online (Global DRO. https://www.globaldro.com/home/indexfor2023. https://www.globaldro.com/home/indexfor2023.)
13. Chou R, McDonagh MS, Nakamoto E, Griffin J. Analgesics for osteoarthritis: an update of the 2006 comparative effectiveness review. *[Internet].* Rockville (MD): Agency for Healthcare Research and Quality (US); 2011 October Report No. 11(12)-EHC076-EF.
14. Mehallo CJ, Drezner JA, Bytomski JR. Practical management: nonsteroidal anti-inflammatory drug (NSAID) use in athletic injuries. *Clin J Sport Med.* 2006;16(2):170–4.
15. Massey T, Derry S, Moore RA, McQuay HJ. Topical NSAIDs for acute pain in adults. *Cochrane Database Syst Rev.* 2010 Jun 16(6):CD007402. Update in: *Cochrane Database Syst Rev.* 2015;6:CD007402. doi:10.1002/14651858.CD007402.pub2
16. Woo WW, Man SY, Lam PK, Rainer TH. Randomized double-blind trial comparing oral paracetamol and oral nonsteroidal anti-inflammatory drugs for treating pain after musculoskeletal injury. *Ann Emerg Med.* 2005;46(4):352–61.
17. Dimmen S, Engebretsen L, Nordsletten L, Madsen JE. Negative effects of parecoxib and indomethacin on tendon healing: an experimental study in rats. *Knee Surg Sports Traumatol Arthrosc.* 2009;17(7):835–9.
18. Schoen RT, Vender RJ. Mechanisms of nonsteroidal anti-inflammatory drug-induced gastric damage. *Am J Med.* 1989;86(4):449–58.
19. Laine L, Curtis SP, Cryer B, Kaur A, Cannon CP. Risk factors for NSAID-associated upper GI clinical events in a long-term prospective study of 34 701 arthritis patients. *Aliment Pharmacol Ther.* 2010;32(10):1240–8.
20. Hooper L, Brown TJ, Elliott R, Payne K, Roberts C, Symmons D. The effectiveness of five strategies for the prevention of gastrointestinal toxicity induced by non-steroidal anti-inflammatory drugs: systematic review. *BMJ.* 2004;329(7472):948.
21. Koch M, Dezi A, Ferrario F, Capurso I. Prevention of nonsteroidal anti-inflammatory drug-induced gastrointestinal mucosal injury. A meta-analysis of randomized controlled clinical trials. *Arch Intern Med.* 1996;156(20):2321–32.
22. Kelly JP, Kaufman DW, Jurgelon JM, Sheehan J, Koff RS, Shapiro S. Risk of aspirin-associated major upper-gastrointestinal bleeding with enteric-coated or buffered product. *Lancet.* 1996;348(9039):1413–16.
23. Coxib and traditional NSAID Trialists' CNT Collaboration, Bhala N, Emberson J, et al. Vascular and upper gastrointestinal effects of non-steroidal anti-inflammatory drugs: meta-analyses of individual participant data from randomised trials. *Lancet.* 2013;382(9894):769–79.
24. Nissen SE, Yeomans ND, Solomon DH, et al. Cardiovascular safety of celecoxib, naproxen, or ibuprofen for arthritis. *N Engl J Med.* 2016;375(26):2519–29.
25. Kiltz U, Zochling J, Schmidt WE, Braun J. Use of NSAIDs and infection with Helicobacter pylori — what does the rheumatologist need to know? *Rheumatology.* 2008;47(9):1342–7.
26. Perazella MA, Tray K. Selective cyclooxygenase-2 inhibitors: a pattern of nephrotoxicity similar to traditional nonsteroidal anti-inflammatory drugs. *Am J Med.* 2001;111(1):64–7.
27. Uhl RL, Roberts TT, Papaliodis DN, Mulligan MT, Dubin AH. Management of chronic musculoskeletal pain. *J Am Acad Orthop Surg.* 2014 Feb;22(2):101–10. doi:10.5435/JAAOS-22-02-101
28. Kroenke K, Krebs EE, Bair MJ. Pharmacotherapy of chronic pain: a synthesis of recommendations from systematic reviews. *Gen Hosp Psychiatry.* 2009 May–Jun;31(3):206–19. doi:10.1016/j.genhosppsych.2008.12.006
29. Cushman DM, Borowski L, Hansen C, Hendrick J, Bushman T, Teramoto M. Gabapentin and tricyclics in the treatment of post-concussive headache, a retrospective cohort study. *Headache.* 2019 Mar;59(3):371–82. doi:10.1111/head.13451
30. Alberti FF, Becker MW, Blatt CR, Ziegelmann PK, da Silva Dal Pizzol T, Pilger D. Comparative efficacy of amitriptyline, duloxetine and pregabalin for treating fibromyalgia in adults: an overview with network meta-analysis. *Clin Rheumatol.* 2022 Jul;41(7):1965–78. doi:10.1007/s10067-022-06129-8
31. Meng FY, Zhang LC, Liu Y, et al. Efficacy and safety of gabapentin for treatment of postherpetic neuralgia: a meta-analysis of randomized controlled trials. *Minerva Anestesiol.* 2014 May;80(5):556–67.
32. Toth C. Pregabalin: latest safety evidence and clinical implications for the management of neuropathic pain. *Ther Adv Drug Saf.* 2014 Feb;5(1):38–56. doi:10.1177/2042098613505614
33. Ferreira GE, Abdel-Shaheed C, Underwood M, et al. Efficacy, safety, and tolerability of antidepressants for pain in adults: overview of systematic reviews. *BMJ.* 2023 Feb 1;380:e072415. doi:10.1136/bmj-2022-072415
34. Ferreira GE, McLachlan AJ, Lin CWC, et al. Efficacy and safety of antidepressants for the treatment of back pain and osteoarthritis: systematic review and meta-analysis. *BMJ.* 2021 Jan 20;372:m4825. doi:10.1136/bmj.m4825
35. van den Driest JJ, Bierma-Zeinstra SMA, Bindels PJE, Schiphof D. Amitriptyline for musculoskeletal complaints: a systematic review. *Fam Pract.* 2017 Apr 1;34(2):138–46. doi:10.1093/fampra/cmw134
36. Ferguson JM. SSRI antidepressant medications: adverse effects and tolerability. *Prim Care Companion J Clin Psychiatry.* 2001 Feb;3(1):22–7. doi:10.4088/pcc.v03n0105

37. Santarsieri D, Schwartz TL. Antidepressant efficacy and side-effect burden: a quick guide for clinicians. *Drugs Context*. 2015 Oct 8;4:212290. doi:10.7573/dic.212290
38. Trindade E, Menon D, Topfer LA, Coloma C. Adverse effects associated with selective serotonin reuptake inhibitors and tricyclic antidepressants: a meta-analysis. *CMAJ (Can Med Assoc J)*. 1998 Nov 17;159(10):1245–52.
39. Hainline B, Derman W, Vernec A, et al. International Olympic Committee consensus statement on pain management in elite athletes. *Br J Sports Med*. 2017 Sep;51(17):1245–58. doi:10.1136/bjsports-2017-097884
40. Charlesworth J, Fitzpatrick J, Perera NKP, Orchard J. Osteoarthritis-a systematic review of long-term safety implications for osteoarthritis of the knee. *BMC Musculoskelet Disord*. 2019 Apr 9;20(1):151. doi:10.1186/s12891-019-2525-0
41. Deckey DG, Doan M, Hassebrock JD, et al. Prevalence of cannabinoid (CBD) use in orthopaedic sports medicine patients. *Orthop J Sports Med*. 2022 Apr 5;10(4):23259671221087629. doi:10.1177/23259671221087629
42. Naik H, Trojian TH. Therapeutic potential for cannabinoids in sports medicine: current literature review. *Curr Sports Med Rep*. 2021 Jul 1;20(7):345–50. doi:10.1249/JSR.0000000000000858
43. Maurer GE, Mathews NM, Schleich KT, Slayman TG, Marcussen BL. Understanding cannabis-based therapeutics in sports medicine. *Sports Health*. 2020 Nov/Dec;12(6):540–6. doi:10.1177/1941738120956604
44. Chou R, Pinto RZ, Fu R, et al. Systemic corticosteroids for radicular and non-radicular low back pain. *Cochrane Database Syst Rev*. 2022;10:CD012450.
45. Eskin B, Shih RD, Fiesseler FW, et al. Prednisone for emergency department low back pain: a randomized controlled trial. *J Emerg Med*. 2014;47(1):65–70.
46. Couppé C, Døssing S, Bülow PM, et al. Effects of heavy slow resistance training combined with corticosteroid injections or tendon needling in patients with lateral elbow tendinopathy: a 3-arm randomized double-blinded placebo-controlled study. *Am J Sports Med*. 2022;50(10):2787–96.
47. Olaussen M, Holmedal O, Lindbaek M, Brage S, Solvang H. Treating lateral epicondylitis with corticosteroid injections or non-electrotherapeutical physiotherapy: a systematic review. *BMJ Open*. 2013;3(10):e003564.
48. Smidt N, Assendelft WJ, van der Windt DAWM, Hay EM, Buchbinder R, Bouter LM. Corticosteroid injections for lateral epicondylitis: a systematic review. *Pain*. 2002;96(1–2):23–40.
49. Coombes BK, Bisset L, Brooks P, Khan A, Vicenzino B. Effect of corticosteroid injection, physiotherapy, or both on clinical outcomes in patients with unilateral lateral epicondylalgia: a randomized controlled trial. *JAMA*. 2013;309(5):461–9.
50. Peters-Veluthamaningal C, van der Windt DAWM, Winters JC, Meyboom-de Jong B. Corticosteroid injection for trigger finger in adults. *Cochrane Database Syst Rev*. 2009;2009(1):CD005617.
51. Green S, Buchbinder R, Glazier R, Forbes A. Interventions for shoulder pain. *Cochrane Database Syst Rev*. 2000;2:CD001156.
52. Vecchio PC, Hazleman BL, King RH. A double blind trial comparing subacromial methylprednisolone and lignocaine in acute rotator cuff tendinitis. *Br J Rheumatol*. 1993;32(8):743–5.
53. Buchbinder R, Green S, Youd JM. Corticosteroid injections for shoulder pain. *Cochrane Database Syst Rev*. 2003;2003(1):CD004016.
54. Faber E, Kuiper JI, Burdorf A, Miedema HS, Verhaar JAN. Treatment of impingement syndrome: a systematic review of the effects on functional limitations and return to work. *J Occup Rehabil*. 2006;16(1):7–25.
55. Plafki C, Steffen R, Willburger RE, Wittenberg RH. Local anaesthetic injection with and without corticosteroids for subacromial impingement syndrome. *Int Orthop*. 2000;24(1):40–2.
56. Speed CA. Fortnightly review: corticosteroid injections in tendon lesions. *BMJ*. 2001;323(7309):382–6.
57. Gottlieb NL, Riskin WG. Complications of local corticosteroid injections. *JAMA*. 1980;243(15):1547–8.
58. Pluim BM, de Hon O, Staal JB, et al. β_2-Agonists and physical performance: a systematic review and meta-analysis of randomized controlled trials. *Sports Med*. 2011;41(1):39–57.
59. Riiser A, Stensrud T, Stang J, Andersen LB. Aerobic performance among healthy (non-asthmatic) adults using beta2-agonists: a systematic review and meta-analysis of randomised controlled trials. *Br J Sports Med*. 2021;55(17):975–83.
60. Guddat S, Fußhöller G, Geyer H, et al. Clenbuterol - regional food contamination a possible source for inadvertent doping in sports. *Drug Test Anal*. 2012;4(6):534–8.
61. Kamalakkannan G, Petrilli CM, George I, et al. Clenbuterol increases lean muscle mass but not endurance in patients with chronic heart failure. *J Heart Lung Transplant*. 2008;27(4):457–61.
62. Prather ID, Brown DE, North P, Wilson JR. Clenbuterol: a substitute for anabolic steroids?. *Med Sci Sports Exerc*. 1995;27(8):1118–21.
63. Davis E, Loiacono R, Summers RJ. The rush to adrenaline: drugs in sport acting on the beta-adrenergic system. *Br J Pharmacol*. 2008;154(3):584–97.
64. Bhasin S, Storer TW, Berman N, et al. The effects of supraphysiologic doses of testosterone on muscle size and strength in normal men. *N Engl J Med*. 1996;335:1–7.
65. Broeder CE, Quindry J, Brittingham K, et al. The Andro Project: physiological and hormonal influences of androstenedione supplementation in men 35 to 65 years old participating in a high-intensity resistance training program. *Arch Intern Med*. 2000;160(20):3093–104.
66. King DS, Sharp RL, Vukovich MD, et al. Effect of oral androstenedione on serum testosterone and adaptations to resistance training in young men: a randomized controlled trial. *JAMA*. 1999;281(21):2020–8.
67. Wallace MB, Lim J, Cutler A, Bucci L. Effects of dehydroepiandrosterone vs. androstenedione supplementation in men. *Med Sci Sports Exerc*. 1999;31(12):1788–92.
68. Morales AJ, Haubrich RH, Hwang JY, Asakura H, Yen SS. The effect of six months treatment with a 100 mg daily dose of dehydroepiandrosterone (DHEA) on circulating sex steroids, body composition and muscle strength in age-advanced men and women. *Clin Endocrinol*. 1998;49(4):421–32.
69. Welle S, Jozefowicz R, Statt M. Failure of dehydroepiandrosterone to influence energy and protein metabolism in humans. *J Clin Endocrinol Metab*. 1990;71(5):1259–64.
70. Gao W, Kim J, Dalton JT. Pharmacokinetics and pharmacodynamics of nonsteroidal androgen receptor ligands. *Pharm Res*. 2006;23(8):1641–58.
71. Handelsman DJ. Indirect androgen doping by oestrogen blockade in sports. *Br J Pharmacol*. 2008;154(3):598–605.
72. Handelsman DJ. Clinical review: the rationale for banning human chorionic gonadotropin and estrogen blockers in sport. *J Clin Endocrinol Metab*. 2006;91(5):1646–53.
73. Thompson PD, Cullinane EM, Sady SP, et al. Contrasting effects of testosterone and stanozolol on serum lipoprotein levels. *JAMA*. 1989;261(8):1165–8.
74. Payne JR, Kotwinski PJ, Montgomery HE. Cardiac effects of anabolic steroids. *Heart*. 2004;90(5):473–5.
75. Stergiopoulos K, Brennan JJ, Mathews R, Setaro JF, Kort S. Anabolic steroids, acute myocardial infarction and polycythemia: a case report and review of the literature. *Vasc Health Risk Manag*. 2008;4(6):1475–80.
76. Gazvani MR, Buckett W, Luckas MJ, Aird IA, Hipkin LJ, Lewis-Jones DI. Conservative management of azoospermia following steroid abuse. *Hum Reprod*. 1997;12(8):1706–8.

77. Knuth UA, Maniera H, Nieschlag E. Anabolic steroids and semen parameters in bodybuilders. *Fertil Steril.* 1989;52(6):1041–7.
78. Pope HG Jr, Wood RI, Rogol A, Nyberg F, Bowers L, Bhasin S. Adverse health consequences of performance-enhancing drugs: an Endocrine Society scientific statement. *Endocr Rev.* 2014;35(3):341–75.
79. Pope HG Jr, Katz DL. Psychiatric and medical effects of anabolic-androgenic steroid use. A controlled study of 160 athletes. *Arch Gen Psychiatry.* 1994;51(5):375–82.
80. Pope HG Jr, Kouri EM, Hudson JI. Effects of supraphysiologic doses of testosterone on mood and aggression in normal men: a randomized controlled trial. *Arch Gen Psychiatry.* 2000;57(2):133–56.
81. U.S. Food and Drug Administration. *Testosterone information* [cited 2025 Feb 28]. Available from: https://www.fda.gov/drugs/postmarket-drug-safety-information-patients-and-providers/testosterone-information.
82. Bhasin S, Brito JP, Cunningham GR, et al. Testosterone therapy in men with hypogonadism: an endocrine society clinical practice guideline. *J Clin Endocrinol Metab.* 2018 May 1;103(5):1715–44. doi:10.1210/jc.2018-00229
83. Meinhardt U, Nelson AE, Hansen JL, et al. The effects of growth hormone on body composition and physical performance in recreational athletes: a randomized trial. *Ann Intern Med.* 2010;152(9):568–77.
84. Berggren A, Ehrnborg C, Rosén T, Ellegård L, Bengtsson BA, Caidahl K. Short-term administration of supraphysiological recombinant human growth hormone (GH) does not increase maximum endurance exercise capacity in healthy, active young men and women with normal GH-insulin-like growth factor I axes. *J Clin Endocrinol Metab.* 2005;90(6):3268–73.
85. Yarasheski KE, Campbell JA, Smith K, Rennie MJ, Holloszy JO, Bier DM. Effect of growth hormone and resistance exercise on muscle growth in young men. *Am J Physiol.* 1992;262(3 Pt 1):E261–7.
86. Holt RI, Sönksen PH. Growth hormone, IGF-I and insulin and their abuse in sport. *Br J Pharmacol.* 2008;154(3):542–56.
87. Bisi G, Podio V, Valetto MR, et al. Acute cardiovascular and hormonal effects of GH and hexarelin, a synthetic GH-releasing peptide, in humans. *J Endocrinol Investig.* 1999;22(4):266–72.
88. Rich JD, Dickinson BP, Merriman NA, Thule PM. Insulin use by bodybuilders. *JAMA.* 1998;279(20):1613.
89. Elliott S. Erythropoiesis-stimulating agents and other methods to enhance oxygen transport. *Br J Pharmacol.* 2008 Jun;154(3):529–41. doi:10.1038/bjp.2008.89
90. Sawka MN, Joyner MJ, Miles DS, Robertson RJ, Spriet LL, Young AJ. American College of Sports Medicine position stand. The use of blood doping as an ergogenic aid. *Med Sci Sports Exerc.* 1996;28(6):i–viii.
91. Eichner ER. Sports anemia, iron supplements, and blood doping. *Med Sci Sports Exerc.* 1992;24(9 suppl):S315–18.
92. Grgic J, Grgic I, Pickering C, Schoenfeld BJ, Bishop DJ, Pedisic Z. Wake up and smell the coffee: caffeine supplementation and exercise performance-an umbrella review of 21 published meta-analyses. *Br J Sports Med.* 2020;54(11):681–8.
93. Raya-González J, Rendo-Urteaga T, Domínguez R, Castillo D, Rodríguez-Fernández A, Grgic J. Acute effects of caffeine supplementation on movement velocity in resistance exercise: a systematic review and meta-analysis. *Sports Med.* 2020;50(4):717–29.
94. Bellar DM, Kamimori G, Judge L, et al. Effects of low-dose caffeine supplementation on early morning performance in the standing shot put throw. *Eur J Sport Sci.* 2012;12:57.
95. Carvalho A, Marticorena FM, Grecco BH, Barreto G, Saunders B. Can I have my coffee and drink it? A systematic review and meta-analysis to determine whether habitual caffeine consumption affects the ergogenic effect of caffeine. *Sports Med.* 2022 Sep;52(9):2209–20. doi:10.1007/s40279-022-01685-0
96. Guest N, Corey P, Vescovi J, El-Sohemy A. Caffeine, CYP1A2 genotype, and endurance performance in athletes. *Med Sci Sports Exerc.* 2018;50(8):1570–8.
97. Institute of Medicine (US) Committee on Military Nutrition Research. *Caffeine for the Sustainment of Mental Task Performance: Formulations for Military Operations.* Washington (DC): National Academies Press (US); 2001. 2. Pharmacology of Caffeine.
98. Higgins JP, Tuttle TD, Higgins CL. Energy beverages: content and safety. *Mayo Clin Proc.* 2010;85(11):1033–41.
99. Naulleau C, Jeker D, Pancrate T, et al. Effect of pre-exercise caffeine intake on endurance performance and core temperature regulation during exercise in the heat: a systematic review with meta-analysis. *Sports Med.* 2022;52(10):2431–45.
100. Killer SC, Blannin AK, Jeukendrup AE. No evidence of dehydration with moderate daily coffee intake: a counterbalanced cross-over study in a free-living population. *PLoS One.* 2014;9(1):e84154.
101. Maughan RJ, Griffin J. Caffeine ingestion and fluid balance: a review. *J Hum Nutr Diet.* 2003;16(6):411–20.
102. Gunja N, Brown JA. Energy drinks: health risks and toxicity. *Med J Aust.* 2012;196(1):46–9.
103. Crippa A, Discacciati A, Larsson SC, Wolk A, Orsini N. Coffee consumption and mortality from all causes, cardiovascular disease, and cancer: a dose-response meta-analysis. *Am J Epidemiol.* 2014;180(8):763–75.
104. Graham AS, Hatton RC. Creatine: a review of efficacy and safety. *J Am Pharm Assoc (Wash).* 1999;39(6):803–77.
105. Safdar A, Yardley NJ, Snow R, Melov S, Tarnopolsky MA. Global and targeted gene expression and protein content in skeletal muscle of young men following short-term creatine monohydrate supplementation. *Physiol Genomics.* 2008;32(2):219–28.
106. Dempsey RL, Mazzone MF, Meurer LN. Does oral creatine supplementation improve strength? A meta-analysis. *J Fam Pract.* 2002;51(11):945–51.
107. Eckerson JM. Creatine as an ergogenic aid for female athletes. *Strength Cond J.* 2016;38:14.
108. Kendall KL, Smith AE, Graef JL, et al. Effects of four weeks of high-intensity interval training and creatine supplementation on critical power and anaerobic working capacity in college-aged men. *J Strength Cond Res.* 2009;23(6):1663–9.
109. Fernández-Landa J, Santibañez-Gutierrez A, Todorovic N, Stajer V, Ostojic SM. Effects of creatine monohydrate on endurance performance in a trained population: a systematic review and meta-analysis. *Sports Med.* 2023 May;53(5):1017–27. doi:10.1007/s40279-023-01823-2
110. Poortmans JR, Francaux M. Long-term oral creatine supplementation does not impair renal function in healthy athletes. *Med Sci Sports Exerc.* 1999 Aug;31(8):1108–10. doi:10.1097/00005768-199908000-00005
111. Lopez RM, Casa DJ, McDermott BP, Ganio MS, Armstrong LE, Maresh CM. Does creatine supplementation hinder exercise heat tolerance or hydration status? A systematic review with meta-analyses. *J Athl Train.* 2009;44(2):215–23.
112. Bizzarini E, De Angelis L. Is the use of oral creatine supplementation safe? *J Sports Med Phys Fitness.* 2004;44(4):411–6.
113. Eichner ER. Stimulants in sports. *Curr Sports Med Rep.* 2008;7(5):244–5.
114. Bergeron MF, Senchina DS, Burke LM, Stear SJ, Castell LM. A-Z of nutritional supplements: dietary supplements, sports nutrition foods

and ergogenic aids for health and performance—Part 13. *Br J Sports Med.* 2010 Oct;44(13):985–6. doi:10.1136/bjsm.2010.078394
115. Gillies H, Derman WE, Noakes TD, Smith P, Evans A, Gabriels G. Pseudoephedrine is without ergogenic effects during prolonged exercise. *J Appl Physiol.* 1996;81(6):2611–7.
116. Sidney KH, Lefcoe NM. The effects of ephedrine on the physiological and psychological responses to submaximal and maximal exercise in man. *Med Sci Sports.* 1977;9(2):95–9.
117. Swain RA, Harsha DM, Baenziger J, Saywell RM Jr. Do pseudoephedrine or phenylpropanolamine improve maximum oxygen uptake and time to exhaustion?. *Clin J Sport Med.* 1997;7(3):168–73.
118. Bell DG, Jacobs I. Combined caffeine and ephedrine ingestion improves run times of Canadian Forces Warrior Test. *Aviat Space Environ Med.* 1999;70(4):325–9.
119. Bell DG, Jacobs I, McLellan TM, Zamecnik J. Reducing the dose of combined caffeine and ephedrine preserves the ergogenic effect. *Aviat Space Environ Med.* 2000;71(4):415–9.
120. Bell DG, Jacobs I, Zamecnik J. Effects of caffeine, ephedrine, and their combination on time to exhaustion during high-intensity exercise. *Eur J Appl Physiol Occup Physiol.* 1998;77(5):427–33.
121. Bailey JA, Averbuch RN, Gold MS. Cosmetic psychiatry. *Dir Psychiatr.* 2009;29:1.
122. Lardon MT. Performance-enhancing drugs: where should the line be drawn and by whom? *Psychiatry (Edgmont).* 2008;5(7):58–61.
123. Haller CA, Benowitz NL. Adverse cardiovascular and central nervous system events associated with dietary supplements containing ephedra alkaloids. *N Engl J Med.* 2000;343(25):1833–8.
124. Combat Methamphetamine Epidemic Act of 2005 (CMEA) [Internet]. United States Department of Justice; [cited 2011 Jan 8]. Available from: http://www.deadiversion.usdoj.gov/meth/index.html
125. Roth TL, Marson A. Genetic disease and therapy. *Annu Rev Pathol.* 2021 Jan 24;16:145–66. doi:10.1146/annurev-pathmechdis-012419-032626
126. Rivera VM, Gao GP, Grant RL, et al. Long-term pharmacologically regulated expression of erythropoietin in primates following AAV-mediated gene transfer. *Blood.* 2005;105(4):1424–30.
127. Battery L, Solomon A, Gould D. Gene doping: Olympic genes for Olympic dreams. *J R Soc Med.* 2011;104(12):494–500.
128. Brzeziańska E, Domańska D, Jegier A. Gene doping in sport — perspectives and risks. *Biol Sport.* 2014;31(4):251–9. doi:10.5604/20831862.1120931
129. Diamanti-Kandarakis E, Konstantinopoulos PA, Papailiou J, Kandarakis SA, Andreopoulos A, Sykiotis GP. Erythropoietin abuse and erythropoietin gene doping: detection strategies in the genomic era. *Sports Med.* 2005;35(10):831–40.
130. Wells DJ. Gene doping: possibilities and practicalities. *Med Sport Sci.* 2009;54:166–75.
131. Li T, Yang Y, Qi H, et al. CRISPR/Cas9 therapeutics: progress and prospects. *Signal Transduct Target Ther.* 2023 Jan 16;8(1):36. doi:10.1038/s41392-023-01309-7
132. Lee SJ. Regulation of muscle mass by myostatin. *Annu Rev Cell Dev Biol.* 2004;20:61–86.
133. Haidet AM, Rizo L, Handy C, et al. Long-term enhancement of skeletal muscle mass and strength by single gene administration of myostatin inhibitors. *Proc Natl Acad Sci USA.* 2008 March 18;105(11):4318–22.

77 Prolotherapy

Aeneas Janze

INTRODUCTION

- Overuse injuries remain a constant challenge for the sports medicine physician. Injuries such as chronic tendinopathies are traditionally treated with corticosteroids or nonsteroidal anti-inflammatory drugs (NSAIDs), although it has been decades since Puddu et al. (1) demonstrated that tendinosis is not an inflammatory condition. Most investigations demonstrate that such treatments provide at best a short-term decrease in pain. With growing concern of complications associated with corticosteroids and chronic NSAID use, the search for other treatment options continues (2).
- Proliferative therapies ("prolotherapy") are a subject of growing interest and research. Although not a new concept, prolotherapy is relatively new to the rigors of evidence-based medicine. As such, early research efforts were largely comprised case reports and had been subject to much skepticism. Over the past 10–15 years, however, a marked increase in quality studies in prolotherapy and regenerative medicine in general has begun to shift this viewpoint, and a growing number of physicians are beginning to incorporate prolotherapy and other regenerative techniques into their musculoskeletal practice.
- Prolotherapy is an injection technique that uses the body's own repair system for treatment of chronic musculoskeletal pain. It is a unique alternative to standard care that can be performed quickly in an outpatient setting. The theoretical basis and state of current evidence regarding prolotherapy are discussed in this chapter.

PROLOTHERAPY DEFINITIONS

- Injection of a solution that stimulates increased collagen formation to strengthen lax ligaments and improve joint stability (3,4)
- Injection of growth factors or growth factor stimulants that cause growth of normal cells or tissues (5,6)

The author would like to acknowledge the work of the first edition authors of the chapter on Prolotherapy, Drs. Keith Scorza and Manik Singh.

COMMON USES

- Commonly used for chronic musculoskeletal pain; most frequently used for chronic tendinopathies, chronic ligament pain, chronic neck and back pain, or any painful condition thought to arise secondary to ligamentous laxity and/or joint instability
- Growing interest in use for osteoarthritis (OA); may contribute to correcting instabilities that contribute to OA. There is emerging evidence that dextrose stimulates chondrocytes to regrow cartilage (see Dextrose section below).

HISTORICAL PERSPECTIVES

- Hippocratic treatises suggested the utilization of scar tissue to add stability to joints, advising the use of a "hot poker" as treatment for recurrent dislocating shoulders.
- During the 1800s, sclerosing agents were used for treatment of varicose veins, hemorrhoids, and nonsurgical hernias.
- Prolotherapy was first described in modern literature by Dr. Louis Schultz (7).
  - Injected sodium psylliate into painful temporomandibular joints (TMJs) and reported effectiveness for treatment of chronic pain
  - Performed animal studies revealing soft-tissue fibrosis within 4–6 days after injections, suggesting that agents might stabilize joints by tightening ligaments
- The term "prolotherapy" was popularized by Dr. George S. Hackett (3,4).
  - Theorized that chronic musculoskeletal pain was secondary to chronic laxity of ligaments and bone-tendon junctions
  - Used the term "prolotherapy" to simplify phrases such as fibroproliferative therapy, proliferant therapy, sclerotherapy, and regenerative injection therapy
  - Note: "Prolotherapy" and "sclerotherapy" have evolved into distinct treatment disciplines. Most current proliferants in prolotherapy aim to stimulate normal tissue growth for musculoskeletal treatments, while sclerotherapy utilizes sclerosing agents to address venous conditions such as varicose veins and hemangiomas.

  - The term "prolo" comes from the word "proliferative" meaning to produce new cells in rapid succession. Dr. Hackett considered prolotherapy the "rehabilitation of an incompetent structure by the generation of new cellular tissue."
  - Published works in 1953 describing the use of prolotherapy for treatment of chronic sacroiliac pain on 253 patients over a 14-year period (3)
- Over the past 20 years, the prevalence of physicians practicing prolotherapy as well as prolotherapy instruction in residency and fellowship curriculums has risen dramatically.
- A 2003 survey of osteopathic physicians identified 95 practitioners in the United States. Only 27% of the surveys were returned; therefore, the prevalence was likely greater (8).
- A 2003–2004 survey of 908 primary care patients using narcotic therapies for chronic musculoskeletal pain revealed that 8.3% of the patients had received prolotherapy treatments in the past, with 5.9% receiving treatment during the previous 12 months (9).
- A 2006 investigation of prolotherapy side effects identified 314 members of the American Academy of Orthopedic Medicine (AAOM) listed as performing prolotherapy in the member directory (10).
- At the 2023 annual International Association for Regenerative Therapy (IART) conference, a presentation by Dubey et al. revealed the preliminary results of a study that investigated the prevalence of prolotherapy instruction across all US residencies and fellowships that were likely to treat musculoskeletal issues such as Family Medicine, Orthopedic Surgery, Pain, Physical Medicine and Rehabilitation (PM&R), Rheumatology, Osteopathic Manipulative Medicine and Neuromusculoskeletal Medicine (OMM/NMM), and Sports Medicine, among others. The overall survey response rate was 47%. Out of the 853 programs that responded, 115 included prolotherapy in their curriculum. OMM/NMM had the highest prevalence of prolotherapy instruction (73.3%), followed by PM&R (38.6%), and Sports Medicine (31.0%) (11).

PROLOTHERAPY AGENTS

Chemical Agents

- Irritants
  - Examples: phenol, guaiacol, and tannic acid
  - Irritants contain a phenolic hydroxyl group that is oxidized to quinone-like derivatives. Such agents are thought to alkylate surface proteins of cells, either damaging the cell wall or making the cell antigenic. The end result is an initiation of an inflammatory cascade (12).
- Osmotics
  - Examples: dextrose, glycerin, and zinc sulfate
  - The theory is that a hyperosmolar injectant causes a net outflow of water from local cells inducing a controlled injury at the injection site. Dead or injured cells release cellular fragments and cytokines which cause an influx of inflammatory cells (macrophages and granulocytes) and initiate the wound healing cascade (12). Historically dextrose, glycerin, and zinc sulfate have presumptively been lumped together in this category despite a lack of evidence demonstrating osmotic stress to be their primary mechanism of action. Since glycerin and zinc sulfate are rarely used in current prolotherapy practice, research on their mechanism of action in the context of prolotherapy is scant. It has been clearly demonstrated however that osmotic stress is at best, an incomplete explanation for how dextrose induces a proliferative response (See Dextrose section below for more details on mechanism of action).
  - In a study examining the impact of proliferant solutions on rat Achilles tendons, three solutions of the same hyperosmolarity (1110 mOsm) were evaluated: 20% dextrose in water, a mix of 5% dextrose in water with NaCl, and a NaCl solution. After injections into the right Achilles tendon, with the left serving as a control, dextrose-injected tendons displayed significant increases in diameter and fibroblast count after 6 weeks. While the hypertonic saline group also had increases, it wasn't statistically significant. No statistically significant difference was observed between the two dextrose groups (13).
- Combined agents
  - Example: P2G (phenol-glycerin-glucose)
  - P2G is still used frequently enough that ongoing research continues to explore its mechanism of action, in addition to its possible irritant and osmotic effects.
  - A 2020 in vitro study on murine cells by Johnston et al. showed that P2G upregulates the cartilage cell proliferation enhancer cytokine fibroblast growth factor 2 (14).
- Chemotactics
  - Examples: Sodium morrhuate is the only agent in this class (included for historical purposes since it is no longer being manufactured).
  - Sodium morrhuate is a fatty salt derived from cod liver oil and is thought to undergo direct conversion into pro-inflammatory mediators such as prostaglandins, leukotrienes, and thromboxanes. Inflammation then triggers the wound healing cascade (12).
- Sclerosing agents
  - Examples: polidocanol, sodium psylliate (Sylnasol), sodium tetradecyl sulphate, and bleomycin
  - Though sclerosing agents were the first agents to be used for prolotherapy in the 1940s and 1950s, they are currently used much more frequently to treat venous issues such as varicose veins, hemangiomas, and vascular malformations and are rarely used as a proliferative agent in contemporary prolotherapy.
  - Most sclerosing agents work by causing endothelial destruction, which leads to inflammation and fibrosis (15).

  - In the first published study on sclerotherapy in 1937, Schultz noted soft-tissue fibrosis 4–6 days after injections of sodium psylliate into the TMJ followed by joint stabilization (7).
  - Hackett injected Sylnasol (5% sodium salts of several fatty acids of psyllium seed with 2% benzyl alcohol) into gastrocnemius and superficial flexor tendons of rabbits and noted an increase in bone formation at tendon junctions at 1–3 months. At 9–12 months, a 40% increase in tendon diameter and 30% increase in thickness of tendon-osseous junctions were noted. Tensile strengths were not tested (4).
- Particulates
  - Example: pumice flour (no longer manufactured/available)
  - Particulates are thought to attract macrophages to the injection site, which ingest them and secrete polypeptide growth factors (16).

Ozone Gas ("Prolozone")

- Since the early 1900s, there have been over 3900 studies evaluating the efficacy and safety of medical ozone for various pathologies spanning all medical specialties. The primary method for systemic administration is major autohemotherapy, which involves mixing ozone with a patient's own blood before reinfusion. Other administration routes include cavity insufflation, topical applications with ozonated oils, ozone saunas, and direct injections into ligaments, tendons, and joints often referred to as "prolozone." The prolozone technique has been in use for approximately 25 years, and due to a significant increase in rigorous research methods in both animal and clinical studies over the last 10 years, much has been learned about ozone's likely mechanism of action.
- The NAD^+/NADH balance is vital for cell energy processes, and an imbalance is associated with metabolic syndrome. In a study by Hwan et al. the oxidation of NADH to NAD^+ notably enhanced mitochondrial fat burning both in lab settings and in living organisms, significantly improving major issues like weight gain, blood sugar irregularities, abnormal lipid levels, and liver fat accumulation (17).
- When injected, ozone reacts ionically with double bonds found in short-chain fatty acids in cell membranes to form peroxides called ozonides. These ozonides, upon entering the cells oxidize NADH into NAD^+ (18).
- Largely through the upregulation of NAD^+ and modulation of local cytokines, prolozone is thought to work by enhancing tissue oxygenation, promoting accelerated utilization of glucose in cellular metabolic processes, optimizing protein metabolism, augmenting erythrocyte functionality, suppressing the production of inflammatory agents, curtailing the synthesis of prostaglandins, and mitigating oxidative stress within joints (19).
  - Ozone has been shown to have anti-inflammatory, anabolic, and salutary metabolic properties.
    - In a 2022 retrospective observational study of 65 patients with chronic knee osteoarthritis (KOA) by Fernandez-Cuadros et al., the anti-inflammatory and anabolic effects of ozone were evaluated by serum levels of interleukin (IL)-6 and insulin-like growth factor (IGF)-1 after patients received 4-weekly intra-articular injections of 20 $\mu g \cdot mL^{-1}$ ozone. Ozone treatment significantly reduced pro-inflammatory IL-6 levels across all patient categories, demonstrated a metabolic effect by decreasing IGF-1 levels in patients with obesity/diabetes, and presented an anabolic effect by increasing IGF-1 in patients without obesity/diabetes. Furthermore, other inflammation biomarkers like C-reactive protein, erythrocyte sedimentation rate, and uric acid were decreased, and improvements in pain, function, and quality of life were observed (20).
- Similar to other proliferative agents, ozone can be used to treat any number of musculoskeletal disorders. The vast majority of peer-reviewed literature on ozone injections, however, has focused on chronic lumbar pain secondary to intervertebral disc herniations. A 2017 study by Giurazza et al. (21) indicated that in excess of 50,000 patients with disc-related lumbar pain have been safely treated with intradiscal ozone injections (see Lower Back Pain section below).

Orthobiologics

- Over the past 15–20 years, there has been a significant surge in the development and application of both autologous and exogenous orthobiologics. This rapid evolution has posed challenges for regulatory agencies trying to keep up. Many clinicians keen on integrating regenerative medicine into their practices find it challenging to navigate the frequently shifting regulatory landscape, particularly due to the substantial variations across countries. While an exhaustive review of the current rules and regulations pertaining to the use of orthobiologics is outside the scope of this chapter, US physicians are advised to consult the Code of Federal Regulations Title 21 for further details and guidance.

Autologous Agents (See Chapter 78, Platelet-Rich Plasma Therapy and Autologous Blood)

- Whole blood, platelet-rich plasma (PRP), platelet releasate, platelet lysate, bone marrow aspirate concentrate, alpha 2 macroglobulin, adipose, and others
  - Autologous agents use specific growth factors, stimulators of growth factors, and/or carriers of growth factors (*e.g.*, platelets) to initiate an inflammatory cascade and/or stimulate healing (22–24).

Exogenous Agents

- Exosomes, peptides, placental/amniotic products, cord blood, and others
- Work in different ways to stimulate healing and regeneration of tissue

Dextrose

- Dextrose is the most commonly utilized proliferative agent in modern prolotherapy and merits specific attention.
- Though traditionally thought of as an osmotic agent, osmotic effects cannot fully explain the proliferative effect of dextrose. See "Osmotics" above (13).
  - Inflammatory effects cannot fully explain the proliferative effect of dextrose.
  - In a study examining the impact of NSAIDs and acetaminophen on Achilles tendon histological changes in a prolotherapy model, 60 rats' right Achilles tendons were injected with 20% dextrose thrice over two weeks while the left tendons remained untreated for control. Following each injection, the first two groups received their respective medications for three consecutive days. The tendons were analyzed at 3 and 6 weeks postinitial injection. Significant growth in transverse diameter and fibroblast count was observed in the injected tendons compared to controls, yet no significant differences were discerned among the medication groups. The findings suggest that prolotherapy promotes fibroblast activity and extracellular matrix development, and short-term NSAID use does not hinder tissue proliferation postprolotherapy (25).
  - Dextrose is not inflammatory at a 10% concentration and yet has been used:
    - to induce subsynovial connective tissue fibrosis in the rabbit carpal tunnel as a potential model to study carpal tunnel syndrome (26).
    - in published studies examining finger OA, thumb OA, and KOA (6,27,28).
- In vitro studies have demonstrated that cells bathed in dextrose show increased expression of genes for growth factors (29).
  - Clarkson et al. observed that human renal mesangial cells exposed to 5–30 mM of dextrose demonstrated increased expression of 200 genes, many encoding for cytoskeleton P-proteins and growth factors (30).
  - Lam et al. observed that renal fibroblasts exposed to dextrose demonstrated increased gene expression of connective tissue growth factor (CTGF) and IGF (31).
  - A concentration as low as 0.6% dextrose causes proliferation of chondrocytes, osteocytes, and fibroblasts and causes release of platelet-derived growth factor, transforming growth factor beta, basic fibroblast growth factor, IGF, epidermal growth factor, and CTGF (5).
  - Sugars in general appear to have a sensorineural effect on C-fibers and have been shown to rapidly decrease neurogenic inflammation and pain (32,33).
- Dextrose is analgesic in the epidural space compared to saline.
  - A 2017 double-blind study by Maniquis-Smigel et al. involving 35 participants compared a 5% dextrose epidural injection versus saline on patients with nonsurgical chronic low back pain. Each participant received a single epidural injection of either 5% dextrose or 0.9% saline. 84% of the dextrose recipients experienced a 50% or more reduction in pain at 4 hours, compared to only 19% in the saline group, suggesting an analgesic effect of dextrose at the level of the dorsal root (34).
  - In a follow-up uncontrolled study, 32 patients with low back pain received an epidural injection of 10 mL D5W (without anesthetic) biweekly for four sessions, and subsequently as required, for a year. 66% of participants experienced a 50% reduction in pain. The study concluded that repeated epidural D5W injections led to consistent pain relief and marked improvements in pain and disability over a year, suggesting dextrose might have a sensorineural effect on neurogenic pain (35).
- There is evidence that dextrose helps decrease pain by tightening lax ligaments and stabilizing joints.
  - In a 2003 case series by Reeves et al., 16 knees with >6 months of chronic pain and anterior cruciate ligament laxity as measured by the KT1000 arthrometer were injected every 2 months for one year with 10% or 25% dextrose and then an average of 4 times per year for an additional 2 years. 6 knees measured normal (no laxity) at 6 months, 9 measured normal after one year, and 10 measured normal after 3 years. Pain also decreased in patients whose knees continued to measure loose (28).
- There is evidence that dextrose is an allosteric modulator of acid-sensing ion channel 1a (ASIC1a) and works with substance P to inhibit the acid-sensing ion channel 3, a channel that has been implicated in long-term hyperalgesia in the mouse model.
  - In a 2022 study by Han et al., the effect of dextrose was evaluated in the fibromyalgia mouse model. One of the key findings was that 5% dextrose and 25% dextrose had equivalent antihyperalgesic effects at high volumes but that at low volumes even 25% dextrose lost its antihyperalgesic properties. The authors surmised that this was likely due to the ASIC1a channel requiring mechanical transduction in addition to dextrose in order to activate. Osmolarity did not play a role. The contralateral noninjected limb also became less painful, likely indicating modulation of central sensitization pathways through an unknown mechanism. The study also built on prior research showing substance P to actually be analgesic peripherally. One of the primary ways substance P is released peripherally is through the transient receptor potential vanilloid 1 (TRPV1) receptor at C-fiber terminals. Blockage of either substance P (but not the TRPV1 receptor) or the ASIC1a channel negated the antihyperalgesic effects of dextrose. Interestingly, the addition of 1% lidocaine also negated the effect. Lower lidocaine concentrations were unfortunately not tested (36).
- There is evidence that dextrose induces chondrogenesis.
  - In a 2016 study, Topol et al. examined the effects of dextrose injection on cartilage growth in KOA. Six participants

with symptomatic KOA underwent 4- to 6-monthly intra-articular injections with 12.5% dextrose. The study employed a blinded arthroscopic evaluation method to assess cartilage growth in specific zones. Results indicated cartilage growth in 19 of 54 zone comparisons. Biopsies revealed active cartilage consistent with fibro- and hyaline-like cartilage types. Additionally, participants showed an improvement in the Western Ontario McMaster University Osteoarthritis Index (WOMAC) scores (37).

    - In a 2023 study by Zahid et al., the effects of prolotherapy on osteoarthritic changes in rat knee joints induced by monosodium iodoacetate (MIA) were examined. Thirty rats were categorized into three groups. The control group (A) showed normal articular cartilage. Group B, injected with MIA, exhibited significant deterioration in cartilage appearance, decreased chondrocyte count, and cartilage thickness. Group C, given MIA followed by prolotherapy injections, displayed notable improvements in cartilage appearance, increased chondrocyte count, and cartilage thickness compared to group B. The findings suggest that prolotherapy can effectively counteract MIA-induced osteoarthritic changes in rat knee joints (38).
- Dextrose is effective in treating muscle contusions in the mouse model.
    - In a 2018 study, Tsai et al. examined the efficacy of dextrose prolotherapy in treating muscle injuries in mice using 10%, 20%, and 30% dextrose concentrations. While untreated muscle injuries displayed elevated levels of various injury markers, introducing dextrose significantly reduced these levels and promoted muscle healing by curbing macrophage response and boosting muscle satellite cell regeneration. The 10% dextrose concentration had a greater effect than the 20% and 30% concentrations (39).

PROLOTHERAPY TECHNIQUE

Prolotherapy Training

- Prolotherapy is not currently regulated, and certification is not required.
- While a single injection of dextrose, PRP, or other proliferant into a painful joint, tendon, or ligament can technically be labeled as "prolotherapy," the classical prolotherapy approach often entails multiple injections at many locations, sometimes distant from the site of pain.
- The authors strongly recommend learning prolotherapy with organizations that teach classical prolotherapy techniques. Organizations such as the AAOM, the Hackett Hemwall Patterson Foundation and their sister organization the IART, and the American Osteopathic Association of Prolotherapy Regenerative Medicine have been teaching classical prolotherapy techniques for decades and often offer 3–4 day workshops or more extended medical missions abroad where novice practitioners can learn directly from experienced prolotherapists.

Choosing the Right Proliferant

- Choice of best agent for injection, volume of agent, or concentration of agent is not clear.
- Most prolotherapists currently use dextrose as their preferred proliferative agent.
- Common concentrations range from 12.5% to 25% dextrose combined with an anesthetic agent and saline. Concentrations above 25% dextrose are thought to be too cytotoxic and are avoided.
- 15% dextrose is typically used for most extra-articular injections, and 25% dextrose is used for most intra-articular injections.
- There have been several successful trials using 10% dextrose as the proliferant as well as some basic science articles suggesting that even concentrations as low as 1% are effective in stimulating a proliferative response. More research is needed (6,27,28,40).
- Ozone is gaining traction as a viable alternative or adjunct to dextrose especially in low back pain associated with disc herniation (21).
- The most common combined agent includes phenol, glycerin, and dextrose (referred to as P2G), commonly with concentrations of 1% phenol, 12.5% glycerin, and 12.5% dextrose. P2G is not recommended for novice prolotherapists since phenol makes P2G less benign/forgiving than dextrose and ozone.
- Prolotherapists often begin with affordable proliferants like dextrose, P2G, or ozone, and only advance to stronger and typically costlier options like PRP if initial treatments are not effective. Starting with an off-the-shelf product like dextrose is beneficial, especially when the initial treatment area is extensive. As treatments progress, the painful area often begins to localize, making it more suitable for a solution like PRP, where typically only 4–5 mL might be available.

The Prolotherapy Physical Exam

- ***The palpatory exam is an essential aspect of all classical prolotherapy treatments.*** The classical prolotherapy technique usually involves injecting multiple tendinous, ligamentous, or fascial structures around the joint(s)/area being treated, usually at the areas that are most tender to palpation. A grade 1 injury to a tendon or ligament, for example, will not be visible on ultrasound (US) or magnetic resonance imaging (MRI) but will be tender to palpation and should be treated.
- A complete prolotherapy treatment of the knee, for example, may include injections all along the lateral collateral ligament, medial collateral ligament, medial patellofemoral ligament, patellar retinaculum, patellar tendon origin and insertion, popliteus insertion, iliotibial band insertion, the proximal anterior tibiofibular ligament, the pes anserine, and intra-articular space (41).

- Classical prolotherapy necessitates a thorough examination of the patient's musculoskeletal pain history and a comprehensive physical assessment to pinpoint and address the primary cause of pain. For instance, treating a patient with shin splints would require an understanding that dysfunction in the tibialis posterior often correlates with a flattening of the plantar arch to include laxity of the spring ligament, the long and short plantar ligaments, and the plantar fascia itself. As a result, treating the underlying issue might entail addressing multiple structures beyond the patient's presenting area of concern.

Needling Technique

- The recommended needling technique for all proliferants, including many of the orthobiologics, is the same. Ozone, however, is an exception. Due to it being a diffusible gas, ozone typically involves fewer injections and requires slightly less precision.
- The classical prolotherapy technique is typically taught using landmark-guided injections though over the past 10–15 years there has been a shift toward the increased use of US and fluoroscopy as supplementary tools. These are particularly useful when targeting deeper or more complex structures or when injecting in high-risk areas.
- Therapeutic injections are often performed at the site of greatest tenderness or along the path of a painful ligament or tendon. For large areas of pain, injections are performed at small intervals (*e.g.*, 1 cm) with an injection of 0.5–1 mL of agent at each site.
- When injecting the insertion sites of ligaments or tendons, a peppering technique is often used to fenestrate the enthesis and stimulate a stronger tissue response.
- Total volume injected varies according to target area. Techniques studied for lower back pain, for example, have ranged anywhere from 10 mL to 80 mL or more depending on how many structures are ultimately injected (facets, transverse processes, iliolumbar ligaments, supraspinous and interspinous ligaments, sacroiliac joints, thoracolumbar fascia, etc.).
- Various needling techniques such as needle redirection and skin sliding are often used to reduce the number of injections through the patient's skin.
- Classical prolotherapy treatments can often exceed 20–30 injections in a single sitting and efforts should be made to prepare the patient for this. Depending on the sensitivity of the targeted area and the needle's gauge, surface anesthesia at each injection site may or may not be necessary. Typically, sensitive regions such as the foot almost always require surface anesthesia, but in less sensitive areas, patients might opt to skip the additional skin injections. Despite the high number of injections, prolotherapy is generally well tolerated, though a minority of patients may require pretreatment with a mild sedative.
- Classical prolotherapy requires most injections to be performed either into the joint or only once the needle contacts bone (the enthesis) for reasons of both increased efficacy and increased safety, since the enthesis is both a common site of pathology and is of typically very low vascularity. If US is available, all pathological structures beyond the enthesis should also be treated.
- Patients should be informed that postinjection soreness is expected and typically lasts between 24 and 72 hours, but can occasionally extend up to two weeks. This soreness is often likened to the feeling after a workout. While most experience mild discomfort, a few might find it more intense. For pain management, acetaminophen or schedule IV narcotics are recommended. Anti-inflammatory medications are usually avoided in dextrose prolotherapy due to the theoretical significance of the inflammatory response and always avoided when injecting with PRP.

Adjusting When Treatments Are Unsuccessful

- Injections are commonly performed at 4- to 6-week intervals though more research is needed to determine optimal frequency. Though immediate symptom improvement may occur from time to time, the patient should be made aware that it may take up to 2 to 3 months before they start noticing sustained benefit. For this reason, the procedure is often performed several times before deciding whether the additional intervention is likely to be of benefit. If after three treatments the patient has not noticed any significant sustained benefit, a change in approach is usually required and would usually involve asking some or all of the following questions:
  - Is the primary driver of the patient's pain functional or structural? If the patient has pain with running due to improper footwear or an inefficient running style (functional), a structural intervention like prolotherapy is unlikely to provide sustained long-term benefit.
  - Is the root cause of pain coming from an as yet untreated structure, either near or distant from the area being treated? Is a lax costotransverse ligament posteriorly causing anterior costochondral pain for example?
  - Is the injury or degenerative area too severe to be treated with prolotherapy?
  - Do I need to use a stronger agent such as PRP or adipose, or should the patient be referred for surgical evaluation?

CURRENT EVIDENCE

- Since there is no commercial incentive to investigate the effects of dextrose prolotherapy, the majority of prolotherapy research has been self-funded by individual practitioners or small group practices. For this reason, prior to 15–20 years ago, most prolotherapy research came in the form of case reports, case series, or small uncontrolled trials with most meta-analyses concluding prolotherapy to be of questionable or unknown benefit. Over the past 10–15 years, however, there has been a marked increase in prolotherapy research, much of it consisting of randomized controlled studies of at least moderate to good quality.

The Knee

- Rabago et al. recruited 90 adults with chronic KOA to compare the effectiveness of dextrose, saline, and at-home exercises over 52 weeks. The injector, assessor, and study participants were all blinded. Both the dextrose and saline groups utilized a classical prolotherapy method where up to 15 sites were injected with up to 0.5 mL of solution using a peppering technique. The study evaluated WOMAC scores, a knee pain scale, postprocedure opioid use, and overall patient satisfaction. The dextrose prolotherapy group showed a significantly greater improvement in WOMAC scores and individual knee pain scores than the saline and exercise groups. Participants were highly satisfied with prolotherapy and there were no reported adverse events (41).
- In a follow-up study, Rabago et al. enrolled 65 of the above 90 study participants in an open label trial to assess long-term outcomes of up to 2.5 years. In the initial 17-week trial period, participants received an average of 4.6-monthly prolotherapy treatments and were then followed for up to a total of 2.5 years. Participants reported consistent improvement in WOMAC scores, surpassing minimal clinical benchmarks, with a 35.8% improvement observed at a mean follow-up of 2.5 years (42).
- In a 2023 study by Yildiz et al., dextrose prolotherapy was compared to conventional physiotherapy (CPT) in treating 60 female patients with KOA. The dextrose group received two rounds of prolotherapy in 1 month, with each round consisting of a 25% intra-articular injection and multiple 15% dextrose injections into all the ligament/bone insertions using a classical prolotherapy technique. The CPT group received hot packs, electrical nerve stimulation, and therapeutic US over 4 weeks. Outcomes were measured at 1- and 3-month posttreatment. Although both treatments showed improvements in pain, functionality, and strength, prolotherapy outperformed CPT in all assessed parameters (43).
- In a 2020 study, Sit et al. conducted a double-blind study comparing 25% dextrose injections to a normal saline control for symptomatic KOA in 76 patients. Four intra-articular injections were performed every 4 weeks for 16 weeks. After 52 weeks, the dextrose group showed significant improvements in pain, function, and overall quality of life based on the WOMAC function score and visual analog scale (VAS) pain scale when compared to the saline group (44).
- A 2017 systematic review of prolotherapy for KOA evaluated 10 studies, all of which showed significant improvements in pain, functionality, and range of motion after prolotherapy treatment, with 82% of patients expressing high satisfaction. The variation in outcome measures and participant groups prevented a meta-analysis. The authors concluded that existing evidence suggests prolotherapy is safe and effective for KOA, but future research should emphasize standardized treatment protocols and larger participant groups (45).
- In a 2011 double-blind Osgood-Schlatter study by Topol et al., 65 knees in 54 athletes aged 9–17 were treated with monthly 12.5% dextrose injections, monthly 1% lidocaine injections, or usual physical therapy care. At 3 months, the study became open label and participants could choose to get dextrose injections if desired. Results at 3 months showed that dextrose-treated athletes were more likely to participate in sports without alteration or symptoms compared to the other groups. By 1 year, dextrose-treated knees had the highest frequency of symptom-free sport participation (46).
- A 2022 double-blind study by Wu et al. compared 12.5% dextrose injections to a saline control for 70 patients with Osgood-Schlatter disease. Injections were administered monthly for 3 months. Outcomes were measured using the Victorian Institute of Sport Assessment-Patella (VISA-P) score. By 12 months, the dextrose group showed significantly better VISA-P scores than the saline group, with rapid improvements suggesting the efficacy of the dextrose injections. Both treatments had a positive clinical impact, but the dextrose group demonstrated superior results at 6-month and 12-month check-ins (47).
- A 2020 double-blind study by Nakase et al. compared 20% dextrose injections to a saline control for 49 knees (38 patients) with Osgood-Schlatter disease. Injections were administered monthly for 3 months. Both the saline and dextrose groups showed significant improvements in VISA-P scores with no discernible advantage of dextrose over saline (48).
- In a 2020 double-blind trial conducted by Orscelik et al., the efficacy of 25% dextrose was compared to PRP in the treatment of patellar chondromalacia. Seventy-five participants with MRI-confirmed grade II to IV OA underwent three injections at 3-week intervals of either 25% dextrose or PRP, following an unsuccessful 3-month period of conservative treatment. By the end of the first 6 weeks, both groups showed significant improvements in stiffness, crepitus, and range of motion though more pronounced improvements were seen in the PRP group. At the 1-year mark, outcomes became comparable between the two groups with VAS scores improving from 7.5 to 1.0 in the PRP group and from 6.9 to 1.2 in the prolotherapy group (49).
- In a single-blind 2020 study involving 60 patients with KOA, Imani et al. evaluated the effects of adding ozone gas to dextrose and somatropin (DSO) compared to dextrose and somatropin (DS) alone. Both groups showed a significant reduction in WOMAC scores after 16 weeks of treatment though the group receiving DSO displayed a more pronounced improvement compared to the DS group (50).

- In a double-blind 2017 study by Lopes et al., the effect of 20 μg · mL^{-1} ozone in KOA was compared to air. Ninety eight participants received weekly intra-articular injections for 8 weeks. Outcomes were measured using the VAS and WOMAC scale among others. After 8 weeks, the placebo group improved from a VAS of 7.3 to a VAS of 4.1, whereas the ozone group improved from 7.2 to 1.7. In most functional measures and quality of life, the ozone group was also statistically superior to the placebo group (51).
- A 2018 double-blind study by Babaei-Ghazani compared the effects of US-guided intra-articular corticosteroid injections (CSI) to ozone injections in patients with KOA. In this study of 62 participants, one group received 40 mg of triamcinolone, while the other group received 15 μg · mL^{-1} of ozone. Both treatments were evaluated using measures such as the WOMAC score, knee flexion range, effusion on US, and VAS. Results indicated improvements in both groups, but the ozone group showed more prolonged benefits in VAS and WOMAC scores than the corticosteroid group. There was no significant difference in knee flexion and joint effusion between the two groups (52).
- In a 2024 unblinded study by Babaei-Ghazani, 72 patients with chronic pes anserine bursitis were grouped to receive corticosteroids, ozone, or 20% dextrose injections under US guidance. Results showed significant pain and symptom relief (measured by VAS and WOMAC scores) in the corticosteroid and ozone groups after 1 week, and in both the ozone and dextrose groups (but not the corticosteroid group) after 8 weeks (53).
- A 2023 double-blind study by Sconza et al. compared the effectiveness of intra-articular ozone injections to hyaluronic acid (HA) injections for pain relief in 52 patients with KOA. At the study's 6-month conclusion, 44 patients remained. Both ozone and HA treatments showed significant improvement in pain, stiffness, and function within a month, and these benefits persisted at 3-month follow-up. By the 6-month mark, both groups had similar outcomes with a slight increase in pain. No significant difference in pain scores between the groups was noted. Both treatments were deemed safe with minimal side effects. Ozone was more cost-effective (54).

The Elbow

- In a 2013 three-arm single-blind pilot study involving 26 adults, Rabago et al. investigated the effectiveness of US-guided dextrose compared to US-guided dextrose and sodium morrhuate in patients with chronic lateral epicondylosis. The third arm received no treatment in a "wait-and-see approach." The primary evaluation metric was the Patient-Rated Tennis Elbow Evaluation (PRTEE) over various time points. Results indicated that both prolotherapy groups experienced significant improvements in elbow pain and function to include grip strength over the 16-week period compared to the nonintervention group (55).
- In a double-blind 2020 study, Akcay et al. compared the effectiveness of dextrose prolotherapy and saline in treating chronic lateral epicondylosis. Sixty participants were divided into two groups, receiving either 15% dextrose or normal saline injections at the start, and then at the end of the 4th and 8th weeks. Evaluations were conducted at the beginning, and then at the end of the 4th, 8th, and 12th weeks. Primary measurements included the VAS for pain and PRTEE. Both groups showed significant improvements in all outcome measures during the study though the dextrose group showed higher improvements in the PRTEE score in certain intervals compared to the saline group. There was no significant difference between groups in VAS, DASH scores, and handgrip strength at any time points. The authors concluded that while dextrose showed slightly better results in specific metrics, saline presented a comparable clinical effect, suggesting the need for further studies (56).
- A 2023 double-blind 3-arm study by Ciftci et al. compared the effectiveness of 5% dextrose, 15% dextrose, and 0.9% saline for chronic lateral epicondylosis in 60 patients. The injections were administered at weeks 0, 3, and 6 at the entheses of the forearm extensors and at the annular ligament. Results showed that the 15% dextrose group exhibited significant improvements in pain, handgrip strength, and pressure pain threshold compared to the other groups. Both dextrose groups demonstrated better outcomes than the saline group by week 12. The study concluded that 5% and 15% dextrose are both more effective than 0.9% saline for chronic lateral epicondylosis. The 15% dextrose group was particularly beneficial for handgrip strength, pain relief, and pressure pain threshold, making it the recommended treatment (57).
- A prospective unblinded 2022 study by Gupta et al. compared 25% dextrose injections to CSI for the treatment of tennis elbow in 260 patients. A single injection of either 1 mL of 25% dextrose or 1 mL triamcinolone (dose unknown) was performed at the extensor carpi radialis brevis tendon 5 mm from its insertion site. Both the corticosteroid group and the dextrose group showed comparable significant benefit at 6, 12, 24, and 52 weeks, with VAS scores improving between 40–45 points on a 100-point scale at one year (58).
- A 2022 systematic review and meta-analysis on the effectiveness of prolotherapy for lateral epicondylitis by Arias-Vázquez et al. reviewed 9 clinical trials and concluded that prolotherapy was effective at reducing pain over the medium to long term and at improving function over the medium term for individuals with lateral epicondylitis. Due to potential biases in the studies, however, the evidence quality was considered moderate (59).
- In a 2019 nonblinded comparison study by Ulusoy et al., 3-weekly CSI were compared to 6-8 ozone injections performed in 3-day intervals in 80 patients suffering from chronic lateral epicondylitis. While both treatments showed comparable initial results, the ozone group displayed superior pain relief at the 3rd, 6th, and 9th months postinjection (60).

The Achilles Tendon

- In a 2010 prospective case series by Ryan et al., 99 patients (and 108 tendons) with recalcitrant Achilles tendinosis were treated with US-guided injections of a 25% dextrose/lidocaine solution and followed for two years, investigating short-term (28 week) sonographic appearance and pain outcomes over a 28.6-month period. After a median of five injection consultations per patient, significant improvements in pain scores (an average drop of 5 points on the 10-point VAS scale during or immediately after sport participation) were observed for both midportion and insertional tendinosis though sonographic improvements were only seen in the midportion tears. Weaknesses include lack of a control group and 32% of patients being lost to follow-up (61).
- Yelland et al. performed a single-blinded randomized study involving 43 patients with Achilles tendinopathy. Subjects were randomized into three groups: prolotherapy only, eccentric exercises only, and combination of prolotherapy and eccentric exercises. The combined group had superior results, whereas the prolotherapy and the eccentric exercise groups were equivalent. Of note, the prolotherapy group achieved maximum improvement more rapidly than the eccentric exercise group (62).
- In a 2017 case series, Chan et al. injected 43 intratendinous Achilles tears with 25% dextrose and 0.25% bupivacaine followed by immobilization and subsequent rehabilitation. Outcomes measured using the VISA-A questionnaire showed that 70% of patients experienced significant improvements in scores at 3 and approximately 12 months posttreatment. Additionally, US taken about 5 weeks after the treatment indicated reduced echogenicity, with 27% of the tears becoming undetectable (63).

Plantar Fascia

- A 2021 systematic review and meta-analysis by Lai et al. reviewed six studies with 388 adult patients with plantar fasciitis. The results indicated that, in the short and medium term, prolotherapy provided superior pain relief compared to placebo or exercise but was less effective than CSI. For functional recovery, prolotherapy outperformed placebo or exercise in the short term but was less effective than corticosteroids and extracorporeal shockwave therapy. In the long term, prolotherapy showed better pain improvement than corticosteroids and exercise and had equivalent outcomes when compared against PRP injections. The study concluded that prolotherapy is a safe and potentially long-term beneficial treatment for plantar fasciitis, warranting more standardized, long-term research (64).
- In a 2020 double-blind study conducted by Mansiz-Kaplin et al., the impact of 15% dextrose was compared to a saline control in 60 patients with chronic plantar fasciopathy. Participants received injections twice, with a 3-week gap, and their pain levels and ultrasonographic progress were assessed after 15 weeks. Results showed that 80% of the patients in the dextrose group had their plantar fascia thickness revert to normal (<4 mm), in contrast to just 13.3% in the control group. Moreover, the dextrose group experienced significantly more pain relief than controls with 90% reporting no pain at rest and 60% reporting no pain with activity by the study's conclusion (65).
- In 2018, Ersen et al. compared the effectiveness of US-guided 15% dextrose prolotherapy (3 series of injections spaced 3 weeks apart) compared to a control group that performed plantar fascia and Achilles tendon stretches three times weekly for 3 months. All participants were also provided heel lifts and advised against heavy activities. Outcome measurements, including the VAS, Foot and Ankle Outcome Score (FAOS), and Foot Function Index (FFI), were taken at specified intervals. By the end of the study, both groups showed significant improvement in all scores. Although there was no significant difference between the groups at 21 days, the prolotherapy group outperformed the control group in terms of VAS and FAOS scores at 42, 90, and 360 days and FFI scores at 42 and 90 days. However, by 360 days, both groups' FFI scores were comparable (66).
- In a 2018 single-blind randomized controlled study, Atlas et al. evaluated the effectiveness of 15% dextrose injections compared to a saline placebo for treating patients with plantar fasciitis. The prolotherapy group (n = 15) received three injections of 15% dextrose and physical therapy, while the control group (n = 15) received saline with physical therapy. Both groups showed improvement in both pain and function but the improvements were significantly greater in the prolotherapy group (67).
- In a double-blind 2019 study by Babaei-Ghazani et al., the efficacy of 15 $\mu g \cdot mL^{-1}$ ozone injections were compared to corticosteroid (triamcinolone 40 $mg \cdot mL^{-1}$) in treating chronic plantar fasciitis in 30 patients. Both treatments were found to be effective in both pain relief and functional measures. While the corticosteroid group experienced quicker relief within 2 weeks postinjection, the ozone group showed more significant improvements after 12 weeks (68).
- In a 2019 double-blinded randomized trial by Bahrami et al. involving 44 adult patients with plantar fasciopathy, the effectiveness of a single 40 mg methylprednisolone injection was compared to a single 15 $\mu g \cdot mL^{-1}$ ozone injection. Pain severity, functional levels, and pressure pain thresholds were assessed before and 1, 4, and 12 weeks postinjection using various metrics. Results indicated that while both treatments were effective in reducing pain and improving function at 1 and 3 months posttreatment, the corticosteroid group showed significant improvement within the 1st week. By the third month, no significant differences were observed between the two treatment outcomes (69).

Thumb and Finger OA

- In a 2000 study, Reeves et al. studied the use of a 10% dextrose solution for OA of the fingers. This study included individuals with at least a 6-month history of pain at the metacarpophalangeal, proximal interphalangeal, or distal interphalangeal joints. Thirteen patients were randomized to the intervention group and 14 to the control group, and injections were performed to the medial and lateral joint lines. Evaluation was performed at 0, 2, and 4 months. The intervention group was noted to have significant improvement in pain with motion and improved flexion range of motion. There was no change in rest pain or grip strength (6).

- In a 2014 double-blind prospective trial, Jahangiri et al. compared the effectiveness of 10% dextrose prolotherapy to CSI in treating OA of the first carpometacarpal joint. Sixty participants were equally divided into two groups: the corticosteroid group received a single dose after two-monthly saline placebo injections, while the dextrose group received monthly injections for 3 months. One month after trial completion, both groups showed improvement, but the CSI group had a notably better response. By 2 months, both groups displayed comparable benefits. At the 6-month mark, however, the dextrose group continued to improve in pain and function, while the CSI group's condition began to regress (27).

Groin Pain

- A 2005 case series by Topol et al. evaluated the effect of prolotherapy in 22 rugby and two soccer players suffering from chronic groin pain due to osteitis pubis and/or adductor tendinopathy, which hindered their sports participation. These athletes had not responded to conventional therapies or gradual reintroduction to sports activities. They were treated with monthly injections of 12.5% dextrose and 0.5% lidocaine into multiple sites along the superior and inferior pubic ramus using classical prolotherapy technique. Athletes were treated until their pain completely subsided or if no improvement was noted for two consecutive sessions. On average, participants received 2.8 treatments. The study found significant pain reduction and functional improvement, with 20 out of 24 participants reporting no pain and 22 being unrestricted in sports activities by the end of the study (70).
- In a similar larger case series in 2008, Topol et al. evaluated the effect of prolotherapy in 75 elite kicking athletes with chronic groin pain. The results indicated a significant improvement in pain, with 82% reduction on the VAS and 78% improvement on the Nirschl pain phase scale (NPPS). Although six athletes showed no improvement, 66 returned to unrestricted sports activities within an average of 3 months (71).
- In a 2020 retrospective cohort study involving elite male soccer players suffering from prolonged anterior and medial groin pain resistant to conservative treatments, the efficacy of dextrose prolotherapy versus PRP injections was examined. Out of the 15 participants, 9 received dextrose and 6 received PRP. Both treatments involved three-weekly injection sessions, followed by 12-week progressive home exercise protocol postinjections. Both treatment groups showed significant improvement in VAS pain (87.5%) and NPPS (80% for dextrose and 89% for PRP) with no notable differences between the groups (72).

Rotator Cuff Tendinopathy

- In a 2023 study, Abd et al. performed a double-blind trial comparing a single 2 mL US-guided injection of either 16.7% dextrose or PRP on 64 patients suffering from supraspinatus tendinopathy who had not seen results from conventional treatments. Both treatments led to clinically significant improvements in shoulder function and pain, and no significant differences between the groups were observed except for a temporary increase in postinjection pain in the PRP group (73).
- In a 2017 randomized controlled trial by Seven et al., 120 patients with chronic rotator cuff lesions were treated with either physical therapy exercises and a home exercise program or with dextrose prolotherapy (from 1 to 6 injections depending on necessity of additional injections) and a home exercise program. The physical therapy group received three sessions weekly for 12 weeks. Both groups saw significant improvements, but the prolotherapy group had notably better VAS scores, improved shoulder function, and better shoulder range of motion. Additionally, 92.9% of the prolotherapy group reported excellent or good outcomes compared to 56.8% in the control group (74).
- A 2016 double-blind study by Bertrand et al. evaluated the effects of dextrose prolotherapy on chronic rotator cuff tendinopathy in 73 participants. Patients were randomly assigned to receive three-monthly injections of either (1) 25% dextrose into painful entheses, (2) saline into painful entheses, or (3) saline above entheses. All participants also underwent programmed physical therapy. Nine months posttreatment, 59% of the dextrose group reported significant pain reduction, compared to 37% in the saline-on-entheses group and 27% in the saline-above-entheses group. The dextrose group also reported higher satisfaction levels. No differences were observed in US findings across groups (75).

TMJ Pain

- A 2021 systematic review and meta-analysis by Sit et al. evaluated the efficacy of dextrose prolotherapy in TMJ pain. Ten RCTs involving 336 participants were included. The primary focus was on pain intensity, with secondary outcomes being maximum interincisal mouth opening (MIO) and disability score. The meta-analysis of five RCTs revealed that prolotherapy significantly reduced TMJ pain at 12 weeks compared to placebo injections. However, there was no significant difference observed for changes in MIO and functional scores. Overall, the evidence suggests that prolotherapy is effective in treating TMJ pain when compared to placebo injections, based on low- to moderate-quality studies (76).

- In a 2022 retrospective study, Pandey et al. compared autologous blood to 25% dextrose for treatment of TMJ dislocation and pain. In a 6-month follow-up, the autologous blood group displayed better outcomes in mouth opening and mandibular movements, whereas the dextrose group had a more significant reduction in pain intensity. Both treatments showed similar effects in reducing dislocation frequency and TMJ sounds (77).
- A 2020 double-blind prospective study by Zarate et al. evaluated the effectiveness of intra-articular dextrose prolotherapy compared to lidocaine for treating TMJ dysfunction. The study involved 29 participants (25 female) experiencing moderate-to-severe jaw or facial pain for at least 3 months. Participants received blinded injections of either 20% dextrose/0.2% lidocaine or lidocaine (0.2% in sterile water) at 0, 1, and 2 months, after which they were unblinded and offered prolotherapy for 9 more months. By 12 months, the prolotherapy group showed greater improvement in both pain and dysfunction, with a significant number experiencing over 50% improvement compared to the lidocaine group (78).
- A 2019 double-blind randomized trial by Louw et al. evaluated the effectiveness of dextrose prolotherapy versus lidocaine in 42 participants (54 joints) with chronic TMJ dysfunction. Participants received three-monthly intra-articular injections of either dextrose with lidocaine or lidocaine alone. By the 3-month mark, the prolotherapy group reported significantly better outcomes in terms of reduced pain, improved jaw function, and increased mouth opening compared to the control group. When both groups were subsequently treated with prolotherapy after the initial 3-month blinding period, the combined data at 12 months indicated marked improvements in pain and jaw function for 70% of the participants (79).
- In a 2022 double-blind study by Haggag et al. involving 30 patients with bilateral disc displacement with reduction (DDWR), the efficacy of dextrose prolotherapy was assessed. Patients were divided into two groups, receiving either a 25% dextrose solution or normal saline injections in the TMJ. Over 6 months, the dextrose group experienced significant improvements in pain, mouth opening capability (MIO), and overall treatment satisfaction compared to the saline group. While joint sounds improved with dextrose treatment, the change was not statistically significant. The study suggests that 25% dextrose injections are a safe and effective treatment for TMJ DDWR-related symptoms (80).
- A 2023 study by Taskesen et al. evaluated the efficacy of dextrose prolotherapy alone versus in combination with arthrocentesis for treating symptomatic TMJ hypermobility. Of the 24 patients studied, half received only prolotherapy, while the other half also underwent an arthrocentesis procedure. Both treatments reduced pain scores, but the combination of prolotherapy and arthrocentesis was more effective in reducing the frequency of TMJ locking episodes in both short- and long-term evaluations. Thus, combining prolotherapy with arthrocentesis might offer superior results in managing TMJ hypermobility compared to prolotherapy alone (81).

Hip OA

- A 2020 randomized study by Gul et al. evaluated the effect of dextrose prolotherapy versus a 12-week progressive resistance exercise program for patients with symptomatic OA due to developmental dysplasia of the hip who were awaiting total hip arthroplasty. The dextrose arm received 15% dextrose injections into all the tender tendinous insertions sites in the anterior and lateral hip and 25% dextrose was injected into the hip joint. The study, which included 46 hips from 44 participants, evaluated pain levels using the VAS and functional outcomes with the Harris Hip Score (HHS) over a year. While both groups experienced notable improvements, from day 21 onward, the dextrose injection group consistently showed better results. By the 6-month mark, the prolotherapy group outperformed the exercise group in both VAS pain change score and HHS change score. The prolotherapy group's VAS score dropped an average of 4.6 points by the 6-month mark compared to 2.8 points for the control arm (82).

Ankle OA

- In a 2019 retrospective comparison study by Akpancar et al., patients with chronic ankle pain due to osteochondral lesions of the talus and resistant to standard treatments were given three injection sessions at 3-week intervals of either PRP or 25% dextrose. Excellent or good outcomes were reported by approximately 89% patients treated with dextrose and 91% patients treated with PRP (83).

Lower Back Pain

- A 2012 systematic review and meta-analysis by Magalhaes et al. evaluated the use of ozone therapy for low back pain secondary to herniated disc. The main outcome was whether patients experienced short-term (at least 6 months) or long-term (more than 6 months) pain relief. The analysis included eight observational studies and four randomized trials. The evidence level for long-term pain relief was II-3 for intradiscal ozone therapy (evidence obtained from diagnostic studies of uncertain quality) and II-1 for paravertebral ozone therapy (evidence obtained from at least one properly conducted study of adequate size). The recommendation grade was 1C for intradiscal therapy (strong recommendation, low-quality evidence), and 1B for paravertebral ozone therapy (strong recommendation, moderate-quality evidence). Some limitations included the absence of precise diagnoses, the use of mixed therapeutic agents, and a lack of placebo-controlled trials (84).
- In a 2014 retrospective study by Buric et al., 107 patients who had been treated with intradiscal ozone injections were followed up with after 5 years. While 19 patients eventually underwent surgery, 82% of those who did not reported continued significant benefit. Sixty of those patients were later able to be reached at the 10-year mark, and 88% reported continued benefit (85).

- In a 2016 double-blind study by Perri et al., the effect of intradiscal injections of ozone plus corticosteroid was compared to corticosteroid alone. Of the 517 participants, half received the combined treatment, while the other half received only the steroid and anesthetic. Procedures were CT-guided, and outcomes were tracked using the VAS Questionnaire over 6 months. Results showed the ozone discolysis treatment was significantly more effective, especially for herniated or protruded discs and mild to moderate disc degeneration than the steroid and anesthetic alone. By the sixth month, 80.9% of the ozone/steroid-treated group were successful (VAS score of 3 or less), compared to 31.5% of patients in the steroid only group. The success rate with extrusions was 41% in the ozone group compared to 3.5% in the control group (86).
- In a 2022 noninferiority randomized trial by Kelekis et al., 49 patients with single-level contained lumbar disc herniations and persistent radicular leg pain were randomized into two treatment groups: 25 received intradiscal ozone therapy, and 24 underwent microdiscectomy. The main measure of success was the improvement in leg pain after 6 months. Additional measures included pain scores and the Roland Morris Disability Index, assessed at various intervals. The results showed that the difference in leg pain improvement between the two treatments was minimal, favoring neither method definitively. Both treatments provided significant and lasting improvements in pain and disability. Notably, 71% of patients who received ozone therapy did not require microdiscectomy. Additionally, the ozone procedure was quicker by 58 minutes and had a significantly shorter recovery time. No major adverse events were reported in either group (87).

Other Conditions

- Case reports have claimed use of prolotherapy for multiple other musculoskeletal complaints to include neck pain, headaches and migraines, and costochondritis, among others. No organized studies are available.

CONTRAINDICATIONS, COMPLICATIONS, AND ADVERSE REACTIONS

- Complications arising from prolotherapy are more likely to stem from needle injuries than they are from the proliferant solution itself. Novice injectors are therefore encouraged to start with areas of the body that pose the least risk such as the knee or elbow. The highest risk areas in landmark-guided prolotherapy injections are the cervical spine and ribs.
- Suggested contraindications include acute illness, infection at proposed injection site, anatomic defects precluding injection, metastatic cancer, systemic inflammation, gouty arthritis, bleeding disorders, inability to perform postprocedure range-of-motion exercises, nonmusculoskeletal pain, whole-body pain, and low pain tolerance.
- Common adverse effects include needle trauma (*e.g.*, pain, bruising, bleeding, fullness, or numbness at injection site), light headedness, local infection, and local nerve damage. For procedures to the spine and neck, risks include pneumothorax, spinal headache, disc injury, and potential spinal nerve/cord injury, although injury rates are similar to other commonly performed back procedures (88).
- Prolotherapy agents are considered relatively safe. Dextrose has been used safely as an intravenous treatment for hypoglycemia for over 50 years. The safety of ozone has been well established in the literature (18). P2G has not been reported in clinical trials to have significant side effects or adverse reactions (89).
- Most dextrose formulations are derived from corn and anaphylaxis to corn-derived dextrose solutions have been described in the literature (90).

SUMMARY

- As we observe the evolving landscape of sports and pain medicine, there appears to be a shift taking place from mere symptom management to seeking root cause solutions.
- Regenerative medicine, albeit in its nascent stage, is hinting at transformative, long-term solutions for chronic pain. And while ongoing research will be critical to optimize the treatments we currently have, and to develop more advanced treatments for the future, current studies appear to suggest that prolotherapy in its current state offers promising outcomes with minimal risks.

REFERENCES

1. Puddu G, Ippolito E, Postacchini F. A classification of Achilles tendon disease. *Am J Sports Med.* 1976;4(4):145–50.
2. Kaeding C, Best TM. Tendinosis: pathophysiology and nonoperative treatment. *Sports Health.* 2009;1(4):284–92.
3. Hackett GS. Joint stabilization through induced ligament sclerosis. *Ohio Med.* 1953;49(10):877–84.
4. Hackett GS, Henderson DG. Joint stabilization: an experimental histologic study with comments on the clinical application in ligament proliferation. *Am J Surg.* 1955;89(5):968–73.
5. Reeves KD, Hassanein K. Randomized prospective double-blind placebo-controlled study of dextrose prolotherapy for knee osteoarthritis with or without ACL laxity. *Altern Ther Health Med.* 2000;6(2):68–80. 68–74, 77–80.
6. Reeves KD, Hassanein K. Randomized, prospective, placebo-controlled double-blind study of dextrose prolotherapy for osteoarthritic thumb and finger (DIP, PIP, and trapeziometacarpal) joints: evidence of clinical efficacy. *J Altern Complement Med.* 2000;6(4):311–20.
7. Schultz L. A treatment for subluxation of the temporomandibular joint. *JAMA.* 1937;190:1032–5.
8. Dorman TA. Prolotherapy: a survey. *J Orthopaed Med.* 1993;15(2):49–50.
9. Fleming S, Rabago DP, Mundt MP, Fleming MF. CAM therapies among primary care patients using opioid therapy for chronic pain. *BMC Complement Altern Med.* 2007;7:15.

10. Dagenais S, Ogunseitan O, Haldeman S, Wooley JR, Newcomb RL. Side effects and adverse events related to intraligamentous injection of sclerosing solutions (prolotherapy) for back and neck pain: a survey of practitioners. *Arch Phys Med Rehabil.* 2006;87(7):909–13.
11. Dubey J, Rabago DP, Andrie J. Prolotherapy in the academy, results of a National survey [Conference presentation]. In: *IART 2023 Annual Conference, Madison, WI, United States*; 2023 Oct 19–21.
12. Banks AR. A rational for prolotherapy. *J Orthop Med.* 1991;13(3):54–9.
13. Kim HJ, Jeong TS, Kim WS, Park YS. Comparison of histological changes in accordance with the level of dextrose-concentration in experimental prolotherapy model. *J Korean Acad Rehabil Med.* 2003;27:935–40.
14. Johnston E, Emani C, Kochan A, et al. Prolotherapy agent P2G is associated with upregulation of fibroblast growth factor-2 genetic expression in vitro. *J Exp Orthop.* 2020 Dec 6;7(1):97.
15. Reddy GS, Reddy GV, Reddy KS, Priyadarshini BS, Sree PK. Intralesional sclerotherapy — A novel approach for the treatment of intraoral Haemangiomas. *J Clin Diagn Res.* 2016 Jan;10(1):ZD13–4.
16. Dagenais S, Yelland MJ, Del Mar C, Schoene ML. Prolotherapy injections for chronic low-back pain. *Cochrane Database Syst Rev.* 2007 Apr 18;2007(2):CD004059.
17. Hwang JH, Kim DW, Jo EJ, et al. Pharmacological stimulation of NADH oxidation ameliorates obesity and related phenotypes in mice. *Diabetes.* 2009 Apr;58(4):965–74.
18. Bocci V, Zanardi I, Travagli V. Oxygen/ozone as a medical gas mixture. A critical evaluation of the various methods clarifies positive and negative aspects. *Med Gas Res.* 2011 Apr 28;1(1):6.
19. Akkawi I. Ozone therapy for musculoskeletal disorders current concepts. *Acta Biomed.* 2020 Nov 12;91(4):e2020191.
20. Fernández-Cuadros ME, Pérez-Moro OS, Albaladejo-Florín MJ, et al. Intra articular ozone modulates inflammation and has anabolic effect on knee osteoarthritis: IL-6 and IGF-1 as pro-inflammatory and anabolic biomarkers. *Processes.* 2022;10:138.
21. Giurazza F, Guarnieri G, Murphy KJ, Muto M. Intradiscal O_2O_3: Rationale, injection technique, short- and long-term outcomes for the treatment of low back pain due to disc herniation. *Can Assoc Radiol J.* 2017 May;68(2):171–7.
22. Creaney L, Hamilton B. Growth factor delivery methods in the management of sports injuries: the state of play. *Br J Sports Med.* 2008;42(5):314–20.
23. Foster TE, Puskas BL, Mandelbaum BR, Gerhardt MB, Rodeo SA. Platelet-rich plasma: from basic science to clinical applications. *Am J Sports Med.* 2009;37(11):2259–72.
24. Sampson S, Gerhardt M, Mandelbaum B. Platelet rich plasma injection grafts for musculoskeletal injuries: a review. *Curr Rev Musculoskelet Med.* 2008;1(3-4):165–74.
25. Kim HJ, Kim SH, Yun DH, Lee KS, Jeong TS. The effects of anti-inflammatory drugs on histologic findings of the experimental prolotherapy model. *J Korean Acad Rehabil Med.* 2006;30:378–84.
26. Oh S, Ettema AM, Zhao C, et al. Dextrose-induced subsynovial connective tissue fibrosis in the rabbit carpal tunnel: a potential model to study carpal tunnel syndrome? *Hand.* 2008;3(1):34–40.
27. Jahangiri A, Moghaddam FR, Najafi S. Hypertonic dextrose versus corticosteroid local injection for the treatment of osteoarthritis in the first carpometacarpal joint: a double-blind randomized clinical trial. *J Orthop Sci.* 2014 Sep;19(5):737–43.
28. Reeves KD, Hassanein K. Long term effects of dextrose prolotherapy for anterior cruciate ligament laxity: a prospective and consecutive patient study. *Altern Ther Health Med.* May–Jun 2003;9(3):58–62.
29. Kim SR, Stitik TP, Foye PM, Greenwald BD, Campagnolo DI. Critical review of prolotherapy for osteoarthritis, low back pain, and other musculoskeletal conditions: a physiatric perspective. *Am J Phys Med Rehabil.* 2004;83(5):379–89.
30. Clarkson M, Murphy M, Gupta S, et al. High glucose-altered gene expression in mesangial cells. Actin-regulatory protein gene expression is triggered by oxidative stress and cytoskeletal disassembly. *J Biol Chem.* 2002;277(12):9707–12.
31. Lam S, van der Geest RN, Verhagen NA, et al. Connective tissue growth factor and IGF-I are produced by human renal fibroblasts and cooperate in the induction of collagen production by high glucose. *Diabetes.* 2003;52(12):2975–83.
32. Bertrand H, Kyriazis M, Reeves KD, et al. Mannitol cream in the treatment of postherpetic neuralgia: randomized, placebo-controlled, crossover pilot study (Abs). *Can Fam Physician.* 2017;63(suppl 1):S106.
33. Moshrif AA, Elwan M. The effect of addition of buffered dextrose solution on pain occurring during local steroid injection for plantar fasciitis. *Ann Rheum Dis.* 2019;78:538–9. ((Moshrif A.A.; Elwan M.) Al Azhar University, Rheumatology, Assiut, Egypt). doi:10.1136/annrheumdis-2019-eular.2008
34. Maniquis-Smigel L, Dean Reeves K, Jeffrey Rosen H, et al. Short term analgesic effects of 5% dextrose epidural injections for chronic low back pain: a randomized controlled trial. *Anesth Pain Med.* 2017;7(1):e42550.
35. Maniquis-Smigel L, Reeves KD, Rosen HJ, et al. Analgesic effect and potential cumulative benefit from caudal epidural D5W in consecutive participants with chronic low-back and buttock/leg pain. *J Altern Complement Med.* 2018 Dec;24(12):1189–96.
36. Han DS, Lee CH, Shieh YD, et al. A role for substance P and acid-sensing ion channel 1a in prolotherapy with dextrose-mediated analgesia in a mouse model of chronic muscle pain. *Pain.* 2022 May 1;163(5):e622–33.
37. Topol GA, Podesta LA, Reeves KD, et al. Chondrogenic effect of intra-articular hypertonic-dextrose (prolotherapy) in severe knee osteoarthritis. *PM R.* 2016;8(11):1072–82.
38. Zahid A, Qamar K, Tabassum A, Abaid M, Bashir Kiani MR, Aslam M. Ameliorative effects of prolotherapy on histomorphology of tibial articular cartilage of chemically induced osteoarthritic knee joint in a rat model. *J Coll Physicians Surg Pak.* 2023 Aug;33(8):836–41.
39. Tsai SW, Hsu YJ, Lee MC, Huang HE, Huang CC, Tung YT. Effects of dextrose prolotherapy on contusion-induced muscle injuries in mice. *Int J Med Sci.* 2018 Jul 30;15(11):1251–9.
40. Woo MS, Park J, Ok SH, et al. The proper concentrations of dextrose and lidocaine in regenerative injection therapy: in vitro study. *Korean J Pain.* 2021 Jan 1;34(1):19–26.
41. Rabago D, Patterson JJ, Mundt M, et al. Dextrose prolotherapy for knee osteoarthritis: a randomized controlled trial. *Ann Fam Med.* 2013 May–Jun;11(3):229–37.
42. Rabago D, Mundt M, Zgierska A, Grettie J. Hypertonic dextrose injection (prolotherapy) for knee osteoarthritis: long term outcomes. *Complement Ther Med.* 2015 Jun;23(3):388–95.
43. Yildiz KM, Guler H, Ogut H, Yildizgoren MT, Turhanoglu AD. A comparison between hypertonic dextrose prolotherapy and conventional physiotherapy in patients with knee osteoarthritis. *Med Int.* 2023 Aug 29;3(5):45.
44. Sit RWS, Wu RWK, Rabago D, et al. Efficacy of intra-articular hypertonic dextrose (prolotherapy) for knee osteoarthritis: a randomized controlled trial. *Ann Fam Med.* 2020 May;18(3):235–42.
45. Hassan F, Trebinjac S, Murrell WD, Maffulli N. The effectiveness of prolotherapy in treating knee osteoarthritis in adults: a systematic review. *Br Med Bull.* 2017 Jun 1;122(1):91–108.
46. Topol GA, Podesta LA, Reeves KD, Raya MF, Fullerton BD, Yeh HW. Hyperosmolar dextrose injection for recalcitrant Osgood-Schlatter disease. *Pediatrics.* 2011 Nov;128(5):e1121–8.
47. Wu Z, Tu X, Tu Z. Hyperosmolar dextrose injection for Osgood-Schlatter disease: a double-blind, randomized controlled trial. *Arch Orthop Trauma Surg.* 2022 Sep;142(9):2279–85.

48. Nakase J, Oshima T, Takata Y, Shimozaki K, Asai K, Tsuchiya H. No superiority of dextrose injections over placebo injections for Osgood-Schlatter disease: a prospective randomized double-blind study. *Arch Orthop Trauma Surg.* 2020 Feb;140(2):197–202.
49. Orscelik A, Akpancar S, Seven MM, Erdem Y, Koca K. The efficacy of platelet rich plasma and prolotherapy in chondromalacia patella treatment. *Turk J Sports Med.* 2020;55(1):28–37.
50. Imani F, Hejazian K, Kazemi MR, Narimani-Zamanabadi M, Malik KM. Adding ozone to dextrose and somatropin for intra-articular knee prolotherapy: a randomized single-blinded controlled trial. *Anesth Pain Med.* 2020 Nov 7;10(5):e110277.
51. Lopes de Jesus CC, Dos Santos FC, de Jesus LMOB, Monteiro I, Sant'Ana MSSC, Trevisani VFM. Comparison between intra-articular ozone and placebo in the treatment of knee osteoarthritis: a randomized, double-blinded, placebo-controlled study. *PLoS One.* 2017 Jul 24;12(7):e0179185.
52. Babaei-Ghazani A, Najarzadeh S, Mansoori K, et al. The effects of ultrasound-guided corticosteroid injection compared to oxygen-ozone (O_2-O_3) injection in patients with knee osteoarthritis: a randomized controlled trial. *Clin Rheumatol.* 2018 Sep;37(9):2517–27.
53. Babaei-Ghazani A, Eftekharsadat B, Soleymanzadeh H, ZoghAli M. Ultrasound guided pes anserine bursitis injection Choices; prolotherapy or oxygen-ozone or corticosteroid: a randomized multicenter clinical trial. *Am J Phys Med Rehabil.* 2024;103(4):310–17.
54. Sconza C, Di Matteo B, Queirazza P, et al. Ozone therapy versus hyaluronic acid injections for pain relief in patients with knee osteoarthritis: preliminary findings on molecular and clinical outcomes from a randomized controlled trial. *Int J Mol Sci.* 2023 May 15;24(10):8788.
55. Rabago D, Lee KS, Ryan M, et al. Hypertonic dextrose and morrhuate sodium injections (prolotherapy) for lateral epicondylosis (tennis elbow): results of a single-blind, pilot-level, randomized controlled trial. *Am J Phys Med Rehabil.* 2013;92(7):587–96.
56. Akcay S, Gurel Kandemir N, Kaya T, Dogan N, Eren M. Dextrose prolotherapy versus normal saline injection for the treatment of lateral epicondylopathy: a randomized controlled trial. *J Altern Complement Med.* 2020 Dec;26(12):1159–68.
57. Ciftci YGD, Tuncay F, Kocak FA, Okcu M. Is low-dose dextrose prolotherapy as effective as high-dose dextrose prolotherapy in the treatment of lateral epicondylitis? A double-blind, ultrasound guided, randomized controlled study. *Arch Phys Med Rehabil.* 2023;104(2):179–87.
58. Gupta GK, Rani S, Shekhar D, Sahoo UK, Shekhar S. Comparative study to evaluate efficacy of prolotherapy using 25% dextrose and local corticosteroid injection in tennis elbow – A prospective study. *J Family Med Prim Care.* 2022 Oct;11(10):6345–9.
59. Arias-Vázquez PI, Castillo-Avila RG, Tovilla-Zárate CA, Quezada-González HR, Arcila-Novelo R, Loeza-Magaña P. Efficacy of prolotherapy in pain control and function improvement in individuals with lateral epicondylitis: a systematic review and meta-analysis. *ARP Rheumatol.* 2022 Apr–Jun;1(2):152–67.
60. Ulusoy GR, Bilge A, Öztürk Ö. Comparison of corticosteroid injection and ozone injection for relief of pain in chronic lateral epicondylitis. *Acta Orthop Belg.* 2019 Sep;85(3):317–24.
61. Ryan M, Wong A, Taunton J. Favorable outcomes after sonographically guided intratendinous injection of hyperosmolar dextrose for chronic insertional and midportion achilles tendinosis. *AJR Am J Roentgenol.* 2010 Apr;194(4):1047–53.
62. Yelland MJ, Sweeting KR, Lyftogt JA, Ng SK, Scuffham PA, Evans KA. Prolotherapy injections and eccentric loading exercises for painful Achilles tendinosis: a randomised trial. *Br J Sports Med.* 2011;45(5): 421–8.
63. Chan O, Havard B, Morton S, et al. Outcomes of prolotherapy for intratendinous Achilles tears: a case series. *Muscles Ligaments Tendons J.* 2017 May 10;7(1):78–87.
64. Lai WF, Yoon CH, Chiang MT, et al. The effectiveness of dextrose prolotherapy in plantar fasciitis: a systemic review and meta-analysis. *Medicine.* 2021 Dec 23;100:e28216.
65. Mansiz-Kaplan B, Nacir B, Pervane-Vural S, Duyur-Cakit B, Genc H. Effect of dextrose prolotherapy on pain intensity, disability, and plantar fascia thickness in unilateral plantar fasciitis: a randomized, controlled, double-blind study. *Am J Phys Med Rehabil.* 2020;99(4):318–24.
66. Ersen Ö, Koca K, Akpancar S, et al. A randomized-controlled trial of prolotherapy injections in the treatment of plantar fasciitis. *Turk J Phys Med Rehabil.* 2018;64(1):59–65.
67. Atlas EU, Askin A, Tosun A. Is hypertonic dextrose injection effective in the treatment of plantar fasciitis: a clinical randomized study. *Med Bull.* 2018;56(3):102–8.
68. Babaei-Ghazani A, Karimi N, Forogh B, et al. Comparison of ultrasound-guided local ozone (O_2-O_3) injection vs corticosteroid injection in the treatment of chronic plantar fasciitis: a randomized clinical trial. *Pain Med.* 2019 Feb 1;20(2):314–22.
69. Bahrami MH, Raeissadat SA, Barchinejad M, Elyaspour D, Rahimi-Dehgolan S. Local ozone (O_2-O_3) versus corticosteroid injection efficacy in plantar fasciitis treatment: a double-blinded RCT. *J Pain Res.* 2019 Jul 24;12:2251–9.
70. Topol GA, Reeves KD, Hassanein KM. Efficacy of dextrose prolotherapy in elite male kicking-sport athletes with chronic groin pain. *Arch Phys Med Rehabil.* 2005 Apr;86(4):697–702.
71. Topol GA, Reeves KD. Regenerative injection of elite athletes with career-altering chronic groin pain who fail conservative treatment: a consecutive case series. *Am J Phys Med Rehabil.* 2008 Nov;87(11): 890–902.
72. Ozkan O, Torgutalp SS, Karacoban L, Donmez G, Korkusuz F. Do pain and function improve after dextrose prolotherapy or autologous platelet-rich plasma injection in longstanding groin pain? *Montenegrin J Sports Sci Med.* 2020;9(2):5–12.
73. Abd Karim S, Hamid MS, Choong A, Ooi MY, Usman J. Effects of platelet-rich plasma and prolotherapy on supraspinatus tendinopathy: a double blind randomized clinical trial. *J Sports Med Phys Fitness.* 2023 May;63(5):674–84.
74. Seven MM, Ersen O, Akpancar S, et al. Effectiveness of prolotherapy in the treatment of chronic rotator cuff lesions. *Orthop Traumatol Surg Res.* 2017 May;103(3):427–33.
75. Bertrand H, Reeves KD, Bennett CJ, Bicknell S, Cheng AL. Dextrose prolotherapy versus control injections in painful rotator cuff tendinopathy. *Arch Phys Med Rehabil.* 2016;97(1):17–25.
76. Sit RW, Reeves KD, Zhong CC, et al. Efficacy of hypertonic dextrose injection (prolotherapy) in temporomandibular joint dysfunction: a systematic review and meta-analysis. *Sci Rep.* 2021 Jul 19;11(1): 14638.
77. Pandey SK, Baidya M, Srivastava A, Garg H. Comparison of autologous blood prolotherapy and 25% dextrose prolotherapy for the treatment of chronic recurrent temporomandibular joint dislocation on the basis of clinical parameters: a retrospective study. *Natl J Maxillofac Surg.* 2022 Sep–Dec;13(3):398–404.
78. Zarate MA, Frusso RD, Reeves KD, Cheng AL, Rabago D. Dextrose prolotherapy versus lidocaine injection for temporomandibular dysfunction: a pragmatic randomized controlled trial. *J Altern Complement Med.* 2020 Nov;26(11):1064–73.
79. Louw WF, Burrils F, Reeves KD, Chang AL, Rabago D. Treatment of temporomandibular dysfunction with dextrose prolotherapy: a

randomized controlled trial with long term follow-up. *Mayo Clin Proc.* 2019;94(5):820–5.

80. Haggag MA, Al-Belasy FA, Said Ahmed WM. Dextrose prolotherapy for pain and dysfunction of the TMJ reducible disc displacement: a randomized, double-blind clinical study. *J Craniomaxillofac Surg.* 2022 May;50(5):426–31.
81. Taşkesen F, Cezairli B. Efficacy of prolotherapy and arthrocentesis in management of temporomandibular joint hypermobility. *Cranio.* 2023 Sep;41(5):423–31.
82. Gül D, Orsçelik A, Akpancar S. Treatment of osteoarthritis secondary to developmental dysplasia of the hip with prolotherapy injection versus a supervised progressive exercise control. *Med Sci Monit.* 2020 Feb 11;26:e919166.
83. Akpancar S, Gül D. Comparison of platelet rich plasma and prolotherapy in the management of osteochondral lesions of the talus: a retrospective cohort study. *Med Sci Monit.* 2019 Jul 30;25:5640–7.
84. Magalhaes FN, Dotta L, Sasse A, Teixera MJ, Fonoff ET. Ozone therapy as a treatment for low back pain secondary to herniated disc: a systematic review and meta-analysis of randomized controlled trials. *Pain Physician.* 2012 Mar–Apr;15(2):E115–29.
85. Buric J, Rigobello L, Hooper D. Five and ten year follow-up on intradiscal ozone injection for disc herniation. *Int J Spine Surg.* 2014 Dec 1;8:17.
86. Perri M, Marsecano C, Varrassi M, et al. Indications and efficacy of O_2-O_3 intradiscal versus steroid intraforaminal injection in different types of disco vertebral pathologies: a prospective randomized double-blind trial with 517 patients. *Radiol Med.* 2016 Jun;121(6):463–71.
87. Kelekis A, Bonaldi G, Cianfoni A, et al. Intradiscal oxygen-ozone chemonucleolysis versus microdiscectomy for lumbar disc herniation radiculopathy: a non-inferiority randomized control trial. *Spine J.* 2022 Jun;22(6):895–909.
88. Dagenais S, Mayer J, Haldeman S, Borg-Stein J. Evidence-informed management of chronic low back pain with prolotherapy. *Spine J.* 2008;8(1):203–12.
89. Rabago D, Slattengren A, Zgierska A. Prolotherapy in primary care practice. *Prim Care.* 2010;37(1):65–80.
90. Guharoy SR, Barajas M. Probable anaphylactic reaction to corn-derived dextrose solution. *Vet Hum Toxicol.* 1991 Dec;33(6):609–10.

Orthobiologic Therapies

78

Andre A. Abadin, Erek W. Latzka, and Kimberly G. Harmon

INTRODUCTION

- Soft-tissue injuries including tendon, muscle, and ligament injuries account for a large proportion of injuries to recreational and elite athletes. Enhancing the healing of these injuries beyond ice, rest, activity modification, and the tincture of time has been the goal of sports medicine physicians.
- It is now known that nonsteroidal anti-inflammatory drugs, commonly prescribed for soft-tissue injury, do not enhance healing, but alleviate pain (1). Furthermore, surgery has not been shown to be effective in treating tendinopathy compared to nonsurgical treatments (2).
- The advent of orthobiologic therapies holds the potential to use the body's own healing ability to speed up and improve tissue repair. A number of different options have been investigated.
- This chapter will explore the pathophysiology of common orthobiologic therapies, examine the human literature to date, and offer conclusions based on the best available data.

AUTOLOGOUS BLOOD

History

- Percutaneous release of extensor tendons of the elbow has been shown to be an effective treatment of lateral epicondylitis (3).
- Theorized by Edwards and Calandruccio that the benefits of this treatment were secondary to the beneficial effect of bleeding in the area, which started an inflammatory reaction that led to a cascade of healing (4)

Definition

- Injection of a small amount (2–3 cc) of the patient's own blood back into a damaged or injured area

Conclusion

- Multiple case series show that autologous blood injection is an effective treatment for tendinosis despite varied techniques, protocols, and rehabilitation between studies (5).
- However, autologous blood appears to be used less frequently with the rise of newer orthobiologic treatments.

PLATELET-RICH PLASMA

History

- The first use was reported in cardiopulmonary bypass surgery (6).
- The use spread to cardiac, plastic surgery, and orthopedic procedures.
- The first use in tendons was documented in 2006 by Mishra and Pavelko (7).

Definition

- A volume of autologous plasma that has a platelet concentration above baseline (8)
- The plasma allows platelets to clot.
- A clot is composed of fibrin, fibronectin, and vitronectin, which are cell adhesion molecules required to promote tissue healing (8).

Terminology

- Platelet-rich growth factors
  - Another term for platelet-rich plasma (PRP)
- Platelet-rich fibrin matrix
  - Typically used to refer to PRP that has been clotted
  - The clot provides substance and is usually used in surgical techniques.
- Platelet concentrate
  - A solid composition of platelets without plasma
  - Will not clot without plasma (no fibrin)
- Platelet releasate
  - The product is created from activated platelets, that is, the released growth factors from the platelets.
  - Typically created by creating a pellet of platelets in plasma and then adding thrombin to activate platelets
- Leukocyte-rich and leukocyte-poor PRP
  - Neutrophil concentrations above (leukocyte-rich) or below (leukocyte-poor) baseline compared to whole blood

Variables to Consider in PRP Product

- Platelet concentration
  - There may be an optimum concentration of platelets above which the concentration may be inhibitory.
  - Graziani et al. demonstrated that 2.5× baseline was the optimal concentration in vitro (9).
  - Han et al. demonstrated that PRP with 50 ng · mL^{-1} TGF-β was more stimulatory than 200 ng · mL^{-1} (10).
  - Other studies have shown that proliferation is dependent on platelet concentration, with higher concentrations being more effective (11).
  - Marx suggested that the minimum effective number of platelets was a concentration of 1,000,000/μL in 6 mL of PRP. Many modern platelet concentrating systems do not achieve this concentration (12).
- Presence or absence of leukocytes
  - There is debate regarding whether white blood cells (WBCs) enhance or are a detriment to healing.
  - There are three subtypes of WBCs.
    - Neutrophils
      - Contain hydrolytic enzymes
      - Release proteases and free radicals
      - In muscle injury, neutrophils promote secondary damage after the initial injury (13,14).
    - Monocytes
      - The primary role is the removal of debris.
      - Balance anti-inflammatory and proinflammatory aspects of healing (15)
    - Lymphocytes
      - Initiate cell-to-cell interactions
      - Play an important role in vessel formation by supporting the proliferation and differentiation of stem cells
- Viability of platelets
  - Once platelets are activated (by thrombin, calcium chloride, or collagen), they release 95% of their growth factors in the first hour (12).
  - Platelets can be damaged during the collection process (mechanical trauma).
- Anticoagulation
  - Anticoagulant citrate dextrose A
    - Reversible
    - Citrate binds to calcium to inhibit the initiation of the clotting cascade.
    - Dextrose and other buffers support the viability of platelets (16).
    - Acidic, which will lower pH, thus making it more painful to inject
    - Some PRP protocols use bicarbonate to buffer back acidity.
    - There is some evidence that the release of platelet-derived growth factors α (and early healing) is enhanced by an acidic environment (17).
  - Citrate phosphate dextrose also binds calcium but is 10% less effective at supporting platelet viability (16).
    - Once anticoagulated, PRP will remain stable and sterile for 8 hours (12).
- How and when PRP is activated
  - Requires exogenous activation prior to injection into target tissue
  - Thrombin
  - Calcium chloride activates the clotting cascade by allowing the polymerization of fibrin fibers required for clotting.
- Exogenous activation
  - When activated, a fibrin clot is formed and the PRP increases in density, forming a globule or membrane.
  - For surgical use, this can allow the product to be incorporated into repairs with sutures.
  - For use with injections, the product will gel and be difficult or impossible to inject.
  - Growth factor release begins as soon as PRP is activated, so products should be used relatively quickly after activation. This will occur with products that use no anticoagulation.
  - Some techniques use double-barreled syringes to inject the PRP and thrombin simultaneously so the activation occurs at the time of the injection.
- Amount of fibrinogen
  - Fibrinogen forms a matrix that enmeshes platelets and supports cell migration.
  - Depending on how PRP is activated, different molecular structures can be formed.
  - Drastic activation from high thrombin concentrations may form a less stable tetramolecule or bilateral junctions, which leads to fibrin monomers that are not favorable for cytokine enmeshment or cell migration (18).
  - Slower activation encourages more stable trivalent or equilateral junctions, which leads to a multifiber assembly that supports cytokine enmeshment and cell migration (18).
  - A study showed that both leukocyte-rich and leukocyte-poor PRP had similar amounts of fibrinogen present (19).

PRP IN TENDINOPATHY

Theory

- Tendon pain that lasts more than 3–6 weeks is not inflammatory.
- Tendinosis or tendinopathy is degenerative on biopsies with an absence of inflammatory cells.

- PRP can stimulate healing by starting an inflammatory reaction.
- Inflammation is the first stage of healing.

Selected Studies

Rotator Cuff Tendinopathy

- Kesikburun et al. (2013) (20)
  - Randomized controlled trial, level 1
  - 40 patients with magnetic resonance imaging (MRI) findings of rotator cuff tendinopathy (RCT) and at least 50% improvement in pain with diagnostic ancestry subacromial injection
  - Patients received an ultrasound (US)-guided subacromial PRP injection or an US-guided subacromial normal saline injection.
  - No statistically significant difference at 1-year follow-up between the two cohorts for improving quality of life, pain, disability, and shoulder range of motion
- Kwong et al. (2021) (21)
  - Randomized controlled trial, level 1
  - 99 patients with MRI findings of RCT
  - Patients received an US-guided supraspinatus and subacromial leukocyte-poor PRP injection or an US-guided subacromial corticosteroid injection.
  - Improvement in pain and patient-reported outcome scores, but no statistically significant difference at 1-year follow-up between the two cohorts
- Schwitzguebel et al. (2019) (22)
  - Randomized controlled trial, level 1
  - 80 patients with symptomatic isolated interstitial tears of the supraspinatus confirmed by MRI
  - Patients received either an US-guided supraspinatus PRP injection or a normal saline injection. Both groups received two injections, 1 month apart.
  - At 7 and 12 months, there was no statistical difference in lesion size or improvement of pain or function.

Common Extensor Tendinopathy

- Gupta et al. (2020) (23)
  - Randomized controlled trial, level 1
  - 80 patients with lateral epicondylosis that failed 3 months of conservative therapy
  - Patients received a palpation-guided PRP or corticosteroid injection at the common extensor origin.
  - At 6 weeks, the corticosteroid group had greater improvement in pain and function. However, at 3 and 12 months, the PRP group had greater improvement in pain and function.
- Tang el al. (2020) (24)
  - Systematic meta-analysis
  - 20 randomized controlled trials reviewed
  - Studies included PRP versus corticosteroid versus autologous blood injection.
  - At 2 months, the corticosteroid group had greater improvement in pain and function. However, after 2 months, PRP had greater improvement in pain and function.
- Karjalainen et al. (2021) (25)
  - Cochrane meta-analysis
  - 32 randomized controlled trials reviewed
  - Studies included PRP injection versus another intervention.
  - At 3 months, PRP does not show clinically significant improvement in pain or function compared to placebo injections.

Gluteus Medius Tendinopathy

- Fitzpatrick et al. (2019) (26)
  - Randomized controlled trial, level 1
  - 80 patients with gluteus medius tendinopathy without tears diagnosed with MRI or US with failed conservative treatments for more than 3 months
  - The patients received either an US-guided intertendinous leukocyte-rich PRP or corticosteroid injection.
  - The PRP group had statistically significant improvements in pain and function compared to the corticosteroid group at 12 weeks and was sustained for 2 years.
- Ali et al. (2018) (27)
  - Systematic review of level 1 studies
  - Three randomized controlled trials and two case series reviewed
  - Studies include PRP for the treatment of gluteus medius tendinopathy, greater trochanteric pain syndrome, or trochanteric bursitis.
  - Improvement in pain and function at 3 months and up to 12 months; however, heterogeneity of pathology limits definitive conclusions

Patella Tendinopathy

- Andriolo et al. (2019) (28)
  - Systematic review and meta-analysis
  - 70 studies including randomized controlled trials, prospective and retrospective studies, and case series
  - Studies included nonoperative treatments for chronic patella tendinopathy, and 15 studies used PRP.
  - PRP, especially multiple injections (2 or greater), resulted in better patient satisfaction, reduced pain, and improved function.
- Barman et al. (2022) (29)
  - Systematic review and meta-analysis
  - 8 studies including randomized and nonrandomized controlled trials
  - Studies included PRP injections versus other injection treatments or noninjection treatments.
  - PRP did not demonstrate a statistically significant difference in pan and function compared to other injection treatments. However, when compared to extracorporeal shockwave therapy there was a statistically significant improvement in pain and function.

Achilles Tendinopathy

- Boesen et al. (2017) (30)
    - Randomized controlled trial, level 1
    - 60 patients with greater than 3 months of midsubstance Achilles pain
    - The patient received either an US-guided high-volume injection (steroid and saline), 4 PRP injections over 2 weeks, or placebo.
    - High-volume injection groups and PRP showed statistically more significant improvement in pain, function, and reduction in tendon thickness and vascularity. However, the PRP group was more effective at reducing pain after 6 weeks.
- Liu et al. (2019) (31)
    - Systematic meta-analysis
    - 5 randomized controlled trials reviewed
    - Studies included PRP versus placebo.
    - There was no statistical difference in pain and function between the two groups. However, the PRP group demonstrated a statistically significant decrease in tendon thickness compared to placebo.

Plantar Fasciopathy

- Khurana et al. (2021) (32)
    - Randomized controlled trial, level 1
    - 118 patients with at least 4 weeks of pain and a clinical diagnosis of plantar fasciopathy
    - The patients received either a palpation-guided PRP injection or a corticosteroid injection.
    - The PRP group had statistically significant improvement in pain and function at 1 month and reached maximum benefits at 6 months postinjection.
- Peerbooms et al. (2019) (33)
    - Randomized controlled trial, level 1
    - 115 patients with at least 6 months of pain and have failed conservative treatment
    - The patients received either a palpation-guided PRP injection or a corticosteroid injection. The investigator who injected the patients were blinded to the treatments.
    - At 12 months, the PRP group showed statistically significant improvement in pain and function compared to the corticosteroid group.

Conclusion

- Multiple level 1 randomized controlled trials showed improvement in pain and function in chronic tendinopathy.
- The most compelling data are the treatment of the common extensor tendon and plantar fasciopathy (34).
- Future randomized controlled trials need to determine the ideal treatment protocol (type of PRP and frequency of injections) and patient characteristics for other tendinopathies.

PRP IN OSTEOARTHRITIS

Theory

- PRP may be able to stimulate chondral anabolism and inhibit the catabolic process.
- PRP may reduce synovial membrane hyperplasia and modulate cytokine levels.
- PRP in vitro is shown to stimulate the synthesis of collagen and proteoglycans, producing histological and biomechanical tissue similar to that within an articular joint.

Selected Studies

Knee Osteoarthritis

- Di Martino et al. (2019) (35)
    - Double-blinded, randomized controlled trial, level 1
    - 192 patients with chronic symptomatic knee degenerative changes and Kellgren-Lawrence grade 0–3
    - The patients received palpation-guided 3-weekly injections of leukocyte-poor or hyaluronic acid injections.
    - The PRP group had greater improvement in pain and function at 2, 6, 12, and 24 months; however, it was not statistically significant.
- Migliorini et al. (2021) (36)
    - Bayesian network meta-analysis, level 1
    - 30 randomized controlled trials reviewed
    - Studies included treatment effectiveness of PRP, corticosteroid, hyaluronic acid, and placebo in the treatment of knee osteoarthritis.
    - PRP demonstrated superior function and pain scores compared to the other intra-articular injections at 3, 6, and 12 months.
- Bennell et al. (2021) (37)
    - Randomized controlled trial, level 1
    - 144 patients, 50 years or older, with symptomatic knee pain and Kellgren-Lawrence grade 2–3
    - The patients received either 3 US-guided leukocyte-poor PRP or normal saline 1 week apart.
    - There was no statistically significant benefit in pain or function at 2 months or 12 months.
- Chu et al. (2022) (38)
    - Double-blinded, randomized controlled trial, level 1
    - 610 patients, between ages 18–80, with symptomatic knee pain, Kellgren-Lawrence grade 1–3
    - The patients received either 3 US-guided leukocyte-poor PRP or normal saline 1 week apart.

- Leukocyte-poor PRP group showed statistically significant benefits in function and pain scores compared to the saline group at 6, 12, 24, and 60 months of follow-up.

Hip Osteoarthritis

- Kraeutler et al. (2021) (39)
  - Randomized controlled trial, level 1
  - 31 patients (33 hips) with hip pain and Kellgren-Lawrence grade 2–3
  - The patient received either three palpation-guided leukocyte-poor PRP or hyaluronic acid 1 week apart.
  - The PRP group had statistically significant improvement in pain and function at 6 months.
- Gazendam et al. (2020) (40)
  - Systematic meta-analysis
  - 11 randomized controlled trials reviewed
  - Studies included treatment effectiveness of PRP, corticosteroid, hyaluronic acid, and normal saline in the treatment of hip osteoarthritis.
  - PRP, corticosteroid, and hyaluronic acid did not show improved pain or function compared to normal saline at 2,4, and 6 months.
- Ye at al. (2018) (41)
  - Systematic meta-analysis
  - 4 randomized controlled trials reviewed
  - Studies included treatment effectiveness of PRP versus hyaluronic acid.
  - The PRP group showed statistically significant improvement in pain at 2 months, but not at 6 or 12 months. There was not a statistically significant improvement in function at 2, 6, and 12 months.

Glenohumeral Osteoarthritis

- There are currently no level 1 randomized controlled trials comparing PRP to another intervention.

Conclusion

- Improvement in pain and function for the treatment of knee osteoarthritis demonstrated with leukocyte-poor PRP compared to corticosteroid and hyaluronic acid
- PRP that has been activated may improve outcomes compared to nonactivated PRP in knee osteoarthritis (42).
- PRP seems to be just as effective as hyaluronic acid and normal saline for reducing pain and improving function in mild to moderate hip osteoarthritis.
- It is difficult to truly compare studies as PRP is often not characterized.
- There is a lack of randomized controlled trials for other joints, so it is difficult to draw conclusions on the effectiveness of PRP within those joints.

PRP IN LIGAMENTOUS INJURY

Theory

- PRP can lead to cell differentiation, proliferation, and collagen expression.
- Increase the amount of type I and type III collagen, which is the predominant collagen in ligaments
- Will improve overall tensile strength and remodeling of fibrillar components

Studies

- Blanco-Rivera et al. (2020) (43)
  - Randomized controlled trial for lateral ankle sprains
  - 21 patients with first-time grade II lateral ankle sprains for no more than 48 hours
  - The patients were all immobilized. One group received a palpation-guided PRP injection. The other group did not receive any injections.
  - The PRP group had a statistically significant improvement in pain at 3, 5, and 8 weeks, but not at 24 weeks. The PRP group had statistically significant improvement in function only at 8 weeks.
- Podesta et al. (2013) (44)
  - Case series for partial ulnar collateral ligament (UCL) tears
  - 34 patients with partial-thickness UCL confirmed by MRI and failed 2 months of conservative treatments
  - The patients received an US-guided PRP injection within the UCL tear.
  - Pain, function, and joint space widening with valgus stress all improved. One patient underwent ligament reconstruction.

Conclusion

- Additional studies, preferably randomized controlled trials, are needed before recommendations can be made.

MESENCHYMAL STROMAL CELLS

History

- Alexander Friedenstein demonstrated the differentiation capabilities of mesenchymal stem cells in vitro and in vivo in the 1960s (45).
- In 1991, Arnold Caplan first coined the term "mesenchymal stem cell" (46).
- Due to further understanding of the capabilities of mesenchymal stem cells, there have been proposed name changes to accurately describe them: mesenchymal stromal cells (MSCs) or medicinal signaling cells (47).

Definition

- MSCs are cells that can differentiate into various tissues such as bone, cartilage, and soft tissue (46).
- The mechanism of action of healing is poorly understood in vivo; however, recent research suggests that autocrine and paracrine activities play a critical role in tissue repair (48).
- Despite animal studies demonstrating cartilage preservation and regeneration, clinical studies have not been able to replicate such results.

Terminology

- MSCs
  - Reported in bone marrow, umbilical cord blood, adipose tissue, and muscle
- Stromal cells
  - Differentiating connective tissue cells found in bone marrow that support blood cell growth
- Embryonic stem cells
  - Pluripotent cells derived from an embryo capable of differentiating into any of the three primary germ cell layers
- Bone marrow aspirate concentration (BMAC)
  - A concentration of bone marrow aspirate that contains a small number of MSCs after it has undergone a centrifuge process
- Adipose-derived mesenchymal stromal cells (AD-MSCs)
  - MSCs harvested from adipose tissue
  - Can be culture expanded
    - Ensures large enough quantity of stromal cells to have a therapeutic effect
    - Creates a consistent and homogenous product
  - AD-MSCs can be processed either enzymatically or mechanically.
    - Enzymatically processed AD-MSCs are referred to as stromal vascular fraction (SVF).
    - Mechanically processed AD-MSCs are referred to as microfat.
- Amniotic-derived stromal cells
  - Stromal cells isolated from birth tissue or fluid (amniotic, umbilical, or placental)

Types of MSCs Preparation

- BMAC (49)
  - Usually obtained from the iliac crest, especially the posterior superior iliac spine
  - A trochar is inserted into the bone and heparin is injected prior to aspiration.
  - After a series of micropipetting and centrifuging, the product is made.
  - Harvest about 60 mL of bone marrow for 6 mL of BMAC.
  - Culture-expanded BMAC may not be used clinically in the United States.
- AD-MSCs
  - The most common source to harvest is abdominal adipose tissue.
    - Can either harvest via resection or liposuction
  - Isolation of MSCs can be completed by enzymatic or mechanical isolation or a combination (50).
  - The end product of enzymatically treated adipose is SVF (51).
    - Contains endothelial, fibroblasts, pericytes, macrophages, and MSCs
    - SVF is considered more than minimally manipulated by the Food and Drug Administration (FDA) and thus illegal in the United States unless used in an FDA-approved Investigational New Drug (IND) study.
  - Mechanically separated fat, often termed microfat, leaves cells intact within native adipose tissue.
    - There are 510K FDA-cleared devices available.
    - It is unclear/debated whether this use of microfat for orthobiologics is acceptable to the FDA (see below).
  - Culture-expanded AD-MSCs may not be used clinically in the United States unless used in an FDA-approved IND study.
- Amniotic-derived stromal cells
  - MSCs are gathered from amniotic fluid or membrane immediately after a live birth (52).
    - Amniotic fluid can also be obtained during an amniocentesis in the second trimester.
    - Recommendations to gather amniotic fluid immediately after a live birth or during second trimester to maximize the number of MSCs obtained
  - Debate if commercial products produce viable MSCs
  - Amniotic MSCs may not be used clinically in the United States unless used in an FDA-approved IND study.

Regulatory Considerations (53,54)

- Therapeutic use of human cells, tissues, and tissue products (HCT/Ps) are regulated by the FDA. They are regulated under a three-tiered risk-based system:
  - Tier 1 (lowest risk): These include blood products, which are required to follow current good tissue practices (CGTP), but are not regulated by the FDA as HCT/Ps (they do not require registration with the FDA or annual reporting).
  - Tier 2 (low risk): These HCT/Ps must meet Title 21 Code of Federal Regulations, Part 1271 criteria. They are regulated as 361 products, which require CGTP, registration with the FDA, and annual reporting.
    - Minimal manipulation: Processing does not alter the original relevant characteristics of the tissue.

        - Homologous use: Repair, reconstruction, replacement, or supplementation of a recipient's cells or tissues with an HCT/P that performs the same basic function
        - Autologous use
        - No systemic effect
        - The Same Surgical Procedure Exception allows the use of HCT/Ps that are removed from an individual and implanted into the same individual during the same surgical procedure.
    - Tier 3 (higher risk): These HCT/Ps do not meet the above criteria. They are regulated as 351 products, which require preclinical trials, pharmacology/toxicity studies, IND approval for human clinical trials, and finally biologics license application prior to marketing.
- PRP is considered a tier 1 blood product
- BMAC is considered a tier 2/361 product unless it is culture expanded, in which case it becomes a tier 3/351 product.
- Amniotic-derived MSCs are considered a tier 3/351 product, as they are neither homologous nor autologous.
- SVF is considered a tier 3/351 product, as it is processed beyond minimal manipulation.
    - Due to the 2022 ruling (USA vs California Stem Cell Treatment Center) against the FDA, there is currently disagreement between California and Florida State Judicial Systems on whether SVF can be considered a 361 product under the Same Surgical Procedure Exception.
- The status of microfat as either a tier 2/361 versus tier 3/351 product is unclear and debated.
    - Although not homologous, microfat has been used as a 361 product under the Same Surgical Procedure Exception.
- Devices can be approved via the 361 pathway or via the 510K pathway, which allows devices equivalent to those already on the market to be grandfathered in.
    - Device approval (*i.e.*, Lipogems) does not equal product approval (*i.e.*, Microfat) for use in orthopedic conditions.
- Orthobiologic treatments "have not been approved for the treatment of any orthopedic condition, such as osteoarthritis, tendonitis, disc disease, tennis elbow, back pain, hip pain, knee pain, neck pain, or shoulder pain" per the FDA's statement to patients and consumers in 2020 (55).
- Physicians using orthobiologic treatments should be familiar and comply with FDA regulations.
    - In 2021, a period of regulatory discretion ended, and since that time, the enforcement of these regulations has increased. This enforcement can come from the FDA, the Federal Trade Commission (FTC), and individual state licensing boards.
    - Specifically, the FTC regulates advertising/fraud
        - cannot advertise "stem cells"
        - cannot suggest a systemic effect
        - cannot advertise off-label uses of devices or products

MSCS IN TENDINOPATHY

Theory

- Chronic tendinopathy is a degenerative process.
- MSCs inhibit the disruption of collagen fibers, reversing an abnormal collagen ratio (56).
- Tenocytes are stimulated leading to the production of collagen fibrils and the restoration of normal tendon anatomy.

Selected Studies

- Culture-expanded AD-MSCs
    - Jo et al. (2020) (57)
        - Retrospective comparative study for RCT with partial-thickness tears
        - 19 patients with partial tears of the rotator cuff tendon confirmed by MRI or US after failing at least 3 months of conservative treatments
        - The patients were placed in one of three groups: low, mid, and high doses of cultured AD-MSCs (based on cell count). No control group. Each patient received an intratendinous injection with US guidance.
        - No adverse effects were reported.
        - 90% improvement in pain at 1- and 2-year follow-up for the mid- to high-dose group. Function and strength improved in the high dose at 2 years.
- SVF
    - Khoury et al. (2021) (58)
        - Pilot study for common extensor tendinopathy
        - 18 tennis players with chronic, recalcitrant common extensor tendinopathy who already failed conservative treatments
        - All patients received an US-guided intratendinous expanded SVF injection.
        - No adverse effects were reported.
        - At 6 months, all patients had improvement in pain, function, and structure of the tendon.
    - Usuelli et al. (2018) (59)
        - Randomized controlled trial for midportion Achilles tendinopathy
        - 44 patients with chronic Achilles tendinopathy for more than 3 months
        - Patients were randomized to receive either an US-guided leukocyte-rich PRP or SVF.
        - At 6 months, both groups had improvement in pain and function; however, there was a statistically significant improvement in pain at 15 and 30 days postinjection in the SVF group.
- Microfat
    - There are currently no peer-reviewed studies comparing microfat to another intervention.

- BMAC
  - Pascual-Garrido et al. (2012) (60)
    - Case series for chronic patellar tendinopathy
    - Eight patients with MRI confirmed tendinopathy and failed 6 months of conservative treatment
    - All patients received an US-guided intratendinous BMAC injection.
    - Statistically significant improvements in pain and function scores at 1-, 2-, and 5-year follow-up
  - Thueakthong et al. (2021) (61)
    - Retrospective case study for midportion and insertional Achilles tendinopathy
    - 15 patients with at least 12 months of symptoms who failed conservative treatments
    - All patients received a palpation-guided BMAC injection.
    - There was a statistically significant improvement in pain at 6, 10, 24, and 48 weeks postinjection with no reported adverse effects.

Conclusion

- No studies reported adverse effects.
- Although studies report improvement in pain and function, the lack of a control group hinders the ability to draw definitive conclusions.

MSCS IN OSTEOARTHRITIS

Theory

- In vitro studies demonstrate chondrogenic potential.
- Through paracrine activity, the release of bioactive molecules can regenerate tissue within a human joint.
- In vivo studies have not demonstrated regenerative activity.

Selected Studies

- Culture-expanded AD-MSCs
  - Freitag et al. (2019) (62)
    - Randomized control trial for knee osteoarthritis
    - 30 patients with grade 2–3 osteoarthritis on Kellgren-Lawrence scale
    - Patients were randomized to conservative management, a single US-guided intra-articular AD-MSC injection, or two US-guided intra-articular AD-MSC injections separated by 6 months.
    - No adverse effects were reported.
    - At 12 months, there was a statistically significant improvement in pain and function in both AD-MSCs groups. At 12 months, there was less progression of articular cartilage degradation in the 2-injection group versus the 1-injection group.
- SVF
  - Garza et al (2020) (63)
    - Double-blinded randomized control trial for knee osteoarthritis
    - 39 patients
    - Patients randomized to receive either autologous SVF or a placebo US-guided injection (both groups received lipoaspiration)
    - At 6 and 12 months, the SVF group had a statistically significant improvement in pain and function. The improvement was dose-dependent.
- Microfat
  - Dall'Oca et al. (2019) (64)
    - Case series on hip osteoarthritis
    - Six patients with 0–2 Tonnis grading and 6 months of hip pain
    - All patients received an intra-articular microfat injection.
    - No adverse effects were reported.
    - All patients had improvement in pain and function scores at 6 months.
  - Kaszynski et al. (2022) (65)
    - Randomized controlled trial for knee osteoarthritis
    - 54 patients with grade 1–3 osteoarthritis on Kellgren-Lawrence scale
    - Patients were randomized to receive either PRP or microfat
    - Both groups had improvement in pain and function compared to their baseline values at 6 and 12 months.
- BMAC
  - Shapiro et al. (2017) (66)
    - Prospective, single-blinded study on knee osteoarthritis
    - 25 patients with bilateral knee pain and bilateral knee osteoarthritis
    - Each patient received an US-guided intra-articular injection of normal saline in one knee and BMAC in the contralateral knee.
    - No adverse effects were reported.
    - Pain improved from baseline in both knees at 1 week, 3 months, and 6 months. However, there was not a statistically significant difference between the injected knee and the uninjected knee.
- General
  - McIntyre et al. (2018) (67)
    - Systematic review on the effectiveness of MSCs on osteoarthritis (knee, ankle, hip)
    - 28 studies were included, but 14 studies were reviewed for osteoarthritis.

- Every study included for osteoarthritis focused on the knee, except one prospective case series that treated ankle, hip, and knee osteoarthritis.
- Conclusion: BMAC and AD-MSCs are safe, but difficult to assess their effectiveness for reducing pain and improving function due to many studies lacking a control group.

- Gong et al. (2021) (68)
  - Systematic review on the effectiveness of MSCs on knee osteoarthritis
  - 13 studies were included (6 BMAC, 4 AD-MSC, 1 umbilical cord–derived, 1 placenta-derived, 1 peripheral blood–derived).
  - 10 studies demonstrated improved cartilage thickness, quality, and repair with MRI and arthroscopy.
  - Unfortunately, the heterogeneity of the patient population of the studies and MSCs preparation limit specific conclusions.

Conclusion

- BMAC and AD-MSCs are safe without reported adverse outcomes when used to treat osteoarthritis.
- Most studies have focused on knee osteoarthritis, with a lack of studies on other joints.
- There was an improvement in pain and function, but there is a lack of evidence in cartilage regeneration or preservation in clinical trials.

MSCS IN LIGAMENTOUS INJURY

- There are no human clinical trials demonstrating the effectiveness of MSCs on ligamentous injuries.

SUMMARY

- Orthobiologics have grown in use and popularity for treatments of a variety of musculoskeletal conditions.
- PRP has the most level 1 randomized controlled trials; common extensor tendon, plantar fasciopathy, and knee osteoarthritis have the most robust data in support of PRP as a treatment option (34).
- While MSCs have been shown to be safe, there lacks definitive evidence to support use in the treatment of arthritis, tendinopathy, and ligamentous injuries.
- A tiered approach regarding the use of orthobiologics is recommended. Proven safety, peer-reviewed trials, and a patient-centered approach are imperative when a decision to use orthobiologics is made to treat chronic musculoskeletal conditions (69).

REFERENCES

1. Kane SF, Olewinski LH, Tamminga KS. Management of chronic tendon injuries. *Am Fam Physician.* 2019 Aug 1;100(3):147–57.
2. Challoumas D, Clifford C, Kirwan P, Millar NL. How does surgery compare to sham surgery or physiotherapy as a treatment for tendinopathy? A systematic review of randomised trials. *BMJ Open Sport Exerc Med.* 2019;5(1):e000528.
3. Baumgard SH, Schwartz DR. Percutaneous release of the epicondylar muscles for humeral epicondylitis. *Am J Sports Med.* 1982;10(4):233–6. doi:10.1177/036354658201000408
4. Edwards SG, Calandruccio JH. Autologous blood injections for refractory lateral epicondylitis. *J Hand Surg Am.* 2003;28(2):272–8. doi:10.1053/jhsu.2003.50041
5. Chou LC, Liou TH, Kuan YC, Huang YH, Chen HC. Autologous blood injection for treatment of lateral epicondylosis: a meta-analysis of randomized controlled trials. *Phys Ther Sport.* 2016;18:68–73. doi:10.1016/j.ptsp.2015.06.002
6. Giordano GF, Rivers SL, Chung GK, et al. Autologous platelet-rich plasma in cardiac surgery: effect on intraoperative and postoperative transfusion requirements. *Ann Thorac Surg.* 1988;46(4):416–19. doi:10.1016/s0003-4975(10)64655-3
7. Mishra A, Pavelko T. Treatment of chronic elbow tendinosis with buffered platelet-rich plasma. *Am J Sports Med.* 2006;34(11):1774–8. doi:10.1177/0363546506288850
8. Marx RE, Carlson ER, Eichstaedt RM, Schimmele SR, Strauss JE, Georgeff KR. Platelet-rich plasma: growth factor enhancement for bone grafts. *Oral Surg Oral Med Oral Pathol Oral Radiol Endod.* 1998;85(6):638–46. doi:10.1016/s1079-2104(98)90029-4
9. Graziani F, Ivanovski S, Cei S, Ducci F, Tonetti M, Gabriele M. The in vitro effect of different PRP concentrations on osteoblasts and fibroblasts. *Clin Oral Implants Res.* 2006;17(2):212–19. doi:10.1111/j.1600-0501.2005.01203.x
10. Han J, Meng HX, Tang JM, Li SL, Tang Y, Chen ZB. The effect of different platelet-rich plasma concentrations on proliferation and differentiation of human periodontal ligament cells in vitro. *Cell Prolif.* 2007;40(2):241–52. doi:10.1111/j.1365-2184.2007.00430.x
11. Marx RE. Platelet-rich plasma: evidence to support its use. *J Oral Maxillofac Surg.* 2004;62(4):489–96. doi:10.1016/j.joms.2003.12.003
12. Marx RE. Platelet-rich plasma (PRP): what is PRP and what is not PRP? *Implant Dent.* 2001;10(4):225–8. doi:10.1097/00008505-200110000-00002
13. Tidball JG. Inflammatory processes in muscle injury and repair. *Am J Physiol Regul Integr Comp Physiol.* 2005;288(2):R345–53. doi:10.1152/ajpregu.00454.2004
14. Best TM, Hunter KD. Muscle injury and repair. *Phys Med Rehabil Clin N Am.* 2000;11(2):251–66.
15. El-Sharkawy H, Kantarci A, Deady J, et al. Platelet-rich plasma: growth factors and pro- and anti-inflammatory properties. *J Periodontol.* 2007;78(4):661–9. doi:10.1902/jop.2007.060302
16. Lucarelli E, Beccheroni A, Donati D, et al. Platelet-derived growth factors enhance proliferation of human stromal stem cells. *Biomaterials.* 2003;24(18):3095–100. doi:10.1016/s0142-9612(03)00114-5
17. Liu Y, Kalén A, Risto O, Wahlström O. Fibroblast proliferation due to exposure to a platelet concentrate in vitro is pH dependent. *Wound Repair Regen.* 2002;10(5):336–40. doi:10.1046/j.1524-475x.2002.10510.x
18. Dohan Ehrenfest DM, Rasmusson L, Albrektsson T. Classification of platelet concentrates: from pure platelet-rich plasma (P-PRP) to leucocyte- and platelet-rich fibrin (L-PRF). *Trends Biotechnol.* 2009;27(3):158–67. doi:10.1016/j.tibtech.2008.11.009

19. Castillo TN, Pouliot MA, Kim HJ, Dragoo JL. Comparison of growth factor and platelet concentration from commercial platelet-rich plasma separation systems. *Am J Sports Med.* 2011;39(2):266–71. doi:10.1177/0363546510387517
20. Kesikburun S, Tan AK, Yilmaz B, Yaşar E, Yazicioğlu K. Platelet-rich plasma injections in the treatment of chronic rotator cuff tendinopathy: a randomized controlled trial with 1-year follow-up. *Am J Sports Med.* 2013;41(11):2609–16. doi:10.1177/0363546513496542
21. Kwong CA, Woodmass JM, Gusnowski EM, et al. Platelet-rich plasma in patients with partial-thickness rotator cuff tears or tendinopathy leads to significantly improved short-term pain Relief and function compared with corticosteroid injection: a double-blind randomized controlled trial. *Arthroscopy.* 2021;37(2):510–17. doi:10.1016/j.arthro.2020.10.037
22. Schwitzguebel AJ, Kolo FC, Tirefort J, et al. Efficacy of platelet-rich plasma for the treatment of interstitial supraspinatus tears: a double-blinded, randomized controlled trial. *Am J Sports Med.* 2019;47(8):1885–92. doi:10.1177/0363546519851097
23. Gupta PK, Acharya A, Khanna V, Roy S, Khillan K, Sambandam SN. PRP versus steroids in a deadlock for efficacy: long-term stability versus short-term intensity-results from a randomised trial. *Musculoskelet Surg.* 2020;104(3):285–94. doi:10.1007/s12306-019-00619-w
24. Tang S, Wang X, Wu P, et al. Platelet-rich plasma Vs autologous blood vs corticosteroid injections in the treatment of lateral epicondylitis: a systematic review, pairwise and network meta-analysis of randomized controlled trials. *PM & R.* 2020;12(4):397–409. doi:10.1002/pmrj.12287
25. Karjalainen TV, Silagy M, O'Bryan E, Johnston RV, Cyril S, Buchbinder R. Autologous blood and platelet-rich plasma injection therapy for lateral elbow pain. *Cochrane Database Syst Rev.* 2021;9(9):CD010951. doi:10.1002/14651858.CD010951.pub2
26. Fitzpatrick J, Bulsara MK, O'Donnell J, Zheng MH. Leucocyte-rich platelet-rich plasma treatment of gluteus medius and minimus tendinopathy: a double-blind randomized controlled trial with 2-year follow-up. *Am J Sports Med.* 2019;47(5):1130–7. doi:10.1177/0363546519826969
27. Ali M, Oderuth E, Atchia I, Malviya A. The use of platelet-rich plasma in the treatment of greater trochanteric pain syndrome: a systematic literature review. *J Hip Preserv Surg.* 2018;5(3):209–19. doi:10.1093/jhps/hny027
28. Andriolo L, Altamura SA, Reale D, Candrian C, Zaffagnini S, Filardo G. Nonsurgical treatments of patellar tendinopathy: multiple injections of platelet-rich plasma are a suitable option — a systematic review and meta-analysis. *Am J Sports Med.* 2019;47(4):1001–1018. doi:10.1177/0363546518759674
29. Barman A, Sinha MK, Sahoo J, et al. Platelet-rich plasma injection in the treatment of patellar tendinopathy: a systematic review and meta-analysis. *Knee Surg Relat Res.* 2022;34(1):22. doi:10.1186/s43019-022-00151-5
30. Boesen AP, Hansen R, Boesen MI, Malliaras P, Langberg H. Effect of high-volume injection, platelet-rich plasma, and sham treatment in chronic midportion achilles tendinopathy: a randomized double-blinded prospective study. *Am J Sports Med.* 2017;45(9):2034–43. doi:10.1177/0363546517702862
31. Liu CJ, Yu KL, Bai JB, Tian DH, Liu GL. Platelet-rich plasma injection for the treatment of chronic Achilles tendinopathy: a meta-analysis. *Medicine.* 2019;98(16):e15278. doi:10.1097/MD.0000000000015278
32. Khurana A, Dhankhar V, Goel N, Gupta R, Goyal A. Comparison of midterm results of Platelet Rich Plasma (PRP) versus Steroid for plantar fasciitis: a randomized control trial of 118 patients. *J Clin Orthop Trauma.* 2021;13:9–14. Erratum in: *J Clin Orthop Trauma.* 2021 Oct;*21*:101559. doi:10.1016/j.jcot.2020.09.002
33. Peerbooms JC, Lodder P, den Oudsten BL, Doorgeest K, Schuller HM, Gosens T. Positive effect of platelet-rich plasma on pain in plantar fasciitis: a double-blind multicenter randomized controlled trial. *Am J Sports Med.* 2019;47(13):3238–46. doi:10.1177/0363546519877181
34. Abadin AA, Orr JP, Lloyd AR, Henning PT, Pourcho A. An evidence-based approach to orthobiologics for tendon disorders. *Phys Med Rehabil Clin N Am.* 2023 Feb;34(1):83–103.
35. Di Martino A, Di Matteo B, Papio T, et al. Platelet-rich plasma versus hyaluronic acid injections for the treatment of knee osteoarthritis: results at 5 Years of a double-blind, randomized controlled trial. *Am J Sports Med.* 2019;47(2):347–54. doi:10.1177/0363546518814532
36. Migliorini F, Driessen A, Quack V, et al. Comparison between intra-articular infiltrations of placebo, steroids, hyaluronic and PRP for knee osteoarthritis: a Bayesian network meta-analysis. *Arch Orthop Trauma Surg.* 2021;141(9):1473–90. doi:10.1007/s00402-020-03551-y
37. Bennell KL, Paterson KL, Metcalf BR, et al. Effect of intra-articular platelet-rich plasma vs placebo injection on pain and medial tibial cartilage volume in patients with knee osteoarthritis: the RESTORE randomized clinical trial. *JAMA.* 2021;326(20):2021–30. doi:10.1001/jama.2021.19415
38. Chu J, Duan W, Yu Z, et al. Intra-articular injections of platelet-rich plasma decrease pain and improve functional outcomes than sham saline in patients with knee osteoarthritis. *Knee Surg Sports Traumatol Arthrosc.* 2022;30(12):4063–71. doi:10.1007/s00167-022-06887-7
39. Kraeutler MJ, Houck DA, Garabekyan T, Miller SL, Dragoo JL, Mei-Dan O. Comparing intra-articular injections of leukocyte-poor platelet-rich plasma versus low-molecular weight hyaluronic acid for the treatment of symptomatic osteoarthritis of the hip: a double-blind, randomized pilot study. *Orthop J Sports Med.* 2021;9(1):2325967120969210. doi:10.1177/2325967120969210
40. Gazendam A, Ekhtiari S, Bozzo A, Phillips M, Bhandari M. Intra-articular saline injection is as effective as corticosteroids, platelet-rich plasma and hyaluronic acid for hip osteoarthritis pain: a systematic review and network meta-analysis of randomised controlled trials. *Br J Sports Med.* 2021;55(5):256–61. doi:10.1136/bjsports-2020-102179
41. Ye Y, Zhou X, Mao S, Zhang J, Lin B. Platelet rich plasma versus hyaluronic acid in patients with hip osteoarthritis: a meta-analysis of randomized controlled trials. *Int J Surg.* 2018;53:279–87. doi:10.1016/j.ijsu.2018.03.078
42. Simental-Mendía M, Ortega-Mata D, Tamez-Mata Y, Olivo CAA, Vilchez-Cavazos F. Comparison of the clinical effectiveness of activated and non-activated platelet-rich plasma in the treatment of knee osteoarthritis: a systematic review and meta-analysis. *Clin Rheumatol.* 2022 Dec 11;42(5):1397–1408. doi:10.1007/s10067-022-06463-x
43. Blanco-Rivera J, Elizondo-Rodríguez J, Simental-Mendía M, Vilchez-Cavazos F, Peña-Martínez VM, Acosta-Olivo C. Treatment of lateral ankle sprain with platelet-rich plasma: a randomized clinical study. *Foot Ankle Surg.* 2020;26(7):750–4. doi:10.1016/j.fas.2019.09.004
44. Podesta L, Crow SA, Volkmer D, Bert T, Yocum LA. Treatment of partial ulnar collateral ligament tears in the elbow with platelet-rich plasma. *Am J Sports Med.* 2013;41(7):1689–94. doi:10.1177/0363546513487979
45. Friedenstein AJ, Piatetzky-Shapiro II, Petrakova KV. Osteogenesis in transplants of bone marrow cells. *J Embryol Exp Morphol.* 1966;16(3):381–90.
46. Caplan AI. Mesenchymal stem cells. *J Orthop Res.* 1991;9(5):641–50. doi:10.1002/jor.1100090504
47. Caplan AI. Mesenchymal stem cells: time to change the name. *Stem Cells Transl Med.* 2017;6(6):1445–51. doi:10.1002/sctm.17-0051
48. Samsonraj RM, Raghunath M, Nurcombe V, Hui JH, van Wijnen AJ, Cool SM. Concise review: multifaceted characterization of human mesenchymal stem cells for use in regenerative medicine. *Stem Cells Transl Med.* 2017;6(12):2173–85. doi:10.1002/sctm.17-0129
49. Chahla J, Mannava S, Cinque ME, Geeslin AG, Codina D, LaPrade RF. Bone marrow aspirate concentrate harvesting and processing technique. *Arthrosc Tech.* 2017;6(2):e441–5. doi:10.1016/j.eats.2016.10.024

50. Alstrup T, Eijken M, Bohn AB, Møller B, Damsgaard TE. Isolation of adipose tissue-derived stem cells: enzymatic digestion in combination with mechanical distortion to increase adipose tissue-derived stem cell yield from human aspirated fat. *Curr Protoc Stem Cell Biol.* 2019;48(1):e68. doi:10.1002/cpsc.68
51. Ramakrishnan VM, Boyd NL. The adipose stromal vascular fraction as a complex cellular source for tissue engineering applications. *Tissue Eng Part B Rev.* 2018;24(4):289–99. doi:10.1089/ten.TEB.2017.0061
52. Riboh JC, Saltzman BM, Yanke AB, Cole BJ. Human amniotic membrane-derived products in sports medicine: basic science, early results, and potential clinical applications. *Am J Sports Med.* 2016;44(9):2425–34. doi:10.1177/0363546515612750
53. Center for Biologics Evaluation and Research. *Important Patient and Consumer Information about Regenerative Medicine Therapies.* U.S. Food and Drug Administration; n.d. Retrieved June 3, 2021, from https://www.fda.gov/vaccines-blood-biologics/consumers-biologics/important-patient-and-consumer-information-about-regenerative-medicine-therapies
54. Center for Biologics Evaluation and Research. *Tissue & Tissue Products.* U.S. Food and Drug Administration; n.d. Retrieved December 9, 2022, from https://www.fda.gov/vaccines-blood-biologics/tissue-tissue-products
55. Center for Biologics Evaluation and Research. *Regulatory Considerations for Human Cells, Tissues, and Cellular and Tissue-Based Products: Minimal Manipulation and Homologous Use.* U.S. Food and Drug Administration; n.d. Retrieved July 1, 2020, from https://www.fda.gov/regulatory-information/search-fda-guidance-documents/regulatory-considerations-human-cells-tissues-and-cellular-and-tissue-based-products-minimal
56. Oshita T, Tobita M, Tajima S, Mizuno H. Adipose-derived stem cells improve collagenase-induced tendinopathy in a rat model. *Am J Sports Med.* 2016;44(8):1983–9. doi:10.1177/0363546516640750
57. Jo CH, Chai JW, Jeong EC, Oh S, Yoon KS. Intratendinous injection of mesenchymal stem cells for the treatment of rotator cuff disease: a 2-year follow-up study. *Arthroscopy.* 2020;36(4):971–80. doi:10.1016/j.arthro.2019.11.120
58. Khoury M, Tabben M, Rolón AU, Levi L, Chamari K, D'Hooghe P. Promising improvement of chronic lateral elbow tendinopathy by using adipose derived mesenchymal stromal cells: a pilot study. *J Exp Orthop.* 2021;8(1):6. doi:10.1186/s40634-020-00320-z
59. Usuelli FG, Grassi M, Maccario C, et al. Intratendinous adipose-derived stromal vascular fraction (SVF) injection provides a safe, efficacious treatment for Achilles tendinopathy: results of a randomized controlled clinical trial at a 6-month follow-up. *Knee Surg Sports Traumatol Arthrosc.* 2018;26(7):2000–10. doi:10.1007/s00167-017-4479-9
60. Pascual-Garrido C, Rolón A, Makino A. Treatment of chronic patellar tendinopathy with autologous bone marrow stem cells: a 5-year-followup. *Stem Cells Int.* 2012;2012:953510. doi:10.1155/2012/953510
61. Thueakthong W, de Cesar Netto C, Garnjanagoonchorn A, et al. Outcomes of iliac crest bone marrow aspirate injection for the treatment of recalcitrant Achilles tendinopathy. *Int Orthop.* 2021;45(9):2423–8. doi:10.1007/s00264-021-05112-3
62. Freitag J, Bates D, Wickham J, et al. Adipose-derived mesenchymal stem cell therapy in the treatment of knee osteoarthritis: a randomized controlled trial. *Regen Med.* 2019;14(3):213–30. doi:10.2217/rme-2018-0161
63. Garza JR, Campbell RE, Tjoumakaris FP, et al. Clinical efficacy of intra-articular mesenchymal stromal cells for the treatment of knee osteoarthritis: a double-blinded prospective randomized controlled clinical trial. *Am J Sports Med.* 2020;48(3):588–98. doi:10.1177/0363546519899923
64. Dall'Oca C, Breda S, Elena N, Valentini R, Samaila EM, Magnan B. Mesenchymal Stem Cells injection in hip osteoarthritis: preliminary results. *Acta Biomed.* 2019;90(1-S):75–80. doi:10.23750/abm.v90i1-S.8084
65. Kaszyński J, Bąkowski P, Kiedrowski B, et al. Intra-articular injections of autologous adipose tissue or platelet-rich plasma comparably improve clinical and functional outcomes in patients with knee osteoarthritis. *Biomedicines.* 2022;10(3):684. doi:10.3390/biomedicines10030684
66. Shapiro SA, Kazmerchak SE, Heckman MG, Zubair AC, O'Connor MI. A prospective, single-blind, placebo-controlled trial of bone marrow aspirate concentrate for knee osteoarthritis. *Am J Sports Med.* 2017;45(1):82–90. doi:10.1177/0363546516662455
67. McIntyre JA, Jones IA, Han B, Vangsness CT Jr. Intra-articular mesenchymal stem cell therapy for the human joint: a systematic review. *Am J Sports Med.* 2018;46(14):3550–63. doi:10.1177/0363546517735844
68. Gong J, Fairley J, Cicuttini FM, et al. Effect of stem cell injections on osteoarthritis-related structural outcomes: a systematic review. *J Rheumatol.* 2021;48(4):585–97. doi:10.3899/jrheum.200021
69. Shapiro SA, Master Z, Arthurs JR, Mautner K. Tiered approach to considering orthobiologics for patients with musculoskeletal conditions. *Br J Sports Med.* 2023 Feb;57(3):179–80.

79 Common Injections in Sports Medicine

Christopher Lutrzykowski, Elizabeth Rothe, Thomas Hoke, Robert Stevens, and James Dunlap

INTRODUCTION

- Injections are a common intervention provided by sports clinicians. Injections can be both diagnostic and therapeutic. If delivered properly and with sound indications, injections can be very rewarding for both the patient and the provider.
- This chapter details the indications, benefits, risks, evidence, and technique for administering common palpation-guided injections in sports medicine. These injections, while in most cases simple to administer, should be done only after proper training and appropriate supervision. Most injections are simple to learn (see one, do one, teach one); judgment on their use, however, takes time and effort to acquire. Ultrasound-guided injections are discussed in Chapter 80.
- Corticosteroid as solute for injection will be the primary agent discussed. Other injection solutes such as proliferants and orthobiologics are discussed in Chapters 77 and 78, respectively.

INDICATIONS

- Injections/aspirations are indicated for both diagnosis and therapy.
  - Diagnostic arthrocentesis:
    - Synovial fluid analysis to rule out infection, traumatic, rheumatic, or crystal-induced etiology (Table 79.1)
    - To perform a therapeutic trial to differentiate various etiologies
    - Imaging studies
    - Synovial biopsy
  - Therapy:
    - To remove tense effusions to relieve pain and improve function
    - To remove blood or pus from a joint
    - For injection of steroids and other intra-articular therapies
    - For therapeutic lavage of joints

Risks/Complications (1) (Table 79.2)

- **Infection** (2–4): The risk of postinjection infection is extremely rare, on the order of one infection per 3000–50,000 injections when sterile technique is used. *Staphylococcus aureus* is the most common organism involved, with recent reports also implicating methicillin-resistant *S. aureus*. Since the initial writing of this chapter, concern has been raised regarding intra-articular steroid injection prior to joint replacement due to increased risk of post-joint replacement infection (5). While still felt to be rare, avoidance of joint replacement for at least 3 months post-corticosteroid injection would be wise (6,7). Pseudoseptic arthritis may occur following hyaluronic acid (HA) injection, but felt to be quite rare (8).
- **Tendon rupture** (9): Collagen atrophy and tendon rupture are rare but have been described in the literature. Injections into tendons should be avoided. In addition, corticosteroid injections into the synovial sheath or peritendinous region of major weight-bearing tendons (Achilles, patellar, and plantar fascia) should be done with extreme caution, and the athlete should be protected from weight-bearing exercise for a period of 2–4 weeks. A systematic review from 202 of injection prior to rotator cuff repair suggests an increased risk of revision surgery due to rupture if an injection was given within 1 year of repair (odds ratio: 1.3-2.8) (10).
- **Postinjection flare:** This entity is seen in 2%–10% of patients. In this setting, the patient develops a flare of pain in the immediate 6- to 12-hour period after an injection. The etiology for this reaction is thought to be secondary to a local reaction to the microcrystalline steroid suspension and is generally self-limited. The postinjection flare has also been attributed to the preservative that accompanies the anesthetic (11). This complication may be treated with activity modification and a short course of a nonsteroidal anti-inflammatory drug (NSAID). Ice has not been shown to be beneficial in a randomized controlled trial (RCT) (12). Patients with pain beyond 36 hours should be evaluated for a septic joint.
- **Skin atrophy/depigmentation/hyperpigmentation:** When steroid is applied too close to the surface of the skin, local atrophy and depigmentation/hyperpigmentation can occur.

Table 79.1 Classification of Synovial Fluid

Classification	Appearance	WBC	PMNs (%)	Crystals	Culture
Normal	Clear to straw colored	<150	<25	None	Negative
Noninflammatory	Yellow	<3000	<30	None	Negative
Inflammatory	Yellow or cloudy	3000–75,000	>50	None	Negative
Infectious	Yellow or purulent	50,000–200,000	>90	None	Positive
Crystal-induced	Cloudy, turbid	500–200,000	<90	Yes	Negative
Hemorrhagic	Red-brown	50–10,000	<50	None	Negative

PMNs, polymorphonuclear leukocytes; WBC, white blood cell.
Source: O'Connell TX. Interpreting tests from joint aspirates. In: Phenninger JL, editor. *The Clinics Atlas of Office Procedures — Joint Injection Techniques.* Vol. 5 (no. 4). Philadelphia (PA): WB Saunders Company; 2002.

These changes may be irreversible. Deeper injections such as intra-articular knee injections are less likely to cause this (13).

- **Hyperglycemia:** In some diabetics, there may be short-term difficulties with glycemic control secondary to the local absorption of corticosteroid. Hyperglycemia has been reported in the literature, but the limited available studies regarding this effect have noted variability in glucose elevation but are usually mild, typically last less than 5 days, and may be preparation dependent (14,15).
- **Cartilage degeneration:** Traditional teaching limits corticosteroid injections into a weight-bearing joint to no more than three injections per year, because there is some concern about weakening articular cartilage or frank chondrotoxicity from studies on postoperative bupivacaine continuous drips (1,16,17). Previous studies indicated that more frequent injections are well tolerated, particularly when used in a disease-specific manner (18). More recent studies have raised some doubts as to the efficacy of repeat injections as this may lead to rapidly progressive idiopathic arthritis (19,20), cartilage loss (21), and that no additional symptom relief was gleaned from repeat injections (20,21). Chondrotoxicity has been reported with multiple anesthetic agents and may potentiate the effects of corticosteroid injection (22). No adverse effects have been reported with repeat HA injection (23).

Table 79.2 Common Adverse Outcomes

Complication	Estimated Incidence (%)
Postinjection flare	2–10
Steroid arthropathy	0.8
Tendon rupture	<1
Facial flushing	<1
Skin atrophy, depigmentation	<1
Iatrogenic infectious arthritis	<0.001–0.072
Transient paresis of injected extremity	Rare
Hypersensitivity reaction	Rare
Asymptomatic pericapsular calcification	43
Acceleration of cartilage attrition	Unknown

Source: Gray RG, Gottleib NL. Intra-articular corticosteroids. An updated assessment. *Clin Orthop Relat Res.* 1983;(177):253–63.

- **Chondrotoxicity:** Prior studies indicated evidence of chondrolysis in postoperative patients treated with continuous intra-articular bupivacaine (24,25). More recent studies looking at the anesthetic class have demonstrated chondrotoxic effects of these agents to a varying degree. A recent systematic review has demonstrated in vitro chondrotoxic effects of lidocaine with a dose- and time-dependent response. Cell death was seen at doses of 0.5%; however, this was negligible. Bupivacaine also demonstrates both a dose- and time-dependent chondrotoxic effect in particular with concentrations greater than .25%. Bupivacaine may also be more chondrotoxic than other preparations, leading the author group to abandon this anesthetic for intra-articular use. Ropivacaine has also been shown to be chondrotoxic but in concentrations greater than .75%. In comparison to lidocaine and bupivacaine, these effects appear to be less. Data on other agents are sparse but seem to follow the pattern of other injectable anesthetics (22). Because no minimum volume has been described, cautious use of intra-articular anesthetic is recommended until this risk has been clearly defined in in vivo settings.
- **Intravascular injection**
- **Traumatic injection:** Possible to cause a pneumothorax and damage articular cartilage, local nerves, or soft-tissue structures
- **Vasovagal reactions**
- **Facial flushing:** Facial flushing after corticosteroid injection may be as common as 15% for all types of injections. This side effect is usually mild (26,27).
- **Intramuscular (IM) injection**

CONTRAINDICATIONS (18)

- Cellulitis or broken skin over the needle entry site would increase the risk for infection.
- Unstable coagulopathy
- Intra-articular fractures
- Septic effusion of a bursa or a periarticular structure

- Lack of response to prior injections
- Difficult to access joints, for example, hip, spine, sternoclavicular (28), and sacroiliac joints
- Joint prostheses — relative contraindication
- Known hypersensitivity to any component of the injection
  - Caution regarding interaction between protease inhibitors and corticosteroid injection causing Cushing syndrome (29–31)

GENERAL PRINCIPLES (32,33)

- **Consent:** Because there are inherent risks and complications associated with corticosteroid injections, informed consent should be obtained, witnessed, and documented.
- **Equipment:** Most injections are performed using an alcohol, chlorhexidine, or povidone-iodine wipe; some authors recommend a sterile scrub before injecting into a large joint (2,18). While recent data suggest that chlorhexidine may be the superior cleansing agent prior to surgery, no studies demonstrating increased antimicrobial protection have been performed for joint injection (34). Sterile versus nonsterile gloves are another area of controversy; as a rule, the authors teach that sterile gloves are used for joints and nonsterile gloves may be used for soft-tissue structures. Some advocate sterile gloves for all injections, whereas others prefer using the one sterile glove technique. In this technique, the physician wears the sterile glove on the noninjecting hand to ensure proper positioning after the local preparation. Finally, the "sterile no touch" technique may be employed as well, with only the needle touching the patient after preparation. Other equipment may include the following:
  - Povidone-iodine wipes and/or alcohol wipes
  - Sterile or nonsterile gloves
  - Sterile drapes: optional
  - 21- to 27-gauge 1.5-in needles for injection
  - 18- to 20-gauge needles for aspirations
  - 1- to 10-mL syringes for injections
  - 3- to 50-mL syringes for aspirations
  - Topical anesthetic spray
  - Anesthetic of choice
  - 2 × 2 gauze sponges
  - Small dressings such as adhesive bandages
  - Access to equipment to treat severe allergic reactions: oxygen; epinephrine 1:1000; diphenhydramine 25–50 mg IM; and advanced cardiac life support equipment

MEDICATIONS

- **Anesthesia:** The three main uses of anesthesia include diminishing pain, aiding in diagnosis, and providing a volume for corticosteroid injections. Although there are many local anesthetics, the two most commonly used are the amide compounds lidocaine and bupivacaine.
  - Lidocaine (Xylocaine) is available commercially as a 0.5%–2% concentration. The most commonly used concentration is 1%; 2% may be used in small areas where a small volume is required. Time from injection to onset of effect is 1–2 minutes, with duration of action of approximately 1–2 hours. The upper limit of dosing is 10 mL for 2% and 20 mL for 1%; above these levels, side effects can be expected.
  - Bupivacaine (Marcaine) is available commercially in 0.25%–0.5% concentrations. Time from injection to onset of effect is 5–30 minutes, with duration of action of approximately 8 hours. The upper limit of dosing is 30 mL for 0.5% and 60 mL for 0.25%; above these levels, side effects can be expected.
  - Ropivacaine (Naropin) is available commercially in 0.2%–1% concentrations. Time of onset is from 3 to 15 minutes and duration is typically 5–6 hours.
  - Side effects including anaphylaxis can occur; resuscitation equipment should be available.
  - When skin anesthesia is necessary prior to injection, an alternative to a local injection is topical anesthetic spray. When used, however, spray lightly to avoid cold injury and secondary skin changes.
  - It is recommended to draw the anesthetic prior to the corticosteroid with multiuse vials to limit anesthetic contamination by the steroid ("clear to cloudy").
- **Corticosteroids** (18): Corticosteroids are commonly used in musculoskeletal medicine. The corticosteroid reportedly treats the local inflammatory response and not the clinical problem. Steroids have both mineralocorticoid and glucocorticoid effects. The mineralocorticoid effects modify salt and water balance, while the glucocorticoid effect suppresses the inflammatory response. The ideal choice is to use a medication that maximizes the anti-inflammatory effect. Steroids also differ in their solubilities, potencies, and duration of action (Table 79.3). The duration of the effect is thought to vary inversely with the drug's solubility. Short-acting agents tend to have a lower incidence of postinjection flare, although studies are lacking. Traditionally, higher solubility agents (*e.g.*, betamethasone [Celestone], dexamethasone, and methylprednisolone) have been thought to be better for soft tissues, whereas lower solubility agents (*e.g.*, triamcinolone hexacetonide) tend to favor joint injections. There are little data to corroborate this in the literature. There is also growing concern regarding the safety of corticosteroid injection on chondrocyte health although much of the data are predominantly from in vitro studies. Combination with amide anesthetics may increase chondrocyte toxicity as well. This has import for repeat intra-articular injections as that may increase the risk further (22,35). Selected dosing is found in Table 79.4.
- **NSAIDs:** Ketorolac (Toradol) intra-articular injection may provide equivalent pain relief with respect to corticosteroid

Table 79.3 Relative Potencies and Solubilities of Corticosteroids

Corticosteroid	Relative Anti-Inflammatory Potency	Equivalent Dose (mg)	Solubility	Concentration (mg·mL^{-1})
Short-Acting				
Cortisone	0.8	25	NA	25, 50
Hydrocortisone	1	20	0.002	25
Intermediate-Acting				
Triamcinolone	5	4	0.0002	20
Hexacetonide				
Methylprednisolone	5	4	0.001	20, 40, 80
Long-Acting				
Dexamethasone	25	0.6	0.01	4, 8
Sodium phosphate				
Betamethasone	25	0.6	NA	6

NA, not applicable.
Source: Genovese MC. Joint and soft tissue injection: a useful adjuvant to systemic and local treatment. *Postgrad Med.* 1998;103(2):125–34.

and HA injection in some joint locations although data are sparse (36–38). Chondrocyte toxicity in vitro may be similar to corticosteroids (38) but has not been born out through in vivo animal model studies (39). Dosage range has not been fully identified but generally from 30 to 60 mg (38–40).

- **Botulinum toxin:** Botulinum toxin A is a neurotoxic protein produced by *Clostridium botulinum* that has medicinal purposes. The mechanism of action is to produce flaccid paralysis by reversibly inhibiting the presynaptic release of neurotransmitters, mainly acetylcholine. Other neurotransmitters affected include substance P, calcitonin gene–related peptide, and glutamate. By affecting these neurotransmitters, botulinum toxin A can result in antinociceptive and analgesic effect and may also produce a local anti-inflammatory action (41). Botulinum toxin A has been proposed and studied for the treatment of chronic adductor–related groin pain,

Table 79.4 Recommended Corticosteroid and Lidocaine Dosages for Injections

Site of Injection	Dose of 1% Lidocaine (mL)	Dose of Triamcinolone (mg)	Dose of Betamethasone (mg)
de Quervain	1–2	40	6
Carpal tunnel	0.5–1	40	6
Trigger finger	1	20	3
Tennis elbow	0.5–1	40	6
Subacromial space	6–8	40	6
Glenohumeral	6–8	40–60	6–9
Acromioclavicular	1–2	40	6
Plantar fascia	1–2	40	6
Anserine bursa	2–3	40	6
Trochanteric bursa	4–5	40–60	6–9
Intra-articular knee	4–6	40–60	6–9
Morton neuroma	1–2	20–40	3–6
Myofascial	1–2	NA	NA
Iliotibial band	1–2	20–40	3–6
Ankle	2–3	40	6

NA, not applicable.
Source: Stankus SJ. Inflammation and the role of anti-inflammatory medications. In: Lillegard WA, Butcher JD, Rucker KS, editors. *Handbook of Sports Medicine.* 2nd ed. Boston (MA): Butterworth-Heinemann; 1999.

plantar fasciopathy, chronic exertional compartment syndrome, popliteal artery entrapment syndrome, and posttraumatic headache. Many of these studies are limited by small cohort size and heterogeneity but do show promise for the treatment of these disorders (42–46).

EVIDENCE-BASED ASSESSMENT

- Since the initial writing of this chapter, there have been well over 100 systematic reviews, meta-analyses, and RCTs and despite this fact, there continues to be conflicting or insufficient quality data to provide a definitive global answer on the efficacy of steroid injections in many locations. With some injection locations, corticosteroid may provide lasting relief, but with others, short-term or no relief has also been found. Data regarding efficacy of corticosteroid injection are listed for each injection site where there are data available. The addition of image-guided injection may help improve efficacy as accuracy of injection improves. Where available, evidence regarding the accuracy and efficacy of specific palpation-guided injection is also included in the descriptions of specific injections that follows.

SPECIFIC INJECTIONS (SEE ONLINE CHAPTER 79, ADDENDUM SPECIFIC INJECTIONS)

REFERENCES

These references are cited only in the online content of the chapter.

1. Turner JL, McKeag DB. Complications of joint aspirations and injections. In: Phenninger JL, editor. *The Clinics Atlas of Office Procedures: Joint Injection Techniques*. Philadelphia (PA): WB Saunders Company; 2002:433–43.
2. Charalambous CP, Tryfonidis M, Sadiq S, Hirst P, Paul A. Septic arthritis following intra-articular steroid injection of the knee — a survey of current practice regarding antiseptic technique used during intra-articular steroid injection of the knee. *Clin Rheumatol*. 2003;22(6):386–90.
3. Murray RJ, Pearson JC, Coombs GW, et al. Outbreak of invasive methicillin-resistant *Staphylococcus aureus* infection associated with acupuncture and joint injection. *Infect Control Hosp Epidemiol*. 2008;29(9):859–65.
4. von Essen R, Savolainen HA. Bacterial infection following intra-articular injection. A brief review. *Scand J Rheumatol*. 1989;18(1):7–12.
5. Avila A, Do MT, Acuña AJ, Samuel LT, Kamath AF. How do pre-operative intra-articular injections impact periprosthetic joint infection risk following primary total hip arthroplasty? A systematic review and meta-analysis. *Arch Orthop Trauma Surg*. 2023 Mar;143(3):1627–35. doi:10.1007/s00402-022-04375-8
6. Kim YM, Joo YB, Song JH. Preoperative intra-articular steroid injections within 3 months increase the risk of periprosthetic joint infection in total knee arthroplasty: a systematic review and meta-analysis. *J Orthop Surg Res*. 2023 Feb 28;18(1):148. doi:10.1186/s13018-023-03637-4
7. Avila A, Acuña AJ, Do MT, Samuel LT, Kamath AF. Intra-articular injection receipt within 3 months prior to primary total knee arthroplasty is associated with increased periprosthetic joint infection risk. *Knee Surg Sports Traumatol Arthrosc*. 2022 Dec;30(12):4088–97. doi:10.1007/s00167-022-06942-3
8. Sedrak P, Hache P, Horner NS, Ayeni OR, Adili A, Khan M. Differential characteristics and management of pseudoseptic arthritis following hyaluronic acid injection is a rare complication: a systematic review. *J ISAKOS*. 2021 Mar;6(2):94–101. doi:10.1136/jisakos-2020-000438
9. Kennedy JC, Willis RB. The effects of local steroid injections on tendons: a biomechanical and microscopic correlative study. *Am J Sports Med*. 1976;4(1):11–21.
10. Puzzitiello RN, Patel BH, Nwachukwu BU, Allen AA, Forsythe B, Salzler MJ. Adverse impact of corticosteroid injection on rotator cuff tendon health and repair: a systematic review. *Arthroscopy*. 2020 May;36(5):1468–75. doi:10.1016/j.arthro.2019.12.006
11. Rhee YG, Cho NS, Kim BH, Ha JH. Injection-induced pyogenic arthritis of the shoulder joint. *J Shoulder Elb Res*. 2008 Jan–Feb;17(1):63–7.
12. An TW, Boone SL, Boyer MI, Gelberman RH, Osei DA, Calfee RP. Effect of ice on pain after corticosteroid injection in the hand and wrist: a randomized controlled trial. *J Hand Surg Eur Vol*. 2016 Nov;41(9):984–9. doi:10.1177/1753193416657678
13. Kumar A, Dhir V, Sharma S, Sharma A, Singh S. Efficacy of methylprednisolone acetate versus triamcinolone acetonide intra-articular knee injection in patients with chronic inflammatory arthritis: a 24-week randomized controlled trial. *Clin Ther*. 2017 Jan;39(1):150–8. doi:10.1016/j.clinthera.2016.11.023
14. Slotkoff A, Clauw D, Nashel D. Effect of soft tissue corticosteroid injection on glucose control in diabetics. *Arthritis Rheum*. 1994;37(suppl 9):s347.
15. Russell SJ, Sala R, Conaghan PG, et al. Triamcinolone acetonide extended-release in patients with osteoarthritis and type 2 diabetes: a randomized, phase 2 study. *Rheumatology*. 2018 Dec 1;57(12):2235–41. doi:10.1093/rheumatology/key265
16. Genovese MC. Joint and soft-tissue injection. A useful adjuvant to systemic and local treatment. *Postgrad Med J*. 1998;103(2):125–34.
17. Pfenninger JL. Joint and soft tissue aspiration and injection. In: Pfenninger JL, Fowler GC, editors. *Procedures for Primary Care Physicians*. St. Louis (MO): Mosby; 1994.
18. Stephens MB, Beutler AI, O'Connor FG. Musculoskeletal injections: a review of the evidence. *Am Fam Physician*. 2008;78(8):971–6.
19. Boutin RD, Pai J, Meehan JP, Newman JS, Yao L. Rapidly progressive idiopathic arthritis of the hip: incidence and risk factors in a controlled cohort study of 1471 patients after intra-articular corticosteroid injection. *Skelet Radiol*. 2021 Dec;50(12):2449–57. doi:10.1007/s00256-021-03815-7
20. Ayub S, Kaur J, Hui M, et al. Efficacy and safety of multiple intra-articular corticosteroid injections for osteoarthritis-a systematic review and meta-analysis of randomized controlled trials and observational studies. *Rheumatology*. 2021 Apr 6;60(4):1629–39. doi:10.1093/rheumatology/keaa808
21. McAlindon TE, LaValley MP, Harvey WF, et al. Effect of intra-articular triamcinolone vs saline on knee cartilage volume and pain in patients with knee osteoarthritis: a randomized clinical trial. *JAMA*. 2017;317(19):1967–75. doi:10.1001/jama.2017.5283
22. Jayaram P, Kennedy DJ, Yeh P, Dragoo J. Chondrotoxic effects of local anesthetics on human knee articular cartilage: a systematic review. *Pharm Manag PM R*. 2019 Apr;11(4):379–400. doi:10.1002/pmrj.12007

23. Altman R, Hackel J, Niazi F, Shaw P, Nicholls M. Efficacy and safety of repeated courses of hyaluronic acid injections for knee osteoarthritis: a systematic review. *Semin Arthritis Rheum.* 2018 Oct;48(2):168–75. doi:10.1016/j.semarthrit.2018.01.009
24. Bailie DS, Ellenbecker TS. Severe chondrolysis after shoulder arthroscopy: a case series. *J Shoulder Elb Res.* 2009;18(5):742–7.
25. Rapley JH, Beavis RC, Barber FA. Glenohumeral chondrolysis after shoulder arthroscopy with continuous bupivacaine infusion. *Arthroscopy.* 2010;26(4):439–40.
26. Cole BJ, Schumacher HR Jr. Injectable corticosteroids in modern practice. *J Am Acad Orthop Surg.* 2005;13(1):37–46.
27. Lee YK, Lee GY, Lee JW, Lee E, Kang HS. Intra-articular injections in patients with femoroacetabular impingement: a prospective, randomized, double-blind, cross-over study. *J Korean Med Sci.* 2016 Nov;31(11):1822–7. doi:10.3346/jkms.2016.31.11.1822
28. Weinberg AM, Pichler W, Grechenig S, Tesch NP, Heidari N, Grechenig W. Frequency of successful intra-articular puncture of the sternoclavicular joint: a cadaver study. *Scand J Rheumatol.* 2009;38(5):396–8.
29. Xiao RC, Walley KC, DeAngelis JP, Ramappa AJ. Corticosteroid injections for adhesive capsulitis: a review. *Clin J Sport Med.* 2017 May;27(3):308–20. doi:10.1097/JSM.0000000000000358
30. Maviki M, Cowley P, Marmery H. Injecting epidural and intra-articular triamcinolone in HIV-positive patients on ritonavir: beware of iatrogenic Cushing's syndrome. *Skelet Radiol.* 2013;42(2):313–5.
31. Albert NE, Kazi S, Santoro J, Dougherty R. Ritonavir and epidural triamcinolone as a cause of iatrogenic Cushing's syndrome. *Am J Med Sci.* 2012;344(1):72–4.
32. Paluska AS. Indications, contraindications, and overview for aspirating or injecting a joint or related structure. In: Pfenninger JL, editor. *The Clinics Atlas of Office Procedures: Joint Injection Techniques*, Vol. 5(4) Philadelphia (PA): WB Saunders; 2002.
33. White RD. Supplies and equipment needed for joint injection. In: Pfenninger JL, editor. *The Clinics Atlas of Office Procedures: Joint Injection Techniques*, Vol. 5(4). Philadelphia (PA): WB Saunders; 2002:403–12.
34. Aftab R, Dodhia VH, Jeanes C, Wade RG. Bacterial sensitivity to chlorhexidine and povidone-iodine antiseptics over time: a systematic review and meta-analysis of human-derived data. *Sci Rep.* 2023 Jan 7;13(1):347. doi:10.1038/s41598-022-26658-1
35. Wernecke C, Braun HJ, Dragoo JL. The effect of intra-articular corticosteroids on articular cartilage: a systematic review. *Orthop J Sports Med.* 2015 Apr 27;3(5):2325967115581163. doi:10.1177/2325967115581163
36. Abrams GD, Chang W, Dragoo JL. In vitro chondrotoxicity of nonsteroidal anti-inflammatory drugs and opioid medications. *Am J Sports Med.* 2017 Dec;45(14):3345–50. doi:10.1177/0363546517724423
37. Bellamy JL, Goff BJ, Sayeed SA. Economic impact of ketorolac vs corticosteroid intra-articular knee injections for osteoarthritis: a randomized, double-blind, prospective study. *J Arthroplast.* 2016 Sep;31(9 suppl l):293–7. doi:10.1016/j.arth.2016.05.015
38. Min KS, St Pierre P, Ryan PM, Marchant BG, Wilson CJ, Arrington ED. A double-blind randomized controlled trial comparing the effects of subacromial injection with corticosteroid versus NSAID in patients with shoulder impingement syndrome. *J Shoulder Elb Res.* 2013 May;22(5):595–601. doi:10.1016/j.jse.2012.08.026
39. Park KD, Kim TK, Bae BW, Ahn J, Lee WY, Park Y. Ultrasound guided intra-articular ketorolac versus corticosteroid injection in osteoarthritis of the hip: a retrospective comparative study. *Skelet Radiol.* 2015 Sep;44(9):1333–40. doi:10.1007/s00256-015-2174-9
40. Ahn JK, Kim J, Lee SJ, Park Y, Bae B, Lee W. Effects of Ultrasound-guided intra-articular ketorolac injection with capsular distension. *J Back Musculoskelet Rehabil.* 2015;28(3):497–503. doi:10.3233/BMR-140546
41. Ahadi T, Nik SS, Forogh B, Madani SP, Raissi GR. Comparison of the effect of ultrasound-guided injection of botulinum toxin type A and corticosteroid in the treatment of chronic plantar fasciitis: a randomized controlled trial. *Am J Phys Med Rehabil.* August 2022;101(8):733–7. doi:10.1097/PHM.0000000000001900
42. Creuzé A, Fok-Cheong T, Weir A, et al. Novel use of botulinum toxin in long-standing adductor-related groin pain: a case series. *Clin J Sport Med.* 2022 Nov 1;32(6):567–73. doi:10.1097/JSM.0000000000001066
43. Charvin M, Orta C, Davy L, et al. Botulinum toxin A for chronic exertional compartment syndrome: a retrospective study of 16 upper- and lower-limb cases. *Clin J Sport Med.* 2022 Jul 1;32(4):e436–40. doi:10.1097/JSM.0000000000000958
44. Isner-Horobeti ME, Dufour SP, Blaes C, Lecocq J. Intramuscular pressure before and after botulinum toxin in chronic exertional compartment syndrome of the leg: a preliminary study. *Am J Sports Med.* 2013 Nov;41(11):2558–66. doi:10.1177/0363546513499183
45. Hislop M, Brideaux A, Dhupelia S. Functional popliteal artery entrapment syndrome: use of ultrasound guided Botox injection as a nonsurgical treatment option. *Skelet Radiol.* 2017 Sep;46(9):1241–8. doi:10.1007/s00256-017-2686-6
46. Yerry JA, Kuehn D, Finkel AG. Onabotulinum toxin a for the treatment of headache in service members with a history of mild traumatic brain injury: a cohort study. *Headache.* 2015 Mar;55(3):395–406. doi:10.1111/head.12495
47. Cole BF, Peters KS, Hackett L, Murrell GA. Ultrasound-guided versus blind subacromial corticosteroid injections for subacromial impingement syndrome: a randomized, double-blind clinical trial. *Am J Sports Med.* 2016 Mar;44(3):702–7. doi:10.1177/0363546515618653
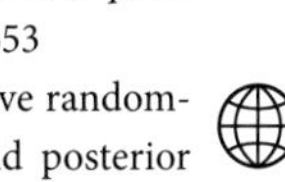
48. Ganokroj P, Matrakool L, Limsuwarn P, et al. A prospective randomized study comparing the effectiveness of midlateral and posterior subacromial steroid injections. *Orthopedics.* 2019 Jan 1;42(1):e44-50. doi:10.3928/01477447-20181109-03
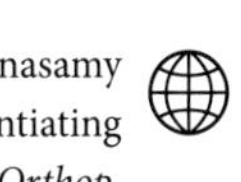
49. Duraiswamy G, Khanna V, Prasad P, Sambandam SN, Mounasamy V. Posterior subacromial injections are superior in differentiating a rotator cuff from a biceps pathology: a cadaveric study. *J Orthop.* 2020;19:89–92. doi:10.1016/j.jor.2019.11.015
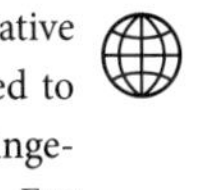
50. Sumanont S, Boonard M, Peradhammanon E, et al. Comparative outcomes of combined corticosteroid with low volume compared to high volume of local anesthetic in subacromial injection for impingement syndrome: systematic review and meta-analysis of RCTs. *Eur J Orthop Surg Traumatol.* 2018 Apr;28(3):397–407. doi:10.1007/s00590-017-2056-z
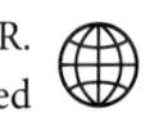
51. Henkus HE, Cobben LP, Coerkamp EG, Nelissen RG, van Arkel ER. The accuracy of subacromial injections: a prospective randomized magnetic resonance imaging study. *Arthroscopy.* 2006;22(3):277–82.
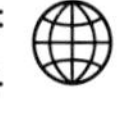
52. Mathews PV, Glousman RE. Accuracy of subacromial injection: anterolateral versus posterior approach. *J Shoulder Elbow Surg.* 2005;14(2):145–8.
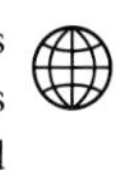
53. Ogbeivor C, Bandaru S, Milton C. A comparison of the effectiveness of lateral versus posterior approach to shoulder injection in patients with subacromial impingement syndrome: a pragmatic randomized controlled trial. *Muscoskel Care.* 2019 Sep;17(3):257–68. doi:10.1002/msc.1416
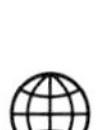
54. Partington PF, Broome GH. Diagnostic injection around the shoulder: hit or miss? A cadaveric study of injection accuracy. *J Shoulder Elbow Surg.* 1998;7(2):147–50.
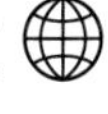
55. Ogbeivor C. Needle placement approach to subacromial injection in patients with subacromial impingement syndrome: a systematic review. *Muscoskel Care.* 2019 Mar;17(1):13–22. doi:10.1002/msc.1375
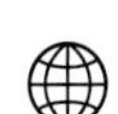
56. Buchbinder R, Green S, Youd JM. Corticosteroid injections for shoulder pain. *Cochrane Database Syst Rev.* 2003;2003(1):CD004016.

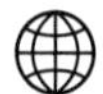
57. Gruson KI, Ruchelsman DE, Zuckerman JD. Subacromial corticosteroid injections. *J Shoulder Elbow Surg*. 2008;17(1 suppl):118S–30S.

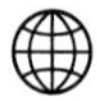
58. Mohamadi A, Chan JJ, Claessen FM, Ring D, Chen NC. Corticosteroid injections give small and transient pain relief in rotator cuff tendinosis: a meta-analysis. *Clin Orthop Relat Res*. 2017;475(1):232–43.

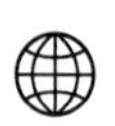
59. Zadro J, Rischin A, Johnston RV, Buchbinder R. Image-guided glucocorticoid injection versus injection without image guidance for shoulder pain. *Cochrane Database Syst Rev*. 2021 Aug 26;8(8):CD009147. doi:10.1002/14651858.CD009147.pub3

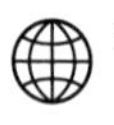
60. Cole BF, Peters KS, Hackett L, Murrell GA. Ultrasound-guided versus blind subacromial corticosteroid injections for subacromial impingement syndrome: a randomized, double-blind clinical trial. *Am J Sports Med*. 2016 Mar;44(3):702–7. doi:10.1177/0363546515618653

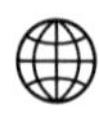
61. Akbari N, Ozen S, Zenlikçi HB, Haberal M, Çetin N. Ultrasound guided versus blind subacromial corticosteroid and local anesthetic injection in the treatment of subacromial impingement syndrome: a randomized study of eLicacy. *Jt Dis Relat Surg*. 2020;31(1):115–22.

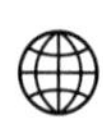
62. Rijs Z, de Groot PCJ, Zwitser EW, Visser CPJ. Is the anterior injection approach without ultrasound guidance superior to the posterior approach for adhesive capsulitis of the shoulder? A sequential, prospective trial. *Clin Orthop Relat Res*. 2021 Nov 1;479(11):2483–9. doi:10.1097/CORR.0000000000001803

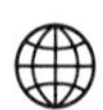
63. Powell SE, Davis SM, Lee EH, et al. Accuracy of palpation-directed intra-articular glenohumeral injection confirmed by magnetic resonance arthrography. *Arthroscopy*. 2015 Feb;31(2):205–8. doi:10.1016/j.arthro.2014.08.013

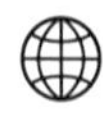
64. Porat S, Leupold JA, Burnett KR, Nottage WM. Reliability of non-imaging-guided glenohumeral joint injection through rotator interval approach in patients undergoing diagnostic MR arthrography. *AJR Am J Roentgenol*. 2008;191(3):W96–9.

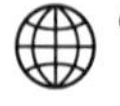
65. Sethi PM, Kingston S, Elattrache N. Accuracy of anterior intra-articular injection of the glenohumeral joint. *Arthroscopy*. 2005;21(1):77–80.

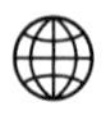
66. van der Heijden GJ, van der Windt DA, Kleijnen J, Koes BW, Bouter LM. Steroid injections for shoulder disorders: a systematic review of randomized clinical trials. *Br J Gen Pract*. 1996;46(406):309–16.

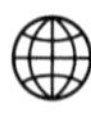
67. Carette S, Moffet H, Tardif J, et al. Intraarticular corticosteroids, supervised physiotherapy, or a combination of the two in the treatment of adhesive capsulitis of the shoulder: a placebo-controlled trial. *Arthritis Rheum*. 2003;48(3):829–38.

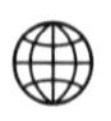
68. Gaujoux-Viala C, Dougados M, Gossec L. Efficacy and safety of steroid injections for shoulder and elbow tendonitis: a meta-analysis of randomised controlled trials. *Ann Rheum Dis*. 2009;68(12):1843–9.

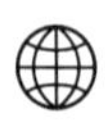
69. Lorbach O, Anagnostakos K, Scherf C, Seil R, Kohn D, Pape D. Nonoperative management of adhesive capsulitis of the shoulder: oral cortisone application versus intra-articular cortisone injections. *J Shoulder Elbow Surg*. 2010;19(2):172–9.

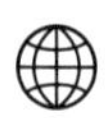
70. Goh GJ, Over KE, Daroszewska A, Whitehouse GH, Bucknall RC. The value of arthrography in steroid injection of the shoulder joint. *Br J Rheumatol*. 1997;36(6):709–10.

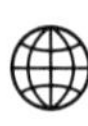
71. Raeissadat SA, Rayegani SM, Langroudi TF, Khoiniha M. Comparing the accuracy and efficacy of ultrasound-guided versus blind injections of steroid in the glenohumeral joint in patients with shoulder adhesive capsulitis. *Clin Rheumatol*. 2017 Apr;36(4):933–40. doi:10.1007/s10067-016-3393-8

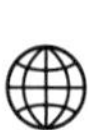
72. Metzger CM, Farooq H, Merrell GA, et al. Efficacy of a single, image-guided corticosteroid injection for glenohumeral arthritis. *J Shoulder Elbow Surg*. 2021 May;30(5):1128–34. doi:10.1016/j.jse.2020.08.008

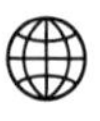
73. Mall NA, Foley E, Chalmers PN, Cole BJ, Romeo AA, Bach BR Jr. Degenerative joint disease of the acromioclavicular joint: a review. *Am J Sports Med*. 2013 Nov;41(11):2684–92. doi:10.1177/0363546513485359

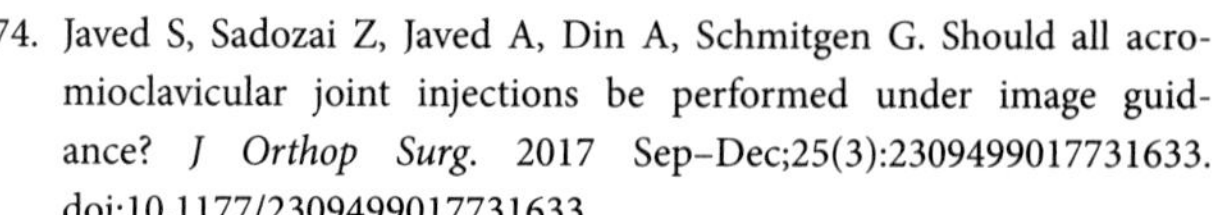
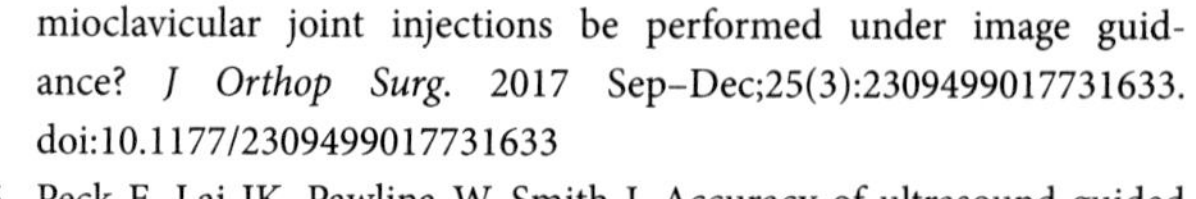
74. Javed S, Sadozai Z, Javed A, Din A, Schmitgen G. Should all acromioclavicular joint injections be performed under image guidance? *J Orthop Surg*. 2017 Sep–Dec;25(3):2309499017731633. doi:10.1177/2309499017731633

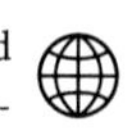
75. Peck E, Lai JK, Pawlina W, Smith J. Accuracy of ultrasound-guided versus palpation-guided acromioclavicular joint injections: a cadaveric study. *Pharm Manag PM R*. 2010;2(9):817–21.

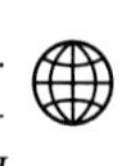
76. Borbas P, Kraus T, Clement H, Grechenig S, Weinberg AM, Heidari N. The influence of ultrasound guidance in the rate of success of acromioclavicular joint injection: an experimental study on human cadavers. *J Shoulder Elbow Surg*. 2012;21(12):1694–7.

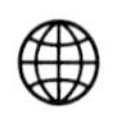
77. Park KD, Kim TK, Lee J, Lee WY, Ahn JK, Park Y. Palpation versus ultrasound-guided acromioclavicular joint intra-articular corticosteroid injections: a retrospective comparative clinical study. *Pain Physician*. 2015 Jul–Aug;18(4):333–41. Erratum in: *Pain Physician*. 2015 Sep–Oct;18(5):517.

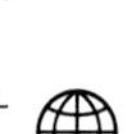
78. Sabeti-Aschraf M, Stotter C, Thaler C, et al. Intra-articular versus periarticular acromioclavicular joint injection: a multicenter, prospective, randomized, controlled trial. *Arthroscopy*. 2013;29(12):1903–10.

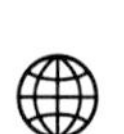
79. Altay T, Günal I, Oztürk H. Local injection treatment for lateral epicondylitis. *Clin Orthop Relat Res*. 2002:2002(398):127–30.

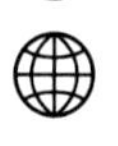
80. Dogramaci Y, Kalici A, Savaş N, Duman G, Yanat AN. Treatment of lateral epicondylitis using three different local injection modalities: a randomized prospective clinical trial. *Arch Orthop Trauma Surg*. 2009;129(10):1409–14.

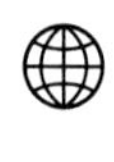
81. Sims SE, Miller K, Elfar JC, Hammert WC. Non-surgical treatment of lateral epicondylitis: a systematic review of randomized controlled trials. *Hand (N Y)*. 2014 Dec;9(4):419–46. doi:10.1007/s11552-014-9642-x

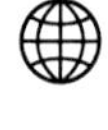
82. Lai WC, Erickson BJ, Mlynarek RA, Wang D. Chronic lateral epicondylitis: challenges and solutions. *Open Access J Sports Med*. 2018 Oct 30;9:243–51. doi:10.2147/OAJSM.S160974

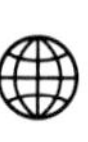
83. Coombes BK, Bisset L, Vicenzino B. Efficacy and safety of corticosteroid injections and other injections for management of tendinopathy: a systematic review of randomised controlled trials. *Lancet*. 2010 Nov 20;376(9754):1751–67. doi:10.1016/S0140-6736(10)61160-9

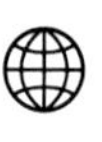
84. Niemiec P, Szyluk K, Jarosz A, Iwanicki T, Balcerzyk A. Effectiveness of platelet-rich plasma for lateral epicondylitis: a systematic review and meta-analysis based on achievement of minimal clinically important difference. *Orthop J Sports Med*. 2022 Apr 8;10(4):23259671221086920. doi:10.1177/23259671221086920

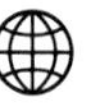
85. Chen XT, Fang W, Jones IA, Heckmann ND, Park C, Vangsness CT Jr. The efficacy of platelet-rich plasma for improving pain and function in lateral epicondylitis: a systematic review and meta-analysis with risk-of-bias assessment. *Arthroscopy*. 2021 Sep;37(9):2937–52. doi:10.1016/j.arthro.2021.04.061

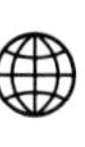
86. Jurado Vélez JA, Colberg RE, Fleisig GS. Percutaneous microtenotomy using a microdebrider coblation wand for the treatment of lateral epicondylitis: a systematic review. *Medicine (Baltim)*. 2022 Aug 5;101(31):e29957. doi:10.1097/MD.0000000000029957

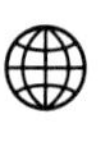
87. Ashraf MO, Devadoss VG. Systematic review and meta-analysis on steroid injection therapy for de Quervain's tenosynovitis in adults. *Eur J Orthop Surg Traumatol*. 2014 Feb;24(2):149–57. doi:10.1007/s00590-012-1164-z

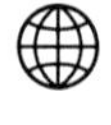
88. Cavaleri R, Schabrun SM, Te M, Chipchase LS. Hand therapy versus corticosteroid injections in the treatment of de Quervain's disease: A systematic review and meta-analysis. *J Hand Ther*. 2016 Jan–Mar;29(1):3–11. doi:10.1016/j.jht.2015.10.004

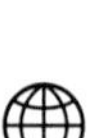
89. Oh JK, Messing S, Hyrien O, Hammert WC. Effectiveness of Corticosteroid Injections for Treatment of de Quervain's Tenosynovitis. *Hand (N Y)*. 2017 Jul;12(4):357–61. doi:10.1177/1558944716681976

90. Peters-Veluthamaningal C, Winters JC, Groenier KH, Meyboom-DeJong B. Randomised controlled trial of local corticosteroid injections for de Quervain's tenosynovitis in general practice. *BMC Muscoskelet Disord.* 2009 Oct 27;10:131. doi:10.1186/1471-2474-10-131

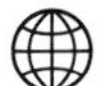
91. Kumar V, Talwar J, Rustagi A, Krishna LG, Sharma VK. Comparison of clinical and functional outcomes after platelet-rich plasma injection and corticosteroid injection for the treatment of de Quervain's tenosynovitis. *J Wrist Surg.* 2023;12(2):135–42. doi:10.1055/s-0042-1760124

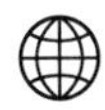
92. Atroshi I, Flondell M, Hofer M, Ranstam J. Methylprednisolone injections for the carpal tunnel syndrome: a randomized, placebo-controlled trial. *Ann Intern Med.* 2013 Sep 3;159(5):309–17. doi:10.7326/0003-4819-159-5-201309030-00004

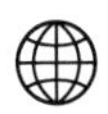
93. Hofer M, Ranstam J, Atroshi I. Extended follow-up of local steroid injection for carpal tunnel syndrome: a randomized clinical trial. *JAMA Netw Open.* 2021 Oct 1;4(10):e2130753. doi:10.1001/jamanetworkopen.2021.30753

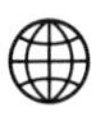
94. Alhindi AK, Ghaddaf AA, Alomari MS, et al. Effect of ultrasound-guided versus landmark-guided local corticosteroid injection for carpal tunnel syndrome: a systematic review and meta-analysis. *Arch Orthop Trauma Surg.* 2023;143(1):545–61. doi:10.1007/s00402-022-04437-x

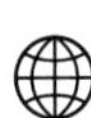
95. Wang H, Zhu Y, Wei H, Dong C. Ultrasound-guided local corticosteroid injection for carpal tunnel syndrome: a meta-analysis of randomized controlled trials. *Clin Rehabil.* 2021 Nov;35(11):1506–17. doi:10.1177/02692155211014702

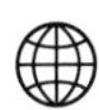
96. Senna MK, Shaat RM, Ali AAA. Platelet-rich plasma in treatment of patients with idiopathic carpal tunnel syndrome. *Clin Rheumatol.* 2019 Dec;38(12):3643–54. doi:10.1007/s10067-019-04719-7

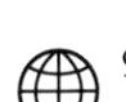
97. Alsaeid MA. Dexamethasone versus hyaluronidase as an adjuvant to local anesthetics in the ultrasound-guided hydrodissection of the median nerve for the treatment of carpal tunnel syndrome patients. *Anesth Essays Res.* 2019 Jul–Sep;13(3):417–22. doi:10.4103/aer.AER_104_19

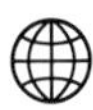
98. Dong C, Sun Y, Qi Y, et al. Effect of platelet-rich plasma injection on mild or moderate carpal tunnel syndrome: an updated systematic review and meta-analysis of randomized controlled trials. *BioMed Res Int.* 2020 Nov 14;2020:5089378. doi:10.1155/2020/5089378

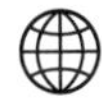
99. Shen PC, Chou SH, Lu CC, et al. Comparative effectiveness of various treatment strategies for trigger finger by pairwise meta-analysis. *Clin Rehabil.* 2020 Sep;34(9):1217–29. doi:10.1177/0269215520932619

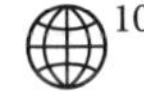
100. Leow MQH, Zheng Q, Shi L, Tay SC, Chan ES. Non-steroidal anti-inflammatory drugs (NSAIDs) for trigger finger. *Cochrane Database Syst Rev.* 2021 Apr 14;4(4):CD012789. doi:10.1002/14651858.CD012789.pub2

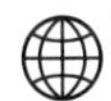
101. Gil JA, Hresko AM, Weiss APC. Current concepts in the management of trigger finger in adults. *J Am Acad Orthop Surg.* 2020 Aug 1;28(15):e642–50. doi:10.5435/JAAOS-D-19-00614

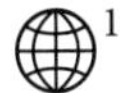
102. Seigerman D, McEntee RM, Matzon J, et al. Time to improvement after corticosteroid injection for trigger finger. *Cureus.* 2021 Aug 3;13(8):e16856. doi:10.7759/cureus.16856

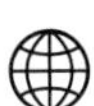
103. Pathak SK, Salunke AA, Menon PH, Thivari P, Nandy K, Yongsheng C. Corticosteroid injection for the treatment of trigger finger: a meta-analysis of randomised control trials. *J Hand Surg Asian Pac Vol.* 2022 Feb;27(1):89–97. doi:10.1142/S242483552250014X

104. Currie KB, Tadisina KK, Mackinnon SE. Common hand conditions: a review. *JAMA.* 2022 Jun 28;327(24):2434–45. doi:10.1001/jama.2022.8481

105. Torres A, Fernández-Fairen M, Sueiro-Fernández J. Greater trochanteric pain syndrome and gluteus medius and minimus tendinosis: nonsurgical treatment. *Pain Manag.* 2018 Jan;8(1):45–55. doi:10.2217/pmt-2017-0033

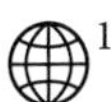
106. Barratt PA, Brookes N, Newson A. Conservative treatments for greater trochanteric pain syndrome: a systematic review. *Br J Sports Med.* 2017 Jan;51(2):97–104. doi:10.1136/bjsports-2015-095858

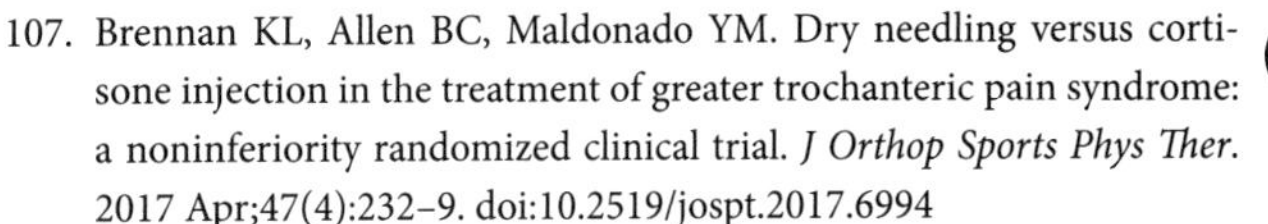
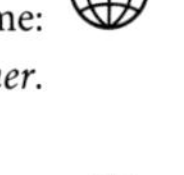
107. Brennan KL, Allen BC, Maldonado YM. Dry needling versus cortisone injection in the treatment of greater trochanteric pain syndrome: a noninferiority randomized clinical trial. *J Orthop Sports Phys Ther.* 2017 Apr;47(4):232–9. doi:10.2519/jospt.2017.6994

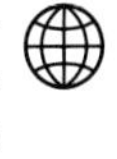
108. Mao LJ, Crudup JB, Quirk CR, Patrie JT, Nacey NC. Impact of fluoroscopic injection location on immediate and delayed pain relief in patients with greater trochanteric pain syndrome. *Skelet Radiol.* 2020 Oct;49(10):1547–54. doi:10.1007/s00256-020-03451-7

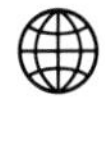
109. Jacobson JA, Yablon CM, Henning PT, et al. Greater trochanteric pain syndrome: percutaneous tendon fenestration versus platelet-rich plasma injection for treatment of gluteal tendinosis. *J Ultrasound Med.* 2016 Nov;35(11):2413–20. doi:10.7863/ultra.15.11046

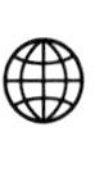
110. Fang WH, Chen XT, Vangsness CT Jr. Ultrasound-guided knee injections are more accurate than blind injections: a systematic review of randomized controlled trials. *Arthrosc Sports Med Rehabil.* 2021 Jun 26;3(4):e1177–87.

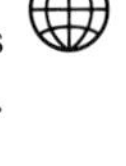
111. Wada M, Fujii T, Inagaki Y, Nagano T, Tanaka Y. Isometric contraction of the quadriceps improves the accuracy of intra-articular injections into the knee joint via the superolateral approach. *JB JS Open Access.* 2018 Oct 23;3(4):e0003.

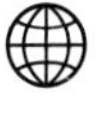
112. Chernchujit B, Tharakulphan S, Apivatgaroon A, Prasetia R. Accuracy comparisons of intra-articular knee injection between the new modified anterolateral Approach and superolateral approach in patients with symptomatic knee osteoarthritis without effusion. *Asia Pac J Sports Med Arthrosc Rehabil Technol.* 2019 Mar 26;17:1–4.

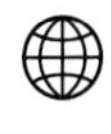
113. Maricar N, Parkes MJ, Callaghan MJ, Felson DT, O'Neill TW. Where and how to inject the knee—a systematic review. *Semin Arthritis Rheum.* 2013 Oct;43(2):195–203.

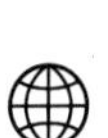
114. Wagner BS, Howe AS, Dexter WW, et al. Tolerability and efficacy of 3 approaches to intra-articular corticosteroid injections of the knee for osteoarthritis: a randomized controlled trial. *Orthop J Sports Med.* 2015 Aug 25;3(8):2325967115600687.

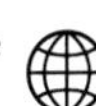
115. Jüni P, Hari R, Rutjes AWS, et al. Intra-articular corticosteroid for knee osteoarthritis. *Cochrane Database Syst Rev.* 2015;10:CD005328.

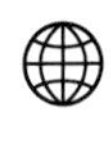
116. Gregori D, Giacovelli G, Minto C, et al. Association of pharmacological treatments with long-term pain control in patients with knee osteoarthritis: a systematic review and meta-analysis. *JAMA.* 2018;320(24):2564–79.

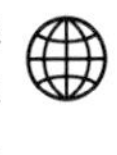
117. Saltychev M, Mattie R, McCormick Z, Laimi K. The magnitude and duration of the effect of intra-articular corticosteroid injections on pain severity in knee osteoarthritis: a systematic review and meta-analysis. *Am J Phys Med Rehabil.* 2020;99(7):617–25.

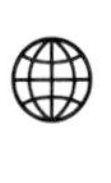
118. Hepper CT, Halvorson JJ, Duncan ST, Gregory AJ, Dunn WR, Spindler KP. The efficacy and duration of intra-articular corticosteroid injection for knee osteoarthritis: a systematic review of level I studies. *J Am Acad Orthop Surg.* 2009;17(10):638–646.

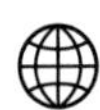
119. Ellis R, Hing W, Reid D. Iliotibial band friction syndrome—a systematic review. *Man Ther.* 2007;12(3):200–8.

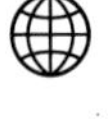
120. Gunter P, Schwellnus MP. Local corticosteroid injection in iliotibial band friction syndrome in runners: a randomised controlled trial. *Br J Sports Med.* 2004;38(3):269–72.

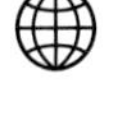
121. Lee JH, Lee JU, Yoo SW. Accuracy and efficacy of ultrasound-guided pes anserinus bursa injection. *J Clin Ultrasound.* 2019 Feb;47(2):77–82. doi:10.1002/jcu.22661

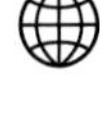
122. Finnoff JT, Nutz DJ, Hennin PT, Hollman JH, Smith J. Accuracy of ultrasound-guided versus unguided pes anserinus bursa injections. *PM&R.* Aug 2010;2(8):732–9.

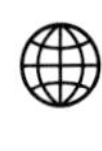
123. Yoon HS, Kim SE, Suh YR, Seo Y, Kim HA. Correlation between ultrasonographic findings and the response to corticosteroid injection in pes anserinus tendinobursitis syndrome in knee osteoarthritis patients. *J Kor Med Sci.* 2005;20(1):109–12.

124. Heidari N, Pichler W, Grechenig S, Grechenig W, Weinberg AM. Does the anteromedial or anterolateral approach alter the rate of joint puncture in injection of the ankle? A cadaver study. *J Bone Joint Surg Br.* 2010;92(1):176–8.
125. Khosla S, Thiele R, Baumhauer JF. Ultrasound guidance for intra-articular injections of the foot and ankle. *Foot Ankle Int.* 2009;30(9):886–90.
126. Wisniewski SJ, Smith J, Patterson DG, Carmichael SW, Pawlina W. Ultrasound-guided versus nonguided tibiotalar joint and sinus tarsi injections: a cadaveric study. *P MR.* 2010;2(4):277–81.
127. Gilliland CA, Salazar LD, Borchers JR. Ultrasound versus anatomic guidance for intra-articular and periarticular injection: a systematic review. *Phys Sportsmed.* 2011 Sep;39(3):121–31. doi:10.3810/psm.2011.09.1928
128. Ward ST, Williams PL, Purkayastha S. Intra-articular corticosteroid injections in the foot and ankle: a prospective 1-year follow-up investigation. *J Foot Ankle Surg.* 2008;47(2):138–44.
129. Vannabouathong C, Del Fabbro G, Sales B, et al. Intra-articular injections in the treatment of symptoms from ankle arthritis: a systematic review. *Foot Ankle Int.* 2018 Oct;39(10):1141–50. doi:10.1177/1071100718779375
130. Boffa A, Previtali D, Di Laura Frattura G, Vannini F, Candrian C, Filardo G. Evidence on ankle injections for osteochondral lesions and osteoarthritis: a systematic review and meta-analysis. *Int Orthop.* 2021 Feb;45(2):509–23. doi:10.1007/s00264-020-04689-5
131. Kubo T, Kumai T, Ikegami H, Kano K, Nishii M, Seo T. Diclofenac-hyaluronate conjugate (diclofenac etalhyaluronate) intra-articular injection for hip, ankle, shoulder, and elbow osteoarthritis: a randomized controlled trial. *BMC Muscoskelet Disord.* 2022 Apr 20;23(1):371. doi:10.1186/s12891-022-05328-3
132. Cole BJ, Schumacher HR Jr. Injectable corticosteroids in modern practice. *J Am Acad Orthop Surg.* 2005;13(1):37–46.
133. Cunnington J, Marshall N, Hide G, et al. A randomized, double-blind, controlled study of ultrasound-guided corticosteroid injection into the joint of patients with inflammatory arthritis. *Arthritis Rheum.* 2010;62(7):1862–9.
134. Crawford F, Atkins D, Young P, Edwards J. Steroid injection for heel pain: evidence of short-term effectiveness. A randomized controlled trial. *Rheumatology.* 1999;38(10):974–7.
135. Tsai WC, Hsu CC, Chen CP, Chen MJ, Yu TY, Chen YJ. Plantar fasciitis treated with local steroid injection: comparison between sonographic and palpation guidance. *J Clin Ultrasound.* 2006;34(1):12–6.
136. Li Z, Xia C, Yu A, Qi B. Ultrasound-versus palpation-guided injection of corticosteroid for plantar fasciitis: a meta-analysis. *PLoS One.* 2014 Mar 21;9(3):e92671. doi:10.1371/journal.pone.0092671
137. Breton A, Leplat C, Picot MC, et al. Prediction of clinical response to corticosteroid or platelet-rich plasma injection in plantar fasciitis with MRI: a prospective, randomized, double-blinded study. *Diagn Interv Imaging.* 2022 Apr;103(4):217–24. doi:10.1016/j.diii.2021.10.008
138. Mosca M, Fuiano M, Massimi S, et al. Ruptures of the plantar fascia: a systematic review of the literature. *Foot Ankle Spec.* 2022 Jun;15(3):272–82. doi:10.1177/1938640020974889
139. Shetty SH, Dhond A, Arora M, Deore S. Platelet-rich plasma has better long-term results than corticosteroids or placebo for chronic plantar fasciitis: randomized control trial. *J Foot Ankle Surg.* 2019 Jan;58(1):42–6. doi:10.1053/j.jfas.2018.07.006
140. Ahadi T, Cham MB, Mirmoghtadaei M, Raissi GR, Janbazi L, Zoghi G. The effect of dextrose prolotherapy versus placebo/other non-surgical treatments on pain in chronic plantar fasciitis: a systematic review and meta-analysis of clinical trials. *J Foot Ankle Res.* 2023 Feb 10;16(1):5. doi:10.1186/s13047-023-00605-3
141. Chutumstid T, Susantitaphong P, Koonalinthip N. Effectiveness of dextrose prolotherapy for the treatment of chronic plantar fasciitis: a systematic review and meta-analysis of randomized controlled trials. *Pharm Manag PM R.* 2023 Mar;15(3):380–91. doi:10.1002/pmrj.12807

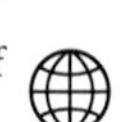
142. Jain SK, Suprashant K, Kumar S, Yadav A, Kearns SR. Comparison of plantar fasciitis injected with platelet-rich plasma vs corticosteroids. *Foot Ankle Int.* 2018 Jul;39(7):780–6. doi:10.1177/1071100718762406

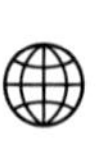
143. David JA, Sankarapandian V, Christopher PR, Chatterjee A, Macaden AS. Injected corticosteroids for treating plantar heel pain in adults. *Cochrane Database Syst Rev.* 2017 Jun 11;6(6):CD009348. doi:10.1002/14651858.CD009348.pub2

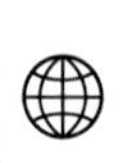
144. Sucuoğlu H, Süzen Özbayrak S, Uludağ M, Tüzün Ş. Short-term efficacy of joint and soft tissue injections for musculoskeletal pain: an interventional cohort study. *Agri.* 2016 Apr;28(2):79–88. doi:10.5505/agri.2015.48802

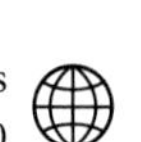
145. Thomson L, Aujla RS, Divall P, Bhatia M. Non-surgical treatments for Morton's neuroma: a systematic review. *Foot Ankle Surg.* 2020 Oct;26(7):736–43. doi:10.1016/j.fas.2019.09.009

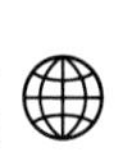
146. Matthews BG, Hurn SE, Harding MP, Henry RA, Ware RS. The effectiveness of non-surgical interventions for common plantar digital compressive neuropathy (Morton's neuroma): a systematic review and meta-analysis. *J Foot Ankle Res.* 2019 Feb 13;12:12. doi:10.1186/s13047-019-0320-7

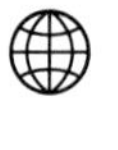
147. Lorenzon P, Rettore C, Scalvi A. Infiltrative therapy of Morton's neuroma. *Acta Biomed.* 2022 Mar 10;92(S3):e2021556. doi:10.23750/abm.v92iS3.12545

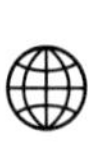
148. Lu VM, Puffer RC, Everson MC, Gilder HE, Burks SS, Spinner RJ. Treating Morton's neuroma by injection, neurolysis, or neurectomy: a systematic review and meta-analysis of pain and satisfaction outcomes. *Acta Neurochir.* 2021 Feb;163(2):531–43. doi:10.1007/s00701-020-04241-9

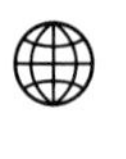
149. Santiago FR, Muñoz PT, Ramos-Bossini AJL, Martínez AM, Olleta NP. Long-term comparison between blind and ultrasound-guided corticoid injections in Morton neuroma. *Eur Radiol.* 2022 Dec;32(12):8414–22. doi:10.1007/s00330-022-08932-y

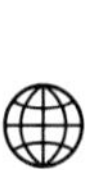
150. Lizano-Díez X, Ginés-Cespedosa A, Alentorn-Geli E, et al. Corticosteroid injection for the treatment of Morton's neuroma: a prospective, double-blinded, randomized, placebo-controlled trial. *Foot Ankle Int.* 2017 Sep;38(9):944–51. doi:10.1177/1071100717709569

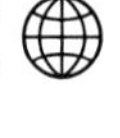
151. Choi JY, Lee HI, Hong WH, Suh JS, Hur JW. Corticosteroid injection for Morton's interdigital neuroma: a systematic review. *Clin Orthop Surg.* 2021 Jun;13(2):266–77. doi:10.4055/cios20256

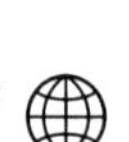
152. Santos D, Morrison G, Coda A. Sclerosing alcohol injections for the management of intermetatarsal neuromas: a systematic review. *Foot.* 2018 Jun;35:36–47. doi:10.1016/j.foot.2017.12.003

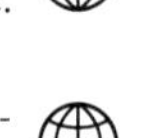
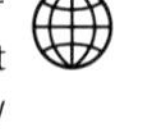
153. Park YH, Lee JW, Choi GW, Kim HJ. Risk factors and the associated cutoff values for failure of corticosteroid injection in treatment of Morton's neuroma. *Int Orthop.* 2018 Feb;42(2):323–9. doi:10.1007/s00264-017-3707-8

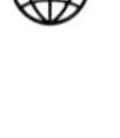
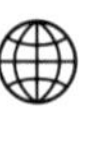
154. Ruiz Santiago F, Prados Olleta N, Tomás Muñoz P, Guzmán Álvarez L, Martínez Martínez A. Short term comparison between blind and ultrasound guided injection in morton neuroma. *Eur Radiol.* 2019 Feb;29(2):620–7. doi:10.1007/s00330-018-5670-1

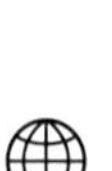
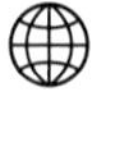
155. Mahadevan D, Attwal M, Bhatt R, Bhatia M. Corticosteroid injection for Morton's neuroma with or without ultrasound guidance: a randomised controlled trial. *Bone Joint Lett J.* 2016 Apr;98-B(4):498–503. doi:10.1302/0301-620X.98B4.36880

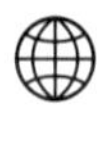
156. Appasamy M, Lam C, Alm J, Chadwick AL. Trigger point injections. *Phys Med Rehabil Clin N Am.* 2022 May;33(2):307–33. doi:10.1016/j.pmr.2022.01.011

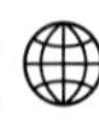
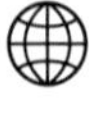
157. Borg-Stein J, Iaccarino MA. Myofascial pain syndrome treatments. *Phys Med Rehabil Clin N Am.* 2014 May;25(2):357–74. doi:10.1016/j.pmr.2014.01.012

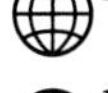
158. Alvarez DJ, Rockwell PG. Trigger points: diagnosis and management. *Am Fam Physician*. 2002 Feb 15;65(4):653–60.

159. Navarro-Santana MJ, Sanchez-Infante J, Gómez-Chiguano GF, et al. Dry needling versus trigger point injection for neck pain symptoms associated with myofascial trigger points: a systematic review and meta-analysis. *Pain Med*. 2022 Mar 2;23(3):515–25. doi:10.1093/pm/pnab188

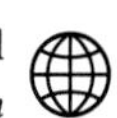
160. Diep D, Chen KJQ, Kumbhare D. Ultrasound-guided interventional procedures for myofascial trigger points: a systematic review. *Reg Anesth Pain Med*. 2021 Jan;46(1):73–80. doi:10.1136/rapm-2020-101898

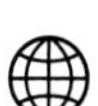
161. Liu L, Huang QM, Liu QG, et al. Effectiveness of dry needling for myofascial trigger points associated with neck and shoulder pain: a systematic review and meta-analysis. *Arch Phys Med Rehabil*. 2015 May;96(5):944–55. doi:10.1016/j.apmr.2014.12.015

80 Ultrasound and Image-Guided Procedures

Haruki Ishii, Salvador E. Portugal, and Yao-Wen Eliot Hu

INTRODUCTION

- Ultrasound has gained popularity as the modality of choice for needle guidance and placement in peripheral articular and other musculoskeletal structures (1). Ultrasound is a reproducible, noninvasive imaging modality, which allows for real-time dynamic assessment of targeted structures (2). In 2015, an American Medical Society for Sports Medicine (AMSSM) position statement supported the use of ultrasound for interventional musculoskeletal procedures, promoting accuracy, efficacy, cost-effectiveness, and potential with new procedures (3). Another benefit of ultrasound over computed tomography and fluoroscopy is the lack of ionizing radiation (4). Musculoskeletal ultrasound use is further detailed in Chapter 21.

STANDARDS FOR TEACHING, PERFORMANCE, AND CREDENTIALING

- Two professional organizations, AMSSM and the American Institute of Ultrasound in Medicine (AIUM), have published position statements, official statements, training guidelines, and practice parameters for performing ultrasound-guided interventional musculoskeletal procedures.
  - In 2014, AIUM published a training guideline for providers who perform ultrasound-guided musculoskeletal interventional procedures, recommending educational standards for clinician performance (5).
  - Furthermore, AIUM in 2016 published practice parameters for selected ultrasound-guided procedures, establishing clinical standards for performance (6).
  - In 2021, AMSSM recommended a sports ultrasound curriculum for fellowships, establishing specific educational guidelines and standards for ultrasound-guided interventional procedures (7).
- There is currently no available certification for the individual clinician with regard to ultrasound-guided interventional procedures. However, clinical practice accreditation for diagnostic musculoskeletal ultrasound, diagnostic peripheral nerve, and ultrasound-guided interventional procedures is individually available through AIUM (8).
- Standards for ultrasound-guided procedures are important to ensure clinical and educational quality. Adherence to these standards, along with accreditation, may be required for financial reimbursement in the future.

ULTRASOUND GUIDANCE FOR ACCURACY IN INTERVENTIONAL PROCEDURES

Shoulder

- **Glenohumeral Joint:** In 2012, Patel et al. (9) conducted a cadaveric study to compare the accuracy of glenohumeral injections between landmark and ultrasound guidance. The study demonstrated that accuracy was significantly higher for ultrasound-guidance, with accuracy being 92.5% versus 72.5% for landmark-based. A 2014 systematic review and meta-analysis demonstrated ultrasound-guided glenohumeral joint injections were more accurate compared to fluoroscopy (93% vs. 80%, respectively); however, this difference was not statistically different (10). In a 2022 retrospective study, accuracy of ultrasound-guided glenohumeral injections using a posterior approach, confirmed using magnetic resonance arthrography (MRA), reached 97% (11).
  - Injection of contrast prior to magnetic resonance arthrography is another indication for ultrasound use. The accuracy of contrast injection under both fluoroscopic and ultrasound guidance are comparable, both achieving 100% accuracy (12).
- **Acromioclavicular Joint:** Multiple studies have demonstrated that an ultrasound-guided acromioclavicular (AC) joint injection is significantly more accurate compared to a landmark-based injection, with reported average accuracy of 90%–100% (13–16). However, there has been no direct comparison of ultrasound versus fluoroscopic-guided AC joint procedures.

- **Sternoclavicular Joint:** Evidence is limited in terms of direct comparison between different methods of intervention at the sternoclavicular (SC) joint; however, a cadaveric study showed 100% accuracy of SC joint injection under ultrasound guidance (17).
- **Subacromial and Subdeltoid Bursa:** Although current evidence demonstrates ultrasound guidance provides more consistently accurate injections to the subacromial and subdeltoid bursa, a definite conclusion regarding superiority of ultrasound-guided injections over palpation-guided injections cannot be drawn at this time, given high variability among the different studies (3).
- **Biceps Tendon Sheath:** One study compared the accuracy of ultrasound-guided biceps tendon sheath injections to landmark-based injections (18). Ultrasound guidance provided accurate injections in approximately 87% of cases, whereas landmark-based injections were accurate only approximately 27% of the time. A more recent study by Yiannakopoulos et al. (19) also compared the accuracy between ultrasound-guided and landmark-based injections at the bicipital groove, revealing superior accuracy of ultrasound-guided injections (100%) over landmark-based injections (68%).

Elbow

- A 2010 double-blinded randomized control trial evaluated the accuracy of an ultrasound-guided injection into the elbow joint (20). Ultrasound guidance provided accurate injections in 91% of cases, whereas landmark-based injections were accurate only 64% of the time; however, this did not reach statistical difference, thereby warranting further research at this time.
- Current literature is lacking when evaluating the accuracy of ultrasound-guided versus landmark-based extra-articular elbow procedures.

Wrist/Hand

- **Distal Radioulnar Joint:** Accuracy rate of ultrasound-guided distal radioulnar joint injections was reported to be 100% (21).
- **Scaphotrapeziotrapezoid Joint:** Smith et al. (22) reported that ultrasound guidance provided accurate injections in 100% of cases, whereas landmark-based injection accuracy was 80%.
- **Proximal Interphalangeal and Metacarpophalangeal Joints:** Raza et al. (23) conducted a study to compare the accuracy of proximal interphalangeal or metacarpophalangeal joint injections under ultrasound guidance versus a landmark-based approach. The study illustrated significantly greater accuracy with ultrasound guidance over a landmark-based approach, with accuracy being 96% versus 59%, respectively.
- **Thumb Carpometacarpal (CMC) Joint:** Umphrey et al. (24) reported in a cadaveric study that the accuracy for ultrasound-guided trapeziometacarpal joint injections was 94%. In addition, To et al. (25) illustrated in a cadaveric study that ultrasound guidance for successful thumb CMC injections was superior compared to landmark-based approaches, with accuracy of 75% and 50%, respectively.
- **Carpal Tunnel:** To et al. (25) conducted a cadaveric study evaluating carpal tunnel injections with and without ultrasound guidance, showing 100% and 90% success with landmark-based and ultrasound-guided injections, respectively, although the results were not statistically significant.
    - Makhlouf et al. (26) showed in a randomized controlled trial that ultrasound-guided carpal tunnel injections provided statistically significant clinical outcomes when compared to landmark-based injections. But the study did not directly evaluate for ultrasound versus landmark-based accuracy.
- **de Quervain Tenosynovitis:** Leversedge et al. (27) and Kang et al. (28) illustrated superior accuracy with ultrasound-guided (100% and 93.3%) versus landmark-based injections (52% and 40%) into the first dorsal compartment of the wrist. However, Shin et al. (29) showed that although ultrasound-guided corticosteroid injections for de Quervain tenosynovitis provided symptomatic improvement and decreased symptom recurrence when compared to landmark-based injections, the study did not investigate ultrasound guidance versus landmark-based accuracy and the clinical improvement was not statistically significant.

Hip

- Several studies have demonstrated that an ultrasound-guided hip joint injection was associated with very high accuracy, ranging from 97%–100% (30–32). A 2016 meta-analysis comparing the accuracy of ultrasound-guided and landmark-based hip injections illustrated superiority of ultrasound-guided injections compared to landmark-based injections, with accuracy being 100% versus 72%, respectively (33).
- **Trochanteric Bursa:** A 2017 cadaveric study examined the accuracy of ultrasound-guided and landmark-based approaches for trochanteric bursa injections and reported higher accuracy with ultrasound guidance over that of landmark-based injections (92% vs. 67%, respectively), but without statistical significance (34).
- **Sacroiliac Joint:** Needle placement with ultrasound guidance into the sacroiliac joint was confirmed successful by fluoroscopic arthrogram in 96% of patients (35).

Knee

- In a 2016 review, Wu et al. (36) examined nine relevant studies, eight of which assessed the accuracy of knee arthrocentesis. The review illustrated that ultrasound guidance achieved greater accuracy when compared to landmark-based approaches. More recently, Fang et al. (37) published a systematic review including 12 level-I human studies, 7 of which conducted a direct comparison of ultrasound-guided versus landmark-based knee injections. In each study, ultrasound technique offered higher accuracy.

- **Pes Anserine Bursa:** Finnoff et al. (38), in a cadaveric ultrasound-guided versus landmark-based pes anserine bursa injection study published in 2010, showed accuracy of 92% in the ultrasound-guided group and that of 17% in the landmark-based group. This result was corroborated by Lee et al. in 2019 (39).

Foot/Ankle

- **Tibiotalar Joint:** Reach et al. (40) and Wisniewski et al. (41) separately published cadaveric studies, demonstrating that the accuracy for tibiotalar joint injection was 100% using ultrasound.
- **Subtalar Joint:** The mean accuracy of ultrasound-guided injections in two cadaveric studies was 95% (40,42).
- **Peroneus Tendon Sheath:** Muir et al. (43) showed in a cadaveric study that the accuracy for ultrasound-guided peroneus tendon sheath injections was 100% when compared to that of landmark-based injections (60%).

ULTRASOUND-GUIDED PERCUTANEOUS TENOTOMY AND MINIMALLY INVASIVE TENDON PROCEDURES

- Tenotomy is accomplished via open surgical debridement, arthroscopy, or more recently, transcutaneous approaches under ultrasound guidance (44–46).
- To date, ultrasound-guided percutaneous needle tenotomy (PNT), also known as fenestration or dry needling, has been shown to be effective in treating tendinopathies at many anatomical sites (47–54).
- During PNT, a needle repeatedly passes through a segment of disrupted tendon approximately 20–50 times (55), causing local trauma that converts a chronic degenerative process into an acute inflammatory process with better healing potential (47). Accurate placement of the needle within the pathological portion of tendon enhances the effectiveness of the PNT, signifying the importance of ultrasound guidance for this procedure (55).
- In 2022, a systematic review conducted by Shomal Zadeh et al. (56) assessed the current literature for the efficacy of ultrasound-guided PNT compared to that of other treatment modalities, including surgical tenotomy, corticosteroid injection, and platelet-rich plasma (PRP) injection, for chronic tendinopathy in various anatomical sites. This systematic review included 12 randomized control trials (RCTs) and concluded that ultrasound-guided PNT is an effective modality for chronic tendinopathy and showed comparable outcomes to the above treatment options. However, there is limited data comparing ultrasound-guided PNT to other modalities such as extracorporeal shock wave therapy, physical therapy, and biological compound injections, thereby warranting further research.
- Ultrasound-guided percutaneous ultrasonic tenotomy (PUT) is another potential minimally invasive modality that has lately evolved for treatment of recalcitrant tendinopathy. With this technique, abnormal tendon tissue identified under ultrasound undergoes phacoemulsification through a small incision via a handheld instrument, where small-amplitude, high-frequency oscillations emulsify necrotic tissue and a tube-within-a-tube irrigation system aspirates the debris (57,58).
- Vajapey et al. (59), in their systematic review of a total of seven studies, concluded that PUT could have the potential to be an effective treatment alternative in those who failed conservative management. However, there is paucity of data on this topic with a limited number of tendons being studied; hence, more studies are needed to accurately assess its effectiveness and comparative efficacy.
- Another percutaneous tendon procedure is prolotherapy, which is a type of regenerative injection-based modality for chronic tendinopathy. Injectate, including dextrose, phenol-glycerin-glucose (P2G), and sodium morrhuate (60), serves as an irritant that begins the inflammatory cascade to promote the proliferation of fibroblasts, collagen tissue synthesis, and healing (61,62). Prolotherapy is further detailed in Chapter 77.
- Other examples of percutaneous tendon injections for treatment of tendinopathy are autologous whole blood and PRP. With PRP injections, wounded tissues are saturated with growth factors that surpass physiological levels to promote healing (56). In 2017, Fitzpatrick et al. (63), in their meta-analysis of 18 studies, compared PRP injections to different types of injections, such as saline, local anesthetic, corticosteroid, or needle tenotomy, for treatment of tendinopathy and concluded that the effectiveness of PRP was variable depending on the method of PRP preparation and injection. Orthobiologic therapies are further detailed in Chapter 78.

ULTRASOUND-GUIDED CARPAL TUNNEL RELEASE

- Carpal tunnel releases (CTRs) are performed to release pressure on the median nerve by transecting the transverse carpal ligament (64). Although CTRs are traditionally done via open (OCTR), endoscopic (ECTR), and mini-open (mini-OCTR) approaches, the procedure has evolved to be potentially performed under ultrasound guidance (USCTR) (65,66), which was first described in a cadaveric study published by Rowe et al. in 2005 (67). With current technological advancements, USCTR only requires a 1–5 mm skin incision, which is up to 10 times smaller than that of ECTR and mini-OCTR (68).

- The goal of most USCTR is to place the device within the transverse safe zone (TSZ) (69), a space bordered radially by the median nerve and ulnarly by the hook of the hamate or ulnar artery (whichever structure is located more radially) (69–71).
- Preoperative localization of the TSZ and at-risk structures, such as the median nerve and its palmar cutaneous branch or the thenar motor branch, the third common palmar digital nerve, the proximal and distal carpal rows, and the ulnar nerve and artery play an important role for successful outcomes (66). Although a recent study found that inexperienced clinicians could be trained to achieve successful USCTR on cadavers with a rapid learning curve (72), identifying these at-risk structures using ultrasound may involve significant training (65).
- Although various USCTR techniques have been described and studied in literature, including but not limited to a hook knife, the MANOS CTR device, surgical grade wire (Guo thread), and the SX-One MicroKnife, there are no direct comparison studies assessing outcomes among the different USCTR methods. Thus, no conclusions can be drawn regarding the method that may be the most effective. Additional randomized controlled trials are warranted to investigate the best device and technique to perform USCTR.
- Although quality of evidence is overall very low, current literature review suggests that USCTR appears to be an effective treatment modality for carpal tunnel syndrome when compared to current standard of care albeit having no significant statistical difference on medium-term outcomes (65). The potential benefits highlighted in the literature include faster recovery with shorter return-to-work times compared to mini-OCTR (73,74), similar functional outcomes after simultaneous bilateral CTR when compared to unilateral and staged bilateral CTR (75), and decreased functional limitations following the procedure for patients with disabilities who are crutch or wheelchair-dependent (76). No permanent neurovascular adverse effects have been reported in the available literature (65).

ULTRASOUND-GUIDED TRIGGER FINGER RELEASE

- Open surgical pulley release is still considered the gold standard for the treatment of trigger finger but ultrasound-guided percutaneous trigger finger release (USTFR) has recently gained popularity (77). USTFR may be accomplished using a large-bore needle, hook knife, needle-knife, minimally invasive surgical knives, or other commercial devices.
- Although there are limited studies on the effectiveness of USTFR with various devices, Colberg et al. (78) in a prospective case series of 60 patients undergoing USTFR via an 18-gauge needle with a special blade tip reported 97% complete symptom resolution. Furthermore, Chopin et al. (79) reported 93.4% and 85.7% complete symptom resolution at 6 and 12 months, respectively, in their case series of 105 patients undergoing USTFR with a 21-gauge needle, and Cromheecke et al. (77) reported 98.7% complete resolution of symptoms in their case series of 78 patients undergoing USTFR with a second-generation minimally invasive surgical knife.
- There is also a paucity of literature directly comparing the efficacy of individual devices but clinical outcomes appear promising. Nikolaou et al. (80) found that USTFR using a hook knife resulted in comparable clinical outcomes, fewer loss-of-work days, and improved cosmetic results when compared to open trigger finger release. In addition, by comparing the efficacy of a needle knife versus a 21-gauge needle in USTFR, Yang et al. (81) found in a cadaveric study that 93.3% of the USTFR procedures using a needle knife resulted in a complete pulley release as opposed to 36.7% with the 21-gauge needle.

ULTRASOUND-GUIDED HYDRODISSECTION

- Hydrodissection (HD) is a relatively new and emerging technique that has been introduced as a safe and effective treatment option for several pathologies, such as entrapment neuropathy (82), chronic tendinopathy (83,84), myofascial injuries, and pain secondary to fibrosis or adhesion (85,86).
- Fascial plane HD is a technique involving the use of injectates to separate targeted structures from fascial planes (87). A cadaver study has demonstrated that even a small amount of the inter-fascicular space injection can spread broadly and penetrate deeper structures (88), allowing for the focalization of injectates (89). Similarly, perineural HD is a procedure where nerves are completely released from their surrounding structures (90) and promotes nerve decompression by lysing fibrotic adhesions with injected solution (87,91). Furthermore, perineural HD has been shown to improve kinematic properties of the entrapped nerve (92).
- Among different types of injectates, including normal saline, local anesthetics, corticosteroids, and 5% dextrose, 5% dextrose appears to be the most commonly used solution given its minimal pharmacological adverse reactions on the surrounding structures (92).
- There are two primary approaches with regard to ultrasound-guided HD of peripheral nerves, including an in-plane approach and an out-of-plane with subsequent in-plane approach (93). There is a paucity of in-depth comparison of the performance between the above two methods in terms of the learning curve, effectiveness, and safety (87).
- Carpal tunnel syndrome (CTS) is the most extensively studied entrapment neuropathy treated by ultrasound-guided HD. Multiple approaches to inject the carpal tunnel exist, including proximal-to-distal, radial, ulnar, and distal-to-proximal methods (94). A 2018 cadaveric study

demonstrated decreased gliding resistance of the median nerve within the carpal tunnel immediately following HD (95). Wu et al. (96) reported that HD treatment resulted in significantly greater reduction in symptoms in patients with mild-to-moderate CTS. Several studies investigated the efficacy of ultrasound-guided perineural HD with 5% dextrose, showing greater short- (97,98) and long-term efficacy (99). About 4 mL of 5% dextrose was reported to provide greater improvement compared to 1 and 2 mL (98). However, Wang et al. (100), in their randomized controlled trial that compared the efficacy of corticosteroid HD versus corticosteroid perineural injection alone, reported that both interventions resulted in clinical and electrophysiological improvement; however, the HD group did not have additional improvement compared to the other group.

- Several case reports have been published reporting successful treatment of peripheral neuropathies with ultrasound-guided HD, such as a case of cubital tunnel syndrome described by Stoddard et al. (101) in 2019, a case of Baxter's neuropathy described by Sahoo et al. (102) in 2020, a case of occipital neuralgia described by Kaga et al. (103) in 2020, a case of posterior interosseous neuropathy described by Tsujino et al. (104) in 2021, and a case of Hunter Canal Syndrome described by Hu and Ridings (105) in 2022. In addition, a few case series have also been published reporting the efficacy of ultrasound-guided HD, such as a case series of pronator syndrome reported by Delzell and Patel (106) in 2019 and a case series of radial tunnel syndrome reported by Gill et al. (107) in 2022, suggesting HD as a possible alternative to operative management. Ultrasound-guided HD of the sciatic nerve prior to corticosteroid injection for the treatment of piriformis syndrome has also been reported to be effective with immediate pain relief following the procedure in a majority of cases (32/38) with continued pain relief in approximately 50% of those who were available for follow-up (89).
- Ultrasound-guided HD can be also safely performed in the cervical region to treat patients with chronic upper back and thoracic neuropathic pain. Lam et al. (108) conducted a retrospective chart review revealing greater than 50% of pain relief in patients who underwent HD with 5% dextrose of the stellate ganglion, brachial plexus, cervical nerve roots, and paravertebral spaces.

ULTRASOUND-GUIDED HYDRODILATATION

- Hydrodilatation with corticosteroid was first described by Andren and Lundberg (109) in 1965 for the treatment of adhesive capsulitis by expansion of the joint capsule. Since then, multiple studies have been published, but evidence has been mixed. A 2018 systematic review concluded that combination of hydrodilatation and corticosteroid injection potentially accelerates recovery with the greatest benefit being within the first 3 months (98). A more recent meta-analysis also highly recommended hydrodilatation as a treatment option for adhesive capsulitis of shoulder given pain relief and functional improvement (110). However, two meta-analyses concluded that the effectiveness of hydrodilatation combined with corticosteroid was similar to that of corticosteroid alone (111,112).
- Capsule-rupturing hydrodilatation is the technique where joint capsule is distended until it ruptures under image guidance (113). Capsule-preserving hydrodilatation is another technique where the intra-articular pressure is measured using a real-time pressure-volume profile monitoring system to preserve the capsule at maximum volume of fluids (114). Two studies suggested that the capsule-preserving technique was more effective than the capsule-rupturing technique when treating adhesive capsulitis of shoulder (114,115).
- Hydrodilatation of the glenohumeral joint can be performed under fluoroscopic or ultrasound guidance. Using ultrasound, hydrodilatation is typically performed via the posterior glenohumeral recess (116). Lately, a new approach via the rotator interval was introduced (117). Wang et al. (116) compared the effectiveness of hydrodilatation for the treatment of adhesive capsulitis of shoulder via the posterior glenohumeral recess versus the rotator cuff interval, illustrating that although improvements were seen in both groups, there was greater reduction of pain during shoulder movement with the rotator cuff interval group.

ULTRASOUND-GUIDED RADIOFREQUENCY ABLATION

- Radiofrequency ablation (RFA) is a modality commonly used to treat musculoskeletal conditions including but not limited to facet arthropathy and knee osteoarthritis. RFA is the targeted thermocoagulation of the sensory nerves, thereby reducing or blocking the sensory input from the painful structure with the intention of alleviating pain (118).
- Historically, RFA has been done under fluoroscopic guidance (119); however, the use of ultrasound has been recently introduced and attempted as a novel alternative technique. Several potential benefits with ultrasound guidance include the lack of radiation exposure, precise needle placement with better soft-tissue visualization (120), and improved cost-effectiveness (119).
- In 2014, Gofeld et al. (119) conducted a cadaver study and reported accurate and rapid placement of radiofrequency cannula at the base of the superior articular processes under ultrasound, utilizing a magnetic positioning system. Since then, a few case reports (118,121) and case series (122,123) have been published, reporting successful treatment of several different musculoskeletal conditions, such as knee osteoarthritis, greater trochanteric pain syndrome, and Morton neuroma with ultrasound-guided RFA. A technique paper was also published recently, describing the use of ultrasound

for cooled RFA with satisfactory outcomes (120). That being said, further clinical studies with larger sample size and prolonged follow-up are warranted at this time to compare the efficacy of ultrasound-guided RFA to RFA using other image modalities, particularly with fluoroscopic-guided RFA procedures.

SUMMARY

- Using ultrasound for guidance in procedures has proven accuracy, efficacy, and cost-effectiveness in various anatomic targets.
- With the advent of new procedures and refinement of traditional procedures, ultrasound may improve clinical access, procedural efficacy, and potential for adverse effects.
- Clinical and educational standards for procedural performance help ensure quality and may be required for financial reimbursement in the future.

REFERENCES

1. Weidner S, Kellner W, Kellner H. Interventional radiology and the musculoskeletal system. *Best Pract Res Clin Rheumatol.* 2004;18(6):945–56.
2. Patel Y, Scillia AJ, Festa A, McInerney VK, Hirsch S. *The Role of Ultrasound-Guided Injections in Orthopaedic Sports Medicine: Upper Extremity.* AAOS Now; 2015. p. 14–17.
3. Finnoff JT, Hall MM, Adams E, et al. American Medical Society for Sports Medicine (AMSSM) position statement: interventional musculoskeletal ultrasound in sports medicine. *PM R.* 2015;7(2):151–68.e12.
4. Patel RP, McGill K, Motamedi D, Morgan T. Ultrasound-guided interventions of the upper extremity joints. *Skeletal Radiol.* 2022;52(5):897–909.
5. American Institute of Ultrasound in Medicine. *Official Statements: Training Guidelines for Physicians and Chiropractors Who Perform Ultrasound-Guided Musculoskeletal Interventional Procedures.* American Institute of Ultrasound in Medicine website; 2014. http://www.aium.org/resources/statements.aspx
6. AIUM practice parameter for the performance of selected ultrasound-guided procedures. *J Ultrasound Med.* 2016 Sep;35(9):1–40. doi:10.7863/ultra.35.9.1-d
7. Hall MM, Bernhardt DT, Finnoff JT, et al. American Medical Society for sports medicine sports ultrasound curriculum for sports medicine fellowships. *Clin J Sport Med.* 2021 Jul 1;31(4):e176–87. doi:10.1097/JSM.0000000000000944
8. American Institute of Ultrasound in Medicine. *Official Statements: Standards and Guidelines for the Accreditation of Ultrasound Practices.* American Institute of Ultrasound in Medicine website; 2020. http://www.aium.org/resources/statements.aspx
9. Patel DN, Nayyar S, Hasan S, Khatib O, Sidash S, Jazrawi LM. Comparison of ultrasound-guided versus blind glenohumeral injections: a cadaveric study. *J Shoulder Elbow Surg.* 2012;21(12):1664–8. doi:10.1016/j.jse.2011.11.026
10. Amber KT, Landy DC, Amber I, Knopf D, Guerra J. Comparing the accuracy of ultrasound versus fluoroscopy in glenohumeral injections: a systematic review and meta-analysis. *J Clin Ultrasound.* 2014;42(7):411–16.
11. Kuratani K, Tanaka M, Hanai H, Hayashida K. Accuracy of shoulder joint injections with ultrasound guidance: confirmed by magnetic resonance arthrography. *World J Orthop.* 2022;13(3):259–66. doi:10.5312/wjo.v13.i3.259
12. Ali AH, Said HG, Abo Elhamd E, Mahmoud MK, Qenawy OK. Shoulder MR arthrography: comparative evaluation of three different contrast injection techniques using an anterior approach. *J Magn Reson Imaging.* 2021;53(2):481–90.
13. Borbas P, Kraus T, Clement H, Grechenig S, Weinberg AM, Heidari N. The influence of ultrasound guidance in the rate of success of acromioclavicular joint injection: an experimental study on human cadavers. *J Shoulder Elbow Surg.* 2012;21(12):1694–7.
14. Peck E, Lai JK, Pawlina W, Smith J. Accuracy of ultrasound-guided versus palpation-guided acromioclavicular joint injections: a cadaveric study. *PM R.* 2010;2(9):817–21.
15. Sabeti-Aschraf M, Lemmerhofer B, Lang S, et al. Ultrasound guidance improves the accuracy of the acromioclavicular joint infiltration: a prospective randomized study. *Knee Surg Sports Traumatol Arthrosc.* 2011;19(2):292–5.
16. Edelson G, Saffuri H, Obid E, Lipovsky E, Ben-David D. Successful injection of the acromioclavicular joint with use of ultrasound: anatomy, technique, and follow-up. *J Shoulder Elbow Surg.* 2014;23(10):e243–50. doi:10.1016/j.jse.2014.01.012
17. Pourcho AM, Sellon JL, Smith J. Sonographically guided sternoclavicular joint injection: description of technique and validation. *J Ultrasound Med.* 2015;34(2):325–31. doi:10.7863/ultra.34.2.325
18. Hashiuchi T, Sakurai G, Morimoto M, Komei T, Takakura Y, Tanaka Y. Accuracy of the biceps tendon sheath injection: ultrasound-guided or unguided injection? A randomized controlled trial. *J Shoulder Elbow Surg.* 2011;20(7):1069–73.
19. Yiannakopoulos CK, Megaloikonomos PD, Foufa K, Gliatis J. Ultrasound-guided versus palpation-guided corticosteroid injections for tendinosis of the long head of the biceps: a randomized comparative study. *Skeletal Radiol.* 2020;49(4):585–91.
20. Cunnington J, Marshall N, Hide G, et al. A randomized, double-blind, controlled study of ultrasound-guided corticosteroid injection into the joint of patients with inflammatory arthritis. *Arthritis Rheum.* 2010;62(7):1862–9. doi:10.1002/art.27448
21. Smith J, Rizzo M, Sayeed YA, Finnoff JT. Sonographically guided distal radioulnar joint injection: technique and validation in a cadaveric model. *J Ultrasound Med.* 2011;30(11):1587–92.
22. Smith J, Brault JS, Rizzo M, Sayeed YA, Finnoff JT. Accuracy of sonographically guided and palpation guided scaphotrapeziotrapezoid joint injections. *J Ultrasound Med.* 2011;30(11):1509–15.
23. Raza K, Lee CY, Pilling D, et al. Ultrasound guidance allows accurate needle placement and aspiration from small joints in patients with early inflammatory arthritis. *Rheumatology.* 2003;42(8):976–9. doi:10.1093/rheumatology/keg269
24. Umphrey GL, Brault JS, Hurdle MFB, Smith J. Ultrasound-guided intra-articular injection of the trapeziometacarpal joint: description of technique. *Arch Phys Med Rehabil.* 2008;89(1):153–6.
25. To P, McClary KN, Sinclair MK, et al. The accuracy of common hand injections with and without ultrasound: an anatomical study. *Hand (N Y).* 2017 Nov;12(6):591–6. doi:10.1177/1558944717692086
26. Makhlouf T, Emil NS, Sibbitt WL Jr, Fields RA, Bankhurst AD. Outcomes and cost-effectiveness of carpal tunnel injections using sonographic needle guidance. *Clin Rheumatol.* 2014 Jun;33(6):849–58. doi:10.1007/s10067-013-2438-5
27. Leversedge FJ, Cotterell IH, Nickel BT, Crosmer M, Richard M, Angermeier E. Ultrasonography-guided de Quervain injection:

accuracy and anatomic considerations in a cadaver model. *J Am Acad Orthop Surg.* 2016 Jun;24(6):399–404. doi:10.5435/JAAOS-D-15-00753
28. Kang JW, Park JW, Lee SH, et al. Ultrasound-guided injection for De Quervain's disease: accuracy and its influenceable anatomical variances in first extensor compartment of fresh cadaver wrists. *J Orthop Sci.* 2017 Mar;22(2):270–4. doi:10.1016/j.jos.2016.11.013
29. Shin YH, Choi SW, Kim JK. Prospective randomized comparison of ultrasonography-guided and blind corticosteroid injection for de Quervain's disease. *Orthop Traumatol Surg Res.* 2020 Apr;106(2):301–6. doi:10.1016/j.otsr.2019.11.015
30. Levi DS. Intra-articular hip injections using ultrasound guidance: accuracy using a linear array transducer. *PM R.* 2013 Feb;5(2):129–34. doi:10.1016/j.pmrj.2012.08.010
31. Pourbagher MA, Ozalay M, Pourbagher A. Accuracy and outcome of sonographically guided intra-articular sodium hyaluronate injections in patients with osteoarthritis of the hip. *J Ultrasound Med.* 2005 Oct;24(10):1391–5. doi:10.7863/jum.2005.24.10.1391
32. Smith J, Hurdle MF, Weingarten TN. Accuracy of sonographically guided intra-articular injections in the native adult hip. *J Ultrasound Med.* 2009 Mar;28(3):329–35. doi:10.7863/jum.2009.28.3.329
33. Hoeber S, Aly AR, Ashworth N, Rajasekaran S. Ultrasound-guided hip joint injections are more accurate than landmark-guided injections: a systematic review and meta-analysis. *Br J Sports Med.* 2016 Apr;50(7):392–6. doi:10.1136/bjsports-2014-094570
34. Mu A, Peng P, Agur A. Landmark-guided and ultrasound-guided approaches for trochanteric bursa injection: a cadaveric study. *Anesth Analg.* 2017;124(3):966–71. doi:10.1213/ANE.0000000000001864
35. De Luigi AJ, Saini V, Mathur R, Saini A, Yokel N. Assessing the accuracy of ultrasound-guided needle placement in sacroiliac joint injections. *Am J Phys Med Rehabil.* 2019;98(8):666–70.
36. Wu T, Dong Y, Song HX, Fu Y, Li JH. Ultrasound-guided versus landmark in knee arthrocentesis: a systematic review. *Semin Arthritis Rheum.* 2016;45(5):627–32. doi:10.1016/j.semarthrit.2015.10.011
37. Fang WH, Chen XT, Vangsness CT Jr. Ultrasound-guided knee injections are more accurate than blind injections: a systematic review of randomized controlled trials. *Arthrosc Sports Med Rehabil.* 2021;3(4):e1177–87. doi: 10.1016/j.asmr.2021.01.028
38. Finnoff JT, Nutz DJ, Henning PT, Hollman JH, Smith J. Accuracy of ultrasound-guided versus unguided pes anserinus bursa injections. *PM R.* 2010;2(8):732–9. doi:10.1016/j.pmrj.2010.03.014
39. Lee JH, Lee JU, Yoo SW. Accuracy and efficacy of ultrasound-guided pes anserinus bursa injection. *J Clin Ultrasound.* 2019 Feb;47(2):77–82. doi:10.1002/jcu.22661
40. Reach JS, Easley ME, Chuckpaiwong B, Nunley JA II. Accuracy of ultrasound-guided injections in the foot and ankle. *Foot Ankle Int.* 2009;30(3):239–42. doi:10.3113/FAI.2009.0239
41. Wisniewski SJ, Smith J, Patterson DG, Carmichael SW, Pawlina W. Ultrasound-guided versus nonguided tibiotalar joint and sinus tarsi injections: a cadaveric study. *PM R.* 2010;2(4):277–81. doi:10.1016/j.pmrj.2010.03.013
42. Smith J, Finnoff JT, Henning PT, Turner NS. Accuracy of sonographically guided posterior subtalar joint injections: comparison of 3 techniques. *J Ultrasound Med.* 2009;28(11):1549–57. doi:10.7863/jum.2009.28.11.1549
43. Muir JJ, Curtiss HM, Hollman J, Smith J, Finnoff JT. The accuracy of ultrasound-guided and palpation-guided peroneal tendon sheath injections. *Am J Phys Med Rehabil.* 2011 Jul;90(7):564–71. doi:10.1097/PHM.0b013e31821f6e63
44. Koh KH, Ahn JH, Kim SM, Yoo JC. Treatment of biceps tendon lesions in the setting of rotator cuff tears: prospective cohort study of tenotomy versus tenodesis. *Am J Sports Med.* 2010;38(8):1584–90.
45. Maffulli N, Testa V, Capasso G, Bifulco G, Binfield PM. Results of percutaneous longitudinal tenotomy for Achilles tendinopathy in middle- and long-distance runners. *Am J Sports Med.* 1997;25(6):835–40.
46. Walch G, Edwards TB, Boulahia A, Nové-Josserand L, Neyton L, Szabo I. Arthroscopic tenotomy of the long head of the biceps in the treatment of rotator cuff tears: clinical and radiographic results of 307 cases. *J Shoulder Elbow Surg.* 2005;14(3):238–46.
47. Bradberry DM, Sussman WI, Mautner KR. Ultrasound-guided percutaneous needle tenotomy for chronic tensor fascia lata tendinopathy: a case series and description of sonographic findings. *PM R.* 2018;10(9):979–83.
48. Chiavaras MM, Jacobson JA. Ultrasound-guided tendon fenestration. *Semin Musculoskelet Radiol.* 2013 Feb;17(1):85–90.
49. Jacobson JA, Rubin J, Yablon CM, Kim SM, Kalume-Brigido M, Parameswaran A. Ultrasound-guided fenestration of tendons about the hip and pelvis: clinical outcomes. *J Ultrasound Med.* 2015;34(11):2029–35.
50. Koh J, Png MA, Howe TS, Lee B, Morrey B, Mohan BAFC. Ultrasound-guided percutaneous tenotomy shows sustained clinical and sonographic outcomes for recalcitrant lateral elbow tendinopathy at 7.5 years. *Orthop J Sports Med.* 2020;8(7_suppl 6):2325967120S00420.
51. Kirschner JS, Cheng J, Hurwitz N, et al. Ultrasound-guided percutaneous needle tenotomy (PNT) alone versus PNT plus platelet-rich plasma injection for the treatment of chronic tendinosis: a randomized controlled trial. *PM R.* 2021;13(12):1340–9.
52. Lavallee M, Bush C. Ultrasound-guided percutaneous tenotomy and its associated pain reduction and functionality outcomes in nonelite active adults. *Am J Phys Med Rehabil.* 2021;100(4):349–53.
53. McShane JM, Nazarian LN, Harwood MI. Sonographically guided percutaneous needle tenotomy for treatment of common extensor tendinosis in the elbow. *J Ultrasound Med.* 2006;25(10):1281–9.
54. Rha DW, Park GY, Kim YK, Kim MT, Lee SC. Comparison of the therapeutic effects of ultrasound-guided platelet-rich plasma injection and dry needling in rotator cuff disease: a randomized controlled trial. *Clin Rehabil.* 2013;27(2):113–22.
55. Jacobson JA, Kim SM, Brigido MK. Ultrasound-guided percutaneous tenotomy. *Semin Musculoskelet Radiol.* 2016 Nov;20(5):414–21.
56. Shomal Zadeh F, Shafiei M, Hosseini N, Alipour E, Cheung H, Chalian M. The effectiveness of percutaneous ultrasound-guided needle tenotomy compared to alternative treatments for chronic tendinopathy: a systematic review. *Skeletal Radiol.* 2023;52(5):875–88.
57. Koh JS, Mohan PC, Howe TS, et al. Fasciotomy and surgical tenotomy for recalcitrant lateral elbow tendinopathy: early clinical experience with a novel device for minimally invasive percutaneous microresection. *Am J Sports Med.* 2013;41(3):636–44. doi:10.1177/0363546512470625
58. Barnes DE. Ultrasonic energy in tendon treatment. *Oper Tech Orthop.* 2013;23(2):78–83. doi:10.1053/j.oto.2013.05.006
59. Vajapey S, Ghenbot S, Baria MR, Magnussen RA, Vasileff WK. Utility of percutaneous ultrasonic tenotomy for tendinopathies: a systematic review. *Sports Health.* 2021;13(3):258–64. doi:10.1177/1941738120951764
60. Banks A. A rationale for prolotherapy. *J Orthop Med.* 1991;13(3):54–9.
61. Lin CL, Huang CC, Huang SW. Effects of hypertonic dextrose injection in chronic supraspinatus tendinopathy of the shoulder: a randomized placebo-controlled trial. *Eur J Phys Rehabil Med.* 2019;55(4):480–7. doi:10.23736/S1973-9087.18.05379-0
62. Lee DH, Kwack KS, Rah UW, Yoon SH. Prolotherapy for refractory rotator cuff disease: retrospective case-control study of 1-year follow-up. *Arch Phys Med Rehabil.* 2015;96(11):2027–32. doi:10.1016/j.apmr.2015.07.011

63. Fitzpatrick J, Bulsara M, Zheng MH. The effectiveness of platelet-rich plasma in the treatment of tendinopathy: a meta-analysis of randomized controlled clinical trials. *Am J Sports Med.* 2017;45(1):226–33.
64. Fajardo M, Kim SH, Szabo RM. Incidence of carpal tunnel release: trends and implications within the United States ambulatory care setting. *J Hand Surg Am.* 2012;37(8):1599–605.
65. Chou RC, Robinson DM, Homer S. Ultrasound-guided percutaneous carpal tunnel release: a systematic review. *PM R.* 2023;15(3):363–79.
66. Wise A, Pourcho AM, Henning PT, Latzka EW. Evidence for ultrasound-guided carpal tunnel release. *Curr Phys Med Rehabil Rep.* 2021;9(1):11–22.
67. Rowe NM, Michaels J V, Soltanian H, Dobryansky M, Peimer CA, Gurtner GC. Sonographically guided percutaneous carpal tunnel release: an anatomic and cadaveric study. *Ann Plast Surg.* 2005;55(1):52–6.
68. Petrover D, Richette P. Treatment of carpal tunnel syndrome: from ultrasonography to ultrasound-guided carpal tunnel release. *Joint Bone Spine.* 2018;85(5):545–52.
69. Nakamichi KI, Tachibana S. Ultrasonographically assisted carpal tunnel release. *J Hand Surg Am.* 1997;22(5):853–62.
70. Nakamichi KI, Tachibana S. Distance between the median nerve and ulnar neurovascular bundle: clinical significance with ultrasonographically assisted carpal tunnel release. *J Hand Surg Am.* 1998;23(5):870–4.
71. Sytsma TT, Ryan HS, Lachman N, Kakar S, Smith J. Anatomic relationship between the hook of the hamate and the distal transverse carpal ligament: implications for ultrasound-guided carpal tunnel release. *Am J Phys Med Rehabil.* 2018;97(7):482–7.
72. Dekimpe C, Andreani O, Camuzard O, et al. Ultrasound-guided percutaneous release of the carpal tunnel: comparison of the learning curves of a senior versus a junior operator. A cadaveric study. *Skeletal Radiol.* 2019;48(11):1803–9.
73. Capa-Grasa A, Rojo-Manaute JM, Rodríguez FC, Martín JV. Ultra minimally invasive sonographically guided carpal tunnel release: an external pilot study. *Orthop Traumatol Surg Res.* 2014;100(3):287–92.
74. Rojo-Manaute JM, Capa-Grasa A, Chana-Rodríguez F, et al. Ultra-minimally invasive ultrasound-guided carpal tunnel release: a randomized clinical trial. *J Ultrasound Med.* 2016;35(6):1149–57.
75. Leiby BM, Beckman JP, Joseph AE. Long-term clinical results of carpal tunnel release using ultrasound guidance. *Hand.* 2022;17(6):1074–81.
76. Henning PT, Yang L, Awan T, Lueders D, Pourcho AM. Minimally invasive ultrasound-guided carpal tunnel release: preliminary clinical results. *J Ultrasound Med.* 2018;37(11):2699–706.
77. Cromheecke M, Haignère V, Mares O, De Keyzer PB, Louis P, Cognet JM. An ultrasound-guided percutaneous surgical technique for trigger finger release using a minimally invasive surgical knife. *Tech Hand Up Extrem Surg.* 2022;26(2):103–9. doi:10.1097/BTH.0000000000000367
78. Colberg RE, Jurado Vélez JA, Garrett WH, Hart K, Fleisig GS. Ultrasound-guided microinvasive trigger finger release technique using an 18-gauge needle with a blade at the tip: a prospective study. *PM R.* 2022;14(8):963–70. doi:10.1002/pmrj.12665
79. Chopin C, Le Guillou A, Salmon JH, Lellouche H, Richette P, Maillet J. Treatment of Trigger finger by ultrasound-guided needle release of a1 pulley: a series of 105 cases. *Joint Bone Spine.* 2022;89(6):105433. doi:10.1016/j.jbspin.2022.105433
80. Nikolaou VS, Malahias MA, Kaseta MK, Sourlas I, Babis GC. Comparative clinical study of ultrasound-guided A1 pulley release *vs* open surgical intervention in the treatment of trigger finger. *World J Orthop.* 2017;8(2):163–9. doi:10.5312/wjo.v8.i2.163
81. Yang J, Ma B, Zhong H, Zhang Y, Zhu J, Ni Y. Ultrasound-guided percutaneous A1 pulley release by acupotomy (needle-knife): a cadaveric study of safety and efficacy. *J Pain Res.* 2022;15:413–22. doi:10.2147/JPR.S349869
82. Jui Su DC, Yeh MC, Chou W. Poster 142 radial tunnel syndrome treated by ultrasound-guided perineural hydrodissection: a case report. *PM R.* 2016;8(9 suppl):S207–8. doi:10.1016/j.pmrj.2016.07.183
83. Chen B, Stitik TP, Foye PM, Roque-Dang CM, Lai LP. Successful treatment of sciatica and associated proximal hamstring tendinopathy with ultrasound-guided hydrodissection. *PM R.* 2013;9(5):S223.
84. Stanford RA, Kingsbury D. Poster 244: hydrodissection of Achilles tendon and fat pad as a treatment of chronic Achilles tendinopathy—a case report. *PM R.* 2017;9:S209–10.
85. Courseault J, Kessler E, Moran A, Labbe A. Fascial Hydrodissection for chronic hamstring injury. *Curr Sports Med Rep.* 2019;18(11):416–20.
86. Piraccini E, Maitan S. Ultrasound-guided rhomboid plane hydrodissection for fascial adhesion. *J Clin Anesth.* 2020;59:13.
87. Lam KHS, Hung CY, Chiang YP, et al. Ultrasound-guided nerve hydrodissection for pain management: rationale, methods, current literature, and theoretical mechanisms. *J Pain Res.* 2020;13:1957–68.
88. Kimura H, Kobayashi T, Zenita Y, Kurosawa A, Aizawa S. Expansion of 1 mL of solution by ultrasound-guided injection between the trapezius and rhomboid muscles: a cadaver study. *Pain Med.* 2020;21(5):1018–24.
89. Burke CJ, Walter WR, Adler RS. Targeted ultrasound-guided perineural hydrodissection of the sciatic nerve for the treatment of piriformis syndrome. *Ultrasound Q.* 2019;35(2):125–9.
90. Cass SP. Ultrasound-guided nerve hydrodissection: what is it? A review of the literature. *Curr Sports Med Rep.* 2016;15(1):20–2.
91. Norbury JW, Nazarian LN. Ultrasound-guided treatment of peripheral entrapment mononeuropathies. *Muscle Nerve.* 2019;60(3):222–31.
92. Chang KV, Wu WT, Özçakar L. Ultrasound imaging and guidance in peripheral nerve entrapment: hydrodissection highlighted. *Pain Manag.* 2020;10(2):97–106.
93. Soneji N, Peng PW. Ultrasound-guided pain interventions – a review of techniques for peripheral nerves. *Korean J Pain.* 2013;26(2):111–24. doi:10.3344/kjp.2013.26.2.111
94. Guo K, McCool L, Wang H, Guo D, Guo D. The modified ultrasound-guided distal-to-proximal carpal tunnel injection with median nerve hydrodissection: a retrospective safety review of 827 procedures. *Hand.* 2021;16(3):407–9.
95. Evers S, Thoreson AR, Smith J, Zhao C, Geske JR, Amadio PC. Ultrasound-guided hydrodissection decreases gliding resistance of the median nerve within the carpal tunnel. *Muscle Nerve.* 2018;57(1):25–32.
96. Wu YT, Chen SR, Li TY, et al. Nerve hydrodissection for carpal tunnel syndrome: a prospective, randomized, double-blind, controlled trial. *Muscle Nerve.* 2019;59(2):174–80.
97. He JJ, Wei XM, Dou ZL, et al. Ultrasound-guided nerve hydrodissection with 5% dextrose 4 weeks after steroid injection in treatment of carpal tunnel syndrome: a retrospective study. *Front Neurol.* 2021;12:782319.
98. Lin MT, Liao CL, Hsiao MY, Hsueh HW, Chao CC, Wu CH. Volume matters in ultrasound-guided perineural dextrose injection for carpal tunnel syndrome: a randomized, double-blinded, three-arm trial. *Front Pharmacol.* 2020;11:625830.
99. Li TY, Chen SR, Shen YP, et al. Long-term outcome after perineural injection with 5% dextrose for carpal tunnel syndrome: a retrospective follow-up study. *Rheumatology.* 2021;60(2):881–7.
100. Wang JC, Hsu PC, Wang KA, Chang KV. Ultrasound-guided triamcinolone acetonide hydrodissection for carpal tunnel syndrome: a randomized controlled trial. *Front Med.* 2021;8:742724.
101. Stoddard JM, Taylor CR, O'Connor FG. Ulnar nerve entrapment at the cubital tunnel successfully treated with ultrasound-guided peripheral nerve hydrodissection: a case report and further evidence for a developing treatment option. *Curr Sports Med Rep.* 2019;18(11):382–6.

102. Sahoo RK, Peng PW, Sharma SK. Ultrasound-guided hydrodissection for Baxter's neuropathy secondary to plantar fasciitis: a case report. *A A Pract*. 2020;14(13):e01339.
103. Kaga M. First case of occipital neuralgia treated by fascial hydrodissection. *Am J Case Rep*. 2022;23:e936475.
104. Tsujino S, Seki Y, Maehara M, Shirasawa S. Palsy of the posterior interosseous nerve treated by targeted ultrasound-guided perineural hydrodissection. *J Ultrason*. 2021;21(87):357–60.
105. Hu YWE, Ridings C. Subsartorius fascial plane hydrodissection as novel treatment for Hunter's canal syndrome. *Clin J Sport Med*. 2022;32(6):e644–6.
106. Delzell PB, Patel M. Ultrasound-guided perineural injection for pronator syndrome caused by median nerve entrapment. *J Ultrasound Med*. 2020;39(5):1023–9.
107. Gill B, Rahman R, Khadavi M. Ultrasound-guided hydrodissection provides complete symptom resolution in radial tunnel syndrome: a case series and scoping review on hydrodissection for radial nerve pathology. *Curr Sports Med Rep*. 2022;21(9):328–35.
108. Lam SK, Reeves KD, Cheng AL. Transition from deep regional blocks toward deep nerve hydrodissection in the upper body and torso: method description and results from a retrospective chart review of the analgesic effect of 5% dextrose water as the primary hydrodissection injectate to enhance safety. *BioMed Res Int*. 2017;2017:7920438.
109. Andren L, Lundberg BJ. Treatment of rigid shoulders by joint distension during arthrography. *Acta Orthop Scand*. 1965;36(1):45–53.
110. Catapano M, Mittal N, Adamich J, Kumbhare D, Sangha H. Hydrodilatation with corticosteroid for the treatment of adhesive capsulitis: a systematic review. *PM R*. 2018;10(6):623–35. doi:10.1016/j.pmrj.2017.10.013
111. Zhang J, Zhong S, Tan T, et al. Comparative efficacy and patient-specific moderating factors of nonsurgical treatment strategies for frozen shoulder: an updated systematic review and network meta-analysis. *Am J Sports Med*. 2021;49(6):1669–79. doi:10.1177/0363546520956293
112. Saltychev M, Laimi K, Virolainen P, Fredericson M. Effectiveness of hydrodilatation in adhesive capsulitis of shoulder: a systematic review and meta-analysis. *Scand J Surg*. 2018;107(4):285–93. doi:10.1177/1457496918772367
113. Wu WT, Chang KV, Han DS, Chang CH, Yang FS, Lin CP. Effectiveness of glenohumeral joint dilatation for treatment of frozen shoulder: a systematic review and meta-analysis of randomized controlled trials. *Sci Rep*. 2017;7(1):10507. doi:10.1038/s41598-017-10895-w
114. Cho JH. Updates on the treatment of adhesive capsulitis with hydraulic distension. *Yeungnam Univ J Med*. 2021;38(1):19–26. doi:10.12701/yujm.2020.00535
115. Kim K, Lee KJ, Kim HC, Lee KJ, Kim DK, Chung SG. Capsule preservation improves short-term outcome of hydraulic distension in painful stiff shoulder. *J Orthop Res*. 2011;29(11):1688–94. doi:10.1002/jor.21446
116. Wang JC, Tsai PY, Hsu PC, et al. Ultrasound-guided hydrodilatation with triamcinolone acetonide for adhesive capsulitis: a randomized controlled trial comparing the posterior glenohumeral recess and the rotator cuff interval approaches. *Front Pharmacol*. 2021;12:686139.
117. Ricci V, Chang KV, Özçakar L. Ultrasound-guided hydrodilatation of the shoulder capsule at the rotator interval: technical tips and tricks. *Pain Pract*. 2020;20(8):948–9. doi:10.1111/papr.12920
118. Chen YT, Olanrewaju CM. A novel treatment approach of ultrasound-guided radiofrequency ablation of the greater trochanteric sensory nerve for recalcitrant greater trochanteric pain syndrome. *Cureus*. 2021;13(11):e19859.
119. Gofeld M, Brown MN, Bollag L, Hanlon JG, Theodore BR. Magnetic positioning system and ultrasound guidance for lumbar zygapophyseal radiofrequency neurotomy: a cadaver study. *Reg Anesth Pain Med*. 2014;39(1):61–6.
120. Lash D, Frantz E, Hurdle MF. Ultrasound-guided cooled radiofrequency ablation of the genicular nerves: a technique paper. *Pain Manag*. 2020;10(3):147–57.
121. Wong J, Bremer N, Weyker PD, Webb CA. Ultrasound-guided genicular nerve thermal radiofrequency ablation for chronic knee pain. *Case Rep Anesthesiol*. 2016;2016:8292450.
122. Ahmed A, Arora D. Ultrasound-guided radiofrequency ablation of genicular nerves of knee for relief of intractable pain from knee osteoarthritis: a case series. *Br J Pain*. 2018;12(3):145–54.
123. Shah R, Ahmad M, Hanu-Cernat D, Choudhary S. Ultrasound-guided radiofrequency ablation for treatment of Morton's neuroma: initial experience. *Clin Radiol*. 2019;74(10):815.e9–e13.

85

Psychological Considerations in Physical Activity, Exercise, and Sport

Jeffrey L. Goodie and Abby N. Diehl

INTRODUCTION

- Physical activity, exercise, and sports influence behaviors, thoughts, and emotions. Similarly, what people do, how they think, and emotional responses influence the participation and performance of individuals in physical activity, exercise, and sports. Promoting participation in physical activity and enhancing performance in exercise and sports requires an understanding of the increasing evidence-base connecting psychology with exercise and sport.
- Only 23% of U.S. adults engage in recommended physical activity levels (1). Healthy adults between 18–65 year old should engage in moderate-intensity aerobic physical activity (*e.g.*, brisk walking) for at least 30 minutes, 5 days a week, or vigorous intensity aerobic physical activity (*e.g.*, jogging) for at least 20 minutes, 3 days each week. Additionally, these adults should engage in physical activity that maintains or increases muscle strength and endurance, at least 2 days a week (2).
- Physical activity and exercise are effective interventions for ameliorating depressive symptoms (3). Exercise was shown to decrease depressive symptoms as much as antidepressant medications (4).
- Exercise and physical activity may improve other behavioral and psychological concerns (*e.g.*, alcohol abuse, anxiety disorders, distress, eating disorders) (5–7). Exercise can improve cognitive functioning in adults of all ages and may reduce the impact on normal and pathological aging (8).

EPIDEMIOLOGY OF MENTAL HEALTH DISORDERS IN ATHLETES

- A systematic review and meta-analysis found that the prevalence of mental health symptoms among current elite athletes ranged from 19% (*i.e.*, alcohol misuse) to 34% (*i.e.*, anxiety and/or depressive symptoms (9).
- The burden of mental health disorders in athletes is extensive, especially with regard to potential impact on recovery from musculoskeletal (MSK) injury (10). For instance, athletes with MSK, particularly if they identify as female, are more likely to report symptoms of depression. Moreover, the relationship is bidirectional as depression symptoms are a predictor of disability in athletes.
- In one sample, over half of elite athletes report a lifetime prevalence of mental health problems (MHPs) of which onset peaks at 19 years of age making recurrent episodes of MHP common (11).
- In contrast, the 'mental health through sport' conceptual model has gained popularity recently, demonstrating that participation in sports is associated with better mental health in adulthood (12), particularly considering anxiolytic and antidepressant effects of physical activity. Team sports may provide additional social benefits, and mechanisms include: pro-social behavior, sense of belonging, and interpersonal communication practice.
- The restrictions and cancellations related to sport, subsequent to the COVID-19 pandemic outbreak, has had a significant impact on the mental health of athletes. The long-term mental health consequences of social isolation/team separation, fear of job loss, and lack of regular structured physical activity/practice are largely unknown; however, a recent review reported rates of anxiety, depression, and general stress are on the rise in athletes (13).

INITIATING PHYSICAL ACTIVITY IN SEDENTARY/LOW ACTIVE ADULTS

- The dominant paradigm for increasing physical activity is social cognitive interventions, which emphasizes internal attitudes, intentions, and self-efficacy toward environmental and social factors for the goal of intentional behavior change. Interventions to increase physical activity have historically involved changing attitudes toward physical activities and/or enhancing environmental opportunities for activity in individual or small group settings. (14).

- Simple interventions can increase physical activity. In one-on-one clinical interventions, several common components, such as practicing/rehearsing physical activity, biofeedback, using heart rate monitors, creating specific activity action plans, use of prompts/cues for behaviors, and providing self-rewards, have been demonstrated to enhance physical activity behaviors. At postintervention, physical activity interventions are effective at changing and maintaining behavior changes at 6-month follow-ups (15).
- Individual behavioral counseling approaches for physical activity could begin as a step-wise approach, specifically, initially targeting goals for less sedentary time, which can facilitate greater success moving toward moderate to vigorous physical activity recommendations (16). At a systemic and policy level, lessons from behavioral science, such as environmental design, methods of informational design, and promoting group cohesiveness toward behavior change, can be utilized to influence physical activity (17). For example, within a sample of young adults, providing normative peer feedback about step-count per day significantly increased daily step-count compared to no feedback control group (18).
- Motivational interviewing (MI), which is a conversational style designed to evoke and enhance one's own internal motivation for behavior change, has been shown to have a small positive effect on increasing self-reported physical activity in individuals with chronic health conditions (19). MI-based interventions positively impact both motivation for and engagement in physical activity behavior among sedentary adults. Wearable fitness trackers (WFTs) are gaining cultural popularity; however, only individuals who are not currently meeting physical activity recommended guidelines have demonstrated effectiveness of WFTs regarding initiation of physical activity (20).
- Digital interventions (*e.g.*, mobile smartphone applications, wearable fitness trackers) have exceptional potential to utilize behavioral change theory to promote physical activities (21). Additionally, review of available evidence suggests that text messaging interventions to promote physical activity enhance step count per day postintervention (22).
- In primary care settings, family medicine clinicians using the 5 As (Ask, Advise, Agree, Assist, Arrange) approach to physical activity for counseling results in immediate improvement in physical activity (23).

COMPETITIVE OR PERFORMANCE ANXIETY

- Although the exact prevalence is unknown, largely due to methodological and terminology differences across studies, performance or competitive anxiety in athletes is believed to be very common. Anxiety is linked to many types of performance, especially when an evaluation of behavioral abilities is present, as is the case in sport (24). Performance or competitive anxiety encompasses a range of cognitive appraisals, observable behaviors, and measurable physiological parameters, which occur in response to a sport situation perceived as potentially stressful by the individual (25). Moreover, dispositional intolerance for uncertainty, reflected in negative beliefs about the implications of uncertainty, is related to increased performance anxiety and lower sport confidence in athletes (26).
- Recent data suggest that few athletes report presence of anxiety disorder (16.8% of females, 6.6% of males) reaching moderate clinical cut off for symptoms of anxiety (GAD-7), which highlights normalization of anxiety in athletes, who have been socialized to receive help for performance anxiety (11).
- Meta-analysis evidence supports the effectiveness (medium to large-sized effect) of psychological interventions that target the thoughts, behaviors, and somatic components that contribute to the maintenance of competitive or performance anxiety in athletes when compared to controls (27).
- Behavioral strategies for performance enhancement include the use of visual imagery, diaphragmatic breathing, progressive muscle relaxation, biofeedback, autogenic training, yoga, mindfulness, meditation, and desensitization (27).
  - Visual imagery may involve imagining a relaxing scene or mental rehearsal of one's performance and a desired course of action.
  - Diaphragmatic breathing is a simple relaxation technique that involves taking slow, deep inhalations, concentrating on only moving the abdomen, holding each inhalation for a few seconds, and then exhaling.
  - Desensitization is the technique in which the athlete gradually diminishes anxiety associated with certain performance aspects (*e.g.*, free-throws in basketball) or specific anxiety disorders (*e.g.*, social phobia) through gradual exposure, either imaginal or in vivo, to the feared or anxiety-eliciting stimuli.
- Cognitive strategies, such as reappraisal and self-talk interventions, can also help athletes develop a greater sense of arousal control, and more importantly, improve performance. This might include encouraging the athlete to replace any sabotaging negative self-statements (*e.g.*, "I will never make this shot.") with reassuring, realistic self-statements (*e.g.*, "I have made this shot before and will try my best to make it again.") (28).
- Mindfulness and experiential acceptance approaches have been suggested to promote performance during sport as these interventions focus on promoting present attention and willingness to experience internal experiences. These interventions show promise in improving performance and lowering competitive anxiety; however, the empirical evidence is limited to make strong claims (29).

BEHAVIORAL HEALTH CONDITIONS ASSOCIATED WITH EXERCISE

- Behavioral health concerns, including alcohol use, tobacco use, sleep problems, disordered eating, and exercise overtraining can all have significant impacts on physical activity and athletic performance.

Alcohol Use and Dependence

- In a 2017 survey of 23,028 college student athletes by the National Collegiate Athletic Association (NCAA) regarding substance use habits, 77.1% reported using alcohol in the preceding 12 months, making it the most abused substance by athletes (30).
  - Alcohol use has declined since 2009. Binge drinking (four or more drinks for women; five or more drinks for men in one sitting) has also declined from 55% to 45% in student athletes (30).
  - Among these athletes, 25% reported that they had done something that they later regretted after drinking (30).
- *The Diagnostic and Statistical Manual of Mental Disorders-Fifth Edition-Text Revision* (*DSM-5-TR*) delineates criteria for alcohol use disorder (see Box 85.1) (31).

85.1 DSM-5-TR Criteria for Alcohol Use Disorder

A. A problematic pattern of alcohol use leading to clinically significant impairment or distress, as manifested by at least two of the following, occurring within a 12-mo period:
1. Alcohol is often taken in larger amounts or over a longer period than was intended.
2. There is a persistent desire or unsuccessful efforts to cut down or control alcohol use.
3. A great deal of time is spent in activities necessary to obtain alcohol, use alcohol, or recover from its effects.
4. Craving, or a strong desire or urge to use alcohol.
5. Recurrent alcohol use resulting in a failure to fulfill major role obligations at work, school, or home.
6. Continued alcohol use despite having persistent or recurrent social or interpersonal problems caused or exacerbated by the effects of alcohol.
7. Important social, occupational, or recreational activities are given up or reduced because of alcohol use.
8. Recurrent alcohol use in situations in which it is physically hazardous.
9. Alcohol use is continued despite knowledge of having a persistent or recurrent physical or psychological problem that is likely to have been caused or exacerbated by alcohol.
10. Tolerance, as defined by either of the following:
    a. A need for markedly increased amounts of alcohol to achieve intoxication or desired effect.
    b. A markedly diminished effect with continued use of the same amount of alcohol.
11. Withdrawal, as manifested by either of the following:
    a. The characteristic withdrawal syndrome for alcohol (refer to Criteria A and B of the criteria set for alcohol withdrawal).
    b. Alcohol (or a closely related substance, such as a benzodiazepine) is taken to relieve or avoid withdrawal symptoms.

Specify if:

In early remission: After full criteria for alcohol use disorder were previously met, none of the criteria for alcohol use disorder have been met for at least 3 mo but for less than 12 mo (with the exception that Criterion A4, "Craving, or a strong desire or urge to use alcohol," may be met).

In sustained remission: After full criteria for alcohol use disorder were previously met, none of the criteria for alcohol use disorder have been met at any time during a period of 12 mo or longer (with the exception that Criterion A4, "Craving, or a strong desire or urge to use alcohol," may be met).

Specify if:

In a controlled environment: This additional specifier is used if the individual is in an environment where access to alcohol is restricted.

Code based on current severity/remission: If an alcohol intoxication, alcohol withdrawal, or another alcohol-induced mental disorder is also present, do not use the codes below for alcohol use disorder. Instead, the comorbid alcohol use disorder is indicated in the 4th character of the alcohol-induced disorder code (see the coding note for alcohol intoxication, alcohol withdrawal, or a specific alcohol-induced mental disorder). For example, if there is comorbid alcohol intoxication and alcohol use disorder, only the alcohol intoxication code is given, with the 4th character indicating whether the comorbid alcohol use disorder is mild, moderate, or severe: F10.129 for mild alcohol use disorder with alcohol intoxication or F10.229 for a moderate or severe alcohol use disorder with alcohol intoxication.

Specify current severity/remission:

(F10.10) **Mild:** Presence of 2–3 symptoms.
(F10.11) **Mild: In early remission**
(F10.11) **Mild: In sustained remission**
(F10.20) **Moderate:** Presence of 4–5 symptoms.
(F10.21) **Moderate: In early remission**
(F10.21) **Moderate: In sustained remission**
(F10.20) **Severe:** Presence of six or more symptoms.
(F10.21) **Severe: In early remission**
(F10.21) **Severe: In sustained remission**

- A helpful screening tool in determining whether the athlete is a problem drinker is the Alcohol Use Disorders Identification Test (AUDIT-C) (32), which has been validated for use among college students (33).
  - The AUDIT-C is scored on a scale of 0–12 (scores of 0 reflect no alcohol use) by summing the circled numbers in each of the four columns, and then summing the values to obtain a total severity score (see Fig. 85.1).
  - In men, a score of 4 or more is considered positive; in women, a score of 3 or more is considered positive.
  - Generally, the higher the AUDIT-C score, the more likely it is that an individual's drinking is affecting their health and safety.
  - If the AUDIT-C score is positive, health care providers should conduct a brief intervention. This includes bringing attention to the elevated level of drinking, informing the athlete about the effects of alcohol on health, recommend limiting use or abstaining, exploring and supporting in choosing a responsible drinking goal, and follow-up and refer for specialty treatment, if indicated.

Tobacco Use and Dependence

- The NCAA 2018 revealed that among all athletes 10.5% had smoked cigarettes, 13.4% had used smokeless tobacco, and 8% used e-cigarettes in the last year (30).
- Every athlete who uses tobacco products should be offered a minimal intervention. An intervention lasting less than 3 minutes can increase overall tobacco abstinence rates (34).
- The 5'A's model is recommended as a brief intervention (see Table 85.1). Intensive tobacco cessation programs are also available to assist individuals in their quit efforts. The more effective interventions are based on a dose-response relation, with four or more sessions yielding higher abstinence rates (34).
- Other substances used by college athletes include amphetamines (4.1%), anabolic steroids (1.2%), cocaine (2.1%), ecstasy (1.1%), ephedrine (2.5%), marijuana (20.3%), and psychedelics (2.4%) (30).
  - Overall, the use of these substances has generally decreased, except for the use of amphetamines, which has increased. The most common reason students report taking amphetamines is for the treatment of attention-deficit hyperactivity disorder; the second most common reason is to increase energy.

Audit-C

1. How often do you have a drink containing alcohol?

Never (0)	Monthly or less (1)	Two or four times a month (2)	Two to three times per week (3)	Four or more times a week (4)

2. How many drinks containing alcohol do you have on a typical day when you are drinking?

1 or 2 (0)	3 or 4 (1)	5 or 6 (2)	7 or 9 (3)	10 or more (4)

3. How often do you have six or more drinks on one occasion?

Never (0)	Less than monthly (1)	Monthly (2)	Weekly (3)	Daily or almost daily (4)

Figure 85.1: AUDIT-C. (Data from Bush K, Kivlahan DR, McDonell MB, et al. The AUDIT Alcohol Consumption Questions [AUDIT-C]: an effective brief screening test for problem drinking. *Arch Internal Med.* 1998;3:1789–95.)

Sleep Disturbance

- Poor sleep among athletes is associated with decreased performance, increased risk of injury, and impaired recovery (35).
- Among athletes, 27%–37% report symptoms of insomnia (35).
- Sleep and behavioral health concerns have a bidirectional relationship among athletes. Poor sleep is associated with an increased risk of behavioral health concerns (*e.g.*, anxiety, depression, eating disorders, suicidal ideation); likewise, behavioral health problems (*e.g.*, depression) can result in sleep problems.
- Clinical diagnostic criteria for primary insomnia as established in the DSM-5-TR include difficulties with sleep onset, sleep maintenance, or nonrestorative sleep that lasts at least 1 month (31). These sleep problems must cause clinically significant impairment in functioning and must not be due to other clinical or substance use problems.
- Expert consensus recommendations for sleep in athletes includes: (1) Provide sleep education. (2) Screen for sleep problems using screen measure validated for athletes (*e.g.*, Athlete Sleep Screening Questionnaire. (3) Encourage naps. (4) Bank sleep before a period of anticipated sleep loss (36).
- Evidence-based interventions for sleep difficulties can include both nonpharmacologic and pharmacologic interventions.
- Cognitive-behavioral interventions, including sleep education, sleep hygiene, sleep restriction, and stimulus control strategies have been well-studied and can lead to long-term benefits (37). For athletes, the use of such strategies may be helpful in the short-term (*e.g.*, before competitions), but has demonstrated a positive impact on performance over the long-term (*i.e.*, weeks or months) (36).
  - Stimulus control interventions assist the patient with associating the bed with sleep. Patients are instructed to only use the bed for sleep and sexual activity (*e.g.*, no reading or watching TV in bed), to go to bed only when sleepy, to get out of bed if not asleep within 10–15 minutes, and to

Table 85.1 The 5 A's Model for Treating Tobacco Use and Dependence

Ask about tobacco use	Identify and document tobacco use status for every patient at every visit.
Advise to quit	In a clear, strong, and personalized manner, urge every tobacco user to quit.
Assess willingness to make a quit attempt	Is the tobacco user willing to make a quit attempt at this time.
Assist in quit attempt	For the patient willing to make a quit attempt, offer medication and provide or refer for counseling or additional treatment to help the patient quit. For patients unwilling to quit, provide interventions designed to increase future quit attempts.
Arrange follow-up	For the patient willing to make a quit attempt, arrange for follow-up contacts, beginning within the first week after the quit date. For patients unwilling to make a quit attempt at the time, address tobacco dependence and willingness to quit at next clinic visit.

Source: U.S. Department of Health and Human Services. *Treating Tobacco Use and Dependence: 2008 Update.* Rockville, MD: Public Health Service; 2008.

stay out of bed until they are sleepy. If, when they return to bed, they still do not fall asleep within 10–15 minutes, they should again get out of bed until they are ready to fall asleep. Each morning patients should wake at the same time and avoid naps throughout the day.

- Sleep restriction therapy requires determining the average amount of sleep an individual obtains at night, setting a consistent wake time, and then setting the time that the individual would go to sleep by working backwards based on the average sleep time and wake time. If someone typically sleeps 6 hours and wants to wake at 5:00 AM, they would go to sleep at 11:00 PM
- There are few studies that have examined the use of pharmacologic sleep aids in athletes. Melatonin, caffeine, and nonbenzodiazepine sleep aids may help to facilitate sleep schedule changes (38).

Feeding and Eating Disordered Behavior

- Disordered feeding and eating behavior can range from that which meets clinical diagnostic criteria for anorexia nervosa (see Box 85.2), bulimia nervosa (see Box 85.3), as established in the DSM-5-TR to subclinical levels of disordered feeding and eating behavior, which might include occasional purging, and/or laxative use, or diet pill use referred to as "other specified feeding or eating disorder" and "unspecified feeding or eating disorder" in the DSM-5-TR. Avoidant/restrictive food intake disorder and binge eating disorder were included in the revised DSM-5-TR; however, there is a paucity of research with regard to these eating behaviors in athletes (39).
- Given the risk to the health and performance of athletes with disordered eating behaviors, the American Medical Society for Sports Medicine (AMSSM) recommended the following for the prevention, detection, and treatment of eating disorders and disordered eating (40):
  - Routine annual screening for eating disorders.
  - Targeted programs that may help reduce the risk of disordered eating behavior among athletes (41).
  - Cognitive behavioral therapy and family therapy as recommended treatments for eating disorders in athletes. Behavioral therapies have the strongest evidence for the treatment of eating disorders.
  - When disordered eating is suspected, health care providers should conduct a thorough physical and psychosocial evaluation. If treatment is indicated, a multidisciplinary treatment team model, which includes medical, dietary, behavioral, coaches, and cognitive interventions, is necessary for effective treatment.
- Disordered eating behaviors are more common among athletes, particularly those in weight-sensitive sports where low body weight confers a competitive advantage, compared to the general population (42).
- Although there have been challenges in determining prevalence rates (43), researchers have demonstrated that in a sample of adolescent elite athletes, the overall prevalence of eating disorders was 7.0%, compared to 2.3% in controls (44).
- Disordered eating is not confined to female athletes, and assessment of eating behavior in both females and males is essential. The combined prevalence estimates for both disordered eating behavior and formally diagnosed eating disorders range in adult collegiate elite athletes from 0% to 19% in males and 6%–45% in females (45). The competitive nature of athletics may increase the risk of disordered eating (46).
- Awareness of a broad array of signs and symptoms of eating disorders in general can facilitate early detection in those athletes who may struggle with disordered eating (39):
  - General physical (rapid changes in weight, failure to gain weight at an appropriate developmental level, fatigue, hypothermia)
  - Psychological/neurological (insomnia, depression, anxiety, self-harm, memory/concentration concerns, obsessive thoughts about eating/food)

85.2 DSM-5-TR Criteria for Anorexia Nervosa

A. Restriction of energy intake relative to requirements, leading to a significantly low body weight in the context of age, sex, developmental trajectory, and physical health. *Significantly low weight* is defined as a weight that is less than minimally normal or, for children and adolescents, less than that minimally expected.

B. Intense fear of gaining weight or of becoming fat, or persistent behavior that interferes with weight gain, even though at a significantly low weight.

C. Disturbance in the way in which one's body weight or shape is experienced, undue influence of body weight or shape on self-evaluation, or persistent lack of recognition of the seriousness of the current low body weight.

Specify whether:

F50.01 Restricting type: During the last 3 mo, the individual has not engaged in recurrent episodes of binge-eating or purging behavior (i.e., self-induced vomiting or the misuse of laxatives, diuretics, or enemas). This subtype describes presentations in which weight loss is accomplished primarily through dieting, fasting, and/or excessive exercise.

F50.02 Binge-eating/purging type: During the last 3 mo, the individual has engaged in recurrent episodes of binge-eating or purging behavior (i.e., self-induced vomiting or the misuse of laxatives, diuretics, or enemas).

Specify if:

In partial remission: After full criteria for anorexia nervosa were previously met, Criterion A (low body weight) has not been met for a sustained period, but either Criterion B (intense fear of gaining weight or becoming fat or behavior that interferes with weight gain) or Criterion C (disturbances in self-perception of weight and shape) is still met.

In full remission: After full criteria for anorexia nervosa were previously met, none of the criteria have been met for a sustained period of time.

Specify current severity:

The minimum level of severity is based, for adults, on current body mass index (BMI) (see below) or, for children and adolescents, on BMI percentile. The ranges below are derived from World Health Organization categories for thinness in adults; for children and adolescents, corresponding BMI percentiles should be used. The level of severity may be increased to reflect clinical symptoms, the degree of functional disability, and the need for supervision.

Mild: BMI $\geq$ 17 kg/m^2.

Moderate: BMI 16–16.99 kg/m^2.

Severe: BMI 15–15.99 kg/m^2.

Extreme: BMI $<$ 15 kg/m^2.

Reprinted with permission from the *Diagnostic and Statistical Manual of Mental Disorders*, 5th ed. Text Revision (Copyright © 2022). American Psychiatric Association.

85.3 DSM-5-TR Criteria for Bulimia Nervosa

A. Recurrent episodes of binge eating. An episode of binge eating is characterized by both of the following:
   1. Eating, in a discrete period of time (e.g., within any 2-h period) an amount of food that is definitely larger than what most individuals would eat during a similar period of time under similar circumstances.
   2. A sense of lack of control over eating during the episode (e.g., a feeling that one cannot stop eating or control what or how much one is eating).

B. Recurrent inappropriate compensatory behaviors in order to prevent weight gain, such as self-induced vomiting; misuse of laxatives, diuretics, or other medications; fasting; or excessive exercise.

C. The binge eating and inappropriate compensatory behaviors both occur, on average, at least once a week for 3 mo.

D. Self-evaluation is unduly influenced by body shape and weight.

E. The disturbance does not occur exclusively during episodes of anorexia nervosa.

Specify if:

In partial remission: After full criteria for bulimia nervosa were previously met, some, but not all, of the criteria have been met for a sustained period of time.

In full remission: After full criteria for bulimia nervosa were previously met, none of the criteria have been met for a sustained period of time.

Specify current severity:

The minimum level of severity is based on the frequency of inappropriate compensatory behaviors (see below). The level of severity may be increased to reflect other symptoms and the degree of functional disability.

Mild: An average of 1–3 episodes of inappropriate compensatory behaviors per week.

Moderate: An average of 4–7 episodes of inappropriate compensatory behaviors per week.

Severe: An average of 8–13 episodes of inappropriate compensatory behaviors per week.

Extreme: An average of 14 or more episodes of inappropriate compensatory behaviors per week.

Unspecified

Reprinted with permission from the *Diagnostic and Statistical Manual of Mental Disorders*, 5th ed. Text Revision (Copyright © 2022). American Psychiatric Association.

  - MSK (stress fractures, low bone density)
  - Dermatology (loss of hair, skin discoloration, lack of skin healing)
  - Oral/dental (dental erosion/caries, recurrent sore throats, oral trauma)
  - Gastrointestinal (abdominal pain, reflux, constipation, diarrhea)
  - Cardiorespiratory (chest pain, hypotension, bradycardia, shortness of breath) (42).
- However, clinicians and coaches should use caution as medical/physiological changes are sometimes not observable in individuals with eating disorders or a disordered eating behavior. Therefore, routine screening and specific targeted questions are key.
- Risk factors for developing disordered eating include (47):
  - Psychological factors, such as body dissatisfaction, negative affect, dieting, and over eating; internalized sociocultural factors, such as thinness ideal and mental health care (48).
  - Sports-specific factors such as participation in a variety of sports, not only sports promoting lean builds (*e.g.*, gymnastics, figure skating). For men, distance running, wrestling, bodybuilding, lightweight football, horse racing, rowing, and ski jumping have been associated with disordered eating (46).
- The "female athlete triad" was coined by the American College of Sports Medicine (ACSM) in 1992 to describe three interrelated conditions of functional hypothalamic amenorrhea, osteoporosis, and low energy available that often occur together in female athletes (49) (see Chapter 131, The Female Athlete for further discussion).
- In the 2007 ACSM position on the female athlete triad, it is recommended that females are screened for symptoms at preparticipation or annual health screening exams. Athletes who demonstrate one of the triad components should be screened for the other components (50).
- According to the ACSM, treatment for those demonstrating the female athlete triad should focus on increasing energy availability (*i.e.*, increasing energy intake and/or reducing energy expenditure) through nutritional counseling and modification of exercise behaviors (50). Resumption of menses and improvement of bone mass/strength is key. A multidisciplinary approach, including a team of primary care and/or sports medicine physician, dietitian, athletic trainer, and psychologist, is recommended.
- Binge eating disorder (BED) is a clinical mental disorder, defined by the American Psychiatric Association as recurrent binge eating without compensatory weight control behavior such as self-induced vomiting, diuretic use, and excessive levels of physical activity (*Diagnostic and Statistical Manual of Mental Disorders* (*DSM-5-TR*)) (51).
- Currently, no guidelines for the management or treatment of BED in athletes exist within the reviewed literature. BED in athletes is likely related to restriction of calories and multimodal stressors (51).

EXERCISE OVERTRAINING "ADDICTION"

- Exercise addiction (EA) is not a DSM-5-TR diagnosis like alcohol and tobacco abuse. Researchers describe EA as a multidimensional phenomenon that involves perceived need for physical activity associated with excessive exercise behavior with tolerance and/or withdrawal and psychological symptoms (52).
- Withdrawal symptoms can encompass mood symptoms, such as anxiousness, irritability, depression, and restlessness, when exercise is impeded or guilt when an exercise session is missed (52).
- Prevalence rates have ranged from 2.7% to 42% of the athlete population and approximately 3% in the leisure exercise population (53). EA has been viewed as a "behavioral addiction," which includes the following: hypothesized mechanisms for exercising dependence include affect regulation (*i.e.*, exercise enhances positive affect and/or reduces negative affect), sympathetic arousal or habituation (*i.e.*, hormonal changes maintain need for repeated exercise), β-endorphin (*i.e.*, opioid peptides produce addictive behaviors), and cytokine overproduction (*i.e.*, exercise provides relief from symptoms associated with overproduction cytokines (*e.g.*, fatigue, poor concentration, anxiety, depression) (54).
- In a 2022 systematic review, the authors highlighted that exercise addiction measurement in athletes may be particularly problematic due to predetermined training schedules, which would be counter to an additive process of urge/craving and resulted in 10× greater prevalence rate of EA in athletes compared with nonathletes (53).
- Researchers argue that "serious conceptual consideration" must be taken. Specifically, elite athletes may assign different interpretations to assessment tools compared with leisure exercisers (55).
- Overtraining syndrome (OTS) is a condition associated with long-term imbalance between training and recovery within athletic performance. OTS involves an accumulation of training stress that results in decrease in performance capacity of an athlete. An example would be a runner who trains at increased distances every day without allowing a day of rest or recovery in between sessions. The ultimate result of overtraining behavior is the opposite of what is pursued, and restoration of performance can take several weeks or months. There are limited data related to OTS due to the lack of clearly reporting of data time frame, given the key component of prolonged maladaptation within this construct (56) (see Chapter 45, Overtraining Syndrome for further discussion).

- OTS is thought to be characterized by fatigue, mood decline, and physiological changes (*e.g.*, resting cortisol levels).
- Mood changes are of the key characteristics of OTS, and, therefore, monitoring an athlete's mood during increased stress may also be helpful.
- In a 2022 review of the literature in OTS, the authors noted that no studies have provided objective evidence of changes in athletic performance precompared with post OTS diagnosis (57). Despite real-world field observations, the scientific base for understanding OTS is lacking.
- OTS Recommendations from AMSSM (56):
  - Individual developed plans for athletes with OTS should include an evaluation for mental health stressors and relative rest depending on the time frame.
  - Ongoing monitoring of training loads, obtaining appropriate rest, optimal nutrition, and hydration plan as part of prevention of OTS.

REHABILITATION

- The success of rehabilitation can be significantly impacted by psychological factors. It is important to not only address these concerns during rehabilitation, but also know when to refer individuals for more intensive specialty behavioral health care.

Injury Rehabilitation

- Over 8.6 million U.S. children, adolescents, and adults (*i.e.*, 34.1 episodes per 1000 persons) endure sports or recreational-related injuries each year (58). The injured athlete may not only present with a concern about the injury itself. Fear of movement (*i.e.*, kinesiophobia) and fear of reinjury are two of the most important factors predicting whether an athlete will return to preinjury activity levels (59).
- Although athletes are not considered to be at higher risk for suicide, those who sustain substantial injuries, particularly traumatic brain injuries, may be at greater risk for suicide (60).
- There are multiple models to guide rehabilitation including the integrated model, the biomedical model, the biopsychosocial model, and the self-determination theory model. (59,61):
  - The biomedical model places the primary focus on the physiological functioning of the athlete, and readiness to play is based on biological markers.
  - The biopsychosocial model applied to injury rehabilitation among athletes requires an understanding of how the physical, behavioral, cognitive, emotional, and social factors influence each other and the recovery process. An understanding of the relations between these factors allows the health care provider to more effectively target areas for treatment (see Table 85.2). The provider may then choose from among several effective interventions to tailor a rehabilitation program to meet the athlete's needs. This might include the use of imagery and other mental devices, increasing social support, pain management, and/or other cognitive-behavioral techniques, such as self-management training.
  - The integrated model proposes that athletes' responses to injury and their rehabilitation outcomes are influenced by both personal and situational factors. Personal factors might include the athlete's personality, mental toughness, and history of stress, while situational factors could include the severity of the injury, social support, and the athlete's perceptions of their medical team. The model also highlights the importance of cognitive appraisal and emotional response, suggesting that how an athlete interprets and emotionally reacts to their injury can greatly influence their rehabilitation process. The initial appraisal is impacted by personal (*e.g.*, age, gender, personality) and social factors (*e.g.*, social support).

Table 85.2 Biopsychosocial Factors in Injury Rehabilitation

Physical Factors	Where is the injury? What is the frequency, intensity, and duration of any associated pain? Are there any other current significant medical problems? What is their energy level? How is their sleep? What is their history of sports injuries?
Behavioral Factors	Are they adhering to the rehabilitation program? Do they put forth their best effort at rehabilitation sessions? Are there any substance abuse issues (*e.g.*, alcohol, tobacco, excessive eating)? How have they changed their life since the injury (*e.g.*, have they skipped important responsibilities?)
Cognitive Factors	What is their attitude about the injury, the treatment they have received, and the rehabilitation process? Do they engage in predominantly positive or negative self-statements?
Emotional Factors	Have they recently felt more sad, anxious, upset, and/or irritated than they would have liked? Do they have any fears about returning to their sport? Are they experiencing grief over the loss of their sport or exercise activity?
Relationship Factors	Do they have an adequate social support system? Have coaches and/or teammates been constructive in the rehabilitation process? Have they changed their behavior toward family and friends (*e.g.*, more isolative)? Are they experiencing any relationship difficulties/stressors as a result of the injury?

Source: Robinson CS. Psychology and the injured runner: recovery enhancing strategies. In: O'Connor FG, Wilder RP, Nirschl R, editors. *Textbook of Running Medicine*. New York: McGraw-Hill; 2001. pp. 621–8.

  - The self-determination theory model suggests that people are more likely to engage in behaviors that they find intrinsically motivating and that satisfy their basic psychological needs for autonomy, competence, and relatedness. In the context of sports rehabilitation, practitioners can use self-determination theory to promote adherence by fostering a sense of autonomy (*e.g.*, by involving athletes in decision-making processes), competence (*e.g.*, by setting achievable goals and providing positive feedback), and relatedness (*e.g.*, by providing social support).
- Regardless of the model used for rehabilitation, a systematic review found that relaxation/guided imagery, positive self-talk and cognitive restructuring, goal setting, counseling, emotional written disclosure, and modeling videos were effective for promoting postinjury recovery among athletes (59).

Psychological Issues and Athlete Return to Play

- Psychological readiness is one important factor to consider in return-to-play decisions and should be considered separately from physical readiness (62).
- Following a significant illness or injury, athletes may experience fear of the illness or injury recurring, worry about their inability to perform at previous levels, increased feelings of isolation, social identity loss, and feeling pressure to return before they are ready (62).
- According to the ACSM, when making return-to-play decisions it is desirable to (62):
  - Monitor the psychological readiness of athletes preparing to or who have returned to play.
  - Encourage and facilitate connections between the athlete and the team.
  - Remain aware of psychological and sociocultural factors that may influence return-to-play decisions.
  - Screen for and monitor psychological factors that have the potential to impact treatment and rehabilitation.
  - Encourage, coordinate, and facilitate specialty behavioral health services as needed to reduce the impact of psychological factors during treatment and return-to-play decisions.

Referral to Specialty Behavioral Health Services

- It is important that health care providers are vigilant of symptoms that may warrant referral for more extensive behavioral health assessment and treatment, and that they are aware of the appropriate professionals to consider when making referrals for athletes (63).
- Athletes may be reluctant to pursue behavioral health services due to concerns about stigma, confidentiality, perceptions of others, fear of impact on career, and/or misunderstanding about such services (62).
- The term "sport psychologist" is not well defined, and it should not be assumed that someone who describes themselves as a sport psychologist is qualified to provide clinical assessment or treatment services.
- The American Psychological Association recognizes sport psychology as a proficiency that is acquired with specialty training after doctoral training in psychology and licensure as a psychologist (63). Some "sport psychologists" may be primarily researchers, and other individuals may have no or limited training in psychology. When making a referral to a psychologist for clinical assessment or treatment services for behavioral health conditions in athletes, ask whether the individual is a "licensed psychologist" with specialized training in sport and performance psychology.

SUMMARY

- Physical activity and exercise are important for improving and maintaining behavioral health.
- Behavioral health concerns can impact athletic performance, hinder rehabilitation, and impact return-to-play decisions.
- It is important for those who work with athletes to monitor for, identify, and treat behavioral health problems.
- When referring individuals for behavioral health care, ensure that the provider qualified to provide behavioral health care services.

REFERENCES

1. Centers for Disease Control and Prevention. National Center for Chronic Disease Prevention and Health Promotion, Division of Nutrition, Physical Activity, and Obesity. *Data, Trend and Maps* [online].
2. Piercy KL, Troiano RP, Ballard RM, et al. The physical activity guidelines for Americans. *JAMA*. 2018;320(19):2020–8.
3. Heissel A, Heinen D, Brokmeier LL, et al. Exercise as medicine for depressive symptoms? A systematic review and meta-analysis with meta-regression. *Br J Sports Med*. 2023;57(16):1049–57.
4. Recchia F, Leung CK, Chin EC, et al. Comparative effectiveness of exercise, antidepressants and their combination in treating non-severe depression: a systematic review and network meta-analysis of randomised controlled trials. *Br J Sports Med*. 2022;56(23):1375–80.
5. Cook BJ, Wonderlich SA, Mitchell JE, Thompson R, Sherman R, McCallum K. Exercise in eating disorders treatment: systematic review and proposal of guidelines. *Med Sci Sports Exerc*. 2016;48(7):1408–14.
6. Lardier DT, Coakley KE, Holladay KR, Amorim FT, Zuhl MN. Exercise as a useful intervention to reduce alcohol consumption and improve physical fitness in individuals with alcohol use disorder: a systematic review and meta-analysis. *Front Psychol*. 2021;12:675285.
7. Singh B, Olds T, Curtis R, et al. Effectiveness of physical activity interventions for improving depression, anxiety and distress: an overview of systematic reviews. *Br J Sports Med*. 2023;57(18):1203–9.
8. Mandolesi L, Polverino A, Montuori S, et al. Effects of physical exercise on cognitive functioning and wellbeing: biological and psychological benefits. *Front Psychol*. 2018;9:509.

9. Gouttebarge V, Castaldelli-Maia JM, Gorczynski P, et al. Occurrence of mental health symptoms and disorders in current and former elite athletes: a systematic review and meta-analysis. *Br J Sports Med.* 2019;53(11):700–706.
10. Marconcin P, Silva AL, Flôres F, et al. Association between musculoskeletal injuries and depressive symptoms among athletes: a systematic review. *Int J Environ Res Publ Health.* 2023;20(12):6130.
11. Åkesdotter C, Kenttä G, Eloranta S, Franck J. The prevalence of mental health problems in elite athletes. *J Sci Med Sport.* 2020;23(4):329–335.
12. Eather N, Wade L, Pankowiak A, Eime R. The impact of sports participation on mental health and social outcomes in adults: a systematic review and the 'Mental Health through Sport' conceptual model. *Syst Rev.* 2023;12(1):102.
13. Shukla A, Dogra DK, Bhattacharya D, Gulia S, Sharma R. Impact of COVID-19 outbreak on the mental health in sports: a review. *Sport Sci Health.* 2023:1–15.
14. Rhodes RE, Janssen I, Bredin SSD, Warburton DER, Bauman A. Physical activity: health impact, prevalence, correlates and interventions. *Psychol Health.* 2017;32(8):942–75.
15. Howlett N, Trivedi D, Troop NA, Chater AM. Are physical activity interventions for healthy inactive adults effective in promoting behavior change and maintenance, and which behavior change techniques are effective? A systematic review and meta-analysis. *Transl Behav Med.* 2019;9(1):147–57.
16. Dogra S, Copeland JL, Altenburg TM, Heyland DK, Owen N, Dunstan DW. Start with reducing sedentary behavior: a stepwise approach to physical activity counseling in clinical practice. *Patient Educ Counsel.* 2022;105(6):1353–61.
17. Gormley L, Belton CA, Lunn PD, Robertson DA. Interventions to increase physical activity: an analysis of candidate behavioural mechanisms. *Prev Med Rep.* 2022;28:101880.
18. Wally CM, Cameron LD. A randomized-controlled trial of social norm interventions to increase physical activity. *Ann Behav Med.* 2017;51(5):642–51.
19. O'Halloran PD, Blackstock F, Shields N, et al. Motivational interviewing to increase physical activity in people with chronic health conditions: a systematic review and meta-analysis. *Clin Rehabil.* 2014;28(12):1159–71.
20. Nuss K, Moore K, Nelson T, Li K. Effects of motivational interviewing and wearable fitness trackers on motivation and physical activity: a systematic review. *Am J Health Promot.* 2021;35(2):226–35.
21. De Santis KK, Jahnel T, Matthias K, Mergenthal L, Al Khayyal H, Zeeb H. Evaluation of digital interventions for physical activity promotion: scoping review. *JMIR Public Health Surveill.* 2022;8(5):e37820.
22. Smith DM, Duque L, Huffman JC, Healy BC, Celano CM. Text message interventions for physical activity: a systematic review and meta-analysis. *Am J Prev Med.* 2020;58(1):142–51.
23. Carroll JK, Winters PC, Sanders MR, Decker F, Ngo T, Sciamanna CN. Clinician-targeted intervention and patient-reported counseling on physical activity. *Prev Chronic Dis.* 2014;11:E89.
24. Rowland DL, Moyle G, Cooper SE. Remediation strategies for performance anxiety across sex, sport and stage: identifying common approaches and a unified cognitive model. *Int J Environ Res Publ Health.* 2021;18(19):10160.
25. Ford JL, Ildefonso K, Jones ML, Arvinen-Barrow M. Sport-related anxiety: current insights. *Open Access J Sports Med.* 2017;8:205–12.
26. Robinson G, Freeston M. Intolerance of uncertainty as a predictor of performance anxiety and robustness of sport confidence in university student-athletes. *J Clin Sport Psychol.* 2015;9(4):335–44.
27. Ong NC, Chua JH. Effects of psychological interventions on competitive anxiety in sport: a meta-analysis. *Psychol Sport Exerc.* 2021;52:101836.
28. Hatzigeorgiadis A, Galanis E, Zourbanos N, Theodorakis Y. Self-talk and competitive sport performance. *J Appl Sport Psychol.* 2014;26(1):82–95.
29. Noetel M, Ciarrochi J, Van Zanden B, Lonsdale C. Mindfulness and acceptance approaches to sporting performance enhancement: a systematic review. *Int Rev Sport Exerc Psychol.* 2019;12(1):139–75.
30. The National Collegiate Athletic Association. *NCAA Study of Substance Use of College Student Athletes.* Indianapolis (IN); 2018.
31. American Psychiatric Association. *Diagnostic and Statistical Manual of Mental Disorders.* 5th ed. 2022. text rev.
32. Bush K, Kivlahan DR, McDonell MB, Fihn SD, Bradley KA. The AUDIT alcohol consumption questions (AUDIT-C): an effective brief screening test for problem drinking. Ambulatory Care Quality Improvement Project (ACQUIP). Alcohol Use Disorders Identification Test. *Arch Intern Med.* 1998;158(16):1789–95.
33. Barry AE, Chaney BH, Stellefson ML, Dodd V. Evaluating the psychometric properties of the AUDIT-C among college students. *J Subst Use.* 2015;20(1):1–5.
34. U.S. Department of Health and Human Services. *Treating Tobacco Use and Dependence: 2008 Update.* Rockville (MD): Public Health Service; 2008.
35. Montero A, Stevens D, Adams R, Drummond M. Sleep and mental health issues in current and former athletes: a mini review. *Front Psychol.* 2022;13:868614.
36. Walsh NP, Halson SL, Sargent C, et al. Sleep and the athlete: narrative review and 2021 expert consensus recommendations. *Br J Sports Med.* 2021;55:356–68.
37. Edinger JD, Arnedt JT, Bertisch SM, et al. Behavioral and psychological treatments for chronic insomnia disorder in adults: an American Academy of Sleep Medicine systematic review, meta-analysis, and GRADE assessment. *J Clin Sleep Med.* 2021;17(2):263–98.
38. Baird MB, Asif IM. Medications for sleep schedule adjustments in athletes. *Sports Health.* 2018;10(1):35–9.
39. Joy E, Kussman A, Nattiv A. 2016 update on eating disorders in athletes: a comprehensive narrative review with a focus on clinical assessment and management. *Br J Sports Med.* 2016;50(3):154–62.
40. Chang C, Putukian M, Aerni G, et al. Mental health issues and psychological factors in athletes: detection, management, effect on performance and prevention—American Medical Society for Sports Medicine Position Statement-Executive Summary. *Br J Sports Med.* 2020;54(4):216–20.
41. Martinsen M, Bahr R, Børresen R, Holme I, Pensgaard AM, Sundgot-Borgen J. Preventing eating disorders among young elite athletes: a randomized controlled trial. *Med Sci Sports Exerc.* 2014;46(3):435–47.
42. Conviser JH, Tierney AS, Nickols R. Essentials for best practice: treatment approaches for athletes with eating disorders. *J Clin Sport Psychol.* 2018;12(4):495–507.
43. Chatterton JM, Petrie TA. Prevalence of disordered eating and pathogenic weight control behaviors among male collegiate athletes. *Eat Disord.* 2013;21(4):328–41.
44. Martinsen M, Sundgot-Borgen J. Higher prevalence of eating disorders among adolescent elite athletes than controls. *Med Sci Sports Exerc.* 2013;45(6):1188–97.
45. Bratland-Sanda S, Sundgot-Borgen J. Eating disorders in athletes: overview of prevalence, risk factors and recommendations for prevention and treatment. *Eur J Sport Sci.* 2013;13(5):499–508.
46. McDonald AH, Pritchard M, McGuire MK. Self-reported eating disorder risk in lean and non-lean NCAA Collegiate Athletes. *Eat Weight Disord.* 2020;25(3):745–50.
47. Arthur-Cameselle J, Sossin K, Quatromoni P. A qualitative analysis of factors related to eating disorder onset in female collegiate athletes and non-athletes. *Eat Disord.* 2017;25(3):199–215.
48. Stice E, Gau JM, Rohde P, Shaw H. Risk factors that predict future onset of each DSM-5 eating disorder: predictive specificity in high-risk adolescent females. *J Abnorm Psychol.* 2017;126(1):38–51.

49. Barrack MT, Ackerman KE, Gibbs JC. Update on the female athlete triad. *Curr Rev Musculoskelet Med.* 2013;6(2):195–204.
50. Nattiv A, Loucks AB, Manore MM, Sanborn CF, Sundgot-Borgen J, Warren MP, American College of Sports Medicine. American College of Sports Medicine position stand. The female athlete triad. *Med Sci Sports Exerc.* 2007;39(10):1867–82.
51. Williams G. Binge eating and binge eating disorder in athletes: a review of theory and evidence. *Sport J.* 2016;19:1.
52. Godoy-Izquierdo D, Ramírez MJ, Díaz I, López-Mora C. A systematic review on exercise addiction and the disordered eating-eating disorders continuum in the competitive sport context. *Int J Ment Health Addiction.* 2023;21(1):529–61.
53. Juwono ID, Tolnai N, Szabo A. Exercise addiction in athletes: a systematic review of the literature. *Int J Ment Health Addiction.* 2022;20(5): 3113–27.
54. Weinstein A, Weinstein Y. Exercise addiction-diagnosis, bio-psychological mechanisms and treatment issues. *Curr Pharm Des.* 2014;20(25):4062–9.
55. Szabo A, Griffiths MD, de La Vega Marcos R, Mervó B, Demetrovics Z. Methodological and conceptual limitations in exercise addiction research. *Yale J Biol Med.* 2015;88(3):303–8.
56. Meeusen R, Duclos M, Foster C, European College of Sport Science, American College of Sports Medicine, et al. Prevention, diagnosis, and treatment of the overtraining syndrome: joint consensus statement of the European College of Sport Science and the American College of Sports Medicine. *Med Sci Sports Exerc.* 2013;45(1):186–205.
57. Weakley J, Halson SL, Mujika I. Overtraining syndrome symptoms and diagnosis in athletes: where is the research? A systematic review. *Int J Sports Physiol Perform.* 2022;17(5):675–81.
58. Sheu Y, Chen LH, Hedegaard H. Sports- and recreation-related injury episodes in the United States, 2011-2014. *Natl Health Stat Report.* 2016(99):1–12. Hyattsville, MD.
59. Gennarelli SM, Brown SM, Mulcahey MK. Psychosocial interventions help facilitate recovery following musculoskeletal sports injuries: a systematic review. *Phys Sportsmed.* 2020;48(4):370–7.
60. Pichler EM, Ewers S, Ajdacic-Gross V, et al. Athletes are not at greater risk for death by suicide: a review. *Scand J Med Sci Sports.* 2023;33(5):569–85.
61. Hess CW, Gnacinski SL, Meyer BB. A review of the sport-injury and-rehabilitation literature: from abstraction to application. *Sport Psychol.* 2019;33(3):232–43.
62. Psychological issues related to illness and injury in athletes and the team physician: a consensus statement-2016 update. *Med Sci Sports Exerc.* 2017;49(5):1043–54.
63. Portenga ST, Aoyagi MW, Cohen AB. Helping to build a profession: a working definition of sport and performance psychology. *J Sport Psychol Action.* 2017;8(1):47–59.

86 Complementary and Integrative Health (CIH)

Preya Y. Patel, Anthony I. Beutler, and Wayne B. Jonas

WHAT IS COMPLEMENTARY AND INTEGRATIVE HEALTH?

- Many different medical systems and medical practices exist in the world today including traditional Oriental medicine, Native American practices, Ayurveda, and Western biomedicine (to name only a few).
- Western biomedicine is the medicine practiced in American hospitals and taught in American medical schools. Western biomedicine is neither the oldest nor the most widely used medical system in the world today. The World Health Organization estimates that a substantial portion of the world's population receives their medical care outside the Western biomedical system (1).
- Integrative health is the pursuit of personal health and well-being foremost while addressing disease as needed, with the support of a health team dedicated to all evidence-based approaches — conventional, complementary and self-care. It is a partnership between the practitioner and patient that looks to a wider set of offerings with proven approaches — approaches that address the underlying causes of disease. A growing body of evidence shows that when patients are integrally involved in managing their own care, they will be healthier and happier. While the constraints in our health care system prohibit rapid, wholesale change to an integrative health approach, physicians can still begin to transform their own practices and incorporate more healing factors into day-to-day practice. Many already include the elements of integrative health care (2) (see Fig. 86.1).

WHO USES COMPLEMENTARY AND INTEGRATIVE HEALTH?

- Many developing countries rely on CIH practices to provide most of the health care for their citizens.
- Americans spend more than $30.2 billion each year (most of it unreimbursed by insurance) on CIH practices (3). Visits to U.S. CIH practitioners rose from 400 million per year in 1990 to 600 million per year in 1996 and have continued to increase steadily. Approximately 40% of the U.S. population (compared with 75% of the population of France) report using a CIH practice at least once during the year (4,5).
- Among Western CIH consumers, 95% use CIH in a "complementary" fashion or in addition to Western biomedicine. Only 5% use CIH exclusively, or as an "alternative" to Western biomedicine (6).
- Studies reveal that CIH users in the United States tend to be more educated, more affluent, more holistic in their view of health care, and more likely to have chronic pain or a chronic disease than nonusers of CIH (5–7). Past reports indicated that some minorities, such as African Americans, were less likely to use CIH. However, a more recent study specifically designed to assess CIH use among minorities found no difference in CIH use among ethnic groups (8). Women consistently use CIH more than men, as they do all medical care. Medical specialists also use CIH often; the percentage of use varies across specialties but an average of 45% of physicians use some type of CIH regularly.
- COVID has increased pain and mental health issues among the population. While no overall survey of CIH use during COVID has been done, a Harris Poll found an increase in supplement use during the pandemic — up to 76% for the general population (9).

DO ATHLETES AND SPORTS MEDICINE PROVIDERS USE COMPLEMENTARY AND INTEGRATIVE HEALTH?

- No comprehensive study of CIH use among athletes is available (10). One study at a single Division I National Collegiate Athletic Association (NCAA) institution found that 56% of athletes (67% of women, 49% of men) used CIH. Eighty percent of these athletes used CIH in addition to traditional Western medicine (11). Common sense and common experience suggest that CIH use should be regarded as the rule, not the exception, in athletes.
- According to the 2002 National Health Interview Survey (NHIS), CIH use is more prevalent in adults who engage in physical activity during leisure time (4).

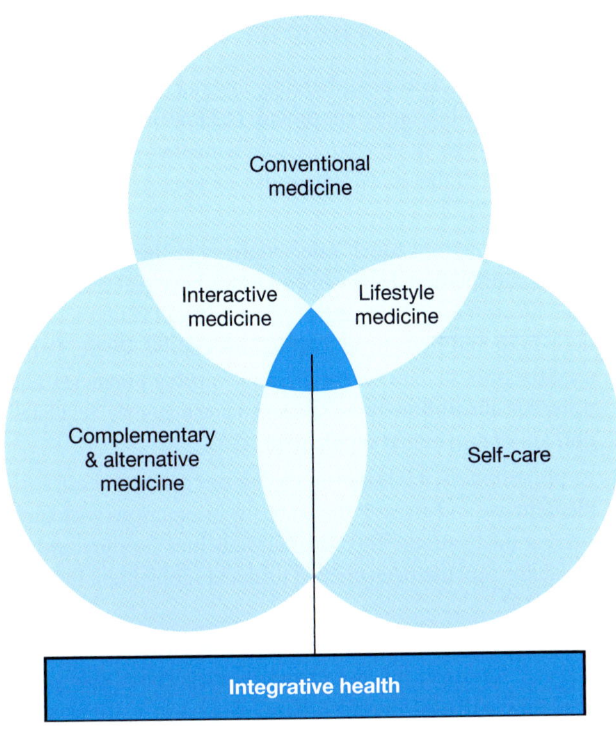

Figure 86.1: Integrative health model. (Reprinted from: https://jamaicahospital.org/newsletter/integrative-care-therapies-that-may-benefit-your-health/.)

- Athletes may use CIH therapies to enhance performance, decrease recovery time after workouts, or speed return to play following an injury.
- According to a survey completed by 257 physicians from members of the American Medical Society for Sports Medicine (AMSSM), about 88% of physicians who responded recommended at least one CIH therapy in the last year. The most common modality recommended was osteopathic manipulation/chiropractic followed by acupuncture and yoga (12).
- The high pressure and high stakes of athletic competition, together with the exceptionally small margin that separates success from failure, demand that sports medicine physicians exercise great vigilance in protecting the athletes entrusted to their care.

WHERE CAN I FIND GOOD EVIDENCE ON COMPLEMENTARY AND INTEGRATIVE HEALTH THERAPIES?

- The best type of evidence to use in evaluating a CIH therapy depends on:
  - Risks posed by the therapy
  - Cost of the therapy
  - Information preference of the individual patient
  - Availability of other proven, effective, and safe therapies for the patient's condition
- Randomized controlled trials (RCTs) are important for evaluating high-risk and/or high-cost therapies because RCTs provide essential safety and risk-benefit data. However, RCTs have some important limitations. RCTs are difficult and expensive to sustain for long periods of study. Additionally, the results of an RCT depend greatly on the careful selection of the all-important "control" group (13).
- Clinical outcomes research is another, less recognized type of research trial that is useful in studying CIH therapies. Outcomes research is more like clinical practice than RCTs: It involves a wider range of patients over longer periods of time and allows for variations in care caused by interactions with multiple providers. Outcomes research examines the probability that a therapy will produce a beneficial effect and provides an estimate of how large that effect will be in everyday clinical practice. For long-term, chronic conditions and their therapies, outcomes research often provides the only relevant evidence (14).
- Table 86.1 lists several sources for obtaining quality evidence on specific CIH therapies and practices.
- The patient's individual beliefs and personality can affect the likelihood of therapeutic efficacy. If a patient believes that a specific therapy will alleviate their condition, this "prior plausibility" has its own therapeutic effect.
- If conventional medicine offers a safe, proven therapy that is acceptable to the patient, any potential CIH therapy must pass equally stringent evidence standards for efficacy and safety before being considered as a viable treatment option.

HOW DO I ADVISE MY PATIENTS ABOUT COMPLEMENTARY AND INTEGRATIVE HEALTH THERAPIES?

- Effective patient-doctor communication about CIH is crucial for appropriate treatment of complex medical conditions. There has been a study showing that 19.9% of the 1067 patients surveyed do not inform their physicians of their CIH therapy use (15). This CIH communication gap results in a wasteful, and potentially dangerous, patient-physician environment.
- Patients who use CIH practices possess character traits that incline them to active participation and partnering in their medical care (5). A physician who refuses to discuss and denies any knowledge of CIH treatments does not alter the patient's need for partnering but merely forces them to seek association elsewhere — thus widening the already precipitous CIH communication gap.
- Many effective strategies can be used to partner with patients on CIH therapies. However, we recommend the strategy proposed by Jonas (16). He suggests using the "Five P" approach — protect, permit, promote, price, and partner with patients. The decision to use CIH in any situation depends on the specific patient and the specific treatment. Physicians should: (1)

Table 86.1 Internet Resources — Reliable Complementary and Integrative Health (CIH) Evidence for Physicians

The Cochrane Library

The library contains a database of systematic reviews featuring randomized controlled trials of CIH and conventional therapies, as well as a controlled trials register that provides bibliographic listings of controlled trials and conference proceedings.

Abstracts of the reviews and trials are available free of charge at http://www.cochrane.org

Full text copies of all materials are available through several subscription services including http://gateway.ovid.com

PubMed

The most comprehensive and popular medical search engine has a new "clinical queries" filter to assist in limiting your search results to CIH. The most comprehensive search is obtained by using the keywords "complementary medicine."

Free access at multiple Web sites including http://www.pubmed.org

National Center for Complementary and Integrative Health (NCCIH) https://www.nccih.nih.gov/

The clinical trials section contains an index of trials by treatment or condition. The index can also be accessed via www.clinicaltrials.govor through PubMed.

National Library of Medicine

Powerful search engine allows searches across all government guidelines, plus PubMed. "Synonym and related terms" search option is very helpful for CIH therapies with multiple common names.

The search engine may be accessed free of charge at https://hstat.nlm.nih.gov

Individual guidelines from many government agencies can be found at http://www.guideline.govor http://www.cdc.gov/publications

Natural Medicines Comprehensive Database

The online database contains comprehensive listings and cross-listings of natural and herbal therapies, including very helpful sections on "all known uses" and "herb-drug interactions." The database also offers an extensive review of the available pharmacologic evidence.

From the publishers of The Prescriber's Letter, the database can be accessed via a purchased subscription at http://www.naturaldatabase.com

Office of Dietary Supplements

This NIH-based website addresses the scientific exploration of dietary supplements and was created to strengthen knowledge and understanding of dietary supplements. It includes a dietary supplement fact sheet database to present information about dietary supplements and their ingredients. These fact sheets can be found at https://ods.od.nih.gov/factsheets/list-all/

prevent the use of therapies that may cause patient harm, (2) permit those that are safe and noncostly if they will engage and empower the patient, (3) promote therapies that have been proven to help, (4) protect the patient from injury and increased prices, and (5) partner with the patient to incorporate CIH therapies in their life using shared decision-making.

Protecting patients from harm and prices

- Many CIH practices are inherently low risk when performed or prescribed by competent providers. However, herbal remedies and high-dose vitamin supplementation (both very popular CIH therapies) can cause serious or fatal consequences (17).
- "Natural" does not equal "safe," contrary to the popular conceived connotation. Herbs and vitamins have real effects, real side effects, and real toxicities. Even without direct toxicity, herb-herb and herb-drug interactions can be severe. Other quality issues such as contamination, varying potencies, and differing absorption rates abound in the poorly regulated domain of nutritional supplements (18).
- As practitioners, it is important to ask our patients about supplement use and assess if there are any interactions with their current medications. The Natural Medicines Comprehensive Database Tool has been created to assess supplement interactions (19).
- Biofeedback, meditation, prayer, and acupuncture pose minimal risk for direct toxicity. However, even these "safe" practices may indirectly result in harm if used in place of more effective treatments. The physician should detail the risks and benefits (both direct and indirect) of all therapeutic options.
- People spend money out of pocket for therapies and there is evidence showing that people will buy supplements instead of food. Price is becoming more important as disparity issues in the country have gotten worse.

Permitting unproven, nontoxic therapies

- Physicians may experience trepidation in allowing patients to engage in unproven practices or therapies. However, if the therapy has no toxicity and is not used in place of a proven effective treatment, the practice can be safely permitted and may be encouraged.
- The physician's ultimate goal should be to relieve patient suffering. Patients welcome relief — and physicians should do likewise — even should relief come through nonquantifiable means (spiritual effect, placebo effect, belief, prior plausibility) (20).
- Homeopathic arnica, acupuncture, spinal manipulation, turmeric and many other CIH therapies can be safely permitted when properly administered and appropriately prescribed.

Promoting Proven Treatments

- Physicians should promote safe, effective treatments regardless of their medical system of origin if they have been proven in good RCTs. Western biomedicine has adopted and should continue to incorporate proven techniques and therapies from other systems of medical care (14).
- Acupuncture is a prime example of a CIH therapy that should be promoted for individuals with knee OA. Massage for the back is another example of a proven CIH therapy to be promoted.

Partnering with the Patient

- Physicians must partner with their patients to provide motivation and guidance on how to incorporate CIH into their lifestyle. There are clinical tools such as the HOPE Note Toolkit that may be used to integrate CIH into the patient's routine practice (16). Shared decision-making to help them be involved in their treatment decisions is an important part of good medical care, including with CIH.

WHAT'S THE CURRENT EVIDENCE FOR OR AGAINST SOME POPULAR COMPLEMENTARY AND INTEGRATIVE HEALTH TREATMENTS?

- Summaries of the evidence for and against a few of the most popular CIH treatments used by athletes and the general population appear in the following sections. They are organized into the sections Prevent, Promote, and Protect.

Prevent Use of the Following

Herbs and Supplements

- Ephedra (Ma Huang, herbal ecstasy, Zhong Mahuang) (21–24)
  - Primary use: Weight loss or enhanced athletic performance and endurance. Less commonly used for respiratory conditions or asthma.
  - Evidence: Ephedra can potentiate a small weight loss of 2–5 kg over 6 weeks to 6 months, but only in patients with body mass index over 30. The weight loss is typically transient and often requires combination with other stimulants (*i.e.*, caffeine or guarana). Multiple studies show no performance-enhancing effect unless combined with caffeine/guarana or used in very high dosages.
  - Toxicity: High dosages and combination with caffeine are known to increase toxicity. High dosages can cause dizziness, restlessness, anxiety, palpitations, hypertension, myocardial infarction, seizure, stroke, and psychosis, among other conditions (24–29). Fatal events have been reported. Newer evidence suggests that toxicity can occur with short-term use in low doses as well (25,26). Capsules have been found to contain many impurities, including banned substances.
  - Regulated/banned: Banned by the Food and Drug Administration (FDA) and the International Olympic Committee (IOC) (30).
  - Conclusion: Ephedra products, especially ephedra/guarana combinations, are banned substances, are not safe, and have been demonstrated to cause considerable harm. As negative publicity builds, "ephedra-free" versions of products appear, but there is no evidence that these will be any safer than the original formulations.
- Chromium picolinate (31–33)
  - Primary use: Increase lean body mass, improve glycemic control in diabetes, enhance athletic performance, and increase energy.
  - Evidence: While earlier, design-flawed studies suggested some beneficial effects, newer studies show no ergogenic or fat-burning effects. Some studies suggest slight, dose-dependent improvements in diabetes control and lipid profiles.
  - Toxicity: Tremor and cognitive, sleep, and mood changes have been reported as side effects. Concern exists for potential DNA mutations with long-term exposure to chromium supplementation.
  - Regulated/banned: No.
  - Conclusion: Although inexpensive and minimally toxic with short-term use, real concern exists for DNA mutations with long-term use or high chromium levels. Since the reported benefits are very small and the risk of long-term toxicity is potentially great, patients should avoid this supplement.
- St. John's wort (SJW) (34–37)
  - Primary use: Antidepressant, anxiolytic, anti-insomnia, and adjunct to weight-loss uses are commonly described.
  - Evidence: Most evidence suggests SJW to be effective for mild to moderate depression. SJW may also be effective in obsessive-compulsive disorders. Severe depression is not reliably treated by SJW, and higher dosages of SJW increase the risk for severe skin reactions.
  - Toxicity: Insomnia, restlessness, and GI distress are common. Hypericin doses over 5 $mg \cdot d^{-1}$ increase the risk for photodermatitis. SJW has fewer side effects than tricyclic antidepressants or selective serotonin reuptake inhibitor antidepressants; however, the potential for severe herb-herb and drug-herb interactions — including serotonin syndrome — is greater with SJW. SJW can accelerate the metabolism of drugs cleared by the P450 enzyme system and should not be used by those on immunosuppressants or antiviral medications without monitoring.
  - Regulated/banned: Not banned by athletic regulatory agencies. However, due to the risk of serious drug interactions, the distribution of SJW was banned in France. The governments of Japan, the United Kingdom, and other European countries are considering similar bans.
  - Conclusion: Due to interactions with commonly used medications, SJW should be prevented to keep the athletes safe from drug-drug interactions.

Other CIH Therapies

- Cranial Electrotherapy Stimulation (CES)
  - Primary Use: Treat chronic pain, depression, anxiety, and insomnia.
  - Evidence: CES is a form of brain stimulation that uses low levels of alternating current delivered via electrodes placed on the earlobes, occipital area, mastoid processes,

or temples. A survey of more than 1000 military personnel who received CES (limited by a less than 20% response to the survey) did report improvement (>25% effectiveness) in depression, anxiety, post traumatic stress disorder, insomnia, or pain in the majority of patients (38).

- Toxicity: No serious side effects have been documented.
- Regulated/banned: No, FDA Class II medical device.
- Conclusion: There are limited studies to show the effectiveness of CES, although in military patients it has been shown to be effective.

Permit Use in This Category

Herbs and Supplements

- Glucosamine sulfate (39–45)
  - Primary use: Relief of stiffness and pain in OA and temporomandibular joint dysfunction (TMJ).
  - Evidence: Despite a high-quality meta-analysis showing no benefit in glucosamine supplementation, multiple trials have demonstrated superior efficacy of glucosamine sulfate to placebo. So why is this issue still not settled? The issue centers around the quality of clinical trials performed to date. While the large NIH-sponsored Glucosamine/chondroitin Arthritis Intervention Trial (GAIT) trial showed no efficacy for glucosamine overall, this trial was hampered by a 60% placebo response rate, far above that seen in clinical practice. Further review of the GAIT trial shows an over-enrollment of patients with very mild OA symptoms and an under-enrollment of patients with more clinically relevant moderate to severe OA symptoms. The subgroup analysis of patients with moderate-severe symptoms showed the glucosamine/chondroitin combination to be significantly more effective than placebo and more effective than celecoxib in relieving OA pain (46). Other studies are hampered by industry sponsorship. The results of the meta-analyses vary greatly depending on which studies they include and how heavily each study result is weighed. Insufficient data exists to determine if glucosamine slows the rate of OA progression. Knee OA is the most widely studied, but efficacy data also exists for glucosamine in TMJ and OA of the hand and spine.
  - Toxicity: Mild GI distress (comparable to placebo levels) has been reported. Concerns for exacerbations of diabetic control or reactions in patients with shellfish allergy appear to be unfounded. Despite disagreement regarding efficacy, all published data show that glucosamine sulfate supplementation is extremely safe for all adults. No data exist regarding use in pregnant women and children. Patients on renal dialysis should not use glucosamine sulfate since metabolites are cleared via the kidney.
  - Regulated/banned: No.
  - Conclusion: Glucosamine may provide effective relief of OA symptoms for some patients with at least moderate symptoms. A 6- to 8-week trial of glucosamine supplementation should be permitted as safe and possibly effective for OA pain, especially in the senior athlete population where comorbidities may limit other treatment options. Glucosamine supplementation should be discontinued if no clinical response occurs after a 6- to 8-week trial due to its moderate cost.
- Chondroitin (45,47–49)
  - Primary use: Improving pain and stiffness from OA.
  - Evidence: Several trials suggest (size and design limiting) that chondroitin and ibuprofen are more effective than ibuprofen alone for improving OA symptoms. Additionally, the drugs have different times to onset of action. Ibuprofen reaches maximum efficacy in a matter of days; chondroitin is maximally effective over a few weeks. Chondroitin is typically sold in varying combinations with glucosamine, manganese, and magnesium. Some data suggest the combination of glucosamine and chondroitin treatment to be more effective than the single agent alone.
  - Toxicity: Mild GI distress is the most common side effect. Combination tablets can exceed safe daily doses of manganese and cause central nervous system irritability. Chondroitin has a heparinoid structure and may predispose to bleeding if used with other anticoagulants.
  - Regulated/banned: No.
  - Conclusion: Although less convincing than glucosamine, some evidence supports chondroitin use in OA. Several studies with 5+ years of follow-up report no adverse events related to chondroitin use. Given the moderately high cost of chondroitin tablets, a 6- to 8-week trial period is advisable. If no clinical effect is noted during this trial, chondroitin should be discontinued due to cost considerations.
- Panax Ginseng (50–53)
  - Primary use: Improve physical stamina, concentration, and memory; stimulate immune function; slow the aging process; and relieve various other health problems, such as respiratory and cardiovascular disorders, depression, anxiety, and menopausal hot flashes. Topical use (applied to the skin) of Asian ginseng as part of a multi-ingredient preparation is promoted for premature ejaculation. Improve cognitive function and athletic performance and increase energy.
  - Evidence: Many studies document that ginseng supplementation has no ergogenic effects. Similarly, Panax ginseng has not been shown to improve memory when used alone but has been demonstrated to have efficacy when combined with ginkgo supplementation in middle-aged individuals.
  - Toxicity: Insomnia, tachycardia, and palpitations become more common with high doses. Mastalgia, vaginal bleeding, and amenorrhea are likely related to the estrogenic effects of ginseng. Long-term use is not well studied.

Ginseng will intensify the effects of other common stimulants (caffeine, guarana, and tea).

- Regulated/banned: No.
- Conclusion: Studies suggest minimal toxicity with short-term use, but long-term use is more difficult to justify since estrogenic risks may outweigh the unclear benefits. However, further studies continue to explore other possible indications for ginseng supplementation.

- Homeopathy (Arnica) (54–58)
  - Primary use: Relief of delayed-onset muscle soreness (DOMS) and low back pain.
  - Evidence: Homeopathic arnica is more properly viewed as an alternative medical system with many distinct, pharmacologic interventions. No single homeopathic treatment has been conclusively proven to be effective in reducing DOMS. Small trials of diverse remedies offer contradictory conclusions for homeopathy in DOMS. Poor design, differing methodologies, and differing definitions of DOMS predictably plague these trials.
  - Toxicity: No side effects above placebo levels have been reported. Reports of severe allergic reactions appear to be rare. Extreme dilution of homeopathic remedies makes direct toxicity highly unlikely.
  - Regulated/banned: No. A few states credential homeopathic physicians.
  - Conclusion: The homeopathic system of medicine is complex and has not yet been adequately evaluated. However, its costs and toxicities are low in the hands of trained professionals. Current research does not support its use for DOMS, although there has been a limited study that demonstrates the possibility of providing pain relief 3 days posteccentric exercise.
- Branch chain amino acids (BCAAs) *i.e.*, leucine, isoleucine, and valine (59)
  - Primary use: Provide energy during exercise.
  - Evidence: Studies have not consistently shown that taking supplements of BCAAs or any of their three constituent amino acids singly enhances exercise and athletic performance, builds muscle mass, or aids in recovery from exercise. Consuming animal foods containing complete proteins — or a combination of plant-based foods with complementary proteins that together provide all essential amino acids — automatically increases the consumption of BCAAs. This is also true of consuming protein powders made from complete proteins, especially whey, which has more leucine than either casein or soy.
  - Toxicity: Up to 20 $g \cdot d^{-1}$ BCAA supplements in divided doses appear to be safe. For leucine alone, studies suggest an upper safe limit of intake of 500 $mg \cdot kg^{-1} \cdot d^{-1}$ in healthy young and elderly men, or about 38 $g \cdot d^{-1}$ for a man weighing 75 kg (165 lb).
  - Regulated/banned: No.
  - Conclusion: BCAAs can be metabolized by mitochondria in skeletal muscle to provide energy during exercise. The BCAAs, especially leucine, might also stimulate protein synthesis in exercised muscle. However, intake of these with foods rather than supplements provides evidence of incorporating the essential amino acids needed.
- Turmeric (60)
  - Primary use: Aids in the management of oxidative and inflammatory conditions, metabolic syndrome, arthritis, anxiety, and hyperlipidemia. It may also help in the management of exercise-induced inflammation and muscle soreness, thus enhancing recovery and performance in active people.
  - Evidence: Its antioxidant and anti-inflammatory mechanisms are best achieved when curcumin is combined with agents such as piperine, which increase its bioavailability significantly. Turmeric and curcumin (the active ingredient in tumeric) are challenging to study because curcumin is unstable (it easily changes into other substances) and has low bioavailability (not much reaches bloodstream) when it's taken orally.
  - Toxicity: Side effects include diarrhea, headache, rash, and yellow stool.
  - Regulated/banned: No.
  - Conclusion: Research suggests that curcumin can help in the management of oxidative and inflammatory conditions, metabolic syndrome, arthritis, anxiety, and hyperlipidemia. It may also help in the management of exercise-induced inflammation and muscle soreness, thus enhancing recovery and subsequent performance in active people. Because the actions of turmeric and its components in people are complex and not well understood, no clear conclusions have been reached about whether these substances have benefits for health conditions.

Other CIH Therapies

- Pulsed electromagnetic field (PEMF) therapy (61–64)
  - Primary use: Decrease pain and stiffness in OA, chronic pain, depression, anxiety, and insomnia.
  - Evidence: The beneficial effect of PEMF therapy in delayed union fractures is well established. Similar magnetic fields have been found to stimulate proteoglycan production in vitro in chondrocytes. Pulsed electromagnetic field (PEMF) therapy is an emerging modality for the treatment of musculoskeletal disorders with a wide range of indications for use and has been approved by the American Food and Drug Administration (FDA). The optimum dosage and frequency of PEMF — as well as acceptable technical standards for the PEMF equipment — remain unknown. The cost of PEMF can exceed $200 per day.
  - Toxicity: Unknown. The effects of pulsed electromagnetic fields on human tissues have not been well studied.
  - Regulated/banned: No.
  - Conclusion: Patients should be advised that PEMF does provide short-term benefits to relieve pain and improve function in patients with OA.

- Transcutaneous electrical nerve stimulation (TENS) (65)
  - Primary use: Relief of low-back pain.
  - Evidence: While RCTs are lacking, a Cochrane review found that TENS is effective at providing pain relief and improving range of motion in patients suffering from chronic low back pain.
  - Toxicity: There is no known toxicity associated with TENS. Patients can experience mild discomfort and involuntary muscle contraction due to the electrical stimulation of the nerves.
  - Regulated/banned: No.
  - Conclusion: Early, poor-quality data indicate this treatment modality is effective with minimal side effects. The cost of TENS devices may be prohibitive, and more studies with improved academic rigor are needed.
- Massage (66–68)
  - Primary use: Relief of low back pain and relief of DOMS.
  - Evidence: A Cochrane review found that when massage is combined with exercises and education, it might be beneficial for the relief of subacute and chronic lower back pain. This review found that acupuncture massage is more effective than traditional massage, but more studies are needed. Another study found two types of massage (deep tissue and relaxation) to be more effective than conventional therapy for low back pain. A review of 17 case series found no consistent evidence that massage improved exercise performance but did find a trend supporting massage as effective in relieving DOMS.
  - Toxicity: None.
  - Regulated/banned: No.
  - Conclusion: While further studies are needed, massage is a low-cost treatment modality with negligible side effects that can be used along with traditional pain relief and rehabilitation modalities for the relief of subacute and chronic low back pain. Current evidence does not support massage to relieve specific sports-related injury or pain.
- The role of expectation in physical performance
  - Primary use: Placebo used in concert with patients' expectations on whether they expect to perform well or not.
  - Evidence: In a review, Pollo et al. (69) provide examples where physiologic or pathologic conditions are altered following the administration of an inert substance with verbal instructions that induce expectations of a change. Placebo effects can extend beyond the clinical setting, in the domain of physical performance, and have implications for sports competitions.
  - Toxicity: Placebo (from negative expectations) may produce adverse effects, and deception is ethically problematic.
  - Regulated/banned: No, but ethical issues can be associated with deception.
  - Conclusion: Despite very different experimental conditions and across many different outcomes measured, data strongly indicate context factors and athletes' expectations as important factors in physical performance to be taken into account in training strategies and exercises.
- Spinal manipulation (46,70–73)
  - Primary use: Relief of low back pain/stiffness, relief of DOMS, and speeding return to play following a low back injury.
  - Evidence: Majority of evidence suggests spinal manipulation to be at least as effective as but not superior to conventional treatment for acute or chronic low back pain. Nine of 10 well-designed RCTs in a review concluded that spinal manipulation provided more pain relief than control treatments. However, differences among manipulation techniques make conclusions difficult to generalize. Additionally, several Cochrane reviews have found that there is no clinically relevant difference in pain reduction between spinal manipulation and other standard therapies. Manipulation may require more physician visits than conventional care, increasing the cost of therapy. Health insurers may reimburse some of this cost.
  - Toxicity: Rare case reports of stroke, paralysis, or spinal cord damage are mostly related to cervical spine manipulation and occur at a frequency of one per million of manipulations. No severe complications have been reported from over 15,000 patients enrolled in monitored RCTs.
  - Regulated/banned: No.
  - Conclusion: Competently performed lumbar spine manipulation is safe and likely effective for low back pain, although it may be at a higher cost than other therapies and may not provide any greater benefit than these lower cost therapies.
- Figure 86.2 is an evidence-based recommendations map that displays a comprehensive view of the Standard Mean Differences (SMD) of each ingredient (x-axis) compared with placebo for pain reduction according to the number of patients pooled across studies at a time point closest to 3 months (y-axis) and the confidence in that effect (higher confidence associated with larger bubble sizes); the resulting evidence-based recommendations are indicated in white (conditional recommendations in favor), light gray (no recommendation), and dark gray (recommendations against current use).

Promote Use from This Category

Herbs and Supplements

- Collagen Hydrosylate (74)
  - Primary Use: To provide an anabolic effect on cartilage tissue.
  - Evidence: A clinical trial of 24 weeks' duration to show improvement of joint pain in athletes who were treated with the dietary supplement collagen hydrolysate. The results of this study have implications for the use of collagen hydrolysate to support joint health and possibly reduce the risk of joint deterioration in a high-risk group.

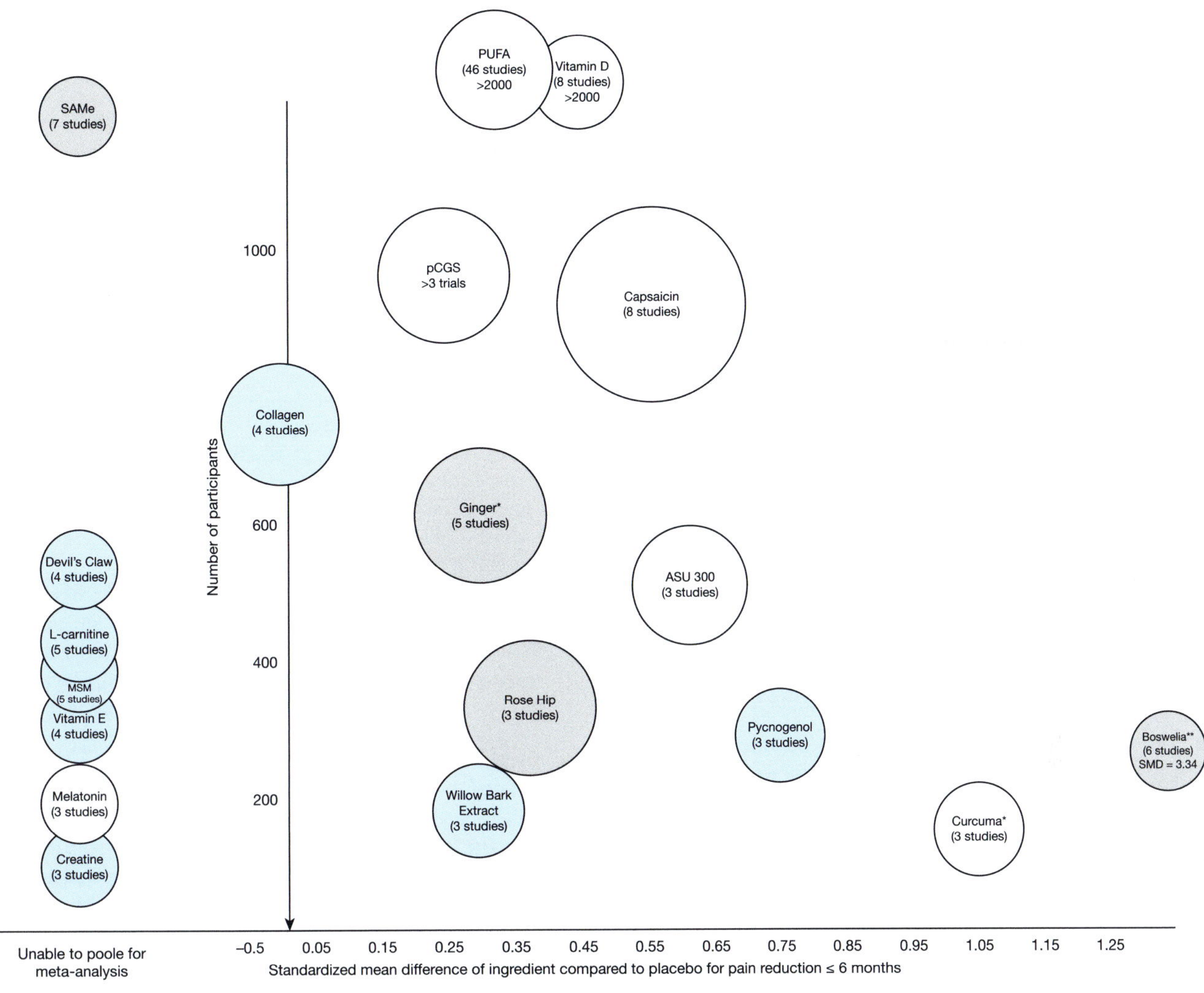

Figure 86.2: CAM evidence-based recommendation map. This is an evidence-based recommendations map that displays a comprehensive view of the Standard Mean Differences (SMD) of each ingredient (x-axis) compared with placebo for pain reduction according to the number of patients pooled across studies at a time point closest to 3 months (y-axis) and the confidence in that effect (higher confidence associated with larger bubble sizes); the resulting evidence-based recommendations are indicated in white (conditional recommendations in favor), light gray (no recommendation), and dark gray (recommendations against current use). *Conditional recommendation for use as a food source, not as a dietary supplement at this time. **Conditional recommendation for additional research, not use as a dietary supplement at this time. ASU, avocado soybean unsaponifiables; MSM, methylsulfonylmethane; pCGS, patented crystalline glucosamine sulfate; PUFA, polyunsaturated fatty acids; SAMe, s-adenoysl-l-methionine (39). (Reprinted from Figure 2 of Crawford C, Boyd C, Paat CF, et al. Dietary ingredients as an alternative approach for mitigating chronic musculoskeletal pain: evidence-based recommendations for practice and research in the military. *Pain Med.* 2019;20(6):1236–47.)

- Toxicity: None.
- Regulated/Banned: No.
- Conclusion: Athletes consuming collagen hydrolysate can reduce parameters (such as pain) that have a negative impact on athletic performance. It also may be beneficial in patients with osteoarthritis.

Other CIH Therapies

- Acupuncture (75–80)
  - Primary use: Relief of acute and chronic low back pain, chronic neck pain, OA, and lateral elbow pain.
  - Evidence: Acupuncture may be considered as a separate medical system or an adjunct to other therapies. There are conflicting data regarding the effectiveness of acupuncture for acute low back pain. However, for the treatment of chronic low back pain, acupuncture has been found to be more effective than no treatment or sham treatments for short-term pain relief and functional improvement. It should be noted that acupuncture has not been found to be more effective than other complementary or alternative treatments for chronic low back pain. There is moderate evidence now showing that acupuncture is effective for immediate pain relief of chronic neck pain, and this relief persists at short-term follow-up. For lateral elbow pain, a recent Cochrane review found insufficient evidence to make any recommendations. RCTs

of acupuncture for low back pain are contradictory and poorly designed. Acupuncture has been proven effective in reducing postoperative pain and relief of nausea.

- Toxicity: Broken needles, pneumothorax, and infectious disease transmission are anecdotally reported, but unlikely in the hands of licensed professionals. Pain, fatigue, bleeding, and fainting are the most common side effects.
- Regulated/banned: No. Over 30 states license acupuncturists. The FDA has approved acupuncture needles as experimental devices.
- Conclusion: There is a growing body of clinical experience and RCT evidence indicating that acupuncture is effective for pain relief. Also, acupuncture is low cost and does not carry with it the side effects or risks of sedation, renal toxicity, GI bleeding, or addiction common to many conventional pain treatments. For these reasons, acupuncture — under the care of a trained professional — can be recommended to patients for pain relief so long as acupuncture is not thought to be a cure for a musculoskeletal injury that needs rehabilitation or surgery. It is most advisable that patients use acupuncture as an adjunct to proven treatments for pain relief.

- The Veteran Health Administration has included the following approaches which have been shown to have evidence of promising or potential benefits: (81)
  - Acupuncture
  - Biofeedback
  - Clinical hypnosis
  - Guided imagery
  - Meditation
  - Tai Chi and Qi Gong
  - Therapeutic massage
  - Yoga

SUMMARY

- Integrative health is a combination of conventional, complementary, and self-care modalities utilized by physicians and patients.
- Physicians should have open discussions about complementary modalities used by patients and provide education regarding modalities that may be safe versus those that have harmful effects.
- Sports medicine physicians have the additional burden of identifying complementary and integrated medicine toxicities and side effects that may cause athletes to run afoul of antidoping regulations or safe sport participation standards.
- Shared decision-making is the most important tool when discussing CIH modalities with athletes and other patients.

REFERENCES

1. Marty AT. Fundamentals of complementary and alternative medicine. *Chest.* 1997;112(6):16.
2. James J. Patient engagement: health affairs Brief. *Health Aff.* 2013 Feb 14. doi:10.1377/hpb20130214.898775
3. National Institute of health. Americans spent $30.2 billion out-of-Pocket on complementary health approaches. In: *National Center for Complementary and Integrative Health.* U.S. Department of Health and Human Services; 2016. Available from: https://www.nccih.nih.gov/news/press-releases/americans-spent-302-billion-outofpocket-on-complementary-health-approaches
4. Barnes PM, Bloom B, Nahin RL. Complementary and alternative medicine use among adults and children: United States, 2007. In: *National Health Statistics Report, No. 12.* Hyattsville (MD): National Center for Health Statistics; 2008. p. 1–23.
5. Eisenberg DM, Davis RB, Ettner SL, et al. Trends in alternative medicine use in the United States, 1990-1997: results of a follow-up national survey. *JAMA.* 1998;280(18):1569–75.
6. Astin JA. Why patients use alternative medicine: results of a national study. *JAMA.* 1998;279(19):1548–53.
7. Beutler AI, Jonas WB. Complementary and alternative medicine for the sports medicine physician. In: Birrer RB, O'Connor FG, editors. *Sports Medicine for the Primary Care Physician.* 3rd ed. Boca Raton (FL): CRC Press; in press.
8. Mackenzie ER, Taylor L, Bloom BS, Hufford DJ, Johnson JC. Ethnic minority use of complementary and alternative medicine (CAM): a national probability survey of CAM utilizers. *Altern Ther Health Med.* 2003;9(4):50–6.
9. Jonas W. *The State of Supplements* – Dr. *Wayne Jonas.* Healing Works Foundation. Available from: https://healingworksfoundation.org/wp-content/uploads/2021/07/Samueli-2021-Supplement-Survey-Report_FNL.pdf,
10. White J. Alternative sports medicine. *Phys Sportsmed.* 1998;26(6):92–105.
11. Nichols AW, Harrigan R. Complementary and alternative medicine usage by intercollegiate athletes. *Clin J Sport Med.* 2006;16(3):232–7.
12. Kent JB, Tanabe KO, Muthusubramanian A, Statuta SM, MacKnight JM. Complementary and alternative medicine prescribing practices among sports medicine providers. *Altern Ther Health Med.* 2020 Sep;26(5):28–32.
13. Jonas WB, Levine JS. How to practice evidence-based complementary medicine. In: Jonas W, Levin J, editors. *Essentials of Complementary and Alternative Medicine.* Philadelphia (PA): Lippincott Williams & Wilkins; 1999. p. 72–87.
14. Walach H, Jonas WB, Lewith G. The role of outcomes research in evaluating complementary and alternative medicine. In: Lewith G, Jonas W, Walach H, editors. *Clinical Research in Complementary Therapies.* London (UK): Churchill Livingston; 2002. p. 29–45.
15. Connor J, Buring JE, Eisenberg DM, Osypiuk K, Davis RB, Wayne PM. Patient disclosure of complementary and integrative health approaches in an academic health center. In: *Global Advances in Health and Medicine.* Thousand Oaks, CA: SAGE Publications; 2020. https://www.ncbi.nlm.nih.gov/pmc/articles/PMC7079303/
16. Jonas WB. Hope note. Dr. *Wayne Jonas.* 27 Sept. 2022. https://healingworksfoundation.org/resources/hope-note/
17. Jonas WB. Alternative medicine — Learning from the past, examining the present, advancing to the future. *JAMA.* 1998;280(18):1616–8.
18. De Smet PA. Herbal remedies. *N Engl J Med.* 2002;347(25):2046–56.
19. Natural Medicines Comprehensive Database Tool. *TRC Healthcare;* 2022. https://natmed-advisor.therapeuticresearch.com/QuickCheck?inputState=interactions.

20. Moerman DE, Jonas WB. Deconstructing the placebo effect and finding the meaning response. *Ann Intern Med.* 2002;136(6):471–6.
21. Bell DG, Jacobs I, McLellan TM, Zamecnik J. Reducing the dose of combined caffeine and ephedrine preserves the ergogenic effect. *Aviat Space Environ Med.* 2000;71(4):415–9.
22. Congeni J, Miller S. Supplements and drugs used to enhance athletic performance. *Pediatr Clin North Am.* 2002;49(2):435–61.
23. Gillies H, Derman WE, Noakes TD, Smith P, Evans A, Gabriels G. Pseudoephedrine is without ergogenic effects during prolonged exercise. *J Appl Physiol.* 1996;81(6):2611–7.
24. Haller CA, Benowitz NL. Adverse cardiovascular and central nervous system events associated with dietary supplements containing ephedra alkaloids. *N Engl J Med.* 2000;343(25):1833–8.
25. Doyle H, Kargin M. Herbal stimulant containing ephedrine has also caused psychosis. *BMJ.* 1996;313(7059):756.
26. Food and Drug Administration. *Proposed Rule: Dietary Supplements Containing Ephedrine Alkaloids.* [cited 2000 Jan 25]. Available from: www.verity.fda.gov
27. Jacobs KM, Hirsch KA. Psychiatric complications of ma-huang. *Psychosomatics.* 2000;41(1):58–62.
28. Morgenstern LB, Viscoli CM, Kernan WN, et al. Use of ephedra containing products and risk for hemorrhagic stroke. *Neurology.* 2003;60(1):132–5.
29. Walton R, Manos GH. Psychosis related to ephedra-containing herbal supplement use. *South Med J.* 2003;96(7):718–20.
30. Food and Drug Administration HHS. Final rule declaring dietary supplements containing ephedrine alkaloids adulterated because they present an unreasonable ris. *Fed Regist.* 2004;69(28):6787–854.
31. Fox GN, Sabovic Z. Chromium picolinate supplementation for diabetes mellitus. *J Fam Pract.* 1998;46(1):83–6.
32. McLeod MN, Gaynes BN, Golden RN. Chromium potentiation of antidepressant pharmacotherapy for dysthymic disorder in 5 patients. *J Clin Psychiatry.* 1999;60(4):237–40.
33. Speetjens JK, Collins RA, Vincent JB, Woski SA. The nutritional supplement chromium(III) tris(picolinate) cleaves DNA. *Chem Res Toxicol.* 1999;12(6):483–7.
34. Brenner R, Azbel V, Madhusoodanan S, Pawlowska M. Comparison of an extract of hypericum (LI 160) and sertraline in the treatment of depression: a double-blind, randomized pilot study. *Clin Ther.* 2000;22(4):411–9.
35. Gaster B, Holroyd J. St John's wort for depression: a systematic review. *Arch Intern Med.* 2000;160(2):152–6.
36. Schrader E. Equivalence of St. John's wort extract (Ze 117) and fluoxetine: a randomized, controlled study in mild-moderate depression. *Int Clin Psychopharmacol.* 2000;15(2):61–8.
37. Woelk H. Comparison of St John's wort and imipramine for treating depression: randomised controlled trial. *BMJ.* 2000;321(7260):536–9.
38. Jonas WB. Cranial electrical stimulation: what is it, and should We Use it in practice?. *Ann Intern Med.* 2018;168(6):446–7. doi:10.7326/M17-3420
39. Crawford C, Boyd C, Paat CF, et al. Dietary ingredients as an alternative approach for mitigating chronic musculoskeletal pain: evidence-based recommendations for practice and research in the military. *Pain Med.* 2019 Jun 1;20(6):1236–47. doi:10.1093/pm/pnz040
40. Clegg DO, Reda DJ, Harris CL, et al. Glucosamine, chondroitin sulfate, and the two in combination for painful knee osteoarthritis. *N Engl J Med.* 2006;354(8):795–808.
41. Foerster KK, Schmid K, Rovati LC. Efficacy of glucosamine sulfate in osteoarthritis of the lumbar spine: a placebo-controlled, randomized, double-blind study. ACR/ARHP scientific abstracts. Arthritis Rheum. 2000;43:S67–15. https://doi.org/10.1002/art.1780432007
42. McAlindon TE, LaValley MP, Gulin JP, Felson DT. Glucosamine and chondroitin for treatment of osteoarthritis: a systematic quality assessment and meta-analysis. *JAMA.* 2000;283(11):1469–75.
43. Pavelká K, Gatterová J, Olejarová M, Machacek S, Giacovelli G, Rovati LC. Glucosamine sulfate use and delay of progression of knee osteoarthritis: a 3-year, randomized, placebo-controlled, double-blind study. *Arch Intern Med.* 2002;162(18):2113–23.
44. Thie NM, Prasad NG, Major PW. Evaluation of glucosamine sulfate compared to ibuprofen for the treatment of temporomandibular joint osteoarthritis: a randomized double blind controlled 3 month clinical trial. *J Rheumatol.* 2001;28(6):1347–55.
45. Wandel S, Jüni P, Tendal B, et al. Effects of glucosamine, chondroitin, or placebo in patients with osteoarthritis of hip or knee: network meta-analysis. *BMJ.* 2010;341:c4675.
46. Andersson GB, Lucente T, Davis AM, Kappler RE, Lipton JA, Leurgans S. A comparison of osteopathic spinal manipulation with standard care for patients with low back pain. *N Engl J Med.* 1999;341(19):1426–31.
47. Leeb BF, Schweitzer H, Montag K, Smolen JS. A metaanalysis of chondroitin sulfate in the treatment of osteoarthritis. *J Rheumatol.* 2000;27(1):205–11.
48. Leffler CT, Philippi AF, Leffler SG, Mosure JC, Kim PD. Glucosamine, chondroitin, and manganese ascorbate for degenerative joint disease of the knee or low back: a randomized, double-blind, placebo-controlled pilot study. *Mil Med.* 1999;164(2):85–91.
49. Towheed TE, Anastassiades TP. Glucosamine and chondroitin for treating symptoms of osteoarthritis: evidence is widely touted but incomplete. *JAMA.* 2000;283(11):1483–4.
50. Allen JD, McLung J, Nelson AG, Welsch M. Ginseng supplementation does not enhance healthy young adult's peak aerobic exercise performance. *J Am Coll Nutr.* 1998;17(5):462–6.
51. Ellis JM, Reddy P. Effects of Panax ginseng on quality of life. *Ann Pharmacother.* 2002;36(3):375–9.
52. Wesnes KA, Ward T, McGinty A, Petrini O. The memory enhancing effects of a Ginkgo biloba/Panax ginseng combination in healthy middle aged volunteers. *Psychopharmacology.* 2000;152(4):353–61.
53. Yun TK, Choi SY. Non-organ specific cancer prevention of ginseng: a prospective study in Korea. *Int J Epidemiol.* 1998;27(3):359–64.
54. Ernst E, Barnes J. Are homeopathic remedies effective for delayed onset muscle soreness? A systematic review of placebo-controlled trials. *Perfusion.* 1998;11:4–8.
55. Tveiten D, Bruset S, Borchgrevnink CF, Norseth J. Effects of the homeopathic remedy Arnica D 30 on marathon runners: a randomized, double-blind study during the 1995 Oslo Marathon. *Complement Ther Med.* 1998;6:71–4.
56. Vickers AJ, Fisher P, Smith C, Wyllie SE, Lewith GT. Homoeopathy for delayed onset muscle soreness: a randomised double blind placebo controlled trial. *Br J Sports Med.* 1997;31(4):304–7.
57. Vickers AJ, Fisher P, Smith C, Wyllie SE, Rees R. Homeopathic Arnica 30x is ineffective for muscle soreness after long-distance running: a randomized, double-blind, placebo-controlled trial. *Clin J Pain.* 1998;14(3):227–31.
58. Pumpa KL, Fallon KE, Bensoussan A, Papalia S. The effects of topical Arnica on performance, pain and muscle damage after intense eccentric exercise. *Eur J Sport Sci.* 2014;14(3):294–300. doi:10.1080/17461391.2013.829126
59. NIH Office of Dietary Supplements. *Office of Dietary Supplements–Dietary Supplements for Exercise and Athletic Performance.* U.S. Department of Health and Human Services. [cited 2024 April 1]. Available from: https://ods.od.nih.gov/factsheets/ExerciseAndAthleticPerformance-HealthProfessional/#antioxidants
60. Hewlings SJ, Kalman DS. Curcumin: a review of its effects on human health. *Foods.* 2017;6(10):92. https://www.ncbi.nlm.nih.gov/pmc/articles/PMC5664031/

61. Aaron RK, Ciombor DM, Jolly G. Stimulation of experimental endochondral ossification by low-energy pulsing electromagnetic fields. *J Bone Miner Res.* 1989;4(2):227–33.
62. Bassett CA, Pawluk RJ, Pilla AA. Augmentation of bone repair by inductively coupled electromagnetic fields. *Science.* 1974;184(4136):575–7.
63. Hulme J, Robinson V, DeBie R, Wells G, Judd M, Tugwell P. Electromagnetic fields for the treatment of osteoarthritis. *Cochrane Database Syst Rev.* 2002;1:CD003523.
64. Markovic L, Wagner B, Crevenna R. Effects of pulsed electromagnetic field therapy on outcomes associated with osteoarthritis: a systematic review of systematic reviews. *Wien Klin Wochenschr.* 2022 Jun;134(11–12):425–33. doi:10.1007/s00508-022-02020-3
65. Gadsby JG, Flowerdew M. Transcutaneous electrical nerve stimulation and acupuncture-like transcutaneous electrical nerve stimulation for chronic low back pain. *Cochrane Database Syst Rev.* 2007;1:CD000210.
66. Furlan AD, Imamura M, Dryden T, Irvin E. Massage for low-back pain. *Cochrane Database Syst Rev.* 2010;6:CD001929.
67. Cherkin DC, Sherman KJ, Kahn J, et al. Effectiveness of focused structural massage and relaxation massage for chronic low back pain: protocol for a randomized controlled trial. *Trials.* 2009;10:96.
68. Best TM, Hunter R, Wilcox A, Haq F. Effectiveness of sports massage for recovery of skeletal muscle from strenuous exercise. *Clin J Sport Med.* 2008;18(5):446–60.
69. Pollo A, Carlino E, Benedetti F. Placebo mechanisms across different conditions: from the clinical setting to physical performance. *Philos Trans R Soc Lond B Biol Sci.* 2011;366(1572):1790–8.
70. Assendelft WJ, Morton SC, Yu EI, Suttorp MJ, Shekelle PG. Spinal manipulative therapy for low back pain. *Cochrane Database Syst Rev.* 2009;1:CD000447.
71. Koes BW, Assendelft WJ, van der Heijden GJ, Bouter LM. Spinal manipulation for low back pain. An updated systematic review of randomized clinical trials. *Spine.* 1996;21(24):2860–73.
72. Rubinstein SM, van Middelkoop M, Assendelft WJ, de Boer MR, van Tulder MW. Spinal manipulative therapy for chronic low-back pain: an update of a Cochrane review. *Spine.* 2011;36(13):E825–46.
73. Walker BF, French SD, Grant W, Green S. Combined chiropractic interventions for low-back pain. *Cochrane Database Syst Rev.* 2011;2:CD005427.
74. Clark KL, Sebastianelli W, Flechsenhar KR, et al. 24-week study on the use of collagen hydrolysate as a dietary supplement in athletes with activity-related joint pain. *Curr Med Res Opin.* 2008;24(5):1485–96. https://pubmed.ncbi.nlm.nih.gov/18416885/.
75. Hazzard ME. Acupuncture. (1997, November 3–5). NIH Consensus Statement, 15 (5), 1–34. Available: consensus. nih. gov. *Altern Health Pract.* 1999;5(2):177–8; [cited 1997 Dec 30].
76. Furlan AD, Van Tulder MW, Cherkin D, et al. Acupuncture and dry-needling for low back pain. *Cochrane Database Syst Rev.* 2005;20:CD001351.
77. Garvey TA, Marks MR, Wiesel SW. A prospective, randomized, double blind evaluation of trigger-point injection therapy for low-back pain. *Spine.* 1989;14(9):962–4.
78. Green S, Buchbinder R, Barnsley L, et al. Acupuncture for lateral elbow pain. *Cochrane Database Syst Rev.* 2002;2002:CD003527.
79. Trinh K, Graham N, Gross A, et al. Acupuncture for neck disorders. *Cochrane Database Syst Rev.* 2010;3:CD004870.
80. Tulder MW VA, Cherkin DC, Berman B, Lao L, Koes BW. Acupuncture for low back pain. *Cochrane Database Syst Rev.* 2000;2:CD001351.
81. Healthcare Analysis and Information Group (HAIG). *FY 2015 VHA Complementary and Integrative Health (CIH) Services (Formerly CAM)*; 2015. Available from: https://sciencebasedmedicine.org/wp-content/uploads/2016/07/FY2015_VHA_CIH_signedReport.pdf.

SECTION VI

Sports-Specific Considerations

Baseball and Cricket

88

Dennis A. Cardone, Matthew T. Kingery, Naina Rao, and Eric J. Strauss

INTRODUCTION/BACKGROUND

- America's pastime continues to be one of the most popular youth sports. An estimated 6.5 million children aged 6–12 play baseball or softball in the United States (1), and 60,000 continue to play competitively in college (2).
    - Over half of youth baseball players experience shoulder or elbow pain over the course of a season (3), and almost 25% report a prior overuse injury (4).
    - Although the vast majority of baseball injuries are secondary to overuse, rare catastrophic injuries can occur secondary to full-speed collisions or players struck by batted balls (5).
- *Youth Baseball*
    - Little League is the most popular youth baseball league, with participation ranging from ages 4–16. There are several other youth leagues in the United States including Babe Ruth League and other local recreational leagues as well.
    - Based on the player's age, youth baseball limits the maximum number of pitches that a player can throw in a single day. In addition, based on the player's age and number of pitches thrown in a day, the league institutes a minimum number of rest days before pitching again.
- Although less common in the United States, Cricket is a similar overhead sport and is the second most popular international sport. It is estimated that over 1.24 billion people worldwide participate in the sport (6).
    - About 3.7% of all sports-related injuries in adolescents are cricket related (7), with 2.6 injuries per 10,000 hours played. Almost half of the injuries come from bowling (8,9).
    - Although serious injuries are associated with blunt chest impact and head and eye trauma, most injuries involve soft-tissue trauma or throwing injuries.

SPORT SPECIFICS (SEE CHAPTER 55, THE THROWING SHOULDER)

- *Anatomy*
    - Shoulder: Includes the sternoclavicular, acromioclavicular, glenohumeral, and scapulothoracic joints. The glenohumeral joint is a complex joint involving many static stabilizers including the joint capsule, glenoid labrum, glenohumeral ligaments, and dynamic stabilizers including the rotator cuff musculature.
    - Elbow: Includes the ulnotrochlear, radiocapitellar, and proximal radioulnar joints. Further stabilizers include the medial and lateral collateral ligament complexes. Musculature of the elbow includes the biceps brachii, brachioradialis, brachialis, triceps, anconeus, supinator, and pronator teres.
- *Biomechanics:* The biomechanics of overhead throwing depend on a carefully coordinated, full body sequence of movements that begin with force generation in the lower extremities and rely on the shoulder to transmit the force to the elbow, wrist, and hand (10).
    - Six phases of overhead throwing:
        - (1) In the wind-up, body weight is transferred entirely to the stance (rear) leg, the torso rotates toward the throwing shoulder, and the elbows are held flexed with the arms at the side.
        - (2) In the early cocking phase, the hands separate, the supraspinatus and deltoid abduct the arm, and the infraspinatus and teres minor externally rotate the shoulder. The lead (stride) leg extends to meet the ground, which generates linear velocity.
        - (3) Late cocking begins when the lead foot strikes the ground. The throwing shoulder continues to externally rotate until the glenohumeral joint reaches maximal external rotation. The pelvis and torso rotate toward the target while the throwing arm lags, creating potential energy. The elbow experiences the highest degree of valgus stress in this phase.
        - (4) In the acceleration phase, the shoulder begins to rotate internally, and the elbow extends. The trunk moves from hyperextension to flexion as the elbow reaches near full extension and the ball leaves the hand.
        - (5) Deceleration occurs after the ball is released. The arm is adducted across the body and powerful eccentric contractions throughout the kinetic chain are required to decelerate the throwing arm.
        - (6) Follow-through involves stabilization of the body over the stride leg, which absorbs the forces of the throwing motion. The rear leg is brought forward to meet the stride leg, and the forward motion is completed.

- Five positions or phases of cricket bowling (11):
  - (1) Starting with the back foot impact, the front arm points out and stretches toward the batsman.
  - (2) During the front foot impact phase/delivery stride, the bowler rotates their shoulder girdle in the transverse plane and abducts and externally rotates their bowling arm with the humerus parallel to the ground (known as the upper arm horizontal position).
  - (3) In the cradle position, the bowler's arms are brought together in front of their body in preparation for the ball release phase.
  - (4) In the ball release stage, the glenohumeral joint undergoes internal rotation while the arm circumducts along with elbow extension (12).
  - (5) Finally, in the follow-through, the bowler extends their front leg and returns to a balanced position with low-range shoulder elevation and moderate elbow flexion.
- Baseball players (particularly pitchers) develop unique patterns in their throwing motions throughout their playing careers that can impart different stresses on different parts of the upper extremity. Similarly, the deliveries of cricket bowlers can vary considerably, resulting in different patterns of stress on the arm, shoulder, and counter-rotating trunk (13).
  - Furthermore, bowlers can be categorized into two broad types that are characterized by different mechanics in their delivery of the ball. Pace bowlers (roughly analogous to a fastball pitcher) emphasize the speed of the ball, while spin bowlers (roughly analogous to a curveball pitcher) emphasize the rotation of the ball.

- *Equipment*
  - Baseball equipment includes batting helmets (with optional face shield), batting gloves, athletic cups, cleats, metal or wood bats, and gloves. Additional optional protective gear includes elbow guards and/or leg guards when batting and sliding mitts worn when base running.
  - Position-specific equipment for baseball includes mask, chest, throat, and shin protectors for catchers; toe guards for batters and catchers; forearm batting protectors; and gloves or mitts for field players.
  - Cricket equipment additionally include batting helmets (with optional face shield), batting gloves, athletic cups, cleats, leg pads, wooden cricket bat, wickets, stumps, bails, and padded gloves.
  - Position-specific equipment includes winged leg pads, chest guards, arm guards, and helmets for batsmen; slim leg pads for wicketkeepers, and gloves for batsmen and wicketkeepers (14).

MUSCULOSKELETAL ISSUES

- **Shoulder Injuries** (see Chapter 51, Shoulder Instability, Chapter 52, Rotator Cuff Syndromes, and Chapter 54, Shoulder Superior Labrum Anterior and Posterior Tears and Biceps Tears)
  - *Superior labral injuries* (including tears of the Superior Labrum from Anterior to Posterior, or SLAP tears) are common overuse injuries in baseball players.
    - Risk factors for symptomatic superior labral injuries include tight posterior shoulder structures, poor throwing mechanics, and changes in throwing or training.
    - Symptoms include painful clicking, pain with overhead actions, and pain with the acceleration phase of throwing.
    - Position players are more likely to return to prior levels of competitive play after operative management compared to pitchers (15).
  - *Posterior labral injuries* are becoming increasingly recognized as a source of pain and dysfunction in baseball players.
    - The injury can be caused by an acute event (*e.g.*, sliding into a base with the arm outstretched), but is more commonly an insidious overuse injury. A posterior labral tear in the context of posterior humeral head subluxation in the lead batting shoulder is known as "batter's shoulder" (16).
    - The presenting issue is typically pain, rather than instability.
    - The labral tear can often be visualized on MRI, but may require diagnostic arthroscopy for adequate evaluation (17).
  - *Instability* can be due to labral injury, trauma, poor mechanics, overuse, or generalized joint laxity.
    - Symptoms include pain during the acceleration phase of throwing.
    - Physical examination findings include a positive apprehension and relocation test, a positive load-and-shift test, and possibly generalized ligamentous laxity.
    - MRI or MRA is the diagnostic modality of choice to evaluate the status of the glenoid labrum.
    - Treatment includes physical therapy with scapular stabilization exercises and a graduated return-to-play program. If symptoms are severe or unresponsive to conservative treatment, surgical repair may be required (18).
  - *Rotator cuff injuries* vary from mild forms of tendonitis and impingement to complete, full-thickness tears.
    - Examination findings include a positive Neer sign, positive Hawkins sign, and pain and weakness with resistive muscle testing.
    - If a tear is suspected, the diagnosis is confirmed with MRI imaging.
    - Physical therapy can be successful for partial-thickness tears, but operative repair is generally required for full-thickness injuries (19).
  - *Posterior internal impingement*, found primarily in pitchers and fast bowlers.

- This injury is characterized by posterior shoulder pain during the late cocking phase and is caused by repetitive contact between the undersurface of the rotator cuff insertion on the greater tuberosity and the posterosuperior glenoid rim.
- Examination findings include a positive clunk test, a positive grind test, and a positive O'Brien test.
- MRI typically demonstrates a posterosuperior labral tear, partial posterior supraspinatus tear, and/or humeral osteochondral lesion.
- Conservative treatment includes physical therapy with an emphasis on stretching of the posterior shoulder structures, rest, and NSAIDs, and surgery if conservative therapies fail (20).

- *Glenohumeral internal rotation deficit* (GIRD) is a loss of passive shoulder internal rotation greater than 20° compared to the nonthrowing shoulder.
  - Due to the stresses placed on the throwing shoulder, players often develop an adaptive shift in the rotational arc of motion of the shoulder with an increase in external rotation ROM and a compensatory decrease in internal rotation ROM (21).
  - Treatment involves posteroinferior capsular stretching and periscapular strengthening (22,23).
- *A Bennett lesion* is a mineralization of the capsulolabral complex at the posterior-inferior glenoid rim.
  - This ossification is closely related to tight posterior capsular structures and GIRD in baseball players.
  - Bennett lesions can be asymptomatic, the direct source of shoulder pain, or the radiographic marker of a concomitant shoulder injury (24).
- *Suprascapular neuropathy* is an injury of the suprascapular nerve that can be caused by chronic traction secondary to overhead throwing or direct compression from a space occupying lesion (*e.g.*, paralabral cyst).
  - Patients present with posterior and lateral shoulder pain and weakness of the supraspinatus and/or infraspinatus.
  - Atrophy of the supraspinatus and/or infraspinatus is variable, but this finding should raise suspicion for nerve entrapment.
  - First-line treatment is physical therapy, but in the presence of an identifiable compressive lesion, surgical decompression is often recommended (25).
- *Thoracic outlet syndrome (TOS)* is caused by compression of the subclavian artery (vascular TOS) or brachial plexus (neurogenic TOS).
  - In throwing athletes, the source of compression is often hypertrophied muscles in the dominant shoulder or fibrous scar tissue from repetitive microtrauma.
  - Presentation is variable and can include arm weakness or early fatigue of the pitching arm.
  - For the vascular variant, the diagnosis is made with CTA or MRA, which can be performed with the arm in the position that provokes the patient's symptoms (26).
- *Thrower's fracture of the humerus* is an atraumatic midshaft or distal third spiral humeral shaft fracture that occurs during the throwing motion.
  - The repetitive stress placed on the humerus over time causes a fatigue injury or stress fracture that ultimately propagates and results in sudden failure of the humerus.
  - If there is suspicion for an impending thrower's fracture in a player with arm pain and negative radiographs, MRI can be obtained to rule out a stress reaction (27).
- *Little Leaguer's shoulder* (proximal humeral epiphysiolysis) is a Salter Harris type 1 injury of the proximal humeral physis in skeletally immature baseball players (rarely seen in cricket bowlers) (28).
  - Radiographs show widening of the physis compared to the contralateral shoulder.
  - Treatment consists of a period of throwing cessation, physical therapy, and graduated return to sport (29).

- **Elbow Injuries** (see Chapter 56, Elbow Instability, Chapter 57, Elbow Articular Lesions and Fractures, and Chapter 58, Elbow Tendinopathies)
  - *Osteochondritis dissecans (OCD)* of the humeral capitellum is often due to repetitive valgus stress across the radiocapitellar joint.
    - Symptoms can include lateral elbow pain associated with throwing, as well as clicking and locking during elbow motion. Crepitus and limited extension may be found on examination, and loose bodies may be seen on plain films.
    - Diagnosis can be made on x-rays or MRI; however, MRI is needed to determine whether the lesion is stable or unstable.
    - Treatment depends on the degree of lesion displacement. Conservative management consists of a period of throwing cessation and physical therapy. For high-grade lesions or those refractory to nonoperative treatment, surgery is indicated.
    - Outcomes are generally more favorable for position players compared to pitchers (30).
  - *Olecranon stress fracture* results from repetitive concentric firing of the triceps muscle, typically occurring during pitching.
    - Physical examination typically shows point tenderness over the olecranon and pain during the throwing motion.
    - If the fracture is not clearly evident on radiographs, the diagnosis can be made on CT or MRI.

- Treatment primarily consists of rest, and repeat imaging can assist with determining when the fracture is healed. When nonoperative management fails, surgery provides good outcomes (31).

- *Ulnar collateral ligament* tears can occur in both pitchers and position players due to the repetitive valgus stress placed on the elbow during the throwing motion.
  - Patients may recall an acute onset of medial elbow pain or may report nonspecific loss of throwing velocity or control.
  - Physical examination findings include decreased elbow extension, tenderness over the course of the ulnar collateral ligament, and laxity and pain with valgus stress testing.
  - MRI demonstrates the specific location and severity of the tear.
  - Partial tears can often be managed with rest and physical therapy, but complete tears in patients who wish to return to sport require operative management (32,33).
- *Ulnar neuritis* can result from the repetitive tensile forces of the throwing motion or compression from hypertrophied muscles in the elbow.
  - Symptoms include pain at the medial elbow, as well as paresthesia in the fourth and fifth digits.
  - Examination shows pain reproduced with cubital tunnel pressure, a positive Tinel sign at the cubital tunnel, and distal hand weakness.
  - Treatment consists of rest and physical therapy. If symptoms recur when throwing is resumed, surgical decompression with or without transposition is generally successful (34).
- *Valgus extension overload and posteromedial* impingement are seen primarily in pitchers and older bowlers.
  - This is caused by repetitive contact between the posteromedial olecranon and the olecranon fossa during the deceleration phase of the throwing motion which, in turn, leads to chondromalacia at the medial aspect of the ulnohumeral articulation, osteophyte formation on the posteromedial olecranon, and secondary injuries to the UCL and radiocapitellar joint.
  - Symptoms include pain with elbow hyperextension and physical exam may show valgus instability if the UCL is also injured.
  - X-rays may reveal osteophytes or loose bodies.
  - Treatment includes rest, throwing modification, ice, and NSAIDs. Surgical treatment to resect the osteophytes and/or loose bodies may be performed if nonoperative management fails (35).
- *Little Leaguer's elbow* is an overuse injury found in skeletally immature pitchers in which the repeated valgus stress results in medial epicondyle traction apophysitis (36).
  - Associated injuries include UCL tears and/or flexor-pronator mass strains.
  - Examination is significant for medial elbow tenderness, often worse with valgus stress.
  - Treatment includes rest and throwing modifications. Pediatric UCL reconstruction is indicated in the setting of a concomitant UCL tear (37).
- *Lateral epicondylitis* (tennis elbow) is an overuse injury due to eccentric overload of the common extensor tendon at the origin of the extensor carpi radialis brevis tendon.
  - This injury is often seen in cricket batsmen due to repetitive strains from wrist extension, forearm supination, and/or wrist deviation.
  - On examination, there is tenderness over the lateral epicondyle that can be reproduced with resisted wrist extension while the elbow is extended and forearm pronated. Pain during resisted extension of the middle finger with an extended elbow also supports the diagnosis (38).
  - Early stages are managed by physical therapy. Chronic tendinopathy and tears may require surgical correction (39).

Hand and Wrist Injuries (see Chapter 59, Soft-Tissue Injuries of the Wrist and Hand, and Chapter 60, Wrist and Hand Fractures)

- *Flexor tendon pulley rupture* involving the A4 pulley of the middle finger is found in fastball-dominant pitchers.
  - Examination demonstrates pain, ecchymosis, and tenderness over the volar aspect of the middle finger.
  - The diagnosis is confirmed with MRI.
  - Treatment involves a specialized pulley ring splint for 4 weeks followed by gradual return to throwing over several weeks. Nonoperative management is generally successful (40).
- *Hypothenar hammer syndrome* is vascular insufficiency of the ulnar artery and/or superficial palmar arch caused by the repetitive trauma of catching a baseball.
  - This occurs more commonly in catchers and presents with pain, weakness, and paresthesias in the ulnar digits.
  - MRI or MRA may demonstrate a thrombosis or aneurysm of the involved vessels.
  - Mild symptoms are treated with equipment modifications including additional padding over the hypothenar eminence. For patients who do not improve with conservative measures, surgery can be pursued (41).
- *Hamate hook fractures* occur due to the repetitive trauma of the lead batting hand against the end of the bat.
  - Patients present with pain and ecchymosis over the hamate, grip weakness, and ulnar nerve paresthesias if a displaced fracture fragment is compressing the ulnar nerve.
  - The fracture is often difficult to assess on plain radiographs, and CT is often required for accurate diagnosis.

- Due to the high incidence of nonunion with nonoperative management, early surgical intervention is generally indicated (42).
- *Dorsal fracture dislocation* of the proximal interphalangeal (PIP) is the most common hand injury in cricket and usually occurs while catching the ball (43).
  - Radiographs should be obtained to rule out fracture. Adequate stabilization requires operative management.
  - Mallet finger can also result from miscatching a cricket or baseball (44).
- **Trunk Injuries** (see Chapter 50, Thoracolumbar Injuries)
  - *Side strain* is an acute tear of the internal or external oblique muscle.
    - This can affect pace bowlers due to the sudden eccentric contraction of the muscle along with lateral trunk flexion when the nonbowling arm is pulled down from the cradle position during the final delivery action (45).
    - In pitchers, this can occur during late cocking and early acceleration stages of throwing when the activity of the abdominal muscles is increased (46).
    - Avulsion fractures may occur at the osteochondral tip of the lower ribs. When chronic, the osteochondral tips of the lower ribs hypertrophy and result in bony or soft-tissue impingement.
    - Pain is located in midaxillary line of the four lower ribs during resisted side flexion on the affected side.
    - Diagnosis can be made clinically but MRI can show tear of internal oblique or transversalis muscle (47).
    - Treatment options are initially conservative with rest, taping, and physical therapy.
  - *Latissimus dorsi avulsion* is a difficult to diagnose and uncommon overuse injury seen in baseball pitchers and cricket fast bowlers.
    - Weakness of adduction or internal rotation, change in posterior axillary fold, pain on resisted shoulder internal rotation, or bruising in the axilla are signs of latissimus dorsi avulsion as the source of injury.
    - MRI can show the injury, granted that the field of view is expanded distal enough.
    - Nonoperative treatment is the mainstay but surgical management is considered if patient is unable to return to sport (48,49).
  - *Lumbar spine injuries* are seen in fast bowlers and occur on the nonbowling side.
    - Most common are stress fractures, usually of the L4 and L5 pars interarticularis, and disc degeneration (50).
    - Lumbar stress fractures are the result of repetitive flexion, hyperextension, and rotation of the lumbar spine.
    - Bowlers specifically have large amounts of contralateral trunk side flexion for ball release.
    - Chronic fractures often lead to disc degeneration, which can be diagnosed via MRI (51,52).

MEDICAL ISSUES

- *Commotio cordis* is dysrhythmia or cardiac arrest occurring after a direct blow to the chest.
  - Batters hit by pitches, or fielders hit by line drives, causing a so-called "R on T" phenomenon where the impact occurs at a specific point in the electrical cycle leading to ventricular dysrhythmia, collapse, and sudden death.
  - Numerous cases reports have heightened awareness and increased advocacy for the use of safer and softer baseballs, particularly in youth baseball (53).
  - Initial treatment is prompt resuscitation and defibrillation.
- *Head injuries* occur often in baseball due to wild pitches, swinging bats, and hit baseballs often striking fans or spectators. The most common mechanism of injury is direct ball impact to players on the field (54).
- *Craniofacial fractures* from cricket account for 6%–7.1% of the total sports-related maxillofacial injuries (39,55).
- *Oral cancer* is a concern in many baseball players using chewing tobacco, which has been commonly used throughout the history of the sport. In 2016, Major League Baseball banned chewing tobacco for all new major league players in an attempt to decrease its prevalence among all levels of play.
- *Eye injuries* are typically the result of wild pitches and struck baseballs. Baseball is the leading cause of sports-related eye injuries in children (56). Because of this, new helmet designs feature an extended face guard, and sports goggles are recommended for runners on base. Eye injuries in cricket are rare and have been more often due to ricocheting bails than impact with a bowled ball (57).
- *Abdominal injuries* have been reported from sliding, collisions, falls, and direct impact of the baseball. Common injuries to the abdomen include muscular contusion, rectus sheath hematoma, and spleen and renal injury. Careful physical examination is important, and CT imaging is often necessary to make a final diagnosis (58).
- *Gastrointestinal illness*, specifically traveler's diarrhea, is common in cricket players due to the international aspect of the sport as well as sport's prevalence in Asian countries (59).
- *Skin lesions* are formed due to infection, friction, and trauma. Common friction injuries that occur on the hands of pitchers and bowlers are friction bullae due to application of torque and the resulting shearing forces. Bullae should be diagnosed with history and physical examination and treated with drainage to reduce pain (6).

- *Aneurysm of midaxillary artery* is rare but has been reported in baseball players and should be considered in the differential diagnosis of a throwing athlete with hand pain and paresthesias. Arterial embolization in the arm or hand may occur and is thought to be due to the forceful downward displacement of the humeral head or pectoralis minor tendon, damaging the arterial intima in throwing athletes. Treatment is often surgical revascularization (60,61).

INJURY PREVENTION

- To minimize overuse injuries, youth baseball players are restricted in their maximum number of pitches per game and adolescent cricket players are limited in the number of consecutive overs in a spell. However, the number of pitches thrown over the course of a game or season that puts youth players at risk of injury has yet to be clearly determined. However, based on the available data, limiting a player's pitch count is a reasonable way to decrease injury rate (62).
- Players, parents, coaches, and physicians should be aware that a player's official pitch count significantly underestimates the number of high-effort throws made (63). This is compounded when playing on two or more teams simultaneously in separate leagues.
- Although it was previously believed that throwing curveballs at a young age increases the risk of injury, the current data does not suggest that throwing breaking balls is associated with added injury risk (64).
- Perhaps more important than absolute pitch count limits or restrictions on types of pitches thrown is the appropriate management of fatigue in youth pitchers. As a player's pitch count increases over the course of a game, lower body and core musculature begins to fatigue. As a player becomes fatigued, there is deviation from proper throwing mechanics and increased risk of arm pain and subsequent injury (65).
- Players should be heavily discouraged from continuing to pitch after developing any shoulder or elbow pain.
- Formal injury prevention programs for youth players consisting of supervised stretching, strengthening, dynamic mobility, balance training, and an emphasis on proper throwing mechanics have been shown to decrease the rate of injuries (66,67).
- Single-leg balance test and Star Excursion Balance Test are used to identify bowlers who are at high risk of sustaining back and trunk injuries and should be educated in prevention methods (68).

American Academy of Pediatrics 2012 Policy Statement on Baseball and Softball (69)

- Baseball and softball for children 5 through 14 years of age should be acknowledged as relatively safe sports. Catastrophic and chronically disabling injuries are rare.
- Preventive measures should be used to protect young baseball pitchers from throwing injuries. These measures include a restriction on the number of pitches thrown in organized and informal settings, as well as instruction in proper training, conditioning, and throwing mechanics. Parents, coaches, and players should be educated about the early warning signs of an overuse injury and encouraged to seek timely and appropriate treatment if evidence of an injury develops.
- Serious and potentially catastrophic baseball injuries can be minimized by the proper use of available safety equipment. This includes the use of approved batting helmets; helmets, masks, and chest and neck protectors for all catchers; and rubber spikes. Protective fencing of dugouts and benches and the use of break-away bases also are recommended, as is the elimination of the on-deck circle. Protective equipment should always be properly fitted and well maintained. These preventive measures should be used in games and practices and in organized and informal participation.
- Baseball and softball (and cricket) players should be encouraged to wear polycarbonate eye protectors on the batting helmets to reduce the risk of eye injury. These eye protectors should be required for functionally one-eyed athletes (best corrected vision in the worst eye of less than 20/50) and for athletes who have undergone eye surgery or experienced severe eye injuries if the ophthalmologists judge them to be at an increased risk for eye injuries. These athletes also should protect their eyes when fielding by using polycarbonate sports goggles (69,70).
- Use of low-impact baseballs and softballs for children 5 to 14 years of age should be considered. In particular, children younger than 10 years should be encouraged to use the lowest-impact balls.
- Developmentally appropriate rule modifications, such as avoidance of headfirst sliding, should be implemented for children younger than 10 years.
- Because current data are limited, the routine use of chest protectors to prevent commotio cordis is not recommended for baseball players other than catchers (71).

REHABILITATION

- Rehabilitation for a baseball player or throwing athlete is often injury specific. Physical therapy should include rehabilitation of the large lower-body muscle groups and the smaller muscle groups of the upper extremity. Strengthening often needs to be directed at the rotator cuff and scapular stabilizing muscles.
- The phases of rehabilitation include the acute, recovery, and maintenance phases.
  - The acute phase concentrates on reducing pain and swelling and improving strength.

- During the recovery phase, treatment is focused on pain-free range of motion, strength, and improved stability and function.
- The maintenance phase of rehabilitation includes increases in power, endurance, strength, and activity-specific function.

- Interval throwing programs (ITPs) are structured to increase a pitcher's strength and endurance before returning to competitive pitching. ITPs are prescribed after an injury or at the start of preseason training. Programs are designed for players to reach specific goals, often over a period of 3 to 4 weeks, and combine periods of exercise and rest. Throwing days start with warm-ups and stretching and are followed by throwing. Throwing distances are gradually increased throughout the program.

REFERENCES

1. Association SFI. *Sports, Fitness, and Leisure Activities Topline Participation Report*. 2022.
2. NCAA. *NCAA Sports Sponsorship and Participation Rates Report*; 2022 Jun 1.
3. Lyman S, Fleisig GS, Andrews JR, Osinski ED. Effect of pitch type, pitch count, and pitching mechanics on risk of elbow and shoulder pain in youth baseball pitchers. *Am J Sports Med*. 2002;30(4):463–8.
4. Makhni EC, Morrow ZS, Luchetti TJ, et al. Arm pain in youth baseball players: a survey of healthy players. *Am J Sports Med*. 2015;43(1):41–6.
5. Boden BP, Tacchetti R, Mueller FO. Catastrophic injuries in high school and college baseball players. *Am J Sports Med*. 2004;32(5):1189–96.
6. Farhadian JA, Tlougan BE, Adams BB, Leventhal JS, Sanchez MR. Skin conditions of baseball, cricket, and softball players. *Sports Med*. 2013;43(7):575–89.
7. Finch C, Valuri G, Ozanne-Smith J. Sport and active recreation injuries in Australia: evidence from emergency department presentations. *Br J Sports Med*. 1998;32(3):220–5.
8. Finch CF, Elliott BC, McGrath AC. Measures to prevent cricket injuries: an overview. *Sports Med*. 1999;28(4):263–72.
9. Stretch RA. Cricket injuries: a longitudinal study of the nature of injuries to South African cricketers. *Br J Sports Med*. 2003;37(3):250–3. discussion 3.
10. Weber AE, Kontaxis A, O'Brien SJ, Bedi A. The biomechanics of throwing: simplified and cogent. *Sports Med Arthrosc Rev*. 2014;22(2):72–9.
11. Mathankar1 A. Overview of biomechanics and movement patterns of cricket spin bowlers. *J Soc Indian Physiother*. 2020;4(2):65–9.
12. Dutton M, Gray J, Prins D, Divekar N, Tam N. Overhead throwing in cricketers: a biomechanical description and playing level considerations. *J Sports Sci*. 2020;38(10):1096–104.
13. Ranson CA, Burnett AF, King M, Patel N, O'Sullivan PB. The relationship between bowling action classification and three-dimensional lower trunk motion in fast bowlers in cricket. *J Sports Sci*. 2008;26(3):267–76.
14. *Australia SM. Cricket - preventing injury* [Web]. Victoria State Government Department of Health: Sports Medicine Australia. updated 28 Feb 2015. Available from: https://www.betterhealth.vic.gov.au/health/healthyliving/cricket-preventing-injury#bhc-content
15. Douglas L, Whitaker J, Nyland J, et al. Return to play and performance perceptions of baseball players after isolated SLAP tear repair. *Orthop J Sports Med*. 2019;7(3):2325967119829486.
16. Wanich T, Dines J, Dines D, Gambardella RA, Yocum LA. 'Batter's shoulder': can athletes return to play at the same level after operative treatment? *Clin Orthop Relat Res*. 2012;470(6):1565–70.
17. Kercher JS, Runner RP, McCarthy TP, Duralde XA. Posterior labral repairs of the shoulder among baseball players: results and outcomes with minimum 2-year follow-up. *Am J Sports Med*. 2019;47(7):1687–93.
18. DeFroda SF, Goyal D, Patel N, Gupta N, Mulcahey MK. Shoulder instability in the overhead athlete. *Curr Sports Med Rep*. 2018;17(9):308–14.
19. Klouche S, Lefevre N, Herman S, Gerometta A, Bohu Y. Return to sport after rotator cuff tear repair: a systematic review and meta-analysis. *Am J Sports Med*. 2016;44(7):1877–87.
20. Spiegl UJ, Warth RJ, Millett PJ. Symptomatic internal impingement of the shoulder in overhead athletes. *Sports Med Arthrosc Rev*. 2014;22(2):120–9.
21. Lubis AM, Wisnubaroto RP, Ilyas EI, Ifran NN. Glenohumeral internal rotation deficit in non-pitcher overhead athletic athletes: case series analysis of ten athletes. *Ann Med Surg*. 2020;58:138–42.
22. Rose MB, Noonan T. Glenohumeral internal rotation deficit in throwing athletes: current perspectives. *Open Access J Sports Med*. 2018;9:69–78.
23. Keller RA, De Giacomo AF, Neumann JA, Limpisvasti O, Tibone JE. Glenohumeral internal rotation deficit and risk of upper extremity injury in overhead athletes: a meta-analysis and systematic review. *Sports Health*. 2018;10(2):125–32.
24. Ferrari JD, Ferrari DA, Coumas J, Pappas AM. Posterior ossification of the shoulder: the Bennett lesion. Etiology, diagnosis, and treatment. *Am J Sports Med*. 1994;22(2):171–6. discussion 5-6.
25. Strauss EJ, Kingery MT, Klein D, Manjunath AK. The evaluation and management of suprascapular neuropathy. *J Am Acad Orthop Surg*. 2020;28(15):617–27.
26. Thorne CM, Yildirim B, Tracci MC, Chhabra AB. Vascular problems in elite throwing athletes. *J Hand Surg Am*. 2023;48(1):68–75.
27. Miller A, Dodson CC, Ilyas AM. Thrower's fracture of the humerus. *Orthop Clin North Am*. 2014;45(4):565–9.
28. Drescher WR, Falliner A, Zantop T, Oehlert K, Petersen W, Hassenpflug J. Little league shoulder syndrome in an adolescent cricket player. *Br J Sports Med*. 2004;38(4):e14.
29. Bednar ED, Kay J, Memon M, Simunovic N, Purcell L, Ayeni OR. Diagnosis and management of little league shoulder: a systematic review. *Orthop J Sports Med*. 2021;9(7):23259671211017563.
30. Sasanuma H, Iijima Y, Saito T, et al. Satisfaction with elbow function and return status after autologous osteochondral transplant for capitellar osteochondritis dissecans in high school baseball players. *Am J Sports Med*. 2020;48(12):3057–65.
31. Smith SR, Patel NK, White AE, Hadley CJ, Dodson CC. Stress fractures of the elbow in the throwing athlete: a systematic review. *Orthop J Sports Med*. 2018;6(10):2325967118799262.
32. Carr JB II, Camp CL, Dines JS. Elbow ulnar collateral ligament injuries: indications, management, and outcomes. *Arthroscopy*. 2020;36(5):1221–2.
33. Torres SJ, Limpisvasti O. Ulnar collateral ligament repair of the elbow-biomechanics, indications, and outcomes. *Curr Rev Musculoskelet Med*. 2021;14(2):168–73.
34. Dowdle SB, Chalmers PN. Management of the ulnar nerve in throwing athletes. *Curr Rev Musculoskelet Med*. 2020;13(4):449–56.
35. Park JY, Yoo HY, Chung SW, et al. Valgus extension overload syndrome in adolescent baseball players: clinical characteristics and surgical outcomes. *J Shoulder Elb Res*. 2016;25(12):2048–56.
36. Mukherjee S. Little league elbow in a prepubertal cricket player. *Curr Sports Med Rep*. 2015;14(6):455–8.
37. Wei AS, Khana S, Limpisvasti O, Crues J, Podesta L, Yocum LA. Clinical and magnetic resonance imaging findings associated with Little League elbow. *J Pediatr Orthop*. 2010;30(7):715–9.

38. Buchanan BK. *Tennis Elbow*. StatPearls; 2022.
39. Pardiwala DN, Rao NN, Varshney AV. Injuries in cricket. *Sports Health*. 2018;10(3):217–22.
40. Gallant GG, Tulipan JE, Rivlin M, Ilyas AM. Baseball injuries of the hand and wrist. *J Am Acad Orthop Surg*. 2021;29(15):648–58.
41. Hui-Chou HG, McClinton MA. Current options for treatment of hypothenar hammer syndrome. *Hand Clin*. 2015;31(1):53–62.
42. Bansal A, Carlan D, Moley J, Goodson H, Goldfarb CA. Return to play and complications after hook of the hamate fracture surgery. *J Hand Surg Am*. 2017;42(10):803–9.
43. Barton N. Sports injuries of the hand and wrist. *Br J Sports Med*. 1997;31(3):191–6.
44. Shafi M. Cricket injuries: an orthopaedist's perspective. *Orthop Surg*. 2014;6(2):90–4.
45. Nealon AR, Kountouris A, Cook JL. Side strain in sport: a narrative review of pathomechanics, diagnosis, imaging and management for the clinician. *J Sci Med Sport*. 2017;20(3):261–6.
46. Fleisig GS, Hsu WK, Fortenbaugh D, Cordover A, Press JM. Trunk axial rotation in baseball pitching and batting. *Sports Biomech*. 2013;12(4):324–33.
47. Humphries D, Jamison M. Clinical and magnetic resonance imaging features of cricket bowler's side strain. *Br J Sports Med*. 2004;38(5):e21.
48. Naidu KS, James T, Rotstein AH, Balster SM, Hoy GA. Latissimus dorsi and teres major tendon avulsions in cricketers: a case series and literature review. *Clin J Sport Med*. 2017;27(3):e24–8.
49. Schickendantz MS, Kaar SG, Meister K, Lund P, Beverley L. Latissimus dorsi and teres major tears in professional baseball pitchers: A case series. *Am J Sports Med*. 2009;37(10):2016–20.
50. Ranson CA, Kerslake RW, Burnett AF, Batt ME, Abdi S. Magnetic resonance imaging of the lumbar spine in asymptomatic professional fast bowlers in cricket. *J Bone Joint Surg Br*. 2005;87(8):1111–6.
51. Alway P, Felton P, Brooke-Wavell K, Peirce N, King M. Cricket fast bowling technique and lumbar bone stress injury. *Med Sci Sports Exerc*. 2021;53(3):581–9.
52. Orchard J, James T, Kountouris A, Farhart P. Cricket injuries. In: Hutson M, Speed C, eds. *Sports Injuries*. Oxford University Press; 2011:0.
53. Curfman GD. Fatal impact--concussion of the heart. *N Engl J Med*. 1998;338(25):1841–3.
54. Pasternack JS, Veenema KR, Callahan CM. Baseball injuries: a Little league survey. *Pediatrics*. 1996;98(3 pt 1):445–8.
55. Lee K. Cricket related maxillofacial fractures. *J Maxillofac Oral Surg*. 2012;11(2):182–5.
56. Miller KN, Collins CL, Chounthirath T, Smith GA. Pediatric sports- and recreation-related eye injuries treated in US emergency departments. *Pediatrics*. 2018;141(2):e20173083.
57. Mann DL, Dain SJ. Serious eye injuries to cricket wicketkeepers: a call to consider protective eyewear. *Br J Sports Med*. 2013;47(10):607–8.
58. Riviello RJ, Young JS. Intra-abdominal injury from softball. *Am J Emerg Med*. 2000;18(4):505–6.
59. O'Donovan CM, Connor B, Madigan SM, Cotter PD, O'Sullivan O. Instances of altered gut microbiomes among Irish cricketers over periods of travel in the lead up to the 2016 World Cup: a sequencing analysis. *Travel Med Infect Dis*. 2020;35:101553.
60. Ishitobi K, Moteki K, Nara S, Akiyama Y, Kodera K, Kaneda S. Extra-anatomic bypass graft for management of axillary artery occlusion in pitchers. *J Vasc Surg*. 2001;33(4):797–801.
61. Todd GJ, Benvenisty AI, Hershon S, Bigliani LU. Aneurysms of the mid axillary artery in major league baseball pitchers—a report of two cases. *J Vasc Surg*. 1998;28(4):702–7.
62. Fleisig GS, Andrews JR, Cutter GR, et al. Risk of serious injury for young baseball pitchers: a 10-year prospective study. *Am J Sports Med*. 2011;39(2):253–7.
63. Wahl EP, Pidgeon TS, Richard MJ. Youth baseball pitch counts vastly underestimate high-effort throws throughout a season. *J Pediatr Orthop*. 2020;40(7):e609–15.
64. Grantham WJ, Iyengar JJ, Byram IR, Ahmad CS. The curveball as a risk factor for injury: a systematic review. *Sports Health*. 2015;7(1):19–26.
65. Erickson BJ, Sgori T, Chalmers PN, et al. The impact of fatigue on baseball pitching mechanics in adolescent male pitchers. *Arthroscopy*. 2016;32(5):762–71.
66. Sakata J, Nakamura E, Suzuki T, et al. Efficacy of a prevention program for medial elbow injuries in youth baseball players. *Am J Sports Med*. 2018;46(2):460–9.
67. Sakata J, Nakamura E, Suzuki T, et al. Throwing injuries in youth baseball players: can a prevention program help? A randomized controlled trial. *Am J Sports Med*. 2019;47(11):2709–16.
68. Ruchi Choudhary M. To evaluate and compare dynamic balance between cricketers and non-cricketers using star excursion balance test. *Int J Physiother Res*. 2019;7(5):3215–9.
69. Rice SG, Congeni JA, Council on Sports Medicine and Fitness, McCambridge T, Brenner J, et al Baseball and softball. *Pediatrics*. 2012;129(3):e842–56.
70. Stuart MJ. *Facial injuries in sports, an issue of clinics in sports medicine*. Elsevier Health Sciences; 2017.
71. Weinstock J, Maron BJ, Song C, Mane PP, Mark Estes NA III, Link MS. Failure of commercially available chest wall protectors to prevent sudden cardiac death induced by chest wall blows in an experimental model of commotio cordis. *Pediatrics*. 2019;117(4):e656–62.

Basketball

89

Chad A. Asplund and Michael Needham

INTRODUCTION/BACKGROUND

- Basketball has been an organized sport since the 1890s and is considered a limited contact sport.
- Played at a variety of levels: Olympic, professional, high school, middle/grade school, and recreation
- Five on five is most popular form of team basketball, although there has been an increase in 3 × 3 play, especially internationally.
- With the great popularity of basketball, most teams at the high school level and beyond have associated physicians or certified athletic trainers who are responsible for injury prevention and medical care; however, care for the athlete falls to the hands of many health care providers because many injuries occur outside of organized play (1,2).
- Injury rates in basketball are increasing as popularity rises and the nature of the sport becomes more aggressive (2,3).

SPECIFIC ISSUES

- Basketball involves a tremendous amount of running with explosive movements and rapid changes in direction and pace. Extreme stresses on the body during play result in many acute musculoskeletal injuries, whereas the ability to play year-round and at most ages leads to many overuse injuries.

Epidemiology of Injuries

- Nearly 1.6 million people are involved in basketball injuries each year in the United States (4).
- College injury rates are 7.9 per 1000 athlete exposures (AEs) for males and 7.6 for females, with game injuries (9.9/1000) being more common than practice injuries (4.4/1000) (Morris).
- High school players are more likely to be injured during competition than college players (3.27/1000 AEs vs. 1.4/1000 AEs) (5).
- Five most common orthopedic sports injuries sustained in the National Basketball Association were:
  - concussions (9.5–14.9 per year)
  - fractures of the hand (3.5–5.5 per year)
  - lower extremity stress fractures (4.8 per year)
  - meniscal tears (2.3–3.3 per year)
  - anterior cruciate ligament (ACL) tears (1.5–2.6 per year) (6).
- Most commonly injured joints are ankle (22%) and knee (18%) (6).
- Sprains are the most common type of injury in basketball. Sprains account for 32%–34% of injuries at the collegiate level (7) and 44% at the high school level (3).
- Children are more susceptible to overuse injuries due to open physes, especially at the elbow, knee, and ankle (8).
- Following European professional players over 2 years, there were 37 surgeries (8.7%) performed on a total of 423 injuries (9); 6.9%–8.1% of U.S. high school basketball injuries required surgery (3) (Table 89.1).

MEDICAL ISSUES

Dermatologic Issues

- Fungal infections are prevalent in athletes, and tinea pedis is the most common dermatophytosis.
  - High-top shoes, perspiration, friction, and poor foot care contribute to recurrent problems.
  - Drying the feet, changing socks, using absorbent powders (without corn starch), and applying over-the-counter and prescription antifungals are effective treatment measures.
  - Similar measures should be taken to treat tinea cruris or "jock itch," which is also common in athletes.
- Blisters are another common problem that can cause significant problems for the basketball athlete.
  - Rigid footwear and significant movement inside of the shoe cause this to occur as the shear stresses between epidermal layers cause fluid to build up.
  - These can be safely drained under sterile conditions if full and tense, and these areas should be protected with Vaseline, moleskin, etc., and treated with topical antibiotics if there are open lesions.
  - Proper footwear, including cushion socks, and conditioning can prevent blisters.

Table 89.1 Common Location of Basketball Injuries (10)

Location	Frequency of Injury
Ankle/foot	39.7%
Knee	14.7%
Head/face/neck	13.6%
Arm/hand	9.6%
Hip/thigh/upper leg	8.4%

Concussion

- Concussion or mild traumatic brain injury (MTBI) occurs in basketball from two mechanisms — player-to-player contact or contact with the floor (3).
- MTBI comprises 3.3% of injuries in male basketball players <20 year old and 5.2% in females <20 year old, which represents a twofold increase in males and a threefold increase in girls over a 10-year period (2) and reflects the higher incidence of MTBI in females of all age groups.
- Player collisions are the most likely etiology, and most of these occur in the open court, not under the basket (11).

Cardiac

- Basketball involves significant physiologic stress as reflected in findings from professional players. Heart rates average 169 bpm and are above 85% predicted maximum for 75% of competitive playing time (12).
- Hypertension is seen in basketball, even though many players are young.
  - Blood pressure elevation over 140 mm Hg systolic and 90 mm Hg diastolic on two separate readings should be investigated.
  - Family history, supplement and medication use, and substance abuse should be considered while investigating other secondary causes.
  - Blood pressure should be controlled before allowing exercise.
    - In mild and moderate hypertension, exercise is often part of a treatment plan, but in severe hypertension, it is contraindicated. When choosing treatment options, medications with negative performance side effects such as diuretics and nonselective β-blockers should be a last resort (13).
- Sudden cardiac death is a rare but serious threat, with an incidence of 1 in 11,394 in National Collegiate Athletic Association basketball players.
  - Incidence is significantly higher in males and in black athletes, with a prevalence of 1 in 3000 Division I male basketball players based on a study from 2004 to 2008 (14).
  - This represents a significantly higher incidence than previously estimated, and basketball players have been found to be at higher risk for sudden cardiac death than any other athletes (14,15).
    - This could be linked to a predisposition for basketball players to be tall and thin, or Marfanoid, or to a predisposition for a higher prevalence of hypertrophic cardiomyopathy (HCM) in young African American athletes (16).
- Preparticipation examination with a focus on history taking is the best method to prevent sudden death but has not been proven to improve morbidity or mortality.
- High-risk individuals with a family history of premature or sudden death, history of exercise-related syncope, or findings of Marfan syndrome should be identified for further testing.

Marfan Syndrome

- Marfan syndrome is a disorder that affects multiple organ systems, including disproportionate overgrowth of the long bones in the musculoskeletal system and valve dysfunction, dilated cardiomyopathy, and predisposition to aortic aneurysm and dissection in the cardiovascular system (17).
- Because people affected with Marfan syndrome tend to be tall with longer extremities, a higher proportion of them are found among basketball players.
- Family history is important because Marfan syndrome is passed on as a dominant trait, but about 25% of cases are sporadic.
- Marfan syndrome diagnostic criteria is a list of features doctors use to diagnose (or decide if someone has) Marfan syndrome. The diagnostic criteria are sometimes called the "Ghent criteria," named after the city in Belgium where doctors decided which features to include on the list (Table 89.2).
- In the 2010 revised Ghent nosology, aortic root aneurysm and ectopia lentis are now cardinal features, and in absence of any family history, the presence of these two manifestations is sufficient for the unequivocal diagnosis of Marfan syndrome.
- In patients who die from Marfan syndrome, the etiology is cardiovascular (aortic dissection, congestive heart failure, or cardiac valve disease) in over 90% of cases (17).
- Marfan syndrome is further discussed in Chapter 30, Cardiology.

Hypertrophic Cardiomyopathy

- HCM accounts for 36% of sudden cardiac death in young athletes and has been noted to occur more commonly in male athletes and approximately twice as often in nonwhites, predominantly blacks (15,16).
- HCM is a relatively common disorder, with an incidence of about 1:500, and can lead to cardiac death by fatal arrhythmias, so thorough evaluation is indicated in those diagnosed with HCM to risk stratify and determine treatment (16).
- Clinical diagnosis of HCM is established most easily and reliably with two-dimensional echocardiography by imaging the hypertrophied but nondilated left ventricular (LV) chamber, in the absence of another cardiac or systemic disease (*e.g.*, hypertension or aortic stenosis) (16).

Table 89.2 Diagnostic Criteria for Marfan Syndrome by Body System (18)

For an *index (new) case*, diagnosis REQUIRES: Major criteria in two categories AND involvement of a third system.

For the *relative of an index case*, diagnosis REQUIRES: One major criterion in family history AND one major criterion in any organ system AND involvement in a second organ system.

Body System	Major Criteria	Minor Criteria
Skeletal	Must have 4 of the following: • Pectus carinatum • Surgical pectus excavatum • Arm span greater than height • Length of torso shorter than length of legs • Positive wrist sign • Scoliosis (>20° curve) • Spondylolisthesis • Pes planus • Protrusion acetabuli	• Nonsurgical pes excavatum • Hypermobile joints • High arched palate • Marfanoid facial appearance (long, thin face; deep set eyes)
Cardiovascular	• Ascending aortic dilation or aneurysm • Aortic dissection	• Mitral valve prolapse • Enlarged pulmonary artery • Calcium deposits on mitral valve • Any aortic aneurysm • Any aortic dissection
Pulmonary	No major criteria	• Spontaneous pneumothorax • Apical blebs
Skin	No major criteria	• Recurrent hernia • Striae
Dura	• Dural ectasia	No minor criteria

- In clinically diagnosed patients, increased LV wall thicknesses range widely from mild (13–15 mm) to massive (≥30 mm) (normal LV thickness ≤12 mm) (16).
- However, in trained athletes, modest segmental wall thickening (*i.e.*, 13–15 mm) raises the differential diagnosis between extreme physiologic LV hypertrophy (*i.e.*, athlete's heart) and mild morphologic expressions of HCM; further imaging may be needed.
- Magnetic resonance imaging (MRI) may be of diagnostic value when echocardiographic studies are technically inadequate or in identifying segmental LV hypertrophy undetectable by echocardiography.
- Because of this potential gray area between physiologically normal "athlete's heart" and mild HCM, clearance and return-to-play decisions should be made by a cardiologist familiar with HCM and athletes.
- HCM is further discussed in Chapter 30, Cardiology.

MUSCULOSKELETAL ISSUES

Facial and Oral Injuries

- Five to 10% of basketball injuries involve the face or scalp (11), and an estimated 7500 eye injuries occur annually in the United States (9).
- Basketball has no accepted regulations regarding the use of mouth guards or protective eyewear, and few players wear face guards or mouth guards for protection against injury.
- There is ample contact between players, and most facial injuries result from contact with elbows or fingers from other players (19).
- Most lacerations occur over bony prominences, and fractures must be suspected when significant force is applied and symptoms extend beyond local mild tenderness and ecchymosis.
- The American Academy of Ophthalmology recommendations state that they "strongly recommend" eye protection for all athletes with risk for eye injury and that eye protection should be mandatory for functionally one-eyed athletes and for athletes after eye surgery or after eye trauma (20).
- Of eye injuries in professional basketball players, eyelid lacerations make up 50%, periorbital contusions make up 28%, and corneal abrasions make up 12% (21,22).
- Dental injuries are often permanent as teeth do not have much ability to heal. Mouth guards absorb force and help prevent tooth fracture, jaw injury, and even neck injury. A 10-year study of the women's basketball team showed a reduction in incidence of dental injury after instituting mandatory mouth guard use from 8.3 injuries per 100 athlete seasons to 2.8 injuries, but the reduction was not statistically significant (23). Custom-molded guards are inexpensive and preferable to off-the-shelf products.
- Dental literature reports injury rates from 1% to 14% (24). Most dental trauma occurs to the upper anterior teeth, especially the upper lip and two central incisors.
- In some studies, mouth guards and protective eyewear have been shown reduce rates of injury (18,22), but an estimated 1%–4% or less of players use these protections (22,25).

Spine and Pelvis

- Back injuries make up more than 5.3% of all basketball injuries (26).
- The dynamic nature of basketball, including fast changes in direction, repetitive jumping, twisting, rapid starts and stops, high velocity, and overhead arm use, produces significant strain on the spine. The vertebral column and intervertebral discs carry 70% of forces, and the posterior spine transmits 30%.
- Cervical injury from acceleration/deceleration injuries (whiplash) occurs in basketball but is less severe than in other contact sports. Pain and muscular dysfunction are common, but radicular symptoms can be a warning of more significant injury.
  - Treatment includes relative rest, motion and strength exercises, nonsteroidal anti-inflammatory drugs (NSAIDs), ice, heat, and modalities.
  - If pain persists, consider facet dysfunction or intervertebral disc degeneration.
- Basketball typically involves repetitive extension and hyperextension from rebounding, guarding opponents, and shooting. This can lead to excessive forces on the lumbar spine and injury. Defects of the posterior portions of the vertebra can lead to significant low back pain exacerbated by extension and axial loading.
- Spondylolysis is the presence of a defect in the pars interarticularis from any etiology including congenital defects, chronic stress, or acute fracture. This is the most common source of back pain in people under age 26 (10).
  - Symptoms include low back pain with radiation into the buttock and hamstrings from resulting spasm. Pain is worse with standing and back extension, and there is an absence of radicular pain.
  - Treatment involves back strengthening with a focus on flexion exercises, avoidance of back extension that produces pain, and analgesia as needed.
  - Radiographs are indicated if symptoms persist in order to detect any instability of the spine.
- Spondylolisthesis is the resulting anterior-posterior subluxation of the one vertebra on another when bilateral defects occur.
  - Slippage greater than 50% may need surgical attention. Otherwise, treat patients conservatively with exercise and follow them closely for development of symptoms of nerve root impingement or spinal stenosis.
  - Many athletes can return to basketball after aggressive strengthening and rehabilitation.
- Sacroiliac (SI) dysfunction is commonly seen, misdiagnosed, and treated as muscular low back pain, and athletes fail to improve significantly.
  - Patients usually cannot find any comfortable position for more than 10–15 minutes and have pain radiating into the posterior thigh. Pain is worse with motion that involves combined back flexion/extension and trunk rotation.
  - Physical examination with focused attention to palpation of SI joints and functional testing (Faber test, Gaenslen test, Gillet test, Trendelenburg test) will allow identification and more appropriate treatment.

Upper Extremity

- In high school players, 10%–12% of all basketball injuries occur to the hand and wrist, and 2%–4% occur to the shoulder (3).
- The most common upper extremity injuries are sprains and dislocations of the proximal interphalangeal (PIP) joints of the finger (27,28).
  - Radiographs should be considered when a PIP joint injury is identified, as an untreated fracture or dislocation at this location may result in significant long-term disability (29).
  - Mallet finger (distal interphalangeal flexion injury) can be seen, which requires a minimum of 6 weeks of continuous splinting and can lead to swan neck deformity if untreated (29).

Lower Extremity

- Lower extremity injuries account for the majority of injuries at every level of competition. Lower extremity injuries account for 51% in recreational players (1) and between 56% and 69% in high school athletes (30,31).
- There is a gender difference, with 56%–64% of male injuries occurring to the lower extremity and 65%–69% of female injuries occurring to the lower extremity (3,7,12). This is thought to be due to higher rates of knee injuries in females compared to males.

Knee

- Twelve percent of all injuries in male collegiate athletes are knee injuries, whereas the knee accounts for 19% of injuries in women (32).
- Although knee injuries are not the most common type of lower extremity injury, they account for most of the lost playing time (21).
- Patellofemoral syndrome is a broad description that characterizes pain and dysfunction of the extensor mechanism of the knee resulting from poor biomechanics (patella tracks laterally) or inflammation that, in athletes, is usually associated with overuse of the knee. Treatment involves modification of training regimen, ice, NSAIDs, and correction of underlying muscle or bony maltracking with quadriceps strengthening and improving landing mechanics. The vastus medialis is responsible for maintaining medial patellar alignment when other forces act to move the patella laterally.

If strength training does not correct the problem, taping or functional braces can be helpful.

- Medial tibial stress syndrome (shin splints) and tibial stress fractures represent two common causes of anterior shin pain in basketball players and two points on a continuum of muscle overuse, leading to periostitis and finally bone degradation.
  - These overuse injuries are characterized by pain on the medial border of the tibia, typically in the lower midportion.
  - Ice, rest, NSAIDs, correcting foot and ankle biomechanics, and adjusting training regimens will usually improve shin splints.
  - Stress fracture symptoms included worsening of typical pain beyond the time of activity and prolonged recovery times from episodes of intense activity or competition.
  - Plain films can show periostitis and stress fractures, but delayed-phase bone scans and MRI are much more sensitive.
  - Treatment involves an initial period of rest that may include use of removable casts or crutches for pain relief.
  - A very gradual reintroduction of activity with close symptom monitoring will allow for recovery in most cases.
- Patellar tendinitis, or jumper's knee, is common in basketball, found in 40%–50% of high-level players (33). It results from excessive forces through the extensor mechanism on the anterior knee.
  - Symptoms include anterior knee pain just below the patella that is worse with sitting, squatting, kneeling, or climbing stairs. Point tenderness on the superior pole of the patellar tendon and pain with hyperextension of the knee are seen.
  - An initial phase of symptom reduction with relative rest, ice, and NSAIDs can be followed by strengthening exercises with postactivity ice application.
  - The use of infrapatellar straps or taping is common.
- Osgood-Schlatter disease is an inflammatory apophysitis resulting from excessive pull by the patellar tendon on the tibial tuberosity. It appears in young players typically age 10–15 years during a period of rapid growth combined with intense physical activity.
- Treatment includes relative rest and analgesia, but pain diminishes when growth ceases. Rupture is rare, so participation in sports should not be limited.
- ACL injuries account for 10% of male basketball knee injuries and 26% of female knee injuries (2).
  - The majority of ACL injuries are noncontact and involve the player planting and pivoting on the knee.
  - ACL injury differences between males and females have been attributed to intrinsic factors such as intercondylar notch size and shape, hormone differences, ACL size, and joint laxity as well as extrinsic factors such as strength, skill, experience, shoe wear, and conditioning.
  - The International Olympic Committee Medical Commission put together a current concepts statement identifying risk factors for female athletes suffering ACL injury that include (a) being in the preovulatory phase of menstrual cycle as opposed to the postovulatory phase, (b) having decreased intercondylar notch width, and (c) developing increased knee abduction movement during impact on landing (34).
  - A prospective cohort study showed that high knee abduction movement during landing conferred increased risk of ACL injury (34). This suggests further that teaching good landing mechanics is important to reduce lower extremity injury in basketball players, particularly in females.
  - Several studies, mostly relatively small, have been done assessing the efficacy of improved landing mechanics with decreased peak tibial shear force, which is a measure of axial loading. These studies have shown that modified mechanics can decrease the risk of ACL injury without compromising performance (34–36).
  - The natural history of ACL tears is early degenerative arthritis to the affected knee. To avoid this, it is generally recommended for athletes to have ACL reconstruction using one of many accepted techniques (patellar autograft, cadaver graft, hamstring autograft, and the like). Return to play within 12 months is seen in 50%–75% of athletes' status post ACL repair, although the numbers tend to be lower in women, and up to two-thirds do not return to the preinjury level of competition (37). If patients are not expecting significant continued activity on the knee, there are times when rehabilitation and bracing are appropriate.

Ankle and Foot

- Ankle injuries make up 87% of lower extremity injuries and are the most common type seen in basketball (2). Inversion sprains to the anterior talofibular ligament comprise 66% of all ligamentous ankle injuries. Many injuries result from a player landing on another player's foot, putting centers and forwards at higher risk than guards.
- Ankle taping has been shown to prevent injury (38), but there is concern that the support from taping declines with time and activity.
- Lace-up and semirigid ankle braces have been shown by prospective trials to reduce incidence of ankle injury (hazard ratio, 0.32) but have not been shown to significantly reduce severity (12).
  - Many players do not like wearing ankle braces, but if given a week-long break-in period, there is no detriment to athletic performance and players feel comfortable (7).
- When considering radiographs for acute ankle injuries, the Ottawa ankle rules have a sensitivity of 98% for ankle fractures and should be used. Specificity of the rules varies greatly from 10% to 70% (39) (Table 89.3).

Table 89.3 Ottawa Foot and Ankle Rules

Ankle X-Rays Needed	Foot X-Rays Needed
Pain in the malleolar zone (tibia and fibula 6 cm above the articulation with the talus) AND any of the below findings: • Bony tenderness at posterior tip or edge of lateral malleolus • Bony tenderness at the posterior edge or tip of medial malleolus • Inability to bear weight both immediately and in the emergency department	Any pain in the midfoot AND any of the below findings: • Bony tenderness at the base of the fifth metatarsal • Bony tenderness at the navicular • Inability to bear weight both immediately and in the emergency department

- Ankle sprains should be treated with relative rest, NSAIDs, weight bearing as tolerated, ice, bracing, and physical therapy with a focus on regaining proprioception that helps prevent repetitive injury. Ankle instability is discussed in detail in Chapter 67, Ankle Instability.
- Navicular stress fractures are the most common stress fractures seen in jumping athletes and present with foot pain that is activity related and may persist to a lesser degree out of activity.
  - Bone scan or MRI is needed for diagnosis because plain films are inadequate.
  - Treatment involves immobilization and non–weight bearing until the navicular is nontender (18).

EVENT COVERAGE

- The majority of basketball games are played indoors; however, for those that take place in outdoor settings, it is important to consider environmental concerns (heat, cold, lightning, wind, etc.).
- Knee and ankle injuries are the most common injuries seen in basketball competitions and the covering physician should be prepared to evaluate and treat acute injuries.
- Lacerations are also very common; it is important that covering providers have supplies for laceration repair.
- Male African American basketball players are at the highest risk for sudden cardiac death; therefore, it is imperative to have a cardiac emergency action plan, and an automated external defibrillator accessible.

REFERENCES

1. Kingma J, ten Duis HJ. Sports members' participation in assessment of incidence rate of injuries in five sports from records of hospital-based clinical treatment. *Percept Mot Skills*. 1998;86(2):675–86.
2. Randazzo C, Nelson NG, McKenzie LB. Basketball-related injuries in school-aged children and adolescents in 1997–2007. *Pediatrics*. 2010;126(4):727–33.
3. Borowski LA, Yard EE, Fields SK, Comstock RD. The epidemiology of US high school basketball injuries, 2005–2007. *Am J Sports Med*. 2008;36(12):2328–35.
4. Stop Sports Injury. https://ncys.org/safety/stop-sports-injuries/. Accessed May 13, 2025.
5. Zynda AJ, Wagner KJ, Liu J, et al. Epidemiology of pediatric basketball injuries presenting to emergency departments: sex- and age-based patterns. *Orthop J Sports Med*. 2022;10(1):23259671211066503.
6. Andreoli CV, Chiaramonti BC, Buriel E, Pochini AC, Ejnisman B, Cohen M. Epidemiology of sports injuries in basketball: integrative systematic review. *BMJ Open Sport Exerc Med*. 2018;4(1):e000468.
7. National Collegiate Athletic Association. *NCAA Injury Surveillance System for All Sports*. Overland Park (KA): National Collegiate Athletic Association; 1998.
8. Caine D, DiFiori J, Maffulli N. Physeal injuries in children's and youth sports: reasons for concern? *Br J Sports Med*. 2006;40(9):749–60.
9. Jones NP. Eye injury in sport. *Sports Med*. 1989;7(3):163–81.
10. Borenstein DG, Wiesel SW, Boden SD. *Low Back Pain: Medical Diagnosis and Comprehensive Management*. Philadelphia (PA): WB Saunders; 1995. p. 735.
11. Powell J. Injury toll in prep sports estimated at 1.3 million. *Athl Train*. 1989;24:360–73.
12. McInnes SE, Carlson JS, Jones CJ, McKenna MJ. The physiological load imposed on basketball players during competition. *J Sport Sci*. 1995;13(5):387–97.
13. Asplund C. Treatment of hypertension in athletes: an evidence-based review. *Phys Sportsmed*. 2010;38(1):37–44.
14. Harmon KG, Asif IM, Klossner D, Drezner JA. Incidence of sudden cardiac death in national collegiate athletic association athletes. *Circulation*. 2011;123(15):1594–600.
15. Maron BJ, Doerer JJ, Haas TS, Tierney DM, Mueller FO. Sudden deaths in young competitive athletes: analysis of 1866 deaths in the United States, 1980–2006. *Circulation*. 2009;119(8):1085–92.
16. Maron BJ. Hypertrophic cardiomyopathy: a systematic review. *JAMA*. 2002;287(10):1308–20.
17. Judge DP, Dietz HC. Marfan's syndrome. *Lancet*. 2005;366(9501):1965–76.
18. Kerr IL. Mouth-guards for the prevention of injuries in contact sports. *Sports Med*. 1986;3(6):415–27.
19. Azodo CC, Odai CD, Osazuwa-Peters N, Obuekwe ON. A survey of orofacial injuries among basketball players. *Int Dent J*. 2011;61(1):43–6.
20. American Academy of Ophthalmology. *Protective Eyewear for Young Athletes*. Joint policy statement of the American Academy of Pediatrics and American Academy of Ophthalmology [Internet]; 2003. Available from: http://one.aao.org/CE/PracticeGuidelines/ClinicalStatements_Content.aspx?cid=1fda605b-97b9-47e3-90d1-11b7a9607797
21. Drakos MC, Domb B, Starkey C, Callahan L, Allen AA. Injury in the national basketball association: a 17-year overview. *Sports Health*. 2010;2(4):284–90.
22. Zagelbaum BM, Starkey C, Hersh PS, Donnenfeld ED, Perry HD, Jeffers JB. The National Basketball Association eye injury study. *Arch Ophthalmol*. 1995;113(6):749–52.
23. Cohenca N, Roges RA, Roges R. The incidence and severity of dental trauma in intercollegiate athletes. *J Am Dent Assoc*. 2007;138(8):1121–6.
24. Kvittem B, Hardie NA, Roettger M, Conry J. Incidence of orofacial injuries in high school sports. *J Public Health Dent*. 1998;58(4):288–93.
25. Spinas E, Savasta A. Prevention of traumatic dental lesions: cognitive research on the role of mouthguards during sport activities in paediatric age. *Eur J Paediatr Dent*. 2007;8(4):193–8.
26. McKay GD, Goldie PA, Payne WR, Oakes BW, Watson LF. A prospective study of injuries in basketball: a total profile and comparison by gender and standard of competition. *J Sci Med Sport*. 2001;4(2):196–211.

27. Wilson RL, McGinty LD. Common hand and wrist injuries in basketball players. *Clin Sports Med.* 1993;12(2):265–91.
28. Zvijac J, Thompson W. Basketball. In: Caine CG, Lindner KJ, eds. *Epidemiology of Sports Injuries.* Champaign (IL): Human Kinetics; 1996. p. 86–97.
29. Micheo W. Head and face considerations. In: McKeag DB, ed. *Olympic Handbook of Sports Medicine: Basketball.* Oxford (UK): Blackwell; 2003.
30. Gomez E, DeLee JC, Farney WC. Incidence of injury in Texas girls' high school basketball. *Am J Sports Med.* 1996;24(5):684–7.
31. Messina DF, Farney WC, DeLee JC. The incidence of injury in Texas high school basketball. A prospective study among male and female athletes. *Am J Sports Med.* 1999;27(3):294–9.
32. Arendt EA, Agel J, Dick R. Anterior cruciate ligament injury patterns among collegiate men and women. *J Athl Train.* 1999;34(2):86–92.
33. Khan K. Lower extremity considerations. In: McKeag D, ed. *Olympic Handbook of Sports Medicine: Basketball.* Oxford (UK): Blackwell; 2003.
34. Renstrom P, Ljungqvist A, Arendt E, et al. Non-contact ACL injuries in female athletes: an International Olympic Committee current concepts statement. *Br J Sports Med.* 2008;42(6):394–412.
35. Lim BO, Lee YS, Kim JG, An KO, Yoo J, Kwon YH. Effects of sports injury prevention training on the biomechanical risk factors of anterior cruciate ligament injury in high school female basketball players. *Am J Sports Med.* 2009;37(9):1728–34.
36. Myers CA, Hawkins D. Alterations to movement mechanics can greatly reduce anterior cruciate ligament loading without reducing performance. *J Biomech.* 2010;43(14):2657–64.
37. Ardern CL, Webster KE, Taylor NF, Feller JA. Return to the preinjury level of competitive sport after anterior cruciate ligament reconstruction surgery: two-thirds of patients have not returned by 12 months after surgery. *Am J Sports Med.* 2011;39(3):538–43.
38. Garrick JG, Requa RK. Role of external support in the prevention of ankle sprains. *Med Sci Sports.* 1973;5(3):200–3.
39. Bachmann LM, Kolb E, Koller MT, Steurer J, ter Riet G. Accuracy of Ottawa ankle rules to exclude fractures of the ankle and mid-foot: systematic review. *BMJ.* 2003;326(7386):417.

90 Boxing

Kevin deWeber and Curtis Papenfuss

INTRODUCTION

- Boxing is a contest between two competitors matched for gender, age group, and weight in which the objective is to land punches using gloved hands to the face, head, or frontal torso of the opponent.
  - The victor is determined by either bout stoppage by a referee for injury or domination or by the total of three judges' scores at the end of the bout.
  - Boxing places extreme demands on the musculoskeletal and cardiovascular systems and requires immense mental toughness.
  - The injuries incurred are broad and can range from minor to life-threatening.

LEVELS OF PARTICIPATION

- Amateur and professional boxing have some similarities but many differences (Table 90.1).
- While the overall objective is the same, the rules and equipment differ.
  - Nearly all amateurs must wear headguards, whereas professionals do not.
  - Professionals' gloves tend to be lighter in weight.
  - Professional bouts have more rounds of longer duration.

EPIDEMIOLOGY

- Injury epidemiology for amateur boxing is based on high-level data, whereas that for professionals is limited to a few cohort studies.
- The most injured body region in boxing is head/face/neck, followed by upper extremity (especially hand), lower extremity, and trunk (Table 90.2).
- The predominant types of injury in competition are facial contusions, abrasions, and lacerations, whereas in training, they are sprains and strains (1).
- Training constitutes the vast majority of time in boxing since competition bouts are infrequent and are of relatively short duration.
- Injury rates are markedly higher in competition, and higher in professional boxers than in amateurs.
  - The competition injury rate in amateurs is 54.7 per 1000 athlete exposures compared to 170–230 per 1000 in professionals (1–4).
  - Injury risk factors include male gender, increasing age, and higher weight class (5).
  - The higher rates of injury in professional competitions are due to longer bouts, higher boxer skill, higher threshold for referee bout stoppage, and absence of headguards.
- The incidence of concussion and other types of acute traumatic brain injury (TBI) in amateur boxing has not been well studied. About 11% of injuries in professional bouts are concussions (3).
- There is no good-quality evidence of association between amateur boxing and chronic TBI (6).
- A link between professional boxing and chronic TBI is likely, but the risk is markedly reduced with modern rules and regulations.
  - Risk factors include longer career, higher age, higher number of bouts and of knockouts, and genetic factors (4).
- Death from boxing is a rare event.
- During professional competition, facial lacerations are the most common injury, comprising about 60% of injuries (3). Headguards in amateurs make facial laceration a rarity.
- Eye trauma is common in professional boxing (30% of injuries) but uncommon in amateurs. Injuries are usually minor (corneal abrasion, subconjunctival hemorrhage, lid and periocular swelling), but vision-threatening ocular injuries such as retinal tear or detachment, cataract, macular lesions, angle injuries, and globe rupture rarely occur.
- Renal contusion, splenic or hepatic injury, and commotio cordis are documented but rare.

SPECIFIC RULES

- Rules for professional boxing vary by state and by promotion (*e.g.*, World Boxing Association and World Boxing Council). The common goal is to make the sport relatively safe, fair, and competitive for all participants.
  - Professional matchmakers strive to match competitors by gender, weight class, experience, and skill level.

Table 90.1 Comparison of Amateur and Professional Boxing

Issue	Amateur	Professional
Governing bodies and rules	USA Boxing, IBA (formerly AIBA)	States, tribes, and countries have their own sanctioning bodies, and rules may be influenced somewhat by promotion (*e.g.*, WBA, WBO, WBC, IBF)
Bout duration	3 rounds of 1.5–3 min, depending on age	4–12 rounds of 3 min, depending on skill
Headguards	Required for all, except elite men (18 and older) in national or international competition	Not allowed
Mouthguards	Required	Required
Gloves	10, 12, or 16 oz depending on weight and age	8 or 10 oz, depending on weight and jurisdiction
Scoring	Three judges, weighted by scoring blows	Three judges, weighted by damage more than scoring
Referee stoppage	Tends to be earlier	Tends to be later
Physician stoppage	Allowed	Permission varies by jurisdiction
Medical suspension after bout	Standardized based on type of stoppage (*e.g.*, knockout, stoppage for head blows)	Minimum durations vary by state and may be lengthened based on physician judgment
Risk of cTBI or CTE	No evidence of link	Low-quality evidence of link

cTBI, chronic traumatic brain injury; CTE, chronic traumatic encephalopathy; IBA, International Boxing Association; IBF, International Boxing Federation; WBA, World Boxing Association; WBC, World Boxing Council; WBF, World Boxing Federation; WBO, World Boxing Organization.

- Rounds are 3 minutes in duration with 4–12 rounds per bout. See Table 90.2.

- Rules for amateur boxing are governed by USA Boxing and International Boxing Association, which govern US and international boxing, respectively.
- Rounds are 1.5–3 minutes long depending on age, and there are 3 rounds per bout. See http://www.usaboxing.org for latest rulebook.
- Equipment: Mouthguards are universally required and should be custom made and tightly fitting on the upper teeth (7).
- Groin guards are required for males to protect the testicles. Properly fitting boxing shoes and gloves are required.
- Glove weight ranges from 10 to 16 ounces and is determined mainly by weight class and amateur/professional designation. Heavier gloves reduce the impact due to their more absorptive nature, leading to less severe injury.
- Headguards are currently required for amateurs except for elite (adult) males in national and international competition. Headguards markedly reduce the risk of lacerations but have not been proven to reduce concussion or other TBI. They also lead to increased risk-taking in boxers, leading to more blows absorbed (8).
- Licensing requirements: Amateur boxers must undergo a comprehensive preparticipation physical evaluation (PPE) annually by a physician. Professional boxing license requirements vary by state but usually include annual PPE and optometric examination and testing for blood-borne infections.
  - Neuroimaging is required in some states for professional boxing. The Association of Ringside Physicians recommends brain magnetic resonance imaging (MRI) at initial licensing in all professional boxers, plus either CT angiogram or magnetic resonance angiogram in boxers 40 years and older.
  - MRI should be repeated at a minimum of every 3 years provided initial/previous imaging had no abnormalities.
  - Imaging should be repeated sooner for any neurocognitive or neurological decline from baseline or prior to the next bout if a boxer sustained a significant head impact exposure (in competition/training) that poses a risk for TBI (9).

Table 90.2 Injury Rates by Body Region in Boxing

Body Region	Amateur Training (%)	Amateur Competition (%)	Professional Training (%)	Professional Competition (%)
Head/Neck	10	73	74–96	71–86
Upper extremity	49	24	0–22	8–22
Lower extremity	23	3	0–2	1.5
Trunk	17	3	0	2

Data taken from Refs. 1–5.

MUSCULOSKELETAL INJURIES

- Sprains and strains are most common during training and occur primarily in the upper extremities though they may also be seen in the lower extremities and trunk.
- Fractures of the nose, face, or teeth comprise about 3% of professional boxing injuries. They are exceedingly rare in amateurs. Hand fractures are rare.
- Dislocations of the shoulder are rare.

Responsibilities of the Ringside Physician

- Prevention and treatment of acute injuries is the primary role of the ringside physician. This is accomplished through a sound medical plan to cover all aspects of the event — the precompetition phase, the ringside observation, and the postbout examination.
- All boxing events are required to have a physician physically present at ringside to allow bouts to occur. One physician per ring is usually sufficient for amateur events.
  - Two or more physicians are recommended for professional events because injuries may be more severe. This also assures that bouts (which may be televised) can continue on schedule with physician supervision at ringside if one physician must leave the area to perform an evaluation or provide treatment.
- The ringside physician(s) should be seated at or close to ringside with an unobstructed view of the ring and quick access to the ring stairs.
- The ringside physician must evaluate the competition site prior to the first bout. An area for prebout and postbout assessments should be designated in advance. This area should be secure, easily accessible, quiet, well-lit, with enough room for a table, a few chairs, and medical equipment and should be easily accessible by the ambulance crew if transportation to a higher level of care is needed.
- Recommended items for the ringside physician include:
  - Blood pressure cuff, stethoscope, thermometer, and penlight for prebout examinations
  - Gauze pads, penlight, and disposable examination gloves for in-ring evaluations
  - Other supplies that would be carried in a typical team physician medical bag should optimally be available nearby, usually in the postbout examination area
- The ringside physician must identify the nearest emergency room with neurosurgical, ophthalmologic, and dental capabilities. Emergency medical service phone numbers and directions to urgent care centers and hospitals should be obtained in advance.
- On-site ambulance is also universally required for professional events.
  - Emergency medical system (EMS) personnel should have oxygen and face mask, as well as cardiac resuscitation equipment and appropriate equipment for spinal stabilization, including cervical collar and an extrication device, which may be a long spine board, scoop stretcher, vacuum mattress, or similar device depending on the jurisdiction.
  - On-site physicians and EMS personnel should review the available equipment and emergency action plan prior to the beginning of the event.

EVENT COVERAGE

- The prebout physical examination should be conducted on the day of competition. All boxers will have already completed a comprehensive licensing PPE and have been ascertained by the promoter and/or sanctioning jurisdiction to be cleared from any prior medical suspensions. Therefore the prebout examination should primarily ascertain that the athlete is fully capable to box — neurologically intact, afebrile, free of acute illness, not under the influence of medications, and free of significant injury.
- The examination should begin with vital signs including blood pressure, pulse, and temperature. It should also include, at a minimum, evaluation for any neurologic condition or musculoskeletal injury that could compromise self-defense. The exam should also include auscultation of the heart and lungs, palpation of the abdomen for organomegaly, inspection of the skin for lesions consistent with contagious disease, as well as a brief neurological assessment, including inspection of the eyes for physiological anisocoria.
  - Examples of disqualifying conditions in the prebout examination are listed in Box 90.1.

Ringside Care (11)

- Close observation during action. The physician's role is to closely observe the individual boxers, looking for injuries or signs of distress during and between rounds.
  - Effective defense is necessary for safety and its absence mandates cessation of a contest. Early signs of a lapse in defense and of the onset of fatigue are lowered punch counts, lowered arms, staggering, or running.
  - Observation of cumulative trauma is also important. Facial swelling, cuts, and epistaxis can lead to impaired vision and mouth breathing, making the boxer susceptible to significant head trauma. The experienced referee will provide a level of safety by closely observing the boxers, administering standing eight counts, and alerting the physician when there is a concern. If the referee is concerned, the ringside physician should be alert and ready to render care.
- Observation between rounds. If there is concern, the physician may "mount the apron" (climb the stairs to the small margin of standing area outside the ropes) and listen to what is being said by the corners (a boxer's coaches and attendants).

90.1 Examples of Disqualifying Conditions on Prebout Physical Examination

- Severe hypertension (SBP ≥ 160 or DBP ≥ 100 in adults despite rest and repeat measurements) (10)
- Fever over 100.4 °F
- Neurological or mental status impairment from drugs or alcohol
- Unresolved symptoms from past concussion
- Acute bacterial or herpetic skin infection
- Facial lacerations that have not completed at least 4 weeks of healing
- Fractures that have not completed required treatment and rehabilitation
- Musculoskeletal conditions that compromise joint range of motion
- Acute respiratory illness causing reduced lung functions (*e.g.*, acute asthma)
- Cardiac arrhythmia
- Liver or spleen enlargement

NOTE: This is not a comprehensive list. Physician judgment should be used. DBP, diastolic blood pressure; SBP, systolic blood pressure.

  - The physician can also go into the ring and stand behind the corners if a closer inspection is required. Physicians should avoid treatment of injuries between rounds.
  - Only "corners" or "cutmen" are allowed to treat injuries between rounds; treatment methods are limited to towels/gauze, cold compression, petroleum jelly, topical epinephrine, and thrombin.
  - Do not interfere in the coaching and treatment taking place during the 1 minute between rounds; this time belongs to the corners.
- Care during action. The physician enters the ring to evaluate an upright boxer during action only at the referee's request. This should occur during a time out or after bout stoppage. However, in the case of a knockout, loss of consciousness, or serious injury, the physician can immediately enter the ring without the referee's request.
- Some jurisdictions allow professional bout stoppage by the ringside physician, whereas some do not. Any amateur bout may be stopped by the ringside physician.
- When entering the ring during the action, the physician should enter calmly, quickly, and confidently, carrying gauze and penlight and wearing exam gloves. They should quickly evaluate the boxer's general condition and any specific injuries without providing treatment (other than wiping blood briefly to evaluate location of lacerations) and promptly render a return-to-play decision to the referee. This should optimally take about 10–30 seconds. If no serious conditions are present, the bout can resume.
- Conditions requiring bout stoppage
  - Loss of consciousness, altered mental status, or obvious concussion
  - Nasal fracture causing airway obstruction or open nasal or facial fracture
  - Loss of vision in one eye for any reason (*e.g.*, hematoma, globe injury, heavy bleeding)
  - Laceration affecting delicate structures such as lacrimal duct, eyelid tarsal plate or lid tissue adjacent to it, or those with exposed cartilage
  - Musculoskeletal injury causing markedly impaired defensive ability
  - Obvious mandible or maxilla fractures
  - A boxer or coach does not want the bout to continue (a corner can "throw in the towel" to request bout stoppage)
- Management of a downed or unconscious boxer
  - The physician should enter the ring quickly and confidently and if the boxer is unconscious, stabilize the cervical spine and, if required, open the airway with a jaw thrust maneuver.
  - Boxers usually regain consciousness quickly without further stimulation. If unconsciousness persists longer than about 60 seconds, the physician should signal the EMS crew to bring emergency equipment including equipment for spinal stabilization, airway equipment, and oxygen into the ring to immediately begin airway support and prepare for transportation to a hospital.
  - Once conscious, the physician should evaluate the boxer's motor function, speech, orientation, and pupillary reaction. When the boxer is moving all extremities and cervical spine injury has been excluded, they should be allowed to sit upright for a few moments. If recovery progresses well, transition the boxer to seated position on the canvas, then to a stool, then to standing, and then help the boxer walk to their corner. Accompany the boxer to the postbout medical area and continue to monitor.
  - Boxers displaying postconcussion seizures, repetitive vomiting, focal neurologic deficits, ataxia, increasing headache, or worsening mental status or cognition should be emergently transported to a hospital via ambulance.
  - If no signs of deterioration are present, the boxer may be released to the supervision of the coach, family, or a responsible adult. They should be instructed regarding where to take the boxer if they display any decline in physical or cognitive function, and it is important to stress the importance of follow-up evaluation and care if concussion has been diagnosed.
- Postbout examination (12)
  - Each boxer must be examined immediately after the bout, whether injury is initially suspected or not.
  - For amateur bouts without obvious injury, a quick evaluation can be performed at ringside after the boxer exits the ring.

- For all professional bouts — and any amateurs requiring a more thorough evaluation — the boxers should be taken to the predetermined medical area away from ringside and crowd.
  - Do not let an event official concerned with keeping the show on schedule prevent a careful evaluation.
- The examination should include observation of gait, speech, and cognition. A quick survey of the face, head, mouth, and upper extremities should be performed; the mouthguard and gloves must be removed and hand wraps cut off.
- Complete any forms required by the sanctioning body to document injuries and any mandatory suspension. Each jurisdiction has different medical suspension duration guidelines based on number of rounds competed or type of bout stoppage, but these durations can be lengthened based on physician judgment.
  - For amateur bouts under USA Boxing rules, suspension durations are predetermined by the type of bout stoppage. For instance, the minimum restriction period for any bout ending by head blows is 30 days of no sparring or competition (13).
  - See latest version of *USA Boxing Medical Handbook* for a complete list of suspensions: https://www.teamusa.org/USA-Boxing/Rulebook/Medical-Handbook.

REFERENCES

1. Alevras AJ, Fuller JT, Mitchell R, Lystad RP. Epidemiology of injuries in amateur boxing: a systematic review and meta-analysis. *J Sci Med Sport.* 2022;25:995–1001.
2. Bledsoe GH, Li G, Levy F. Injury risk in professional boxing. *South Med J.* 2005;98(10):994–8.
3. Zazryn TR, McCrory PR, Cameron PA. Injury rates and risk factors in competitive professional boxing. *Clin J Sport Med.* 2009;19(1):20–5.
4. Zazryn TR, Cameron PA, McCrory PR. A prospective cohort study of injury in amateur and professional boxing. *Br J Sports Med.* 2006;40(8):670–4.
5. Loosemore M, Lightfoot J, Palmer-Green D, Gatt I, Bilzon J, Beardsley C. Boxing injury epidemiology in the Great Britain team: a 5-year surveillance study of medically diagnosed injury incidence and outcome. *Br J Sports Med.* 2015;49(17):1100–7.
6. Loosemore M, Knowles CH, Whyte GP. Amateur boxing and risk of chronic traumatic brain injury: systematic review of observational studies. *BMJ.* 2007;335(7624):809.
7. deWeber K, Hindagolla V. Mouth guard use in combat sports. A position statement from the association of ringside physicians. *J Combat Sports.* 2022;4(1). https://ringsidearp.org/wp-content/uploads/2022/06/Mouth-Guard-Position-Paper-2021_b.pdf
8. deWeber K, Parlee L, Nguyen A, Lenihan MW, Goedecke L. Headguard use in combat sports: position statement of the Association of Ringside Physicians. *Phys Sportsmed.* 2024 Jun;52(3):229–38.
9. Sethi N, Neidecker J. Neuroimaging in professional combat sports: consensus statement from the Association of Ringside Physicians. *Phys Sportsmed.* 2022;13:1–8.
10. deWeber K, Ota KS, Dye C. Pre-bout hypertension in the combat sports athlete: clearance recommendations. *Phys Sportsmed.* 2022;12:1–7.
11. Sethi N, Bascharon R. Medical evaluation of a fighter during a competition. In: *Association of Ringside Physician's Manual of Combat Sports Medicine.* Vol A7. Union City (NJ): Writer's Republic; 2022. p. 97–106.
12. Davidson J, Hoang V, Bascharon R. Post-fight protocols and procedures. In: *Association of Ringside Physician's Manual of Combat Sports Medicine.* Vol A8. Union City (NJ): Writer's Republic; 2022. p. 107–12.
13. *USA Boxing Medical Handbook for Ringside Physicians.* Updated2021Oct 3. p. 14–5. Available from: https://www.teamusa.org/USA-Boxing/Rulebook/Medical-Handbook. Last accessed 2022 Dec 19.

Mixed Martial Arts

91

Stephanie F. Alessi-LaRosa and Michael B. Schwartz

INTRODUCTION

- Mixed martial arts (MMA) is the fastest-growing segment of combat sports — contests that are won solely on the basis of causing direct injury to the opponent.
- Participants vary in age, weight, gender, and fighting styles, which can present a challenge for the ringside physician.
- Common styles of MMA combat include wrestling, boxing, kickboxing, Brazilian jiu-jitsu, karate, bare knuckle and Muay Thai.
- There are both amateur and professional classifications but no unified governing body for the sport. Currently, independent organizations govern their own athletes. However, medical requirements for participation are based on individual jurisdictions without any uniform guidelines.
- The safety of the contest is heavily dependent on the competence of the ringside physician.

RULES AND REGULATIONS (1)

- MMA contests consist of between three and five rounds, lasting 3–5 minutes each.
- The contest may be held in a cage or standard boxing ring.
- A contest may end by knockout, technical knockout, or submission, a process by which a fighter taps either his opponent or the mat three times to signify that they concede the match.
- It is imperative that ringside physicians have the authority to end a contest at any time if they believe a fighter is too severely injured to continue. However, this is not a standard rule and should be explored by the physician before agreeing to participate in an event.

RINGSIDE PHYSICIAN'S ROLE

- The responsibilities of the ringside physician are best divided into three phases: prefight, ringside, and post fight.

Prefight Responsibilities

- The preparticipation examination (PPE) is a vital aspect in determining fitness, preventing deaths, and minimizing injuries.
- The PPE consists of multiple evaluations including:
  - Review of previous fight results when available.
  - Proposed weight loss based on information included on the fighter's physical examination.
  - Collection and analysis of prefight medical requirements (Table 91.1). The medical requirements listed were developed by the American Association of Professional Ringside Physicians and the Association of Boxing Commissions.
  - Medical history
  - Physical examination
- The medical history should begin with completion of a simple but comprehensive medical history and exam.
- The standard PPE for athletics is described in Chapter 18. But unique to MMA-questions specifically related to a history of laser-assisted in situ keratomileusis (LASIK) surgery or cataracts should be noted.
- Physical examination: The prefight examination allows the ringside physician an opportunity to identify potential physical limitations.
- The examination must be brief and focused. Variation from these criteria may lead to disqualification. Essential elements include:

Table 91.1 Preparticipation Medical Requirements for Mixed Martial Arts

Medical Requirements	Interval of Time
CT scan/MRI brain scan	Baseline
Dilated eye exam (ophthalmologist)	1 yr
Hepatitis B surface antigen, hepatitis C antibody, HIV blood testing	180 d
CT, MRI, or complete neurologic exam	1 yr
Electrocardiogram (with interpretation)	Initial only (if normal)
Complete history and physical examination	1 yr (commission approved form)
Final prefight mini-physical	At the venue
Serum or urine pregnancy test	14 d
Complete gynecologic examination	6 mo

CT, computed tomography; HIV, human immunodeficiency virus; MRI, magnetic resonance imaging.

- Vital signs: blood pressure <140/100 mm Hg, pulse <100, afebrile.
- Skin: look for surgical or traumatic scars, rashes
- Visual acuity: <20/40 bilaterally near or <20/100 distant
- Eyes: signs of radial keratotomy or LASIK procedures, cataracts
- Ears: ruptured tympanic membranes
- Nose: rhinitis, deviation
- Throat/glands: exudate, lymphadenopathy
- Respiratory: prolonged expiration, wheezing
- Cardiac: arrhythmias, murmurs
- Abdominal: distension, tenderness
- Genitourinary: hernias, testicular exam
- Musculoskeletal: range of motion, joint deformities
- Neurologic: pupils, fundi, cognitive, motor, cerebellar, sensory

- Female fighters:
  - Have female present
  - Previous surgeries including breast augmentation
  - On-site urine pregnancy testing
- Special considerations include:
  - Copied medical reports: The physician must be alert to falsified documents.
  - Rapid weight loss: This is a major problem in MMA because of significantly fewer weight classes compared to boxing. Cutting weight rapidly may lead to hyperthermia, arrhythmia, seizures, renal failure, rhabdomyolysis, or death.
  - Electrocardiogram (ECG): Many athletes have ECG tracings that may appear abnormal, which may be due to genetics, habitus, or athletics-related changes in their hearts. A comparative study is important along with an echocardiogram and/or additional testing (exercise stress test, cardiopulmonary exercise testing, cardiac MRI, etc.) as indicated.
  - Radial keratotomy: Can result in traumatic rupture of the cornea.
  - LASIK: May result in dislocation of the corneal flap; a history of photorefractive keratectomy (PRK) is acceptable
  - Breast implants: May deflate or rupture with trauma.

Ringside Responsibilities

- Arrive at least 1.5–2 hours before the first bout.
- Inspect the ring/cage. Be sure the physicians working at ringside have easy access to the ring/cage. Physicians should familiarize themselves with how the cage entry mechanisms operate. Two physicians (Minimum) should be present at the ringside for each contest.
- Meet with the emergency medical services (EMS) personnel. No bout should be held without availability of an ambulance. If an ambulance must leave, the fight should be delayed until it is replaced.
- Emergency equipment should be stored under the ring, thus allowing for easy access. Necessary items include:
  - Backboard
  - Emergency kit with resuscitation equipment including: AED, bag-valve mask, oropharyngeal and nasopharyngeal airways, mask, and rigid cervical collars as well as a method for spinal motion control and extrication and transfer of an athlete with potential spinal injury (*i.e.*, long spine board, scoop stretcher, or vacuum mattress. The kit should also have gloves, gauze, a blood pressure cuff, ophthalmoscope, and otoscope.
  - Oxygen tank with appropriate tubing and mask
- Communication among the physicians and referees at ringside is imperative. The physicians should meet with the referees beforehand to discuss where each physician will be located at ringside in the event that the referee would like consultation during the fight.
- Emergency action plan and plans for emergency egress should be prearranged in advance, taking into consideration the potential for confusion at ringside.
- Referees are essential to the success of the contest, and all participating referees should have their blood pressure and pulse checked before the fights begin. Upper limits of 150/100 for blood pressure are generally acceptable.
- At ringside, a physician should have gloves, gauze, a penlight, and a stethoscope on their person at all times.
- During MMA competitions where the fighters may be grappling on the mat for an extended period of time, maintaining visibility is crucial. The physician should not hesitate to move around to get a better view of the action. The jumbotron, monitor, or other projection device in the arena, can often be a useful means of observing a fighter's activity.
- "Tapping out" provides an honorable way for an MMA combatant to end a match. Experienced participants know when they are helpless and will not hesitate to tap out. Less experienced, amateur combatants require careful attention when they are subject to a chokehold in particular; often they will not tap out and may lose consciousness.
- The most difficult ringside decision is whether the fight should continue. This decision can be made at several points during the contest:
- During a round:
  - A fighter's inability to adequately protect him/herself from an opponent's attacks, along with loss of coordinated footwork and punching, is indicative of brain injury.
  - Lacerations near the eye may cause bleeding or damage to surrounding nerves, which may lead to obstructed vision.
  - Repeated kicks/trauma to the lateral knee may cause foot drop due to the common fibular nerve location leading to difficulty walking and excessive tripping/falling.
- Time out:
  - The referee may choose to call a timeout and ask the physician to evaluate the fighter based on suspicion of injury.

This evaluation should last no more than a few seconds to determine if the fight should continue.

- Between rounds:
  - In the corner, between rounds, is a perfect time to chat with the fighter and his corner man. Asking the fighter and corner people if they wish to continue is important. The fighter should respond to questions quickly, clearly, and accurately. Pupillary response and extraocular movements should also be assessed at this time.

Post-fight Evaluation

- After each bout, both fighters must be examined. The examination should take place in a private area. Having three physicians at ringside allows for one to perform a detailed examination while the next fight begins.
- The examination should include observation of the fighter's gait, ability to converse, pupillary examination, and examination of the hands and any areas suspected of injury based on the action during the bout.
- EMS personnel should accompany the physician in case emergency transport is required.
- Referral to a medical center is indicated for:
  - Brain or spinal injury
  - Musculoskeletal injuries requiring immobilization or assisted ambulation
  - Difficulty breathing
  - Severe fatigue or dehydration
  - Severe lacerations
- Documentation of the post-fight examination is important to determine any medical suspensions necessary. The fighter should sign off on the exam after any findings have been explained.
- Directions to a local trauma center and head injury instructions should be provided in the event that symptoms develop later that night.

MMA INJURIES

- Although MMA has been promoted as a ruthless "blood" sport, a recent study evaluated injuries incurred during competition and found an overall incidence rate of 22.9–28.6 per 100 bouts.
- Head and face injuries are more common in the striking predominant styles of MMA participation (boxing, karate, Muay Thai), whereas the joint injuries are more common in the grappling predominant styles (Brazilian jiu-jitsu, judo, wrestling) (2).
- The distribution of injuries is best described by a meta-analysis published in 2014 that reviewed studies of MMA injuries from multiple study databases up to May 2013. The study encompassed an overall incidence rate of 228.7 per 1000 athlete exposures. Most frequent injuries were those of the head and accounted for 66.8%–78.0% with wrist/hand injuries next at a rate of 6%–12%. The injuries included lacerations, fractures, and concussions (3).
- Although concussions are less common in MMA compared with boxing, a high level of vigilance on the part of the ringside physician is imperative. The evaluation and treatment of head injuries is covered in Chapter 48.

REFERENCES

1. Mohegan Tribe Department of Athletic Regulation. *Rules and Regulations Regarding Boxing and Mixed Martial Arts*. Uncasville (CT): Mohegan Tribe Department of Athletic Regulation; 2022 Jun 30.
2. Jensen AR, Maciel RC, Petrigliano FA, Rodriguez JP, Brooks AG. Injuries sustained by the mixed martial arts athlete. *Sports Health*. 2017;9(1):64–9.
3. Lystad RP, Gregory K, Wilson J. The epidemiology of injuries in mixed martial arts: a systematic review and meta-analysis. *Orthop J Sports Med*. 2014;2(1):2325967113518492.

92 Cheerleading

Luke Zabawa and Mark Hutchinson

INTRODUCTION

- Cheerleading is one of the most popular sports in the United States, with more than 3 million participants annually (1).
  - However, only 29 state high school athletic associations recognize cheerleading as a sport (2).
- The National Collegiate Athletic Association (NCAA) does not include competitive cheerleading as a sponsored sport.
  - This limits access to safety resources and regulations, certified athletic trainers, team physicians, and mandated preparticipation physical examinations.
- Cheerleading competitions are held at regional and national levels, and training is a year-round activity.
- Cheerleaders perform through three seasons, then peak for national competitions in the spring.
  - This constant "in-season" state limits appropriate time for recuperation or conditioning, which in turn magnifies the risk of overuse injuries (3).
- Routines can include gymnastic elements, tumbling runs, partner stunts, pyramid formations, and dance routines.
- The sport requires that all extremities be completely functional for stunts and tumbling runs.
  - Cheerleaders often lift a partner, perform a tumbling run, perform a dance routine, and balance atop a pyramid — all within the span of a few minutes.
- Despite the indisputable risks of cheerleading, the sport receives less attention in the medical literature compared with other sports of similar or lower risk level (4).
  - A lack of awareness of the physical demands of the sport may contribute to the limited cheerleading-related research, with multiple studies incorrectly characterizing cheerleading as a noncontact, individual (as opposed to team) sport (5,6).

CHEERLEADING-SPECIFIC ISSUES AND RULES

Definitions (7)

- Base — A person who is in direct contact with the performing surface and is supporting another person's weight
- Cradle — Dismount from a stunt/pyramid/toss in which the top person lands in a face-up, semipiked position
- Cupie/awesome — A stunt in which both of the top person's feet are in one hand of the base
- Dive roll — An aerial forward roll where the feet of the performer are at or above the performer's waist prior to the hands making contact with the performing surface
- Flatback — A stunt in which the top person is in a face-up, straight-body position parallel to the performing surface
- Flip — When a person is airborne while the feet pass over the head
- Height-increasing apparatus — Any type of equipment that increases the height of a skill
- Inverted/inversion — A body position where the shoulders are below the waist
- Loading position — Any intermediate position below shoulder level that uses continuous motion to put a top person in a stunt or pyramid
- Middle — A person who is being supported by a base while also supporting a top person
- Primary weight — Fifty percent or more of a top person's weight (*e.g.*, a middle layer holding the foot of a hitched leg would not be considered primary weight)
- Pyramid — A skill in which a top person is being supported by a middle layer person
- Rewind — Skill in which the top person starts with at least one foot on the ground, is tossed into the air, and performs a forward, backward, or side flip into a stunt, pyramid, loading position, or cradle
- Spotter — A person who is responsible for assisting or catching the top person in a partner stunt or pyramid. This person cannot be in a position of providing primary support for a top person but must be in a position to protect the top person coming off of a stunt or pyramid.
- Stunt — A skill in which a top person is supported by a base or bases

USA Cheer General Restrictions (7)

- The use of any height-increasing apparatus (*e.g.*, mini-trampoline, etc.) other than a spring floor is prohibited for performance.

- The top person in a partner stunt, pyramid, or transition cannot be released from bases or leave the floor unassisted with the intent to land or be caught in an inverted body position.
- An individual may not jump, flip, or dive over, under, or through partner stunts, pyramids, or individuals from basket tosses, similar tosses, partner stunts, or other tosses from hands.
- Drops (knee, seat, thigh, front, back, and split) from a jump, stand, or inverted position are prohibited unless most of the weight is first borne on the hands/feet, which breaks the impact of the drop.
- Soft-soled athletic shoes must be worn while cheering or competing. Gymnastics shoes, jazz shoes, and/or boots are prohibited.
- Supports, braces, and soft casts that are unaltered from the manufacturer's original design/production do not require any additional padding. Supports/braces that have been altered from the manufacturer's original design/production must be padded with a closed-cell, slow-recovery foam padding no less than one-half inch thick if the participant is involved in partner stunts, pyramids, or tosses. A participant wearing a plaster cast or a walking boot must not be involved in partner stunts, pyramids, tosses, jumps, or tumbling.

Surface Restrictions (7)

- The following skills are only allowed on a mat, grass (real or artificial), or rubberized track surface:
  - Basket tosses, elevator/sponge tosses, and other similar multi-based tosses
  - Inversion releases from the ground or a skill (*e.g.*, handspring loads, hand-to-hand releases)
  - Flipping skills into or from stunts, tosses, or pyramids
  - Two and one-half high pyramids. Mounts or dismounts to and from 2 ½ high pyramids may not flip or twist on a rubberized track surface.
- At football games, kick double baskets and baskets that flip AND twist are only allowed during pregame or half-time situations while on grass (real or artificial) or a matted surface with dimensions of at least 10′ × 10′.
- At basketball, volleyball, and other indoor games, the following skills are prohibited for all timeouts (regardless of matting) and for pregame, half-time, or postgame performances without matting.
  - Basket tosses, elevator/sponge tosses, and other similar multi-based tosses.
  - Partner stunts in which the base uses only one arm to support the top person. Exception: Cupies/awesomes are allowed with an additional spotter.
  - Flips into or from partner stunts.
  - Inversions. Exception: High school level inversions are allowed. (For college, braced flips can be braced by single-based skills with a spotter).
  - Twisting dismounts greater than 1¼ rotation. Twisting dismounts up to 1¼ rotation on the court require an additional spotter.
  - Two and one-half person high pyramids
  - Airborne twisting and tumbling skills (Arabians, full twisting layouts, etc.) are allowed, along with cartwheels, roundoffs, and aerial cartwheels.
- At basketball, volleyball, and other indoor games during pregame, half-time, or postgame performances where sufficient matting is used, there are no additional restrictions to the standard rules. (Sufficient matting varies by skill. In general, there should be at least two to three feet of clearance between nontumbling skills and the edge of the mat.)

PHYSIOLOGY OF CHEERLEADING

- The physical fitness of a collegiate cheerleader is similar to that of any other college sport athlete (8).
  - The mean level of body fat is 15.5% for female subjects and 16.4% for male subjects.
  - VO_{2max} scores are 48.8 ± 6.6 $mL·kg^{-1}·min^{-1}$ for men and 40.7 ± 5.8 $mL·kg^{-1}·min^{-1}$ for women.
  - Bench press maximum scores are 102.7 ± 19.2 kg for men and 37.0 ± 7.7 kg for women.
  - Abdominal muscular endurance scores as determined by the total number of curl-ups performed nonstop without a break in form are 55.8 ± 24.0 for men and 64.7 ± 18.7 for women.
  - Men scored 40.3 ± 11.9 for the total number of push-ups performed nonstop without a break in form, and women scored 24.3 ± 7.6.
  - Isokinetic quadriceps strength (60° peak % body weight) results were 84.7 ± 21.8% for men and 75.1 ± 6.9% for women.

EPIDEMIOLOGY OF INJURIES

- In 2012, approximately 37,344 pediatric cheerleading-related injuries presented to emergency departments nationwide, corresponding to a rate of 64 injuries per 100,000 children and adolescents (9).
- Cheerleading presents a high risk of catastrophic injury (10–12).
- The number of catastrophic injuries related to cheerleading has increased from 1.5 per year from 1982 to 1992 to 4.8 per year from 2003 to 2009 (13).
- Rising incidence of catastrophic injury related to:
  - Increasing participation
  - Incorporation of more complex skills including pyramids, partner stunts, and tossing
  - Better reporting of injuries

- The overall injury rate in cheerleading across all age groups is 1.0 per 1,000 athletic exposures (14).
  - An athletic exposure is defined as 1 athlete participating in one practice or competition session.
- College cheerleaders have the highest injury rate (2.4), followed by elementary school (1.5), high school (0.9), all-star (0.8), middle school (0.5), and recreational (0.5) cheerleaders (15).
- The overall injury rate in high school cheerleading is lower than in other girls' high school sports (13).

MECHANISM

- The most common mechanisms of injury are:
  - Stunting (42%–60%) (14,16)
  - Basing/spotting (23%) (14)
  - Tumbling (14%–26%) (14)
  - Falls from heights (14%–25%) (14)
- Stunting accounts for 96% of concussions and closed-head injuries (14,16).
- Pyramid stunts are responsible for most head/neck injuries (50%–66%) (17).

TYPES OF INJURIES

- When all age groups are considered together, lower extremity injuries are most common (30%–37% of all cheerleading injuries), followed by injuries to the upper extremities (21%–26%), head/neck (16%–19%), and trunk (7%–17%) (13,14,16,18). Table 92.1 describes body parts injured by different team categories.
- Younger cheerleaders are more likely to experience upper extremity injuries (41 vs. 25% of all injuries for 6- to 11-year-olds vs. 12- to 17-year-olds, respectively) (14).
- Older cheerleaders are more likely to have lower extremity injuries (38% vs. 29% of all injuries for 12- to 17-year-olds vs 6- to 11-year-olds) (14). Table 92.2 describes injury types by different team categories.
- Incidence:
  - Sprains and strains are the most common types of injuries (48%–53% of all cheerleading injuries).
  - Abrasions/contusions/hematomas (13%–18%)
  - Fractures/dislocations (9%–16%)
  - Lacerations/punctures (4%)
  - Concussion/head injuries (3.5%–4%) (14)
- Sprain and strains are the most common injury to cause time loss from sport (3).
- There is a single case report of a cheerleader with a splenic rupture after being thrown in the air and caught by a fellow cheerleader in a cradle (19).
- Younger cheerleaders (5–11-year-olds) are 1.6 times more likely to suffer a fracture or dislocation compared with older cheerleaders (12–18-year-olds) (20).
- Older cheerleaders are 1.2 times more likely to suffer a sprain or strain than are younger cheerleaders (20).

HEAD INJURIES

- Concussion rates in cheerleading (0.06 per 1000 exposures) are relatively low compared with other girls' high school sports, such as soccer (0.36), basketball (0.16–0.21), lacrosse (0.20), softball (0.07–0.11), and field hockey (0.10) (21). Table 92.3 compares head injury and catastrophic injury rates between cheerleading and other sports.
- Concussion rates increase with age and competitive level, likely because of the increasing difficulty of stunts (14).
- From 2010 to 2019, the incidence of concussions and closed head injuries increased by 44%, and patients requiring hospital admission from a head injury increased by 118% (22).

Table 92.1 Body Part Injured by Team Category (16)

Body Part Injured	All Star (%)	Collegiate (%)	High School (%)	Middle School (%)	Recreation League (%)	Total (%)
Head	6	14	10	0	8	10
Face	33	13	17	11	23	19
Neck	7	6	12	22	15	10
Trunk	12	26	25	22	15	22
Upper extremity	23	18	15	33	8	17
Lower extremity	19	24	22	11	31	22

Adapted from Table 4, Shields BJ, Fernandez SA, Smith GA. Epidemiology of cheerleading stunt-related injuries in the United States. *J Athl Train*. 2009;44(6):586–94.

Table 92.2 Type of Injury by Team Category (16)

Type of Injury	All Star (%)	Collegiate (%)	High School (%)	Middle School (%)	Recreation League (%)	Total (%)
Abrasion, contusion, or hematoma	13	17	19	22	15	17
Concussion or closed head injury	1	13	6	0	8	7
Fracture or dislocation	12	10	9	0	8	9
Laceration or puncture	16	3	5	0	8	7
Strain or sprain	38	44	53	67	46	48
Other	20	13	9	11	15	12

Adapted from Table 4, Shields BJ, Fernandez SA, Smith GA. Epidemiology of cheerleading stunt-related injuries in the United States. *J Athl Train.* 2009;44(6):586–94.

CATASTROPHIC INJURIES

- From 1982 to 2009, the National Center for Catastrophic Sports Injury Research recorded 76 direct catastrophic injuries in high school cheerleaders and 34 in collegiate cheerleaders (13).
- Because of the much larger number of high school cheerleaders, the rate of catastrophic injuries was 5 times higher for collegiate versus high school cheerleaders (2.0 vs. 0.4 per 100,000 participants, respectively) (23).
- From 1982 to 2009, cheerleading accounted for 65.0% of all direct catastrophic injuries to girl athletes at the high school level and 70.8% at the college level (13).

RISK FACTORS FOR INJURY

- Higher body mass index (17)
- Previous injury (17)
- Cheering on harder surfaces (24)
- Performing stunts (17)
- Supervision by a coach with low level of training and experience (17)
- Critical height is defined as the approximate fall height below which a life-threatening injury would not be expected to occur.
  - Critical height is much higher for a landing mat on a foam floor (11 ft) and for a spring floor (10.5 ft) than for concrete or vinyl tile floor (0.5 ft) (24).
  - Critical heights for natural grass, artificial turf, and a wood gym floor are 3.5 ft, 4 ft, and 4.5 ft, respectively.
  - The most serious cheerleading injuries occur at or above the critical height for the surface on which the cheerleader is performing at the time of injury (25).

Prevention

- The American Association of Cheerleading Coaches and Advisors and the National Federation of State High School Associations have enacted rules and recommendations (26,27).
  - Required coaches training and certification
  - Proper strength and conditioning for all cheerleaders
  - Avoiding stunts and tumbling on hard surfaces
  - Specific rules for execution of technical skills

Table 92.3 Overall Injury Rates in Girls' High School Sports (13)

Sport	Overall Injury Rate (per 1000 Exposures)	Catastrophic Injury Rate (per 100 000 Exposures)
Cheerleading	0.9	0.50–1.62
Gymnastics	8.5	0.44
Soccer	5.3	0.03
Basketball	4.4	0.03
Field hockey	3.7	0.00
Softball	3.5	0.02
Volleyball	1.7	0.00

Adapted from Table 1, Mueller FO, Cantu RC. Catastrophic sports injury research. *27th Annual Report, Fall 1982–Spring 2009.* Chapel Hill, NC: National Center for Catastrophic Sport Injury Research; 2009.

- Rules for execution of technical skills:
  - Pyramid height limited to no more than two persons
  - Top cheerleaders must be supported by one or more bases in direct weight-bearing contact with the performing surface.
  - Bases must be stationary and maintain constant contact with suspended cheerleaders.
  - Basket toss should be limited to four throwers, the toss should start from ground level, and 1 thrower must be behind the flyer during the toss.
  - Spotters must be present for every person extended above shoulder level.
  - Suspended persons are not to be inverted or rotated on dismount.
- Cheerleaders supervised by coaches with the most education, qualifications, and training had a nearly 50% reduction in injury risk compared with cheerleaders supervised by coaches with the lowest amount of education, qualifications, and training (17).

SUMMARY

- Cheerleading should be designated a sport so that it is subject to rules and regulations set forth by a sport's governing body (28).
- Cheerleaders should have a preparticipation physical examination before participating in a cheerleading program and should have access to appropriate strength and conditioning programs (28).
- Cheerleaders should be trained in proper spotting techniques and should only attempt stunts after they have demonstrated appropriate skill progression and proficiency required to complete the stunt (28).
- Spotters and bases should have adequate upper body and core strength and balance to support flyers (28).
- Technical skills, such as pyramids, mounts, tosses, and tumbling, should not be performed on hard (*e.g.*, concrete, asphalt), wet, or uneven surfaces or surfaces with obstructions.
- Pyramids should not be more than two people high and should only be performed with spotters (28).
- Concussion protocols should be followed in response to a possible head injury.

REFERENCES

1. Outdoor Foundation. *2019 Outdoor Participation Report*. Accessed September 5, 2022.
2. National Federation of State High School Associations.
3. Hutchinson MR. Cheerleading injuries: patterns, prevention, case reports. *Phys Sportsmed*. 1997 Sep;25(9):83–96.
4. Bagnulo A. Cheerleading injuries: a narrative review of the literature. *J Can Chiropr Assoc*. 2012;56(4):292–8.
5. Pfister T, Pfister K, Hagel B, Ghali WA, Ronksley PE. The incidence of concussion in youth sports: a systematic review and meta-analysis. *Br J Sports Med*. 2016;50(5):292–7.
6. McCarthy MM, Bihl JH, Frank RM, Salem HS, McCarty EC, Comstock RD. Epidemiology of clavicle fractures among US high school athletes, 2008-2009 through 2016-2017. *Orthop J Sports Med*. 2019;7(7):2325967119861812.
7. USA Cheer. 2022-23 *USA Cheer College Cheer Rules*. Accessed September 5, 2022.
8. Thomas DQ, Seegmiller JG, Cook TL, Young BA. Physiologic profile of the fitness status of collegiate cheerleaders. *J Strength Cond Res*. 2004;18(2):252–4.
9. Naiyer N, Chounthirath T, Smith GA. Pediatric cheerleading injuries treated in emergency departments in the United States. *Clin Pediatr*. 2017;56(11):985–92.
10. Boden BP, Prior C. Catastrophic spine injuries in sports. *Curr Sports Med Rep*. 2005;4(1):45–9.
11. Mueller FO. Catastrophic head injuries in high school and collegiate sports. *J Athl Train*. 2001;36(3):312–5.
12. Luckstead EF, Patel DR. Catastrophic pediatric sports injuries. *Pediatr Clin North Am*. 2002;49(3):581–91.
13. Mueller FO, Cantu RC. Catastrophic sports injury research. In: *27th Annual Report, Fall 1982–Spring 2009*. Chapel Hill, NC: National Center for Catastrophic Sport Injury Research; 2009.
14. Shields BJ, Smith GA. Cheerleading-related injuries in the United States: a prospective surveillance study. *J Athl Train*. 2009;44(6):567–77.
15. Caine D, Caine C, Maffulli N. Incidence and distribution of pediatric sport-related injuries. *Clin J Sport Med*. 2006;16(6):500–13.
16. Shields BJ, Fernandez SA, Smith GA. Epidemiology of cheerleading stunt-related injuries in the United States. *J Athl Train*. 2009 Nov–Dec;44(6):586–594. doi:10.4085/1062-6050-44.6.586
17. Schulz MR, Marshall SW, Mueller FO, et al. Incidence and risk factors for concussion in high school athletes, North Carolina, 1996-1999. *Am J Epidemiol*. 2004 Nov 15;160(10):937–944.
18. Jacobson BH, Hubbard M, Redus B, et al. An assessment of high school cheerleading: injury distribution, frequency, and associated factors. *J Orthop Sports Phys Ther*. 2004 May;34(5):261–5.
19. Fort GG, Fort FG. Cheerleading as a cause of splenic rupture. *Am J Emerg Med*. 1999 Jul;17(4):432–3.
20. Shields BJ, Smith GA. Cheerleading-related injuries to children 5 to 18 years of age: United States, 1990-2002. *Pediatrics*. 2006 Jan;117(1):122–9.
21. Lincoln AE, Caswell SV, Almquist JL, Dunn RE, Norris JB, Hinton RY. Trends in concussion incidence in high school sports: a prospective 11-year study. *Am J Sports Med*. 2011 May;39(5):958–63.
22. Xu AL, Suresh KV, Lee RJ. Progress in cheerleading safety: update on the epidemiology of cheerleading injuries presenting to US emergency departments, 2010-2019. *Orthop J Sports Med*. 2021 Oct 13;9(10):23259671211038895.
23. Boden BP, Tacchetti R, Mueller FO. Catastrophic cheerleading injuries. *Am J Sports Med*. 2003 Nov–Dec;31(6):881–8.
24. Shields BJ, Smith GA. The potential for brain injury on selected surfaces used by cheerleaders. *J Athl Train*. 2009 Nov–Dec;44(6):595–602.
25. Shields BJ, Smith GA. Epidemiology of cheerleading fall-related injuries in the United States. *J Athl Train*. 2009 Nov–Dec;44(6):578–85.
26. American Association of Cheerleading Coaches and Administrators. 2011-2012 *School Cheerleading Rules*.
27. National Federation of State High School Associations. *2012–2013 spirit rule book*.
28. LaBella CR, Mjaanes J, Council on Sports Medicine and Fitness. Cheerleading injuries: epidemiology and recommendations for prevention. *Pediatrics*. 2012 Nov;130(5):966–71.

Martial Arts

93

Robert B. Patton and Garry W. K. Ho

INTRODUCTION

- Martial arts include combative and noncombative sports with complex cultural, social, and geographical elements that result in diverse participation that is as old as human history. This presents a challenge to the covering physician who must be aware of these elements to best care for these athletes.
- The specific origins of martial arts are often closely tied to the history and culture of the regions where they developed. For example, karate, which originated in Okinawa, Japan, has roots in traditional Okinawan martial arts and was influenced by the various styles of Chinese kung fu. Judo, which also originated in Japan, was developed from traditional Japanese jujutsu and incorporates elements of grappling and throws.
- There are more than 190 recognized martial arts, of which three are Olympic sports (judo, 1964; taekwondo, 2000; and karate, 2020).
- Behind soccer, judo is the second most practiced sport in the world.
- Martial arts are practiced by people of all ages and backgrounds around the world and are often taught in specialized schools or studios, called kwoons, kwans, dojos, dojangs, or other culturally informed names.
- Participation occurs under a variety of contexts — as a health practice, therapeutic exercise, performance art, for cultural expression, self-defense method, combative skill, or competitive sport.
- Some schools accept athletes as young as 3 years old (1), while other athletes do not start participating until well into their 80s.
- There are classifications for visually impaired athletes in Paralympic judo, and the World Karate Federation (WKF) formed a Para-Karate Commission to develop the ancient discipline of "kata" for wheelchair athletes, as well as athletes with visual impairment and cognitive disabilities.
- As diverse as the population are the ways martials arts can be practiced. The physical form practiced may be differentiated as striking versus grappling, hard versus soft, armed versus unarmed, and individual (solo) versus sparring.
- Injury rates are difficult to accurately and reliably quantify and report, due to variations in injury definitions (*i.e.*, cessation of match, observed injury, reported injury, time loss injury); differences in study methods (competition injuries [more commonly studied] vs. training injuries [less commonly studied]); lack of consistency in the use of protective equipment; and lack of certain study populations (*e.g.*, pediatric and adolescent) (2).
- Mixed martial arts (MMA) is covered separately in Chapter 91.

INJURY PATTERNS

- In karate, common injuries include contusions, abrasions, strains, and sprains of the extremities, arms, legs, and neck, as well as fractures of the hand and foot.
    - During kata (prearranged patterns of movements), injuries are likely to be due to repetitive motions and overuse.
    - Head injuries, including concussions, epistaxis, and skull fractures, also occur as a result of strikes to the head during sparring.
        - A rule change by the WKF in 2000 discouraged or penalized blows to the head, resulting in a significant overall decrease in head injuries (3).
- In taekwondo, injuries to the legs and feet are particularly common, due to the high kicks and fast movement involved in the sport.
    - Strains and sprains of the arms, neck, and back are also common.
    - Fractures, lacerations, and head injuries can occur as well.
    - Arms are often used for blocking, which can reduce head injury but increase injuries to the upper extremity.
- In judo and Brazilian jiu-jitsu, injuries to the arms and shoulders are common, due to the grappling and submission techniques used in these sports.
    - Strains and sprains of the legs, neck, and back are also possible.
    - Dental injuries can occur due to the proximity of the opponents' heads, and head injuries can result from falls or strikes.
    - Chokeholds confer a high risk of asphyxia, and the American Academy of Pediatrics strongly discourages child and adolescent participation in martial arts that include these techniques (4).

- In boxing and kickboxing, head injuries, including concussions, lacerations, epistaxis, and skull fractures, are a major risk due to the repeated strikes to the head.
  - Hand and wrist fractures (boxer's fracture) can also occur due to the high impact of punches.
  - Strains and sprains of the arms, legs, and neck are also common.
- In Muay Thai, injuries to the legs and shins are common due to the use of kicks and knee strikes, as well as the use of hard shin guards.
  - Fractures, strains, and sprains of the arms, neck, and back can also occur. Head injuries, including lacerations, concussions, and skull fractures, are a risk due to the use of strikes to the head.
- It is important to note that while protective gear — such as mouthguards, hand wraps, and headgear — may help reduce the risk of injury in all collision and full-contact martial arts, there is a lack of data supporting the use of protective headgear (including padded helmets) to reduce the incidence or severity of concussions, specifically.
  - Additionally, an unintended consequence of using head protection in youths may result from a false sense of security, leading to more aggressive strikes, risky maneuvering, and potentially higher risk of injury (limited evidence) (4).
  - Proper training technique, conditioning, and supervision can also help prevent injuries.

MARTIAL ARTS IN HEALTH AND MEDICINE

- Studies have demonstrated beneficial outcomes in a wide array of social, health, and behavioral domains.
- In pediatrics, a meta-analysis indicated that aggression is not increased, but rather decreased by practicing martial arts (5), and individual studies have shown that the combination of traditional Chinese martial art skill set and moral philosophical training can decrease school violence (6).
  - However, this is balanced with some concern that early MMA training may lead to increased aggressive behavior, particularly with the media exposure to higher risk strikes and maneuvers (7).
- Other benefits in pediatric/adolescent populations are an increased overall physical fitness level; increased muscle strength, flexibility, and balance; improved self-esteem/self-awareness; improved self-respect; and improved overall cognitive function (2).
- Martial arts practice has also been suggested to improve stereotypic behaviors, social-emotional functioning, cognition, and attention in individuals with autism spectrum disorder/condition (8).
- In adults, martial arts practice can improve social function, reduce cancer-related fatigue, and improve function in patients with cancer (9).
- Tai chi, in particular, has been the focus of many studies including meta-analysis demonstrating its effectiveness as an alternative or adjunctive treatment for chronic conditions such as osteoarthritis, osteoporosis, headache, and low back pain (8), and studies indicating its superiority to conventional lower extremity training in preventing falls in older adults (10). Importantly, no studies have demonstrated any harm in practicing tai chi.

RULES AND REGULATIONS

- The differences in rules and governing bodies are greater even than the variety of the arts themselves, participants, and methods of participation.
- Olympic governing bodies for the three Olympic martial arts include:
  - Judo: International Judo Federation
  - Taekwondo: World Taekwondo
  - Karate: WKF
- There are many other governing bodies both nationally and internationally.

EVENTS

- Karate: The word karate is a Japanese term that means "empty hand." The WKF has established specific rules and regulations for karate competition, which are designed to ensure the safety and fairness of the sport.
  - Matches are held on a 20 × 20 ft matted area, called a tatami, with a central competition area marked off by a line.
  - Competitors are rank stratified by belt color. Kyu is a term used to describe the lower ranks in karate, typically from white belt to brown belt, and dan is a term used to describe the higher ranks in karate, typically from black belt to red-and-white belt.
  - Competitors wear traditional karate uniforms (karate gi) and protective gear, including padded gloves, foot protectors, and a mouthguard.
  - Matches are divided into rounds, with a break in between rounds. The duration of the rounds and the number of rounds in a match depend on the age and gender of the competitors or the type of competitive event.
  - Points (ippon: full point; or waza-ari: half point) are awarded for clean (unimpeded), accurate techniques that land on the legal target areas of the body. Illegal techniques, such as kicks to the head, below the knee, to the groin, or strikes with fingertips, are not allowed and may result in

disqualification. These illegal strikes are often referred to as "forbidden techniques." The specific illegal strikes and targets in karate competition vary depending on the governing body and the level of play. The amount of force allowed on contact or collision also varies. Keikoku, Chui, and Hansoku are penalties of increasing infraction severity.

- If a competitor is unable to continue the match due to injury or other reasons, the match will be stopped, and the other competitor will be declared the winner — as long as the other competitor has not incurred a disqualifying penalty.
- The competitor with the most points at the end of the match is declared the winner. If the match is tied, the judges may use a tie-breaking system to determine the winner.

- Judo: The word "judo" is a Japanese term that means "gentle way." This is a martial art that emphasizes throws, joint locks, and other techniques to control and or submit an opponent. The International Judo Federation has established specific rules and regulations for judo competition.
  - Matches are held on a mat called a tatami, with a central competition area marked off by a line.
  - Competitors wear traditional judo uniforms (judogi) and may also wear protective gear, such as a mouthguard and headgear.
  - Matches are divided into periods, with a break in between periods. The duration of the periods and the number of periods in a match depend on the age and gender of the competitors. For adult males, there are usually two periods, each lasting 4 minutes. If the match is tied at the end of the two periods, a third period may be held, lasting up to 3 minutes.
  - Points (ippon: full point; or waza-ari: half point) are awarded for clean, accurate techniques that result in an opponent being thrown or controlled. Illegal techniques, such as strikes or kicks, are not allowed and earn a disqualification penalty (hansoku-make). A "shido" is a minor penalty that may be awarded to a competitor for infractions such as stalling or not using proper technique.
  - If a competitor is unable to continue the match due to injury or other reasons, the match will be stopped and the other competitor will be declared the winner.
  - The competitor who scores the most points or throws their opponent to the mat with a clean technique is declared the winner. If the match is tied, the judges may use a tie-breaking system to determine the winner.

ROLE OF THE RINGSIDE OR COVERING EVENT PHYSICIAN

- Prior to event:
  - Understand rules (especially stoppage), equipment, protective gear, and venue.
  - Explore authority to stop the contest at any time if the athlete is too severely injured to continue the contest. This is not standardized and should be considered prior to agreeing to cover the event.
  - Explore athletes' ability to stop even if they feel they are unable to continue (*e.g.*, tapping out).
  - Preparticipation examination (PPE). Though there are no standardized requirements for PPE, requirements can be extrapolated from those of MMA as appropriate (see Chapter 90 of this text), with particular attention to:
    - Ocular — laser assisted in situ keratomileusis, photorefractive keratectomy, retinal detachments, and contact lenses
    - Neurological — traumatic brain injury (TBI) and concussions
    - ENT
    - Special considerations for female athletes include on site pregnancy testing and surgical history including breast augmentation surgery.
    - Other medical history and prior fight history as appropriate
  - Prepare and make accommodations for needed equipment, supplies, and personnel.
  - Communicate with other medical personnel and local emergency medical services (EMS) familiar with the event/area to develop a comprehensive emergency action plan (EAP).
- Preevent:
  - Arrive at least 2 hours before the contest.
  - Inspect competition area/ring/cage, ensuring access to competition area.
  - Meet with EMS and medical personnel to review EAP. Rehearsals of ingress and egress routes are useful.
  - Meet with referees, judges, or arbitrators. Suggest that all essential personnel have blood pressure and heart rate checked prior to event (BP < 150/100 is generally acceptable).
  - Prepare/inspect medical kit.
- During event:
  - Observe carefully and monitor. Move around to maintain an unobstructed view of the event.
    - Often large events have video displays that are helpful in maintaining close observation.
  - During quick assessments and triages on the mat, personal protective equipment with gloves, face mask, and eye protection should be worn. Consider bleeding precautions.
  - Gauze, flashlight, and stethoscope are essential and should be kept on person throughout the contest.
  - Clearance decisions to safely continue or not should consider an athlete's ability to protect themselves in the setting of concussion/TBI or any other injuries.
  - In larger or mass precipitation events, there should be a triage mechanism to provide fast-track treatment.

- Postevent:
  - Postfight evaluation (PFE), single versus multiple bouts, consider escalation to higher level of care/local trauma center PRN.
  - Multiple physicians present allows for PFE to be conducted while other contests are continued.
  - Consider referral to a medical center for severe lacerations, injuries requiring immobilization, TBI, spinal injuries, or airway injuries.
  - Explanation of injuries to athlete, safety netting (for evolving or developing injuries), and documentation of PFE are essential.

CONCLUSION

- It is important to recognize that martial arts carry a risk of injury, and the role of the sports medicine physician is crucial in providing medical support and care to participants.
- This chapter highlighted the importance of understanding the risks and benefits of martial arts and the role of medical professionals in promoting safe and healthy participation in the sport.
- There remains significant need for research on the long-term effects of martial arts participation and the sequelae of injury.
- Finally, although not discussed in this chapter, the physician must also consider the importance of media representation, both of themselves condoning a sport and of the sport in its relation to aggressive behavior.

REFERENCES

1. Hill K. *Century's Lil' Dragons*. About Web site. Available from: https://www.century-europe.eu/Lil-Dragon_1?srsltid=AfmBOoowjf0ZoKaaKUNgKbYySGxgcT41p2-cZVGth74fSm7VMk4fnMvF. Accessed 2025 May 12.
2. Koutures C, Demorest RA. Participation and injury in martial arts. *Curr Sports Med Rep*. 2018 Dec;17(12):433–8. doi:10.1249/JSR.0000000000000539
3. Macan J, Bundalo-Vrbanac D, Romić G. Effects of the new karate rules on the incidence and distribution of injuries. *Br J Sports Med*. 2006 Apr;40(4):326–30. discussion 330.
4. Demorest RA, Koutures C, Council on Sports Medicine and Fitness. Youth participation and injury risk in martial arts. *Pediatrics*. 2016 Dec;138(6):e20163022. doi:10.1542/peds.2016-3022
5. Moore B, Dudley D, Woodcock S. The effect of martial arts training on mental health outcomes: a systematic review and meta-analysis. *J Bodyw Mov Ther*. 2020 Oct;24(4):402–12. doi:10.1016/j.jbmt.2020.06.017
6. Fung ALC, Lee TKH. Effectiveness of Chinese martial arts and philosophy to reduce reactive and proactive aggression in schoolchildren. *J Dev Behav Pediatr*. 2018 Jun;39(5):404–14. doi:10.1097/DBP.0000000000000565
7. Council on Communications and Media. Virtual violence. *Pediatrics*. 2016;138(2):e20161298.
8. Bremer E, Crozier M, Lloyd M. A systematic review of the behavioural outcomes following exercise interventions for children and youth with autism spectrum disorder. *Autism*. 2016 Nov;20(8):899–915. doi:10.1177/1362361315616002
9. Sur D, Sabarimurugan S, Advani S. The effects of martial arts on cancer-related fatigue and quality of life in cancer patients: an up-to-date systematic review and meta-analysis of randomized controlled clinical trials. *Int J Environ Res Public Health*. 2021 Jun 6;18(11):6116.
10. Huang ZG, Feng YH, Li YH, Lv CS. Systematic review and meta-analysis: Tai Chi for preventing falls in older adults. *BMJ Open*. 2017 Feb 6;7(2):e013661. doi:10.1136/bmjopen-2016-013661

Extreme Sports

Justine Ko, Matthew D. Sedgley, and Jaron Santelli

94

INTRODUCTION

- Extreme sports is a broad term used to describe a wide range of sporting activities played in extreme conditions that tests the physical and mental limits of an athlete.
- This is a growing subgroup of sports characterized by high speeds and high risk, and often performed in areas with limited or no access to medical care (1).
- Extreme sports include a wide variety of sports and terrains. The following list contains some of the most popular extreme sports grouped by terrain:
  - Land:
    - Mountain biking (MTB)
    - Skateboarding
    - Ultramarathon
    - Rock climbing (described in further detail in Chapter 108)
  - Water
    - Rafting/Kayaking
    - Sea/SCUBA diving (described in further detail in Chapter 100)
    - Surfing (described in further detail in Chapter 119)
  - Snow and Ice
    - Skiing/Snowboarding (described in further detail in Chapter 113)
      - Big Mountain Skiing and Snowboarding
    - Ice Climbing (described in further detail in Chapter 108)
  - Air
    - BASE jumping
    - Skydiving
    - Paragliding
- Please note that this chapter focuses primarily on those sports that are not otherwise covered elsewhere in this text.

LEVELS OF COMPETITION

- Amateur/Recreational
  - Local groups and recreational teams may host events and practices.
  - Often have little or no access to on-site medical care.
- Professional
  - X-Games have been held annually since 1998 and continue to contribute to the growing interest in extreme sports.
  - Professional extreme sport series now exist all over the world and vary significantly in medical support and access.
  - A handful of extreme sports have been included at the Olympic level including alpine skiing, snowboarding, skateboarding, white water rafting.

EPIDEMIOLOGY

- There are limited data on the injury frequency and epidemiology related to extreme sports, in part due to the wide variety of sporting events classified under this umbrella term and the variety of governing bodies. Also, there may be variable consistency in reporting of injury.
- Similar to traditional sports, there is a higher injury rate in competition and in novice athletes (1).
- Although new extreme sports have emerged, this chapter focuses on the more popular sports and their sport-specific conditions.
  - New extreme sports are constantly on the rise, such as volcano surfing and ice swimming; however, they will not be covered in this chapter.

EVENTS

Mountain Biking

- Introduction/Epidemiology
  - MTB is a subdivision of cycling that is classified by courses on unpaved terrain (2).
  - Currently, the Union Cycliste Internationale (UCI) recognizes seven classes of MTB including cross country, downhill, four-cross, enduro, pump track, alpine snow bike, electric MTB (2).
  - The bicycle frame and fit varies based on the type of biking (please see Chapter 98 Cycling for additional detail) (3).
  - Popularity is growing for MTB with an estimated 30 million people practicing the sport worldwide (4).

- Specific Issues
  - Common safety equipment for riders include: helmets (both open and full face), spinal protection, knee pads, and gloves/wrist protection.
  - Helmet use has decreased concussion, head and facial injuries (5).
    - Currently, USA Cycling and UCI have mandatory helmet requirements during training sessions and competitions.
  - Competition categories (6):
    - Downhill biking involves timed trial runs on a downhill course that is premarked between two lines.
    - Cross-country biking had its Olympic debut in 1996. Its courses consist of uphill, downhill, and flat terrain of varying lengths, usually 3–9 km long.
    - Enduro races consist of a series of downhill and technical riding stages and time-limited uphill rides. The winner is determined by the fastest time cumulatively for all stages on the course (7).
    - Pump track courses are designed to have banked turns and terrain that allows riders to complete the circuit by "pumping" or generating forward motion through their up and down body movements without the use of pedaling.
- Medical Issues
  - These races are often held in more extreme conditions.
    - Environmental exposures must be considered, including: heat, cold, and wind.
  - Friction-related injuries, such as chafing and blisters, are common.
    - These should be treated with barrier protection, drying powder, and antibiotic ointment as needed.
    - Properly fitted clothing and equipment are also crucial in preventative measures (3).
  - Skin wounds from crashes are also very common and should be assessed for possible repair and infection.
  - Genitourinary-related medical conditions, such as neuropathies and erectile dysfunction require specialty assessment.
    - Oftentimes these are related to poorly fitted bicycles, poor saddle fit, and poor riding habits such as prolonged seating times (3).
    - Discussion and correction of these bad habits should be attempted whenever possible.
  - Serious falls or accidents and contact with the handlebar can place the riders at risk for penetrating or blunt abdominal injuries, such as splenic rupture and pancreatic/duodenal hematomas (3).
    - A high level of suspicion may be required to pick up these injuries when penetrating injuries are not present.
- Musculoskeletal Issues
  - Estimated injury risk rate of 0.6% (4).
  - Most common orthopedic injuries include fractures (up to 85%) followed by ligamentous injuries and sprains (4).
  - Many of the common injuries overlap with those of cycling, including concussion, upper extremity injuries, and handlebar injuries. Please see Chapter 98 Cycling for further details.

Skateboarding

- Epidemiology
  - Interest in the sport has continued to grow since the opening of the first skate parks in 1976 (8). There are an estimated 12.5 million participants in the sport worldwide.
  - Skateboarding made its Olympic debut at the 2020 Tokyo Olympics (held in 2021 due to the COVID-19 pandemic).
  - A wide range of age groups participate in this sport, including children and adolescents. For children and adolescents, those aged 11–14 were most commonly injured (8).
- Specific Issues
  - Skating competitions occur in street, park, vert/halfpipe, slalom and downhill venues.
    - Street competitions consist of a course that may include urban features such as handrails or benches. Pedestrians, uneven surfaces, and traffic can influence skating in this capacity.
    - Park competitions take place on a man-made course that combines features of "vert skating" (halfpipe and quarterpipe) and "street skating" (handrails and stairs). The course will likely be better maintained and free of traffic or other potential urban hazards.
      - Participants in park and vert/halfpipe competitions generally have two to three runs from 45–60 seconds where they can perform tricks that are then graded based on criteria such as height, originality, speed, and execution.
    - Slalom events require rides to travel at high speeds around set gates.
    - Downhill skateboarding is a speed event where athletes can travel in excess of 90 mph. Athletes usually travel on a closed road course.
  - Equipment:
    - Helmet: Currently, helmets are only required in competition for skaters under the age of 18.
    - Wrist guards and knee guards are recommended. Wrist guards have been shown to prevent and decrease the incidence of wrist injuries.
    - Skateboards are made of three main parts: the board, the wheels, and the truck that holds the wheels to the board. Variations in boards exist which account for

changes in the top speed and stability of the skateboard. Generally speaking, larger wheels provide greater speed and wider boards provide greater stability (8).

- Medical Issues
  - Head and facial injuries are less common; however, concussions do occur.
  - Dermatologic
    - Abrasions and lacerations
    - Bruising
    - Treat with symptom control, ice, irrigation, and repair as needed.
  - Pediatric skateboarders
    - The American Academy of Pediatrics recommends that children age 5 and less should not participate in skateboarding (8). Those aged 6–10 should be closely supervised.
- Musculoskeletal Issues
  - Upper extremity injuries
    - FOOSH injuries are common. Most upper extremity injuries involve the forearm and the wrist (9).
    - Scaphoid fractures: prophylactic splinting and reimage at 7–10 days if needed, given the high incidence of FOOSH injuries.
    - "Skateboarder's elbow" is caused by direct impact from landing on one's elbow. It generally results in a comminuted fracture of the olecranon process (9).
    - Clavicular fractures: treat with sling and pain control. Early range of motion is beneficial.
  - Lower extremity injuries are less common among skateboarders, but can include abrasions and sprains. Among these injuries, ankle injuries are the most common.
  - Physeal injuries (pediatrics and adolescents)
    - Special attention should be given to physeal injuries. Up to 33% of injuries in the children and adolescent skating population involve the physis (1).
    - Forearm and ankle fractures are most common in the pediatric population (10). Protective equipment is recommended for the pediatric population.

Ultramarathon

- Introduction/Epidemiology
  - Defined as a footrace that exceeds the traditional 42 km marathon. Most races are between 50 and 161 km (11). Terrain is often in austere environments.
  - The sport has been gaining popularity in recent years.
- Medical Issues
  - Environmental exposures
    - Given the length of these races, runners may experience a wide variety of environmental exposures (see Chapter 48 for further discussion of environmental emergencies).
      - Heat stroke: many runners are at risk for increased core temperatures
        - Treatment includes rapid on-site cooling through ice baths and cooling packs.
        - Failure to treat appropriately may lead to multi-organ dysfunction and/or death.
      - Hypothermia may be a risk on cold and/or wet courses and can lead to death as well.
        - This is a particular risk on remote or trail courses where athletes may get disoriented or where there may be long distances between aid stations.
        - Complications include frostbite to extremities, cardiac arrhythmias, and death.
        - Treatment includes passive external rewarming, and internal rewarming in severe cases.
      - Encounters with animals may lead to envenomations, bites, and wounds. Geography determines species-specific dangers. Medical personnel often must be prepared with antivenoms, supportive care, or egress from rural areas to higher levels of care when appropriate.
  - Exercise-associated hyponatremia (EAH)
    - Defined as a sodium level $<135\ \text{mmol} \cdot \text{L}^{-1}$
    - Risk factors for exercise-associated hyponatremia includes prolonged running times, inexperienced runners, excessive water intake during the marathon (12).
      - Ultramarathon runners may be at increased risk for hyponatremia given the longer run times and need for prolonged/excessive water consumption.
      - Runners should continue to drink to thirst to avoid hyponatremia. Muscle breakdown may increase chemical triggers such as IL-6 that may drive more antidiuretic hormone and thus increase the frequency of EAH.
      - Treatment depends on the severity. For mild cases, salt and broth can be used to correct the sodium imbalance. For severe cases or symptoms, IV hypertonic (3%) saline should be utilized.
  - Exercise-associated collapse (EAC)
    - This is thought to be caused by a sudden decrease in venous return when a runner suddenly stops running after the race.
    - This collapse occurs after a runner has stopped and not during the act of running.
    - Treatment includes laying the patient supine and lifting their legs to aid in venous return.
  - Gastrointestinal issues (11)
    - Many ultramarathon runners experience GI motility issues, nausea/vomiting, diarrhea. This is thought to be multifactorial including variations in GI motility,

gut vasoconstriction, and changes to caloric/water intake.
    - Ondansetron can be used to help relieve nausea.
    - Ibuprofen should be avoided during these races/runs given the increased risk for GI bleeding, GI upset, and renal dysfunction.
  - Exertional Rhabdomyolysis (11)
    - Defined as an elevated creatinine kinase (CK) level over 5× the upper limit of normal.
    - It is related to increased muscle breakdown and decreased clearance.
    - Treatment includes hydration and monitoring of levels, renal clearance, and urinary output.
    - Failure to treat appropriately may lead to acute kidney injury. See Chapter 39 Hematology for a detailed discussion of exertional rhabdomyolysis.
- Musculoskeletal injuries: Many of these overlap with those seen with running. For specific running-related injuries, please see Chapter 113 Running.

Whitewater Rafting/Kayaking

- Introduction/Epidemiology
  - There are an estimated 2.6 million participants in the sport of whitewater rafting (13).
- Specific Issues
  - Most of the competitions take place on rivers with whitewater conditions. The International Scale of River Difficulty helps rate the degree of difficulty, from small waves in Class I to extreme unpredictability in the most difficult Class VI (13).
  - In competition, there is usually a course that runs at least 200 m. For canoe and kayak slalom, participants are required to navigate a series of gates in an upstream or downstream direction (depending on a predetermined designation). A winner is determined based on the fastest time.
  - Equipment
    - Kayak
    - Two-ended paddles are used to help the kayaker navigate the water
    - Helmet
- Medical Issues
  - Submersion Injuries
    - Drowning is the leading cause of fatalities in the sport (13).
    - Hypothermia
  - Environmental exposure, including exposure to the heat and cold, are common (see Chapter 48 for further discussion of environmental considerations).
  - Dermatologic
    - Abrasions and blisters of the hands from repeated rowing motions.
    - External auditory canal exostosis: growths that develop in the external auditory canal related to epithelial damage from recurrent cold water exposure. These can lead to hearing problems and may require surgical removal in extreme cases (13).
    - Trench foot is a nonfreezing cold injury that results from repeated and prolonged exposure to wet and cold conditions (14). Treatment includes gentle rewarming and wound care.
    - Particular attention should be paid to the skin for fungal and staphylococcus infections. Given the moist conditions and propensity for minor fissures and wounds, these are relatively common. Treat with topical and oral antibiotics/antifungals as indicated.
  - Gastrointestinal (13)
    - Whitewater rafting exposes participants to a number of pathogens in the water.
    - Giardia has been reported in up to 14% in this athlete population. Symptoms include diarrhea, flatulence, and generally develop 1–2 weeks after exposure. Treatment is tinidazole (2 g orally single dose) or metronidazole (500 mg twice daily for 5–7 days).
    - Leptospirosis, although rare, must also be considered. Usually patients have fevers, myalgias, rigors. However, this can develop into kidney failure, uveitis, and more serious sequelae (15). Most cases are self-limiting; however, antibiotics may be required in more severe cases. Doxycycline 100 mg twice daily for 7 days or azithromycin 500 mg daily for 3 days can be used.
- Musculoskeletal Issues
  - Although fatal injuries are rare in the sport, acute musculoskeletal injuries are more common in novice rafters and overuse injuries are more common in experienced participants (13).
  - Acute injuries account for about 58% of injuries.
    - Often related to direct trauma by paddles, objects in the river, or other participants.
    - Injuries also occur from swimming or recovering from a capsized raft.
    - Upper extremity injuries are most common.
      - Shoulder injuries include shoulder dislocations, AC separation, labral tears, pectoralis major ruptures (13).
  - Overuse injuries
    - Most commonly in the upper arm from paddling. Tendinopathies of the rotator cuff and wrist extensor tendinopathies.
  - Core and back injuries are also common, although one study showed that these injuries were often more related to lifting and loading rafts rather than direct rafting injuries (13).
    - Paraspinal and lumbosacral injuries from repetitive and heavy rotational loads (15)

BASE Jumping

- Epidemiology
  - There are an estimated 3000 BASE jumpers around the world (16).
  - Guidelines for BASE jumping were written in 1997 by the Cliff Jumpers Association of America (CJAA) (16).
- Specific Issues
  - BASE jumping or "Building, Antenna, Span, Earth" jumping consists of fixed objects jumps using a parachute.
    - The starting height and parachute release is much lower than skydiving jumps. There is a much shorter canopy flight due to the elevation difference with most canopy flights lasting 10–15 seconds (17).
  - Most participants have significant skydiving experience.
  - Equipment: There are four categories within BASE jumping, each using different attire (18).
    - Normal clothes
    - Track suit
    - One-piece track suit
    - Wingsuit
  - Although BASE jumping equipment originates from skydiving parachutes, there are a number of differences, mainly to account for the more rapid deployment and shorter jump distances (16).
    - BASE jumpers utilize a one-parachute system, unlike skydiving. This is in part related to the lack of time to deploy a second parachute and in part related to increased risk with entanglement.
    - Certain points, such as the bridle points and the rib attachment points, are reinforced due to the abrupt parachute releases that exert extra forces.
    - Main canopy/parachute release is initiated by the "pilot chute" or smaller round chute attached to the main parachute. Timing of this release is key, given the short distance and canopy time.
    - Some jumps may utilize a "pilot chute assist" so that the pilot chute is released at the time of exit, meaning there is no free fall time.
  - Exiting is defined as the time/point when a jumper leaves the surface they are jumping from. Body position is crucial during this time as jumpers have less time to establish aerodynamic stability (16).
- Medical Issues
  - Overall BASE jumping is considered one of the most dangerous recreational sports with an estimated 1 in 60 fatality rate.
  - Frequency of injury correlates with the amount of time spent BASE jumping (4).
  - The two most common causes of severe injury are object strike and poor landing (17).
    - Surrounding objects and potential points of interference must be assessed during flight planning.
    - Fatal injuries are largely related to low or no pull events during which the parachute was not opened or had a delayed opening.
  - Visceral injuries
    - BASE jumping places the participants at higher risk for visceral injuries during falls or crash landings.
    - Pneumothorax
      - Presents with decreased breath sounds of the lung, respiratory distress, tracheal deviation.
      - Consider tension pneumothorax if hypotension or cardiopulmonary arrest occurs. Advanced trauma life support guidelines should be followed.
      - An extended focused assessment with sonography in trauma (EFAST) exam can help diagnose chest injuries if a portable ultrasound is present.
      - Needle decompression/thoracostomy should be performed. This can be performed in the second and third intercostal space at the midclavicular line or in the fourth and fifth intercostal space at the mid-axillary line. A large gauge needle such as 14 g should be utilized.
    - Intra-abdominal hemorrhage
      - In blunt injury, the spleen is most commonly injured.
      - Hollow organs may also be injured and will have a more delayed presentation. Advanced imaging and a high level of suspicion will be needed to make this diagnosis.
      - A EFAST exam can be performed onsite if a portable ultrasound is available to assess for bleeding. Serial abdominal/FAST exams should be performed if extrication or transportation is delayed.
  - Blunt chest trauma
    - BASE jumpers are at risk for blunt chest trauma from direct impact and from the abrupt stress from the harness during parachute deployment.
  - Concussion and closed head injuries
    - Although many BASE jumpers wear helmets, concussions, and minor head injuries are still seen. Rates of head injuries are not reported in the literature.
    - Similar to other sports, these athletes should refrain from contact sports during their injury period and undergo progressive return to sport once symptoms resolve.
  - Chapter 15 Field Side Emergencies further discusses emergency management strategies of these and other injuries that may occur in base jumping.
- Musculoskeletal issues
  - Although not well studied, one reports that lower limb and thoracolumbar injuries were most common among serious BASE injuries (1).
  - Rib injuries
    - These may result from the forces sustained through the harness during parachute release.

- Providers should assess for pneumothorax in the setting of rib fracture.
- The mainstay of treatment for rib fractures is pain control and incentive spirometry.
- Flail chest is defined as multiple rib fractures in two or more parts with associated paradoxical lung movements.
- Multiple rib fractures and flail chest often require prolonged observation and oxygen support.

Skydiving

- Introduction/Epidemiology
  - Skydiving is one of the aerial sports governed by the World Air Sports Federation.
  - The first world championship was held in 1951. Currently, there are an estimated 1 million skydivers across the world (19).
- Specific Issues
  - There are a number of sport skydiving categories (19,20):
    - Formation: Teams of 4, 8, 10, or 16 build predetermined formations to score points. Canopy formation competitions also exist for formations created under parachute during the canopy period.
    - Free-flying: Artistic free fall moves are performed by two or more skydivers and scored based on technical and artistic categories.
    - Accuracy landing: This event is judged based on individual or team accuracy in landing on a predetermined target.
    - Speed skydiving: Participants try to achieve the highest terminal velocity, often in a head-first formation.
  - Exit altitude tends to be around 4000 m (19).
  - Overall injury rate of 17.4 in 10,000 jumps (20). Most injuries occurred during parachute flight.
  - Equipment (19)
    - Parachute: manual release of a smaller pilot chute that pulls out the main parachute.
    - Reserve parachute: works independently in the event of failure of the main parachute release. There is an altitude margin between the lowest altitude for release for the primary parachute and the lowest altitude for release for the reserve parachute. In recent years, there has been development of automatic reserve activation devices.
- Medical Issues
  - Hypoxia due to the altitude exposure is thought to be minimal due to the short duration spent above 3000 m (19). However, for flights above 4000 m, participants should be warned that the effects of hypoxia can include delayed reaction time and impaired coordination (19).
  - Skydiving drop zones are often located near hospitals and EMS services can be coordinated.
    - It has been suggested that EMS should be on standby at skydiving drop zones. More direct coordination could be considered for competitions.
- Musculoskeletal Issues
  - Injuries frequently occur on landing due to miscalculations.
  - The most common injuries requiring presentation to the emergency department after a skydiving injury are lower extremity injuries including fractures and ligamentous injuries (20).
  - Large incidence of thoracolumbar injuries (4). Cervical spine precautions and spinal motion control procedures should be initiated on any landing injury.

Paragliding

- Introduction/Epidemiology
  - Paragliding is another sport that is governed by the World Air Sports Federation.
- Specific Issues
  - Equipment (21)
    - Paraglider: This consists of two sails that are connected by "ribs" that create cells. The leading edges of the cells are open to the air, whereas the trailing edges are closed off. Incoming air or "ram air" helps keep the cell compartments of the paraglider open and the paraglider in air.
    - GPS: allows for tracking
    - Variometer: a device that detects rise/fall in altitude
    - Radio: communication with other pilots
  - Types of competition
    - Cross country: trying to fly the greatest distance
    - Acro or acrobatics: performing certain movements or tricks
    - Accuracy: landing on a specific target
    - Comps or competitive: performing predetermined tasks during flight
  - Wind and weather play a major factor in flight and safety.
- Musculoskeletal Issues
  - Incidence of injury in paragliding has been cited by Feletti et al. as 12.5 injuries/1000 participants/year.
  - Accidents often result from poor landing or collapse of the airfoil.
  - Similar to skydiving, lower extremity and thoracolumbar injuries are the most common in paragliding (4). Soft-tissue and ligamentous injuries of the lower extremity are also prevalent in this aerial sport (22).
  - Novices had greater incidence of injury during take-off and landing (4).

EVENT COVERAGE

- Emergency Action Planning
  - Many of these sports are performed in remote areas and difficult terrain that make it challenging to coordinate care plans.
    - As the field of extreme sports continues to grow, the demand for medical coverage will also expand. It is important to understand the needs and expectations of the competitors.
  - Ideally, the medical team and planning teams will consist of those with experience in event/sports medicine, prehospital medicine, emergency medicine, and wilderness medicine (23).
  - An understanding of personnel skill sets, course arrangements, medical equipment, weather, and resource availability including government and transportation resources, is imperative.
  - For expedition length races or endurance races, medical care can/should be offered at transition points and set distances throughout the race (23).
  - Race day communication and command structures should be in place and trialed before race day to avoid confusion on the day of the event.
    - Recall that cellular phone service can be poor in some of these locations. Having back up communications (radio, satellite phones, etc.) is very important.
  - Providers should ensure that proper insurance has been obtained not only for themselves, but also for traveling athletes and other staff.
    - Insurance should include medical evacuation and out-of-country care (care provided out of the United States).
    - Other considerations may include natural disaster, war or civic unrest, and pandemic insurance coverage as well.
  - Providers may consider contacting the consulate prior to travel both for travel tips, local medical contacts, and to inform the proper authorities of team location and travel plans.
- Extrication
  - With these sports occurring in extreme environments, communication methods and extrication plans should be considered when developing emergency action plans (EAPs).
  - Communication is imperative between the medical director, local wilderness agencies, and local emergency medical personnel. Travel options (with back up plans for weather) and times should be included in EAPs.
  - Consider involvement of local search and rescue teams. Ski patrol and terrain-specific agencies should be included in the planning process.
  - Support from insurance agencies and government agencies should be considered.

REFERENCES

1. Laver L, Pengas IP, Mei-Dan O. Injuries in extreme sports. *J Orthop Surg Res*. 2017;12(1):59. doi:10.1186/s13018-017-0560-9
2. Arriel RA, Souza HLR, Sasaki JE, Marocolo M. Current perspectives of cross-country mountain biking: physiological and mechanical aspects, evolution of bikes, accidents and injuries. *Int J Environ Res Public Health*. 2022;19(19):12552. doi:10.3390/ijerph191912552
3. Ansari M, Nourian R, Khodaee M. Mountain biking injuries. *Curr Sports Med Rep*. 2017;16(6):404–12. doi:10.1249/JSR.0000000000000429
4. Bigdon SF, Hecht V, Fairhurst PG, Deml MC, Exadaktylos AK, Albers CE. Injuries in alpine summer sports—types, frequency and prevention: a systematic review. *BMC Sports Sci Med Rehabil*. 2022;14(1):79. doi:10.1186/s13102-022-00468-4
5. Olivier J, Creighton P. Bicycle injuries and helmet use: a systematic review and meta-analysis. *Int J Epidemiol*. 2017;46(1):278–92. doi:10.1093/ije/dyw153
6. Becker J, Moroder P. Extreme mountain biking injuries. In: Feletti F, editor. *Extreme Sports Medicine*. Cham, Switzerland: Springer International Publishing; 2017. p. 139–50. doi:10.1007/978-3-319-28265-7_12
7. Palmer D, Florida-James G, Ball C. Enduro world series (EWS) mountain biking injuries: a 2-year prospective study of 2010 riders. *Int J Sports Med*. 2021;42(11):1012–18. doi:10.1055/a-1320-1116
8. Lustenberger T, Demetriades D. Skateboarding injuries. In: Feletti F, editor. *Extreme Sports Medicine*. Cham: Springer International Publishing; 2017. p. 163–75. doi:10.1007/978-3-319-28265-7_14
9. Fountain JL, Meyers MC. Skateboarding injuries. *Sports Med*. 1996;22(6):360–6. doi:10.2165/00007256-199622060-00004
10. Zalavras C, Nikolopoulou G, Essin D, Manjra N, Zionts LE. Pediatric fractures during skateboarding, roller skating, and scooter riding. *Am J Sports Med*. 2005;33(4):568–73. doi:10.1177/0363546504269256
11. Khodaee M, Ansari M. Common ultramarathon injuries and illnesses: race day management. *Curr Sports Med Rep*. 2012;11(6):290–7. doi:10.1249/JSR.0b013e318272c34b
12. Almond CSD, Shin AY, Fortescue EB, et al. Hyponatremia among runners in the Boston Marathon. *N Engl J Med*. 2005;352(15):1550–6. doi:10.1056/NEJMoa043901
13. Spittler J, Gillum R, DeSanto K. Common injuries in whitewater rafting, kayaking, canoeing, and stand-up paddle boarding. *Curr Sports Med Rep*. 2020;19(10):422–9. doi:10.1249/JSR.0000000000000763
14. Bush JS, Lofgran T, Watson S. Trench foot. In: *StatPearls*. Treasure Island (FL): StatPearls Publishing; 2022. Accessed 2023 March 19. Available from: http://www.ncbi.nlm.nih.gov/books/NBK482364/
15. Wilson I, Folland J, McDermott H, Munir F. White-water paddlesport medicine. In: Feletti F, editor. *Extreme Sports Medicine*. Cham: Springer International Publishing; 2017. p. 139–50. doi:10.1007/978-3-319-28265-7_12
16. Feletti F, Westman A, Mei-Dan O. BASE jumping and wingsuit flying injuries. In: Feletti F, editor. *Extreme Sports Medicine*. Cham: Springer International Publishing; 2017. p. 139–50. doi:10.1007/978-3-319-28265-7_12
17. Mei-Dan O. BASE jumping. In: Mei-Dan O, Carmont MR, editors. *Adventure and Extreme Sports Injuries: Epidemiology, Treatment, Rehabilitation and Prevention*. London: Springer; 2013. p. 91–112. doi:10.1007/978-1-4471-4363-5_5
18. Bouchat P, Brymer E. BASE jumping fatalities between 2007 and 2017: main causes of fatal events and recommendations for safety. *Wilderness Environ Med*. 2019;30(4):407–11. doi:10.1016/j.wem.2019.07.001

19. Westman A. Skydiving. In: Mei-Dan O, Carmont MR, editors. *Adventure and Extreme Sports Injuries: Epidemiology, Treatment, Rehabilitation and Prevention*. London: Springer; 2013. p. 69–90. doi:10.1007/978-1-4471-4363-5_4
20. Mills TJ. Skydiving injuries. In: Feletti F, editor. *Extreme Sports Medicine*. Cham: Springer International Publishing; 2017. p. 197–208. doi:10.1007/978-3-319-28265-7_16
21. Laver L, Mei-Dan O. Paragliding. In: Mei-Dan O, Carmont MR, editors. *Adventure and Extreme Sports Injuries: Epidemiology, Treatment, Rehabilitation and Prevention*. London: Springer; 2013. p. 247–72. doi:10.1007/978-1-4471-4363-5_12
22. Cevik AA, Kaya FB, Acar N, Sahin A, Ozakin E. Injury, hospitalization, and operation rates are low in aerial sports. *Turk J Emerg Med*. 2017;17(3):81–4. doi:10.1016/j.tjem.2016.11.004
23. Ernst R, Townes D. Medical support for expedition-length adventure races. In: Feletti F, editor. *Extreme Sports Medicine*. Cham: Springer International Publishing; 2017. p. 65–76. doi:10.1007/978-3-319-28265-7_7

Rowing

Genevra L. Stone and Kristine A. Karlson

95

INTRODUCTION

- Rowing, sometimes called crew, is a sport in which athletes power a boat using oars. It is pursued at the competitive and recreational level by athletes ranging in age from preteens to nonagenarians. Rowing has been a part of the summer Olympics since the advent of the modern games.
- Boats have one, two, four, or eight rowers, and the rowers have either one oar each (sweep rowing) or two oars each (sculling). In the bigger boats (four and eight rowers), there is often a coxswain, a person to steer the boat and to direct the rowers. Each rower sits on a sliding seat, and feet are placed in a pair of fixed shoes. The oar is held in a pivoting oarlock on an outrigger that can be adjusted in multiple ways to vary the height, position, angle, and load per stroke.
- Most rowing injuries are overuse injuries, related to the volume of training and the repetitive nature of the sport.
- Different disciplines:
  - At the collegiate and elite level, some rowers compete in the lightweight category (internationally defined as women less than 57 kg and men less than 70 kg).
  - Rowing is accessible to para-athletes, and there are a variety of classifications based on disability: arms/shoulders, arms/trunk, and arms/trunk/legs.
  - Recently, coastal rowing and beach sprints have gained popularity. In these disciplines, races include running along a beach, and rowers race in wider, more stable boats to handle the range of water conditions seen in open seas.
- Levels of competition include youth, scholastic, collegiate, under 23, club, elite, and masters racing. Masters rowing includes all rowers who turn 27 year old in the calendar year of competition, and it is further broken down into age groups every 3–7 years (1).
- Spring and summer are the main racing seasons for rowing, and 2000 m is the standard length of a rowing race at levels from high school through elite competition.
  - Masters rowers race 1000 m.
  - In these races, boats race side by side, typically six lanes across.
- In the fall, rowers of all ages compete in "head races," which are roughly 3 miles long, take roughly 15–18 minutes, and have boats racing single file for the fastest time in their division.

FUNDAMENTALS OF ROWING

- The rowing stroke includes four phases:
  - The stroke begins at the *catch,* where the back and legs are maximally flexed and the arms extended. It is at this point that the oar enters the water.
  - During the *drive* (power) phase of the stroke, the legs are extended, the back opened, and the arms flexed to the chest.
  - At the *finish,* the oar is removed from the water, and the blade is feathered (turned parallel to the water).
  - Finally, during the *recovery* phase, the body returns to the catch position by extending the arms, flexing the hips, and then flexing the knees.
- Whether an athlete is rowing with one oar or two determines the nature of the load placed on the athlete's torso. In sweep rowing (single oar), the athlete both rotates toward their oar and tilts toward the oar at the catch in order to extend the length of the stroke (2). The rotation and tilt lead to different loading on the torso and a slightly different injury pattern compared to sculling (two oars), in which the athlete maintains their center over the middle of the boat as both arms extend outward.
- Standard rowing races demand a vigorous anaerobic start (roughly 250 m) followed by near maximal aerobic exertion (1500 m) and conclude with an exhaustive anaerobic sprint (roughly 250 m).
- Rowers' training volumes significantly exceed time spent racing with the ratio becoming more lopsided as the athlete advances in ability. The majority of time spent training is by rowing on the water though many rowers incorporate core strengthening, weight training, the rowing machine (ergometer or "erg"), and cross training. These other training modalities are used more frequently when weather limits the ability to row on the water.
- The erg is a stationary, on-land fitness device that imitates the rowing stroke. Like a boat, it has fixed feet and a sliding seat with a handle that the athlete pulls against resistance. There are many varieties of ergs on the market, and they use different methods of resistance (flywheel, water, etc.). The erg is popular among many athletes without on-water rowing experience in addition to being used frequently by rowers

for training and fitness testing. Coaches value it for comparing athletes as it provides an impartial (ie, not impacted by weather or the performance of the other athletes in a boat) and measurable evaluation of a rower's individual fitness.

MEDICAL ISSUES

- Cardiac:
  - Atrial fibrillation is more common in former endurance athletes when compared with age-matched controls (3). The risk increases with accumulation of lifetime hours training and male sex, but atrial fibrillation can be seen in young and middle-aged endurance athletes (4). From animal models, it appears that this risk is related to increased fibrosis of both atria, causing increased susceptibility to ectopy, in addition to autonomic nervous system imbalance (5).
  - Symptoms of atrial fibrillation include abnormal fatigue, dyspnea, palpitations, and lightheadedness.
  - Diagnosis is made by EKG and, if intermittent, longer term cardiac monitoring via a rhythm capture device such as a Zio Patch. Other precipitating medical conditions such as hyperthyroidism should be considered.
  - Treatment options include rate control, rhythm control, and/or anticoagulation. For the younger population, drug therapy is poorly tolerated and ablation may be the appropriate strategy (5).
  - Once treated, athletes, including the older athletes and those on anticoagulant medications, may return to rowing.
- Dermatologic: The skin of the rower is subject to repetitive trauma of the hands, feet, and the buttock due to friction with the oar handle, shoes, and seat, respectively.
  - Blisters on the hand are considered a badge of honor by experienced rowers and, with good care and continued rowing, will develop into calluses. Rowers rarely wear gloves as they interfere with the ability to feel the oar. It is important to keep blisters in both locations clean and not to intentionally break them open.
  - Blisters may become secondarily infected, occasionally requiring topical or oral antibiotics (6). Rarely, infection of open hand wounds spreads hematogenously requiring immediate medical care and IV antibiotics.
  - Treatment of buttock chafing and abrasions includes changing the seat to one of a different shape, use of a butt pad (usually made of foam), and use of an antichafing cream can help to prevent and to alleviate symptoms.
- Endocrine: As mentioned above, some rowers compete in lightweight divisions, and as in other sports with weight divisions, efforts to meet weight cutoffs can lead to disordered eating and/or to an eating disorder. If disordered eating persists, it can lead to development of Relative Energy Deficiency in Sport in both the male and female athlete populations (7) and/or the Female Athlete Triad. This is described in depth in Chapters 12 (Nutrition) and 131 (Female Athlete) of this text.
- Overtraining: As endurance athletes, many rowers may develop overtraining syndrome, which is a maladaptive response to exercise without adequate recovery.
  - This maladaptive response leads to disruptions in neurologic, endocrine, immunologic, and psychiatric systems (8).
  - Signs of overtraining include depression or mood lability, severe exhaustion, frequent injuries and/or illnesses, inability to gain muscle mass, and decreased performance without another possible cause.
  - The differential includes anemia, infection, malnutrition, and hypothyroidism.
  - Treatment involves rest with gradual, stepwise return to participation. Temporary use of selective serotonin reuptake inhibitors can be considered though one must be aware of the potential negative impact of antidepressants on performance (9).
  - Overtraining syndrome is discussed in depth in Chapter 45 of this text.

MUSCULOSKELETAL ISSUES

- Low back pain: Not only are lower back injuries common in rowing but also rowers are more likely than athletes of other sports to complain of lower back injuries (10,11).
  - At the catch, the boat speed is at the slowest point of the stroke; thus, when the rower begins exerting force on the blade, the load is the highest. The flexed back is the connection in that transfer of power (12).
  - Risk factors for lower back injury include a steep increase in training volume (particularly on the ergometer), reduced flexibility (anterior and posterior lower chain, hip joints), and prior history of lower back pain (13). Within a practice, fatigue leads to decreased use of stabilizing muscles and increased susceptibility to lower back injury (14).
  - When assessing lower back pain, it is important to evaluate for neurologic signs and symptoms, which can be a clue to discogenic pain (15).
  - MRI is the preferred study for definitive diagnosis but should be reserved to athletes with injuries so significant that the imaging will influence management (13).
  - Treatment includes rest, a course of anti-inflammatory medications, and physical therapy to strengthen the core muscles. Rehabilitation should include work on hip range of motion and trunk extensor strength (14). Second-line therapy for discogenic pain includes ultrasound-guided steroid injections, while surgery is reserved for refractory disc injuries.
  - When returning to rowing, errors of distance, technique, or intensity should be addressed. A search for mechanical

errors should occur with modification of equipment as needed to decrease load per stroke, adjust oar/foot height, or switch side rowed (for sweep rowers) (16,17).

- Rib:
  - Rib stress fractures are common in rowing and are reported to be the injury causing the most time lost from sport-specific training (18). The injury results from a multifactorial etiology, likely including serratus anterior tension, heavy equipment loading, and bone mineral properties. All of which occur in a setting of repeated microdamage and cyclic loading (19).
  - Most injuries occur between ribs 4 and 8. Precursors to stress fracture include costochondral pain and intercostal muscle strain. Point tenderness that localizes to a dime-sized area on a rib reproduced with anterior-posterior chest wall compression is concerning for a rib stress fracture. Athletes frequently will also have pain with coughing, sneezing, and rolling over in bed.
  - Definitive diagnosis was classically made by bone scan though MRI has become the modality of choice.
  - Diffuse pain in the mid ribs should be a presumed warning sign and treated with rest, cross-training, gentle stretching, and ice. Once a rib stress fracture is diagnosed, the athlete should avoid rowing and limit activity with the affected side's upper extremity for roughly 6 weeks before a graduated return to training. Cross-training can begin when pain-free.
  - Preventative measures include core stability, trunk mobility, strengthening the pectoral muscles, and identifying and correcting any risk factors related to low bone density (20).
- Knee: The rowing stroke maximally loads the knee when it is in the fully flexed position. As a result, patellofemoral pain is a common complaint.
  - As with patellofemoral problems in other sports, this is more common in women and in those with anatomy that predisposes them to abnormalities in patellar tracking. Tracking problems can be exacerbated by the position of the shoes fixed in the rowing shell. Their height, spacing, or orientation may be mechanically inappropriate for the rower's anatomy (16).
  - Treatment focuses on strengthening of the vastus medialis muscle to improve patellar tracking. Braces do not work well as they limit the flexion required of the knee at the catch.
  - Technical interventions include increasing the height of the seat versus the shoes by using a seat pad, attention to knee tracking during the stroke, and adjusting shoe height, spacing, and orientation if possible (depending on how the shoes are affixed and if the boat is shared equipment).
  - The iliotibial band (ITB) may also be a location of pain in rowers, and ITB friction syndrome results from significant time and load spent in hip flexion with no time spent at complete hip extension.
    - Rehabilitation includes stretching the ITBs bilaterally and strengthening the hip abductors.
- Hip: At the catch of each stroke, the rower is in maximal hip flexion and then begins to extend against a heavy load. This repeated maximal flexion puts rowers at risk of hip injuries.
  - As with other athletes with suspected hip impingement, rowers typically experience deep groin pain without palpable tenderness. They may complain that the pain limits their compression at the catch.
  - The physical exam is likely to reproduce pain in the FADIR (flexion, adduction, internal rotation) position.
  - Plain radiographs may reveal a cam and/or pincer lesion. MRI is used for further diagnosis and surgical planning.
  - In a review of cases, roughly half of rowers studied returned to rowing postoperatively (21). Intra-articular steroid injection may be pursued but are not typically successful over the long term.
- Forearm:
  - The rowing stroke predisposes to forearm tendinopathy in the dorsal wrist, both from tightly gripping the oar during the stroke and from wrist extension on feathering the oar (turning it 90° at the finish).
    - Rowers may complain of pain in the dorsal wrist, specifically at the intersection of the first and second dorsal wrist compartments (16,22). "Intersection syndrome" makes it difficult to feather and, thus, keeps a rower out of the boat.
    - Physical examination will reveal pain and swelling at this location, and, in severe cases, crepitus may be noted.
    - Treatment involves rest as well as technique modification by employing a looser grip with a flatter wrist position when feathering. Medical modalities, such as ice, brief immobilization, nonsteroidal anti-inflammatory medications, and on occasion, local steroid injection into the affected tendon sheath, may all be employed (22).
  - Compartment syndrome may be seen in the rower's forearm as a response to a tight grip with lack of relaxation on the recovery. Rowing frequently in rough water conditions where it is imperative to hold onto the handle may increase the risk of developing compartment syndrome in the forearm. Rowing on the erg is a separate risk factor as the tension on the cord prevents rowers from relaxing their grip on the recovery.
    - Compartment syndrome is characterized by burning exertional pain that escalates in severity with use and resolves quickly with cessation of activity.
    - Treatment is similar to that of forearm tendinopathy. Technique modifications may include changing the grip size. On the erg, rowers may use weightlifting straps to keep their hands on the handles with a looser grip. In refractory cases, the definitive treatment is surgical fasciotomy for compartment release (23).

- Shoulder/thoracic outlet: As athletes who use their upper bodies in a repetitive motion, rowers are susceptible to thoracic outlet syndrome (TOS), both neurogenic and vascular.
  - A rower with TOS may complain of unilateral (more common in sweep rowing) or bilateral upper extremity pain, paresthesias, numbness, weakness, and swelling (24).
  - On a physical exam in an athlete with neurogenic TOS, the Roos test (or the elevated arm stress test) will result in severe pain to the extent that the athlete is not able to complete 3 minutes of the arms in abduction with elbow flexion while opening and closing the hands (25).
  - Confirmatory diagnosis is made with nerve conduction velocity and electromyography studies (25). Ultrasound is the recommended diagnostic modality for vascular TOS, and, if not conclusive, recommendations are to proceed with CT or MR venogram (26).
    - Vascular TOS is a risk factor for upper extremity deep vein thrombosis, which is seen in rowers.
  - Initial treatment of neurogenic TOS consists of physical therapy with range of motion in addition to tendon and nerve gliding techniques. Medical modalities include anti-inflammatories, nerve stimulation, and/or botulinum injections (25). Second-line treatment is surgical decompression.
    - For vascular TOS, treatment begins with anticoagulation therapy prior to definitive surgical management to decompress the thoracic outlet.
  - Neurogenic and vascular TOS is further discussed in Chapter 61, Upper Extremity Nerve Entrapment.

EVENT COVERAGE

- Event coverage for rowing is complicated by the venue: an outdoor body of water in which the athletes are in narrow racing shells.
- Typically, rowers cover a large geographical area (rowing 8–12 miles in a typical practice).
- Many clubs require an athlete to pass a swim test prior to rowing.
- Weather conditions, including precipitation, temperature, and wind speed, are frequently unpredictable as are water conditions, which range from smooth to white caps.
  - Particular risks include extremes of air temperature, cold water temperatures, bodies of water with strong current, and lightning storms.
  - Like other athletes, rowers are susceptible to heat stroke in hot and humid conditions.
  - In cold weather, special care must be taken to protect the distal extremities, including "pogies" to wear over the hands and handles.
  - Many rowing clubs have rules prohibiting members from rowing in small (less stable) boats when the water temperature drops below 50 °F.
  - All boaters should land as soon as possible in the case of lightning in the vicinity.
- In some bodies of water, other watercrafts, ranging from kayaks to commercial vessels, add an additional element of potential danger.
- Development of an emergency action plan is critical and must include a plan for water rescue and the extraction of a collapsed, acutely ill, or injured athlete from the rowing shell onto a coaching launch and how to best get that athlete to a location accessible by emergency medical services providers.
  - If the medical provider is on shore, it will likely be impossible to see what is happening on the water, and a verbal communication system is necessary.
  - If a rowing boat capsizes, each oar is a flotation device, and in many countries, the coxswain must wear a personal flotation device as they do not have their own oar.

REFERENCES

1. *World Rowing — Masters Rowing. World Rowing.* date unknown; [cited 2023 Feb 15] Available from: https://worldrowing.com/events/masters-rowing/
2. Strahan AD, Burnett AF, Caneiro JP, Doyle MM, O'Sullivan PB, Goodman C. Differences in spinopelvic kinematics in sweep and scull ergometer rowing. *Clin J Sport Med.* 2011;21(4):330–6.
3. Baldesberger S, Bauersfeld U, Candinas R, et al. Sinus node disease and arrhythmias in the long-term follow-up of former professional cyclists. *Eur Heart J.* 2008;29(1):71–8.
4. Sanchis-Gomar F, Perez-Quilis C, Lippi G, et al. Atrial fibrillation in highly trained endurance athletes — description of a syndrome. *Int J Cardiol.* 2017;226:11–20.
5. Wilhelm M. Atrial fibrillation in endurance athletes. *Eur J Prev Cardiol.* 2014;21(8):1040–8.
6. Knapik JJ, Reynolds KL, Duplantis KL, Jones BH. Friction blisters. Pathophysiology, prevention and treatment. *Sports Med.* 1995;20(3):136–47.
7. Mountjoy M, Sundgot-Borgen JK, Burke LM, et al. IOC consensus statement on relative energy deficiency in sport (RED-S): 2018 update. *Br J Sports Med.* 2018;52(11):687–97.
8. Kreher JB, Schwartz JB. Overtraining syndrome: a practical guide. *Sports Health.* 2012;4(2):128–38.
9. Pearce PZ. A practical approach to the overtraining syndrome. *Curr Sports Med Rep.* 2002;1(3):179–83.
10. Hosea TM, Hannafin JA. Rowing injuries. *Sports Health.* 2012;4(3):236–45.
11. Trompeter K, Fett D, Platen P. Prevalence of back pain in sports: a systematic review of the literature. *Sports Med.* 2017;47(6):1183–207.
12. Reid DA, Mcnair PJ. Factors contributing to low back pain in rowers. *Br J Sports Med.* 2000;34(5):321–2.
13. Wilson F, Thornton JS, Wilkie K, et al. 2021 consensus statement for preventing and managing low back pain in elite and subelite adult rowers. *Br J Sports Med.* 2021;55(16):893–9.
14. Nugent FJ, Vinther A, McGregor A, Thornton JS, Wilkie K, Wilson F. The relationship between rowing-related low back pain and rowing biomechanics: a systematic review. *Br J Sports Med.* 2021. bjsports-2020-102533.

15. Maurer M, Soder RB, Baldisserotto M. Spine abnormalities depicted by magnetic resonance imaging in adolescent rowers. *Am J Sports Med.* 2011;39(2):392–7.
16. Karlson KA. Rowing injuries: identifying and treating musculoskeletal and nonmusculoskeletal conditions. *Phys Sportsmed.* 2000;28(4):40–50.
17. Rumball JS, Lebrun CM, Di Ciacca SR, Orlando K. Rowing injuries. *Sports Med.* 2005;35(6):537–55.
18. Coburn P, Wajswelner H, Bennell K. A survey of 54 consecutive rowing injuries. In: *National Annual Scientific Conference in Sports Medicine*; 1993. pp. 26–31.
19. Warden SJ, Gutschlag FR, Wajswelner H, Crossley KM. Aetiology of rib stress fractures in rowers. *Sports Med.* 2002;32(13):819–36.
20. Evans G, Redgrave A. Great Britain Rowing Team Guideline for diagnosis and management of rib stress injury: Part 1. *Br J Sports Med.* 2016;50(5):266–9.
21. Boykin RE, McFeely ED, Ackerman KE, Yen Y-M, Nasreddine A, Kocher MS. Labral injuries of the hip in rowers. *Clin Orthop Relat Res.* 2013;471(8):2517–22.
22. Fulcher SM, Kiefhaber TR, Stern PJ. Upper-extremity tendinitis and overuse syndromes in the athlete. *Clin Sports Med.* 1998;17(3):433–48.
23. Harrison JWK, Thomas P, Aster A, Wilkes G, Hayton MJ. Chronic exertional compartment syndrome of the forearm in elite rowers: a technique for mini-open fasciotomy and a report of six cases. *Hand.* 2013;8(4):450–3.
24. Chandra V, Little C, Lee JT. Thoracic outlet syndrome in high-performance athletes. *J Vasc Surg.* 2014;60(4):1012–8.
25. Kuhn JE, Lebus GFV, Bible JE. Thoracic outlet syndrome. *JAAOS - Journal of the American Academy of Orthopaedic Surgeons.* 2015;23(4):222–32.
26. Mustafa J, Asher I, Sthoeger Z. Upper extremity deep vein thrombosis: symptoms, diagnosis, and treatment. *Isr Med Assoc J.* 2018;20(1):53–7.

96 Cross-Country Skiing

Janus D. Butcher

INTRODUCTION

- Cross-country skiing is one of the three Nordic skiing disciplines along with ski jumping and Nordic combined (skiing and jumping). Most historic references to Nordic skiing discuss its military use. Indeed, the sport of biathlon (skiing and shooting) has its origin in this historic relationship.
- Cross-country skiing is generally associated with a low injury rate, and it is considered to be one of the highest aerobic demand activities.
- Although generally confined to the northern tier and mountain states, its popularity in the United States continues to grow.
- Cross-country skiing had remained relatively unchanged from its remote beginnings until dramatic innovations in equipment and technique were widely introduced in the 1980s.
- Currently, two very distinct techniques are used, the diagonal stride (classic) and ski skating (freestyle).

BIOMECHANICS

Diagonal (Classic) Technique

- The diagonal stride technique has been used for centuries and remains a popular style for ski touring and back-country skiing.
- In the diagonal stride, forward propulsion is accomplished through alternating kick and glide actions of the skis. This requires a full stop of the kick ski to propel the skier forward. Backward slip of the planted ski is limited by the application of high-friction kick wax on the cambered portion of the ski surface. The requirement to plant the ski to generate thrust limits the maximum speeds obtainable (1).
- In the diagonal stride, the poles are used primarily for balance but can contribute up to 30% of forward thrust in higher level skiers (1). Double poling (planting both poles simultaneously) is used to maintain forward momentum as increasing tempo limits the effectiveness of the kick and glide action, but increases the proportion of propulsion from the poling action.

Skating Technique

- Developed in the late 1970s, this new technique has rapidly evolved and become the method of choice for most non-elite competitors. Skating is the only technique used in both biathlon and Nordic combined competitions.
- The skating technique generates forward momentum by driving the skis at an angle to the direction of travel in a motion analogous to speed skating. There is no kick phase and thus no stopping of the ski during the cycle. Several different strides or techniques are used: V1, V2, V2 alternate, and free skate (for details, see Nordic Ski Lab video (2)). The transitions between techniques are very dynamic and the choice is dependent upon terrain and skier tempo.
- Double poling is used in most skating strides to transfer upper body energy to the skiing surface and can provide up to 60% of the forward propulsive force (3).

Biomechanical Comparison of the Techniques

- Skating is much more energy efficient than the diagonal stride technique (4). In addition, with skating, there is no need for a high-friction kick wax; so low-friction glide waxes can be used along the entire surface of the ski.
- These factors, combined with the use of extremely lightweight composite construction materials as well as improvements in skiing surface preparation, have resulted in a 10%–30% increase in average speed since the 1950s (4,5).
- Environmental variables such as snow condition, temperature, and relative humidity dictate skier efficiency and speed. Certain conditions will favor one technique over the other. Because of these variables, each event is quite unique. Events using the same technique at the same venue will often have very different outcomes.

COMPETITION

Elite-Level Competition

- The International Ski Federation (FIS) governs international competition. The FIS establishes race rules, schedules, doping control systems, athlete injury surveillance, and most other aspects of World Cup and World Championship racing.

- The specific events held at elite competitions are varied in both distance and technique. Formats include sprint (1 km), sprint relay, middle distance (5, 10, and 15 km), team relay (4 × 5 km, 4 × 10 km), long distance (30 and 50 km), classic/skate pursuit, and others.
- One unique aspect of elite cross-country skiing is that the athletes frequently compete as both sprinters (1 km) as well as marathon skiers (30 or 50 km) within the same race schedule.
    - Historically, most competitors trained and raced in both the classical and skating techniques as well, as demonstrated in the 2022 Winter Olympics when the American Jessie Diggins won the bronze medal in the freestyle team sprint event and days later won the silver medal in the 30 km classic technique distance event.

Non-FIS Competition

- Marathon distance races are held in nearly all of the countries of Northern, Central, and Eastern Europe as well as Japan, North America, and Australia.
- In the United States, a full calendar of local, regional, and national marathon races are scheduled throughout the winter months.
    - The largest of these, the American Birkebeiner, is 52 km long with over 7000 participants and is held in February in northern Wisconsin.
- High school and college cross-country ski teams are common in the Northeast, upper Midwest, and Western states. These competitions include races 5–15 km in length with both classic stride and skating formats.

INJURY EPIDEMIOLOGY AND PATHOPHYSIOLOGY

Overall Incidence

- Historically, the injury rates in cross-country skiing are reported to be between 0.1 and 5.63 injuries per 1000 skiers (6,7). Recent studies have confirmed this reported incidence, with Worth et al reporting a rate of 3.8 injuries per 1000 skiers (8).
    - Younger skiers have a higher rate of injuries, 8.9%, during the course of the season (9). However, the true incidence is difficult to determine because skiing is not generally limited to a confined venue.
    - Injuries tend to be mild and self-limited.
- In the limited data available from more controlled circumstances, such as endurance races, the incidence was found to be substantially higher at 10–35 per 1000 skiers (1,10).
    - The majority of these injuries were fatigue related.
- Studies evaluating injury patterns in elite-level skiers report higher injury rates.
    - One study reported a rate of 11% in World Cup competitors (11).
    - In a 12-month study, the annual rate of injury in a group of elite Finnish skiers was 62%. However, the majority of those injuries occurred in nonskiing training activities (12).
    - Overall, cross-country skiing has been shown to have a lower risk of injury than running among elite participants (9).

Changing Injury Patterns

- As the technique and equipment have changed, several equipment-injury relationships have been suggested although data supporting these associations have been scant at best (13–18).
    - Increased pole length with the skating technique accentuates demands on the shoulder and elbow.
    - Stiffer bindings and rigid boot construction with heel-ski fixation devices in skating equipment may increase the risk of both acute and chronic ankle and knee injuries.
- The biomechanics of the skating (freestyle) technique are also suggested in the changing injury patterns.
    - The skating stride places significantly greater demands on the hip adductors and external rotators (1).
    - A greater emphasis on upper body strength in the double poling action has been implicated in increasing upper extremity overuse injuries (15).
    - Chronic exertional compartment syndrome (ECS) has been associated with the skating technique as ski recovery at the end of the skate cycle places greater demand on the lateral and anterior compartment of the lower extremity (14).

Comparison of Techniques

- Initial reports suggested greater incidence of injury in the skating technique; however, this remains unsubstantiated (10,13,15). Though in one report of injuries occurring during a long-distance event where the skating technique was the dominant style used, the injury rate was found to be higher than reported for similar races in the years prior to the adaptation of the skating technique (10).

Injury Distribution and Type

- Studies describing the distribution of musculoskeletal injuries in mass participation events demonstrated that lower extremity injuries are somewhat more common than upper extremity injuries (55% vs. 35%) (7,9).

Injury types

- Sprains/twists — 40.4%
- Fracture — 27.4%

- Contusions — 16.4%
- Lacerations — 9.3%
- Dislocations — 5.8%
- Other — 0.7%
- The most frequently encountered acute orthopedic complaints include thumb ulnar collateral ligament strain, knee medial collateral ligament sprain, and plantar fascia strain.
- The most common overuse injuries include sacroiliitis, first metatarsophalangeal (MTP) degenerative joint disease/synovitis, lateral ankle pain, ECS, and wrist tendinitis.

COMMON MEDICAL CONDITIONS

- Common medical illnesses reported are similar to those seen in many other endurance sports and include exhaustion/dehydration, bronchospasm gastrointestinal symptoms, and environmental exposure/injury (particularly cold). Many of these are described in depth elsewhere in this text (Chapter 12 Nutrition and Hydration, Chapter 41 Gastroenterology, Chapter 42 Pulmonary, Chapter 47 Environmental Injury).

Photokeratitis

- Also known as snow blindness, this a condition that may be seen in sports where UV light reflects off of the surface snow, ice, or water.
- This is a painful, superficial keratopathy with symptoms that may include redness of the eye as well as eye pain, photophobia, tearing, swollen lids, headache, blurred vision, and/or temporary loss of vision.
- The use of appropriate eyewear including sunglasses or goggles with UV protection may prevent or lessen the severity of this condition.

Exercise-Induced Asthma

- Incidence: Exercise-induced asthma (EIA) affects up to 42% of winter sports athletes, with the highest incidence found in cross-country skiers (19–25).
  - One study reported that 50% of elite cross-country skiers have EIA (23).
- Pathophysiology: EIA refers to an inflammatory-mediated bronchial response precipitated by exercise. Exercise is a common trigger of symptoms in athletes with classic asthma. There does appear to be a separate population of athletes who exhibit symptoms only with extreme exercise. Etiologic factors are low humidity and temperature of the inspired air and extremely high minute volume.
- Typically, the athlete with true EIA will develop symptoms only in relatively extreme circumstances. The likelihood of developing symptoms increases with exercise involving a higher minute volume and cold, dry conditions (22).
- Exposure to chemicals in the wax room is also associated with reactive airway disease (24); in particular, the use of fluorocarbons in the ski wax.
  - This has led to significant changes in the wax industry and a total ban on fluorocarbon use by FIS beginning in the 2021 ski season.
- History: It is common for these athletes to exhibit symptoms intermittently. The usual symptoms include shortness of breath with exercise that is out of proportion to effort, burning chest pain, postexercise cough, and wheezing.
  - Other red flags include a history of childhood asthma, frequent upper respiratory illnesses, and a chronic cough.
- Physical examination: When the athlete is symptomatic, they may demonstrate wheezing; otherwise, the examination is typically normal.
- Diagnostic testing: The majority of testing protocols use running as the exercise challenge with preexercise and postexercise pulmonary function test change as the measured variable, and as such, the protocols have significant limitations when evaluating the cross-country skier (24,26–34). Ski-specific protocols have been described and are used commonly in the evaluation of elite skiers (33).
- Treatment: With EIA, the main goal is prevention of airway irritation and bronchospasm through preexercise administration of medications. Typically, a stepped approach is undertaken, beginning with a single bronchodilator prior to exercise and adding additional medications as needed.
  - Preventative medications
    - Short-acting β-agonists (albuterol, pirbuterol) are usually effective and have the advantage of low cost, ease of use, and high compliance.
    - Leukotriene inhibitors (montelukast sodium) should be reserved as a second-line treatment and should always be used with a β-agonist as a rescue medication.
    - Cromolyn sodium is rarely effective when used alone.
- Moderate to severe symptoms:
  - Athletes who require second-line medications should be further evaluated.
  - Addition of inhaled corticosteroid (budesonide, fluticasone) or β-agonist/corticosteroid combinations
    - Inhaled corticosteroid is effective in alleviating the postexercise cough brought on by late-phase inflammatory effects of EIA.
  - Doping control: Care must be taken to ensure compliance with doping control measures in elite-level skiers.
  - Most asthma medications are restricted, and appropriate procedures for documenting their use is required. Currently, the International Olympic Committee and FIS require documented testing of these athletes prior to the use of asthma medications.
  - The U.S. Anti-Doping Agency hotline is a useful resource for any questions regarding the use of these medications (1-800-223-0393) (www.usada.org).

COMMON MUSCULOSKELETAL PROBLEMS

Sacroiliitis

- *Pathophysiology:* The sacroiliac (SI) joint is a biconcave articulation of the hemipelvis to the sacrum. It has relatively small rotational motion but functions primarily to transmit force from the lower extremity to the spine. SI dysfunction is the most common cause of low back pain in the skier (17).
  - Injury can result from direct trauma associated with a fall, but more commonly arises from repetitive loading. Contributing factors in this injury include SI joint hypermobility, excessive shear forces, and relative core strength deficits.
- *Clinical features:* Symptoms stem from inflammation in the SI joint and include local pain at the SI joint that is exacerbated with walking, running, or skiing.
  - The athlete will often have associated lateral hip pain and pain at the gluteal prominence.
  - Radicular symptoms are unusual and are associated with piriformis spasm, facet irritation, or concomitant lumbar spine disease.
- *Examination:* will typically reveal the following: tenderness at the SI joint and relative hypomobility on the affected side with a standing knee-to-chest test. FABER test (flexion, abduction, and external rotation) will usually elicit symptoms. Neurologic examination is normal.
- *Diagnostic testing:* Radiographs may demonstrate arthrosis or degenerative disease of the lower spine.
- *Treatment:* Pain relief strategies include oral analgesics/anti inflammatory medications, short pulse oral corticosteroids, osteopathic manipulation or chiropractic treatment, ice, massage, and stretching.
  - Long-term management aims at improving SI function through core stabilization and muscle balance training (Theraball program, Pilates, or similar).
  - Technique and equipment issues should also be reviewed.

LOWER EXTREMITY

Retropatellar Knee Pain (Patellofemoral Dysfunction)/Iliotibial Band Friction Syndrome

- See detailed descriptions in Chapters 65 and 66, respectively.

Exertional Compartment Syndrome

- Pathophysiology: In cross-country skiers, ECS typically affects the anterior or lateral compartments, representing injury to the tibialis anterior or peroneus brevis muscles, respectively.
  - ECS is precipitated by exercise-induced swelling of the soft tissue in the confined compartment, leading to ischemic pain in the affected muscle.
  - This is most common in skating technique where the foot is dorsiflexed and everted during ski recovery (14).
  - This injury was very prevalent when the technique was first introduced due to the excessive length of the ski and relatively soft binding used with the classic stride. As equipment has been developed specifically for the skating technique, this has become less common. It is now most commonly seen with the use of combination equipment (designed for both skating and classic technique), acute overtraining (early season transition), and poorly fitting equipment.
- Clinical features: See detailed description of symptoms in Chapters 27 and 69.
- Diagnostic testing: Preexercise and postexercise compartment pressure testing may be helpful, although it is difficult to reproduce the specific conditions of skiing in the laboratory (see Chapter 26).
- Treatment: Includes decreasing compartment inflammation using anti-inflammatory medications and improving function through a balanced stretching and strengthening program
  - Equipment modifications should be made to use a skating-specific boot-binding-ski system. A stiffer binding and shorter ski may also help.
  - In resistant cases, a surgical fasciotomy may be necessary.

Peroneus Tendon Injury

- Pathophysiology: Injury to the peroneus tendon can occur with an acute inversion dorsiflexion injury or can develop through repetitive overload that leads to tendinitis. With an acute injury, the peroneus tendon can be torn or may be subluxed from the fibular groove with disruption of the overlying retinaculum. Acute injuries occur with both classic and skating techniques, whereas chronic tendinitis is usually seen in the skating technique.
- Clinical features: Acute injuries will present with pain, swelling, and bruising along the posterior and inferior fibula. The athlete will often report a pop in association with an appropriate mechanism, as described earlier.
  - Following the acute phase, a chronic clicking sensation may be present, representing subluxation of the peroneal tendon.
  - Peroneal tendinitis will usually present with pain and swelling along the posterior and inferior fibula. Pain will be worse after skiing and will interfere with other activities, such as running and walking.
- Physical examination may demonstrate subluxation of the affected peroneus tendon when compared to the contralateral ankle. Resisted eversion of the foot will reproduce pain.
- Diagnostic testing: In most acute injuries, an ankle x-ray rules out associated fracture.

- In an acute peroneal tear or subluxation, magnetic resonance imaging (MRI) or musculoskeletal ultrasound evaluation may be helpful to evaluate the extent of injury.
- Treatment: Acute strain injuries without a complete tear can be treated with immobilization in a controlled ankle movement (CAM) walker boot. This is typically continued for 4–6 weeks.
  - Complete tear of the tendon or avulsion of the retinaculum is best managed surgically.
  - Tendinitis is managed with temporary immobilization in a CAM walker followed by active rehabilitation incorporating passive stretching and eccentric overload exercise.
  - Anti-inflammatory medications may be helpful for pain management. Corticosteroid injection may also address the athlete's discomfort.
  - An ankle brace or taping may allow the athlete to continue active training during the rehabilitation process.

Skier's Toe

- Pathophysiology: Skier's toe is a term frequently used to describe pain in the first MTP joint.
  - This may represent either an acute injury (turf toe or acute sesamoid injury) or chronic problem (hallux rigidus, MTP synovitis, or sesamoiditis).
    - In skiers, the chronic form stemming from degenerative joint disease and synovitis is most common and is associated almost exclusively with the classical technique. The mechanism of injury is repetitive extreme extension of the MTP joint.
- Clinical features: Athlete complains of pain, swelling, and limited motion at the great MTP joint.
  - Symptoms are exacerbated with classical skiing, running, and other activities involving repetitive forced extension of the toe.
- Physical examination may reveal obvious degenerative changes on inspection of the joint. Tenderness and erythema are common. Pain is exacerbated with passive extension/flexion.
- Diagnostic testing: Radiographs typically demonstrate first MTP degenerative disease.
  - If a stress fracture or sesamoiditis is suspected, a three-phase bone scan or limited MRI study may be useful.
  - Analysis of joint aspirate may demonstrate uric acid crystals if degeneration is caused by gouty arthritis.
- Treatment: Temporary exclusion of the classic technique helps to alleviate symptoms.
  - Modifying nonskiing footwear to eliminate flexion with a spring steel insert or rigid orthotic is also beneficial.
  - Severe cases may require temporary use of a rocker-bottom boot. Nonsteroidal anti-inflammatory drugs are often helpful.
  - In cases with substantial degeneration, the athlete may benefit from surgical intervention.

UPPER EXTREMITY

De Quervain Tenosynovitis

- Pathophysiology: The repetitive gripping and ulnar/radial deviation motion associated with double poling can lead to tendinitis of the extensor pollicis brevis or abductor pollicis longus. Both tendons occupy the first dorsal wrist compartment and are generally both involved. Chronic pain is common if untreated.
- Clinical features: Typical symptoms include pain and swelling along the radial aspect of the wrist. Symptoms can be insidious in onset or may arise acutely with a traumatic event.
  - Pain is precipitated by gripping and rotational motions (removing the lid from a jar or opening a door).
- Examination reveals tenderness along the extensor surface of the thumb, radial wrist, and forearm. Pain is precipitated with resisted thumb abduction or extension.
  - The patient may demonstrate a positive Finkelstein test (see Chapter 55).
- Treatment: Pain modification via the principles of PRICEMM (protection, rest, ice, elevation, medication, and modalities)
  - Corticosteroid injection may also be beneficial.
  - Protective bracing with a thumb spica splint is helpful and may allow the skier to continue to ski while being treated.
  - Physical or occupational therapy is often useful to address strength and flexibility issues.
  - Surgical treatment (synovectomy) may be necessary in persistent cases.
- Return to skiing when symptom free or if symptom free in appropriate brace.

Skier's Thumb (Ulnar Collateral Ligament)/ Extensor Tenosynovitis/Intersection Syndrome

- See detailed descriptions in Chapter 59.

Acromioclavicular Joint Injury

- See detailed descriptions in Chapter 53.

REFERENCES

1. Renstrom P, Johnson RJ. Cross-country skiing injuries and biomechanics. *Sports Med.* 1989;8(6):346–70.
2. Nordic Ski Lab. *Skate Skiing Techniques Explained. {Video}.* YouTube; 2021 Nov 4. Accessed April 1, 2023. Available from: https://www.youtube.com/watch?v=QEJnPtrtri4
3. Smith GA. Biomechanical analysis of cross-country skiing techniques. *Med Sci Sports Exerc.* 1992;24(9):1015–22.
4. Hoffman MD, Clifford PS. Physiological responses to different cross country skiing techniques on level terrain. *Med Sci Sports Exerc.* 1990;22(6):841–8.

5. Street GM. Technological advances in cross-country ski equipment. *Med Sci Sports Exerc.* 1992;24(9):1048–54.
6. Boyle JJ, Johnson RJ, Pope MH. Cross-country ski injuries. A prospective study. *Iowa Orthop J.* 1981;1:41–8.
7. Sherry E, Asquith J. Nordic (cross-country) skiing injuries in Australia. *Med J Aust.* 1987;146(5):245–6.
8. Worth SGA, Reid DA, Howard AB, Henry SM. Injury incidence in competitive cross-country skiers: a Prospective Cohort Study. *Int J Sports Phys Ther.* 2019 Apr;14(2):237–52.
9. von Rosen P, Floström F, Frohm A, Heijne A. Injury patterns in adolescent elite endurance athletes participating in running, orienteering, and cross-country skiing. *Int J Sports Phys Ther.* 2017 Oct;12(5):822–32.
10. Butcher JD, Brannen SJ. Comparison of injuries in classic and skating Nordic ski techniques. *Clin J Sport Med.* 1998;8(2):88–91.
11. Flørenes TW, Nordsletten L, Heir S, Bahr R. Injuries among World Cup ski and snowboard athletes. *Scand J Med Sci Sports.* 2012;22(1):58–66.
12. Ristolainen L, Heinonen A, Turunen H, et al. Type of sport is related to injury profile: a study on cross country skiers, swimmers, long-distance runners and soccer players. A retrospective 12-month study. *Scand J Med Sci Sports.* 2010;20(3):384–93.
13. Bovard R. The new ski-skating poles: a role in fracture risk? *Phys Sportsmed.* 1994;22(1):41–7.
14. Calvelli N, Vergès S, Rousseaux-Blanchi MP, Edouard P, Guinot M. Features of chronic exertional compartmental syndrome of the leg in elite nordic skiers. *Int J Sports Med.* 2020 Mar;41(3):196–202.
15. Dorsen P, Murphy P, Nash HL, Duda M. Brief reports. *Phys Sportsmed.* 1986;14(2):34–40.
16. Lawson SK, Reid DC, Wiley JP. Anterior compartment pressures in cross-country skiers. A comparison of classic and skating skis. *Am J Sports Med.* 1992;20(6):750–3.
17. Lindsay DM, Meeuwisse WH, Vyse A, Mooney ME, Summersides J. Lumbosacral dysfunctions in elite cross-country skiers. *J Orthop Sports Phys Ther.* 1993;18(5):580–5.
18. Schelkun PH. Cross-country skiing: ski skating brings speed and new injuries. *Phys Sportsmed.* 1992;20(2):168–74.
19. Larsson K, Ohlsén P, Larsson L, Malmberg P, Rydström PO, Ulriksen H. High prevalence of asthma in cross country skiers. *BMJ.* 1993;307(6915):1326–9.
20. Lennelöv E, Irewall T, Naumburg E, Lindberg A, Stenfors N. The prevalence of asthma and respiratory symptoms among cross-country skiers in early adolescence. *Can Respir J.* 2019 Sep 15;2019:1514353.
21. Mäki-Heikkilä R, Karjalainen J, Parkkari J, Valtonen M, Lehtimäki L. Asthma in competitive cross-country skiers: a systematic review and meta-analysis. *Sports Med.* 2020 Nov;50(11):1963–81.
22. Mäki-Heikkilä R, Karjalainen J, Parkkari J, Huhtala H, Valtonen M, Lehtimäki L. High training volume is associated with increased prevalence of non-allergic asthma in competitive cross-country skiers. *BMJ Open Sport Exerc Med.* 2022 May 12;8(2):e001315.
23. Pohjantähti H, Laitinen J, Parkkari J. Exercise-induced bronchospasm among healthy elite cross country skiers and non-athletic students. *Scand J Med Sci Sports.* 2005;15(5):324–8.
24. Rundell KW, Wilber RL, Szmedra L, Jenkinson DM, Mayers LB, Im J. Exercise-induced asthma screening of elite athletes: field versus laboratory exercise challenge. *Med Sci Sports Exerc.* 2000;32(2):309–16.
25. Sue-Chu M, Larsson L, Bjermer L. Prevalence of asthma in young cross-country skiers in central Scandinavia: differences between Norway and Sweden. *Respir Med.* 1996;90(2):99–105.
26. Rundell KW, Smoliga JM, Bougault V. Exercise-induced bronchoconstriction and the air we breathe. *Immunol Allergy Clin North Am.* 2018 May;38(2):183–204.
27. Anderson SD, Daviskas E. The mechanism of exercise-induced asthma is. *J Allergy Clin Immunol.* 2000;106(3):453–9.
28. Carlsen KH, Engh G, Mørk M. Exercise-induced bronchoconstriction depends on exercise load. *Respir Med.* 2000;94(8):750–5.
29. de Bisschop C, Guenard H, Desnot P, Vergeret J. Reduction of exercise-induced asthma in children by short, repeated warm ups. *Br J Sports Med.* 1999;33(2):100–4.
30. Eggleston PA. Methods of exercise challenge. *J Allergy Clin Immunol.* 1984;73(5 pt 2):666–9.
31. Garcia de la Rubia S, Pajarón-Fernandez MJ, Sanchez-Solís M, Martinez-Gonzalez Moro I, Perez-Flores D, Pajarón-Ahumada M. Exercise-induced asthma in children: a comparative study of free and treadmill running. *Ann Allergy Asthma Immunol.* 1998;80(3):232–6.
32. Mannix ET, Manfredi F, Farber MO. A comparison of two challenge tests for identifying exercise-induced bronchospasm in figure skaters. *Chest.* 1999;115(3):649–53.
33. Ogston J, Butcher J. A sport-specific protocol for diagnosing exercise-induced asthma in cross-country skiers. *Clin J Sport Med.* 2002;12(5):291–5.
34. Randolph C, Fraser B, Matasavage C. The free running athletic screening test as a screening test for exercise-induced asthma in high school. *Allergy Asthma Proc.* 1997;18(2):93–8.

97 Fencing Injuries

Lee Kiefer, Gerek Meinhardt, and Steven J. Svoboda

INTRODUCTION

- Fencing is a combat sport that occurs between two athletes who fight against each other with bladed weapons (1).
- Fencing began as a form of military training in 14th-century Europe (2).
- Fencing has been a part of the modern Olympic Games since its beginning in 1896 (3).
- Scoring in fencing traditionally occurred through the subjective opinion of referees. In 1936, the first electrical scoring system was introduced to assist the referee's decision (3,4).
- The international governing body for fencing is the Federation Internationale d'Escrime (FIE) (5).
  - As of 2018, the FIE had 153 member countries (6).
- USA Fencing is the national governing body for amateur fencing in the United States and has 40,000 members from 700+ clubs across all 50 states with about 15,000 members 15 and under (5,7).
  - National competition categories range from 10-year-old to 80+ categories (5).
- NCAA Fencing held their first collegiate championship in 1941 (8).
  - There are currently 33 men's NCAA programs, 43 women's NCAA programs, and 107 college clubs as of 2022 (9).
- The format of NCAA fencing is different from a normal international competition. At championships, males and females combine their individual victories toward a combined team tally. There were 26 teams who participated in this format in 2019 (8).

DISCIPLINES AND PARTICIPATION

- There are three different disciplines in fencing with specific weapons and rules: foil, epee, and saber (3). Table 97.1 shows a comparison of the different fencing disciplines.
- Foil
  - To score, the tip of the weapon requires at least 4.90 N or more of pressure to depress (3).
  - Valid target area includes the lamé, a metal vest covering the torso, and an electric bib covering the neck (3).
  - If a fencer hits a nonvalid target, it is called "off-target" (3).
  - Both fencers can register their touch on a scoring box if it occurs within 300 ms (3).
  - Two fencers cannot score at the same time. When both fencers hit, a point is determined by "right-of-way," which are rules that dictate how one obtains priority (3).
- Epee
  - To score, the tip of the weapon requires 7.36 N or more of pressure to depress (3).
  - Valid target includes the entire body (3).
  - Both fencers can register their touch on a scoring box if it occurs within 40 ms (3).
  - Two fencers can score at the same time. There is no "right-of-way" (3).
- Saber
  - To score, one can hit with any part of the blade with no minimum pressure (3).
  - Valid targets include the lamé, a metal vest that covers the torso and both arms, a conductive glove on the saber-holding hand, and a conductive mask (3).
  - Both fencers can register a touch on a scoring box if it occurs within 170 ms (3).
  - Two fencers cannot score at the same time. "Right-of-way" mentioned above also applies, but there are different nuances (3).
- Female participation
  - Individual foil was the first women's fencing event contested at the Olympic Games in 1924 (3).
  - In the 2004 Olympic Games, all three disciplines were included for women (3).
  - Women's fencing was first contested at NCAA championships in 1982 and all three disciplines were included in 2000 (8).
  - Local and regional tournaments are the only play where mixed-gender events occur (10).
- Parafencing
  - Parafencing also known as wheelchair fencing was established in 1948 as rehabilitation for WWII veterans with spinal cord injuries and was introduced into the Paralympic Games in 1960 (3,11).
  - The international governing body is the International Wheelchair and Amputee Sports Federation (IWAS).
  - Parafencing occurs in wheelchairs mounted to special stabilizing frames (3) (Fig. 97.1).

Table 97.1 Characteristics of Three Fencing Disciplines

	Foil	Epee	Saber
Maximum weight (g)	500	770	500
Maximum blade length (cm)	90	90	88
How to register a hit	Tip of weapon	Tip cf weapon	Side or tip of the weapon
Force required for hit (N)	>4.90	>7.36	Any contact
Valid target area	Trunk and neck	Entire body	Everything above waist
Right-of-way scoring[a]	Yes	No	Yes

Citations:
- Max weights and forces: (3,4).
- Target area images: https://www.sandiegofencing.com/fencing.
- Weapon photos: https://www.researchgate.net/figure/Sports-fencing-weapons-foil-top-epee-middle-sabre-bottom-source-215_fig12_332465274.

[a]Right-of-way scoring is a set of rules that dictates which fencers get a point when they both register a hit, based on who is the aggressor, if there was blade contact and other nuances.

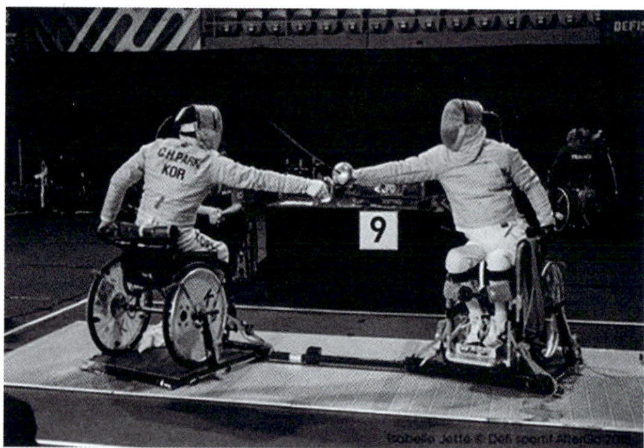

Figure 97.1: Para-athletes participating in a World Cup Saber bout. (© Isabelle Jetté - Défi Sportif AlterGo 2018.)

  - The three disciplines and scoring are the same as in able-bodied fencing, but athletes are not permitted to rise out of the chair (3).
  - There are three classifications based on disability. "A" fencers have the most mobility with torso and arm movements intact; this often includes athletes who are amputees. "B" fencers can have spinal cord injuries with paresis of the legs and sometimes arms. "C" fencers are tetraplegic with the least mobility (11).
- Fencing occurs on a fencing strip, a metal rectangle with dimensions between 4.9 and 6.6 ft wide and 46 ft long (Fig. 97.2).
  - The bout starts with each fencer at an "en garde" line, which are delineated marks 6.5 ft from the middle of the strip (3,4).
- At competitions, there is typically a preliminary round called pools where groups of six or seven fencers will fence in a round-robin to five points or 3 minutes if five points are not reached.
  - Results of pool-play determines seeding for the next round called direct elimination where fencers will move forward in the bracket if they win or be eliminated if they lose.
  - In this round for foil and epee, bouts are fenced to 15 touches or three 3-minute periods with 1 minute of rest in between each period.
  - In saber, bouts are also fenced to 15 touches with a 1-minute break when the leading fencer reaches eight points (3,4).

EPIDEMIOLOGY OF INJURIES

- General epidemiology considerations
  - Injury severity
    - Most fatal injuries since the 1930s have occurred by penetration force after a blade breakage (4).
    - Since an accidental death at the 1982 World Championships due to a broken foil blade puncturing a fencer's mask and into his brain, the safety and testing standards for fencing equipment have been made more rigorous, and no deaths have occurred in high-level fencing (4,12).
    - Punctures, penetrations, and lacerations that result in permanent disability or death are now extremely rare (10).
  - Overall injury rates
    - Figure 97.3 describes injury rates by time and type.
    - Lower extremity injuries are the most common (72.4%) reason for withdrawal from FIE competition,

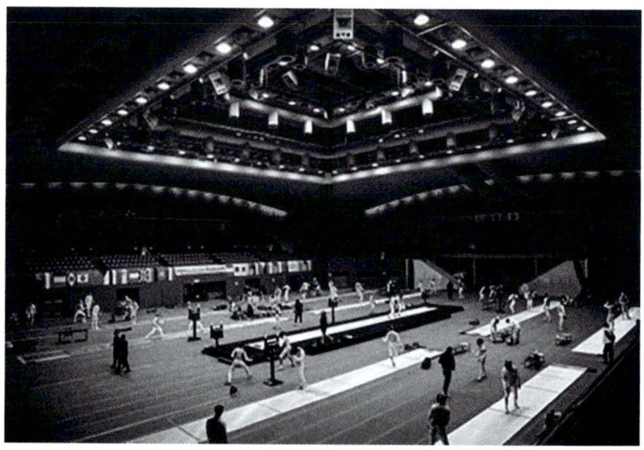

Figure 97.2: Typical fencing venue.

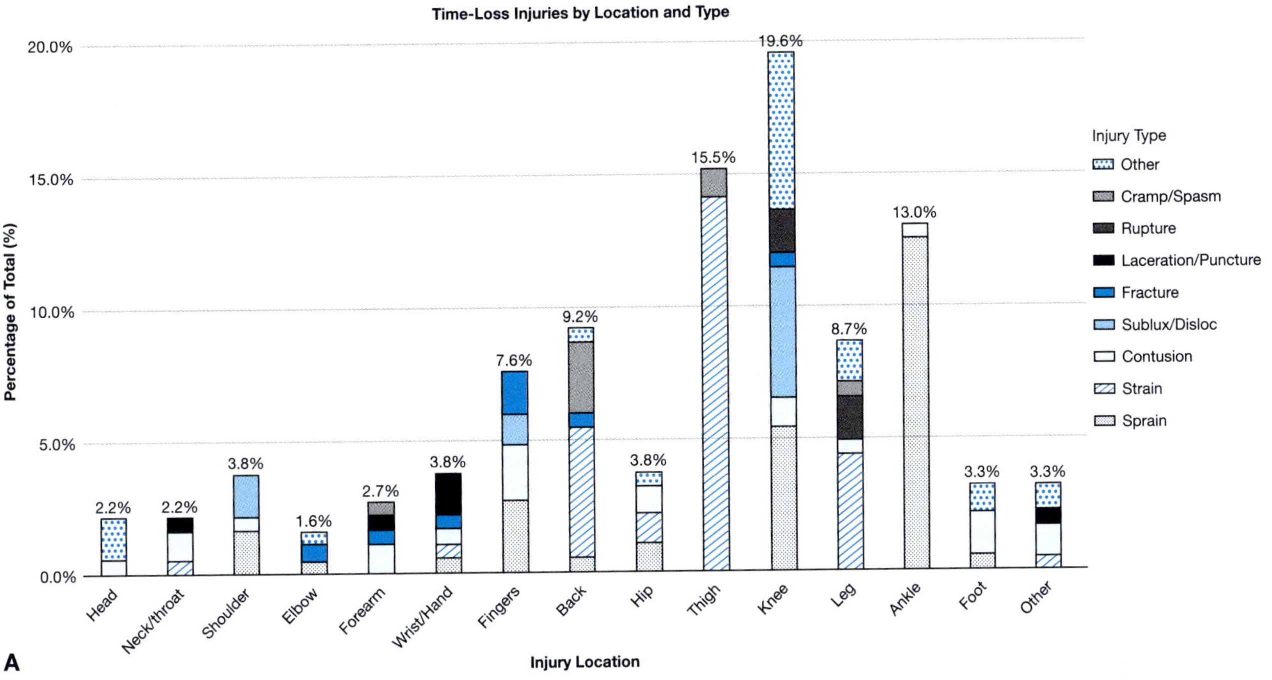

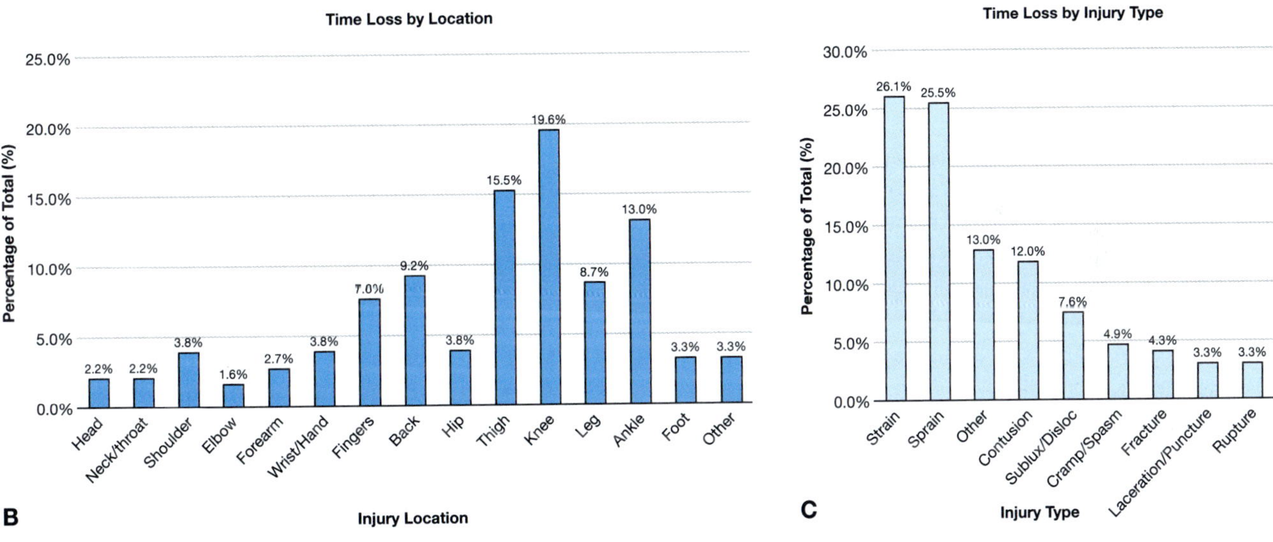

Figure 97.3: A–C: Fencing time-loss injuries by location and type. (Adapted from Harmer PA. Incidence and characteristics of time-loss injuries in competitive fencing: A prospective, 5-year study of National competitions. *Clinical J Sport Med*. 2008;18(2): 137–42. doi: 10.1097/JSM.0b013e318161548d)

with ankle (26.4%), knee (23.6%), and thigh (14.4%) as the most common areas of injury.

- More specifically, first and second-degree lower-extremity strains (40.8%) and sprains (20.1%) are the most common, followed by third-degree sprains/strains (9.8%), and laceration/puncture injuries (2.9%).

- The most common upper extremity injury involved the wrist, hand, or fingers and accounted for 9.2% of injuries (6).

- In the USA Fencing competition, 30.2% of recorded exposures were time-loss injuries and approximately 52% of reported injuries were first or second-degree strains and sprains.
  - Lower limb injuries were most common, specifically in the knee (19.6%), thigh (15.2%), and ankle (13.0%) (13).
- In a study on U.S. Olympic team members and national team members, 69% of fencers had at least one injury in the lead leg (dominant) knee.

- The most common knee injury was undiagnosed knee pain followed by a meniscus tear. 24% reported one or more dominant hip injuries.
- Muscle strains were the most common injury in dominant hips and muscle strains and labral tears were the most common in non-dominant hips. 20% reported ankle sprains (14).

- National team-level fencers incur an average of 3.3 injuries per year, with 52.6% reported as mild (1–3 days of treatment) and 95% occurring in training (15).
- Among 98,000 competitors at USA Fencing domestic events from 2015 to 2019, 70 mild TBIs were reported with 49 requiring withdrawal from competition (16).
- Contusions account for >25% of all recorded injuries (4).

- Injuries by discipline
  - Saber fencers have higher overall injury rates than foil and epee fencers and have the highest number of lower extremity injuries (14,15).
  - Foil and saber fencers have a significantly greater risk of withdrawal from international competition due to injury than epee fencers (6).
- Injuries by sex
  - Female fencers have a greater overall injury risk than males (10,15).
  - Males are more likely to have mild (1–3 days of treatment) injuries than females while females are more likely to have moderate (4–7 days of treatment) and severe (8+ days of treatment) injuries (15).
  - In international competition specifically, males have a significantly greater risk (42.6%) of withdrawal due to injury and are more likely to incur a strain injury than females, especially in the thigh (6).
  - Among U.S. Olympic and national team members, females had more hip and knee injuries than males (14).
  - Females have increased rates of patellofemoral pathology (17).
- Injuries by age
  - Senior (open-age category) fencers have a significantly higher risk (74.3%) of time-loss injury than junior (Under 20) and cadet (Under 17) fencers (6).
  - Senior fencers specifically have a much greater risk of knee sprains and thigh strains than junior and cadet fencers (6). This is likely due to the chronic nature of many fencing injuries, the longer training hours, as well as the increased speed and force of their fencing.
- Parafencing injuries
  - Parafencers are more likely to have a higher injury incident rate compared to able-bodied fencers, especially parafencers with less trunk control (18).
  - Upper extremity injuries account for 73.8% of injuries. Elbow injuries account for 32.6% and shoulder injuries account for 15.8% of this number (18).
- Mechanisms of injury
  - Noncontact injuries (intrinsic effort of fencers) were the most common mechanism of time-loss injury for international fencers withdrawing from competition due to injury, accounting for 47.1% of cases. The next most common mechanisms included the fencer slipping or tripping (28.2%), contact with the opponent (19.5%), and injury by the opponents blade (5.2%) (6).
  - Female fencers have a greater patellofemoral contact force during a lunge compared to male fencers, which suggests the reason for increased rates of patellofemoral pathology (17).

EQUIPMENT

- USA Fencing requires that all fencers at USA Fencing competitions wear full fencing clothing and equipment which conforms with USA Fencing regulations while competing or training. During individual lessons with a coach, the fencer must wear at least a mask and glove, and the coach must wear at least a fencing coach jacket, a glove, and a mask (19). This equipment is shown in Figure 97.4.

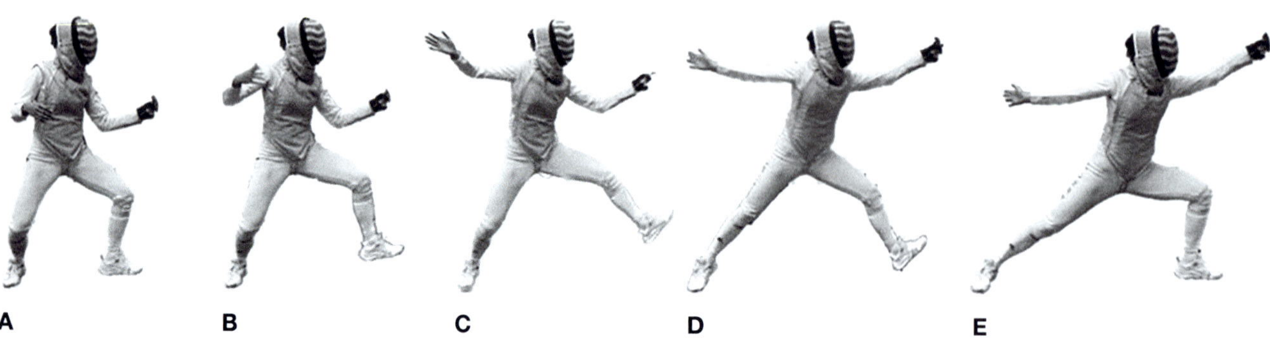

Figure 97.4: A sequence of movement for a foil fencer performing a lunge: (A) en garde position; (B) lead leg lifts off ground; (C) back leg propels fencer forward as lead leg continues to extend; (D) lead leg lands heel first and the dominant arm extends; and (E) final lunge position.

- At all USA Fencing and FIE-sanctioned events, athletes must submit their equipment for checking prior to competition. All passed equipment will receive a label such as a stamp. Referees will check for these verification labels prior to the beginning of each bout (20).
- In official FIE events, all blades, points, jackets, under-arm protectors, knickers, masks, and gloves must bear the FIE homologation certification mark indicating that the equipment manufacturer has passed quality and safety testing (20).
- Weapons (19,20)
  - Weapon blades must be able to withstand high levels of exertion, have a high resistance to breaking, and have a low susceptibility to corrosion, which is proven through mandatory testing for manufacturers.
  - The specifications for the weapons in each discipline are listed in Table 97.1.
  - In international competition, weapon blades must be made of maraging steel which is a higher quality steel than mandatory for local and national competitions (21).
- Uniform (19,20)
  - The jacket, under-plastron (layer that covers half of the torso and sword arm), and knickers (fencing pants) must be made of cloth that can resist 800 Newtons of pressure.
  - The jacket must include a double-thickness lining on the sleeve down to the elbow of the sword arm, have a lower edge that overlaps the knickers by at least 10 cm, and be completely done up and void of buckles or openings that could catch an opponent's weapon.
  - Females must wear a chest/breast protector made of metal or a rigid material like plastic with the outside layer covered by a soft material that is 4 mm thick and 22 kg · m^{-3} dense.
  - Knickers must be fastened below the knees such as by an elastic cuff, and socks must cover the legs up to the knickers.
  - A glove is required on the sword arm only, should have a gauntlet that covers approximately half of the forearm, and should have no holes in the hand.
- Mask
  - The mask must be made from high-quality carbon stainless steel wires that are a minimum 1 mm in diameter, form a mesh that has a maximum of 2.1 mm between wires, withstand the introduction of a conical instrument at a pressure of 12 kg, have two different safety/fastening systems at the rear, and have a bib that can withstand 1600 N of pressure (19).
  - The mask covers the face and side of the head but not the back of the head.
- Field of play
  - The fencing strip is often on an elevated platform of up to 20 in during the final rounds (19). There have been several occurrences of athletes rolling ankles on the sides of strips or falling off the sides/ends of platforms.

PHYSIOLOGY OF FENCING

- Basic movements
  - Fencing is an asymmetrical sport, which typically produces asymmetrical anthropometric characteristics. Fencers have a greater cross-sectional area in the dominant forearm, arm, thigh, and calf (4).
  - Fencers typically start their bout in the "en garde position." The lead foot is aligned parallel to the strip and pointed at the opponent with the knee joint flexed at 20°–30° while the back foot is situated perpendicular to the front foot with the back knee flexed at 90°. This stance provides stability and a launching point for a lunge (4,13).
  - A common footwork maneuver is called a lunge. In a lunge, the feet remain perpendicular to each other as in the en garde position with the back knee extending fully and the front knee flexing to be in a vertical plane above the front foot on landing. Figure 97.4 shows the progression of the lunge maneuver.
  - Fencers hold their weapon in the hand that is the same side as the "lead leg" *i.e.*, right right-handed fencers have their right leg in front (14).
  - For the lead leg, the heel is predominantly loaded during an advance (forward step) and lunge, while the hallux and forefoot are predominantly loaded during a retreat (backward step). For the back leg, the hallux is also predominantly loaded during retreat movements, but the forefoot is predominantly loaded during advance and lunge movements (22).
- Energy expenditure
  - The duration of an international competition is between 9 and 11 hours with the effective combat time falling between 17 and 48 minutes and a single point occurring between 1 and 60 seconds. Athletes lunge 66–210 times over the course of a competition (1,4).
  - Fencing requires short phases of maximal or supramaximal intensity, recruiting both aerobic and anaerobic systems during a bout (1).
  - Fencers' VO_{2max} is expectedly lower than endurance activities. Studies show contradictory evidence on the relationship between VO_{2max} and performance (4).
  - A fencer might cover 250–1000 m during a bout, attack 140 times, and change direction around 170 times during a bout (23).
  - An athlete's heart rate during a fencing bout is dependent on intensity but typically higher during saber bouts compared to other weapons (4).

MEDICAL ISSUES

- **General**
  - Heat illness and exhaustion have been reported and are caused by the quantity of protective gear (4).

- **Infection**
  - There is a low probability of transmitting HIV or Hep B from punctures (10).
  - Transmitting upper respiratory tract infections can occur after shaking hands, which is a required act at the end of each bout (10).
  - Equipment sharing (gloves, masks, jackets) is common at clubs. Skin infections and MRSA outbreaks have been reported (10).
- **Dermatologic**
  - Friction blisters on the hand from contact with the grip of the weapon and under the head of the first metatarsal on the rear foot from the stance to facilitate lunging are common (10).
  - Subungual hematomas are common. It occurs in the fingers from being hit by the opponent's blade and on the toes by being stepped on or wearing ill-fitting shoes (10).
  - Contusions from the opponent's weapon are very common, accounting for more than 25% of all recorded injuries (4).
  - Laceration and puncture injuries account for 2.9% of injuries leading to withdrawal from international competition (6).
- **Ocular**
  - Contact of an opponent's weapon with the mask can cause small pieces of the mask's paint to get into a fencer's eye.
- **Concussions**
  - The two primary mechanisms for diagnosed mild traumatic brain injury are indirect head trauma caused by an opponent's weapon guard contacting the mask and posterior head trauma caused by falling backwards on the strip (16).

MUSCULOSKELETAL ISSUES

- **Shoulder**
  - Shoulder injuries account for 3% of reported injuries (10).
  - Impingement of the shoulder is a common chronic/overuse problem (10).
  - Reported shoulder injuries include sprains, strains, and subluxation/dislocation (6).
  - Evaluation, treatment, and return to play considerations for these conditions are similar to management in other sports.
- **Elbow**
  - Lateral epicondylitis in the dominant arm is a common chronic/overuse problem in fencers and has been documented as a reason for withdrawal from international competition (6).
  - Radial tunnel syndrome is also reported and suspected to be caused by repetitive fencing movements called parries.
  - Impact on the elbow from an opponent's blade can cause bursitis.
  - Evaluation, treatment, and return to play considerations for these conditions are similar to management in other sports.
- **Wrist, hand**
  - The most common upper extremity injuries (7.6% of total injuries) involve the finger (sprains, contusions, fracture, and subluxation/dislocation). Hand injuries were tied for second at 3% (10).
- **Chest**
  - Being the primary target in foil and epee, the chest is a common area for contusions.
  - Most contusions can be managed conservatively with analgesics, ice, and padding for return to play as needed.
- **Back**
  - Low back sprains, strains, and spasms account for 9% of total time loss injuries (10).
  - Lower back injuries can occur from trunk rotation or being off balance (15).
  - Evaluation, treatment, and return to play considerations for these conditions are similar to management in other sports.
    - Persistent or "red flag" symptoms should prompt further evaluation for neurogenic etiology
    - Persistent pain or pain with extension should prompt evaluation for pars injury, though these are rare in fencing.
- **Abdomen**
  - Abdominal strains can be caused by trunk rotation (15).
  - Evaluation, treatment and return to play considerations for these conditions are similar to management in other sports.
- **Thigh, groin, and hamstring**
  - Thigh strains were the second most common specific injury among international fencers withdrawing from competition due to injury (12.6%). The lead leg was injured in 90.1% of thigh strains, and the hamstrings were involved in 90.0% of lead leg thigh strains. 77.3% of thigh strains were non-contact, 18.2% were due to slipping or tripping, and 4.5% involved contact with the opponent (6).
  - Fencing strips can be slippery from dirt, sweat, or loss of traction from wear. It is not uncommon to see an athlete fall into the splits after slipping.
  - Although there is no extensive epidemiological data, the externally rotated position of the hip and extension of the rear leg in the final lunge position (Fig. 97.4E) puts the adductors in a vulnerable position, and injuries may occur here, especially if the leg is over-extended during the execution of the lunge maneuver.
- **Hip**
  - Lead leg hip injuries are more common than nondominant hip injuries (14).

- Athletes reporting time-loss injuries of 3–6 months for the hip include labral tears and impingement. Hip injuries reported by high-level athletes included muscle strain, labral tear, osteoarthritis, fracture, snapping hip syndrome, general pain, and bursitis. Reported injuries requiring operative treatment included labral tear, osteoarthritis, snapping hip syndrome, and impingement (14).
- Fencers may experience a combination of concomitant conditions, such as sacroiliac joint syndrome, hamstring injury, and abdominal strain (15).

Knee

- Knee injuries are the most common time-loss injury for American fencers and include meniscal lesions, ACL and MCL rupture, patellar tendon pain, patellar subluxation/dislocation, and nonspecific knee pain (10).
- Lead leg knee injuries are more common than nondominant knee injuries (14). However, the externally rotated position of the rear leg in the final lunge position (Fig. 97.4E) can lead to valgus forces on the knee, putting the structures of the medial knee, the MCL in particular, in a vulnerable position for injury as well.
- In fencers withdrawing from international competition due to injury, 64.7% of all ruptures involved the knee, with the ACL damaged in 72.7% of these cases.
  - Other knee ruptures involved the medial collateral ligament, lateral collateral ligament, and patella tendon (6).
- Patellar tendon and medial tibial stress syndrome are common chronic/overuse problems (10).
- The longest time-loss injuries among U.S. Olympic and national team members included meniscus injury, patellar/quadriceps tendonitis/bursitis, and ligament injury.
  - Other injuries reported included undiagnosed knee pain, meniscus tear, patellofemoral pain syndrome, IT band syndrome, osteoarthritis, patellar/quad tendinitis/bursitis, loose bodies-osteochondral lesion, patellar instability, Osgood-Schlatter, ligament injury, and fracture.
  - Reported injuries requiring operative treatment included undiagnosed knee pain, ACL injury, meniscus tear, synovial cyst, patellar chondromalacia, osteochondral lesion, patellar fracture, and loose bodies (14).
- Evaluation, treatment, and return to play considerations for knee injuries are similar to their management in other sports.

Ankle

- Ankle sprains were the most common specific injury among international fencers withdrawing from competition due to injury (25.3%). 68.1% of ankle sprains involved the lead leg.
  - The most common mechanism of injury for ankle sprains is slipping or tripping, accounting for 56.8% of cases. Other mechanisms include contact with the opponent (25.0%) and noncontact incidents (18.2%) (6).
  - It is common for fencers to sprain their ankle landing on their opponent's foot or rolling it on the edge of the metal fencing strip.
- Evaluation, treatment, and return to play considerations for ankle injuries are similar to management in other sports, though attention must be paid to the different stresses placed on each ankle during routine movements.

Foot

- Friction blisters are common on the Achilles tendon and under the head of the first metatarsal on the rear foot (10).
- Achilles tendon rupture has occurred when athletes slip from the elevated lip of the strip to the floor underneath (10).
- Achilles and plantar fascia tendonitis are common chronic/overuse problems (10).
  - During a lunge, a peak pressure of 551.8 kPa is exerted on the heel of the lead leg (5). It is common to place a protective heel cup in the lead leg shoe to prevent bruising of the calcaneus or fat pad.

Confusion with nonaccidental trauma (NAT):

- There are numerous anecdotal reports of children below 18 with bruising on the chest, arms, and legs, which is common in fencing, and being misconstrued as nonaccidental trauma by medical professionals. More data is needed in this regard to develop a policy on how to balance both the interests of preventing nonaccidental trauma with protecting the athletes and their parents from incorrect NAT diagnosis.

INJURY PREVENTION

- Recommendations to decrease lower extremity injuries include appropriate warm-up, stretching, proprioceptive training programs, and prophylactic strength training. Increasing education on this topic to athletes and coaches is important (15,24).
- Fencing requires repetitive eccentric contractions during lunging and change of direction. To reduce the change of muscle damage in the lead leg, it is recommended that fencers include high eccentric loads (*i.e.*, Olympic lifts or plyometrics) in their strength and conditioning programs. High-intensity interval training (HIIT) is also recommended during practice to increase the body's tolerance to hydrogen ion accumulation (22).
- Concerns about overtraining, especially in elite populations, were found in a USA Fencing Survey.
  - Recommendations were released to incorporate appropriate and balanced strength and conditioning into athletes' training (15).

EVENT COVERAGE

- All USA Fencing national competitions have a sports medicine booth covered by a team of medical personnel that evaluate, and treat when possible, any athlete needing assistance. Information is obtained and entered into an electronic health record for each athlete.
- Medical personnel covering their first USA Fencing competition will be trained in person about any unique fencing procedures by experienced staff at the beginning of the event.
- The sports medicine team may be called over the intercom to a fencing strip if a fencer gets hurt during a bout. In this case, the team at the booth will send someone with a first aid kit to the strip for evaluation, making sure that the booth is still manned.
- In competition, athletes are allowed one 5-minute "time-out" due to injury or another medical reason as determined by the medical overseer evaluating the injury (19,21).
- A fencer can only have one 5-minute break per competition unless they are allowed another break by medical personnel for a different injury or medical reason (19,21).
- Typically, athletic trainers and physicians who travel with Team USA to international competitions will first have experience covering national events and familiarity with fencing.
- FIE competitions must have a medical doctor on-site for the complete duration of the competition to oversee medical services and supervise antidoping procedures (19).
- USA Fencing medical policies and procedures are overseen by its Sports Medicine Resource Team led by the Director of Sports Medicine while the FIEs are directed by the FIE Medical Commission.
- Most NCAA competitions are covered by athletic trainers for triage of injuries and treatment when possible.

REFERENCES

1. Milia R, Roberto S, Pinna M, et al. Physiological responses and energy expenditure during competitive fencing. *Appl Physiol Nutr Metab.* 2014;39(3):324–8. doi:10.1139/apnm-2013-0221
2. International Olympic Committee. *Fencing.* [cited 2025 Aug 1]. https://olympics.com/en/sports/fencing.
3. Evangelista N, Granet E. *The Editors of Encyclopaedia Britannica.* Chicago, IL: Fencing – Organized Sport. [cited 2025 Aug 1]. https://www.britannica.com/sports/fencing/Organized-sport.
4. Roi GS, Bianchedi D. The science of fencing: implications for performance and injury prevention. *Sports Med.* 2008;38(6):465–81. doi:10.2165/00007256-200838060-00003
5. Jomantas N. *USA Fencing: Celebrating 130 Years of Fencing in America*; 2021. https://www.usafencing.org/news_article/show/1159718
6. Harmer PA. Epidemiology of time-loss injuries in international fencing: a prospective, 5-year analysis of Fédération Internationale d'Escrime competitions. *Br J Sports Med.* 2019;53(7):442–8. doi:10.1136/bjsports-2018-100002
7. USA Fencing. *Membership*; 2023. https://member.usafencing.org/search/members
8. Masin G. *NCAA History. Museum of American Fencing*; 2023. http://museumofamericanfencing.com/wp/ncaa-history/
9. USA Fencing. *College Programs*; 2023. https://www.usafencing.org/college-programs
10. Harmer PA. Getting to the point: injury patterns and medical care in competitive fencing. *Curr Sports Med Rep.* 2008;7(5):303–7. doi:10.1249/JSR.0b013e318187083b
11. Borysiuk Z, Nowicki T, Piechota K, Błaszczyszyn M. Neuromuscular, perceptual, and temporal determinants of movement patterns in wheelchair fencing: preliminary study. *BioMed Res Int.* 2020;2020:6584832. doi:10.1155/2020/6584832
12. Portable Press. *The Tragic Fencing Death of Vladimir Smirnov*; 2015. https://www.portablepress.com/blog/2015/07/tragic-fencing-death-vladimir-smirnov
13. Harmer PA. Incidence and characteristics of time-loss injuries in competitive fencing: a prospective, 5-year study of national competitions. *Clin J Sport Med.* 2008;18(2):137–42. doi:10.1097/JSM.0b013e318161548d
14. Thompson K, Chang G, Alaia M, Jazrawi L, Gonzalez-Lomas G. Lower extremity injuries in U.S. national fencing team members and U.S. fencing Olympians. *Phys Sportsmed.* 2022;50(3):212–17. doi:10.1080/00913847.2021.1895693
15. Park KJ, Brian Byung S. Injuries in elite Korean fencers: an epidemiological study. *Br J Sports Med.* 2017;51(4):220–5. doi:10.1136/bjsports-2016-096754
16. Thompson A, Summers J, Freedman A. The epidemiology of traumatic brain injuries within USA Fencing, 2015-2020: prevention, care, and return to play considerations. *Br J Sports Med.* 2021;55:A41–2.
17. Sinclair J, Bottoms L. Gender differences in patellofemoral load during the epee fencing lunge. *Res Sports Med.* 2015;23(1):51–8. doi:10.1080/15438627.2014.975813
18. Chung WM, Yeung S, Wong AY, et al. Musculoskeletal injuries in elite able-bodied and wheelchair foil fencers – A pilot study. *Clin J Sport Med.* 2012 May;22(3):278–80. doi:10.1097/JSM.0b013e31824a577e
19. USA Fencing. *USA Fencing Rules for Competition.* USA Fencing; 2022. https://cdn1.sportngin.com/attachments/document/0b4e-2752049/USA_Fencing_Rules_2022-08_.pdf#_ga=2.163203964.1783499607.1672265432-1253964151.1662303441
20. FIE. *Material Rules.* Lausanne, SUI: Fédération Internationale d'Escrime; 2022. https://fie.org/fie/documents/rules
21. FIE. *Technical Rules.* Lausanne, SUI: Fédération Internationale d'Escrime; 2022. https://fie.org/fie/documents/rules
22. Trautmann C, Martinelli N, Rosenbaum D. Foot loading characteristics during three fencing-specific movements. *J Sports Sci.* 2011;29(15):1585–92. doi:10.1080/02640414.2011.605458
23. Turner A, James N, Dimitriou L, et al. Determinants of olympic fencing performance and implications for strength and conditioning training. *J Strength Cond Res.* 2014;28(10):3001–11. doi:10.1519/JSC.0000000000000478
24. de Vasconcelos GS, Cini A, Lima CS. Proprioceptive training on dynamic neuromuscular control in fencers: a clinical trial. *J Sport Rehabil.* 2020;30(2):220–5. doi:10.1123/jsr.2019-0469

Fishing

98

Gitansh Bhargava, Lauren E. Juliano, and Alexander R. Kheradi

INTRODUCTION

- Fishing as an activity has existed for millions of years, primarily as a means of sustenance and survival, but over the past several decades, fishing has progressed beyond a commercial endeavor and has developed into a recreational activity, which is sometimes turned into a competition.

SCOPE OF PARTICIPATION

- In 2018, 49.4 million people went out to a body of water to engage in both recreational and commercial fishing, and there are now more individuals who fish than those who play golf and tennis combined (1).
- The four types of fishing competitions most commonly observed are fly-fishing, deep-sea fishing, bass fishing (the most popular), and ice fishing.
- Sport fishing is governed by its own regulatory bodies, which set specific rules and regulations to ensure the sustainability and fairness of the activity.
- Recreational fishing, a hobby enjoyed by a broad spectrum of individuals across all ages and demographics, has simpler requirements:
  - At its most basic level, recreational fishing necessitates the use of a fishing rod — a pole equipped with a reel and attached line — and a fishhook, as well as a suitable body of water.
  - This straightforward equipment setup and the wide accessibility of water bodies make recreational fishing an appealing activity to a vast range of people.

COMPETITION

- All types of marine fishing in the United States are governed by the National Oceanic and Atmospheric Administration (2).
- The International Gaming Fish Association (IGFA) handles all the rules and guidelines for competition and other group angling activities.
- Competitions have specific rules on rod length, types of hooks, and the use of power accessories, etc., which can all be found in both the IGFA handbook and in the handbook for each specific tournament.
- Once a fish takes the bait or lure, the goal is for the angler to bring the fish back to the boat without any additional help or device beyond personal skill.

Fishing Tournaments

- The growing popularity of fishing has led to an exponential increase in the number of fishing tournaments held per year for anglers at every level (3).
- Many types of fishing tournaments exist — bass, catfish, marlin, fly-fishing, ice, etc. However, bass fishing is by far the most popular and exists at the professional, collegiate, high school, and club levels.
- Tournaments can span multiple days and each day of the tournament can last 6–10 hours depending on the time of year and geographic location.
- The collegiate fishing circuit is incredibly popular with three major series — Bass Pro Shops Collegiate Bass Fishing Series, Strike King Bassmaster College Series, and Abu Garcia Fishing Circuit. Though the National Collegiate Athletic Association and the National Association of Intercollegiate Athletics do not recognize bass fishing as an official sport, the governing body for collegiate fishing is the Association of College Anglers (4) and collegiate anglers can compete alongside professionals and win cash prizes without consequences (5).

PROFESSIONAL FISHING

- Professional-level fishing exists throughout the year with many tournaments, the majority of tournaments being centered around bass fishing.
- Ever since Ray Wilson Scott founded the Bass Anglers Sportsman Society (B.A.S.S.) and held the first bass fishing tournament that same year at Beaver Lake, Arkansas, the number of fishing tournaments has steadily been increasing (6).

- The B.A.S.S. Bassmaster Classic is considered the "Super Bowl of Fishing" — an invite-only event with a grand prize worth more than $1 million dollars (7).
- A few of the other notable professional tournaments are the Bass Pro Tour, the FLW Pro Circuit, and the Bassmaster Elite Series.

COMMON INJURIES IN FISHING

- As sport fishing has become more popular, the number of reported injuries has increased (8).
- Data are limited as not all injured patients present for formal evaluation and medical care following a fishing injury.
  - There tend to be more visits to the emergency department for fishing-related injuries during the warmer months.
  - There is no significant difference between the incidence of injury between pediatric and adult populations; however, there is a higher incidence of injuries in males compared to females (9).
- Fishing-related injuries tend to fall into several broad categories:
  - Trauma such as mechanical falls or penetrating trauma from fish hooks, fish spines, or bites during handling
  - Environmental injuries and exposures such as zoonotic infections, envenomations, and sun exposure
  - Overuse injuries similar to those seen in other overhead sports
  - The most affected joint with pain is the shoulder (44.7%), followed by the elbow (16.0%) and hand (16.0%); multiple studies support this distribution of injuries (10,11).

BIOMECHANICS

Bass Fishing Mechanics

- There are a series of motions involved with casting:
  - During the *cocking phase,* the angler brings the rod and reel to a ~10-o'clock position.
  - During the *acceleration phase*, the angler brings the rod and reel overhead to ~3-o'clock position during which the lure is released.
  - The *deceleration phase* occurs after the lure is released from the rod.
  - The partial follow-through phase occurs as the elbow brings the wrist to follow through, causing a valgus stress on the elbow (12).

Fly-Fishing Mechanics

- The biomechanical demands of fly-fishing, such as repetitive motion, utilizing various fly-casting techniques, casting styles, and equipment, are likely what lead to injuries (10,13).
- Many, if not most, anglers tend to have some upper extremity pain, but will not seek medical attention leading to skewed data on the prevalence of injuries.
- Casting styles that include an elliptical or sidearm cast lead to a higher likelihood of injury compared to an overhead casting style (14–16). Most pain was felt in the elbow or wrist (10).
- Adding weight to any aspect of equipment — the rod, line, head, etc. — increases mechanical stress to an angler's arm and hence increases the incidence of injury (10,11).
- A grip that involves a finger on top of the rod leads to a higher likelihood of injury compared to a "V-style" grip or with a thumb on top (10).
- Anglers who attempt to fish for heavy saltwater fish have a higher reported likelihood of injury compared to other anglers fishing for smaller species (16).

Overuse Injuries

- Like overhead throwing sports such as baseball, sport fishing involves a great deal of repetitive overhead motions, which can lead to injury.
- In comparison to baseball pitchers who generally throw approximately 100 pitches a game followed by several days of rest between appearances, pro anglers can cast 8–12 hours daily for weeks at a time (9). A bass fisherman can average more than 960 casts in a single session or approximately 1620 casts/tournament.
- Fly-fishing days can be long, consecutive, and rigorous with an average fly fisherman casting approximately 200 casts per session and sometimes casting for 3 consecutive days (10).
- Mechanics play a role in injuries. Skill and practice are key to handling the increased physical demands of casting longer fishing lines (11,13).
  - Experienced anglers maintain efficient casting form even with "long line lengths," referring to the extended distance of line, often 40 to over 100 feet, cast from the rod tip.
    - Experienced anglers transfer velocity from the shoulder down the arm, allowing precise control and reducing strain.
  - However, less experienced anglers struggle with longer line lengths, often resorting to a "full-arm waving" motion.
    - This inefficient technique reduces control, decreases accuracy, and increases the risk of shoulder, elbow, and wrist injuries due to excessive strain.
- The repetitive strain from casting leaves kids vulnerable to overuse injuries, especially considering their skeletal immaturity and the fact that they often begin competing as early as 13 years old (12).
- Most common injury patterns include ligament tears or tendonitis, which frequently involve the shoulder/rotator cuff, elbow, and wrist.

INJURIES UNIQUE TO FISHING

Fishhook Injuries

- The most reported fishing injury occurs while handling the fishhook, typically while baiting the line or removing the hook from the fish, resulting in the fishhook penetrating the fingers (17).
- Most fishhooks contain a barb which is a backward sharp projection that impedes the fish from freeing itself once it is "hooked." See Figure 98.1.
- Prior to removing a fishhook, the following should be performed (14,17–19):
  - Regardless of whether or not the fishhook has a barb, the initial step to take is to stabilize the lure to avoid further injury;
  - Radiograph of the affected area can help identify depth of penetration, presence barbs, and any bony injury and also guide a plan for removal;
  - Remove any accessory parts (*i.e.*, bait, fishing line) from the fishhook to make removal easier;
  - Perform neurovascular exam proximal and distal to the injury;
  - Clean the injury site with a povidone-iodine or hexachlorophene solution ± an irrigation wash;
  - Consider performing a local or regional anesthetic block to aid in comfort and ease of removal.

Fishhook Removal

- The presence of a barb can lead to further tissue damage if the fishhook is attempted to be pulled out, so careful considerations should be made.
- The techniques that cause the least trauma during removal are the retrograde technique and the string pull techniques, which are typically used for removal of simple hooks without barbs (17).
- **The String Yank Method:** This method works well for fishhooks that are small or medium size and those that are deeply embedded in soft tissue. It does not work particularly well for larger hooks or those that are very superficial. You cannot use this method if the part of the body where the fishhook is embedded is not fixed (*i.e.*, the earlobe) (17–19). See Figure 98.2.
  - A string should be tied around the midpoint of the fishhook bend so there is tension parallel to the fishhook;
  - Pressure should be placed perpendicular/downward to the shank to disengage the barb — ideally, this will move the barb into the original insertion pathway;
  - The string should be pulled parallel to the direction of insertion — if successful, this should allow the hook to come out the same way the barb was inserted; be careful not to get stuck as this does act like a projectile.
- **The Retrograde Method:** The lower the amount of tissue trauma, the much lower the success rate will be, but it works well for barbed and superficially embedded hooks (18,19). See Figure 98.3.
  - Downward pressure should be placed on the fishhook's shank — to disengage the barb from surrounding tissue;
  - The downward pressure should be continued such with an attempt to remove the hook along its original path;
  - Stop if there is any resistance or the patient cannot tolerate the removal attempt. If this occurs, consider another method of removal.
- **Needle Cover Method:** The goal with this method is to cover the barb of the fishhook with a needle. This method works well when the point of fishhook is superficially embedded and the fishhook has a single barb (18,19). See Figure 98.4.
  - Local anesthetic should be administered and an 18-gauge needle should be guided parallel to the shank of the hook until it covers the hook (the bevel should be aimed toward the inside of the curve of the fishhook so it can properly engage the barb);
  - With the bevel covering the barb, the hook and needle should be removed together along the original path of the fishhook (an 11-gauge blade can replace a needle if a needle is not available).
- **Advance and Cut Method:** This is the most used and most frequently successful method, though it does produce some additional trauma to surrounding tissues. (18,19). See Figure 98.5.
  - Local anesthesia should be administered in the area where you believe the barb will advance through the skin when it proceeds along its current course.

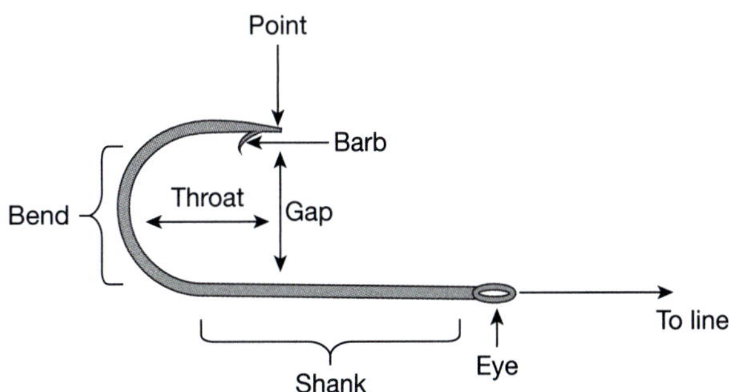

Figure 98.1: Anatomy of a fishhook. (Courtesy of Gitansh Bhargava, DO & Korin Hudson, MD.)

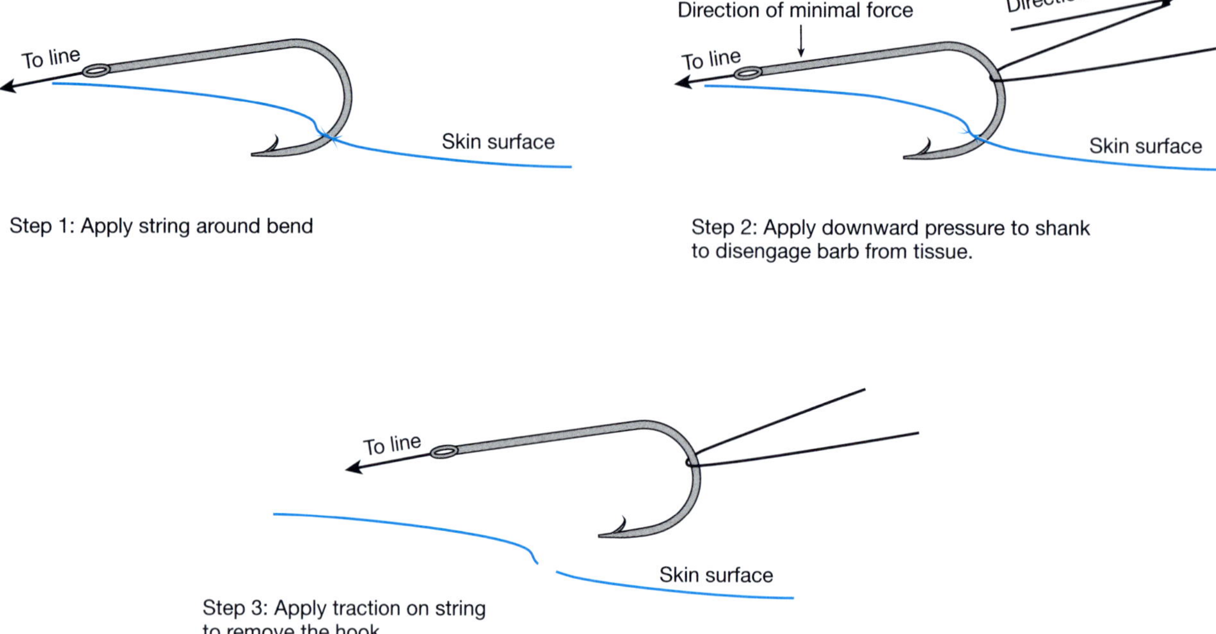

Figure 98.2: Fish hook removal, the String Yank Method. (Courtesy of Gitansh Bhargava, DO & Korin Hudson, MD.)

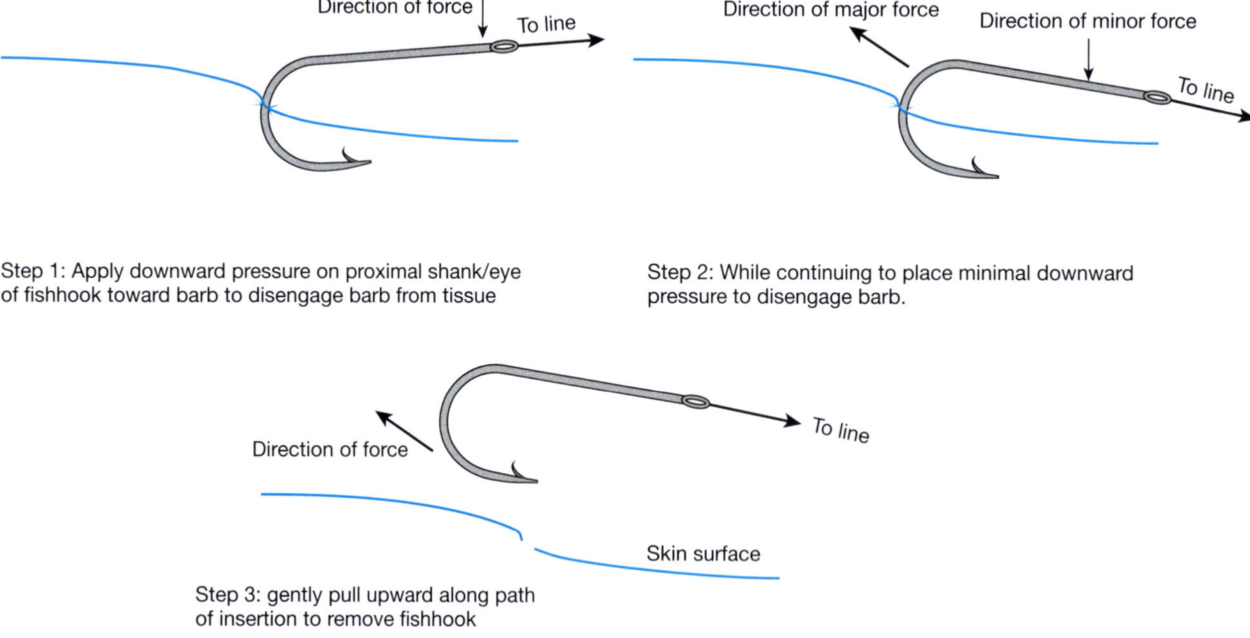

Figure 98.3: Fish hook removal, the Retrograde Technique. (Courtesy of Gitansh Bhargava, DO & Korin Hudson, MD.)

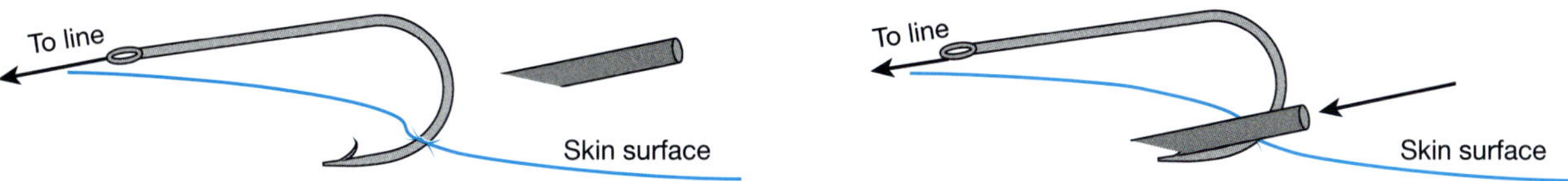

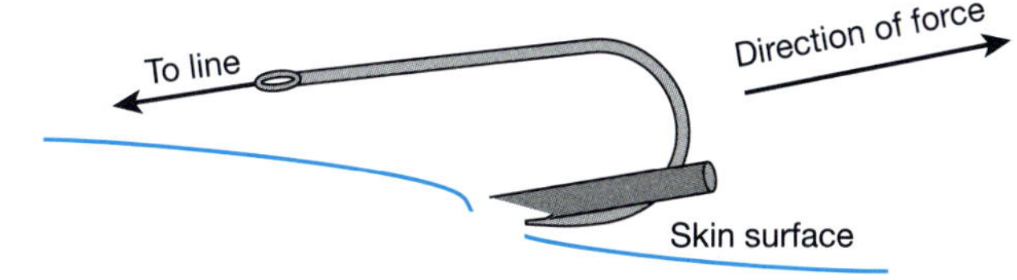

Figure 98.4: Fish hook removal, the Needle Cover Method. (Courtesy of Gitansh Bhargava, DO & Korin Hudson, MD.)

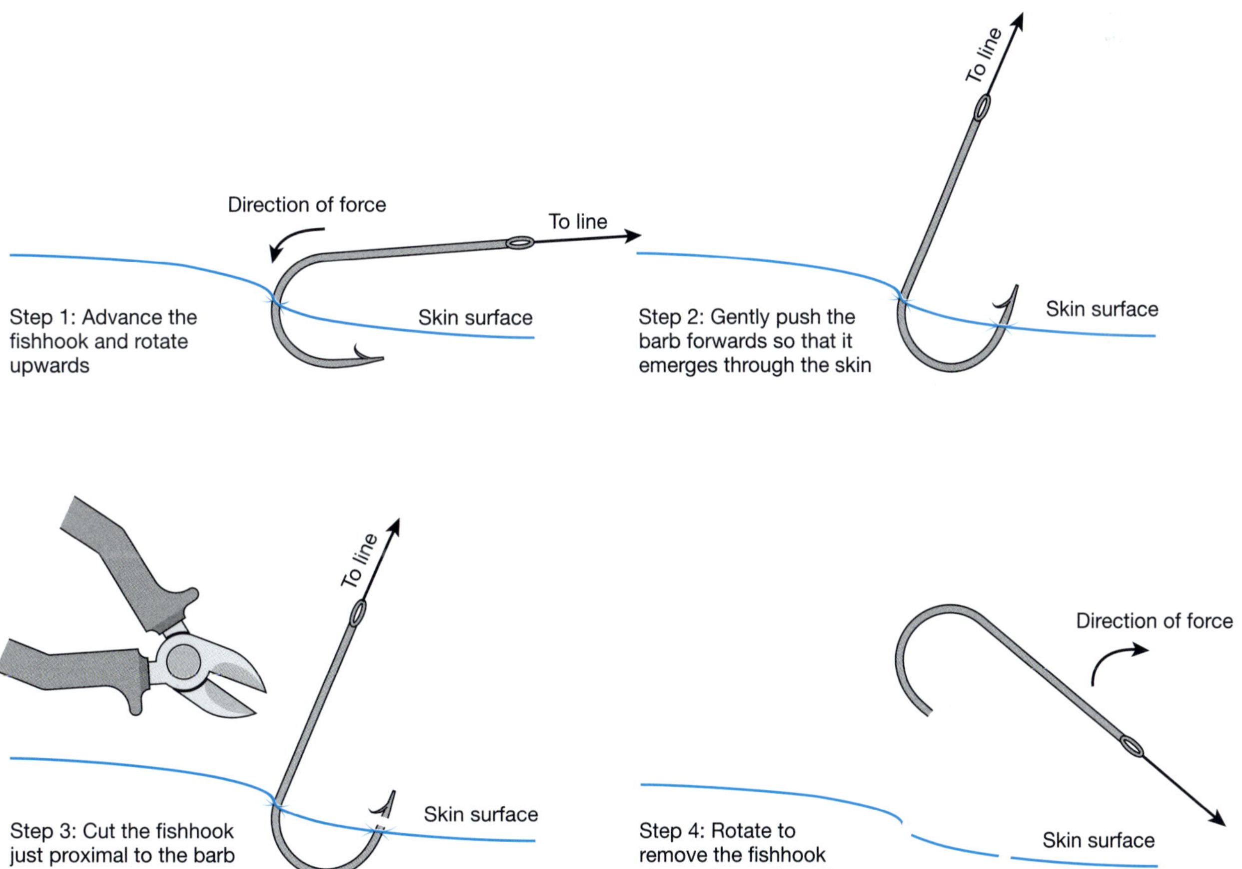

Figure 98.5: Fish hook removal, the Advance and Cut Method. (Courtesy of Gitansh Bhargava, DO & Korin Hudson, MD.)

- Utilize a hemostat or needle driver to grasp the hook and apply pressure to advance the fishhook through the skin while passing through as little tissue as possible.
- Once the barb has emerged through the surface of the skin, stabilize the point/throat of the hook with a second hemostat, proximal to the barb, and cut the tip of the fishhook, including the entire barb, off using wire cutters or similar device. Take care that the point may become a projectile and eye protection for those in the room is advised. The remainder of the fishhook should be removed in a retrograde fashion back toward the wound entry site.
- For a multiple barbed fishhook, instead of cutting the tip of the barb and advancing retrograde, consider cutting the eye of the fishhook and advancing the entire hook through the wound. Take care however to control the end of the hook at all time so the hook does not become a foreign body lost in the wound.

- **Post-Fishhook Removal Considerations**
  - Thoroughly explore the wound for the presence of any foreign bodies (17–19).
  - Copious high-pressure irrigation.
  - Do not perform primary closure or pack wounds.
  - Strongly consider prophylactic antibiotics, especially in an immunocompromised patient or grossly contaminated water source (17).
  - Apply topical antibiotics (*i.e.*, bacitracin) and a simple dressing.
  - Ensure that tetanus vaccination status is up to date.

Ocular Injuries

- Any penetration of the eye should lead to an emergency ophthalmology consultation.
- While waiting for the ophthalmologist to evaluate the patient, cover the affected eye with a plastic or foam cup or ask the patient to wear safety glasses to ensure that the hook does not cause further tissue trauma. Do not apply a pressure dressing or patch over the eye (9,14).
- Commonly associated injuries with ocular trauma are corneal abrasions/lacerations and traumatic cataracts.
  - Traumatic cataracts are caused by the penetration of the lens, which will ultimately require a cataract extraction — with reported cases showing good recovery of vision (20).
- Other ocular injuries that can occur are vitreous hemorrhage, retinal tear or detachment, and endophthalmitis.
- An ocular fishhook removal is usually performed under anesthesia with the advance-and-cut technique commonly utilized (15).
- If the fishhook is isolated to an eyebrow, no formal ophthalmology consultation is needed. Follow the same removal techniques previously discussed.

ZOONOSES

- The most concerning zoonotic infections are bacterial in nature and typically occur secondary to bacteria entering through puncture wounds or exposed wounds while handling fish or fomites exposed to contaminated water (21).

Atypical Mycobacteriosis

- The most notable fish-borne zoonotic bacteria are *Mycobacterium marinum*, *Mycobacterium fortuitum*, and *Mycobacterium ulcerans* (21).
- These are gram positive, aerobic, non–spore-forming, acid-fast positive, nonmotile rods that are slow growing and present in marine and freshwater environments (especially found in stagnant water).
- Infection is usually caused by direct injury from fish fins/bites or wound exposure to contaminated water.
- Symptoms commonly present in extremities resulting in nodular, tender, erythematous swellings in the skin and joints of extremities.
- 95% of cases involve the upper extremities (22).
- Immunocompromised patients can progress to severe infections that are fatal.
- Combinations of treatment drugs include rifampin with ethambutol, clarithromycin with ethambutol, clarithromycin with minocycline, or minocycline monotherapy (22).
- Drug coverage should be for 3–4 months and for 1–2 months after lesion resolution (22).

Fish-Handler's Disease (23)

- Also known as fish tank granuloma or fish fancier's finger.
- A disease that is caused by bacteria (*Erysipelothrix rhusiopathiae* and *M. marinum*) being exposed to open skin wounds.
- The *E. rhusiopathiae* form will generally cause a local cellulitis that can disseminate and lead to bacteremia, infective endocarditis, encephalitis, meningitis, endophthalmitis, necrotizing fasciitis, or suppurative arthritis.
- The *M. marinum* form generally causes a superficial granulomatous inflammation of the extremities. If deeper tissues are involved, tenosynovitis, bursitis, arthritis, and osteomyelitis can result.
- Diagnosis is based on PCR testing or culturing the lesions.
- The treatment is antibiotics.
- *E. rhusiopathiae* form is sensitive to penicillins, carbapenems, cephalosporins, fluoroquinolones, daptomycin, and clindamycin.
- *M. marinum* form often requires rifampin, streptomycin, sulfamethoxazole, trimethoprim, or tetracyclines.

Aeromonas

- This is a gram-negative bacteria found in freshwater, brackish water, marine environments, sewage, and drinking water (21).
- This is the most common bacteria seen in alligator and crocodile bites, but also should be considered in koi and goldfish (23).
- Gastroenteritis, skin/soft-tissue infections, and bacteremia can all occur with infection.
- Most commonly causes cellulitis, which can form a subcutaneous abscess.
- Severe infections are associated with immunosuppressed states (ie, malignancy or cirrhosis) (22).
- Aeromonas is known to have high resistance patterns. Empiric treatment is recommended with fluoroquinolones, a third-/fourth-generation cephalosporin, or a carbapenem.
- In the setting of a severe infection, an aminoglycoside should be added.

Vibrio spp.

- Predominant deep seawater bacteria that is pathogenic in humans; found primarily in brackish and saltwater, but also in freshwater (21,22)
- Infection occurs more commonly through the ingestion of infected shellfish, but can also occur through open skin wounds (22).
- There are three forms of disease: gastroenteritis, skin/soft-tissue infection, or primary bacteremia (the most lethal form).
  - Wound infections can progress rapidly from cellulitis to necrotizing soft-tissue infection.
    - Cellulitis can be treated with antibiotics alone, but necrotizing soft-tissue infection requires aggressive emergent surgical debridement.
  - Early symptoms after exposure can start developing after 12 hours. Death from *Vibrio* sepsis has been seen to occur within 24–48 hours of initial injury (22).
  - Vibrio bacteremia does have an average mortality rate >50%, so should be treated promptly.
- Underlying conditions that cause severe disease include liver disease, alcoholism, diabetes, and malignancies.
- The antibiotic preference for bacteremia and severe soft-tissue infection is IV cefotaxime 2 g q6h + IV minocycline 100 mg q12h.

Venomous Fish Stings

- Envenomation usually occurs secondary to handling the fish (ie, catfish, stonefish, lionfish, stingrays, etc) during fishing or cooking (24).
- Venoms can lead to systemic toxic effects or local inflammatory reactions secondary to heat-labile, high-molecular-weight proteins and low-molecular-weight amines, respectively.
- Common complaints in order of prevalence are pain at the site of sting, wound swelling, erythema, and numbness.
- Catfish stings lead to severe local pain and numbness, which spreads proximally. The venom glands on a catfish can be found on the integumentary sheath that is located on the bony spines of the dorsal and pectoral fins (25,26).
- Stingray stings can lead to bluish-grayish discoloration around the wound, disproportionate pain, muscle cramping, weakness, seizures, hypotension, cardiovascular toxicity, deep wounds, and lacerations.

Management

- Hot water immersion (42 °C) of the affected area for 30–90 minutes inactivates the venoms, which are high-molecular-weight heat-labile proteins.
- Pain relief with oral or parenteral analgesics. Consider peripheral nerve block if needed (26).
- X-rays or ultrasound should be utilized to check for the presence of any foreign body (ie, spine fragments).
- Irrigation and exploration of wound — any remnant of a venomous spine should be removed (26)
- Consider antibiotic and tetanus prophylaxis.

DROWNING

- Drowning is defined as "the process of experiencing respiratory impairment from submersion/immersion in liquid" (27). While submersion refers to the airway below water leading to drowning and immersion refers to the airway above water more likely leading to hypothermia (28).
- Pathophysiology: exposure to water in the lower airway leads to hypoxia and eventually cardiovascular collapse and cardiopulmonary arrest. Most commonly due to destruction of pulmonary surfactant in the alveoli, leading to atelectasis and resulting in ventilation-perfusion mismatch in the lungs. However, other causes of death in drowning can include cardiac dysrhythmias and hypothermia (27).
- Approximately 360,000 deaths globally are attributed to drowning every year according to the World Health Organization.
- Globally, commercial fishing is well known to be among the most dangerous of professions, popularized by movies and television programs. According to the International Labor Organization, more than 100,000 fishing-related deaths occur annually, with many being related to drowning or submersion injuries (29).
- However, far less data are available on recreational fishing related drowning. One estimate, from the Canadian Red Cross Society in the last decade, states there were 5900 water-related deaths in Canada; of that total, 889 (15%) died while fishing (30).

- The Royal Society for the Prevention of Accidents in the United Kingdom estimates in the last decade that of the 1029 people who died in accidental drownings, 91 (8%) were fishermen (31).
- Most water-related injuries and drowning occur while boating. When looking at fishing specifically, it is not the body of water (*i.e.*, river, lake, ocean) or type of transport (*i.e.*, canoeing, kayaking, boating, walking) that is correlated to increased risk of drowning, but rather the consumption of alcohol or lack of personal flotation device that contributes most to risk of death (30).
- Drowning injuries can be categorized based on the aquatic environment where they occur: on-water activities such as boating or kayaking, near-water activities like beach or stream fishing and wading, or ice water sports such as ice fishing. Each of these categories encompasses a distinct set of potential injuries.

Rescue

- Scene safety and safety of the rescuer is the first step in success.
- It is recommended that lay persons should only attempt rescue from safe locations (by reaching, throwing, or rowing to the victim). However, for those who are professionally trained, entering the water for rescue can be considered and should only be attempted according to level of training and with appropriate safety and protective equipment.
- In drowning victims without a pulse, CPR should be attempted as early as possible but only once the victim has been extricated and is in a safe environment for the rescuer (27).

Preventative Measures and Education

- Preventative measures should be focused on public education, including bystander hands-only CPR, abstinence of alcohol use in water-related activities, adequate parental/guardian supervision, personal flotation devices, and self-rescue instruction for both children and adults (27).

SUN EXPOSURE

- All outdoor sportsmen experience greater overall sun exposure (32). However, those who participate in intense UVR exposure water sports (swimming, surfing, boating, sailing) are at an increased risk of basal cell carcinoma (33). While recreational fishing has not been specifically looked at for all skin cancers, it is possible to make a generalization based on these data. Furthermore, a study of a combination of recreational fisherman and boaters has shown an increased risk of melanoma (34).
- Sun exposure is defined as excess exposure to UVB and UVA light leading to sunburn, carcinogenesis, photoaging, photo immune suppression, and photosensitivity (35).
- The first step in reducing injury from the sun's harmful rays is education on the importance of avoiding exposure. The midday sun (10 a.m.–4 p.m.) is the highest index of UV light and is when multiple protective measures should be used. This includes photoprotective clothing/hats/sunglasses, shade or avoidance of direct sunlight, and sunscreens (35).
- Sunscreen-active ingredients form a film or coating over the stratum corneum, filtering the UV wavelengths to absorb or scatter the radiation/photons before it penetrates the epidermis and dermis surface. Efficacy is measured in SPF or sun protective factor and UV filtering levels off at SPF 30 and above (36).
- Sunscreen products contain a combination of ingredients that work through several mechanisms including organic "chemical" agents (water or oil soluble) that absorb photons versus inorganic metal oxide "physical" agents (insoluble) that scatter photons. Sunscreen should be applied 15 minutes before exposure and reapplied every 2 hours (36).
- Treatment: cool compresses, cool baths, NSAIDs, and aloe vera for pain relief (35).

REFERENCES

1. *2019 Special Report on Fishing" (PDF).* Outdoor Industry Association. 30 July 2019. Archived from the original (PDF) on 2019 Oct 14.
2. *Fishing.* Rookie Road; n.d. Retrieved 2022 Oct 9, from https://www.rookieroad.com/fishing/
3. *Fishing Tournaments.* Takemefishing.org; n.d. Retrieved 2022 Dec 23, from https://www.takemefishing.org/how-to-fish/when-to-fish/fishing-tournaments/#:~:text=Types%20of%20Fishing%20Tournaments&text=There%20are%20kids%20fishing%20tournament,you%20most%20like%20to%20do
4. *Information on Colleges with Varsity Bass Fishing Teams: Scholarship stats.Com. Scholarship Stats.Com | Play Your Sport in College!* 2022, Oct 20. Retrieved 2022 Dec 28, from https://scholarshipstats.com/bassfishing
5. Schonbrun Z. Collegiate fishing's added lure: cash on the line. *The New York Times.* 2014 Oct 17. Retrieved 2022 Dec 28, from https://www.nytimes.com/2014/10/18/sports/a-paycheck-for-college-athletes-join-the-fishing-team.html
6. Hicks M. The 50-year evolution' of tournament bass fishing. *Game & Fish.* 2017 Feb 2. Retrieved 2022 Nov 28, from https://www.gameandfishmag.com/editorial/50-year-evolution-of-tournament-bass-fishing/192993
7. Steven. *The 10 Best Bass Fishing Tournaments*; 2022 Oct 13. Retrieved 2022 Nov 13, from https://www.baitcloud.com/blogs/news/test
8. *Is There an Injury Crisis in Pro Fishing?* BassFan. 2010 Sep 15. Retrieved 2022 Dec 23, from https://www.bassfan.com/news_article/3728/is-there-an-injury-crisis-in-pro-fishing
9. Gil JA, Elia G, Shah KN, Owens BD, Got C. Epidemiology of fishing related upper extremity injuries presenting to the Emergency Department in the United States. *Phys Sportsmed.* 2018;46(3):319–23. doi:10.1080/00913847.2018.1462650
10. Kuhn AW, Kuhn JE. Upper extremity pain and overuse injuries in fly-fishing: a North American cross-sectional survey and implications for injury prevention. *Orthop J Sports Med.* 2020;8(10):2325967120959303. doi:10.1177/2325967120959303
11. Mitchell T. *Fishing.* Gone Fishing; n.d. Retrieved 2023 Jan 8, from https://easna.org/WorkingWell/Fishing.html

12. Read CR, Watson SL, Perez JL, Estes AR. Competitive bass anglers: a new concern in sports medicine. *Phys Sportsmed.* 2017;45(3):309–15. doi:10.1080/00913847.2017.1321947
13. Rosenbauer TH. *Avoiding Casting Pains, with* Dr. *Jason Smith [Audio Podcast]*; 2022 Sep 17. Retrieved from https://podcasts.apple.com/us/podcast/the-orvis-fly-fishing-podcast/id278930814?i=1000579789759
14. Dudkiewicz I, Salai M, Blankstein A, Chechik A. Fishing penetration injuries. *Br J Sports Med.* 2000;34(6):459–61. doi:10.1136/bjsm.34.6.459
15. Bartholomew RS, Macdonald M. Fish hook injuries of the eye. *Br J Ophthalmol.* 1980;64(7):531–3. doi:10.1136/bjo.64.7.531
16. McCue TJ, Guse CE, Dempsey RL. Upper extremity pain seen with fly-casting technique: a survey of fly-casting instructors. *Wilderness Environ Med.* 2004;15(4):267–73. doi:10.1580/1080-6032(2004)015[0267:uepswf]2.0.co;2
17. James V, Manickam S, Yee NW, Ganapathy S. Fish hook injuries in children. *Austin Pediatr.* 2018;5(1):1064.
18. Prats M, O'Connell M, Wellock A, Kman NE. Fishhook removal: Case reports and a review of the literature. *J Emerg Med.* 2013;44(6):e375–80. doi:10.1016/j.jemermed.2012.11.058
19. Gammons M, Jackson E. Fishhook removal. *Am Fam Phys.* 2001;63(11):2231–6. Retrieved 2022 Dec 5, from https://www.aafp.org/pubs/afp/issues/2001/0601/p2231.html
20. Ahmad SS, Seng CW, Ghani SA, Lee JF. Cut-it-out technique for ocular fish-hook injury. *J Emerg Trauma Shock.* 2013;6(4):293–5. doi:10.4103/0974-2700.120384
21. Boylan S. Zoonoses associated with fish. *Vet Clin North Am Exot Anim Pract.* 2011;14(3):427–38. doi:10.1016/j.cvex.2011.05.003
22. Finkelstein R, Oren I. Soft tissue infections caused by marine bacterial pathogens: epidemiology, diagnosis, and Management. *Curr Infect Dis Rep.* 2011;13(5):470–7. doi:10.1007/s11908-011-0199-3
23. Schwartz BS, Nydick JA, Abzug JM. Aquatic hand injuries. *J Hand Surg Am.* 2014;39(8):1623–7. doi:10.1016/j.jhsa.2014.06.001
24. Chan HY, Chan YC, Tse ML, Lau FL. Venomous fish sting cases reported to Hong Kong Poison Information Centre: a three-year retrospective study on Epidemiology and Management. *Hong Kong J Emerg Med.* 2010;17(1):40–4. doi:10.1177/102490791001700107
25. Mckinstry DM. Catfish stings in the United States: case report and review. *J Wilderness Med.* 1993;4(3):293–303. doi:10.1580/0953-9859-4.3.293
26. Dorooshi G. Catfish sings: a report of two cases. *J Res Med Sci.* 2012;17(6):578–781.
27. Schmidt AC, Sempsrott JR, Hawkins SC, Arastu AS, Cushing TA, Auerbach PS. Wilderness medical society clinical practice guidelines for the treatment and prevention of drowning: 2019 update. *Wilderness Environ Med.* 2019;30(4 suppl):S70–86. doi:10.1016/j.wem.2019.06.007
28. World Health Organization. *Preventing Drowning: An Implementation Guide.* Geneva. 2017.
29. https://static1.squarespace.com/static/634cbf73ee2d4b58a718c0db/t/63d1ad0be58971179187d965/1674685709886/Final+Published+Marine+Policy+Paper+101222.pdf
30. Picard A. Fishing: The cause of more drowning deaths. *The Globe and Mail.* 2009 [cited 2023 Jan 11]. Available from: https://www.theglobeandmail.com/life/health-and-fitness/fishing-the-cause-of-more-drowning-deaths/article785939/
31. Mail, Angler's. Latest figures highlight the risk of drowning for anglers. *Adventure.Com.* 2019 [cited 2023 Jan 11]. Available from: https://www.advnture.com/news/drowning-warnings-anglers
32. Snyder A, Valdebran M, Terrero D, Amber KT, Kelly KM. Solar ultraviolet exposure in individuals who perform outdoor sport activities. *Sports Med Open.* 2020 Sep 3;6(1):42. doi:10.1186/s40798-020-00272-9
33. Rosso S, Zanetti R, Martinez C, et al. The multicentre south European study 'Helios'. II: different sun exposure patterns in the aetiology of basal cell and squamous cell carcinomas of the skin. *Br J Cancer.* 1996;73(11):1447–54.
34. Holman CD, Armstrong BK, Heenan PJ. Relationship of cutaneous malignant melanoma to individual sunlight exposure habits. *J Natl Cancer Inst.* 1986;76(3):403–14.
35. Fitzpatrick JE, High WA. *Urgent Care Dermatology: Symptom-Based Diagnosis, Chapter 19.* Philadelphia PA: Elsevier, Inc.; 2018.
36. Bolognia JL, Schaffer JV, Cerroni L, eds. *Dermatology.* 4th ed. Elsevier; 2017 Oct 22.

99 Cycling

Chad A. Asplund

INTRODUCTION/BACKGROUND

- Participation in bicycling is rapidly growing.
  - In 2020, 52.7 million Americans aged 6 and older were estimated to have ridden a bicycle six times or more (1).
- There are many different ways to participate in bicycling: road cycling, mountain biking, touring/commuting, cyclocross, and bicycle motocross (BMX).
- With the increased participation, there has been an increase in both traumatic and overuse injuries:
  - Each year, more than 600,000 people in the United States are treated in emergency departments, and more than 1000 people die as a result of bicycle-related injuries (2).
- Most common areas for overuse injuries in bicycling are the knee, neck, and back (3,4).
- Many of these overuse injuries occur secondary to improper bicycle fit or training errors.
- This chapter will outline the different ways people can participate in bicycling, the anatomy and fit of the bicycle, injury epidemiology, traumatic and overuse injuries, cycling-related equipment, and common training errors.

SPECIFIC ISSUES

Different Modes of Cycling

Road Cycling

- Road racing: Open road 25–100 miles.
- Criterium: Multiple laps around a short course.
  - Very popular in the United States
  - High potential for crashing/injury
- Time trial: Race against the clock with wave start with 1–5 minutes between riders.

Mountain Biking

- Cross-country: Longer races over variable terrain.
- Downhill: Steep downhill race where focus is on speed; injuries occur as safety is sacrificed for speed.
- Dual slalom: Two racers compete in downhill ski-style slalom course.

Touring/Commuting

- Long-distance road riding for recreation. Riders may be carrying panniers/saddlebags.

Cyclocross

- Off-road race on road-style bikes, in which riders complete multiple short (1–2 mile) loops in a set time period. Obstacles require the rider to dismount, remount, and carry the bicycle over the course.

BMX/Trick Cycling

- Riders compete against other riders over dirt courses of varied terrain or individually on ramps with stairs and railings with aerial stunts. There is a high risk for injury with aerial acrobatics.
  - Fastest-growing segment of U.S. cycling with 60,000 riders (5).
  - Largest portion of child and adolescent cyclists.

Bicycle Anatomy

- Although there are many different modes of bicycling, the general anatomy of the bicycle is similar (Fig. 99.1).

Bicycle Frame Types

- Standard road: Traditional upright geometry with top tube parallel to ground.
- Compact road: Sloping top tube allows the rider to fit a smaller frame; this maximizes stiffness and minimizes weight.
- Mountain/hybrid: Flatter geometry, heavier bicycle, may have front and/or rear suspension to absorb shock.

Fit

- Most important attribute in the evaluation of overuse bicycling injuries.
- Bicycle fit may be done at local bike shops with bicycle purchase or available for a fee.
- Fit Kit and Serotta "Size Cycle" have been used (6).
- Best frame size for cyclists is as small vertically as possible with enough length horizontally to allow a stretched-out out relaxed upper body. This frame will be lighter and stiffer and handle better (7).

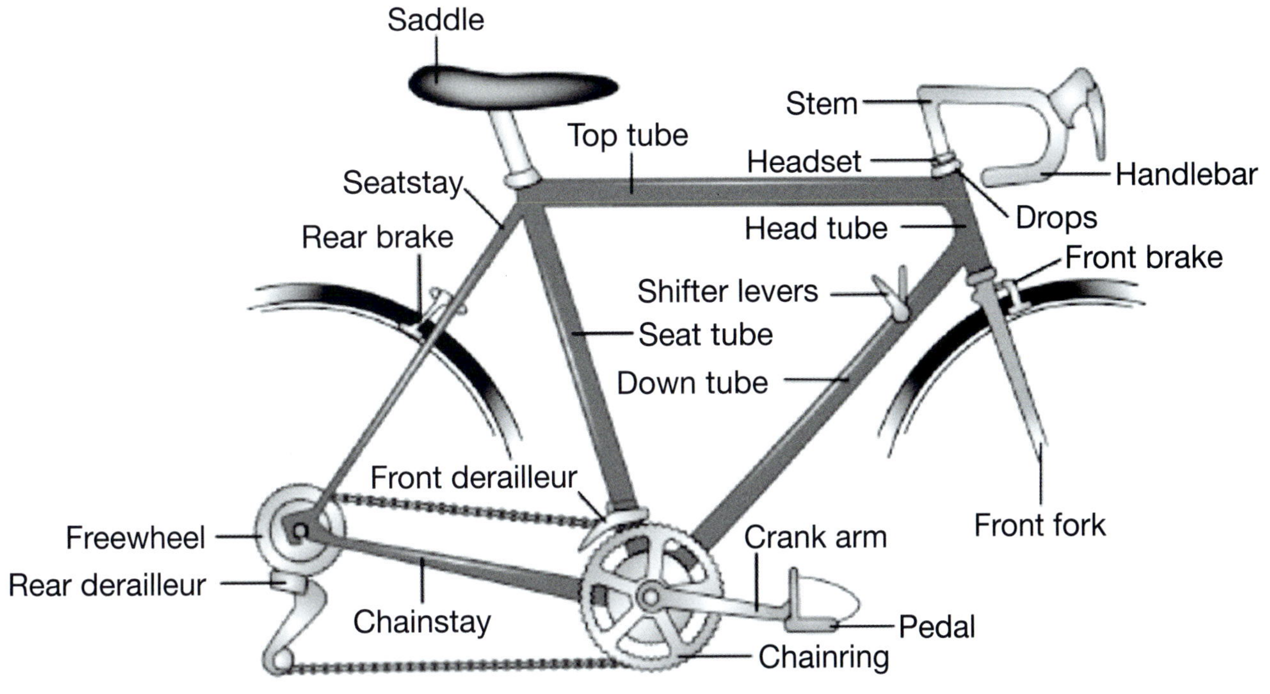

Figure 99.1: Bicycle anatomy.

Frame Size

- Most important attribute for appropriate frame size is top tube length.

Top Tube Length

- The ideal position varies here more than anywhere else for cyclists, depending on riding style, flexibility, body proportions, and frame geometry, among others.
- Upper body position may change as riding style evolves.
- May be measured by placing the elbow at the fore end of the saddle; outstretched fingers should touch the handlebars.
- May also have riders, while in the drops, look straight down; the hub of the front wheel should be obscured by the handlebar.

Seat Height

- Optimal saddle height has been estimated based on maximal power output and caloric expenditure (8).
- Calculate height, which will be within a centimeter of 0.883 × inseam length, measured from the center of the bottom bracket to the low point of the top of the saddle. This allows full leg extension, with a slight bend in the leg at the bottom of the pedal stroke.
- When seated on the bike with the pedal at the 6 o'clock position, there should be 20°–25° of flexion of the knee.
- Alternatively, the seat may be raised until the hips start rocking when pedaling and then the seat is lowered until the rocking disappears.

Saddle Position

- Check the position of the forward knee relative to the pedal spindle; for a neutral knee position, you will be able to drop a plumb line from the tibial tubercle and have it bisect the pedal spindle (knee over pedal spindle position) (8).

Handlebar Position

- Most cyclists select a bar that is just as wide as their shoulders.
  - A wider bar opens the chest for better breathing and more leverage but sacrifices aerodynamics.
  - A narrower bar increases aerodynamics but sacrifices stability.
- Handlebar height should be at or below the saddle height; how far below depends on the flexibility and experience of the cyclist.

Crank Arm Length

- Length is based on size and riding style. Shorter crank arm length is better for quick acceleration. Long crank arms are better for pushing larger gears at a lower cadence (7).
- To minimize oxygen consumption, crank arm length is dependent on femur length.
- 2.33 × femur length +55.8 cm (9). This roughly translates to:
  - Frame size <54 cm: 170-cm crank arm
  - Frame size 55–61 cm: 172.5-cm crank arm
  - Frame size >61 cm: 175-cm crank arm

Gearing

- Chain wheels: Large chainring (usually 52–53 teeth) and small chainring (usually 36–39 teeth); recently, a more compact 50/34 chainring combination has become more popular to allow riders to climb hills and spin at higher cadence.
- Cassette: Cluster of gears (cogs) mounted to the right of the rear wheel, typically 10, 11, or 12 cogs.
- Gear ratio: Number of teeth on chainring divided by number of teeth on selected cog.
- Higher ratio requires more strength, endurance, and technique.
- Lower gear ratio allows for more spinning and higher cadence; without proper technique will yield less power.

Cadence

- Optimal cadence determined by type of race (time trial, climbing, criterium), body type, muscle fiber type, and training level (10).
- Higher cadences put less strain on trained leg muscles.
- Low cadences increase intramuscular pressure, reducing blood flow to the muscles during the power phase of the pedal stroke.
- High-cadence/low-resistance training reduces the incidence of overuse injuries. Cyclists beginning a season or returning from injury should return with this type of training.
- Cadence is individual and should be determined on a rider-by-rider basis.

MEDICAL ISSUES

Common Training Errors Leading to Injury

- Inadequate rest: overreaching to overtraining (see Chapter 45 Overtraining Syndrome)
- Rapid increase in distance or intensity: muscle tightness or microtrauma, which may lead to tendinopathy (most commonly patellar or quadriceps tendon)
- Excessive hill work: anterior knee pain
- Pushing a high-gear ratio: anterior or medial knee pain

Epidemiology

- Each year, more than 600,000 bicyclists in the United States are treated in emergency departments, and more than 1000 people die as a result of bicycle-related injuries (2).
- Children are at particularly high risk for bicycle-related injuries. In 2020, children 15 years and younger accounted for 69% of all bicycle-related injuries seen in U.S. emergency departments (2).
- Peak incidence of bicycle-related injuries is in the 9- to 15-year-old age group.
- Bicycle crashes are the second leading cause of sports-associated serious injury (riding animals is the leading cause) (11).
- Risk factors for injury include not wearing a helmet, crashes involving motor vehicles, unsafe riding environment, and male sex (11).
- Conspicuous (brightly colored) clothing may reduce crash-related injury in cyclists (12).
- Mountain bikes account for 6% of overall injuries, but 70%–85% of mountain bikers sustain injuries each year (2).
- BMX bikers are frequently injured doing stunts; 6.3% of all BMX riders sustain injury in competition (13).

Equipment and Safety

- Helmet: reduces risk of head injuries 74%–85% (13,14).
- Should be worn snugly in a horizontal position on the head with the straps forming a "V" around the ears and held in place with buckle fastened.
- Only 15%–25% of children wear helmets correctly (13). Common errors include wearing helmets that are sized incorrectly, worn too far back on the head, or with straps that are adjusted incorrectly.
- Helmet use increases with mandatory legislation (15).
  - Possible barriers to use of helmets: discomfort, poor fit, cost, underestimation of risk of injury, peer pressure
- Protective eyewear: protects from ultraviolet radiation, flying objects, and irritants
- Cycling gloves: cushion hands from road shock, protect hands in falls
- Cycling shorts: protect inner thigh, groin, and perineum from chafing and pressure trauma

Environmental Injuries (16–18)

- Cyclists may be predisposed to heat and cold injuries and altitude sickness, underscoring the importance of proper clothing, nutrition, hydration, and acclimatization.
- For more information, see Chapter 47 on environmental injuries.

Skin

- Abrasions (road rash): graded as first degree (superficial), second degree (partial thickness), or third degree (full thickness).
- Wound irrigation, debridement, protection from further trauma and bacterial contamination, creation of a moist wound environment, and judicious use of antibiotics (when indicated) will help achieve optimal outcomes.
- Topical lidocaine cream may be applied 15 minutes prior to debridement to facilitate thorough wash-out/cleaning of wound.

- Treated with hydroactive dressing and silvadene or mupirocin ointment.
- Polymeric dressings may be useful for larger wounds (19).
- Large third degree: silvadene cream three times daily or wet to dry dressings.

Visceral Injuries

- Mostly caused by blunt trauma from crashes and/or impaling handlebars:
  - Abdominal wall hematomas (15)
  - Liver, spleen, pancreas hematoma

Bowel Perforation

- These injuries are true emergencies and should be treated as such with rapid evaluation and treatment in a facility capable of cross-sectional imaging and surgical intervention if required.

MUSCULOSKELETAL ISSUES

Traumatic Injuries

Upper Extremity

- Fall on outstretched hand
  - Scaphoid fracture
  - Distal radius (Colles) fracture
  - Fractures of the radial head
- Acromioclavicular joint separation; usually direct trauma to shoulder
  - First- and second-degree may resume riding as tolerated.
  - Third-degree may take 4–6 weeks to heal.
- Clavicle fracture
  - If non-displaced, may resume riding in 48 hours.
  - Athletes with displaced fractures may return in 4–6 weeks as bone heals or as pain dictates.
  - Fractures with >2 cm of displacement may benefit from surgical fixation (11).

Head

- Head injuries account for most bicycle-related deaths (1000/y).
- Generally, head injuries are preventable with helmets (severity reduced 85%–90%) (20).
- Helmet wear reduces incidence of skull fracture and reduces severity of head injury but does not reduce the incidence of concussion (20).
- Mandatory legislation increases helmet use among cyclists, particularly in younger age groups (21).
- Bicycle-related mortality in children age 1–15 dropped significantly with mandatory helmet legislation (21).

Overuse Injuries

- The most common site for overuse injuries in the bicyclist is the knee (3).
- Location of knee pain:
  - Anterior
    - Patellar pain syndrome, quadriceps tendinopathy, chondromalacia patella, patellar tendinopathy
    - Causes: training errors: rapid increase in mileage, high gearing, and excessive hills
    - Bicycle fit problems: seat too low or too far forward, malpositioned cleats, crank arm too long
    - Anatomic issues: genu valgum, genu varum, hyperpronation
    - Treatment: review and adjust training program, improve bike fit, correct anatomic abnormalities as possible, quadriceps strengthening
  - Medial
    - Irritation of medial patellofemoral ligament, plica, or pes anserine bursitis
    - Causes: training errors
    - Bicycle fit problems: cleats with toes pointing out, feet too far apart
    - Treatment: review and adjust training program; adjust cleats or shorten bottom bracket axle; rehabilitation and knee strengthening
  - Lateral
    - Iliotibial band (ITB) friction syndrome/tendinopathy
    - Causes: two mechanisms have been proposed for this syndrome:
    - Excessive friction resulting as the ITB slides back and forth over the lateral femoral epicondyle.
    - Changing tension in the anterior and posterior fibers of the ITB compresses the fat between the tract and a bursa, creating inflammation and merely the illusion of movement (22).
    - Bicycle fit problems: improper cleat placement; seat too high or too posterior; anatomic—hyperpronation, genu varum, tight ITB, leg length discrepancy
    - Treatment: adjust cleats, lower seat, move saddle forward, consider cycling orthotics, ITB stretching, hip girdle strengthening
  - Posterior
    - Biceps femoris tendinopathy, semimembranosus tendinopathy, posterior capsule strain
      - Causes: overly aggressive training
      - Bicycle fit problems: saddle too high or too far forward, improper cleat position
      - Treatment: review and adjust training plan, move seat up and/or back, adjust cleats; rehabilitation of hamstring, quadriceps strengthening

Neck

- Second most common location of bicycling-related overuse injuries (4)
- Common; present in among 60% of riders (23)
- Bicyclists may develop myofascial trigger points in the neck (levator scapulae, splenius capitis, trapezius, sternocleidomastoid, infraspinatus, supraspinatus, and rhomboid muscles).
  - Causes: most commonly caused by increased load on the arms and shoulders necessary to support the rider and the hyperextension of the neck in the horizontal riding position (4).
  - Bicycle fit problems: saddle too far aft, effective top tube length too long, handlebars too far below saddle.
  - Treatment: may be treated by raising handlebars, shortening stem to reduce hyperextension of the neck. Strength and flexibility exercises may also be used.

Back

- The low back muscles are primarily what the cyclist uses for control and generation of power.
  - Causes: chronic pain and fatigue may develop due to prolonged position on the bike. In older cyclists, may be secondary to some degree of degenerative changes.
  - Bicycle fit problems: saddle too far aft.
  - Treatment:
  - On bike: change positions frequently, push lower gears, use higher cadence, and rise from the saddle on climbs.
  - Management: strength, flexibility of lumbar musculature.
  - May need to move the saddle forward as excess forward reach may exaggerate lordotic lumbar posture (4).

Hands

- Ulnar neuropathy: ulnar nerve may be compressed in Guyon canal, causing pain, numbness, and tingling in lateral fourth and fifth fingers due to compression of the ulnar nerve
  - May be treated with padded gloves, increased handlebar padding, and frequent change of hand positions while riding
- Carpal tunnel syndrome: compression of the median nerve causing numbness and tingling in the index, middle, and ring fingers
- Tenosynovitis: tendons of the extensor pollicis brevis and abductor pollicis longus (De Quervain tenosynovitis); caused by tight grip on handlebars (24)

Foot/Ankle

- Paresthesias: numbness/tingling in feet
  - Causes: tight shoe straps and increased pressure on pedals
  - Course: usually self-limited
  - Management: loosen straps on shoes, ride at higher cadence to reduce foot pressure
- Metatarsalgia
  - Causes: poor foot position, increased pedal pressure; may be caused by pes planus or hyperpronation
  - Management: adjust cleats or consider cycling orthotics

Hip

- Trochanteric bursitis: friction causes repetitive sliding of fascia lata over greater trochanter
- Iliopsoas tendinopathy: pain in medial proximal thigh; usually caused by saddle that is too high; may lower seat and/or evaluate frame size

Perineum

- Saddle sores: caused by friction and pressure that may then result in infection; may be prevented with chamois cream
- Crotchitis (tinea cruris): more common in women; try to minimize time off bike spent in sweat-soaked cycling shorts
- Ischial tuberosity (sit bones) tenderness: eases with continual riding; may also consider wearing padded cycling shorts or adding a padded seat cover
- Erectile dysfunction: when adjusted for age and other comorbidities, cyclists are 2.0× more likely to have erectile dysfunction than noncyclists (25)
- Pudendal neuropathy: compression of dorsal branch of pudendal nerve between bike seat and pubic symphysis (26,27)
  - May be prevented by adjusting seated position every 5–10 minutes, tilting saddle slightly downward, or changing saddle design
  - May be minimized by rising out of the saddle for 10–15 seconds every 15–20 minutes

Vascular

- External iliac artery endofibrosis (28–30)
  - Progressive stenotic intimal thickening of the external iliac artery
  - Presents with pain/cramps in buttocks, thighs, or calves; may also present with sensation of swollen leg with maximal effort or strenuous cycling
  - Prevalence as high as 20% in professional cyclists (30)
  - Majority in men; 85% unilateral (30)
  - Diagnosis:
    - Ultrasound with continuous wave Doppler
    - Systolic humeral and posterior tibial arterial pressures with oscillometer
    - Exercise test with decrease in ankle blood pressure measurement
    - Arteriography with femoral Seldinger technique

EVENT COVERAGE

- Most common injuries during recreational cycling events or races include:
  - Traumatic injuries (see above)
  - Concussions (see above)
  - Dermatologic issues (see above)
- Medical plan
  - Coordinating appropriate medical resources reduces response time to an incident and can allow you to focus on the race operations while someone else is dedicated to the medical needs of the event (31).
  - Coordinate with the team to determine if you will need basic or advanced life support training.
  - Have members of the medical team walk the course before the event to determine the best locations for personnel. Focusing on:
    - Anticipated "trouble spots" on course (*i.e.*, tricky corner or fast downhill)
    - Ingress/egress routes for ambulances and staff

REFERENCES

1. Statistica. 2006. Available from: https://www.statista.com/statistics/191204/participants-in-bicycling-in-the-us-since-2006/
2. Centers for Disease Control and Prevention. *Web-Based Injury Statistics Query and Reporting System (WISQARS)*. Atlanta (GA): Centers for Disease Control and Prevention, National Center for Injury Prevention and Control; [Accessed 2022 Sept 15]. Available from: cdc.gov/injury/wisqars.
3. Asplund C, St Pierre P. Knee pain and bicycling: fitting concepts for clinicians. *Phys Sportsmed*. 2004;32(4):23–30.
4. Asplund C, Webb C, Barkdull T. Neck and back pain in bicycling. *Curr Sports Med Rep*. 2005;4(5):271–4.
5. Grubb C. BMX builds racers. *Velonews*. 2003;1(1):11.
6. Christiaans HH, Bremner A. Comfort on bicycles and the validity of a commercial bicycle fitting system. *Appl Ergon*. 1998;29(3):201–11.
7. Colorado Cyclist. *Bike Fit: How to Fit Your Custom Bicycle*. [cited 2025 June 14]. Available from: https://www.owascoveloclub.com/Education_files/Colorado%20Cyclist%20Bike%20Fit%20Tips.pdf
8. Burke ER. Proper fit of the bicycle. *Clin Sports Med*. 1994;13(1):1–14.
9. Too D. Biomechanics of cycling and factors affecting performance. *Sports Med*. 1990;10(5):286–302.
10. Burke ER. Serious cycling. In: *Champaign: Human Kinetics*; 1995, p. 13, 47–50, 160–8, 179–204.
11. Wiesel BB, Getz CL. Current concepts in clavicle fractures, malunions and non-unions. *Curr Opin Orthop*. 2006;17(4):325–30.
12. Thornley SJ, Woodward A, Langley JD, Ameratunga SN, Rodgers A. Conspicuity and bicycle crashes: preliminary findings of the Taupo Bicycle Study. *Inj Prev*. 2008;14(1):11–8.
13. Thompson MJ, Rivara FP. Bicycle-related injuries. *Am Fam Physician*. 2001;63(10):2007–14.
14. Stephens-Stidham S, Mallonee S. The prevention of traffic deaths and injuries: the role of physicians. *J Okla State Med Assoc*. 2001;94(6):192–3.
15. Holmes JH 4th, Hall RA, Schaller RT Jr. Thoracic handlebar hernia: presentation and management. *J Trauma*. 2002;52(1):165–6.
16. Bailey DM. Acute mountain sickness: the "poison of the pass." *West J Med*. 2000;172(6):399–400.
17. Baker A. *Bicycling Medicine: Cycling Nutrition, Physiology and Injury Prevention and Treatment for Riders of All Levels*. New York (NY): Simon & Schuster; 1998.
18. Helzer-Julin M. Sun, heat and cold injuries in cyclists. *Clin Sports Med*. 1994;13(1):219–34.
19. Seiffert JG, Ebnet T. The healing effects of polymeric dressings on road rash abrasions in a racing cyclist. *MSSE*. 2008;40(5):S138–9.
20. Olivier J, Radun I. Bicycle helmet effectiveness is not overstated. *Traffic Inj Prev*. 2017 Oct 3;18(7):755–60.
21. Hoye A. Recommend or mandate? A systematic review and meta-analysis of the effects of mandatory bicycle helmet legislation. *Accid Anal Prev*. 2018;120:239–49.
22. Barber FA, Sutker MJ. The iliotibial band syndrome: diagnosis and surgical management. *Tech Knee Surg*. 2008;7(2):102–6.
23. Mellion MB. Neck and back pain in bicycling. *Clin Sport Med*. 1994;13(1):137–64.
24. *National Sporting Goods Association Web Site*. [cited 2010 Aug 6]. Available from: http://www.nsga.org/i4a/pages/index.cfm?pageID=3482
25. Gan ZS, Ehlers ME, Lin FC, Wright ST, Figler BD, Coward RM. Systematic review and meta-analysis of cycling and erectile dysfunction. *Sex Med Rev*. 2021 Apr;9(2):304–11.
26. Asplund C, Barkdull T, Weiss BD. Genitourinary problems in bicyclists. *Curr Sports Med Rep*. 2007;6(5):333–9.
27. Leibovitch I, Mor Y. The vicious cycling: bicycling related urogenital disorders. *Eur Urol*. 2005;47(3):277–87.
28. Abraham P, Saumet JL, Chevalier JM. External iliac artery endofibrosis in athletes. *Sports Med*. 1997;24(4):221–6.
29. Morelli MJ, Stone DA. Bicycling. In: Fu FH, Stone DA, editors. *Sports Injuries, Mechanisms, Prevention and Treatment*. 2nd ed. Philadelphia: Lippincott Williams & Wilkins; 2001. p. 312–9.
30. Peake LK, D'Abate F, Farrah J, Morgan M, Hinchliffe RJ. The investigation and management of iliac artery endofibrosis: lessons learned from a case series. *Eur J Vasc Endovasc Surg*. 2018;55(4):577–83.
31. USA Cycling. [cited 2025 June 14]. Available from: https://usacycling.org/event-organizer/toolkit/operations/event-safety/medical.

100 Dance and Performing Arts

Devin P. McFadden and Melody R. Hrubes

INTRODUCTION/BACKGROUND

- Performing arts athletes are dancers, actors, vocalists, musicians, circus athletes, and so on. Many performers participate in multiple genres, such as the "triple threat": actor, dancer, and singer.
- Performing arts is an aesthetic sport, with success not determined by score, speed, or measure of strength as in traditional sports.
- Performing artists practice or perform almost every day, face extreme competition, play/perform through pain, and compete in challenging environments. There is often no off-season, so these athletes are at high risk for overuse injuries and mental fatigue.
- Many musicians practice 6–8 $h \cdot d^{-1}$, while a Broadway show schedule is typically 2 hours 45 minutes, 8 shows per week with only a single day off.
- To attain a professional level, most musicians dedicate at least 10,000 hours to deliberate practice over 10 years in addition to developing communication skills and expressive gesturing attributed to publicly acclaimed musicians (1,2).
- Within the art forms of music and dance, there are many genres with diverse demands
  - Music: brass, wind, percussion, drum corp
  - Dance: classical ballet, modern, tap, jazz, breaking, hip-hop, Irish dance, Latin, and ballroom, although this list is far from exhaustive

EPIDEMIOLOGY

- Although they may suffer acute conditions, musicians, and dancers are at increased risk for insidious, chronic, overuse injuries caused by repetitive microtrauma, rather than traumatic injuries with a definable onset.
  - Diagnosis and management are more challenging in this setting, and treatment frequently requires activity modification or restriction to allow healing to occur.
- Music: Studies consistently indicate that greater than 80% of musicians experienced pain or injuries that interfered either with playing their instrument or participating in normal orchestral rehearsals and performances.
  - The most common sites affected were the trunk (primarily the back), the right upper limb and neck, the left upper limb and neck, and the neck alone, but the relative proportions varied by instrument (3–5).
- Dance: The annual incidence of injury in professional dancers ranges from 67% to 95% (6).
  - Dancers more commonly suffer from overuse injuries (65%), but acute/traumatic injuries remain a significant issue, accounting for 35% of all injuries (7).
  - The majority of dance injuries are found in the lower extremity.
  - Foot and ankle injuries represent approximately 40% of dance injuries, whereas knee and back injuries each represent approximately 20% (8).

SPECIFIC ISSUES

- Music terminology
  - Tempo: speed of the music
  - Dynamics: volume of the music
  - Crescendo: gradual increase in volume
  - Embouchure: use of lips, facial muscles, tongue, and teeth when playing a wind instrument
  - Intermission: a break between the parts of a performance
  - Score: music notes written on paper
- Dance terminology
  - Positions: positions of the feet, legs, and arms, which all classical ballet techniques are based on, numbered first to fifth
  - En pointe: dancing on the tip of the toes, in footwear called pointe shoes
  - Parallel: both knees and feet with toes pointing forward
  - Pirouette: complete turn of the body on one foot
  - Plié: bending at the knee
  - Relevé: heel raise to the ball of the foot/metatarsal head in flat shoes, or going en pointe in pointe shoes
  - Turnout: rotation of the lower extremity that causes the toes to point laterally

MEDICAL ISSUES

- **Disordered eating/Relative Energy Deficiency in Sport (RED-S):** Although disordered eating is more prevalent in female ballet dancers, anorexia nervosa also occurs in male ballet dancers (9). Therefore, it is important to screen for RED-S in all dancers, paying particular attention to restrictive diets, menstrual irregularity or delayed menses, and history of stress injuries or fractures.
- **Mental health:** Psychological variables are known to affect the outcome of dance injuries in both student and professional dancers, so it must also be addressed when treating a dancer with a physical injury (10). Times of stress, such as an injury, can exacerbate preexisting mental health conditions or prolong the length of recovery (11). For professional dancers, an injury increases the likelihood of losing a company position (12).
- **Hearing loss:** Hearing loss awareness is rising in the musician population. In one study, 45% of student musicians demonstrated noise-induced hearing loss, compared to 11.5% of the general population (13).
- **Eyestrain:** An additional environmental risk factor faced by musicians is eye strain, resulting from reading small-print sheet music in poorly lit rooms on music stands positioned too far away (14).
- **Cardiovascular fitness:** Dance class has lower cardiovascular demands than performance and thus does not adequately prepare dancers for repetitive rehearsals or performances (15). This potentially leads to risk of fatigue and injury (16,17).

MUSCULOSKELETAL ISSUES – MUSICIANS

- Historically, musicians are more prone to injury when learning a new technique, practicing a particularly challenging piece, or using a new instrument (18).
- Musculoskeletal injuries and tendinopathies are common in musicians and tend to present in the same way that they would in nonmusicians.
- Neurologic injuries are vastly more prevalent than in nonmusical populations, making them important diagnoses to recognize and maintain in your differential diagnosis.
  - *Cervical radiculopathy*: Due to the lateral (often leftward) rotation and lateral flexion of the neck required to cradle an instrument, cervical radiculopathy is common in string musicians. This posture causes loading of the facet joints and anatomic narrowing of the ipsilateral neural foramen.
  - On physical examination, one should perform a Spurling test (also known as the quadrant test) where downward pressure is placed on the top of the rotated and extended head. A positive test is defined by pain and paresthesias spreading distally in the distribution of a cervical nerve root on the compressed side. Multiple studies have shown the Spurling test to be a reliable diagnostic tool with specificities ranging from 92% to 100%, although with sensitivities of only 28%–60%, it should not be used for screening purposes (19).
  - Consequently, even without suggestive exam findings, a magnetic resonance imaging (MRI) or nerve conduction studies/electromyography (NCS/EMG) should be considered if clinical suspicion is high.
- *Thoracic Outlet Syndrome (TOS):* This condition results from compression of the neurovascular structures passing through the superior thoracic outlet. The brachial plexus, subclavian artery, and subclavian vein are all at risk of compression while passing between the anterior and middle scalene muscles.
  - Compression may be functional, due to shifts of the clavicle in relation to the shoulder girdle during performance or from external causes such as a neck strap for a baritone saxophone. Compression may also be static, as in the case of those with a cervical rib. Symptoms typically begin as vague paresthesias and pain located in the medial forearm and hand (C7, C8, or T1 dermatomes).
  - Multiple exam maneuvers have been developed to identify the condition, but retrospective studies have found that the Adson test, Wright hyperabduction test, Roos test, and the costoclavicular maneuver all have high false-positive rates (19).
  - Clinical diagnosis must be made with a thorough history guiding a focused radiographic exam.
  - Treatments of choice are postural training and physical therapy. However, when rehabilitation fails, surgical decompression is sometimes necessary.
- Peripheral neuropathies
  - *Cubital tunnel syndrome:* With the elbow maintained in a constant state of flexion during prolonged periods of play, ulnar neuropathy at the elbow is a common injury resulting from the strain of supporting a string instrument.
    - Diagnosis is suspected based on history and can be confirmed if a Tinel sign is present at the cubital tunnel. NCS/EMG can confirm diagnosis.
    - Treatment can include occupational therapy, ergonomic assessment of instrument playing posture, night-time elbow splints, and nonsteroidal anti-inflammatory drugs (NSAIDs), in addition to relative or complete rest. With proper adherence, symptoms frequently resolve within weeks.
    - In recalcitrant cases operative ulnar transposition is the definitive management.
  - *Carpal tunnel syndrome:* Often seen in pianists and keyboardists, carpal tunnel syndrome can result from repetitive flexion and extension of the wrist. The condition can also develop in the bow or pick hand of string instrumentalists.

- Typical symptoms include numbness, tingling, pain, and, in severe cases, weakness of the lateral three and a half fingers, which are supplied by the median nerve.
- The Phalen test is a good screening exam with poor specificity reported but a sensitivity of about 80% (20). Meanwhile, a positive Tinel sign at or just distal to the carpal tunnel is virtually diagnostic with specificities approaching 100%, but it should not be used for screening due to poor sensitivity (20). NCS/EMG can confirm diagnosis.
- Treatment can include occupational therapy, ergonomic assessment of instrument playing posture, neutral wrist splints, and NSAIDs in addition to relative or complete rest. Steroid injections can alleviate symptoms temporarily.
- In recalcitrant cases surgical release is necessary for definitive management.

- *Focal neuropathies:* Trumpet player's neuropathy is a focal neuropathy of the neurovascular supply to the lip due to playing woodwinds with leaky valves or pads that increases the effort required to produce a note. The condition is seen primarily in brass and woodwind players (21).

- *Focal motor dystonia* is commonly reported in musicians. The condition is characterized by the loss of previously highly skilled movements that devolve into involuntary painless spasm during task-specific, finely coordinated movements.
  - Two major forms are *focal hand dystonia* (FHD) and *embouchure dystonia* (ED). The fourth and fifth digits are most commonly affected, with keyboard players, string musicians, and woodwind players being at the highest risk in one study (20).
  - This condition is widely considered to be a consequence of prolonged repetitive daily practice, often when exposed to other risk factors such as genetic predisposition to motor disturbance.
  - The onset of the disorder is often marked by subtle loss of control in fast passages, trill irregularity, fingers sticking to keys, or loss of embouchure control in certain registers.
  - A common response by musicians is to increase rehearsal time to improve their technique, but this only exacerbates the problem.
  - Although focal motor dystonia is highly disabling among musicians and frequently terminates professional careers, retraining programs have shown promise as a treatment (22,23).

MUSCULOSKELETAL ISSUES – DANCE

- Range of Motion (ROM), flexibility, and hypermobility: Although hypermobility can be an occupational advantage for some dancers, it may increase the risk of injury (24–26).
  - Excessive joint mobility may be due to a benign tendency toward increased laxity of the ligaments, or it can indicate more serious conditions such as Ehlers-Danlos or Marfan Syndrome (27).
  - The nine-point Beighton Assessment of Hypermobility (Box 100.1) is used as a quick screen. Hypermobility is a score (greater than or equal to) 4/9 and associated with an increase in recovery time when compared to dancers with non–joint hypermobility syndrome (28).
- Turnout: Turnout is a fundamental position in ballet in which each lower extremity is externally rotated 90°. Forced turnout, and improper technique utilized to compensate for inadequate hip ROM, consists of increased anterior pelvic tilt, 'screwing' into the knees with excess external tibial torsion at the knee, and overpronation at the subtalar joint.
  - Traditionally, the range of motion necessary for proper turnout has been accepted as 70° from the femoral-acetabular joint (29); however, many recent studies have suggested the actual range of motion of the typical ballet dancer hip is between 39.7° and 52.0° (30–32). This suggests there is more range of motion obtained than the traditional understanding of 5° from the tibial external rotation at the knee and 15° from the ankle and foot. Turnout discs that remove the ability to use ground friction can be helpful in determining functional turnout accurately.
- En pointe: When dancing en pointe the majority of the dancer's weight is borne through 1st MTP, and this technique has been demonstrated to increase force through the foot to 12 times the body weight (33).
  - Pointe readiness screens, usually conducted between ages 10 and 13 years, include criteria such as flexibility, range of motions, maturity, and technique.

100.1 Beighton Scoring System for Hypermobility (28)

Score 1 point for each of the following:

1. Forward flexion at the waist, placing flat hands on the floor with knees extended
2. Left knee hyperextension >10°
3. Right knee hyperextension >10°
4. Left elbow hyperextension >10°
5. Right elbow hyperextension >10°
6. Left thumb touching forearm
7. Right thumb touching forearm
8. Left pinky finger extending >90°
9. Right pinky finger extending >90°

Foot/Ankle

- *Dancer's fracture:* A dancer's fracture is a spiral fracture of the shaft of the fifth metatarsal. It is the most common acute, traumatic fracture encountered in dancers, and frequently results from an inversion injury while dancing en pointe.
- *Lisfranc injury:* A Lisfranc injury can occur when a downward force is applied simultaneously to a twisting motion of the foot, resulting in a sprain injury with or without an associated fracture/dislocation to the ligaments between the first and second metatarsals and the medial and middle cuneiforms.
  - Diagnosis requires bilateral weight-bearing or stressed films to compare the injured joint space to the contralateral side. The Fleck sign is an avulsion fracture off the metatarsal base.
  - Sprains can usually be managed conservatively with 4–6 weeks of non–weight-bearing immobilization in a controlled ankle movement (CAM) walker boot, whereas fractures/dislocations require open reduction and internal fixation.
- *Anterior impingement syndrome:* Affects the anterior ankle during dorsiflexion or plié in ballet. Impingement occurs between the anterior tibia and the dorsum of the talus and is sometimes associated with radiographically visible spurring of the tibial ridge and talar neck.
  - Conservative treatment, which is usually effective, involves physical therapy to address posterior chain restrictions, heel wedges to decrease dorsiflexion, biomechanical optimization, activity modification, and graduated return to dance.
  - Surgical intervention can be pursued to remove spurs if nonoperative management fails, particularly if mechanical symptoms persist.
- *Posterior impingement syndrome:* Posterior impingement syndrome, conversely, is characterized by posterolateral ankle pain during plantarflexion as during pointe work in ballet.
  - Symptoms occur when full plantarflexion is not achieved because of a fixed obstruction such as an os trigonum, which causes increased stress on the tendinous structures and bony impingement.
  - An os trigonum occurs when the posterolateral process of the talus does not fuse during puberty. It is a congenital variant that is found in 7%–11% of the population. Presence of an os trigonum, however, does not inevitably lead to impingement, as many dancers with this variant are asymptomatic (34).
  - In this setting, an ankle sprain and the resulting shift in ankle mechanics can unmask a previously asymptomatic anatomic variant.
  - Nonoperative treatment with activity modification, physical therapy to address foot rigidity and biomechanics, NSAIDs, and therapeutic injections is nearly always successful, and surgical intervention is rarely warranted.
- *Flexor hallucis longus (FHL) tendonitis:* Dancer's FHL tendonitis, occurs from overuse and microtrauma resulting from repetitive dorsiflexion and plantarflexion.
  - The FHL travels through the fibro-osseous tunnel above the posterior talar tubercle and can be injured by compressive forces during full plantarflexion and stretching between the talar tubercle and sustentaculum tali during dorsiflexion, as well as by increased pressure from dancing en pointe.
  - Cumulative stress leads to posteromedial ankle pain, inflammatory changes, nodular tendinopathy, and potentially tissue degeneration.
- *Achilles tendinopathy:* Achilles tendinopathy is commonly encountered in dancers and is considered a chronic process rather than an acute inflammatory injury. The Achilles tendon arises from the gastrocnemius-soleus complex and is subject to excessive forces during activities such as dance (35).
  - Earlier studies have demonstrated forces of up to six times the body weight transmitted through the Achilles during running and dance, whereas a study in 2010 showed ankle contact forces of 14 times body weight during the "rock step" in Irish dancers (34,36). Another study of Irish dancers demonstrated that 75% had evidence of pathologic changes to the Achilles on MRI, with only half of those demonstrating radiographic changes actually manifesting symptoms (37). This suggests that the impact of dancing causes subclinical injury in the majority of participants even when not perceived by the dancer.
  - As in other overuse injuries, the onset of Achilles tendinopathy is insidious, with pain most commonly experienced at the insertion of the Achilles tendon onto the calcaneus.
  - Symptoms can be recalcitrant to treatment, so physicians should encourage a multidisciplinary approach including physical therapy, myofascial release of the posterior chain, addressing underlying training errors or biomechanical deficits leading to increased load, and progressive loading exercises to improve tendon vascularity and collagen synthesis to promote healing (37).
- *Hallux Valgus (bunions):* Hallux valgus is a deformity of medial deviation of the first metatarsal with associated lateral deviation of the great toe.
  - This is more common in female dancers than in the general population (38). This is thought to be associated with constrictive shoes such as pointe shoes, along with pes planus, first ray hypermobility, Achilles tendon contracture, and MTP joint hypomobility (39,40). Although technique may play a role, female gender, and genetic predisposition have also been implicated (40–42).
  - Proper technique and pointe shoe fit are suggested for the prevention of hallux valgus in addition to use of toe spacers, stretching of the ankle plantar flexors, and strengthening the intrinsic foot musculature (41).
  - Additional treatment such as injections can be utilized in recalcitrant cases.

- *Hip labral tear:* The repetitive compression and shearing forces on the labrum due to the repetitive rotation at end range of motion in dance can lead to added stress on the anterior labrum, and one study demonstrated 40% of dancers who were assessed and treated for hip pain were found to have labral tears (43).
    - Dancers may complain of hip clicking or pain in the groin with hip flexion, adduction and internal rotation (FADIR), or the examiner may feel a click or pop with hip scour.
    - MRI is the diagnostic test of choice. The probability of a labral tear is greatly increased when femoral acetabular impingement (FAI) is also present (44).
    - Many young dancers diagnosed with labral tears do not require surgery and return to sport with physical therapy and the addition of intra-articular injections, when necessary.
- *Snapping hip syndrome:* Snapping hip syndrome, sometimes referred to as dancer's hip, is characterized by a snapping sensation and frequently an audible pop as the hip is flexed and extended. The cause in dancers is usually friction of the iliopsoas tendon as it passes over the anterior inferior iliac spine, lesser trochanter of the femur, or iliopectineal ridge. This should be differentiated from the more common form of snapping hip syndrome, most frequently encountered by runners, which results from the iliotibial band or tensor fascia lata snapping over the greater trochanter of the femur.
    - Relative rest, stretching of the hip flexors and rotators, and strengthening exercises are the mainstays of rehabilitation. Corticosteroid injections can also be employed if there is an associated bursitis.
- *Spondylolisthesis:* A spondylolisthesis is a common and potentially disabling injury in dancers, causing low back pain with strenuous exercise, rotation, and hyperextension. The cumulative stress of repetitive hyperextension at end-range of motion sometimes results in a stress fracture of the pars interarticularis, a condition known as spondylolysis.
    - Spondylolysis can occur bilaterally, compromising anterior-posterior stability of the spine. If bilateral pars defects are found, spondylolisthesis or anterior slippage of the superior vertebrae can occur.
    - Nearly 90% of spondylolistheses occur at the L5–S1 level, whereas the next most common site of injury is the L4–L5 level (14).
    - X-ray, MRI, and at times CT, are necessary to diagnose acuity. Injury is graded according to the degree of slippage.
    - Grade 1 and 2 injuries are typically managed conservatively with rest, spine-strengthening exercises, and occasionally bracing. Meanwhile, grade 3 and 4 injuries, which represent a minimum of a 50% slippage, are often managed surgically.

CHALLENGES SPECIFIC TO SPORT

- Rehabilitation of a performing arts injury should be a team-based approach with an understanding of both musculoskeletal medicine and the specific demands placed on a performer's body and psyche (45).
- To discover the biomechanics of injury, physicians who care for these specialized performers must commit to understanding the art form of their patients. When possible, observe them in your clinic, their rehearsal space, or onstage with their instrument or in their costume when appropriate.
- Working to understand the vocabulary and art form of each individual artist and coordinating with a multidisciplinary team including the patient's teachers, coaches, therapists, dietitian, and agents is often the best way to achieve success in caring for these unique and talented individuals.
- Musicians: Poor lighting, proximity to speakers (ear plugs), and smoke-filled rooms are common hazards.
- Dancers: Raked stages (those that are at an incline), costumes, bright spotlight and dark off-stage, turning (particularly after concussion), partnered lifting/being lifted, and audience noise are all sources of risk.
- As with many athletes, artists losing the ability to perform forfeit not only their livelihood, but also a source of positive reinforcement.
- Making music is frequently linked to highly positive emotions, which enhance brain adaptations and can even lead to addictive behaviors. This has been proposed as one of many reasons that musicians sometimes over-practice and ignore their bodily signals of fatigue and pain (46). These findings are likely true and should be applied to all performing artists.

REFERENCES

1. Ericsson KA, Krampe RT, Tesch-Römer C. The role of deliberate practice in the acquisition of expert performance. *Psychol Rev.* 1993;100(3):363–406.
2. Hallam S. Culture, musicality, and musical expertise. In: Barrett M, editor. *A Cultural Psychology of Music Education*. Oxford (UK): Oxford University Press; 2010. p. 201–24.
3. Ackermann B, Driscoll T, Kenny DT. Musculoskeletal pain and injury in professional orchestral musicians in Australia. *Med Probl Perform Art.* 2012;27(4):181–7.
4. Silva AG, Lasã FM, Afreixo V. Pain prevalence in instrumental musicians: a systematic review. *Med Probl Perform Art.* 2015;30(1):8–19.
5. Fishbein M, Middlestadt SE, Ottati V, Ellis A. Medical problems among ICSOM musicians: overview of a national survey. *Med Probl Perform Art.* 1988;3(1):1–8.
6. Ojofeitimi S, Bronner S. Injuries in a modern dance company: effect of comprehensive management on injury incidence and cost. *J Dance Med Sci.* 2011;15(3):116–22.
7. Solomon R, Micheli L, Solomon J. The 'cost' of injuries in a professional ballet company. *Med Probl Perform Art.* 1995;10(1):3–10.

8. Shah S. Determining a young dancer's readiness for dancing on pointe. *Curr Sports Med Rep*. 2009;8(6):295–9.
9. Marra M, Sammarco R, De Filippo E, et al. Resting energy expenditure, body composition and phase angle in anorectic, ballet dancers and constitutionally lean males. *Nutrients*. 2019;11(3):502.
10. Mainwaring L, Finney C. Psychological risk factors and outcomes of dance injury, a systematic review. *J Dance Med Sci*. 2017;21(3):87–96.
11. Thomas J, Keel P, Heatherton T. Disordered eating and injuries among adolescent ballet dancers. *Eat Weight Disord*. 2011;16(3):e216–22.
12. Garrick J, Requa R. Ballet injuries. An analysis of epidemiology and financial outcome. *Am J Sports Med*. 1993;21(4):586–90.
13. Phillips SL, Henrich VC, Mace ST. Prevalence of noise-induced hearing loss in student musicians. *Int J Audiol*. 2010;49(4):309–16.
14. Hansen PA, Reed K. Common musculoskeletal problems in the performing artist. *Phys Med Rehabil Clin N Am*. 2006;17(4):789–801.
15. Wyon M, Abt G, Redding E, Head A, Sharp NCC. Oxygen uptake during modern dance class, rehearsal, and performance. *J Strength Cond Res*. 2004;18(3):646–9.
16. Liederbach M, Schanfein L, Kremenic I. What is known about the effect of fatigue on injury occurrence among dancers? *J Dance Med Sci*. 2013;17(3):101–8.
17. Wyon MA, Koutedakis Y. Muscular fatigue: considerations for dance. *J Dance Med Sci*. 2013;17(2):63–9.
18. Ostwald PF, Baron BC, Byl NM, Wilson FR. Performing arts medicine. *West J Med*. 1994;160(1):48–52.
19. Landes P, Malanga GA, Nadler S, Farmer J, PhyscMalanga GA, Nadler SF. Physical examination of the spine. In: Malanga GA, Nadler S, editors. *Musculoskeletal Physical Examination — an Evidence-Based Approach*. Philadelphia (PA): Elsevier Mosby; 2006. p. 33–57.
20. Newmark J, Hochberg FH. Isolated painless manual incoordination in 57 musicians. *J Neurol Neurosurg Psychiatry*. 1987;50(3):291–5.
21. Lederman RJ. Peripheral nerve disorders in instrumentalists. *Ann Neurol*. 1989;26(5):640–6.
22. Altenmüller E, Jabusch HC. Focal dystonia in musicians. *Eur J Neurol*. 2010;17(suppl 1):31–6.
23. Ackermann B, Altenmüller E. The development and use of an anatomy-based retraining program (MusAARP) to assess and treat focal hand dystonia in musicians-a pilot study. *J Hand Ther*. 2021;34(2):309–14.
24. McCormack M, Briggs J, Hakim A, Grahame R. Joint laxity and the benign joint hypermobility syndrome in student and professional ballet dancers. *J Rheumatol*. 2004;31(1):173–8.
25. Hamilton W, Hamilton L, Marshall P, Molnar M. A profile of the musculoskeletal characteristics of elite professional ballet dancers. *Am J Sports Med*. 1992;20(3):267–73.
26. Micheli L, Gillespie W, Walaszek A. Physiologic profiles of female professional ballerinas. *Clin Sports Med*. 1984;3(1):199–209.
27. Knight IA. *A Guide to Living with Hypermobility Syndrome; Bending Without Breaking*. London (UK): Kingsley Publishers; 2011. p. 22–3.
28. Briggs J, McCormack M, Hakim A, Grahame R. Injury and joint hypermobility syndrome in ballet dancers – a 5-year follow-up. *Rheumatology (Oxford)*. 2009;48(12):1613–4.
29. Thomasen E. *Diseases and Injuries of Ballet Dancers*. Aarhus (Denmark): Aarhus University; 1982.
30. Bauman P, Singson R, Hamilton W. Femoral neck anteversion in ballerinas. *Clin Orthop Relat Res*. 1994;302:57–63.
31. Gilbert C, Gross M, Klug K. Relationship between hip external rotation and turnout angle for the five classical ballet positions. *J Orthop Sports Phys Ther*. 1998;27(5):339–47.
32. Khan K, Roberts P, Nattrass C, et al. Hip and ankle range of motion in elite classical ballet dancers and controls. *Clin J Sport Med*. 1997;7(3):174–9.
33. Spilken T. *The Dancers Foot Book*. Princeton (NJ): Princeton Tec Publishers; 1990.
34. Hamilton WG. Posterior ankle pain in dancers. *Clin Sports Med*. 2008;27(2):263–77.
35. Hodgkins CW, Kennedy JG, O'Loughlin PF. Tendon injuries in dance. *Clin Sports Med*. 2008;27(2):279–88.
36. Shippen JM, May B. Calculation of muscle loading and joint contact forces during the rock step in Irish dance. *J Dance Med Sci*. 2010;14(1):11–8.
37. Walls RJ, Brennan SA, Hodnett P, O'Byrne JM, Eustace SJ, Stephens MM. Overuse ankle injuries in professional Irish dancers. *Foot Ankle Surg*. 2010;16(1):45–9.
38. van Dijk CN, Lim LS, Poortman A, Strübbe EH, Marti RK. Degenerative joint disease in female ballet dancers. *Am J Sports Med*. 1995;23(3):295–300.
39. Inman VT. Hallux valgus: a review of etiologic factors. *Orthop Clin North Am*. 1974;5(1):59–66.
40. Coughlin MJ. Hallux valgus. *J Bone Joint Surg Am*. 1996;78(6):932–66.
41. Davenport KL, Simmel L, Kadel N. Hallux valgus in dancers: a closer look at dance technique and its impact on dancers' feet. *J Dance Med Sci*. 2014;18(2):86–92.
42. Piqué-Vidal C, Solé MT, Antich J. Hallux valgus inheritance: pedigree research in 350 patients with bunion deformity. *J Foot Ankle Surg*. 2007;46(3):149–54.
43. Kern-Scott R, Peterson JR, Morgan P. Review of acetabular labral tears in dancers. *J Dance Med Sci*. 2011;15(4):149–56.
44. Cianci A, Sugimoto D, Stracciolini A, Yen YM, Kocher MS, d'Hemecourt PA. Nonoperative management of labral tears of the hip in adolescent athletes: description of sports participation, interventions, comorbidity, and outcomes. *Clin J Sport Med*. 2019;29(1):24–8.
45. Hrubes M, Janowski J. Rehabilitation of the dancer. *Phys Med Rehabil Clin N Am*. 2021;32(1):1–20.
46. Altenmüller E, Kopiez R, Grewe O. A contribution to the evolutionary basis of music: lessons from the chill response. In: Altenmüller E, Schmidt S, Zimmermann E, editors. *Evolution of Emotional Communication from Sounds in Nonhuman Mammals to Speech and Music in Man*. Oxford (UK): Oxford University Press; 2013. p. 13–35.

101 Dive Medicine

Jonathan D. Bailey and James Lynch

INTRODUCTION

- SCUBA is an acronym for self-contained underwater breathing apparatus, the delivery system that makes it possible to breathe compressed gas from a portable supply while underwater.
- Recreational SCUBA diving is a growing sport with approximately 3 million SCUBA divers in the United States and an estimated 6 million divers worldwide (1).
- In the United States, diving is not limited to coastal areas. It is increasingly popular to dive in inland bodies of water like pools, lakes, and quarries (2).
- The sports medicine physician must be aware of "fitness to dive" recommendations for patients of all ages who are seeking medical clearance to dive.
- Improper diagnosis and treatment of some diving injuries can result in catastrophic outcomes, particularly involving the brain and spinal cord.
- The underwater environment and hazards place the SCUBA diver at an increased risk for injury or illness.
- Increased ambient pressure is the most significant environmental exposure in the dive environment.
  - Ambient pressure increases in a linear fashion with depth underwater (Table 101.1) (3).
  - Exposure to increased pressure can result in several pathophysiologic changes as described by the common gas laws (4).
- There are many different types of SCUBA diving
  - Open water diving is the most common form of recreational SCUBA diving and it is usually far from shore and obstacles.
  - As experiences increase, SCUBA divers will increase depth and complexity, diving at night or with the current, incorporating wrecks or other obstacles, diving under frozen surfaces or diving as part of their profession: military diving, rescue diving, or commercial diving.
  - Freediving is not a type of SCUBA diving, but it involves holding one's breath as they dive under the surface of the water. The world record for the deepest free dive is 253 m (5).
- US and Canada morbidity and mortality for recreational diving (6).
  - The mean age for injuries among male and female divers is 37 and 41, respectively.
    - 75% of divers presenting to the Emergency Department (ED) are male.
    - Males make up 64% of the diving population and are 72% of the divers that dive greater than seven times per year.
  - It is estimated that 1 out of 10,000 emergency department presentations is due to SCUBA-related injuries.
  - Most SCUBA-related injuries presenting to the ED are minor with 80% being discharged following treatment or with no treatment at all.
  - Ears are the most commonly affected body part.
  - There are 47 deaths per 1000 SCUBA-related ED visits.
  - There are 1.8 deaths per million recreational dives.
  - The most common cause of death is drowning followed by heart disease (7).

SPECIFIC ISSUES

Equipment (2)

- SCUBA: Self-contained underwater breathing apparatus
  - The diver uses a metal cylinder with compressed air connected to a regulator which provides the air mixture to the diver on inhalation. Expired air is exhaled into the water.
  - Some divers use a rebreather or closed-circuit which recycles exhaled gas and recaptures exhaled oxygen.

Dive Profile Terminology (8)

- Descent: Diving deeper involves increases in pressure of 1 atmosphere per 33 feet of seawater. Equilibration of pressure in gas-filled spaces is critical during this phase.
- Bottom time: The amount of time spent underwater (traditionally referred to as time spent at the lowest depth). Bottom time influences the amount of gas absorption in tissues.

Table 101.1 Effects of Depth on Ambient Pressure

fsw	ata	mm Hg	psi
0 (sea level)	1	760	14.7
33	2	1520	29.4
66	3	2280	44.1
99	4	3040	58.8
132	5	3800	73.5

ata, absolute pressure in atmospheres; fsw, feet of seawater; mm Hg, millimeters of mercury; psi, pounds per square inch.
Source: Reproduced, with permission, from Lynch JH, Bove AA. Diving medicine: a review of current evidence. *J Am Board Fam Med.* 2009;22:399–407. Available from: doi:10.3122/jabfm.2009.04.080099.

- Ascent: Moving up toward the surface involves decreases in pressure and the release of absorbed gas back into local tissues and the bloodstream.
- Surface interval: Time between dives. This time allows the body to reacquire homeostasis, especially with respect to tissue gas concentration. Dive injuries may not present until the diver surfaces.
- Decompression stop: A pause in ascent following a deep dive that allows for absorbed inert gas bubbles to be safely eliminated from tissues.
- No-decompression dive: A dive profile that does not require decompression based on limited depth and bottom time. Most sport divers perform no-decompression dives to mitigate the risk of decompression sickness.

Gas Laws (9,10)

- Boyle Law — the volume of a gas varies inversely to the pressure.
  - Example — The volume of a gas (*i.e.*, in the lungs, sinuses or ears) increases as the diver ascends and the pressure decreases.
  - Associated Pathology — barotrauma.
- Dalton Law — In a mixture of gases, the total pressure exerted is equal to the sum of the partial pressures of the individual gas.
  - Example — The diver breathes compressed surface air, 0.79% nitrogen and 21% oxygen. As the diver descends, nitrogen and oxygen partial pressure increases. There is an increase in systemic nitrogen absorption which can affect the diver's mental abilities.
  - Associated Pathology — nitrogen narcosis.
- Henry Law — The amount of dissolved gas is proportional to the gas's partial pressure in the gas phase.
  - Example — As depth and pressure increase, the more a gas is absorbed into the tissues. On ascent, bubble formation (likely from nitrogen) occurs when the rate of pressure reduction exceeds gas washout.
  - Associated Pathology — decompression illness.

COMMON MEDICAL DISORDERS AND DIVING

Barotrauma

- Ear and sinus barotrauma.
  - Middle ear — the most common injury related to diving (9).
    - Occurs in 30% of first-time divers and 10% of experienced divers.
    - Presentation — acute pain, which may be associated with vertigo and hearing loss.
    - Clinical Findings — range from tympanic membrane (TM) injection to hemotympanum, with or without rupture (11).
    - Treatment — decongestants, analgesics, consider antibiotics when TM rupture is present. TM must heal completely before diving again.
    - Prevention — careful use of Valsalva maneuver during descent.
      - Slow, feet-first descent
      - Nasal and/or systemic decongestants prior to dive may be helpful. As the medication effect diminishes, rebound congestion may occur causing ostial blockage and pain with ascent (12).
      - Avoid diving with an upper respiratory infection (13).
  - Sinus Barotrauma — results from transient nasal pathology or sinusitis.
    - A relative negative pressure during decent that is followed by engorgement and mucosal edema, which may cause bleeding into the sinuses.
    - Clinical findings — facial pain with epistaxis (14).
    - Treatment and Prevention — similar to middle ear barotrauma.
  - Inner Ear Barotrauma — related to middle ear barotrauma and occurs after forceful attempts to equalize the middle ear with the Valsalva maneuver.
    - Rupture of the round or oval window causing hearing loss, tinnitus and vertigo.
    - Dive history will help differentiate barotrauma versus decompression sickness (15).
    - Treatment — bed rest, head elevation, avoid straining, and ENT referral
- Pulmonary barotrauma
  - If the diver breathing compressed air at depth does not allow the compressed air to escape by exhaling, or if air empties slowly from a lung segment due to obstructive pulmonary conditions, then the gas will expand on the ascent (as ambient pressure falls). This causes the alveoli to rupture.

- The greatest change in lung volume occurs near the surface and it is possible to obtain pulmonary barotrauma in water as shallow as 4 feet (16).
- After alveoli trauma, the air under pressure will then escape the alveoli and rush into surrounding tissue resulting in mediastinal or subcutaneous emphysema or pneumothorax.
- In the most severe cases, air will enter the bloodstream via the pulmonary veins, traveling through the left heart as an arterial gas embolism (AGE).
  - Almost all cases of AGE present within 5 minutes of ascent and result in stroke-like events (17).
  - Clinical findings — stupor, bilateral or unilateral motor or sensory changes, unconsciousness, visual disturbance, vertigo, convulsions, and (in about 5% of cases) complete cardiovascular collapse (Table 101.2) (18).
  - Treatment — ACLS, 100% oxygen, hydration and recompression using US Navy Diving Manual Table 6 algorithm with decompression to 60 feet in a hyperbaric chamber while breathing oxygen (Fig. 101.1). Contact local emergency services. Consult DAN for the nearest chamber (18,19).
  - The majority of individuals with AGE fully recover with prompt recompression therapy (17).

- Other barotrauma
  - Dental barotrauma (9)
    - Barodontalgia is the most common dental complaint during a dive and is caused by gases trapped in the tooth from a cavity which then puts pressure on the trigeminal nerve.
    - Clinical presentation — tooth pain with referred otalgia.
    - Divers should also know what type of fillings they have, as some are more likely to lead to fracture, odontocrexis, of the tooth than others.
    - Treatment — dental referral.
  - Mask squeeze (2)
    - Facial barotrauma from failure to equalize the air in the diving mask.
    - Clinical presentation — facial edema, conjunctival hemorrhage and facial ecchymosis in the distribution of the mask.
    - Treatment — none required.
  - Abdominal barotrauma (2)
    - Swallowed air in the stomach during the dive can lead to distention on ascent with possible stomach rupture.
    - Clinical presentation — abdominal pain during the ascent increases as depth becomes shallower.
    - Treatment — surgical repair.

Decompression Sickness

- Decompression sickness (DCS) is caused by bubble formation in the blood and tissues.
  - As ambient pressure increases at depth, the partial pressures of inspired gases increase proportionally.
  - Inert gases, primarily nitrogen, are dissolved in the tissue which creates a supersaturated state in the body.

Table 101.2 Summary of Diving-Related Conditions and Associated Treatments

Condition	Presentation	Dive History	Prevention/Treatment
Barotrauma			
Middle ear	Acute ear pain, vertigo, tympanic membrane rupture	Usually during descent	Slow equalization on descent; decongestants, consider antibiotics for tympanic membrane perforation
Inner ear	Acute vertigo, nausea, vomiting, hearing loss	Usually during descent	Bed rest, elevated head, avoidance of Valsalva, otolaryngology consult
Sinus	Acute facial pain, epistaxis	Usually during descent	Slow equalization on descent; decongestants
Arterial gas embolism	Stupor, coma, focal weakness, visual disturbances	Immediately upon surfacing or during ascent	100% oxygen, supportive care, recompression using US Navy Table 6 Algorithm (Fig. 101.1)
Decompression Sickness			
Type I	Poorly localized joint pain, rash, itching	Significant time at depth; 50% develop symptoms within 1 h of surfacing, 90% within 6 h	100% oxygen, supportive care, recompression using US Navy Table 6 Algorithm (Fig. 101.1)
Type II	Numbness, dizziness, weakness, gait abnormality, hypoesthesia	Significant time at depth; 50% develop symptoms within 1 h of surfacing, 90% within 6 h	100% oxygen, supportive care, recompression using US Navy Table 6 Algorithm (Fig. 101.1)

In an emergency, contact local emergency services and then contact DAN at +1 (919) 684-9111 for the closest recompression chamber.
Source: Reproduced, with permission, from Lynch JH, Bove AA. Diving medicine: a review of current evidence. *J Am Board Fam Med.* 2009;22(4):399–407.

Treament Table 6

1. Descent rate - 20 ft./min.
2. Ascent rate - Not to exceed 1 ft/min. Do not compensate for slower ascent rates. Compensate for faster rates by halting the ascent.
3. Time on oxygen begins on arrival at 60 feet.
4. If oxygen breathing must be interrupted because of CNS Oxygen Toxicity, allow 15 minutes after the reaction has entirely subsided and resume schedule at point of interruption (see paragraph 20-7.11.1.1).
5. Table 6 can be lengthened up to two additional 25-minute periods at 60 feet (20 minutes on oxygen and 5 minutes on air), or up to two additional 75-minute periods at 30 feet (15 minutes on air and 60 minutes on oxygen), or both.
6. Tender breathes 100 percent O_2 during last 30 min. at 30 fsw and during ascent to the surface for an unmodified table or where there has been only a single extension at 30 or 60 feet. If there has been more than one extension, the O_2 breathing at 30 feet is increased to 60 minutes. If the tender had a hyperbaric exposure within the past 18 hours an additional 60-minute O_2 period is taken at 30 feet.

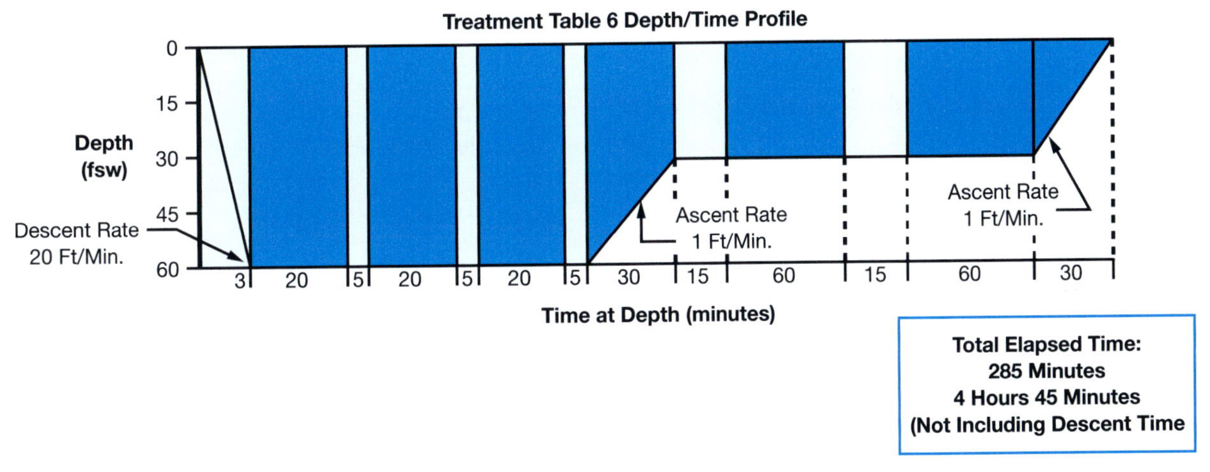

Figure 101.1: US Navy diving manual. (*Source:* Figure 17–5. Treatment Table 6. Page 17–44. Available from: https://www.navsea.navy.mil/Portals/103/Documents/SUPSALV/Diving/US%20DIVING%20MANUAL_REV7.pdf?ver=2017-01-11-102354-393.)

- If the ascent is too rapid, the dissolved nitrogen in the blood and tissues will become supersaturated and form bubbles.
- Bubbles cause tissue injury through mechanical effects, vascular occlusion, and activation of the clotting cascade and inflammatory mediators.
- Bubbles are often detected initially in the venous system and can enter the arterial circulation through a patent foramen ovale (PFO) which then produces symptoms similar to AGE (20).

- Incidence of DCS — 2–3 per 10,000 dives (21).
  - DCS in recreational divers is extremely rare, occurring only after 0.005%–0.08% of dives.
  - Of those with DCS, 60% will develop symptoms within 3 hours and 98% will have symptoms within 24 hours (19).
- DCS type I
  - Type I (nonsystemic or musculoskeletal DCS) is characterized by the absence of neurological and systemic symptoms.
  - Clinical presentation — *musculocutaneous symptoms*, such as a throbbing and poorly localized joint pain, with the shoulder and the elbow the most common. *Cutaneous symptoms* include rash or pruritus, and less commonly cutis marmorata or skin marbling.
  - Treatment — recompression. Contact local emergency services. Consult DAN for the nearest chamber (see Table 101.2).
  - Joint pain rapidly improves with recompression.
  - Cutaneous symptoms improve in 12–24 hours (22).
- DCS Type II
  - Type II (neurologic or systemic DCS) affects the neurologic, vestibular, or pulmonary systems.
  - Neurological involvement is the most common and can be due to either spinal cord or cerebral involvement.
    - Clinical presentation — numbness, dizziness, weakness, gait abnormality, and hypoesthesia (18).
  - Inner Ear DCS (the staggers) — likely from bubble formation in the semicircular canals.

- Clinical presentation — acute vertigo, nystagmus, tinnitus, and nausea with vomiting.
- Pulmonary DCS (the chokes) —likely from a massive pulmonary gas embolism after rapid ascent.
  - Clinical Presentation — substernal pain, cough, cardiovascular schlock resembling adult respiratory distress syndrome (23).
- Treatment — hydration, 100% oxygen, and recompression. Contact local emergency services. Consult DAN for the nearest chamber (Table 101.2).

Flying After Diving (24)

- The Divers Alert Network (DAN) 2002 Consensus Guidelines for Flying After Recreational Diving are summarized below. They apply to air dives followed by flights at cabin altitudes of 2000–8000 ft for divers without DCS symptoms.
  - For a single no-decompression dive, one should wait at least 12 hours prior to flying.
  - For multiple dives per day or multiple days of diving, 18 hours are suggested.
  - For any decompression dive, "substantially longer than 18 hours."

MEDICAL DISORDERS AND FITNESS TO DIVE

- Detailed "fitness to dive" resources are listed in Box 101.1

Cardiovascular Disease

- The number two cause of death during diving, but the most common disabling injury leading to death (7).
- Cardiovascular contraindications to diving are listed in Box 101.2.
- Diving places the following unique stresses on the heart:
  - Increased myocardial oxygen demands from swimming.
  - Preload is increased due to immersion-induced increased central venous return.
  - Afterload is increased from cold-induced peripheral vasoconstriction.
- DAN, UHMS, and South Pacific Underwater Medicine Society (SPUMS) recommend a cardiovascular medical assessment starting for asymptomatic candidates at age 45 (27).
  - Exercise stress testing may be recommended for asymptomatic divers with multiple cardiovascular risk factors (28).
  - Fitness to dive is optimal when a diver can reach a maximum capacity of 13 metabolic equivalents (METS) or stage four of the Bruce protocol while remaining free of chest pain. This peak capacity allows a diver to exercise comfortably at 8–9 METS (29).
  - After successful treatment, divers with some of the disorders listed in Box 101.2 may be able to return to diving after appropriate clearance.
- After a period of stabilization (6–12 months) and a thorough cardiovascular evaluation, individuals with known coronary artery disease, previous heart attacks, and revascularization procedures may return to low-stress sport diving (30).

PFO

- The relationship between PFO and DCS is controversial. Although causality is still unproven, there appears to be an increased relative risk of developing DCS with a PFO versus without.
- The most widely quoted odds ratio for serious DCS with PFO versus without PFO is 2.52 (95% confidence interval, 1.5–4.25) as determined by a meta-analysis in 1998 (31).
- Evidence supports that the average recreational sport diver need not be screened for PFO (27).
- For those already diagnosed as having PFO, this is not an absolute contraindication for diving.
  - A safe strategy would be to reduce the venous bubble load when diving by avoiding dives requiring decompression stops, by limiting bottom time, or by the appropriate use of oxygen-enriched breathing mixes (32).

Asthma

- Despite the theoretical risk, the evidence for the actual risk of pulmonary barotrauma or DCS among divers with asthma is equivocal.

101.1 Detailed Resources for Determining Fitness to Dive.

- DAN Website at https://www.diversalertnetwork.org.
- *Diving Medicine* (25).
- *Bennett and Elliott's Physiology and Medicine of Diving* (26).
- Undersea & Hyperbaric Medical Society (UHMS) https://www.uhms.org/resources/recreational-diving-medical-screening-system.html
- DAN is available for phone consultation:
  - Non-emergency (919) 684-2928 M-F 830 AM – 5 PM ET OR
  - Emergency: (919) 684-9111

101.2 Cardiovascular Contraindications for Diving (27)

- Arrhythmia:
  - Paroxysmal arrhythmias
  - Long QT syndrome
  - Presence of implanted cardiac defibrillator
- Structural:
  - Complex congenital heart disease
  - Left ventricular dysfunction
  - Moderate to severe valvular lesions
  - Hypertrophic cardiomyopathy
  - Congestive heart failure
- Vascular:
  - Uncontrolled hypertension >160/100
  - Pulmonary hypertension
- Other:
  - Untreated/symptomatic cardiovascular disease
  - Poor exercise capacity of cardiac origin
  - Anticoagulation
  - Recurrent syncope

  - A comprehensive review of the literature in 2003 found no epidemiological evidence for an increased relative risk of pulmonary barotrauma, DCS, or death among divers with asthma (33).
  - The theoretical risk to the diver with asthma includes bronchospasm which could lead to airway obstruction preventing gas elimination period expansion of the distal airway could then lead to barotrauma or AGE (34).
- When considering fitness to dive, asthma should not be viewed as a single disease.
  - With such variation among patients of precipitating factors, pulmonary function, degree of airway obstruction, and reversibility, this condition demands individualized consideration based on each specific divers history and disease syndrome (17).
  - When evaluating candidates who have asthma, obtain a thorough history and physical, spirometry, and an exercise challenge (34).
    - The candidate should be well-controlled with no current cardio-pulmonary symptoms.
    - Spirometry should be normal.
    - The candidate should successfully complete a bronchial provocation challenge (34).
    - Cold-, exercise-, or emotion-induced asthmatics should not dive (34).
    - If the diver has used rescue medication in the last 48 hours, the diver should not dive.
    - Conduct an annual review for fitness to dive.
  - Divers with a history of COPD, reduced exercise capacity, and significant obstruction should not be advised to dive (2).

Diabetes

- For those without significant comorbidities or secondary complications, diabetes is a relative contraindication for diving when following consensus guidelines (35).
- Type I and type II diabetic divers should demonstrate knowledge in control of their medical condition, and undergo an annual medical evaluation with an additional focus on cardiovascular health (35).
- Multiple studies have demonstrated that select diabetics can safely participate in recreational diving and that evidence is lacking for a widespread ban on diving for all diabetics (36,37).
- Proposed guidelines for recreational divers with diabetes (35).
  - These guidelines stipulate that adults with diabetes may qualify as fit to dive during their annual medical review if they have:
    - Hemoglobin A1c less than or equal to 8% (35).
    - No symptomatic long-term diabetic complications (cardiovascular, nephropathy, neuropathy, or substantial retinopathy) (35).
    - No significant episodes of hypoglycemia within the past year that required third-party intervention (35).
    - No hypoglycemia unawareness (35).
    - Knowledge of diabetes disease management, glucose monitoring, insulin dose adjustment, and preactivity glucose intake (35).
    - Continuous glucose monitoring prior to diving and for subsequent evaluations of outcomes (35).
  - Additionally, these guidelines provide considerations for the management of hypoglycemia during a dive, patient obligations, and considerations for divers less than 16 years old (physical ability, mental maturity, and disease management skills) (35).

Spontaneous Pneumothorax (38)

- Individuals who have experienced spontaneous pneumothorax should not dive.
- The average probability of a primary spontaneous pneumothorax recurrence is 22 ± 15% with most recurrences (63 ± 39%) occurring in the first 12 months.
- Even if high-resolution computed tomography scanning shows no evidence of pulmonary blebs, recurrence is still high at 33%.

- Surgical treatment (including video-assisted thoracoscopic surgery, wedge apical resection with pleurodesis or thoracotomy) after the first episode of spontaneous pneumothorax may reduce the risk of recurrence but does not protect against pulmonary barotrauma. Recommendations remain to avoid diving.

Elderly and Diving

- The median age of diving victims has increased as a reflection of the aging diving population (7).
- In 2018, 67% of recorded diving fatalities involved individuals aged 50 or older; the oldest was 73 years old (7).
- Order divers are more likely to have chronic medical conditions, and recommendations for diving should be based on the presence of acute or chronic illnesses and the physical conditioning of the individual rather than based on age alone.
- Divers 45 years of age, or those with two or more cardiovascular risk factors, should have a fitness-to-dive medical evaluation every 5 years (39).
- Divers 65 years of age, or those with pre-existing diseases, should have an annual fitness-to-dive medical evaluation (39).
- With careful evaluation, elderly athletes in good health can undertake a safe recreational diving program (40).
- Concerning exercise for older adults, regular physical activity improves psychological well-being, reduces the risk of cognitive decline and dementia, induces favorable metabolic and cardiovascular adaptations, and improves VO_{2max}. (41).

TREATMENT

- Table 101.2 summarizes common diving-related conditions and their associated treatments.

REFERENCES

1. 2022 Diving Fast Facts. *The Diving Equipment & Marketing Association* 2022. Accessed September, 19 2022. https://www.dema.org/store/download.aspx?id=7811B097-8882-4707-A160-F999B49614B6
2. Bove AA. Diving medicine. *Am J Respir Crit Care Med.* 2014;189(12):1479–86. doi:10.1164/rccm.201309-1662CI
3. Lynch JH, Bove AA. Diving medicine: a review of current evidence. *J Am Board Fam Med.* 2009;22(4):399–407. doi:10.3122/jabfm.2009.04.080099
4. Taylor L. Diving physics. In: Bove AA, Davis JC, editors. *Diving Medicine.* 4th ed. Saunders; 2004. pp. 11–35.
5. Deepest No-limit Freedive (Male). *Guinness World Records.* Accessed September 19, 2022. https://www.guinnessworldrecords.com/world-records/673884-deepest-no-limit-freedive-male
6. Buzzacott P, Schiller D, Crain J, Denoble PJ. Epidemiology of morbidity and mortality in US and Canadian recreational SCUBA diving. *Public Health.* 2018;155:62–8. doi:10.1016/j.puhe.2017.11.011
7. Tillmans F, editor. *DAN Annual Diving Report 2020 Edition: A Report on 2018 Diving Fatalities, Injuries, and Incidents.* Durham (NC): Divers Alert Network; 2021.
8. Morris G. SCUBA diving. In: Madden C, Putukian M, Young C, McCarty E, editors. *Netter's Sports Medicine.* Philadelphia: Saunders; 2010. pp. 538–45.
9. Anderson W, Murray P, Hertweck K. Dive medicine: current perspectives and future directions. *Curr Sports Med Rep.* 2019;18(4):129–35. doi:10.1249/JSR.0000000000000583
10. Bosco G, Rizzato A, Moon RE, Camporesi EM. Environmental Physiology and diving medicine. *Front Psychol.* 2018;9:72. Published 2018 Feb 2. doi:10.3389/fpsyg.2018.00072
11. Clenney TL, Lassen LF. Recreational SCUBA diving injuries. *Am Fam Physician.* 1996;53(5):1761–74.
12. Kay E. The diver's ear—under pressure. Doc's Diving Medicine. Updated 2022 Mar 11. Accessed October 6, 2022. http://www.divingdoc.com
13. Cheshire WP. Headache and facial pain in SCUBA divers. *Curr Pain Headache Rep.* 2004;8(4):315–20. doi:10.1007/s11916-004-0015-y
14. Parell GJ, Becker GD. Neurological consequences of SCUBA diving with chronic sinusitis. *Laryngoscope.* 2000;110(8):1358–60. doi:10.1097/00005537-200008000-00026
15. Hunter SE, Farmer JC. Ear and sinus problems in diving. In: Bove AA, Davis JC, editors. *Diving Medicine.* 4th ed. Saunders; 2004. pp. 431–59.
16. Bove AA. Medical aspects of sport diving. *Med Sci Sports Exerc.* 1996;28(5):591–5. doi:10.1097/00005768-199605000-00009
17. Neuman TS. Pulmonary barotrauma. In: Bove AA, Davis JC, editors. *Diving Medicine.* Saunders; 2004. pp. 185–94.
18. Newton HB. Neurologic complications of SCUBA diving. *Am Fam Physician.* 2001;63(11):2211–18.
19. *Diagnosis and Treatment of Decompression Sickness and Arterial Gas Embolism.* U.S. Navy Diving Manual, Revision 7. 2016 Dec 1. Accessed October 6, 2022. https://www.navsea.navy.mil/Portals/103/Documents/SUPSALV/Diving/US%20DIVING%20MANUAL_REV7.pdf?ver=2017-01-11-102354-393
20. Vann RD. Mechanisms and risks of decompression. In: Bove AA, Davis JC, editors. *Diving Medicine.* 4th ed. Philadelphia: Saunders; 2004. pp. 127–64.
21. Pollock N. *DAN Annual Diving Report.* 2008 Edition. Durham (NC): Divers Alert Network; 2008.
22. Moon RE. Treatment of decompression illness. In: Bove AA, Davis JC, editors. *Diving Medicine.* 4th ed. Philadelphia: Saunders; 2004. pp. 195–217.
23. Francis TJ, Mitchell SJ. Pathophysiology of decompression sickness. In: Bove AA, Davis JC, editors. *Diving Medicine.* 4th ed. Philadelphia: Saunders; 2004. pp. 165–83.
24. Sheffield P, Vann R. Flying after diving. In: *Proceedings of the DAN Flying after Diving Workshop*; 2004. Durham (NC).
25. Bove AA. Medical evaluation for sport diving. In: Bove AA, Davis JC, editors. *Diving Medicine.* 4th ed. Philadelphia: Saunders; 2004. pp. 519–32.
26. Brubakk AO, Neuman TS, Bennett PB, Elliot DH. *Bennett and Elliott's Physiology and Medicine of Diving.* 5th ed. London (UK): Saunders; 2003.
27. Jepson N, Rienks R, Smart D, Bennett MH, Mitchell SJ, Turner M. South Pacific Underwater Medicine Society guidelines for cardiovascular risk assessment of divers. *Diving Hyperb Med.* 2020;50(3):273–7. doi:10.28920/dhm50.3.273-277
28. Harrison D, Lloyd-Smith R, Khazei A, Hunte G, Lepawsky M. Controversies in the medical clearance of recreational SCUBA divers: updates on asthma, diabetes mellitus, coronary artery disease,

and patent foramen ovale. *Curr Sports Med Rep.* 2005;4(5):275–81. doi:10.1097/01.csmr.0000306222.19714.33

29. Pendergast DR, Tedesco M, Nawrocki DM, Fisher NM. Energetics of underwater swimming with SCUBA. *Med Sci Sports Exerc.* 1996;28(5):573–80. doi:10.1097/00005768-199605000-00006
30. Caruso J. *Cardiovascular Fitness and Diving.* Divers Alert Network. Accessed 2022 Oct 6. https://dan.org/health-medicine/health-resources/diseases-conditions/cardiovascular-fitness-and-diving/
31. Bove AA. Risk of decompression sickness with patent foramen ovale. *Undersea Hyperb Med.* 1998;25(3):175–8.
32. Moon RE, Bove AA. Transcatheter occlusion of patent foramen ovale: a prevention for decompression illness? *Undersea Hyperb Med.* 2004;31(3):271–4.
33. Koehle M, Lloyd-Smith R, McKenzie D, Taunton J. Asthma and recreational SCUBA diving: a systematic review. *Sports Med.* 2003;33(2):109–16. doi:10.2165/00007256-200333020-00003
34. Coop CA, Adams KE, Webb CN. SCUBA diving and asthma: clinical recommendations and safety. *Clin Rev Allergy Immunol.* 2016;50(1):18–22. doi:10.1007/s12016-015-8474-y
35. Jendle JH, Adolfsson P, Pollock NW. Recreational diving in persons with type 1 and type 2 diabetes: advancing capabilities and recommendations. *Diving Hyperb Med.* 2020;50(2):135–43. doi:10.28920/dhm50.2.135-143
36. Scott DH, Marks AD. Diabetes and diving. In: Bove AA, Davis JC, editors. *Diving Medicine.* 4th ed. Philadelphia: Saunders; 2004. pp. 507–18.
37. Pollock NW, Uguccioni DM, Dear G. Diabetes and recreational diving: guidelines for the future. In: *Proceedings of the Undersea Hyperbaric Medical Society/Divers Alert Network Workshop: June 19, 2005*; 2005. Durham (NC).
38. Villela MA, Dunworth S, Harlan NP, Moon RE. Can my patient dive after a first episode of primary spontaneous pneumothorax? A systematic review of the literature. *Undersea Hyperb Med.* 2018;45(2):199–208.
39. *Guidelines for Lifelong Medical Fitness to Dive.* Divers Alert Network. 2020. Accessed 2022 Sep 19. https://dan.org/safety-prevention/diver-safety/divers-blog/schedule-for-lifelong-medical-fitness-to-dive-evaluation/
40. Bove AA. Diving in the elderly and the young. In: Bove AA, Davis JC, editors. *Diving Medicine.* 4th ed. Philadelphia: Saunders; 2004. pp. 411–20.
41. American College of Sports Medicine, Chodzko-Zajko WJ, Proctor DN, Fiatarine Singh MA, et al. American College of Sports Medicine position stand. Exercise and physical activity for older adults. *Med Sci Sports Exerc.* 2009;41(7):1510–30. doi:10.1249/MSS.0b013e3181a0c95c

102 Esports

Melita N. Moore, Lindsey Migliore, and Khizer Khaderi

INTRODUCTION AND BACKGROUND

- The organized, competitive video gaming industry, known as esports, encompasses a wide range of video game genres that can be played at various levels, including amateur, high school, collegiate, and professional.
- There are over 3 billion gamers worldwide with the average age of 18–34 years old
- Esports consists of several disciplines, such as first-person shooters (FPS), multiplayer online battle arenas (MOBA), real-time strategy (RTS), sports simulation, and fighting games, among others.
- As with traditional sports, esports participants are susceptible to injuries, although the nature of these injuries differs. The majority of these injuries are upper extremity tendinopathies related to overuse as esports athletes can perform 400–600 actions per minute (1).
- The overall injury rates in esports have not been comprehensively studied; however, emerging research indicates a need for improved ergonomic practices, injury prevention strategies, and recovery protocols.
- A complete gaming history should be included in the medical history taking.
- General epidemiological concerns in esports include the potential for long-term musculoskeletal, visual and hearing issues, as well as mental health challenges related to the high-pressure, competitive environment (1).

SPECIFIC ISSUES

- Ergonomics
  - A gaming setup traditionally consists of a desk, gaming chair, monitor, and either a mouse and keyboard for PC gaming or controller for console gaming.
  - Ergonomics of the gaming setup is key to prevention, including proper desk and chair height, monitor positioning, mobile device distance, and regular movement breaks.
- Gaming Peripherals
  - PC gaming utilizes a mouse and keyboard
  - Console-based games use a console and controller
  - Mobile games use a smartphone, tablet, or handheld gaming device
  - "Keybinds" refers to specific button mapping on the keyboard or controller that coordinates with in-game movements. For example, the letters "WASD" on the keyboard typically involves moving the character forward, left, back, and right, respectively
  - Keybinds may place undue stress on specific digits, especially the 5th digit, and vary significantly between individuals due to personal preference (Fig. 102.1).
  - There are three typical grips used with gaming mice (1).
    - Palm: The palm is in contact with the proximal mouse and fingertips are in full contact with the distal mouse
    - Claw: Metacarpophalangeal flexion coupled with wrist extension puts less of the palm in contact with the mouse and uses only the distal phalanges
    - Tip: The palm is completely lifted from the mouse, with only the distal tips of the fingers being used
  - The anatomy of a gamepad controller varies by brand; however, the dual analog stick is the most popular configuration. These are controlled by the thumbs and typically function in movement control (Fig. 102.2).
  - "The Claw" is also a term for a style of grip used with a controller. This grip involves the index finger abducted and maximally flexed at the PIP and DIP while keeping the thumbs on the analog stick (Fig. 102.3).
- Inconsistency in sport science understanding
  - Unlike traditional sports, which involves a gradual introduction to coaching staff, support services, and medical professionals as a player progresses from intramural sports to professional over multiple years, esports does not have a defined "path to professional."
  - Understanding and acceptance of fitness, nutrition, prevention, and rehabilitation is inconsistent.

MEDICAL ISSUES

Altered Body Mass Composition

- When compared to non-esports players, collegiate esports players have a higher body-fat percentage, lower lean body

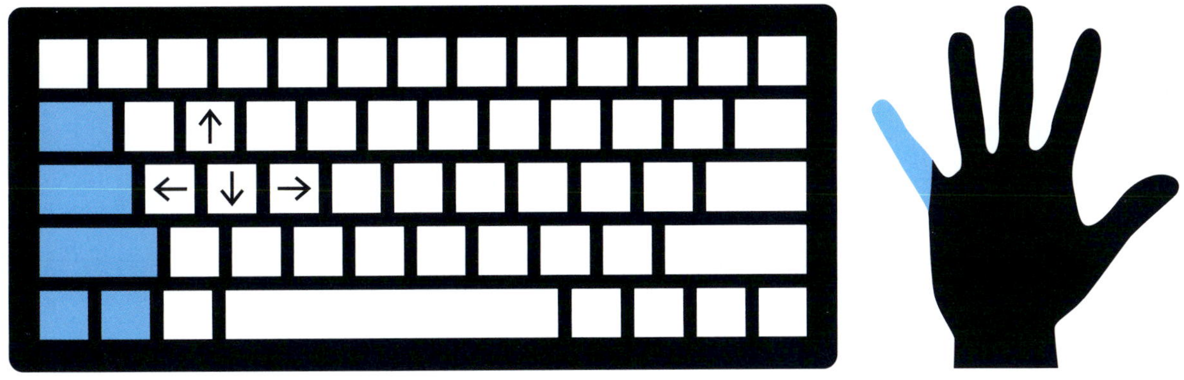

Figure 102.1: WASD Keybind showing undue stress on the 5th digit. (*Source:* Migliore L, McGee C, Moore MN. *Handbook of Esports Medicine*. Springer Nature; 2021. Fig. 2.3.)

mass (LBM) and lower bone mineral content, whereas body mass index (BMI) was comparable (2).

Sedentary Lifestyle

- Prolonged sitting has been associated with a higher risk of mortality (3).
- Gamers meet physical activity guidelines less as compared to nongaming peers.
- The promotion of physical activity is paramount in this population, and as little as a 6-minute walk breaking up prolonged gaming sessions has been linked to improved gaming performance (4).

Deep Vein Thrombosis

- Also called Gaming Thrombosis or Gamer's Thrombosis.
- Results from long gameplay sessions with periods of prolonged immobility put the gaming population at elevated risk.
- Modifiable risk factors include cigarette use, being overweight, birth control use, and prolonged immobility (5).
- Preventive measures include regular breaks in game play, frequent movement, and for elevated risk individuals, the use of compression socks.

Sleep Dysfunction

- Early research suggests esports athletes have decreased total sleep time, poorer quality of sleep, and a higher incidence of insomnia.
- Causes of sleep dysfunction may be attributed to increased stress levels, blue light, competition travel, and extended practice hours.
- Some of the key benefits of sleep for the gaming population include:
    - decreased stress level
    - improved speed, accuracy, and reaction time
    - decreased risk of heart disease and stroke
    - improved concentration, memory, and problem-solving

Nutrition

- The diet of gamers typically includes fewer fruits and vegetables and higher amounts of sweetened beverages.
- The esports ecosystem is fueled by unhealthy beverage sponsorship. Consumption of energy drinks has been linked to other unhealthy food choices, such as high-fat and high-sugar snacking (6).

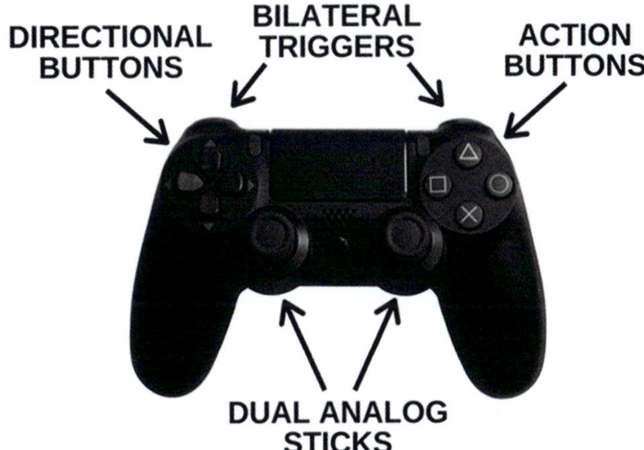

Figure 102.2: Anatomy of a dual analog stick controller. (*Source:* Migliore L, McGee C, Moore MN. *Handbook of Esports Medicine*. Springer Nature; 2021. Fig. 1.2.)

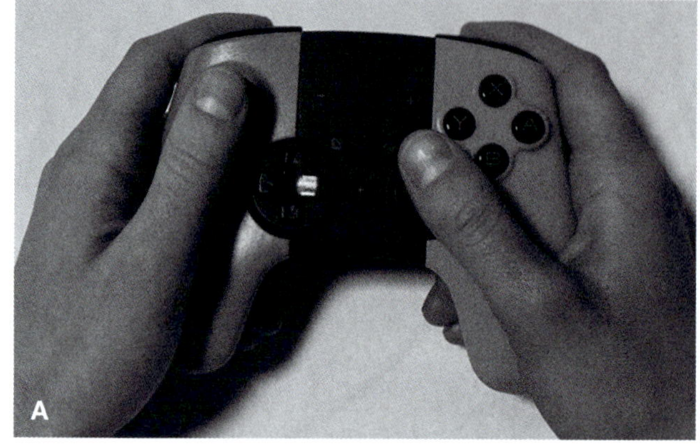

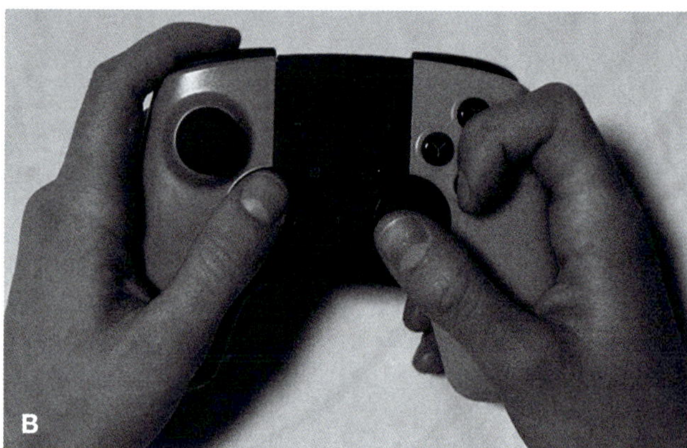

Figure 102.3: A demonstrates a traditional controller grip. B demonstrates "The Claw" grip. (*Source:* Migliore L, McGee C, Moore MN. *Handbook of Esports Medicine*. Springer Nature; 2021.)

- As with all athletes, proper nutrition should be encouraged among esport athletes.
  - Key nutrients that can improve eye health include: Omega-3 fatty acids; vitamins A, C, E; zinc; and lutein.
  - Key nutrients that can improve brain health include: Vitamins B, E, D; magnesium; and antioxidants

Nootropics

- Nootropics are a class of supplements believed to enhance cognitive function and include substances such as caffeine, L-theanine, creatine, *Rhodiola rosea*, and *Ginkgo biloba*.
- Nootropic usage by the esports population is not well understood but heavily marketed, with potential risks and side effects largely unknown.

Gaming Disorder

- Gaming disorder is a pattern of pervasive gaming characterized by impaired control over gaming, increasing priority given to gaming over other activities and interests, and continuation or escalation despite negative consequences that last for at least 12 months.

Doping

- Clean esports is a fairly new topic of interest for the gaming and anti-doping community.
- Unlike traditional sport, currently, there is not a regulatory body in esports to define a prohibited substance list, perform testing, or enforce consequences of doping.
- There is a well-known and widespread issue of amphetamine and stimulant abuse, more specifically, Adderall.
  - Other prominent substances of abuse are caffeine and marijuana.
- Anti-doping education, awareness, and research are paramount in this population.

Hearing Health

- Gamers tend to wear headphones for prolonged periods of time at high volume during gameplay.
- Over a billion young people worldwide could be at risk of hearing loss due to unsafe listening practices (7).
- Regulating exposure to loud sounds and implementation of safe listening practices can help prevent sound induced hearing loss.

Mental Health

- Gaming has traditionally been thought to have a deleterious impact on mental health with social isolation, depression, and loneliness. However, with the evolution of Esports Medicine and research, there is more focus on the mental health benefits of gaming, including increased socialization, improvement of cognitive skills, critical thinking, visuospatial skills, problem-solving, and increased attention.

- Professional and collegiate esports teams utilize Sports Psychologists and Esports Performance Coaches to focus on mental performance.

VISION ISSUES

Vision Health

- Vision health is a major concern in esports as athletes can play greater than 12–16 hours a day with extended screen time.
- Digital Eye Strain: A constellation of symptoms associated with extended screen use.
  - Commonly referred to as Computer Vision Syndrome.
  - Results from prolonged periods of staring at a screen without taking breaks.
  - Symptoms include dry, red, tired, sore and/or watery eyes; headaches; blurred or double vision; and neck, shoulder, or back pain (8).
- Dry Eye Syndrome: Reduced blink rate when focusing on screens, which leads to a decrease in tear production and causing the eyes to dry out.
  - This drying may lead to discomfort, itching, and possibly blurred vision.
  - Use of artificial tears or similar lubricating eye drops may help alleviate these symptoms.
- Myopia: Extended hours of screen time, especially at a close distance, can increase the risk of nearsightedness, especially in younger individuals (9).
- Asthenopia: Also known as eye strain, this includes symptoms such as tired eyes, itching, burning sensations, blurred vision, and headaches including mild retro-orbital headaches to migraines.
- Accommodative Spasm: This is a condition where the eye's focusing muscle, the ciliary muscle, goes into spasm after long periods of intense focus, causing blurred vision, especially at distance.
- Circadian Rhythm Disruption: Overexposure to screens, especially at night, can interfere with the body's sleep-wake cycle, potentially impacting eye health and overall wellness (10).
- Ocular Misalignment: Extended screen time can lead to eye misalignment, which can present as symptoms of double vision.

Strategies to Mitigate Vision Health Issues

- 20-20-20 Rule: Every 20 minutes, look at a stationary object 20 ft away for at least 20 seconds.
- Proper Screen Distance and Position: A good rule of thumb for distance would include the screen being slightly below or at eye level and approximately at an arm's length away.
- Adequate Lighting: Adjusting the lighting to reduce glare and reflections on the screen.
- Regular Eye Exams: Recommend regular check-ups to help detect any eye problems at an early stage, which can then be treated accordingly.
- Use of Eyewear: There are a variety of options to help reduce eye strain, from computer glasses for intermediate distance viewing, to prism glasses to reduce asthenopia, to blue-light blockers, which help filter out high-energy blue light from screens to help prevent circadian rhythm disruption.
  - More research is needed to confirm the effectiveness of these options, but preliminary results are promising.
- Maintaining a Healthy Lifestyle: Regular exercise, outdoor activities, a balanced diet, and adequate sleep can contribute to overall eye health.
- The Stanford Vision Performance Center has introduced the Vision Performance Index (VPI) as a measure to understand the effects of lifestyle factors on visual, mental, and physical performance. The VPI can be implemented in video games and has shown positive correlations in the amount of sleep and physical activity on overall performance (11,12) (Figs. 102.4 and 102.5).

MUSCULOSKELETAL ISSUES

Radial Styloid Tenosynovitis

- De Quervain tenosynovitis, gamer's thumb, selfie thumb
- Chronic overuse caused by stenosing tenosynovitis of the first dorsal compartment at the wrist containing the abductor pollicis longus (APL) and extensor pollicis brevis (EPB).
- Presents with nonspecific pain in the radial wrist that may radiate into the thumb or down the forearm.
- Symptoms are often aggravated by thumb or wrist movement, including rotatory and gripping movements, and when using a controller's analog stick. With advanced disease, patients may complain of weakness with grip. With most overuse injuries, the onset is often gradual, with no clearly defined inciting injury.
- Can be diagnosed on physical examination using Finkelstein test.
- Depending on severity of symptoms, treatment can involve activity modification (decreasing analog stick length), immobilization of the thumb, or corticosteroid injection (13).

Intersection Syndrome

- Due to repetitive wrist extension causing inflammation and aggravation of the first and second dorsal wrist compartments at their intersection point, where the APL and EPB cross over the extensor carpi radialis (ECRL) and brevis (ECRB).

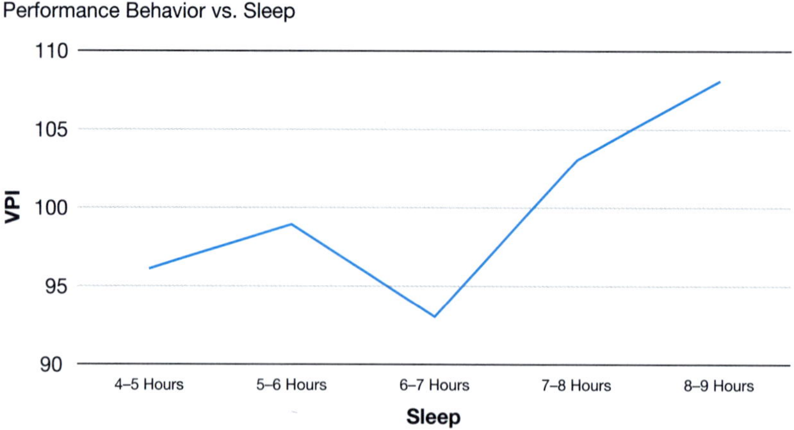

Figure 102.4: Vision Performance Index positive correlation of amount of sleep on overall performance. (Permission from Syed Khizer Rahim Khaderi.)

- Presents with dorsal wrist and forearm pain or "squeaking sound" around 4 cm proximal to Lister tubercle.
- Examination may reveal pinpoint tenderness or swelling over intersection point or crepitus with wrist or thumb extension.
- Can be misdiagnosed as radial styloid tenosynovitis.

Radial Sensory Neuritis

- Can occur in isolation or in conjunction with radial styloid tenosynovitis.
- Near the terminal end, the superficial branch of the radial nerve (RSN) courses close to the skin and is susceptible to compression.
- A purely sensory nerve, symptoms consist of radiating pain and paresthesias across the thumb and dorsoradial hand, and may be worsened with wrist flexion and ulnar deviation.
- Symptoms can be aggravated by superficial compression from watches, long sleeve shirts, or bracelets.

Extensor Carpi Ulnaris Tendonitis

- Part of the common extensor tendon, the extensor carpi ulnaris (ECU) passes through a fibrous sheath prior to inserting on the base of the 5th metacarpal.
- Repetitive wrist movements and non-neutral wrist positioning from keyboards and mice result in ulnar-sided wrist pain that is improved with "keyboard holidays," extended periods away from gaming.
- Can be difficult to distinguish from injury to the triangular fibrocartilage complex.
- Positive ECU Synergy test on physical examination.
- Treatment can involve adjusting the thickness and slope of the keyboard, splinting, and physical therapy.

Ulnar Neuropathy at the Elbow

- *Cubital tunnel syndrome*
- The ulnar nerve is the largest unprotected nerve in the human body and is susceptible to compression or trauma in the elbow.

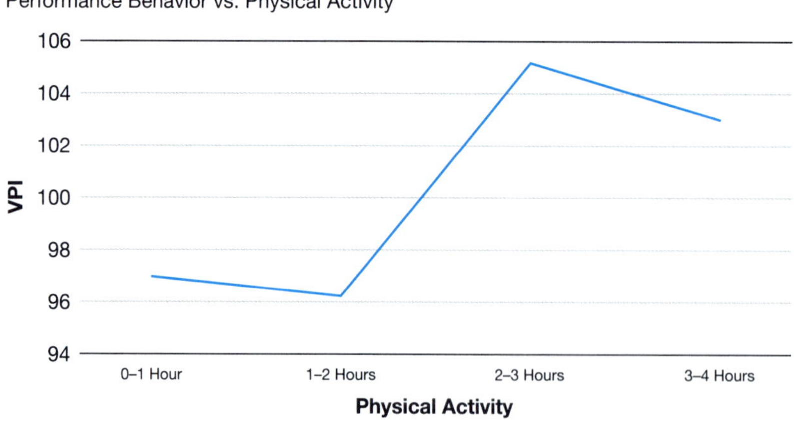

Figure 102.5: Vision Performance Index positive correlation of physical activity on overall performance. (Permission from Syed Khizer Rahim Khaderi.)

- Pressure from armrests and desks can cause compression as the nerve courses superficially between the medial epicondyle and olecranon.
- Sensory and motor symptoms distal to the source of the compression most commonly present with numbness and paresthesia that radiates from the medial forearm into the fourth and fifth digits.
- Untreated symptoms can result in weakness of the ulnar-innervated muscles.
- On physical examination, a positive Tinel test at the cubital tunnel or Froment sign indicates pathology. Electromyogram (EMG) and nerve conduction study (NCS) can confirm diagnosis.
- Treatment involves avoiding compression and excessive flexion, and surgical release may be necessary for refractory cases.

Lateral Epicondylitis

- The lateral epicondyle serves as the origin point for the common extensor tendons.
- Chronic tendinosis results from repetitive eccentric motions that include repeated gripping and wrist extension.
- The most common presenting symptom is pain in the lateral elbow exacerbated by wrist and elbow movements.
- Can be diagnosed on physical examination by Cozen tests.
- Treatment involves avoidance of aggravating movements, forearm counterforce strap, cock-up wrist splint, Occupational therapy and injection therapy for recalcitrant cases.

Proximal Hamstring Tendinopathy

- Prolonged sitting, excessive static stretching, and repetitive hamstring contraction with a flexed hip are most common causes.
- Bent-knee stretch test can aid in the diagnosis.
- Treatment involves physical therapy with progressive loading from isometric to isotonic, soft-tissue mobilization, ergonomic changes, and shaped cushions to offload the affected area.

Sacroiliac Joint Pathology

- Dysfunction is more commonly seen in the obese and sedentary population.
- Pain is localized to the posterior aspect of the joint, back pain that radiates down the posterior thigh that does not cross the knee.
- Clinical tests include: Gaenslen, Yeoman, FABER, and SI joint compression test.
- Treatment involves a multifactorial approach with physical therapy, joint mobilization, core stabilization, postural retraining, and ergonomic modifications.

Compressive Neuropathies of the Lower Extremity

- Seen more commonly in the gaming population.
- Understanding of gaming ergonomics, preferred postures, and type and size of the chair is integral.
  - Common Peroneal Nerve
    - Most common compressive neuropathy in the lower extremity
    - Symptoms include foot drop, numbness, and paresthesias over lateral lower leg and dorsum of the foot
    - Prolonged crossing of the leg or knee flexion can be a contributing factor
  - Sciatic Nerve
    - Can result from prolonged pressure or sitting
    - Symptoms present with numbness, paresthesias, and pain in the buttock and along the posterolateral leg

Postural Dysfunctions

- Forward Head Posture
  - A pattern of upper thoracic and lower cervical flexion coupled with upper cervical and occipital extension.
  - Commonly seen with sitting positions for console and mobile gaming.
  - Ergonomic assessment of the gaming setup should be performed.
- Excessive Postural Thoracic Kyphosis
  - A pattern of tight pectoralis major and minor, weakened/lengthened thoracic extensors and scapular retractors, decreased thoracic intervertebral mobility (14)
  - Due to sustained poor positioning
  - Postural retraining and strengthening are key areas of treatment.
- Upper Cross Syndrome
  - A pattern of tightness of the upper trapezius and levator scapula on the dorsal side crosses with tightness of the pectoralis major and minor. Weakness of the deep cervical flexors, ventrally, crosses with weakness of the middle and lower trapezius (15).
  - Posture includes forward head posture, increased cervical lordosis and thoracic kyphosis, elevated and protracted shoulders, and rotation or abduction and winging of the scapulae.
  - Functional movement and postural retraining can be beneficial for treatment.

EVENT COVERAGE

- The majority of esports injuries are chronic and due to overuse, therefore, on-site event coverage is rare.

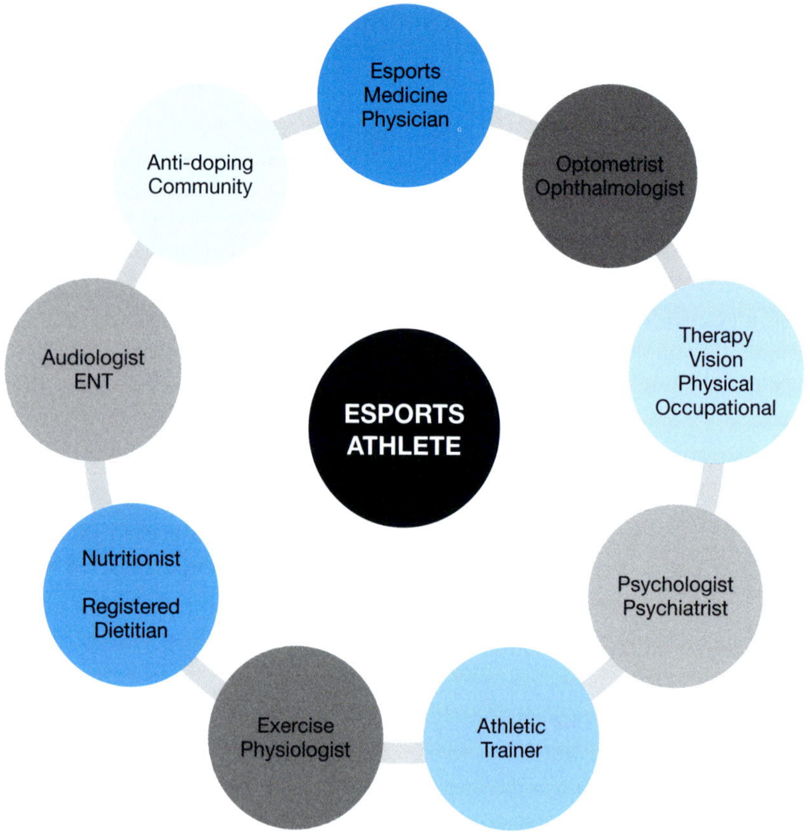

Figure 102.6: Multidisciplinary care of the esports athlete.

- Competitive esports typically is played with teams, leagues, and individual competitions.
  - Professional and collegiate teams compete against each other throughout a season.
  - For non–team-based titles, individuals compete in tournaments.
    - Leagues and tournaments can be regional or international.
- Esports Medicine is in its infancy and most professional and collegiate teams do not have a sports medicine physician, athletic trainer, or physical therapist.
- As esports continues to evolve and gaming becomes more popular, the demand for healthcare providers to be educated about the unique injuries and concerns of gamers is paramount.
- A multidisciplinary team approach is required to meet the needs of esports athletes overall health and wellness (Fig. 102.6).

REFERENCES

1. Migliore L, McGee C, Moore MN. *Handbook of Esports Medicine.* Springer Nature; 2021.
2. DiFrancisco-Donoghue J, Werner WG, Douris PC, Zwibel H. Esports players, got muscle? Competitive video game players' physical activity, body fat, bone mineral content, and muscle mass in comparison to matched controls. *J Sport Health Sci.* 2022;11(6):725–30. doi:10.1016/j.jshs.2020.07.006
3. Young DR, Hivert MF, Alhassan S; Physical Activity Committee of the Council on Lifestyle and Cardiometabolic Health; Council on Clinical Cardiology; Council on Epidemiology and Prevention; Council on Functional Genomics and Translational Biology; and Stroke Council, et al. Sedentary behavior and cardiovascular morbidity and mortality: a science advisory from the American heart association. *Circulation.* 2016;134(13):e262-79. doi:10.1161/CIR.0000000000000440
4. DiFrancisco-Donoghue J, Jenny SE, Douris PC. Breaking up prolonged sitting with a 6 min walk improves executive function in women and men esports players: a randomised trial. *BMJ Open Sport Exercise Medicine.* 2021;7:e001118. doi:10.1136/bmjsem-2021-001118
5. Rambaran KA, Alzghari SK. Gamer's thrombosis: a review of published reports. *Ochsner J.* 2020;20(2):182–6. doi:10.31486/toj.19.0058
6. Bragg MA, Roberto CA, Harris JL, Brownell KD, Elbel B. Marketing food and beverages to youth through sports. *J Adolesc Health.* 2018;62(1):5–13. doi:10.1016/j.jadohealth.2017.06.016
7. Recommendation ITU-T H.870. *Guidelines for Safe Listening Devices/systems*; 2022.
8. Bali J, Neeraj N, Bali RT. Computer vision syndrome: a review. *J Clin Ophthalmol Res.* 2014 Jan–April;2(1):61–8. doi:10.4103/2320-3897.122661
9. Zhu Z, Chen Y, Tan Z, Xiong R, McGuinness MB, Müller A. Interventions recommended for myopia prevention and control among

children and adolescents in China: a systematic review. *Br J Ophthalmol.* 2023;107(2):160–6.

10. Rossoni A, Vecchiato M, Brugin E, et al. The eSports medicine: pre-participation screening and injuries management — an update. *Sports.* 2023;11(2):34. doi:10.3390/sports11020034
11. Ahmed SF, McDermott KC, Burge WK, et al. Visual function, digital behavior and the vision performance index. *Clin Ophthalmol.* 2018;12:2553–61. doi:10.2147/OPTH.S187131
12. Ahmed Y, Reddy M, Mederos J, et al. Democratizing healthcare in the Metaverse. How video games can monitor eye conditions using the Vision Performance Index: a pilot study. *Ophthalmol Sci.* 2024;4(1):100349. doi:10.1016/j.xops.2023.100349
13. Ashraf MO, Devadoss VG. Systematic review and meta-analysis on steroid injection therapy for de Quervain's tenosynovitis in adults. *Eur J Orthop Surg Traumatol.* 2014;24(2):149–57. doi:10.1007/s00590-012-1164-z
14. Sahrmann S, Azevedo DC, Dillen LV. Diagnosis and treatment of movement system impairment syndromes. *Braz J Phys Ther.* 2017 Nov-Dec;21(6):391–9. doi:10.1016/j.bjpt.2017.08.001
15. Physiopedia contributors. Upper-crossed syndrome. *Physiopedia.* 2022 April 1. http:///index.php?title=Upper-Crossed_Syndrome&oldid=299512

103 Equestrian Sports

Kelly Ryan and Jason Pothast

INTRODUCTION/BACKGROUND

- Equestrian sports are immensely popular globally and can attract large television audiences of millions of people for major events such as the Olympics, Melbourne Cup, and Kentucky Derby.
- Equestrian sports can be split into two main and different categories:
  - Eventing — Olympic sport consisting of three disciplines
    - Dressage — Execution of precise movements by a trained horse in a show arena
    - Cross-country — Navigating a long course with varied obstacles and terrain
    - Show jumping — Clearing a course of fences within an arena
  - Horse racing:
    - Flat — Racing on turf, dirt, or synthetic surfaces at lengths usually between 4 furlongs (1 furlong = 1/8 of a mile) and 2 miles
    - Steeplechase — Racing in open fields and navigating obstacles on a predetermined course of usually 2–6 miles and requires horses to jump over either hurdles (3.5 ft high) or steeplechase fences (4.5 ft high)
- The focus of this chapter is on racing and jockeys that compete in flat and steeplechase, though many of the overuse and acute injuries seen in jockeys are seen in other equestrian athletes and are evaluated and managed in a similar manner.
- Flat racing generally takes place over a 12-month season, whereas steeplechase racing tends to be limited to winter or spring months when the ground is softer.
- Professional jockeys can generally start race riding at the age of 16 and are usually referred to as "apprentice jockeys" at the beginning of their careers.
- Steeplechase jockeys retire around the age of 40, but flat jockeys can continue past 50 years of age.
- Male and female jockeys compete on equal terms. The male:female jockey ratio tends to be closer to 50:50 in amateur racing, though there is a higher proportion of male jockeys in professional racing.

EPIDEMIOLOGY

- Concussion rates in horseracing are the highest in the recorded literature when compared to other sports (1).
- Flat jockeys fall approximately once every 250 rides.
  - 0.41% of rides result in a fall and 40% of falls result in an injury (2).
  - Concussion rates among flat jockeys have been described to be as high at 17.1/1000 participant hours (2).
- Steeplechase jockeys fall approximately once every 16 rides.
  - 6.1% of rides result in a fall and 17% of falls result in an injury.
  - Concussion rates among steeplechase jockeys have been described to be as high as 25/1000 participant hours (2).
- Fatality rates among jockeys are on the order 460–900/100 million rides.
  - This is comparable to many so-called extreme sports.
  - Comparable fatality rates/100 million participant days in other sports are as follows: >780 for mountaineering, > for 640 air sports (skydiving, etc.), 146 for motor sports, 67.5 for water sports, 15.7 for rugby union, and 3.8 for football (soccer) (3).
- In addition to the trauma caused by falls, the horse can inflict injuries by biting, pulling, kicking, standing, or rolling on the jockey, as well as hitting the rider in the face with a sudden movement of the head (4).

SPECIFIC ISSUES

- Horses weigh 1000–1200 lbs (450–550 kg) and horse can achieve speeds of up to 40 miles $\cdot$ h^{-1} (32–64 km $\cdot$ h^{-1}) (5).
- When riding, the equestrian/jockey's head is approximately 8–9 ft off the ground (6).
- While there is no weight restriction for the eventing disciplines, flat and steeplechase jockeys adhere to riding weights that vary depending on type of racing.
  - Steeplechase jockeys will typically weigh about 135–140 lbs.
  - Flat jockeys typically weigh between 112 and 119 lbs.

- All equestrians should wear helmets when riding. Professional jockeys are required to wear both helmets and safety vests.
  - Helmets are designed to attenuate energy on impact by deformation of the helmet and in particular the inner lining, which is usually constructed from expanded polystyrene foam.
  - To date, no helmet has been proven to prevent concussion, but as in other sports, their use may prevent skull fracture and severe traumatic brain injury (TBI). Research is ongoing to develop a tangential impact test with a view to reducing concussions.
  - Current helmet standards must comply with minimum safety standards, such as American Society for Testing and Materials (ASTM 1163) (7).
  - Safety vests are purely designed to reduce chest wall injuries (*i.e.*, rib fractures) and are not capable of preventing spinal injuries.
    - Lightweight vests (level 1) are licensed for use during race riding only with several European countries (Ireland, the United Kingdom, France, and Germany) requiring level 2 vests. Heavier vests (levels 2 and 3) are required while riding out/barrier trials/breeze ups, etc. (3).
    - Current safety vest standards must comply with the minimum safety standards, such as American Society for Testing and Materials (F1781-08 or F1937).
- There are currently no equestrian goggle standards, but high-impact plastic or polycarbonate lenses are recommended to reduce the risk of shattering and resultant eye injury.

MEDICAL ISSUES

- During races, the jockey is positioned over the horse in a crouched forward stance, in a state of continuous quasi-isometric movement — an activity that is extremely physically demanding (8) and requires significant enduring strength with their gluteal muscles, hamstrings, and quadriceps to provide stabilization.
- Jockeys require excellent strength and cardiovascular fitness.
  - Flat racing jockeys' heart rates can reach peaks of 190 beats · min^{-1} (9).
- Concussion:
  - After any fall, consider the use of clinical decision rules (such as the Canadian Head CT Rule or New Orleans Head CT Rule (10,11)) as jockeys will likely fall from a height greater than 6 ft off the ground, going anywhere from a still position to 40 miles · h^{-1}.
  - Concussion management is described in depth in Chapters 40 and 48 of this text, and basics principles of head injury management apply. However, there are some return criteria specific to equestrians that will be discussed here (12).
    - The athlete should not be allowed back on a horse until asymptomatic and back to their neurologic baseline.
  - "Return to ride" protocol can include the following steps:
    - Stage 1 — No sporting activity is allowed, but cognitive rest with symptom-limited light physical activity is permitted
    - Stage 2 — Light aerobic exercise, grooming, and feeding horses
    - Stage 3 — Equine-specific exercises, such as jumping jacks, squats, box jumps, and short trials on the Equicizer
    - Stage 4 — Noncontact riding on Equicizer, a mechanical/simulated horse used by riders to work on strength, form, and endurance without the threat of falling of a real animal
    - Stage 5 — Reintroduction to horse — no faster than light galloping
    - Stage 6 — Return to all competition
- Weight management (13–18):
  - Professional racing requires jockeys to meet weight requirements.
  - Depending on natural body weight and size of the jockey, they may have to "cut weight" on race days, which can include fasting, induced vomiting, calorie restriction, or dehydration through the use of saunas and sweatsuits.
  - Unlike other "weight-making sports," jockeys are not able to rehydrate as they get "weighed out" after winning a race, so they must maintain their weight the entire day while riding.
  - Large number of jockeys fail to reach daily requirements of micronutrients and carbohydrates.
  - As racing occurs year round, jockeys may have chronic caloric deficits, which can compromise muscle and liver glycogen stores.
  - Relative Energy Deficiency in Sports can be commonplace, more so in males due to the fact many female jockeys are generally lighter and do not need to participate in caloric restriction as often as their male counterparts.
  - Year-round energy availability mismatch can lead to a variety of physiological adaptations (13,19,20).
    - Reduced testosterone in males
    - Depression/irritability
    - Altered immune system
    - Decreased bone density
    - Severe and prolonged deficits may lead to impaired judgment, decreased coordination, and decreased performance
- Bone health (12,21–24):
  - Racing jockeys often have lower bone density and elevated rates of bone loss.

- Male jockeys tend to have lower bone density than female counterparts when compared to sex-matched controls.
- Low bone mass is highly concerning in a sport with high rates of traumatic falls from heights and high speeds.
- Consider calcium and vitamin D supplementation.

- Mental health (19,25):
  - High performance pressure
  - Injury may lead to greater risk of depression due to physical pain, loss of income, and missed opportunities to participate in high-profile contests.
  - Some jockeys accumulate multiple traumatic injuries throughout their career, which has led some to drug and alcohol abuse.
  - Often chronically undernourished, which can also affect mental health
  - Jockeys often have dysfunctional schedules affecting their ability to sleep.
    - Frequent travel from track to track in order to ride on back-to-back days may leave jockeys with disrupted or dysfunctional sleep schedules.

MUSCULOSKELETAL ISSUES (2,12,26–28)

- Very few overuse injuries. Jockeys are well trained to be on a horse for a short period of time. However, overuse injuries can occur with their regular nonequestrian training such as cycling, weight lifting, running, etc.
- Most injuries are caused by falls and can differ depending on fast flat racing versus steeplechase racing.
- Falls are often categorized by cause:
  - Being thrown from horse
  - Horse reared/spooked
  - Horse breakdown/injury to the animal
  - Jockey error
  - Involvement in another accident
  - Bad behavior by the horse
- Most frequent injuries:
  - Soft-tissue injuries
  - Fractures — 10%–18%
  - Dislocations — 1%–4%
  - Concussions 4%–8% in professional racing (18% in amateur racing)
- Common injuries:
  - Head/neck — Concussion, cervical strains, cervical spine fracture, and spinal cord injury
  - Upper limb — Fractured clavicle, shoulder dislocations, acromioclavicular and sternoclavicular joint issues, and wrist fractures/sprains
  - Torso/back — Thoracic fractures, organ lacerations, and spinal cord injury
  - Hip pelvis — Pelvic fractures and hip fractures
  - Lower limb — Tibia/fibula fractures, ankle dislocations, and foot fractures
- Career-ending injuries:
  - In Great Britain, from 1991 to 2005, there were approximately 1,113,500 rides, 32,445 falls, and 555 injuries. Of these injuries, 45 (8.1%) were career ending (including 4 fatalities).
- Type of injuries: 24.3% torso/pelvis, 22.1% upper limb, 20% head, 17.7% lower limb, and 13.3% neck and spinal cord. Figure 103.1
- shows injury rates (27).
- Locations where injuries occur on the racetrack:
  - Approximately 30%–40% of injuries occur in and around the starting gate.
  - Another 35% of injuries occur in the final turn, homestretch, finish line, and gallop out. Figure 103.2 shows injury incidence based on track location (27).

EVENT COVERAGE

- All jockeys are required to have a preparticipation physical exam.
  - Baseline concussion evaluation may be required and should be considered for all equestrian athletes given the risk of injury.
- In almost all countries, a minimum of two ambulances follow the riders. In many countries, it is standard to have two physicians on track as well.
  - However, in some countries such as New Zealand and Japan, only paramedics work on track.
  - In United States, it is recommended there is a medical director at all tracks; however, actual race-day coverage is highly variable with each state having their own requirements for race-day coverage. Thus, the number and type of emergency medical services that are available may vary as well.
- Diagnostic equipment on track varies from the very basic to full scope medical facilities, many including diagnostic x-ray facilities.
- Injuries are common and medical staff providing coverage at racing events must be prepared to deal with fractures, dislocations, concussion, head injuries, and acute spinal trauma.
- All medical staff must be suitably trained in prehospital care and have the appropriate equipment on site to manage the anticipated trauma.

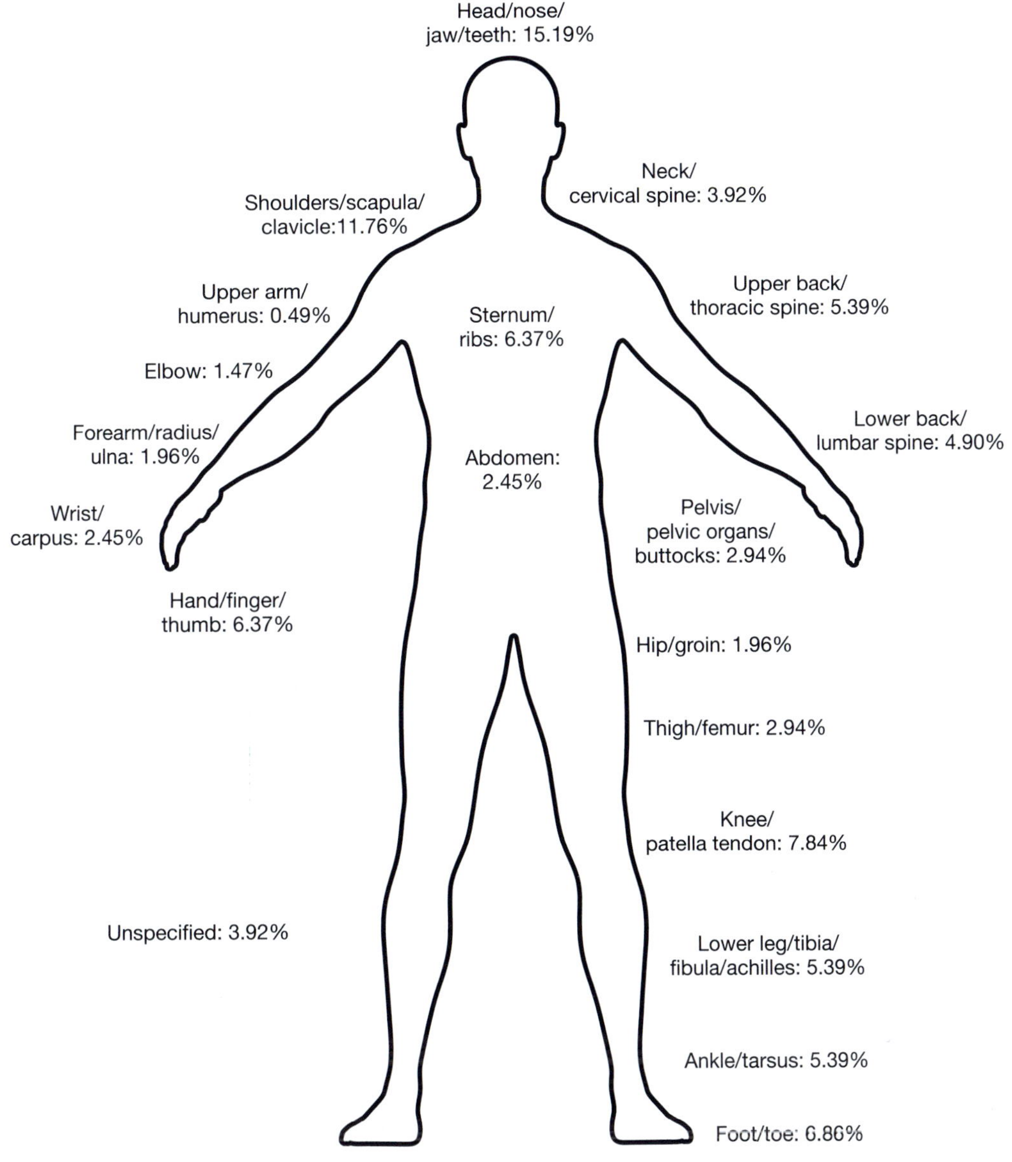

Figure 103.1: Injury rates in flat track racing by body part/region. (*Source:* Ryan K, Garruppo G, Alexander K, Hluchan CM, Lincoln AE. Injuries among Maryland jockeys during thoroughbred racing: 2015-2019. *BMJ Open Sports Exerc Med.* 2020;6(1):e000926.)

- This should include access to a rapid method of transportation for critically injured jockeys (*e.g.*, a fully equipped advanced life support ambulance/air ambulance).

- Ensure medical staff are familiar with locations of local trauma centers and hospitals.
- When covering races, the physician can usually stand by at the starting gate or near the finish line, which statistically is where most injuries will occur.
- All medical staff must have suitable medical malpractice insurance if they wish to provide medical support on a racecourse.
- Jockeys are typically covered by workman's compensation insurance, and in cases of injury, the physician will have to be familiar with local laws and rules in order to provide the best and most timely care to the athlete.

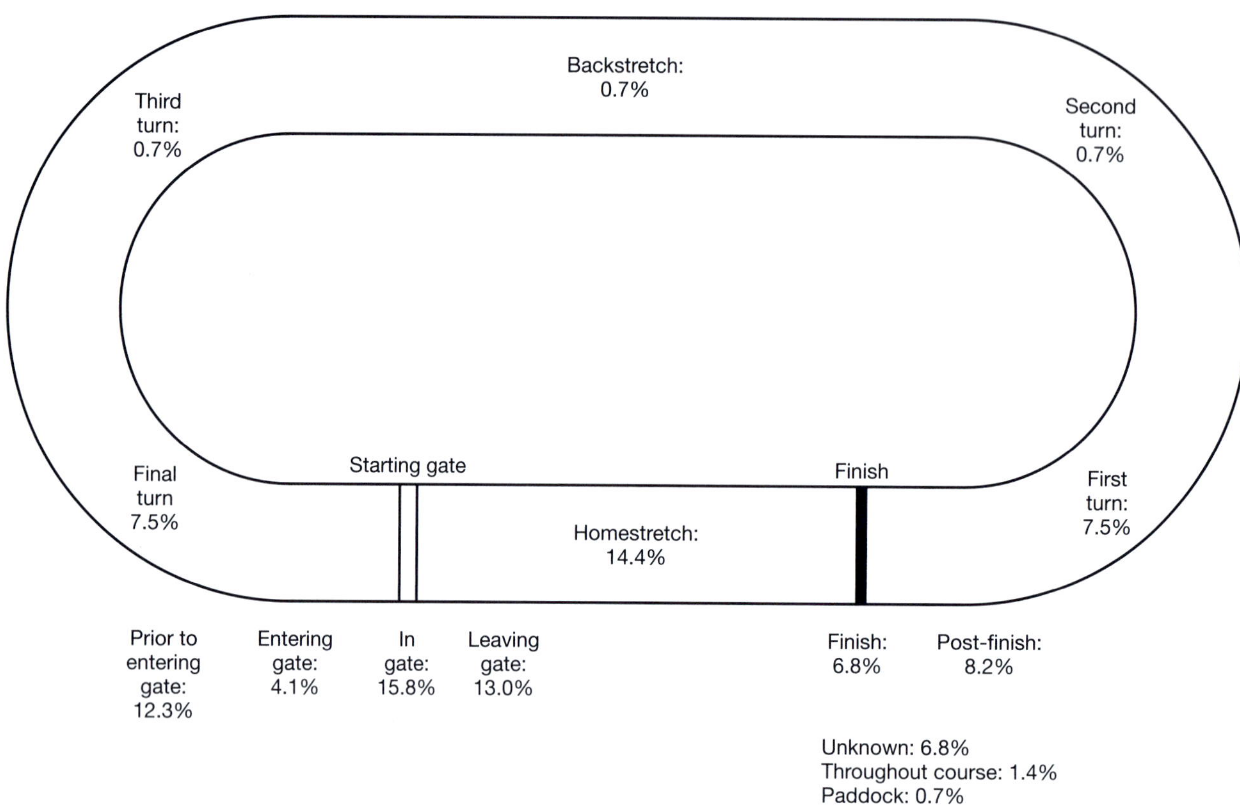

Figure 103.2: Injury rates in flat track jockey based on location of fall/trauma. (*Source:* Ryan K, Garruppo G, Alexander K, Hluchan CM, Lincoln AE. Injuries among Maryland jockeys during thoroughbred racing: 2015–2019. *BMJ Open Sports Exerc Med.* 2020;6(1):e000926.)

REFERENCES

1. Winkler EA, Yue JK, Burke JF, et al. Adult sports-related traumatic brain injury in United States trauma centers. *Neurosurg Focus.* 2016;40(4):E4.
2. O'Connor S, Warrington G, McGoldrick A, Cullen S. Epidemiology of injury due to race-day jockey falls in professional flat and jump horse racing in Ireland, 2011-2015. *J Athl Train.* 2017 Dec;52(12):1140–6. doi:10.4085/1062-6050-52.12.17
3. Madden C, Putukian M, McCarty E, Young C. *Netter's Sports Medicine, E-Book.* Elsevier; 2021.
4. Turner M, McCrory P, Halley W. Injuries in professional horse racing in Great Britain and the Republic of Ireland during 1992-2000. *Br J Sports Med.* 2002 Dec;36(6):403–9. doi:10.1136/bjsm.36.6.403
5. Connor TA, Clark JM, Jayamohan J, et al. Do equestrian helmets prevent concussion? A retrospective analysis of head injuries and helmet damage from real-world equestrian accidents. *Sports Med Open.* 2019 May 24;5(1):19.
6. Havlik HS. Equestrian sport-related injuries: a review of current literature. *Curr Sports Med Rep.* 2010 Sep;9(5):299–302.
7. Gates JK, Lin CY. Head and spinal injuries in equestrian sports: update on epidemiology, clinical outcomes, and injury prevention. *Curr Sports Med Rep.* 2020 Jan;19(1):17–23.
8. Cullen S, O'Loughlin G, McGoldrick A, Smyth B, May G, Warrington GD. Physiological demands of flat horse racing jockeys. *J Strength Cond Res.* 2015 Nov;29(11):3060–6.
9. O'Reilly J, Cheng HL, Poon ETC. New insights in professional horse racing; "in-race" heart rate data, elevated fracture risk, hydration, nutritional and lifestyle analysis of elite professional jockeys. *J Sports Sci.* 2017;35(5):441–8.
10. Stiell IG, Wells GA, Vandemheen K, et al. The Canadian CT Head Rule for patients with minor head injury. *Lancet.* 2001 May 5;357(9266):1391–6.
11. Haydel MJ, Preston CA, Mills TJ, Luber S, Blaudeau E, DeBlieux PM. Indications for computed tomography in patients with minor head injury. *N Engl J Med.* 2000 Jul 13;343(2):100–5.
12. Ryan KD, Brodine J, Pothast J, McGoldrick A. Medicine in the sport of horse racing. *Curr Sports Med Rep.* 2020;19(9):373–9.
13. Ryan K, Brodine J. Weight-making practices among jockeys: an update and review of the emergent scientific literature. *Open Access J Sports Med.* 2021;12:87–98.
14. Dolan E, O'Connor H, McGoldrick A, O'Loughlin G, Lyons D, Warrington G. Nutritional, lifestyle, and weight control practices of professional jockeys. *J Sports Sci.* 2011 May;29(8):791–9.
15. Wilson G, Drust B, Morton JP, Close GL. Weight-making strategies in professional jockeys: implications for physical and mental health and well-being. *Sports Med.* 2014;44(6):785–96.
16. Statuta SM, Asif IM, Drezner JA. Relative energy deficiency in sport (RED-S). *Br J Sports Med.* 2017;51(21):1570–1.
17. von Hippel PT, Rutherford CG, Keyes KM. Gender and weight among thoroughbred jockeys: underrepresented women and underweight men. *Socius.* 2017;3. doi:10.1177/2378023117712599

18. Dolan E, McGoldrick A, Davenport C, et al. An altered hormonal profile and elevated rate of bone loss are associated with low bone mass in professional horse-racing jockeys. *J Bone Miner Metab.* 2012 Sep;30(5):534–542.
19. Losty C, Warrington G, McGoldrick A, et al. Mental health and wellbeing of jockeys. *J Human Sport Exerc.* 2019;14:147–58.
20. Wilson G, Hill J, Sale C, Morton JP, Close GL. Elite male flat jockeys display lower bone density and lower resting metabolic rate than their female counterparts: implications for athlete welfare. *Appl Physiol Nutr Metab.* 2015;40(12):1318–20.
21. Poon ET, O'Reilly J, Sheridan S, Cai MM, Wong SHS. Markers of bone health, bone-specific physical activities, nutritional intake, and quality of life of professional jockeys in Hong Kong. *Int J Sport Nutr Exerc Metab.* 2018;28(4):440–6.
22. Waldron-Lynch F, Murray BF, Brady JJ, et al. High bone turnover in Irish professional jockeys. *Osteoporos Int.* 2010;21(3):521–5.
23. Dolan E, Crabtree N, McGoldrick A, et al. Weight regulation and bone mass: a comparison between professional jockeys, elite amateur boxers, and age, gender and BMI matched controls. *J Bone Miner Metab.* 2012;20:164–70.
24. Silk LN, Greene DA, Baker MK, Jander CB. The effect of calcium and vitamin D supplementation on bone health of male jockeys. *J Sci Med Sport.* 2017;20(3):225–9.
25. Mackinnon AL, Jackson K, Kuznik K, et al. Increased risk of musculoskeletal disorders and mental health problems in retired professional jockeys: a cross-sectional study. *Int J Sports Med.* 2019;40(14):e5–8.
26. Hitchens PL, Hill AE, Stover SM. Jockey falls, injuries, and fatalities associated with thoroughbred and quarter horse racing in California, 2007-2011. *Orthop J Sports Med.* 2013;1(1):2325967113492625.
27. Ryan K, Garruppo G, Alexander K, Hluchan CM, Lincoln AE. Injuries among Maryland jockeys during thoroughbred racing: 2015-2019. *BMJ Open Sport Exerc Med.* 2020;6(1):e000926.
28. Balendra G, Turner M, McCrory P. Career-ending injuries to professional jockeys in British horse racing (1991-2005). *Br J Sports Med.* 2008 Jan;42(1):22–4. doi:10.1136/bjsm.2007.038950

104 Ice Skating-Figure Skating, Speed Skating

Roger Kruse, Gretchen Mohney, and Peter Gerbino

INTRODUCTION

- Ice Skating is a broad category of sports that can be divided into: speed skating and figure skating, as well as being a significant part of a number of other on ice sports such as ice hockey (discussed in Chapter 108) among others.
- The earliest sharpened steel blades with edges were developed by the Dutch in the 13th or 14th century and were used for both transportation as well as recreation (1).
- Figure Skating is the oldest sport within the Olympic Games (2) and U.S. Figure Skating is the national governing body for the sport, as recognized by the U.S. Olympic and Paralympic Committee (USOPC) and International Skating Union (ISU).
- In 2022, there were approximately 223,000 members, 800 full members, collegiate, and school-affiliated clubs.
  - Females comprise 72% and males comprise 25% of the total membership (3).
- U.S. Speed Skating is also part of USOPC and ISU.
  - U.S. Speed Skating has won 84 Olympic medals, more than any other winter sport (4).

SPEED SKATING

- Long track: typically simply referred to as "speed skating" involves athletes racing around a 400 m circuit.
- Short track speed skating, sometimes called simply "short track," is contested on a 111 m oval, often in a hockey rink.
- During individual competitions, only two competitors are on the ice at a time and there are no "heats" or "finals" as in many other racing sports. Instead the competitors are ranked based on time.
- Short track speed skating, sometimes called simply "short track," is contested on a 111 m oval, often in a hockey rink.
- Distances in Olympic competition include 500, 1000, 1500, 3000 m (women), 5000 m, and 10,000 m (men).
- Team Pursuit and Mass Start events also occur in which several athletes are competing simultaneously. This increases the risk of collision and injury and most organizations require helmets, full body cut-resistant suit, cut-resistant gloves, and eye protection.

FIGURE SKATING DISCIPLINES

- *Singles skaters'* complete multi-revolution jumps and spins, spiral sequences, moves, and footwork.
- Pairs skaters skate as a traditional couple, performing synchronous multi-revolution jumps, spins, and incorporate numerous high-risk maneuvers such as throw jumps, overhead lifts.
- Ice dancers skate as a traditional couple, perform intricate deep-edged footwork, varied dance holds, spins, unique acrobatic lifts, and are based on the artistic interpretation of the music. The rules restrict height of overhead lifts and jumps of more than 1 revolution (3).
- Synchronized skating is a technical form of team skating characterized by speed, accuracy, intricate formations, and transitions. Elements may include partner lifts and synchronized spins. Teams may have 12 to 20 athletes who perform side-by-side, most often as 16 skaters (5).

FIGURE SKATING COMPETITION

- The competitive levels are based on the proficiency of skating skills tests, which progress from juvenile, intermediate, novice, junior, and senior.
  - At the junior and senior levels, women's singles, men's singles, pairs, ice dance, and synchronized skating may all qualify and compete at the international level.
- The Olympic Games includes women's singles, men's singles, pairs, ice dance, and a combined discipline team event with one competitor representing each discipline.
  - Synchronized skating continues to bid for inclusion in the Olympic Games (2,5).
- Competitors perform the *short* program, 2 minutes and 40 seconds in length, and the *long program*, 4 minutes, that are combined to determine final standings (3,5).

- Competitors are scored by a judging panel and awarded points for the technical evaluation of program elements, skating skill, and presentation (3,5).
- Historically, competition level is dictated by ability/test level and not age, although competitors must be at least 15 years of age by July 1 for the following 2022/2023 season, with an increase to 16 years of age for the 2023/2024 season, and an increase to 17 years for the season 2024/2025 and subsequent seasons (6).

EQUIPMENT

- Competitive figure skaters purchase boots and blades separate from one another that are selected according to discipline, skill level, boot stiffness, blade length, and pick type.
- The skate is fitted to conform around the foot and ankle, limiting subtalar joint movement. The ankle rests in a plantarflexed position due to the elevated heel and should have a padded tongue to alleviate friction on the anterior foot tendons. Ice dancers typically have an Achilles cut out increasing the available range of motion at the mortise joint.
- To improve the biomechanical advantage for multi-revolution jumps and to facilitate responsiveness to achieve the completion of increasingly complex elements, synthetic materials have replaced traditional leather boots.
    - Customizable heat moldable internal footbed options have become standard among competitive boot manufacturers over the past 10 years.
- Newest construction includes the utilization of 3D custom boot mapping and the integration of a custom carbon fiber boot shell and carbon fiber blades (7–10). Researchers continue to investigate force dampening technology in the boot and/or blade to influence impact force reduction (11–13).
- Speed skating boots are very different. Short track boots are low-cut with flexible ankles and have 16–18 in long, very sharp, fixed blades that are set at an angle to offset the extreme leaning to the left as the skaters race counterclockwise (14). Long track skaters can use either fixed-blade or clap skates, but all long track skaters now use clap skates.
- Clap skates are hinged at the toe so that the heel can rise while the blade remains longer in contact with the ice for greater speed. The blades are 38–45 cm long and about 1.25 mm thick. The edges are kept extremely sharp for maximum bite. The short leather boot is very stiff at the heel.

SKILL DEVELOPMENT

- To perform the increasingly difficult triple and quadruple jumps, the athletes are rotating faster, not necessarily jumping higher. Flight times for single, double, and triple jumps are very similar due to nearly identical vertical velocity at takeoffs (15). However, athletes who have mastered higher revolution jumps, such as triple and quadruple jumps, generate greater vertical velocity at takeoff of lower revolution jumps (16).
- To successfully complete a quadruple jump (quad), the skater must jump up to at least 24 inches in the air and spin faster than 5 revolutions per second. This has been estimated to require generating 150 foot-pounds of torque and 300 lb of force on take-off. The spinning generates 180 lb of centrifugal force, requiring that much force to hold the arms tight to the body. Landing requires transmitting torque and force through the ankle, knee, hip, and back. Peak landing forces from jumping have been measured as high as almost 10 times body weight (17).
- **Spinning** typically requires greater energy expenditure than jumping. The athlete rotates three to six revolutions per second, creating 200–300 lb of centrifugal force, and when the athlete changes position during the spin, these forces can go up. Upper body, lower body, and core strength are all required to keep the arms and legs close to the axis of rotation to counteract the centrifugal force.
- Performing the increasingly difficult throw twists, similar to triple and quadruple jumps, the pair teams use primarily increased rotational rates and, to a lesser degree, increased flight time due to delayed or lower catches (15,17). In pairs skating, the female partner can be thrown great distances by the male. This could result in even higher peak forces on landing.
- Short track skaters are skating very close together and reach speeds in excess of 50 km/h (31 mph) (14). Ideal biomechanics involve modifying skating position (18), mechanics (19), and other factors. Long track skaters can reach speeds of 59 km/h (37 mph) (20) and use similar techniques to improve mechanics, endurance, and speed.

TRAINING

- Figure skaters often begin rigorous training as early as 5 years of age, and some are performing jumps requiring two or three revolutions by the age of 8.
- Elite athletes can spend up to 45 hours a week dedicated to their sport: roughly 15–30 hours per week on the ice and 5–15 hours performing off-ice conditioning.
- Elite figure skaters commonly attend school online and sport specialize, however some balance their training by integrating dance training.

MEDICAL CONSIDERATIONS

Physical

- Most singles and pairs figure skaters are right-leg dominant, rotate counter-clockwise, and land on their right leg.

- The effort required for a long program in figure skating can be compared to running a 4-minute mile. The increasing complexity of the technical elements being performed in all disciplines of skating is comparative to the acrobatics of gymnastics and aerial arts.
- Athletes may interpret a requirement for leanness to increase their potential to achieve multi-revolution jumps and/or lightness for partner lifts, throws, and on-ice acrobatic skill challenges (21).
- Athletes may restrict caloric intake during maturation and/or training, which may contribute to the prevalence of RED-S, with or without ED (19,21).
- The most common dietary issues encountered are inadequate caloric intake and hydration, as well as suboptimal food choices and poor timing of nutrition (22,23).
- Intake of some micronutrients, including vitamin D, vitamin E, magnesium, potassium, folate, pantothenic acid, phosphorus, and calcium, in females was shown to be less than two-thirds of the recommended daily allowance (24).
- Prepubertal figure skaters' bone mineral density of the spine and lower extremities has been shown to be significantly higher than in nonskaters, suggesting that intense weight-bearing exercise may protect bone mass in younger athletes, despite inadequate nutritional intake (25).
- Later age of menarche is common among female figure skaters, particularly in elite pair skaters (26). Later onset of menarche and irregularities of menstrual cycle can be attributed to familial resemblance, as well as to a high level of training, which is associated with inadequate caloric intake with relation to activity level, consistent with RED-S (21,27).
- The incidence of exercise-induced bronchospasm (EIB) ranges from 35% to 50% in elite skaters in the United States (28,29).
- Relatively cold air temperatures in combination with exposure to carbon monoxide and nitrogen dioxide secondary to the Zamboni are the major triggers. EIB is treated the same way as talked about in Chapter 43.
- Vocal cord dysfunction is an important alternative consideration in the differential of EIB in figure skaters.

MUSCULOSKELETAL CONSIDERATIONS

- Acute injuries are most common in pairs skating and ice dancing, possibly due to lift-related injuries and risk for contact and collision with a partner.
- Overuse injuries are more common among singles skaters, who commonly focus on multi-revolution jump repetition and complex spin positioning.
- Lower extremity injuries are more common than upper extremity injuries, across all figure skating disciplines. Head injury is a growing area of research and includes concussions (30–34).

Lower Extremity

Foot

- *Bursitis* is the most common skating problem related to the foot and is caused by boot pressure points causing excessive compression and shear forces.
  - Both malleoli can be affected, although medial malleolar bursitis is more common. The fibula at the top of the boot and the area over the anterior tibialis tendon are also commonly affected.
  - Bursitis is generally well tolerated, but can easily become exacerbated with minor irritation or boot changes.
  - This is treated by operating on the boot, not the skater. Focal stretching/punching out of the boot in rub areas and/or padding placed to distribute compressive forces around the malleoli will typically alleviate the problem.
  - Aspiration and subsequent injection with cortisone and a compressive wrap are tempting, although *infrequently* indicated or beneficial. Surgery is *rarely* required.
- *Haglund deformity or a "pump bump" of the calcaneal tuberosity* is caused by a boot heel that is too wide for the skater's heel. This allows the skater's heel to slide up and down within the boot, resulting in callus and bursa inflammation.
  - For nearly all cases, the skate fit should be addressed. It is important that the heel of the boot be sufficiently narrow to prevent up and down motion of the heel. This can be done with padding medial and lateral to the Achilles tendon region, paying attention not to compress the structure. *Very small heel lifts may be beneficial.*
- *"Lace Bite" is very common in skaters. This is caused primarily by Tibialis anterior and extensor hallux tendinosis or tenosynovitis.* This happens from repetitive dorsiflexion and plantarflexion of the ankle, *excessive compression of crossing laces, and abnormal creasing* of the boot tongue across the anterior foot.
  - Crepitus over the tendon structures and nodules are a common clinical finding.
  - To prevent *anterior compression* injuries, the boot tongue should be in a neutral position or slightly medial, especially when the boots are being broken in. If the tongue is properly centralized, tibialis anterior tendonitis can still occur, but it can be prevented by padding the boot tongue.
- *Achilles tendinitis, partial tears, and nodules of the Achilles tendon* can occur from compression of the tendon from plantar flexion of the foot against the boot. They also can occur with overuse during off-ice training with running and jumping.
  - The Achilles tendon is generally protected by the height of the boot heel, although in some cases the posterior portion of the boot can cause irritation.
  - Boot modification may be helpful in this case.
  - Ice dancers often have boots with low-cut areas for the Achilles tendon to improve their line and their ability to bend their knees.

- *Plantar fasciitis is common in figure skaters because of the repetitive pounding.* It is treated in the usual manner with ice, relative rest, stretching, night splint, and physical therapy.
- *Stress Fractures* commonly occur in the metatarsals and tarsal navicular and are caused by the cumulative effect of jumping, repetitively training a new element, and just plain overuse. Working on foot strength is very important because a rigid boot often causes weakness.
  - Other areas that can be irritated include the base of the fifth metatarsal and the tarsal navicular.
- Corns and calluses are seen frequently. Typically, these issues occur as a result of boot fit. The calluses and corns need to be trimmed and modifying the boot should be considered (35).

Ankle

- *Ankle Sprains/poor ankle proprioception, inversion, and eversion strains are significant issues* among skaters due to the stiffness of the boot and the many hours skaters spend on ice. Over the last 10 years, there has been much more attention placed on optimizing foot and ankle strength in off-ice programs.
- *Lower Leg medial tibial syndrome, peroneal tendonitis, and/or fibular stress syndrome* often develop in figure skaters. These syndromes are typically attributed to the weakness of the tibialis posterior and peroneal muscles and the relative inflexibility of the gastroc-soleus complex. Treatment and prevention include optimizing flexibility of the gastroc-soleus complex, strengthening ankle inverters and evertors, and evaluation of the boot and the skater's position in the boot (35).

Knee

- *Anterior Knee Pain* is one of the most frequent problems and typically occurs in the landing leg. Etiologies are multiple and include relative hip weakness, quadriceps weakness, inadequate flexibility of the hip, thigh musculature, and patella issues. Skaters may also experience patella contusions from falling directly on the ice, but rarely experience patella fractures.
- *Patellar tendinosis and infrapatellar tendinosis are seen in skaters* and are very often difficult to treat because of the length of the competitive season. Activity modifications, strapping, and physical therapy with blood flow restriction are used. In addition, platelet rich plasma injections with ultrasound guidance and ultrasound-guided percutaneous needle tenotomy have recently produced great results.
- *Meniscus and ligament injuries* are relatively rare in figure skaters, likely due to the lack of fixation of the blade on the ice. However, with increasing technical demands and complexity of the pairs and ice dance element in particular, these injuries are increasing.

Core Injuries

- *Core injuries* (rectus abdominis-hip adductor strain), hip flexor, and external and internal oblique injuries continue to grow at an alarming rate. These types of injuries are some of the most common debilitating injuries sustained by figure skaters and often occur during rapid growth spurts and as a result of fatigue or suboptimal conditioning as new technical elements are introduced and lack of attention is paid to the complexities of periodized training. *Hip impingement* and *labral tears* are being seen more frequently.
- *Avulsion fractures* of the ischium, lesser tuberosity, and iliac crest have increasingly been reported. The young, underdeveloped athlete is asked to perform increasingly difficult, double, triple, and quadruple jumps. Proactive evaluation in an athlete for hip strength, flexibility, and endurance can be preventive.
- As the technical difficulty increases, so will injury rates. This is often attributed to the focus on triple and quadruple revolution jumps, increasing complex choreography, and dynamic footwork sequences.
  - The mechanics are multifaceted as the skaters perform greater than 45–60 practice jumps daily. They often have tight hip flexors and asymmetrically strong musculature in their hip stabilizers. In addition, many elements require extreme amounts of hip external rotation, which can lead to impingement, instability, or both (36).

Spine

- Many skating elements and jump landings require an arched or hyperextended back, placing the posterior elements of the lumbar spine at increased risk for causing potential lumbar strain, facet pain, posterior iliac crest injury, spondylolysis, and spondylolisthesis.
- The new scoring system requires the athlete to jump more, land more throws, spin in compromised positions, and perform more dynamic footwork sequences that place accumulative load on the posterior elements of the spine.
- Spondylolysis is often missed by clinicians and a high level of suspicion is important to diagnose this injury in skaters. A young skater with persistent back pain should be evaluated with x-rays, followed by an MRI with special protocol for spondylolysis with particular attention to the pars interarticularis.
- Appropriate therapy includes strengthening the core musculature to provide control of the trunk and pelvis to assist and maintain alignment of the body during jumps, spins, and lifts, as well as strengthening of the ankles supporting musculature.

Upper Extremity

- In the pairs discipline, shoulder strength and stability is challenged during partner lifts, exacerbating the potential for pathology related to multidirectional instabilities, to include muscular strain, tendonitis, and labral injury.
- Shoulder stability strengthening would be beneficial as a preventative measure for all disciplines.

- Repetitive cervical rotation combined with the demands to execute increasingly difficult acrobatic lifts may be contributing to increased cervical and thoracic dysfunction to include disc pathology, facet injury, and/or radiculopathies among elite skaters.

Concussions, Lacerations, Contusions, Facial Trauma

- Skaters involved in pairs skating, ice dancing, and synchronized skating suffer a higher rate of concussions, contusions, and lacerations as compared with single skaters.
- Injury may result from the blade (technique requiring positional blade retrieval or contact/collision trauma), from costume abrasions (lacerations on the partners ear from pairs twist), or rapid contact partner ice surface shards. Frequently, multiple skaters are injured at the same time in synchronized skating.
- Speed skating has a special problem with lacerations. This is especially true in short track where skaters are so close together with the long, sharp skate blades. The ISU has required that all competitors must wear a cut-resistant suit, knee and shin guards, cut-resistant gloves, cut-resistant neck and ankle protection, and an approved helmet. In addition, the front and rear parts of the skate blade must be rounded off with a radius of 1 cm (14,37).

FUTURE

- As the technical elements of skating are becoming more difficult, the kinetic energy involved increases and injury risk increases as well. Quadruple jumps have become almost mandatory and people are talking about "quints" on the horizon. Ice dancers continue to push creative acrobatics combinations and synchronized skaters are doing more lifts and aggressive skating as well.
- Interventions continue to be explored with a goal of both reducing injury and improving performance. Such interventions include wearable jump monitors (1,4), assessment of Y-balance (38) comparing different boot types for kinematics and shock absorption (5), evaluating joint laxity (39), video analysis (40,41), and thorough analysis of the science of figure skating jumps (17).
- Particular attention will continue to be paid to the exclusion of performance-enhancing drugs since the doping scandal involving a Russian skater at the 2022 Beijing Olympics.
- U.S. Figure Skating developed SKATESAFE® - a safe environment for its members that is free of misconduct and harassment, including avenues for athletes to report any and all forms of misconduct.
- The ISU raised the age limit from 15 to 17 for the senior level. This will gradually be phased in by the 2024–2025 season. This was a terrific decision as it allows our athletes to slowly develop the mental and physical capacity to do all that is asked of them in the sport.

REFERENCES

1. Brokaw I. *The Art of Skating, Its History and Development With Practical Directions, original Publication 1910.* current publication Ulan Press; 2012.
2. *Olympic figure skating.* Accessed 2023 12 Feb. https://olympics.com/en/sports/figure-skating
3. U.S. Figure Skating. *U.S. Figure Skating Media Guide* 2022-2023 *Fact Sheet.* Accessed 2023 Feb 28. https://www.usfigureska28ting.org/about/media
4. U.S. Speed Skating. Accessed 2023 Dec 12. https://www.teamusa.org/us-speedskating
5. U.S. Figure Skating. *U.S. Synchronized Skating Media Guide* 2022-2023. Accessed 2023 Feb 28. https://www.usfigureska28ting.org/about/media
6. ISU Skating News. *Age Limits.* Accessed 2023 Jan 2. https://www.isu.org/figure-skating/news/news-fsk/14236-new-rules-for-new-development
7. Aura Skates. Accessed 2023 Feb 26. https://auraskates.com/about-aura/
8. Edea Skates. Accessed 2023 Feb 26. https://edeaskates.com
9. Jackson Skates. Accessed 2023 Feb 26. https://jacksonskates.com
10. MK Blades. Accessed 2023 Feb 26. https://mkblades.com
11. Acuña SA, Smith DM, Robinson JM, et al. Instrumented figure skating blade for measuring on-ice skating forces. *Meas Sci Technol.* 2014;25:125901.
12. Bruening DA, Reynolds RE, Adair CW, Zapalo P, Ridge ST. A sport-specific wearable jump monitor for figure skating. *PLoS One.* 2018;13(11):e0206162.
13. Spiegl O., Tarassova O., Lundgren L.E, Neuman D., Arndt A. Comparison of lightweight and traditional figure skating blades, a prototype blade with integrated damping system and a running shoe in simulated figure skating landings and vertical countermovement jumps, and evaluation of dampening properties of the prototype blade. *Sports Biomech.* 2022;2022:1–22. doi:10.1080/14763141.2022.2063757
14. Quinn A, Lun V, McCall J, Overend T. Injuries in short track speed skating. *Am J Sports Med.* 2003;31(4):507–10.
15. King DL, Arnold AS, Smith SL. A kinematic comparison of single, double and triple axels. *J Appl Biomech.* 1994;10:51–60.
16. King DL, Smith SL, Higginson BK, Muncasy B, Scheirman GL. Characteristics of triple and quadruple toe-loops performed during the Salt Lake City 2002 Winter Olympics. *Sports Biomech.* 2004;3(1):109–23.
17. King D. *The Science of Figure Skating: Jumps.* ACSM Blog; 2018.
18. Richard P, Billaut F. Combining chronic ischemic preconditioning and inspiratory muscle warm-up to enhance on-ice time-trial performance in elite speed skaters. *Front Physiol.* 2018;9:1036.
19. Oleson CV, Busconi BD, Baran DT. Bone density in competitive figure skaters. *Arch Phys Med Rehabil.* 2002;83(1):122–8.
20. Huebsch T. (2018). How much faster is speed skating than running? In: *Canadian Running.* https://runningmagazine.ca/the-scene/olympic-speedskating-running-comparison/. Accessed 2020 3 Feb.
21. Macine RP, Gufsa DW, Moshrefi A, Kennedy SF. Prevalence of disordered eating in athletes categorized by emphasis on leanness and activity type-as systematic review. *J Eat Disord.* 2020;8:47. doi:10.1186/s40337-020-00323-2
22. Ziegler PJ, Jonnalagadda SS, Lawrence C. Dietary intake of elite figure skating dancers. *Nutr Res.* 2001;21(7):983–92.
23. Ziegler PJ, Jonnalagadda SS, Nelson JA, Lawrence C, Baciak B. Contribution of meals and snacks to nutrient intake of male and female elite figure skaters during peak competitive season. *J Am Coll Nutr.* 2002;21(2):114–9.
24. Jonnalagadda SS, Ziegler PJ, Nelson JA. Food preferences, dieting behaviors, and body image perceptions of elite figure skaters. *Int J Sport Nutr Exerc Metab.* 2004;14(5):594–606.

25. Slemenda CW, Johnston CC. High intensity activities in young women: site specific bone mass effects among female figure skaters. *Bone Miner.* 1993;20(2):125–32.
26. Vadocz EA, Siegel SR, Malina RM. Age at menarche in competitive figure skaters: variation by competency and discipline. *J Sports Sci.* 2002;20(2):93–100.
27. Dwyer J, Eisenberg A, Prelack K, Song W, Sonneville K, Ziegler P. Eating attitudes and food intakes of elite adolescent female figure skaters: a cross sectional study. *J Int Soc Sports Nutr.* 2012;9(1):53. http://www.jissn.com/content/9/1/53
28. Provost-Craig MA, Arbour KS, Sestili DC, Chabalko JJ, Ekinci E. The incidence of exercise-induced bronchospasm in competitive figure skaters. *J Asthma.* 1996;33(1):67–71.
29. Wilber RL, Rundell KW, Szmedra L, Jenkinson DM, Im J, Drake SD. Incidence of exercise-induced bronchospasm in Olympic winter sport athletes. *Med Sci Sports Exerc.* 2000;32(4):732–7.
30. Dubravcic-Simunjak S, Kuipers H, Moran J, Simunjak B, Pecina M. Injuries in synchronized skating. *Int J Sports Med.* 2006;27(6):493–9.
31. Dubravcic-Simunjak S, Pecina M, Kuipers H, Moran J, Haspl M. The incidence of injuries in elite junior figure skaters. *Am J Sports Med.* 2003;31(4):511–7.
32. Han JS, Geminiani ET, Micheli LJ. Epidemiology of figure skating injuries: a review of the literature. *Sports Health.* 2018;10(6):532–7.
33. King DL, DiCesaro SF, Getzin AR. Self-reported injuries of US figure skaters. *Cogent Medicine.* 2017;4(1). doi:10.1080/2331205X.2017.1419420
34. Kowalczyk AD, Geminiani ET, Dahlberg BW, Micheli LJ, Sugimoto D. Pediatric and adolescent figure skating injuries: a 15-year retrospective review. *Clin J Sport Med,* 2021;31(3):295–303. doi:10.1097/JSM.0000000000000743
35. Bradley MA. Prevention and treatment of foot and ankle injuries in figure skaters. *Curr Sports Med Rep.* 2006;5(5):258–61.
36. Weber AE, Bedi A, Tibor LM, Zaltz I, Larson CM. The hyperflexible hip: managing hip pain in the dancer and gymnast. *Sports Health.* 2015;7(4):346–58.
37. ISU. *Speed skating. 2020 ISU communication No. 2195.* Retrieved December 12, 2022. https://www.isu.org/speed-skating
38. Slater LV, Vriner M, Schuyten K, Zapalo P, Hart JM. Sex differences in Y-balance performance in elite figure skaters. *J Strength Condit Res.* 2018;34(5):1.
39. Okamura S, Wada N, Tazawa M, et al. Injuries and disorders among young ice skaters: relationship with generalized joint laxity and tightness. *OAJSM.* 2014;5:191–5.
40. Knox CL, Comstock RD. Video analysis of falls experienced by paediatric iceskaters and roller/inline skaters. *Br J Sports Med.* 2006;40(3):268–71.
41. Knox CL, Comstock RD, McGeehan J, Smith GA. Differences in the risk associated with head injury for pediatric ice skaters, roller skaters, and in-line skaters. *Pediatrics.* 2006;118(2):549–54.

105 Football

John M. MacKnight and Jared Astrow

INTRODUCTION

- More than 5 million individuals in the United States play American/tackle football each year, with organized tackle football beginning at age 5 in the Pop Warner league.
- Football is also played in a variety of alternative forms including touch football, flag football, and no-tackle football, which is flag football with players wearing helmets and shoulder pads.
- Although soccer (referred to worldwide as football) is still more prominent internationally, American football is gaining popularity as a participation option throughout the world, especially in Europe.
- Multiple levels of participation from Pop Warner to higher youth leagues, high school, college, and professional. Multiple professional football leagues now exist with subtle differences in venue and rules (*i.e.*, Arena football vs traditional American football). Although the nature of the game is consistent throughout the various levels, the speed and power of the game increase with player age and physical development.
- Given the traumatic nature of football, football players utilize extensive protective equipment including a football helmet, shoulder pads, padding for protection of thighs, knees, iliac crests, and sacrum/coccyx. A variety of protective braces are utilized as well, which are position-specific.
- Sports medicine coverage of American football places unique demands on the sports medicine practitioner. A wide variety of football-specific conditions demand that those responsible for the care of football teams be well versed in an array of both medical and orthopedic issues.
- Appropriate planning can minimize the likelihood of athlete injury and help ensure that athletes are protected and returned to play safely and in a timely manner.

MUSCULOSKELETAL INJURIES

- Reported injury rates in football vary but most studies indicate an injury rate in excess of 50% of players in any given season (1). The majority of these injuries involve the lower extremity, with sprains, contusions, and strains being most common. Fractures account for approximately 10% of injuries (1).

Lower Extremity Injuries

Medial Collateral Ligament Sprain, Knee

- The most common knee injury seen in football, typically resulting from a valgus load to the knee by another player during blocking or tackling.
- Grading of medial collateral ligament (MCL) sprains:
  - Grade I injuries have stretched, but not disrupted, the ligament, and the knee examination (valgus loading of the knee at 0° and 30° of flexion) reveals no laxity compared to the uninjured side.
  - Grade II injuries have partial ligament disruption with discernible laxity and increased excursion on valgus testing but preservation of an endpoint.
  - Grade III injuries represent full ligament tears with gross laxity and no discernible endpoint.
- All three grades are generally managed conservatively with icing, nonsteroidal anti-inflammatory drugs (NSAIDs), and protective bracing. Even athletes with grade III injuries may resume sport in protective braces if symptoms allow.
- Many football programs now use protective medial stabilizing braces to decrease the incidence of MCL injury, particularly in interior linemen. Although data have not clearly proven their efficacy, braces may enhance proprioceptive function (and thus allow the player to avoid high-risk knee positions) and are a reasonable preventative measure for at-risk players (2).

Meniscal Tears

- An injury to the medial or lateral meniscal cartilage typically resulting from a rotational load applied to the flexed knee.
- Pain may be acute or chronic, and the athlete commonly complains of mechanical symptoms including a sense of locking and/or giving way of the knee.
- Meniscal tears are classically characterized by small effusions that develop gradually over 6–24 hours, focal joint line tenderness to palpation, normal ligament testing, and positive McMurray and Apley grind tests. Pain and dysfunction may also be elicited by squatting. Lack of effusion does not necessarily rule out meniscus damage.
- Definitive diagnosis is usually via magnetic resonance imaging (MRI), which demonstrates characteristic signal changes in the affected meniscus.

- Most meniscal tears are amenable to arthroscopic debridement with resumption of football activities in as few as 2 weeks. If a complex or large radial tear is present in the meniscus requiring meniscal repair, a longer recovery process is generally needed (6 weeks).

Anterior Cruciate Ligament Tear

- The most devastating knee injury commonly seen in football, anterior cruciate ligament (ACL) tears generally result from valgus loading of the slightly flexed knee, creating significant shear forces on the ACL with resultant tearing. The majority are noncontact injuries, but the ACL may be torn in a similar contact mechanism to that of the MCL as noted earlier. As such, simultaneous injury of both ligaments is common.
- The injury is accompanied by significant pain, often an audible "pop" or a sense of tearing inside the knee, immediate swelling, subjective instability of the knee, and laxity on the Lachman, anterior drawer test, or pivot shift.
- For competitive athletes, ACL tears generally require surgical reconstruction. Graft options include patellar tendon, hamstring and gracilis tendon, quadriceps tendon, or cadaveric grafts. Patellar tendon grafts are generally preferred in athletes but may lead to earlier patellofemoral arthritis than the alternatives. Caution must also be used with patellar grafting in athletes with prior patellar tendon dysfunction. After 6–9 months of aggressive rehabilitation, functional bracing to protect the reconstructed ACL is generally desirable to aid safe return to full football activities.

Hamstring Strain

- A common injury typically of the mid-substance of the hamstring musculature characterized by partial tearing, edema, and ecchymosis.
- Clinically presents with acute onset of posterior thigh pain in association with sprinting, explosive acceleration or deceleration, or change in direction.
- Physical exam reveals focal tenderness over the injured muscle belly. There may be a discernible muscular defect present. Mild warmth and edema may be present. Ecchymosis is common and can be impressive.
- The athlete typically limps, holds the knee in mild flexion, and has obvious loss of knee extension range of motion.
- Management focuses on acute injury modalities followed by general restoration of range of motion and full strength before resuming running or football activities.
- Significant hamstring strains may take 6 weeks or longer to fully heal. Typically, the closer the hamstring strain is to the ischial tuberosity, the longer the rehabilitation process.

Thigh/Quadriceps Contusion

- The most common soft-tissue injury in football, resulting from blunt trauma.
- Treatment focuses on limitation of hemorrhage and inflammation while maintaining range of motion and strength. Ice and NSAIDs are appropriate initial interventions. Some practitioners advocate immobilizing the knee in 120° of flexion to limit hemorrhage and hematoma formation.
- Massage and ultrasound should be avoided early in the treatment course to allow for early stabilization of the damaged muscle and to minimize the risk of developing myositis ossificans. This complication is characterized by calcific changes in areas of damaged muscle and occurs in up to 20% of cases if treated inadequately.
- Athletes may return to play when they have full range of motion and strength equivalent to that of the uninjured leg.

Turf Toe

- A sprain of the plantar-capsular ligament complex with associated articular cartilage damage to the metatarsal heads or base of the proximal phalanx.
- The first metatarsophalangeal (MTP) joint is the primary area of injury, typically resulting from forced dorsiflexion of the planted toe on the turf. Athletes experience significant pain, have local swelling, and often limp.
- Artificial turf surfaces, lighter and more flexible shoes, and pes planus have been implicated in a rising incidence of turf toe injuries.
- Management centers on protection of the area with a rigid insert in the shoe to protect against dorsiflexion, donut padding, taping, ice, and NSAIDs. Activity status is dictated by pain.

Hip Pointer

- Contusion or separation of attached muscle fibers at the superior aspect of the iliac crest as a result of blunt trauma, generally resulting in a significant degree of pain and dysfunction.
- X-rays are generally unnecessary at the time of diagnosis but should be performed for symptoms that are prolonged or increasing.
- Management includes aggressive icing, stretching of the low back and flank muscles, and additional protective padding at the time of return to play.
- Local modalities such as ultrasound, corticosteroid injections, or platelet-rich plasma injections may speed up the healing response as well.

Upper Extremity Injuries

Glenohumeral Instability

- Glenohumeral instability is a common shoulder malady in football athletes occurring when the glenohumeral joint is partially or completely destabilized as a result of repetitive blows to the shoulder or the unique acute loading that may arise with blocking and tackling.
- Frank dislocations occur anteriorly in 95% of cases and result from excessive abduction, extension, and external rotational forces.
- Physical examination classically reveals apprehension when the humeral head is moved anteriorly or posteriorly in the glenoid.

- Instability events should prompt an early x-ray evaluation to assess for bony injury to the glenoid (Bankart lesion) or impaction injury to the humeral head from sliding across the glenoid (Hill-Sachs lesion).
- Single or recurrent instability episodes may predispose to labral cartilage tears. These typically arise in the **S**uperior portion of the **L**abrum and extend **A**nterior to **P**osterior. This common pattern gives rise to the term "**SLAP**" tear.
- Although surgery to correct shoulder instability is a frequent consideration because of the high relative recurrence rate for subluxations or dislocations, aggressive rotator cuff strengthening coupled with functional bracing may provide excellent results.
- Evidence from randomized controlled trials has not shown a statistically significant difference in redislocation rates, time to return to activity, or functional outcomes between arthroscopic and open repair surgical groups (3).
- SLAP tears in association with mild instability may be addressed arthroscopically without performing a stabilization procedure.
- Offensive linemen may also develop posterior instability from blocking with outstretched arms and repetitively loading the posterior capsule of the glenohumeral joint. Except in extreme cases, aggressive rehabilitation and modification of weightlifting techniques are generally adequate for management.

Acromioclavicular Sprain

- This common shoulder injury, also referred to as a "separated shoulder," is a sprain of the supporting ligaments of the acromioclavicular (AC) joint.
- The typical mechanism of injury is either striking another player with the point of the shoulder or landing directly on the point of the shoulder, often when being tackled.
- Initial presentation reveals exquisite point tenderness over the AC joint. A bony "step-off" with inferior displacement of the acromion relative to the clavicle may be appreciated.
- X-rays are indicated to evaluate for concomitant clavicle fracture and to assess the degree of AC separation. Bilateral AC x-rays are often performed for side-to-side comparison. Weighting of the injured arm may help determine if there is widening of the AC joint with downward distraction.
- Management focuses on control of inflammation and pain, protection of the AC joint via padding, early restoration of active shoulder range of motion, and preservation of shoulder strength.
- Even high-grade AC sprains generally do not require surgery, and most heal completely in 6 weeks. Elite athletes may opt for surgical stabilization to speed their return to play.

Mallet Finger

- Force applied to the distal interphalangeal (DIP) joint of the finger may result in a flexion injury, which either results in injury to the extensor tendon or in an avulsion fracture at its attachment point on the dorsal aspect of the distal phalanx.
- Mallet finger classically presents as an "extension lag" of the DIP joint with drooping and an inability to fully actively extend the DIP joint.
- X-rays may reveal a fracture of the dorsal base of the distal phalanx on lateral view or may be normal with a pure tendon injury.
- Standard management is to splint the DIP joint in mild hyperextension continuously for 6 weeks using a Stax splint or equivalent.
- If recognized and managed early, surgery is often unnecessary.

Jersey Finger

- Forced extension of the actively flexed finger, as in attempting to grasp an opponent for a tackle, may result in avulsion of the flexor digitorum profundus or superficialis from its insertion on the volar side of the distal or middle phalanx, respectively.
- The ring finger is most commonly involved, followed by the middle finger.
- The athlete will feel a pop, and the retracted tendon may be palpable proximally in the finger. Examination will demonstrate loss of independent flexion of the DIP joint or PIP joint.
- Early surgical repair is the treatment of choice.

SPINAL AND NEUROLOGIC INJURIES

Cervical Spine Injury

- Historically, head trauma had been the most common source of morbidity and mortality in football, most commonly from subdural hematomas. Better helmet construction decreased such head injuries but fostered technique changes in play that favored leading with the head and neck for tackling and blocking, so-called "spearing." This dangerous technique led to a marked increase in cervical spine injuries until rule changes were instituted to outlaw spearing in football.
- Reviews of cervical spine injuries in football have documented axial loading of the cervical spine as the major mechanism of catastrophic cervical spine injuries (4).
- The normal cervical spine consists of an arc of vertebral bodies that is able to withstand substantial loading by dissipating forces evenly across each vertebral level. However, when the neck is flexed forward 30°, it becomes a straight-segmented column of bones that cannot dissipate force evenly. Axial loading of the neck in this flexed position may result in excessive forces on the vertebral bodies leading to bony failure, fracture, and cervical spinal cord injury.

Cervical Cord Neurapraxia

- Transient, reversible deformation of the spinal cord resulting from significant trauma to the neck
- The etiology of transient quadriplegia

- Athletes may experience transient bilateral (differentiating this entity from a brachial plexus neurapraxia — see below) sensory changes, frank sensation loss, and variable motor changes including complete paralysis.
- Episodes typically last less than 15 minutes but may persist up to 2 days.
- A ratio of spinal canal to vertebral body widths (as determined by lateral radiographs of the cervical spine) of <0.8 has been found reliably in athletes suffering cervical cord neurapraxia (5). Although this measure has a high sensitivity for cervical cord neurapraxia, it has a low specificity and low positive predictive value and should not be used as a screening tool. In addition, caution must also be used in the interpretation of this ratio in football players because their large vertebral bodies may falsely decrease the ratio in the absence of true cervical spinal stenosis. Advanced imaging modalities have also provided improved screening parameters. The mean subaxial cervical space available for the spinal cord (MSCSAC) on an MRI has been shown to be a reliable tool to screen for the risk of chronic stingers. A cutoff value of 4.3 mm for the MSCSAC can serve as a confirmatory test, with a specificity of 96% and 13.3 positive likelihood ratio for stingers (6).
- Management of the football player with known cervical spinal stenosis remains controversial because leading authorities in this area have expressed differing opinions with respect to return-to-play criteria. Some authorities have suggested that cervical spinal stenosis is an absolute contraindication to return to contact sport. This belief is based on a known predisposition to spinal cord injury in these patients and a higher incidence of permanent neurologic sequelae in this group as compared to those with normal spinal canal volumes.
- Others contend that, despite its association with transient quadriplegia, cervical spinal stenosis is not reliably associated with catastrophic spinal cord injury and does not mandate exclusion from participation in all cases. The following guidelines have been proposed for participation in this group of athletes (7,8):
    - Canal to vertebral body ratio of 0.8 or less in asymptomatic individuals — no contraindication
    - Ratio of 0.8 or less with one episode of cervical cord neurapraxia — relative contraindication
    - Documented episodes of cervical cord neurapraxia associated with intervertebral disc disease and/or degenerative changes — relative contraindication
    - Documented episode of cervical cord neurapraxia associated with MRI evidence of cord defect or cord edema — relative/absolute contraindication
    - Documented episode of cervical cord neurapraxia associated with ligamentous instability, symptoms of neurologic findings lasting more than 36 hours, and/or multiple episodes — absolute contraindication

Brachial Plexus Neurapraxia

- Commonly referred to as a "stinger" or "burner," brachial plexus neurapraxia results from traction or compression of the brachial plexus with violent lateral flexion of the neck.
- The most common nerve injury in football, with defensive players most commonly affected.
- Athletes note unilateral burning or stinging pain, numbness, or tingling radiating from the supraclavicular area down to the fingers, most commonly in a C5 or C6 distribution. There may be weakness, most commonly of the deltoid, but no neck pain. Symptoms typically resolve in minutes. Symptoms that persist suggest more substantial injury to the brachial plexus, including cervical root avulsion, and mandate imaging and appropriate neurologic consultation.
- Athletes may resume competition when they demonstrate full range of motion, full strength, and a normal neurologic examination of the upper extremity.
- Prospective analysis of college football players revealed that a favorable overall spinal canal to vertebral body ratio (>0.9) is associated with a low initial incidence of brachial plexus injury. Players with multiple such injuries have been shown to have significantly smaller ratios than those suffering only one event (6).

Spear Tackler's Spine

- Characterized by developmental narrowing of the cervical canal (a canal to vertebral body ratio of <0.8), straightening or reversal of the normal cervical lordosis, and posttraumatic radiographic abnormalities.
- These individuals are at great risk for permanent spinal cord injury and should be precluded from participation in tackle football (8).

Management of the Potential Cervical Spine Injury (9)

- All unconscious athletes and any conscious athlete complaining of neck pain must have the cervical spine immobilized prior to removal from the playing field. This is accomplished by coordinated sports medicine care with a lead care provider at the head and neck to provide traction and stability, particularly if the athlete must be rolled onto their back prior to receiving additional care.
- The helmet should never be removed on the field without simultaneously removing the shoulder pads as the presence of shoulder pads will favor passive hyperextension of the cervical spine and may contribute to further cervical spine or spinal cord injury. If the helmet remains on, the face mask should be removed to allow control of the athlete's airway. Prior to every football game, care providers should coordinate their protocol for helmet and shoulder pad management in the setting of acute cervical spine injury.
- Evaluation includes cervical spine x-rays in several planes and may require computed tomography (CT) scanning to rule out fracture in equivocal cases. It is acceptable to

perform the initial radiographic evaluation in the emergency department or athletic training room either with or without equipment in place.

- Every potential cervical spine injury must be treated with the same conservative approach and proper technique to prevent unnecessary neurologic compromise.

Lumbar Spine Injury

Spondylolysis

- Stress injury to the pars interarticularis in the posterior aspect of the spine as a result of repetitive extension loading. Offensive and defensive linemen are most commonly affected (10).
- Athletes complain of deep pain in the low back, which is exacerbated by active or passive extension, particularly when standing on one leg. X-rays may reveal a fracture in the pars interarticularis on oblique views although bone scan or MRI may be required to make the diagnosis definitively.
- Most athletes respond well to conservative management including rest and rehabilitative activities. Thoracolumbar bracing may be used for additional spinal stability but is often unnecessary.
- Most athletes may return in 6–8 weeks if asymptomatic.

Spondylolisthesis

- Displacement ("slippage") of one vertebral body over another as a result of a stress injury to the pars interarticularis (spondylolysis).
- Approximately 1% of both professional and collegiate football players have a spondylolisthesis (11).
- The presence of a spondylolisthesis is not a contraindication to playing football but may predispose to pain and associated dysfunction and may also lead to worsening of the anatomic changes in the spine over time.
- Pathologic forces on both lumbar discs and pars interarticularis have been demonstrated in blocking linemen. The mechanics of repetitive blocking, most notably loaded extension of the lumbar spine, may be responsible for the increased incidence of such injuries in football linemen.

Concussion

General

- Concussion is defined as a complex pathophysiological process affecting the brain, induced by traumatic biomechanical forces.
- Concussion is estimated to occur at a rate of at least 250,000 events per year in football players, although it is generally accepted that concussions are grossly underreported. Concussion incidence has been found to be highest at the high school (5.6%) and Division III collegiate levels (5.5%), suggesting an association between the level of play and risk of injury (12,13).
- Mechanisms of injury include a direct blow to the head by an opposing player, whip-like motion of the head and neck in response to a blow delivered to another part of the body, or a blow to the head from hitting the ground. Brain shearing and acceleration/deceleration forces result in a cascade of neurochemical changes including local glucose depletion, edema, and local vascular effects.
- Many athletes either do not realize they have suffered a concussion or fail to report it to their sports medicine staff.
- The majority of concussed football players suffer recurrent concussive injuries, which may place them at risk for long-term neurologic complications.
- Although concussion in football players is discussed below, the reader is additionally directed to Chapter 31 Neuropsychological Testing in Concussion and Chapter 40 Neurology for a further discussion.

Evaluation

- Concussed athletes are often dazed and disoriented and may have loss or alteration in consciousness. These manifestations may be mild and transient or prolonged and profound. They may complain of dizziness, headache, vision disturbance, and nausea, and they often display changes in personality and behavioral patterns.
- Physical examination is generally within normal limits. In addition to an abbreviated neurologic examination to rule out gross neurologic dysfunction (cranial nerve assessment and gross motor, sensory, and cerebellar testing), sideline neuropsychological tests should be performed to screen for impairment in general orientation (person, place, time of day, and situation — game, game location, quarter, score, and opponent), short- and long-term memory/recall, and complex processing tasks such as reciting the months of the year in reverse order. Athletes should always be assessed for the presence of antegrade (since the time of injury) and retrograde (prior to the injury) amnesia. Antegrade amnesia is generally considered to be a more worrisome finding.
- Commonly applied sideline tools to assess these parameters include the Standardized Assessment of Concussion (SAC) and the Sport Concussion Assessment Tool 6 (SCAT-6).
- There is no consistent correlation between the degree of impairment in neuropsychological testing and the anticipated time to return to play from a concussive injury.
- Emphasis should be placed on the description of the concussion's characteristics (presence and duration of antegrade or retrograde amnesia, headache, vomiting, vision change, persisting confusion or disorientation, sleep disturbance) as opposed to a specific grade, which had previously dictated a rigid course of management. Concussions are sufficiently heterogeneous that they require flexibility in their diagnosis and management, particularly with respect to contact sports such as football.

- Brain imaging via CT scan or MRI is generally unnecessary in the evaluation of an uncomplicated concussion. Clinical factors that warrant urgent imaging, typically via CT scanning, include:
  - initial prolonged (>30 seconds) loss of consciousness
  - progressive decline in level of consciousness
  - worsening headache
  - development of a frank neurologic deficit
  - late-onset vomiting
- In these circumstances, imaging should be used to assess for intracranial hemorrhage and/or skull fractures.

Management

- As outlined in recently updated consensus statements, return to play from concussion should follow a consistent algorithm (14).
- It is now standard of care to remove any football player with a concussion from participation for the remainder of the game or practice. No concussed player should return to play on the day of injury regardless of circumstances.
- Complete absence of symptoms both at rest and with exertion, normal neurologic examination, and return to baseline neurocognitive and emotional states are the key features to the determination of suitability to return to play.
- Using these guidelines in a stepwise fashion ensures that the concussed football player has adequate time to heal from the event prior to resuming contact activities.
- Once asymptomatic at rest, the athlete must then demonstrate a return to the normal baseline of their neurocognitive status. This is ideally shown by comparative testing with baseline data obtained prior to the concussion, generally before preseason workouts begin.
- Balance testing has also been shown to aid in the evaluation and management of concussion. This testing modality is again most powerful when compared to a preinjury baseline (15).
- Vestibular ocular motion screening (VOMS) tests should be administered as part of the concussion evaluation as well. This important additional means of screening for subtle neurologic changes or symptom provocation includes eye testing including smooth pursuits, convergence, horizontal and vertical saccades, vestibulo-ocular reflex (VOR) and visual motion sensitivity (VMS).
- Once symptom and neurocognitive criteria are satisfied, the athlete is allowed to advance noncontact activity in a stepwise fashion over several days. If the athlete remains asymptomatic with increasing activity, the athlete is then released to resume full football activities.

Complications

- The most feared complication of concussion is the "second-impact syndrome," a generally fatal cascade of cerebral hemorrhage and edema resulting from a second concussive blow following incomplete resolution of a first concussive event. Although exceedingly rare, the potential for second-impact syndrome absolutely dictates disqualification from all contact activities until the concussed athlete has completely recovered from their initial injury.
- Systematic review of potential long-term effects of sport-related concussion revealed that former high school American football players do not appear to be at increased risk for later-life neurodegenerative diseases. Retired professional American football players may be at increased risk for mild cognitive impairment (16).
- Repeated head trauma from sport has been associated with chronic traumatic encephalopathy (CTE), which is characterized by progressive pathologic changes including deposition of tau protein within the brain and a clinical presentation consistent with dementia.
- Studies have linked the presence of apolipoprotein E4 (apoE4) genotype and risk for cognitive impairment with head injury (17). The resultant cognitive status of such athletes with repeated head trauma appears to be influenced by this genetic predisposition as well as age and cumulative exposure to contact.
- Although its utilization as a screening tool is still under study, apoE4 and similar genetic markers may become a practical means of determining an athlete's relative risk for permanent neurocognitive loss in association with head injury in sport.

Headache

- Football-related headache is common, with 85% of sampled high school and college football players reporting a history of headache as a result of hitting (18).
- Defensive backs (25%), defensive linemen (19%), and offensive linemen (18%) were most likely to have headache related to hitting. Given the high rate of headache and the low rate of serious complications (cerebral hemorrhage, second-impact syndrome), the presence of headache, unless persistent or accompanied by other symptoms, does not mandate disqualification from competition.

Heat Illness

- Heat-related illness in football is common as a result of practice and play in warm weather months coupled with impaired heat dissipation from extensive body coverage with heavy padding and helmets.
- Heat illness may manifest as a broad spectrum of conditions including heat cramps, heat syncope, heat exhaustion, and potentially lethal heat stroke.
- Heat cramps, syncope, and exhaustion are characterized by heat-associated physiologic changes that do not result in significant elevations in core body temperature or in central nervous system dysfunction. Heat cramps and syncope may be treated safely with aggressive oral hydration, external cooling measures, electrolyte supplementation, and rest.

- Heat exhaustion is heralded by complaints of dizziness, headache, nausea and vomiting, and generalized weakness and malaise. Core body temperature (measured rectally) is below 104 °F, and athletes generally continue to sweat to dissipate heat. Management includes removal from participation, removal of helmet and padding, external cooling measures (cool water immersion, fanning), and intravenous fluids. Resolution of associated symptoms, normal hydration status, and restoration of baseline body weight (BW) are necessary prior to resumption of physical activity.
- Heat stroke is defined as core body temperature in excess of 104 °F coupled with central nervous system dysfunction characterized by disorientation, confusion, personality change, and even coma. Although the pathophysiology of classic heat stroke includes absence of sweating, athletes with exertional heat stroke may sweat profusely, an important fact to be remembered by care providers.
- Heat stroke is a medical emergency requiring immediate cooling measures such as ice bath immersion and immediate activation of the emergency medical system for rapid transport to a hospital setting where additional aggressive cooling measures may be employed. Recent research supports the concept of "cool first, transport second" to emphasize the importance of rapidly cooling the heat stroke athlete on-site rather than risking a delay in cooling that may result from the logistics of transport. Consequences of heat stroke may include irreversible brain damage, renal failure, rhabdomyolysis, and death.
- Stimulant supplements and medications as well as "energy drinks" containing stimulants have been implicated in precipitating heat stroke and death in highly competitive athletes. Their detrimental effects are the result of sympathomimetic activity and resultant vasoconstriction during activities that require vasodilation for appropriate heat dissipation.
- Football players must have free access to water. Thirst is a poor measure of hydration status, so athletes must consume fluids regularly during activity regardless of their sense of need to drink.
- The general hydration goal is for fluid consumption sufficient to prevent decreases in total BW of 2% or more (19).
- To optimize preexercise status, players should consume 5–10 mL · kg^{-1} BW 2–4 hours prior to exercise. Consumption of beverages with sodium (20–50 mEq · L^{-1}) and/or small amounts of salted snacks or sodium-containing foods at meals will help stimulate thirst and retain the consumed fluids (20).
- During exercise, the goal is to prevent excessive dehydration (>2% BW loss from water deficit) and excessive changes in electrolyte balance that may compromise exercise performance. It is recommended that individuals monitor their BW changes during training/competition to estimate their sweat losses during particular exercise tasks and weather conditions. Measurement of preexercise and post-exercise BWs is useful for determining sweat rates and customized fluid replacement programs. Differences in metabolic requirements, exercise duration, clothing, equipment, and weather all influence sweat rate and fluid loss.
- American football players wearing full equipment in hot weather may lose sweat >8 L · d^{-1}.
- After exercise, the consumption of normal meals and snacks with sufficient volume of plain water will restore euhydration, provided the food contains sufficient sodium to replace sweat losses (21). More rapid restoration may be accomplished with consumption of 1.25–1.5 L of fluid per kilogram of BW lost (20).
- Diet can be used to ensure adequate salt and electrolyte replacement, which will aid in overall water balance.
- Weights should be monitored to screen for subclinical dehydration, and participation should be precluded for athletes who are greater than 1%–2% below their preexercise baseline weight.
- Appropriate guidelines for practice duration and attire should be based on wet bulb globe temperature (WBGT), which accounts for the heating effects of temperature, humidity, and intensity of sunlight exposure.

SUDDEN DEATH

- Sudden death in football players is a rare but devastating occurrence.
- The primary causes of nontraumatic death in athletes include:
  - hypertrophic cardiomyopathy
  - malignant cardiac arrhythmias
  - heat stroke
  - asthma
  - complications of sickle cell disease
- Screening measures should focus on the identification of such potential conditions or a familial predisposition to them, accepting that such screening methods at present are limited in their yield.
- The presence of an automated external defibrillator (AED) and appropriate training for its use by the sports medicine staff is essential in enhancing survival for athletes with cardiac etiologies of sudden death.
- AEDs and trained staff to use them should be present at all football practices and games whenever logistically feasible.

REFERENCES

1. Saal JA. Common American football injuries. *Sports Med.* 1991 Aug;12(2):132–47. doi:10.2165/00007256-199112020-00005
2. Salata MJ, Gibbs AE, Sekiya JK. The effectiveness of prophylactic knee bracing in American football: a systematic review. *Sports Health.* 2010 Sep;2(5):375–9. doi:10.1177/1941738110378986

3. Godin J, Sekiya JK. Systematic review of arthroscopic versus open repair for recurrent anterior shoulder dislocations. *Sports Health.* 2011 Jul;3(4):396–404. doi:10.1177/1941738111409175
4. Rihn JA, Anderson DT, Lamb K, et al. Cervical spine injuries in American football. *Sports Med.* 2009;39(9):697–708. doi:10.2165/11315190-000000000-00000
5. Torg JS. Cervical spine injuries and the return to football. *Sports Health.* 2009 Sep;1(5):376–83. doi:10.1177/1941738109343161
6. Presciutti SM, DeLuca P, Marchetto P, Wilsey JT, Shaffrey C, Vaccaro AR. Mean subaxial space available for the cord index as a novel method of measuring cervical spine geometry to predict the chronic stinger syndrome in American football players: clinical article. *J Neurosurg Spine.* 2009;11(3):264–71.
7. Kepler CK, Vaccaro AR. Injuries and abnormalities of the cervical spine and return to play criteria. *Clin Sports Med.* 2012 Jul;31(3):499–508. doi:10.1016/j.csm.2012.03.005
8. Cantu RV, Cantu RC. Current thinking: return to play and transient quadriplegia. *Curr Sports Med Rep.* 2005 Feb;4(1):27–32. doi:10.1097/01.CSMR.0000306068.21649.da
9. Waninger KN, Swartz EE. Cervical spine injury management in the helmeted athlete. *Curr Sports Med Rep.* 2011 Jan;10(1):45–9. doi:10.1249/JSR.0b013e3182073767
10. Shurley JP, Newman JK. Spondylolysis in American football players: etiology, symptoms, and implications for strength and conditioning specialists. *Strength Cond J.* 2016 Oct;38(5):40–51. doi:10.1519/SSC.0000000000000244
11. Choi JH, Ochoa JK, Lubinus A, Timon S, Lee YP, Bhatia NN. Management of lumbar spondylolysis in the adolescent athlete: a review of over 200 cases. *Spine J.* 2022 Oct;22(10):1628–33. doi:10.1016/j.spinee.2022.04.011
12. Baugh CM, Kiernan PT, Kroshus E, et al. Frequency of head-impact-related outcomes by position in NCAA division I collegiate football players. *J Neurotrauma.* 2015 Mar 1;32(5):314–26. doi:10.1089/neu.2014.3582
13. Dompier TP, Kerr ZY, Marshall SW, et al. Incidence of concussion during practice and games in youth, high school, and collegiate American football players. *JAMA Pediatr.* 2015 Jul;169(7):659–65. doi:10.1001/jamapediatrics.2015.0210
14. Patricios JS, Schneider KJ, Dvorak J, et al. Consensus statement on concussion in sport: the 6th International Conference on Concussion in Sport-Amsterdam, October 2022. *Br J Sports Med.* 2023 Jun;57(11):695–711.
15. Murray NG, Reed-Jones RJ, Szekely BJ, Powell DW. Clinical assessments of balance in adults with concussion: an update. *Semin Speech Lang.* 2019 Feb;40(1):48–56. doi:10.1055/s-0038-1676451
16. Manley G, Gardner AJ, Schneider KJ, et al. A systematic review of potential long-term effects of sport-related concussion. *Br J Sports Med.* 2017;51(12):969–77.
17. Kutner KC, Erlanger DM, Tsai J, Jordan B, Relkin NR. Lower cognitive performance of older football players possessing apolipoprotein E epsilon4. *Neurosurgery.* 2000;47(3):651–8. discussion 657–8.
18. Evans RW. Sports and headaches. *Headache.* 2018 Mar;58(3):426–37. doi:10.1111/head.13263
19. Riebl SK, Davy BM. The hydration equation: update on water balance and cognitive performance. *ACSMs Health Fit J.* 2013 Nov;17(6):21–8. doi:10.1249/FIT.0b013e3182a9570f
20. Thomas DT, Erdman KA, Burke LM. American College of Sports Medicine joint position statement. Nutrition and athletic performance. *Med Sci Sports Exerc.* 2016 Mar;48(3):543–68. doi:10.1249/MSS.0000000000000852
21. Périard JD, Eijsvogels TMH, Daanen HAM. Exercise under heat stress: thermoregulation, hydration, performance implications, and mitigation strategies. *Physiol Rev.* 2021 Oct 1;101(4):1873–979. doi:10.1152/physrev.00038.2020

106 Golf

Benjamin J. Ingram and Bradley A. Redick

INTRODUCTION

Background

- Golf was invented in the 12th century in Northern Europe (1).
- Today over 60 million people play golf worldwide, on over 30,000 courses, across 200 countries (2,3).
- The first golf course was built in the United States in 1888 (4).
- Currently, more than one-half of the world's courses are in the United States (5).
- In total, 25.6 million Americans played golf in 2022, with a 36% increase in youth aged 6–17 years old, a 17% increase in minority diversity, and a 15% increase in female golfers since 2019 (6,7).
- Most golf injuries result from the golf swing, the equipment, or objects, including the ball, on the course. Injury site locations and frequency differ for amateur and professional golfers (2).

Health Benefits

- As a sport, golf is traditionally classified as a noncontact, low-intensity sport. However, newer evidence categorizes golf as a sport with the potential for moderate-intensity physical activity, suggesting that there may be benefits in cardiovascular, respiratory, and metabolic fitness (3,8).
- MET values for golf range between 2.5 and 8.0 with a mean estimate of 4.5 METs (8).
- Golfers walking the golf course take more steps than those who ride in carts suggesting that the style of play impacts the health benefits conferred by the sport (8)
  - However, golf cart usage increased from 45% to 69% between 1984 and 2006, suggesting fewer players enjoy the full physical activity benefits of golf (9).
  - A caddy in golf is a person who accompanies the golfer during play with typical roles, including carrying the golfer's bag and attending to flag sticks at the hole. Evidence for health benefits from caddying is currently poor, but likely to mirror or exceed the golfer (10).
- Spectating golf involves physical activity while following golfers through the course of play, although the health benefits of this activity are unknown (8).
- Unlike high-contact and high-intensity sports such as soccer and rugby, golfers more frequently continue to play into their middle and older ages, suggesting any health benefits of playing golf can continue into later life (3,8).

The Golf Swing

- For definition in this chapter, the right-handed golfer's dominant side is the right or trailing side and the nondominant side is the left or leading side. The left-handed golfer would reverse left and right regarding dominance.
- There are two types of swings in golf: "modern" (in common use since the 1960s) and "classic" (11).
- The modern swing comprises multiple coordinated movements of different parts of the body: the hands, wrists, arms, trunk, and legs. The modern swing ends in the "reverse C" position (11).
- There are four phases:
  - *Backswing* or take away: Rotation of the trunk, raising the arms, and cocking the wrists while drawing the club head away from the ball. This is often called coiling.
  - *Downswing* or forward swing: Movement of the club head toward the ball using the shoulders and uncocking of the wrists. This is often called uncoiling.
  - *Acceleration* and ball strike: The arms and trunk continue to rotate back toward the ball and the wrists are uncocked. The leading wrist also supinates while the trailing wrist pronates. This is the fastest portion of the swing.
  - *Follow through*: Momentum of the swing continues with rotation of the shoulders and trunk while raising the arms (11).

Epidemiology

- The annual injury rate can approach 40% (11).
- About 46.2% of injuries occur during the swing, particularly with ball impact (12).
- Injuries are different for professional and amateur golfers.
  - Amateur golfers most often injure the lower back and elbow with conflicting evidence on the most common site (13–15).
  - In amateurs, 25% of injuries are from overuse, 21% are from hitting the ground with the club during the swing, and 19% are from poor swing mechanics (16).

- Professional golfers most frequently injure the lower back, followed by nondominant wrist and shoulder injuries. Professional golfers report fewer elbow injuries than their amateur counterparts (13,14).
- About 85% of professional injuries occurred secondary to overuse, 12% occurred from hitting the ground during the swing, and 5% occurred from twisting the trunk (excessive torque) during the swing (17).

- It is unclear whether stretching for increased flexibility prevents golf injury (18).
- Data supporting golf-specific warm-up regimens are lacking. Expert opinion recommends dynamic stretching or activity during warm-up while avoiding static stretching (19).
- Golfers walk between 8 and 11 km during 18 holes of golf, although the individual course may affect the total distance walked. Riding in a golf cart reduces the distance walked to 3 km (3).

SPECIFIC ISSUES

Environmental Risks

- Long grass areas along the course and the edges of woods where the ball may land increase the risk of contact with snakes, ticks, and certain plants known to cause hypersensitivity reactions (such as poison ivy) (20).
- Golf course water hazards in certain areas may harbor bacteria that can cause illnesses such as leptospirosis (20).
- Golf is an outdoor sport; therefore, heat and cold injuries can and do occur on the course.
- Poorly heat-acclimated golfers traveling to warmer environments are at higher risk for heat-related illnesses (20).
  - Alcohol consumption while playing golf can increase the risk of heat injury (18).
- Golfers die from lightning strikes more than any other sport except for fishing (21,22).
  - When the risk of lightning strikes is elevated, golfers should seek shelter in a closed, covered building (clubhouse) or closed vehicle (car) and play should not resume until the threat of lightning has passed.
  - Actions to avoid include sheltering under isolated groups of trees (particularly single trees), standing under or holding metal poles (clubs), remaining in open fields or near open water, sheltering in open vehicles (golf carts), or sheltering in open shelters (sheds, umbrellas).
  - Most lightning strike deaths occur due to cardiac arrest; therefore, Advanced Cardiac Life Support (ACLS) with early defibrillation should be employed (21).

Golf Cart Injuries

- Golf carts as an optional component of play are unique to golf; however, their use for non–golf-related purposes is increasing. Data from 2007 to 2017 estimates over 150,000 golf cart-related injuries, although many injuries do not occur on the golf course (23).
- Current models can reach 20–25 miles · h^{-1} and may be legal on public roads in certain areas. However, safety regulations and golf cart safety features (lack of seat belts and helmets, rear brakes only with rolling front tires) are not tightly regulated (24,25).
- Falling or jumping from the golf cart comprised 47.0% of injuries, followed by struck/run over (14.3%), cart overturning (13.0%), and collision (11.8%) (23).
- The mean and median ages for golf cart injuries is 35 and 28 respectively; however, children (under 16) made up 36.5%–42.9% of golf cart injuries (23,24).
  - Child injuries most frequently involve the head and neck (42.6%), involving face, mouth, head, or neck injuries.
  - Ejection from the golf cart is the mechanism for 61.7% of injuries in children (24).
- Golf cart-related adult injuries frequently involve excessive alcohol intake during the course of play (24,25).

MEDICAL ISSUES

Eye and Head Injuries

- Golf accounts for 1.2%–7.7% of sports-related eye injuries but up to 13.8% of sports-related enucleations, suggesting that golf-related eye injuries are uncommon but can be severe when they occur (26).
- Environmental factors (tree branches, sand, dirt, grass, and rocks) accounted for the majority (37.7%) of golf eye injuries, followed by strikes from golf balls (22.3%) and strikes from golf clubs (18.8%) (27).
- In the pediatric population, golf club strikes encompassed 44.1% of injuries (27). This is believed to be due to children playing too close together or being inadequately supervised during play (26).
- Contusions or corneal abrasions accounted for 50.4% of golf eye injuries, followed by foreign body 9.0% and irritation/inflammation (8.0%) (27).
- The wearing of polycarbonate lenses during golf has been suggested for protection against eye injury during play, but this recommendation is not well established (26).
- The word "fore" is typically yelled by golfers to alert others to the potential of a ball heading the way of another golfer. The typical response, turning toward the person yelling "fore," is not recommended. Turning away and crouching down with the hands covering the face is recommended (13).

Skin Disorders

- Golf is a sport played in an outdoor setting with minimal sun protection available on the course. Golfers spend the majority of their time in sunny locations on the course and often play in the middle of the day when the ultraviolet (UV) light is most damaging to the skin (28).

- Reflection of UV rays from surfaces varies across the golf course: grass (1%–2%), water (5%–7%), and sand (20%–30%) (28).
- Prevention recommendations include golfers protecting exposed skin with sunscreens (SPF of 15 or higher) and protective clothing that blocks these harmful UV rays (long-sleeve shirts, pants, and wide-brim hats).
  - Tightly woven fabrics provide increased sun protection.
  - Baseball-style caps do not protect the ears or the back of the neck (28,29).
- UV radiation is most intense during midday hours of 10 AM–4 PM (daylight savings) or 9 AM–3 PM (standard time) and exposure can be further reduced by limiting play during peak UV radiation hours (midday), staying in the shade when possible, and reapplying sunscreen every 2 hours (or more often with heavy sweating or toweling off (28,29).
- Eye sun exposure risk can be reduced with UV-blocking sunglasses during play (29).

Neurologic and Psychological Disorders

- The yips or "golfer's cramps" are intermittent involuntary motor disturbances that can affect both amateur and professional golfers. This disorder is described as jerking, tremors, or spasms, most commonly present during putting or chipping (30).
- The pathophysiology of yips is not well understood. Traditional thought attributes yips to performance anxiety, although there is growing evidence that yips are a focal task-specific dystonia. No medications have strong evidence of benefit. Botulinum toxin injections have been proposed to treat hand dystonias; however, high-quality data are lacking (30–32).
- A Japanese survey-based study with 1497 respondents (92% response) found that 39% of the golfers in the study reported prior yips. Those with yips had statistically significantly more time playing golf and more severe musculoskeletal issues than those without yips. Putting was the most common club and situation for yips (54%) (31).

MUSCULOSKELETAL ISSUES

Lower Back Injuries

- The lower back is a common injury location in professional and amateur golfers (prevalence 15%–35% in amateurs and 55% in professionals) (33).
- The lumbar spine rotates, side bends, compresses, flexes, and hyperextends during the golf swings, applying asymmetric stress to the spine. These movements result in lateral bending, shear, compression, and torque forces. The shear and torque forces are 80% higher in the amateur compared to the professional golfer (4,12,14).
- Despite professional golfers having a more efficient and smoother swing than their amateur counterparts, professional golfers still have the highest incidence of lower back pain of all professional sports (14).
- The biomechanics behind golf-related lower back pain is not currently well understood (33,34). Although the modern swing ends the follow-through phase in the "reverse C" (lumbar hyperextension) and the so-called "Crunch factor" describes the lumbar lateral bending that takes place during the swing (11,35).
  - Both reverse C and "crunch factor" can be more pronounced in amateur golfers. Explanations for this difference include inadequate weight transfer during the swing, a more varied stance, leaning away from the ball at impact and follow-through, and less hip turn than allowed in the classic swing (4,11,13,14).
- The golf swing can produce eight times the body weight loads on the lumbar spine. These forces put golfers at risk for muscle strains, herniated nucleus pulposus (HNP), facet arthropathies, and spondylosis/spondylolisthesis (36).
- Golf bags are traditionally carried on one shoulder, leading to asymmetric loading (18).
- Newer bags have the ability for two-shoulder carry or the use of a rolling pull cart. In additional, most golf carts have an area for carrying golf bags.
- Most golf-related lower back injuries can be managed conservatively, with greater than 90% of patients recovering in 4 weeks after injury; however, typical "red flags" in the evaluation of back pain should prompt a more complete workup (4,11,35).
- As part of conservative management of golf-related lower back pain, consider core-strengthening exercises with or without formal physical therapy and review golf swing mechanics on return to play. Care by a physician, therapist, and professional golf instructor at return to play has been shown to produce a 98% rate of no new golf injuries at year on return (35).
- Changing to a more classic swing may also remove some of the problematic forces that result from the modern swing (11).
- Stress fractures of the ribs, attributed in literature to the weakness of the serratus anterior, have been reported in golfers (35).
- Two small survey-based case series (*N* = 34 and *N* = 13) revealed that 50% of golfers returned to play 12 months after spinal fusion surgery, with approximately 50% returning to practice by around 6 months (36–38).

Shoulder Injuries

- Shoulder injuries account for 8%–12% of golf injuries, with overuse injuries predominating. The nondominant shoulder is typically affected due to its range of motion going through internal rotation, adduction, abduction, and external rotation during the swing (8,14).

- The acromioclavicular (AC) joint is the most often injured area, followed by impingement and rotator cuff tendinopathy, posterior glenohumeral subluxation, rotator cuff tears, and glenohumeral arthritis (10,14).
- The AC joint is compressed during the backswing on the nondominant side and may cause shoulder pain. This is especially true in older golfers (20).
- Treatment of the degenerative AC joint includes shortening the backswing and weight training with a focus on the rotator cuff muscles. Reviewing swing mechanics may also be beneficial (20).
- The nondominant shoulder is more sensitive than the dominant shoulder to impingement and rotator cuff damage that will negatively affect the golf swing (20).
- A systematic review meta-analysis including 859 athletes, including golfers in the pooled data, revealed that 85% of athletes undergoing rotator cuff repair returned to sports, with 65% returning to an equivalent level of play. However, among professional and competitive athletes, only 50% returned to the same level of play (39).
- Golfers who undergo total shoulder arthroplasty (TSA) to either the dominant or nondominant shoulder or both shoulders may return to sport safely as early as 6 months post-procedure with a mean visual analog scale improvement of 4.3 points. In one study, 75% of patients returned to golf pain-free (5).
- The effect on improved play is most pronounced with TSA on the dominant shoulder compared to the nondominant shoulder, with small but statistically significant improvements in driving distance and stroke handicap (12.5 yards and 1.4 strokes) (5,40).
- Golf may be resumed after shoulder hemiarthroplasty (HA) and reverse shoulder arthroplasty (RSA), although sports-specific outcomes do not appear as positive as with TSA (5).
- Shoulder instability is a rare problem in golfers and is usually found in the younger golfer with generalized joint laxity (1).

Elbow Injuries

- Amateur golfers are more likely to have elbow injuries compared to professionals (41).
- The term "golfer's elbow" refers to medial epicondylosis, usually in the dominant hand, although most amateur golfing elbow injuries occur in the lateral nondominant elbow ("tennis elbow"). Eighty-five percent of all golf elbow injuries occur in the lateral aspect (13).
- Minimal stress is placed on the elbows and forearms during the swing take away. Most stress on the elbow occurs during the impact with the ball (or the ground in the event of a fat shot) (41).
- Reasons for injury include overuse, poor swing mechanics, and contact with objects other than the ball, such as the ground and rocks (13).
- Medial epicondylitis can occur for a variety of reasons, including striking the ground before the ball and hitting off of hard surfaces and practice mats (14).
- Tennis elbow is associated with gripping the club too tightly and forceful contraction of nondominant extensors during the impact phase of the swing (14).
- Three common therapies for these elbow injuries are counterforce bracing, equipment modification, and physical therapy.
    - Counterforce bracing can help provide a reactive force against the contractile muscle, and either spread the force over a wider area or decrease the contractile pull on the epicondyle (14,41).
    - Equipment changes such as graphite shafts can help decrease the force applied to the forearm by decreasing the amount of vibration at impact (41).
    - Physical therapy can focus on forearm muscle strength, flexibility, and endurance (41).

Hand and Wrist Injuries

- The nondominant hand and wrist are injured more frequently than the dominant wrist because of increased stress during the swing with more forceful impact when ground contact occurs (1,12,42).
- Overuse tendinopathies are the most common problems seen in the golfer's wrist and are typically secondary to the repetitive movements generated during the golf swing and stress at impact.
    - Higher-level golfers tend to experience overuse from frequent swing repetition during practice sessions. In contrast, amateur golfers experience overuse from poor swing mechanics and traumatic injuries from striking the ground or trees during the swing (42).
- De Quervain tenosynovitis involving the first dorsal compartment is a common condition affecting golfers, even those with good swing mechanics. Ulnar deviation of the nondominant wrist at ball impact and repeated impact between the club and the ground may trap the nondominant thumb between the trailing hand and shaft, thus stressing the tendons in the first dorsal compartment. Poor swing mechanics may also lead to premature uncocking of the wrist at the beginning of the downswing rather than during acceleration and ball strike resulting in ulnar deviation of the nondominant wrist too early in the swing (2,41).
    - Treatment of de Quervain tenosynovitis usually involves swing modification and conservative therapy, with corticosteroid injections and surgery reserved for when conservative measures have failed (2).
- Improper swing mechanics may injure other tendon groups, including the extensor carpi ulnaris of the nondominant

arm and flexor carpi radialis and ulnaris of the dominant arm (1,14).

- Amateurs are more likely to hit a "fat" shot, defined as the club head striking the ground too far behind the ball, specifically impacting these tendon groups. Disruption of the extensor carpi ulnaris (ECU) tendon sheath in the nondominant wrist, most commonly occurs with fat shots (13,42).
- Triangular fibrocartilage complex (TFCC) tears occur due to repetitive rotational movements of the wrist or with the striking of the wrist during the swing (2,42).
- Hook of the hamate fractures, the most common fracture in golf, occur with impingement between the hand and the club handle (butt of the club), more common in the nondominant hand, occurring most commonly when the club strikes the ground (42).
  - Accounting for only 2% of all wrist fractures, 33% of hamate fractures are found in golfers (41,43).
  - The "carpal tunnel view" is the best x-ray to visualize a hamate fracture. If it is not visible on plain film and is still suspected, then a computed tomography (CT) scan is the image of choice. Preventive measures include proper club length with the butt of the club extending slightly beyond the palm of the leading hand rather than digging into the hypothenar eminence (42).
- Peripheral nerve compression can occur at the carpal tunnel and Guyon canal due to repetitive impingement from the club handle (butt of the club), particularly in the nondominant hand (2).

Hip Injuries

- There is minimal literature on hip injuries in golf.
- In one survey study involving 703 professional and amateur golfers, hip injuries accounted for only 2.8% of all injuries reported. The study did not comment further on the nature of those injuries (44).
- Golf can be safely played following total hip arthroplasty (45).

Knee Injuries

- Despite being a low-impact sport, knee injuries make up 3%–18% of golf injuries with poor technique and overuse being the cause of many golf-related knee injuries (12,46).
- The dominant knee receives peak force during the backswing, followed by the transfer of force to the nondominant knee during the impact and follow-through (14).
- Osteoarthritis of the knees needs to be taken into consideration during the evaluation of the knee pain with older golfers (14).
- Golf can safely be played with decreased pain following dominant or nondominant knee arthroplasty, although some patients may have continued pain while or after playing golf (14,46).
- The low-impact nature of golf makes the sport a favorable sport following arthroplasty, although post-surgical rates of return to golf may be as low as 30%–57% (46).
- For those who do return to playing golf, there may be a slight increase in the average number of plays per month. The effect of arthroplasty on handicap strokes and drive length is unclear (46,47).
- Patients undergoing unicompartmental arthroplasty may return to golf at higher rates (46).
- Lower extremity fatigue may place golfers, particularly older or poorly conditioned participants, at risk of injury during later holes; therefore, decreased walking or avoiding uneven terrain may be recommended in selected individuals (46).
- Other knee injuries, such as strains, can be caused by a combination of environmental factors, such as hilly terrain and wet grass, causing a player to slip while walking.

Event Management

- Golf matches and tournaments may be multiple-day events, starting early in the day and ending in the late afternoon or dusk, on courses that can exceed 100 acres in size (21).
- Injuries to the golfers may be acute or acute exacerbations of existing chronic injuries. Treatment and return-to-play considerations for golfers are no different from other sports, with the athlete's safety being paramount.
  - At higher-level events, secure areas should be available for athletes, with staffing appropriate for the expected injuries, which are more commonly overused in higher-level competition (21).
- Event coverage planning must account for all players, caddies, and spectators at the event, as caddies and spectators frequently move along the course with the players.
  - Players, caddies, and spectators are all exposed to the same environmental conditions (*e.g.*, heat, cold, lightning, sun exposure, and wet conditions) and contingencies must be in place should environmental injuries occur (21).
- Lightning is of particular concern for spectators as there is little protection on golf courses, and encouraging large groups to seek adequate shelter voluntarily can be difficult (21).
  - Because lightning can be up to 10 miles before or after rain, lightning detection systems are recommended, especially if large crowds are expected. Sirens and air horns may be employed to warn of impending dangers.
  - The 30-30 rule states that individuals should seek shelter when thunder is heard within 30 seconds of seeing lightning (6 miles away), and activity should resume only 30 minutes after the last thunder or lightning is noted. The adage that lightning is one mile away for every second between seeing lightning and hearing thunder is inaccurate and should not be used (48).

- All should seek shelter as per the environmental hazards section earlier in the chapter (Chapter 48 of this text). Buses can be considered for shelter if building space is inadequate for the crowd.
- Particularly in large event preparations, arrangements will need to be made for dedicated medical team communication and mobility capabilities appropriate for large crowds (bicycles, golf carts, etc.) (21).
- The need for automated external defibrillators (AED) and coordination with local emergency services before the event is no different from other sporting events (21).
- Alcohol consumption is common for spectators and sometimes for athletes during the course of play (21).

REFERENCES

1. Mellion MB, Walsh WM, Shelton GL. *The Team Physician's Handbook*. 2nd ed. Philadelphia (PA): Mosby; 1996. 910 p.
2. Woo SH, Lee YK, Kim JM, Cheon HJ, Chung WH. Hand and wrist injuries in golfers and their treatment. *Hand Clin*. 2017 Feb;33(1):81–96.
3. Luscombe J, Murray AD, Jenkins E, Archibald D. A rapid review to identify physical activity accrued while playing golf. *BMJ Open*. 2017 Nov 28;7(11):e018993.
4. Fu FH, Stone DA. *Sports Injuries*. 2nd ed. Philadelphia (PA): Lippincott Williams & Wilkins; 2001. 1264 p.
5. Salem HS, Park DH, Thon SG, et al. Return to golf after shoulder arthroplasty: a systematic review. *Am J Sports Med*. 2021 Mar;49(4):1109–15.
6. National Golf Foundation. *Participation Rises Again*. Accessed 2023 Mar 12. Available from: https://www.ngf.org/participation-rises-again/
7. National Golf Foundation. *Golf's Biggest Participation Jump*. Accessed 2023 Mar 12. Available from: https://www.ngf.org/golfs-biggest-participation-jump/
8. Murray AD, Daines L, Archibald D, et al. The relationships between golf and health: a scoping review. *Br J Sports Med*. 2017 Jan;51(1):12–19.
9. Puterbaugh JS. A good walk spoiled: on the disappearance of golf as an active sport in America. *Curr Sports Med Rep*. 2011 Jul;10(4):228–32.
10. Sorbie GG, Beaumont AJ, Williams AK, Lavallee D. Golf and physical health: a systematic review. *Sports Med*. 2022 Dec;52(12):2943–63.
11. Gluck GS, Bendo JA, Spivak JM. The lumbar spine and low back pain in golf: a literature review of swing biomechanics and injury prevention. *Spine J*. 2008;8(5):778–88.
12. Zouzias IC, Hendra J, Stodelle J, Limpisvasti O. Golf injuries: epidemiology, pathophysiology, and treatment. *J Am Acad Orthop Surg*. 2018 Feb 15;26(4):116–23.
13. McHardy A, Pollard H, Luo K. Golf injuries: a review of the literature. *Sports Med*. 2006;36(2):171–87.
14. Wadsworth LT. When golf hurts: musculoskeletal problems common to golfers. *Curr Sports Med Rep*. 2007;6(6):362–5.
15. Wiesler ER, Lumsden B. Golf injuries of the upper extremity. *J Surg Orthop Adv*. 2005;14(1):1–7.
16. McCarroll JR, Rettig AC, Shelbourne KD. Injuries in the amateur golfer. *Phys Sportsmed*. 1990;18(3):122–6.
17. McCarroll JR, Gioe TJ. Professional golfers and the price they pay. *Phys Sportsmed*. 1982;10(7):64–70.
18. Brandon B, Pearce PZ. Training to prevent golf injury. *Curr Sports Med Rep*. 2009;8(3):142–6.
19. Ehlert A, Wilson PB. A systematic review of golf warm-ups: behaviors, injury, and performance. *J Strength Cond Res*. 2019 Dec;33(12):3444–62.
20. Flaherty G, Udoeyop I, Whooley P, Jones M. Avoiding the rough: travel health risks facing golf tourists. *J Travel Med*. 2017 May 1;24(3):taw100.
21. Wadsworth LT. Sideline and event management in golf. *Curr Sports Med Rep*. 2011 May-Jun;10(3):131–3.
22. Cherington M. Lightning injuries in sports: situations to avoid. *Sports Med*. 2001;31(4):301–8.
23. Horvath KZ, McAdams RJ, Roberts KJ, Zhu M, McKenzie LB. Fun ride or risky transport: golf cart-related injuries treated in U.S. emergency departments from 2007 through 2017. *J Safety Res*. 2020 Dec;75:1–7.
24. Miller B, Yelverton E, Monico J, Replogle W, Jordan JR. Pediatric head and neck injuries due to golf cart trauma. *Int J Pediatr Otorhinolaryngol*. 2016 Sep;88:38–41.
25. Sciarretta JD, Harris T, Romano A, Davis BD, Pepe A. Golf cart-related injuries: a community at risk. *Am Surg*. 2016 Jan;82(1):E36–7.
26. Crane ES, Kolomeyer AM, Kim E, Chu DS. Comprehensive review of golf-related ocular injuries. *Retina*. 2016 Jul;36(7):1237–43.
27. Kim EJ, Ganga A, Rana V, et al. A 20-year nationwide analysis of golf-associated eye injuries in the United States. *Am J Emerg Med*. 2022 Nov;61:175–8.
28. U.S. Department of Health and Human Services. *The Surgeon General's Call to Action to Prevent Skin Cancer; U.S. Department of Health and Human Services*. Washington (DC): Office of the Surgeon General; 2014.
29. Weikert AE, Pagoto SL, Handley E, Courtney JB, Brunke-Reese D, Conroy DE. Golfers' interest in multilevel sun-protection strategies. *Int J Environ Res Public Health*. 2021 Jul 7;18(14):7253.
30. Dhungana S, Jankovic J. Yips and other movement disorders in golfers. *Mov Disord*. 2013 May;28(5):576–81.
31. Gon Y, Kabata D, Kawamura S, et al. Association of the yips and musculoskeletal problems in highly skilled golfers: a large scale epidemiological study in Japan. *Sports (Basel)*. 2021 May 21;9(6):71.
32. Adler CH, Temkit M, Crews D, et al. The yips: methods to identify golfers with a dystonic Etiology/Golfer's cramp. *Med Sci Sports Exerc*. 2018 Nov;50(11):2226–30.
33. Cole MH, Grimshaw PN. The biomechanics of the modern golf swing: implications for lower back injuries. *Sports Med*. 2016 Mar;46(3):339–51.
34. Quinn SL, Olivier B, McKinon W, Dafkin C. Increased trunk muscle recruitment during the golf swing is linked to developing lower back pain: a prospective longitudinal cohort study. *J Electromyogr Kinesiol*. 2022 Jun;64:102663.
35. Reed JJ, Wadsworth LT. Lower back pain in golf: a review. *Curr Sports Med Rep*. 2010;9(1):57–9.
36. Shifflett GD, Hellman MD, Louie PK, Mikhail C, Park KU, Phillips FM. Return to golf after lumbar fusion. *Sports Health*. 2017 May/Jun;9(3):280–4.
37. Luxenburg D, Bondar KJ, Cohen LL, Constantinescu D, Barnhill S, Donnally CJ III. Return to golf following cervical and lumbar spinal fusion: a systematic review. *World Neurosurg*. 2021 Dec;156:4–10.
38. Jain NS, Lin CC, Halim A, et al. Return to recreational sport following lumbar fusion. *Clin Spine Surg*. 2020 May;33(4):E174–7.
39. Klouche S, Lefevre N, Herman S, Gerometta A, Bohu Y. Return to sport after rotator cuff tear repair: a systematic review and meta-analysis. *Am J Sports Med*. 2016 Jul;44(7):1877–87.
40. Papaliodis D, Richardson N, Tartaglione J, Roberts T, Whipple R, Zanaros G. Impact of total shoulder arthroplasty on golfing activity. *Clin J Sport Med*. 2015 Jul;25(4):338–40.
41. McCarroll JR. Overuse injuries of the upper extremity in golf. *Clin Sports Med*. 2001;20(3):469–79.
42. Ek ET, Suh N, Weiland AJ. Hand and wrist injuries in golf. *J Hand Surg Am*. 2013 Oct;38(10):2029–33.
43. Bayes MC, Wadsworth LT. Upper extremity injuries in golf. *Phys Sportsmed*. 2009;37(1):92–6.

44. Gosheger G, Liem D, Ludwig K, Greshake O, Winkelmann W. Injuries and overuse syndromes in golf. *Am J Sports Med*. 2003;31(3):438–43.
45. Swanson EA, Schmalzried TP, Dorey FJ. Activity recommendations after total hip and knee arthroplasty: a survey of the American Association for Hip and Knee Surgeons. *J Arthroplasty*. 2009;24(6 suppl l):120–6.
46. Baker ML, Epari DR, Lorenzetti S, Sayers M, Boutellier U, Taylor WR. Risk factors for knee injury in golf: a systematic review. *Sports Med*. 2017 Dec;47(12):2621–39.
47. Gorbaty JD, Rao AJ, Varkey DT, Muña K, Saltzman BM, Hamid N. Total joint arthroplasty and golf play: analysis of regional golf handicap database. *J Am Acad Orthop Surg*. 2021 May 15;29(10):e513–17.
48. Thomson EM, Howard TM. Lightning injuries in sports and recreation. *Curr Sports Med Rep*. 2013 Mar-Apr;12(2):120–4.

Gymnastics

Joey Bonanno, Ian Thomas, Ellen Casey, and Marcia Faustin

107

INTRODUCTION

- Gymnastics is a popular sport in the United States and worldwide. USA Gymnastics club membership (level 3–10 + elite) statistics report a total of 128,465 participants during the 2020–2021 season (1).
  - Women's Artistic Program: ~105,000
  - Men's Artistic Program: ~10,600
  - Rhythmic Program: ~3800
  - Acrobatic Program: ~2000
  - Trampoline & Tumbling Program: ~6000
  - Gymnastics for Adults Program: ~1800
- ~1500 athletes participate in the National Collegiate Athletic Association gymnastics each year (NCAA Sports Sponsorship and Participation Rates Report) (2).
- Gymnastics training begins at a very young age, typically involving rigorous hours. The average age at onset is 5–6 years for girls and 6–7 years for boys (3).
  - Most girls reach their highest competitive level by age 16. Caine et al. postulated that female gymnasts peak at an earlier age than athletes in most other sports due to the biomechanical demands for a small, lean, and prepubertal physique (4). However, the average age of female artistic gymnasts continues to increase, with the median age for the 2020 Olympics being in their 20s (5), suggesting that prior expectations of peaking at early ages may have been due to tradition and beliefs rather than based on science and physiology.
  - Peak performance for males is often at a later age because of the requirements for greater levels of strength that occur after puberty (6).

EPIDEMIOLOGY

- Table 107.1 highlights many of the epidemiologic considerations across the various gymnastics disciplines.

EVENTS

- Gymnastics involves seven disciplines recognized by Fédération Internationale de Gymnastique (FIG; International Gymnastics Federation): Men's Artistic, Women's Artistic, Rhythmic, Aerobic, Tumbling & Trampoline, Acrobatic, Aerobic, and Parkour (20).
  - Men's artistic gymnastics:
    - Involves six events: floor exercise, pommel horse, still rings, vault, parallel bars, and horizontal bar.
  - Women's artistic gymnastics involves four events: vault, uneven bars, balance beam, and floor exercise.
  - Trampoline & tumbling:
    - Four events: power tumbling, trampoline, synchronized trampoline, and double-mini trampoline.
    - Trampoline first became an Olympic sport at the 2000 Olympic Games (1); however, double-mini trampoline and power tumbling are not competed at the Olympic level.
  - Rhythmic:
    - Six events: rope, hoop, ball, clubs, ribbon, and group.
    - Rhythmic gymnastics requires significant flexibility, artistry, and agility, and only involves female competitors only at the Olympic level (1).
    - Given the simultaneous hyperextension and rotation seen in rhythmic gymnastics elements, these athletes are at a unique risk for spine-related injuries (21).
  - Acrobatic
    - Five events: women's pair, men's pair, mixed pair, women's group, and men's group.
    - Acrobatic gymnastics is not currently an Olympic sport but involves various acrobatic and dance elements performed with choreography (1).
  - Aerobic
    - Performance by individuals and groups; emphasis on strength, flexibility, and aerobic fitness.
    - Aerobic gymnastics is not currently an Olympic sport.

Table 107.1 Epidemiologic Considerations in Gymnastics

Discipline	Epidemiologic Considerations

Men's Artistic	• Overall prevalence: 0.7 injuries per gymnast (7).
	• Among elite male gymnasts:
	  • Training injury rate: 27.1 injuries per 1000 gymnasts (8).
	  • Competition injury rate: 58.5 per 1000 gymnasts (8).
	  • Additionally, data has shown a 3.2 times greater injury rate at the USA National Championships and Olympic trials compared to National Championships Qualifier meets (8).
	• Men's collegiate injury rate: 8.78 injuries per 1000 athlete exposures (9).

Women's Artistic	Female Artistic:
	• Overall injury rate: 0.3–3.6 injuries per gymnast (7).
	  • The competition injury rate is 1.67 times the practice injury rate (10).
	• Woman's collegiate injury rate: 9.37 per 1000 athlete exposures (11).
	  • 2nd highest injury rates (6.1 injuries per 1000 athlete exposures) (12).
	  • Highest rates of ACL injury (0.33 per 1000 AEs, equal to football) (13) and stress fractures (25.6 per 1000 AEs) (14).
	Highest rates of Achilles tendon injuries (15,16).

Rhythmic[a]	• Injury rate: 73.4 (±30.2) per 1000 gymnasts (At the Olympic level) (17).
Trampoline &Tumbling[a]	Injury rate: 52.6 (±44.9) injuries per 1000 trampoline athletes (At the Olympic level) (17).
Parkour[a]	• 50% of injuries involve the upper and lower extremities (18).
Gender Differences	Female gymnasts are more likely to undergo surgery and have longer time to return to sport compared to their male counterparts (11,16).
Injury Location	• Lower-limb injuries are more common than upper-limb injuries in both men's and women's gymnastics (7,8,17).
Specific Events	• Floor exercise and vaulting are associated with the highest injury rates in artistic gymnastics (7,8,10,19). Floor exercise has the greatest association with acute injuries (7,10).

[a]More research and data collection are needed to further define injury prevalence in the disciplines of rhythmic gymnastics, tumbling & trampoline, acrobatic gymnastics, and parkour.

- Parkour
  - Parkour is rooted in military obstacle course training and martial arts, and involves various acrobatic movements to get from point A to point B (22).
  - Parkour was first developed in France in the 1990s as a method to overcome obstacles in urban and natural environments (22). The sport was officially recognized as a discipline by the FIG Executive Committee in 2017.
  - In 2020, USA Gymnastics participated in the first FIG Parkour World Championship (1).
  - The events in parkour include men and women's speed and freestyle divisions (1).

RULES AND EQUIPMENT

- In gymnastics, the code of points dictates the degree of difficulty for each skill and evolves with the sport. It is revised every 4 years, increasing the level of difficulty.
- Special equipment used by gymnasts includes grips with or without wooden dowels for uneven bars, high bars and rings, beam shoes, and wrist supports. Gymnasts may also train using varied cushioned mats, foam pits, beam and bar pads, low balance beams, Tumble Trak, rod floor, and twisting or spotting belts.

RISK FACTORS FOR INJURY

- Gymnastics is a sport with historically accepted early specialization, which can lead to excessive training loads and a lack of periodization are proposed risk factors for injury. Gymnastics training also has physiological benefits.

Intrinsic Risk Factors

- Age and Adolescent growth spurt: Rapid changes in height alter the moment of inertia of certain skills, requiring gymnasts to make gradual adjustments to technique.
  - Two early studies indicated an increased risk of gymnastics injury during age or maturity periods associated with rapid growth affecting articular cartilage and physes (23,24).
  - These studies have since been corroborated by multiple studies both within and without the sport of gymnastics (25–27).
- Sex: In both men's and women's gymnastics lower-limb injuries are more common than upper-limb injuries (7,8,17), but the distribution of injuries varies by gender, with male gymnasts having a greater proportion of upper extremity injuries (42.8%) than female gymnasts (30.8%) (20) likely a result of differences in the competitive events.
  - A recent study by Tisano in 2022 studying pediatric gymnastics injuries reported in United States Emergency Medicine Departments demonstrated upper extremity injuries predominating among childhood gymnasts,

particularly female gymnasts, and in adolescence, the rates of concussion, foot, and ankle injuries increased (28).

- Female artistic gymnastics had the highest rates of ACL injury (13), stress fracture (14), and Achilles tendon injuries (11,15), and female gymnasts were more likely to undergo surgery and have a longer recovery compared to male gymnasts (11,16).

- Previous injury: A 2010 study by Kolt and Caine reported 24.5%–32.3% of all injuries affected female artistic gymnasts. Caine reported reinjury rates of 32.7% in 1 year (29), and as many as one in four injuries is a reinjury (4).
- Prior injury was implicated as a significant predictor of overuse injury in young female gymnasts (30), with the lumbar back as the most common site of recurrent injury in female gymnasts (29).
  - The high rates of reinjury in gymnasts are felt to be due to premature return to training and inadequate rehabilitation (29).
- Psychosocial factors: Gymnastics training often involves many hours as well as years of commitment.
  - Studies have reported increased life stress was associated with the number and severity of injuries (31,32) as well as higher negative life stress among those who are injured compared to their noninjured counterparts (33).
  - More recently, studies have shown an increased correlation between anxiety and depression in individual-oriented sports as compared to team-oriented sports (34).
  - In addition, collegiate gymnastics, which places greater emphasis on team success over individual performance, may be protective (34).

Extrinsic Factors

- Biomechanics
  - Gymnasts perform over 200 landings and dismounts weekly, placing significant loads on the athletes' bodies, predisposing them to injury (35).
  - Due to the forces of repetitive loading, floor exercise has been shown to be associated with the most injuries in both men's and women's artistic gymnastics (7,8,10,19).
  - Biomechanical studies have demonstrated that the spring floor can place forces up to 15 times the gymnast's body weight on the lower extremity (36,37).
  - Specifically, studies have shown most spontaneous Achilles ruptures occur on the back-tumbling back handspring take-off (15).
  - In addition to floor exercise, twisting-associated landings pose a significant risk for lower-extremity injury, especially where there is incomplete rotation while landing (12).
- Competition: Previous studies have demonstrated that the incidence, when calculated per exposure, is two to three times higher for competition (23,38,39). More recently, studies demonstrated competition injury rates of 1.67 times that of practice injury rates in women's artistic gymnastics and a competition injury rate of 58.5 per 1000 elite male gymnasts (compared to a training injury rate of 27.1 per 1000 gymnasts), respectively (8,10). O'Kane cited higher pressure to perform, travel, different equipment, and environment inherent in traveling to a competition, as additional potential factors contributing to higher competition injury rates (19).
- Early sport specialization: Specialization in any single sport prior to puberty is an independent risk factor for injury (9).
  - The majority of gymnasts specialize by age 8 (40).
  - More research regarding the potential detrimental effects of early sport specialization in gymnasts is still needed.
- High training volume: Jayanthi et al report that training in any single sport for more hours per week than the athlete's chronological age confers an increased risk of overuse injuries than those who train fewer hours (9).
  - Preadolescent and adolescent gymnasts frequently train 20+ $h \cdot wk^{-1}$ (29,41), while Level 9 and 10 athletes often train from 24 to 36 $h \cdot wk^{-1}$, and elite athletes train 30–42 $h \cdot wk^{-1}$
  - A retrospective study of USA Gymnastics (USAG) National Team elite-level athletes comparing training interruptions due to COVID-19 by Casey et al. reported a mean training time of 23.2 ± 9.2 $h \cdot wk^{-1}$ before the pandemic (42).
- Lack of periodization: The year-round training associated with gymnastics and involvement of skills that require early technical development increases the risk of gymnastics-related injury (43,44).
- Level of competition: Prior studies have found that gymnasts at advanced or elite levels suffer more injuries (23,29,38,39,45) possibly due to an increased number of training hours and increased skill difficulty (17,33). A 2015 study by Saluan et al demonstrated the injury rate per 1000 exposure hours in female gymnasts was 2.86 for elite gymnasts, 2.82 for high-level gymnasts, 1.67 for intermediate gymnasts, and 0.69 for novice gymnasts (46).

INJURY PREVENTION

- Many of the recommendations for minimizing injuries are adapted from early specialization research done in other sports and may be challenging to follow these recommendations due to the nature of the sport of gymnastics (minimal cross-training).
  - Train fewer hours per week than athlete's chronological age (41).
  - Encourage cross-training before puberty (41).
  - Alternating swinging and support-type movements may reduce wrist loading (47).

- Periodize conditioning regimens:
  - Goal is to maximize training adaptations and prevent the onset of overtraining syndrome (48).
  - Periodized stretch training was more advantageous to increasing flexibility and improving performance (49).
  - Increases in training loads should be very gradual and perhaps reduced during periods of rapid growth (24).

MEDICAL ISSUES

Low Energy Availability/Female Athlete Triad/Relative Energy Deficiency in Sport

- The female and male athlete triad (Triad) was originally defined in 1992 and 2017, respectively by the interplay between low energy availability, hypothalamic-pituitary-gonadal suppression, and impaired bone health (50–52).
- In 2014 the International Olympic Committee (IOC) introduced "Relative Energy Deficiency in Sport" (RED-S), which aimed to expand the triad to include impairments in metabolic rate, immunity, protein synthesis, and cardiovascular health (53).
- Risk factors include lean and aesthetic sports participation, perfectionism, early sport specialization, drive for thinness, and inadequate nutrition (40,54).
- Although the exact prevalence is unknown, female gymnasts, similar to other female athletes in sports (especially if aesthetics and leanness are emphasized), are at risk for developing low energy availability and the related conditions within the spectrum of the triad (51,55,56).
  - It is important to note that many gymnasts with the Triad/RED-S still have normal bone mineral density despite chronically low energy availability and menstrual dysfunction (see bone accrual below).
  - RED-S is further elaborated upon in Chapters 12 (Nutrition) and 131 (The Female Athlete).

Bone Accrual

- Gymnastics training also has physiological benefits, which have been shown to be osteogenic for bone development and which may overcome the negative influence of high training volume and low energy balance (57,58).
  - After 1 year of specific gymnastics training, there were favorable effects in prepubertal female gymnasts (59).
  - Early puberty seems to be the most sensitive period for maximizing bone mineral gain.
    - Recreational gymnastics, attainable by most children, has a positive influence on bone development (60).
    - Dose-response relationship between gymnastics exposure and bone mass (61).
    - 40% of peak bone was accrued in a 5-year window surrounding the attainment of peak height velocity (62).
  - Health benefits more marked after menarche in females (63).
    - Higher peak bone mineral content velocity during adolescence associated with decreased fracture risk later in life (64,65).
  - Skeletal benefits were found to be maintained 10 years after retirement from gymnastics training (66).

Disordered Eating/Eating Disorders

- Studies of gymnasts have found a high prevalence of disordered eating behaviors and weight control behaviors (67,68).
  - A cross-sectional survey study in the United States among former female collegiate gymnasts found that 34% of the participants reported a history of disordered eating (40).
    - A greater number of in-season injuries has been found among female college gymnasts who reported a higher drive for thinness (69).
    - Further research among female collegiate gymnasts showed a higher proportion of time-loss injury and osteoporosis during college, and worse pain/physical function postcollege for those with disordered eating during college (40).
- Eating disorders in males:
  - Body image issues and eating disorders are less prevalent in male gymnasts (70); however, some concerning behaviors surrounding disordered eating have been noted in this population as well (70). Early research has demonstrated that 5%–10% of eating disorders affect males (71–75).

Mental Health

- The culture of sport contributes to the stigma against mental health issues in the athletic population (76). Stigma, low mental health literacy, negative past experiences, busy schedules, and hypermasculinity all contribute to the hesitation of athletes to seek treatment for mental health (76).
- Furthermore, as gymnastics is primarily an individual sport at the club and elite level, the pressure placed on these athletes can be monumental. Studies have shown that those in individual sports are more likely to suffer from anxiety and depression compared to those in team-oriented sports (13% vs. 7%) (34).
- Collegiate gymnastics involves a greater emphasis on team success and may be protective against mental health issues among gymnasts (34).
- At the elite level of gymnastics, mainstream media coverage of high-profile events (*e.g.*, Olympic Games) can place significant external pressure on athletes, and the psychological impact can be detrimental (77).
- There has been a recent shift in the concern for the mental health of athletes, represented by the position statements published by the American Medical Society of Sports Medicine and the IOC, emphasizing a multidisciplinary approach to treatment (78,79).

- The Sport Mental Health Assessment Tool 1 and the Sport Mental Health Recognition Tool 1, developed by the IOC, aim to facilitate early recognition of mental health symptoms in athletes, to ensure timely referral for appropriate treatment (80).

COMMON AND UNIQUE INJURY TYPES IN GYMNASTS

Ankle Sprains

- Lateral ankle sprains, typically caused by inversion injuries, are the most common acute injuries in gymnastics (29,45,81). One study found an alarming number of ankle injuries from gymnasts landing with their foot inside a crack in the floor or between mats (82).
- Gymnasts also sustain deltoid ligament sprains secondary to short landings at higher rates than other collegiate sports (83).
- Evaluation and treatment of gymnasts' ankle injuries follow rehabilitation protocols similar to those seen in other sports.

Achilles Injuries

- The eccentric loading on the Achilles tendon places gymnasts at an increased risk for spontaneous Achilles ruptures, especially during back-tumbling (back handspring take-offs) performed on the floor exercise (15,16,84).
- Among all levels and disciplines, female collegiate gymnasts experience the highest rates of Achilles tendon injuries (15,16).
  - Compared to other college sports, women's gymnastics had the highest rate of spontaneous Achilles tendon ruptures (16.73/100,000 athlete exposures) (16). Men's basketball had the second-highest rate (4.26/100,000 athlete exposures) (16).
- Risk factors for spontaneous Achilles' tendon ruptures in collegiate female gymnasts include elite training prior to college, performance of difficult floor skills and vaults, competing as an all-around gymnast, use of retinoid medications (Accutane), and identification as Black or African American (15).

Concussion

- Concussions are more common among male artistic gymnasts compared to female artistic gymnasts (11).
  - The incidence of concussions in gymnastics has been shown to reach 5.7 concussions per 1000 male gymnasts (8).
- Concussions occur more commonly in adolescents compared to childhood gymnasts (28).
- In collegiate gymnastics, concussions comprised 8.4% of all injuries and were most often attributed to contact with a surface/equipment (85).
- Former collegiate gymnasts with a history of concussions had a higher incidence of anxiety during their collegiate career for which they sought treatment (40).
- Once a gymnast is medically cleared to return to gymnastics, a gymnastics-specific return-to-play program can be employed (1).

Spondylolysis

- Spondylolysis is a stress fracture of the pars interarticularis and a common cause of lower back pain in young gymnasts (19,85–87).
- In the general pediatric and adolescent population, the prevalence of spondylolysis ranges from 4.4% to 4.7% (88), but in gymnasts, it reaches 11% (89,90).
- Proposed mechanisms for the development of spondylolysis in gymnastics are the focus on elements requiring repetitive extension-based movements, which place significant mechanical stress on the pars interarticularis (85,91–94).
- Most commonly diagnosed injuries in club gymnasts (19).
- Micheli et al. demonstrated that out of 100 adolescent athletes with a chief complaint of low back pain, 47% were diagnosed with spondylolysis (86).
- Given the simultaneous hyperextension and rotation seen in rhythmic gymnastics elements, these athletes are at a unique risk for spine-related injuries, with spondylolysis affecting approximately 8% of the normal population but up to 20% of rhythmic gymnasts (21).

Physical Exam

- Gymnasts with spondylolysis typically have axial lumbar spine pain and may be unilateral or central. The pain typically increases with activity (especially lumbar extension) and decreases with rest. Physical examination may find tenderness to palpation of the posterior elements or paravertebral muscles of the lower lumbar spine.
- Historically, a single-leg standing hyperextension test (Stork Test) has been used in the past to assess for spondylolysis; however, Masci et al. found the test was neither sensitive nor specific for the detection of active spondylolysis (95).
- The overhead mobility test and bridge test can be used to assess a gymnast's shoulder, thoracic spine, lumbar spine, and hip range of motion and target areas of hypomobility to address in physical therapy (96).

Diagnostic Testing for Suspected Spondylolysis

- Diagnostic testing begins with anteroposterior and lateral plain radiographs to assess bony pathology (97). Oblique views are no longer recommended as they lead to increased radiation and do not increase the sensitivity or specificity for lumbar spondylolysis (98).

- In recent years, magnetic resonance imaging (MRI) has replaced computed tomography (CT) and single photon emission computed tomography (SPECT) as the first-line imaging modality after radiographs.
  - MRI has been shown to accurately detect early stage stress reactions, visualize soft tissue, and also identify potential causes of low back pain other than spondylolysis (7,97,99).
  - MRI is particularly useful in skeletally immature athletes as it avoids the radiation exposure associated with CT (97).
  - A combination of MRI and CT can be useful in determining fracture acuity and the chance of bony union.
    - SPECT will detect early stress fracture, but there is increased cost, radiation, and risk of false negative & positive results (97).
    - 86.7% of athletes with early spondylolysis on CT and high signal intensity on T2 MRI images and 60% of athletes with progressive spondylolysis on CT and high signal intensity on T2 MRI images demonstrated bony healing. However, 0% of athletes with progressive spondylolysis on CT without high signal intensity on T2 MRI or with terminal spondylolysis demonstrated bony healing (100).
    - Similar results were seen in athletes with very early and progressive spondylolysis on CT demonstrated 100%, 93%, and 80% bony healing rates, but no athletes with terminal spondylolysis demonstrated bony union (101).

Spondylolysis Prognosis and Management

- Conservative management for lumbar spondylolysis includes rest, avoidance of sports or exacerbating activities, use of a lumbosacral orthosis, and physical therapy focused on spine stabilization, abdominal muscle strengthening, and hamstring flexibility for ~12 weeks (97,101).
- In a recent study exploring the outcomes of pediatric spondylolysis, the treatment period ranged from 1 to 7 months with a mean range of 2.5–3.6 months (101).
- Bilateral spondylolysis can lead to isthmic spondylolisthesis. Progression of spondylolisthesis is most likely to occur during times of peak growth velocity during puberty (102).
- Spondylolysis is further elaborated upon in Chapter 50 (Thoracic and Lumbar Spine).

ACL Tears

- ACL tears are a devastating lower extremity and female collegiate gymnasts are at greater risk than many other collegiate sports (13,103,104).
  - Hootman et al. found female collegiate gymnasts have one of the highest rates of ACL injury (0.33 per 1000 AEs) (13).
- Additionally, female gymnasts have the second-highest graft tear rate after surgical reconstruction, behind football (104).

Growth Center Injuries in Gymnasts

- Osgood-Schlatter disease is a common form of apophyseal traction injury at the tibial tubercle apophysis seen in children and adolescents (105). Onset is usually atraumatic and insidious with pain and swelling around the tibial tubercle during and after sports activities (106). It occurs more commonly in males (3:1) with an age of onset of 10–15 years in boys and 8–13 years in girls (106). Additional risk factors include decreased flexibility of the rectus femoris, external tibial rotation, increased posterior tibial slope, and elongated patellar tendons (106).
  - Gymnasts typically present with anterior knee pain, tibial tubercle tenderness, and pain during events or skills that require running and jumping (107).
  - Osgood-Schlatter disease is typically managed conservatively as the disease is self-limited and resolves with skeletal maturity (108,109).
  - Operative management may be necessary in more severe cases that persist into adulthood or those that progress to tibial avulsion fracture (105,108).
- Sinding-Larsen-Johansson syndrome is an apophyseal injury of the inferior pole of the patella at the origin of the patellar tendon (110). Sinding-Larsen-Johansson syndrome is a common apophyseal injury in young gymnasts. Clinical presentation, evaluation, and treatment are similar to Osgood-Schlatter disease, see above.
- Ischial apophysitis develops in the setting of repetitive tension on the ischial tuberosity from the proximal hamstring tendons (111). Repetitive flexion forces of the hip with simultaneous knee flexion, such as sprinting for a vault or floor, play a major role in the development of these injuries (111).
  - A complication of ischial apophysitis includes an avulsion fracture that often presents with a sudden pop during activity, followed by swelling and ecchymosis along the posterior thigh (111,112).
  - Conservative management of ischial apophysitis includes rest from gymnastics until the pain resolves, physical therapy, and gradual return to sport; however, surgical management may be required in the case of an avulsion fracture with displacement (112).
- Sever injury to the calcaneal apophysis is common in gymnasts and typically occurs between 7 and 14 years old (82). The main finding on examination is tenderness at the insertion of the Achilles tendon onto the calcaneus or the medial or lateral aspect of the calcaneal body. Traditionally considered traction apophysitis, newer evidence has indicated that Sever injury may result from repetitive compression to the actively remodeling metaphysis (113).
  - Similar to apophysitis in other areas, Sever injury is a self-limited condition.
  - Treatment includes relative rest, ice, heel cups used on a short-term basis, stretching, and strengthening exercises (114).
- Distal radial epiphysitis:
  - Chronic wrist pain affects 46%–87% of young gymnasts, more common during adolescent growth spurt (115,116).

Factors associated with wrist pain include training hours, skill level, and age at initiation of training (24).

- Distal radial epiphysitis, also known as "gymnast's wrist," is an overuse injury resulting in irritation and inflammation of the growth plate of the distal radius due to repetitive stress, and cross-sectional surveys indicate that approximately 45% of gymnasts report pain of at least 6 months in duration (24,116).
- Gymnast's wrist is characterized by dorsal wrist pain with loaded wrist dorsiflexion without acute trauma or swelling (117).
- Radiographs may reveal distal radial physeal injury (24), and cases of stress-related premature closure of the distal radial physis have been reported (30,118–120). Premature closure of the distal radial growth plate may result in positive ulnar variance (23,116,121), which can increase the risk of ulnar-sided wrist pathology.
- The mainstay treatment is reduction of loading to the wrist, then focusing on strengthening of the wrist and upper extremity.
- Current evidence supports the use of wrist guards with/or without palmar pads in the prevention of gymnasts' wrist pain and injury by limiting dorsiflexion and ulnocarpal joint intra-articular peak pressures (122).
  - Most commonly used wrist guards are a dorsal-support brace without palmar padding or volar support (122).
- One study found a volar carpal force dissipation wrist guard to be an effective method for reducing pain in more than 50% of younger lower-level male gymnasts after 3 weeks of use (123).
- Knowledge regarding wrist guard design, most effective indications, and application to gymnasts is lacking.
  - Recent studies have demonstrated that wrist guards may decrease wrist pain, but more studies are needed to determine whether wrist guards prevent wrist pain or injury (123,124).
- In skeletally mature gymnasts, if ulnar-sided wrist pain develops as a result of positive ulnar variance, an ulnar shortening procedure may be indicated to treat this condition.

- Elbow dislocations in gymnasts are typically the result of a fall on an outstretched hand injury (56). At a young age, gymnasts are taught the appropriate ways to fall, to decrease the risk of elbow dislocations and other injuries. Elbow joint dislocations require a thorough neurovascular examination, x-rays, and, in most cases, closed reduction of the dislocation (125).
- Osteochondritis dissecans (OCD) is osteonecrosis of subchondral bone, most specifically OCD of the capitellum can occur due to repetitive loads placed on the elbow joint during the performance of gymnastics elements (126). It occurs in young gymnasts with open growth plates, typically aged 10–15, from repeated valgus stress to the elbow. One study conducted in the setting of a tertiary children's hospital found that 73% of females with elbow OCD were competitive gymnasts, typically level 7 (127).
  - Initial evaluation includes history, physical exam, x-ray, and MRI if high suspicion. Literature has also shown that in female gymnasts, OCD of the elbow tends to occur in the non-dominant arm and at a younger age compared to male athletes (127).
  - Symptoms include the gradual onset of lateral elbow pain that worsens with activity, inability to fully extend the elbow, and possibly locking or clicking.
  - Management depends on the severity of symptoms and imaging results.
- Griplock is an injury unique to gymnastics that occurs when the gymnast's handgrip (used on horizontal bars and rings) inappropriately catches on the bar, and the athlete's momentum carries him or her around the bar, the hand and forearm are kept in a locked position. The injuries associated with griplock include open or closed fractures of the distal radius and ulna and extensor tendon injuries that may lead to residual extensor tendon lag (128,129). Griplock is more common in male gymnasts, who use a bar with a smaller circumference, and in gymnasts whose grips are overused and stretched out (128,129). One study in male gymnasts found that 36%–38% of coaches across a 10-year period reported having a gymnast who sustained a griplock injury (128).
- Gymnasts frequently train with blisters or *rips* on their hands caused by the friction created between skin and bars. These areas should be kept clean to avoid infection. Once an open lesion has dried, the application of a topical antibiotic ointment or vitamin C can be used at night to prevent both infection and painful cracking of the lesion.
- Heel pad contusions develop after trauma to the fat pad or calcaneus, from a landing onto the beam or floor, or directly hitting them on the bars. If symptoms continue to worsen, radiographs and/or MRI should be performed to rule out an occult fracture or a calcaneal stress fracture.
  - Management: rest, ice, pain medication, and/or a heel cushion.

EVENT COVERAGE

- The majority of U.S. gymnastics competitions are sanctioned by USAG.
  - *Rules and Policies Manual* governs various disciplines and all sanctioned USAG competitions.
- FIG governs international competition even when hosted in the United States.
  - Other governing bodies include the NCAA, YMCA, AAU, NFHS, and USAIGC, and have different competitive rules and competition procedures than USAG.

Table 107.2 Suggested Protocol for Accessing and Removing an Injured Gymnast from a Loose Foam Pit

1. Control the helpers.
   - Well-intentioned coaches and athletes should be told to stay out of the pit unless directed by the medical staff to enter the pit due to disturbing the blocks and potentially making the injury worse or making it more difficult to remove the athlete.
2. Talk to the athlete and observe from outside of the pit.
   - Avoid entering the pit unless it is necessary.
3. If the injury appears to be life-threatening, enter the pit directly without the use of a mat.
   - Assign an individual to alert EMS.
   - Removing an injured gymnast from the pit takes four to six adults.
   - Take off your shoes and socks since they can impede your progress and increase the disturbance of the foam blocks.
   - Use slow and steady movements.
   - Attempt to stabilize the cervical spine if possible.
   - Assess the airway, respiratory status, and level of consciousness.
   - Avoid moving the foam from underneath the gymnast as this may cause the gymnast to sink further into the pit.
   - Attempt to place the gymnast directly on a backboard (if available) or on a mat placed gently in the pit.
4. If the injury appears non–life-threatening, use a 4-in mat to enter the pit.
   - Gently place the mats in front of the gymnast's head and on his or her sides.
   - A ladder placed across the pit may be used as an alternative means to reach the gymnast and stabilize the neck.
   - Slowly crawl toward the gymnast.
   - One person should attempt to stabilize the cervical spine.
   - Using a coordinated effort, transfer the gymnast to the mat or directly onto a backboard, if available.
5. Practice with medical staff and EMS, and meet personnel prior to the competition.
   - It is surprisingly difficult to maneuver in a loose foam pit, much less attempt to rescue an athlete from this environment, without prior experience.

EMS, emergency medical services.
Source: Hecht SS, Burton MS. Medical coverage of gymnastics competitions. *Curr Sports Med Rep*. 2009;8(3):113–8.

COMPETITION LOGISTICS AND CONSIDERATIONS

- Gymnastics discipline and level of competition; number of competitors.
- Dates, location, venue (training and competition).
- Administrative body responsible for meet organization.
- Meet director responsibilities.
  - Meet organization.
  - Equipment safety.
  - Correct application of the competition policies and procedures as outlined in the USAG Rules and Policies Manual.

VENUE CONSIDERATIONS

- Club meets.
  - Practice venues or competitive events hosted at a gymnastics club may have unstable surfaces such as loose foam pits and resi pits.
  - Protocol (Table 107.2) (130) for accessing and removing injured gymnasts from unstable surfaces should be in place.
- Collegiate/Elite (Podium Meets).
  - Podium: Raised competition surface for placement of all competitive equipment rather than the equipment set up directly on the arena floor.
    - National and International meets.
  - Logistical issues.
    - Increased distance and time it may take the medical staff to reach an injured athlete (130).
    - An injured gymnast has 30 seconds after he/she stands up from a fall to restart the routine (130).
- Precompetition Recommendations.
  - Review medical services planning checklist (130).
  - Meet with the medical team, meet the director, and stakeholders.
- Competition Recommendations.
  - Main responsibility is to be readily available to assess and treat injured or ill gymnasts, coaches, and officials.
  - Sports medicine staff members should station themselves in close proximity to each apparatus and with extra attention to the floor exercise and vault events, along with tumbling and dismounting activities where injuries are more likely to occur (130).
- Postcompetition Recommendations.
  - Check in with the meet director.
  - Solicit input from other medical staff for ideas for future improvement.
  - Clean up the training room and any equipment used and properly dispose of medical waste (130).

REFERENCES

1. *USA Gymnastics*; 2022. Available from: https://usagym.org/
2. *NCAA Sports Sponsorship and Participation Rates Report:* 1981-2007 [Internet]. [cited 2010 December 20]. Available from: http://www.ncaapublications.com/productdownloads/PR2008.pdf
3. McNitt-Gray JL. Gymnastics. In: Garrett WE, Lester GE, McGowan J, et al, editors. *Women's Health in Sports and Exercise*. Rosemont (IL): AAOS; 2001. p. 209–28.
4. Caine D. Injury epidemiology. In: Sands WA, Caine DJ, Borms J, editors. *Scientific Aspects of Women's Gymnastics*, Vol. 45. Basel (Switzerland): Karger; 2003. p. 72–104.

5. Zaccardi N, Omatiga M. *Olympic women's gymnastics median age in 20s for first time in decades.* OlympicTalk | NBC Sports. 2021 July 14. [Retrieved November 24, 2022]. Available form: https://olympics.nbcsports.com/2021/07/14/olympic-gymnastics-average-age/
6. Kreipe RE. Normal somatic adolescent growth and development. In: McAnarney ER, Kreipe RE, Orr DP, et al, editors. *Textbook of Adolescent Medicine.* Philadelphia: WB Saunders; 1994. p. 44–67.
7. Campbell RA, Bradshaw EJ, Ball NB, Pease DL, Spratford W. Injury epidemiology and risk factors in competitive artistic gymnasts: a systematic review. *Br J Sports Med.* 2019;53(17):1056–69. doi:10.1136/bjsports-2018-099547
8. Kruse DW, Nobe AS, Billimek J. Injury incidence and characteristics for elite, male, artistic USA gymnastics competitions from 2008 to 2018. *Br J Sports Med.* 2021;55(3):163–8. doi:10.1136/bjsports-2019-101297
9. Jayanthi NA, LaBella CR, Fischer D, Pasulka J, Dugas LR. Sports-specialized intensive training and the risk of injury in young athletes: a clinical case-control study. *Am J Sports Med.* 2015;43(4):794–801.
10. Kerr ZY, Hayden R, Barr M, Klossner DA, Dompier TP. Epidemiology of National collegiate athletic association women's gymnastics injuries, 2009-2010 through 2013–2014. *J Athl Train.* 2015;50(8):870–8. doi:10.4085/1062-6050-50.7.02
11. Westermann RW, Giblin M, Vaske A, Grosso K, Wolf BR. Evaluation of men's and women's gymnastics injuries: a 10-year observational study. *Sports Health.* 2015;7(2):161–5. doi:10.1177/1941738114559705
12. Hunter LY, Torgan C. Dismounts in gymnastics: should scoring be reevaluated?. *Am J Sports Med.* 1983;11(4):208–10. doi:10.1177/036354658301100404
13. Hootman JM, Dick R, Agel J. Epidemiology of collegiate injuries for 15 sports: summary and recommendations for injury prevention initiatives. *J Athl Train.* 2007;42(2):311–9.
14. Rizzone KH, Ackerman KE, Roos KG, Dompier TP, Kerr ZY. The epidemiology of stress fractures in collegiate student-athletes, 2004-2005 through 2013-2014 academic years. *J Athl Train.* 2017;52(10):966–75. doi:10.4085/1062-6050-52.8.01
15. Bonanno J, Cheng J, Tilley D, Abutalib Z, Casey E. Factors associated with Achilles tendon rupture in women's collegiate gymnastics. *Sports Health.* 2022;14(3):358–68. doi:10.1177/19417381211034510
16. Chan JJ, Chen KK, Sarker S, et al. Epidemiology of Achilles tendon injuries in collegiate level athletes in the United States. *Int Orthop.* 2020;44(3):585–94. doi:10.1007/s00264-019-04471-2
17. Edouard P, Steffen K, Junge A, Leglise M, Soligard T, Engebretsen L. Gymnastics injury incidence during the 2008, 2012 and 2016 Olympic Games: analysis of prospectively collected surveillance data from 963 registered gymnasts during Olympic Games. *Br J Sports Med.* 2018;52(7):475–81. doi:10.1136/bjsports-2017-097972
18. Rossheim ME, Stephenson CJ. Parkour injuries presenting to United States emergency departments, 2009-2015. *Am J Emerg Med.* 2017;35(10):1503–5. doi:10.1016/j.ajem.2017.04.040
19. O'Kane JW, Levy MR, Pietila KE, Caine DJ, Schiff MA. Survey of injuries in Seattle area levels 4 to 10 female club gymnasts. *Clin J Sport Med.* 2011;21(6):486–92. doi:10.1097/JSM.0b013e31822e89a8
20. Thomas RE, Thomas BC. A systematic review of injuries in gymnastics. *Phys Sportsmed.* 2019;47(1):96–121. doi:10.1080/00913847.2018.1527646
21. Gram MCD, Clarsen B, Bo K. Injuries and illnesses among competitive Norwegian rhythmic gymnasts during preseason: a prospective cohort study of prevalence, incidence and risk factors. *Br J Sports Med.* 2021;55(4):231–6. doi:10.1136/bjsports-2020-102315
22. FIG. *Parkour: FIG – Discipline*; n.d. Retrieved November 24, 2022, from.https://www.gymnastics.sport/site/pages/disciplines/hist-pk.php
23. Caine D. Injury and growth. In: Sands WA, Caine DJ, Borms J, editors. *Scientific Aspects of Women's Gymnastics*, Vol. 45. Basel (Switzerland): Karger; 2003. p. 46–71.
24. DiFiori JP, Puffer JC, Aish B, Dorey F. Wrist pain, distal radial physeal injury, and ulnar variance in young gymnasts: does a relationship exist? *Am J Sports Med.* 2002;30(6):879–85.
25. Arnold A, Thigpen CA, Beattie PF, Kissenberth MJ, Shanley E. Overuse physeal injuries in youth athletes: risk factors, prevention, and treatment strategies. *Sports Health.* 2017;9(2):139–47.
26. Johnson D, Williams S, Bradley B, Sayer S, Murray Fisher J, Cumming S. Growing pains: maturity associated variation in injury risk in academy football. *Eur J Sport Sci.* 2020;20(4):544–52.
27. Caine D, Maffulli N, Caine C. Epidemiology of injury in child and adolescent sports: injury rates, risk factors, and prevention. *Clin Sports Med.* 2008;27(1):19–50.
28. Tisano B., Zynda AJ, Ellis HB, Wilson PL. Epidemiology of pediatric gymnastics injuries reported in US emergency departments: sex- and age-based injury patterns. *Orthop J Sports Med.* 2022;10(6):23259671221102478. doi:10.1177/23259671221102478
29. Caine D, Cochrane B, Caine C, Zemper E. An epidemiologic investigation of injuries affecting young competitive female gymnasts. *Am J Sports Med.* 1989;17(6):811–20.
30. Caine DJ, Daly RM, Jolly D, Hagel BE, Cochrane B. Risk factors in young competitive female gymnasts. *Br J Sports Med.* 2006;40:90–1.
31. Kerr GA, Minden H. Psychological factors related to the occurrence of athletic injuries. *J Sport Exerc Psychol.* 1988;10:167–73.
32. Kolt G, Kirkby R. Injury in Australian female competitive gymnasts: a psychological perspective. *Aust J Physiother.* 1996;42(2):121–6.
33. Petrie TA. Psychosocial antecedents of athletic injury: the effects of life stress and social support on female collegiate gymnasts. *Behav Med.* 1992;18(3):127–38.
34. Pluhar E, McCracken C, Griffith KL, Christino MA, Sugimoto D, Meehan WP 3rd. Team sport athletes may be less likely to suffer anxiety or depression than individual sport athletes. *J Sports Sci Med.* 2019;18(3):490–6.
35. Ozgüven HN, Berme N. An experimental and analytical study of impact forces during human jumping. *J Biomech.* 1988;21(12):1061–6.
36. Bruggemann G. Mechanical load in artistic gymnastics and its relation to apparatus and performance. In: *Symposium Medico-Technique.* Lausanne, Switzerland: International Gymnastics Federation; 1999. p. 17–27.
37. Sands WA, Shultz BB, Newman AP. Women's gymnastics injuries. A 5-year study. *Am J Sports Med.* 1993;21(2):271–6.
38. Caine D, Knutzen K, Howe W, et al. A three-year epidemiological study of injuries affecting young female gymnasts. *Phys Ther Sport.* 2003;4:10–23.
39. Marshall SW, Covassin T, Dick R, Nassar LG, Agel J. Descriptive epidemiology of collegiate women's gymnastics injuries: National Collegiate Athletic Association Injury Surveillance System, 1988-1989 through 2003-2004. *J Athl Train.* 2007;42(2):234–40.
40. Sweeney E, Howell DR, Seehusen CN, Tilley D, Casey E. Health outcomes among former female collegiate gymnasts: the influence of sport specialization, concussion, and disordered eating. *Phys Sportsmed.* 2021;49(4):438–44. doi:10.1080/00913847.2020.1850150
41. Kolt GS, Kirkby RJ. Epidemiology of injury in elite and subelite female gymnasts: a comparison of retrospective and prospective findings. *Br J Sports Med.* 1999;33(5):312–18.
42. Casey E, Bonanno J, Cheng J, et al. Return to sport in elite gymnastics: unprecedented training interruptions provide lessons for the future. *Pharm Manag PM R.* 2023;15(7):881–90. doi:10.1002/pmrj.12880

43. Myer GD, Jayanthi N, Difiori JP, et al. Sport specialization, part I: does early sports specialization increase negative outcomes and reduce the opportunity for success in young athletes? *Sports health.* 2015;7(5):437–42. doi:10.1177/1941738115598747
44. Bell D.R, Post E.G, Biese K., Bay C., Valovich McLeod T. Sport specialization and risk of overuse injuries: a systematic review with meta-analysis. *Pediatrics.*2018 Sept;142(3):e20180657. doi:10.1542/peds.2018-0657
45. Lindner KJ, Caine DJ. Injury patterns of female competitive club gymnasts. *Can J Sport Sci.* 1990;15(4):254–61.
46. Saluan P, Styron J, Ackley JF, Prinzbach A, Billow D. Injury types and incidence rates in precollegiate female gymnasts: a 21-year experience at a single training facility. *Orthop J Sports Med.* 2015;3(4):2325967115577596. doi:10.1177/2325967115577596
47. Sands WA. Injury prevention in women's gymnastics. *Sports Med.* 2000;30(5):359–373.
48. Lorenz DS, Reiman MP, Walker JC. Periodization: current review and suggested implementation for athletic rehabilitation. *Sports Health.* 2010;2(6):509–18.
49. Lima CD, Brown LE, Li Y, Herat N, Behm D. Periodized versus non-periodized stretch training on gymnasts flexibility and performance. *Int J Sports Med.* 2019;40(12):779–88. doi:10.1055/a-0942-7571
50. De Souza MJ, Nattiv A, Joy E, et al. 2014 Female Athlete Triad Coalition Consensus Statement on Treatment and Return to Play of the Female Athlete Triad: 1st International Conference held in San Francisco, CA, May 2012, and 2nd International Conference held in Indianapolis, IN, May 2013. *Clin J Sport Med.* 2014;24(2):96–119. doi:10.1097/JSM.0000000000000085
51. Nattiv A, Loucks AB, Manore MM, et al. American College of Sports Medicine position stand. The female athlete triad. *Med Sci Sports Exerc.* 2007;39(10):1867–82.
52. Fredericson M, Kussman A, Misra M, et al. The male athlete triad-A consensus statement from the Female and Male Athlete Triad Coalition part II: diagnosis, treatment, and return-to-play. *Clin J Sport Med.* 2021;31(4):349–66. doi:10.1097/JSM.0000000000000948
53. Mountjoy M, Sundgot-Borgen J, Burke L, et al. The IOC consensus statement: beyond the female athlete triad--relative energy deficiency in sport (RED-S). *Br J Sports Med.* 2014;48(7):491–7.
54. Gibbs JC, Nattiv A, Barrack MT, et al. Low bone density risk is higher in exercising women with multiple triad risk factors. *Med Sci Sports Exerc.* 2014 Jan;46(1):167–76. doi:10.1249/MSS.0b013e3182a03b8b
55. Nattiv A, Mandelbaum BR. Injuries, and special concerns in female gymnasts. *Phys Sportsmed.* 1993;21(7):66–82. Available from: "http://www.ncaa.org!sports3cience">http://www.ncaa.org!sports3cience
56. Ott SM. Gymnastics. In: Ireland ML, Nattiv A, editors. *The Female Athlete.* Philadelphia (PA): Saunders; 2002. p. 669.
57. Dowthwaite JN, DiStefano JG, Ploutz-Snyder RJ, Kanaley JA, Scerpella TA. Maturity and activity-related differences in bone mineral density: Tanner I vs. II and gymnasts vs. nongymnasts. Bone 39, 895-900. *Pediatr Exerc Sci.* 2006;22:21–33.
58. Maïmoun L, Georgopoulos NA, Sultan C. Endocrine disorders in adolescent and young female athletes: impact on growth, menstrual cycles, and bone mass acquisition. *J Clin Endocrinol Metab.* 2014;99(11):4037–50.
59. Cassell C, Benedict M, Specker B. Bone mineral density in elite 7- to 9-yr-old female gymnasts and swimmers. *Med Sci Sports Exerc.* 1996;28(10):1243–6.
60. Jürimäe J, Gruodyte-Raciene R, Baxter-Jones ADG. Effects of gymnastics activities on bone accrual during growth: a systematic review. *J Sports Sci Med.* 2018(17):245–58.
61. Erlandson MC, Kontulainen SA, Baxter-Jones AD. Precompetitive and recreational gymnasts have greater bone density, mass, and estimated strength at the distal radius in young childhood. *Osteoporos Int.* 2011;22(1):75–84.
62. Baxter-Jones ADG, Faulkner RA, Forwood M, Mirwald RL, Bailey DA. Bone mineral accrual from 8 to 30 years of age: an estimation of peak bone mass. *J Bone Miner Res.* 2011;26:1729–39.
63. Maïmoun L, Coste O, Philibert P, et al. Peripubertal female athletes in high-impact sports show improved bone mass acquisition and bone geometry. *Metabolism.* 2013;62(8):1088–98.
64. Weaver CM, Gordon CM, Janz KF, et al. The National Osteoporosis Foundation's position statement on peak bone mass development and lifestyle factors: a systematic review and implementation recommendations. *Osteoporos Int.* 2016;27(4):1281–386.
65. Xu J, Lombardi G, Jiao W, Banfi G. Effects of exercise on bone status in female subjects, from young girls to postmenopausal women: an overview of systematic reviews and meta-analyses. *Sports Med.* 2016;46(8):1165–82.
66. Erlandson MC, Kontulainen SA, Chilibeck PD, Arnold CM, Faulkner RA, Baxter-Jones AD. Higher premenarcheal bone mass in elite gymnasts is maintained into young adulthood after long-term retirement from sport: a 14-year follow-up. *J Bone Miner Res.* 2012;27(1):104–10. doi:10.1002/jbmr.514
67. Petrie TA, Stoever S. The incidence of bulimia nervosa and pathogenic weight control behaviors in female collegiate gymnasts. *Res Q Exerc Sport.* 1993;64(2):238–41.
68. Rosen DS, Hough DO. Pathogenic weight-control behavior of female college gymnasts. *Phys Sportsmed.* 1988;16:141–4.
69. Scheid JL, Stefanik ME. Drive for thinness predicts musculoskeletal injuries in division II NCAA female athletes. *J Funct Morphol Kinesiol.* 2019;4(3):52.
70. Pinto AJ, Dolan E, Baldissera G, et al. "Despite being an athlete, I am also a human-being": male elite gymnasts' reflections on food and body image. *Eur J Sport Sci.* 2020 Aug;20(7):964–72. doi:10.1080/17461391.2019.1682059
71. Murray SB, Nagata JM, Griffiths S, et al. The enigma of male eating disorders: a critical review and synthesis. *Clin Psychol Rev.* 2017 Nov;57:1–11.
72. Sharp CW, Clark SA, Dunan JR, Blackwood DHR, Shapiro CM. Clinical presentation of anorexia nervosa in males: 24 new cases. *Int J Eat Disord.* 1994 Mar;15(2):125–34.
73. Fairburn CG, Beglin SJ. Studies of the epidemiology of bulimia nervosa. *Am J Psychiatry.* 1990 Apr;147(4):401–8.
74. Carlat DJ, Camargo CA, Herzog DB. Eating disorders in males: a report on 135 patients. *Am J Psychiatry.* 1997 Aug;154(8):1127–32.
75. Andersen AE. *Males with Eating Disorders.* New York & London: Routledge; 1990.
76. Castaldelli-Maia JM, Gallinaro JGd ME, Falcão RS, et al. Mental health symptoms and disorders in elite athletes: a systematic review on cultural influencers and barriers to athletes seeking treatment. *Br J Sports Med.* 2019;53(11):707–21. doi:10.1136/bjsports-2019-100710
77. Faustin M, Burton M, Callender S, Watkins R, Chang C. Effect of media on the mental health of elite athletes. *Br J Sports Med.* 2022;56(3):123–4. doi:10.1136/bjsports-2021-105094
78. Chang C, Putukian M, Aerni G, et al. Mental health issues and psychological factors in athletes: detection, management, effect on performance and prevention. American Medical Society for Sports Medicine position statement-executive summary. *Br J Sports Med.* 2020;54(4):216–20. doi:10.1136/bjsports-2019-101583

79. Reardon CL, Hainline B, Aron CM, et al. Mental health in elite athletes: international olympic committee consensus statement (2019). *Br J Sports Med.* 2019;53(11):667–99. doi:10.1136/bjsports-2019-100715
80. Gouttebarge V, Bindra A, Blauwet C, et al. International Olympic Committee (IOC) sport mental health assessment tool 1 (SMHAT-1) and sport mental health recognition tool 1 (SMHRT-1): towards better support of athletes' mental health. *Br J Sports Med.* 2021;55(1):30–7. doi:10.1136/bjsports-2020-102411
81. Dixon M, Fricker P. Injuries to elite gymnasts over 10 yr. *Med Sci Sports Exerc.* 1993;25(12):1322–1329.
82. Mackie SJ, Taunton JE. Injuries in female gymnasts. *Phys Sportsmed.* 1994;22(8):40–45.
83. Kopec TJ, Hibberd EE, Roos KG, Djoko A, Dompier TP, Kerr ZY. The epidemiology of deltoid ligament sprains in 25 National Collegiate Athletic Association Sports, 2009-2010 through 2014-2015 academic years. *J Athl Train.* 2017 Apr;52(4):350–9. doi:10.4085/1062.6050-52.2.01
84. Wertz J, Galli M, Borchers JR. Achilles tendon rupture: risk assessment for aerial and ground athletes. *Sports health.* 2013;5(5):407–9.
85. Dietrich M, Kurowski P. The importance of mechanical factors in the etiology of spondylolysis. A model analysis of loads and stresses in human lumbar spine. *Spine.* 1985;10(6):532–42. doi:10.1097/00007632-198507000-00007
86. Micheli LJ, Wood R. Back pain in young athletes: significant differences from adults in causes and patterns. *Arch Pediatr Adolesc Med.* 1995;149(1):15–8. doi:10.1001/archpedi.1995.02170130017004
87. Selhorst M, Fischer A, MacDonald J. Prevalence of spondylolysis in symptomatic adolescent athletes: an assessment of sport risk in nonelite athletes. *Clin J Sport Med.* 2019;29(5):421–5. doi:10.1097/JSM.0000000000000546
88. Standaert CJ, Herring SA. Spondylolysis: a critical review. *Br J Sports Med.* 2000;34(6):415–22. doi:10.1136/bjsm.34.6.415
89. Fawcett L, James S, Botchu R, Martin J, Heneghan NR, Rushton A. The influence of spinal position on imaging findings: an observational study of thoracolumbar spine upright MRI in elite gymnasts. *Eur Spine J.* 2022 Feb;31(2):225–32. doi:10.1007/s00586-021-06997-9
90. Bennett DL, Nassar L, DeLano MC. Lumbar spine MRI in the elite-level female gymnast with low back pain. *Skelet Radiol.* 2006 Jul;35(7):503–9. doi:10.1007/s00256-006-0083-7
91. Rossi F. Spondylolysis, spondylolisthesis and sports. *J Sports Med Phys Fitness.* 1978;18(4):317–40.
92. Tertti M, Paajanen H, Kujala UM, Alanen A, Salmi TT, Kormano M. Disc degeneration in young gymnasts. A magnetic resonance imaging study. *Am J Sports Med.* 1990;18(2):206–8.
93. Hellström M, Jacobsson B, Swärd L, Peterson L. Radiologic abnormalities of the thoraco-lumbar spine in athletes. *Acta Radiol.* 1990;31(2):127–32.
94. Jackson DW, Wiltse LL, Cirincoine RJ. Spondylolysis in the female gymnast. *Clin Orthop Relat Res.* 1976;117:68–73.
95. Masci L, Pike J, Malara F, Phillips B, Bennell K, Brukner P. Use of the one-legged hyperextension test and magnetic resonance imaging in the diagnosis of active spondylolysis. *Br J Sports Med.* 2006;40(11):940–6. doi:10.1136/bjsm.2006.030023
96. Bonanno J, Casey E, Faustin M. *The Youth Athlete: Practitioner's Guide to Providing Comprehensive Sports Medicine Care.* 1st ed. Chapter 76. Elsevier; 2023.
97. Chung CC, Shimer AL. Lumbosacral spondylolysis and spondylolisthesis. *Clin Sports Med.* 2021;40(3):471–90. doi:10.1016/j.csm.2021.03.004
98. Beck NA, Miller R, Baldwin K, et al. Do oblique views add value in the diagnosis of spondylolysis in adolescents? *J Bone Joint Surg Am.* 2013 May 15;95(10):e65. doi:10.2106/JBJS.L.00824
99. Dunn AJ, Campbell RS, Mayor PE, Rees D. Radiological findings and healing patterns of incomplete stress fractures of the pars interarticularis. *Skelet Radiol.* 2008;37(5):443–50. doi:10.1007/s00256-008-0449-0
100. Sairyo K, Sakai T, Yasui N. Conservative treatment of lumbar spondylolysis in childhood and adolescence: the radiological signs which predict healing. *J Bone Joint Surg Br.* 2009;91(2):206–9. doi:10.1302/0301-620X.91B2.21256
101. Sakai T, Tezuka F, Yamashita K, et al. Conservative treatment for bony healing in pediatric lumbar spondylolysis. *Spine.* 2017;42(12):E716–20. doi:10.1097/BRS.0000000000001931
102. Tsirikos AI, Garrido EG. Spondylolysis and spondylolisthesis in children and adolescents. *J Bone Joint Surg Br.* 2010;92(6):751–9.
103. Agel J, Rockwood T, Klossner D. Collegiate ACL injury rates across 15 sports: National collegiate athletic association injury surveillance System data update (2004-2005 through 2012-2013). *Clin J Sport Med.* 2016;26(6):518–23. doi:10.1097/JSM.0000000000000290
104. Gans I, Retzky JS, Jones LC, Tanaka MJ. Epidemiology of recurrent anterior cruciate ligament injuries in National Collegiate Athletic Association Sports: the injury surveillance program, 2004-2014. *Orthop J Sports Med.* 2018;6(6):2325967118777823.
105. Ladenhauf HN, Seitlinger G, Green DW. Osgood-schlatter disease: a 2020 update of a common knee condition in children. *Curr Opin Pediatr.* 2020;32(1):107–12. doi:10.1097/MOP.0000000000000842
106. Lucenti L, Sapienza M, Caldaci A, Cristo C, Testa G, Pavone V. The etiology and risk factors of Osgood-Schlatter disease: a systematic review. *Children.* 2022 Jun 2;9(6):826. doi:10.3390/children9060826
107. Hart E, Meehan WP 3rd, Bae DS, d'Hemecourt P, Stracciolini A. The young injured gymnast: a literature review and discussion. *Curr Sports Med Rep.* 2018;17(11):366–75. doi:10.1249/JSR.0000000000000536
108. Circi E, Atalay Y, Beyzadeoglu T. Treatment of Osgood-Schlatter disease: review of the literature. *Musculoskelet Surg.* 2017;101(3):195–200. doi:10.1007/s12306-017-0479-7
109. Vaishya R, Azizi AT, Agarwal AK, Vijay V. Apophysitis of the tibial tuberosity (Osgood — Schlatter disease): a review. *Cureus.* 2016;8(9):780.
110. Medlar RC, Lyne ED. Sinding-Larsen-Johansson disease. Its etiology and natural history. *J Bone Joint Surg Am.* 1978;60(8):1113–16.
111. Yeager KC, Silva SR, Richter DL. Pelvic avulsion injuries in the adolescent athlete. *Clin Sports Med.* 2021;40(2):375–84. doi:10.1016/j.csm.2020.12.002
112. Kaila R, French SR, Wood DG. Outcomes following adolescent athlete proximal hamstring apophyseal avulsion bone fragment excision and direct tendon-ischial tuberosity reattachment. *J Pediatr Orthop B.* 2023;32, 3, 278, 86. doi:10.1097/BPB.0000000000000978
113. Ogden JA, Ganey TM, Hill JD, Jaakkola JI. Sever's injury: a stress fracture of the immature calcaneal metaphysis. *J Pediatr Orthop.* 2004;24(5):488–92.
114. Gillespie H. Osteochondroses and apophyseal injuries of the foot in the young athlete. *Curr Sports Med Rep.* 2010;9(5):265–8.
115. Caine D, Roy S, Singer KM, Broekhoff J. Stress changes of the distal radial growth plate. A radiographic survey and review of the literature. *Am J Sports Med.* 1992;20(3):290–8.
116. DiFiori JP, Puffer JC, Mandelbaum BR, Mar S. Factors associated with wrist pain in the young gymnast. *Am J Sports Med.* 1996;24(1):9–14.
117. McAuley E, Hudash G, Shields K, et al. Injuries in women's gymnastics. The state of the art. *Am J Sports Med.* 1987;15(6):558–565.
118. Albanese SA, Palmer AK, Kerr DR, Carpenter CW, Lisi D, Levinsohn EM. Wrist pain and distal growth plate closure of the radius in gymnasts. *J Pediatr Orthop.* 1989;9(1):23–28.
119. Caine D, DiFiori J, Maffulli N. Physeal injuries in children's and youth sports: reasons for concern? *Br J Sports Med.* 2006;40(9):749–70.

120. Caine D, Howe W, Ross W, Bergman G. Does repetitive physical loading inhibit radial growth in female gymnasts? *Clin J Sport Med.* 1997;7(4):302–8.
121. DiFiori JP, Puffer JC, Mandelbaum BR, Dorey F. Distal radial growth plate injury and positive ulnar variance in nonelite gymnasts. *Am J Sports Med.* 1997;25(6):763–8.
122. Choo S, Smith P, Cook J. Use of wrist guards for gymnasts – A systematic review. *Sport J.* 2022. Available from: https://thesportjournal.org/article/use-of-wrist-guards-for-gymnasts-a-systematic-review/
123. Trevithick B, Mellifont R, Sayers M. Wrist pain in gymnasts: Efficacy of a wrist brace to decrease wrist pain while performing gymnastics. *J Hand Ther.* 2020 Jul-Sep;33(3):354–60. doi:10.1016/j.jht.2019.03.002
124. Choo S, Cook JL. Wrist support does not prevent wrist injury or pain but may be therapeutic for existing wrist pain in female gymnasts. *Sports Injr Med.* 2022;6:185. doi:10.29011/2576-9596.100185
125. Morrey B.F. *Morrey's the Elbow and its Disorders.* 4th ed. New York, Ny: Elsevier; 2009. p. 436–49.
126. Hastings H. *Capitellar Osteochondrosis Dessicans (OCD) in Gymnasts.* Bloomington, Indiana: Indiana University, Indiana Hand to Shoulder Center; 2012.
127. Eisenberg K, Wu M, Hart E, Williams K, Bae DS. Differences in clinical presentation of osteochondritis dissecans of the capitellum in males and females. *Orthop J Harvard Med School.* 2017;18:25–31.
128. Bezek EM, Vanheest AE, Hutchinson DT. Grip lock injury in male gymnasts. *Sports Health.* 2009;1(6):518–21. doi:10.1177/1941738109347965
129. Samuelson M, Reider B, Weiss D. Grip lock injuries to the forearm in male gymnasts. *Am J Sports Med.* 1996;24(1):15–8. doi:10.1177/036354659602400104
130. Hecht SS, Burton MS. Medical coverage of gymnastics competitions. *Curr Sports Med Rep.* 2009;8(3):113–18.

Ice Hockey

Naina Bouchereau-Lal and Peter H. Seidenberg

108

INTRODUCTION

- Ice hockey is an extremely fast-paced, high-contact game that requires the mastery of many skills (1). Many of these skills (skating, stick handling, body checking, shooting, and goaltending) are unique to the sport (2).
- The sport dates back to the 1850s, with formal rules first established in Canada in 1881 (3).
- It is a National Collegiate Athletic Association (NCAA), international, and Olympic sport that made its debut in the Antwerp Olympic Games in 1920 (3).
- Its popularity is increasing every year in the United States. USA Hockey, the governing body for the sport, saw a 74% increase in adult membership from 103,533 in 2007 to 180,400 in 2016 (4).
- During the 2021–2022 season, there were 630,561 registered players, coaches, and officials in USA Hockey.
  - USA Hockey is the governing body for amateur hockey in the United States (3).
- Women are active participants in all roles in ice hockey (3).
  - Females were involved in Canada as early as 1892.
  - The International Ice Hockey Federation coordinated women's world ice hockey tournaments in 1992, 1994, and 1997, and it first appeared as a medal sport in the 1998 Olympic Games.
  - Currently, the NCAA continues to consider female ice hockey as emerging sport, and USA Hockey registrants include 87,971 female players (3).
  - Many women play on men's teams, even up to the minor league level.
- The physician providing medical care for ice hockey athletes needs to be proficient in treating a wide variety of traumatic and atraumatic problems that range in severity from mild to life-threatening.

EQUIPMENT (5–12)

- All leagues require helmets with properly fastened chip strap, which should fit snugly and use a four-point fit (like football helmets).
  - The hockey helmet must be able to withstand low-mass, high-velocity impacts from the puck and high-mass, low-velocity forces from running into the boards.
- All players on the players' and the penalty bench must wear the protective helmet/facemask while in the bench area.
- USA Hockey requires in all age classes, except the adult class, the use of Hockey Equipment Certification Council (HECC)—approved helmets, full face masks, and full mouthpieces for all players during both practices and games.
- The mouthpiece should be internal and should cover all the remaining teeth of one jaw, customarily the upper jaw. It is required to be colored (not clear) in age 19 and under leagues. A form-fitting, customized mouthpiece is recommended.
  - International play does not require mouthpieces; however, it is strongly recommended that all players wear a mouthguard, preferably the custom-made variety.
  - The purpose of mouthguards is to protect dentition.
  - They may also prevent or decrease the severity of concussion, although this is controversial.
- Full face masks with chin straps properly fastened are mandatory for all youth and college leagues and continue to gain popularity on the professional level.
- Kevlar throat protectors are required in many leagues and countries.
- Gloves, elbow pads, shin pads, shoulder pads, hip pads or padded hockey pants, protective cup, and tendon pads are recommended.
  - There is a trend of wearing hockey gloves with shorter cuffs for the purpose of allowing increased wrist motion.
    - This may be at the cost of increased risk of wrist and forearm injury.
  - Hockey pants have padding to protect from the hips to the top of the knees.
  - Shin pads should cover from the top of the knees to the ankles.
- All protective equipment except helmets, facemask, padded hockey gloves, padded hockey pants, and goalie leg pads are worn under the uniform.
- Goalkeeper protective equipment
  - Blocker worn on stick hand.

- Trapper glove worn on the nonstick hand looks similar to a baseball mitt with protective padding extending up the forearm.
- Leg guards up to 11 in in width worn on each leg.
- Full face masks are required. Form-fitting masks are not permitted and are illegal except in Adult leagues. Use of the masks in adults requires signing a waiver.
- Approved HECC helmets are required unless the above form-fitting mask includes a back skull plate.
- Throat/neck laceration protectors are recommended.
- Chest protector
- Cup
- Goalie skates

- Skates have a protective heel tip (not required for the goalie).
  - Probably the most important piece of equipment used by the hockey player.
  - Speed skates and figure skates are prohibited.
  - Many players prefer leather skates that have external plastic shields for ankle support and protection.
  - Athletes usually prefer ice skates to be snuggly fit and may not wear socks to improve the feel of the ice.
- The puck is made of vulcanized rubber or other approved material and weighs between 5.5 and 6.0 ounces. It is 1-in thick and 3 in in diameter. It is black in color.
  - A 4.0- to 4.5-ounce puck is recommended for the 8 and under (Youth) and 8 and under girls age classifications as well as for Midget League play.
- Except for adults, no player or goalkeeper is permitted on ice while wearing jewelry unless it is completely covered by equipment or taped to the body.
- The wearing of casts or splints made of hard or unyielding materials is prohibited even if padded unless directed in writing by a licensed medical physician.
- Equipment that is in poor condition or under repair or has been altered with a purpose of causing harm to other players is prohibited. Use of such equipment results in penalization of the offending player.

PHYSIOLOGY OF ICE HOCKEY

- Skating during a game involves repeated accelerations, decelerations, turning, and stopping (13).
- The players skate forward, backward, and side to side, often with some changes in direction (13).
- During competition, the players typically work at >70% of their VO_{2max} with a substantial amount of play at >90% VO_{2max} (14).
  - However, with the frequent stoppage of play per shift (on average 2–3 minutes) and with 3–4 minutes of rest between shifts, the resulting mean VO_2 consumed per game is 55%–66% of maximum.
- Players can lose 4.5–6.5 lb of weight via sweat per game (15).
- If games are played on consecutive days, glycogen stores are often not replenished (15).
- Elite ice hockey players lose on average 10% body fat (15).
- Physiologic differences by position (15,16)
  - Energy expenditure
    - Playing time
    - Goalies have the least number of substitutions and may play an entire game.
    - Goaltending requires quick, short explosive movements interspersed with periods of relative rest.
    - High reliance on adenosine triphosphate (ATP)-phosphocreatine system.
    - Defense players have more playing time than forwards and typically have less rest time between shifts.
    - Forwards and defense players have a high reliance on both glycolytic and aerobic metabolism.
    - During games, adult forwards and defense players skate greater than 4 miles.
    - Energy expenditure is one-third aerobic and two-thirds anaerobic; postgame lactate increases over eight times the pregame level.
  - Forwards have greater anaerobic activity and typically skate faster than defense players or goalies.
  - Despite the above differences by position, muscle fiber composition remains equivalent between positions.
- Flexibility (17)
  - Goalkeepers are significantly more flexible than forwards or defense players.
  - Forwards and defense players have been found to have equal flexibility.
- Shooting (13)
  - Properly coordinated acceleration and deceleration of motion of body segments produces maximum velocity.
  - Motion is concentrated in the lower arm.
  - However, maximum velocity is produced through maximal use in full rotation of the trunk.
  - Accuracy of the shot is enhanced via trunk stabilization and restricted use of body segments.

EPIDEMIOLOGY OF INJURIES

- Ice hockey is classified as a collision sport by the American Academy of Pediatrics (18,19).
- There are many opportunities for an injury in this aggressive, fast-paced sport.
  - Contact/collision occurs with a hard ice surface, unpadded boards, goal posts, equipment from other players (skate blades, sticks), the puck, and the bodies and, at times, fists of the opponents (20).

- In elite hockey, the puck can travel at speeds up to 120 miles · h^{-1}, producing impact forces >1250 lb.
- Professional players can skate at speeds up to 30 miles · h^{-1}.
- Sliding on the ice after a fall can occur at speeds up to 15 miles · h^{-1}.

- Psychosocial factors, including low vigor, high fatigue, and athletic identity, have been shown to play a role in risk factors for injury (21–23).
  - Studies have shown that psychosocial, psychologic, and psychiatric factors such as perceived vulnerability, willingness to report, incidence, symptom reports, time loss, playing style, and mental health issues influence rates of sports-related concussion.
- Equipment that is in poor repair also places the athlete at increased risk for injury; however, even when adequate protection is worn, injury is still possible. Studies have found that 58% of injuries occur on body parts that were covered with protective equipment (24).

- Overall injury rates
  - Aggregation of injury data are limited by varying definitions and methods for reporting in the literature.
  - Data from injuries presenting to U.S. emergency departments demonstrate the following distribution of injury location (4):
    - Upper extremity: 36%–43.8%
    - Head: 12.3%–16.3%
    - Lower extremity: 16.1%–19.1%
    - Trunk: 9.3%–13.8%
    - Face: 10.0%–23.0%
    - The above data are limited by the fact that not all ice hockey injuries result in a visit to the local emergency department.
  - Overall injury rate is 5.93 injuries per 1000 player-hours (1), with 1.5–2.2 per 1000 hours during practice, 13.8–54 per 1000 hours during games (25). Due to difficulty quantifying player-hours, many studies instead describe injury rates per athlete exposure.
  - Injury is more common in the game setting (65%–76%) than in practice, although practice represents significantly more time. Injuries are thus 5–25 times more common in game settings (25,26).
  - Acute and traumatic injuries account for 85% of injuries, whereas overuse injuries represent 8%–52% of all injuries (26).
  - Illegal play accounts for an estimated 26.3%–66% of total injuries (27).
  - During games, Pelletier et al. (28) found that 27.1% of injuries occur during the first period, 35.6% occur during the second period, and 26.6% occurred during the third period. In McKay et al. (29), injuries were significantly more frequent in the first period than the second or third periods. In contrast, other investigators suggest that third-period injuries are roughly equal to first- and second-period injuries combined (24) or that injuries are twice as common in the third period (30).
- Age-specific injury rates: Injuries appear to increase with increasing age, with a peak in early adulthood (Table 108.1).
- Studies suggest that injury rates in youth hockey show a dramatic increase during the first year that body checking is permitted, regardless of the age that checking is instituted (31).
- Mechanisms of injuries (26)
  - Collisions: 6.6%–51% of all injuries (26).
  - Puck: 3%–20% of injuries. Puck velocity may reach 120 miles · h^{-1} at professional levels (26).
  - Stick: 8%–29% of injuries (26).
  - Skate: 5%–11% of injuries, often related to lacerations from sharp steel blades (30).
  - Fighting: 3%–6.5% of injuries (30).
  - Overuse: 8%–52% of all injuries (26).
  - Falls: 4%–7% (26).
  - Foul play or illegal play: 9%–16% (24).
  - Noncontact injuries: 2.2% (28).
- Types of injury
  - Sprain/strain: 17.7% (4).
    - Average number of days lost from play due to sprains = 13.61 (28).
  - Contusion: 13.5% (4).
  - Laceration: 26% (4).
  - Fracture: 14.7% (4).
    - Average number of days lost from play due to fractures = 22.22
  - Concussion: 7%–18.6% (26,28).
  - General trauma: 5.9% (28).
- Rates of injury per anatomic site are listed in Table 108.2.
- Injuries related to position on ice (25,32)
  - Goalkeeper: 3.5%–5.8%.
  - Defense player: 31.2%–36.8%.
  - Center: 18.5%.

Table 108.1 Injury Rates by Age of Athlete (30)

Age of Athlete	Rate of Injury per 1000 Player-Hours	
	Practice Time	Game Time
Youth (ages)		
Squirt (9–10)	1.2	0
Pee Wee (11–12)	2.2	0
Bantam (13–14)	2.5	10.9
Junior A (17–19)	3.9	96.1
Intercollegiate (18–21)	2.3	84.3
Swedish Elite (19–33)	1.4	78.4

Table 108.2 Anatomic Location of Hockey Injuries (28)

Anatomic Site of Injury	Percentage of Total Injuries Reported
Head and neck	10.6%
Face, eye, ear, jaw, teeth	17.6%
Shoulder and clavicle	14.9%
Chest and back	4.8%
Arm, elbow	3.7%
Forearm, wrist, hand	6.9%
Hip, groin, abdomen	6.4%
Hamstring, thigh	9.0%
Knee	18.6%
Ankle	3.2%
Foot	1.6%

- Wing: 36%.
- Missing position data: 8.5%.
- However, position played has no statistical relationship to days lost from an injury.
  - Majority of injured players return to play in 1 week (33).
- Injuries by sex: NCAA injury data analysis shows the following differences between injury rates in male versus female ice hockey athletes (34,35):
  - Rate of injury in games was eight (males) and five (females) times higher than in practice.
  - Preseason practice injury rates were approximately twice those of in-season practice injury rates (males and females).
  - Most common injuries in games:
    - Male = knee internal derangement (13.5%), concussion (9%), acromioclavicular joint injury (8.9%).
    - Female = concussion (21.6%), knee internal derangement (12.9%), acromioclavicular joint injury (6.8%)
  - Most common injuries in practice:
    - Male = pelvis and hip strain (13.1%), knee internal derangement (10.1%), ankle ligament sprains (5.5%)
    - Female = concussion (13.2%), pelvis and hip strains (12%), foot contusion (7.2%)
  - More research is needed to determine why women hockey players have a higher rate of concussions than men.
    - Despite the prohibition of body checking in women's ice hockey, women continue to experience concussions at an alarming rate and with greater frequency than is reported in men's games (34).
    - These differences may be due to anatomic and biomechanical differences such as neck strength and head mass differences or rule differences (*e.g.*, no checking in women's ice hockey). However, it also may be related to greater willingness to self-report a neck or head injury (35).
    - In one study, checking-related concussions were less common in women than men overall but more common in division I women than division III women (35).

INJURIES BY LOCATION

- **Ocular:** 38% to 47% of sports-related eye injuries occur in hockey (36).
  - Most common injuries are soft tissue (34%), hyphema (27%), other intraocular injuries (23%), corneal damage (9%), orbital fracture (4%), and ruptured globes (3%).
  - Pashby (37) found that approximately 15% of all eye-injured hockey athletes were left with an injury resulting in a legally blind eye.
  - However, 58% of these injuries would have been prevented with face shields (37).
- **Concussion:** Management should be as in any other sport. No concussed athletes should be allowed to return to competition.
  - Hockey players sustain head trauma impact forces from axial loading in a similar mechanism as football players (36).
  - Unlike football, the hockey athlete is also at risk of traumatic brain injury through contact with a hockey puck, which as previously mentioned can reach speeds of up to 120 miles $\cdot$ h^{-1} (38).
  - Concussions account for 18.6% of all hockey injuries (25).
    - This percentage is likely underestimated, because many injury reporting studies have only looked at injuries that have resulted in time lost from play (33). In addition, it is suggested that, especially in youth hockey organizations, there is a trend of underreporting concussions. As such, many concussions may not have been identified (38).
  - Benson et al. (39) included mild concussions in their head and neck injury study and found a concussion incidence of 1.53–1.57 per 1000 athlete exposures.
  - National Hockey League (NHL) studies have found the concussion rate to be 1.04–1.81 per 1000 athlete exposures (40).
  - NCAA data show an overall concussion rate of 0.74 per 1000 athlete exposures (41).
  - Emergency department data suggest that the percentage of traumatic brain injuries increases as age decreases (19).
- **Maxillofacial:** When abrasions and lacerations are excluded, maxillofacial trauma represents 11.5% of hockey injuries (42).
  - Ice hockey accounts for roughly 40% of all sports-related dental injuries (43).

- Blows from the stick represent 39%–54% of maxillofacial and dental injuries, whereas contact with the puck represents 14.2%–30% of injuries in the same area (44,45).
- Facial injuries (85%) outnumber head and neck injuries (13% and 6%, respectively) (45).
- Of these injuries, 69.9% occur during games with the remainder occurring during practice sessions (42).
- The most commonly diagnosed dental injury was an uncomplicated crown fracture, and the most common cause being a hit with a hockey stick, which accounted for 52.7% and 40.3% of dental injuries in games and practices, respectively (46).
- Injury to teeth and alveolar processes represents 84.5% of injuries (42).
- Face and head injuries account for 20%–40% of all hockey-related injuries (44,47,48) and dental injuries up to 11.5% (42)
- Maxillofacial injuries have been drastically reduced since the introduction of mandatory face masks at many levels of the sport (3).
  - In 2014, the NHL implemented new regulations making visor use mandatory for all incoming players, a change that felt initial pushback but has since been shown to significantly decrease the rate of eye injury among professional athletes (49).
- Despite face masks, facial lacerations still occur, and the team physician should be prepared to evaluate and repair these injuries appropriately.

- **Cervical spine**
  - The number of catastrophic cervical spine injuries in ice hockey is low compared to other sports; however, the incidence per 1000 participants is relatively high (50).
    - In one study of injury data from the 2001–2002 NCAA Ice hockey season, 9% of all hockey injuries occurred to the spine (51).
  - Mechanism of injury is axial loading caused by a blow to the head from collision with the boards, other players, the ice, or the goal post (51).
  - These injuries generally occur in the lower cervical region: C-5 through C-7 levels. Checking from behind is the most common cause of injury; the player being checked is looking down and not anticipating the check, which sends them hurtling crown first into the boards, axially loading the cervical spine (51).
  - The effect of helmet and face mask use on cervical spine injuries is controversial.
    - After the increased use of helmets with a facemask in ice hockey, there retrospectively appears to be an increasing incidence of cervical spine injury. Several investigators hypothesize that this is caused as a result of the player wearing a helmet adopting a more aggressive style of play, resulting in more cervical injury. It has been proposed that the protective devices have also altered how officials perceive game situations, leading them to be more lenient in penalization. The net result has been an increase in illegal and injurious behaviors, such as checking from behind (an activity associated with catastrophic cervical spine injury) (27).
    - However, the prospective study by LaPrade et al. of intercollegiate athletes and face mask use showed no increase in head and neck injuries (52).
  - Many of the reported cervical spine injuries were a result of either illegal play or high-risk aggressive behavior. New rules have been instituted by both the Canadian Amateur Hockey Association and USA Hockey in an attempt to reduce the number of spinal cord injuries. These new rules have moved action away from the boards and restricted checking. Data from the Canadian registry suggest that fewer cases of major spinal column trauma and complete quadriplegia have been caused by illegal playing techniques since the rule changes have been instituted (53).
- **Shoulder:** Clavicle fractures, acromioclavicular joint sprain/separation (59%), and glenohumeral subluxation/dislocation and tear (40%) are relatively common in ice hockey (25).
  - They usually are high-velocity injuries that result from the shoulder being driven into the boards following aggressive body checks.
- **Elbow:** A player who does not wear elbow pads may receive a traumatic olecranon bursitis and/or elbow fracture during collision with the ice or the boards (54).
- **Wrist, hand**
  - When hockey players fight (which occurs frequently at higher levels of play), the gloves are typically thrown down, and blows are exchanged using bare hands. The typical street fighter hand injuries can then occur (12).
  - Gamekeeper's thumb (ulnar collateral ligament injury) has been reported and is typically due to the player's thumb being hyperabducted when the stick handle is suddenly forced toward the body during a collision with the boards (12).
  - Wartenberg syndrome (55): In hockey, direct trauma to the superficial radial nerve at the wrist can occur when an opponent strikes the distal forearm with the stick. The athlete complains of pain and/or paresthesias shooting up the thumb and dorsal wrist in a radial distribution. Players who use gloves with shorter cuffs (to increase wrist mobility) are at increased risk for this injury.
  - Scaphoid fracture: Mechanism of injury usually is a fall on an outstretched hand or a dorsiflexed wrist colliding with the boards. The gloves provide some protection against this injury (12).
- **Chest:** Commotio cordis has been reported in youth ice hockey. League organizers and physicians should have an automated external defibrillator (AED) available at the rink because there is a 16% survival rate with rapid defibrillation (20).

- **Back**
  - Back strain and sprain — Players skate in forward flexed position. This position, combined with the frequent trunk rotation that accompanies shooting and passing, can place the player at risk for these injuries.
  - Spondylolysis has been reported in ice hockey athletes.
- **Abdomen**
  - Because of the abrupt and sudden changes in movement, hockey players are at risk for abdominal muscle strain (27).
  - Athletes can sustain traumatic abdominal injury, especially when the handle of the stick is forced into the abdomen during a collision into the boards (which is typically the result of illegal checking) (4).
- **Thigh, groin**
  - Anterior thigh hematoma may occur from a collision with the boards or from blocking a shot puck. These hematomas are at risk of myositis ossificans (27), and treatment should be directed at preventing this complication.
    - If the hematoma is identified immediately after the game, the athlete can be placed in fixed knee flexion for 24 hours in an attempt to tamponade the bleeding, thereby decreasing the size of the hematoma.
    - Old hematomas should not be passively stretched, as this may increase the risk of myositis ossificans.
  - Adductor strains are common enough that studies have been performed in attempt to determine if certain players are at increased risk for this injury and to ascertain what prevention measures can be implemented in attempt to decrease the lost playing time. Hockey players are at risk for this injury due to explosive starts and changes in direction (27).
  - Osteitis pubis has also been reported in hockey players. There is thought to be an increased risk for this disorder due to abrupt and sudden change in the movement (27).
  - Core muscle injury (previously known as sports hernias) is also reported.
- **Knee:** Most common significant lower extremity injury.
  - Knee and leg injuries account for 22% of all ice hockey injuries (25).
  - Although anterior cruciate ligament (ACL) and meniscal injuries have been reported, medial collateral ligament (MCL) injuries account for 56% of knee injuries (25).
  - The mechanisms of MCL injury are both contact and noncontact valgus stress to the knee.
  - The ACL appears to be spared because the foot does not lock in position on the ice (25).
- **Ankle:** Ankle sprain — Mechanism of injury is dorsiflexion, eversion, and external rotation (27), producing deltoid ligament sprain.
  - This is in contrast to most other sports where the typical mechanism is plantar flexion, inversion, and internal rotation, producing lateral ligament (especially anterior talofibular ligament) injury.
  - The mechanism of injury also places the hockey athlete at risk for syndesmotic injury (high ankle sprain) (25) and Maisonneuve fracture (due to transmittal of the force out through the fibula).
  - Ankle sprain result in 12% of major injuries in ice hockey (defined as absence from sport >28 days) (25).
  - In attempt to prevent these debilitating injuries, many hockey players prefer skates that have added external ankle support (11).
  - Boot lace lacerations — The ice skate blade is essentially a 10- to 12-in shaped scalpel. The anterior ankle is at risk for lacerations of tendons and neurovascular structures because of its proximity to the skates of others. A relatively small laceration can cause damage to these underlying superficial structures (17).
    - However, most athletes are relatively protected from this injury because of the thickly padded skate tongue over the interior angle. Athletes who turn their skate tongue downward (out of personal preference) place themselves at increased risk.
- **Foot:** Lace bite is nagging dorsal foot pain and/or paresthesias (27).
  - Some players do not wear socks and prefer tight-fitting skates because this is thought by athletes to improve performance and speed on the ice. The compression of the laces in such situations can cause extensor tendon and nerve injuries of the dorsum of the foot.
  - To prevent this injury, the tongue of the boot should remain in a neutral position.

MEDICAL ILLNESSES

- Indoor ice rinks have ice-resurfacing machines, commonly referred to as Zambonis, which are gas or propane powered. The emissions from the machine coupled with poor ventilation can create increased carbon monoxide levels on the ice.
- Nitrogen dioxide-induced lung injury and other indoor air quality syndromes.
- Cold-induced vasomotor rhinitis (56,57).
  - Profuse watery rhinorrhea that typically begins within minutes of skating on the ice. It is thought to be the result of an overly sensitive cholinergic reflex in response to exposure to the cold air and change and humidity.
  - The athlete has little nasal itching, ocular pruritus, or sneezing, but increased nasal secretions, post-nasal drip; sinus headaches, anosmia, and sinusitis are common.
  - It is a diagnosis of exclusion. Rhinitis caused by infection, allergy, anatomic abnormalities, and eosinophilia should first be ruled out.

- Many athletes self-medicate with decongestants for this disorder; however, this category of medicine is on the banned substance list for the international Olympic Committee (IOC). There has been some promise in treating this disorder with ipratropium bromide nasal spray, a medication that is not on the prohibited list.

PREVENTION

- Youth hockey programs need to educate players, coaches, and parents of the importance of knowing and following the rules (22).
- Body checking should not be allowed in youth hockey for children ages 12 and under, girls/women classifications, and all non-check adult classifications (5).
- Fair-play rules should be used to decrease the incidence of injury in youth hockey. This system gives teams credit for sportspersonship in the final standings of the league in tournament play. Teams have points added to their totals for staying under a preestablished limit of penalties per game, whereas teams that rely on intimidation and foul play have points subtracted. Implementation of this style of play was shown to reduce the number of high school hockey injuries (22).
- Players, coaches, parents, and officials should be educated on the dangers of checking another player from behind (22).
- The officials and coaches should be encouraged to strictly enforce the rules against illegal body checking.
  - These forms of checking include boarding, charging, checking from behind, cross-checking, elbowing, and roughing.
- Contact with an opposing player made above the shoulder using the fist, forearm, elbow, shoulders, knees, or stick must be penalized. If such an act was deliberate, the stiffest sanctions should be used.
- Deliberate attempts to injure other players are illegal and should be heavily penalized.
- Rules against high-sticking should be strictly enforced.
  - Frequently occurs during a slap shot or when attempting to bat down airborne puck.
    - During a slap shot, it is considered high sticking if the stick comes above the level of the waist on the backswing; slap shots are illegal in midget play.
    - Batting a puck down with the stick above the shoulders is also considered high sticking.
- Fighting needs to be discouraged by officials, coaches, players, and players' parents.
- Players should be encouraged or mandated to wear helmets with full-coverage facemasks at any level of play for both game and practice situations.
- USA Hockey has enacted a "Heads Up, Don't Duck" initiative to decrease the frequency of cervical spine and spinal cord injuries. Players are taught to make contact with the boards with any body part except the head. For example, if head contact is unavoidable the player should lift the head (not duck) to prevent an axial load to the top of the head. Fortunately, the number of catastrophic and potentially catastrophic injuries among USA Hockey players continues to decline (2).
- In 2014, the NHL implemented new regulations making visor use mandatory for all incoming players, a change that felt initial pushback but has since been shown to significantly decrease the rate of eye injury among professional athletes (49).
- The importance of developing more effective primary prevention strategies for commotio cordis — such as effective chest protectors and safety balls — and promoting their widespread use is needed (20).
- Arena characteristics, such as flexible boards and glass, appear to reduce the risk of injury (31).
- Ensure adequate ventilation and monitoring of air quality in indoor ice rinks.
- The medical team providing coverage for ice hockey should have the availability of medical equipment for the stabilization of potentially devastating injury at the ice rink. This should include a spine board, cervical collar, and cardiopulmonary resuscitation equipment (58). The logistics of how to get this equipment to the injured athlete on the ice should be preestablished. An emergency plan should be in place and practiced prior to the beginning of the season so that in the event of a devastating injury, morbidity due to delay and stabilization can be reduced.

REFERENCES

1. Ornon G, Ziltener JL, Fritschy D, Menetrey J. Epidemiology of injuries in professional ice hockey: a prospective study over seven years. *J Exp Orthop*. 2020 Dec;7(1):1–8.
2. Anderson GR, Melugin HP, Stuart MJ. Epidemiology of injuries in ice hockey. *Sports Health*. 2019 Nov;11(6):514–9.
3. USA Hockey Web Site [Internet]. 2022 [cited 2022 Oct 1]. Available from: https://www.usahockeyrulebook.com/
4. Morrissey PJ, Maier SP II, Zhou JJ, et al. Epidemiology and trends of adult ice hockey injuries presenting to United States emergency departments: a ten-year analysis from 2007-2016. *J Orthop*. 2020 Nov 1;22:231–6.
5. Ice Hockey Rules Changes — 2024-25 [Internet]. Nfhs.org. 2024. Available from: https://www.nfhs.org/sports-resource-content/ice-hockey-rules-changes-2024-25/
6. Clark JM, Post A, Hoshizaki TB, Gilchrist MD. Protective capacity of ice hockey helmets against different impact events. *J Bioeng*. 2016 Dec;44(12):3693–704.
7. International Ice Hockey Federation (IIHF): 2021-2022 Official Rulebook, from the IIHF Web Site [Internet]. 2022 [cited 2022 Oct 1]. Available from: http://www.iihf.com
8. Maeda Y, Kumamoto D, Yagi K, Ikebe K. Effectiveness and fabrication of mouthguards. *Dent Traumatol*. 2009 Dec;25(6):556–64.

9. Joyner D, Snouse S. Skiing, speed skating, ice hockey. In: Ireland M, Nattiv A, editors. *The Female Athlete*. Philadelphia: Saunders; 2002, p. 769–75.
10. DeLee JC, Drez D. Etiology of injury to the foot and ankle. *Orthopa Sports Med Principles Practice*. 2003;2:2224–74.
11. Green H, Bishop P, Houston M, McKillop R, Norman R, Stothart P. Time-motion and physiological assessments of ice hockey performance. *J Appl Physiol*. 1976;40(2):159–63.
12. Tedesco LJ, Swindell HW, Anderson FL, et al. Evaluation and management of hand, wrist and elbow injuries in ice hockey. *Open Access J Sports Med*. 2020;11:93–103.
13. Hajek F, Keller M, Taube W, von Duvillard SP, Bell JW, Wagner H. Testing-specific skating performance in ice hockey. *J Strength Cond Res*. 2021 Dec 1;35(suppl 12):S70–75.
14. Roczniok R, Adam M, Przemysław P, Stanula A, Gołaś A. On-ice special tests in relation to various indexes of aerobic and anaerobic capacity in polish league ice hockey players. *Procedia Soc Behav Sci*. 2014 Mar 19;117:475–81.
15. Bigg JL, Gamble AS, Vermeulen TF, Bigg LM, Spriet LL. Sweat loss and fluid intake of female varsity ice hockey players during on-ice practices and games. *J Strength Cond Res*. 2020 Feb 1;34(2):389–95.
16. Roczniok R, Stanula A, Maszczyk A, et al. Physiological, physical and on-ice performance criteria for selection of elite ice hockey teams. *Biol Sport*. 2016 Jan 1;33(1):43–8.
17. Sim FH, Simonet WT, Melton LJ III, Lehn TA. Ice hockey injuries. *Am J Sports Med*. 1988 Jan;16(suppl 1):S86–96.
18. Council on Sports Medicine and Fitness, Brooks A, Loud KJ, Brenner JS, et al. Reducing injury risk from body checking in boys' youth ice hockey. *Pediatrics*. 2014 Jun;133(6):1151–7.
19. Kontos AP, Elbin RJ, Sufrinko A, et al. Incidence of concussion in youth ice hockey players. *Pediatrics*. 2016 Feb 1;137(2):e20151633.
20. Madias C, Maron BJ, Weinstock J, Estes NAM 3rd, Link MS. Commotio cordis—sudden cardiac death with chest wall impact. *J Cardiovasc Electrophysiol*. 2007 Jan;18(1):115–22.
21. McKay C, Campbell T, Meeuwisse W, Emery C. The role of psychosocial risk factors for injury in elite youth ice hockey. *Clin J Sport Med*. 2013 May 1;23(3):216–21.
22. Smith AM, Alford PA, Aubry M, et al. Proceedings from the ice hockey summit III: action on concussion. *Curr Sports Med Rep*. 2019 Jan 1; 18(1):23–34.
23. Smith AM, Stuart MJ, Wiese-Bjornstal DM, Gunnon C. Predictors of injury in ice hockey players: a multivariate, multidisciplinary approach. *Am J Sports Med*. 1997 Jul;25(4):500–7.
24. Mölsä J, Airaksinen O, Näsman O, Torstila I. Ice hockey injuries in Finland: a prospective epidemiologic study. *Am J Sports Med*. 1997 Jul;25(4):495–9.
25. Tucker C, Dhawan A. Ice hockey injuries. *Sports Med Update*. 2018;Winter(4):4–8.
26. Donskov AS, Humphreys D, Dickey JP. What is injury in ice hockey: an integrative literature review on injury rates, injury definition, and athlete exposure in men's elite ice hockey. *Sports*. 2019 Oct 23;7(11):227.
27. Mosenthal W, Kim M, Holzshu R, Hanypsiak B, Athiviraham A. Common ice hockey injuries and treatment: a current concepts review. *Curr Sports Med Rep*. 2017 Sep 1;16(5):357–62.
28. Pelletier RL, Montelpare WJ, Stark RM. Intercollegiate ice hockey injuries: a case for uniform definitions and reports. *Am J Sports Med*. 1993 Jan;21(1):78–81.
29. McKay CD, Tufts RJ, Shaffer B, Meeuwisse WH. The epidemiology of professional ice hockey injuries: a prospective report of six NHL seasons. *Br J Sports Med*. 2014 Jan 1;48(1):57–62.
30. Stuart MJ, Smith A. Injuries in Junior A ice hockey. A three-year prospective study. *Am J Sports Med*. 1995;23(4):458–61.
31. Black AM, Hagel BE, Palacios-Derflingher L, Schneider KJ, Emery CA. The risk of injury associated with body checking among Pee Wee ice hockey players: an evaluation of Hockey Canada's national body checking policy change. *Br J Sports Med*. 2017 Dec 1;51(24):1767–72.
32. Tuominen M, Stuart MJ, Aubry M, Kannus P, Parkkari J. Injuries in men's international ice hockey: a 7-year study of the international ice hockey federation adult world championship tournaments and olympic winter games. *Br J Sports Med*. 2015 Jan 1;49(1):30–6.
33. Schneider KJ, Nettel-Aguirre A, Palacios-Derflingher L, et al. Concussion burden, recovery, and risk factors in elite youth ice hockey players. *Clin J Sport Med*. 2021 Jan 1;31(1):70–7.
34. Abbott K. Injuries in women's ice hockey: special considerations. *Curr Sports Med Rep*. 2014 Dec 1;13(6):377–82.
35. Rosene JM, Raksnis B, Silva B, et al. Comparison of concussion rates between NCAA Division I and Division III men's and women's ice hockey players. *Am J Sports Med*. 2017 Sep;45(11):2622–9.
36. Popkin CA, Nelson BJ, Park CN, et al. Head, neck, and shoulder injuries in ice hockey: current concepts. *Am J Orthop*. 2017 May;46(3):123–34.
37. Pashby TJ. Ocular injuries in hockey. *Int Ophthalmol Clin*. 1988 Oct 1; 28(3):228–31.
38. Pauelsen M, Nyberg G, Tegner C, Tegner Y. Concussion in ice hockey — a cohort study across 29 seasons. *Clin J Sport Med*. 2017 May 1;27(3):283–7.
39. Benson BW, Mohtadi NG, Rose MS, Meeuwisse WH. Head and neck injuries among ice hockey players wearing full face shields vs half face shields. *JAMA*. 1999;282(24):2328–32.
40. Wennberg RA, Tator CH. Concussion incidence and time lost from play in the NHL during the past ten years. *Can J Neurol Sci*. 2008 Nov;35(5):647–51.
41. Kerr ZY, Roos KG, Djoko A, et al. Epidemiologic measures for quantifying the incidence of concussion in national collegiate athletic association sports. *J Athl Train*. 2017 Mar;52(3):167–74.
42. Sane J, Ylipaavalniemi PE, Leppänen HE. Maxillofacial and dental ice hockey injuries. *Med Sci Sports Exer*. 1988 Apr 1;20(2):202–7.
43. Häyrinen-Immonen R, Sane J, Perkki K, Malmström M. A six year follow up study of sports related dental injuries in children and adolescents. *Dent Traumatol*. 1990;6(5):208–12.
44. Lahti H, Sane J, Ylipaavalniemi P. Dental injuries in ice hockey games and training. *Med Sci Sports Exerc*. 2002 Mar 1;34(3):400–2.
45. Rampton J, Leach T, Therrien SA, Bota GW, Rowe BH. Head, neck, and facial injuries in ice hockey: the effect of protective equipment. *Clin J Sport Med*. 1997 Jul 1;7(3):162–7.
46. Willimon SC, Gaskill TR, Millett PJ. Acromioclavicular joint injuries: anatomy, diagnosis, and treatment. *Phys Sportsmed*. 2011 Feb 1;39(1):116–22.
47. Flik K, Lyman S, Marx RG. American collegiate men's ice hockey: an analysis of injuries. *Am J Sports Med*. 2005 Feb;33(2):183–7.
48. Moslener MD, Wadsworth LT. Ice hockey: a team physician's perspective. *Curr Sports Med Rep*. 2010 May 1;9(3):134–8.
49. Keshen S, Easterbrook M, Micieli JA. Ocular and facial injuries sustained by goaltenders in the National Hockey League: a preventable problem. *Can J Ophthalmol*. 2020 Feb 1;55(1):68–70.
50. Mueller FO, Cantu RC. *National Center for Catastrophic Sports Injury Research: Twentieth Annual Report, Fall 1982–Spring 2002*. Chapel Hill (NC): National Center for Catastrophic Sports Injury Research; 2002. p. 1–25.
51. Boden BP, Jarvis CG. Spinal injuries in sports. *Phys Med Rehabil Clin N Am*. 2009 Feb 1;20(1):55–68.
52. LaPrade RF, Burnett QM, Zarzour R, Moss R. The effect of the mandatory use of face masks on facial lacerations and head and neck injuries in ice hockey: a prospective study. *Am J Sports Med*. 1995 Nov;23(6):773–5.

53. Banerjee R, Palumbo MA, Fadale PD. Catastrophic cervical spine injuries in the collision sport athlete, part 1: epidemiology, functional anatomy, and diagnosis. *Am J Sports Med.* 2004 Jun;32(4):1077–87.
54. Melvin PR, Souza S, Mead RN, Smith C, Mulcahey MK. Epidemiology of upper extremity injuries in NCAA men's and women's ice hockey. *Am J Sports Med.* 2018 Aug;46(10):2521–9.
55. Nuber GW, Assenmacher J, Bowen MK. Neurovascular problems in the forearm, wrist, and hand. *Clin Sports Med.* 1998;17(3):585–610.
56. Ayars G. Nonallergic rhinitis. *Immun and Allergy Clin.* 2000 May 1; 20(2):179–92.
57. Bousquet J, Van Cauwenberge P, Bachert C, et al. Requirements for medications commonly used in the treatment of allergic rhinitis. European Academy of allergy and clinical immunology (EAACI), allergic rhinitis and its impact on asthma (ARIA). *Allergy.* 2003 Mar 24;58(3):192–197.
58. Ghiselli G, Schaadt G, McAllister DR. On-the-field evaluation of an athlete with a head or neck injury. *Clin Sports Med.* 2003;22(3):445–65.

109 Rock and Mountain Climbing

Erin Anne Miller and Winston J. Warme

INTRODUCTION

- Climbing began as an ascension to the summit of a mountain — Mt. Everest, the tallest peak on the planet at 29,035 ft, was a goal of climbers for generations and finally succumbed to Sir Edmund Hillary and Tenzing Norgay in 1953.
  - Once the tallest peak was reached, the focus shifted from simply summiting peaks to increasingly difficult and complex routes on them.
  - The increased technical skill required for these steep, sustained climbs led to focused sport-specific training and overtraining injuries.
- While climbing began as a lifestyle defined as the pursuit of a summit, it has diversified into a widely varied sport consisting of multiple disciplines and defies a succinct definition.
- The 2020 Olympics in Tokyo marked the debut of rock climbing as an Olympic discipline and highlights the degree to which climbing has become a mainstream sport.
- Indoor gyms evolved to prepare for the demands of this physical sport and novel indoor training techniques were developed.
  - The first climbing gym in the United States was established in Seattle in 1987, and by 2023, IBISWorld reported 486 climbing gyms in the United States. Gyms have artificial climbing walls that allow climbing in urban environments and have created widespread access, with even small cities boasting several indoor gyms.
  - With this accessibility, the profile of a climber has significantly changed. While 25 years ago climbers were thought of as reckless fringe elements taking extreme risks, the climbers of today range from kids on climbing teams to professionals and executives.
- While in 1989 the estimated number of active climbers in the United States was 100,000 (1), the Statista 2020 report estimates 10.28 million climbers.
  - Some climbers may never leave the relatively safe confines of a climbing gym, whereas others live in a van to climb outdoors as many days as possible.
  - Participants with no experience will often drop-in to a gym to climb, and "weekend warriors" with demanding day jobs abound.
  - Professional and sponsored climbers are featured in the mainstream media, and a dedicated subset of "dirtbag" climbers live out of their vans and travel to different climbing sites year-round.
  - This has made readily apparent the most notable division in climbing, that being recreational outdoor and competitive indoor climbing.
    - Competitive climbing is undertaken in a controlled gym environment to set a reproducible standard and has numerous competitions and structured practice through gym teams.
    - Recreational and some professional climbers pursue outdoor routes with a variety of objectives and see the gym primarily as a training ground for their other objectives.
    - Training for climbing ranges from the simple maxim of "climb more" to improve, to World Cup, Olympic, and professional athletes with highly structured training schedules including periodization focusing on power, power/endurance, and endurance while utilizing specialized training tools.

TYPES OF CLIMBING

- Multiple subdivisions of climbing exist, all with unique features that should be considered when treating the climbing athlete. Understanding these different disciplines allows assessment of the risks associated with each type.
- The first two disciplines discussed — bouldering and sport climbing — can be found either in a gym or outside; the remainder are exclusive to the outdoors.
  - *Bouldering:* Athletes climb without ropes or harnesses on short routes, which typically involve tricky, gymnastic moves.
    - The routes are referred to as "problems," as they frequently require learning or practicing unique moves.
    - Most climbing gyms have bouldering walls that average 15 ft in height; outdoor bouldering may potentially be much higher when climbers attempt "highball" problems that can reach 50 ft in height.

    - When bouldering outside, boulderers use thick foam mats termed "crash pads" to cushion their falls, and other participants serve as "spotters" to help them land safely.
- *Sport climbing:* The climber wears a harness connected to a rope that they clip into bolts that are drilled into the wall; a belayer with a friction belay device holds the other end of the rope to limit the length of a fall.
    - Routes vary widely in length from 50 to several hundred or even several thousand feet.
    - The protection of the bolts allows the climber to push physical limits as a fall is safer.
    - Sport climbing may be performed indoors or outdoors.
- *Traditional ("Trad") climbing:* Similar to sport climbing, harnesses and ropes are used on long routes, frequently involving multiple "pitches or rope lengths." Historically, metal pitons were hammered into cracks, but the transition to sustainable climbing has obviated their use.
    - Instead of clipping the rope to bolts that are fixed to the wall, removable stoppers and camming devices are placed into natural features in the rock to provide protection and limit the length of falls.
    - There is an additional level of knowledge and skill required compared to sport climbing, as knowing how to safely place the gear (called protection or "pro") is critically important.
        - Poor placement of gear can lead to its dislodgement in the event of a fall and increase the chance of injury.
    - Trad climbing is exclusively practiced outdoors and makes larger and more remote objectives possible for the climber.
- *Aid climbing:* For those routes that are too difficult to ascend the features on the rock with hands and feet alone, aid climbing allows a means to the top.
    - Small hooks with sling ladders ("etriers") attached are placed on rock edges or in cracks of the rock that are too small to place hands or feet; the climber steps up on the slings to ascend the rock.
- *Ice climbing:* Ascension of ice formations (waterfalls or icefalls) using ice axes, crampons (spikes fastened onto mountaineering boots), and ice screws.
    - The ice screws are used to clip in the rope to allow a belay; the degree of protection offered is dependent on ice quality and weather conditions.
- *Alpine, big wall, and mountaineering:* This is a broad generalization of traditional climbing pursuits with longer, multiday or week endeavors frequently involving multiple disciplines of climbing and may involve long hikes to "approach" the climb.
    - Alpine climbers often haul gear behind them and take folding "portaledges" that clip onto the protection placed in the wall to use as a sleeping surface.

- Within each of the climbing disciplines detailed above, there are multiple ways the route can be ascended, detailed below in order of increasing risk.
    - *Top roping:* The rope is clipped into an anchor above the climber the entire time, minimizing the distance of any fall.
    - *Lead climbing:* The climber goes up with the rope below them, clipping into bolts or gear along the route until they get to the top "anchor." There is a potential for large falls between bolts or placed gear.
    - *Speed climbing:* Most of the above disciplines can have the additional goal of speed added; extra risk may be taken to save time.
    - *Solo climbing* ("Soloing"): Climbing alone without a belayer; variations are listed below in ascending level of risk:
        - Top-rope solo: The climber has a rope attached to an anchor at the top and wears a self-locking device to catch a fall.
        - Lead solo: The climber wears a self-locking device and trails a rope behind them that is clipped into the wall as with trad climbing. Falls are significantly longer as the fixed point of the rope is always below them.
        - Deep-water soloing/psicobloc: The climber ascends routes over water without any rope; the water is used to cushion falls.
        - Free solo: The climber has no form of protection.
- The Olympic disciplines of climbing are all indoor climbing. There are currently three disciplines, and athletes are required to compete in each of them:
    - *Competition bouldering:* All participants climb the same novel bouldering routes; the winner is the one who completes the most routes with the least attempts.
    - *Speed climbing:* A standardized route is used in every competition and athletes race up the route protected by a top rope; the fastest climber wins.
    - *Lead climbing:* Different novel routes up 50-ft walls are set a priori and the climber must figure out the moves as they ascend the route, clipping their rope into bolts as they go; the climber who ascends highest or the fastest climber to the top wins.
- Climbing has several different scales to rate the difficulty of climbs, and climbers have varied skill sets that make certain routes more difficult than others. Therefore, ratings are subjective, and there is often disagreement on the actual difficulty.
    - Routes that climbers see as harder than they expect based on the stated rating are termed "sandbagged."
- The most common rating scales are:
    - *Yosemite Decimal System:* Initially created to describe all types of terrain, climbing requiring a rope for protection is considered class 5. The number after the decimal represents the relative difficulty. Climbs are rated from 5.1

(easy, suitable for beginners) to the hardest route that has been climbed at 5.15. Additional subdivisions begin at 5.9 with plus or minus, and 5.10–5.15 have subdivisions of A through D. An "A" designation indicates aid climbing is required, and grading of aid climbing difficulty is from 1 to 5.

- Most athletes can climb up to a 5.6–5.9 grade with little training; specific climbing experience is typically needed for more difficult climbs.
- Serious, dedicated climbers climb in the 5.10–5.12 range.
- Very few recreational climbers, but most professionals, are able to complete routes above 5.13.

- *Bouldering V scale:* Rates difficulty of boulder problems from V0 to V17.
- *Font scale:* Used in Europe instead of the decimal system. It runs from 1 to 9, starting with grade 6. There are subdivisions of A, B, and C with an optional + that may be added.

EPIDEMIOLOGY

- Contrary to conventional wisdom, many types of climbing are relatively safe, and catastrophic injuries are rare.
- True injury rate is difficult to establish; overall, injuries are roughly split by thirds into chronic overuse, acute supraphysiologic loading, and fall from height/rockfall.
  - 37% of injuries require evaluation by an orthopedist, and 43% of those patients undergo surgical intervention (2,3).
- Several studies have reviewed emergency department (ED) visits for climbing injuries.
  - From 2008 to 2016, the average yearly number of US ED visits was 3816.
    - Fractures were found in 27% of these patients, with lower extremities involving 47% of visits and upper extremities only 25% (4).
  - Over a 4-year period in the United States, the admission rate for climbing injuries was 11%, and less than 1% of climbing injuries resulted in death (5).
  - Only 0.6% of climbing injuries are reported from equipment failure (2,6).
- This presents a skewed picture of overall climbing injuries, however, as the subset of chronic and perceived minor injuries are not captured by ED visits.
  - In a survey study of 394 climbers, the fracture rate was only 8%, and tendon injuries were the most common at 56% (7).
  - A larger survey of 808 climbers found that, compared to ED data, lower extremity injuries only accounted for 21% of climbing injuries, finger injuries were the most common at 39%, fractures occurred in only 5%, and dislocations in 3%. Concussion was the least common injury at <1% (3).
- Minor injuries, however, are common. The injury rate in the 2018 Youth Olympics was 2%, the lowest of all the sports in the games (8).
  - The injury rate at the 2005 Climbing World Championships was 3.1 per 1000 hours, and multiple additional studies found rates from 0.2 to 2.95 per 1000 hours (9–11).
  - In comparison to other sports, such as cycling with 13.5, football with 31, ice hockey with 83, and rugby with 286 injuries per 1000 hours, the climbing injury rate is relatively low (11).
  - The unique grips and gymnastic body movements found in most commonly in bouldering, competition, and sport climbing yield more hand, hip, and knee injuries, compared to mountaineering, traditional, and alpine climbing where injuries from falls from a greater height are more common.
  - Injury rates in climbing disciplines are reported with wide variation across multiple studies, and it is impossible to say if one form is "riskier" or even differentiate between indoor and outdoor climbing.
  - Of the climbing disciplines, bouldering has the highest injury rate — likely due to the limited protection, the more demanding gymnastic nature of the routes, and the reality that every fall involves a landing on the ground or fairly limited padding (3,8).
  - Additional risk factors include:
    - Gender — Female climbers have a higher risk of shoulder and upper arm injuries with an odds ratio of 2.05; no other significant differences in male/female injury patterns have been reported (12).
    - Young age — Pediatric patients with open growth plates are susceptible to growth plate injuries in the fingers; physeal stress fractures were found in 20% of youth climbers in one study. As climbing gains popularity and youth teams proliferate, the incidence has risen from 0.8% in 1998 to 3.4% in 2012 (13).
    - Increased age — Athletes older than 35 sustain a greater proportion of finger and shoulder overuse injuries, including subacromial bursitis (8).
    - Experience level — The experience level of a climber increases the risk of a finger injury, with beginners, leisure, and amateur climbers having odds ratios of 0.19, 0.18, and 0.26, respectively, compared to professional climbers (12).

EQUIPMENT

- It is important to recognize that falls are an expected and accepted part of climbing, and protection is used to manage risk and decrease the rate of injury.

- Excluding bouldering, ground falls — that is, falling from a height onto the ground, or other hard surface, such as a ledge — are avoided at all costs as injury is frequently unavoidable in this scenario.
- Most falls are caught by the belayer with the rope and do not result in any injury.
- To mitigate risk of falls and other injuries, the sport requires a large amount of specialized equipment and training.
  - Climbing shoes (Figure 109.1A and B) — Rubber-soled shoes are used to allow the climber to obtain grip on the rock. The toes are stiff, narrow, and pointed to allow the toe to be placed on subcentimeter edges while supporting the entire body weight. Shoes are often purposefully sized small, causing metatarsophalangeal joint and interphalangeal joint flexion to maximize load bearing (2).
  - Chalk — Used on the hands to provide better friction and absorb sweat.
  - Gloves — Climbers do not wear traditional gloves for protection on their hands, but will wear commercial "crack gloves" or fashion a thick layer of tape to protect the sensitive skin on the back of the hand from abrasions when "jamming" — putting the hand into a crack in the rock.
  - Fall prevention
    - Harnesses are worn by both the climber and belayer for all climbing except bouldering and soloing. A strap goes around the waist with two leg loops.
    - Ropes are 8–11 mm thick and made with elasticity to absorb some of the force in a fall; while ropes are typically designed to hold 1000 kg, the care of the rope is critical as time, multiple falls, sharp rock edges, sunlight, and even dirt decrease the integrity of the rope.
    - Belay devices are used by the climber's partner to hold the rope in the case of a fall with minimal force on the belayer; there are multiple variations with more modern "autolocking" devices that decrease the risk of user error. All depend on creating a bend in the rope to increase friction.
    - Helmets are recommended outside to protect in the case of rockfall or an upside-down fall; however, these are not universally worn.
    - Protection or "pro" (Figure 109.1C and D) refers to the bolts or gear placed in cracks in the wall, the carabiners or "quick draws" (two carabiners connected by a short sling) are used to clip into them, and the cams, stoppers, and nuts that are placed into the rock when bolts are not available.
      - Indoor climbers require relatively less equipment as the infrastructure is built into the walls of many climbing gyms.
      - Climbing outdoors requires additional gear or "pro."

TRAINING

- While acute injuries in the form of catastrophic accidents readily come to mind, overuse injuries are somewhat more common. Understanding the training dedicated climbers

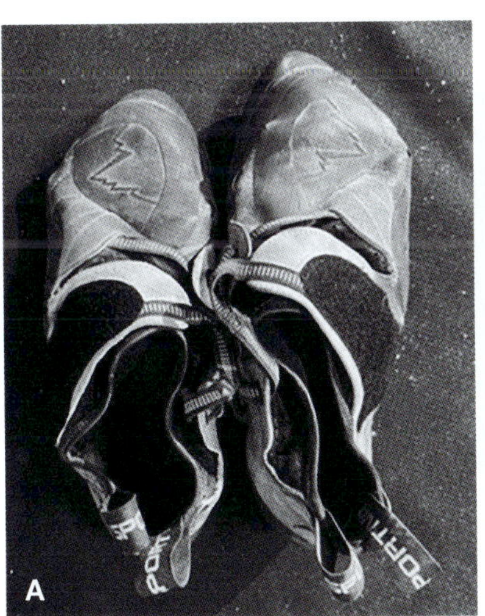

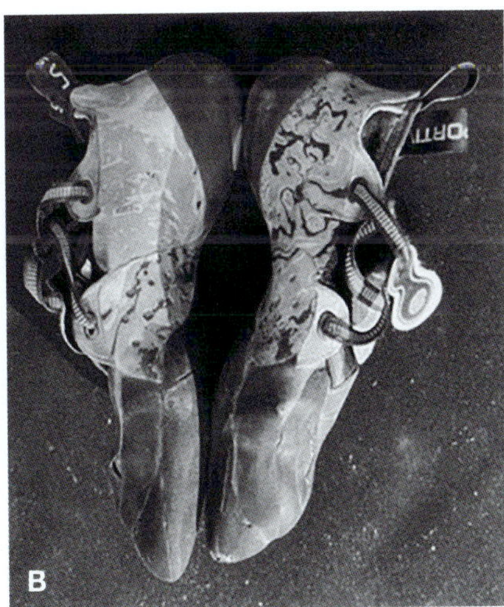

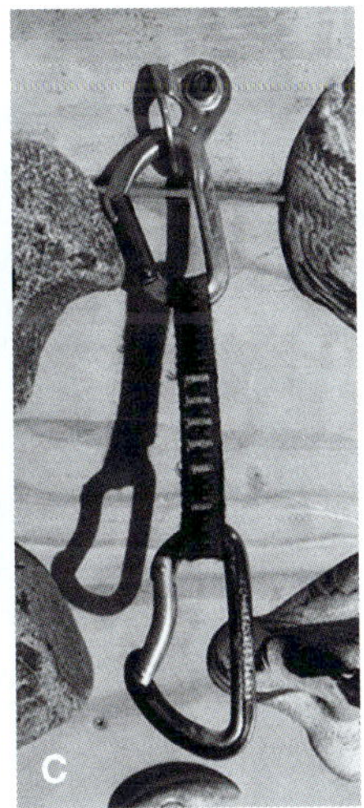

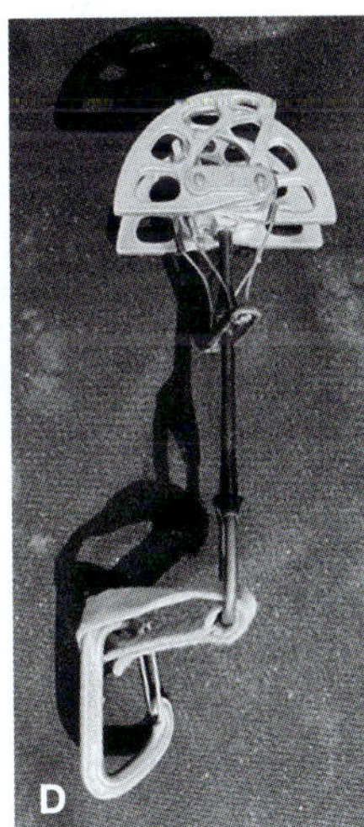

Figure 109.1: Climbing equipment. A and B: Climbing shoes are worn snugly to the climber's foot and the rubber further molds over time. Thick rubber is used around the toe and heel. A: AP view of the narrow, pointed toe box. B: Lateral view demonstrates a high arch and aggressive cup around the heel. C and D: Climbing protection or "pro" C: Equipment used in sports climbing, including bolts that link carabiner pairs called quickdraws to the rope, which is subsequently clipped to the lower carabiner. D: Equipment used in traditional climbing, which uses a variety of devices placed into the crack to allow clipping of the rope; a Camelot or "cam" is shown.

undertake is important to help guide the treatment and rehabilitation of the numerous climbing-specific injuries.

- Core strength training — Frequently gymnastic techniques, such as front levers, are used to improve core strength.
- Flexibility — Climbers often work on stretching and will cross-train with yoga to improve their ability to reach into odd positions to use the best holds.
- Grip strength training — Specific training to improve grip is undertaken to allow the climber to generate high loads through the fingers.
    - Hang board — A series of increasingly smaller edges that climbers practice holding their body weight on.
        - Serious athletes will wear additional weight when hanging.
        - Different grips are also practiced, which place variable amounts of strain through the fingers, including hanging by just two or even one finger in "pockets."
- Rice bucket — A bucket filled with rice to provide resistance where climbers work the antagonistic muscles for finger and wrist extension.
    - Campus board — A series of ledges a fixed distance apart on an overhanging ledge on which climbers practice dynamic and explosive movements, typically without using footholds.
    - Standardized interactive climbing training boards include MoonBoards, Tension Boards, Kilter Boards, Lattice Boards, System Boards — allow climbers to attempt progressively difficult standardized problems to increase their strength and power.

INJURIES

- Climbing-specific injuries that are unique to the sport are primarily found in the hand and discussed in detail below. These unique injuries are the result of the variation of hand positions the climber uses (Figure 109.2).
- Hand/finger injuries
    - *Pulley rupture*
        - The annular pulleys, which keep the flexor tendons opposed to the bone, are **the most commonly injured structure in climbers.**
            - Sudden dynamic loading can cause a closed pulley rupture, most commonly at the A2 pulley, which lies over the proximal phalanx.
            - The greatest stress on the A2 pulley is when the climber is using the "crimp" position with the hand (PIPs flexed with distal interphalangeal joint [DIPs] extended), which generates forces up to 450 N — the accepted load failure of the A2 pulley is 400 N (2).
            - The A4 pulley lies over the middle phalanx and is more commonly injured with the open-hand grip.
            - Multiple pulley ruptures are less common but cause acute bowstringing that is often evident clinically.
            - Chronic pulley attenuation is more rare.
        - On history, patients may report hearing a "pop" at the time of injury, and on exam, there is tenderness over the pulley site.
            - Patients with multiple pulley ruptures may have visible bowstringing of the tendon along the finger

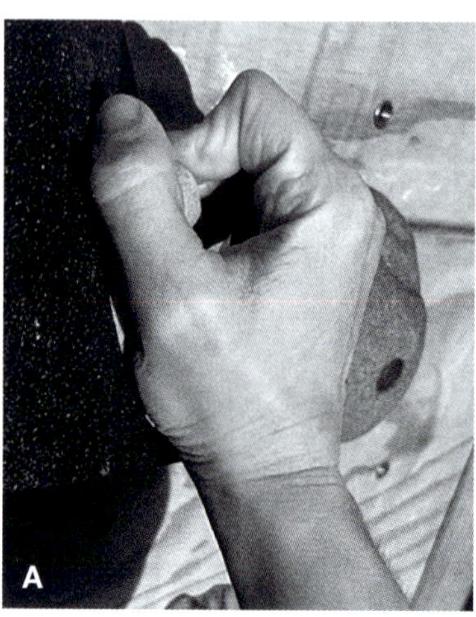

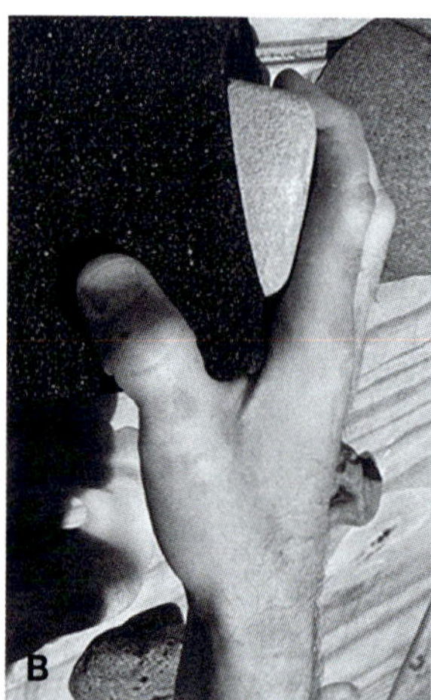

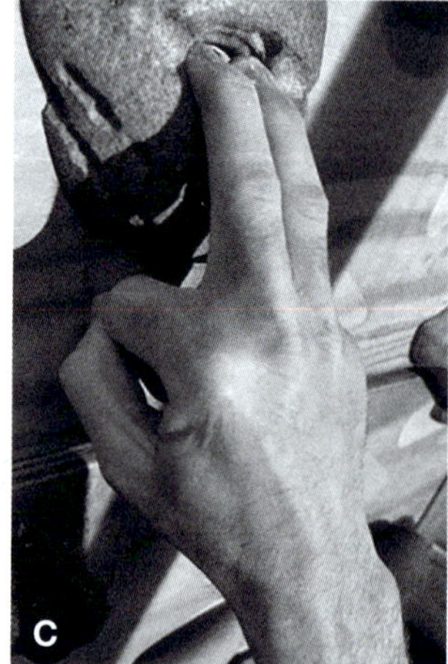

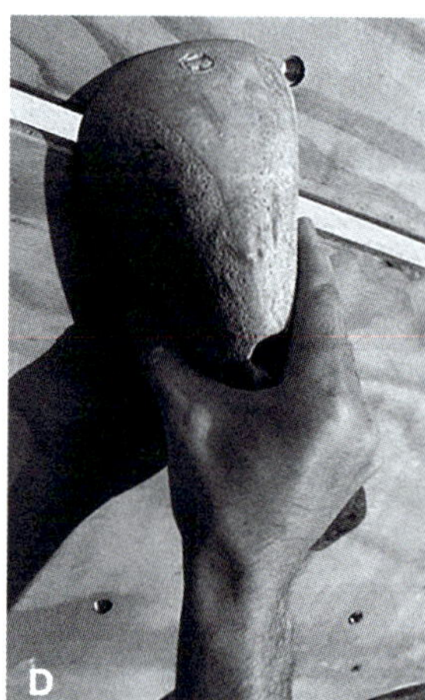

Figure 109.2: Grip positions are unique to climbing and subject the hand to a wide variety of forces. A: The crimp position has the proximal interphalangeal joints flexed and DIPs extended, leading to maximal force on the A2 pulley. B: An open-hand position decreases the load on the pulleys. C: A pocket only allows one or two fingers to be placed and leads to differential glide on flexor digitorum profundus tendons and strain on the lumbricals. D: The pinch grip loads the thumb carpometacarpal joint.

with resisted flexion and are often unable to achieve full finger flexion.

- Definitive diagnosis can be obtained with ultrasound — greater than 2 mm of space between the tendon and bone is consistent with rupture (10,14). MRI may also demonstrate increased space but is more costly than ultrasound (Figure 109.3)
- Grading of pulley injuries is on a one to four scale (14):
    - Grade 1 — Pulley strain, no increased space on ultrasound
    - Grade 2 — Partial A2 rupture or complete A4 rupture, <2 mm space on ultrasound
    - Grade 3 — Complete A2 rupture, >2 mm space on ultrasound
    - Grade 4 — Multiple pulley ruptures or complete A2 rupture with concomitant injury
- Treatment of grades 1–3 is with conservative management — a custom pulley ring splint (made by a hand therapist or from a custom kit available online) should be worn around the finger, and active range of motion may continue unrestricted.
    - The finger should be non–weight bearing for 6–8 weeks with grade 1 and 2 injuries and 2–3 months for grade 3 with subsequent gradual return to load-bearing activities (8,11,14).
    - At the time of return to climbing, a custom ring splint should still be worn for the next 8 weeks.
- In multiple pulley ruptures, when bowstringing is clinically apparent, or in patients who cannot generate full flexion of the finger after conservative treatment, surgical pulley reconstruction is undertaken by a hand surgeon. Palmaris longus tendon autograft is used to re-create the A2 pulley. Stiffness is a frequent complication (14). Return to climbing occurs between 3 and 6 months after surgical intervention.

- *Tenosynovitis* of finger flexors
    - This is the second most common finger climbing injury. Inflammation of the flexor tendons or pulley system, often after a pulley injury, is common and extremely frustrating for climbers. Synovitis and scar formation around the pulleys are seen similar to the changes found in trigger finger; however, climbers do not experience catching/locking/triggering of the finger (11,14). It is difficult to differentiate on history and exam from a pulley injury.
    - Patients usually deny any acute injury, hearing a pop, or any excessive loading, but may report pain beginning after an intense training session or increasing frequency of sessions. On exam, diffuse tenderness over the volar fingers is apparent, most commonly affecting the middle and ring fingers (14).
    - Ultrasound may demonstrate synovitis as fluid around the tendon, termed the "halo" sign, but bowstringing is absent (8).
    - Conservative management with decreased intensity, avoiding crimping, and anti-inflammatories are recommended, and the use of a supportive ring splint; symptoms may be recurrent, lasting more than a year but eventually resolve. This is often a point of intense frustration for climbers (11,14,15).
        - Steroid injections are controversial; we do not recommend them in climbers given the risk, albeit very low, of tendon rupture. A retrospective study demonstrated no complications in 42 climbers injected with steroids (16); however, given the high forces climbers place through their tendons, any level of increased risk of tendon injury is deemed

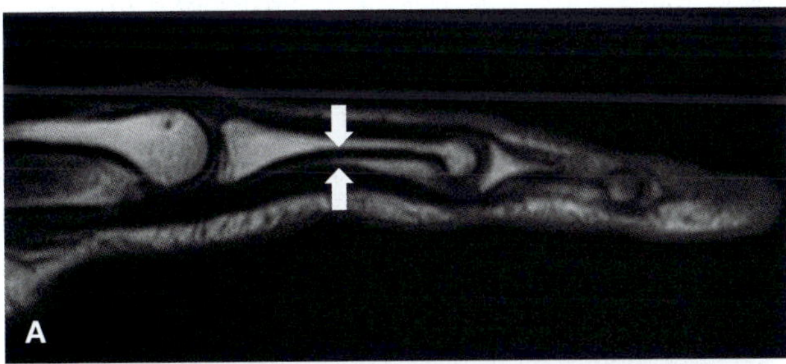

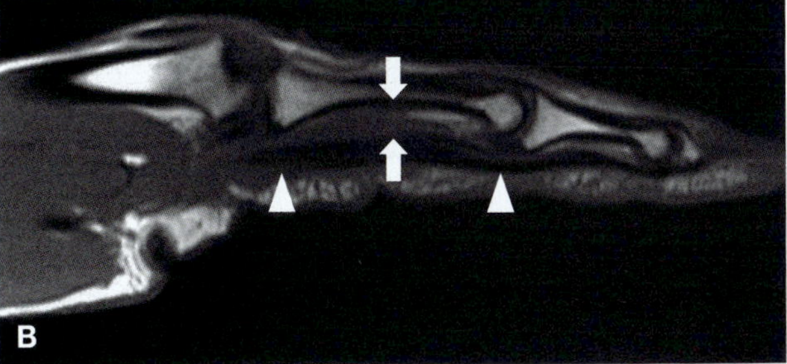

Figure 109.3: Flexor tendon bowstringing seen on MRI. A: Lateral view of a finger demonstrating an intact pulley system — in this view, the dark tendon is nicely opposed to the proximal phalanx along the majority of the bone. B: Bowstringing seen in a finger with an A2 pulley rupture — the tendon does not contact the proximal phalanx except at the base and head.

unacceptable. Hyaluronic acid injections may be preferable, but more data are needed (15).

- *Proximal interphalangeal (PIP) joint injuries*
  - The PIP joint is supported by strong collateral ligaments as well as bony structure that gives it stability through motion. Lateral stress on the finger can lead to tearing of these collateral ligaments, often seen during "crack climbing" where the climber's fingers are inserted into a small seam on the rock and a sudden, unexpected torsional force is applied — such as if a foot slips. If the force is enough, dislocation or even fracture may occur (11).
  - Evaluation of the joint should be completed by a hand surgeon to assess collateral ligament stability; three-view radiographs of the finger are obtained to ensure joint congruency and rule out fracture.
  - Stable, congruent joints are treated conservatively with buddy taping, early motion, and avoidance of load bearing.
  - Complete collateral ligament injuries with an unstable joint require operative intervention with repair of the ligament or reconstruction with tendon graft in the case of chronic injury.
- *Lumbrical shift syndrome*
  - An intrinsic muscle of the hand, the lumbricals originate on the flexor digitorum profundus (FDP) tendons and insert on the extensor mechanism. The origin of this muscle on the tendon exposes it to unique injury in climbing — when using a "pocket" hold, one or two fingers are extended and the rest flexed in the palm, creating differential motion between the FDP tendons and causing injury ranging from strain to musculotendinous avulsion. The third lumbrical is most commonly affected (11,14).
  - On history, the patient reports sudden, sharp pain in the palm. Exam is normal when the fingers are loaded in concert but demonstrates palmar pain when the finger associated with the injured lumbrical is loaded individually.
  - Treatment is conservative with early stretching and motion exercises — failure to initiate treatment can lead to scarring in the muscle and further injury. Buddy taping to the adjacent finger can prevent stress of the injured muscle. Severe injuries may take up to 5 months for recovery (14).
- *Finger growth plate injuries*
  - Epiphyseal fractures occur in pediatric patients whose growth plates remain open.
    - Closure of the growth plates/ossification completes between ages 14 and 16 in females and 17 and 19 in males.
    - Repeated stress via dynamic loading, such as overtraining or regular campus board training, commonly causes Salter-Harris I, II, or III type fractures through the growth plate as the epiphysis is the weakest part of the bone (8,10,14) (Figure 109.4).
    - 87.5% of climbers younger than 14 with finger pain were found to have epiphyseal fractures (17).
  - The ring and middle fingers are most commonly affected.
  - Patients do not report a specific injury to the finger but often have increased their training frequency or volume of climbing.
  - On exam, there is tenderness over the dorsal PIP.
  - Diagnosis is made with three-view plain radiographs of the finger; if x-rays are negative and pain persists more than 2 weeks, MRI should be obtained.
  - Chronic growth plate injuries risk premature closure: Thus, any epiphyseal injury should be treated promptly.
  - Treatment is conservative in acute, nondisplaced fractures — The finger should be non–weight bearing (no climbing!) and undergo range-of-motion exercises several times daily until radiographs demonstrate fracture healing (8). Splinting is not required unless needed for patient compliance.
  - Displaced fractures usually require surgical reduction and stabilization with Kirschner wires by a hand surgeon.
  - Chronic or fractures may have evidence of sclerosis on x-rays or advanced imaging, and surgical treatment is recommended (8).
  - Patients who continue climbing despite fracture are at risk for necrosis of the fracture fragment and early growth plate closure, with consequences of a foreshortened finger, axial-deviation, chronic joint deformity, and stiffness (11); the severity of these injuries should be stressed to patients and parents.
- *Hook of hamate fracture*
  - Rather than direct impact on the hook of the hamate, in climbers this fracture pattern is caused by an avulsion injury due to excess pressure of the ring and small finger FDP tendons, which are highest with an "under-cling" grip position where the hand is fully supinated and ulnarly deviated while grasping a hold (2,14).
  - Patients infrequently recall a specific injury; they complain of ulnar-sided wrist pain and possible ring and small finger paresthesia. On exam, there is pain on palpation over the ulnar palm and reproduction of pain with the wrist in ulnar deviation and resisted flexion of the ring and small fingers (14).
  - Radiographs of the wrist should include a carpal tunnel view to visualize the hook of the hamate as it is not seen on standard wrist views; CT is obtained if the diagnosis is unclear.

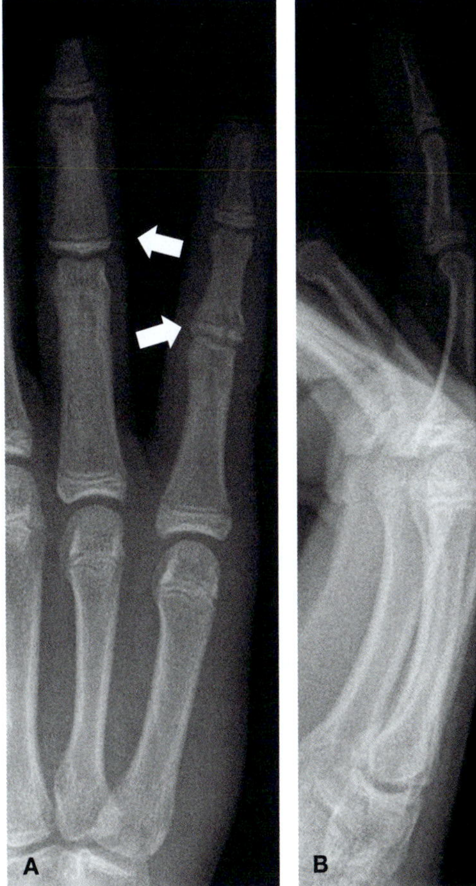

Figure 109.4: X-rays of a small finger physeal injury. A: AP view demonstrates loss of visualization of the growth plate when compared to adjacent digits. B: Lateral view depicts a Salter-Harris type III fracture with mild extension through the injury.

- Conservative treatment with cast immobilization and non–weight bearing is recommended for climbers; while other athletes return to play quicker with hook of hamate excision, this has been shown to decrease grip strength up to 15% and is not recommended in a high-level climber (14).
- In the case of nonunion, surgical excision is recommended despite the consequence of decreased grip strength.

- *Retinacular cysts*
  - Microtears in the pulley system, typically over the A1 or A2 pulleys, can allow synovial fluid to leak out creating a firm, hard cyst limited to a few mm in size. These may be painful with direct loading during climbing. A hand surgeon can offer rupture in office or surgical excision.
- *Nerve compression*
  - Carpal tunnel syndrome may be seen in climbers; it is managed as in nonclimbers with no notable deficits despite concerns in the literature for flexor tendon bowstringing after transverse carpal ligament release (11).
  - Radial tunnel syndrome is uncommon but may have a slightly increased incidence in climbers given forearm muscle hypertrophy; it presents with pain dorsally and distal to the lateral elbow, reproduced with resisted middle finger extension and weakness with finger extension. If conservative therapy with stretching fails, a hand surgeon may consider a radial tunnel release (11).

- Upper arm/shoulder
  - *AC separation* is typically caused by a fall on the point of the shoulder or a sudden load with the arm externally rotated and abducted overhead.
    - Lower-grade separations may be treated conservatively in a sling with range-of-motion exercises, while higher-grade injuries are considered for surgical intervention.
  - *Rotator cuff tears* in middle-aged climbers may be acute or chronic. Impingement, positive Jobe test, or positive belly-press test should raise suspicion, and MRI can confirm the diagnosis (11); referral to a shoulder surgeon is recommended.
    - Acute cuff tears are usually repaired surgically whereas chronic tears conservative management may be effective as the surrounding muscles have compensated to some degree (14).

- *Glenohumeral dislocation* is often managed conservatively in the ED with relocation; however, close follow-up with an orthopedist is warranted — many surgeons will recommend arthroscopic stabilization in the setting of anterior dislocation and Bankart lesion (tear of the anterior labrum often with a bony defect in the glenoid socket) to prevent recurrence in the climbing athlete (2). Climbing athletes over 40 years of age who sustain a dislocation may concomitantly injure their rotator cuff tendons, so thorough evaluation is important.
- *Superior labral anterior to posterior tears*, in contrast, are more frequent and result from repetitive microtrauma while loading the arm overhead while internally rotated. Crank and O'Brien tests are positive (14). MRI is diagnostic.
  - Treatment is conservative with physical therapy to work on shoulder stabilization (11). Referral is warranted for persistent symptoms, as biceps tenodesis yields good results in chronic injuries (13).
- *Brachialis tendonitis* is also termed "*climber's elbow.*" It results from an imbalance in the upper arm musculature — most hand positions while climbing are in pronation, which offloads the biceps and transfers the entire load to the brachialis. This may be the entire body weight if the climber is in a "lock-off" position, and chronically loading in this fashion causes tears in the musculotendinous junction of the brachialis (2). Climbers may also develop medial or lateral epicondylitis, which are not specific to climbing. Diagnosis of brachialis tendonitis can be made with reproduction of pain with resisted elbow flexion in the pronated position that resolves in the supinated position (14). Treatment is conservative with rest, anti-inflammatories, and eccentric muscle strengthening.

- Back
  - *Climber's back* is a chronic posture deformity, consisting of thoracic kyphosis, lumbar lordosis, and hunched shoulders — it stems from an imbalance of the anterior and posterior chain muscles.
    - Overdevelopment of the pectoralis minor leads to shortening of the tendon and anterior displacement of the shoulders.
    - Flexibility training and balanced strengthening of pushing and pulling muscles should be used to prevent as well as treat this deformity and decrease the risk of spondylosis, chronic back pain, and thoracic outlet syndrome (2).
  - *Vertebral compression fractures* are uncommon but should be considered in any climber with back pain who reports a fall from height.
- Lower extremity
  - *Foot and ankle fractures* are common in the lower extremity after a fall from height onto the feet.
    - Climbers have a particularly high rate of sustentaculum tali fracture of the calcaneus (2).
      - Any athlete with a calcaneal injury following a fall from height should also be evaluated for concomitant lumbar spine injury, as the force of impact is often transmitted proximally, leading to coexistent injuries.
    - Bimalleolar and trimalleolar ankle fractures, ankle sprains, and ankle and subtalar dislocations are also common after a significant fall, and appropriate referral to an orthopedist is warranted.
  - *Hamstring strain* may be sustained by a climber using a heel-hook position (Figure 109.5A) — eccentric muscle contraction may even create a hamstring avulsion (18). Treatment is conservative in most cases, but severe avulsions may need surgical repair.
  - *Knee injuries*
    - *Posterior lateral corner and lateral collateral injuries* may also be created by the heel-hook position as the hip is externally rotated with additional external rotation and varus stress transferred to the knee (2,18).
      - Orthopedic referral is recommended.
    - *Meniscus tears and medial collateral ligament injuries* are common with the drop-knee position (Figure 109.5B) — as the hip is internally rotated and the knee deeply flexed, the force is transferred medially (2).
      - Evaluation by an orthopedic surgeon is warranted in the patient with knee pain who describes a drop-knee mechanism.
  - *Foot injuries* — As previously noted, climbing shoes are designed to maximize load bearing at the toes to allow use along small edges and are fitted snugly to prevent slippage between the foot and the shoe.
    - This can cause multiple climbing-shoe–related foot complaints, including plantar fasciitis, metatarsalgia, hallux valgus, hallux rigidus, metatarsophalangeal (MTP) joint sesamoiditis, interdigital neuroma (Morton neuroma), deep peroneal neuritis, and retrocalcaneal bursitis (2,11).
    - Treatment involves active rest, cross-training, the use of larger and stiffer shoes for a period of time, stretching, anti-inflammatories, and/or orthotic use until symptoms improve.
    - Ingrown toenails as well as chronic fungal foot infections are also common and may be treated in a standard fashion.
    - Retrocalcaneal bursitis may be triggered by shoes but exacerbated with certain climbing moves, such as the heel hook. Avoidance of this position should be counseled while the foot is symptomatic.
    - As mentioned above, climbers have an increased incidence of sustentaculum tali fractures, which are often missed on radiographs; a high index of suspicion should be maintained in patients with heel pain and a fall from height. The fracture may be

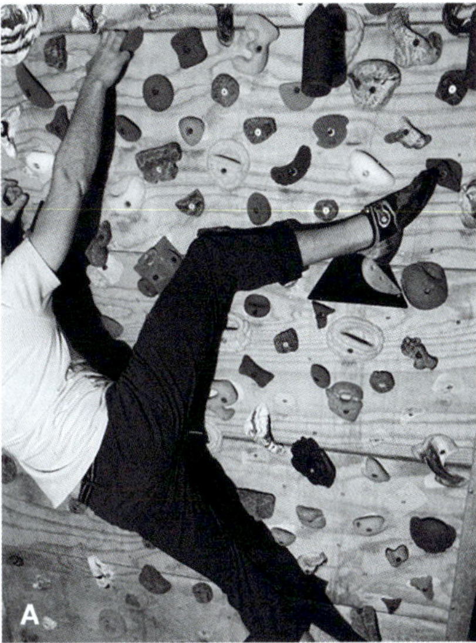

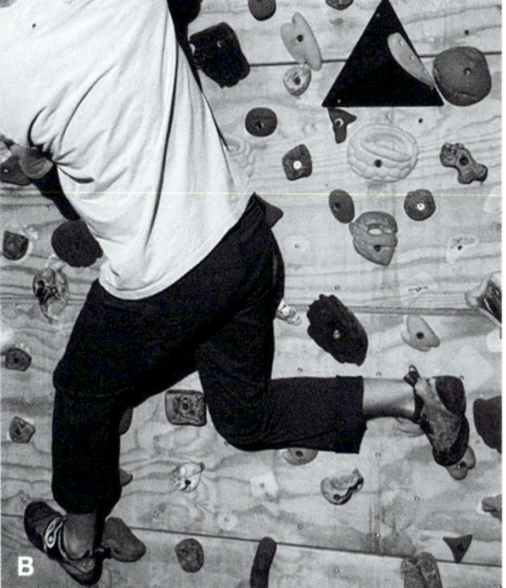

Figure 109.5: Lower body positions pose a risk for hip and knee injuries; variation in technique and upper body position may relatively increase or decrease the risk. A: In a heel hook, the climber's weight is suspended from the heel with the hip externally rotated and the knee experiences a varus stress. B: In the drop-knee position, the hip is internally rotated, and the knee experiences a valgus stress.

bilateral and concomitant lumbar injury should be suspected (2).

- Radiographic Harris heel view should be obtained to ensure this injury is not missed, and prompt referral to a foot and ankle surgeon made once this fracture is diagnosed.

- *Head injuries*
  - While head injuries are uncommon, they can occur both indoors and outdoors, most frequently as a result of a ground fall from a height, resulting from failure of safety equipment, or free solo climbing.
    - Less frequently, rockfall can cause major head injuries, including skull fractures and intracranial hemorrhage.
    - More minor head injuries can be caused by the climber dropping gear on the belayer's head.
- Frostbite
  - In alpine climbers and mountaineers, exposure to extreme cold in remote locations far from civilization may lead to exposure injuries such as frostbite.
  - This is most commonly seen on the toes, but also may involve the fingers, nose, and ears.
  - Initial treatment consists of rapid rewarming and transfer to a burn center for consideration of thrombolytic agents.
  - If there is persistent necrotic tissue after rewarming, amputation may be undertaken.

INJURY PREVENTION

- The physician plays an important role in both education and prevention. As a large proportion of injured climbers experience recurrent injury within the year of the index injury, there is an opportunity to intervene with appropriate counseling.
- General precautions
  - Climbers should be aware of safety hazards in the environment, keeping in mind environmental risks, including rockfall and weather.
  - Proper safety equipment should be used at all times.
  - Rings should never be worn while climbing as a devastating ring avulsion injury could occur if the ring catches on an edge or in a crack during a fall.
- Taping
  - Many climbers routinely tape their fingers as prevention for pulley injuries; there are several studies that show this does not decrease the risk of pulley injury and in fact, climbers who taped preventatively were more prone to injury with an odds ratio of 5 (19).
  - Taping is beneficial to prevent skin damage when crack climbing but is ineffective at injury prevention despite being often recommended by climbers. Postinjury during the rehabilitation period, it does play a role; however, more effective is the use of a custom ring splint to support the pulleys as the climber returns to full activity (11).

- Balanced training
  - Warming up is an important tenet of most sports; however, it has been shown to be especially beneficial in climbing.
    - The first 100–120 moves lead to an increase in physiologic bowstringing of the tendons up to 30%, which decreases the force and subsequent risk of pulley injury (11).
      - The crimp position should be avoided until after the first 120 moves.
  - The use of campus boards leads to massive forces on the pulleys and tendons predisposing to injuries. Therefore, it is recommended that their use in training should be limited to no more than once a week and avoided in adolescents.
  - Brachialis tendonitis risk may be decreased if adequate strengthening of the brachialis muscle in the controlled setting — pull-ups should be done with the forearm in the pronated position to train the brachialis rather than the biceps.
  - Lumbrical tears may be avoided by more symmetric loading of the fingers in flexion — when using pocket holds, if possible, the uninvolved fingers should be kept partially extended rather than fully flexing them into the palm to avoid the differential motion of the FDPs that shears the lumbrical origin. In many cases, this is not practical, so training these finger pairs, usually ring and middle or index and middle on a hang board with incrementally increased loading can allow the lumbrical muscles to stretch out to accommodate this position.
  - It is important for training to be balanced; ensure training days are a mix of power, endurance, and aerobic capacity.
  - After high-intensity training or climbing days, it is important to take appropriate rest days to prevent overuse injuries.
- Footwear
  - Many of the foot pathologies seen in climbers stem from shoes being too small; encouraging the use of appropriate fitting shoes and choosing newer shoe models that provide less stress to the MTPs may be beneficial.
  - Climbers should be encouraged to avoid all-day wear of tight-fitting shoes and remove shoes between climbs.
- Safety equipment
  - Belayers should be appropriately trained and knowledgeable in the equipment they are using to avoid dropping their climber during a fall.
  - Appropriate maintenance of equipment, including ropes, is critical in preventing catastrophic failure.
  - Ground fall injuries may be minimized by placing adequate protective gear lower on the climb when "trad climbing."
  - Self-reported helmet use in climbers is extremely low, but given the dangers of rockfall and other hazards, their use outdoors should be encouraged.
- Pediatric climbers
  - Many athletes are unaware of the unique risk for epiphyseal injuries climbing with open growth plates presents, and thus do not seek treatment for unexplained finger pain. Educating patients, parents, and coaches on this risk is important.
    - Adolescents should train with an open grip as much as possible and avoid repetitively using the crimp position as this increases the load on the middle phalanx dorsally, where the risk of growth plate injury is highest (11,17).
    - Campus boards should be avoided in skeletally immature athletes.

SUMMARY

- Climbers are known for pushing the limits and accepting a high degree of suffering to achieve their goals.
- There are numerous sport-specific injuries, particularly related to the large forces that may be generated on the hands.
- Many climbers do not believe physicians are knowledgeable of these injuries and turn to other climbers or physiotherapists for advice, often leading to delayed presentations for definitive care.
- Physicians who have knowledge and understanding of common climbing injuries and the high commitment level of many climbers may be more likely to gain their confidence and improve compliance.

REFERENCES

1. Addiss DG, Baker SP. Mountaineering and rock-climbing injuries in US national parks. *Ann Emerg Med.* 1989;18(9):975–9. doi:10.1016/S0196-0644(89)80463-9
2. Cole KP, Uhl RL, Rosenbaum AJ. Comprehensive review of rock climbing injuries. *J Am Acad Orthop Surg.* 2020;28(12):e501–9. doi:10.5435/JAAOS-D-19-00575
3. McDonald JW, Henrie AM, Teramoto M, Medina E, Willick SE. Descriptive epidemiology, medical evaluation, and outcomes of rock climbing injuries. *Wilderness Environ Med.* 2017;28(3):185–96. doi:10.1016/j.wem.2017.05.001
4. Buzzacott P, Schöffl I, Chimiak J, Schöffl V. Rock climbing injuries treated in US emergency departments, 2008-2016. *Wilderness Environ Med.* 2019;30(2):121–8. doi:10.1016/j.wem.2018.11.009
5. Forrester JD, Tran K, Tennakoon L, Staudenmayer K. Climbing-related injury among adults in the United States: 5-year analysis of the National Emergency Department Sample. *Wilderness Environ Med.* 2018;29(4):425–30. doi:10.1016/j.wem.2018.05.006

6. Neuhof A, Hennig FF, Schöffl I, Schöffl V. Injury risk evaluation in sport climbing. *Int J Sports Med.* 2011;32(10):794–800. doi:10.1055/s-0031-1279723
7. Nelson NG, McKenzie LB. Rock climbing injuries treated in emergency departments in the U.S., 1990-2007. *Am J Prev Med.* 2009;37(3):195–200. doi:10.1016/j.amepre.2009.04.025
8. Lutter C, Tischer T, Schöffl VR. Olympic competition climbing: the beginning of a new era — a narrative review. *Br J Sports Med.* 2021;55(15):857–64. doi:10.1136/bjsports-2020-102035
9. Schöffl VR, Kuepper T. Injuries at the 2005 World Championships in rock climbing. *Wilderness Environ Med.* 2006;17(3):187–90. doi:10.1580/PR26-05
10. Jones G, Johnson MI. A critical review of the incidence and risk factors for finger injuries in rock climbing. *Curr Sports Med Rep.* 2016;15(6):400–9. doi:10.1249/JSR.0000000000000304
11. Schweizer A. Sport climbing from a medical point of view. *Swiss Med Wkly.* 2012;142:w13688. doi:10.4414/smw.2012.13688
12. Nelson CE, Rayan GM, Judd DI, Ding K, Stoner JA. Survey of hand and upper extremity injuries among rock climbers. *Hand (N Y).* 2017 Jul;12(4):389-394.
13. Schöffl V, Morrison A, Schöffl I, Küpper T. The epidemiology of injury in mountaineering, rock and ice climbing. *Med Sport Sci.* 2012;58:17–43. doi:10.1159/000338575
14. Sims LA. Upper extremity injuries in rock climbers: diagnosis and management. *J Hand Surg Am.* 2022;47(7):662–72. doi:10.1016/j.jhsa.2022.01.009
15. Mohn S, Spörri J, Mauler F, Kabelitz M, Schweizer A. Nonoperative treatment of finger flexor tenosynovitis in sport climbers — a retrospective descriptive study based on a clinical 10-year database. *Biology.* 2022;11(6):815. doi:10.3390/biology11060815
16. Schöffl V, Strohm P, Lutter C. Efficacy of corticosteroid injection in rock climber's tenosynovitis. *Hand Surg Rehabil.* 2019;38(5):317–22. doi:10.1016/j.hansur.2019.07.004
17. Schöffl V, Lutter C, Woollings K, Schöffl I. Pediatric and adolescent injury in rock climbing. *Res Sports Med.* 2018;26(suppl 1):91–113. doi:10.1080/15438627.2018.1438278
18. Lutter C, Tischer T, Cooper C, et al. Mechanisms of acute knee injuries in bouldering and rock climbing athletes. *Am J Sports Med.* 2020;48(3):730–8. doi:10.1177/0363546519899931
19. Larsson R, Nordeman L, Blomdahl C. To tape or not to tape: annular ligament (pulley) injuries in rock climbers — a systematic review. *BMC Sports Sci Med Rehabil.* 2022;14(1):148. doi:10.1186/s13102-022-00539-6

110 Lacrosse

Kyle W. Zittel and William F. Postma

INTRODUCTION

History (1)

- Lacrosse is considered to be the oldest sport in North America first played by Native Americans.
- The sport was derived from *baggataway*, a game French observed Native Americans playing in 17th century Canada. One of the original purposes of the game was to keep men fit and prepared for war.
- The term *lacrosse*, describing the stick used in the game, comes from appearance similar to bishop's crosier or crosse.
- In 1879, Canada formed the National Lacrosse Association (now the Canadian Lacrosse Association). Lacrosse is the National Summer Sport of Canada.
- Eleven U.S. men's college and club teams formed the National Lacrosse Association in 1879. By 1950, over 200 teams existed in the United States.

BACKGROUND

Demographics (2)

- U.S. Lacrosse Participation Survey in 2017 collected data from US Lacrosse Membership, National Collegiate Athletic Association (NCAA), National Federation of State High School Associations, and Laxpower. com.
  - Estimated that 826,000 people played organized lacrosse in 2017
  - Youth, 447,213; high school, 324,689; college, 42,508; professional, 390; and postcollege, 12,183
  - Over 183,000 men at 2900 high schools have school-sponsored programs (24% rise since 2012).
  - Over 65,000 women at 2717 high schools have school-sponsored programs (28.3% growth since 2012).
  - Over 25,000 men participated in over 370 universities with sanctioned programs.
  - Nearly 500 universities have sanctioned women's programs for 17,331 women athletes.
- Though growth has slowed some in recent years, since 2001, total participation has increased 226%, and has been referred to as the fastest growing team sport in the United States at all levels.
- There are currently two men's professional leagues: The National Lacrosse League (indoor or box) and the Premier Lacrosse League (PLL, outdoor or field). The PLL's inaugural season debuted in June of 2019, originally in competition with the established Major League Lacrosse League. In December 2020, the two leagues merged under the banner of the PLL.
- There are currently two women's professional leagues in the United States: Athletes Unlimited and Women's Professional Lacrosse League.
- Currently, both men and women teams also compete at the international level.
- The USA Lacrosse organization is recognized as the governing body in the United States.
- World Lacrosse, formerly the Federation of International Lacrosse, is the international governing body with 77 international members/teams.

Game Play

- Men's field lacrosse (3)
  - The men's game is played with 10 players per side:
    - Three attackmen (offense), three defensemen (defense), three midfielders (both), and one goalie (defense)
    - Teams may allow a maximum of six players on the offensive half and seven on the defensive half.
  - The field is 110 × 60 yards.
    - Goals are 6-feet square with a 9-feet diameter circular *crease* around them.
  - Substitutions may occur during play stoppage or during play.
  - Players may pass the ball or run while cradling the ball in their stick, or *crosse*.
  - The object is to score more points than the opponent by putting the ball into the opposition's goal.
  - Players may hit an opposing player who controls the ball or is within 5 yards of the ball.
  - Players may hit an opponent's stick or gloved hand with their own stick.
  - Players may use their body to contact opposing players.

  - Recently, the introduction of a shot clock at various levels of play has increased the pace of the game.
- Women's field lacrosse (4)
  - The women's game is played with 12 players.
  - One goalie, four attackers, four defenders, and three midfielders
  - The field is 120 × 70 yards.
  - No direct contact between players or checking is permitted per the rules, though significant incidental contact does occur during play.
- Men's box lacrosse
  - Six players per side, smaller net 4 × 4 ft (1.2 × 1.2 m)
  - Played in enclosed area (hockey rink/arenas)
  - More contact allowed than field lacrosse

Equipment (5,6)

- *Crosse* or stick
  - Length varies by position
  - Head: made of mesh or string
  - Shaft-made of wood, laminated wood, or synthetic material
    - Typically, metal alloy or carbon composite
    - Solid wood shafts are generally disallowed in organized play.
  - Attackmen's and midfielders' sticks must be 40–42 in long.
  - Defensemen's sticks must be 52–72 in long.
  - Head size of a goalie's stick is 10 and 12 in wide under NCAA rules.
  - The sticks for all other positions have head sizes that are smaller at 6–10 in (15–25 cm) wide at its widest point.
- Ball
  - Made of solid rubber
  - 7.75–8 in in circumference and weighing 5–5.25 ounces
- Personal equipment
  - While personal equipment varies by different game and position played, required equipment includes:
    - All players are required to wear mouthguards.
    - In men's game, helmet with full face mask, shoulder pads, elbow pads, and gloves
    - Women are currently only required to wear mouthguards and eye protection, although they may wear helmets (goalies are a notable exception).
  - Goalies
    - Both men's and women's goalies are also require head, chest, and throat protection.
    - Athletic cup and groin protection are highly recommended for male athletes.
  - Attackmen
    - Frequently wear lager elbow pads/arm guards, shoulder pads, and optional rib protectors
    - Sticks are shorter.
  - Defensemen
    - Frequently wear less or smaller protective gear in the men's game
    - Have a much longer stick than other players
  - Midfielders
    - Offensive, defensive, and face-off specialists
    - Often wear less protection than attackmen
    - May have longer or shorter sticks depending on position (defensive midfielders have longer sticks)

EPIDEMIOLOGY

- The NCAA Injury Surveillance System was developed by the NCAA in 1982 to monitor collegiate athlete injury patterns (7).
  - The latest data were presented in 2021 as a summary of injury patterns from the 2014–2015 season through the 2018–2019 season in all three NCAA divisions. (8,9)
  - Includes both time loss (TL) and non-time loss (NTL) injuries
- Injury rate in the men's game is overall reported to be 4.90 per 1000 athlete exposures (AEs) (8).
- The overall Division I injury rate is 4.34 per 1000 AEs, Division II injury rate is 3.68 per 1000 AEs (injury rate ratio [IRR] = 1.18; 95% confidence interval [CI] = 1.04, 1.33), while the overall Division III injury rate is 6.70 per 1000 AEs.
  - The competition IRR is higher than the practice injury rate (IRR = 2.59; 95% CI = 2.35, 2.84). A higher overall rate of injuries occurs during preseason than the regular season (IRR = 1.22) and postseason (IRR = 2.18).
  - Contact injuries (practice-related) were higher in preseason than regular season.
- Overall injury rate for NCAA women's lacrosse is 4.99 per 1000 athlete.
  - Competition injury rate was higher than the practice injury rate.
  - Overall preseason injury rates were higher than regular season and postseason injury rates.
  - Similar to the men's game, injury rates were highest in Division III 7.27 per 1000 AEs.
  - Table 110.1 shows injury frequency by body part (8).

INJURY PATTERNS AND MEDICAL CONSIDERATIONS

- Men's overall injuries (8)
  - Strains (23.3%), sprains (21.4%), and contusions (16.1%)
  - Knee injuries (15.1%), thigh injuries (12.3%), and ankle injuries (11.6%) accounted for the largest proportions of

Table 110.1 Injury Frequency by Body Part for Men's and Women's Lacrosse in Both Games and Practices

Men	Women
Game • Head/face/neck: 15% • Shoulder/Arm/Elbow/Hand/Wrist: 25% • Trunk/back: 7.3% • Lower extremity: 52%	Game • Head/face/neck: 16.2% • Shoulder/Arm/Hand/Wrist: 17.3% • Trunk/back: 6.4% • Lower extremity: 59.6%
Practice • Head/face/neck: 9.6% • Shoulder/Arm/Elbow/Hand/Wrist: 15.1% • Trunk/back: 9.1% • Lower extremity: 63.6%	Practice • Head/face/neck: 10.5% • Upper extremity: 6.5% • Trunk/back: 7.4% • Lower extremity: 74.2%

Source: D'Alonzo BA, Bretzin AC, Chandran A, Boltz AJ, Robison HJ, Collins CL, Morris SN. Epidemiology of injuries in National Collegiate Athletic Association men's lacrosse: 2014-2015 through 2018-2019. *J Athl Train*. 2021;56(7):758–65.

all reported injuries, with rates comparable in both practice and competition.
    - Ankle injuries (11.6%) accounted for the largest proportions of all reported injuries, with rates comparable in both practice and competition.
    - Ankle sprains (7.7%)
  - Hamstring tears (6.9%)
  - Concussions (8.0%)
  - Ball handling accounted for a larger proportion of competition injuries (13.8%) than practice injuries (4%).
  - Larger proportion of practice injuries than competition injuries were attributed to general play (39.0% vs. 27.4%) and running (13.7% vs. 6.8%).
  - TL
    - 27.9% of all reported injuries were NTL
    - 50.1 resulted in TL of >1 day
    - 29.3% resulted in TL of 10 or more days
  - In men's professional lacrosse, injury data from a single season (2019) revealed that an overall injury rate over the course of a professional lacrosse season was 43.87%. (10)
    - Three players (1.9%) underwent surgery and two players (1.2%) sustained season-ending injuries.
- Women's overall injuries (9)
  - Sprains (19.9%), strains (19.2%), inflammatory conditions (15.3%), and contusions (12.8%)
  - Knee injuries (17.4%) and ankle injuries (13.2%) accounted for the largest proportions of all women's lacrosse injuries reported, with comparable proportions of injuries reported during practice and competition.
    - Partial or complete lateral ligament complex tears (ankle sprains; 9.1%)
    - Partial or complete hamstring tears (3.8%)
  - Concussions (7.2%; overall rate = 3.58 per 10 000 AEs)
  - Injuries are most commonly attributed to noncontact (26.6%) and overuse (25.2%) mechanisms.
  - Similar proportions of injuries occurred during competition (33.5%) and practice (36.2%) during general play. However, a higher proportion of injuries in the practice setting were attributed to running (21.3%).
  - TL
    - 40.1% of all reported injuries were NTL.
    - 29.7% resulted in TL > 1 day.
    - 35.0% resulted in TL of 10 or more days.
  - Catastrophic injuries
    - Data were collected from 1982 to 2009 (11).
      - Seven fatalities (0.73 per 100,000 participants) have occurred as a result of indirect contact while playing lacrosse (exertional injury or complication of a nonfatal injury). Two fatalities (1.24/100,000 participants) have occurred as a result of indirect contact while playing lacrosse (exertional injury or complication of a nonfatal injury).
    - 1980 to 2008 high school and college mortality rate associated with lacrosse was 1.46 deaths per 100,000 person-years.
    - In men's high school lacrosse:
      - Two fatalities (0.21 fatalities per 100,000 participants)
      - Four nonfatal (permanent severe functional disability) injuries (0.42/100,000 participants)
      - Seven serious injuries (0.63/100,000 participants) were reported as a result of direct competition or practice. These injuries are defined as significant, though without permanent disability.
    - In men's collegiate lacrosse:
      - Four fatalities (2.49 fatalities per 100,000 participants)
      - Five nonfatal (permanent severe functional disability) injuries (1.86/100,000 participants)
      - Two serious injuries (1.24/100,000 participants) were reported as a result of direct competition or practice.
  - Commotio cordis and sudden death are known to occur but are rare (12).

Musculoskeletal Injuries

- Noncontact (13–16)
  - Lower extremity
    - Muscle strains of groin, hamstring, and low back strains
      - Associated with twisting motion of the torso, which is common motion during passing, shooting, checking, and scooping ground balls. These motions are often performed at high speeds and with rapid changes in direction.
      - Treatment includes cryotherapy and strengthening of affected regional musculature as part of a gradual return-to-play plan and to reduce the risk of repeat injuries (17).

- Knee
  - Knee injuries account for fewer than 20% of lacrosse injuries, and, similar to other field sports, anterior cruciate ligament and medial collateral ligament (MCL) injuries are common (18).
    - These may be the result of a lateral blow, but more often result from planting the foot during change of direction, resulting in intolerable stresses on ligaments.
  - The MCL is more commonly affected than lateral collateral ligament, typically the result of force on the lateral aspect of knee at full extension, with foot planted.
    - Because of the MCL's deep attachment to the medial meniscal periphery, meniscal tears should be suspected with higher grade MCL injuries.
    - Grades I, II, and most grade III MCL tears may be treated nonsurgically.
    - Treatment typically includes cryotherapy, hinged braces, and hamstring and quad strengthening, which are mainstays of rehabilitation.
    - Recovery may take up to 6 weeks, with hinged brace used in competition for 1–2 months for protection.
- Patellofemoral syndrome
  - Often seen in female players aged 12–15, due to anatomic stresses
  - Typically presents as anterior knee pain without any physical findings (*i.e.*, instability or effusion)
  - Theoretic risk factors include foot pronation, genu valgus, rotated or tilted patellae, or an increased dynamic Q-angle.
  - This is almost always treated nonoperatively. In the past, focus has been on strengthening of medial quadriceps (vastus medialis oblique) and hamstrings for prevention and treatment, but now it is recognized that excessive femoral anteversion as the result of relatively weak hip external rotators and abductors may also contribute to maltracking of the patella, particularly in women (19).
- Prepatellar bursitis is a common complication, especially in adolescent athletes.
  - Padding and protection of the area may decrease injury.
  - As with olecranon bursitis, discussed below, drainage or injection carries risks and should be considered carefully.
- Medial tibial stress syndrome
  - Overuse injury associated with fatigue of the tibialis anterior, which is associated with eccentrically deceleration of the forefoot, leads to irritation of fascia or the anterior border of the tibia.
  - Prevention revolves around proper stretching and activity modification may be required.
- Ankle
  - The majority of ankle injuries result from inversion mechanisms.
  - Slight inversion and plantar flexion are the state of least stability and the point when injury most often occurs.
  - Ligamentous injuries are most common.
    - Anterior talofibular ligament, followed by calcaneofibular ligament, and then posterior talofibular ligament
    - Deltoid ligament injuries are associated with eversion mechanism.
  - Avulsion fractures should be suspected with higher grade ligamentous injuries (grade II or higher).
  - Most sprains will recover in 1–3 weeks.
  - Early mobilization for nonfractures is the key to rapid return to healthy play.
  - Consider non–weight-bearing exercises (*i.e.*, aqua jogging).
  - Strengthening of evertors, invertors, plantar flexors, and dorsiflexors, as well as hip abductors and adductors and extensors.
  - Final rehabilitation should include dynamic strengthening focusing on proprioception (*i.e.*, slide board, figure-eight running drills).
- Fifth metatarsal fractures (20)
  - Fifth metatarsal base fractures are the most common foot fractures and predisposed to poor bone healing secondary to watershed vascular supply.
  - Zone 1 and 2 fractures can be treated with weight bearing as tolerated in surgical shoes or walking boots. Consideration for surgical management is patient specific in athletes.
  - Zone 1 — proximal avulsion fracture
  - Zone 2 (Jones fracture) — metaphyseal-diaphyseal junction
    - Increased risk of nonunion
  - Zone 3 — proximal diaphyseal fracture
    - Commonly seen in athletes as stress fractures
    - Associated with cavo-varus foot (high arch)
    - Commonly treated operatively
- Turf toe
  - Sprain of the plantar capsuloligamentous complex of the hallux metatarsophalangeal joint. This occurs due to hyperextension of the first metatarsal associated with rapid deceleration, commonly on artificial turf.
  - Prevention includes proper shoe fit, allowing some toe and forefoot movement.
  - Limiting hyperextension by taping is the appropriate treatment to allow for return to play.

- Upper extremity
  - Blocker's exostosis
    - This is a benign overgrowth of bone in the humerus that results in reaction to repeated direct trauma.
    - Most often occurs with repetitive stick-to-body contact at deltoid insertion.
    - The use of appropriate shoulder protection (deltoid cup) is important in prevention.
    - Monitoring for myositis ossificans is important (see below).
  - Goal keeper's thumb (21)
    - Fracture of distal or proximal phalanx of thumb
    - Typically results from impact of ball directly on extending thumb as goalie is attempting to save shot on goal
    - May require surgical fixation or immobilization
    - May be prevented with rigid covering over distal end of thumb
  - Medial and lateral epicondylitis
    - Usually result of cradling motion in the throwing arm. This cradling motion requires rapid pronation/supination and flexion/extension of the arm.
    - Stretching of affected muscle groups along with braces to reduce strain at tendinous insertions has proven effective in treating this injury.

- Contact
  - Lower extremity contact injuries are less common and are most often associated with stick-to-body or ball-to-body contact.
  - Contusions are common and may result from contact with a hard rubber ball, which may be propelled at up to 100 miles per hour.
    - Player controlling the ball is often repeatedly hit in the upper torso and extremities by the defender's stick.
    - Contusions are treated by standard PRICEMM protocol (protection, rest, ice, compression, elevation, modalities, medication) and may be covered with donut padding to help distribute future forces around the injured area.
    - May be complicated by *myositis ossificans*, which is the inflammatory bony deposition in muscle from repetitive trauma. Often occurs in vastus lateralis and deltoid insertion of humerus. Areas receiving repeated trauma should be protected with donut and hard plate over area.
  - Upper extremity
    - Olecranon bursitis
      - Often stick-to-body or body-to-ground contact
      - Many players do not wear elbow pads and are thus more susceptible to this injury.
      - Drainage of bursal fluid allows for improvement of symptoms and can be performed.
      - Bursitis may also respond to steroid injection into the bursal sac. However, this treatment carries increased risk of infection and is not routinely recommended.
      - Light compression and protective gear (*i.e.*, elbow pads) may help symptom relief and reduce risk of further complications.
    - AC separation
      - Associated with checks into the boards (box lacrosse), stick-to-body contact with a downward blow to the outer aspect of the shoulder, and fall on the outstretched hand (FOOSH) mechanisms.
      - Specific taping systems have been used to allow for reduction in pain with movement to encourage earlier mobilization.
      - AC immobilizers can be helpful in limiting movement of the joint to reduce pain.
      - Activity without pain is a key factor in determining readiness for return to play.
    - Clavicle fracture
      - Frequently the result of a direct blow from an opponent's *crosse*.
      - Most clavicle fractures can be treated with a sling for comfort, although some experts encourage fixation, especially when significant shortening (>2 cm) has occurred (22).
    - Scaphoid fracture
      - Most often from FOOSH injury
      - Immobilization is the appropriate treatment.
    - Hamate fracture (23)
      - Typically, the "hook" of the hamate is fractured due to a sudden deceleration of the *crosse* stick within the grip of the hand, such as when a player's stick is stopped by another's while shooting or passing.
      - Best identified with a "carpal tunnel view" on plain film or computed tomography.
      - Often heals with time and symptomatic treatment, but cases with chronic pain may improve with surgical excision of the avulsed tip (24).
    - Metacarpal, phalangeal, and interphalangeal joint dislocations (25)
      - Immediate traction and reduction are ideal.
      - Often associated with stick checking or falls where the stick traps the hand/fingers in a pathologic manner.
    - Gamekeeper's or skier's thumb (26)
      - Associated typically with falls in which the thumb is trapped by the stick
      - Hyperextension results in a tear of the ulnar collateral ligament.
      - May be complicated by retraction of the ulnar collateral ligament under the adductor aponeurosis,

thus impairing reattachment to the proximal phalanx (Stener lesion) (27)

- Forearm fractures
  - Either from stick-to-body contact during checking or from FOOSH injuries
  - Immobilization is the mainstay of treatment.
  - Surgical reduction and fixation may be required depending on the severity of injury.
- Shoulder subluxation/dislocation
  - Anterior instability is the most common and most often occurs when a significant force is applied to an abducted and externally rotated shoulder (as when a player is passing or shooting).
  - Although rare (2%–4% of dislocations), posterior instability can also occur, especially when a force is applied as the shoulder is flexed, adducted, and internally rotated, which occurs especially with defensive players as they push an attacker out of position (16).
  - An experienced practitioner may attempt a manual relocation on the sideline, as this may be easier prior to the posttraumatic spasming of the musculature. It is essential to assess for neurovascular integrity after relocating the joint, and it is highly advisable to get plain films to assess for any bony fracture (*i.e.*, Hill-Sachs deformity or bony Bankart lesion) (28).
  - Treatment should start with aggressive physical therapy to strengthen the stabilizing muscles around the joint, although some surgeons have recommended surgical stabilization even for first-time dislocators, because the rate of redislocation is high. Risks and benefits should be discussed with the patient (29).
- Shoulder burners (stingers)
  - Commonly result from stick-to-body contact with a check to the shoulder or a fall onto head or shoulder
  - Downward, forward depression of the shoulder
  - Often present with acute, shooting, shock-like pain in extremity
  - May have some transient motor deficits
  - Typically resolve without complication
  - Bilateral burners are almost exclusively the result of a more central spinal cord injury and should be evaluated as such.

Medical Considerations

- Exertional heat illness (EHI) and exertional heat stroke (EHS) can and does occur in lacrosse as with any sporting environment in summer months and/or elevated temperatures.
  - EHI lacrosse rates = 0.6 per 100,000 AEs during training and competition in NCAA
  - May occur in both field and box lacrosse
  - EHS is a true medical emergency with potential for organ injury and death (30).
  - Players with more protective equipment (*i.e.*, goalies) are at higher risk.
  - Hydration is essential and athletes should be provided with adequate hydration and electrolyte replacement during practices and games.
  - Anticipate problems with acclimation in different climates/altitudes.
    - Avoid conditions where EHI is more likely, such as when the wet bulb globe temperature is elevated.
    - Identify players at greater risk (higher body mass index, slower long-distance run times).
    - Players should be monitored for signs/symptoms of EHI.
    - Consider screening for sickle cell trait in higher risk ethnicities because mortality is higher in EHI with those carrying the trait.
  - Players showing signs of EHI should be immediately removed from play, equipment should be removed, and measures should be taken to decrease body temperature.

Other Common Injures

- Concussions (31)
  - Lacrosse helmets are designed to deflect blows from a stick or ball but are not meant to protect against high-velocity impacts, like being thrust into the boards (box lacrosse) or impact into the ground.
  - Also common when players are crouched down for scooping ground balls and are struck by another player.
  - Recommendations for concussion management encourage abandoning grading of concussions.
  - When in doubt, withhold player from play until symptom-free and a graded exercise progression is completed without resumption of symptoms.
- Eye injuries (32,33)
  - These are much more common in women's lacrosse due to minimal protective gear. However, the addition of eye protection, recently mandated by the NCAA, has significantly reduced the number of injuries (4).
  - It is felt that appropriate enforcement of the rules for contact will minimize eye and facial injuries.
  - May be the result of contact with ball or inadvertent stick contact
  - Traumatic eye injuries should be referred for immediate ophthalmologic examination.
  - Sunken eyes or extraocular muscle deficiencies may represent periorbital skull fractures.
  - Assessment for associated closed head injury may be warranted.
- Thoracic and abdominal trauma
  - Most commonly occur from stick checking.

- Injuries to abdominal organs are uncommon but should be considered in cases of significant abdominal pain or tenderness on exam.
- Rib padding may offer some protection.

- Trauma to the anterior neck
  - Usually results from the ball striking the throat
  - Goalies are most at risk.
  - Throat deflectors significantly reduce the incidence of injury.
- Lacerations are common and may be due to contact with the ball, stick, or shear forces from the chin strap on the face.
  - These should be treated as any other laceration with attention to hemostasis, and wound cleaning and closure, with sutures if needed.
- Epistaxis
  - If related to direct trauma, the athletes should be assessed for possible nasal fracture, associated facial fractures, dental injuries, and/or concussion.
  - Bleeding should be controlled by having the athlete hold their head forward (to avoid swallowing blood which can lead to nausea and/or vomiting).
  - Have the athlete hold firm pressure on the lower two-thirds of the nose, pinching the nostrils.
  - Packing may aid in tamponading bleed. Packing may be soaked with a vasoconstrictor (*i.e.*, oxymetazoline) to aid in hemostasis. If packing is left in place, antibiotic prophylaxis should be considered.
- Abrasions/turf burns
  - More common in box lacrosse or competition on artificial surfaces
  - Padding and lubrication with petroleum jelly should be used on at-risk areas to reduce incidence.
  - Ensure antiseptic cleansing of wounds and clean dressings to reduce infection risk.
- Blisters
  - Occur in areas of increased friction
  - Petroleum jelly, powders, moleskin, and nylon socks under thick socks may all help to reduce friction.
  - Treatment with donut pads to distribute forces away from the blister; appropriate cleansing of blister (especially if it has opened)

REFERENCES

1. *US Lacrosse Web site* [Internet]. Baltimore (MD): US Lacrosse. [cited 14 May 2011]. Available from: http://www.lacrosse.org
2. *US lacrosse Participation Survey* 2017 [Internet]. Baltimore (MD). [cited april 1]. Available from: http://www.uslacrosse.org
3. Sherbondy PS. Lacrosse. In: Mellion MB, Walsh WM, Madden C, Putukian M, Shelton GL, editors. *Team Physician's Handbook* 3rd ed. Philadelphia: Hanley & Belfus; 2002:759–65.
4. *NCAA Web site* [Internet]. Indianapolis (IN): NCAA Publications; [cited 16 May 2011]. Available from: http://www.ncaapublications.com/productdownloads/WLC09.pdf
5. *NCAA Web site* [Internet]. Indianapolis (IN): NCAA Publications; [cited 14 May 2011]. Available from: http://www.ncaapublications.com/productdownloads/LC12.pdf
6. Bakus C, Beil C, Bassett AJ, Bishop ME. Gender-specific injury patterns in the lacrosse athlete. *J Cartil Jt Preserv*. 2022:2(4):100084.
7. Dick R, Agel J, Marshall SW. National collegiate athletic association injury surveillance system commentaries: introduction and methods. *J Athl Train*. 2009;44(2):173–82.
8. D'Alonzo B.A, Bretzin AC, Chandran A, et al. Epidemiology of injuries in National collegiate athletic association men's lacrosse: 2014-2015 through 2018-2019. *J Athl Train*. 2021;56(7):758–65.
9. Bretzin AC, D'Alonzo BA, Chandran A, et al. Epidemiology of injuries in National collegiate athletic association women's lacrosse: 2014-2015 through 2018-2019. *J Athl Train*. 2021;56(7):750–7.
10. Warner TS, Buckley PS, Logan CA. Epidemiology of injuries in men's professional lacrosse among 158 athletes in a single season. *J Cartil Jt Preserv*. 2022;2(4):100086.
11. *National Center for Catastrophic Sport Injury* [Internet]. Chapel Hill (NC): NCCSIR Data Tables; [cited 16 May 2011]. Available from: http://www.unc.edu/depts/nccsi/index.htm
12. Maron BJ, Doerer JJ, Haas TS, Estes NA, Hodges JS, Link MS. Commotio cordis and the epidemiology of sudden death in competitive lacrosse. *Pediatrics*. 2009 Sep;124(3):966–71. Epub 2009 Aug 10. doi:10.1542/peds.2009-0167
13. Bartlett B, Cress D, Bull RC. Lacrosse. In: Bull RC, ed. *Handbook of Sports Injuries*. New York: McGraw-Hill, Health Professions Division; 1991:423–51.
14. Casazza BA, Rossner K. Baseball/lacrosse injuries. *Phys Med Rehabil Clin N Am*. 1999;10(1):141–57. vii.
15. Matthews LS, Hinton RY, Burke N. Lacrosse. In: Fu FH, Stone DA, editors. *Sports Injuries: Mechanisms, Prevention and Treatment*. Philadelphia: Lippincott Williams & Wilkins; 2001:568–82.
16. Ring D, Jupiter JB. Injuries to the shoulder girdle. In: Browner BD, Jupiter JB, Levine AM, Trafton PG, Krettek C, editors. *Skeletal Trauma: Basic Science, Management and Reconstruction*. New York: Saunders; 2008:1767–9.
17. Arner JW, McClincy MP, Bradley JP. Hamstring injuries in athletes: evidence-based treatment. *J Am Acad Orthop Surg*. 2019 Dec 1;27(23):868–77. doi:10.5435/JAAOS-D-18-00741
18. Yadav S, Dhakshanamoorthy R, Kumar I, Prakash A, Nagarajan R. Bone bruise patterns in ligamentous injuries of the knee with focus on anterior cruciate ligament. *Cureus*. 2022 Dec 1;14(12):e32113. doi:10.7759/cureus.32113
19. Petersen W, Ellermann A, Gösele-Koppenburg A, et al. Patellofemoral pain syndrome. *Knee Surg Sports Traumatol Arthrosc*. 2014 Oct;22(10):2264–74. doi:10.1007/s00167-013-2759-6
20. Roche AJ, Calder JDF. Treatment and return to sport following a Jones fracture of the fifth metatarsal: a systematic review. *Knee Surg Sports Traumatol Arthrosc*. 2013;21(6):1307–15. doi:10.1007/s00167-012-2138-8
21. Elkousy HA, Janssen H, Ferraro J, Levin LS, Speer K. Lacrosse goalkeeper's thumb. A preventable injury. *Am J Sports Med*. 2000;28(3):317–21.
22. Woltz S, Stegeman SA, Krijnen P, et al. Plate fixation compared with nonoperative treatment for displaced midshaft clavicular fractures: a multicenter randomized controlled trial. *J Bone Joint Surg Am*. 2017 Jan 18;99(2):106–12. doi:10.2106/JBJS.15.01394
23. Ingari JV. Wrist and hand. In: DeLee JC, Drez D, Miller MD, editors. *DeLee & Drez's Orthopaedic Sports Medicine: Principles and Practice*. New York: Saunders; 2009:1340–7.

24. Tian A, Goldfarb CA. Hook of hamate fractures. *Hand Clin.* 2021 Nov;37(4):545–52. doi:10.1016/j.hcl.2021.06.013
25. Elfar J, Mann T. Fracture-dislocations of the proximal interphalangeal joint. *J Am Acad Orthop Surg.* 2013 Feb;21(2):88–98. doi:10.5435/JAAOS-21-02-88
26. Bowers AL, Horneff JG, Baldwin KD, Huffman GR, Sennett BJ. Thumb injuries in intercollegiate men's lacrosse. *Am J Sports Med.* 2010 Mar;38(3):527–31. doi:10.1177/0363546509348754
27. Pulos N, Shin AY. Treatment of ulnar collateral ligament injuries of the thumb: a critical analysis review. *JBJS Rev.* 2017 Feb 21;5(2):e3. doi:10.2106/JBJS.RVW.16.00051
28. Visser CP, Coene LN, Brand R, Tavy DL. The incidence of nerve injury in anterior dislocation of the shoulder and its influence on functional recovery. A prospective clinical and EMG study. *J Bone Joint Surg Br.* 1999 Jul;81(4):679–85. doi:10.1302/0301-620x.81b4.9005
29. Verweij LPE, Sierevelt IN, van der Woude HJ, Hekman KMC, Veeger HEJD, van den Bekerom MPJ. Surgical intervention following a first traumatic anterior shoulder dislocation is worthy of consideration. *Arthroscopy.* 2023 Aug 39(12):2577–86, S0749-8063(23)00667-9. doi:10.1016/j.arthro.2023.07.060
30. Roberts WO, Armstrong LE, Sawka MN, Yeargin SW, Heled Y, O'Connor FG. ACSM expert consensus statement on exertional heat illness: recognition, management, and return to activity. *Curr Sports Med Rep.* 2021;20(9):470–84.
31. McCrory P, Meeuwisse W, Johnston K, et al. Consensus statement on concussion in sport 3rd International Conference on Concussion in Sport held in Zurich, November 2008. *Clin J Sport Med.* 2009;19(3):185–200.
32. Waicus KM, Smith BW. Eye injuries in women's lacrosse players. *Clin J Sport Med.* 2002;12(1):24–9.
33. Webster DA, Bayliss GV, Spadaro JA. Head and face injuries in scholastic women's lacrosse with and without eyewear. *Med Sci Sports Exerc.* 1999;31(7):938–41.

111 Motor Sports

Luke Bennett and Scott Epsley

INTRODUCTION

- The term "motorsport" is most commonly used to describe four-wheeled automobile racing, or two-wheeled motorcycle racing, both of which are conducted over a wide range of categories and disciplines.
- Other niche motorized-sporting pursuits may be encountered (*e.g.*, powerboat racing, snowmobile racing), while they are not considered in detail here — analogous principles of medical management will apply, in addition to any specific environmental considerations present (*e.g.*, drowning risk and cold exposure, respectively, for these examples).
- Motorsport has traditionally assumed the use of an internal combustion engine, and such propulsion still dominates worldwide, however electrical and hybrid motors are now commonly employed in many international racing categories. High-voltage electrical components may impose specific considerations around safety, including for medical and rescue interventions (1).

COMPETITION AND GOVERNANCE

- The majority of global motorsport is governed by the Federation Internationale de l'Automobile (FIA) and the Federation Internationale de Motorcyclisme (FIM), both headquartered in Switzerland.
- Detailed regulations — around medical fitness for athletes, car and equipment design, circuit specifications and safety — are well established and evolving constantly.
- Motorsports are notable for their reliance on a technically sophisticated conveyance (the race-car or motorcycle) upon which athletic performance is superimposed, and for the ergonomic interfaces between athlete and machine, around which injuries may be significant.
- Motorsports are also unique (in many cases) by the conduct of a concurrent "engineering" and "athletic" competition within the same event, usually represented by distinct but parallel "team" and "individual" championships (respectively). This arrangement can impose strategic and (occasionally) ethical conflicts in the domains of both sport and medicine.
- The extended team of engineers, mechanics and others who support a motorsports athlete may also come under the care of the sports physician, and a working knowledge of relevant family and travel medicine for these personnel is valuable.
- In the USA, motorsport tends to be regulated in a more fragmented fashion across a variety of series ownership structures, although event safety procedures are broadly comparable to wider international standards at the elite level.
- Motorsports may be conducted upon a dedicated circuit (with variable levels of safety design); on closed public roads (both sealed and unsealed, mostly with exposed road-side fixtures); or off-road on public and private land.
- Circuit racing is commonly conducted on a sealed tarmac oval (typically high-speed and simple layouts) or road course (a more variable and longer circuit format).
- A competition course may vary in length from a few hundred feet (in drag-racing) to hundreds of miles (for endurance off-road events), with wide variations in the distribution and sophistication of safety and retrieval services available to attend an incident.
- In addition to race or competition periods, many motorsports employ a format of practice or reconnaissance sessions, along with timed qualifying to determine a starting order, in the hours or days before racing. Such periods may extend the risk window for incidents and injury to occur.
- Grassroots motorsport can be surprisingly accessible to participants with a minimum of mandatory safety equipment designed to encourage participation and reduce competitor costs.
  - Event medical facilities might be rudimentary in some such locations, commonly consisting of a single local ambulance crew without specific motorsports training.
- Conversely, the highest levels of international competition are regulated in every detail of circuit, vehicle, and equipment design to mitigate the risk of injury to athletes, officials, and spectators (2).
  - International-level drivers and riders are subject to intensive physical preparation and medical scrutiny, and event medical services may provide a specialist prehospital trauma response within seconds of an incident.

EPIDEMIOLOGY

- Although most motorsport involves only a single driver or rider, some categories utilize two (or occasionally more) occupants (*e.g.*, a navigator in rally and off-road events, or a motorcycle sidecar passenger). The presence of multiple occupants can increase the complexity of a medical incident response.
- Most motorsport disciplines are conducted in an open format and have historically been dominated by male competitors, partly due to an enormous preponderance in the male participation rate at all levels.
  - Female participation is increasing steadily from a very-low base, especially in grassroots categories, with dedicated programs in many regions attempting to rectify this gender participation imbalance.
- Karting and other forms of entry-level motorsport (including circuit and motorcycle racing) welcome pediatric competitors of various ages, with specific classes in karting commonly catering to 6-year-old children onward.
  - An international karting license is available from 12 years, and children may also navigate in some national rally competitions after attaining this age (3).
  - In the USA, karting, dirt oval racing and motocross competition are also available to children as young as 5 years (4).
- Many motorsport categories also cater to older competitors, commonly aged into their 60s or 70s. Indeed, the middle to retirement age can be prime competition years for drivers who have accumulated sufficient wealth to compete at a national or international level, often in very sophisticated vehicles.
  - More strict medical requirements may apply to race licensing for older competitors, especially in terms of cardiac screening, vision testing and control of comorbidities.
- Drivers in more elite categories tend to exhibit greater physical fitness on a variety of standard measures (5,6). Semi-professional or amateur competitors more commonly display medical fitness comparable to the general population.
- Athletes with significant physical disability are often approved to compete in motorsports on a case-by-case basis, subject to safe modifications in-car controls, and the ability to self-extricate from the vehicle within a defined timeframe (2,7).
- The FIA collects global statistics on fatalities and severe injuries into a closed database.
  - Worldwide fatalities had approximately halved from 79 deaths in 2001 to 41 deaths in 2019 (before pandemic closures).
  - Closed-road events (*i.e.*, rallies and similar formats, most with two vehicle occupants) produce approximately double the number of global fatalities as circuit racing and were also far more likely to produce spectator fatalities.
  - Conversely, a small but persistent number of officials are killed each year, mostly at circuit events (8).
- There is little coherent public data on non-fatal injuries, outside of attempts at smaller national-level safety projects (9–11). Observational studies of clinical presentations to large trauma centers have concluded that motorsports produce worse injury outcomes than other sports (12,13).

ATHLETE EQUIPMENT

- A full-face helmet, designed and engineered to one of several impressive minimum standards (usually FIA/FIM internationally, or Snell homologation in the USA) is mandatory in most motorsport competitions. Open-face helmets are less frequently used, but still legal in some categories.
- Helmet construction is usually of carbon composite or a material of equivalent hardness. The current international FIA helmet standard includes rigorous testing to prevent intrusion from projectiles or crash debris, especially around the vulnerable visor area (14).
- A specific Snell/FIA helmet standard has been developed for pediatric use, with an adapted shell shape and reduced weight to minimize rotational inertia (15).
- The frontal head restraint (FHR) device tethers the helmet to limit neck movement in a crash impact and has dramatically reduced the incidence of high cervical injuries and skull base fractures under extreme cervical hyperflexion forces (16).
  - The HANS device (Head and Neck Support Device) (17) is the most common FHR used in four-wheeled motorsport worldwide.
- Most motorsport categories mandate the use of fire-protective apparel, including underwear, overalls, balaclava, gloves, socks, and footwear. FIA regulations mandate overlap zones for each fireproof garment, especially around ankles, wrists and neck, and even extend to the specification of fireproof stitching material for attachment of sponsor labels at the international level (18).
- Jewelry, including rings and/or facial and body piercings, are prohibited under FIA regulations (18). Foreign metallic objects in contact with skin are considered to produce a heat transmission hazard (in case of fire), an airway foreign body (if detached around the face or tongue), and/or create a risk of additional trauma to the digits (for rings), or pinna and other facial parts (during emergency helmet removal). Some categories and jurisdictions may be more liberal in permitting the wearing of jewelry during competition.
- Drivers in both IndyCar and Formula One now wear approved monitoring sensors for rescue team monitoring on-scene after an incident: a biometric glove in Formula One; and a medical sensor vest in IndyCar (19). Additionally, in both categories an accelerometer contained within the molded radio earpiece allows post-incident interrogation of impact forces immediately adjacent to the brain.

- Karting competitors are relatively exposed and unrestrained (*i.e.*, no seat belt harness is used) compared to other four-wheeled motorsports. Rigid chest protection is employed in addition to traditional safety apparel (20).
- Motorcycle competitors in all categories are significantly more vulnerable to both axial and peripheral injury than their four-wheeled counterparts. At the highest levels, a new suite of safety equipment has been progressively introduced including automated personal airbag protection (activated from within the race suit) around torso, neck and clavicles; various items of rigid central and peripheral armor, specialized protective leather race suits and gloves, plus durable exoskeleton boots offering reinforced (but mobile) ankle and heel protection (21).
  - Specialized helmets for motorcycles allow multi-planar movement of the head within the helmet shell in order to mitigate dangerous rotational forces in an oblique impact (including with the ground).

VEHICLE AND MOTORCYCLE SAFETY FEATURES

- Four-wheeled racing vehicles exhibit a wide array of integrated safety design features across an exhaustive number of competition categories worldwide. Such features might typically include some combination of the following:
  - frontal impact zones for energy absorption and driver foot protection
  - a carbon-fiber driver safety cell/chassis or integrated welded metallic-tube roll cage.
  - energy-absorbing side and/or rear impact structures
  - integrated overhead protection for open-cockpit categories (*e.g.*, "halo" or aero-screen)
  - energy-absorbing lateral head protection structures, and a high-sided cockpit to limit head exposure
  - impregnable protection for fuel tanks or high-voltage batteries
  - high-specification safety belts
  - cockpit oxygen supply and fire-suppression systems
  - roof access hatch for medical rescue team use
- In the case of electrical propulsion, additional measures (such as electrical status warning lights, cut-off circuits and procedures for high-voltage battery systems) are necessary to protect drivers, mechanics, and officials from potentially fatal electrical discharge, especially after a crash impact.
- By contrast, racing motorcycles are necessarily limited in their inherent safety design, with most impact mitigation served by rider apparel. Basic motorcycle safety features might include:
  - handlebar/hand protection
  - aerodynamic forward screens for airborne debris
  - external coverage of moving or hot mechanical parts
  - traction control, in some categories

CIRCUIT SAFETY

- Circuit design (*i.e.*, appropriate matching of circuit characteristics to the velocity, direction of travel and design of the race vehicles) makes an enormous contribution to reducing injury rates. Some of the philosophy of fixed circuit safety infrastructure can also be adapted to temporary closed-road courses (albeit with the increased danger of collision with fixed roadside objects).
- Circuit designs (whether permanent or temporary facilities) might incorporate the following features:
  - generous run-off areas with either gravel traps or high-friction pavement
  - energy absorbing barriers protecting concrete walls in likely impact zones
  - debris catch fencing of appropriate height and integrity to protect officials and spectators
  - access points for fire and medical teams, as well as removal of immobile race vehicles
  - electronic light/flag systems for incident control
  - well-designed pit entry and exit sectors, merging slower and faster traffic

ATHLETE PERFORMANCE AND PHYSIOLOGY

- Motorsport athletes are exposed to a complex mixture of physical, cognitive, and psychological demands during competition. They must navigate the racing course with precision at the limits of (ever-evolving) tire adhesion, usually while concurrently processing streams of verbal and strategic data, in close proximity to other competitors, under intense media scrutiny and with enormous physical and physiological stress.
- There remains a paucity of systematically collected live data for motorsport athletes, with most insights being limited to small enthusiast studies over several decades (22–28). Any biometric sensor attached to the skin is required to meet specific FIA testing standards compatible with fireproofing, which greatly limits live data gathering at the elite level (19).
- Nevertheless, basic observations regarding driver physiology in competition are as follows:
  - Heart rate elevation in the range of 140–180 beats · min^{-1} is commonly observed during competition (22–25), although this represents an additive combination of both physical exertion and psychological arousal. Heart rate is higher in sessions which are hotter, or more competitive (*e.g.*, race conditions vs. practice sessions, or in proximity to other vehicles).
  - Significant heat stress is a feature of closed-cockpit racing in most climates (22–26). This phenomenon appears to

be of similar magnitude in female drivers (27) regardless of menstrual phase (28).

- Motorsport athletes are known to possess considerably faster-than-average reaction times (29), compared to the general population.
- Driver weight has been a perennial concern in some categories, with pressure to maintain very low driver body weight as an inexpensive performance saving for any engineering team. The FIA introduced a minimum driver weight, recorded separately from the defined car regulations to elite open-wheel categories in 2019 (30), with great success in terms of driver health.
- Driver seat position can be critical to performance but is often compromised by engineering considerations, especially if multiple drivers of different sizes must share the same vehicle (such as in endurance events).
  - In the worst case, poor seat fitting can contribute to spinal fractures in an impact (31).
  - There is an effort to make seat specifications and positioning more flexible in junior categories (32), and for female drivers (33,34).
- Fine-grade EMG studies are beginning to demonstrate considerable performance benefits for both drivers and riders resulting from subtle changes in seating posture (35), and at the same time uncover nuances related to visual tracking around the halo device, and while following another vehicle (36,37).

MOTORSPORT INJURIES

- To a remarkable degree, the steady increase in safety around motorsport nowadays produces generally minor medical outcomes from the great majority of incidents. Analysis by Patalak et al of the 2011 to 2015 seasons demonstrated that NASCAR drivers experienced 134 times the number of crashes per mile compared to road-going passenger vehicles, but experienced 9.3 times fewer injuries per crash (38).
- A prospective survey of three MotoGP (elite motorcycle circuit racing) events in the USA found a crash prevalence of 9.7 per 100 rider hours, mostly involving a less injurious "low-side" loss of control (39).
  - A larger European paper covering the 2014 MotoGP/Moto2/Moto3 seasons found a rate of around 4 injuries per 1000 km of race and practice sessions (mostly fractures and joint dislocations) (40).
- Trackside physicians working in the prehospital context will be trained to collaborate as a team with paramedics, and event officials according to local procedures.
  - Whenever possible, this group should coordinate with highly trained fire rescue crews with specialty training in vehicle extrication and motorsports.
  - This is a specialized context that differs not only from the clinic-based environment, but also from highway vehicle crash management, encompassing scene safety and control, effective communications, and unique time-sensitivity.
- As a general rule, the safest possible extrication, with minimal patient intervention on-scene, followed by rapid transport of the patient to definitive emergency care is favored. Interventions at the scene should not delay immediate transfer unless necessary for safe transportation (41).
- Recognized trauma guidelines (*e.g.*, ATLS or similar frameworks) should be employed in the management of all motorsport patients (41). It is important to recognize, however:
  - Traditional trauma care based upon road vehicle accidents may not transfer directly to the motorsport context, where speeds are higher and mitigation measures will modify the clinical presentation (38,42).
  - Even when a single isolated injury is apparent, primary and secondary surveys remain critically important.
  - When an athlete is released into outpatient care post-incident, vigilant tertiary surveillance by their support team for occult injury in the following hours and days is very important (and often unexpectedly fruitful)
- As referenced above, reliable data on injury frequency and incidence in motorsports are sparse, however, the following injury classes (in approximately ascending order of typical severity) are observed across the most common categories in automobile sports:
  - peripheral soft tissue contusions to exposed aspects of ankles, knees, and elbows
  - hand and wrist strains/fractures (often in conflict with violent steering wheel movements at impact)
  - seat or seat harness-related contusion
  - concussion — often mild or subtle
  - rib contusion or fracture
  - lower limb fracture
  - isolated burns
  - spinal injury (stable)
  - pelvic fracture
  - spinal fracture (unstable)
  - abdominal organ injury
  - closed head injury/traumatic brain injury (43)
  - chest injury (including pneumothorax, hemothorax and/or aortic injury)
  - severe polytrauma
- Musculoskeletal injuries are discussed in more detail separately below.
- The presence of some features might produce a higher index of suspicion for clinicians caring for a driver post-incident:
  - visible damage to helmet
  - rotational impact

- impact with exposed concrete barriers and fixed roadside objects
- very-high speed, especially in dry weather and race-day conditions
- forces recorded upon the race vehicle over 25 G, and especially over 40 G
- multiple impact
- front-to-side impact

- The mode of extrication (10) can be a useful (if unproven) prognostic signpost for injury severity in four-wheeled motorsport — in ascending order of seriousness:
  - driver self-extricated from the vehicle unaided
  - driver self-extricated from the vehicle with assistance, or with visible difficulty
  - "controlled" extrication by rescue crew (patient *stable* but injured — *e.g.*, spinal pain or limb fractures)
  - "emergency" or "rapid" extrication by rescue crew (patient *unstable*, or external factors such as fire)
  - disincarceration (dismantling of the vehicle to access injured driver)
- As in many contact sports, concussion has been the subject of increased attention and caution in motorsports in both Europe and North America (44,45). Initial assessment and progress should always be monitored with the SCAT tool or other valid alternative, and return to competition guided conservatively according to local clinical guidelines (understanding that drivers/riders may function to a higher baseline of cognitive ability compared to other athletes) (45). Head injuries are discussed at length in Chapter 49 of this text.
- Management of all motorsport injuries should be undertaken with the appropriate and timely specialist input. Return to competition should be contemplated only when the athlete can control their vehicle with full function, to avoid endangering themselves, fellow competitors, and trackside workers. Reintegration after serious injury is typically approved in consultation with medical representatives of the relevant championship series, via a formal certification process.

MUSCULOSKELETAL ISSUES

Musculoskeletal Demands

- Drivers — physical demands of driving are influenced by the unique aspects of each racing series including track type, car design, and G forces imparted on the body.
- Track type:
  - Oval racing (American stock car & IndyCar) requires the body to resist lateral G forces while turning in the same direction (typically anti-clockwise) for 200–250 laps.
  - Road and street course racing imposes both lateral and anteroposterior G forces due to intense braking and acceleration zones (46).
  - The nature of the terrain in rally courses may require increased levels of grip and dexterity on the steering wheel with faster and more versatile wrist work (47).
- Car design:
  - Formula 1 and IndyCars reach speeds in excess of 360 km · h^{-1} creating large forces on the body when braking, accelerating, and cornering (46).
  - Unlike Formula 1 cars, IndyCars do not possess power steering. Thus, drivers must apply a force pulling down with one hand and up with the other of around 35 lb through the steering wheel, on average greater than 1100 times per race.
  - IndyCar drivers have been shown to apply 135 lb of force through the brake pedal over 250 times during a race (48).
- G forces & vibration:
  - Open wheel drivers experience 4–6 G during braking and cornering maneuvers. Due to the torso being so tightly strapped in, forces are mostly transmitted to the head and neck. Due to the weight of the helmet plus the HANS device, a driver cornering at 4 G will experience 26 kg of centrifugal force on the neck (46). Furthermore, at 4 G neck muscles may reach ipsilateral tolerance of 100% MVC in some drivers (49).
  - Respiratory, upper limb and vastus lateralis muscle activation is also significantly increased as a result of the G forces acting on the body (49). Lower body strength is important in bracing the body against the cockpit to resist lateral G forces (50).
  - Stock car drivers frequently cite vibration as a cause of upper limb issues (51). Vibration through the steering wheel has also been shown to increase upper limb muscle activity (49).
- As a result of these physical demands, drivers develop musculoskeletal adaptations through a combination of driving and training. These adaptations can be unique between racing series' and are listed below:
  - Rally drivers possess increased grip strength, ankle plantar flexion strength, and trunk extension strength than open-wheel drivers (47).
  - Isometric neck strength has been shown to be stronger in Formula 1 drivers than in Indycar drivers, followed by NASCAR and sports car drivers respectively (5).
  - In open-wheel drivers isometric neck extension is strongest (~40–55 kg), followed by lateral flexion (~30–45 kg), and flexion (~20–30 kg) (5,47).
  - Formula 1 drivers demonstrate 10% stronger leg extension strength than basketball players (47).
  - Stock car drivers described upper body strength as the most important physical demand, with wheel-to-wheel contact creating sudden unexpected upper limb/wrist demands. Neck, core, and leg strength were also rated highly important by drivers (50).

- High trunk flexion and extension strength were reported in rally and open-wheel drivers, necessary to create high intra-abdominal pressure to assist in stabilizing the spine against shear and compression forces.
- Both rally and Formula 1 drivers demonstrate up to 40% higher shoulder muscle endurance than controls (47).

- Pit crew
  - Musculoskeletal demands and associated injuries in motor racing are not only limited to drivers but extend to mechanics and pit crew. To meet the physical demands pit crew train up to 7 d · wk^{-1} for around 10 months of the year, with individualized programs designed for the physical requirements of specific tasks (51).
  - As with drivers the physical requirements and musculoskeletal issues that arise as a result are highly variable between racing series', with some examples listed below.
- American Stock Car/NASCAR
  - Five members of the crew are allowed to service the car during a pit stop with roles being assigned to two tire changers, a refueler, and a jackman.
  - Equipment needs to be lifted over the pit wall after the car comes to a stop in the pit box, and service is carried out in 12–15 seconds.
  - The weight of the equipment includes a 25 lb jack, 70 lb tires, and 95 lb fuel cans carried on the refueler's shoulder.
  - Upper and lower body strength is of prime importance (51).
- Formula 1
  - Pit crew are usually mechanics who assist during races as pit crew, with assigned tasks based on physical characteristics.
  - Roles are divided between up to 22 people with highly coordinated tasks. For example, three people are assigned to each tire change, with tires weighing approximately 25 lb.
  - There is no refueling, and pit stops usually occur in under 3 seconds, with 1.82 seconds being the record.
  - Speed, agility, and precision are key characteristics of Formula 1 pit crew (52).

Musculoskeletal Issues

- Drivers
  - There is a paucity of information in the literature on motor racing drivers' injuries (53). Injury type and severity may differ between racing categories due to different vehicle performance, physical demands, and safety features (54). The risk of injury has been shown to be greater in professional drivers, those spending more than 10 days per month testing, and those competing in long-distance races (53).
  - Musculoskeletal issues for drivers, broken down by body region, are listed below.
- Upper limb
  - Upper extremity fractures.
    - Distal radius and scaphoid (NASCAR) (51).
    - Hand, forearm, and wrist (multiple racing categories) (53).
    - Clavicle — both racing and training incidents such as cycling accidents (55–57).
  - Joint pain
    - Wrist (50) 63% of Formula 1 drivers and 32% of rally drivers report wrist pain (47).
    - Thumb (50)
    - Shoulder (50) 47% of rally drivers report shoulder pain (47) and 11% of drivers across multiple categories incurred a shoulder injury (53).
  - DeQuervain tenosynovitis (54).
  - Forearm compartment syndrome (54).
    - In a wearable EMG study it was found that drivers may not relax their grip at parts of this course where in-car telemetry suggests high steering wheel grip is not necessary. Thus, the ability to relax the grip may be as important to performance conservation as training grip strength (58).
  - Neuropathies (26% of NASCAR drivers).
    - Cubital tunnel syndrome
    - Carpal tunnel syndrome
    - Digital neuromas in the digit in contact with the spoke of the steering wheel (51)
- Lower limb
  - Fracture
    - Tibia/leg (54)
    - Foot and ankle
    - Knee (53)
  - Ligament injuries/sprain
    - Ankle
    - Knee (53)
  - Contusions of the legs (50,54)
- Neck and trunk
  - Back pain (22.5% stock car, 88% Formula 1) (47, 50)
  - Neck pain (15% stock car, 63% Formula 1) (47, 50)
  - Neck sprain
    - Decreased from 34%–53% between 1996 and 2000 (54) to 5% in a 2017 report likely due to the introduction of the HANS device (53).
  - Spinal fracture
    - Burst fractures (lumbar) (54)
    - Crush fractures (thoracic and lumbar) (59,60)
    - Lumbar spine (53)
    - Cervical spine (rally drivers) (53)
  - Spinal cord injury (61)

  - Blunt trauma or hyperflexion/extension to the trunk and spine (39% of Karting hospital admissions) (62)
- Pit crew
  - The carrying of heavy equipment such as tires and fuel cans, use of high torque impact guns in tire changing, as well as speed and agility requirements and repetition of the task, make the pit crew susceptible to injury.
  - In a study of NASCAR pit crew injuries over 10 years, 42% were found to occur in tire changers (51). Furthermore, there is a risk of accidental contact with a car.
- Musculoskeletal issues as reported by pit crew members are outlined below by body region.
- Upper limb
  - Medial or lateral elbow epicondylitis — 26%
  - TFCC tears (due to 847 nm of torque with the impact gun) — 14%
  - Finger crush injuries, including the nail bed and distal phalanx — 29%
  - Hook of hamate fracture (from contact with the impact gun)
  - Tendinopathy (tire changers and refuelers) — 23%
  - Biceps and triceps tendon ruptures (refuelers) (51)
- Lower limb
  - Fracture
    - Contact with cars either through miscalculation, brake locking, or mechanical issues (63).
  - Knee ligament injury (contact with cars) (64)
    - ACL rupture
    - MCL sprains
  - Femoroacetabular impingement
    - Rear tire changers in NASCAR due to repetition (7–10 years of doing the job) (65)
- Neck and trunk
  - Neck ligament strains (hit by a car) (64)
  - Lower back injury (lifting heavy objects such as tires and fuel cans, especially when performed at speed) (66)

MEDICAL CONSIDERATIONS IN MOTORSPORT

Medical Screening and Competition Licensing

- Pre-participation medical screening is commonly undertaken for motorsport athletes, and may be a mandatory component of competition licensing.
- Race licensing requirements vary with national jurisdiction (or championship series in the USA), and the sports physician will typically be presented with specific documentation relevant to the license category of the athlete. The FIA "Appendix L" Chapter 2 sets a detailed baseline standard for various categories of race license, with which issuing national authorities are expected to conform (2). These standards include the following for international and national competition licenses:
  - annual history and examination
  - periodic EKG for drivers under 50 years, plus exercise stress test for older drivers
  - visual testing including acuity, fields and color perception
  - case-by-case consideration of well-controlled comorbidities such as diabetes, epilepsy, cardiac disease, mental health disorders, and amputations
- Pre-participation cardiac screening of athletes (especially young athletes) is the subject of both North American and European consensus statements, which include detailed history and examination plus EKG (optional in the USA) (67).
  - These statements have not been updated for some years, and cardiac screening has become significantly more aggressive for athletes in the post-SARS CoV2 pandemic period in many nations (68,69). For motorsports, where patient preference dictates, it is common practice to add echocardiography to the screening ECG.
- Although there is no evidence for such practice, it might also be reasonable to screen for relevant vascular, musculoskeletal and/or organ anomalies for a young professional motorsports athlete in anticipation of future traumatic incidents — at the same time establishing baseline imaging for future comparison post-incident. The following might be considered in discussion with the patient (and/or their guardian):
  - comprehensive screening/annual blood tests
  - plain chest radiograph
  - MRI/CT of brain and/or cervical spine
  - MRI/CT of thoracic and lumbar spine
  - ultrasound of abdominal organs and large vasculature

General Practice and Travel Medicine

- The physician who travels with a motorsport team or championship may tend to inherit the routine general medical care for motorsport athletes — and also their family members, managers, mechanics, engineers and other team personnel. Depending on the intensity and geographical distribution of the Championship calendar (and therefore the potential isolation from routine healthcare services), provision for the supply of common general practice medications, plus basic emergency supplies, should be considered.
- For international championships, a familiarity with basic travel medicine might be required, including:
  - infectious disease hygiene and prevention (respiratory and gastrointestinal)
  - travel vaccination and other regional prophylaxis requirements (*e.g.*, malaria)
  - sleep and circadian (jetlag) management

Alcohol and Anti-Doping Regulations in Motorsport

- Most motorsport globally is conducted under FIA and FIM supervision, and subject to World Anti-doping Agency Regulations, including the WADA list of prohibited substances and WADA testing protocols (Appendix A) (2). Separately, the FIA and FIM regulate alcohol testing for motorsport athletes (Appendix C), which mandates zero blood alcohol content (with margins of 0.02% FIA and 0.01% FIM) for drivers and officials trackside (2).
- Motorsport in the USA is conducted under somewhat less rigorous anti-doping policies, according to each championship's regulations (including those governed internally by the NASCAR and IndyCar organizations respectively).
    - Like the FIA, both of these organizations also prohibit blood alcohol concentrations over 0.02% for competitors and track-side officials, and consumption within 12 hours before on-track activity (70).

REFERENCES

1. Danger, high voltage. *Auto+Medical: FIA International Journal of Motorsport Medicine Issue 2*. 2014:13–7.
2. FIA International Sporting Code and Appendices. https://www.fia.com/regulation/category/123
3. Motorsport UK. 6-13 years old (webpage). Motorsport UK [cited 2023 Mar 17]. Available from: https://www.motorsportuk.org/6-13-years-old/
4. Families New to Youth Racing (webpage). Youth Racers of America. [cited 2023 Mar 17]. Available from: https://youthracersofamerica.com/families-new-to-youth-racing/
5. McKnight PJ, Bennett LA, Malvern JJ, Ferguson DP. VO2peak, body composition, and neck strength of elite motor racing drivers. *Med Sci Sports Exerc*. Dec 2019;51(12):2563–9.
6. Barthel SC, Buckingham TM, Haft CE, Bechtolsheimer JE, Bechtolsheimer TA, Ferguson DP. A comparison of the physiological responses in professional and amateur sports car racing drivers. *Res Q Exerc Sport*. 2020;91(4):562–73.
7. Racing Enabled. *Auto+Medical: FIA International Journal of Motorsport MedicineIssue 13*; 2018:10–17.
8. Vision Zero. *Auto+Medical: FIA International Journal of Motorsport Medicine Issue 22*; 2021:12–19.
9. Aiming Wide. *Auto+Medical: FIA International Journal of Motorsport Medicine Issue 23*; 2021:20–3.
10. Trafford P, Henderson M, Trammell T. Spinal Injuries and Motorsport.*Auto+Medical: FIA International Journal of Motorsport Medicine Issue 1*. 2014;2014:30–41.
11. Deakin ND, Roberts I, Collett A, Fraser D, Hutchinson PJ. Keeping competitors safe: A four-year study. *Auto+Medical: FIA International Journal of Motorsport Medicine Issue 6*. 2015 Nov;2015:38–51.
12. Andrew NE, Gabbe BJ, Wolfe R, et al. Twelve-month outcomes of serious orthopaedic sport and active recreation-related injuries admitted to level 1 trauma centers in Melbourne, Australia. *Clin J Sport Med*. Sep 2008;18(5):387–93.
13. Hassan AH, Gharooni AA, Mee H, Geffner J, Anwar F. Sports injuries: a 5-year review of admissions at a major trauma center in the United Kingdom. *J Trauma Inj*. 2023;36(1):39–48.
14. FIA Reveals Ultra-protective Helmet for F1 (Webpage). Federation Internationale de l'Automobile. 2018 [cited 2023 Mar 18]. Available from: https://www.fia.com/news/fia-reveals-ultra-protective-helmet-f1
15. SNELL/FIA CM2016 Standard For Protective Headgear. *For Use in Children's Motor Sports Activities [Internet Document]*. Snell Foundation. [cited 2023 Mar 18]. Available at: https://smf.org/standards/cmh/CM2016.pdf
16. Kaul A, Abbas A, Smith G, Manjila S, Pace J, Steinmetz M. A revolution in preventing fatal craniovertebral junction injuries: lessons learned from the Head and Neck Support device in professional auto racing. *J Neurosurg Spine*. 2016;25(6):756–61.
17. Head and Neck Restraints (webpage). HANS. [cited 2023 Mar 18]. Available at: https://www.hansdevice.com/head-and-neck-restraints
18. Appendix L. *International Sporting Code. [webpage]*. Federation Internationale de l'Automobile. [cited 2023 Mar 18]. Available at: https://www.fia.com/appendix-l-international-drivers-licences-medical-examinations-drivers-equipment-and-conduct-2019
19. Body of Data. *Auto+Medical: FIA International Journal of Motorsport Medicine Issue 18*. Nov 2019:12–17.
20. *First FIA-Standard Karting Body Protection Delivered (webpage)*. Federation Internationale de l'Automobile. [cited 2023 Mar 18]. Available at: https://www.fia.com/news/first-fia-standard-karting-body-protection-delivered
21. Holding J. *Safety Devices in MotoGP: Airbags, Helmets, Boots and Other Gear (Webpage)*. Autosport Magazine; April 24, 2021. Available at: https://www.autosport.com/motogp/news/safety-devices-in-motogp-airbags-helmets-boots/6438518/
22. Jacobs PL, Olvey SE, Johnson BM, Cohn K. Physiological responses to high-speed, open-wheel racecar driving. *Med Sci Sports Exerc*. 2002 Dec;34(12):2085–90.
23. Brearley MB, Finn JP. Responses of motor-sport athletes to v8 supercar racing in hot conditions. *Int J Sports Physiol Perform*. 2007 Jun;2(2):182–91.
24. Potkanowicz ES. A real-time case study in driver science: physiological strain and related variables. *Int J Sports Physiol Perform*. 2015 Nov;10(8):1058–60.
25. Turner AP, Richards H. Physiological and selective attention demands during an international rally motor sport event. *BioMed Res Int*. 2015 Oct;2015:638659.
26. Carlson LA, Ferguson DP, Kenefick RW. Physiological strain of stock car drivers during competitive racing. *J Therm Biol*. 2014 Aug;44:20–6.
27. Potkanowicz E. Physiological Responses of Female Motorsport Athletes to the Environment of the Cockpit: A Case Study. *Auto+Medical: FIA International Journal of Motorsport Medicine Issue 9*. 2016 Dec. pp. 48–59.
28. Ferguson D. Study Shows Female Drivers Just as Fit as Male.*Auto+Medical: FIA International Journal of Motorsport Medicine Issue 17*. 2019 Aug. 5 p.
29. Baur H, Müller S, Hirschmüller A, Huber G, Mayer F. Reactivity, stability, and strength performance capacity in motor sports. *Br J Sports Med*. 2006 Nov;40(11):906–11.
30. Rimmer L. *How Much Does an F1 Car Weigh in 2023 and What's Included in the Limit? (Webpage)*. Motorsport.com; 2023 Mar 2. Available at: https://au.motorsport.com/f1/news/how-much-does-an-f1-car-weigh-in-2023/10437687/
31. Seating Pains. *Auto+Medical: FIA International Journal of Motorsport Medicine Issue 214*. 2018 Aug. pp. 10–17.
32. New Safety Features on Gen 2 Formula 4 Car (News Item). *Auto+Medical: FIA International Journal of Motorsport Medicine Issue 23*. Aug 2021. p. 4.

33. Rosalie S, Rosalie S. Customizing female racing drivers' seat fit can improve their performance. *Auto+Medical: FIA International Journal of Motorsport Medicine Issue 23*; 2021 Aug. pp. 32–49.
34. Physical Examination. *Auto+Medical: FIA International Journal of Motorsport Medicine Issue 22*. 2021 Apr; pp. 26–31.
35. Rosalie SM, Malone JM. Effect of Halo-type Frontal Cockpit protection on Overtaking. *Case Reports*. 2018 Sep 7. 2018:bcr-2018.
36. Rosalie SM, Malone JM. Effect of a halo-type structure on neck muscle activation of an open-cockpit race car driver training under qualifying conditions. *BMJ Case Rep*. 2018 May;2018:bcr2017224013. 2018:bcr-2017.
37. Rosalie S, Malone J. Do racing drivers practice racing? The effect of intentional following on formula car drivers' steering behaviour. *J Expert*. 2019;2(3):164–83.
38. Patalak JP, Harper MG, Weaver AA, Dalzell NM, Stitzel JD. Estimated crash injury risk and crash characteristics for motorsport drivers. *Accid Anal Prev*. 2020 Mar 1;136:105397.
39. Bedolla J, Santelli J, Sabra J, Cabanas JG, Ziebell C, Olvey S. Elite motorcycle racing: crash types and injury patterns in the MotoGP class. *Am J Emerg Med*. 2016;34(9):1872–5.
40. Zasa M, Schiavi P, Polo R, et al. Epidemiology of injuries in the 2014 MotoGP World championship: the "Clinica mobile" experience. *Sport Orthop Traumatol*. 2016;32:289–94.
41. MacPartlin M. Motorsport Resuscitation Review. *Auto+Medical: FIA International Journal of Motorsport Medicine Issue 8*. 2016 September. pp. 40–53.
42. Missed Spinal Fracture in Motorsport. *Auto+Medical: FIA International Journal of Motorsport Medicine Issue 18*. 2019 November. pp. 36–43.
43. Olvey S. Traumatic Brain Injury in Motorsport. *Auto+Medical: FIA International Journal of Motorsport Medicine. Issue 2*. 2014. pp. 36–45.
44. Hutchinson P, Olvey S. Concussion in Motorsport. *Auto+Medical: FIA International Journal of Motorsport Medicine. Issue 5*. 2015 Aug. pp. 36–45.
45. Deakin ND, Cronin T, Trafford P, et al. Concussion in motor sport: a medical literature review and engineering perspective. *Concussion*. Oct 2017;2(3):CNC43.
46. Williams JA *Review of the Physiological Responses to Open-Wheeled Racing with Current Trends in Testing and Strength Training*. Www. Researchgate.Net. Feb 2021. Accessed 2023 Apr 2. www.researchgate.net/profile/Jackson-Williams-4/publication/349443803_Review_of_the_Physiological_Responses_to_Open-Wheeled_Racing_with_Current_Trends_in_Testing_and_Strength_Training/links/603053d8299bf1cc26d981c4/Review-of-the-Physiological-Responses-to-Open-Wheeled-Racing-with-Current-Trends-in-Testing-and-Strength-Training.pdf
47. Backman J, Häkkinen K, Ylinen J, Häkkinen A, Kyröläinen H. Neuromuscular performance characteristics of open-wheel and rally drivers. *J Strength Cond Res*. 2005;19(4):777–84.
48. Pruett M. *Dario Franchitti: So You Think Driving an Indy Car Is Easy? Try Braking—Part 1*. Roadandtrack.Com. 13 Aug 2012. Accessed 2023 Mar 31. www.roadandtrack.com/motorsports/news/a9140/dario-franchitti-so-you-think-driving-an-indy-car-is-easy-try-braking-part-1-37898/
49. Backman J. *Acute Neuromuscular Responses to Car Racing*. Jyx. Jyu, 2005 Sep 1. Accessed 2023 Mar 31. jyx.jyu.fi/bitstream/handle/123456789/12567/URN_NBN_fi_jyu-2005484.pdf?sequence=1.
50. Ebben WP, Suchomel TJ. Physical demands, injuries, and conditioning practices of stock car drivers. *J Strength Cond Res*. 2012;26(5):1188–98.
51. Wertman G., Gaston RG, Heisel W. Upper extremity injuries in NASCAR drivers and pit crew: an epidemiological study. *Orthop J Sports Med*. 2016;4(2):2325967116629427.
52. Martinetti A, Awadhpersad P, Singh S, van Dongen LAM. Gone in 2s: a deep dive into perfection analysing the collaborative maintenance pit-stop of Formula 1. *J Qual Mainten Eng*. 2021;27(3):550–64.
53. Koutras C., Antoniou SA, Jäger M, Heep H. Acute injuries sustained by racing drivers: a cross-sectional study. *Acta Orthop Belg*. 2017;83(4):512–20.
54. Minoyama O, Tsuchida H. Injuries in professional motor car racing drivers at a racing circuit between 1996 and 2000. *Br J Sports Med*. 2004;38(5):613–16.
55. Foster M. *Aitken Suffered Broken Collarbone, Fractured Vertebra*. Planetf1.Com. 2021 Aug 1. Accessed 2023 Apr 2. www.planetf1.com/news/jack-aitken-spa-crash/
56. *IndyCar Driver Josef Newgarden Racing with Broken Collarbone, Hand at Road America*. Autoweek.Com, 2016 Jun 24. Accessed 2023 Apr 1.www.autoweek.com/racing/indycar/a1848611/indycar-driver-josef-newgarden-racing-broken-collarbone-hand-road-america/
57. *Lance Stroll Reveals Full Extent of Cycling Accident Injuries*. Espn.Com, 2023 Mar 8. Accessed 2023 Apr 14. www.espn.com/f1/story/_/id/35809881/lance-stroll-reveals-full-extent-cycling-accident-injuries
58. Kataoka Y, Douglas J. Mining muscle use data for fatigue reduction in IndyCar. In: *11th Annual MIT Sloan Sports Analytics Conference*; 2017.
59. Franchitti D. *IndyCar Champion Fractures Spine in Crash*. Bbc.Com, 2013 Oct 7.Accessed 2023 Apr 14. www.bbc.com/sport/motorsport/24425701. .
60. *IndyCar: Will Power Has Fractured Back, No Surgery Required*. Autoweek.Com. 2011 Oct 24. Accessed 2023 Mar 31. www.autoweek.com/racing/indycar/a1990286/indycar-will-power-has-fractured-back-no-surgery-required/
61. *IndyCar Driver Robert Wickens Has Rods, Screws Placed into Spine*. SI.Com. 2018 Aug 22, Accessed 2023 Apr 14. www.si.com/racing/2018/08/22/robert-wickens-screws-spine-surgery-indycar. .
62. Eker HH, Van Lieshout EM, Den Hartog D, Schipper IB. Trauma mechanisms and injuries associated with go-karting. *Open Orthop J*. 2010 Feb 17;4:107–10.
63. *Crew Members Injured in Pit Collision at IndyCar Practice*. Jacksonville.Com, 2012 Jul 6. Accessed 2023 Apr 18. www.jacksonville.com/story/sports/motorsports/2012/07/07/crew-members-injured-pit-collision-indycar-practice/15861717007/
64. *No. 38 Jackman Treated and Release from Hospital after Being Hit on Pit Road*. Speedwaydigest.Com, 2010 Oct 30. Accessed 2023 Apr 18. www.speedwaydigest.com/index.php/news/nascar-cup-series-news/3140-no-38-jackman-treated-and-released-from-hospital-after-being-hit-on-pit-road
65. Stewart L. *Rookie Stripe: Why Pit Crews Are Susceptible to Injury Based on Position*. Skirtsandscuffs.Com. Accessed 2023 Apr 21. www.skirtsandscuffs.com/2017/06/rookie-stripe-why-pit-crews-are.html
66. *NASCAR Injuries and Safety Measures*. Resurgens.Com, 2021 Feb 11. Accessed 2023 Apr 7. www.resurgens.com/news/nascar-injuries-and-safety-measures
67. Link MS, Pelliccia A. *Screening to prevent sudden cardiac death in athletes*. UpToDate. Waltham (MA). Accessed 2023 Mar 19. Available at: http://www.uptodate.com.
68. Phelan D, Kim JH, Drezner JA, et al. When to consider cardiac MRI in the evaluation of the competitive athlete after SARS-CoV-2 infection. *Br J Sports Med*. 2022 Apr 1;56(8):425–6.
69. Writing Committee, Gluckman TJ, Bhave NM, Allen LA, et al. 2022 ACC expert consensus decision pathway on cardiovascular sequelae of COVID-19 in adults: myocarditis and other myocardial involvement, post-acute sequelae of SARS-CoV-2 infection, and return to play: a report of the American College of Cardiology Solution Set Oversight Committee. *J Am Coll Cardiol*. 2022 May 3;79(17):1717–56.
70. *IndyCar 2019 Substance Abuse Policy*. Indycar; [cited 2023 Mar 19] Available at: https://hardcards.indycar.com/Resources/pdfs/2019/2019 INDYCARSubstanceAbusePolicy.pdf

Rugby

112

Daniel Poole and Peter H. Seidenberg

INTRODUCTION

- Rugby is a fast-paced contact-collision game with the continuous pace of soccer combined with contact situations similar to those seen in American football.
- It is played by both sexes in a broad age range (1).
- Rugby is currently played in a variety of formats (7, 10, 12, and 15s), with the most popular variations being the 7 and 15s (1).
- There are 7.69 million rugby players worldwide (2).
- World Rugby membership spans 128 countries (3).
- There are more than 100,000 members in USA Rugby (3).
  - The USA national men's team (the Eagles) was established in 1975, and the women's team was established in 1987.
  - Major League Rugby, the professional form of men's 15s, began in 2018.
  - The Women's Premier League, the top annual competition for women's rugby (15s), was established in 2008 (4).
- World Cup competition occurs every 4 years.

HISTORY

- Invented in 1832 when William Webb Ellis picked up the ball and advanced it in a soccer match at Rugby College in England. The only way to stop the runner was to tackle them (4).
- American football is thought to have been birthed from rugby in the late 19th century.
- Rugby 15s was an Olympic sport in 1900, 1908, 1920, and 1924 (5).
- Rugby sevens returned to the Olympics in 2016 (6).

MATCH (7)

- Whereas American football is a game of yardage, rugby is a game of possession.
  - The player with possession of the ball is the front most player on the attacking team. They may advance the ball by running with the ball, kicking it forward, or passing it backward or laterally to another person on their team.
  - All teammates are behind the ball carrier.
  - Blocking for the ball carrier is not permitted.
- The objective is to maintain control of the ball and touch it down in the try zone (the rugby equivalent of the American football end zone).
- Once crossing the try line, the player must touch the ball down on the ground in order to register a try, which is worth five points.
- The try entitles the scoring team to attempt to kick the ball through the goalposts directly back from the point the ball was touchdown in the try zone, which is worth another two points.
- An offensive player may also attempt to drop kick the ball through the goalposts during open play, which is worth three points.

POSITIONS (7)

- In rugby 15s, there are 15 players on each team with specific positions and responsibilities and each team may name up to eight substitutes.
- The players numbered 1 through 8 are the forwards.
  - They generally are responsible for gaining and maintaining possession of the ball.
- Players numbered 9 through 15 are the backs.
  - They are generally responsible for advancing the ball down the field and defending the open field.
- Props — 3 players of the front row, which includes two props on either side of a hooker, who are responsible for the stability and strength of the front row.
  - Position 1 is the loosehead prop.
  - Position 3 is the tighthead prop.
  - Position 2 is the hooker, who is responsible for hooking (securing the ball with feet) during the scrum.
    - Hooker is in the middle position of the front row of the scrum and is tightly supported by the props on either side, who support the hooker so their feet are off the ground. This enables the hooker to hook the ball backward during the scrum.
    - Hooker is usually slightly shorter and lighter than the props to ride a stable front row platform; however, at elite levels, this stereotype is not necessarily true.

- Second row/locks
  - Positions 4 and 5 are responsible for providing the driving force to the front row of the scrum.
  - Typically, they are the jumpers for the line out.
  - Generally, they are the tallest players on the pitch.
- Flanker/wing forward
  - Positions 6 and 7 may be either openside or blindside.
  - Openside lines up in the scrum furthest from the touch-line, while blindside lines up on the narrower side.
  - Typically, they are the first players to leave a scrum.
  - Generally, they are the best tacklers and all-around athletes on the team.
  - The ideal flanker has both size and speed.
- Eightman
  - Position 8 is at the rear end of the scrum and has their head between the second-row players, providing stability and drive to the scrum
  - Generally, the eighth man is the tallest loose forward.
- Scrumhalf
  - Position 9 acts as the quarterback of the forwards and is responsible for offensive and defensive strategy of the forwards during loose play.
  - Secures the ball from the scrum, rucks, mauls, and tackles
  - Responsible for placing the ball in the tunnel (see scrum below)
  - The scrumhalf is usually small and quick and has a fast and accurate pass.
- Flyhalf
  - Position number 10 acts as the quarterback of the backs, responsible for calling back plays and is the first player in the back line.
  - Generally, the flyhalf is smaller and lighter than other backs with good passing and kicking ability.
- Centers
  - Position 12 inside and 13 outside, these are generally larger and more physical backs
  - Often called upon to crash into the competition by intentionally running into defenders to establish a ruck or maul
- Wings
  - Positions 11 and 14, generally the quickest and most elusive players on the team, they are required to outrun the opposition in open-field play
- Fullback
  - Position 15, the "last line of defense" in rugby
  - Essential skills include being able to field a kicked ball, kick for distance and accuracy, and consistently tackle in the open field.
- Rugby sevens has fewer positions and are not noted by numbers.
  - Forwards include the hooker, loosehead prop, and tighthead prop.
  - Backs include the scrumhalf, flyhalf, center, and wing.

FORMATIONS (7)

- Scrum
  - This aspect of the game is tightly controlled by the referee to prevent injury.
    - In preparation for the scrum, each pack assembles under the directions of their individual hooker.
    - When both sides are square, stable, and stationary, the referee calls "crouch." Next, when both sides are again square, stable, and stationary, the referee calls "bind." Finally, when both sides are again square, stable, and stationary, with the hooker still applying the brake foot, the referee calls "set." At this point, the scrum-half introduces the ball into the tunnel and the hooker attempts to hook (kick) the ball backward to their own team.
    - After the ball has traveled to the rear of the scrum, the ball can be picked out for advancement.
    - The scrum is used to restart play after the referee has stopped play for minor infringements and at other points in the match.
- Line out
  - Used to restart play after the ball has gone into touch (out of bounds).
  - Two to seven forwards from each team are arranged in parallel lines that are perpendicular to the touch line. The hooker throws the ball into the tunnel formed by the standing forwards of both teams.
  - Each team has jumpers who will fight for possession of the thrown ball.
  - The jumper is assisted by lifters — two players who grab the jumper above the knees (usually by the shorts) and lift them into the air. The lifters also ensure a controlled return to the ground after the jumper has caught the ball. Afterward, a maul is usually formed.
- Maul
  - Formed when the ball carried is stopped by a defender but not taken to the ground.
  - Players from both teams attempt to drive the maul down the field by binding to each other and giving a unified push.
  - Both sides attempt to grab the ball out of the maul to restart open-field play.
- Ruck
  - Formed when a player is tackled and brought to the ground
  - The tackled player releases the ball on the ground.
  - The opposing team comes together over the top of the ball in an attempt to drive the other team backward away from the ball.
  - One team must drive the other team completely off the ball before the ball can be picked up.

EQUIPMENT (7)

- Ball: ovoid ball that is somewhat larger and rounder than an American football
- Boots: the rugby cleats
  - Typically have removable studs or molded multi-studded rubber soles and have cleats similar to soccer. Single-toe cleats as in baseball are not permitted.
- Prohibited equipment
  - Any item contaminated by blood
  - Any sharp or abrasive item
  - Any items containing buckles, clips, rings, hinges, zippers, screws, bolts, or rigid material or projection not otherwise permitted
  - Jewelry
  - Gloves
  - Shorts or leggings with padding sewn into them
  - Any item that is normally permitted but, in the referee's opinion, is liable to cause injury
  - Communication devices
- Optional equipment:
  - Shoulder pads: generally, a padded pullover top with a maximum thickness of 1/2 inch of foam padding
  - Mitts: fingerless gloves
  - Soft headgear: scrum cap for ear protection to prevent ear trauma
  - Goggles
  - Mouth guard: The relative risk of making a dental injury claim for nonwearers was estimated to be 4.6 times that of wearers (8).
  - Shin guards: thin, 0.5 cm of padding only (no hard plastic)
- Some authors suggest a lack of regulation mandating protective equipment has resulted in an injury rate three times that of American football (9,10).

INJURY RISK

- Athletes average a distance of 6.9 km per game.
  - Of this, 37% is spent standing or walking, 27% jogging, 10% cruising, 14% striding, 5% high-intensity running, and 6% (approximately 420 m) sprinting (11).
  - In addition, the rugby player is involved in more than one to two episodes of collision contact per minute.
  - This equals approximately 40 tackles and up to 70 rucks and mauls per game.
  - Forwards may sustain an additional 30 scrums and 40 line outs per game (11).
  - There are few substitutions allowed and the mean duration of high-intensity work (sprinting or contact) is 38 seconds · min^{-1} with an average workload of 51 minutes per 80-minute match.
    - By comparison, the average American football game has only 10 minutes of contact or significant exertion per game (12).

EPIDEMIOLOGY

- Current studies on rugby injury incidents demonstrates a lack of standardized definition for injury, resulting in the discrepancy seen in the literature with reports ranging from 30 to 91 or even 120 per 1000 match hours (13).
- In 2007, the International Rugby Board (IRB) developed definitions and procedures to improve the quality of data collection (14).
- Injury rates for youth rugby (<18 years) is about 24 per 1000 player hours (15,16).
- Concussion is the most common head or neck injury with an incidence of 0.2–6.9 per 1000 game hours.
- Youth athletes with a concussion must undergo 14 days rest and be symptom free before beginning the 5-day graduated return-to-play protocol (4).
- Injuries in women occur with less frequency.
  - Exception may be anterior cruciate ligament (ACL) injury (17,18).
- Incidence rate of injury in amateur players is lower than that in professional players, but higher than adolescent and youth rugby players (19).
- Gameplay produces a greater number and severity of injuries compared to practice (20–23).
- Higher body mass index has been associated with a higher injury rate (24).
- Tackling has been cited as the major cause of injury (13).
  - The player being tackled is more likely to be injured than the tackler (21,22).
  - The player with the lower momentum is four times more likely to be injured than the player with a higher momentum (21).
  - There is a high rate of tackling injury when two or more tacklers simultaneously make contact with the ball carrier (25).
  - The location of injuries varies based on sex, age, and level of play (1,12,13,15,20,22,24,26–34). However, it should be noted that the quality of the data is limited due to lack of standardization.
  - The type of injury varies widely and includes sprains, strains, contusions, abrasions, and lacerations, which are to be expected in rugby (13,20,22,29).
    - Sprains, strains, and other soft-tissue injury: 74%
    - Laceration or abrasion: 10%
    - Fracture: 7%

- Closed head injury: 5%
- Other: 4%

- Head and upper spinal injuries (14%–30%) (13)
  - Lacerations and concussions are the most common, followed by facial fractures.
  - Concussion is often unreported due to lack of knowledge of the symptoms of concussion and/or a delay in diagnosis (35,36).
  - Spinal injuries can lead to catastrophic neurological consequences (tetraplegia) and deaths have been reported (37).
    - Permanent neurological damage from spinal cord injuries is estimated to be 4.25/100,000, comparable to other contact sports such as American football (38).
- Upper limb injuries (15%–20%) (13)
  - The shoulder was involved in the greatest number of upper limb injuries, and the damage was disproportionately severe.
  - Acromioclavicular (AC) joint sprain and rotator cuff strain are the most common, but shoulder instability and dislocation caused the longest absence from participation.
- Lower limb injuries (30%–55%)
  - Not only accounts for the highest number of injuries but also the most severe injuries (measured by time lost from participation)
  - The knee seemed to have the most injuries of the lower limb with the medial collateral ligament (MCL), meniscus, and extensor mechanism injuries being the most common.
  - ACL and MCL injury resulted in longest periods of absence from sport.
  - Thigh injuries were predominantly hematomas and hamstring strains.
  - Ankle injuries were mostly lateral ligament sprains and Achilles tendon injuries.
- Cervical spine injuries
  - In the United States, Wetzler et al. (39) published a retrospective study of cervical spine injuries that occurred during the rugby scrum from 1970 to 1994.
    - 58% of rugby cervical spine injuries occurred during the scrum.
    - 64% of above injuries occurred during engagement.
    - 36% of above injuries occurred when the scrum collapsed.
    - Hookers accounted for 78% of injured players, and props accounted for 19% of injured players. Second row players accounted for the remaining 3%.
  - In the United States, 47.5% of all rugby cervical spine injuries occurred in hookers versus 18.6% outside of the United States (39).
  - In the United States, 57.6% of catastrophic rugby injuries occurred in the scrum, in contrast to 41.5% outside of the United States (3,40).
    - It is theorized that the discrepancy may be because most rugby players in the United States learn to play the sport at college age or older, while athletes in other countries learn rugby skills and techniques at a much younger age (3).
  - Swain et al. (41) prospectively evaluated neck injury in Australian amateur rugby. Their data show that the majority of neck injuries occur in the tackling phase of play.
    - This is true of all positions, with the exception of the front row (especially hooker), where the majority of neck injuries occur during the scrum.
    - There was no statistical difference between the phase of play and the severity of neck injury (42).
    - The greatest number of neck injuries occurred during the game play rather than training (85.6%) (41).

INJURIES BY POSITION

- The front row is most susceptible to an injury during a scrum.
  - When the ball is put into play during a scrum, the necks of the front row are already in position of slight flexion.
  - The two opposing scrums are applying an axial force on the cervical spines that is equivalent to 5–1.5 tons (36,40).
    - Collapse is often related to the following (43):
      - Inappropriately vertical force vectors during engagement
      - Poor field conditions with poor traction
      - Inexperience
      - Fatigue
      - Playing with injury
      - Opposing scrum mismatch in terms of size, ability, strength, and experience
- The second row is susceptible to other specific injuries:
  - Neck injury — for the same reasons as the front row but to a lesser extent
  - Auricular hematomas, ear avulsions, and head lacerations because their heads are positioned between the thighs of the front row players
    - Scrum caps or an electrical tape headband are often worn to secure their ears to the side of their head.
  - Fall-related injuries — due to being lifted during line outs
  - Flanker/wing forward
    - Susceptible to injuries in the tackling situation
    - High incidence of AC joint injuries
  - Eightman: susceptible to similar head and facial injuries as the locks because of their head position between the locks
  - Scrumhalf: susceptible to contact injuries while attempting to secure the ball
  - Pack (positions 1–9): at risk for contact knee injuries (40)
  - Backs (positions 10–15)

- At risk for contact and noncontact knee injuries
- Susceptible to injury of the head, neck, and shoulders during tackling
- Injury incidence between forwards and backs is similar; however, forwards tend to have more severe injuries when they do occur (13).
- In rucks, the players are on the ground or at risk for abrasions, lacerations, contusions, and orofacial trauma from the cleats of other players.
- In mauls and rucks, all players are susceptible to hand and finger injuries from binding to each other's jerseys.
- During tackling, players are at risk for the same injuries as other collision sports.

INJURY PREVENTION

- Rules have been instituted to decrease the incidence of head injury. The following actions are illegal (7):
  - A player requiring a head injury assessment (HIA) must be temporarily replaced. If the player is not available to return to the field of play after 12 minutes, the replacement becomes permanent.
  - Players must not do anything that is reckless or dangerous to others, including leading with the elbow or forearm, or jumping into, or over, a tackler.
  - A player must not tackle an opponent early, late, or dangerously. Dangerous tackling includes, but is not limited to, tackling or attempting to tackle an opponent above the line of the shoulders even if the tackle starts below the line of the shoulders.
  - A player must not tackle an opponent who is not in possession of the ball.
  - A player must not lift an opponent off the ground and drop or drive that player so that their head and upper body make contact with the ground.
  - A player must not tackle, charge, pull, push, or grasp an opponent whose feet are off the ground.
  - A player must not charge or knock down an opponent carrying the ball without attempting to grasp that player.
- Many players have additional equipment to decrease injury risk, such as scrum caps or electrical tape headbands to secure their ears to the side of their head to prevent ear injuries or shoulder pads to attempt to prevent AC joint injuries.
  - There are currently limited studies to date that show that these measures have prevented injuries. However, Marshall et al. (44) found that proper use of mouth guards and padded headgear reduces orofacial and scalp injuries.
  - The use of padded headgear has no effect on concussion incidence (44–46).
  - Taping, shin guards, and grease showed no change in injury rates (44).
  - Support sleeves may decrease sprains and strains (44).
  - The referee conducts a safety inspection of the pitch and all players prior to the match (7).
    - Toe cleats (often used in baseball) are not allowed as tackled players are frequently on the ground underneath players from both teams who are attempting to secure the ball with their feet and toe cleats would increase the risk of laceration injuries.
    - The referee may prohibit a player from participating if unsafe footwear, uniform, illegal equipment, or long fingernails are found.
    - Medical personnel are encouraged to join the referee for the inspection.
- Because tight five players have the highest incidence of cervical spine injury in the United States, they should have extensive practice and instruction prior to the competition.
- Depowering the scrum or having uncontested scrums in less experienced play is a technique used to decrease the risk of injury (47).
- Because fatigue is thought to be a risk factor for injury, all players should maintain a high level of fitness (43).
- USA Rugby encourages all coaches to complete a series of coaching clinics. These clinics will arm coaches with techniques to provide proper instruction on some of the more complex skills and techniques of the game.
- The laws of the game are updated frequently to improve the safety of the players with recent focus on reducing the risk of injury during the scrum.
- A standardized coach and referee education program has been shown in New Zealand to decrease catastrophic neck injuries (48).
- More research is required to make better recommendations regarding prevention strategies and best practices.

EVENT COVERAGE

- There is only one referee to monitor play and play is stopped only for a penalty, the ball leaving the field of play, a score, or for a serious injury (in the judgment of the referee) (7).
- The referee may summon a medical attendant onto the pitch or may allow the player to temporarily leave the pitch for medical evaluation (7).
  - Even though a medical attendant may be on the pitch evaluating an injured player, the referee may also choose to allow play to continue around the injured player.
  - The medical attendant does not have the power to stop play but does have the ability to determine whether an injured player is allowed to continue to play.
- Sideline preparedness
  - Because the spectrum of injury is wide, the physician covering the sport must be well rounded and prepared to handle a variety of acute injuries.

- The nature of substitution rules of rugby places more pressure on a sideline position to make a timely decision on fitness to play. Prompt and accurate evaluation is therefore critical (7).
  - The game continues without a substitution while the physician is evaluating the injured athlete.
  - If another player replaces the injured rugger, they cannot return to the match even if physically capable. Therefore, the coach relies on the physician to tell them whether to play one man down until the injured person returns or whether a permanent substitution needs to be made. Except in the following cases:
    - A player be substituted for a maximum of 15 minutes for control of bleeding from an injury. After bleeding is controlled, they may return to play. This is commonly referred to as a blood sub.
    - A referee may permit a substituted tight five player to return to the match to replace an injured player if no eligible player on the team is experienced in these skilled positions.
    - A player requiring an HIA (evaluation for potential concussion) must be temporarily replaced. If the player is not available to return to the field of play after 12 minutes, the replacement becomes permanent.
- Therefore, there is a delicate balance between not prematurely removing an athlete from play versus minimizing the time the team competes one man short while the physician is performing the evaluation.
- Lacerations deserve special mention because the team physician's proficiency in attending to a bleeding wound within the allotted "blood sub" time of 15 minutes will determine whether an athlete is able to return to play.
- Proper training in evaluating concussion is paramount with increasing emphasis on education and protection over the past several years (49,50).
- Although rare, catastrophic injury has been reported in rugby union play. An emergency response plan should be preestablished in case of such a situation (51).
- The USA Rugby and the IRB websites have sections for medical providers that provide good information for those interested in providing sideline coverage for rugby union (https://usa.rugby/player-welfare and https://www.world.rugby/the-game/player-welfare).

REFERENCES

1. Viviers PL, Viljoen JT, Derman W. A review of a decade of rugby Union injury epidemiology: 2007-2017. *Sports Health.* 2018;10(3):223–7.
2. World Rugby. *Year in Review—Global Participation Numbers.* 2021. [cited 2007 September 27]. Available from: http://publications.worldrugby.org/yearinreview2021/en/46-1.
3. USA Rugby Member Stats. n.d. [cited 2022 October 4]. Available from: http://membershipstats.usa.rugby/
4. Rugby 101 – How the sport works: USA rugby. *How the Sport Works.* USA Rugby; n.d. [cited 2022 October 4]. Available from: https://usa.rugby/rugby101
5. The Olympic Studies Centre. RUGBY history of rugby at the Olympic Games. *OSC Reference Collection.* 2017. [cited 2022 October 4]. Available from: http://www.olympic.org/studies
6. History of Rugby Sevens Olympics.com. n.d. [cited 2022 October 4]. Available from: https://olympics.com/en/sports/rugby-sevens/.
7. Worldrugby.org. Laws of the game: world rugby laws. *Laws of the Game World Rugby Laws.* n.d. [cited 2022 October 4]. Available from: https://www.world.rugby/the-game/laws/home
8. Quarrie KL, Gianotti SM, Chalmers DJ, Hopkins WG. An evaluation of mouthguard requirements and dental injuries in New Zealand rugby union. *Br J Sports Med.* 2005;39(9):650–1.
9. Marshall SW, Waller AE, Dick RW, Pugh CB, Loomis DP, Chalmers DJ. An ecologic study of protective equipment and injury in two contact sports. *Int J Epidemiol.* 2002;31(3):587–92.
10. Willigenburg NW, Borchers JR, Quincy R, Kaeding CC, Hewett TE. Comparison of injuries in American collegiate football and club rugby: a prospective cohort study. *Am J Sports Med.* 2016;44(3):753–60.
11. Cunniffe B, Proctor W, Baker JS, Davies B. An evaluation of the physiological demands of elite rugby union using global positioning system tracking software. *J Strength Cond Res.* 2009;23(4):1195–203.
12. Dexter WD. Rugby. In: Mellion MB, Putukian M, Madden C, editors. *Sports Medicine Secrets.* Philadelphia: Hanley and Belfus; 2003.
13. Jakoet I, Noakes TD. A high rate of injury during the 1995 Rugby World Cup. *S Afr Med J.* 1998;88(1):45–7.
14. Fuller CW, Molloy MG, Bagate C, et al. Consensus statement on injury definitions and data collection procedures for studies of injuries in rugby union. *Br J Sports Med.* 2007;41(5):328–31.
15. Freitag A, Kirkwood G, Scharer S, Ofori-Asenso R, Pollock AM. Systematic review of rugby injuries in children and adolescents under 21 years. *Br J Sports Med.* 2015;49(8):511–9.
16. Haseler CM, Carmont MR, England M. The epidemiology of injuries in English youth community rugby union. *Br J Sports Med.* 2010;44(15):1093–9.
17. Levy AS, Wetzler MJ, Lewars M, Laughlin W. Knee injuries in women collegiate rugby players. *Am J Sports Med.* 1997;25(3):360–2.
18. Peck KY, Johnston DA, Owens BD, Cameron KL. The incidence of injury among male and female intercollegiate rugby players. *Sport Health.* 2013;5(4):327–33.
19. Yeomans C, Kenny IC, Cahalan R, et al. The incidence of injury in amateur male rugby union: a systematic review and meta-analysis. *Sports Med.* 2018;48(4):837–48.
20. Bathgate A, Best JP, Craig G, Jamieson M. A prospective study of injuries to elite Australian rugby union players. *Br J Sports Med.* 2002;36(4):265–9.
21. Brooks JH, Fuller CW, Kemp SPT, Reddin DB. A prospective study of injuries and training amongst the England 2003 Rugby World Cup squad. *Br J Sports Med.* 2005;39(5):288–93.
22. Targett SG. Injuries in professional rugby union. *Clin J Sport Med.* 1998;8(4):280–5.
23. Kaplan KM, Goodwillie A, Strauss EJ, Rosen JE. Rugby injuries: a review of concepts and current literature. *Bull NYU Hosp Jt Dis.* 2008;66(2):86–93.
24. Quarrie KL, Alsop JC, Waller AE, Bird YN, Marshall SW, Chalmers DJ. The New Zealand rugby injury and performance project. VI. A prospective cohort study of risk factors for injury in rugby union football. *Br J Sports Med.* 2001;35(3):157–66.
25. McIntosh AS, Savage TN, McCrory P, Fréchède BO, Wolfe R. Tackle characteristics and injury in a cross section of rugby union football. *Med Sci Sports Exerc.* 2010;42(5):977–84.

26. Fuller CW, Taylor A, Douglas M, Raftery M. Rugby World Cup 2019 injury surveillance study. *S Afr J Sports Med.* 2020;32(1):v32i1a8062.
27. Fuller CW, Taylor A, Kemp SP, Raftery M. Rugby world cup 2015: world rugby injury surveillance study. *Br J Sports Med.* 2017;51(1):51–7.
28. Garraway WM, Lee AJ, Hutton SJ, Russell EBAW, Macleod DAD. Impact of professionalism on injuries in rugby union. *Br J Sports Med.* 2000;34(5):348–51.
29. Gerrard DF, Waller AE, Bird YN. The New Zealand Rugby Injury and Performance Project: II. Previous injury experience of a rugby-playing cohort. *Br J Sports Med.* 1994;28(4):229–33.
30. Ma R, Lopez V Jr, Weinstein MG, et al. Injury profile of American women's rugby-7s. *Med Sci Sports Exerc.* 2016;48(10):1957–66.
31. Quarrie KL, Cantu RC, Chalmers DJ. Rugby union injuries to the cervical spine and spinal cord. *Sports Med.* 2002;32(10):633–53.
32. Quarrie KL, Handcock P, Toomey MJ, Waller AE. The New Zealand rugby injury and performance project. IV. Anthropometric and physical performance comparisons between positional categories of senior A rugby players. *Br J Sports Med.* 1996;30(1):53–6.
33. Quarrie KL, Handcock P, Waller AE, Chalmers DJ, Toomey MJ, Wilson BD. The New Zealand rugby injury and performance project. III. Anthropometric and physical performance characteristics of players. *Br J Sports Med.* 1995;29(4):263–70.
34. Waller AE, Feehan M, Marshall SW, Chalmers DJ. The New Zealand Rugby Injury and Performance Project: I. Design and methodology of a prospective follow-up study. *Br J Sports Med.* 1994;28(4):223–8.
35. Kirkwood G, Parekh N, Ofori-Asenso R, Pollock AM. Concussion in youth rugby union and rugby league: a systematic review. *Br J Sports Med.* 2015;49(8):506–10.
36. Marshall SW, Spencer RJ. Concussion in rugby: the hidden epidemic. *J Athl Train.* 2001;36(3):334–8.
37. Kaux JF, Julia M, Delvaux F, et al. Epidemiological review of injuries in rugby union. *Sports.* 2015;3(1):21–9.
38. Brown JC, Lambert MI, Verhagen E, Readhead C, Van Mechelen W, Viljoen W. The incidence of rugby-related catastrophic injuries (including cardiac events) in South Africa from 2008 to 2011: a cohort study. *BMJ Open.* 2013;3(2):e002475.
39. Wetzler MJ, Akpata T, Albert T, Foster TE, Levy AS. A retrospective study of cervical spine injuries in American rugby, 1970 to 1994. *Am J Sports Med.* 1996;24(4):454–8.
40. Dietzen CJ, Topping BR. Rugby football. *Phys Med Rehabil Clin N Am.* 1999;10(1):159–75.
41. Swain MS, Pollard HP, Bonello R. Incidence, severity, aetiology and type of neck injury in men's amateur rugby union: a prospective cohort study. *Chiropr Osteopat.* 2010;18(1):18–12.
42. Kuster D, Gibson A, Abboud R, Drew T. Mechanisms of cervical spine injury in rugby union: a systematic review of the literature. *Br J Sports Med.* 2012;46(8):550–4.
43. Milburn PD. Biomechanics of rugby union scrummaging. Technical and safety issues. *Sports Med.* 1993;16(3):168–79.
44. Marshall SW, Loomis DP, Waller AE, et al. Evaluation of protective equipment for prevention of injuries in rugby union. *Int J Epidemiol.* 2005;34(1):113–18.
45. Mcintosh AS, McCrory P, Finch CF, Best JP, Chalmers DJ, Wolfe R. Does padded headgear prevent head injury in rugby union football?. *Med Sci Sports Exerc.* 2009;41(2):306–13.
46. Stokes KA, Cross M, Williams S, et al. Padded headgear does not reduce the incidence of match concussions in professional men's rugby union: a case-control study of 417 cases. *Int J Sports Med.* 2021;42(10):930–5.
47. Wetzler MJ, Akpata T, Laughlin W, Levy AS. Occurrence of cervical spine injuries during the rugby scrum. *Am J Sports Med.* 1998;26(2):177–80.
48. Quarrie KL, Gianotti SM, Hopkins WG, Hume PA. Effect of nationwide injury prevention programme on serious spinal injuries in New Zealand rugby union: ecological study. *BMJ.* 2007;334(7604):1150.
49. Harmon KG, Clugston JR, Dec K, et al. American Medical Society for Sports Medicine position statement on concussion in sport. *Br J Sports Med.* 2019;53(4):213–25.
50. McCrory P, Meeuwisse W, Dvořák J, et al. Consensus statement on concussion in sport—the 5th international conference on concussion in sport held in Berlin, October 2016. *Br J Sports Med.* 2017;51(11):838–47.
51. Bergfeld J. Sideline preparedness for the team physician: a consensus statement. *Med Sci Sports Exerc.* 2001.

113 Running

Robert P. Wilder and Francis G. O'Connor

EPIDEMIOLOGY OF RUNNING INJURIES (1)

- There are over 30 million runners, of whom more than 10 million run on more than 100 $d \cdot y^{-1}$.
- One million enter competitive races per year (1–3).
- Yearly injury incidence rate ranges from 29.5% to 56% (1–6).
- Injury rate ranges from 2.5 to 5.8 injuries per 1000 hours of running (1,3,4).
  - The lower rate of 2.5 per 1000 hours is seen in long-distance and marathon runners.
  - Sprinters have the highest rate of 5.8 injuries per 1000 hours (4).
  - Middle-distance runners are between the two at 5.6 injuries per 1000 hours (4).
- Despite the relatively high incidence rate of running injuries per runner per year, this incidence rate is still two to six times lower than that in other sports (1,3).

Common Injury Sites (7–12)

- Most running injuries are musculoskeletal overuse syndromes (Table 113.1); 70%–80% occur from the knee down (1,10,11).
  - Back: 5%
  - Hip and groin: 15%
  - Knee: 40%
  - Lower leg: 16%–20%
  - Foot and ankle: 20%–26%
- Although there are no overall age- or gender-related differences, females have slightly increased rates of hip, knee, and bone stress injury and males slightly increased risk of foot, ankle, and Achilles injury (11,12).
- There are differences in injury pattern between sprinters, middle-distance runners, and long-distance runners. Hamstring strains and tendinitis are more commonly seen in sprinters; backache and hip problems are more commonly seen in middle-distance runners; and foot problems are more common among long-distance and marathon runners (4,10).

Risk Factors for Running Injuries (1,11,13–24)

- Important risk factors (for which a clear association with injury has been identified)
  - Training miles per week (risk increases at 19 miles $\cdot$ wk^{-1} and increases more sharply at 40 miles $\cdot$ wk^{-1}) (15,17)
  - Previous running injury (within past 12 months) (17)
  - Inexperienced runner (running <3 years)
  - Recent transition in training
  - Training intensity
  - Cavus feet, leg length inequality, hip abductor weakness
  - Age >50 in females
- Equivocal risk factors (for which evidence demonstrating a clear link with injury is unclear)
  - Hyperflexibility or hypoflexibility
  - Stretching exercises (25,26)
  - Running shoes (27,28)
  - Shoe orthotics
  - Roadside running
  - Malalignment problems (genu varum and valgus, high Q-angle, femoral neck anteversion, pelvic obliquity, knee and patella alignment, rearfoot valgus, leg length discrepancy)
  - Body morphology (slight protective effect in men with body mass index >26 $kg \cdot m^2$)
  - Age
  - Foot strike pattern (rearfoot, midfoot, forefoot)
- Unrelated risk factors (have not been associated with increase in running injuries)
  - Gender
  - Running surface
  - Cross-training
  - Time of day
  - Warm-up or cool-down period

Table 113.1 Top Running Injuries (7–9)

Diagnosis	Percentage
Patellofemoral pain syndrome	32.2
Tibial stress syndrome, "shin splints"	17.3
Achilles tendinitis	7.2
Stress fractures	7.2
Patellar tendinitis	5.7
Iliotibial band syndrome	6.3
Metatarsal stress syndrome	3.3
Adductor strain	3
Hamstring strain	2.6
Posterior tibial tendinitis	2.6
Ankle sprain	2.4
Peroneus tendinitis	1.9
Iliac apophysitis	1.6

BIOMECHANICS OF RUNNING

The Running Gait Cycle

- During walking, the stance phase occupies 40% of the gait cycle. The stance phase is decreased to approximately 30% while running and 20% while sprinting (29).
- Walking differs from running in that walking has two double support periods in stance, whereas running has two periods of double float in swing. Running does not have a period of double support (29).
- See Chapter 25 Gait Analysis for further discussion.

Kinematics

- Generally, there is an increase in joint range of motion (ROM) as velocity increases. However, there are no major differences between walking and running kinematics in the coronal and transverse planes. Most kinematic differences occur in the sagittal plane (29,30). The body lowers its center of gravity with increased speed by increasing flexion at the hips and knees and by increased dorsiflexion at the ankle (29,31).
- The hip
  - The hip demonstrates an overall increase in ROM as velocity increases. The most significant motion occurs in the sagittal plane. Most of this increase occurs in flexion, and the amount of extension actually decreases slightly. Overall ROM was determined to be 43° with maximum flexion and extension, measuring 37° and 6°, respectively, for normal walking. In running, however, overall ROM was increased to 46°, with the hip flexing and never quite returning past neutral into extension (29,32).
- The knee
  - As in the hip, the most significant motion occurs in the sagittal plane. The knee joint demonstrates increased flexion as velocity increases, but extension is, as in the hip, decreased. Maximum flexion in walking reaches 64°, and extension is −8° (8° of flexion). In running, maximum flexion reaches 79°, and extension is −16° (16° of flexion) (29,31).
- The ankle and foot
  - Overall ROM at the ankle during walking is estimated to be 30°, with maximum plantarflexion of 18° and maximum dorsiflexion of 12°. Running produces a greater overall ankle ROM of 50° due to increased hip and knee flexion during running (29).
  - At initial contact, due to the increased hip and knee flexion, the ankle undergoes rapid dorsiflexion during the absorption phase.
    - In running, because the ankle never quite reaches the amount of plantarflexion that it undergoes while walking, the amount of supination in the subtalar joint is limited, but the degree of pronation is increased (21,29).
    - Subtalar motion is determined by muscular activity as well as response to ground reactive forces. Midtarsal joint motion, however, is determined by subtalar position (21,29).
  - When the calcaneus and the talus are supinated, the axis is such that an increased obliquity is produced across the oblique and longitudinal midtarsal joints, which serves to lock the midtarsal joint functionally, thereby resulting in a decrease in available motion and allowing the foot to become a "rigid lever." This occurs during late terminal stance and preswing.
- When the calcaneus and talus are pronated, the axis is such that an increased parallelism exists between the oblique and longitudinal midtarsal joints, resulting in an increased available motion in these joints, serving to unlock the midtarsal joint and allowing an increased ROM for adaptation to the ground surface as well as absorbing the ground reactive forces, which lets the foot become a "mobile adapter." This occurs during the midstance (29).
  - As the foot makes contact with the floor, the pelvis, femur, and tibia begin the process of internal rotation. This internal rotation lasts through loading response and into midstance, resulting in eversion and unlocking of the subtalar joint. This results in subtalar pronation, which allows unlocking of the oblique and longitudinal midtarsal joints, resulting in further pronation. The pelvis, femur, and tibia then begin to rotate externally, which causes inversion and locking of the subtalar joint (29).

Kinetics

- Walking produces vertical ground reactive forces equal to 1.3–1.5 times body weight. During running, vertical ground reactive forces spike sharply at contact to produce an impact peak, may slightly decrease, and then continue to an active peak measuring 2.2–2.6 times body weight. It is thus during midstance when ground reactive forces are greatest, with peak internal joint moments generating peak mechanical stress on tissues (33,34).

- It is unclear whether increased impact forces lead to injury or affect performance (33,35–38).
- The percentage of muscle activity increases throughout the stance phase during running. It is rare to see a muscle group active for more than 50% of the stance phase during walking, but in running, activity is noted for 70%–80% of the stance phase (39).
- During walking, the *gluteus maximus* is active from the end of the swing phase until the foot is flat on the floor. This serves to decelerate the limb and stabilize the hip joint for initial contact. During running, however, it is active from terminal swing through 40% of the stance phase. This helps produce hip extension (29).
- The *hip abductors* function during the terminal swing and throughout 50% of the stance phase during walking and running. This serves to stabilize the stance leg pelvis at initial contact, which prevents excessive sagging of the swing leg (29,40).
- The *hip adductors* are active during the last one-third of the stance phase during walking. During running, they are active during the entire stance and swing phases (29,39).
- The *quadriceps* are active at the end of the swing phase to bring about terminal knee extension and to aid in hip flexion, through a concentric contraction. They also help stabilize the knee joint at initial contact, through an eccentric contraction. In running, they are highly active during the absorption phase of stance to deal with the greater requirements of weight acceptance. They are continually active throughout knee flexion eccentrically to limit the rate at which knee flexion occurs. They are active for 50%–60% of the running stance phase and for only 25% of the walking stance phase (29).
- During walking, the *hamstrings* are active at the end of swing phase and into stance phase until the foot is in full contact with the ground. This occurs in about 10% of the walking gait cycle. During running, they are active during the last third of the swing phase during hip and knee extension. Here they are acting concentrically across the hip joint but eccentrically across the knee joint. This action initiates hip extension and resists knee extension simultaneously (29).
- During walking, the *anterior tibial muscle* group is active from late stance phase through the swing phase and then for the first 10%–15% of the next stance phase. This produces dorsiflexion of the ankle during the swing phase through concentric contraction. It also helps control plantarflexion by initial contact through eccentric contraction, thereby preventing foot slap. During running, these muscles are active from the late stance phase through the swing phase and for the first 50%–60% of the next stance phase. For their duration of activity, they are undergoing concentric contraction. During walking, they decelerate foot plantarflexion at initial contact; however, during running they appear to accelerate movement of the leg over the fixed foot. In heel strikers, a greater degree of activity is found in the anterior tibial muscle group than in midfoot strikers (29).
- Activity of the *posterior leg musculature* begins during terminal swing of gait. During walking, these muscles act to resist forward movement of the tibia over the fixed foot during the stance phase. They are active from 25% to 50% of the stance phase through mostly eccentric contraction. During their last 25% of activity, they undergo concentric contraction to initiate active plantarflexion. During running gait, initial contact is a period of rapid dorsiflexion. Here, the triceps undergo eccentric contraction, again to resist this motion. They are active for approximately 60% of the stance phase. Initially, they serve to stabilize the ankle joint at initial contact, and then to provide for propulsion (29).
- Although a decrease in impact peak force has been observed as one moves from a rearfoot to midfoot to forefoot strike pattern, the effect on injury rates and pattern is unknown (41–43).

COMMON RUNNING INJURIES

Patellofemoral Syndrome (7,44–48)

- Definition
  - Pain associated with the articular surface of the patella and femoral condyles
  - "Runner's knee"; number 1 presenting complaint to runners' clinics
  - Number 1 cause of lost time in basic training in military recruits
- Diagnosis (46,49)
  - Anterior, peripatellar, subpatellar pain
  - Increased pain following prolonged sitting (theater sign) as well as running downhill and walking downstairs
  - Apprehension (shrug) sign
  - Abnormal patella tilt (tilt <5° in males and <10° in females)
  - Abnormal patella glide (medial glide < two quadrants, lateral glide > three quadrants)
- Contributing factors (44,46,49–51)
  - Femoral dysplasia
  - Patellar facet asymmetry
  - Malalignments contributing to excessive pronation
    - Femoral anteversion
    - External tibial torsion
    - Varus ankle, foot
  - Patella alta, baja
  - Increased Q-angle

- Muscle and soft-tissue imbalances
  - Weak vastus medialis oblique (VMO)
  - Tight lateral structures (iliotibial band [ITB], lateral retinaculum)
  - Weakness of hip abductors, extensors, external rotators
- Treatment (48,49,52)
  - Correct biomechanical factors that lead to compensatory subtalar pronation and obligatory internal tibial rotation: genu valgum, tibia vara, hindfoot varus, forefoot pronation
  - Flexibility: ITB, hamstrings, quadriceps, gastrocnemius
  - Manual therapy to stretch tight retinaculum: medial glide and tilt
  - Strengthening: quadriceps with emphasis on VMO, hip abductors, extensors, external rotators
  - McConnell taping
  - Bracing (patellar straps and braces) (53)
  - With persistent symptoms, consider:
    - Magnetic resonance imaging (MRI) (osteochondritis, cartilage injury)
    - Injections (steroid, viscosupplementation)
    - Surgery: lateral release if tight retinaculum; realignment

Iliotibial Band Syndrome (44,54–58)

- Definition
  - An overuse tendinopathy of the ITB most commonly as it passes over the lateral femoral condyle.
  - ITB syndrome is the most common cause of lateral knee pain in runners, accounting for up to 12% of all running-related overuse injuries (59–62).
  - ITB syndrome results from repetitive friction of the ITB at the lateral femoral epicondyle. The ITB moves anterior to the epicondyle as the knee extends and posterior as the knee flexes, remaining tense in both positions (56,63,64). Specifically, the posterior edge of the ITB impinges against the lateral femoral epicondyle of the femur just after foot strike. This "impingement zone" occurs at or at slightly less than 30° of knee flexion (64). Fairclough et al. (65) have alternatively proposed that ITB syndrome results from compression of the ITB against the lateral femoral epicondyle as a consequence of internal tibial rotation after foot strike as opposed to friction. Repetitive irritation can lead to chronic inflammation, especially beneath the posterior fibers of the ITB, which are thought to be tighter against the lateral femoral condyle than the anterior fibers (56,64).
  - The ITB is a continuation of the tendinous portion of the tensor fascia lata (TFL) muscle, with some contribution from the gluteal muscles. It is connected to the linea aspera via the intermuscular septum. Distally, the ITB spans out and inserts on the lateral border of the patella, the lateral retinaculum, and Gerdy's tubercle of the tibia. The ITB is free from bony attachment between the superior aspect of the lateral femoral epicondyle and Gerdy's tubercle (56,66,67).
  - Functioning as abductors during open-chain activity, the TFL, gluteus medius, and gluteus minimus provide important function through the support phase of the gait cycle, eccentrically lengthening while stabilizing the pelvis and controlling femoral adduction (56,68).
- Diagnosis
  - Lateral pain and crepitus at lateral femoral condyle (or insertion at Gerdy's tubercle)
  - Tight ITB on Ober test
  - Abductor weakness
- Contributing factors (54,56,59,61,69–72)
  - Varus positioning of knee, tibia, and foot
  - Increased hip adduction and internal rotation
  - Internal tibial torsion
  - Excessive supination or pronation
  - Abductor tightness and weakness
  - Higher knee flexion at heel strike
  - Downhill running
  - Running on crowned roads
  - Excessive running in same direction on track
- Treatment
  - PRICEMM (protection, rest, ice, compression, elevation, modalities, medication); iontophoresis
  - ITB strap or dual-action strap
  - Foam roller exercise for soft-tissue work
  - Myofascial release
  - Flexibility and strength (hip abductors, adductors, rotators, flexors, extensors)
  - Gait modification (increased stride frequency, increased step width)
- With persistent symptoms, consider:
  - Injection (steroid, platelet rich plasma (PRP))
  - MRI to rule out lateral meniscus, other

Shin Splints/Medial Tibial Stress Syndrome

- Definition
  - Medial Tibial Stress Syndrome (MTSS) is a clinical entity characterized by diffuse tenderness over the posteromedial aspect of the distal third of the tibia. Shin splints have been reported to account for 12%–18% of running injuries (73–75) and to occur in 4% of all military recruits in basic training (76). Women appear more frequently affected than men.
  - MTSS should be differentiated from stress fractures and exertional compartment syndrome. Although different entities, they may coexist.
    - Plain films are negative (except in cases of previous or coexistent stress fracture). Bone scans demonstrate

characteristic vertical linear increased activity along the tibial periosteum, which differs from the more focal fusiform increased radiotracer uptake exhibited by stress fractures.

- MTSS is felt by most to represent a periostalgia or tendinopathy along the tibial attachment of the tibialis posterior or soleus muscles. Other proposed etiologies have included posterior compartment syndrome and fascial inflammation.
  - Detmer (77) proposed a classification scheme for MTSS based on etiology. Type 1 includes local stress fractures, type 2 includes periostitis/periostalgia, and type 3 includes deep posterior compartment syndrome.

- Diagnosis
  - Dull ache in medial shaft with activity
  - Tenderness to palpation along the shaft
  - Normal neurovascular exam and x-ray
- Contributing factors
  - Factors that increase valgus forces and pronation, which then increase eccentric contraction of the soleus and tibialis posterior: femoral anteversion, genu varum, tibia and forefoot varus, excessive Q-angle.
  - Excessive pes planus or pes cavus
  - Tarsal coalition
  - Leg length inequality
  - Muscle imbalances: inflexibility of plantarflexors; weakness of dorsiflexors, plantarflexors, invertors
  - Extrinsic risk factors include improper shoe wear, a rapid transition in training, inadequate warm-up, running on uneven or hard surfaces, running in cold weather, and low calcium intake.
- Treatment (76)
  - Flexibility: gastrocnemius-soleus, tibialis posterior
  - Strength: concentric and eccentric, including tibialis posterior soleus, tibialis anterior, flexor hallucis, and flexor digitorum longus
  - Orthotics to control compensatory pronation
  - Shin sleeve
- With persistent symptoms, consider:
  - Bone scan/MRI to rule out stress fracture
  - Compartment testing to rule out compartment syndrome
  - Consider lumbar radiculopathy

Exertional Compartment Syndrome

- Definition
  - Chronic exertional compartment syndrome (CECS) is defined as reversible ischemia secondary to a noncompliant osseofascial compartment that is unresponsive to the expansion of muscle volume that occurs with exercise. Most commonly seen in the lower leg, exertional compartment syndrome in athletes has also been described in the thigh and medial compartment of the foot (78–80).
  - There are four major compartments in the leg. Each is bound by bone and fascia, and each contains a major nerve.
    - The anterior compartment contains the extensor hallucis longus, extensor digitorum longus, peroneus tertius, and anterior tibialis muscles, as well as the deep peroneal nerve.
    - The lateral compartment contains the peroneus longus and brevis as well as the superficial peroneal nerve.
    - The superficial posterior compartment contains the gastrocnemius and soleus muscles and the sural nerve.
    - The deep posterior compartment contains the flexor hallucis longus, flexor digitorum longus, and posterior tibialis muscles, as well as the posterior tibial nerve. Some authors believe that the posterior tibialis should be considered a separate compartment because it is surrounded by its own fascia (81).
  - Anterior compartment syndrome is most common (45%), followed by the deep posterior compartment (40%), lateral compartment (10%), and superficial posterior compartment (5%) (82).
- Diagnosis
  - Recurrent exercise-induced leg discomfort that occurs at a well-defined and reproducible point and increases if the training persists. Pain is usually described as a tight, cramp-like, or squeezing ache over a specific compartment of the leg. Relief of symptoms only occurs with discontinuation of activity. Examination may or may not demonstrate fascial hernias. In some cases, the classic exertional component is not as evident, and patients complain of pain at rest or with daily activities as well.
  - A neurologic and vascular examination should also be performed with reproduction of the symptoms. Understanding the distribution of nerves and functions of muscles in relation to symptoms can help identify the affected compartment in cases where the pain is not well localized to one specific compartment, or it may help determine the compartments that are more severely affected in cases where more than one compartment is involved.
    - Anterior compartment: weakness of dorsiflexion or toe extension; paresthesias over the dorsum of the foot; numbness in the first web space; or even transient or persistent foot drop.
    - Lateral compartment: sensory changes over the anterolateral aspect of the leg and weakness of ankle eversion. An inversion and equinus deformity may also be present.
    - Superficial posterior compartment: dorsolateral foot hypoesthesia and plantarflexion weakness.
    - Deep posterior compartment: paresthesias in the plantar aspect of the foot and weakness of toe flexion and foot inversion.
  - The gold standard diagnostic tool is intra-compartment pressure monitoring (83). This is discussed further in Chapter 26 of this text.

- One or more of the following pressure criteria must be met in addition to a history and physical examination that is consistent with the diagnosis of CECS:
  - Preexercise pressure ≥15 mm Hg;
  - 1-minute post-exercise pressure ≥30 mm Hg; or
  - 5-minute post-exercise pressure ≥20 mm Hg
- Diagnosis may require the *sport-specific activity* to induce symptoms and raise intra-compartment pressure (84).
  - Other tools that have been used in the diagnosis of compartment syndrome include the triple-phase bone scan, MRI, near-infrared spectroscopy, methoxyisobutylisonitrile (MIBI) perfusion imaging, and thallous chloride scintigraphy (85–98).
- Contributing factors
  - Enclosure of compartmental contents in an inelastic fascial sheath, increased volume of the skeletal muscle with exertion due to blood flow and edema, muscle hypertrophy as a response to exercise, and dynamic contraction factors due to the gait cycle.
  - It has also been proposed that myofiber damage as a result of eccentric exercise causes a release of protein-bound ions and a subsequent increase in osmotic pressure within the compartment. The increase in osmotic pressure increases capillary relaxation pressure, thus decreasing the blood flow.
  - Rapid increases in muscle size due to fluid retention are also believed to play a role in the development of chronic exertional compartment syndrome in athletes taking the popular supplement creatine (99).
- Treatment (98)
  - Conservative measures include relative rest (limiting activity to that level that avoids any more than minimal symptoms), anti-inflammatories, stretching and strengthening of the involved muscles, gait retraining (change to a ball-of-foot strike from heel strike), and orthotics (particularly in cases of excessive pronation) (100).
  - Botox injections can be used in cases with limited number of compartment involvement (101).
  - Should symptoms persist despite 6–12 weeks of conservative care, in cases of extreme pressure elevation or progressive neurologic deficit, surgical remediation (fasciotomy of the involved compartments with or without fasciectomy) should be undertaken (102–107).
  - Single and double incision as well as endoscopic techniques have been described. Regardless of the technique, any fascial hernias must be included in the fascial incision.
  - Surgical treatment generally has good success with return to running without significant symptoms.
    - Anterior compartment fasciotomy success rates usually exceed 85%. Deep posterior success rates are lower, approximately 70%.
    - Due to a high rate of coexistence, some authors advocate release of the lateral compartment whenever a procedure for anterior compartment syndrome is performed. Others have stated that this dual release may not be necessary if clinical evaluation and compartment pressure testing fail to demonstrate lateral compartment involvement.
    - When performing a deep posterior compartment release, attention must be paid to adequate decompression of the tibialis posterior (97,108,109).
  - There is emerging evidence for use of ultrasound guided fasciotomy (110).

Achilles Tendinopathy

- Definition (98,111–117)
  - A spectrum of tissue disorders involving the Achilles tendon and sheath: tendinitis, tendinosis, peritendinitis, and tear
- Diagnosis
  - Tenderness at myotendinous junction or insertion
- Contributing factors
  - Pronation
  - Lower extremity varus
  - Tight heel cord
  - Weak dorsiflexors/plantarflexors
  - Ankle instability
- Treatment (114)
  - Heel lifts
  - Control pronation
  - Flexibility (include gastrocnemius and soleus)
  - Strength (particularly eccentric strength) (117,118)
  - Modalities (iontophoresis, cross-friction massage)
- If persistent, consider:
  - Retrocalcaneal bursitis
  - MRI (evaluate tears)
  - Immobilization
  - Lidocaine or saline hydrodissection for paratenonitis
  - Nitro-DUR patches (119,120)
  - Platelet-rich plasma (controversial) (121–124)
  - Extracorporeal shock-wave therapy (ESWT) (125,126)

PLANTAR FASCIITIS

- Definition
  - An overload injury including inflammation, degeneration, and tearing of the plantar fascia, most commonly at its calcaneal insertion
- Contributing factors (8,127–130)
  - Tight gastrocnemius-soleus, plantar fascia
  - Rigid rear foot
  - Overpronation or oversupination

- Decreased ankle strength
- Obesity
- Excessive time on one's feet

- Diagnosis (8,131–133)
  - Pain in plantar heel worse in morning and with activity
  - Tenderness in plantar medial heel
  - Normal neurologic exam
  - No bony (calcaneal) tenderness
- Treatment
  - Phase 1: nonsteroidal anti-inflammatory drugs, Medrol (if severe)
    - Device (*i.e.*, Counterforce [CTF] arch brace) or low dye taping
    - Stretch (gastrocnemius-soleus, plantar fascia, hamstrings, ITB)
    - Strength (foot intrinsic, ankle, lower quarter stability)
  - Phase 2: Physical therapy (phonophoresis/iontophoresis, massage, manual therapy to improve ankle and subtalar mobility)
    - Continue exercise
    - Different device (*i.e.*, heel cushion)
    - Night splint or sock (134–138)
  - Phases 3 and 4: Injections (three maximum) (136,139–142), orthotics (143–146)
- If persistent, consider:
  - MRI to rule out calcaneal stress injury
  - Electromyography/nerve conduction studies to rule out medial calcaneal, plantar neuropathy (first branch of lateral plantar nerve), and radiculopathy
  - Immobilization (147)
  - Emerging therapies: shockwave therapy (symptoms >12 months) (148–156), platelet-rich plasma/autologous blood (157,158), Botox injection (9,158,159), percutaneous ultrasonic tenotomy (160).
  - Surgery if conservative care fails (6–12 months)

Stress Fractures

- Definition
  - Failure of bone to adapt adequately to mechanical loads (ground reaction forces and muscle contraction) experienced during physical activity
  - Tibial stress fractures predominate in distance runners. Navicular stress fractures predominate in track athletes.
- Diagnosis (161)
  - Focal tenderness
  - Recent transition in training
  - X-ray (often negative, especially early)
  - Bone scan (acute all three phases with increased uptake vs chronic [delayed only])
  - MRI (periosteal and marrow edema T2 > T1)
- Risk factors
  - Prior stress fracture (162,163)
  - Rapid transition in training (164)
  - Low energy availability (165,166)
  - Low bone mineral density (in women) (162,167,168)
  - Menstrual irregularities; in particular, amenorrhea >6 months
  - Smaller cross-sectional bone geometry (169–172)
  - Low calcium and vitamin D intake (173–175)
  - Lesser thigh and calf muscle size (167,176)
  - Leg length difference >0.5 cm (176)
  - Excessive pes cavus (femoral, tibial) or pes planus (metatarsals)
  - Varus forefoot (177–179)
  - Higher loading rate, but not peak force magnitude of ground reaction force (179,180)
  - Femoral anteversion
  - Hip adduction, rearfoot eversion (tibial)
  - Poor shoe wear (shoes >5 months old) (181)
  - Early sport specialization (182)
- Treatment
  - Noncritical: Noncritical stress fractures can be treated with 6–8 weeks of relative rest and include the following: medial tibia, metatarsals 2, 3, and 4; fifth metatarsal avulsion. Athletes may benefit from a short period (*i.e.*, 3 weeks) in a walking boot.
  - Critical stress fractures require more specific attention due to slower healing and higher rates of nonunion and include the following: femoral neck, anterior tibia, medial malleolus, navicular, base of fifth metatarsal.
    - Femoral neck (183)
      - Normal x-ray, no cortical break: conservative treatment, partial weight bearing to weight bearing as tolerated. Follow clinically and serial MRI 8–12 weeks. Cortical break: orthopedic referral.
      - Superior (distraction) fractures have a higher incidence of worsening and nonunion than inferior (compression) fractures.
    - Anterior tibia (184,185)
      - Conservative care can take up to 6–8 months. Options include pneumatic leg brace ± bone stimulator, casting, and relative rest
      - If no healing: orthopedic referral (transverse drilling, grafting, medullary fixation)
    - Medial malleolus (186,187)
      - Nondisplaced: boot or air cast for 6 weeks
      - Displaced or nonunion: orthopedic referral
    - Navicular (188)
      - Non–weight-bearing for 6–8 weeks
      - Progressive activity over 6 more weeks
    - Proximal fifth metatarsal (189–191)

- Jones fracture of proximal diaphysis: cast, non-weight-bearing for 6–10 weeks
- Nonunion: orthopedic referral consider orthopedic early in competitive athletes.
- Emerging evidence for PRP (192) and ESWT (193)

PRACTICAL GUIDELINES FOR CLINICIANS

- Certain injuries require the runner to refrain from running (stress fractures, radiculopathy). With most overuse injuries, however, some level of training may be permitted following the "Relative Activity Modification Guidelines" (194).
  - Pain/discomfort should not exceed the mild level (<3/10 on the 10-point pain scale).
  - Pain that eases after a warm-up is generally benign. Do not run if pain progressively worsens.
  - Do not run if you are limping or changing your gait mechanics.
- Supplement lost run training with cross-training (aqua running, bike, elliptical).
- Do not increase mileage more rapidly than 10% per week.
- Long run of the week increases no more than 2 miles · wk^{-1} and should not exceed 30% of one's weekly mileage.
- Change shoes every 350–400 miles.

REFERENCES

1. Epperly T, Atkinson B, Fields KB. Epidemiology of running injuries. In: Wilder R, O'Connor F, Magrum E, editors. *Running Medicine*. CA: Healthy Learning, Monterey; 2025. pp. 17–24.
2. Jacobs SJ, Berson BL. Injuries to runners: a study of entrants to a 10,000 meter race. *Am J Sports Med*. 1986;14(2):151–5.
3. van Mechelen W. Running injuries. A review of the epidemiological literature. *Sports Med*. 1992;14(5):320–35.
4. Lysholm J, Wiklander J. Injuries in runners. *Am J Sports Med*. 1987;15(2):168–71.
5. Taunton JE, Ryan MB, Clement DB, McKenzie DC, Lloyd-Smith DR, Zumbo BD. A prospective study of running injuries: the Vancouver Sun Run "In Training" clinics. *Br J Sports Med*. 2003;37(3):239–44.
6. Walter SD, Hart LE, McIntosh JM, Sutton JR. The Ontario cohort study of running-related injuries. *Arch Intern Med*. 1989;149(11):2561–64.
7. Davis IS, Powers CM. Patellofemoral pain syndrome: proximal, distal, and local factors, an international retreat, April 30–May 2, 2009, Fells Point, Baltimore, MD. *J Orthop Sports Phys Ther*. 2010;40(3):A1–16.
8. Cole C, Seto C, Gazewood J. Plantar fasciitis: evidence-based review of diagnosis and therapy. *Am Fam Physician*. 2005;72(11):2237–42.
9. Babcock MS, Foster L, Pasquina P, Jabbari B. Treatment of pain attributed to plantar fasciitis with botulinum toxin A: a short-term, randomized, placebo-controlled, double-blind study. *Am J Phys Med Rehabil*. 2005;84(9):649–54.
10. Pinshaw R, Atlas V, Noakes TD. The nature and response to therapy of 196 consecutive injuries seen at a runners' clinic. *S Afr Med J*. 1984;65(8):291–8.
11. Francis P, Whatman C, Sheerin K, Hume P, Johnson MI. The proportion of lower limb running injuries by gender, anatomical location and specific pathology: a systematic review. *J Sports Sci Med*. 2019;18(1):21–31.
12. Hollander K, Rahlf AL, Wilke J, et al. Sex-specific differences in running injuries: a systematic review with meta-analysis and meta-regression. *Sports Med*. 2021;51(5):1011–39. doi:10.1007/s40279-020-01412-7
13. Cowan DN, Jones BH, Frykman PN, et al. Lower limb morphology and risk of overuse injury among male infantry trainees. *Med Sci Sports Exerc*. 1996;28(8):945–52.
14. Cowan DN, Jones BH, Robinson JR. Foot morphologic characteristics and risk of exercise-related injury. *Arch Fam Med*. 1993;2(7):773–7.
15. Fredericson M. Common injuries in runners. Diagnosis, rehabilitation, and prevention. *Sports Med*. 1996;21(1):49–72.
16. Jones BH, Cowan DN, Tomlinson JP, Robinson JR, Polly DW, Frykman PN. Epidemiology of injuries associated with physical training among young men in the army. *Med Sci Sports Exerc*. 1993;25(2):197–203.
17. Macera CA, Pate RR, Powell KE, Jackson KL, Kendrick JS, Craven TE. Predicting lower-extremity injuries among habitual runners. *Arch Intern Med*. 1989;149(11):2565–68.
18. Taunton JE, Ryan MB, Clement DB, McKenzie DC, Lloyd-Smith DR, Zumbo BD. A retrospective case-control analysis of 2002 running injuries. *Br J Sports Med*. 2002;36(2):95–101.
19. van Gent R, Siem D, van Middelkoop M, van Os AG, Bierma-Zeinstra SM, Koes BW. Incidence and determinants of lower extremity running injuries in long distance runners: a systematic review. *Br J Sports Med*. 2007;41(8):469–80.
20. Wen DY, Puffer JC, Schmalzried TP. Lower extremity alignment and risk of overuse injuries in runners. *Med Sci Sports Exerc*. 1997;29(10):1291–8.
21. Yeung EW, Yeung SS. Interventions for preventing lower limb soft-tissue injuries in runners. *Cochrane Database Syst Rev*. 2001;3:CD001256.
22. Breathnach O, Ng K, Spindler K, Wasserstein D. Pathophysiology and epidemiology of stress fractures. In: *Stress Fractures in Athletes*. Cham: Springer; 2020. p. 29–39.
23. Fuller JT, Thewlis D, Buckley JD, Brown NA, Hamill J, Tsiros MD. Body mass and weekly training distance influence the pain and injuries experienced by runners using minimalist shoes: a randomized controlled trial. *Am J Sports Med*. 2017 Apr;45(5):1162–70. doi:10.1177/0363546516682497
24. Jungmalm J, Nielsen RØ, Desai P, Karlsson J, Hein T, Grau S. Associations between biomechanical and clinical/anthropometrical factors and running-related injuries among recreational runners: a 52-week prospective cohort study. *Inj Epidemiol*. 2020;7(1):10. doi:10.1186/s40621-020-00237-2
25. Amako M, Oda T, Masuoka K, Yokoi H, Campisi P. Effect of static stretching on prevention of injuries for military recruits. *Mil Med*. 2003;168(6):442–6.
26. Thacker SB, Gilchrist J, Stroup DF, Kimsey CD Jr. The impact of stretching on sports injury risk: a systematic review of the literature. *Med Sci Sports Exerc*. 2004;36(3):371–8.
27. Bergstra SA, Kluitenberg B, Dekker R, et al. Running with a minimalist shoe increases plantar pressure in the forefoot region of healthy female runners. *J Sci Med Sport*. 2015 Jul;18(4):463–8. doi:10.1016/j.jsams.2014.06.007
28. Malisoux L, Chambon N, Urhausen A, Theisen D. Influence of the heel-to-toe drop of standard cushioned running shoes on injury risk in leisure-time runners: a randomized controlled trial with 6-month follow-up. *Am J Sports Med*. 2016 Nov;44(11):2933–40. doi:10.1177/0363546516654690

29. Birrer RB, Buzermanis S, DellaCorte MP, Grisalfi PJ. Biomechanics of running. In: O'Connor F, Wilder R, editors. *The Textbook of Running Medicine*. New York: McGraw-Hill; 2001.
30. Ounpuu S. The biomechanics of running: a kinematic and kinetic analysis. *Instr Course Lect*. 1990;39:305–18.
31. Mann RA, Hagy J. Biomechanics of walking, running, and sprinting. *Am J Sports Med*. 1980;8(5):345–50.
32. Ounpuu S. The biomechanics of walking and running. *Clin Sports Med*. 1994;13(4):843–63.
33. Dicharry J. Kinematics and kinetics of gait: from lab to clinic. *Clin Sports Med*. 2010;29(3):347–64.
34. Rodgers MM. Dynamic biomechanics of the normal foot and ankle during walking and running. *Phys Ther*. 1988;68(12):1822–30.
35. Hreljac A. Impact and overuse injuries in runners. *Med Sci Sports Exerc*. 2004;36(5):845–9.
36. Hreljac A, Marshall RN, Hume PA. Evaluation of lower extremity overuse injury potential in runners. *Med Sci Sports Exerc*. 2000;32(9):1635–41.
37. Nigg BM. The role of impact forces and foot pronation: a new paradigm. *Clin J Sport Med*. 2001;11(1):2–9.
38. O'Connor JA, Lanyon LE, MacFie H. The influence of strain rate on adaptive bone remodelling. *J Biomech*. 1982;15(10):767–81.
39. Mann RA. Biomechanics of running. In: Nicholas JA, Hershman EB, editors. *The Lower Extremity and Spine in Sports Medicine*, Vol. 1. St. Louis: The C.V. Mosby Company; 1986. p. 395–411.
40. Inman VT. Functional aspects of the abductor muscles of the hip. *J Bone Joint Surg Am*. 1947;29(3):607–19.
41. Hamill J, Gruber A. Biomechanics of running. In: Wilder R, O'Connor F, Magrum E, editors. *Running Medicine*. CA: Healthy Learning, Monterey; 2025. pp. 25–32.
42. Anderson LM, Bonanno DR, Hart HF, Barton CJ. What are the benefits and risks associated with changing foot strike pattern during running? A systematic review and meta-analysis of injury, running economy, and biomechanics. *Sports Med*. 2020;50(5):885–917.
43. Gruber AH, Edwards WB, Hamill J, Derrick TR, Boyer KA. A comparison of the ground reaction force frequency content during rearfoot and non-rearfoot running patterns. *Gait Posture*. 2017;56:54–9.
44. Kuwabara A, Fredericson M. The knee. In: Wilder R, O'Connor F, Magrum E, editors. *Running Medicine*. CA: Healthy Learning, Monterey; 2025. pp. 199–212.
45. Dierks TA, Manal KT, Hamill J, Davis IS. Proximal and distal influences on hip and knee kinematics in runners with patellofemoral pain during a prolonged run. *J Orthop Sports Phys Ther*. 2008;38(8):448–56.
46. Fredericson M, Yoon K. Physical examination and patellofemoral pain syndrome. *Am J Phys Med Rehabil*. 2006;85(3):234–43.
47. Fulkerson JP. Diagnosis and treatment of patients with patellofemoral pain. *Am J Sports Med*. 2002;30(3):447–56.
48. Powers CM, Ward SR, Chen YJ, Chan LD, Terk MR. The effect of bracing on patellofemoral joint stress during free and fast walking. *Am J Sports Med*. 2004;32(1):224–31.
49. Collado H, Fredericson M. Patellofemoral pain syndrome. *Clin Sports Med*. 2010;29(3):379–98.
50. Messier SP, Davis SE, Curl WW, Lowery RB, Pack RJ. Etiologic factors associated with patellofemoral pain in runners. *Med Sci Sports Exerc*. 1991;23(9):1008–15.
51. Thomeé R, Renström P, Karlsson J, Grimby G. Patellofemoral pain syndrome in young women. I. A clinical analysis of alignment, pain parameters, common symptoms and functional activity level. *Scand J Med Sci Sports*. 1995;5(4):237–44.
52. Noehren B, Davis I. The effect of gait retraining on hip mechanics, pain and function in runners with patello-femoral pain syndrome. In: *PFPS Retreat*. Baltimore (MD): University of Delaware; 2009 May.
53. Powers CM, Shellock FG, Beering TV, Garrido DE, Goldbach RM, Molnar T. Effect of bracing on patellar kinematics in patients with patellofemoral joint pain. *Med Sci Sports Exerc*. 1999;31(12):1714–20.
54. Fredericson M, Cookingham CL, Chaudhari AM, Dowdell BC, Oestreicher N, Sahrmann SA. Hip abductor weakness in distance runners with iliotibial band syndrome. *Clin J Sport Med*. 2000;10(3):169–75.
55. Fredericson M, Weir A. Practical management of iliotibial band friction syndrome in runners. *Clin J Sport Med*. 2006;16(3):261–8.
56. Fredericson M, Wolf C. Iliotibial band syndrome in runners: innovations in treatment. *Sports Med*. 2005;35(5):451–9.
57. Fulkerson JP, Kalenak A, Rosenberg TD, Cox JS. Patellofemoral pain. *Instr Course Lect*. 1992;41:57–71.
58. Grau S, Krauss I, Maiwald C, Axmann D, Horstmann T, Best R. Kinematic classification of iliotibial band syndrome in runners. *Scand J Med Sci Sports*. 2011;21(2):184–9.
59. Barber FA, Sutker AN. Iliotibial band syndrome. *Sports Med*. 1992;14(2):144–8.
60. Clement DB, Taunton JE, Smart GW, McNicol KL. A survey of overuse running injuries. *Phys Sportsmed*. 1981;9(5):47–58.
61. Lidenburg G, Pinshaw R, Noakes TD. Iliotibial band friction syndrome in runners. *Phys Sports Med*. 1984;12(5):118–30.
62. Noble CA. Iliotibial band friction syndrome in runners. *Am J Sports Med*. 1980;8(4):232–4.
63. Evans P. The postural function of the iliotibial tract. *Ann R Coll Surg Engl*. 1979;61(4):271–80.
64. Orchard JW, Fricker PA, Abud AT, Mason BR. Biomechanics of iliotibial band friction syndrome in runners. *Am J Sports Med*. 1996;24(3):375–9.
65. Fairclough J, Hayashi K, Toumi H, et al. Is iliotibial band syndrome really a friction syndrome?. *J Sci Med Sport*. 2007;10(2):74–8.
66. Martens M, Libbrecht P, Burssens A. Surgical treatment of the iliotibial band friction syndrome. *Am J Sports Med*. 1989;17(5):651–4.
67. Terry GC, Hughston JC, Norwood LA. The anatomy of the iliopatellar band and iliotibial tract. *Am J Sports Med*. 1986;14(1):39–45.
68. Gottschalk F, Kourosh S, Leveau B. The functional anatomy of tensor fasciae latae and gluteus medius and minimus. *J Anat*. 1989;166: 179–89.
69. MacMahon JM, Chaudhari AM, Adriacchi TP. *Biomechanical Injury Predictors for Marathon Runners: Striding Towards Iliotibial Band Syndrome Injury Prevention*. Hong Kong (HK): International Society of Biomechanics; 2000.
70. Messier SP, Edwards DG, Martin DF, et al. Etiology of iliotibial band friction syndrome in distance runners. *Med Sci Sports Exerc*. 1995;27(7):951–60.
71. Messier SP, Pittala KA. Etiologic factors associated with selected running injuries. *Med Sci Sports Exerc*. 1988;20(5):501–5.
72. Meardon SA, Campbell S, Derrick TR. Step width alters iliotibial band strain during running. *Sports Biomech*. 2012;11(4):464–72. doi:10.1080/14763141.2012.699547
73. Briner WW Jr. Shin splints. *Am Fam Physician*. 1988;37(2):155–60.
74. Gudas CJ. Patterns of lower-extremity injury in 224 runners. *Compr Ther*. 1980;6(9):50–9.
75. James SL, Bates BT, Osternig LR. Injuries to runners. *Am J Sports Med*. 1978;6(2):40–50.
76. Andrish JT, Bergfeld JA, Walheim J. A prospective study on the management of shin splints. *J Bone Joint Surg Am*. 1974;56(8):1697–700.
77. Detmer DE. Chronic shin splints. Classification and management of medial tibial stress syndrome. *Sports Med*. 1986;3(6):436–46.
78. Birnbaum J. Recurrent compartment syndrome in the posterior thigh. *Am J Sports Med*. 1983;11(1):48–9.

79. Mollica MB, Duyshart SC. Analysis of pre- and post-exercise compartment pressures in the medial compartment of the foot. *Am J Sports Med.* 2002;30(2):268–71.
80. Raether PM, Lutter LD. Recurrent compartment syndrome in the posterior thigh. Report of a case. *Am J Sports Med.* 1982;10(1):40–3.
81. Albertson KS, Dammann GG. The leg. In: O'Connor FG, Wilder RP, editors. *The Textbook of Running Medicine.* New York: McGraw-Hill; 2001. p. 647–54.
82. Edwards P, Myerson MS. Exertional compartment syndrome of the leg: steps for expedient return to activity. *Phys Sportsmed.* 1996;24(4):31–46.
83. Hutchinson MR, Ireland ML. Chronic exertional compartment syndrome: gauging pressure. *Phys Sportsmed.* 1999;27(5):101–2.
84. Padhiar N, King JB. Exercise induced leg pain-chronic compartment syndrome. Is the increase in intra-compartment pressure exercise specific? *Br J Sports Med.* 1996;30(4):360–2.
85. Amendola A, Rorabeck CH, Vellett D, Vezina W, Rutt B, Nott L. The use of magnetic resonance imaging in exertional compartment syndromes. *Am J Sports Med.* 1990;18(1):29–34.
86. Awbrey BJ, Sienkiewicz PS, Mankin HJ. Chronic exercise-induced compartment pressure elevation measured with a miniaturized fluid pressure monitor. A laboratory and clinical study. *Am J Sports Med.* 1988;16(6):610–5.
87. Breit GA, Gross JH, Watenpaugh DE, Chance B, Hargens AR. Near-infrared spectroscopy for monitoring of tissue oxygenation of exercising skeletal muscle in a chronic compartment syndrome model. *J Bone Joint Surg Am.* 1997;79(6):838–3.
88. Eskelin MK, Lötjönen JM, Mäntysaari MJ. Chronic exertional compartment syndrome: MR imaging at 0.1 T compared with tissue pressure measurement. *Radiology.* 1998;206(2):333–7.
89. Hayes AA, Bower GD, Pitstock KL. Chronic (exertional) compartment syndrome of the legs diagnosed with thallous chloride scintigraphy. *J Nucl Med.* 1995;36(9):1618–24.
90. Jimenez C, Allen T, Hwang I. Diagnostic imaging of running injuries. In: O'Connor F, Wilder R, eds. *The Textbook of Running Medicine.* New York: McGraw-Hill; 2001. p. 67–84.
91. Kaplan PA, Helms CA, Dussault R. *Musculoskeletal MRI.* 1st ed. Philadelphia (PA): WB Saunders; 2001.
92. Matin P. Basic principles of nuclear medicine techniques for detection and evaluation of trauma and sports medicine injuries. *Semin Nucl Med.* 1988;18(2):90–112.
93. Mattila KT, Komu ME, Dahlström S, Koskinen SK, Heikkilä J. Medial tibial pain: a dynamic contrast-enhanced MRI study. *Magn Reson Imaging.* 1999;17(7):947–54.
94. Owens S, Edwards P, Miles K, Jenner J, Allen M. Chronic compartment syndrome affecting the lower limb: MIBI perfusion imaging as an alternative to pressure monitoring. Two case reports. *Br J Sports Med.* 1999;33(1):49–51.
95. Rowden GA, Abdelkarim B, Vaca F. *Compartment Syndromes.* eMedicine from WebMD, Medscape [Internet]. 2008 [cited 2008 Oct 29]. Available from: http://emedicine.medscape.com
96. Samuelson DR, Cram RL. The three-phase bone scan and exercise induced lower-leg pain. The tibial stress test. *Clin Nucl Med.* 1996;21(2):89–93.
97. Wilder RP, Magrum E. Exertional compartment syndrome. *Clin Sports Med.* 2010;29(3):429–35.
98. Wilder RP, Sethi S. Overuse injuries: tendinopathies, stress fractures, compartment syndrome and shin splints. *Clin Sports Med.* 2004;23(1):55–81, vi.
99. Glorioso J, Wilckens J. Exertional leg pain. In: O'Connor F, Wilder R, eds. *The Textbook of Running Medicine.* New York: McGraw Hill; 2001. p. 181–98.
100. Zimmermann WO, Hutchinson MR, Van den Berg R, Hoencamp R, Backx FJG, Bakker EWP. Conservative treatment of anterior chronic exertional compartment syndrome in the military, with a mid-term follow-up. *BMJ Open Sport Exerc Med.* 2019 Mar 19;5(1):e000532.
101. Charvin M, Orta C, Davy L, et al. Botulinum toxin A for chronic exertional compartment syndrome: a retrospective study of 16 upper- and lower-limb cases. *Clin J Sport Med.* 2022;32(4):e436–40.
102. Leversedge FJ, Casey PJ, Seiler JG 3rd, Xerogeanes JW. Endoscopically assisted fasciotomy: description of technique and in vitro assessment of lower-leg compartment decompression. *Am J Sports Med.* 2002;30(2):272–78.
103. Mouhsine E, Garofalo R, Moretti B, Gremion G, Akiki A. Two minimal incision fasciotomy for chronic exertional compartment syndrome of the lower leg. *Knee Surg Sports Traumatol Arthrosc.* 2006;14(2):193–7.
104. Raikin SM, Rapuri VR, Vitanzo P. Bilateral simultaneous fasciotomy for chronic exertional compartment syndrome. *Foot Ankle Int.* 2005;26(12):1007–11.
105. Slimmon D, Bennell K, Brukner P, Crossley K, Bell SN. Long-term outcome of fasciotomy with partial fasciectomy for chronic exertional compartment syndrome of the lower leg. *Am J Sports Med.* 2002;30(4):581–8.
106. Tzortziou V, Maffulli N, Padhiar N. Diagnosis and management of chronic exertional compartment syndrome (CECS) in the United Kingdom. *Clin J Sport Med.* 2006;16(3):209–13.
107. Wittstein J, Moorman CT 3rd, Levin LS. Endoscopic compartment release for chronic exertional compartment syndrome. *J Surg Orthop Adv.* 2008;17(2):119–21.
108. Davey JR, Rorabeck CH, Fowler PJ. The tibialis posterior muscle compartment. An unrecognized cause of exertional compartment syndrome. *Am J Sports Med.* 1984;12(5):391–7.
109. Schepsis AA, Gill SS, Foster TA. Fasciotomy for exertional anterior compartment syndrome: is lateral compartment release necessary? *Am J Sports Med.* 1999;27(4):430–5.
110. Lueders DR, Sellon JL, Smith J, Finnoff JT. Ultrasound-guided fasciotomy for chronic exertional compartment syndrome: a cadaveric investigation. *PM R.* 2017;9(7):683–90.
111. Aström M, Rausing A. Chronic Achilles tendinopathy. A survey of surgical and histopathologic findings. *Clin Orthop Relat Res.* 1995;316:151–64.
112. Järvinen M, Józsa L, Kannus P, Järvinen TL, Kvist M, Leadbetter W. Histopathological findings in chronic tendon disorders. *Scand J Med Sci Sports.* 1997;7(2):86–95.
113. Kader D, Saxena A, Movin T, Maffulli N. Achilles tendinopathy: some aspects of basic science and clinical management. *Br J Sports Med.* 2002;36(4):239–49.
114. Khan KM, Cook JL, Bonar F, Harcourt P, Astrom M. Histopathology of common tendinopathies. Update and implications for clinical management. *Sports Med.* 1999;27(6):393–408.
115. Paavola M, Kannus P, Järvinen TA, Khan K, Józsa L, Järvinen M. Achilles tendinopathy. *J Bone Joint Surg Am.* 2002;84(11):2062–76.
116. Puddu G, Ippolito E, Postacchini F. A classification of Achilles tendon disease. *Am J Sports Med.* 1976;4(4):145–50.
117. Silbernagel KG, Thomeé R, Thomeé P, Karlsson J. Eccentric overload training for patients with chronic Achilles tendon pain — A randomised controlled study with reliability testing of the evaluation methods. *Scand J Med Sci Sports.* 2001;11(4):197–206.
118. Mafi N, Lorentzon R, Alfredson H. Superior short-term results with eccentric calf muscle training compared to concentric training in a randomized prospective multicenter study on patients with chronic Achilles tendinosis. *Knee Surg Sports Traumatol Arthrosc.* 2001;9(1):42–7.

119. Hunte G, Lloyd-Smith R. Topical glyceryl trinitrate for chronic Achilles tendinopathy. *Clin J Sport Med*. 2005;15(2):116–7.
120. Paoloni JA, Appleyard RC, Nelson J, Murrell GA. Topical glyceryl trinitrate treatment of chronic noninsertional Achilles tendinopathy. A randomized, double-blind, placebo-controlled trial. *J Bone Joint Surg Am*. 2004;86(5):916–22.
121. deVos RJ, Weir A, van Schie HTM, et al. Platelet-rich plasma injection for chronic Achilles tendinopathy: a randomized controlled trial. *JAMA*. 2010;303(2):144–9.
122. Monto RR. Platelet rich plasma treatment for chronic Achilles tendinosis. *Foot Ankle Int*. 2012;33(5):379–85.
123. Gaweda K, Tarczynska M, Krzyzanowski W. Treatment of Achilles tendinopathy with platelet-rich plasma. *Int J Sports Med*. 2010;31(8):577–83.
124. Owens RF Jr, Ginnetti J, Conti SF, Latona C. Clinical and magnetic resonance imaging outcomes following platelet rich plasma injection for chronic midsubstance Achilles tendinopathy. *Foot Ankle Int*. 2011;32(11):1032–9.
125. Taylor J, Dunkerley S, Silver D, et al. Extracorporeal shock-wave therapy (ESWT) for refractory Achilles tendinopathy: a prospective audit with 2-year follow up. *Foot*. 2016;26:23–9.
126. Wei M, Liu Y, Li Z, Wang Z. Comparison of clinical efficacy among endoscopy-assisted radio-frequency ablation, extracorporeal shockwaves, and eccentric exercises in treatment of insertional Achilles tendinosis. *J Am Podiatr Med Assoc*. 2017;107(1):11–6.
127. Fredericson M, Bergman AG. A comprehensive review of running injuries. *Crit Rev Phys Med Rehab*. 1999;11:1–34.
128. Kibler WB, Goldberg C, Chandler TJ. Functional biomechanical deficits in running athletes with plantar fasciitis. *Am J Sports Med*. 1991;19(1):66–71.
129. Pfeffer GB. Plantar heel pain. In: Baxter DE, editor. *The Foot and Ankle in Sport*. St. Louis: Mosby-Year Book; 1995. p. 195–206.
130. Riddle DL, Pulisic M, Pidcoe P, Johnson RE. Risk factors for plantar fasciitis: a matched case-control study. *J Bone Joint Surg Am*. 2003;85(5):872–7.
131. DiMarcangelo MT, Yu TC. Diagnostic imaging of heel pain and plantar fasciitis. *Clin Podiatr Med Surg*. 1997;14(2):281–301.
132. Gill LH. Plantar fasciitis: diagnosis and conservative management. *J Am Acad Orthop Surg*. 2004;350:2159–66.
133. Kravitz SR, Medicino RW, Thomas JL, et al. The diagnosis and treatment of heel pain. *J Foot Ankle Surg*. 2001;40(5):329–40.
134. Barry LD, Barry AN, Chen Y. A retrospective study of standing gastrocnemius-soleus stretching versus night splinting in the treatment of plantar fasciitis. *J Foot Ankle Surg*. 2002;41(4):221–7.
135. Batt ME, Tanji JL, Skattum N. Plantar fasciitis: a prospective randomized clinical trial of the tension night splint. *Clin J Sport Med*. 1996;6(3):158–62.
136. Crawford F, Thomson C. Interventions for treating plantar heel pain. *Cochrane Database Syst Rev*. 2003;3:CD000416.
137. Petrizzi MJ, Petrizzi MG, Roos RJ. Making a tension night splint for plantar fasciitis. *Phys Sportsmed*. 1998;26(6):113–4.
138. Powell M, Post WR, Keener J, Wearden S. Effective treatment of chronic plantar fasciitis with dorsiflexion night splints: a crossover prospective randomized outcome study. *Foot Ankle Int*. 1998;19(1):10–8.
139. Acevedo JI, Beskin JL. Complications of plantar fascia rupture associated with corticosteroid injection. *Foot Ankle Int*. 1998;19(2):91–7.
140. Chandler TJ. Iontophoresis of 0.4% dexamethasone for plantar fasciitis. *Clin J Sport Med*. 1998;8(1):68.
141. Kane D, Greaney T, Bresnihan B, Gibney R, FitzGerald O. Ultrasound guided injection of recalcitrant plantar fasciitis. *Ann Rheum Dis*. 1998;57(6):383–4.
142. Kruse RJ, McCoy RL, Erickson T. Diagnosing plantar fascia rupture. *Phys Sportsmed*. 1995;23(1):65–9.
143. Karageanes SJ. What type of orthosis is most effective in treating chronic plantar fasciitis? *Clin J Sport Med*. 2007;17(3):227–8.
144. Pfeffer G, Bacchetti P, Deland J, et al. Comparison of custom and prefabricated orthoses in the initial treatment of proximal plantar fasciitis. *Foot Ankle Int*. 1999;20(4):214–21.
145. Roos E, Engström M, Söderberg B. Foot orthoses for the treatment of plantar fasciitis. *Foot Ankle Int*. 2006;27(8):606–11.
146. Winemiller MH, Billow RG, Laskowski ER, Harmsen WS. Effect of magnetic vs sham-magnetic insoles on plantar heel pain: a randomized controlled trial. *JAMA*. 2003;290(11):1474–78.
147. Tisdel CL, Harper MC. Chronic plantar heel pain: treatment with a short leg walking cast. *Foot Ankle Int*. 1996;17(1):41–2.
148. Böddeker R, Schäfer H, Haake M. Extracorporeal shockwave therapy (ESWT) in the treatment of plantar fasciitis — A biometrical review. *Clin Rheumatol*. 2001;20(5):324–30.
149. Haake M, Buch M, Schoellner C, et al. Extracorporeal shock wave therapy for plantar fasciitis: randomised controlled multicentre trial. *BMJ*. 2003;327(7406):75.
150. Moretti B, Garofalo R, Patella V, Sisti GL, Corrado M, Mouhsine E. Extracorporeal shock wave therapy in runners with a symptomatic heel spur. *Knee Surg Sports Traumatol Arthosc*. 2006;14(10):1029–32.
151. Ogden JA, Alvarez R, Levitt R, Cross GL, Marlow M. Shock wave therapy for chronic proximal plantar fasciitis. *Clin Orthop Relat Res*. 2001;387:47–59.
152. Ogden JA, Alvarez RG, Marlow M. Shockwave therapy for chronic proximal plantar fasciitis: a meta-analysis. *Foot Ankle Int*. 2002;23(4):301–08.
153. Rompe JD, Decking J, Schoellner C, Nafe B. Shock wave application for chronic plantar fasciitis in running athletes. A prospective, randomized placebo-controlled trial. *Am J Sports Med*. 2003;31(2):268–75.
154. Rompe JD, Schoellner C, Nafe B. Evaluation of low-energy extracorporeal shock-wave application for treatment of chronic plantar fasciitis. *J Bone Joint Surg Am*. 2002;84(3):335–41.
155. Speed CA, Nichols D, Wies J, et al. Extracorporeal shock wave therapy for plantar fasciitis. A double blind randomised controlled trial. *J Orthop Res*. 2003;21(5):937–40.
156. Weil LS Jr, Roukis TS, Weil LS, Borrelli AH. Extracorporeal shock wave therapy for the treatment of chronic plantar fasciitis: indications, protocol, intermediate results, and a comparison of results to fasciotomy. *J Foot Ankle Surg*. 2002;41(3):166–72.
157. Sneed D, Wong C. Platelet-rich plasma injections as a treatment for Achilles tendinopathy and plantar fasciitis in athletes. *PM R*. 2023 Mar;15(11):1493–506. doi:10.1002/pmrj.12965
158. Logan LR, Klamar K, Leon J, Fedoriw W. Autologous blood injection and botulinum toxin for resistant plantar fasciitis accompanied by spasticity. *Am J Phys Med Rehabil*. 2006;85(8):699–703.
159. Placzek R, Deuretzbacher G, Meiss AL. Treatment of chronic plantar fasciitis with botulinum toxin A: preliminary clinical results. *Clin J Pain*. 2006;22(2):190–2.
160. Vajapey S, Ghenbot S, Baria M, Magnussen RA, Vasileff WK. Utility of percutaneous ultrasonic tenotomy for tendinopathies: a systematic review. *Sports Health*. 2021;13(3):258–64.
161. Harrast MA, Colonno D. Stress fractures in runners. *Clin Sports Med*. 2010;29(3):399–416.
162. Bennell KL, Malcolm SA, Thomas SA, et al. Risk factors for stress fractures in track and field athletes. A twelve-month prospective study. *Am J Sports Med*. 1996;24(6):810–8.
163. Wright AA, Taylor JB, Ford KR, Siska L, Smoliga JM. Risk factors associated with lower extremity stress fractures in runners: a systematic review with meta-analysis. *Br J Sports Med*. 2015;49(23):1517–23.

164. Sullivan D, Warren RF, Pavlov H, Kelman G. Stress fractures in 51 runners. *Clin Orthop Relat Res.* 1984;187:188–92.
165. Barrack MT, Gibbs JC, De Souza MJ, et al. Higher incidence of bone stress injuries with increasing female athlete triad-related risk factors: a prospective multisite study of exercising girls and women. *Am J Sports Med.* 2014;42(4):949–58.
166. Tenforde AS, Parziale AL, Popp KL, Ackerman KE. Low bone mineral density in male athletes is associated with bone stress injuries at anatomic sites with greater trabecular composition. *Am J Sports Med.* 2018;46(1):30–6.
167. Beck TJ, Ruff CB, Shaffer RA, Betsinger K, Trone DW, Brodine SK. Stress fracture in military recruits: gender differences in muscle and bone susceptibility factors. *Bone.* 2000;27(3):437–44.
168. Kelsey JL, Bachrach LK, Procter-Gray E, et al. Risk factors for stress fracture among young female cross-country runners. *Med Sci Sports Exerc.* 2007;39(9):1457–63.
169. Crossley K, Bennell KL, Wrigley T, Oakes BW. Ground reaction forces, bone characteristics, and tibial stress fracture in male runners. *Med Sci Sports Exerc.* 1999;31(8):1088–93.
170. Franklyn M, Oakes B, Field B, Wells P, Morgan D. Section modulus is the optimum geometric predictor for stress fractures and medial tibial stress syndrome in both male and female athletes. *Am J Sports Med.* 2008;36(6):1179–89.
171. Popp KL, Hughes JM, Smock AJ, et al. Bone geometry, strength, and muscle size in runners with a history of stress fracture. *Med Sci Sports Exerc.* 2009;41(12):2145–50.
172. Koltun KJ, Sekel NM, Bird MB, et al. Tibial bone geometry is associated with bone stress injury during military training in men and women. *Front Physiol.* 2022;13:803219.
173. Lappe J, Cullen D, Haynatzki G, Recker R, Ahlf R, Thompson K. Calcium and vitamin D supplementation decreases incidence of stress fractures in female navy recruits. *J Bone Miner Res.* 2008;23(5):741–9.
174. Nieves JW, Melsop K, Curtis M, et al. Nutritional factors that influence change in bone density and stress fracture risk among young female cross-country runners. *PM R.* 2010;2(8):740–94.
175. Välimäki VV, Alfthan H, Lehmuskallio E, et al. Risk factors for clinical stress fractures in male military recruits: a prospective cohort study. *Bone.* 2005;37(2):267–73.
176. Bennell KL, Malcolm SA, Thomas SA, Wark JD, Brukner PD. The incidence and distribution of stress fractures in competitive track and field athletes. A twelve-month prospective study. *Am J Sports Med.* 1996;24(2):211–7.
177. Hughes LY. Biomechanical analysis of the foot and ankle for predisposition to developing stress fractures. *J Orthop Sports Phys Ther.* 1985;7(3):96–101.
178. Korpelainen R, Orava S, Karpakka J, Siira P, Hulkko A. Risk factors for recurrent stress fractures in athletes. *Am J Sports Med.* 2001;29(3):304–10.
179. Matheson GO, Clement DB, McKenzie DC, Taunton JE, Lloyd-Smith DR, Macintyre JG. Scintigraphic uptake of 99mTc at non-painful sites in athletes with stress fractures. The concept of bone strain. *Sports Med.* 1987;4(1):65–75.
180. Davis IF, Milner CE, Hamill JF. Does increased loading during running lead to tibial stress fractures? A prospective study. *Med Sci Sports Exerc.* 2004;36:S58.
181. Gardner LI Jr, Dziados JE, Jones BH, et al. Prevention of lower extremity stress fractures: a controlled trial of a shock absorbent insole. *Am J Public Health.* 1988;78(12):1563–7.
182. Rauh MJ, Tenforde AS, Barrack MT, Rosenthal MD, Nichols JF. Sport specialization and low bone mineral density in female high school distance runners. *J Athl Train.* 2020;55(12):1239–46.
183. Fullerton LR Jr. Femoral neck stress fractures. *Sports Med.* 1990;9(3):192–7.
184. Batt ME, Kemp S, Kerslake R. Delayed union stress fractures of the anterior tibia: conservative management. *Br J Sports Med.* 2001;35(1):74–7.
185. Rettig AC, Shelbourne KD, McCarroll JR, Bisesi M, Watts J. The natural history and treatment of delayed union stress fractures of the anterior cortex of the tibia. *Am J Sports Med.* 1988;16(3):250–5.
186. Schils JP, Andrish JT, Piraino DW, Belhobek GH, Richmond BJ, Bergfeld JA. Medial malleolar stress fractures in seven patients: review of the clinical and imaging features. *Radiology.* 1992;185(1):219–21.
187. Shelbourne KD, Fisher DA, Rettig AC, McCarroll JR. Stress fractures of the medial malleolus. *Am J Sports Med.* 1988;16(1):60–3.
188. Khan KM, Brukner PD, Kearney C, Fuller PJ, Bradshaw CJ, Kiss ZS. Tarsal navicular stress fracture in athletes. *Sports Med.* 1994;17(1):65–76.
189. Portland G, Kelikian A, Kodros S. Acute surgical management of Jones' fractures. *Foot Ankle Int.* 2003;24(11):829–33.
190. Vu D, McDiarmid T, Brown M, Aukerman DF. Clinical inquiries. What is the most effective management of acute fractures of the base of the fifth metatarsal? *J Fam Pract.* 2006;55(8):713–7.
191. Zwitser EW, Breederveld RS. Fractures of the fifth metatarsal; diagnosis and treatment. *Injury.* 2010;41(6):555–62.
192. Le HM, Stracciolini A, Stein CJ, Quinn BJ, Jackson SS. Platelet rich plasma for hallux sesamoid injuries: a case series. *Phys Sportsmed.* 2022;50(2):181–4.
193. Leal C, D'Agostino C, Gomez Garcia S, Fernandez A. Current concepts of shockwave therapy in stress fractures. *Int J Surg.* 2015;24(Pt B):195–200.
194. O'Connor F, Wilder R, Nirschl R. Basic treatment concepts. In: O'Connor F, Wilder R, Nirschl R, editors. *Textbook of Running Medicine.* New York: McGraw-Hill; 2001. p. 505–16.

114 Alpine Skiing and Snowboarding

Devin P. McFadden and Brian F. Merrigan

INTRODUCTION/BACKGROUND

- Alpine skiing and snowboarding are two of the most popular winter sports throughout the world.
- The popularity of skiing and snowboarding continues to grow throughout the world, with 200 million participants worldwide and 12 million in the United States alone (1,2).
- Skiing has been a mode of transportation in colder climates for thousands of years and modern alpine skiing has been a form of recreation since the mid-19th century.
- By contrast, snowboarding is a relatively newer sport, tracing its origin to the United States in the 1960s.
- Snowboarders tend to be younger than skiers and have a reputation for greater risk taking.

EPIDEMIOLOGY

- Historical injury rates of 7.6 per 1000 skier days were quoted as early as the 1950s (2,3).
- Although modern equipment has led to a reduction in injury volume, the severity of injuries has increased because new equipment allows for greater speeds and sharper turns.
- Injury patterns are distinct to each specific sport, with predominantly lower extremity injuries in skiing and predominantly upper extremity injuries in snowboarding.
- Injury rates have improved over the years, which is attributed to helmet use, hard-shelled ski boots, release bindings, and better grooming of slopes (4).
  - Helmets, now required in most skiing and snowboarding competitions, and wrist guards have both been proven to be effective in preventing injury.
- Current data among professional winter athletes suggests injury rates of 3.5 per 1000 athlete-days, with freestyle skiers and snowboarders having the highest injury incidence rates (5).
- Among recreational skiers and snowboarders, the injury rate averages 2.2 per 1000 ski/snowboarder days with male snowboarders accounting for 1/3 of all injuries (6).
- Catastrophic injuries still occur, however, with an average of 38 fatalities yearly in the United States alone, or 0.67 fatalities per 1 million skier visits (7).

BIOMECHANICS

- The different biomechanics and equipment used for skiing and snowboarding result in their vastly different injury patterns.
- Skiers are capable of sharp, quick turns and high-velocity collisions.
  - Fall on outstretched hand (FOOSH) injury is relatively uncommon, leading to a greater percentage of lower extremity injuries.
  - In addition, a skier who has lost control can find his/her skis advancing in diverging directions, which causes a rotational torque and leads to a high incidence of knee injuries.
  - Downhill skiers tend to fall forward after losing control or colliding with something and have a greater incidence of lumbar burst fractures compared to other back/spine injuries (2).
  - Lacerations have been noted to account for 8% of all injuries in skiers, where released bindings expose athletes to the sharpened ski edge (8).
- Snowboarders, by comparison, have both feet strapped to a single board, and the large surface area of the board and comparative difficulty making sharp turns result in lower velocity falls. This allows the athlete to extend his/her arms and brace for impact.
- Subsequently, snowboarders have a significantly increased risk of injury to the hand, wrist, and arm.
- These falls also result in less torsion and fewer injuries to the knees.
- Lacerations occur less frequently than in skiers as the feet stay strapped to the board and bindings do not release during falls.
- Snowboarders more frequently injure their backs while falling backward after a missed jump, causing axial loading and an increased incidence of compression fractures in the thoracolumbar spine (2).

MEDICAL ISSUES

Head and Spinal Cord Injury

- The leading cause of death in both skiing and snowboarding is traumatic brain injury, usually following a collision with a tree, chairlift pole, or another person (9).
- Studies indicate that head injuries make up 9%–19% of all snow-sport injuries reported by ski patrols and emergency departments, with neck and spinal cord injuries representing 1%–4% (10).

Environmental and Altitude Injury

- Exercise-induced bronchospasm (EIB), acute mountain sickness (AMS), and hypothermia can all be encountered when skiing or snowboarding.
- EIB is a transient, reversible narrowing of the distal airways caused by strenuous activity. EIB is more common in cool conditions, as cold air itself can trigger airway hyperresponsiveness.
  - Rapid respiratory rates, cool air temperatures, and low-humidity environments contribute to airway drying and bronchial spasm.
  - Some estimate that EIB affects up to 50% of winter athletes (11).
  - Common symptoms include post-exercise dyspnea, cough, burning chest pain, and rarely wheezing.
  - Symptoms peak 10–20 minutes after exercise, with a late phase occurring at 2–12 hours and lasting up to 2 days in some athletes.
  - The eucapnic voluntary hyperventilation challenge (EVHC) seems to be the most accurate method of making a diagnosis, although a laboratory-based or sport-specific competition-based exercise challenge is also a viable alternative.
  - Treatment is similar to that of mild asthma, with albuterol used as a rescue medication at the onset of symptoms or 20–40 minutes prior to activity as a prophylactic measure.
  - Physicians of competitive athletes must be aware of the World Anti-Doping Agency (WADA) regulations, which set limits on the amount of B2 agonists an athlete can inhale.
    - Currently, athletes are permitted to administer inhaled albuterol (in divided doses not exceeding 1600 μg in 24 h and 600 μg in 8 h), formoterol (≤54 μg in 24 h), and salmeterol (≤200 μg in 24 h) (12).
- AMS, or altitude sickness, is the pathologic response of the human body to acute increases in elevation to levels greater than 2500 m.
  - Oxygen levels decrease as altitude increases, leading to elevated respiratory rates, heart rates, and stroke volumes.
  - Common symptoms include throbbing headaches, anorexia, nausea, fatigue, dizziness, and insomnia and can easily be mistaken for a viral illness, hangover, or allergic response.
  - AMS can progress to high-altitude cerebral edema (HACE) and/or high-altitude pulmonary edema (HAPE) if not promptly recognized and treated. Both HACE and HAPE are potentially fatal conditions.
  - Improper hydration, fitness, and rate of ascent are risk factors for developing symptoms, and proper acclimatization can take up to a week (13).
  - Hypothermia is defined as a core body temperature less than 35 °C. The mortality rate from hypothermia is estimated to be 0.18 deaths per 1 million skier days (14,15). And although this is a rare cause of injury in recreational skiers, due to its potential morbidity, it deserves mention here.
  - With every 1000 meters of altitude ascended, the environmental temperature drops by 5.5 °C.
  - Death by hypothermia is usually a secondary sequela of an injury, avalanche, or altitude sickness that prevents the athlete from escaping from the elements (14).
  - When hypothermic patients are evacuated, they should immediately be dressed in warm, dry clothing.
  - A Bair Hugger or similar commercial warming device is one way to provide external rewarming, whereas heated intravenous fluids and exposure to heated, humidified air have been shown to be effective in rewarming even severely obtunded patients.

MUSCULOSKELETAL ISSUES

Ski Injuries

- As noted above, upper extremity injuries are uncommon in skiing, representing only an estimated 14% of alpine ski injuries (7).
- Shoulder injuries occur at a rate of 0.2–0.5 per 1000 skier days and represent 4%–11% of alpine ski injuries, with the most common injury types being: glenohumeral joint subluxations, rotator cuff strains, acromioclavicular joint separations, proximal humeral fractures, and clavicle fractures (7,16).
- Although less common than in snowboarders, wrist and hand injuries do occur in skiing, typically as a consequence of a FOOSH injury. The most common fracture in the forearm is the distal radius or Colles fracture.
  - The diagnosis is usually made based on plain radiographs, and for fractures that are not displaced, immobilization is all that is needed.
  - However, if the fracture is significantly displaced, if the joint space is compromised, or if the neurovascular supply is injured, then surgical intervention is often required.

- The thumb is the most frequently injured digit of the hand in skiing, and the injury almost universally results from the traction caused when an isolated thumb is pulled away from the rest of the hand in a skier using poles.
  - This results in extension and forced abduction at the metacarpophalangeal (MCP) joint and the aptly named *skier's thumb* — a sprain injury to the ulnar collateral ligament (UCL) of the first MCP joint.
  - Injury characterized by pain and tenderness to palpation over the ulnar aspect of the thumb and clinical diagnosis is made based on UCL laxity noted on exam.
  - Conservative management with thumb spica casting followed by splinting is recommended when less than 30° of valgus laxity is noted.
  - A complete disruption of the UCL with retraction of the ligament to the adductor aponeurosis is known as a Stener lesion and is characterized by a palpable mass. In this case, or if a bony avulsion is present, surgical management is preferred.
  - The UCL can also be injured through chronic stress rather than an acute, violent force and, in this case, is commonly referred to as gamekeeper's thumb.
  - Although UCL injury is undoubtedly the most common and most recognized injury pattern, dislocations, subluxations, and Bennett fractures of the base of the first metacarpal are also quite common in skiers (1).
- Traumatic knee injuries represent 27%–41% of all injuries in skiers, making them the most frequently reported ski injury (7). The classic explanation for these injuries focuses on the torque generated by the diverging skis of a skier who has lost control and the resultant external rotation and valgus stress placed on the knee as the primary causes of medial collateral ligament and anterior cruciate ligament (ACL) injury.
  - Other injury patterns have also been noted; however, such as an airborne skier landing with his center of gravity too far back, resulting in the anterior displacement of the tibia when levered against the static ski boot in what has been referred to as an "anterior drawer effect."
  - Finally, a skier whose weight is too far back on his skis will experience simultaneous flexion and internal rotation at the knee joint if he catches his inside edge on the snow, yielding perhaps the most common cause of ACL disruption (8).
  - ACL injuries are more common in cold environments, likely due to the reduced capacity of cold knee flexor muscles to counter the knee extensor muscles, which cause anterior shear force on the tibia (5).
- Tibia and fibula fractures, as well as boot-top hematomas, can occur due to the continued momentum of the lower legs if the skis are rapidly slowed or stopped.
- Achilles tendon ruptures can also result from a similar mechanism, as the force is translated through the stronger proximal tibia distally to the ankle (17).
- Ankle and foot injuries remain possible but are relatively rare since the advent of hard-shelled boots.

Snowboarding Injuries

- Snowboarders are 13 times more likely than skiers to sustain a wrist injury (18), and wrist injuries represent 28% of all snowboarding injuries (19).
- Ankle injuries are also much more common in snowboarders, with a more than twofold increase in risk compared to skiers (1).
- Snowboarder's ankle is a rare but potentially disabling fracture of the lateral process of the talus and can lead to avascular necrosis and chronic nonunion if mistaken for a routine ankle sprain.
  - Although the exact mechanism of injury is not clearly understood, a high-energy axial load of the lateral ankle is required and results in pain of the anterolateral ankle that can mimic a severe ankle sprain (8).
  - Up to 40% of these lesions are missed by standard radiography; thus, diagnosis requires a high index of suspicion and can often only be made by computed tomography scan (18,20).
  - Treatment for fractures with displacement of less than 2 mm is casting, whereas comminuted fractures or those with a greater degree of displacement should be referred for possible surgical management.

INJURY PREVENTION

- Helmet use has been shown to reduce the incidence and severity of many types of injuries.
  - From ski patrol data related to both skier/snowboarder self-reported head injuries and to medically diagnosed lacerations, fractures, and traumatic brain injuries, helmets have proven to be an effective means of injury prevention (7,10).
  - A well-designed meta-analysis of 12 studies suggested that helmet use could potentially prevent 35% of all head injuries without increasing the risk of neck injury (10).
  - In addition, studies have shown that helmets do not increase the risk of compensation behavior among skiers and snowboarders (21).
- The effectiveness of wrist guards in preventing snowboarding injuries has also been evaluated and has demonstrated a promising reduction in wrist injuries in those who wore protection.
  - For every 50 snowboarders who wear a wrist guard, one wrist injury will be prevented.
  - Evidence is mixed as to whether wrist guards decrease or increase the risk of shoulder injuries (22).
- Educational campaigns focusing on alpine sport safety and sun protection use have been met with moderate success but are resource-intensive and thus unlikely to find widespread acceptance (23,24).

SUMMARY

- Skiing and snowboarding are fun yet potentially dangerous snow sports.
- Injuries usually involve the upper extremity in snowboarders and the lower extremity in skiers.
- Environmental injuries are frequently overlooked due to the prevalence of orthopedic trauma; nonetheless, their importance within the sport cannot be underestimated by the treating physician.
- Preventative measures and improvements in equipment have come a long way in helping to reduce injury rates; however, helmets and wrist guards can only be effective to the extent that they are used.

REFERENCES

1. Hunter RE. Skiing injuries. *Am J Sports Med.* 1999;27(3):381–9.
2. Kary JM. Acute spine injuries in skiers and snowboarders. *Curr Sports Med Rep.* 2008;7(1):35–8.
3. Earle AS, Moritz JR, Saviers GB, Ball JD. Ski injuries. *JAMA.* 1962;180:285–8.
4. Davidson TM, Laliotis AT. Alpine skiing injuries. A nine-year study. *West J Med.* 1996;164(4):310–4.
5. Fu XL, Du L, Song YP, Chen HL, Shen WQ. Incidence of injuries in professional snow sports: a systematic review and meta-analysis. *J Sport Health Sci.* 2022;11(1):6–13.
6. Dickson TJ, Terwiel FA. Injury trends in alpine skiing and a snowboarding over the decade 2008-09 to 2017-18. *J Sci Med Sport.* 2021;24(10):1055–60.
7. Davey A, Endres NK, Johnson RJ, Shealy JE. Alpine skiing injuries. *Sports Health.* 2019;11(1):18–26.
8. Abu-Laban RB. Snowboarding injuries: an analysis and comparison with alpine skiing injuries. *CMAJ (Can Med Assoc J).* 1991;145(9):1097–103.
9. Ackery A, Hagel BE, Provvidenza C, Tator CH. An international review of head and spinal cord injuries in alpine skiing and snowboarding. *Inj Prev.* 2007;13(6):368–75.
10. Russell K, Christie J, Hagel BE. The effect of helmets on the risk of head and neck injuries among skiers and snowboarders: a meta-analysis. *CMAJ (Can Med Assoc J).* 2010;182(4):333–40.
11. Butcher JD. Exercise-induced asthma in the competitive cold weather athlete. *Curr Sports Med Rep.* 2006;5(6):284–8.
12. Allen H, Backhouse SH, Hull JH, Price OJ. Anti-doping policy, therapeutic use exemption and medication use in athletes with asthma: a narrative review and critical appraisal of current regulations. *Sports Med.* 2019;49(5):659–68.
13. Eichner ER. Sports medicine pearls and pitfalls: going higher. *Curr Sports Med Rep.* 2008;7(6):310–1.
14. Windsor JS, Firth PG, Grocott MP, Rodway GW, Montgomery HE. Mountain mortality: a review of deaths that occur during recreational activities in the mountains. *Postgrad Med J.* 2009;85(1004):316–21.
15. Sherry E, Richards D. Hypothermia among resort skiers: 19 cases from the Snowy Mountains. *Med J Aust.* 1986;144(9):457–61.
16. Roberts WO. *Bull's Handbook of Sports Injuries.* 2nd ed. New York (NY): McGraw-Hill; 2004.
17. Pećina M. Injuries in downhill (alpine) skiing. *Croat Med J.* 2002;43(3):257–60.
18. Sacco DE, Sartorelli DH, Vane DW. Evaluation of alpine skiing and snowboarding injury in a northeastern state. *J Trauma.* 1998;44(4):654–9.
19. Kim S, Endres NK, Johnson RJ, Ettlinger CF, Shealy JE. Snowboarding injuries: trends over time and comparisons with alpine skiing injuries. *Am J Sports Med.* 2012;40(4):770–6.
20. Kramer IF, Brouwers L, Brink PR, Poeze M. Snowboarders' ankle. *BMJ Case Rep* [Internet]. 2014 [cited 2023 Jan 06];2014:2014(10). bcr2014204220. Available from: https://www.ncbi.nlm/pmc/articles/PMC4216907/. https://doi.org/10.1136/bcr-2014-204220
21. Haider AH, Saleem T, Bilaniuk JW, Barraco RD, Eastern Association for the Surgery of Trauma Injury ControlViolence Prevention Committee. An evidence-based review: efficacy of safety helmets in the reduction of head injuries in recreational skiers and snowboarders. *J Trauma Acute Care Surg.* 2012;73(5):1340–7.
22. Russell K, Hagel B, Francescutti LH. The effect of wrist guards on wrist and arm injuries among snowboarders: a systematic review. *Clin J Sport Med.* 2007;17(2):145–150.
23. Josse JM, Cusimano M. The effect of a skiing/snowboarding safety video on the increase of safety knowledge in Canadian youths — a pilot study. *Int J Circumpolar Health.* 2006;65(5):385–8.
24. Walkosz BJ, Buller DB, Andersen PA, et al. Increasing sun protection in winter outdoor recreation a theory-based health communication program. *Am J Prev Med.* 2008;34(6):502–9.

115 Rodeo

Craig R. Denegar

INTRODUCTION

- Rodeo, unlike many of the sports addressed in this section, is not a single sport or event. In rodeo, cowboys and cowgirls compete in one or more individual competitions that constitute a performance. In addition to the competitors, bull fighters, and to a lesser other arena personnel, risk injury and may require medical care.
- A rodeo is often made up of several performances over several days. Many rodeos also have "slack" where competitors in the timed events compete before the performance because there are more entrees in the timed events than can be accommodated in a typical 2–3 hour performance.
- Rodeo is not solely a professional sport. Youth, high school, college, and professional rodeo organizations sponsor competitions. Although rodeo is associated with the American West, there are rodeos across the United States and Canada as well as South America, Central America, and Australia.
- The events in *professional* rodeo include the rough stock competitions and timed events.
  - Rough stock competitions consist of: bareback riding, saddle bronc riding, and bull riding.
  - The timed events include: tie-down calf roping, steer wrestling, steer roping, team roping, barrel racing, and breakaway roping.
- In *youth, high school, and college rodeo*, additional timed events may be on a schedule, but our focus will be on the primary events listed in Table 115.1.
- For the most part, the rough stock events, tie-down roping, steer wrestling, steer roping, and team roping are cowboy events, whereas cowgirls compete in barrel racing and breakaway roping. However, these gender roles are not absolute across all levels of rodeo.

HISTORY

- Rodeo did not begin as an athletic competition but grew from the work of cowboys and cowgirls working with livestock on ranches. The events of bareback and saddle bronc riding are the extension of work done to break horses at a time when the horse was the fastest means of transportation. The care of cattle required the roping and tying of the animal to administer medical care. Tie-down calf roping and steer wrestling are offshoots of this work.
- Bull riding, however, emerged from the cowboy spirit rather than the work of the cowboy. At the end of the trail or a long day of work, cowboys began to develop competitions among themselves or cowboys from other outfits to see who the best rider, best roper, and all-around best ranch hands were. From these informal competitions and our fascination with the life of the cowboy, Wild West shows and true rodeo competitions evolved.
- Although the Wild West shows have vanished, rodeo has grown into a business, drawing large crowds to events and allowing the professional to earn a living through rodeo competition.
  - As noted hereinbefore, there are rodeos for young cowboys and cowgirls, high school and college athletes, and professionals. Box 115.1. offers a partial list of the organizations that sponsor or sanction rodeos.
  - Unlike many sports where athletes are a part of a team or identified athletic organization, the rodeo athlete, for the most part, stands alone. Rodeo athletes usually pay an entry fee to compete and earn only what they win in competition or through sponsorship. In reality, the opportunity to earn money requires that the rodeo athlete compete. These athletes travel extensively, and the sports medicine provider may have little knowledge of the athlete's medical history and little opportunity for follow-up care.

RODEO SPORTS MEDICINE

- The history of rodeo sports medicine is as unique as the sport itself. Although local practitioners may have provided care to rodeo athletes who came to town to compete, a formal program to provide and coordinate care only appeared in the United States through a program developed in 1980 with the support of the Justin Boot Company.
- The Justin Sports Medicine Team (www. http://justinsportsmedicineteam.com) now coordinates care at major rodeos across the United States. In Canada, the Canadian Pro Rodeo Sport Medicine Team (https://www.prorodeosportmed.com) has grown over the past 25 years to coordinate volunteer coverage of Canadian Professional Rodeo Association events.

Table 115.1 Events of Professional Rodeo and Associated Injuries

Event	Description	Injuries and Risk
Rough stock	Must ride 8 s, scored 0–100, 50 points for animal performance, 50 points for cowboy. Protective vests are common or required in bull riding and bareback riding.	Accounts for a majority of injuries. Concussion and fractures account for a large portion of serious injuries.
Bull riding	Cowboy maintains position on the animal using a bull rope. Helmets worn by some contestants.	Accounts for nearly half of injuries and a large portion of fatalities. High incidence of concussion and fractures.
Bareback	Cowboy maintains position on animal with a handle-shaped rigging. Cowboys wear protective vests but not helmets.	Second highest risk of serious injury. Injuries to the elbow caused by hyperextension are common.
Saddle bronc	Cowboy sits in a saddle and maintains control holding a bronc rein (rope). Considered the most technically demanding rough stock event. Cowboys wear protective vests but not helmets.	Lower risk of serious injury of rough stock events. Knee injuries (posterior cruciate ligament) occur with landing on fully flexed knee following dismount.
Timed events	Performance is judged on time to complete the event.	Lower risk of injury, especially concussion and crush/impact mechanism injury, compared to rough stock events.
Tie-down roping	Cowboy must rope calf, dismount, flank (lay on side) calf, and tie three legs.	Thumb, shoulder, and lower extremity injuries during dismount are most common.
Steer roping	Cowboy must rope and trip steer, dismount, and tie 3 legs	Similar to tie-down roping
Steer wrestling	Cowboy dismounts, grabbing the horns of a running steer and then throws the steer with all four legs pointed in the same direction.	Shoulder and lower extremity sprains are the most common injuries.
Team roping	Two cowboys attempt to rope the head and hind legs of the steer.	Shoulder and hand injuries are most common.
Women's barrel racing	Horses run a cloverleaf pattern around 3 barrels.	Primary risk or serious injury occurs if horse falls
Women's breakaway roping	Cowgirls must rope the calf and is timed based on when the rope breaks away from the saddle	General risk of roping- and riding-related injuries

- However, the Justin Sports Medicine Team and the Canadian Pro Rodeo Sports Medicine Team are not present at all professional rodeo events in the United States and Canada. At many professional and other rodeo competitions at all levels, care for the rodeo athlete is dependent on local providers.
- Bull riding is the event in rodeo that draws the most attention. In 1994, a group of rodeo cowboys formed Professional Bull Riders (PBR) and the associated risks of this single event led to efforts to provide well-coordinated care to bull riders at the top level in their sport.
- The PBR brought increased attention to medical care through the Justin Sports Medicine program and more recently through partnership with Extreme Sports Medicine Inc.
- There has also been an increased focus on injury prevention through improved safety equipment and conditioning.
- Today, the growing network of providers has greatly improved sports medicine care for the rodeo athlete.

EVENTS AND RULES

- The rules and equipment differ between the events in professional rodeo, although there are some commonalities.
- In the *rough stock* events, cowboys must stay on the animal for 8 seconds without touching the animal with their free arm. Cowboys are awarded a score from 0 to 100 by a team of judges if they are successful in staying on for the 8 seconds. One-half of the score is based on the performance of the animal and one-half on the ability of the rider.
- In bareback and saddle bronc events, the cowboy must mark out the animal, meaning that the cowboy's spurs must be in contact with the point of the horse's shoulder until the horse's front feet hit the ground once the chute gate is opened.

115.1 Websites That May Assist in Locating Information on Age Groups, Rules, and Events

Youth Rodeo Association (http://www.yratx.com/).
National High School Rodeo Association (http://www.nhsra.com/)
National Intercollegiate Rodeo Association (http://www.collegerodeo.com/)
Professional Rodeo Cowboys Association (http://www.prorodeo.com/)
Women's Professional Rodeo Association (http://www.wpra.com/)
Professional Bull Riders (http://www.pbrnow.com/)

- In bareback riding, the cowboy's hand is inserted into a rigging that resembles the handle of a suitcase, whereas in saddle bronc, the cowboy holds onto a rein attached to a halter.
- In bull riding, there is no requirement for a mark out. The bull rider wraps one hand in a bull rope wrapped around the chest of the bull. In bull riding, the cowboy wears a protective vest, and the use of helmets has become widespread in the past decade.
- In bull riding, the cowboy wears a protective vest. The use of helmets has become widespread in the past decade, although their use is not mandatory at the professional level. Several manufacturers offer certified helmets designed for bull riders.
- Many bareback and saddle bronc riders also wear protective vests, but beyond the vests, helmets, and a mouthpiece, the cowboys have little to protect them from injury.
- In the *timed events*, the goal is to complete the required task in the shortest amount of time.
- In barrel racing, the cowgirl rides her horse in a cloverleaf pattern around three barrels. Penalties are assessed if a barrel is knocked over, with the fastest total time winning.
- In the *roping* events and steer wrestling, the animal is given a head start into the arena.
  - In tie-down calf roping, the cowboy must rope the calf from the back of his horse, dismount and reach the calf, flank or throw the calf to the ground, and tie any three legs.
  - The steer roper must rope and trip the steer, and while the horse maintains tension on the rope, dismount and tie any three legs.
  - In team roping, two cowboys, a header and a heeler, chase the steer. The header's job is to rope the steer around the head and turn the steer so that the heeler can throw his rope around the two back feet. The clock is stopped when the ropes are tensioned and the riders face each other.
  - In tie-down roping, steer roping and team roping the cowboy must wrap the rope around the horn on the saddle (dally) to secure the animal.
  - The steer wrestler must chase and ride alongside the steer. The hazer, a cowboy riding on the opposite side of the steer, guides the animal into position. The cowboy dismounts onto the head of the steer, grasping around the horns. The cowboy must stop the steer and throw it to the ground with all four feet pointing in the same direction.
  - In breakaway roping the cowgirl ropes the calf and is timed based on when the rope pulls taut and breaks away from the saddle

INJURIES AND EPIDEMIOLOGY

- Working around livestock carries inherent risks, and the medical team providing care at a rodeo must anticipate the possibility of injury to rodeo athletes, bull fighters, and those who handle and manage the horses, bulls, calves, and steers.
- Overall injury rates of 14.7–16.6 (1,2) injuries per 1000 exposures (an attempt in a rodeo event) have been reported in professional rodeo. An injury rate of 10.98 per 1000 exposures has been reported in collegiate rodeo competition (3).
- The incidence of catastrophic and fatal injuries has been reported to be 9.5–19.7 and 4.05–7.29 per 100,000 exposures, respectively, with the greatest risk occurring in bull riding (4).
- Overall, more injuries occur in rough stock competitions (1–4) and more injuries occur in professional bull riding than bareback and saddle bronc events (1–5).
  - Rough stock events also account for the greatest portion of injuries in high school rodeo (6).
  - Of the rough stock events, bull riding is the most dangerous, and many injuries are severe (7,8).
  - The incidence rate of injury in professional and high school bull riding has been estimated to be 48.1 (1)–32.2 (2) and 28.5 (3) per 1000 exposures, respectively.
  - Incidence rates in professional bareback and saddle bronc riding of 41.2 and 23.1 per 1000 exposures are reported (1). Similar rates have been reported in high school athletes (3).
  - In a survey of 100% bull riders, compared to 24% of tie-down ropers, reported a rodeo-related injury (9).
- Steer wrestlers have the highest injury rate of timed event competitors (1–3) and had the highest injury rate in a study of collegiate rodeo (3).
- Contusions, sprains, concussions, strains, and fractures were most commonly reported injuries (1), with collision with the ground or animal and being stepped on by an animal the three most common mechanisms of injury.
- Similar distributions, types, and mechanisms of injury have been reported in adolescent rodeo athletes treated in emergency departments (8).
  - The head and spine were the most common sites of injury in a case series of rodeo athletes treated in trauma centers (7).
- Injuries to the hand, wrist, elbow, and shoulder may result from a cowboy being "hung-up" where their hand does not release from the bull rope or bareback rigging. Elbow injuries are very common in bareback riders because of the stresses to the joint during the ride.
- In rough stock events, concussion and injury to the cervical spine can occur when the cowboy is thrown from the animal.
- In saddle bronc riding, there is a greater risk of injuries to the knee, particularly the cruciate ligaments during the dismount.
- Injuries in tie-down calf roping and steer wrestling often involve the lower extremity, with the knee being most susceptible.
- Severe hand/finger injuries and traumatic amputation can occur in the roping events when the competitor wraps the rope around the saddle horn. Breakaway roping does not require the competitor to dally the rope.
- Team roping, breakaway roping, and barrel racing carry the lowest risk of injury.

- Rodeo athletes are also susceptible to muscle strains, particularly involving the groin.
- Roping cowboys can suffer from nontraumatic or repetitive use injuries to the shoulder and arm.
- A significant concern in rodeo is the care of open wounds. These can occur at any point before, during, and after a rodeo. The sports medicine team must recognize that the rodeo arena and livestock holding areas are inherently dirty. All wounds must be thoroughly cleansed and closely monitored for infection.

EVENT PREPARATION

- Providing sports medicine care to rodeo athletes is a unique experience. The first reaction when one witnesses an injury to an athlete is to wait until play stops and run to the assistance of the athlete. However, bulls and horses do not stop play when an injury occurs.
  - The livestock in and around the arena pose a significant risk to sports medicine personnel, and the provider must be certain that the arena is safe to enter before attending to an injury and take care not to become a second victim.
- Rodeo athletes are a unique group of athletes. The cowboy culture is one of toughness bred from the demands of the working ranch where medical assistance is often far away and care for the livestock is paramount.
- Rodeo athletes may not readily seek attention for an injury or may choose not to follow the advice of the sports medicine professional. However, the expansion of rodeo sports medicine has increased the bond of trust between athlete and provider. Still, developing a professional relationship can take time.
- Once one is aware of the environment and culture of rodeo, planning for sports medicine coverage is similar to other sports that pose a high risk of traumatic injury. The provider must be prepared to assess injuries that are both orthopedic and nonorthopedic in nature.
- Some of these injuries can be life-threatening, so a well-planned and practiced emergency action plan must be in place.
- The sports medicine team should practice caring for a rodeo athlete wearing a protective vest and helmet.
- The rodeo ground is often rough, and access by emergency medical assistance can be limited by fencing and seating. A plan for the equipment to be brought to the injured athlete should also be developed as it is often impossible to roll a stretcher over the soft ground found in a well-prepared arena.
- A plan to transport an injured athlete from the arena must be developed at each venue as access, egress points, and specific personnel and plan details will vary between locations.
- Emergency medical personnel should be on-site during competition and should be reminded of the danger posed by livestock. These professionals should only enter the arena when directed by the medical staff in charge.

INJURY PREVENTION

- Unlike team sports and individual sports where coaches and strength and conditioning specialists are available to athletes, rodeo athletes rely on themselves and fellow athletes for the management of their conditioning and rehabilitation from minor injuries.
- These athletes often ask event medical staff for advice and recommendations. In general, the sports medicine team should promote the use of safety equipment and be prepared to provide recommendations regarding strength and flexibility training. The safety equipment requirements differ between rodeo organizations, and helmets are not required for all riders at the professional level.
- Rodeo athletes earn their living on the road and may not have access to strength training and other exercise equipment. The sports medicine provider may need to adapt recommended exercises to the athlete's schedule and environment. Moreover, the sport-specific demands of the athlete's event must be considered.

SUMMARY

- Rodeo is an exciting sport, and the rodeo athlete is genuinely appreciative of sports medicine professionals willing to learn about the sport and provide care. There is certainly a need to continue to expand and coordinate care of the rodeo athlete.
- Although the rodeo arena is a unique setting, the athletes and officials for rodeo are willing to share their knowledge and help the sports medicine professional to both understand the sport and feel welcome in what is often a new world of athletic health care.

REFERENCES

1. Sinclair Elder AJ, Nilson CJ, Elder CL. Analysis of 4 years of injury in professional rodeo. *Clin J Sport Med.* 2020;30(6):591–7.
2. Butterwick DJ, Hagel B, Nelson DS, LeFave MR, Meeuwisse WH. Epidemiologic analysis of injury in five years of Canadian professional rodeo. *Am J Sports Med.* 2002;30(2):193–8.
3. Watts M, Bobo L, Whitehead MT, Dompier TP, Oliver GD. Characteristics of injury in collegiate rodeo. *Clin J Sport Med.* 2022;32(2):e145–50.
4. Butterwick DJ, Lafave MR, Lau BH, Freeman T. Rodeo catastrophic injuries and registry: initial retrospective and prospective report. *Clin J Sport Med.* 2011;21(3):243–8.

5. Butterwick DJ, Meeuwisse WH. Bull riding injuries in professional rodeo: data for prevention and care. *Phys Sportsmed.* 2003;31(6):37–41.
6. Sinclair AJ, Smidt C. Analysis of 10 years of injury in high school rodeo. *Clin J Sport Med.* 2009;19(5):383–7.
7. Seifert CL, Rogers M, Helmer SD, Ward JG, Haan JM. Rodeo trauma: Outcome data from 10 Years of injuries. *Kans J Med.* 2022;15(2):208–11.
8. Forrester MB. Rodeo-related injuries among adolescents treated at emergency departments. *J Emerg Med.* 2021;61(4):387–95.
9. Crichlow R, Williamson S, Geurin M, Heggem H. Self-reported injury history in Native American professional rodeo competitors. *Clin J Sport Med.* 2006;16(4):352–4.

Shooting Sports

Bjørn Bakken, Rebecca Peebles, and Chris G. Pappas

116

INTRODUCTION

- Shooting sports are competitive and recreational activities that challenge various forms of rifle, shotgun, and pistol marksmanship.
- Shooting sports are held at recreational, collegiate, national, international, and Olympic levels.
- Shooting sports were included in the first Olympic Games in 1896 (1–5). An ancient version of biathlon, Military Patrol, was added to the 1924 Winter Olympics (4,6) and then evolved into the current sport of Biathlon in 1960 (6).
- International rifle, shotgun, pistol competitions are largely governed by the International Shooting Sport Federation (ISSF), formerly known as the International Shooting Union (ISU), and Biathlon is governed by the International Biathlon Union (IBU).
- Women were first allowed to compete in Olympic shooting sports in 1968. In 1992, mixed gender fields were discontinued and women's specific events were added. However, in 2017, the IOC reinstated mixed events in place of three existing men's only divisions (1,3,4).
- The incidence of acute injuries within shooting sports is relatively low; however, the treating physician should be familiar with the various biomechanical, environmental, and psychosocial factors that can influence a shooting athlete's health (1,7–15).

DISCIPLINES

- The various disciplines within shooting sports are typically defined by the type of firearm that is used and, in some instances, whether there is an additional athletic component involved, as in biathlon, which combines rifle marksmanship and cross-country skiing (2,5,6,16).
- *Rifle* competitions include high power rifle, precision rifle, small bore rifle, and air rifle.
  - Competitors shoot in multiple positions (standing, kneeling, prone) at fixed targets of varying distances (5).
  - Depending on the event, competition is held at an indoor or outdoor range with varying exposure to the elements.
- *Shotgun* competitions include trap, skeet, and sporting clay competitions.
  - Competitors shoot at clay targets either thrown from standardized positions and angles (trap and skeet) or from variable angles and distances (sporting clay).
  - Competitors typically use 12 gauge shotguns and competitions are held at outdoor ranges (2,5,17).
- *Pistol* competitions include rapid fire and single-shot events.
  - Athletes are typically required to shoot with one hand, unsupported, at targets of fixed distances (5).
  - Olympic events use small-caliber firearms at indoor shooting ranges; however, some non-Olympic events are held at outdoor ranges.
- *Running Target* competitions involve shooting either an air-rifle or .22 caliber rifle at horizontally moving targets of fixed distances (3).
- *Biathlon* combines the physical exertion of cross-country ski racing with rifle marksmanship and races are held during the winter months at outdoor cross-country ski venues equipped with outdoor shooting ranges.
  - Athletes shoot a .22 caliber rifle at fixed metal targets at 50 m in both the prone and standing positions following multiple loops of cross-country skiing (6,16).

EQUIPMENT

- Shooting sports involve the use of different types of firearms (rifle, shotgun, and pistol) of varying sizes and calibers/gauges.
- Rifle competitions offer the greatest variability in the size of firearm used between Olympic and non-Olympic events, ranging from low-velocity rifles in the Olympics (air rifle and .22 caliber) to high-velocity, high-caliber rifles in non-Olympic competition (2,3,5).
- Olympic pistol events utilize low-velocity firearms for competitions (air pistol or .22 caliber pistol); however, there are other, non-Olympic outdoor events that utilize higher-caliber handguns (3).
- Shotgun competitions are generally limited to a 12-gauge shotgun of various sizes and weights depending on the desired spread of the fired pellets (3,5).

- Depending on the type of competition, shooting jackets made of thick, nonslip material are worn to aid in maintaining shooting positions and counteract the recoil of the firearm (5).
- Shooters are allowed to wear shooting-specific shoes that help stabilize their stance; however, in Olympic events, shoes must meet standards set by the ISSF (5).
- Biathletes wear athletic clothing and equipment appropriate for cross-country skiing. During competition, biathletes do not remove their skiing equipment during shooting.
- Blinders are sometimes used to improve focus and prevent distractions within the visual field (5).

PHYSIOLOGY OF SHOOTING/PHYSICAL FITNESS REQUIREMENTS

- Shooting requires athletes to hold static positions for extended periods of time, requiring high degrees of isometric strength and balance (5,12,18,19).
- Biathlon requires both the cardiovascular fitness needed for cross-country skiing, but also upper body strength for maintaining a stable shooting position (6,16,20).
- Cardiovascular fitness is also important as a lower heart rate is favored for precision shooting (21).
- Relative effect of age (RAE) is the concept that athletes whose birthdays are in the beginning of the defined age range represent the dominance of the age group and least discontinuation rate.
  - RAE does not appear to play a significant role in shooting sports as it does in sports where size, strength, and cognitive development are an advantage.
    - Among the French Federation for Shooting Sports participants, a notable exception to this is seen in late adolescent males and adults.
  - It is hypothesized that this is because athletes who have less size or strength advantage self-select into sports such as shooting where they do not need this to be competitive.
  - In the case of adults, previously high-performing athletes from other sports may select disciplines such as shooting once they have lost their competitive edge due to age or injury (22).
- Psychological stressors play a large role in athlete health and performance (23–27). There is evidence that psychological stress related to competition alters HPA axis function in competitive shooters (26), highlighting the importance of identifying psychosocial factors and management strategies that can affect an athlete's health and performance.

MEDICAL ISSUES

- Shooting, particularly at indoor firing ranges, has been associated with higher levels of lead in the blood. Lead levels vary widely depending on the type, quality, and caliber of the ammunition as well as the ventilation of the facility (28,29).
  - Athletes are exposed to lead when fumes from ignition (firing) of ammunition generate airborne lead dust and microparticles. Lead levels are also high at the target due to fragmentation of the bullet on impact. Shooters can inhale lead or contaminate hands, clothing, hair, face, etc. on retrieval of their target. Last, lead exposure can occur while cleaning the firearm (29).
  - Long-term health effects of lead exposure include renal dysfunction, hypertension, increased CVD mortality, hypochromic microcytic anemia, cognitive dysfunction, mood changes, and neurological changes including disrupted layering of myelin (28,29).
  - There is evidence that shooters with higher blood lead levels demonstrate higher levels of hostility (but not verbal or physical aggression) when compared to their archery peers, particularly when blood lead levels are >10 μg/dL (28).
  - Adolescents are at particular risk for long-term health consequences related to lead exposure as myelinogenesis continues until age 25 (29).
  - Female shooters of child-bearing age are also at risk of exposing a fetus or infant to lead via storage of lead in bones that is later mobilized during pregnancy and lactation (29).
  - To minimize the risk of toxic lead levels, shooting athletes should wear protective clothing while shooting, avoid eating and drinking at the firing range, and wash their hands and face thoroughly after leaving the firing range (29).
- Shooting at outdoor firing ranges with protective shooting clothing can potentially subject athletes to thermal stress that can affect health and shooting performance (30).
  - In competition, this is rarely seen as outdoor pistol and rifle events generally shield the athlete under a protective overhang. Therefore, shotgun (high power rifle and long range rifle) athletes are the most exposed to the elements.
  - Heat acclimatization several days prior to competition is recommended to improve exercise-heat tolerance in hot, outdoor conditions (31).
- Biathletes are at risk of cold-related injuries such as frostbite and hypothermia (31,32).
  - Athletes typically use gloves made of thin material to achieve maximal tactile sensation of the trigger for improved shooting accuracy, which puts them at risk for thermal injury (32).
  - Frostbite risk is also higher for support staff, coaches, and officials as their metabolic activity is considerably lower than athletes during competition and are often exposed to the cold for prolonged periods of time (31).
- Exposure to gastrointestinal and upper respiratory infections during travel and competition represent the majority of illness associated with shooting sports (30).
- Hearing loss related to frequent exposure to loud gunfire has previously been reported in the literature (33). The Occupational Safety and Health Administration recommends minimizing exposure to rapid impulse noises greater

than 140 dB. Sound generated by weapons used in competitive shooting sports range from 140 to 160 dB (34).

- Hearing protection should be worn by athletes during training and competition.
- Potential hearing damage in the fetus is another reason why pregnant women may want to avoid shooting.

- Ocular injuries are uncommon in shooting sports. Dry eyes and irritation from dusty environments are the most common ocular issues addressed during event coverage.

MUSCULOSKELETAL ISSUES

- Acute musculoskeletal injuries are relatively uncommon in shooting sports and are typically limited to mild sprains and strains (7–15).
- Overuse injuries account for the vast majority of musculoskeletal injuries seen both in competition and training. These are likely underreported as most injury data collection is done during competition (9).
- Lower back pain is common within rifle disciplines. This is due to the biomechanical stress of holding a shooting stance for a prolonged period of time, particularly in the standing position, which places high load on the facet joints (1,9,12).
  - Kneeling and prone positions are generally better tolerated during back pain flares and can allow an athlete to continue to practice while seeking treatment.
  - However, discogenic back pain may be aggravated by the prone position and may better tolerate the kneeling position until symptoms are controlled.
- Calf and thigh strains can occur from prolonged use during stabilization for shooting stances without appropriate stretching and recovery between shooting sessions (9).
- Foot and ankle sprains are uncommon but occasionally seen during competition when traversing unfamiliar terrain between shooting sessions (14).
- Posterior knee pain can also occur from prolonged hyperextension in standing positions.
- Shoulder pain is a common source of musculoskeletal injury in shotgun athletes, usually caused by the repetitive recoil from the gun (1,9,15,35).
  - Athlete's using over/under shotguns are particularly prone to shoulder pain due to the heavy nature of this firearm when compared to other types of shotguns.
  - The effect of repetitive recoil can also predispose an athlete to shoulder fatigue (35).
- Hand/wrist pain is less frequent than low back and shoulder pain, but commonly seen in pistol athletes (1,9).
  - Rare cases of hypothenar atrophy have been reported in pistol shooters presumably from ulnar nerve entrapment or injury (9).
- The various shooting events place different physiologic and physical demands on the athletes resulting in higher injury rates in males during Winter Olympics and females during Summer Olympics (1).
- Focal dystonia, uncontrollable abnormal movements, or muscle contractions during specific tasks, has been reported in shooting sports.
  - The exact prevalence of dystonia is unknown as this condition is often misdiagnosed.
  - Dystonia most commonly occurs with prolonged or repetitive muscle contractions.
  - Although very rare in shooting sports, the stances and duration of time spent shooting during practice sessions and competitions in shooting sports do increase the risk of dystonia development (36).

INJURY PREVENTION AND TRAINING

- There is no consensus on strength and cardiovascular fitness training in shooting athletes (11). Similar to other sports, the type, frequency, and duration of training programs varies widely and it is unknown how this training translates functionally to improvements in the sport (11,20).
- Studies have shown muscular control on marksmanship score is most significant for standard pistol events with impact of 67%–79% for .22 caliber pistol at 50 feet compared to 15% for shotgun on 48-shot course and 1%–3% for 9.0 mm caliber air pistol at 10 m (11).
- It is well established that decreased postural sway improves performance for shooting athletes. Postural stability is thought to be derived from a combination of core strength, proprioception, and limb strength (upper and lower) (20).
- Likewise, lower resting heart rates are advantageous for maintaining stance stability in shooting sports. Routine cardiovascular exercise can help achieve lower heart rates.

PSYCHOLOGICAL FACTORS

- Stress and anxiety are considered to be beneficial in shooting events as they contribute to a heightened level of alertness. Despite this, if excessive, stress and anxiety can produce elevated heart rate, tremor, and altered concentration, which can all have a detrimental effect on marksmanship (24).
- Routine use of psychological training such as meditation, visualization, breathing techniques, listening to music, etc. have been shown to improve performance in shooting sports. Use of professional psychological support varies in shooting sports but could prove beneficial for athletes that experience high levels of anxiety or poor self-image and confidence (24).
- Although injury rates are low in shooting sports, recovery and return to sport after injury are positively impacted by psychological support from professionals and coaches during the recovery process (24).

MEDICATIONS AND SUPPLEMENTS

- International Shooting Sports Federation, Intercollegiate Pistol Competition (United States and World Anti-Doping Agencies) and National Collegiate Athletic Association ban β-blockers in shooting competitions entirely as they are considered performance-enhancing drugs (37,38) due to the ability to lower an athlete's heart rate and improve postural sway and stability.
- Caffeine is the most widely used stimulant in the general population.
  - Athletes traveling across time zones to compete, much like military and law-enforcement officers, are often faced with decreased marksmanship (performance) from sleep deprivation. Caffeine can be ergogenic when timing and dosing are optimal.
  - A systematic review by Torres and Kim showed that caffeine improves reaction time, particularly during sleep deprivation or stressful environments, but in general did not improve accuracy. Caffeine did seem to mitigate performance decline with fatigue over time such as long events (39).
  - Side effects of caffeine can include increased blood pressure and heart rate causing shakiness and anxiety, which can negatively impact marksmanship (39,40).
  - Optimal caffeine dosing appears to be 3–5 mg/kg. Dosing >5 mg/kg increases the risk of unwanted side effects and can impair performance (39,40).
  - Optimal timing depends on the length of the event. Peak effect occurs about 60 minutes after consumption and the half-life is 4–5 hours (39,40).
  - NCAA has banned guarana-based caffeine and regulates the quantity used to <15 μg/mL in urine samples. WADA has caffeine listed on its watch list for possible performance-enhancing substances (37,38).
- There is rising interest in using purine alkaloids as they have similar effects as caffeine without the unwanted increase in heart rate and blood pressure, thus limiting jitteriness.
  - One study showed a synergistic effect of methylliberine, theacrine and caffeine to achieve a more rapid peak onset that would be sustained over a longer duration. This combination showed similar improvements as caffeine alone in reaction time and sustained performance in marksmanship but without unwanted hemodynamic stress (40).
  - These substances have not specifically been addressed by any of the anti-doping guidelines (37,38).

EVENT COVERAGE

- Medical providers should be familiar with the specific safety protocols and emergency action plans (EAP) for each shooting range.
  - A list of the local hospitals should be obtained and EAPs should be coordinated with EMS prior to larger events.
  - On-site medical supplies for common sports and environmental injury, illness, and trauma should be arranged (provided by the event or the medical team).
- If providing medical coverage for outdoor events, medical providers should dress appropriately according to the weather, for example, light breathable clothing for outdoor events during the summer (skeet and trap shooting) compared to thick jackets and warm boots for events during the winter months (biathlon).
  - Hearing protection and sunglasses are highly recommended regardless of the season.

REFERENCES

1. Harr MR, Mansfield CJ, Urbach B, Briggs M, Onate J, Boucher LC. Prevalence and Incidence of Injury during Olympic-style Shooting Events: A Systematic Review. *Int J Sports Phys Ther.* 2021;16(5):1235–49. Published online October 1, 2021 doi:10.26603/001c.28231
2. ISSF–International Shooting Sport Federation. www.issf-sports.org. https://www.issf-sports.org/theissf/history.ashx
3. *Shooting | sport.* Encyclopedia Britannica. https://www.britannica.com/sports/shooting
4. *Shooting and Para shooting | Olympic & Paralympic Sports.* United States Olympic & Paralympic Museum. Accessed 8, Aug 2023. https://usopm.org/hall-of-fame/shooting/#:~:text=SHOOTING%20%26%20PARA%20SHOOTING
5. Lokegaonkar J. *Gunning for glory: Know everything about shooting at the Olympics.* Olympics.com. Published February 11, 2023. https://olympics.com/en/news/olympic-shooting-air-rifle-3-positions-rapid-fire-air-pistol-shotgun-trap-skeet
6. *A Quick Look at Biathlon through the Years.* International Biathlon Union - IBU. Published January 4, 2022. Accessed August 8, 2023. https://www.biathlonworld.com/news/biathlon-through-the-years/3RgwCwR2wmrfuh52QrcHez
7. Soligard T, Palmer D, Steffen K, et al. New sports, COVID-19 and the heat: sports injuries and illnesses in the Tokyo 2020 Summer Olympics. *Br J Sports Med.* 2022;57(1):46–54. doi:10.1136/bjsports-2022-106155.https://doi.org/10.1136/bjsports-2022-106155
8. Laoruengthana A, Poosamsai P, Fangsanau T, Supanpaiboon P, Tungkasamesamran K. The epidemiology of sports injury during the 37th Thailand National Games 2008 in Phitsanulok. *J Med Assoc Thai.* 2009;92(suppl 6):S204–10.
9. Kabak B, Karanfilci M., Ersöz T., Kabak M. Analysis of sports injuries related with shooting. *J Sports Med Phys Fit.* 2016;56(6):737–43.
10. Soligard T, Steffen K, Palmer D, et al. Sports injury and illness incidence in the Rio de Janeiro 2016 Olympic Summer Games: a prospective study of 11274 athletes from 207 countries. *Br J Sports Med.* 2017;51(17):1265–71. doi:10.1136/bjsports-2017-097956
11. Mon-López D, Moreira da Silva F, Calero Morales S, López-Torres O, Lorenzo Calvo J. What do olympic shooters think about physical training factors and their performance? *Int J Environ Res Public Health.* 2019;16(23):4629. doi:10.3390/ijerph16234629
12. Noormohammadpour P, Rostami M, Mansournia MA, Farahbakhsh F, Pourgharib Shahi MH, Kordi R. Low back pain status of female university students in relation to different sport activities. *Eur Spine J.* 2016;25(4):1196–203. doi:10.1007/s00586-015-4034-7

13. Palmer D, Cooper DJ, Emery C, et al. Self-reported sports injuries and later-life health status in 3357 retired Olympians from 131 countries: a cross-sectional survey among those competing in the games between London 1948 and PyeongChang 2018. *Br J Sports Med.* 2021;55(1):46–53. doi:10.1136/bjsports-2019-101772
14. Engebretsen L, Soligard T, Steffen K, et al. Sports injuries and illnesses during the London summer olympic games 2012. *Br J Sports Med.* 2013;47(7):407–14. doi:10.1136/bjsports-2013-092380
15. Watts M, Densie IK. Duck shooting injuries in Southland, New Zealand. *N Z Med J.* 2013;126(1374):78–9.
16. Köykkä M, Laaksonen MS, Ihalainen S, Ruotsalainen K, Linnamo V. Performance-determining factors in biathlon prone shooting without physical stress. *Scand J Med Sci Sports.* 2022;32(2):414–23. Published online November 2, 2021. doi:10.1111/sms.14087
17. Association NR. An NRA shooting sports journal | 10 interesting facts about the history of the shooting sports. *An NRA Shooting Sports Journal.* Accessed August 8, 2023. https://www.ssusa.org/content/10-interesting-facts-about-the-history-of-the-shooting-sports/
18. Raffalt PC, Fillingsnes Marker I, Adler AT, Alkjaer T. Dynamics of Postural Control in Elite Sport Rifle Shooters. *J Mot Behav.* 2021;53:20–9. Published online February 11, 2020. doi:10.1080/00222895.2020.1723478
19. Era P, Konttinen N, Mehto P, Saarela P, Lyytinen H. Postural stability and skilled performance—a study on top-level and naive rifle shooters. *J Biomech.* 1996;29(3):301–6. doi:10.1016/0021-9290(95)00066-6
20. Zemková E, Zapletalová L. The role of neuromuscular control of postural and core stability in functional movement and athlete performance. *Front Physiol.* 2022;13:796097. doi:10.3389/fphys.2022.796097
21. Sobhani V, Rostamizadeh M, Hosseini SM, Hashemi SE, Refoyo Román I, Mon-López D. Anthropometric, physiological, and psychological variables that determine the elite pistol performance of women. *Int J Environ Res Public Health.* 2022;19(3):1102. doi:10.3390/ijerph19031102
22. Delorme N, Raspaud M. Is there an influence of relative age on participation in non-physical sports activities? The example of shooting sports. *J Sports Sci.* 2009;27(10):1035–42. doi:10.1080/02640410902926438
23. Bühlmayer L, Birrer D, Röthlin P, Faude O, Donath L. Effects of mindfulness practice on performance-relevant parameters and performance outcomes in sports: a meta-analytical review. *Sports Med.* 2017;47(11):2309–21. doi:10.1007/s40279-017-0752-9
24. Moreira da Silva F, Malico Sousa P, Pinheiro VB, López-Torres O, Refoyo Roman I, Mon-López D. Which are the most determinant psychological factors in olympic shooting performance? A self-perspective from elite shooters. *Int J Environ Res Public Health.* 2021;18(9):4637. doi:10.3390/ijerph18094637
25. Park SH, Lim BS, Lim ST. The effects of self-talk on shooting athletes' motivation. *J Sports Sci Med.* 2020;19(3):517–21. Published 2020 Aug 13.
26. Lee JK, Park JK, Kim H, et al. Association of the HPA axis response to upcoming competition and shooting outcomes in elite junior shooting players. *Stress.* 2020;23(2):153–61. doi:10.1080/10253890.2019.1660871
27. Loch F, Ferrauti A, Meyer T, Pfeiffer M, Kellmann M. Acute effects of mental recovery strategies in simulated air rifle competitions. *Front Sports Act Living.* 2023;5:1087995. doi:10.3389/fspor.2023.1087995
28. Naicker N, de Jager P, Naidoo S, Mathee A. Is there a relationship between lead exposure and aggressive behavior in shooters? *Int J Environ Res Public Health.* 2018;15(7):1427. doi:10.3390/ijerph15071427
29. Goldman RH, Woolf AD, Karwowski MP. Gun marksmanship and youth lead exposure: a practice-oriented approach to prevention. *Clin Pediatr.* 2017;56(11):1068–71. doi:10.1177/0009922817701177
30. Tikuisis P, Keefe AA, Keillor J, Grant SW, Johnson RF. Investigation of rifle marksmanship on simulated targets during thermal discomfort. *Aviat Space Environ Med.* 2002;73(12):1176–83.
31. Bergeron M, Bahr R, Bärtsch P, et al. International Olympic Committee consensus statement on thermoregulatory and altitude challenges for high-level athletes. *Br J Sports Med.* 2012;46(11):770–9. doi:10.1136/bjsports-2012-091296
32. Urakov A, Urakova N. *Finger Temperature when Shooting from a rifle in the Cold: thermal Recommendations.* Faculty of Education; 2020:135.
33. Nondahl DM, Cruickshanks KJ, Wiley TL, Klein R, Klein BE, Tweed TS. Recreational firearm use and hearing loss. *Arch Fam Med.* 2000;9(4):352–7. doi:10.1001/archfami.9.4.352
34. Golob J. *Shooting While Pregnant.* Accessed August 8, 2023. https://www.juliegolob.com/wp-content/uploads/2014/01/Ebook_Shooting_While_Pregnant_Resource_for_Expecting_Moms_Julie_Golob.pdf
35. Monzoni R. *Assessment of Effort and Pain after Compak Sporting Competition Using Three Different Over&under Shotguns.* Published online January 1, 2018.
36. Lenka A, Jankovic J. Sports-related dystonia. *Tremor Other Hyperkinet Mov.* 2021;11(1):54. doi:10.5334/tohm.670
37. NCAA. *NCAA Banned Substances.* NCAA.org. Published July 14, 2022. https://www.ncaa.org/sports/2015/6/10/ncaa-banned-substances.aspx
38. *World Anti-Doping Code International Standard Prohibited List 2023.* https://www.wada-ama.org/sites/default/files/2022-09/2023list_en_final_9_september_2022.pdf
39. Torres C, Kim Y. The effects of caffeine on marksmanship accuracy and reaction time: a systematic review. *Ergonomics.* 2019;62(8):1023–32. doi:10.1080/00140139.2019.1613572
40. Cintineo HP, Bello ML, Chandler AJ, Cardaci TD, McFadden BA, Arent SM. Effects of caffeine, methylliberine, and theacrine on vigilance, marksmanship, and hemodynamic responses in tactical personnel: a double-blind, randomized, placebo-controlled trial. *J Int Soc Sports Nutr.* 2022;19(1):543–64. doi:10.1080/15502783.2022.2113339

117 Soccer

Nicholas A. Piantanida, Richard A. Francesco, and Hamish A. Kerr

INTRODUCTION

- Soccer is the most popular sport in the world with an estimated 300 million registered players, which approximates 4% of the world's population (1), and many countries reporting increased participation over the last 20 years.
- Krustrup et al. reported evidence for the health benefits of playing soccer and describe it as a "joyful, social and popular sporting activity" that effectively trains multiple types of fitness and can have a positive benefit across the lifespan (2–6).

BACKGROUND

- The rules of soccer (football) were officially codified by the Football Association (FA) in 1863 in London, England. In 1869, Princeton and Rutgers played the first American intercollegiate football game played by the FA rules.
- The enactment of Title IX in 1972 within the National Collegiate Athletic Association (NCAA) formed the initial American catalyst of soccer growth with a direct effect on the creation of female soccer programs. The 1991 U.S. women's soccer team World Cup victory in China was a second stimulus for growth.
- The soccer World Cup was held in the United States for men and women in 1994 and 1999, respectively, and men will host again in 2026. This local spectacle of sport propelled and elevated the caliber of play of soccer in the United States, which culminated in strong World Cup with the US women's national team winning the tournament in 1991, 1999, 2015, and 2019 and achieving Olympic Gold Medal performances for women's soccer in 1996, 2004, 2008, and 2012. The men's team have had successes, reaching the World Cup quarter finals in 2002, and winning the CONCACAF Gold Cup 7 times.
- The U.S. Soccer Federation is the governing body of soccer in the United States. The professional first divisions for men's and women's soccer in the United States are Major League Soccer (MLS) and National Women's Soccer League (NWSL) respectively. Currently, the MLS is composed of 30 teams, and the NWSL is composed of 14 teams with further expansion to 16 in 2026.

PHYSICAL DEMANDS

- Soccer is classified as a high-to moderate-intensity contact/collision sport by the American Academy of Pediatrics.
- Soccer is classified as a low-static, high-dynamic sport (7).
- Soccer demands change of direction or cutting maneuvers followed by deceleration and jumping with major muscle movement and proprioception through the trunk and lower extremity.
- The aerobic challenges of soccer infuse the endurance requirements of a distance runner with the abrupt acceleration demands of a sprinter. The average distance covered by an elite midfield male player is in the 10-km range, with the strikers, full-backs, and center-backs covering less distance. Sprinting makes up significantly 10% of the total distance (8).
- The physiologic demands of soccer present unique challenges to hydration. Several sport-specific factors expose soccer players to risk of heat injury, including limited stoppage times with periods of intense aerobic activity, large fields with limited to no shade, and numerous games or practice sessions occurring in a day with limited attention to environmental stressors of heat and/or humidity.
- Particular attention must be paid to proper fueling and hydration and to the risk of heat illness.
- In 2006, the U.S. Soccer Federation published its "Youth Soccer Heat Stress Guidelines" based on research conducted at the University of Connecticut (9).
  - As little as 2% body weight drop in young competitors in hot conditions not only generates impairments in performance but also causes a compounded reduction in the ability to dissipate heat, resulting in accelerated heat-related injury.
  - Most experts agree that a 5% drop in body weight during or following a soccer match or practice should sideline that athlete for 24 hours to recuperate fluid losses and to identify an intrinsic etiology such as poor acclimatization, supplement usage, or illness (10,11).
- It has been demonstrated that 30–60 mg of carbohydrate ingestion in the fluids before and during soccer activity can delay muscle glycogen depletion. In one study, indoor soccer athletes who drank a glucose polymer enhanced work output

and increased time to exhaustion when compared to controls (12). Nutrition needs in athletes are discussed in depth in Chapter 12 of this text.

EPIDEMIOLOGY

- The overall injury incidence in soccer varies across studies because of differences in study designs, populations, and injury definitions.
- Soccer has a higher injury rate than many contact sports, including field hockey, rugby, basketball, and football (13) although the severity of injuries may be lower than rugby/football.
- Soccer injury incidence varies based on age, sex, level of participation, and type of exposure (practice vs. game) (13–17).
  - In male soccer athletes, comparison of male elite youth finds game time injuries of 9.5–48.7 injuries/1000 hours compared to practices injuries 3.7–11.4 injuries/1000 hours. Male professional soccer players' injuries for game time participation are 8.7–65.9 injuries/1000 hours compared to practice injuries of 1.4–5.8 injuries/1000 hours.
  - Female youth and female adult soccer players combined as one group, injury incidence ranges from game time injuries of 12.5–30.3 injuries/1000 hours compared to practice injuries of 1.2–3.8 injuries/1000 hours. NCAA injury surveillance reported 8.3 injuries/1000 athletic exposures for 2014–2019 (18).
- Lower extremity injuries are the most common, with non-body contact composing the majority of the injuries (13,14,18–20).
  - Ankle injuries represent 16%–29% of these injuries and predominate among male players.
  - Knee injuries occur in 16%–29% of players and occur more frequently in females.
- Ankle sprain is the single leading injury in soccer and is implicated as a reinjury 56% of the time (21).
- Head injuries represent 1.2%–8% of all injuries, depending on the study (22). The higher head injury rates in youth soccer are thought to be attributed to underdeveloped neck muscles to absorb the impact shock, increased ball weight to head weight ratio, and, more importantly, improper technique heading the ball (23,24).
- There are differences in injury rates between women and men seen for both serious anterior cruciate ligament (ACL) tear injury and concussion-type injuries. Women soccer players sustain more concussions than men, at a ratio of 4.3:1, and more ACL injuries, at ratios of 1.8:1 (practice) and 5.78:1 (games) (25–28).
- Indoor versus outdoor soccer injury rates are similar in severity and type (26).
- Soccer in some countries has migrated to artificial turf. In 2005, Fédération Internationale de Football Association (FIFA) accepted the use of third-generation artificial turf for official tournaments. Research on injury risk on third-generation artificial turf is limited but indicates small differences in injury pattern between artificial turf and natural grass (29).

SOCCER INJURY CHARACTERISTICS

Ankle Injury

- The mechanism of a lateral ankle sprain is often an inversion stress, as the subtalar joint tilts in plantarflexion to manage tasks such as pivoting, jumping, and hard turns while controlling the soccer ball. In this position, the anterior talofibular ligament (ATFL) is at maximal tension and most vulnerable to injury because the stability of the subtalar joint is deviated from the neutral mortise position. The calcaneofibular ligament (CFL) and posterior talofibular ligament follow in order of injury as the magnitude of stress is increased to the ATFL. Ankle injuries are discussed in depth in Chapter 69 of this text.
- Medial ankle ligament injuries are uncommon due to the dominant strength of the deltoid ligament. Therefore, a medial ankle disruption denotes a high-energy impact injury mechanism with a greater likelihood of contact with an opponent and will possibly demonstrate ankle mortise alteration requiring surgical repair and extensive rehabilitation.
- The mechanism of injury for high ankle injuries in soccer players occurs during collisions or player-to-player impact for contested balls. The ankle position during impact can be in the talar neutral position, with or without a slight lateral talar tilt. This predisposes the athlete to greater stresses across the CFL and the inferior anterior tibiofibular ligament.
  - On a clinical exam, performing a proximal tibial-fibular "squeeze test" with distal referred pain at the ankle or instability with external foot rotation is sensitive for a high ankle sprain.
- Talar dome lesions such as osteochondral fractures or a fracture to the lateral process of the talus must be considered in the ankle with persistent pain and swelling beyond 2 weeks.
  - If clinical suspicion is high, magnetic resonance imaging (MRI) can assist in assessing this injury.
- Chronic anterior ankle pain extending on to the midfoot in an injured soccer player who had an acute axial loading of the forefoot and midfoot (kick into the turf) should be evaluated for a bifurcate ligament injury, impingement syndrome (especially for repeat ankle injuries), or Lisfranc fracture.
  - If weight-bearing x-rays of the ankle/foot are normal, then an MRI of the ankle/foot should be done.
- Severs' disease (calcaneal apophysitis) and retrocalcaneal bursitis are commonly seen in young indoor soccer players with ankle pain or hindfoot pain (13,20,21,23) secondary to a pattern of repetitive heel trauma against the sideboards. Achilles tendinopathy and medial calf strains are typically seen in soccer players older than 18 years. Achilles tendinopathy differs from the above two conditions by presenting

several centimeters proximally to the tendon insertion into the calcaneus.

- The use of diagnostic ultrasound helps evaluate Achilles tendinopathy and retrocalcaneal bursitis (30).

- Chronic posterior ankle pain should raise concern for a calcaneal stress fracture as evident by calcaneal squeeze test or an os trigonum fracture. Both can be verified by MRI or triple-phase nuclear bone scan.

Knee Injury

- Soccer players can experience the spectrum of overuse and acute knee problems.
  - Youth players are susceptible to Osgood-Schlatter disease or any other patellofemoral anterior knee tracking maladies seen in all running sports.
  - Senior soccer players incur collateral ligament and meniscal injuries, along with the pain of degenerative osteoarthritis or patellar chondromalacia.
- Meniscal and/or knee ligament injuries are vulnerable during dynamic passing sequences as the grounded cleats of the soccer shoe fixate the leg and support both rapid rotational and flexion changes of the trunk or lower leg. This sports-specific motion produces a sudden rotation of the femur relative to the fixed leg. As mentioned earlier, tackling is a high-risk maneuver where knee ligament strain often occurs when a player is tackled with the loaded leg secured to the ground.
- Soccer athletes can tear their ACL through direct contact or noncontact. Noncontact/non-collision ACL tears are the predominant means for ACL injury in most sports other than skiing. Male collegiate soccer players have an equal rate of contact versus noncontact ACL injuries (31–33). Female collegiate soccer players, however, have higher rates of ACL injury than their male counterparts, and follow the usual trend for noncontact ACL injury. ACL injuries are described in depth in Chapter 61 of this text.
- Contact ACL injuries in male soccer players follow a pattern of collision with a valgus stress to the knee. These injuries are often complicated by associated injuries to the menisci, the collateral ligaments, and the articular cartilage.
- In chondral injuries, soccer maneuvers that require repetitive pivoting and deceleration produce extreme stress on the articular cartilage, generating abrasive wear or the acute disruption of the deep cartilage ultrastructure by large shear forces. Chondral lesions are more often found on the femoral condyle.
  - Acute x-ray imaging for a swollen knee should include tunnel views to investigate an osteochondral fracture, and if present, the fracture should be staged by knee MRI and comanaged with an orthopedic surgeon.

Lower Leg Injury

- A soccer player's lower leg is vulnerable to abrasions, contusions, and fractures. Shin guards have become the only mandatory protective devices in soccer, but serve primarily to protect the leg from minor soft-tissue injuries. Soccer tibial and fibular fractures occur at high rates despite athletes wearing shin guards (34). Robertson et al describe an injury rate of 0.64–0.71/1000 player hours for tibial fractures in soccer (35).
- The soccer player with both a tibia and fibula fracture is sidelined, on average, for 40 weeks. Players with individual fibula and tibia fractures return to competitive play on average in 18 and 35 weeks, respectively (34,36).
  - Nondisplaced tibial diaphyseal fractures may be best managed with primary operative repair, which has improved rate of return and time to return to soccer compared to nonoperative management (35,36).
- The broad differential for exertional lower leg pain incorporates many overuse injuries to the lower extremity. The more common exertional lower leg ailments include chronic exertional compartment syndrome, medial tibial stress syndrome (MTSS), and stress fractures. Less common includes popliteal artery entrapment (37).
- Chronic exertional compartment syndrome is insidious and effort-dependent, with pain associated with running that reduces performance over several months to years. This syndrome is described in depth in Chapter 27 of this text. By contrast, acute compartment syndrome may occur when a player sustains a high-velocity kick to the protected or unprotected portion of the leg.
  - In both cases, the player typically describes lower leg pain with tingling and/or weakness extending to the dorsum of the foot. Diagnostic measurement of compartment pressures with a handheld device and comanagement with an orthopedic surgeon should follow. Nonoperative solutions have also become favored (38).
- Injury patterns for MTSS and stress fractures are multifactorial (intrinsic or extrinsic sources of overuse) and represent maladaptive versions of cyclic tissue and bone recovery.
  - Stress fractures and MTSS are best differentiated by triple-phase bone scan or MRI and treated with phased degrees of activity modification. MRI results depicting a stress fracture have both diagnostic and prognostic recovery parameters.

Hamstring Injury

- Hamstring injuries make up one of the most common musculoskeletal injuries reported by male and female soccer players. Between 2014 and 2019, the most commonly reported injury among Major League Soccer players were hamstring strains (12.3%). Sex, injury setting, and playing surface can contribute to injury type and injury reporting during matches was four times greater than that during periods of training (39,40).
- With hamstring injury, the athletes will generally report an acute sensation of a muscle pull and/or audible pop. The mechanism is most often noncontact in nature and will cause an immediate hindrance to running gait and the ambulatory cycle.

- A palpable and/or physical defect within the muscle belly of the posterior thigh can often be appreciated on initial examination. Paresthesia and sciatica-like pain may also be reported in the following days given the adjacent proximity of the sciatic nerve within the posterior thigh musculature. A decrease in hip extension and knee flexion power is commonly reported. Early swelling and ecchymosis are also common.
- There are two types of injuries that lead to hamstring strain.
  - Type 1 injuries are due to maximum eccentric muscle activation with simultaneous muscle lengthening. This may be observed during explosive bouts of running or jumping. The biceps femoris long head is the most common muscle to be damaged in type 1 hamstring strains.
  - Type 2 injuries appear with excessive lengthening of the hamstrings muscle while the hip is flexed and knee extended. Type 2 injuries occur during the late swing phase of kicking (41).
- The majority of hamstring injuries recover with conservative management. Surgical intervention is indicated for tendon avulsion injury in athletes who suffer compromised performance on healing.
- Return to play is based on equal lower extremity strength, range of motion, and proprioception. Eccentric strengthening exercises of the hamstring muscle group are key to aid prevention of future or repeat injury.
- Given the complexity of hamstring injuries, it is crucial to utilize an individualized approach in evaluating the soccer athlete. Multi-method approaches are paramount to identify determinants of injury severity and recovery within the competitive soccer athlete (41).

Groin Injury

- Although less common, groin and torso injuries may be the most challenging to treat as there is a broad differential diagnosis and clinical presentations often overlap in signs and symptoms (42,43).
- The mechanism of groin injury in the soccer athlete is associated with a force at the groin while the hip is abducted and externally rotated, sometimes against an opposing force such as the ground or the opponent. This process of strain or overstretching compromises the adolescent's apophyseal pelvic ring or pubic attachments or, in the case of the senior player, the muscular-tendinous attachments (44).
- Adductor muscle tendinopathy is a form of overuse strain where groin pain gradually develops after advancing play intensity or frequency of workouts. These cases should be differentiated from osteitis pubis and "sports hernias" (athletic pubalgia), which can present with a similar pain pattern (45).
- Hip flexor strain to the iliopsoas/bursitis is seen in soccer and is clinically defined by deep groin pain with an occasional slapping hip sensation or pain extension onto the anterior thigh.
  - Treatment consists of relative rest with a prescribed stretching program for hip flexors and rotators. In addition, an iliopsoas strengthening program should precede the return to competitive play (46).
- Gilmore groin, or groin disruption, was clinically defined in 1980 following the successful treatment of three professional soccer players who had been sidelined with pain for 3 months. Clinical symptoms of groin disruption include insidious unilateral pain in the adductor region that progresses with activity and follows a course of post-activity aggravation getting out of bed or the car.
  - Exam findings are evasive and variable but may include tenderness and dilation of the internal inguinal ring on scrotal hernia palpation. The anatomic features of this condition include torn external oblique aponeurosis, torn conjoined tendon, conjoined tendon tear from the pubic tubercle, dehiscence between conjoined tendon and inguinal ligament, and no hernia.
  - Diagnosis should include Stork radiographs to evaluate pelvic stability and MRI (43), with arthrography often added to exclude labral tears which can coexist. Diagnostic musculoskeletal ultrasound has also been reported to be useful.
  - Treatment failures after a 2- to 4-week rehabilitative process should proceed to surgery for repair according to Gilmore (47) although more recent review suggests 2 months nonoperative management (48).

Heading and Head Injury

- Most of the head impacts sustained while playing soccer are subconcussive, and as such do not result in symptoms (49,50). When concussions do occur, they typically arise from elbow-to-head, head-to-head, and head-to-ground events (22,24).
- Soccer players with a history of concussion tend to perform worse on computerized neurocognitive testing and baseline preseason neurocognitive testing should be considered (51). Female soccer players with a concussion may perform more poorly than males in neurocognitive testing and have more symptoms (52,53).
  - There are concerns that repeated concussions, and possibly cumulative load of subconcussive blows, may predispose professional soccer players with long careers to degenerative neurological diseases such as motor neuron disease and/or chronic traumatic encephalopathy (54,55). These concerns, although not based on prospective longitudinal investigation, have prompted some soccer federations to limit the exposure to heading the ball at young ages (56).
- One of the challenges identifying concussion in soccer is that 70% of collegiate soccer players experience concussion-like symptoms during a defined season, but only 20% were aware that they sustained an injury (57). Concussions are discussed in depth in Chapter 41 of this text.
- Cervical muscle strength has been suggested may lower head accelerations experienced (58,59). There are strategies being developed to improve soccer-specific neck strength to help prevent injury (60–62).

- Although head injuries and subconcussive impacts in soccer may predispose players to future musculoskeletal injury as well as repeated concussions (63–65), headgear in soccer has not been shown to be protective against concussion (66–70).
- Teaching correct technique for heading should be encouraged (71). Heading is a skill inherent to soccer. Heading technique is a complex synchronized motion whereby the forehead strikes forcefully through the ball as the trunk goes into flexion, which requires coaching and practice. Maintaining a rigid neck during impact diminishes potential injury from angular head and neck acceleration (58).

Facial and Oral Injuries

- The mechanism for eye injuries is usually blunt trauma caused by a kicked ball or the kicking foot. Early referral to an ophthalmologist is crucial, as visual sequelae may manifest in a delayed manner regardless of initial presence of external injury or ocular complaints (72).
  - A hyphema is the most common injury type and can occur in up to 50% of all blunt eye traumas in soccer (13). A hyphema is an injury to the anterior chamber and should be comanaged with an ophthalmologist as there can be complications and long-term consequences.
  - Blunt trauma to the orbital region of the athlete also has the potential to cause significant damage to the posterior segment of the eye. The most common fundoscopic finding is peripheral commotio retina, although retinal injury may also include retinal tear, vitreous hemorrhage, retinal detachment, and/or macular hole.
  - The frequency of eye injuries in soccer has prompted the recommendation by the American Academy of Pediatrics Committee on Sports Medicine and Fitness and the American Academy of Ophthalmology Committee on Eye Safety and Sports Ophthalmology that protective sports eye equipment using polycarbonate lenses be worn during both soccer practice and competition (73,74).
  - Eye injuries are discussed in depth in Chapter 35 of this text.
- Orofacial and dental injuries in soccer rank second behind basketball (75,76) but are exceedingly rare events. Widespread use of protective mouthguards has been advocated in the dental literature to reduce the number of such injuries (77), but this practice is not supported in the sports medicine literature.
  - Maxillofacial and dental injuries are discussed further in Chapters 36 and 37 of this text.

PREVENTION

- Educating soccer players on the importance of fair play, compliance with the rules and proper technique, especially with heading is paramount. Enforcement of infringements for dangerous play, such as leading with an elbow, has been championed by FIFA.
- Injury prevention and optimizing sport performance is closely related, and up to 75% of soccer injuries can be reduced by 75% by the implementation of a multilevel preventative approach (78). FIFA 11+ is a 20-minute warm-up exercise program, developed in 2006, which has shown improvement in both injury and performance metrics. This includes a greater than 50% reduction in overuse injuries as well as significant improvement in measurements of balance and strength in the intervention group (79,80).
- Attention to equipment utilization, including shin guards and mouthguards, and optimal field conditions pays dividends on injury prevention.
- Use of wet bulb globe temperature (WBGT) in accordance with American College of Sports Medicine guidelines should direct periods of play or practice and hydration standards.
- Prophylactic ankle taping or bracing benefits players with clinical instability or history of previous ankle strain, although certain player demographics have been found to benefit from prophylactic bracing without prior ankle injury. Acute lateral ankle sprains are the single most often diagnosed injury in female soccer players, and a 50% reduction of such injuries has been seen with prophylactic soccer-specific ankle bracing in amateur women players (81).
- Arnason et al. have demonstrated a significant reduction in hamstring strains in elite soccer players through eccentric hamstring strengthening (82).
- Neuromuscular training (NMT) programs designed to increase dynamic strength, agility, and balance offer significant protective benefits in risk reduction from ankle sprain injury (83).
  - Those with a history of ankle instability will benefit most from proprioceptive training of the lower extremity. Grimm et al. underscore the utility of such ankle injury prevention programs in the athletic soccer player (84).
- NMT programs can decrease the incidence of ACL injuries in youth soccer players (85). Female soccer players are in a position to receive the most benefit from such programs. However, recent research shows male athletes undergoing NMT programs reporting a reduction in similar injuries. NMT should be incorporated early in the athlete's career under the guidance from a qualified health or physical education professional.
- Players with significant knee instability do not benefit from bracing, as the movements inherent to soccer (pivoting, cutting, acceleration and deceleration) cannot be adequately controlled (86–88). To avoid the risk of ACL injury, exclusion from soccer participation is worthy of discussion.
- Prophylactic strengthening to the hip adductor muscle group to prevent groin injury is best accomplished utilizing the Copenhagen Adduction exercise. Prior hip adduction strengthening regimens had not shown a significant reduction in groin strain (89).
- Educate players and staff on the early identification and management of concussions. Preseason standardized neuropsychological testing should be done in patients at risk.

- Team physicians should prescribe a supervised and progressive rehabilitative process. Return-to-play decisions after injury should come directly from the team physician and physical therapist.
  - End-state rehabilitation and functional goals include full range of motion, 90% strength, and dynamic agility testing (90).

REFERENCES

1. Khan KM, Thompson AM, Blair SN, et al. Sport and exercise as contributors to the health of nations. *Lancet*. 2012;380(9836):59–64.
2. Krustrup P, Aagaard P, Nybo L, Petersen J, Mohr M, Bangsbo J. Recreational football as a health promoting activity: a topical review. *Scand J Med Sci Sports*. 2010;20(suppl 1):1–13.
3. Krustrup P, Bangsbo J. Recreational football is effective in the treatment of non-communicable diseases. *Br J Sports Med*. 2015;49(22):1426–7.
4. Krustrup P, Hansen PR, Andersen LJ, et al. Long-term musculoskeletal and cardiac health effects of recreational football and running for premenopausal women. *Scand J Med Sci Sports*. 2010;20(suppl 1):58–71.
5. Krustrup P, Krustrup BR. Football is medicine: it is time for patients to play. *Br J Sports Med*. 2018;52(22):1412–4.
6. Krustrup P, Williams CA, Mohr M, et al. The "Football is Medicine" platform-scientific evidence, large-scale implementation of evidence-based concepts and future perspectives. *Scand J Med Sci Sports*. 2018;28(suppl 1): 3–7.
7. Levine BD, Baggish AL, Kovacs RJ, Link MS, Maron MS, Mitchell JH. Eligibility and disqualification recommendations for competitive athletes with cardiovascular abnormalities: task force 1—classification of sports—dynamic, static, and impact—a scientific statement from the American Heart Association and American College of Cardiology. *J Am Coll Cardiol*. 2015;66(21):2350–5.
8. Reilly T, Thomas V. An analysis of work-rate in different positional roles in professional football match-play. *J Hum Movement Sci*. 1976;2:87–97.
9. Soccer U. *U.S. Soccer Federation Youth Soccer Heat Stress Guidelines*; 2007. Available from: https://onthepitch.org/wp-content/uploads/2007/08/ussf_hydration_guide.pdf
10. Casa DJ, Armstrong LE, Hillman SK, et al. National athletic trainers' association position statement: fluid replacement for athletes. *J Athl Train*. 2000;35(2):212–24.
11. Maughan RJ, Shirreffs SM, Merson SJ, Horswill CA. Fluid and electrolyte balance in elite male football (soccer) players training in a cool environment. *J Sports Sci*. 2005;23(1):73–9.
12. Foster C, Thompson NN, Dean J, Kirkendall DT. Carbohydrate supplementation and performance in soccer players. *Med Sci Sports Exerc*. 1986;18:12.
13. Koutures CG, Gregory AJ, American Academy of Pediatrics Council on Sports Medicine and Fitness. Injuries in youth soccer. *Pediatrics*. 2010;125(2):410–4.
14. Junge A, Rösch D, Peterson L, Graf-Baumann T, Dvorak J. Prevention of soccer injuries: a prospective intervention study in youth amateur players. *Am J Sports Med*. 2002;30(5):652–9.
15. Pfirrmann D, Herbst M, Ingelfinger P, Simon P, Tug S. Analysis of injury incidences in male professional adult and elite youth soccer players: a systematic review. *J Athl Train*. 2016;51(5):410–24.
16. Junge A. Epidemiology in female football players. In: Volpi P, editor *Football Traumatology* 2nd ed. Switzerland: Springer International Publishing; 2015:21–8.
17. López-Valenciano A, Ruiz-Pérez I, Garcia-Gómez A, et al. Epidemiology of injuries in professional football: a systematic review and meta-analysis. *Br J Sports Med*. 2020;54(12):711–8.
18. Chandran A, Morris SN, Boltz AJ, Robison HJ, Collins CL. Epidemiology of injuries in national collegiate athletic Association Women's soccer: 2014-2015 through 2018-2019. *J Athl Train*. 2021;56(7):651–8.
19. Engström B, Johansson C, Törnkvist H. Soccer injuries among elite female players. *Am J Sports Med*. 1991;19(4):372–5.
20. Schmidt-Olsen S, Jørgensen U, Kaalund S, Sørensen J. Injuries among young soccer players. *Am J Sports Med*. 1991;19(3):273–5.
21. Emery CA, Meeuwisse WH, Hartmann SE. Evaluation of risk factors for injury in adolescent soccer: implementation and validation of an injury surveillance system. *Am J Sports Med*. 2005;33(12):1882–91.
22. Putukian M, Echemendia RJ, Chiampas G, et al. Head injury in soccer: from science to the field; summary of the head injury summit held in April 2017 in New York City, New York. *Br J Sports Med*. 2019;53(21):1332.
23. Sullivan JA, Gross RH, Grana WA, Garcia-Moral CA. Evaluation of injuries in youth soccer. *Am J Sports Med*. 1980;8(5):325–7.
24. Watson A, Mjaanes JM, Council On Sports M, Fitness. Soccer injuries in children and adolescents. *Pediatrics*. 2019;144(5):e20192759.
25. Arendt E, Dick R. Knee injury patterns among men and women in collegiate basketball and soccer. NCAA data and review of literature. *Am J Sports Med*. 1995;23(6):694–701.
26. Emery CA, Meeuwisse WH. Risk factors for injury in indoor compared with outdoor adolescent soccer. *Am J Sports Med*. 2006;34(10):1636–42.
27. Hewett TE, Myer GD, Ford KR. Anterior cruciate ligament injuries in female athletes: Part 1, mechanisms and risk factors. *Am J Sports Med*. 2006;34(2):299–311.
28. Kiani A, Hellquist E, Ahlqvist K, Gedeborg R, Michaëlsson K, Byberg L. Prevention of soccer-related knee injuries in teenaged girls. *Arch Intern Med*. 2010;170(1):43–9.
29. Fuller CW, Dick RW, Corlette J, Schmalz R. Comparison of the incidence, nature and cause of injuries sustained on grass and new generation artificial turf by male and female football players. Part 2: training injuries. *Br J Sports Med*. 2007;41(suppl 1):i27–32.
30. Konarski W, Poboży T. The utility of ultrasound in the diagnostic evaluation of the posterior ankle joint. *Med Ultrason*. 2021;23(2):226–30.
31. Boden BP, Dean GS, Feagin JA Jr, Garrett WE Jr. Mechanisms of anterior cruciate ligament injury. *Orthopedics*. 2000;23(6):573–8.
32. Delfico AJ, Garrett WE Jr. Mechanisms of injury of the anterior cruciate ligament in soccer players. *Clin Sports Med*. 1998;17(4):779–85. vii.
33. Yu B, Garrett WE. Mechanisms of non-contact ACL injuries. *Br J Sports Med*. 2007;41(suppl 1):i47–51.
34. Boden BP. Leg injuries and shin guards. *Clin Sports Med*. 1998;17(4):769–77. vii.
35. Robertson GAJ, Ang KK, Jamal B. Fractures in soccer: the current evidence, and how this can guide practice. *J Orthop*. 2022;33:25–30.
36. Boden BP, Lohnes JH, Nunley JA, Garrett WE Jr. Tibia and fibula fractures in soccer players. *Knee Surg Sports Traumatol Arthrosc*. 1999;7(4):262–6.
37. Sirico F, Palermi S, Gambardella F, et al. Ankle Brachial index in different types of popliteal artery entrapment syndrome: a systematic review of case reports. *J Clin Med*. 2019;8(12):2071.
38. Zimmermann WO, Hutchinson MR, Van den Berg R, Hoencamp R, Backx FJG, Bakker EWP. Conservative treatment of anterior chronic exertional compartment syndrome in the military, with a mid-term follow-up. *BMJ Open Sport Exerc Med*. 2019;5(1):e000532.
39. Forsythe B, Knapik DM, Crawford MD, et al. Incidence of injury for professional soccer players in the United States: a 6-year prospective study of major League soccer. *Orthop J Sports Med*. 2022;10(3): 23259671211055136.

40. Chandran A, Elmi A, Young H, DiPietro L. Determinants of lower-extremity injury severity and recovery in U.S. High School Soccer Players. *Res Sports Med.* 2022;30(3):272–82.
41. Garcia AG, Andrade R, Afonso J, Runco JL, Maestro A, Espregueira-Mendes J. Hamstrings injuries in football. *J Orthop.* 2022;31:72–7.
42. Poor AE, Roedl JB, Zoga AC, Meyers WC. Core muscle injuries in athletes. *Curr Sports Med Rep.* 2018;17(2):54–8.
43. de Sa D, Hölmich P, Phillips M, et al. Athletic groin pain: a systematic review of surgical diagnoses, investigations and treatment. *Br J Sports Med.* 2016;50(19):1181–6.
44. Serner A, Tol JL, Jomaah N, et al. Diagnosis of acute groin injuries: a prospective study of 110 athletes. *Am J Sports Med.* 2015;43(8):1857–64.
45. Taylor R, Vuckovic Z, Mosler A, et al. Multidisciplinary assessment of 100 athletes with groin pain using the Doha agreement: high prevalence of adductor-related groin pain in conjunction with multiple causes. *Clin J Sport Med.* 2018;28(4):364–9.
46. Morelli V, Smith V. Groin injuries in athletes. *Am Fam Physician.* 2001;64(8):1405–14.
47. Gilmore J. Groin pain in the soccer athlete: fact, fiction, and treatment. *Clin Sports Med.* 1998;17(4):787–93. vii.
48. Hopkins JN, Brown W, Lee CA. Sports hernia: definition, evaluation, and treatment. *JBJS Rev.* 2017;5(9):e6.
49. Basinas I, McElvenny DM, Pearce N, Gallo V, Cherrie JW. A systematic review of head impacts and acceleration associated with soccer. *Int J Environ Res Public Health.* 2022;19(9):5488.
50. Caccese JB, Lamond LC, Buckley TA, Kaminski TW. Reducing purposeful headers from goal kicks and punts may reduce cumulative exposure to head acceleration. *Res Sports Med.* 2016;24(4):407–15.
51. Mihalik JP, Lynall RC, Teel EF, Carneiro KA. Concussion management in soccer. *J Sport Health Sci.* 2014;3(4):307–13.
52. Colvin AC, Mullen J, Lovell MR, West RV, Collins MW, Groh M. The role of concussion history and gender in recovery from soccer-related concussion. *Am J Sports Med.* 2009;37(9):1699–704.
53. Caccese JB, Bryk KN, Porfido T, CARE Consortium Investigators, et al. Cognitive and behavioral outcomes in male and female NCAA Soccer athletes across multiple years: a CARE consortium study. *Med Sci Sports Exerc.* 2023;55(3):409–17.
54. Mackay DF, Russell ER, Stewart K, MacLean JA, Pell JP, Stewart W. Neurodegenerative disease mortality among former professional soccer players. *N Engl J Med.* 2019;381(19):1801–8.
55. Myer GD, Barber Foss K, Thomas S, et al. Altered brain microstructure in association with repetitive subconcussive head impacts and the potential protective effect of jugular vein compression: a longitudinal study of female soccer athletes. *Br J Sports Med.* 2019;53(24):1539–51.
56. Lalji R, Snider H, Chow N, Howitt S. The 2015 U.S. Soccer Federation header ban and its effect on emergency room concussion rates in soccer players aged 10-13. *J Can Chiropr Assoc.* 2020;64(3):187–92.
57. Delaney JS, Frankovich R. Head injuries and concussions in soccer. *Clin J Sport Med.* 2005;15(4):216–13. discussion 2-3.
58. Dezman ZD, Ledet EH, Kerr HA. Neck strength imbalance correlates with increased head acceleration in soccer heading. *Sports Health.* 2013;5(4):320–6.
59. Gutierrez GM, Conte C, Lightbourne K. The relationship between impact force, neck strength, and neurocognitive performance in soccer heading in adolescent females. *Pediatr Exerc Sci.* 2014;26(1):33–40.
60. Peek K, Andersen J, McKay MJ, et al. The effect of the FIFA 11 + with added neck exercises on maximal isometric neck strength and peak head impact magnitude during heading: a pilot study. *Sports Med.* 2022;52(3):655–68.
61. Müller C, Zentgraf K. Neck and trunk strength training to mitigate head acceleration in youth soccer players. *J Strength Cond Res.* 2021;35(suppl 12):S81–9.
62. Becker S, Berger J, Backfisch M, Ludwig O, Kelm J, Fröhlich M. Effects of a 6-week strength training of the neck flexors and extensors on the head acceleration during headers in soccer. *J Sports Sci Med.* 2019;18(4):729–37.
63. Kakavas G, Malliaropoulos N, Blach W, Bikos G, Migliorini F, Maffulli N. Ball heading and subclinical concussion in soccer as a risk factor for anterior cruciate ligament injury. *J Orthop Surg Res.* 2021;16(1):566.
64. Biese KM, Kliethermes SA, Watson AM, et al. Musculoskeletal injuries and their association with previous concussion history: a prospective study of high school volleyball and soccer players. *Am J Sports Med.* 2021;49(6):1634–41.
65. Brooks MA, Peterson K, Biese K, Sanfilippo J, Heiderscheit BC, Bell DR. Concussion increases odds of sustaining a lower extremity musculoskeletal injury after return to play among collegiate athletes. *Am J Sports Med.* 2016;44(3):742–7.
66. McGuine T, Post E, Pfaller AY, et al. Does soccer headgear reduce the incidence of sport-related concussion? A cluster, randomised controlled trial of adolescent athletes. *Br J Sports Med.* 2020;54(7):408–13.
67. Naunheim RS, Ryden A, Standeven J, et al. Does soccer headgear attenuate the impact when heading a soccer ball? *Acad Emerg Med.* 2003;10(1):85–90.
68. Delaney JS, Al-Kashmiri A, Drummond R, Correa JA. The effect of protective headgear on head injuries and concussions in adolescent football (soccer) players. *Br J Sports Med.* 2008;42(2):110–5. discussion 5.
69. Broglio SP, Ju YY, Broglio MD, Sell TC. The efficacy of soccer headgear. *J Athl Train.* 2003;38(3):220–4.
70. Mansell J, Tierney RT, Sitler MR, Swanik KA, Stearne D. Resistance training and head-neck segment dynamic stabilization in male and female collegiate soccer players. *J Athl Train.* 2005;40(4):310–9.
71. Caccese JB, Kaminski TW. Minimizing head acceleration in soccer: a review of the literature. *Sports Med.* 2016;46(11):1591–604.
72. Leshno A, Alhalel A, Fogel-Levin M, Zloto O, Moisseiev J, Vidne-Hay O. Pediatric retinal damage due to soccer-ball-related injury: results from the last decade. *Eur J Ophthalmol.* 2021;31(1):240–4.
73. Vinger PF, Capão Filipe JA. The mechanism and prevention of soccer eye injuries. *Br J Ophthalmol.* 2004;88(2):167–8.
74. American Academy of Pediatrics Committee on Sports Medicine and Fitness. Protective eyewear for young athletes. *Pediatrics.* 2004;113(3 pt 1):619–22.
75. Flanders RA, Bhat M. The incidence of orofacial injuries in sports: a pilot study in Illinois. *J Am Dent Assoc.* 1995;126(4):491–6.
76. Tesini DA, Soporowski NJ. Epidemiology of orofacial sports-related injuries. *Dent Clin North Am.* 2000;44(1):1–18. v.
77. Powers JM, Godwin WC, Heintz WD. Mouth protectors and sports team dentists. Bureau of health education and audiovisual services, council on dental materials, instruments, and equipment. *J Am Dent Assoc.* 1984;109(1):84–7.
78. Ekstrand J, Gillquist J. Soccer injuries and their mechanisms: a prospective study. *Med Sci Sports Exerc.* 1983;15(3):267–70.
79. Thorborg K, Krommes KK, Esteve E, Clausen MB, Bartels EM, Rathleff MS. Effect of specific exercise-based football injury prevention programmes on the overall injury rate in football: a systematic review and meta-analysis of the FIFA 11 and 11+ programmes. *Br J Sports Med.* 2017;51(7):562–71.
80. Vlachas T, Paraskevopoulos E. The effect of the FIFA 11+ on injury prevention and performance in football: a systematic review with meta-analysis. *BioMed.* 2022;2(3):328–40.
81. Thijs K, Huisstede B, Goedhart E, Backx F. The preventive effect of a soccer-specific ankle brace on acute lateral ankle sprains in girls amateur soccer players: study protocol of a cluster-randomised controlled trial. *Inj Prev.* 2019;25(3):152–6.

82. Arnason A, Andersen TE, Holme I, Engebretsen L, Bahr R. Prevention of hamstring strains in elite soccer: an intervention study. *Scand J Med Sci Sports*. 2008;18(1):40–8.
83. Owoeye OBA, Palacios-Derflingher LM, Emery CA. Prevention of ankle sprain injuries in youth soccer and basketball: effectiveness of a neuromuscular training program and examining risk factors. *Clin J Sport Med*. 2018;28(4):325–31.
84. Grimm NL, Jacobs JC Jr, Kim J, Amendola A, Shea KG. Ankle injury prevention programs for soccer athletes are protective: a level-I meta-analysis. *J Bone Joint Surg Am*. 2016;98(17):1436–43.
85. Campbell CJ, Carson JD, Diaconescu ED, Canadian Academy of Sport and Exercise Medicine, et al. Canadian Academy of Sport and Exercise Medicine position statement: Neuromuscular training programs can decrease anterior cruciate ligament injuries in youth soccer players. *Clin J Sport Med*. 2014;24(3):263–7.
86. Trojian TH, Mohamed N. Demystifying preventive equipment in the competitive athlete. *Curr Sports Med Rep*. 2012;11(6):304–8.
87. Rishiraj N, Taunton JE, Lloyd-Smith R, Regan W, Niven B, Woollard R. Effect of functional knee brace use on acceleration, agility, leg power and speed performance in healthy athletes. *Br J Sports Med*. 2011;45(15):1230–7.
88. Rishiraj N, Taunton JE, Lloyd-Smith R, Woollard R, Regan W, Clement DB. The potential role of prophylactic/functional knee bracing in preventing knee ligament injury. *Sports Med*. 2009;39(11):937–60.
89. Harøy J, Clarsen B, Wiger EG, et al. The Adductor Strengthening Programme prevents groin problems among male football players: a cluster-randomised controlled trial. *Br J Sports Med*. 2019;53(3):150–7.
90. Maestroni L, Turner A, Papadopoulos K, et al. Comparison of strength and power characteristics before ACL rupture and at the end of rehabilitation before return to sport in professional soccer players. *Sports Health*. 2023 May;15(6):814–23. doi:10.1177/19417381231171566

118 Softball Injuries

Lindsay J. DiStefano, Brandon Bentley, and Allison Schafer*

INTRODUCTION

- Competitive fast-pitch softball is a sport predominantly played by women, though many co-ed and men's leagues exist as well. Slow-pitch softball is also seeing a rise in popularity around the world; however, the majority of the literature surrounding softball is centered around fast-pitch softball, which will remain the focus of this chapter.
- Softball has been an National Collegiate Athletic Association (NCAA) sport since 1982 and was an Olympic sport from 1996 to 2008 and returned as an Olympic sport in 2020 (held in 2021 due to the COVID-19 pandemic).
- During the 2018–2019 academic years, high school fast-pitch softball was the fifth most popular sport, with 368,640 participants (1).

RULES AND REGULATIONS

- Softball is frequently compared to baseball as the overall structure is quite similar. When appropriate, references to the rules and regulations of baseball will be provided for comparison.
- Softball, like baseball, has nine field positions: Pitcher, catcher, first base, second base, third base, shortstop, left field, center field, and right field.
- Regulation games consist of seven innings *(Baseball: nine innings)*.
- Distance between bases: 18.29 m (60 ft) *(Baseball: 60 ft [Little League] to 90 ft)*.
- Distance between the pitcher's mound and home plate: 13.11 m (43 ft) (14 and under: 12.19 m [40 ft]; 12 and under: 10.66 m [35 ft]) *(Baseball: 46 ft [Little League] to 60.5 ft)*.
- In contrast to baseball, the pitching mound in softball is not elevated.
- The ball size is 30.5 cm (12 in) *(Baseball: 23 cm [9 in])*.

*Authors acknowledge the late Dr. Jeffrey Anderson and his contribution to an earlier version of this chapter in the first edition of this text. The sports medicine community is forever grateful for his contributions and friendship.

INJURY EPIDEMIOLOGY

- The rate of injuries in softball, both high school and collegiate, has increased over the last 10 years. This increase could be secondary to better-reporting mechanisms or changes with the game and training.
- Injuries requiring medical disqualification for a season are relatively uncommon in softball. Knee sprains/strains, fractures, and concussions are the most common reasons for disqualification in high school softball (2).

High School Softball

- From 2004–2005 through 2013–2014 season, the overall injury rate for high school softball is 1.16/1000 athlete exposures (AE) (3).
- The most injured body parts were the head and face (3).
- Most shoulder and elbow injuries in the high school population are due to overuse, with a rate of shoulder injuries: 1.4/10,000 AEs and a rate of elbow injuries: 0.41/10,000 AEs (4).

NCAA Softball

- The intercollegiate injury data come from studies using the NCAA Injury Surveillance Program (ISP) from 2014–2015 to 2018–2019 seasons (5).
- Softball accounts for 9% of all female NCAA athletes.
- The overall injury rate from 2014 to 2019 is reported at 3.92/1000 AEs with preseason injury rates being higher (5.23/1000 AEs) than regular season (3.49/1000 AEs) and postseason being the lowest (2.58/1000 AEs).
- Shoulder injuries have the highest prevalence rate (15.2%), followed by hand/wrist (11.8%), knee (11.2%), and head/face injuries (11.2%) with the majority of these reported as contusions, sprains, and inflammatory conditions.
- Overuse injuries account for 29.4% of injuries.
- Head and face injuries account for just over 7% of collegiate injuries, and contact with a pitched or batted ball is the common mechanism of injury (6).
- Although time loss from injury fluctuates, on average, about one-third of NCAA softball-related injuries result in time loss from sport.

- Overall, the position of outfielder seems to account for the greatest proportion of injuries (23.76%), followed by middle infielder (17.27%) and pitchers (15.55%).

Professional Softball

- Although few studies exist, initial data report an overall injury rate of 3.78/1000 AEs per professional season with the majority of injuries occurring during competition.
- Over 70% of injuries account for <1 week out of sport.
- Position players are more likely to injure lower extremities while pitchers have equal rates of lower extremity and upper-extremity injuries (7).

Time Loss

- Softball injury epidemiology has primarily focused on time-loss (TL) injuries, or those injuries requiring >24 hours away from softball participation. Non-time-loss (NTL) injuries also represent a significant impact on sports medicine health-care as the volume of NTL injuries among softball players is more prevalent than TL injuries among high school athletes.
- NTL injuries in softball are often less severe than TL injuries.
  - When counting both TL and NTL injuries, Snyder Valier et al. reported an overall injury rate of 7.56/1000 AEs between 2011 and 2014 (8).
  - Between 2011 and 2014, the rate of NTL softball-related injuries in US secondary schools was 6.32/1000 AEs, accounting for 83% of all injuries (8).
  - NTL injuries were more common during preseason activity versus regular season or postseason, and most frequently affected the shoulder, hands/fingers, elbow, and ankle.
  - Contusions, abrasions, and strains were the most common NTL injury diagnoses.

Mechanism of Injury

- Most data come from the NCAA, and injury rates and patterns vary by position. Veillard et al. (5) reported overall injuries by position from the NCAA ISP data. This is shown in Figure 118.1.
- Batting and pitching account for more competition injuries, while throwing and general play accounts for most practice injuries (5).
- The most common mechanism of injury during games is contact with something (*e.g.*, ground, base, ball, and wall) other than a person (5,6,9), and in high school softball, this is usually due to base running (9).
- The majority of practice injuries are due to noncontact mechanisms (no contact with anything external to the body) (*e.g.*, throwing and running) (6,9).
- Base running is responsible for <10% of all collegiate game injuries (5) but 32.7% of all high school game injuries (9).
- 11% of collegiate game-related injuries are the result of being struck by a ball (6).

Pitching

- Pitchers are more likely to be injured by a batted ball (22.4% of acute injuries in pitchers) than by other causes.
- The pitcher is more likely to sustain a facial fracture than other players on the field.
- Regular-season game injuries to the shoulder in pitchers cause 11.2% of game injuries.
- The windmill pitch makes softball unique compared to baseball and other upper-extremity sports. The windmill pitch requires the pitcher to circumduct his or her extended arm 485° around the body and release the ball below the hip with an underarm motion.

SPECIFIC INJURIES

Shoulder

- Shoulder injury rate in high school softball between 2005 and 2017 was 1.14/10,000 AEs.
- Shoulder injuries most frequently occurred in competition versus practices, and greater than 50% were due to overuse/insidious mechanisms of injury (4).

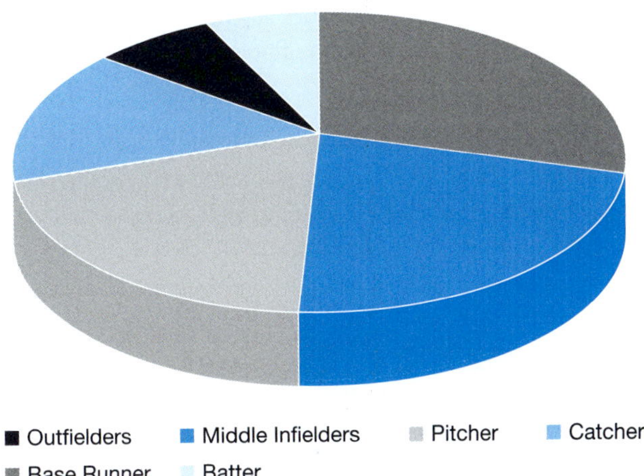

Figure 118.1: Injury rates by position in fast-pitch softball. (From the NCAA Injury Surveillance Program Veillard KL, Boltz AJ, Robison HJ, Morris SN, Collins CL, Chandran A. Epidemiology of injuries in National Collegiate Athletic Association women's softball: 2014–2015 through 2018–2019. *J Athl Train*. 2021;56(7): 734–41.)

- In practices, throwing — not including pitching — caused more than half of softball injuries (68.2%) as compared with competition injuries (23.5%); injury proportion ratio [IPR]: 2.90.
  - Though perhaps counterintuitive, less than 20% of shoulder injuries in high school softball occur in pitchers.
- Muscle strain/incomplete tears are the most common shoulder injuries in softball (35.0%) (10).
- Biceps-labral complex injuries are considered the most common shoulder injury in overhead athletes.
  - Examination should include O'Brien active compression test, resisted throwing test, and palpation of the bicipital tunnel. These three maneuvers result in a more sensitive result than the traditional Speed, Yergason, and full and empty can tests (11).
  - Rehabilitation should focus on glenohumeral and scapulothoracic strength and mobility.
- 5.3% of softball athletes sustained shoulder injuries that required surgery, which is less than the 10% reported prevalence among baseball athletes. Although the literature does not specify specific injury surgery rates, rotator cuff, labral, and bicep surgeries are most common.
  - Injuries that were sustained while the athlete was on the pitcher's mound were significantly more likely to result in surgery than any other field position (10).
- Adolescent softball athletes with upper-extremity pain are more likely to have decreased external rotation and decreased total range of motion in the shoulder, as well as restricted hip range of motion (12).
  - Evaluation and management of hip restriction should not be missed, as it has implications on throwing mechanics and recovery.
- ROM deficits in softball athletes do not appear to be predictive of subsequent shoulder or elbow injury (13).
- The Functional Arm Scale for Throwers (FAST, Figure 118.2) is a validated and reliable patient-reported outcome scale in softball athletes (13).
  - Patients answer questions and are given scores related to pain, throwing, activities of daily living (ADLs), psychological health, and advancement.
  - This distinguishes between pitchers and field positions.
  - The FAST can be used to track and monitor progress made during rehabilitation and readiness to return to sport.

Elbow

- From the 2005–2006 season through 2015–2016 season, the overall rate of elbow injuries in high school softball was roughly 0.40/10,000 AEs (4,14).
- Elbow injuries most frequently occurred in competition versus practices, and greater than 50% were due to overuse/insidious mechanisms of injury (4).
- Pitchers accounted for less than 20% of elbow injuries in high school softball elbow injuries in softball are less likely to require surgery than in baseball (14).
- The majority of elbow injuries in softball occur while throwing (nonpitching).
  - Outfielders have the highest rate of elbow injuries, accounting for 27.1% of all elbow injuries in high school softball (14).
  - Literature is lacking on specific injury diagnosis; however, the extensor mechanism (both strains and tendinosis) is typically the most frequent elbow complaint.
- Elbow injuries requiring surgery are rare and most can be resolved utilizing rehabilitation and evaluation of throwing mechanics.
- X-rays can be diagnostic in certain pediatric cases of apophysitis but will often be nondiagnostic for ligament and intra-articular conditions. Because of this deficiency, MRI and MRI arthrograms are often utilized for elbow injury diagnosis.

Ulnar Diaphyseal Stress Fractures

- The postulated mechanism of development of the stress injury includes repetitive flexion of the wrist (15) or recurrent pronation of the wrist (16).
- Athletes will present with vague pain in the ulnar associated with specific repetitive activity. Pain is often reproduced with resisted pronation, wrist flexion, and flexion of the ulnar-sided digits of the hand (17,18). Workup is similar to other stress injuries, including radiographs, magnetic resonance imaging, and radionuclide bone scans.

Lower Extremity Injuries

- Similar to concussions, the incidence rates of anterior cruciate ligament (ACL) injuries (0.74/10,000 AEs) and ankle sprain injuries (3.2/10,000 AEs) in softball are relatively low compared to other intercollegiate sports (19,20).
- However, both injuries are more frequent in softball compared to baseball (ACL injuries: 0.11/10,000 AEs; ankle sprains: 2.3/10,000 AEs).
- These data suggest that a sex discrepancy in ACL injuries between softball and baseball does exist, which correlates with other sports such as basketball and soccer.
- Despite the overall relatively low injury rate for ACL injuries in softball, knee internal derangement injuries still account for nearly 10% of overall injuries in the sport (ACL injuries account for 33% of these injuries) (6).

Concussions

- Although concussions are not extremely common in softball compared to contact and collision sports, concussion rates are nearly twice as high as those reported in high school baseball (21).
- The reason for this higher incidence of injury may be due to possible sex differences in concussion pathology or the closer distances between bases and the pitcher's position relative to home plate.
- Concussions in NCAA softball typically occur due to catching, fielding, or pitching. A much lower proportion of

1. How satisfied are you with the way your arm is now functioning?
☐ Completely ☐ Extremely ☐ Moderately ☐ Slightly ☐ Not satisfied at all

2 How much pain do you have prior to your start, following your warm-up?
☐ None ☐ Mild ☐ Moderate ☐ Severe ☐ Extreme

3. How much strength have you lost in your arm as a result of your injury?
☐ None ☐ Mild ☐ Moderate ☐ Severe ☐ Extreme

4. How much strength have you lost in your arm as a result of your arm injury?
☐ None ☐ Mild ☐ Moderate ☐ Severe ☐ Extreme

5. How much pain or discomfort do you have in your arm with daily activities involving reaching?
☐ None ☐ Mild ☐ Moderate ☐ Severe ☐ Extreme

6. How much pain or discomfort do you have in your arm if you use it for activities that last longer than 30 minutes?
☐ None ☐ Mild ☐ Moderate ☐ Severe ☐ Extreme

7. How much has your arm injury limited your ability to advance in baseball or softball?
☐ Not at all ☐ Slightly ☐ Moderately ☐ Severely ☐ Extremely

8. How much have you modified your behavior to avoid making your arm injury worse?
☐ Not at all ☐ Slightly ☐ Moderately ☐ Severely ☐ Extremely

9. Since your arm injury, do you have a more negative outlook on life?
☐ Not at all ☐ Slightly ☐ Moderately ☐ Severely ☐ Extremely

10. How much does your arm injury interfere with the things that are important, other than sports?
☐ Not at all ☐ Slightly ☐ Moderately ☐ Severely ☐ Extremely

11. How stiff is your arm at night?
☐ Not at all ☐ Slightly ☐ Moderately ☐ Severely ☐ Extremely

12. How much has your playing time gone down since the injury to your arm?
☐ Not at all ☐ Slightly ☐ Moderately ☐ Severely ☐ Extremely

13. How much are you limited when lifting your arm overhead to get dressed?
☐ Not at all ☐ Slightly ☐ Moderately ☐ Severely ☐ Extremely

14. Has your enjoyment of life decreased since your arm injury?
☐ Not at all ☐ Yes, slightly ☐ Yes, moderately ☐ Yes, severely ☐ Yes, extremely

15. Has your arm injury decreased how long you can continue throwing during a single game or practice?
☐ Not at all ☐ Yes, slightly ☐ Yes, moderately ☐ Yes, severely ☐ Yes, extremely

16. Have your sports accomplishments decreased since your arm injury?
☐ Not at all ☐ Yes, slightly ☐ Yes, moderately ☐ Yes, severely ☐ Yes, extremely

17. Has your life been more stressful because of your arm injury?
☐ Not at all ☐ Yes, slightly ☐ Yes, moderately ☐ Yes, severely ☐ Yes, extremely

18. How much has your arm injury limited your ability to throw "long toss"?
☐ Not at all ☐ Slightly ☐ Moderately ☐ Severely ☐ Unable to Throw

19. How much has your throwing accuracy decreased since your arm injury?
☐ Not at all ☐ Slightly ☐ Moderately ☐ Severely ☐ Unable to Throw

20. How weak does your arm feel during throwing?
☐ Not at all ☐ Slightly ☐ Moderately ☐ Severely ☐ Unable to Throw

21. How painful is your arm during "game speed" throwing?
☐ Not at all ☐ Slightly ☐ Moderately ☐ Severely ☐ Unable to Throw

22. How painful is your arm during 50–75% effort throwing?
☐ Not at all ☐ Slightly ☐ Moderately ☐ Severely ☐ Unable to Throw

Pitchers Only:

1. How much has your arm injury limited the speed of your pitches?
☐ Not at all ☐ Slightly ☐ Moderately ☐ Severely ☐ Unable to perform

2. How much has your arm injury limited your ability to throw "bullpen" sessions?
☐ Not at all ☐ Slightly ☐ Moderately ☐ Severely ☐ Unable to perform

3. How much has your arm injury limited your ability to "hit your spots"?
☐ Not at all ☐ Slightly ☐ Moderately ☐ Severely ☐ Unable to perform

4. How limited is your ability to pitch your turn in the rotation?
☐ Not at all ☐ Slightly ☐ Moderately ☐ Severely ☐ Unable to perform

5. How much have your overall pitching statistics been hurt since your arm injury?
☐ Not at all ☐ Slightly ☐ Moderately ☐ Severely ☐ Unable to perform

6. How much has your pitch count decreased since your arm injury?
☐ Not at all ☐ Slightly ☐ Moderately ☐ Severely ☐ Unable to perform

7. How much has your arm injury limited your ability to throw different types of pitches?
☐ Not at all ☐ Slightly ☐ Moderately ☐ Severely ☐ Unable to perform

8. Has your "feel" for pitching decreased since your arm injury?
☐ Not at all ☐ Slightly ☐ Moderately ☐ Severely ☐ Unable to perform

9. Do you need more time to recover between outings since your arm injury?
☐ Not at all ☐ Slightly ☐ Moderately ☐ Severely ☐ Unable to perform

Note: 22 questions for all throwers with nice additional questions specifically for pitchers. Each question is scored on a Likert Scale, 1 point – 5 points. Score may be broken down into categories for Pain, Throwing, ADLs, Psychological Health, and Advancement. (adapted from https://orthotoolkit.com/fast/)

Figure 118.2: The Functional Arm Scale for Throwers (FAST). There are 22 questions for all throwers with nine additional questions specifically for pitchers. Each question is scored on a Likert Scale, 1 point–5 points. Score may be broken down into categories for Pain, Throwing, ADLs, Psychological Health, and Advancement. (Permission from Sauers EL, Bay RC, Snyder Valier AR, Ellery T, Huxel Bliven KC. The functional arm scale for throwers (FAST)—Part I: the design and development of an upper extremity region-specific and population-specific patient-reported outcome scale for throwing athletes. *Orthopa J Sports Med*. 2017;5(3). doi:10.1177/2325967117698455)

concussions occur during batting compared to baseball (22). However, the mechanism of sport related concussion in both sports is due to equipment/apparatus contact (23).

- Concussion rates in high school and college are reported between 2 and 3/10,000 AEs. Rates are slightly higher during competition play than during practice (23,24).

Head and Face Injuries

- In softball, the most common injuries presenting to the Emergency Department are head and neck injuries (25).
  - Among head, neck, and face injuries, contusions, abrasions, and lacerations are the most prevalent (26), with the most common mechanism being contact with a ball (27).
  - Facial fractures account for roughly 15% of head and face injuries with the vast majority of these resulting from a ball strike (27).
  - Orbital blowout fractures are one of the most common facial fractures (28).
    - On-field assessment should evaluate for step-off, extraocular eye movement (to assess for entrapment), testing of cranial nerves, and bruising (specifically Battle sign, which would indicate skull fracture).
    - Providers should have a high level of suspicion for a facial fracture when an athlete is struck by a ball. Often, emergency room evaluation is warranted.
      - Tonometry should be utilized to evaluate intraocular pressure.
      - CT is the gold standard for initial imaging.
      - Ophthalmology consultation may be required.
- There are over 600,000 sports-related eye injuries reported to the emergency department each year. Softball accounts for 4.1% of these with 25% of the injuries being corneal/scleral abrasion (29).
  - It is reported nationally that roughly 19,000 pediatric eye injuries occur each year and 20% of these occur in recreational softball/baseball (second only to basketball).
    - 71% of these were due to being struck with the ball (30).
  - The sideline physician should consider carrying fluorescein dye for evaluation of ocular abrasions, particularly corneal injuries, and when evaluating for potential globe rupture.
  - Point-of-care ultrasound can also be used to evaluate traumatic eye injuries, such as vitreous hemorrhage, retinal detachment, and lens dislocation.
- 12.4% of the 22,000 annual dental injuries in pediatric patients are attributed to baseball/softball (31,32).

Peripheral Nerve Injuries

- Although peripheral nerve injuries, such as carpal and cubital tunnel-related injuries, account for a small proportion of injuries in high school softball (0.57 per 100,000 AEs), these injuries are often due to overuse and have the highest rate of being recurrent (33).

INJURY PREVENTION

Training and Mechanics

- No formal injury prevention pitching programs have been studied in softball, but recommendations for exercise-based prevention and pitching mechanics exist.
- Poor trunk and pelvic control place increased loads on the throwing shoulder and are associated with pain (34–37).
  - Trunk positioning and rotation are important to facilitate a straight and smooth throwing arm circle and allow the efficient transfer of energy.
  - Pelvic and core stability exercises are recommended (37).
  - Trunk positioning and rotation are important to facilitate a straight and smooth throwing arm circle and allow the efficient transfer of energy.
  - Position of the center of mass and stride length at foot contact are also associated with upper-extremity pain in softball pitchers, which may be due to poor balance.
- Proper conditioning must be emphasized in all levels of softball due to the high prevalence of overuse injuries and preseason injuries.
- Neuromuscular training programs, such as ACL injury prevention programs, have demonstrated success with other sports, but have yet to be studied in softball. These programs may be beneficial for reducing a variety of noncontact injuries (*e.g.*, muscle strains, ankle sprains, and knee pathologies).
- Sliding in softball, both headfirst and feet first, demonstrates higher injury rates than baseball at 42.0/1000 versus 4.9/1000 slides (38). Therefore, the American Academy of Orthopaedic Surgeons has recommended the following regarding sliding (39).
  - Sliding is prohibited with players under 10 years old.
  - Proper instruction in sliding technique should be provided, and players should practice their technique using a sliding bag.
  - The runner should slide to avoid a collision at home plate.

Field Equipment

- Breakaway bases should be encouraged at all levels of softball.
  - Traditional stationary bases are bolted to a metal post and sunk into the ground. In contrast, breakaway bases are snapped onto grommets attached to anchored rubber mats, which hold them in place. Sliding will dislodge this attachment, but normal running will not disrupt the attachment.
  - Janda et al. (40) demonstrated that breakaway bases in recreational softball games reduced sliding injuries by 98% and associated medical costs by 99%.
  - These bases are currently allowed by most softball governing bodies (NCAA, National Federation of State High School Associations [NFHS], Amateur Softball Association of America [ASA]), but are not mandatory.

- The American Academy of Orthopaedic Surgeons has supported the use of breakaway bases to prevent injuries and reduce health care costs (39).

- A double base for first base (runner's base) should be considered for all levels of softball.
  - Currently required in International Softball Federation championships and the ASA, allowed by the NFHS, but not allowed by the NCAA.
  - The American Academy of Orthopaedic Surgeons recommends the double base to prevent ankle and foot injuries (39).

Player Equipment

- Batting helmet face masks should be encouraged, if not mandated, by all levels of softball to protect the batter and base runner.
  - These face masks are currently required by USA Softball and NFHS, but not NCAA.
  - Face masks for fielders should also be considered to help prevent facial injuries in the field.
    - May be most beneficial for pitchers.
    - Currently allowed, but not required by the NFHS, NCAA, and USA.

Pitcher Safety

- The windmill method of pitching does not reduce the stress on pitchers' shoulders, so pitch counts and interval-throwing programs should be used to help reduce shoulder injuries.
- Pitch distance increased from 40 to 43 feet by NFHS and ASA for high school softball to reduce pitching injuries in 2010–2011.
- Pitch counts appear to be directly associated with shoulder pain and injury risk in high school-aged softball pitchers (41).
- Youth softball pitchers are reported to throw as many as 1200 pitches during a 3-day tournament (42).
- Pitch counts are not required to be followed in softball, but recommendations exist.
- The American Orthopaedic Society for Sports Medicine recommends the following (www.stopsportsinjuries.com):
  - Softball pitchers <13 years old avoid pitching on more than two consecutive days.
  - Softball pitchers >13 years old avoid pitching more than three days in a row.
  - Specific maximum pitch counts per age (Table 118.1).

Sliding Safety

- Sliding is prohibited with players under 10 years old.

Table 118.1 Recommended Maximum Pitch Counts for Softball

Age	Pitches/Game	Pitches/Day Days 1 and 2	Pitches/Day Day 3
8–10	50	80	0
10–12	65	95	0
13–14	80	115	80
15 and older	100	140	100

Source: Adapted from AOSSM, https://ncys.org/wp-content/uploads/2022/02/2022_ST_Softball-Injuries-2.pdf

- Proper instruction in sliding technique should be provided, and players should practice their technique using a sliding bag.
- The runner should slide to avoid a collision at home plate.

COVERAGE CONSIDERATIONS

- An emergency action plan (EAP) should be developed, reviewed, and practiced at each institution for each specific location of sports activity by all stakeholders present (*e.g.*, healthcare providers, coaches, and officials) to optimize the chain of survival.
- Associated coordinated care plans and procedures for specific injuries and medical conditions should accompany the institution's EAPs.
- Environmental conditions should be closely monitored for safety by the healthcare team. Specifically, heat and lightning are common environmental concerns for softball.
- The Plan & Procedure for Heat-Related Conditions should include the following (44):
  - Event guidelines for hot, humid weather conditions, with consideration of wet-bulb globe temperature (WBGT).
  - Signs and symptoms of heat illness can include dizziness, headache, nausea, weakness, cramps, fatigue, and decreased cognitive function.
  - Heat stroke should be suspected in individuals with central nervous system dysfunction and a core body (rectal) temperature >105°F (40.5°C). Immediate cooling via cold water immersion should occur.
- The Plan & Procedure for Lightning should include the following:
  - Seek shelter in an enclosed building or metal car/bus (dugouts are not appropriate).
  - Resumption of sport can occur after 30 minutes from the last sign of lightning (lightning seen or thunder heard).

REFERENCES

1. Association NCS. *High School Sports*; 2022. Available from: https://www.ncsasports.org/articles-1/high-school-sports
2. Tirabassi J, Brou L, Khodaee M, Lefort R, Fields SK, Comstock RD. Epidemiology of high school sports-related injuries resulting in medical disqualification: 2005-2006 through 2013-2014 academic years. *Am J Sports Med.* 2016;44(11):2925–32.
3. Wasserman EB, Register-Mihalik JK, Sauers EL, et al. The first decade of web-based sports injury surveillance: descriptive epidemiology of injuries in US high school girls' softball (2005-2006 through 2013-2014) and National Collegiate Athletic Association women's softball (2004-2005 through 2013-2014). *J Athl Train.* 2019;54(2):212–25.
4. Oliver GD, Saper MG, Drogosz M, et al. Epidemiology of shoulder and elbow injuries among US high school softball players, 2005-2006 through 2016-2017. *Orthop J Sports Med.* 2019;7(9):2325967119867428.
5. Veillard KL, Boltz AJ, Robison HJ, Morris SN, Collins CL, Chandran A. Epidemiology of injuries in National Collegiate Athletic Association women's softball: 2014–2015 through 2018–2019. *J Athl Train.* 2021;56(7): 734–41.
6. Marshall SW, Hamstra-Wright KL, Dick R, Grove KA, Agel J. Descriptive epidemiology of collegiate women's softball injuries: National Collegiate Athletic Association Injury Surveillance System, 1988-1989 through 2003-2004. *J Athl Train.* 2007;42(2):286–94.
7. Patel N, Bhatia A, Mullen C, Bosman E, Lear A. Professional women's softball injuries: an epidemiological cohort study. *Clin J Sport Med.* 2021;31(1):63–9. doi:10.1097/jsm.0000000000000698
8. Snyder Valier AR, Bliven KCH, Gibson A, et al. Non–time-loss and time-loss softball injuries in secondary school athletes: a report from the National Athletic Treatment, Injury and Outcomes Network (NATION). *J Athl Train.* 2020;55(2):188–94.
9. Powell JW, Barber-Foss KD. Sex-related injury patterns among selected high school sports. *Am J Sports Med.* 2000;28(3):385–91.
10. Krajnik S, Fogarty KJ, Yard EE, Comstock RD. Shoulder injuries in US high school baseball and softball athletes, 2005-2008. *Pediatrics.* 2010;125(3):497–501. doi:10.1542/peds.2009-0961
11. Calcei JG, Boddapati V, Altchek DW, Camp CL, Dines JS. Diagnosis and treatment of injuries to the biceps and superior labral complex in overhead athletes. *Curr Rev Musculoskelet Med.* 2018 Mar;11(1):63–71.
12. Martin CL, Pobocik K, Hannah M, Faherty MS, Christopher S, Vallabhajosula S. Clinical measures of adolescent softball players with and without upper-extremity pain: a preliminary study. *J Sport Rehabil.* 2022;31(8):971–7.
13. Shanley E, Rauh MJ, Michener LA, Ellenbecker TS, Garrison JC, Thigpen CA. Shoulder range of motion measures as risk factors for shoulder and elbow injuries in high school softball and baseball players. *Am J Sports Med.* 2011;39(9):1997–2006.
14. Pytiak AV, Kraeutler MJ, Currie DW, McCarty EC, Comstock RD. An epidemiological comparison of elbow injuries among United States high school baseball and softball players, 2005-2006 through 2014-2015. *Sports Health.* 2018;10(2):119–24.
15. Mutoh Y, Mori T, Suzuki Y, Sugiura Y. Stress fractures of the ulna in athletes. *Am J Sports Med.* 1982;10(6):365–7.
16. Tanabe S, Nakahira J, Bando E, Yamaguchi H, Miyamoto H, Yamamoto A. Fatigue fracture of the ulna occurring in pitchers of fast-pitch softball. *Am J Sports Med.* 1991;19(3):317–21.
17. Grossfeld SL, Van Heest A, Arendt E, House J. Pitcher's periostitis. A case report. *Am J Sports Med.* 1998;26(2):303–7.
18. Verhey JT, Verhey E, Holland D, Baker JC, Long JR. Ulnar shaft stress fractures in fast-pitch softball pitchers: a case series and proposed mechanism of injury. *Skeletal Radiol.* 2021;50(4):835–40.
19. Hootman JM, Dick R, Agel J. Epidemiology of collegiate injuries for 15 sports: summary and recommendations for injury prevention initiatives. *J Athl Train.* 2007;42(2):311–19.
20. Stanley LE, Kerr ZY, Dompier TP, Padua DA. Sex differences in the incidence of anterior cruciate ligament, medial collateral ligament, and meniscal injuries in collegiate and high school sports:2009-2010 through 2013-2014. *Am J Sports Med.* 2016;44(6):1565–72. doi:10.1177/0363546516630927
21. Kerr ZY, Chandran A, Nedimyer AK, Arakkal A, Pierpoint LA, Zuckerman SL. Concussion incidence and trends in 20 high school sports. *Pediatrics.* 2019;144(5):e20192180.
22. Gessel LM, Fields SK, Collins CL, Dick RW, Comstock RD. Concussions among United States high school and collegiate athletes. *J Athl Train.* 2007;42(4):495–503.
23. Chandran A, Boltz AJ, Morris SN, et al. Epidemiology of concussions in National Collegiate Athletic Association (NCAA) sports: 2014/15-2018/19. *Am J Sports Med.* 2022;50(2):526–36.
24. Pierpoint LA, Collins C. Epidemiology of sport-related concussion. *Clin Sports Med.* 2021;40(1):1–18.
25. Lee A, Farooqi AS, Talwar D, Maguire KJ. Pediatric softball injuries presenting to emergency departments. *Pediatr Emerg Care.* 2022;10:1097.
26. Kim M, Moeller E, Thaller SR. Sports-related craniofacial injuries among pediatric and adolescent females: a National Electronic Injury Surveillance System database study. *J Craniofac Surg.* 2021;32(4):1603–6.
27. Strickland JS, Crandall M, Bevill GR. A retrospective analysis of softball-related head and facial injuries treated in United States emergency departments, 2013-2017. *Orthop J Sports Med.* 2019;7(2):2325967119825660.
28. Boyette JR, Pemberton JD, Bonilla-Velez J. Management of orbital fractures: challenges and solutions. *Clin Ophthalmol.* 2015 Nov;9:92127–37.
29. Patel V, Pakravan P, Mehra D, Watane A, Yannuzzi NA, Sridhar J. Trends in sports-related ocular trauma in United States emergency departments from 2010 to 2019: multi-center cross-sectional study. *Semin Ophthalmol.* 2023;9:333–7.
30. Miller KN, Collins CL, Chounthirath T, Smith GA. Pediatric sports-and recreation-related eye injuries treated in US emergency departments. *Pediatrics.* 2018;141(2):e20173083.
31. Montero E, Kistamgari S, Chounthirath T, Michaels NL, Zhu M, Smith GA. Pediatric sports-and recreation-related dental injuries treated in US emergency departments. *Clin Pediatr.* 2019;58(11–12):1262–70.
32. Jowett AD, Brukner PD. Fifth metacarpal stress fracture in a female softball pitcher. *Clin J Sport Med.* 1997;7(3):220–1.
33. Zuckerman SL, Kerr ZY, Pierpoint L, Kirby P, Than KD, Wilson TJ. An 11-year analysis of peripheral nerve injuries in high school sports. *Phys Sportsmed.* 2019;47(2):167–73.
34. Kibler WB, Kuhn JE, Wilk K, et al. The disabled throwing shoulder: spectrum of pathology—10-year update. *Arthroscopy.* 2013;29(1):141.e26–61.e26.
35. Oliver GD, Dwelly PM, Kwon Y-H. Kinematic motion of the windmill softball pitch in prepubescent and pubescent girls. *J Strength Cond Res.* 2010;24(9):2400–7.
36. Oliver GD, Gilmer GG, Anz AW, et al. Upper extremity pain and pitching mechanics in National Collegiate Athletic Association (NCAA) division I softball. *Int J Sports Med.* 2018;39(12):929–35.
37. Wasserberger KW, Friesen KB, Downs JL, Bordelon NM, Oliver GD. Comparison of pelvis and trunk kinematics between youth and

collegiate windmill softball pitchers. *Orthop J Sports Med.* 2021;9(8): 23259671211021826.
38. Stovak M, Parikh A, Harvey AT. Baseball and softball sliding injuries: incidence and correlates during one high school league varsity season. *Clin J Sport Med.* 2012;22(6):501–4.
39. American Academy of Orthopaedic Surgeons. Position statement: use of breakaway bases in preventing recreational baseball and softball injuries. *Am Acad Orthop Surg.* 2010;1140.
40. Janda DH, Wojtys EM, Hankin FM, Benedict ME, Hensinger RN. A three-phase analysis of the prevention of recreational softball injuries. *Am J Sports Med.* 1990;18(6):632–5.
41. Gooch B, Lambert BS, Goble H, McCulloch PC, Hedt C. Relationship between pitch volume and subjective report of injury in high school female fast-pitch softball pitchers. *Sports Health.* 2022;14(5):702–9. doi:10.1177/19417381211051381
42. Lear A, Patel N. Softball pitching and injury. *Curr Sports Med Rep.* 2016;15(5):336–41. doi:10.1249/jsr.0000000000000293
43. Huxel Bliven KC, Snyder Valier AR, Bay RC, Sauers EL. The Functional Arm Scale for Throwers (FAST)—part II: reliability and validity of an upper extremity region-specific and population-specific patient-reported outcome scale for throwing athletes. *Orthop J Sports Med.* 2017;5(4):2325967117700019.
44. Casa DJ, DeMartini JK, Bergeron MF, et al. National Athletic Trainers' Association position statement: exertional heat illnesses. *J Athl Train.* 2015;50(9):986–1000.

119 Sailing

Joanne B. "Anne" Allen

INTRODUCTION

- Sailing was a mode of transportation and trade until the 1600s, when yachts were built for King Charles I and were raced along the Thames.
- Competitive sailboat racing became more popular with the start of the first "America's Cup" Race in 1851 off the Isle of Wight. It is now the oldests continuously contested trophy in the world.
- The modern-day sport of sailboat racing takes many forms with different event types, sailboat classes, crew positions, venues, and competitive scenarios.
- Events include team and solo global circumnavigation races, such as The Ocean Race, the Around Alone Race, and the Fastnet, in addition to the Olympic and Paralympic Games.
- In addition to professional racing, amateur sailors of all ages also compete in world and national class championships, college and high school events, and local race weeks and club regattas.
- High-performance sailboat racing with faster speeds requires the sports medicine team to increase attention to emergency management, safety, and injury prevention.

BACKGROUND

- Sailing as a sport is governed by the International Federation of World Sailing and respective national governing bodies. They follow the Racing Rules of Sailing which may vary according to each event and are overseen by race officials.
- The "playing field" is a body of water and the racecourse varies depending on the environment, geography, wind, waves, current visibility, temperatures, and weather patterns. The event itself may be racing around buoys, or may cover vast distances and long periods of time.
  - The courses may even include ice, for ice boating.
- Racing is inclusive of all genders, races, ethnicities, and ages from Juniors to Great Grand Masters, with some events classified as "open," and others as men's/women's/mixed.
- Similar to motorsports, sailing races are usually won by the first boat to cross the finish line that has properly completed the course.
  - In a regatta, there can be multiple races, with cumulative times or points to determine victory.
- Types of races
  - Fleet races — The most common form of competitive sailing; this involves boats racing around a set course for time. Handicap ratings may be assigned, and ultimately the fastest adjusted time wins (Figure 119.1).
  - Match races — Involve two boats racing head-to-head against each other on a course, and the first across the finish line wins, though penalties for rule infractions may be assigned during the race.
  - Team races — Typically two teams of three boats each competing against each other. Points are awarded for finishing position, and the team with the most points wins. Teams use tactics not only to finish first but also to attempt to slow their opponents.
  - Distance races — Vary in duration and distance, racing from point A to point B, and sometimes around the globe.
- Understanding sailing terminology such as port/starboard, windward/leeward, and sailing maneuvers such as tacking and jibbing, as well as the right of way rules, is necessary for medical and safety providers.

SAILBOATS/EQUIPMENT

- Sailing races also vary in boat classes and equipment, crew numbers and positions, and physical and mental demands (1).
- The basic parts of a sailboat are shown in Figure 119.2.
- Several types of sailboats are used in racing at different levels:
  - Keelboat — It has a weighted keel that counter-balances the force on the sails. These larger boats are often raced competitively, but offer a larger deck for stability.
  - Dinghy — Generally, dinghies are under 22 feet in length and are lighter in weight. Though there may be a range of designs, these boats typically have centerboards or daggerboards rather than a deep, heavy keel. Because of their size

Figure 119.1: Racing of lightning class sailboats. A: Spinnaker sailing downwind. B: Lightning Class racing.

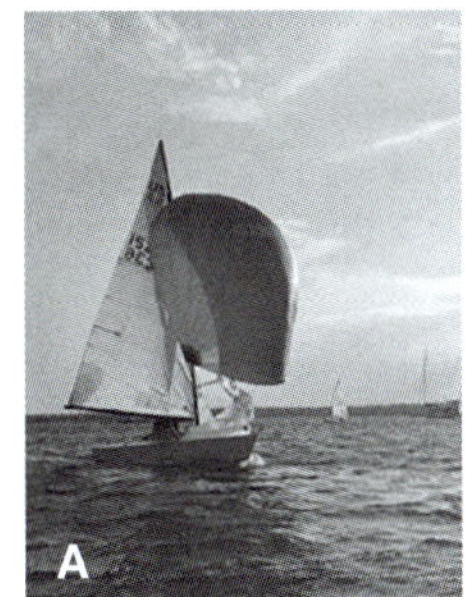

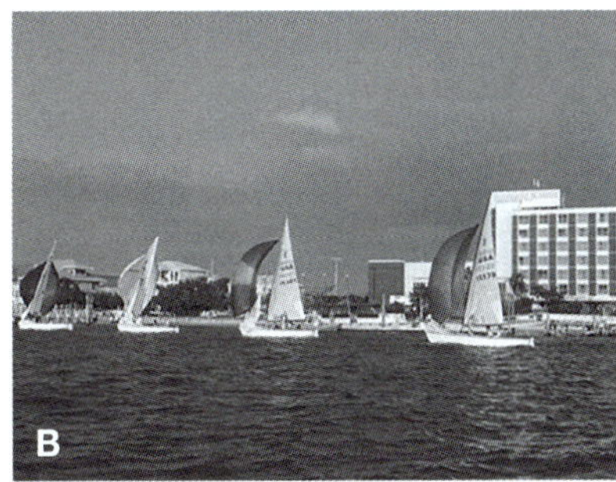

and simplicity, many dinghies can be sailed by just one or two people and are often used to teach beginners to sail. The International Laser Class Association class (formerly called Laser) is a type of single-handed dinghy commonly used in racing both in club regattas and at the Olympic level.

- Skiff — These are lightweight dinghies mostly sailed by two people with a "rack" that extends the sailor's bodies outside the smaller central hull. The sailors are also attached to the boats with a trapeze wire and harness that allow the sailors to project their bodies well outside of the hull to counterbalance the power of the sails.
- Catamaran — These are boats with two hulls connected by a trampoline. The sailors use trapeze wires/harnesses to project their bodies outboard with their feet on the edge of the windward hull for counterbalance. These boats have no keel or daggerboards to prevent side slippage.
- Windsurfer — These are single sails attached to a surfboard via a universal joint. The windsurfer controls the sail via a wishbone that functions similarly to the boom of a traditional boat.
- Kite boards — These boats are simply small-sized "surfboards" that are propelled across the water. The sailor is attached to a large kite by a harness and lines. The kite direction, and therefore the board direction, is controlled by varying the tension along four lines, via a bar. Different kite sizes may be used depending on the wind strength. There are generally two types of kites — pump kites and foil kites. Pump kites have air bladders that need to be pumped up, and these bladders retain the aerofoil shape of the kite. Whereas foil kites do not have air bladders, and it is the directed flow of the air around the kite that helps the kite hold its shape. Unlike the older disciplines, kite boarders can do jumps into the air by directing the kite swiftly upward (Figure 119.3).
- Foil sailing involves a hydrofoil attached beneath a monohull, a catamaran, or a board. Hydrofoils are wing-like structures mounted under the hull or board, lifting it out of the water as the speed increases. This decreases drag and increases speed further, often in excess of the wind speed. In kite foiling, the hydrofoil is attached to a kiteboard; in wind foiling, the hydrofoil is attached to a

Figure 119.2: The Anatomy of a Sailboat: 1 — mainsail, 2 — staysail, 3 — spinnaker, 4 — hull, 5 — keel, 6 — rudder, 7 — skeg, 8 — mast, 9 — spreader, 10 — shroud, 11 — sheet, 12 — boom, 13 — mast, 14 — spinnaker pole, 15 — backstay, 16 — forestay, 17 — boom vang. (*Source:* https://en.wikipedia.org/wiki/Stays_(nautical)#/media/File:Sailingboat-lightning-num.svg.)

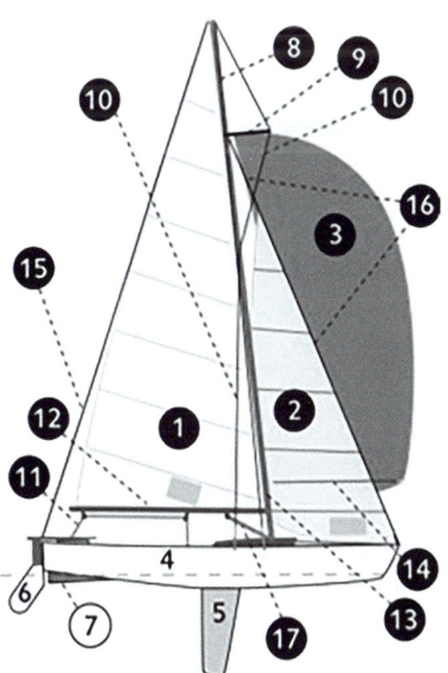

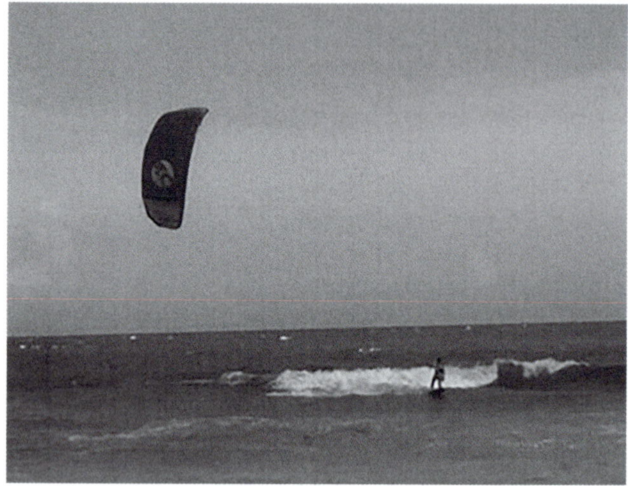

Figure 119.3: Kite sailing.

windsurf board, and the sailor stands on the board holding a wing (handheld sail). Foiling was introduced in the Olympics in Brazil in the North American Catamaran Racing Association class 2016, and in the America's Cup in 2021, and has grown in popularity. The America's Cup Class is currently sailed professionally in a 75-ft hydrofoiling monohull with foil cant arms and a 26.5 m mast, which can reach speeds up to 50 knots and is crewed by an eight-person team (Figure 119.4).

- The Olympic and Paralympic classes vary. They currently include one and two person dinghies, foiling board/kite sailing, foiling multihulls, and high-performance skiffs.
  - Inclusion of sailors with impairments on an even playing field with able-bodied sailors has been well demonstrated in multiple classes with adaptive equipment.
- Protective gear, such as personal flotation devices (PFDs), impact vests, helmets, foul weather gear, and safety harnesses, is needed depending on the type of racing and weather conditions.
  - As extreme sailing and high-performance boats have been increasing in popularity, water safety helmet, and body armor use (in high-speed sailing) has also become more common.
  - Proper sunscreen and eye protection are also strongly recommended (1).

BIOMECHANICS

- Whether a high school sailor in a local series, a grand-master racing in a national championship, a team who is racing in a world championship, or a crew of 12 racing in a trans-pacific ocean race, a wide variety of skills are required and the biomechanics differ with each crew position and boat type, and risk of injury is thus different with each sailing maneuver (2).
  - These skills include the physical demands of:
    - Helming the boat-steering, either with a large wheel or tiller.
    - Trimming the sails (sometimes on large "coffee grinder" winch handles on larger keelboats) — optimizes the shape and position of the sails relative to the wind.
    - Hiking is the action of moving the crew's body weight as far to the windward (upwind) side as possible, in order to decrease the extent to which the boat heels (leans away from the wind). This is shown in Figure 119.5.
    - Trapeze work involves a wire that comes from a point high on the mast where the shrouds are fixed to a hook on a crew member's harness at waist level. The position when extended on the trapeze is outside the hull,

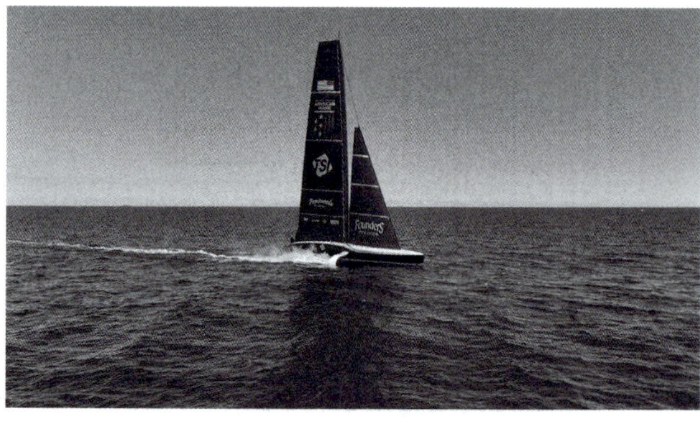

Figure 119.4: America's Cup Class boat on hydrofoils. (Used with permission from American Magic Media Center.)

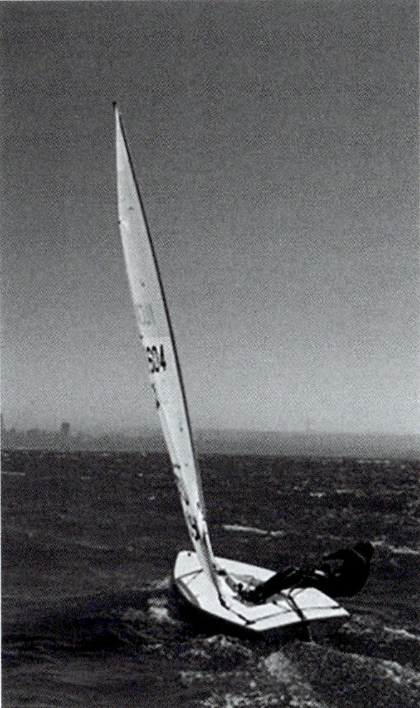

Figure 119.5: Example of hiking out on a laser in full foul weather gear.

braced against the hull, giving the crew member more leverage to keep the boat flat.

- Hoisting and dousing sails involves raising and lowering sails such that they can be changed during the race.
- Managing the spinnaker involves maneuvering a sail designed specifically for sailing downwind. Either symmetrical or asymmetrical spinnakers may be used with differing wind angles. Raising and lowering the spinnaker may be performed while the boat is already under motion and may be a very difficult operation.
- Managing foiling systems involves hydrofoil or hydrosail sailboats and wing-link foils mounted under the hull. These lift the hull out of the water as speeds increase. This decreases drag and increases speed further. In foiling crafts, height control is an added dimension/skill.
- Mental demands include concentration and focus for navigation and racing tactics.

- Sailors may be at high risk while performing explosive, powerful moves, such as grinding on a pedestal winch during a tacking or jibing maneuver.
- Falls on the deck or companionway and being hit by objects (including the boom) are also common mechanisms of injury (1,3).
- Inherent postures such as the physical stress of dynamic hiking, which involves maximal voluntary contraction of the quadriceps, isometric endurance, and tolerance of muscular fatigue, put the sailor at further risk (4).
- A study of the 2002 Danish Olympic team showed that Laser (now called ILCA) sailors had the highest VO_{2max} at 58.3 ± 4.2 mL · kg^{-1} · min^{-1}, consistent with endurance athletes (5).
  - Board and kite sailing are also physiologically demanding endurance events, and biomechanics may involve both sustained isometric contractions and constant pumping of the sail, depending on conditions, while balancing on a foiling board. Helmsman and crew on trapeze boats have had VO_{2max} results of 55.3 ± 4.0 and 57.3 ± 3.7 mL · kg^{-1} · min^{-1}, respectively (5).

EPIDEMIOLOGY

- The medical issues and musculoskeletal issues in sailing have been evaluated in multiple regattas and different environments, and vary based on the specific event.
- Overall injury rates have been estimated to be between 0.29 (novice dinghy) and 4.61 (heterogeneous group)/1000 days of athlete exposure (6).
- The incidence of injury in an America's Cup team was reported by Neville to be between 2.2 and 8.6 per 1000 hours in sailboat racing and training, with the most common injury being sprains and strains (7).
- A study of the 635 nautical mile Newport-to-Bermuda race found an injury rate of 12 per 1000 races per sailor (8).

MEDICAL ISSUES

- Nathanson reported fatality rates of 1.19 deaths per million sailing person-days, which is comparable to those in US football.
  - The US Coast Guard (USCG) reported 23 deaths/year related to sailing, most often due to drowning, usually without a life jacket.

- Alcohol and other substances that cause impairment also increase the risk of mortality and morbidity in boating accidents (9).
- Severe weather may also play a significant factor contributing to illnesses, injuries, and even fatalities, such as in the offshore 1998 Sydney to Hobart race, and in a 2023 lightning strike to a Sail GP boat.

- Medical issues that should be considered include underlying conditions that may require attention in a pre-participation evaluation.
  - Sailors with seizure disorders have at least a 15-fold increased risk of drowning compared with the general population (10), and should always wear a life jacket. They should not sail in solo events.
  - Cardiac issues should also be addressed as they may be factors in drowning events, especially in cold water immersion.
  - Patients with severe asthma or chronic obstructive pulmonary disease may be at increased risk of triggering pulmonary issues in certain sailing environments and should have inhalers on hand (6).
- Marine life exposure causing wounds is of come concern, especially from *Vibrio* species, and should be prevented and treated accordingly. The immunocompromised are likely at increased risk of infection.
- Environmental issues such as hypothermia, heat illness, dehydration, seasickness, poor nutrition, and sun-related problems are also prevalent within the sport of sailing.
- Seasickness was the most common illness reported in the Newport to Bermuda offshore races from 1998 to 2006 and is often preventable with seasickness bands or scopolamine patches in susceptible sailors (8).
- Dermatological conditions such as cracked skin, skin sores, and fungal rashes were the most common illnesses reported during the Whitbread Round the World Yacht Race 1997–1998 (11).
  - The importance of sunscreen to prevent long-term skin damage and skin cancer is important to reinforce to athletes.
- Although there are no "weight classes" like there are in other sports, combined crew weight may be limited in certain boat classes to optimize boat performance. It is possible this may change with the new foiling boats/boards.
  - Team members may dehydrate to "cut weight" for weigh-in purposes, much like wrestling and boxing.
  - Awareness of problems associated with relative energy deficiency in sport (RED-S) in sailors is also critical because they are often required to "make weight," which can lead to disordered eating and related conditions.
  - America's Cup sailors have been found to average 56 kcal · kg^{-1} of body weight in daily energy expenditure, supporting the importance of proper nutrition and hydration during racing events (7,12).
- Because most events require sailors to be on the water for extended periods without access to land-based facilities, it is necessary to also consider gastrointestinal issues, bladder problems in some disabled sailors, diabetic/blood sugar management, adequate nutrition, and the ability to readily manage minor emergencies on the water (6,13).
- Additionally, medical personnel should be aware that the world anti-doping agency anti-doping rules may apply in certain sailing events, and a therapeutic use exemption may be required. For example, beta blockers are banned in match-racing helms.

MUSCULOSKELETAL CONDITIONS

- Although most musculoskeletal conditions seen in sailing can be classified as overuse injuries, acute injuries are also common. These are often related to accidents involving boat equipment and have been increasing due to the newer high-speed foiling boats (14–16).
  - Lacerations from hitting sharp metal edges on the rig or hydrofoil, abrasions from mishandling sheets, finger fractures from problems with winch overrides, contusions from free-flying winch handles, concussions from contact with an accidentally jibing boom, or slips and falls on a wet foredeck have all been documented (1–3,6–8,14–16).
  - Fisher reported previously that although head injuries make up just 10% of sailing-related injuries, many of these are severe, with >50% of them being fatal on larger racing yachts, usually caused by boom-related injuries (8).
    - However, more concussion data are being gathered, as foiling boats are becoming more mainstream.
    - It is uncertain if helmet use while sailing will prevent concussions, but more athletes have been using helmets as concussion awareness has increased in all sports.
- Overuse musculoskeletal injuries are boat size/type and crew position specific, and are primarily represented by low back pain and knee pain, especially in Olympic classes. Table 119.1 reviews the different injury types in different sailing disciplines (1–3,15,17).
- Small boat/dinghy sailing often requires a dynamic effort in heavy air conditions and will vary with the sailor and boat class.
  - The hiking strap placement and foot position on the straps have been shown to be factors in forces generated at the knee and should be observed in any sailor with knee pain (18).
    - The different hiking styles and torques placed on the knee when tacking the boat from a hiked-out position may affect the development of meniscal injuries or patellofemoral injuries in these athletes.
    - Hiking crew members are also susceptible to lumbar spine disk problems, and core stability is essential to preventing injury.
  - In boats that use a trapeze, the harness fit may play a role in preventing low back pain, suggesting that custom-fit harnesses should be considered (1).

Table 119.1 Injury Patterns in Sailing

Smaller boats, Olympic classes	Lower back (52.9%) Other back areas (41.2%) Knees (25%–32%) Thigh/leg (26.5%) Neck (23.5%) Shoulder (23.5%) Forearm or elbow (20.6%)
Larger boats, America's Cup Class, and Offshore racing boats	Lumbar spine (16%) Shoulder (16%) Knee (10%) Cervical spine (8%) Hand (7%)
Disabled sailors (Paralympic classes)	Upper extremity (60%) Spine (20%) Lower extremities (44.6%)
Boardsailing (Windsurfers)	Upper extremity (18.5%) Head and neck (17.8%) Trunk (16.0%)

Source: Allen JB. Sailing. In: Madden CC, Putukian M, McCarty EC, Young CC, editors. *Netter's Sports Medicine*. 3rd ed. Philadelphia (PA): Elsevier; 2023. pp. 664–71.

- Larger yachts have been noted to have crew position-specific injuries that include the following: (1–3,6–8,11,14,15).
  - Helm: Carpal tunnel syndrome, lateral epicondylitis, and postural strain issues due to prolonged sustained positioning on long tacks may occur.
  - Grinders: Lateral epicondylitis, rotator cuff tendinopathy, and lumbar disk issues may develop due to the biomechanics of the sailors positioning on the pedestal winches, which can affect both potential injury and peak performance if not addressed properly.
  - Mast: Shoulder injuries are common due to repetitive halyard hoisting at the mast. Proper hand-over-hand technique, using the legs and trunk for strength and stability, may reduce overhead injuries to the shoulder.
  - Trimmer: The angle of cervical rotation and extension required to visualize the sail and trim for speed can cause a "trimmer's neck," a cervical strain that can lead to more complicated cervical spine issues.
  - Bow: This crew position requires advanced mobility and agility skills, who may be jibing the spinnaker pole downwind, climbing the mast to fix mechanical issues, or changing headsails in heavy seas, making the bow crew increasingly susceptible to injuries, especially concussions. Usually, the bow crew is clipped into a safety harness to avoid falling overboard in heavy seas.
- Board sailing, kite sailing, and foil sailing all have increased injury risk due to high speeds and more difficulty controlling the vessel in heavy wind and seas.
  - A high level of concentration is required to effectively steer these boats that require appropriate physical and psychological training to reduce fatigue.
  - With hydrofoils in particular, the technology exposes crews to high speeds and accelerations (over 40 knots, 46 mph, and 74 km · h^{-1}) that increase the risk of high-energy trauma, with lofting or wind-shear dropping, especially in the case of collisions between boats/boards or boat capsizing (6,16,19).
    - In a recent study, the prevalence of illnesses and overuse injuries during the foiling regatta week were 6.5% and 18.2%, respectively, while the incidence of acute injuries was 16/1000 sailor-hours.
    - Upper limbs, lower limbs, and lumbar spine were involved in 34.6%, 26.9%, and 15.4% of cases of musculoskeletal injuries, respectively (16,19). Cervical spine and clavicular injuries are common in wind foiling (20).
  - The adoption of wearing sailing gloves may prevent hand injuries, and their use is crucial in cold climate conditions and when handling ropes under high tension (7,16).
  - Helmets are used more frequently in these classes, and concussion data collection in these classes is ongoing.
- The Olympic classes 49erFX, 49er, and Nacra 17, in a 2014 survey, reported more injuries that were mainly traumatic events, compared with overuse injuries in the other classes (20).

EVENT COVERAGE

- Event coverage for the sport of sailing includes both on and off-the-water care.
- Knowledge about the sport is critical for the successful care of the sailors.
- Prevention is the cornerstone to a healthy sailing team through proper nutrition, adequate hydration, strength and endurance training, cardiovascular fitness, mental preparedness, and use of environmentally appropriate clothing and equipment.
- Preparation by the medical team through safety and medical awareness, preparticipation evaluation, proper injury assessment, and treatment are keys to the success of the sailor and to the team's performance.
- Also, other key safety factors include prevention of illness and injury from environmental factors such as dehydration and heat/cold, or traumatic and overuse injuries on the boat, to water immersion with near-drowning or contact with marine life (1).
- Safety in a water environment requires specific emergency management plans (including extrication and evacuation), and personnel with seamanship skills who are familiar with water rescues and resuscitation in cases of capsizes, collisions, and man overboard situations (1).
  - Emergency plans should also include plans for foul weather, including heat, cold, lightning, and rough water.

- Sailing is evolving rapidly as a sport, with the advent of foiling, as well as with changes in racing formats that favor faster and shorter races and medical personnel need to anticipate the accompanying medical implications.

REFERENCES

1. Madden C, Putukian M, McCarty E, Young C. *Netter's Sports Medicine.* 3rd ed. Philadelphia, PA: Elsevier. 2022. Madden.
2. Allen JB. Sports medicine and sailing. *Phys Med Rehabil Clin N Am.* 1999;10(1):49–65.
3. Allen JB, De Jong MR. Sailing and sports medicine: a literature review. *Br J Sports Med.* 2006;40(7):587–93.
4. Mackie H. Useful biomechanics for sailing: development of technique analysis protocol for Europe and Laser sailors. In: Legg SJ, editor. *Human Performance in Sailing Conference Proceedings: Incorporating the 4th European Conference on Sailing Sports Science and Sports Medicine and the 3rd Australian Sailing Science Conference.* Palmerston North, New Zealand: Massey University; 2003.
5. Bojsen Moller J, Larsson B, Magnusson SP, Aagaard P. Strength and endurance profiles of elite Olympic class sailors. In: Legg SJ, editor. *Human Performance in Sailing Conference Proceedings: Incorporating the 4th European Conference on Sailing Sports Science and Sports Medicine and the 3rd Australian Sailing Science Conference.* Palmerston North, New Zealand: Massey University; 2003. p. 97–111.
6. Nathanson A, Baird J, Mello M. Sailing injury and illness: results of an online survey. *Wilderness Environ Med.* 2010;21(4):291–7.
7. Neville V, Molloy J, Brooks J, Speedy DB, Atkinson G. Epidemiology of injuries and illnesses in America's Cup yacht racing. *Br J Sports Med.* 2006;40(4):304–12.
8. Nathanson A, Fischer E, Mello M, Baird J. Injury and illness at the Newport-Bermuda race 1998-2006. *Wilderness Environ Med.* 2008;19(2):129–32.
9. *2011 USCG National Recreational Boating Survey Report.* Web site. [Accessed 2024 Oct 6]. http://www.uscgboating.org/assets/1/workflow_staging/AssetManager/671.PDF.
10. Bell GS, Gaitatzis A, Bell CL, Johnson AL, Sander JW. Drowning in people with epilepsy How great is the risk? *Neurology.* 2008;71(8):578–82.
11. Spalding T, Malinen T, Tomson M, Goertzen M, Sinclair R, Allen J. Analysis of medical problems during the 2001-2002 Volvo Ocean Race. *N Z J Sports Med.* 2006;33(2):38.
12. Bernardi M, Fontana G, Rodio A, et al. Physiological characteris-tics of America's cup sailors. In: Legg SJ, editor. *Human Performance in Sailing Conference Proceedings: Incorporating the 4th European Conference on Sailing Sports Science and Sports Medicine and the 3rd Australian Sailing Science Conference.* Palmerston North, New Zealand: Massey University; 2003. p. 31–5.
13. Allen JB, Alison B. Safety in Paralympic Sailing. In: *Vista Conference Proceedings of the International Paralympic Committee.* Paper accepted for publication; 2006.
14. Allen JB, Dent D, Andrews JR, et al. Sports medicine injuries in the America's Cup 2000. *N Z J Sports Med.* 2006;33(2):43–7.
15. Neville V, Folland JP. The epidemiology and aetiology of injuries in sailing. *Sports Med.* 2009;39(2):129–45.
16. Feletti F, Aliverti A. Extreme sailing medicine, injuries and illnesses. In: Feletti F, editor. *Extreme Sports Medicine.* Switzerland: Springer International Publishing; 2017. p. 275–87.
17. Shephard RJ. Injuries in sailing: International Olympic Committee Medical Commission. In: Renstrom PAFH, editor. *Clinical Practice of Sports Injury Prevention and Care.* Oxford: Blackwell Scientific Publications; 1994. p. 641–54.
18. Tan B, Aziz AR, Spurway NC, et al. Determinants of maximal hiking performance in laser sailors. In: Legg SJ, editor. *Human Performance in Sailing Conference Proceedings: Incorporating the 4th European Conference on Sailing Sports Science and Sports Medicine and the 3rd Australian Sailing Science Conference.* Palmerston North, New Zealand: Massey University; 2003. p. 25–30.
19. Feletti F, Brymer E, Aliverti A, Alivert A. Injuries and illnesses related to dinghy-sailing on hydrofoiling boats. *BMC Sports Sci Med Rehabil.* 2021;13(1):118. DOI:10.1186/s13102-021-00343-8
20. Tan B, Leong D, Vaz Pardal C, Lin CY, Kam JW. Injury and illness surveillance at the International Sailing Federation Sailing World Championships 2014. *Br J Sports Med.* 2016 Jun;50(11):673–981.

Surfing

120

Jason Guo, Reid Collis, and Robert P. Wilder

INTRODUCTION

- Surfing is an ancient sport that originated in the South Pacific and eventually became an integral part of Hawaiian culture.
- The practice of surfing in Hawaii was discouraged by missionaries in the 1800s but was subsequently revived as a sport by Hawaiian Olympic swimmer Duke Kahanamoku who introduced the sport to California and Australia in the 1920s (1).
- There are now approximately 2.8 million surfers in the United States and 37 million worldwide (2).
- The International Surfing Association is recognized by the International Olympic Committee as the leading authority on surfing, and surfing became an official Olympic sport at the 2020 Tokyo Olympic Games.
- Surfing competitions typically involve 20- to 40-minute elimination heats in which surfers are scored by a group of judges with high scorers advancing on to further rounds.
    - Athletes are judged on degree of difficulty, control, power, speed, style, and originality.
    - Points for individual surfing contests are accumulated throughout the year to determine the overall tour rankings.

ACTIVITY PROFILE

- Surfing is a sport that is characterized by intermittent periods of high-intensity exercise interspersed with low-intensity activity and rest periods (3).
- During competition, surfers spend 55% of the time paddling, 34% stationary, and 3%–8% of the time wave riding; they may perform up to 2000 strokes in a 2-hour session (2).
- Paddling is performed with the surfer lying in the prone position with the back and neck in hyperextension and with the arms alternating, pulling through the water alongside the board.
    - Paddling biomechanics differ from freestyle swimming because long axis rotation is diminished while lying prone on the board and kicking is eliminated as a means of forward propulsion (3).
    - While paddling out, a maneuver called "duck diving" is used to dive nose first under oncoming waves in order to continue away from shore.
- When a suitable wave is identified, surfers attempt to match the speed of the oncoming wave in order to ride along the wave front.
    - In big-wave surfing, surfers may be towed to the wave front by a motorized watercraft in order to match a larger wave's higher velocity.
- Once the surfer is pulled toward shore by the wave, they explosively transition from a prone to a standing position and ride down the face of the wave.

ATHLETE ATTRIBUTES

- The mean age of professional surfers is 27.5 and 26.7 years for men and women, respectively (4).
- Elite male and female surfers tend to be shorter and lighter when compared to age-matched swimmers and water polo players.
    - Shorter stature may be an advantage because a lower center of gravity allows for greater dynamic balance (4).
- Elite surfers have aerobic fitness, as measured by maximal oxygen consumption during arm exercise, that is significantly greater than untrained subjects and comparable to athletes in other aquatic endurance sports (5).
- Lactate threshold during arm exercise is significantly greater in elite versus nonelite surfers. Higher lactate threshold has a positive correlation with surfing performance (5).

EQUIPMENT

- Surfboards are categorized as shortboards or longboards based on length. Some overlap exists, but in general, shortboards are 6–7 ft long, and longboards are 9–10 ft long.
    - Shortboards have a pointed nose, whereas longboards have a rounded nose. Longboards are more buoyant but less maneuverable.
- Modern surfboards are constructed with an inner core of polyurethane or polystyrene foam with a fiberglass shell.

The naturally slippery surface is treated with surf wax for traction (2).

- Most surfboards are affixed with fins on their underside that act as stabilizing struts.
- Wetsuits are utilized to allow athletes to surf in cooler climates and to surf during a greater portion of the year (2).
- Ankle leashes are elastic ropes that tether the surfboard to the surfer via an ankle strap. Shorter leashes increase the risk of board-induced self-injury via a recoil mechanism, whereas longer leashes increase the risk of the board injuring other surfers.
- Surfers recognize the risk of head injury as moderate to high, but only 2% of surfers wear protective headgear. The most commonly cited reason for not wearing a helmet is "no need." Other reasons include discomfort, claustrophobia, and effects on balance (6).
  - Helmets consist of shatterproof plastic shells with a molded foam lining that is secured with a chin strap.
  - Other protective amenities include shatterproof, ultraviolet protectant visors, and ear cups to protect against tympanic membrane rupture.

INJURY EPIDEMIOLOGY

- Acute injuries occur at a rate of 0.74–1.79 injuries per 1000 hours surfed across recreational and professional surfers (7,8).
- Surfboard-related injuries are the most common cause of injury in recreational surfers, accounting for 39% of acute surfing injuries, followed by maneuvering while surfing or approaching a wave (20% of injuries) (7).
- For recreational surfers, lacerations are the most common form of acute injury, accounting for 41%–46% of injuries (1,7,8).
  - The most common locations are the face and lower extremity (1,7,9).
- In contrast, among competitive surfers, sprains and strains are the most common form of acute injury during competition, accounting for 39% of injuries, with the most commonly injured body part being the lower extremity (1).
  - Knee strains account for a majority of these injuries and occur during aggressive turning and aerial maneuvering.
- Chronic musculoskeletal injuries account for up to 39% of all chronic-surfing-related health problems.
  - The most common injuries occur to the back/spine and shoulder, followed by knee and elbow (3,6).

SPECIFIC INJURIES

- *Lacerations* are common among surfers and occur due to direct contact with the board, rocks, coral, fellow surfers, and other objects.
  - Wounds should be cultured for aerobic, anaerobic, and marine organisms.
  - Common pathogens involved in marine soft-tissue injuries include *Streptococcus* species, *Escherichia coli, Pseudomonas aeruginosa, Mycobacterium marinum, Staphylococcus aureus,* and *Vibrio* species (10).
  - Outpatient oral antibiotic therapy should include coverage directed at *Vibrio* species including ciprofloxacin or trimethoprim-sulfamethoxazole. Parenteral choices include cefotaxime, ceftazidime, ceftriaxone, and tobramycin (10,11).
  - When lacerations are secondary to envenomation, they should be allowed to heal by secondary intention or delayed primary closure (12).
- *Tympanic membrane rupture* occurs with head trauma from a strong wave or when the head contacts the water during a fall.
  - Symptoms and signs include ear pain, conductive hearing loss, tinnitus, vertigo, and bloody otorrhea (13).
  - Antibiotic therapy is only indicated with concomitant infection (14).
  - Athletes should be advised not to return to play until the perforation is healed. If necessary, ear plugs can be placed to keep out water while the healing process continues (6).
- *Surfer's myelopathy* refers to spinal cord infarction that occurs more frequently in novice surfers.
  - The mechanism of infarction is thought to be related to prolonged hyperextension during paddling in novice, unconditioned athletes that leads to either avulsion of the artery of Adamkiewicz, inferior vena cava obstruction, or fibrocartilaginous embolism (15).
  - Overall prevalence is unknown, but case reports exist in the literature. For individuals affected by surfer's myelopathy, the majority achieve complete resolution of symptoms (15).
  - Surfers most commonly complain of progressive lower-extremity pain, paresthesia, and urinary retention that progresses rapidly over several hours. Recovery is reported to occur over months, though in rare cases permanent neurological deficits, including quadriplegia, have been reported (2,16).
  - Magnetic resonance imaging (MRI), including T2- and diffusion-weighted imaging, is the most sensitive study for finding areas of spinal cord infarction. In published cases, ischemic MRI changes were localized to the distal thoracic watershed zone (15).
  - Initial management entails rapid evaluation with MRI, empiric intravenous steroid administration, aggressive hydration, and permissible hypertension.
  - Patients with incomplete resolution of symptoms will likely benefit from acute inpatient rehabilitation after medical stabilization. Long-term care may include intermittent catheterization and urodynamic studies, scheduled bowel regimens, pressure relief, deep vein thrombosis prophylaxis, and physical and occupational therapy.

MEDICAL ISSUES

- *Surfer's ear or external auditory exostosis (EAEs)* typically presents as multiple, bilateral broad-based growths of lamellar bone obstructing the external auditory canal leading to complications such as cerumen impaction, conductive hearing loss, and otitis externa.
  - Overall, the prevalence of EAE among surfers is 38%–73% (17,18).
  - A dose-dependent relationship between length of exposure to cold water and the prevalence of EAE has been identified (18); cold water surfers are 2.6 times more likely to have EAE than warm water surfers (17).
  - If medical management of EAE complications fails, surgical excision can be performed.
  - Prevention of EAE entails decreasing exposure to cold water by means of ear plugs, ear molds, or hoods, though the effectiveness of these interventions is inconclusive (19–21).
- *Otitis externa* may be caused by EAE, trauma, and chronic moisture.
  - Common organisms include *P. aeruginosa* and *S. aureus*, whereas fungal species such as *Candida* and *Aspergillus* may be found in persons with diabetes (22).
  - Treatment includes a 1-week course of topical antibacterial drops with systemic antibiotics indicated if a persistent case develops or if otitis media is suspected (23).
  - Prevention includes application of acetic acid into the external canal after surfing and use of ear plugs (22).
- *Sun exposure* increases the risk for skin cancer and pterygiums among surfers (2).
  - Consistent use of sunscreen is recommended to mitigate risk of skin cancer.
  - Pterygiums are fibrous growths over the cornea that are associated with long-term sun exposure.
    - The majority of pterygiums are benign. However, atypical pterygiums may be associated with an increased risk of ocular surface neoplasia.
    - The main risk factor of pterygium progression is UV radiation exposure (24–26).
    - For patients requiring surgical intervention, conjunctival or conjunctival-limbal autografting is the preferred technique for ophthalmologists (25).
    - Given the direct association with wind, particle, and UV exposure and the development of pterygiums, use of protective eyewear such as polarized goggles or sunglasses during surfing is recommended.
- *Gastroesophageal reflux disease* (GERD) is significantly more prevalent in surfers (21%) than in nonsurfing athletes (7%).
  - Higher surfing frequency is correlated with higher prevalence of GERD symptoms (27).
  - Mechanisms that lead to a higher risk of GERD in the surfing population include increased intra-abdominal pressure secondary to lying prone on a hard surface during heavy exertion (27).
  - Shortboard surfing has a higher prevalence of GERD than longboard surfing.
    - Longboards have a greater surface area, allowing surfers to distribute their body mass over a greater area and thus allowing less pressure to be focused along the abdomen (27).
  - A small meal of 400–500 kcal 2–4 hours prior to surfing that is free of fatty foods, peppermint, chocolate, alcohol, and acidic beverages will help maintain glycogen stores while decreasing the risk of GERD.
  - If refractory to lifestyle modifications, a trial of a proton pump inhibitor or H_2 blocker should be initiated for acid suppression.
- Marine envenomations are also a risk for surfers, given their significant exposure to the ocean and marine wildlife.
  - *Seabather's eruption*, also known as "sea lice," is a hypersensitivity reaction to larval toxins of certain coelenterates, most notably *Linuche unguiculata* and *Edwardsiella lineata*, in Bermuda, the Caribbean region, and the East Coast of the United States (28).
    - Symptoms include an urticarial maculopapular rash in the area covered by a swimsuit that appears immediately or may be delayed by 1.5 days (22).
    - Treatment includes topical corticosteroids, oral antihistamines, and if necessary, oral steroids. Bathing suits should be thoroughly washed to avoid re-envenomation (18).
  - *Coelenterates* are marine invertebrates including jellyfish, Portuguese man-of-war, and box jellyfish that have tentacles filled with venomous cells called nematocysts that typically cause a local response but can rarely cause multiorgan damage (22).
    - Jellyfish stings present with burning pain, erythema, edema, urticaria, and bullae formation, which may progress to skin necrosis (22).
    - Tentacles and other retained animal parts should be removed and washed off with seawater, not freshwater (29).
    - No consensus exists for appropriate jellyfish toxin treatment, but anecdotal evidence exists for application of hot or cold packs and irrigation with vinegar, urine, or baking soda (22,29).
    - Topical treatment with an anesthetic agent such as benzocaine or lidocaine have been found to provide symptomatic relief (29).
    - Alcohol, methylated spirits, and freshwater should be carefully avoided, since they may massively discharge nematocysts.

- Pressure immobilization bandaging should be avoided, as laboratory studies have shown that it stimulates additional venom discharge from nematocysts (30).
- An antivenom exists for the box jellyfish toxin.

- *Stingrays* are commonly encountered when entering or exiting the water. Their sting is caused by a sharp spine located on their tail that can penetrate wet suits and booties (6).
  - Patients stung by stingrays often present with pain out of proportion to wound appearance (6).
  - Treatment includes removing retained animal parts and hot water immersion to inactivate the heat-labile toxin (6).
  - Careful wound exploration and irrigation is recommended as stings are occasionally associated with bacterial contamination.
    - In significant stingray stings, a course of prophylactic oral antibiotics is recommended, with attention to marine bacteria coverage, including *Vibrio sp* and others (31,32).
    - Antibiotics to consider include, but are not limited to, trimethoprim-sulfamethoxazole, doxycycline, or ciprofloxacin (32).
  - Prevention involves shuffling one's feet through the sand to scare away stingrays and avoiding times and areas where they are known to congregate.
- *Coral envenomation* usually consists of toxins from multiple sources such as urchins and sea cucumbers (6).
  - Acetic acid can alleviate the pain associated with coral envenomation (10).

EVENT COVERAGE

- Physicians covering a surfing event should be prepared with an appropriate emergency action plan.
- Such plans should include treatment for the conditions outlined above, but must also include specific plans for rapidly extricating the injured surfer from the water and bringing them safely to shore for evaluation and treatment.
- As many surfing events may be somewhat remote, an appropriate emergency transport plan must be in place and should include emergency medical services as well as aeromedical, when appropriate, and the nearest trauma center.
- A protocol should also exist for poor weather and should include under what circumstances the event will be postponed or canceled, and who has the authority to make this decision.

REFERENCES

1. Nathanson A, Haynes P, Galanis D. Surfing injuries. *Am J Emerg Med.* 2002;20(3):155–60. doi:10.1053/ajem.2002.32650
2. Minasian B, Hope N. Surfing on the world stage: a narrative review of acute and overuse injuries and preventative measures for the competitive and recreational surfer. *Br J Sports Med.* 2022;56(1):51–60. doi:10.1136/bjsports-2021-104307
3. Hanchard S, Duncan A, Furness J, Simas V, Climstein M, Kemp-Smith K. Chronic and gradual-onset injuries and conditions in the sport of surfing: a systematic review. *Sports (Basel).* 2021;9(2):23. doi:10.3390/sports9020023
4. Mendez-Villanueva A, Bishop D. Physiological aspects of surfboard riding performance. *Sports Med.* 2005;35(1):55–70. doi:10.2165/00007256-200535010-00005
5. Mendez-Villanueva A, Bishop D, Hamer P. Activity profile of world-class professional surfers during competition: a case study. *J Strength Cond Res.* 2006;20(3):477–82. doi:10.1519/16574.1
6. Taylor KS, Zoltan TB, Achar SA. Medical illnesses and injuries encountered during surfing. *Curr Sports Med Rep.* 2006;5(5):262–7. doi:10.1097/01.csmr.0000306426.16414.52
7. McArthur K, Jorgensen D, Climstein M, Furness J. Epidemiology of acute injuries in surfing: type, location, mechanism, severity, and incidence — a systematic review. *Sports (Basel).* 2020;8(2):25. doi:10.3390/sports8020025
8. Lowdon BJ, Pateman NA, Pitman AJ. Surfboard riding injuries. *Med J Aust.* 1983;2(12):613–16. doi:10.5694/j.1326-5377.1983.tb122722.x
9. Muhonen EG, Kafle S, Torabi SJ, Abello EH, Bitner BF, Pham N. Surfing-related craniofacial injuries: a NEISS database study. *J Craniofac Surg.* 2022;33(8):2383–7. doi:10.1097/scs.0000000000008769
10. Auerbach PS, Auerbach PS. Marine envenomations. *N Engl J Med.* 1991;325(7):486–93. doi:10.1056/nejm199108153250707
11. Diaz JH, Lopez FA. Skin soft tissue and systemic bacterial infections following aquatic injuries and exposures. *Am J Med Sci.* 2015;349(3):269–75. doi:10.1097/maj.0000000000000366
12. McGoldrick J, Marx JA. Marine envenomations; Part 1: vertebrates. *J Emerg Med.* 1991;9(6):497–502. doi:10.1016/0736-4679(91)90223-3
13. Richmond DR, Yelverton JT, Fletcher ER, Phillips YY. Physical correlates of eardrum rupture. *Ann Otol Rhinol Laryngol Suppl.* 1989;140(5 suppl 1):35–41. doi:10.1177/00034894890980s507
14. Kerr AG. Trauma and the temporal bone. The effects of blast on the ear. *J Laryngol Otol.* 1980;94(1):107–10. doi:10.1017/s0022215100088538
15. Thompson TP, Pearce J, Chang G, Madamba J. Surfer's myelopathy. *Spine.* 2004;29(16):E353–6. doi:10.1097/01.brs.0000134689.84162.e7
16. Bickley RJ, Belyea CM, Harpstrite JK, Min KS. Surfing injuries: a review for the orthopaedic surgeon. *JBJS Rev.* 2021;9(4). doi:10.2106/jbjs.rvw.20.00152
17. Kroon DF, Lawson ML, Derkay CS, Hoffmann K, McCook J. Surfer's ear: external auditory exostoses are more prevalent in cold water surfers. *Otolaryngol Head Neck Surg.* 2002;126(5):499–504. doi:10.1067/mhn.2002.124474
18. Wong BJF, Cervantes W, Doyle KJ, et al. Prevalence of external auditory canal exostoses in surfers. *Arch Otolaryngol Head Neck Surg.* 1999;125(9):969–72. doi:10.1001/archotol.125.9.969
19. DiBartolomeo JR. Exostoses of the external auditory canal. *Ann Otol Rhinol Laryngol Suppl.* 1979;88(6 pt 2 suppl 61):2–20. doi:10.1177/00034894790880s601
20. Chaplin JM, Stewart IA. The prevalence of exostoses in the external auditory meatus of surfers. *Clin Otolaryngol Allied Sci.* 1998;23(4):326–30. doi:10.1046/j.1365-2273.1998.00151.x
21. Attlmayr B, Smith IM. Prevalence of 'surfer's ear' in Cornish surfers. *J Laryngol Otol.* 2015;129(5):440–4. doi:10.1017/s0022215115000316
22. Zoltan TB, Taylor KS, Achar SA. Health issues for surfers. *Am Fam Physician.* 2005;71(12):2313–17.
23. Sander R. Otitis externa: a practical guide to treatment and prevention. *Am Fam Physician.* 2001;63(5):927–42.
24. Lin AD, Miles K, Brinks MV. Prevalence of pterygia in Hawaii: examining cumulative surfing hours as a risk factor. *Ophthalmic Epidemiol.* 2016;23(4):264–8. doi:10.3109/09286586.2015.1119284

25. Shahraki T, Arabi A, Feizi S. Pterygium: an update on pathophysiology, clinical features, and management. *Ther Adv Ophthalmol.* 2021;13:25158414211020152. doi:10.1177/25158414211020152
26. Mackenzie FD, Hirst LW, Battistutta D, Green A. Risk analysis in the development of pterygia. *Ophthalmology.* 1992;99(7):1056–61. doi:10.1016/s0161-6420(92)31850-0
27. Norisue Y, Onopa J, Kaneshiro M, Tokuda Y. Surfing as a risk factor for gastroesophageal reflux disease. *Clin J Sport Med.* 2009;19(5):388–93. doi:10.1097/jsm.0b013e3181b8ef41
28. Tomchik RS, Russell MT, Szmant AM, Black NA. Clinical perspectives on seabather's eruption, also known as "sea lice". *J Am Med Assoc.* 1993;269(13):1669–72. doi:10.1001/jama.269.13.1669
29. Montgomery L, Seys J, Mees J. To pee, or not to pee: a review on envenomation and treatment in European jellyfish species. *Mar Drugs.* 2016;14(7):127. doi:10.3390/md14070127
30. Cegolon L, Heymann WC, Lange JH, Mastrangelo G. Jellyfish stings and their management: a review. *Mar Drugs.* 2013;11(2):523–50. doi:10.3390/md11020523
31. Clark AT, Clark RF, Cantrell FL. A retrospective review of the presentation and treatment of stingray stings reported to a poison control system. *Am J Ther.* 2017;24(2):e177–80. doi:10.1097/mjt.0000000000000365
32. Cevik J, Hunter-Smith DJ, Rozen WM. Infections following stingray attacks: a case series and literature review of antimicrobial resistance and treatment. *Travel Med Infect Dis.* 2022;47:102312. doi:10.1016/j.tmaid.2022.102312

121 Swimming

Justine Ko, Korin B. Hudson, and Nancy Rolnik

INTRODUCTION

- Swimming remains one of the most popular forms of physical activity in the United States. It is a lifetime activity and enjoyed by participants of all ages (1).
- The world governing body for all aquatics is World Aquatics, formerly known as Fédération Internationale de Natation.
- Swimming competitions may take place either in pools or in open water such as lakes, rivers, or the ocean, and they may range in length from sprint distances (25 m) to marathon distance swims of 20–50 km or more.
- Swimming provides many health benefits without age limitations such as in other competitive sports. It is an excellent option for cardiovascular exercise for all ages.
  - It has been shown to improve cardiorespiratory fitness through VO_{2max} and improve body fat percentage (1).
- Many master's swimming clubs and fitness groups offer programs for beginner adult swimmers, making the sport available for everyone.

EPIDEMIOLOGY

- Swimming is an all-year sport that can result in overuse injuries.
  - Collegiate and elite training programs include cross-training and strength training programs that can affect injury patterns.
  - The majority of injuries in swimming are due to overuse, with the most frequently injured body part being the shoulder (2).
  - Knee and lower back injuries are also commonly found (2).
- It has been a part of the Olympic games since 1896 (3) and has included both individual and team events.
- Swimming has an overall low incidence of injury, ranging from two to three injuries/1000 hours of exposure (2).
- Injuries are higher in competition than in training and are generally related to overuse rather than acute injury.
- Training can range from 9 to 110 $km \cdot wk^{-1}$ depending on the competition level.

SPECIFIC ISSUES

- **Gear/equipment**
  - Equipment includes swimsuit, swim cap, ear plugs, and goggles. Swimsuit and swim caps aid in decreasing drag while swimming. Goggles help with visibility during the swim and to prevent water entry/eye irritation.
  - Notably, high-tech swimsuits were banned in 2009 after findings showed it directly affected athlete performance.
  - Pool details (4)
    - An Olympic-sized swimming pool is 50 m long, 25 m wide, and has 10 lanes. The minimum depth is 2 m, but 3 m is recommended.
    - 15-m marks must be visible to the competitor and officials on both ends of the pool.
    - Starting platforms
      - The front edge of the starting platform may not exceed 30 in above the water.
- **Stroke mechanics**
  - The four competitive strokes include: *freestyle*, *backstroke*, *breaststroke*, and *butterfly*.
  - Swimming velocity is determined by stroke rate and stroke length and optimization of each affects performance (5).
  - A breakdown in stroke mechanics can predispose swimmers to injury, so it is important for the clinician and coach to focus attention on fundamental stroke mechanics.
    - Bilateral breathing helps the swimmer develop equal pulling strength in both arms and helps ensure equal body roll on each side.
  - Regardless of the swimmer's chosen stroke, most training is done in freestyle or drills alternating with freestyle such as freestyle/backstroke combos.
  - The freestyle stroke consists of four phases: *entry/catch*, *pull phase*, *push phase*, and *recovery phase*.
    - Entry/catch phase: This is described as the phase when the swimmer's hand enters the water. The swimmer extends their arm to its maximum length. To keep the elbow high, the swimmer must roll the body approximately 45° on the swimmer's long axis. In mechanical studies, the body roll angle can vary due to the athlete's fatigue or breathing side (6).

- Pull phase: The shoulder internally rotates and adducts as the arm follows an S-shaped path to propel the body forward. The elbow should point toward the sidewall during this phase.
- Push phase: This phase maximizes the propulsion forward as the shoulder/arm gets ready to exit the water.
- Recovery phase: The swimmer's arm comes out of the water to bring the arm forward and prepare for the next cycle. The torso rotates on the body's longitudinal axis as the shoulder exits the water in an abducted and externally rotated position. The elbow should remain high above the hand until the hand enters the water, fingers first, just in front and outside the line of the shoulder.
- The upper trapezius, rhomboids, supraspinatus, and deltoid all function in combination to position the scapula and humerus for hand entry and exit. It is important that the neck be extended around 30°–45° to decrease drag and reduce cervical strain.

- Studies have suggested that 11.7% of forward propulsion is produced from kicking (7). The flutter kick helps stabilize the swimmer's trunk. This kick starts at the hip and simulates a motion similar to kicking off a loose shoe.
  - The knees should flex only 30°–40°. Flexion at the hip is minimal.
  - The swimmer must focus on the coordinated motion of both the upper and lower extremity.
  - If the swimmer fails to kick throughout the stroke, the body will lose some of its buoyancy, and more drag is created. The upper extremity will then compensate, placing more stress at the shoulders.
- When stroke mechanics need correction, the use of an underwater video can help clarify the errors. Working with a qualified coach is important.

Training

- Many competitive swimmers engage in rigorous training schedules, often performing two workouts a day, averaging between 8000 and 20,000 yards · d^{-1}.
  - Swimmers should gradually increase training volume and intensity to allow muscle adaptations and prevent overuse.
- Training should also incorporate injury prevention. Unlike many sports, swimming largely utilizes the shoulders for force, with the shoulder producing about 90% of forward propulsion. As an intrinsically unstable joint, strengthening of the dynamic muscle groups of the shoulder is crucial.
  - Swimmers who perform specific shoulder strengthening exercises, such as shoulder external rotation and scapular stabilization exercises, have a lower incidence of shoulder injuries (8).
  - Performing a thorough warm-up before swimming, including shoulder-specific stretches and exercises, can improve shoulder function and reduce the risk of injury. (8). Active warm-up routines have shown a positive effect on swimming performance (9).
- Coaches can monitor training volume and intensity to reduce the risk of overuse injuries. Swimmers can use training diaries and wearable technology to monitor recovery and training durations (10).
  - Wearables can help coaches monitor stroke volume.
  - Current technology attempts to combine the functions of an accelerometer, gyroscope, and magnetometer to assess speed and function (10).
- Training aids
  - Kickboard workouts can allow the swimmer to maintain their fitness level while resting the shoulders. The elbow should be flexed to minimize irritation at the shoulder.
  - Pull buoys are foam pieces that are placed between the legs. They help increase buoyancy of the swimmer and allow focus on core strength and strokes. They can also be used when there is a lower extremity injury that requires rest for recovery.
  - Swim paddles increase the workload for the upper body. It allows the shoulders and muscles to work harder. This should be managed carefully to not overload the shoulder and cause injury.
- Breathing training
  - Controlled frequency breathing
    - Commonly used technique in swimming training during which swimmers utilize prolonged breath holds to induce a hypercapnic effect. The training is to decrease respiratory muscle fatigue, which is thought to improve swimming times (11).
      - This method is thought to recruit certain thoracic musculature as trainers are placed in the "struggle" phase of breath-holding for certain periods.
  - Intermittent hypoxic training
    - This training remains controversial. It involves intermittent exposure to normobaric hypoxia.
    - It is thought to improve anaerobic capacity and swimming performance (12).
- Resistance training (5)
  - Overall traditional resistance training helps to improve performance. It aids in isolated training of swimming-specific muscles.
    - Low-volume, high-velocity resistance training showed improvements in swimming performance.
    - High-volume resistance training showed no effect on swimming performance.
  - Land-based training
    - Swim bench: no significant improvement in maximal power but improvement in swimming performance

- **Competition**
  - Participants reach peak performance around 21–26 years of age (13).
  - Competition levels
    - Young children can start competitively swimming around 6 years of age.
    - It is thought that 8 years of experience is needed to reach elite performance in any given stroke.
    - Master's swimmers age rules include athletes aged 25 years and older.
      - Master's individual events include athletes in 5-year age intervals (*e.g.*, age 25–29, age 30–34, etc.).
      - Master's relay events are based on total age of team members in whole years (*e.g.*, total age 100–119 years, 120–159 years, etc) continued in 40-year increments as high as is necessary.
  - Athletes compete in one of the four strokes — *freestyle, breaststroke, backstroke, or butterfly* — or a combination of the four (medley). The medley event can be done as an individual or group relay.
  - Master's swimmers, triathletes, and other competitive athletes enjoy the instruction and group training benefits of masters swimming programs as a safe and enjoyable fitness option.

MEDICAL ISSUES

- **Life-threatening issues**
  - Drowning is a global problem, with more than 236,000 global drowning fatalities annually as estimated by the World Health Organization (14). It is the 3rd leading cause of unintentional injury/death.
  - Drowning prevention includes teaching people how to swim, encouraging swimming in lifeguarded areas, avoiding swimming in dangerous conditions such as in situations where rip tides or a strong undertow is present, and limiting exposure to very cold water.
  - Most resuscitations occur at the water side, so it is important that lifeguards are taught basic life support techniques, including the use of the bag valve mask, oral and nasopharyngeal airways, high-quality CPR, and automated external defibrillators (AEDs) to further reduce deaths.
    - Even basic training in "hands-only" CPR and AED use by laypersons/bystanders can be lifesaving in such situations.
  - Weather events can also create potential life threats. Lifeguards, coaches, and team physicians must be aware of storms, lightning, and rough water, especially during outdoor events.
- **Environmental exposures**
  - Hypothermia
    - Hypothermia is a well-known risk in open water swimming. The International Triathlon Union and World Aquatics introduced a minimum water temperature for competition.
  - Heat injury
    - While less common, exertional heat stroke must be considered (please see Chapter 48 for additional information on environmental exposure).
    - Factors that contribute to exertional heat stroke include water temperature, ambient sunlight, race distance, and race suits.
      - Wetsuits are made to prevent hypothermia and cold injury but can trap heat in warmer temperatures.
  - Sun exposure
    - For swimmers training in open water or outdoors, it is important to pay close attention to the skin to prevent sunburn.
    - Twenty to thirty minutes prior to swimming, waterproof sunscreen should be liberally applied.
    - Sunscreen should be applied immediately after swimming or at 2-hour intervals (15).
- **Asthma/exercise-induced bronchoconstriction (EIB)**
  - Please see Chapter 43 Pulmonary for more in-depth discussion on pulmonary conditions in athletes.
  - In most of the world, swimmers train in enclosed pools that are both warm and humid.
  - A diagnosis of asthma is commonly found in elite athletes, especially endurance sports athletes (16).
    - The activation of the parasympathetic response is thought to contribute to bronchial constriction and the pathogenesis of asthma in this population (16).
    - A study involving the 1998 Winter Olympic Games swimmers revealed that 22.4% of swimmers reported either use of asthma medications or diagnosis of asthma or both (17).
    - It appears that athletes with asthma may gravitate to this environment because it is less asthmogenic (8). However, there is some evidence that inhaling chlorine by particles causes bronchospasm.
      - Chlorine is a bronchial irritant and contributes to the EIB/asthma in swimmers.
  - Coaches and trainers need to be aware of the asthmatic swimmer and have appropriate, athlete-specific emergency action plans (EAPs) including availability of their rescue inhaler.
- **Ear conditions**
  - Otitis externa
    - Also known as "swimmer's ear," this is one of the most common medical problems encountered by daily swimmers. The many hours swimmers spend submerging their ears in pool or open water may lead to ear canal maceration and infection.
      - Topical treatment with antibiotic drops is generally effective. Some providers opt for a combination treatment of topical antibiotic and topical steroid.

    - The swimmer should remain out of the pool for 2–3 days. Alternately, swimmers should use ear plugs that effectively keep water out of the ear canal for that time.
    - Preventive measures include maintaining a dry ear. Drying agents such as Vosol otic drops or a homemade mixture of 50% vinegar and 50% alcohol can be used. Using a hair dryer on the cool setting is another option.
    - In severe cases, an ear wick may be required to properly instill the treatment drops. Most ear wicks fall out on their own. If they do not, swimmers should be advised to have it removed in 2–3 days. The swimmer should be advised to avoid further trauma to the ear canal with cotton swabs.
  - External auditory canal exostosis
    - Also known as "surfer's ear"
    - It is caused by cold-water exposure. They are benign growths that develop in the external auditory canal.
      - In severe cases, they can cause hearing problems from physical obstruction and conductive hearing loss. Surgical excision may be required in severe cases.
- **Conjunctivitis**
  - Bacterial, viral, and chemical conjunctivitis present as a red eye with drainage.
    - Bacterial: more commonly unilateral. Treatment includes antibiotic ointment or drops. Erythromycin ointment may be used in noncontact lens wearers. Fluoroquinolone drops should be used in those who wear contacts.
    - Viral: most commonly bilateral, self-resolving
    - Chemical: generally related to an irritant, self-resolving with removal of the offending agent
  - Chemical/allergic conjunctivitis is most commonly related to the chlorine in pools.
    - The use of goggles while swimming can help prevent chemical conjunctivitis, which is a self-limiting problem (18).
- **Dermatologic conditions**
  - Swimmer's xerosis
    - After hours submersed in the water, the skin becomes dehydrated and pruritic.
      - Prevention is the key. The postswim shower should be short with warm water instead of hot water. Swimmers should apply lotion or body oil to their lightly patted skin after showering (19).
      - Barrier protection/artificial skin can be used to prevent water loss.
  - Contact dermatitis
    - Swimmers may develop dermatitis from contact with goggles and other equipment. Hydrocortisone cream can be used.
  - Cutaneous granulomas
    - Usually, self-resolves
    - Linked to *Mycobacterium marinum*
    - Antibiotic treatment with clarithromycin and trimethoprim-sulfamethoxazole can also be used.
  - Swimmers can also develop bacterial and fungal infections.
    - Please see Chapter 32 for additional details on dermatologic conditions.
- **Green hair**
  - Although not harmful, green hair can cause the swimmer undue anxiety (15).
    - Application of 2% hydrogen peroxide to the hair and rinsing this out in 30 minutes will help remove the discoloration.

MUSCULOSKELETAL ISSUES

Upper Extremity Injuries

Shoulder

- The shoulder is the most injured joint in swimmers. It accounts for a reported 16%–76% of all injuries (2).
- Shoulder injuries are a common problem in swimmers, particularly those who engage in high-volume training or competition. Shoulder pain is the most common complaint in competitive swimmers. In one survey of athletes, up to 91% of swimmers reported shoulder pain (20).
- Swimmer's shoulder
  - Swimmer's shoulder covers a wide range of shoulder injuries in swimmers, including rotator cuff tendinopathy, shoulder impingement, and labral pathology.
    - Typically, the swimmer feels maximum pain at the beginning of the pull-through phase. Often, the swimmer will swim through this pain for weeks until the pain is present throughout the entire freestyle stroke.
  - Typical treatment includes ice, training regimen modification, physical therapy, anti-inflammatory medication, and occasionally subacromial or glenohumeral corticosteroid injection. Rarely is surgery necessary.
  - Fatigue, muscle imbalance, and shoulder laxity contribute to the development of a swimmer's shoulder. Land and in-water training can each play a factor in injury development.
    - The swimmer should limit the total weekly mileage and swim with various strokes.
    - Swimmers have been shown to have greater shoulder adduction and internal rotation strength, which can lead to an imbalance in the shoulder. The swimmer should focus on creating a balance by strengthening the external rotators (21,22).
    - Therapy should be aimed at increasing the strength of the serratus anterior, a key scapular stabilizer, and

one of the most important muscles involved in the freestyle stroke. Any scapular dyskinesis should be addressed (8,23).

- Shoulder laxity and instability
  - Excessive shoulder mobility can functionally allow the athlete to have a more powerful stroke, but this excessive motion can also lead to overstretching of the supporting shoulder structures. Ultimately, this may result in pain and decreased performance.
    - Glenohumeral laxity can be beneficial up to a certain point as it allows for a longer stroke length and subsequent performance improvements (23).
    - It is a fine balance. A stretched shoulder capsule can lead to subluxation and repeat injury, keeping the athlete poolside. The more unstable the glenohumeral joint, the greater the risk of developing a labral tear, a Hill-Sachs lesion, or a Bankart lesion.
  - Instability can be anterior, posterior, inferior, or a combination.
  - Radiographs, including an axillary view, should be obtained. If a labral tear is suspected, magnetic resonance imaging can be ordered.
  - The mainstay of treatment is rotator cuff muscle strengthening and scapular stabilization.
    - If instability is persistent despite rehabilitation, surgery to tighten the capsule may be warranted. Athletes should be warned that a more stable shoulder may limit their performance, as their arm reach will likely be reduced after surgery.

Elbow

- Triceps tendinitis can develop as a result of the full extension necessary in the backstroke.
- The ulnar collateral ligament may be stressed in the recovery phase of the freestyle leading to sprain.
- Treatment is with rest, nonsteroidal anti-inflammatory drugs (NSAIDs), and ice as appropriate.

Lower Extremity Injuries

Hip and Groin Issues

- Hip and groin issues are most commonly seen in breaststrokers given their repetitive hip adduction movements (18).
- These injuries tend to include adductor strains, iliopsoas injuries, and sports hernias. Adductor strains have been reported in up to 41% of breaststroke swimmers (8).
- Treatment includes stretching and a core strengthening program.

Knee Issues

- Knee pain is the second most common musculoskeletal complaints among swimmers (8).
- The incidence is highest amount breaststroke swimmers with an incidence as high as 86%.
- Breaststroker's knee (8)
  - Swimmers complain of anterior and medial knee pain thought to be related to the repetitive valgus stress on the knee from the breaststroke kick.
    - The unique whip kick done in the breaststroke places a valgus stress at the knee. Due to these mechanics, breaststrokers have more knee complaints than swimmers competing in the other strokes.
    - The valgus force created at the knee may contribute to medial collateral ligament sprain. The swimmer needs instruction on proper technique for prevention.
  - The mainstays of treatment include rest, ice, and anti-inflammatory medications. Biomechanical errors should be identified and corrected.
  - Prevention is also key.
    - Emphasis is on lower extremity and core strengthening.
    - It is recommended that breaststrokers take a break from breaststroke at least 2 months of the year (8).
- Patellofemoral pain
  - The symptoms typical of patellofemoral syndrome also occur in swimmers usually due to the flutter kick, the dolphin kick used in the butterfly stroke, and wall push off after flip turns.
  - Treatment includes rest, ice, NSAIDs, and quadriceps strengthening. Swimmers should be encouraged to train using a foam buoy between the thighs in order to rest the knees.
  - Some swimmers may benefit from a neoprene patella stabilizing brace, which would substitute for McConnell taping.

Foot/Ankle Problems

- Extensor tendinitis may occur from the flutter kick or dolphin kick.
- Treatment includes rest, ice, and NSAIDs. Rest from the flutter kick is best achieved using a foam pull buoy. A lower extremity stretching program focusing on improved range of motion at the ankle will help in the recovery and also in prevention.
- Local foot injury can occur if the swimmer kicks the side of the pool or gutter. This usually results in abrasions or contusions but occasionally may cause a fracture. Proper flip turn technique will prevent foot injuries.

Neck and Back Injuries

Low Back Strain

- The butterfly and breaststroke require hyperextension of the lower back to maintain body position and complete the stroke. The body roll done by freestyle and backstroke swimmers can also cause strain, especially when the swimmer fatigues (2,8,18). The athlete will tend to roll less at the hip and more at the shoulder, increasing the strain at the lumbar spine. High-level swimmers or master's swimmers have shown to have an increased risk of developing degenerative disc disease (8).

- The flip turn may also contribute to lumbar pain given the frequent flexion and rotation involved.
- Treatment includes core strengthening and return to fundamental stroke techniques.

Cervical Strain

- Swimmers can develop strain at the neck if head rotation is exaggerated during the breathing cycle.
- The head rotation during the breathing cycle should only be enough to allow a breath, not bringing the face fully out of the water as some athletes do. As the swimmer moves forward, the water edge next to the mouth is cupped, allowing minimal rotation to achieve a sufficient breath.
- The athlete should maintain head position along the long axis without lifting the head or tucking the chin down when taking a breath.
- During the breaststroke, the head and neck should remain in the same position throughout the stroke. The cervical spine should be aligned with the back.
- Treatment involves stroke corrections (8).
  - Proper body roll reduces excess rotation at the neck during breathing cycles.

Spondylolysis/Spondylolisthesis

- The hyperextension of the back required specifically in the butterfly and breaststroke can predispose a swimmer to the development of a spondylolysis. The swimmer will often complain of pain during flip turns and starts. Spondylolysis rarely progresses to spondylolisthesis.
- Rest, training load and modification, and physical therapy are the mainstay of treatment. Rarely will the athlete require surgery.

EVENT COVERAGE

- Coverage should ideally include providers familiar with common swimming injuries.
- As with any event coverage, AEDs should be readily available should a cardiac event occur.
- A lifeguard and personnel familiar with CPR should be present at all practices and competitions.
- Open water and outdoor events (18)
  - In open water or outdoor events, weather must be considered. An EAP should be in place when severe weather and lightning occurs.
  - Additional lifeguards/medical personnel may need to be stationed on boats to allow easier access to participants should the need arise.

REFERENCES

1. Lahart IM, Metsios GS. Chronic physiological effects of swim training interventions in non-elite swimmers: a systematic review and meta-analysis. *Sports Med.* 2018;48(2):337–59. doi:10.1007/s40279-017-0805-0
2. Trinidad A, González-Garcia H, López-Valenciano A. An updated review of the epidemiology of swimming injuries. *PM R.* 2021;13(9):1005–20. doi:10.1002/pmrj.12503
3. Hill L, Mountjoy M, Miller J. Non-shoulder injuries in swimming: a systematic review. *Clin J Sport Med.* 2022;32(3):256–64. doi:10.1097/JSM.0000000000000903
4. *NCAA Publications* – 2021-22 & 2022-23 *Men's and Women's Swimming and Diving Rules.* [Accessed 2023 July 5]. Available from: https://www.ncaapublications.com/p-4637-2021-22-2022-23-mens-and-womens-swimming-and-diving-rules.aspx
5. Crowley E, Harrison AJ, Lyons M. The impact of resistance training on swimming performance: a systematic review. *Sports Med.* 2017;47(11):2285–307. doi:10.1007/s40279-017-0730-2
6. Psycharakis SG, Sanders RH. Body roll in swimming: a review. *J Sports Sci.* 2010;28(3):229–36.
7. Ichikawa H, Shimojo H, Baba Y, Mise T, Nara R, Shimoyama Y. The difference of propulsive force between water surface and underwater conditions in flutter kick swimming. *Proceedings.* 2020;49(1):167. doi:10.3390/proceedings2020049167
8. Nichols AW. Medical care of the aquatics athlete. *Curr Sports Med Rep.* 2015;14(5):389–96. doi:10.1249/JSR.0000000000000194
9. Neiva HP, Marques MC, Barbosa TM, Izquierdo M, Marinho DA. Warm-up and performance in competitive swimming. *Sports Med.* 2014;44(3):319–30. doi:10.1007/s40279-013-0117-y
10. Morais JE, Oliveira JP, Sampaio T, Barbosa TM. Wearables in swimming for real-time feedback: a systematic review. *Sensors.* 2022;22(10):3677. doi:10.3390/s22103677
11. Burtch AR, Ogle BT, Sims PA, et al. Controlled frequency breathing reduces inspiratory muscle fatigue. *J Strength Cond Res.* 2017;31(5):1273–81. doi:10.1519/JSC.0000000000001589
12. Czuba M, Wilk R, Karpiński J, Chalimoniuk M, Zajac A, Langfort J. Intermittent hypoxic training improves anaerobic performance in competitive swimmers when implemented into a direct competition mesocycle. *PLoS One.* 2017;12(8):e0180380. doi:10.1371/journal.pone.0180380
13. Born DP, Stäcker I, Romann M, Stöggl T. Competition age: does it matter for swimmers?. *BMC Res Notes.* 2022;15(1):82. doi:10.1186/s13104-022-05969-6
14. WHO. *Drowning*; [Accessed 2023 July 5]. Available from: https://www.who.int/news-room/fact-sheets/detail/drowning
15. Blattner CM, Kazlouskaya V, Coman GC, Blickenstaff NR, Murase JE. Dermatological conditions of aquatic athletes. *World J Dermatol.* 2015;4(1):8–15. doi:10.5314/wjd.v4.i1.8
16. Carlsen KH. Asthma in olympians. *Paediatr Respir Rev.* 2016;17:34–5. doi:10.1016/j.prrv.2015.08.013
17. Weiler JM, Ryan EJ 3rd. Asthma in United States olympic athletes who participated in the 1998 olympic winter games. *J Allergy Clin Immunol.* 2000;106(2):267–71.
18. Khodaee M, Edelman GT, Spittler J, et al. Medical care for swimmers. *Sports Med Open.* 2015;2(1):27. doi:10.1186/s40798-016-0051-2
19. Freiman A, Barankin B, Elpern DJ. Sports dermatology part 2: swimming and other aquatic sports. *CMAJ.* 2004;171(11):1339–41. doi:10.1503/cmaj.1040892

20. DeFroda SF, Goyal D, Patel N, Gupta N, Mulcahey MK. Shoulder instability in the overhead athlete. *Curr Sports Med Rep*. 2018;17(9):308–14. doi:10.1249/JSR.0000000000000517
21. Davis DD, Nickerson M, Varacallo M. Swimmer's shoulder. In: *StatPearls*. Treasure Island: StatPearls Publishing; 2023. [Accessed 2023 Jul 5]. Available from: http://www.ncbi.nlm.nih.gov/books/NBK470589/
22. Matzkin E, Suslavich K, Wes D. Swimmer's shoulder: painful shoulder in the competitive swimmer. *J Am Acad Orthop Surg*. 2016 Aug;24(8):527–36. doi:10.5435/JAAOS-D-15-00313
23. De Martino I, Rodeo SA. The swimmer's shoulder: multi-directional instability. *Curr Rev Musculoskelet Med*. 2018;11(2):167–71. doi:10.1007/s12178-018-9485-0

Tennis and Other Racquet Sports

122

Kinsley Pierre and Marc R. Safran

- Racquet sports encompass a variety of distinct competitive games such as squash, badminton, racquetball, padel, pickleball, and, of course, tennis. Collectively, these games are enjoyed by individuals from diverse backgrounds and skill levels, both in the United States and around the world.
  - Tennis holds a prominent position globally as one of the most popular sports and stands out as the most widely recognized among all racquet sports.
- Racquet sports are enjoyed by people from all walks of life, ranging from recreational players to professionals, who can actively participate in these sports.
- Racquet sports offer a suitable form of exercise for individuals of varying levels of fitness and age, presenting an opportunity for both physical activity and social interaction. These games can be enjoyed in singles play or cooperatively with peers in doubles, fostering a social environment alongside the physical health benefits they provide.

TENNIS

- According to the International Tennis Federation, globally, 87 million people actively play tennis (1).
- The dimensions of a standard tennis court vary depending on whether the game being played is singles or doubles.
  - For singles, competitive and recreational play, the court is 78 feet long and 27 feet wide.
  - In doubles, the court is 78 feet long; however, the width extends to 36 feet to account for the additional players.
- The tennis ball is pressurized and is composed of rubber and fabric, with a hollow center.
  - Tennis balls have a diameter of 2.575–2.7 in (6.54–6.86 cm) and a circumference of 8.09–8.48 in (20.6–21.5 cm).
  - The mass of a tennis ball must be between 1.975–2.095 oz (56–59.4 g).
- There are many different types of racquets used in tennis. An adult tennis racquet typically measures 27 in (68.58 cm) long.
  - Most are made with titanium, graphite, or fiberglass and weigh, on average, 300 g or 10.6 oz.
  - The strings on a standard tennis racquet are usually composed of natural gut, synthetic gut, nylon, multifilament, and hybrid, and may vary in thickness (gauge).
- A net is positioned at the center of the court, dividing it into two sides for the opposing players. When a player is unsuccessful at returning the ball within the legal dimensions of the court, a point is awarded to their opponent. To win a game, a player must score a minimum of four points. To win a set, a player must win at least six games (seven games if they cannot win six games before their opponent wins five games). To win the match, a player must win two out of three sets.

SQUASH

- The World Squash Federation estimates that 25 million people play squash worldwide.
- The standard length for a squash court is 32 feet long and about 21 feet wide. However, court size varies in North America and International play, and by the number of players on the court.
  - Similar to tennis, squash can be played as singles or doubles. In doubles, the courts may be larger, up to 45 feet long and about 25 feet wide.
- Squash balls are composed of raw rubber and other synthetic materials. Squash balls have a diameter of 1.56–1.59 in (3.95–4.05 cm) and a circumference of 4.89–5 in (12.41–12.72 cm).
  - The mass of a squash ball is between 0.8–0.9 oz (23–25 g).
  - There are four types of squash balls that are designated by a small colored dot. A blue dot is used for an introductory (beginner) squash ball, a red dot for a progress squash ball, a yellow dot for a competition play squash ball, and a double yellow dot for a professional play squash ball.
    - The beginner balls play faster and progress from blue > red > yellow > double yellow, with blue being the fastest and double yellow the slowest
- Adult squash racquets also vary in styles, but the average length typically measures about 27 in long.
  - Squash racquets are typically composed of graphite and aluminum, weighing between 135 and 190 g or 4.8 and 6.7 oz.

- The strings on a standard squash racquet are composed of nylon, natural gut, synthetic gut, or multifilament.
- Unlike tennis, there is no net, so players are next to each other on the court. Additionally, the squash court is surrounded by four walls, and the walls are used in play.
- To win a game, a player must score 11 points before their opponent. To win the match, the player must win three games.

RACQUETBALL

- Racquetball is estimated to have 20 million players worldwide.
- In North America, the standard dimensions for a racquetball court are 40 feet in length and 20 feet in width. However, the size of the court may vary internationally. Like most racquet and ball sports, games can be played in either singles or doubles play.
- Balls used in racquetball are hollow and composed primarily of rubber. Racquetballs have a diameter of 2.25 in (5.7 cm) and a circumference of 7.07 in (18 cm). The mass of a racquetball is 1.4 oz (40 g).
- The standard racquet for an adult measures about 19–22 in long, with most made of titanium or graphite.
  - The average weight of a racquet is 150–185 g or 5.3–6.5 oz.
  - The strings differ depending on the type of racquet used and can be composed of either nylon, gut, plastic, monofilament, graphite, or metal.
- Courts for racquetball can be three- or four-sided in a rectangular room. Thus, like squash, there is no net and players on next to each other on the court.
- To win a game of racquetball, a player must score a designated, predetermined, and agreed-upon score (usually 15) before the opposing player. To win the match, a player must win two out of three games.

BADMINTON

- With an estimated global average of around 220 million active players, badminton stands as one of the most widely played sports in the world.
- The average size for a badminton court is 44 feet long and 17–20 feet wide, depending on if played in singles or doubles.
- Unlike other racquet sports, badminton does not involve the use of a ball. The projectile used in a game of badminton is called a birdie or shuttlecock. The shuttlecock is composed of 16 feathers from a duck, arranged and organized around a plastic and cork base.
- The racquets used in badminton are smaller and lighter than racquets used in tennis. The standard racquet for an adult is approximately 26 in long.
  - Although there is a range of styles available for racquets in badminton, most are composed of graphite, steel, or aluminum, weighing 100 g or 3.52 oz, on average.
  - The strings of most badminton racquets are composed of nylon, natural gut, and other synthetic materials.
- A net is placed in the middle of the court to divide it into two halves.
- To win a game of badminton, a player must score 21 points before their opponent and must win two out of three games to win a match.

PICKLEBALL

- According to the Sports and Fitness Industry Association, pickleball is played by approximately 8.9 million players around the world.
  - In the last few years, it has increased in popularity and gained 159% more players (2). At the time of this publication, pickleball is considered the fastest-growing sport, and recently, two professional pickleball leagues have started.
- The average length of the court is 44 feet long and is 20 feet wide. It can be played in singles or doubles.
- The balls used in pickleball are hollow, composed of plastic, and are perforated with several holes. The size of the holes varies based on whether pickleball is being played indoors (larger holes) or outdoors (smaller holes). Pickleballs have a diameter of 2.874″–2.972 in (7.3–7.55 cm) and a circumference of 9.03–9.34 in (22.93–23.72 cm). The mass of a pickleball is between 0.78 and 0.935 oz (22–26.5 g).
- The racquets used in pickleball are not true racquets and are considered paddles.
  - These paddles are much smaller than racquets used in other racquet and ball sports.
  - On average, the paddles are 15.5–17 in long and are composed of aluminum, graphite, and other synthetic materials.
- Like tennis and badminton, a net is placed in the middle of the court that separates into two distinct sections for opposing players.
- Points are only awarded on the serve; a point cannot be scored by the receiving side until the ball has been touched by both teams. Points are awarded if the ball hits the net or bounces out of bounds on the opposing side.
  - To win a game of pickleball, a player must reach 11 points before the opposing player and win by 2. To win a match, typically a player must win two out of three games.

SPECIFIC CONSIDERATIONS

- Each of these sports is a unilateral arm dominant sport, resulting in asymmetric forces to the upper and lower extremities and rotational forces on the spine.
- Racquet sports require bursts of activity lasting seconds to less than a minute with periods of relative inactivity between points.

- Certain racquet sports, such as squash and racquetball, carry a significant risk of eye injury due to the size, shape, and hardness of the ball, and as a result of turning around quickly to see the opponent hitting the ball. Protective goggles are usually required.
- Squash and racquetball also have a higher risk of contact injuries, especially lacerations from racquet contact, as players are in close proximity to their opponent in a confined space (the enclosed court).

INJURY INCIDENCE

- Determining the precise occurrence of injuries in tennis and other racquet sports is challenging due to significant variations in definitions, methodologies, and study populations among different research endeavors (3).
- Number of investigations have reported tennis injury incidence to be anywhere from 2 to 20 injuries per 1000 hours of tennis played (4–6).
  - In a comprehensive review of 28 epidemiologic studies on tennis injury that have been published since 1966, Pluim et al. (7) reported the incidence as ranging from 0.04 to 21.5 injuries per 1000 hours played (7).
  - This same investigation found that most injuries occurred in the lower extremity (31%–67%), followed by the upper extremity (20%–49%), and lastly the trunk (3%–21%). The anatomic location of injuries was supported by a recent investigation of the injury profile of Swedish tennis players over a 2-year period (8).
    - Other studies have confirmed that lower extremities predominate for the acute injuries, whereas chronic complaints are more common in the upper extremities.
- In an investigation of elite junior tennis players (15–18 years of age) at the United States Tennis Association (USTA) National Junior Championships (9), based on a questionnaire, only 23% of girls and 45% of boys reported no injury that prevented them from playing for 1 week or longer.
  - 53% of girls and 29% of boys noted more than one injury in the past.
  - Low back pain was the most common ailment for both genders (47% of girls, 31% of boys), followed by shoulder pain.
  - 35% of junior tennis players complained of shoulder pain at some point in time, whereas more than 50% of older players and elite athletes note shoulder pain at some point in their career (9,10).
  - Although there was no significant difference in the overall injury rate between boys and girls, there was a difference in the distribution of injuries. Girls sustained more injuries to the feet, leg, and wrist, whereas boys more commonly injured the ankle, groin, and hand (9).
- Nahn and colleagues found that lower extremity injuries were the most common presenting injuries to emergency rooms in the United States for squash, racquetball, and badminton participants (11).
  - In squash, racquetball, and badminton, sprains and strains were the most common injuries to the trunk and extremities.
  - Lacerations accounted for nearly half of all head and neck injuries from these sports presenting to the emergency room.
  - Nearly 25% of head and neck injuries seen in squash, racquetball, and badminton are ocular injuries.

BACK INJURIES

- Trunk rotation is an essential factor in generating power within racquet sports. Hyperextension and rotation are important in generating power for the tennis serve and the overhead smash (Fig. 122.1). Improper technique and insufficient equipment can result in injuries.
- Back pain is very common in tennis players and was identified as the most common injury in junior tennis players (8).
  - Forty-seven percent of female and 31% of male tennis players reported low back pain (currently or in the past), and low back pain has been reported in up to half of all professional players (10).
- Many causes of low back pain in players are muscular in nature.
  - These players often complain of a shorter duration of pain, with discomfort usually localized in the paraspinal musculature away from the midline.
  - Rest, physical therapy, and anti-inflammatory medications are appropriate treatment options for muscular discomfort in the back.
- Neurologic complaints, such as numbness, tingling, or weakness of the legs, are not seen with muscular-type discomfort and should warrant further investigation if noted.
  - Persistent back pain or back pain that is not responsive to conservative measures also warrants further investigation.
  - In older athletes, intervertebral disk degeneration, disk herniation, and facet arthrosis may occur, leading to radicular symptoms.
  - In the younger player, spondylolysis or spondylolisthesis is more common.
    - Overuse and in particular, back extension, such as seen during the service motion, is thought to be a main contributor to the development of pars lesions.
    - The reported incidence of symptomatic defects of the pars ranges from 15% to 47% in the younger athletic population (12).

SPONDYLOLYSIS

- Players with spondylolysis will often complain of axial/midline low back pain, and some will report radiation to the gluteal area or proximal lower extremity.

Figure 122.1: Professional tennis player serving the ball, with the photograph at the early acceleration phase. Note the shoulder moving from maximal external rotation. The trunk position is noted to be hyperextended and rotated toward the dominant side, causing significant asymmetric forces on the spine. (Figure used with permission from Marc R. Safran, MD.)

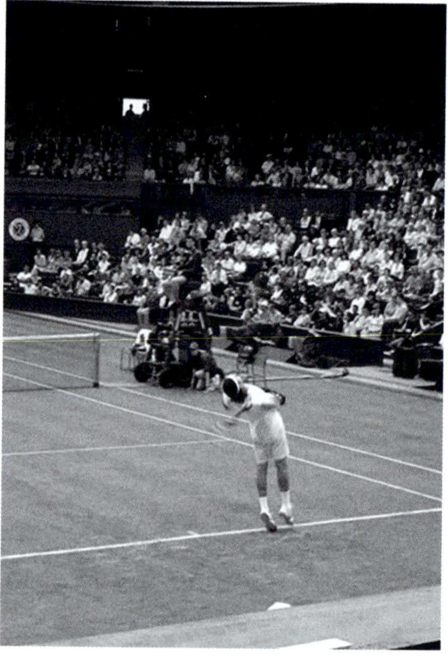

- The onset of pain may begin after an acute injury; however, it is more often gradual, with mild symptoms being present for some time. Pain is often exacerbated by back extension during the service motion.
- Treatment of spondylolysis and low-grade spondylolisthesis in the tennis player is typically nonoperative and includes prolonged periods of rest in addition to physical therapy.
- Some clinicians prefer to place athletes with spondylolysis in a thoracolumbosacral orthosis or Boston brace to immobilize the low back to theoretically improve healing rates. This is controversial, however, because some evidence does support improved healing rates, whereas other studies do not, and compliance can be challenging in this group.
- Players who do not respond to nonoperative treatment, as well as those with high-grade spondylolisthesis, may be surgical candidates.

ABDOMINAL MUSCLE STRAINS

- Abdominal muscle strains are not infrequent in sports like tennis and occur at all levels of competitive play. These injuries generally occur during the tennis serve and are the result of the forceful trunk rotation and flexion required to generate force.
- Those athletes who do not efficiently use the kinetic chain to serve (using power from the legs) tend to be more susceptible to abdominal muscle strains, usually involving the nondominant side — the rectus abdominis or the obliques.
  - Poor iliopsoas muscle strength is associated with a higher risk of lower abdominal muscle strain.
- Most abdominal muscle injuries in tennis involve the rectus abdominis contralateral to the dominant arm (13), usually occurring during the tennis serve.
- With the open stance strokes now prevalent in tennis, there is an increased incidence of oblique muscle injuries reported as well (14).
- Trunk rotation and flexion, and lumbar extension are critical components of the serve, placing large forces on the abdominal wall musculature. Consequently, the most common injury mechanism of the abdominal muscles in tennis players involves a forced concentric contraction of the abdominal musculature when the spine is completely hyperextended, as seen during the tennis serve (14).
- Open stance mechanics also lead to more abdominal muscle activity that is used for racquet speed generation and force to hit the ball harder, placing great strain on the abdominal muscles, putting these muscles at risk of strain injury.
- The typical presentation for an abdominal wall muscle injury is a competitive player complaining of acute nondominant abdominal wall pain worsened by the service motion.
- Treatment of abdominal muscle injury in the tennis player includes rest with or without cryotherapy, followed by rehabilitation exercises (14).

SHOULDER

- The dominant shoulder is highly susceptible to injury and is often a source of pain in fast-paced racquet sports.
- Of upper extremity injuries, the shoulder is the most commonly injured in tennis (15).
- Anatomically, the shoulder joint offers the greatest range of motion (ROM) among all major joints in the body, but this extensive mobility comes at the cost of stability.
- The shoulder is also particularly susceptible to injury in racquet sports due to the required acceleration and deceleration

of the arm to its maximum potential while maintaining precise control over the racquet during ball strike (Fig. 122.2).

- A careful balance between mobility and stability is necessary to maximize performance. While increased range of motion, particularly shoulder external rotation, is beneficial for the tennis player who is trying to generate maximal velocity and spin with their strokes, too much motion may result in increased reliance on soft tissues for stability, which may break down and result in shoulder instability.

Rotator Cuff Syndrome

- Rotator cuff syndrome is common in tennis players of all levels (15). It usually occurs as a result of repetitive overhead serving motions.
- Symptoms include lateral shoulder pain with activity or at rest, pain with active arm abduction, or pain with internal/external rotation of the shoulder.
  - Tennis players particularly complain of pain while serving and hitting overheads or high volleys.
- Although rotator cuff syndrome may be the result of overuse, or outlet impingement, it may also be seen in other situations, such as rotator cuff tears, instability or microinstability, superior labral anterior to posterior (SLAP) injuries, internal impingement, glenohumeral internal rotation deficit (GIRD), SICK scapula (see below), shoulder stiffness, os acromiale, or scapular dyskinesis.
- It is incumbent upon the tennis physician to determine the cause of rotator cuff pain and correct the cause.
- Initial treatment includes rest and rehabilitation, with specific emphasis not only on shoulder motion (usually posterior capsular tightness), but also on rotator cuff strengthening and scapular stabilization muscle exercises (discussed later).
- Analgesics, including nonsteroidal anti-inflammatory medications, may help with the pain to assist in rehabilitation, as can injectable corticosteroids.
- Aggressive treatment of rotator cuff tears is important in tennis players; Sonnery-Cottet et al. (16) have shown that repair of smaller rotator cuff tears results in a higher rate of return to tennis play as compared with players who have undergone repair of larger rotator cuff tears.

Biceps Tendinitis

- Biceps tendinitis is another common complaint in tennis and other racquet sport athletes and may be due not only to the overhead service motion but also the pronation/supination motions of the forearm required for forehands and backhands.
  - The biceps tendon may also become inflamed when the rotator cuff is inflamed and/or there is rotator cuff dysfunction as a result of strain, tendinopathy, or tearing.
  - The biceps tendon may become impinged by the humeral head and acromion or due to its proximity to the inflamed rotator cuff.
  - Symptoms in the biceps tendon may also arise when there is a concomitant SLAP lesion and/or coracoid impingement.
- Athletes may complain of pain in the anterior aspect of the shoulder and be point tender in this area.
- Treatment again consists of rest and shoulder rehabilitation. Oral anti-inflammatory medications have a role in the treatment of biceps tendonitis, whereas the use of injectable corticosteroids remains controversial.

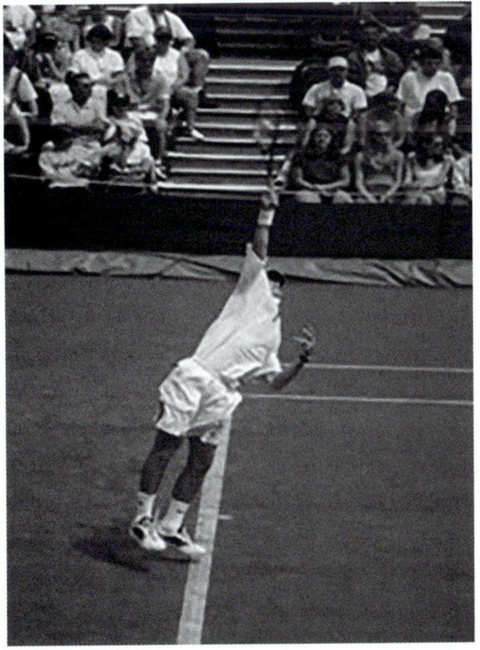

Figure 122.2: Professional tennis player serving the ball, with the photograph at the time of contact with the ball. This is in the acceleration phase, where the shoulder has gone from maximal external rotation while the body was rotated maximally to the dominant side, to full overhead reach and the body/trunk moving to the nondominant side. This requires precise motion and timing to allow for the serve to be hard and accurate. (Figure used with permission from Marc R. Safran, MD.)

The Tennis Player's Shoulder

- Although scapular dyskinesis and capsulolabral changes within the overhead athlete's shoulder usually do not directly cause symptoms, they can combine in various ways to cause dysfunction and pathology in the shoulder.
- Alterations in scapular motion or position can significantly affect overall glenohumeral biomechanics, as the scapula is critical in shoulder function.
  - These changes take time to develop and are therefore usually seen in players who participate in tennis on a frequent basis and over a long period of time.
- The term "SICK scapula" was introduced to describe a pathologic state of the scapula seen in overhead athletes that is characterized by:
  - **S**capular malposition,
  - **I**nferior medial border prominence,
  - **C**oracoid pain and malposition, and
  - **K**inesis abnormalities of the scapula (17,18).
- Clinically, this syndrome can be recognized by a drooping shoulder on the player's dominant side, along with scapular asymmetry on inspection.
  - This scapular asymmetry can be further elucidated by slowly adducting the abducted shoulder or with repeated slow forward elevation as the hands are brought from the side to eye level and back down again.
- Patients may complain of anterior, posterior, or superolateral shoulder pain, and a careful history and physical exam should be undertaken to recognize this constellation of findings instead of attributing the player's pain to other isolated lesions.
- It has been recognized that tennis players develop an increase in external rotation of the dominant shoulder at the expense of internal rotation, leaving the total arc of shoulder rotation unchanged (19).
- When there is a greater loss of internal rotation than gain in external rotation *and* the difference between the dominant and nondominant arm in internal rotation is greater than 25°, then the potential for injury is considered greater and falls under the umbrella of GIRD (17,20).
  - Kvitne and Jobe (21) initially proposed that repetitive loading in the 90/90 position (late cocking phase of the tennis serve) caused microtrauma to the anterior shoulder capsular structures and the anterior labrum, causing subtle anterior instability.
    - This instability allows the humeral head to translate anteriorly, bringing the greater tuberosity of the humerus and the rotator cuff in close proximity to the posterior glenoid.
  - This was one theoretical etiology of internal impingement (22), where the undersurface of the posterosuperior rotator cuff (supraspinatus and infraspinatus) may impinge between the humeral head and the posterosuperior rim of the glenoid. This damages the rotator cuff tendons and may also lead to posterior superior labral pathology.
  - Players with this pathology usually complain of pain in the posterior shoulder with overhead activity.
- Alternatively, this anterior instability could also cause overuse of the rotator cuff by trying to maintain shoulder stability.
- More recent research has shown that posterior capsular contracture results in posterior shoulder tightness and internal rotation contracture, and this contracture results in altered humeral head motion, resulting in internal impingement (20).
  - Posterior capsular contracture as a result of posterior rotator cuff inflammation or hypertrophy of the posterior inferior glenohumeral ligament (IGHL) results in altered humeral head motion in the 90/90 position.
  - The humeral head moves in a posterior and superior direction in the 90/90 position with posterior IGHL contracture, leading to increased posterior superior labral wear (including SLAP tears), internal impingement, and possibly SLAP tears through the "peel back" mechanism (17,20).
- Overhead athletes, such as the tennis player (who serves overhead), may also develop a variant of SLAP lesion where there is labral damage superiorly and posteriorly.
  - Brockmeyer and colleagues have introduced a treatment algorithm for SLAP tears, which is based on a classification system (23). They recommend:
    - Type I tears should be treated conservatively or through arthroscopic debridement.
    - Type II tears can be addressed through SLAP repair or biceps tenotomy/tenodesis.
    - Type III involves resection of the unstable bucket-handle tear.
    - Type IV treatment includes SLAP repair, with biceps tenotomy/tenodesis recommended if more than 50% of the biceps tendon is affected.
    - Type V lesions should be repaired using a Bankart repair and SLAP repair.
    - Type VI treatment involves the resection of the flap and SLAP repair.
    - Type VII are treated through refixation of the anterosuperior labrum and SLAP repair (23).
- The time of greatest risk for progression of pathology is when the player's GIRD exceeds the external rotation gain (17).
- Initial treatment for each of these shoulder pathologies is usually nonoperative.
  - Rehabilitation exercises should focus on the inciting factors, such as the posterior capsular tightness and any scapular dyskinesis that may be present.
    - Posterior capsular stretching exercises include the "sleeper stretch" and "cross-body stretch" (24), whereas scapular dyskinesis can be addressed by a number of exercises that specifically target the scapular stabilizers (25).

  - Restoration of rotator cuff muscle balance and proprioceptive exercises are also important parts of the rehabilitation protocol (24).
- Should nonoperative management fail to improve symptoms, surgical management includes repairing the SLAP lesions, if present (17), and possibly cutting the posterior IGHL to gain internal rotation.
  - Good outcomes have been reported in patients undergoing combined SLAP and rotator cuff repair (26), though overall results are inconsistent.

ELBOW

Lateral Epicondylitis

- The common term for lateral epicondylitis is "tennis elbow," although tennis is only involved in approximately 5%–10% of cases (27).
- The pathology is caused by degeneration of the deeper fibers of the extensor carpi radialis brevis (ECRB) and is attributable to overuse of wrist extension and excessive pronation/supination.
- There is no acute inflammation, and thus "epicondylitis" is a misnomer (28).
- Causes of lateral epicondylitis in tennis include overuse of wrist extensors, weak forearm and shoulder muscles, vibration resulting from string tension and racquet stiffness effects, undersized or oversized grips, and use of a one-handed backhand with poor form.
- Treatment of lateral epicondylitis is primarily nonoperative, with 90% of patients responding to conservative measures, including rest, anti-inflammatory medications, cock-up wrist splints, physical therapy focusing on stretching and eccentric strengthening of the wrist extensor, and use of counterforce bracing when returning to activity (29).
- Injection of corticosteroids has been a mainstay of treatment for some time (30), but corticosteroid injections *alone* have not been shown to be efficacious in prospective randomized trials.
  - The use of corticosteroid injections in lateral epicondylitis should be considered primarily analgesic.
  - This modality should be used sparingly, and only as an adjunct to physical therapy — reducing the pain so the player can perform the rehabilitation exercises.
- Iontophoresis has been shown to have benefit in the management of the player with tennis elbow (31), and there has been some interest in topical nitric oxide as preliminary prospective randomized control trials have supported both these therapies (32).
- Platelet-rich plasma (PRP) has also been used as a mode of treatment for elbow injuries in tennis, although the widespread use of PRP is still a subject of controversy (See Chapter 78, Orthobiologic Therapies).
- Recalcitrant cases may be treated with debridement of the disease tissue either through an open technique (33) or arthroscopically (34,35).

Medial Epicondylitis

- Although tennis elbow is common in the recreational tennis player, medial epicondylitis is seen more often in the high-level player, likely as a result of overuse of the wrist flexor/pronator muscles from hitting top spin and snapping the wrist into flexion during the service motion. Also, repeatedly hitting the ball late can result in increased stresses to the medial elbow.
- The flexor carpi radialis and pronator teres are most frequently affected, and the pathology looks the same as lateral epicondylitis.
- Treatment is similar to lateral epicondylitis, although caution should be taken with a counterforce brace because that may compress the ulnar nerve.

Ulnar Collateral Ligament Injury

- Tennis players place tremendous tensile strain on the medial elbow, particularly the ulnar collateral ligament (UCL), although injuries in these areas are uncommon in tennis. These forces are highest during the late cocking and early acceleration phases of the service motion and may also be notable during the forehand groundstroke, especially when hitting the ball late (36).
- The most common cause of UCL injury in the tennis player is chronic attenuation due to repetitive performance of the service motion.
- However, UCL injuries may occur as a result of altering kinematics due to pain or injury proximally in the kinetic chain, such as the shoulder, back, or hip.
- A detailed history and examination of the player with medial elbow pain is important because pain in this location may be due to a number of pathologies.
- Players with UCL injuries will typically complain of a loss of "pop" or "zip" on the serve (loss of power/velocity) and have pain during the late cocking or early acceleration phases.
- Most tears in adults are within the midsubstance of the ligament, whereas in adolescents, they often are avulsions from the humerus.
- Treatment of UCL injury may include both operative and nonoperative measures.
  - Nonoperative measures include rest/cessation of overhead sport activities, anti-inflammatory medications, and physical therapy, including an intensive elbow program that excludes exercises that place valgus stress on the elbow.
- Average rates of return to sport with nonoperative treatment range from 42% to 50% (37).

- Operative treatment consists of reconstruction of the torn ligament, usually using a free graft. There have been many modifications since the original technique described by Jobe et al. (38).
- Return to sport (including tennis) following operative intervention has been reported to be 80%–90% (39).

Valgus Extension Overload

- Valgus extension overload (VEO) is an elbow condition that is almost exclusively seen in overhead athletes, involving the formation of posteromedial osteophytes, posteromedial chondromalacia, and risk of olecranon stress fractures.
- During the serving or overhead throwing motion, the medial aspect of the elbow (UCL) experiences tensile forces while compressive forces are seen in the lateral portion of the elbow (radiocapitellar joint), and posteriorly, the olecranon is compressed within the tight-fitting olecranon fossa.
- Repetitive and forceful shearing and abutting of the olecranon within its fossa leads to VEO and can be exacerbated by forceful elbow extension in follow-through and/or UCL insufficiency (40).
- Athletes commonly complain of posteromedial elbow pain during both the acceleration and follow-through phases of the overhead motion. Complaints of locking or catching and an inability to straighten the elbow fully may also be encountered due to loose bodies.
- Although VEO may occur as an isolated phenomenon, it more often occurs in the presence of laxity due to UCL attenuation; thus, the clinician should have a high index of suspicion for UCL injury.
- Initial treatment begins with rest and anti-inflammatory medications, followed by an evaluation of serving or throwing mechanics to identify areas for technique improvement (41).
- Failure of nonoperative management is an indication for surgery in those with VEO. Classically, an open procedure to remove olecranon osteophytes and loose bodies was performed; however, an increasing proportion of VEO is now being treated arthroscopically because this is less invasive and allows assessment of the anterior elbow as well (40).
- Assessment of the UCL is mandatory, and reconstruction (if needed) should be considered in the setting of a torn or severely attenuated ligament.

WRIST

Tendonitis

- Wrist complaints are common in tennis players (9). Nondominant wrist pain is particularly common in players using a two-handed backhand.
- One investigation of female junior tennis players found 29% and 25% prevalence rates of dominant and nondominant wrist pain, respectively (10).
- Tendonitis of the wrist may develop in tennis players who place large amounts of spin and/or velocity on the ball because this places extra demand on the muscles and tendons of the upper extremity.
- Improper technique in novice players may also be a contributing factor to the development of tendonitis.
- Wrist extensors are more commonly involved, but wrist flexor tendonitis may also be present.
    - Of the wrist extensors, the extensor carpi ulnaris (ECU) is often involved, presenting as ulnar-sided wrist pain. As with other forms of wrist tendonitis, overuse and/or improper technique is usually the cause.
    - Subluxation or complete rupture of the ECU tendon can also be seen in the tennis player (42). As such, one should elicit a history of snapping about the wrist.
    - ECU subluxation and/or ECU rupture usually requires surgical correction for return to play.
    - ECU tendonitis is frequently associated with triangular fibrocartilage complex (TFCC) tears (the ECU subsheath is a part of the TFCC) or ulnocarpal abutment (10).
- Other tendons involved in the development of wrist tendonitis in the tennis player include extensor pollicis brevis (EPB)/abductor pollicis longus (APL) (de Quervain tenosynovitis), extensor digitorum communis (EDC), and wrist flexors.
    - de Quervain tenosynovitis likely develops from mechanical irritation of the EPB and APL tendon sheaths near the radial styloid of the radius.
    - Treatment involves cessation of activity, anti-inflammatory medication, thumb spica immobilization, corticosteroid injection, and, in recalcitrant cases, surgical debridement with release of the sheath.
- Rest, anti-inflammatory medications, and immobilization are typically also successful in the treatment of EDC and wrist flexor tendonitis.

Triangular Fibrocartilage Complex Injury

- TFCC injuries in tennis players remain a well-recognized cause of ulnar-sided wrist pain in racquet sport athletes (43).
- Players may report ulnar-sided wrist pain of a mechanical nature, swelling, weakness, or a sense of instability that is increased with the performance of forehands or backhands. The nondominant wrist may also be involved in players with two-handed backhands.
- Although somewhat controversial, most clinicians recommend a magnetic resonance imaging (MRI) arthrogram to confirm the diagnosis of a TFCC tear.
- Occasionally, TFCC tears are accompanied by instability of the distal radioulnar joint (DRUJ). Piano key assessment of the DRUJ for side-to-side instability can help confirm this diagnosis.
- When a TFCC tear is seen with a DRUJ instability, acute surgical treatment is needed.

- Without DRUJ instability, initial management of TFCC injury is nonsurgical, although high-level athletes may opt for initial surgical management in order to return to play more quickly.
- Standard nonsurgical treatments include temporary splint immobilization of the wrist and forearm, oral nonsteroidal anti-inflammatory medication, corticosteroid joint injection, and physical therapy (44).
- Surgical management includes arthroscopic techniques of repair or debridement, depending on the pathology present. Open techniques may be needed when ligament reconstruction is indicated in the setting of DRUJ instability.
- Prognosis for return to play is excellent following treatment of TFCC injuries (45).

Other Causes of Wrist Pain

- Other causes of wrist pain may include fracture of the hook of the hamate (from impaction of the wrist against the bottom of the racquet handle), chondromalacia of the pisiform, radiocarpal arthritis, triquetrolunate ligament injury, ulnar nerve compression in Guyon canal, medial nerve entrapment at the wrist (carpal tunnel syndrome), and ulnar artery thrombosis.
- A recent report has also documented a group of tennis players with stress injury to the lunate (46).
- Falling on an outstretched hand in tennis may result in any number of acute injuries to the hand and wrist.
- Lastly, stress fractures of the nondominant ulna (two-handed backhand players) and stress fractures of the distal radius and ulna of the dominant wrist may also present as wrist pain.

LOWER EXTREMITY INJURIES

Hip/Thigh

- In games like squash, racquetball, and tennis, players frequently perform decisive actions and forceful movements at varying degrees of flexibility, such as swiftly changing their direction, explosive jumping, and abruptly stopping (Fig. 122.3). These movements can be physically strenuous and may exert significant force on the hip and thigh.
- The muscles surrounding the hip play a vital role in transferring forces from the lower extremities to the racquet as part of the kinetic chain in tennis. Consequently, the hip is impacted by various motions in the game such as flexion when lunging for a low ball, extension during the late cocking phase of a serve, and rotation, particularly in the serve motion or strokes that commonly employ open stance mechanics (47).
- The most common injuries in the hip joint are associated with inflammation of musculoskeletal tissues around the hip joint and muscle strains. The likelihood of muscle strain rises when attempting to strike the ball with greater force, especially as fatigue sets in toward the conclusion of a match.

Muscle Strain

- Hip and thigh injuries account for anywhere between 6%–14% and 11%–29% of all tennis injuries, respectively (10). Most of these injuries are muscle strains, with hip adductor muscles and hamstrings being the most commonly involved.
  - As with quadriceps, Achilles, and rotator cuff tears in the general population, older racquet sport athletes are more susceptible to these tendon ruptures.
- Hamstring injuries may occur at either the proximal or distal end of the muscle and are usually associated with explosive accelerations.
- Although less common, hip flexor and quadriceps strains/tears may also occur.
- Adductor muscle strains are usually caused by sudden lateral changes in direction or sliding on clay courts when players' legs may be at maximum abduction ("doing the splits"). These movements place the adductors on maximum stretch and thus predispose them to strains or tears.
  - Those with decreased hip range of motion have been shown to be at increased risk for groin injury (48,49).

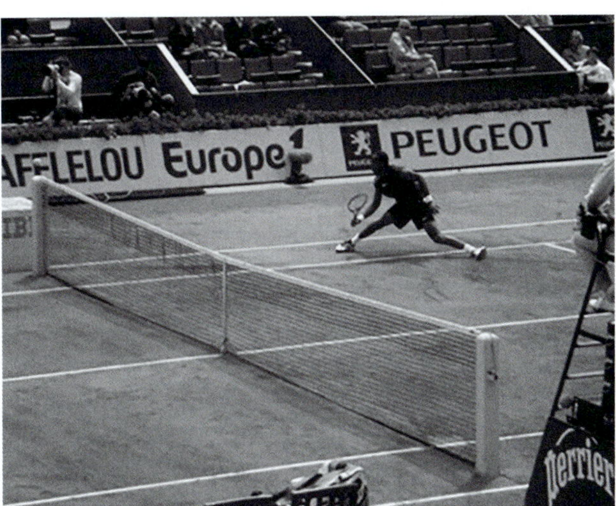

Figure 122.3: Professional tennis player sliding on a clay court with hips abducted and valgus forces on the knee. Players actually slide on hard court surfaces as well as clay and grass courts. These are just some of the forces players are subject to during tennis play that may result in hip injuries (such as adductors) and knee (meniscus and medial collateral ligament). (Figure used with permission from Marc R. Safran, MD.)

   - Players may present with medial thigh or groin pain and may or may not recall a specific inciting event.
   - Among the adductor group, the adductor longus is most commonly injured (50).
   - In cases where the history and physical examination are equivocal, MRI may be helpful to confirm the diagnosis and differentiate between other causes of groin pain, such as osteitis pubis and sports hernia (51).
   - Management of adductor strains is almost always nonoperative, with rest, ice, and physical therapy when tolerated.
   - There is controversy about the treatment of the acute rupture/avulsion, although currently, the pendulum favors nonoperative management.

Femoroacetabular Impingement

- Since the initial description in 1994, femoroacetabular impingement (FAI) has become an increasingly recognized cause of hip pain in athletes and tennis players in particular (52).
- The typical presentation is that of a tennis player reporting groin pain or anterolateral hip pain that is worsened during activity. Onset is usually insidious without a specific precipitating event.
- Players may complain of pain when putting on their socks/shoes, as well as lunging for a low ball. Eventually, the pain may affect the power of their serve, putting other structures in the kinetic chain at risk.
- Examination for FAI includes limited hip internal rotation (as measured in 90° of flexion), as well as pain in flexion (to 90°), adduction, and internal rotation. Labral stress or scour tests also may result in pain and/or clicking.
- Initial imaging should include plain radiographs, which may show the presence of the cam or pincer lesion. Further imaging should include a magnetic resonance arthrogram (MRA) of the involved hip to delineate intra-articular pathology, such as labral tears, that may be present. Many clinicians also inject anesthetic into the hip at the time of MRA.
- If patients have pain relief following injection, then intra-articular hip pathology can be confirmed as the source of pain.
   - Intra-articular sources of pain in tennis players include labral tears, chondral injury, synovitis, and ligamentum teres tears, which may be the result of FAI, hip instability, or trauma.
   - Rarely, do atraumatic labral tears occur without bony dysmorphology or instability.
- Treatment of confirmed FAI with intra-articular pathology is usually surgical. The key to surgical treatment is to address the cause of the pathology (either the cam and/or pincer lesions), as well as any damage to the cartilage or labrum that has resulted, which may be done through open surgical dislocation or arthroscopically (53,54).
- Return to sport for professional athletes, including tennis players, after FAI treatment has been documented (51).

KNEE

- Injuries to the knee in racquet sports are well documented, many stemming from frequent stopping and starting in tennis, with sudden changes in direction, lunging, straightening the bent knee when serving, and the knee-flexed ready position.
   - Data from the USTA national teams show that 19% of all injuries are knee injuries, with 70% of the injuries being traumatic and 30% being overuse (8).
   - Knee injuries, such as meniscus tears and ligament sprains, are less common in the tennis player but do occur due to the twisting demands of the knee during play (55).
   - In middle-aged and elderly players, the most common injuries are meniscus injuries and degenerative cartilage problems.
   - In younger athletes, patellofemoral pain syndrome is the most common etiology of knee complaints (56).
      - The patellofemoral joint in particular is susceptible to overuse injuries, including patellar tendonitis (jumper's knee), patellar instability, and patellofemoral syndrome or chondromalacia patellae.

Patellar Tendinitis

- Patellar tendinitis or jumper's knee is a frequently observed injury that develops due to the high intensity of the game and the physical demands placed on the knee from explosive movements such as sudden changes in direction, pivot, jumping, and sprinting (57) (Fig. 122.4).
- Players with patellar tendonitis typically relate a history of a recent period of increased playing time or intensity. Discomfort is usually during sports participation but may occur with activities of daily living as the disease progresses.
- Treatment for patellar tendonitis incorporates cessation or limitation of play, anti-inflammatory medication, and physical therapy for strengthening of the muscles about the knee (58).

Patellar Instability

- Although an acute patellar dislocation is typically dramatic and infrequent, patellar instability is another common cause of anterior knee pain in the tennis player.
- Athletes may not be able to recall a discrete dislocation event but rather multiple individual episodes of anterior knee pain. Players may complain of pain near the medial facet of the patella or on the lateral aspect of the medial femoral condyle if the medial patellofemoral ligament (MPFL) has been compromised (59).
- Initial treatment of patellar instability and nonspecific patellofemoral pain in the tennis player is nonoperative and should focus on quadriceps (especially vastus medialis oblique) and hip external rotator strengthening.

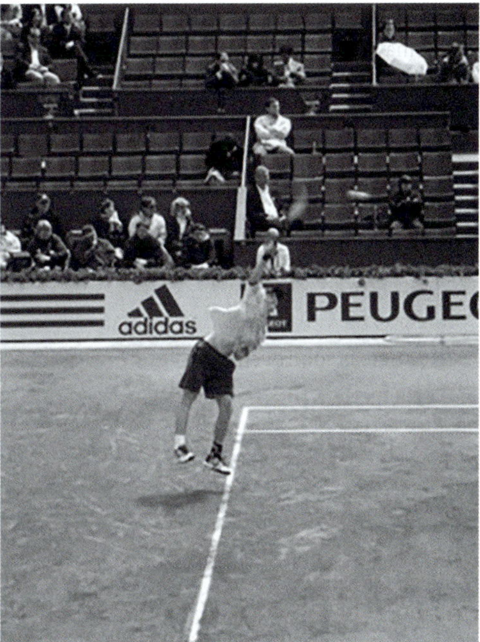

Figure 122.4: Professional tennis player serving the ball, with the photograph just after contact with the ball, in the follow-through phase. Note this player's feet are off the ground. Jumping and landing, along with sudden stops and starts and changing of direction, puts a lot of force on the knee extensor mechanism. This may result in chronic overload, resulting in patellar tendinopathy and patellofemoral pain. (Figure used with permission from Marc R. Safran, MD.)

- Patellar stabilization braces, particularly those with an active system to prevent lateral subluxation, and/or McConnell taping may be beneficial.
- For those with pes planus, orthotics (usually off-the-shelf) should also be considered to help dynamic, weight-bearing alignment.
- If physical therapy is not successful and chronic instability or dislocation occurs, a number of surgical options exist, including lateral release, MPFL repair/reconstruction, tibial tubercle osteotomy, and/or trochleoplasty, although these latter bony procedures may affect the ability to return to high-level play.

LEG/ANKLE/FOOT

Tennis Leg

- Tennis leg is described as a strain or partial tear of the medial head of the gastrocnemius muscle (60). The condition typically occurs when a player forcefully pushes off to begin a sprint to the ball.
- Players will report an acute episode of pain in the back of the lower leg at the calf muscle, and some have described it as though they were hit with a tennis ball on the back of the calf.
- Treatment involves rest, ice, elevation, and physical therapy. Specifically, stretching of the injured muscle is initiated, and as pain allows, strengthening of the gastrocnemius muscle is begun. Walking with a heel lift is used initially, and then the lift is worn when first returning to play. Return to play is guided by the resolution of symptoms.

Ankle Sprains

- Ankle sprains are the most common macrotrauma injury occurring in tennis and other racquet sports due to the frequent starting, stopping, and pivoting motions required (10) (Fig. 122.5).
- The term "ankle sprain" is a general term and may refer to injury to the lateral, medial, or syndesmotic ankle ligaments. Injuries to the syndesmotic ligaments are termed "high ankle sprains."
- Of these types, injuries to the lateral ankle ligaments are most common (61). The lateral ankle ligaments include the anterior talofibular ligament (ATFL), calcaneofibular ligament (CFL), and the posterior talofibular ligament (PTFL).
- Those with previous ankle sprains are at the highest risk of sustaining another. In addition, those with incompletely rehabilitated ankle sprains are at higher risk of recurrent sprain than those who have undergone a complete rehabilitation program that includes strengthening and proprioception exercises.
- Players will note an acute event where the foot usually becomes plantarflexed and experiences a supination moment, therefore placing stretch on the lateral ankle ligaments and the ATFL in particular. They will often report immediate swelling and pain in the area depending on the severity of the injury.
- Initial treatment of ankle sprains includes a combination of rest, ice, elevation, compression, immobilization, and initiation of physical therapy to restore ankle strength, flexibility, and proprioception (62).
- Although this is the general treatment for all grades of ankle sprains in the United States, there is a trend in some European countries to treat acute grade III sprains operatively with ligament repair (63).

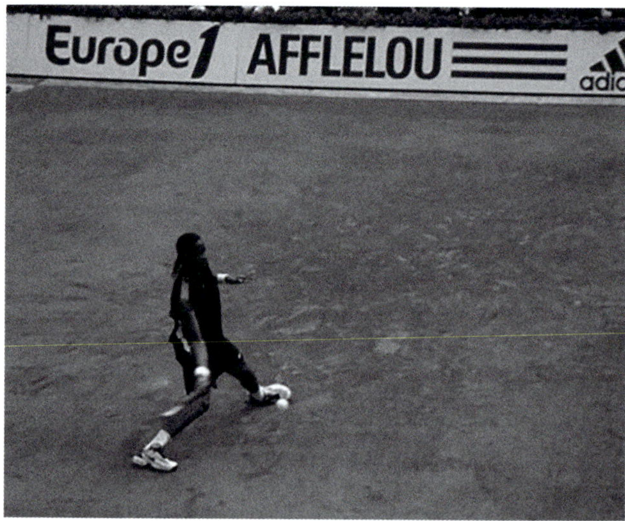

Figure 122.5: Professional tennis player sliding on a clay court with one ankle inverted and the other everted. Ankle sprains are some of the most common injuries in racquet sports, regardless of playing surface. Inversion injuries are more common. Also, as a result of the sudden stops and starts, as well as changes in direction, muscle fatigue of the lower extremities may occur. (Figure used with permission from Marc R. Safran, MD.)

- Taping or bracing of players who sustained a previous ankle sprain may help reduce the recurrence of ankle sprain.
- High ankle sprains take longer to heal, and those with instability of the distal tibiofibular joint may require surgery to stabilize this joint.

Tennis Toe

- The feet are subject to many maladies in tennis, including plantar fasciitis, metatarsalgia, metatarsal stress fractures, blisters, and corns. Another foot injury in tennis is the tennis toe, which though it is not seen only in tennis, will be discussed here as it is named after the sport.
- Tennis toe is an injury to the great toe or second toe from forceful and repetitive abutment of these toes against the toe box of the shoe.
- This can lead to subungual hematomas, nail bed injuries, or injury to the interphalangeal or metatarsophalangeal (MTP) joints.
- This injury is more common when the shoe is too big or too small for the player's foot. Severe subungual hematoma may result in nail dislocation.
- In some cases, decompression of the hematoma, usually by drilling (or burning) a hole in the toenail, is beneficial when there is significant pain.
- Adequate padding of the toe box and well-fitting shoes are important in the prevention of this problem.

ADOLESCENT TENNIS INJURIES

- Muscle and ligament strains and sprains from overuse are the predominant injuries in the young player.
  - Injuries to the lower extremity are twice as common as injuries to the spine and upper extremity.
  - Injuries to the foot, leg, and wrist prevail in the female adolescent player, whereas injuries to the ankle, groin, hand, abdomen, and back prevail in the male adolescent player.

Physeal Injuries

- Wrist epiphysitis.
  - Repeated hyperextension and rotation of the wrist caused inflammation of the distal radius epiphysis.
  - This is commonly seen in adolescent players who attempt to put topspin on the ball.
  - Premature closure of the growth plate is a potential complication of this injury.
  - Players note a warm, swollen bump on the distal radius that is tender to palpation.
  - Radiographs of the distal radius may assist in making the diagnosis.
  - Treatment strategies range from activity modification and wrist immobilization to surgery for treatment of an associated fracture or for premature physeal closure.
  - Players with wrist epiphysitis should avoid push-ups and should flatten their strokes, avoiding top spin.
- Apophysitis of the proximal humerus:
  - This occurs due to traction on the apophysis at the greater/lesser tuberosity of the humerus.
    - Rest and activity modification are the mainstays of treatment.
    - Upon return to play, the player should start with ground strokes only. High volleys and serves should be gradually incorporated.
- Humeral medial epicondyle apophysitis (adolescent medial tennis elbow):
  - Overuse injury resulting from the repetitive muscular contractions of the forearm and wrist flexors during forehands and serves.

- Players note a mildly swollen, tender prominence of the medial elbow.
- Players may sense a decrease in their ability to serve at full speed and to fully straighten the elbow.
- Use of a racquet with vibratory dampening characteristics, an oversized/light/stiff head, flexible shaft, a large cushioned grip (that is comfortable to the player), and low-tensioned strings of gut or high-quality synthetic strings, is recommended.
- Activity modification with limitations on the intensity of conditioning/play and amount of serving, overhead play, throwing, and heavy lifting is encouraged.

- Osgood-Schlatter disease
  - Apophysitis of the tibial tubercle due to traction on the patellar tendon.
  - Shoe wear modification for increased shock absorption and stability, stretching of the quadriceps and hamstring musculature to decrease the tension of the muscles pulling on the patellar tendon, training on soft surfaces (clay or sandy surfaces), and use of a patellar tendon strap are recommended.
- Sever's disease
  - Apophysitis of the calcaneus at the insertion of the Achilles tendon.
  - This is the most common cause of heel pain in the adolescent player.
  - Prevention and treatment involve proper stretching and the use of a heel support that provides cushioning, shock absorption, and decreased tension on the Achilles tendon.

SUMMARY

- Tennis and other racquet sports are enjoyed by millions of people around the world. There are a multitude of injuries that are particular to tennis and overhead sports athletes.
- Injuries in tennis and other racquet sports can stem from acute traumatic incidents during games or practice sessions; however, the majority of cases are attributed to overuse injuries.
  - Lower extremity injuries, such as ankle sprains, are the most common acute injuries, while upper extremity injuries are the more frequent chronic injuries.
- Overuse injuries in racquet sports may affect prominent musculoskeletal tissues such as bone, ligaments, tendons, and muscle in the upper or lower extremity of the body.
  - These injuries arise from a range of factors but in most cases, they develop insidiously due to repetitive microtrauma, excessive strain and loading of the tendons and joints, inadequate rest, and insufficient training and conditioning.

REFERENCES

1. *International Tennis Federation: ITF Global Tennis Report.* 2019. Retrieved from http://itf.uberflip.com/i/1169625-itf-global-tennis-report-2019-overview/39?
2. Vitale K, Liu S. Pickleball: review and clinical recommendations for this fast-growing sport. *Curr Sports Med Rep.* 2020;19(10):406–13.
3. Abrams GD, Renstrom PA, Safran MR. Epidemiology of musculoskeletal injuries in the tennis player. *Br J Sports Med.* 2012;46(7):492–8.
4. Beachy G, Akau CK, Martinson M, Olderr TF. High school sports injuries. A longitudinal study at Punahou School: 1988 to 1996. *Am J Sports Med.* 1997;25(5):675–81.
5. Hjelm N, Werner S, Renstrom P. Injury profile in junior tennis players: a prospective two year study. *Knee Surg Sports Traumatol Arthrosc.* 2010;18(6):845–50.
6. Silva RT, Takahashi R, Berra B, Cohen M, Matsumoto MH. Medical assistance at the Brazilian juniors tennis circuit—a one-year prospective study. *J Sci Med Sport.* 2003;6(1):14–8.
7. Pluim BM, Staal JB, Windler GE, Jayanthi N. Tennis injuries: occurrence, aetiology, and prevention. *Br J Sports Med.* 2006;40(5):415–23.
8. Hutchinson MR, Laprade RF, Burnett QM II, Moss R, Terpstra J. Injury surveillance at the USTA boys' tennis Championships: a 6-yr study. *Med Sci Sports Exerc.* 1995;27(6):826–30.
9. Kibler WB, Safran MR. Musculoskeletal injuries in the young tennis player. *Clin Sports Med.* 2000;19(4):781–92.
10. Kibler WB, Safran MR. Tennis injuries. *Med Sport Sci.* 2005;48:120–37.
11. Nhan DT, Klyce W, Lee RJ. Epidemiological patterns of alternative racquet-sport injuries in the United States, 1997-2016. *Orthop J Sports Med.* 2018;6(7):2325967118786237.
12. Debnath UK, Freeman BJ, Gregory P, de la Harpe D, Kerslake RW, Webb JK. Clinical outcome and return to sport after the surgical treatment of spondylolysis in young athletes. *J Bone Joint Surg Br.* 2003;85(2):244–9.
13. Maquirriain J, Ghisi JP, Kokalj AM. Rectus abdominis muscle strains in tennis players. *Br J Sports Med.* 2007;41(11):842–8.
14. Maquirriain J, Ghisi JP. Uncommon abdominal muscle injury in a tennis player: internal oblique strain. *Br J Sports Med.* 2006;40(5):462–3.
15. Bylak J, Hutchinson MR. Common sports injuries in young tennis players. *Sports Med.* 1998;26(2):119–32.
16. Sonnery-Cottet B, Edwards TB, Noel E, Walch G. Rotator cuff tears in middle-aged tennis players: results of surgical treatment. *Am J Sports Med.* 2002;30(4):558–64.
17. Burkhart SS, Morgan CD, Kibler WB. The disabled throwing shoulder: spectrum of pathology. Part II—evaluation and treatment of SLAP lesions in throwers. *Arthroscopy.* 2003;19(5):531–9.
18. Kibler WB. The role of the scapula in athletic shoulder function. *Am J Sports Med.* 1998;26(2):325–37.
19. Bigliani LU, Codd TP, Connor PM, Levine WN, Littlefield MA, Hershon SJ. Shoulder motion and laxity in the professional baseball player. *Am J Sports Med.* 1997;25(5):609–13.
20. Burkhart SS, Morgan CD, Kibler WB. The disabled throwing shoulder: spectrum of pathology. Part I—pathoanatomy and biomechanics. *Arthroscopy.* 2003;19(4):404–20.
21. Kvitne RS, Jobe FW. The diagnosis and treatment of anterior instability in the throwing athlete. *Clin Orthop Relat Res.* 1993;291:107–23.
22. Walch G, Boileau P, Noel E, Donell ST. Impingement of the deep surface of the supraspinatus tendon on the posterosuperior glenoid rim: an arthroscopic study. *J Shoulder Elb Surg.* 1992;1(5):238–45.

23. Brockmeyer M, Tompkins M, Kohn DM, Lorbach O. SLAP lesions: a treatment algorithm. *Knee Surg Sports Traumatol Arthrosc.* 2016;24(2):447–55.
24. Cools AM, Declercq G, Cagnie B, Cambier D, Witvrouw E. Internal impingement in the tennis player: rehabilitation guidelines. *Br J Sports Med.* 2008;42(3):165–71.
25. Burkhart SS, Morgan CD, Kibler WB. The disabled throwing shoulder: spectrum of pathology Part I—pathoanatomy and biomechanics. *Arthroscopy.* 2003;19(4):404–20.
26. Voos JE, Pearle AD, Mattern CJ, Cordasco FA, Allen AA, Warren RF. Outcomes of combined arthroscopic rotator cuff and labral repair. *Am J Sports Med.* 2007;35(7):1174–9.
27. Gruchow HW, Pelletier D. An epidemiologic study of tennis elbow. Incidence, recurrence, and effectiveness of prevention strategies. *Am J Sports Med.* 1979;7(4):234–8.
28. Wittenberg RH, Schaal S, Muhr G. Surgical treatment of persistent elbow epicondylitis. *Clin Orthop Relat Res.* 1992;278:73–80.
29. Nirschl RP, Ashman ES. Elbow tendinopathy: tennis elbow. *Clin Sports Med.* 2003;22(4):813–36.
30. Lewis M, Hay EM, Paterson SM, Croft P. Local steroid injections for tennis elbow: does the pain get worse before it gets better? Results from a randomized controlled trial. *Clin J Pain.* 2005;21(4):330–4.
31. Nirschl RP, Rodin DM, Ochiai DH, Maartmann-Moe C, DEX-AHE-01-99 Study Group. Iontophoretic administration of dexamethasone sodium phosphate for acute epicondylitis. A randomized, double-blinded, placebo-controlled study. *Am J Sports Med.* 2003;31(2):189–95.
32. Paoloni JA, Appleyard RC, Nelson J, Murrell GA. Topical nitric oxide application in the treatment of chronic extensor tendinosis at the elbow: a randomized, double-blinded, placebo-controlled clinical trial. *Am J Sports Med.* 2003;31(6):915–20.
33. Nirschl RP, Pettrone FA. Tennis elbow. The surgical treatment of lateral epicondylitis. *J Bone Joint Surg Am.* 1979;61(6A):832–39.
34. Baker CLJ, Murphy KP, Gottlob CA, Curd DT. Arthroscopic classification and treatment of lateral epicondylitis: two-year clinical results. *J Shoulder Elb Surg.* 2000;9(6):475–82.
35. Lo MY, Safran MR. Surgical treatment of lateral epicondylitis: a systematic review. *Clin Orthop Relat Res.* 2007;463:98–106.
36. Elliott B, Fleisig G, Nicholls R, Escamilia R. Technique effects on upper limb loading in the tennis serve. *J Sci Med Sport.* 2003;6(1):76–87.
37. Rettig AC, Sherrill C, Snead DS, Mendler JC, Mieling P. Nonoperative treatment of ulnar collateral ligament injuries in throwing athletes. *Am J Sports Med.* 2001;29(1):15–7.
38. Jobe FW, Stark H, Lombardo SJ. Reconstruction of the ulnar collateral ligament in athletes. *J Bone Joint Surg Am.* 1986;68(8):1158–63.
39. Dines JS, ElAttrache NS, Conway JE, Smith W, Ahmad CS. Clinical outcomes of the DANE TJ technique to treat ulnar collateral ligament insufficiency of the elbow. *Am J Sports Med.* 2007;35(12):2039–44.
40. Ahmad CS, Park MC, Elattrache NS. Elbow medial ulnar collateral ligament insufficiency alters posteromedial olecranon contact. *Am J Sports Med.* 2004;32(7):1607–12.
41. Aguinaldo AL, Chambers H. Correlation of throwing mechanics with elbow valgus load in adult baseball pitchers. *Am J Sports Med.* 2009;37(10):2043–8.
42. Montalvan B, Parier J, Brasseur JL, Le Viet D, Drape JL. Extensor carpi ulnaris injuries in tennis players: a study of 28 cases. *Br J Sports Med.* 2006;40(5):424–9.
43. Nagle DJ. Triangular fibrocartilage complex tears in the athlete. *Clin Sports Med.* 2001;20(1):155–66.
44. Henry MH. Management of acute triangular fibrocartilage complex injury of the wrist. *J Am Acad Orthop Surg.* 2008;16(6):320–9.
45. McAdams TR, Swan J, Yao J. Arthroscopic treatment of triangular fibrocartilage wrist injuries in the athlete. *Am J Sports Med.* 2009;37(2):291–7.
46. Maquirriain J, Ghisi JP. Stress injury of the lunate in tennis players: a case series and related biomechanical considerations. *Br J Sports Med.* 2007;41(11):812–5.
47. Maffey L, Emery C. What are the risk factors for groin strain injury in sport? A systematic review of the literature. *Sports Med.* 2007;37(10):881–94.
48. Vad VB, Gebeh A, Dines D, Altchek D, Norris B. Hip and shoulder internal rotation range of motion deficits in professional tennis players. *J Sci Med Sport.* 2003;6(1):71–5.
49. Verrall GM, Slavotinek JP, Barnes PG, Esterman A, Oakeshott RD, Spriggins AJ. Hip joint range of motion restriction precedes athletic chronic groin injury. *J Sci Med Sport.* 2007;10(6):463–6.
50. Tibor LM, Sekiya JK. Differential diagnosis of pain around the hip joint. *Arthroscopy.* 2008;24(12):1407–21.
51. Schilders E, Bismil Q, Robinson P, O'Connor PJ, Gibbon WW, Talbot JC. Adductor-related groin pain in competitive athletes. Role of adductor enthesis, magnetic resonance imaging, and entheseal pubic cleft injections. *J Bone Joint Surg Am.* 2007;89(10):2173–8.
52. Philippon M, Schenker M, Briggs K, Kuppersmith D. Femoroacetabular impingement in 45 professional athletes: associated pathologies and return to sport following arthroscopic decompression. *Knee Surg Sports Traumatol Arthrosc.* 2007;15(7):908–14.
53. Byrd JWT, Jones KS. Prospective analysis of hip arthroscopy with 10-year followup. *Clin Orthop Relat Res.* 2010;468(3):741–6.
54. Ganz R, Parvizi J, Beck M, Leunig M, Nötzli H, Siebenrock KA. Femoroacetabular impingement: a cause for osteoarthritis of the hip. *Clin Orthop Relat Res.* 2003;417:112–20.
55. Plancher KD, Steadman JR, Briggs KK, Hutton KS. Reconstruction of the anterior cruciate ligament in patients who are at least forty years old. A long-term follow-up and outcome study. *J Bone Joint Surg Am.* 1998;80(2):184–97.
56. Renström AF. Knee pain in tennis players. *Clin Sports Med.* 1995;14(1):163–75.
57. Dan M, Parr W, Broe D, Cross M, Walsh WR. Biomechanics of the knee extensor mechanism and its relationship to patella tendinopathy: a review. *J Orthop Res.* 2018;36(12):3105–12.
58. Peers KH, Lysens RJ. Patellar tendinopathy in athletes: current diagnostic and therapeutic recommendations. *Sports Med.* 2005;35(1):71–87.
59. Steensen RN, Dopirak RM, McDonald WG III. The anatomy and isometry of the medial patellofemoral ligament: implications for reconstruction. *Am J Sports Med.* 2004;32(6):1509–13.
60. Blue JM, Matthews LS. Leg injuries. *Clin Sports Med.* 1997;16(3):467–78.
61. Safran MR, Benedetti RS, Bartolozzi AR III, Mandelbaum BR. Lateral ankle sprains: a comprehensive review—part 1—etiology, pathoanatomy, histopathogenesis, and diagnosis. *Med Sci Sports Exerc.* 1999;31(7 Suppl):S429–37.
62. Safran MR, Zachazewski JE, Benedetti RS, Bartolozzi AR III, Mandelbaum R. Lateral ankle sprains: a comprehensive review—part 2—treatment and rehabilitation with an emphasis on the athlete. *Med Sci Sports Exerc.* 1999;31(7 suppl):S438–47.
63. Pijnenburg AC, Bogaard K, Krips R, Marti RK, Bossuyt PM, van Dijk CN. Operative and functional treatment of rupture of the lateral ligament of the ankle. A randomised, prospective trial. *J Bone Joint Surg Br.* 2003;85(4):525–30.

123

Triathlon

Bradford Bindas, Shawn F. Kane, and Fred H. Brennan Jr

INTRODUCTION

- A triathlon is a unique multidisciplinary event, consisting of sequential swim, bike, and run legs. The concept was initially developed as an alternative to standard marathon or 10-km training programs.
    - In 1974, members of the San Diego Track Club hosted a first-of-its-kind swim-bike-run event in and around the waters of California's Mission Bay. That three-event race was called a triathlon, and to this day, the triathlon remains one of the most popular participation and spectator endurance events worldwide.
    - John Collins, a veteran of the first Mission Bay Triathlon, was influential in the further development of the sport. He is responsible for combining three endurance events — the Waikiki Roughwater Swim, the Around-Oahu Bike Ride, and the Honolulu Marathon — into one of the world's most recognized and demanding competitions, The Ironman.
    - Popularity and growth led to the establishment of the International Triathlon Union and the inaugural World Triathlon Championship competition in 1980, the 1994 Goodwill Games in Leningrad, 1995 Pan Am Games in Argentina, and the 2000 Summer Olympic Games in Sydney.
    - The popularity and growth of triathlons continue. USA Triathlon (USAT) now reports more than 400,000 members. There are over 4300 sanctioned USAT competitions each year (1) and over 90,000 athletes competed in an IRONMAN events around the world in 2019 (1,2). The International Triathlon Union has 122 member nations, and Australia alone has over 160,000 Australians participating annually in the sport (3).

DISCIPLINES

- Triathlons are a unique sport that encompasses all fitness-related variables: cardiorespiratory endurance, body composition, muscular strength, endurance, and flexibility.
- Triathlon governing bodies recognize four standard race types based on distance (4). The races are sometimes listed by the total number of kilometers (*e.g.*, Ironman is 225.8).
    - Sprint (0.75-km swim, 22-km bike, 5-km run)
    - Olympic (1.5-km swim, 40-km bike, 10-km run)
    - Half-Ironman (1.9-km swim, 90-km bike, 21-km run)
    - Ironman (3.8-km swim, 180-km bike, 42-km run)
- The popularity of the sport has led to the introduction of short- or fun-distance triathlons, usually about half the distance of a sprint triathlon (3).

TRIATHLON VERBIAGE

- Like all sports, triathlons and triathletes have a unique vocabulary. A few of the more common terms are included here to aid in the understanding of these athletes.
    - Bonking — a reference to when a competitor begins to lose the ability to concentrate, feels disoriented and overly fatigued, and at times, is unable to continue in a race. Bonking occurs when energy intake does not meet energy expenditure and glycogen stores are depleted. The regular intake of carbohydrates during prolonged competitions can prevent this condition from occurring.
    - Transition zone — an area of controlled chaos where athletes change from swimmer to cyclist and from cyclist to runner (T1 and T2, respectively).
    - Traumatic tattooing — skin discoloration resulting from debris that was deeply embedded in the skin following an abrasion from skidding on the pavement.
    - Brick (Bike-Run-Ick) — a training method or workout used to simulate race conditions. It involves training on the bike and running on the same day and is used to simulate the bike-run transition, which many feel is the toughest part of the race.

EPIDEMIOLOGY

- Triathletes compete and train in three distinct events, each of which predisposes the athlete to its own set of injuries.

- Running injuries account for 65%–78% of the total injuries, cycling injuries account for 16%–37% of the total injuries, and swimming accounts for 11%–21% of the injuries experienced by triathletes (4,5). Injuries specific to an individual component event of the triathlon will be covered in that specific chapter.

- Injury incidence: 2.5–5.4 injuries per 1000 hours of triathlon training and 4.6–20.1 injuries per 1000 hours of triathlon competition have been reported. These rates are higher than the reported incidences of 3.9 and 2.5 injuries per 1000 hours of training for track and field and marathon running, respectively (3,6). Acute injury incidence has been reported to be 0.97/1000 hours (7).
- Theoretically, it is possible that triathletes would have fewer overuse injuries compared to other one-sport endurance athletes because triathletes spend much of their time cross-training. The contrary may also be true; triathletes suffer from the cumulative effect of three distinct injury-producing events and are susceptible to more injuries (8).
- Research has demonstrated injury rates among triathletes to be anywhere from 37% to 90% annually, with roughly 50% of injuries occurring solely during the preseason, 37% occurring in-season, and the remainder overlapping between seasons.
  - Overuse injuries are the primary reason for triathlete injury and comprise 68% and 78% of the injuries sustained during preseason and in-season, respectively. Acute injuries due to trauma make up the difference and may comprise up to 24%–27% of injuries in long-distance triathlons compared to 15%–56% on shorter-distance triathlons.
  - Both overuse and acute injuries occur at a higher rate in non-elite athletes compared to elite athletes (5). Up to 87% of athletes may sustain an overuse injury over a 26-week training period (9).
    - Overuse injuries are more common with running and acute injuries are more common with cycling, however, catastrophic injury, namely death, is more likely with swimming portions of the race (5).
- Athletes often continue to train while an injury is healing, or may exacerbate an area already injured, therefore healing and injury exposure are often occurring simultaneously, leading to the proposal of a multistate model to define injuries.
- Overall, there are a limited number of studies reporting the epidemiology of musculoskeletal injuries in long-distance triathlons, as well as inconsistent reporting and definitions of injury in this field (5). Schwellnus et al. defined terms for injury, severity, diagnosis, and methods of recording data for mass participation events and are in the process of conducting a 20-year international longitudinal study using these terms to better understand injury epidemiology (9,10).

INJURY CONSIDERATIONS

- The most common sites for injury in Ironman athletes were the knee, lower leg, and low back, followed by the shoulder (9). It is unclear if cycling or running accounts for most of the lower leg injuries, as these related injuries often cannot be separated (11).
- Neck pain and stiffness caused by prolonged sitting with the shoulders hunched, the neck hyperextended, and the arms tucked tightly in underneath the chest. This is a complaint that many triathletes have after or during the cycling portion of the race in a condition known as "aeroneck."
- Low back pain, patellofemoral pain, quadricep strains, and calf strains are common cycling injuries (9,11,12).
- Iliotibial band syndrome, patellofemoral pain syndrome, hamstring strain, and patellar and Achilles tendinosis are common injuries from running (9).
- Corneal abrasions frequently result from having the goggles kicked off the face at the congested start of the swim phase (13).

PREDICTORS OF INJURY

- The most significant predictor of injury in the preseason is the number of years of experience in triathlons. More experienced triathletes have a higher injury rate (14).
- The most significant predictor of injury during the season was a history of previous injury and high preseason running mileage (>20 miles · wk^{-1}) (9,15,16)
- Training for less than 8 or more than 15 hours · wk^{-1} increases the risk of injury (9).
- Despite differences in the number of training sessions, weekly total mileage, and workout duration, there has been no reported difference in the injury prevalence, distribution, or severity among triathletes who vary in skill from elite to recreational (9,17).
- Total weekly training distance, weekly cycling distance, swimming distance, and total number of workouts (swimming, cycling, and running) per week, but surprisingly not running distance per week, are all associated with an increased incidence of running injuries (13,18).
- The total amount of time spent running and cycling, but not total distance, negatively influences the incidence of cycling injuries (19). Running-related injuries are the most prevalent injuries seen in triathletes. Athletes who spend greater amounts of time training in cycling and swimming are at higher risk for running-related injuries. This may be because there is less time for overall muscle recovery (16).
- Overuse injuries have been correlated with time spent on speed training. Achilles injuries were positively correlated with time on hill running and negatively correlated with

time on long runs. Low back injuries are correlated with time spent cycling. Therefore, it may be recommended athletes limit speed work close to a race and focus on distance (9).

- Total run training time the week before starting to taper for a highly competitive race has been found to be positively correlated with injury in Ironman athletes (20).
- Increased load has been shown to increase injury risk up to 4 weeks after the increase, however, higher training loads may also be protective against injury. Workload may therefore be positive or negative, increasing fitness or risk of injury. It may be recommended to evaluate an athlete's intrinsic risk factors for injury on a multistate model and workload as an extrinsic factor of injury incidence (9).
- Training errors, most specifically improper technique, have been frequently associated with injuries related to cycling and swimming. However, having a coach has not been found to be positively or negatively correlated with injury incidence (20).

MEDICAL CONSIDERATIONS

- Cardiovascular — cardiac muscle fatigues and is stressed while performing endurance events, similarly to skeletal muscle.
  - Troponin T levels are elevated in 27% of Ironman Triathlon finishers, and echocardiograms have demonstrated a 24% reduction in postrace ejection fractions compared to prerace values (10).
  - For the study period of 1985–2016, in triathlons there were a total of 135 sudden deaths, with a majority occurring during the swim event, followed by the run, bike, and postrace recovery. The overall incidence of death was 1 per 76, 000 to 1.74 per 100, 000 participants. The average incidence of sudden death in all endurance events is reported to be between 0.4 and 3.3 per 100,000 entrants (10)
  - The most prominent age group for death was 40–49, however, incidence increased with age and those 60 years and older had an incidence of 18.6 per 100, 000.
  - Rate of death was significantly higher for males compared to females at 2.4 compared to 0.74 per 100, 000, respectively.
  - Detailed autopsy was not available, although data indicates the mode to be primarily sudden cardiac death (SCD).
  - The rate of SCD was not related to race length, swim venue, or swim start. The rate of death is increasing proportionally to the rate of growth in participation each year. SCD is most likely related to undiagnosed coronary artery disease or hypertrophic cardiomyopathy (21–23).
- Gastrointestinal — athletes participating in triathlon are at risk for severe gastrointestinal conditions which can range from mild to severe.
  - Gastrointestinal bleeding — 8%–30% of marathoners have evidence of intra-race or postrace gastrointestinal bleeding (24).
  - Blood shunting to exercising muscles causes relative intestinal ischemia and combined with elevated core body temperatures, leads to cellular death and gastrointestinal bleeding.
  - Abdominal cramping — may be associated with competitors who consume a diet high in fiber before the race. Also seen with the excess consumption of carbohydrates before or during the race.
  - Diarrhea (runner's trots) — abdominal pain and diarrhea associated with prolonged running or biking. This condition is caused by ischemic changes in the bowel due to the shunting of blood to exercising muscles. This may occur during or shortly after the completion of the race.
  - Nausea and vomiting — eating 30 minutes before a triathlon is highly associated with vomiting during the swim. A diet high in fat or protein and the consumption of hypertonic beverages result in a higher rate of nausea and vomiting among competitors.
- Hematology — 30% of triathletes demonstrate microscopic hematuria and 95% have a decrease in haptoglobin after an event (25). These numbers demonstrate that foot-strike hemolysis, renal ischemia, and bladder contusions are frequent occurrences.
- Infectious diseases — freshwater swimming in high-risk areas has resulted in triathletes developing leptospirosis. Lyme disease in endemic areas may also raise the potential risk to triathletes competing in non-traditional, off-road or wilderness extreme-course triathlons.
- Dermatologic — sunburn may affect athletes, particularly during prolonged outdoor events. Sun protection factor (SPF) sunscreen of at least 15, a hat or visor, SPF-rated clothing, and ultraviolet protective sunglasses are recommended to prevent the burning effects of the sun during training and competition.
- Pulmonary-SIPE — swimming-induced pulmonary edema (SIPE) has been reported during triathlon races.
  - SIPE is caused by immersive water pressure shifting fluid volume from venous to arterial circulation resulting in increased diastolic pressures.
  - May be prevented by avoiding over-hydration prior to the swim sequence, immersing oneself in the water prerace if allowed, and avoiding starting the race with maximum effort (26).

TRAINING CONSIDERATIONS

- Triathlons are unique and demanding events that require a dedicated, well-organized training program. Proper training will prepare a competitor for successful completion of the race and minimize the risk of injury while training and competing.

- Training programs need to be customized to meet the competitors' needs; what works for one athlete may not work for another. We recommend that novice competitors consider hiring a USAT-certified coach to learn the sport and maximize available training time. There are also training-related resources on the internet and in triathlon magazines to help develop a suitable and safe program. Advice from more experienced athletes can be helpful.
- Wright et al. have proposed a zone training regimen, which may be used in running or all phases. Zone 1 is easy running, with 75% weekly mileage. Zone 2 is tempo training, 5%–10% of weekly mileage. Zone 3 is high intensity, such as interval or hill training, comprising the final 15%–20% of weekly mileage (27).
- Consider an acute:chronic workload (1 week average:4-week average) ratio of less than 1.5, ideally 0.8–1.35. This has not been formally tested in triathletes, but it may assist in linking training with injury, and therefore reduce injury risk (9).
- Manipulation of the swim discipline (specifically the swimming velocity) provides a metabolic reserve and has been shown to significantly impact performance in the subsequent disciplines. The overall triathlon time is statistically significantly faster when the swim is completed at 80%–90% of maximum velocity (28).
- General triathlon training recommendations:
  - Increase training distance and time by no more than 10% per week, however up to 30% per week may be tolerable in novice runners. Little is known about training progression in experienced endurance athletes (29).
  - Although there is no evidence to demonstrate improved performance or decreased injury rates, consider incorporating a regular stretching program as part of training.
  - Ensure proper amounts of sleep and appropriate nutrition.
  - Listen to your body; if you start a workout and feel tired or run down, change it to a shorter distance. Pushing yourself through fatigue (a sign of overtraining) and completing the longer workout may do you more harm in the long run.
  - Swim, bike, and run distances a little further than the race distance; this builds confidence that you will be able to complete the race.
  - Open-water swimming is much different than lap swimming in a pool (crowded with competitors, fluctuating water conditions, sitting buoys, etc.). Athletes should train in open water as much as possible to acclimate to these differences. Training will require some extra personnel because solo open-water swimming is not recommended.
  - Train on the actual race course if possible.
  - Begin to taper training 1–2 weeks prior to the triathlon. This will allow for adequate recovery and glycogen storage prior to the race.
  - Strive for 8 hours of quality sleep two nights before the race and the night prior to the race. Prerace sleep may be of a lesser quality due to anticipation of the race.
- Brick training
  - A combination bike-run workout that is used to help train for the toughest part of the race — getting off the bike and running.
  - Bricks are demanding workouts that push the triathlete and are thought to have a positive training effect.
  - Brick workouts are very demanding and should not be a routine part of a triathlete's workout.
  - Brick workouts should be incorporated 4–6 weeks before race day.
- Strength training
  - Roughly 50% of triathletes report participating in a strength training program, with significantly more men compared to women participants (29).
  - The main limitations to participation in strength training were time constraints and lack of knowledge on exercise progression and form. Notably, muscle hypertrophy or increasing muscle mass were not limitations to participation (29).
  - A professional strength and conditioning coach improves athlete compliance with strength training (29).
  - Strength training has been shown to reduce injury in triathletes (29).
  - Resistance training may ease the burden of running on aging joints. Exercises focused on power and eccentric exercises may reduce injury potential, especially in master athletes (30).
- Transition zone training
  - "One sport, three disciplines, and two transitions" has been used to define triathlons. This is meant to imply that the two transitions — T1 (transition from swim to bike) and T2 (transition from bike to run) — are just as much part of the competition as the swim, bike, and run.
  - The T1 transition has been shown to have negligible impact on race outcome. The T2 transition has been shown to impact the final race outcome, especially in the longer races. Biomechanics and breathing are the two areas that impact the triathletes' performance in the transition zones. It is recommended that triathletes incorporate transition zone training into their program (31).
- Overtraining
  - A state of persistent mental and/or physical fatigue and a feeling of "staleness" that leads to a decline in training and race performance.
  - Symptoms include loss of interest, insomnia, fatigue, irritability, depression, loss of appetite and weight fluctuations, increased muscle soreness, illness, and a persistent increase in resting pulse rate.
  - Multiple theories exist, including glycogen depletion theory (due to a negative energy balance from inadequate

nutrition), autonomic imbalance theory, neuroendocrine dysfunction, and many more (32).

- Prevention is the best treatment. Structured training programs with built-in relative rest cycles every 4 weeks of training and at least one rest day per week help minimize the risk of overtraining.
- A short decrease in training intensity or up to a 2-week cessation of all training may be the best treatment depending on the severity of symptoms. If this fails to improve the situation, a referral to a sports psychologist may be warranted.
- For further discussion see Chapter 45: Overtraining Syndrome.

NUTRITIONAL CONSIDERATIONS

- The gut plays an important role in training, competition, and recovery that few athletes take into consideration. Proper training and nutrition can help minimize the negative impact of gastrointestinal issues while participating in endurance events.
  - Gastric emptying is impeded by high-intensity exercise (70% of O_{2max}) and further impeded by dehydration and hyperthermia. Gastric emptying is believed to be responsible for most exercise-related gastrointestinal complaints. The gut can be trained to maximize fuel and fluid absorption (33).
- Sports nutrition is discussed in depth in Chapter 12 of this text, but it is important to recall that energy expenditure depends on the duration, frequency, and intensity of the exercise and that energy expenditure and energy intake need to be balanced and appropriate for the specific activity and level of training or competition.
- Triathlons require tremendous energy expenditure, with the average male Ironman competitor using 9000 kcal during a race and 3000–6000 kcal during each training session (34).
  - Of a triathlete's energy expenditure, 99% is from the body's endurance or aerobic system.
  - After approximately 2 minutes of exercise, the body switches from anaerobic systems to aerobic systems for energy.
  - If carbohydrates are not continued during endurance activities, glycogen stores are depleted in approximately 60–90 minutes.
  - Training does not impact the total amount of energy expended during practice or competition. However, it can affect the fuel source used for energy.
    - Overall carbohydrates in the stored form of glycogen are used as the major fuel source for exercising muscles.
- Athletes are always looking for something that will give them an advantage over their competitors. There are many ergogenic aids that are available, both legal and illegal, to athletes to improve their performance.
- Caffeine ingestion of 3–5 g · kg^{-1} also improves endurance performance for many athletes. This dose typically has an ergogenic effect without exceeding serum levels banned in competition by the International Olympic Committee (20).
- Carbohydrate loading has been shown to increase the glycogen stores in the muscles being exercised and improve performance in events that last longer than 90 minutes.
  - The older method of depleting glycogen stores, which involved 1 week of exhaustive exercise in conjunction with 3 days of a low-carbohydrate (<100 g · d^{-1}) diet prior to 3 days of carbohydrate loading with minimal exercise, is no longer recommended due to significant undesired side effects (irritability, hypoglycemia, stiffness and heaviness of muscles, diarrhea, dehydration, and chest pain in older athletes) (14).
  - The current recommendations for muscle glycogen loading include ingesting a 60%–70% carbohydrate diet, combined with a decrease in training volume and intensity for 3 days prior to competition (35).
  - Athletes need to experiment with an individualized pre-event and intra-event "performance fuel source" that will minimize glycogen depletion and dehydration. Triathletes should never initiate a new hydration/nutrition regimen on race day.
  - 200–300 g of carbohydrates ingested in any form are recommended 3–4 hours prior to the race, and high-fat and high-protein foods should be avoided in this time frame.
  - Some competitors recommend, based on anecdote, up to 1 g · kg^{-1} of body weight of carbohydrate 1 hour before the competition, but there is no evidence that this will improve performance, and individual competitors may experience the possible detrimental effects of rebound hypoglycemia and hyperinsulinemia (35).
  - The consumption of foods and/or fluids with low-glycemic indices may provide more sustained blood glucose and insulin responses, reducing the potential metabolic disturbances associated with a rapidly absorbed carbohydrate load.
  - During events that last longer than 1 hour, ingestion of 30–60 g · h^{-1} of carbohydrate has a proven beneficial effect on performance. Glucose and sucrose should be the primary carbohydrates ingested because they provide more energy with fewer side effects than fructose. Newer studies suggest that ingesting a small amount of protein along with carbohydrates may have a synergistic effect on endurance performance (36).
  - After post-event rehydration, ingestion of foods high in carbohydrates, along with a moderate amount of protein, will help with the repair of muscle and other tissue damaged by exercise.
  - A 3:1–4:1 carb:protein shake should be consumed 30–60 minutes after exercise, and glycogen replacement may be achieved in 1–2 days (30).

- Hydration
  - Hydration is the most important factor affecting performance. As little as 2%–4% dehydration has been shown to negatively affect performance (37).
  - Water loss occurs primarily through sweat. Ambient temperature, relative humidity, exercise intensity, acclimatization, and rate of fluid intake all play a role in the overall hydration status of a competitor. Competitors can lose up to 11%–12%% of their body weight during an Ironman race because of sweating (37). Athletes, both trained and untrained, can lose 0.5–2.0 L of sweat per hour (12).
    - Many competitors may not consume enough fluid to negate the fluid lost. Consuming beverages while biking is a little easier and more productive than drinking while running. Elite runners may consume as little as 200 mL of fluid during distance events that last over 2 hours.
    - Minimal dehydration (>2% body weight) increases core temperature, heart rate, and perceived exertion and decreases aerobic capacity and cognitive and mental performance. Worsening dehydration, especially in a hot environment, predisposes an athlete to more serious and possibly life-threatening conditions such as exertional heat stroke, heat cramps, and heat exhaustion (12,37).
  - Starting an event hydrated or slightly overhydrated will be beneficial to the competitor because we know that by the end they will be dehydrated. Competitors need to hydrate themselves the day prior to the competition and consume 400–600 mL up to 2 hours prior to the event (26) or 5–10 mL · kg^{-1} bw (body weight) or 2–4 mL · lb^{-1} 2–4 hours before exercise (38)
  - Ideally, athletes will replace fluids at a rate that nearly approximates their loss. A loss of 500 mL of fluid equates to about a 1-lb decrease in body weight. This can be an excellent guide to post-competition fluid replacement needs (14). The replacement may be generalized to about 3 cups per pound of body weight lost and maybe water or electrolyte based (30).
  - The frequency and amount of fluid consumed by an endurance athlete is a topic of great interest, with recommendations changing as more research on the topic is published. Underhydration or overhydration may result in symptomatic hypovolemia or hyponatremia, respectively. Consuming the proper amount of fluids at the right time is paramount to maximizing performance.
    - American College of Sports Medicine guidelines recommend that competitors replace adequate fluids to nearly match sweat losses. An athlete sweating 400–1000 mL · h^{-1} would consume 150–300 mL every 20 minutes of exercise (39). Slower competitors with lower sweat rates may overhydrate, and conversely, athletes with a high sweat rate or who consume less than 200 mL of fluid an hour during a standard endurance event may develop severe and symptomatic hypovolemia (36).
    - Noakes proposes that all competitors drink *ad libitum* (no more than 400–800 mL · h^{-1}) instead of the traditional "drink as much as possible/forced hydration" model. In his opinion, this method will maintain competitors' vascular status and minimize their risk for dilutional hyponatremia. The International Marathon Medical Directors Association guidelines, authored by Noakes, ACSM, and a mathematical model designed to decipher the etiology of hyponatremia recommend limiting fluid intake to 400–800 mL · h^{-1} when thirst is not an adequate guide (37,38,40).
    - Before a race, athletes should get a baseline weight, obtained by averaging dry weight with minimal clothing each morning over 5–7 days prior to the event to help with rehydration goals after the race (37).
  - Which fluids should be consumed by athletes while training or competing?
    - Competitions lasting less than 1 hour: Water is the recommended fluid replacement (37).
    - Competitions lasting greater than 1 hour: A carbohydrate/electrolyte replacement beverage may improve performance (37).
    - A 4%–8% carbohydrate solution is optimal to maximize the quick absorption of carbohydrates and minimize potential side effects, with 10% carbohydrates being the maximum, but often intolerable, concentration.
    - Ingestion of glycerol pre-exercise has inconclusive evidence for a positive ergogenic benefit. Ingestion is typically 1.2 mg · kg^{-1}. Theoretically, it is used to decrease the rate of dehydration. However, it should be noted that it may predispose the athlete to hyponatremia (37).

COMPETITION COVERAGE CONCERNS

- The coverage of mass participation events is addressed in Chapter 16 of this text. Focus here will remain on issues unique to triathlon as compared to other mass participation or endurance events.
- As with other endurance events, most race-day injuries will be minor and self-limited, but it is important to quickly diagnose and treat the more serious problems, such as heat stroke, hyponatremia, rhabdomyolysis, dehydration, and cardiac disorders.
- In addition to monitoring standard environmental issues (ambient temperature, humidity level, wet bulb globe temperature, lightning, etc.) that may impact the health and safety of the competitors, water conditions must also be taken into account.

- Permitting the use of wetsuits should be considered at cooler water temperatures or for longer events, as discussed below.
- Rescue teams should be staged in boats, kayaks, etc., for rapid access to swimmers who may need immediate assistance.

- The size of the medical staff depends on the number of competitors, type of events, distances covered, and length of time competitors are on the course.
  - Two to three physicians and seven to eight nurses/other paramedical volunteers per every 100 athletes is a reasonable planning guide to support a triathlon. You will also need at least one spotter per 300 participants.
  - One ambulance per 1000 competitors is a reasonable guide when estimating support for an endurance event (41).
- Location of medical services — after the proper resources have been secured, they need to be placed in a location where they are most accessible and effective.
  - Main medical tent — located near the finish line. Most medical incidents occur shortly after the finish line (40).
  - Transition area medical tent — a small, modestly equipped team, able to handle routine injuries as well as stabilize and transport severe injuries, located where the competitors change disciplines, is recommended.
  - Mobile medical teams — depending on the course length and layout, it may be advisable to have teams out on the course that can handle situations that arise a prolonged distance away from medical care.

MEDICAL CONSIDERATIONS

- Review historical casualty data/numbers from previous events.
  - Historically, during Ironman-distance triathlons, 25%–30% of starters receive medical attention; one in four competitors requires transport to a higher level of care (4).
  - Rate of serious medical encounters, hypothermia, hyponatremia, heat exhaustion, etc., occur up to 100 times more frequently than SCD, reported between 16 and 155 per 100,000 entrants (10).
  - Medical utilization rates for shorter distance races are 17–50 encounters per 100 race starters, and 100 to 375 per race starters for longer distances (1).
- Hyperthermia — exercise-associated heat stroke (EHS), a potentially fatal condition characterized by a core temperature of greater than 40°C and end-organ dysfunction (typically identified by mental status changes), is a medical emergency. EHS is described in depth in Chapter 48 Environmental Emergencies.
  - In the triathlon, athletes tend to develop heat stroke toward the middle to end of the run portion of the triathlon (42).
- Hypothermia — colder water and longer swim distances increase the risk of developing hypothermia during the swimming phase.
  - Age-group triathletes are allowed to wear a wetsuit without penalty in water temperatures up to 78°F; between 78°F and 84°F, they can wear a wetsuit but are not eligible for an award; and at temperatures greater than 84°F, wetsuits are not permitted.
  - Professional triathletes are allowed to wear wetsuits when the water temperature is less than 68.0°F and 71.6°F in races less than and greater than 3000 m, respectively.
  - All wetsuits must be less than 5 mm thick (18).
- Exercise-associated collapse (EAC) — EAC is the most common medical problem experienced at the finish line and is believed to be the result of significant postural hypotension and secondary tachycardia, not hyperthermia or dehydration. Treatment consists of elevating the legs and encouraging competitors to keep moving after finishing (43).
- Hyponatremia (44) — hyponatremia is believed to occur in 10%–40% of endurance athletes. Athletes may be hypovolemic or hypervolemic. Exercise-associated hyponatremia is discussed in depth in Chapter 39 endocrinology and sports.
  - Serum sodium above 130 $mg \cdot dL^{-1}$ is usually asymptomatic. Symptoms often occur at levels less than 130 $mg \cdot dL^{-1}$, and may include headache, vomiting, frothy sputum, difficulty breathing, pulmonary edema, and altered mental status.
  - Serum sodium levels measuring less than 125 $mg \cdot dL^{-1}$ are more concerning and may manifest with altered mental status, lethargy, cramps, or seizures.
  - A rapid intravenous infusion of 100 mL of 3% hypertonic saline will begin to correct the symptomatic hyponatremia, although more than one bolus may be required.
- Rhabdomyolysis — extreme muscle breakdown due to intense, prolonged exercise. It is often exacerbated by dehydration and hyperthermia.
  - Elevated serum creatine kinase with brown or reddish (cola-colored) urine and a urine dipstick positive for blood without red blood cells on microscopy makes the diagnosis likely.
  - Elevated serum or urine myoglobin levels help confirm the diagnosis.
  - Treatment includes the administration of intravenous fluids administered to maintain a urine output of 200–300 $mL \cdot h^{-1}$ is recommended to help prevent acute tubular necrosis and subsequent renal failure.
  - Patients with suspected rhabdomyolysis should be transferred for further evaluation and care.

REFERENCES

1. Asplund CA, Miller TK, Creswell L, et al. Triathlon medical coverage: a guide for medical directors. *Curr Sports Med Rep*. 2017;16(4):280–8. doi:10.1249/JSR.0000000000000382

2. USA Triathlon Statistics [Internet]. [cited 2022 Oct 2]. Available from: https://www.teamusa.org/usa-triathlon/about/usat
3. Gosling CM, Forbes AB, McGivern J, Gabbe BJ. A profile of injuries in athletes seeking treatment during a triathlon race series. *Am J Sports Med.* 2010;38(5):1007–14.
4. Korkia PK, Tunstall-Pedoe DS, Maffulli N. An epidemiological investigation of training and injury patterns in British triathletes. *Br J Sports Med.* 1994;28(3):191–6.
5. Rhind J-H, Dass D, Barnett A, Carmont M. A systematic review of long-distance triathlon musculoskeletal injuries. *J Hum Kinet.* 2022;81:123–34. doi:10.2478/hukin-2022-0011
6. Zwingenberger S, Valladares RD, Walther A, et al. An epidemiological investigation of training and injury patterns in triathletes. *J Sports Sci.* 2014;32(6):583–90. doi:10.1080/02640414.2013.843018
7. Andersen CA, Clarsen B, Johansen TV, Engebretsen L. High prevalence of overuse injury among iron-distance triathletes. *Br J Sports Med.* 2013;47(13):857–61. doi:10.1136/bjsports-2013-092397
8. Collins K, Wagner M, Peterson K, Storey M. Overuse injuries in triathletes. A study of the 1986 Seafair Triathlon. *Am J Sports Med.* 1989;17(5):675–80.
9. Kienstra CM, Asken TR, Garcia JD, Lara V, Best TM. Triathlon injuries: transitioning from prevalence to prediction and prevention. *Curr Sports Med Rep.* 2017;16(6):397–403. doi:10.1249/JSR.0000000000000417
10. Schwellnus M, Kipps C, Roberts WO, et al. Medical encounters (including injury and illness) at mass community-based endurance sports events: an international consensus statement on definitions and methods of data recording and reporting. *Br J Sports Med.* 2019;53(17):1048–55. doi:10.1136/bjsports-2018-100092
11. Cushman DM, Dowling N, Ehn M, Kotler DH. Triathlon considerations. *Phys Med Rehabil Clin N Am.* 2022;33(1):81–90. doi:10.1016/j.pmr.2021.08.006
12. American College of Sports Medicine, Sawka MN, Burke LM, et al. American College of Sports Medicine position stand. Exercise and fluid replacement. *Med Sci Sports Exerc.* 2007;39(2):377–90.
13. Hellemans J. Maximizing Olympic distance triathlon performance — a sports medicine perspective [Internet]. [cited 2010 Sep 23]. Available from: http://fulltext.ausport.gov.au/fulltext/1999/triathlon/john.hellemans.pdf
14. Fieseler CM. The ultramarathoner. In: O'Connor FG, Wilder RP, editors. *Textbook of Running Medicine.* New York (NY): McGraw-Hill; 2001:469–77.
15. Cosca DD, Navazio F. Common problems in endurance athletes. *Am Fam Physician.* 2007;76(2):237–44.
16. Williams MM, Hawley JA, Black R, Freke M, Simms K. Injuries amongst competitive triathletes. *N Z J Sports Med.* 1988:25;2–6.
17. Thompson MJ, Rivara FP. Bicycle-related injuries. *Am Fam Physician.* 2001;63(10):2007–14.
18. USA Triathlon Competitive Rules (n.d.) [Internet]. Available from: https://www.teamusa.org/usa-triathlon/about/multisport/competitive-rules
19. Vleck VE, Bentley DJ, Millet GP, Cochrane T. Triathlon event distance specialization: training and injury effects. *J Strength Condit Res.* 2010;24(1):30–6.
20. Paluska SA. Caffeine and exercise. *Curr Sports Med Rep.* 2002;2(4):213–19.
21. Dayer MJ, Green I. Mortality during marathons: a narrative review of the literature. *BMJ Open Sport Exerc Med.* 2019;5(1):e000555. doi:10.1136/bmjsem-2019-000555
22. Harris KM, Creswell LL, Haas TS, et al. Death and cardiac arrest in U.S. Triathlon participants, 1985 to 2016: a case series. *Ann Intern Med.* 2017;167(8):529–35. doi:10.7326/M17-0847
23. USA Triathlon Medical Report [Internet]. [cited 2022 Oct 2]. Available from: https://www.teamusa.org/USA-Triathlon/News/Articles-and-Releases/2012/October/25/102512-Medical-Panel-Report
24. Moses FM. The effect of exercise on the gastrointestinal tract. *Sports Med.* 1990;9(3):159–72. doi:10.2165/00007256-199009030-00004
25. O'Toole ML, Hiller WD, Roalstad MS, Douglas PS. Hemolysis during triathlon races: its relation to race distance. *Med Sci Sports Exerc.* 1988;20(3):272–5. doi:10.1249/00005768-198806000-00010
26. Bove AA. Cardiovascular concerns in water sports. *Clin Sports Med.* 2015;34(3):449–60. doi:10.1016/j.csm.2015.02.003
27. Wright VJ. Masterful care of the aging triathlete. *Sports Med Arthrosc Rev.* 2012;20(4)231–6.
28. Peeling PD, Bishop DJ, Landers GJ. Effect of swimming intensity on subsequent cycling and overall triathlon performance. *Br J Sports Med.* 2005;39(12):960–4.
29. Luckin KM, Badenhorst CE, Cripps AJ, et al. Strength training in long-distance triathletes: barriers and characteristics. *J Strength Condit Res.* 2021;35(2):495–502.
30. Loudon JK. The master female triathlete. *Phys Ther Sport.* 2016;22:123–8. doi:10.1016/j.ptsp.2016.07.010
31. Millet GP, Vleck VE. Physiological and biomechanical adaptations to the cycle to run transition in Olympic triathlon: review and practical recommendations for training. *Br J Sports Med.* 2000;34(5):384–90.
32. Kuipers H. Training and overtraining: an introduction. *Med Sci Sports Exerc.* 1998;30(7):1137–9. doi:10.1097/00005768-199807000-00018
33. Murray R. Training the gut for competition. *Curr Sports Med Rep.* 2006;5(3):161–4.
34. DiMarco NM, Samuels M. Nutritional considerations. In: O'Connor FG, Wilder RP, editors. *Textbook of Running Medicine.* New York (NY): McGraw-Hill; 2001:477–89.
35. Robins A. Nutritional recommendations for competing in the ironman triathlon. *Curr Sports Med Rep.* 2007;6(4):241–8.
36. Convertino VA, Armstrong LE, Coyle EF, et al. American College of Sports Medicine position stand. Exercise and fluid replacement. *Med Sci Sports Exerc.* 1996;28(1):i-x.
37. Armstrong LE. Rehydration during endurance exercise: challenges, research, options, methods. *Nutrients.* 2021;13(3):887. doi: 10.3390/nu13030887
38. Thomas DT, Erdman KA, Burke LM. American College of sports medicine joint position statement. Nutrition and athletic performance. *Med Sci Sports Exerc.* 2016 Mar;48(3):543–68. Erratum in: *Med Sci Sports Exerc.* 2017;49(1):222. doi:10.1249/MSS.0000000000000852
39. American College of Sports MedicineAmerican Dietetic AssociationDietitians of Canada. Joint position statement: nutrition and athletic performance. American College of sports medicine, American dietetic association, and dietitians of Canada. *Med Sci Sports Exerc.* 2000;32(12):2130–45.
40. Noakes T, International Marathon Medical Directors Association. Fluid replacement during marathon running. *Clin J Sport Med.* 2003;13(5):309–18.
41. Cianca JC, Roberts WO, Horn D. Distance running: organization of the medical team. In: O'Connor FG, Wilder RP, editors. *Textbook of Running Medicine.* New York (NY): McGraw-Hill; 2001:489–504.
42. Bouchama A, Knochel JP. Medical progress: heat stroke. *N Engl J Med.* 2002;346(25):1978–88.
43. Anley C, Noakes T, Collins M, Schwellnus MP. A comparison of two treatment protocols in the management of exercise-associated postural hypotension: a randomised clinical trial. *Br J Sports Med.* 2011;45(14):1113–8. doi:10.1136/bjsm.2010.071951
44. Noakes T. Hyponatremia in distance runners: fluid and sodium balance during exercise. *Curr Sports Med Rep.* 2002;1(4):197–207.

Volleyball

Mark Hopkins, Erika Williams, and Thomas Heckman

124

INTRODUCTION

- Volleyball is a popular sport, both recreationally and competitively and is one of the big five international sports: soccer, cricket, field hockey, tennis, and volleyball.
- The Fédération Internationale de Volleyball (FIVB) claims that it is the largest international sporting federation in the world with 220 affiliated national federations.
- Volleyball became an Olympic sport in 1964, and beach volleyball was added in 1996 (1).
  - Women's court volleyball is the second most-sponsored collegiate team sport and women's beach volleyball is the fastest growing Division 1 sport (2).
- Although considered a noncontact sport, play requires quick, forceful movements of the entire body in multiple planes simultaneously, making injuries inevitable.
  - The rate of injury was found to be 2.6 in 1000 hours of play. Fortunately, the incidence of serious injury is relatively low (3).
- There are a variety of sport-specific skills, with each having specific activity-related injuries. Serving, passing, and setting have not been associated with high numbers of injuries. While spiking, or attacking, has been associated with a fairly high incidence of injuries, and blocking has been implicated in causing the highest rate of injury.
- The hand, shoulder, knee, and ankle are among the most commonly injured areas (4).
- Injuries have been found to occur at a higher rate in practice than during competition (2).
- Because volleyball is played on a variety of surfaces, such as wood, grass, concrete, and, in particular, sand, consideration must also be given to injuries common to these surfaces.

INDOOR VOLLEYBALL

- Standard games are on hardwood courts and have six players per side, including a setter, hitter/spikers, blockers, and passers. Each player rotates through different positions and serves.
  - Injury surveillance data found indoor volleyball to have nearly three times the rate of injury compared to beach volleyball (1.8 vs. 5.3 injuries per 1000 hours played).
    - Knee injuries and concussions were in particular more common (2,4).
- Play generally continues through the end of each set without breaks, unless a team takes a time-out. The two teams then switch sides before the next set. Matches are best of five sets, with rally scoring (every point counts) to 25 each set, although this may vary based on level of competition.

BEACH VOLLEYBALL

- Beach volleyball is played barefoot on sand, with two players on each team with no substitutions allowed. The court is smaller for beach volleyball (16 × 8 m) compared with indoor volleyball (18 × 9 m).
- Professional matches are best of three sets.
  - Players switch sides every 7 points in sets to 21 (the first two sets) and every 5 points in sets to 15 (the third set, if necessary), with 1 time-out per team per set.
  - Coaching and medical treatment are limited to these stoppages. This may vary depending on level of play.
- Although injury rates are lower, injury surveillance data showed that time lost from participation was significantly longer in beach versus indoor volleyball for knee, low back, and shoulder injuries, with more chronic injuries as well (2).
- Similar to indoor volleyball, the ankle, knee, fingers, and low back have the highest rate of acute injury in beach volleyball. However, the rate of ankle sprains in beach volleyball is almost half that of indoor volleyball. This is most likely related to fewer players blocking and to a softer court surface (5).
- Consideration should also be given to weather conditions, which play a factor in beach volleyball.

LOWER EXTREMITY

- Lower extremity injuries account for the majority of volleyball injuries.

- In a review of collegiate women's volleyball players, the lower extremity accounted for more than 55% of all game and practice injuries, with ankle ligament sprains representing 44.1% of game injuries and 29.4% of practice injuries (6).
- Many lower extremity injuries in volleyball are due to repetitive motions, such as jumping, landing, and twisting during play.
- The majority of lower extremity injuries occur when the athletes are playing in the front three positions. Studies suggest that 63% of the musculoskeletal injuries result from jumping and landing, which most often occur in these positions (3). In a review of collegiate women's volleyball players, the lower extremity accounted for more than 55% of all game and practice injuries, with ankle ligament sprains representing 44.1% of game injuries and 29.4% of practice injuries (6).

Knee

- The most common overuse injury is *patellar tendinosis* or *jumper's knee.*
  - Players tend to have pain at the lower pole of the patella and, less frequently, at the upper pole and tibial tuberosity. It often has an insidious onset with pain seen with hyperextension of the knee.
  - Initial treatment includes rest, ice, compression with a neoprene sleeve, and nonsteroidal anti-inflammatory drugs (NSAIDs). Long-term management should include vastus medialis strengthening (7).
- Acute knee injuries ranging from mild sprains of the collateral ligaments to more serious anterior cruciate ligament and meniscal tears tend to be caused by quick changes in direction with landing, cutting, and pivoting on the court. This most frequently occurs while landing near the net after an attack.
- Players frequently wear knee pads in indoor volleyball to prevent abrasions or contusions given the amount of diving performed on the hard court surface

Foot and Ankle

- Ankle injuries are the most common acute volleyball injury and were found to account for 44% of all volleyball-related injuries (5). They are typically inversion sprains involving the lateral ligaments and are often a result of a blocker landing on the foot of an attacker from the opposing team under the net (7).
  - Treatment of an acutely injured ankle will vary based on the severity. The player should be removed from play if there is a suspected fracture or excessive swelling or the athlete is unable to bear weight.
  - Ankle injury rehabilitation should include physical therapy, with a focus on regaining joint proprioception to prevent re-injury, in addition to relative rest, NSAIDs, ice, and bracing.
  - Many volleyball teams use ankle braces prophylactically to prevent inversion-type ankle sprains at all levels of competition. Although sprains do still occur, studies have shown some benefit to this practice (8,9).
  - Coaching blockers and attackers on technique for more vertical travel at the net has been shown to decrease the incidence of ankle sprains (7).
  - Metatarsal, navicular, and sesamoid stress fractures present with insidious onset of pain and point tenderness. These are typically diagnosed with X-ray or magnetic resonance imaging (MRI) and require removal from participation until they are healed.
  - *"Sand toe" is* an injury unique to beach volleyball, which is played barefoot. It involves a hyperplantarflexion injury to the metatarsophalangeal joint. Pain typically occurs with motions involving running, jumping, and pushing off.
    - Treatment is similar to "turf toe" and includes relative rest, ice, NSAIDs, stiff shoes or orthotics, and toe strengthening. This condition may take 6 months for complete recovery (4).

UPPER EXTREMITY

Shoulder

- The shoulder is frequently injured as it is subject to repetitive abduction and external rotation followed by forceful extension and internal rotation during serving and spiking.
  - Chronic overuse injuries of the rotator cuff and long head biceps tendon are commonly seen due to this repetitive overhead hitting and/or joint instability (4).
- Injuries of the rotator cuff can vary from mild forms of tendinitis and impingement to complete tears of the muscles of the rotator cuff. Treatment can vary from NSAIDs and physical therapy focusing on scapular stabilization to surgery, depending on severity.
- *Impingement syndrome* occurs when the supraspinatus tendon becomes irritated and painful as it passes through the subacromial space.
  - Players with anatomic variances, such as a "hooked acromion," may be more prone to problems. In addition, further narrowing of the space may be secondary to depression of the dominant shoulder caused by capsular instability and muscular imbalance in volleyball attackers. Painful shoulder motion, in addition to night pain, is a result of these muscular imbalances, overuse, and variances.
  - Conservative therapy includes rest, NSAIDs, and potentially subacromial corticosteroid injections. Surgical decompression may be necessary if this fails to allow return to play.
- *Glenohumeral internal rotation deficit* (GIRD) can occur in players who spend a significant amount of time with their

shoulder in positions of extreme external rotation, specifically while hitting or serving. As a result the posterior capsule may become contracted. A posterior superior shift of the humeral head may be seen in the cocking position. Internal rotation may be limited compared to the nondominant arm.

- Treatment includes the sleeper stretch (4).

- Chronic overload on the shoulder may result in lateralization and depression of the scapula in the dominant arm and a group of symptoms referred to as the "SICK scapula." These include scapular malposition, inferior medial border prominence, coracoid pain, and scapular dyskinesis.
  - Chronic instability and altered kinematics of the scapula may result in rotator cuff pathology and chronic pain (5).
- *Suprascapular neuropathy* is encountered on a surprisingly frequent basis in elite volleyball players. The suprascapular nerve is typically compressed at the spinoglenoid notch resulting in atrophy and weakness of the infraspinatus muscle.
  - Up to 25% loss of external rotation strength may be seen in the affected shoulder.
  - Electromyography is useful in diagnosis, and conservative treatment is generally effective.
  - Rehabilitative exercises should be aimed at strengthening external rotation.
  - Surgery may be considered in cases of persistent pain, because ganglion cysts may also cause similar presentation (4).
- Prevention strategies for shoulder injury in volleyball may include a stretching program to address internal rotation deficits and posterior capsule tightness, core stability and strength, as well as eccentric resistance training to maintain scapular and rotator cuff strength and function. Additionally, mindfulness of training load and volume of repetitive overhead activity may be beneficial (5).

Finger, Hand, and Wrist

- Wrist injuries are commonly related to passing and digging the ball and to contacting the floor or sand after diving.
- Fractures of the pisiform may require axial or "carpal tunnel" views on radiographs in order to make the diagnosis and often require casting.
- Kienböck disease, or aseptic necrosis of the lunate, can be seen with repetitive wrist trauma in volleyball players. MRI that shows sclerosis or collapse of the lunate, rotation of the scaphoid, or degeneration of adjacent intercarpal joints should prompt consultation with an orthopedic/hand surgeon (10).
- Most injuries to the fingers and hands occur as a result of contact with the ball during play at the net, especially during blocking. Sprains and strains are most frequently seen, especially of the proximal interphalangeal joint. Fractures, dislocations, and contusions are less common. The thumb metacarpophalangeal joint is also frequently injured (4).
- Most finger sprains are minor and can be managed conservatively with taping and splinting.
  - Collateral ligament injuries to the interphalangeal joints should be "buddy taped" to an adjacent finger for adequate support.

Low Back

- When a player attacks the ball, lumbar spine strains and sprains can occur, due to the extension followed by forced flexion and rotation, and then landing.
- Suspicion should be high for stress fracture in cases of prolonged pain despite conservative treatment.
  - Focal tenderness to palpation and prolonged pain despite treatment should raise concern.
- Athletes with radiating leg symptoms in the setting of low back pain should be held from play until further evaluation is completed.

OTHER INJURIES

- Contusions over the anterior superior iliac spines or "hip pointers," in addition to contusions over the medial and anterior aspect of the knee, are frequently noted after defensive diving onto a hard court.
  - Kneepads, more often than hip pads, are typically worn for protection.
  - Icing and anti-inflammatory medications can be used in reducing pain and swelling.
- Concussions have been reported to occur in youth volleyball at a rate of approximately 7 per 100 athletes per 12-month period and have been found to occur more in indoor than beach volleyball, most commonly from ball-to-head contact (2,11).

REFERENCES

1. *The Game* [Internet]. [cited2022Dec 15]. Available from: https://www.fivb.com/en/volleyball/thegame_glossary/history
2. Juhan T, Bolia IK, Kang HP, et al. Injury epidemiology and time lost from participation in women's NCAA division I indoor versus beach volleyball players. *Orthop J Sports Med.* 2021;9(4):23259671211004546. doi:10.1177/23259671211004546
3. Verhagen EA, Van Der Beek AJ, Bouter LM, Bahr RM, Van Mechelen W. A one season prospective cohort study of volleyball injuries. *Br J Sports Med.* 2004;38(4):477–81.
4. Eerkes K. Volleyball injuries. *Curr Sports Med Rep.* 2012 Sep/Oct;11(5):251–6. doi:10.1249/JSR.0b013e3182699037
5. Reeser JC, Verhagen E, Briner WW, Askeland TI, Bahr R. Strategies for the prevention of volleyball related injuries. *Br J Sports Med.* 2006 Jul;40(7):594–600.
6. Bahr R, Reeser JC, Fédération Internationale de Volleyball. Injuries among world-class professional beach volleyball players. The Fédération Internationale de Volleyball beach volleyball injury study. *Am J Sports Med.* 2003;31(1):119–25.

7. Agel J, Palmieri-Smith RM, Dick R, Wojtys EM, Marshall SW. Descriptive epidemiology of collegiate women's volleyball injuries: national collegiate athletic association injury surveillance system, 1988–1989 through 2003–2004. *J Athl Train*. 2007;42(2):295–302.
8. Lian OB, Engebretsen L, Bahr R. Prevalence of jumper's knee among elite athletes from different sports: a cross-sectional study. *Am J Sports Med*. 2005;33(4):561–7.
9. Pedowitz DI, Reddy S, Parekh SG, Huffman GR, Sennett BJ. Prophylactic bracing decreases ankle injuries in collegiate female volleyball players. *Am J Sports Med*. 2008;36(2):324–7.
10. Ansari MT, Chouhan D, Gupta V, Jawed A. Kienböck's disease: where do we stand? *J Clin Orthop Trauma*. 2020 Jul-Aug;11(4):606–13.
11. Meeuwisse DW, MacDonald K, Meeuwisse WH, et al. Concussion incidence and mechanism among youth volleyball players. *Br J Sports Med*. 2017;51:A62–3.

125

Water Polo Injuries

Michelle E. Szczepanik and Christopher D. Meyering

INTRODUCTION (1)

- Water polo is a team aquatic sport played throughout the United States and in many countries around the world, particularly in Europe.
- It is a fast-paced, physically demanding game requiring both strength and skill as a swimmer combined with excellent hand-eye coordination to facilitate ball handling, passing, and scoring.
- During a typical match, a player will swim short distances with high-energy bursts lasting 10–18 seconds. For some players, these short distances can add up to 1000 m over the course of a match. These sprints are separated by 30- to 40-second intervals of "eggbeater" leg work to keep the head above the water surface (2).
- In general, water polo is an intensely physical game, with players swimming at a sprint pace in immediate proximity to one another for control of the ball and for defensive maneuvers. The result of such activity and a limited amount of protective equipment is a propensity for many different types of injuries.
  - Statistics from the 2004 Olympic Games demonstrated that an injury occurred once in every two to three matches, with the total incidence being 63 injuries per every 1000 player hours. All injuries were caused by contact with another player, with the head and upper extremities being the most affected (3).
  - Water polo had the highest incidence of injury in the 2009 Fédération Internationale de Natation Amateur (FINA) World Aquatics Championships (4).

HISTORY

- Although the exact origins are unclear, the first documented rules were codified in 1877 by William Wilson, a Scottish aquatics enthusiast. Initially, the game more closely resembled an aquatic form of rugby football.
- The game was altered into its modern-day form by the turn of the 20th century, when it was incorporated into the modern Olympic Games in Paris, France, in 1900.
- Water polo is governed internationally by FINA and within the United States by USA Water Polo, a not-for-profit organization under the aegis of the US Olympic Committee.

REQUIRED EQUIPMENT (5)

- Although it could be played in any suitably sized body of water, water polo is most often played in swimming pools. Known as "the field," the dimensions of the pool will vary depending on the age and gender of the players, ranging from 20 to 30 m long by 10–20 m wide by 2–4 m deep.
- The goals are rectangular, centered at both ends of the field, and 3 m wide by 0.9 m high.
- The ball is spherical, weighing between 400 and 450 g, and coated with a high-friction rubber to facilitate grip. The circumference and pressure have ranges based on gender.
- Individual equipment includes a swimsuit and a swim cap with cupped ear protectors.

GAME PLAY (5)

- The game is divided into four quarters, which are 8 minutes in length for collegiate and professional play; youth leagues through high school have shorter periods, which range from 5 to 7 minutes.
- The object is to throw the ball into the opposing team's goal fully crossing the goal line, thereby scoring 1 point. The team that scores the greatest number of points before regulation time has expired is the winner. If there is a tie at the end of a game, a penalty shootout is necessary to determine the winner.
- The ball may be passed around the field in any direction, but a team may not possess the ball for more than 30 seconds without attempting a shot on goal, or else they forfeit the ball.
- Teams are composed of seven players: six in the field of play and one goalkeeper; teams are designated by the required color of their uniform swim caps, which also serve to protect players' ears.
- All players may use either hand but must use only one hand at a time to handle, pass, and shoot the ball. However, the

goalkeeper, when within the goalkeeper's 6-meter area, may use both hands.

- Players will use the "eggbeater" kick, which combines the clockwise motion of one leg and a counterclockwise motion of the other leg in order to stay afloat.

Fouls (5)

- There are three types of fouls: ordinary, penalty, and exclusion.
  - Ordinary fouls are minor infractions of gameplay; examples of ordinary fouls are listed in Table 125.1; ordinary fouls result in a change of possession by means of a free throw.
  - Penalty fouls are ordinary fouls committed within the 6-m goal area and result in a penalty throw (exclusion fouls in this area also result in a penalty throw).
  - Exclusion fouls are more grievous violations and the penalty for exclusion fouls is removal from play for 20 seconds or if a goal has been scored, the player's team has retaken possession of the ball, or if the excluded player's team is awarded a free throw or goal throw. The official may determine if there was malicious intent to harm another player, in which case the player is removed from the game and the team must play one man down for 4 minutes.

INJURIES

Head Injuries

- Mountjoy et al. reported that concussions were found to make up 1.9% of injuries out of 8904 matches from the Olympic Games and World Championships (6). Similar rates of concussion have been found in some studies; however, other studies have not found concussions to be a typical injury. Furthermore, the out-of-competition concussion rate has not been studied. This is significant and represents a gap in knowledge, as concussions typically have worse return-to-play outcomes compared with other injuries (2,7).

Table 125.1 Examples of Fouls in Water Polo

Examples of Ordinary Fouls	Examples of Exclusion Fouls
• holding the ball underwater or tucking inside swimsuit • using two hands • pushing off pool floor • striking the ball with a closed fist • swimming within 2 m of the opposing goal ahead of the ball • pushing or pushing off	• using two hands to block a pass or shot • exiting the pool without permission • intentionally splashing water in an opponent's face • intentionally striking an opponent (elbow, punch, kick, etc.)

Data from: https://usawaterpolo.org/documents/2024/6/7/LevonUSAWPRulesEdit2024_Update1_.pdf

Eye Injuries

- Annett et al. found that eye injuries accounted for 6.1% of acute injuries in water polo (8).
- The most common eye complaints in water polo are eye irritation or lacerations from direct trauma. Due to the severity of some uncommon injuries, they are also included in this section.

Corneal Abrasion (2,9,10)

- Common mechanism: Excoriation from fingernail, toenail, or trapping of debris under contact lens.
  - Signs/symptoms: Severe eye pain and photophobia.
  - Treatment: If you suspect corneal abrasion, this may require transfer to a facility capable of performing slit lamp examination and fluorescein staining to confirm the diagnosis. This is especially important when looking for any foreign body remnants.
    - The athlete should be advised to keep the eye closed and to avoid rubbing/touching.
    - Topical anesthetic drops may be used temporarily to relieve pain and facilitate exams.
    - Treatment ultimately consists of topical antibiotic ointment or drops for 3–5 days.
  - Return to play: Athletes should not be allowed to return to play until the abrasion has healed.

Laceration of Eyelid, Eyebrow, Lip, and Cheek (2,9)

- Common mechanism: Direct trauma to skin.
- Signs/symptoms: Bleeding from laceration, pain.
- Treatment: Cleanse/irrigate the wound, assess the depth/severity of laceration, and repair via approximation of skin edges. The primary care provider should be skilled in simple laceration repair, although if there is concern about cosmetic results or involvement of the eyelid, particularly if subcutaneous fat is visible, or injuries that involve the lacrimal sac or duct, then consultation with the plastic surgeon and/or ophthalmologist is warranted.
  - Sterile adhesive bandages (*e.g.*, Steri-strips) and adhesive glue (*e.g.*, DERMABOND) may be used for small, superficial repairs with minimal active bleeding.
- Return to play: Athlete may return to play if bleeding is controlled and there has been no change in vision.

Chemical Irritation (2,9)

- Common mechanism: Excessive exposure to chlorine or other disinfectants.
- Signs/symptoms: Discomfort/burning of eyes, scleral injection.
- Treatment: Saline eye drops, limit exposure to chlorinated water.
- Return to play: No restrictions, though try to limit exposure to the irritant.

Hyphema

- Definition: Hemorrhage into the anterior chamber from ruptured trabecular blood vessels (2,9–11).

- Common mechanism: Direct trauma to the globe from fist, elbow, ball, etc.
- Signs/symptoms: Blood pooling in the inferior portion of the anterior chamber of the eye can be seen in the inferior portion of the iris.
- Treatment: This is an ophthalmologic emergency and should be evaluated as quickly as possible. Protect the eye with loose, occlusive dressing (*e.g.*, Fox shield) and seek immediate evaluation by ophthalmology; if untreated, it could result in glaucoma or permanent corneal staining.
- Return to play: As guided by the ophthalmologist, but likely no contact for sports for at least a week for even minor hyphemas.

Blowout Fracture of Orbital Floor

- Occurs because the orbital floor is weaker relative to surrounding bones (2,9,10).
- Common mechanism: Direct trauma to the globe resulting in fracture of the orbital floor.
- Signs/symptoms: Periorbital hematoma, protruding or sunken globe; herniation of inferior contents can cause entrapment, which will manifest as an inability to gaze upward in the affected eye, producing diplopia and/or maxillary numbness.
- Treatment: This is an emergency and should be evaluated as soon as possible by an ophthalmologist. Protect the eye with a loose, occlusive dressing (*e.g.*, Fox shield) and seek immediate evaluation by ophthalmology to rule out intraocular trauma. It is essential to perform a thorough neurologic exam to rule out entrapment of inferior orbital contents.
- Return to play: Only once cleared by the ophthalmologist

Ear Injuries/Conditions

- Many ear injuries, especially traumatic auricular hematoma ("cauliflower ear"), can be avoided through the proper wear of special cupped ear protector swim caps, which are a required part of personal equipment.

Otitis Externa (Swimmer's Ear) (2,10,12)

- Common mechanism: Bacterial infection (often *Pseudomonas* species) from excessive moisture in the external auditory canal, which removes cerumen and creates optimal pH for bacterial growth.
- Signs/symptoms: Inflamed, erythematous, tender external auditory canal; exudates may be present.
- Treatment: *Best treatment is prevention* with alcohol-based drops, which provide antiseptic treatment via desiccation.
    - If infection is present, use antibiotic ear drops with or without steroids for severe inflammation. There are a number of available preparations, but fluoroquinolones such as ofloxacin and ciprofloxacin have the broadest coverage and are typically only dosed twice daily as opposed to 3–4 times daily for other otic antibiotic preparations.
    - Proper technique is important to increase the effectiveness of any otic drops. The athlete should tilt his or her head to the shoulder opposite the affected ear, and the auricle is then grasped and pulled superiorly and posteriorly. Instill drops until the external auditory canal is filled, and then have the athlete lay on his or her side for 15–20 minutes with the affected ear still facing upward to allow for maximal time and surface area exposure.
- Return to play: The athlete should be fever-free and have normal movement of the eardrum without signs of tearing or perforation.

Traumatic Perforation of Tympanic Membrane (2,10,12,13)

- Common mechanism: Compression of the external ear via a slap on the side of the head with a cupped hand, producing a transient high pressure within the canal.
- Signs/symptoms: Immediate pain and loss of hearing in the affected ear; bleeding from the ear may be present; ruptured TM will be evident on an otoscopic exam.
- Treatment: The athlete should be reassured that the TM will heal spontaneously and without hearing loss; however, the athlete *should not* be allowed to swim/submerge their head in water until healed. Individually tailored wax earplugs can be manufactured and used to completely occlude the external auditory canal from water entry in cases where clinical judgment would deem it reasonable for the athlete to return to play before the injury has completely healed.

UPPER EXTREMITY INJURIES

Shoulder

- Mountjoy et al reported a shoulder injury rate of just over 11% in 8904 player matches at the FINA World Championships and the Olympic Games (4).
- A systematic review of the literature showed that the incidence of shoulder injuries can range anywhere from 24% to 80% (14).
- Subacromial/coracoacromial impingement and bursitis, biceps tendinitis, acromioclavicular joint sprains or arthritis, dislocations, rotator cuff injuries, and tears are common shoulder injuries among water polo players (10,14).
- Traumatic dislocations and subluxations are not common injuries in water polo. When they do occur, these injuries typically result during the act of shooting or passing the ball. Shoulder dislocations are the most common injury in water polo to require operative intervention.
- The majority of shoulder injuries that occur are from overuse or are minor injuries such as impingement or bursitis, compared to major injuries involving tears or requiring surgery (2).
- Webster et al. (15) performed a systematic review of the literature showing that shoulder injuries in water polo

players resulted from a variety of factors, including increased mobility, muscle strength imbalance, and altered throwing techniques.

- McMaster et al. (1) demonstrated isokinetic torque imbalances in the rotator cuff of water polo players. The study showed that elite water polo players have significant adductor and internal rotator muscle strength when compared to muscles for abduction and external rotation. This imbalance within the rotator cuff likely increases the propensity for shoulder injuries.
- No other throwing athlete deals with water as their sole base of support for throwing, and unlike other throwing athletes, the water polo player has no fixed point from which to throw. The forceful abduction and external rotation of the glenohumeral joint to achieve the "cocked" throwing position followed by the throw itself places a great strain on the anterior shoulder stabilizing muscles. In addition, the shoulder undergoes large forces when absorbing the impact when blocking a shot, which is unique compared to other water sports (2).
- The majority of shoulder injuries can be rehabilitated through physical therapy, rest, and anti-inflammatory medications. Specifically, rehabilitation should focus on the multifactorial nature of this problem and include strengthening of the scapular stabilizers and rotator cuff, core strengthening, and stretching of the posterior rotator cuff, posterior capsule, scapular stabilizers, and pectoralis muscles (2,16).

Elbow

- The majority of elbow pain in water polo players occurs along the medial aspect of the elbow.
- Most common injuries include ulnar collateral ligament (UCL) injuries, valgus extension overload syndrome with olecranon osteophytes and posteromedial impingement, and osteochondritis dissecans of the capitellum (2,10).
- The overhead throwing motion of a water polo player places great stress on the UCL complex. The ligament can fail at an average load of 260 N or 58 lb. This tension load can be exceeded in elite water polo competitions.
- Mild pain after throwing or a change in activity level is most often associated with overuse injuries. If a "pop" sensation is felt, a UCL injury should be suspected. Mechanical symptoms of catching or locking are often caused by osteophytes and loose bodies.
- Part of the workup for elbow pain should include anteroposterior, lateral, and axial olecranon x-ray views. Magnetic resonance imaging is the study of choice for evaluating potential damage to the UCL complex.
- The majority of elbow injuries can be treated through nonoperative measures, including rest, ice, a short course of bracing to limit extension and physical therapy (2). Any physical therapy should include core body strengthening exercises, with arm flexibility and secondary dynamic stabilizer strengthening.
- Upon completion of rehabilitation, athletes should be enrolled in a throwing program to effectively rehab the elbow.
  - Overuse injuries can take anywhere from 3 to 6 months before an athlete is ready for full competition (10).
  - An injury that involves UCL instability or reconstructive surgery can result in 9–18 months of rehabilitation before an athlete is able to return.

Hand and Fingers

- A player's hand and arm are considered part of the ball during active play and are often hit by opposing players in an attempt to gain possession of the ball. The hand and fingers are also used for shot blocking and grabbing onto other players to maintain position. With the ball being grabbed, thrown, and caught at high speeds, hand and finger injuries are common.
- The most common injuries include lacerations, dislocations, fractures, and overuse injuries, including the following. (As in other sports, water polo players are susceptible to mallet finger, jersey finger, and de Quervain tenosynovitis.)

Web Space Tear

- The most common laceration in water polo (2,10).
- Common mechanism: Occurs when two fingers are forcibly abducted apart. This can occur when players attempt to block or catch balls thrown at high speeds.
- Signs/symptoms: Notable tear and pain between two fingers.
- Treatment: Small tears will heal with time and conservative treatment. The lacerations involving ligaments of the fingers may require reconstructive surgery.
- Return to play: Athletes may return to play if bleeding is controlled and there is no concern for injury to deeper structures.

Dislocations of the Fingers (PIP and DIP) (2,10)

- Common mechanism: Due to a hyperextension of the joint.
- Signs/symptoms: A dislocated finger is usually obvious. The finger appears crooked and swollen and is very painful. It may be bent upward or at strange angles. Bending or attempted straightening of the finger may be difficult.
- Treatment: Athletes and athletic trainers are usually successful with reducing these dislocations poolside. X-rays after a dislocation and reduction are recommended to rule out fractures. Many joints can be treated with "buddy taping" to the healthy finger next to it; however, some dislocations may require surgery.
- Return to play: Depending on the degree of injury, if the finger can be buddy taped and pain is controlled, then the player may return as tolerated. More significant injuries may require weeks or months before return to play, especially if surgery is required.

"Gamekeeper's Thumb" (2)

- Common mechanism: Involves injury to the UCL of the thumb. This can occur when the ball strikes the thumb, causing a hyperabduction of the joint and injuring or tearing the UCL.

- Signs/symptoms: Pain at the base of the thumb in the web space between thumb and index finger; noted swelling or ecchymosis of the thumb or inability to grasp using the thumb and index finger; often tenderness to touch along the index finger side of the thumb.
- Treatment: May include a thumb spica brace or cast, with some injuries requiring surgery.
- Return to play: Data are limited and based off of expert recommendations, but typically return to play will happen no earlier than 4 weeks and may take up to 3 months before it can occur.

LOWER EXTREMITY INJURIES

Thigh, Groin, and Hips

- Injuries to the thigh and hips are not as common as upper extremity injuries, but can still occur in water polo players. The majority of injuries stem from the "eggbeater" kick that is unique to the game of water polo and can cause overuse adductor tendinopathies and muscle strains (2,14).
- Injury to the thigh muscles can occur during the act of throwing when a player is trying to propel out of the water to gain a height advantage over the opposing player. Most often, this involves the adductors, given the mechanism of propelling out of the water.
- Physical play among players can often result in bruised quadriceps and hamstring muscles.
- Athletic pubalgia and femoral-acetabular impingement should be considered as well for sources of groin pain (14).
- Treatment most often involves relative rest and physical therapy to include eccentric strengthening; surgery is reserved for those who do not respond to an adequate trial of conservative modalities (10).

Knee

- Medial knee pain is most often due to overuse. These injuries may include patellofemoral pain syndrome, medial collateral ligament sprains, ligament tears, and meniscus tears (2).
- The aforementioned "eggbeater" kick combines the clockwise motion of one leg and the counterclockwise motion of the other leg in order to stay afloat, which leads to a significant valgus force along the medial aspect of the knee joint, especially to the medial collateral ligament and medial patellar retinaculum (14).
- The force from the eggbeater kick with compression on the medial aspect of the joint can cause degenerative changes (10).
- Most knee injuries can be rehabilitated through physical therapy focusing on strengthening the core muscles as well as the quadriceps, hamstrings, and pelvis.

SPINAL INJURIES

- Although not common, spinal cord injuries can occur. All pools should have cervical collars and spine boards or similar extrication devices available for spinal motion control, as well as qualified personnel to remove players with suspected spine injuries from the water (2).
- Medical personnel should recognize key red flags, including profound muscle weakness and/or reflex loss, bowel and/or bladder incontinence or retention, and saddle numbness and/or sensory changes when dealing with patients complaining of back pain.

Cervical

- Given that players constantly rotate their cervical spine when either breathing in freestyle swimming or for rotation to follow the game, degenerative cervical spine changes, or complaints can occur.
- Water polo players will often have to keep their heads afloat with periods of sustained extension and protraction, causing common muscle aches, cervicalgia, and radiculopathies (2).
- Players are trained to alternate the rotation of their head when swimming, so symptoms are often bilateral.
- Acceleration and deceleration injuries and whiplash can also be common cervical injuries with physical play (2,10).
- Conservative treatment and physical therapy are often successful in the rehabilitation of cervical injuries.

Lumbar

- The lumbar spine can see significant force during the throwing and passing of the ball (10). This can cause many athletes to have hypertrophied latissimus muscles along the dominant arm side.
- Lower back pain can include many different types of injuries, with examples being facet joint syndromes, lumbar disc slips, muscle strains, and overuse injuries (10).
- Physicians must first rule out red flag symptoms before prescribing treatment. Plain film x-rays are usually not required with acute injuries. The majority of low back pain can be rehabilitated with physical therapy and analgesics. Pain that worsens or is not improved with physical therapy may warrant further imaging and testing (2,10).

ENVIRONMENTAL AND MISCELLANEOUS INJURIES

Environmental Injuries

- These injuries can include sunburns, hypothermia, warts, and swimmer's exanthema.

- Sunburns, which increase a person's risk for skin cancer, can occur with outdoor water polo matches (2).
  - International water polo rules forbid players from wearing sunblock or sunscreen during play due to causing the ball to be greasy and slippery.
  - When allowed in outdoor competition or practice, players should wear sun-protective agents on higher risk areas such as the face and shoulders.
- Hypothermia is defined as having a core body temperature less than 95°F or 35°C. Exhaustion, wind, and wetness are all risk factors for hypothermia. Depending on the competition environment, hypothermia can occur in all water sports, including water polo.
- Warts are small, painless skin growths caused by a viral infection. Swimming is a known risk factor for warts.
  - There are numerous treatments for warts, including medications, ointments, cryotherapy, burning (electrocautery), surgical removal, and laser treatment.
- Swimmer's xerosis can be caused by hours of submersion in the water, causing the skin to become dehydrated and pruritic.
  - Treatment includes using mild soaps when bathing, avoiding rubbing the skin dry after a shower or bath, and applying an oil-based protective emollient shortly after a shower or bath.

Lacerations (10)

- Lacerations to the face, forehead, and hands are very common in water polo.
- As previously mentioned, the web space tear (when two fingers are forcibly abducted apart) is the most common laceration in water polo.
- Most lacerations can be repaired with Steri-strips or plastic-based waterproof spray. Some lacerations may require sutures.
- Players' fingernails and toenails are usually inspected by the referee before the start of the game in hopes of decreasing the risk of lacerations.

COVERAGE CONSIDERATIONS

- Physicians covering water polo matches should be prepared to cover medical emergencies and catastrophic injuries such as cardiac events or cervical spine injuries similar to any sporting event.
  - Extra caution should be taken with automated external defibrillator use in the wet poolside environment
  - Additional personnel and specialized training is required for spinal motion control and extrication of the athlete with suspected spinal injury.
- Given that eye injuries are frequently encountered in water polo, having an "eye tray" should be considered if covering this sport regularly. Items to consider in the eye tray include an eye chart, penlight, light source with a blue or cobalt blue filter, fluorescein dye, ophthalmoscope, loupes or magnifying glass, sterile saline, and a contact lens remover. Medications to consider having in the aid bag include anesthetic drops and mydriatic drops.
- Concussions may occur both in competition and practice. Assessing an athlete for a concussion at the poolside using a sideline evaluation tool would be beneficial.
- A poolside laceration repair kit with suture material and plastic-based waterproof spray is also useful when trying to get an athlete back into competition.

REFERENCES

1. McMaster WC, Long SC, Caiozzo VJ. Isokinetic torque imbalances in the rotator cuff of the elite water polo player. *Am J Sports Med.* 1991;19(1):72–5.
2. Stromberg JD. Care of water polo players. *Curr Sports Med Rep.* 2017 Sep 1;16(5):363–9.
3. Junge A, Langevoort G, Pipe A, et al. Injuries in team sport tournaments during the 2004 Olympic Games. *Am J Sports Med.* 2006;34(4):565–76.
4. Mountjoy M, Junge A, Alonso JM, et al. Sports injuries and illnesses in the 2009 FINA World Championships (Aquatics). *Br J Sports Med.* 2010;44(7):522–7.
5. *FINA/USA Water Polo Rules,* 2019-2022 [Internet]. [cited 2022 Sep 21]. Available from: http://www.usawaterpolo.org
6. Mountjoy M, Miller J, Junge A. Analysis of water polo injuries during 8904 player matches at FINA World Championships and Olympic games to make the sport safer. *Br J Sports Med.* 2019;53(1):25–31.
7. Blumenfeld RS, Winsell JC, Hicks JW, Small SL. The epidemiology of sports-related head injury and concussion in water polo. *Front Neurol.* 2016 Jun 24;7:98.
8. Annett P, Fricker P, McDonald W. Injuries to elite male waterpolo players over a 13 year period. *N Z J Sports Med.* 2000;28(4):78–83.
9. Cass SP. Ocular injuries in sports. *Curr Sports Med Rep.* 2012 Jan 1;11(1):11–5.
10. Franíc M, Ivkovíc A, Rudíc R. Injuries in water polo. *Croat Med J.* 2007;48(3):281–8.
11. Barr A, Baines PS, Desai P, MacEwen CJ. Ocular sports injuries: the current picture. *Br J Sports Med.* 2000;34(6):456–8.
12. Wang MC, Liu CY, Shiao AS, Wang T. Ear problems in swimmers. *J Chin Med Assoc.* 2005;68(8):347–52.
13. Spittler J, Keeling J. Water polo injuries and training methods. *Curr Sports Med Rep.* 2016;15(6):410–6.
14. Croteau F, Brown H, Pearsall D, Robbins SM. Prevalence and mechanisms of injuries in water polo: a systematic review. *BMJ Open Sport Exerc Med.* 2021 Jun 1;7(2):e001081.
15. Webster MJ, Morris ME, Galna B. Shoulder pain in water polo: a systematic review of the literature. *J Sci Med Sport.* 2009;12(1):3–11.
16. Nichols AW. Medical care of the aquatics athlete. *Curr Sports Med Rep.* 2015;14(5):389–96.

Weightlifting

126

Devin K. Kelly, Christopher M. Kuenze, Christopher D. Ingersoll, and Joe M. Hart

INTRODUCTION

- In this chapter, the terms weightlifting and resistance training refer to exercises aimed at increasing muscular strength, power, and endurance (1).
- Resistance training may be performed in traditional and home gym settings. Participants may utilize bodyweight exercises, or equipment, including free weights (*e.g.*, barbells and dumbbells), weight machines, medicine balls, kettlebells, resistance bands, and fitness mirrors or smart devices (1).
- Regular resistance training is beneficial to the health of individuals, across sex and ages, in many ways. It results in increases in lean muscle mass, decreases in fat mass, increases in resting metabolic rate, improves insulin sensitivity, reduces resting blood pressure, improves cardiovascular health, increases strength, and improves functional capabilities. Regular resistance training also benefits mental health as it reduces symptoms of anxiety and depression, and improves self-esteem and cognitive abilities (2).
- Apart from resistance training to improve general health, there are distinct weightlifting sports: Olympic lifting, powerlifting, CrossFit, Strongman, Scottish Highland games, and bodybuilding (3).
- Olympic weightlifting lifts (events) are the snatch and the clean-and-jerk. The goal of the competition is to lift the maximum weight in each event for one repetition. The total weight an athlete lifts is determined by combining the greatest weight lifted in each event. There must be one successful lift out of three attempts on each event (3,4).
- Powerlifting events include the squat, bench press, and deadlift. Like Olympic lifting, the goal of the competition is to lift the maximum weight in each event for one repetition (4).
- CrossFit is a high-intensity exercise program in which athletes complete a "workout of the day" consisting of a combination of Olympic and powerlifting, gymnastics, and functional movements. The exercises are performed quickly with minimal rest periods. In the CrossFit games, athletes complete the workout of the day in the least amount of time to win (3,5).
- Strongman competitions and the Scottish Highland games consist of events focused on showing strength during historical farming and military tasks. Strongman events include lifting and carrying stones, flipping tires, overhead pressing logs and stones, and pulling sleds and trucks. The Highland games include throwing events like a caber, stone put, hammer throw, sheaf toss, weight for height, and weight for distance (3).
- Competitive bodybuilding involves high-intensity resistance training to achieve maximal muscle mass, symmetry, and definition. Athletes are judged on their appearance in these categories (1,3).
- Resistance training can improve sports performance. High-velocity concentric phase movements improve endurance performance (*e.g.*, running, cycling, and swimming). Focusing on muscle groups used in sport-specific movements and adding resistance to sport-specific movements is best for improved performance (6,7).
- Weightlifting sports have a similar injury incidence as team sports (1.1–4.4/1000 hours of training). Several studies have identified that CrossFit has a greater injury incidence compared to traditional weightlifting (4,5,8).
- The most common areas of injury from weightlifting are the shoulder, back, and knee (4,5).

BASIC MUSCLE PHYSIOLOGY

Skeletal Muscle Contraction

- Motor units activate the muscle to produce force.
- A motor unit consists of an α-motor neuron, its axon, and the muscle fibers it innervates.
- Several bundles of muscle fibers, called fascicles, comprise a skeletal muscle.
- A muscle fiber is composed of several myofibrils bundled together. Myofibrils contain a series of sarcomeres arranged end-to-end (9).
- Sarcomeres are the functional and contractile components of skeletal muscle that produce force through a dynamic interaction between the proteins, actin, and myosin.
- According to the sliding filament theory, actin and myosin slide past each other to produce sarcomere shortening. Ca^{++} is released in the sarcomere in response to an action potential that exposes myosin cross-bridge binding sites on actin. Myosin cross-bridges bind to actin and pull actin filaments

closer to the center of each sarcomere, producing force and stiffness within the skeletal muscle (9,10).

- The force that a muscle fiber produces depends on the overlap between myosin and actin with the greatest amount of force production resulting from the greatest number of cross-bridges formed (9,10).
- Force production by a skeletal muscle can be voluntarily graded. However, the muscle fibers innervated by one motor neuron (*i.e.*, a motor unit) act in an all-or-none fashion (9).
- The isometric force produced by a motor unit increases to a plateau with increasing frequency of activation. This is known as the force-frequency relationship (11).
- Increase in skeletal muscle force production can be achieved via motor unit recruitment (increasing the number of motor units) and rate coding (increasing motor unit discharge rate) (9,12).
- The minimum force at which a motor unit will discharge action potentials repetitively is called the recruitment threshold. Recruitment thresholds are not fixed (13).
- Henneman size principle states that motor neurons are recruited in order of increasing size (orderly recruitment) (14). There is an inverse relationship between the discharge rate and recruitment threshold of motor units. Earlier recruited motor units have greater discharge rates than later recruited motor units. This is referred to as "The Onion-Skin scheme" due to the appearance of discharge rates versus time plots (15–18).

Skeletal Muscle Fiber Types

- There are several different muscle fiber types based on structure (myosin heavy chain isoform, sarcomere length) and function (metabolic capacity). Different classification techniques exist with varying nomenclature. We will use Type I, Type IIA, and Type IIB as described below. Note that Type IIA is also referred to as IIax and IIB as IIx (see Chapter 6 Exercise Physiology for additional information).
- Type I muscle fibers (slow-twitch, oxidative fibers) have high mitochondria content and a rich blood supply. These fibers are generally smaller in size (diameter) and innervated by smaller diameter axons. Type I fibers contract slowly and are resistant to fatigue because their method of energy metabolism is aerobic. However, Type I fibers produce less tension, resulting in less force production.
- Type IIA muscle fibers (fast-twitch and oxidative-glycolytic fibers) also have high mitochondria content and are moderately capable of performing aerobic and anaerobic metabolism. This fiber type exhibits the performance and metabolic characteristics of both Type I and IIB fibers.
- Type IIB muscle fibers (fast-twitch and glycolytic fibers) have sparse mitochondrial content and blood supply. They fatigue easily but are capable of producing higher force and tension. Type IIB fibers act in an anaerobic capacity during activity.
- While muscle fibers are typed as Type I, IIA, and IIB (IIX), a spectrum of types exists, including hybrid fibers I/IIA, IIA/IIB, and I/IIA/IIB. The proportion of hybrid to pure muscle fiber types is variable among muscles (19,20).
- All muscle fibers within a motor unit have the same metabolic characteristics (*i.e.*, motor units are homogenous based on fiber type). Therefore, motor units can be classified as slow contracting/fatigue resistant (Type I), fast contracting/fatigue resistant (Type IIA), and fast contracting/fatigable (Type IIB). In general, fast-twitch/fatigable motor units are the largest (contain the greatest number of innervated fibers) and have the highest recruitment threshold, whereas slow-twitch/fatigue-resistant motor units are the smallest (contain the fewest number of innervated fibers) and have the lowest recruitment threshold.
- Muscle fiber type composition in a particular human skeletal muscle is largely genetically determined (9); however, some studies suggest fibers transition in the direction of type IIB to type IIA to type I, and that fiber type composition adaptations are due to changes in the proportion of Type IIA and Type IIB fibers (21).
- Specific training programs have been shown to be effective in targeting improvements in the performance of specific fiber types. Heavy resistance training has been shown to cause increased Type IIA fibers and decreased Type IIB fibers, whereas Type I fiber composition in human skeletal muscle was unchanged (22). Low-resistance, high-volume training caused improved muscular endurance, which is thought to indicate an improvement in Type I fiber performance (23,24). Generally, exercise shifts muscle fibers toward slower fiber types, but depends on training (19).
- Structural and genetic characteristics of muscle fiber types have been modulated with fiber-specific stimulation in vitro (25). However, it is unknown whether such changes occur in all muscle fiber types or if the transformation will be sustained over time in vivo.
- Because muscle fiber composition is largely genetically determined, athletes may participate in sports or activities that involve muscle contractions that are more "natural." Whether a distance runner can train to be a successful powerlifter or vice versa is an issue that has not yet been clearly elucidated (20).

Types of Skeletal Muscle Contraction

- The contribution of a muscle to a movement depends on the torque that it exerts. The ratio of muscle torque to load torque determines how muscle length changes during a contraction and, therefore, the type of contraction that is performed.
- Skeletal muscle can produce joint movements through concentric and eccentric contractions.
- Concentric contractions describe a movement that involves the shortening of a muscle against a load, whereas eccentric contractions involve the controlled lengthening of a muscle against a load.

- Eccentric muscle contractions produce greater muscle force and more myofibrillar disruption than concentric exercise (26,27).
- Eccentric muscle contractions (often referred to as "negatives" in weightlifting) are more effective in producing strength gains and hypertrophy than concentric contractions, but they are more likely to cause delayed-onset muscle soreness (27–29). However, both eccentric (negative) and concentric (positive) contractions elicit gains in skeletal muscle strength and size (29).
- Isometric muscle contractions produce muscle tension without joint movement—for example, pushing against a wall or contracting the quadriceps muscle while holding the knee motionless at a particular point in the knee range of motion. Isometric contractions occur when the muscle torque and load torque are equal.
- Isotonic muscle contractions produce muscle tension and joint movement against a constant load where the rate of movement is variable. For example, a dumbbell curl is a contraction against a constant load that can be voluntarily moved at a self-selected rate. This is the most typical contraction in weightlifting.
- Isokinetic muscle contractions involve a constant rate of joint displacement that is maintained by varying amounts of resistance based on muscle effort. This is uncommon in weightlifting or athletic settings. Isokinetic exercise requires expensive machinery and is usually most applicable in the rehabilitation setting.
- Isotonic and isokinetic muscle movements can be performed through concentric or eccentric muscle contractions.

RESPONSES TO RESISTANCE TRAINING

Neural Adaptations

- Early in resistance training programs, improvements in strength are due to neural changes. The increase in maximal voluntary contraction is greater than the increase in muscle cross-sectional area (hypertrophy) (30,31). This is one of the main factors for improving strength in beginners (32).
- Coordinated joint movements are improved by altering activation patterns, decreasing antagonist muscle activity, and increasing synergist muscle activity (30).
- Decreasing antagonist muscle activity and co-contraction reduces energy expenditure and increases joint torque in the direction of movement (33–35).
- Resistance training increases synergist muscle activity contributing to training specificity and gains specific to the exercise trained.
- There are also long-term neuromuscular adaptations to resistance training. Healthy adults who participated in 100 days of resistance training adapted differently based on training modality. Electromyography activity decreased at a greater rate with resistance training compared to endurance exercise (36).
- The strength production of bilateral contractions is less than that of the sum of unilateral contractions. This is termed a bilateral deficit (37). With unilateral contractions, there is cross-education resulting in the contralateral limb strength increasing 10%–15% of the ipsilateral limb strength increase (38).
- Maximal voluntary contractions during resistance training can be increased by additional means, including cueing (39) and mental imagery (40–42). The cross-education training effect can be accomplished by mental imagery (43).

Muscular Adaptations

- Improvements in muscle strength, power, or endurance are best achieved by overloading the muscle(s) being trained. The *overload* principle states that when a muscle is exposed to a stress or load that is greater than what it usually experiences, it will adapt so that it is able to handle the greater load (9,44,45).
- Similarly, the *SAID* principle (specific adaptations to imposed demands) states that a muscle or body tissue will adapt to the specific demands imposed on it. For example, if a muscle is overloaded, its fibers will grow in size so it is able to produce enough force to overcome the imposed load (9,45). Human skeletal muscle hypertrophy occurs when the cross-sectional area of a muscle fiber increases (46,47). As skeletal muscle hypertrophies, contractile proteins are synthesized more than they are degraded. Therefore, skeletal muscle is capable of producing more tension (48). Type IIA fibers exhibit the greatest potential for growth, whereas Type IIB and Type I fibers exhibit the least amount of growth in response to heavy resistance training (48). Muscle hypertrophy is more common in fast-twitch than slow-twitch muscles.
- Strength gains with muscle hypertrophy are due in part to changes in muscle fiber architecture in the pennate muscle (49) and increased fascicle length allowing more sarcomeres in series (50). Muscle fiber lateral force transmission has been shown to contribute to increased strength (51), but more research is required to understand the lateral pathway (52). Muscle fiber hyperplasia does not appear to play a role in increased muscle cross-sectional area or strength gains in resistance-trained men (53).
- Strength training leads to muscle hypertrophy, which increases muscle mass (47). Volume, intensity, and the consistent application of progressive overload are the important factors to induce hypertrophy. Strength gains are specific to the action or the range of motion completed during training; therefore, it is best to train through a full range of motion to optimize strength gains (54).
- Muscle hypertrophy is typically observed with resistance training after 6–7 weeks of strength training (44,48).

- There appears to be a sex difference in the rate at which muscles hypertrophy favoring males (55). Additionally, females lose muscle mass quicker than males when detrained (55).
- In general, it is thought that strengthening exercises using a resistance that is greater than the 6-repetition maximum (RM) are best for muscle hypertrophy, whereas those at a resistance of less than the 20-RM are best for endurance training (56). Simply stated, fewer repetitions using higher weights are best for strength gains, whereas more repetitions using lower weights are best for endurance gains.

BASIC WEIGHTLIFTING PROGRAMS

- There are several different weightlifting programs that can be customized to an individual or their strength training and athletic goals. An effective program balances muscle overloading with recovery time to facilitate strength gains. Sample weightlifting sets based on the DeLorme and daily adjusted progressive resistance exercise (DAPRE) methods are presented in Table 126.1.

The DeLorme Method

- The DeLorme method is a progressive resistance exercise program based on the overload principle (48,57). This method is based on the 10-RM. First, a weight that the athlete can lift 10 times (with the desired muscle group[s]) is determined. A total of 3 sets of 10 repetitions are performed per session for each muscle at 50%, 75%, and 100% of the 10-RM. The athlete is encouraged to perform more than 10 repetitions during the third set to serve as an overload to the muscle group being trained. As the athlete's 10-RM increases, so does the resistance in each set (see Table 126.1).

Daily Adjusted Progressive Resistance Exercise

- The DAPRE method of strength training guides the athlete through four sets of exercises per muscle group or other desired task. DAPRE guidelines provide recommendations for when to increase resistance and how much added resistance is appropriate based on individual performance (see Table 126.1) (58,59).
- A total of four sets of repetitions are performed per muscle group.
  - First and second sets: Perform 10 repetitions at 50% and six repetitions at 75% of the predetermined 6-RM (the maximum weight that can be successfully "lifted" for six repetitions). The 6-RM is termed the "working weight."
  - Third set: 100% of the working weight is used, and repetitions are performed until failure is reached (as many repetitions as safely possible).

Table 126.1 Weightlifting Programs

	DeLorme (49)	DAPRE (50,51)
Set 1	50% 10-RM[a] × 10 reps	50% 6-RM[b] × 10 reps
Set 2	75% 10-RM × 10 reps	75% 6-RM × 6 reps
Set 3	100% 10-RM × 10 reps	100% 6-RM to failure
Set 4	—	Adjusted[c] weight to failure

[a]10-RM = maximum amount of weight with which one can perform 10 consecutive repetitions.
[b]6–RM = maximum amount of weight with which one can perform 6 consecutive repetitions.
[c]Adjusted weight: Add 5 lb if >7 repetitions in third set; subtract 5 lb if <4 repetitions in third set; no change if four to seven repetitions performed in third set.

  - Fourth set: An "adjusted weight" is used, and repetitions are performed until failure is reached. To calculate the "adjusted weight" for the fourth set in this program, the number of repetitions performed in the third set is considered. If five to seven repetitions were performed in the third set, "adjusted" resistance for the fourth set remains the same. If less than five repetitions were performed, the adjusted weight is reduced for the fourth set; if more than seven repetitions were performed, the adjusted weight in the fourth set is increased. For example, if the athlete performs 12 repetitions of 100 lb in the third set, the weight for the fourth set can be increased to 105 lb. If only three repetitions are performed in the third set using 100 lb, the fourth set adjusted weight should be reduced to 90 or 95 lb.
  - Next session guidelines: The "working weight" for the next day of resistance training is adjusted based on the number of repetitions achieved in the fourth set similar to the method used to adjust the weight for the fourth set. Using the example above, if the athlete can perform 10 repetitions during the fourth exercise set using 105 lb, he or she can adjust the working weight for the next day to 105 or 110 lb.
- The DAPRE method can be adjusted for each individual based on his or her training goals. Manipulating the amount of weight added to the adjusted weight for the fourth set or the modified working weight for the next day's lift can change the pace of individual programs.

Periodization

- Periodization is a specific approach to strength training and conditioning that is intended to bring about peak performance at a desired time, typically at the time of competition (44,45,48).
- A macrocycle is a long-term plan of exercise progression with the goal of achieving peak performance at the time of competition. Commonly, macrocycles are composed of preparation, competitive, and transition phases. For seasonal sports participants, a macrocycle will include a calendar year that is divided into the following mesocycles: Preseason, in-season, and off-season.

- A mesocycle is a shorter phase of training that makes up a portion of a macrocycle with variable length depending on the training goals and length of the macrocycle. The volume and intensity of an activity during these cycles should be determined by the goals of the macrocycle and the response of the individual.
- Over the course of an athlete's macrocycle of periodization, training intensity, volume, and mode will change to allow for maximum performance and minimum risk for injury and overuse. For an Olympic athlete, a macrocycle may be 4 years, where periodized training regimens are tailored to maximize performance at the desired time(s).
- In preparation for athletic competition, linear periodization begins in the athletic off-season, where training volume is high, but intensity is low. Initially, strength gains and muscle hypertrophy are the goals of this phase. As training intensity gradually increases through the postseason and into the preseason, training volume decreases. This progression continues through the preseason, where sport-specific skill training is maximized to facilitate the transition to competition.
- Undulating periodization has been shown to be more effective in producing strength gains and muscle hypertrophy when compared with traditional linear paradigms. This method includes the use of varied resistance (*e.g.*, 3- to 5-RM, 8- to 10-RM, and 12- to 15-RM) while completing multiple sets of the same exercise within a single training session (60). It remains unclear how the implementation of this paradigm may affect functional performance goals or the transition from preseason training to in-season performance (60).

Sample Exercises for Major Muscle Groups

- There are several exercises that can be used for each muscle group. The appropriate exercise depends on equipment availability, experience or preference of the weightlifter, and training goals. Isolated muscle exercises are appropriate for strengthening muscles. Whole-body strength exercises that require coordinated, multiple-body segment movements are appropriate to develop power and athletic skill.

Upper Body/Trunk

- Seated military press (deltoid): In the seated position, weighted dumbbells or a bar are lifted above the head and then returned to the anterior shoulders/upper chest.
- Bench press (pectoralis major): While supine on a bench, weighted dumbbells or a bar are lifted off the chest until the arms are fully extended and then lowered slowly back to the chest.
- Bicep curls (biceps brachii): In the seated or standing position, weighted dumbbells or a bar are lifted through the full elbow range of motion from the extended to flexed position and then returned slowly back to the extended position
- Triceps extension (triceps brachii): While in the supine position, with shoulders flexed to 90° and elbows extended, resistance is lowered by flexing the elbow, followed by concentric elbow extension.
- Rows (trapezius/rhomboids): In the seated or standing position and with shoulders flexed to 90°, arms are drawn back by extending the shoulders and flexing the elbows. Visualize "squeezing" the back blades (scapula) together. This exercise can be done with free weights, resistive bands, or a machine.

Lower Body

- Squats (quadriceps): In the standing position with resistance fixed at the shoulders, the body is lowered by flexing the hips and knees while maintaining upright upper body posture.
- Hamstring curls (hamstrings): In the prone position, resistance fixed at the distal lower leg is curled toward the hips by flexing the knee. This is usually done with the assistance of a pulley-style machine, or it can be done in standing with ankle weights.
- Calf raises (triceps surae): In the standing or seated position, the body, with added resistance (if desired), is elevated by plantarflexing the ankle joint.

GUIDELINES FOR EXERCISE PRESCRIPTION (TABLE 126.2)

Training Volume and Intensity

- It is important to consider training volume and intensity of training when designing an effective weightlifting program. The goal of a weightlifting program is to achieve maximal or desired gains while allowing for an appropriate amount of time between sets and between sessions for muscle and body recovery.
- Training volume is determined by multiplying the number of repetitions performed in an exercise session by the resistance used (44). It is the total quantity of work performed. Therefore, similar training volumes are achieved when light resistance is used for high repetitions and when heavy resistance is used for low repetitions. In periodized programs, it is appropriate to begin with high training volumes (off-season) and progress to lower volumes at higher intensity (preseason), leading to more sport-specific skills, with concurrent programs aimed at maintaining strength and conditioning while in-season.
- In addition to training volume, volume load has a dose-response relationship between weekly sets and muscle strength gains (61–63). Volume load is equal to the number of sets times the number of repetitions times load in kilograms (64).
- There are two models for prescribing volume load progression: %1RM and RM Zone. The %1RM method increases the volume load when the number of repetitions to failure

increases. The RM Zone method has a set zone of repetitions, and the load is adjusted so that muscle failure occurs in the repetition zone (61). The RM Zone method has been shown to result in greater volume load progression rate and muscle cross-sectional area gains than the %1RM method (64).

- Intensity is analogous to power and is therefore dependent on the amount of resistance and the speed of the movement (65). Intensity can be expressed as a percentage of 1-RM.
- Athletes should focus on foundational strengthening exercises before advancing to power training (66).
- Overtraining can result in decreases in muscle strength and function. It usually occurs when either training volume or intensity is too great, and the body cannot appropriately adapt (67).
- When designing an exercise or weightlifting program, it is important to include activities that are specific to the athlete's goals. The training goal should be accomplished by manipulating the number of sets, reps, and rest periods. For example, if an athlete wants to perform movements that require high muscle strength and power, the athlete should train with weights that are closer to their 1-RM and perform fewer repetitions per set (45). Likewise, if an athlete wants to perform movements that require endurance, the athlete should use less weight with higher repetitions. The athletic year is divided into in-season, postseason, off-season, and preseason segments. During the postseason and off-season, training should concentrate on recovery from the competitive season and maintain fitness and strength. Strength training can begin in the off-season and gradually progress to power training and sport-specific training during the preseason. Strength, endurance, and power maintenance should be performed in-season.

Rest Periods

- Structured rest periods between sets are important to maximize the effectiveness of a resistance training program. Appropriate rest frequency and duration can allow for maximal performance during each set of a specific task and positively affect the metabolic effects of resistance training (68,69).
- Rest time should increase as the intensity of the exercise increases. Currently, there is no gold standard for rest time between sets. It has been suggested that for low resistance (11- to 13-RM), a 1- to 2-minute rest is appropriate; however, for moderate-resistance (8- to 10-RM) and high-resistance exercise (<5-RM), rest times of 3–5 and >5 minutes, respectively, may be better (56).

Interval Training

- Interval training consists of sets (intervals) of varying-intensity exercises.
- High-intensity interval training (HIIT) is an exercise involving short bursts of vigorous activity interspersed with rest or low-intensity activity periods, intended to improve aerobic function (70). High-intensity functional training (HIFT) is similar to HIIT but includes anaerobic, muscle-strengthening activity. HIFT is an exercise involving short bursts of vigorous activity that focus on functional, multi-joint movement aimed at improving parameters of physical fitness (*e.g.*, strength) and performance (*e.g.*, power), interspersed with rest or low-intensity activity periods (71–73). Note that HIFT is also referred to as high-intensity power training, multimodal high-intensity training, and functional high-intensity training, among others (73).
- Functional exercises are whole-body movements that occur in multiple planes (*e.g.*, squats and deadlifts). When functional exercises are performed in an interval format, they result in improvements not only in anaerobic but also in aerobic fitness (74). Specifically, HIFT has resulted in changes in body composition (75), muscle mass, muscle strength and power (72), and aerobic capacity (71–73).
- HIFT rest periods are not predetermined. They are individually dependent on the training level of the individual (73).
- Injury rates from HIFT are similar to those for other physical activities, including running (73,76).

Other General Recommendations

- Strength describes the maximum force that can be generated by a muscle, whereas power is the ability of a muscle to generate large forces quickly. Endurance is the ability of a muscle to contract repeatedly and generate forces for long periods of time.
- Training for muscle strength should include training with resistance that is closer to maximum ability with lower repetitions. This type of training is most appropriate in the athletic off-season.
- Training for muscle power involves coordinated movements that encourage speed, accuracy, and fluency. Power training is most appropriate in the athletic preseason and gradually progresses to the competitive season (in-season).
- Strength training in both the anterior and posterior musculature or training both agonist and antagonist muscle groups is important in an effective strength-training program. It may improve sport- or activity-specific performance and reduce the risk of injury (77).
- It is important to incorporate gradual warm-up, cool-down, and flexibility exercises into a strength-training regimen to maintain muscle health and fitness, reduce the likelihood of injury or postexercise soreness, and improve athletic and weightlifting performance. Dynamic activity-specific warm-up and cool-down plans are commonly used to prepare the athlete for resistance training while including specific activities from the athlete's sport (78).
- Supervised and guided strength-training programs yield greater strength gains than those that are unsupervised (79). Recruiting assistance from certified strength and

conditioning specialists (CSCSs), exercise physiologists, certified personal trainers (CPTs), or certified athletic trainers (ATCs) may facilitate strength gains and improve overall outcomes and sport-specific preparedness.

- Finally, athletes are encouraged to participate in weightlifting programs with at least one partner. Weightlifting partners can motivate each other, provide constructive feedback on technique and form, and provide "spotting" for heavy or potentially dangerous lifts. An athlete should never participate in weightlifting alone.

INJURY PATTERNS

- Athletes reportedly sustain one to two injuries per year (3).
- Injury incidence differs across weightlifting sports. Olympic Weightlifting injury incidence is 2.4–3.3 injuries/1000 training hours. Powerlifting injury incidence is 1.1–4.4/1000 training hours. CrossFit athletes are 2.26 times more likely to be injured than traditional weightlifters, accounting for age and sex (8).
- 60%–75% of weightlifting injuries are acute and 25%–40% are chronic (80).
- Acute and chronic injuries are the result of technical error, fatigue, overloading, and dropping weights (80).
- The most common sites of injury for weightlifters are the shoulder, back, and knee (3).
- The most common injury types for weightlifters are strains, sprains, tendinitis, and cartilage damage (3). Sprains and strains account for 46% of all resistance training injuries (80).
- When accounting for age and training type, men are 1.80 times more likely to be injured than women (8). Males have higher total injuries, higher acute injuries, and higher chest injuries compared to women. Women have a higher rate of knee injuries than men (3).
- Chronic injuries are more common in older athletes (80).
- There are no differences in injury rates between those who use supplements versus those who do not use supplements. The reported supplement use includes multivitamins, protein powder, protein bars, branched-chain amino acids, creatine, preworkout energy, dehydroepiandrosterone (DHEA), anabolic steroids, caffeine, fat burner, and others (8).
- Upper Extremity Injuries
  - Upper extremity resistance training exercises can create a shoulder imbalance between the internal and external rotators if there is not a dedicated focus on the smaller shoulder stabilizing muscles. This imbalance and repetitive loading can make the shoulder susceptible to injury, specifically instability and labral injuries.
  - 6%–36% of injuries in weightlifting injuries are shoulder injuries (3).
  - Shoulder injuries are prevalent in powerlifters likely due to the bench press that places high compressive forces at the end-range of external rotation (3,4).
  - Common injuries of the shoulder in weightlifters include pain, inflammation, rotator cuff lesions, impingement, bursitis, arthrosis, dislocation, and instability (81).
  - Common elbow injuries in weightlifters include pain, inflammation, arthrosis, dislocation, instability, bursitis, and muscle and tendon/nerve disorders (81).
  - Common hand and wrist injuries in weightlifters include pain, tendovaginitis, and ganglion cysts (81).
  - Pectoralis tendon and distal biceps tendon are soft tissues susceptible to rupture with weightlifting. Pectoralis tendon ruptures typically occur during the bench press (47%–70%) due to forced abduction of the upper arm in the end-range of motion. Distal biceps tendon ruptures typically occur during bicep curls with eccentric contraction using 68 kg or more (80).
- Lower Extremity Injuries
  - Knee injuries are among the most common weightlifting injuries. They tend to be more common in Olympic lifters than powerlifters, and in females than males (3,4).
  - Knee injuries in weightlifters include pain, arthrosis, inflammation, femur fracture, ligamentous instability, meniscus injury, cruciate ligament rupture, and disorder of the patella (81).
  - Greater incidence of knee injuries with high-bar and front squats than low-bar squats due to higher mechanical stress and compressive patellofemoral forces (3).
  - Hip injuries in weightlifters include pain, arthrosis, inflammation, instability, impingement, and strain (81).
  - Foot and ankle injuries in weightlifters include flatfoot/splayfoot, ligament instability, and fracture (81).

MEDICAL CONSIDERATIONS

Aging

- There is a decrease in power performance starting at age 35 (82). For weightlifting sports, the peak performance age for men is 26 and women is 25 (83).
- Resistance training can delay age-related declines in muscle weakness (dynapenia) and muscle mass loss (sarcopenia) (79), neuromuscular function (84), and cognitive function (85).
- Older adults have similar training adaptations as younger adults. Similar recommendations may apply to older adults as to young adults, *e.g.*, low-to-moderate loads performed for moderate-to-high repetitions (10–15 or more), for enhancing muscular endurance (Table 126.2) (61).
- Increasing power in healthy older adults includes (a) training to improve muscular strength and (b) the performance of both single- and multiple-joint exercises for 1–3 sets per exercise using light-to-moderate loading (30%–60% of 1-RM) for 6–10 repetitions with high-repetition velocity (Table 126.2) (61).

Table 126.2 Summary of Progressive Resistance Training Recommendations From the ACSM Position Stand (53) Each Recommendation is Listed With an A, B, C, or D Indicating the Quality or Quantity of Research Supporting That Statement; A is the Best

Evidence Statement	Grade
Strength training	
CON, ECC, and ISOM actions should be included for novice, intermediate, and advanced training.	A
Training with loads ~60%–70% of 1-RM for 8–12 repetitions for novice to intermediate individuals and cycling loads of 80%–100% of 1-RM for advanced individuals.	A
When training at a specific RM load, it is recommended that a 2%–10% increase in load be applied when the individual can perform the current workload for 1–2 repetitions over the desired number on two consecutive training sessions.	B
It is recommended that 1–3 sets per exercise be used by novice individuals.	A
Multiple-set programs (with systematic variation of volume and intensity) are recommended for progression to intermediate and advanced training.	A
Unilateral and bilateral single- and multiple-joint exercises should be included, with emphasis on multiple-joint exercises for maximizing strength in novice, intermediate, and advanced individuals.	A
Free-weight and machine exercises should be included for novice to intermediate training.	A
For advanced strength training, it is recommended that emphasis be placed on free-weight exercises with machine exercises used to complement program needs.	C
Recommendations for sequencing exercises for novice, intermediate, and advanced strength training include large muscle group exercises before small muscle group exercises, multiple-joint exercises before single-joint exercises, higher intensity exercises before lower intensity exercises, or rotation of upper and lower-body or opposing exercises.	C
It is recommended that rest periods of at least 2–3 min be used for core exercises using heavier loads for novice, intermediate, and advanced training. For assistance exercises, a shorter rest period length of 1–2 min may suffice.	B, C
For untrained individuals, it is recommended that slow and moderate CON velocities be used.	A
For intermediate training, it is recommended that moderate CON velocity be used.	A
For advanced training, the inclusion of a continuum of velocities from unintentionally slow to fast CON velocities is recommended and should correspond to the intensity.	C
It is recommended that novice individuals train the entire body 2–3 d a week.	A
It is recommended that for progression to intermediate training, a frequency of 3–4 d a week be used (based on how many muscle groups are trained per workout).	B
It is recommended that advanced lifters train 4–6 d a week.	C
Muscle hypertrophy	
It is recommended that CON, ECC, and ISOM muscle actions be included.	A
For novice and intermediate training, it is recommended that moderate loading be used (70%–85% of 1-RM) for 8–12 repetitions per set for 1–3 sets per exercise.	A
For advanced training, it is recommended that a loading range of 70%–100% of 1-RM be used for 1–12 repetitions per set for 3–6 sets per exercise in a periodized manner such that the majority of training is devoted to 6- to 12-RM and less training devoted to 1- to 6-RM loading.	A
It is recommended that single- and multiple-joint free-weight and machine exercises be included in novice, intermediate, and advanced individuals.	A
For exercise sequencing, an order similar to strength training is recommended.	C
It is recommended that 1- to 2-min rest periods be used in novice and intermediate training; for advanced training, length of rest period should correspond to the goals of each exercise such that 2- to 3-min rest periods may be used with heavy loading for core exercises and 1- to 2-min rest periods may be used for other exercises of moderate to moderately high intensity.	C
It is recommended that slow-to-moderate velocities be used by novice and intermediate-trained individuals; for advanced training, it is recommended that slow, moderate, and fast repetition velocities be used depending on the load, repetition number, and goals of the particular exercise.	C
It is recommended that a frequency of 2–3 d a week be used for novice training.	A
For intermediate training, the recommendation is similar for total-body workouts or 4 d a week when using an upper/lower-body split routine.	B
For advanced training, a frequency of 4–6 d a week is recommended.	C
Muscle power	
The use of predominantly multiple-joint exercises performed with sequencing guidelines similar to strength training is recommended for novice, intermediate, and advanced power training.	B

Table 126.2 Summary of Progressive Resistance Training Recommendations From the ACSM Position Stand (53) Each Recommendation is Listed With an A, B, C, or D Indicating the Quality or Quantity of Research Supporting That Statement; A is the Best (*Continued*)

Evidence Statement	Grade
It is recommended that concurrent to a typical strength-training program, a power component is incorporated consisting of 1–3 sets per exercise using light-to-moderate loading (30%–60% of 1-RM for upper body exercises, 0%–60% of 1-RM for lower-body exercises) for 3–6 repetitions, not to failure.	A
Various loading strategies are recommended for advanced training. Heavy loading (85%–100% of 1-RM) is necessary for increasing force, and light-to-moderate loading (30%–60% of 1-RM for upper body exercises, 0%–60% of 1-RM for lower-body exercises) performed at an explosive velocity is necessary for increasing fast force production.	B
A multiple-set (3–6 sets) power program integrated into a strength-training program consisting of 1–6 repetitions in a periodized manner is recommended.	A
Rest periods of at least 2–3 min between sets for core exercises are recommended when intensity is high. For assistance exercises and those of less intensity, a shorter rest interval (1–2 min) is recommended.	D
The recommended frequency for novice power training is similar to strength training (2–3 d a week).	A
For intermediate power training, it is recommended that either a total-body or upper/lower-body split workout be used for a frequency of 3–4 d a week.	C
For advanced power training, a frequency of 4–5 d a week is recommended using predominantly total-body or upper/lower-body split workouts.	C
Local muscular endurance	
It is recommended that unilateral and bilateral multiple- and single-joint exercises be included using various sequencing combinations for novice, intermediate, and advanced local muscular endurance training.	A
For novice and intermediate training, it is recommended that relatively light loads be used (10–15 repetitions) with moderate-to-high volume.	A
For advanced training, it is recommended that various loading strategies be used for multiple sets per exercise (10–25 repetitions or more) in a periodized manner, leading to a higher overall volume using lighter intensities.	C
It is recommended that short rest periods be used for muscular endurance training, *e.g.*, 1–2 min for high-repetition sets (15–20 repetitions or more) and less than 1 min for moderate (10–15 repetitions) sets. For circuit weight training, it is recommended that rest periods correspond to the time needed to get from one exercise station to another.	C
Low frequency (2–3 d a week) is effective in novice individuals when training the entire body.	A
For intermediate training, 3 d a week is recommended for total-body workouts, and 4 d a week is recommended for upper/lower-body split routine workouts.	C
For advanced training, a higher frequency may be used (4–6 d a week) if muscle group split routines are used.	C
It is recommended that intentionally slow velocities be used when a moderate number of repetitions (10–15) are used.	B
If performing a large number of repetitions (15–25 or more), then moderate-to-faster velocities are recommended.	B
Motor performance	
It is recommended that multiple-joint exercises be performed using a combination of heavy and light-to-moderate loading (using fast repetition velocity) with moderate-to-high volume in periodized fashion 4–6 d a week for maximal progression in vertical jumping ability. The inclusion of plyometric training (explosive form of exercise involving various jumps) in combination with resistance training is recommended.	B
It is recommended that the combination of heavy resistance and ballistic resistance exercise (along with sprint and plyometric training) be included for progression in sprinting ability.	B
Older adults	
For further improvements in strength and hypertrophy in older adults, the use of both multiple- and single-joint exercises (free weights and machines), with slow-to-moderate lifting velocity, for 1–3 sets per exercise with 60%–80% of 1-RM for 8–12 repetitions with 1–3 min of rest in between sets for 2–3 d a week, is recommended.	A
Increasing power in healthy older adults includes (a) training to improve muscular strength and (b) the performance of both single- and multiple-joint exercises for 1–3 sets per exercise using light-to-moderate loading (30%–60% of 1-RM) for 6–10 repetitions with high-repetition velocity.	B
Similar recommendations may apply to older adults as to young adults, *e.g.*, low-to-moderate loads performed for moderate-to-high repetitions (10–15 or more), for enhancing muscular endurance.	B

CON, concentric; ECC, eccentric; ISOM, isometric; RM, repetition maximum.
American College of Sports Medicine. American College of Sports Medicine position stand. Progression models in resistance training for healthy adults. *Med Sci Sports Exerc.* 2009;41(3):687–708.

- For further improvements in strength and hypertrophy in older adults, the use of both multiple- and single-joint exercises (free weights and machines), with slow-to-moderate lifting velocity, for 1–3 sets per exercise with 60%–80% of 1-RM for 8–12 repetitions with 1–3 minutes of rest in between sets for 2–3 days a week, is recommended (Table 126.2) (61).
- Other recommendations to increase muscle size and strength in older adults propose a training period of 50–53 weeks, a frequency of 3 sessions per week, a training volume of 2–3 sets per exercise, 7–9 repetitions per set, a training intensity from 51% to 69% of the 1RM, total time under tension of 6 seconds, a rest of 120 seconds between sets and 2.5 seconds between repetition (86).
- Ultimately, individual responses to resistance training vary (87) and may be related to changes in muscle contractility with age (88). Resistance training programs should follow recommendations but be tailored to the individual.

Sex

- Males and females can benefit from resistance training, including improvements in muscle size and strength (89).
- Males and females have similar muscle damage and protein synthesis with resistance training (90–93).
- Physiological differences exist between sexes. Females tend to have a larger proportion of type I fibers, less lean muscle mass, greater body fat percentage, and smaller muscle cross-sectional area compared to males (94–98).
- When participating in the same resistance training program, males have greater absolute increases in hypertrophy and strength than females, but relative gains are similar between sexes for hypertrophy and lower-body strength and greater in females for upper body strength (95).
- Menstrual cycle can affect resistance training adaptations due to changes in estrogen and progesterone. Greater strength gains are achieved with resistance training during the follicular phase, and recovery time is longer during the luteal phase. Therefore, follicular phase resistance training will optimize outcomes in females (98).
- Minimal research has been done on weightlifting in people who are pregnant; however, research in this area shows that resistance training can improve insulin dosage, and rate of insulin injection, and reduce the incidence of macrosomia in those with gestational diabetes mellitus (99).
- There is an age-related accelerated decline in weightlifting performance in females in perimenopausal to menopausal years (45–55 years). The decline in performance with age is similar to males at all other times due to a decrease in androgens and estrogen. Testosterone in females decreases by 15% from pre- to postmenopause, along with a decline in muscle mass and strength (82).
- Resistance training programs are effective in increasing muscle mass in postmenopausal women (100).
- Overall, further research is necessary to determine what specific training parameters should be prescribed on the basis of sex, if any.

Youth

- Resistance training is safe for children and adolescents if properly designed and supervised and the child is able to follow directions (101,102).
- Youth resistance training can improve strength and coordination, confidence in physical abilities, mental health, and well-being, and lead to a more active life into adulthood (103). Resistance training also reduces overuse and acute sports-related injuries by up to 66% (104).
- Initially, the focus should be on developing proper technique and safety using submaximal loads (101).
- The choice of machine-based, free-weight, or functional resistance training should be variable and dependent on goals. Machines may be safer for children and adolescents; however, they may also be inappropriately sized as they are typically designed for adult use, and they have large incremental weight increases. Free weights allow for a full range of motion that allows for more gradual weight increases and are effective in improving strength and agility in youth (101,105).
- Effective training parameters for strength improvements in youth athletes include training periods of more than 23 weeks, 5 sets per exercise, 6–8 repetitions per set, a training intensity of 80%–89% of the 1RM, and 3–4 minutes of rest between sets (105).
- Alternative guidelines for effective resistance training for youth athletes are 1–3 sets of 6–15 repetitions performed 2–3 times per week on nonconsecutive days (106).
- In general, resistance training should focus on a full range of motion, beginning with larger muscle exercises followed by smaller muscle exercises, and weight should be increased gradually. Additionally, varying types of training and programs may help to avoid plateaus and overtraining (101).
- Strength, agility, and sport-specific performance outcomes of resistance training are not different between pre- and post-pubertal athletes, or across ages of children and adolescents. However, girls have greater improvements in sport-specific performance compared to boys (105).

Nutrition

- Higher-volume resistance training sessions may require higher dietary carbohydrate intake to optimize performance (107,108).
- If the training volume is 11 or more sets per muscle group or an athlete has another high-intensity session planned that day for the same musculature, an increase in carbohydrate intake of up to $1.2 \text{ g} \cdot \text{kg}^{-1} \cdot \text{h}^{-1}$ may support training adaptations (108).

- Protein supplementation is related to increased muscle mass and strength during prolonged resistance training postexercise or before sleep (109,110).
- Postexercise whey protein supplementation, and a combination of casein and whey high-protein milk supplementation, may increase abdominal fat loss, fat-free mass, strength, power, and altered serum concentrations of skeletal muscle regulatory markers adaptations in response to resistance training (111,112).
- Although protein supplementation supports training adaptations, higher protein intake does not affect resistance training outcomes or disease biomarkers moreso than moderate protein intake (113).
- Creatine monohydrate supplementation with resistance training results in a greater increase in fat-free mass and strength compared to training alone (114).
- Keto diet may help to decrease fat mass and maintain fat-free mass, but does not support increases in fat-free mass (115).
- A high-protein plant-based diet is similar to a protein-matched mixed diet in increasing muscle strength with resistance training (116).
- Weightlifting athletes use supplementation to enhance training effects, which may or may not include anabolic steroids.
- A reported 76% of male bodybuilders use anabolic steroids and 100% use dietary supplements to increase or preserve muscle mass. Bodybuilders who do not use performance-enhancing drugs, including anabolic steroids, are considered natural bodybuilders (117). Natural bodybuilders are more likely to supplement with creatine monohydrate, and bodybuilders who use performance-enhancing drugs are more likely to supplement with branched-chain and essential amino acids (118).

Disease Processes

- Resistance training can serve as both a preventative measure and an intervention strategy for the development and progression of several diseases. This section reviews a few examples but is not intended as an exhaustive list.

Hypertension

- Resistance training performed according to American College of Sports Medicine (ACSM) guidelines reduces blood pressure in normotensive and hypertensive adults (119).
- Resting systolic and diastolic blood pressures across all blood pressure categories because of progressive resistance training. Although small, these reductions in blood pressure can reduce coronary heart disease by 5%–9%, stroke by 8%–14%, and all-cause mortality by 4% (119).
- Combined and isometric resistance exercise improves arterial stiffness (pulse wave velocity, a vascular health biomarker) in adults with hypertension (120).
- Resistance training and combined training have even been shown to result in postexercise systolic and diastolic hypotension in adults with resistant hypertension (121).
- Dynamic resistance training is proposed for adults with high-normal blood pressure (−3.0 to −4.7 mm Hg systolic and −3.2 to −3.8 mm Hg diastolic). Isometric resistance training is recommended for adults with normal blood pressure but risk of hypertension with an expected reduction in blood pressure of −5.4 to −8.3 mm Hg systolic and −1.9 to −3.1 mm Hg diastolic (122).

Type 2 Diabetes Mellitus

- In individuals with impaired fasting glucose (blood glucose levels of 100–125 mg · dL^{-1}), resistance exercise results in lower fasting blood glucose levels 24 hours after exercise, with greater reductions in response to both volume (multiple- vs. single-set sessions) and intensity of resistance exercise (vigorous compared with moderate). ACSM evidence category C (123).
- A combination of aerobic and resistance exercise training may be more effective in improving blood glucose control than either alone; however, more studies are needed to determine if total caloric expenditure, exercise duration, or exercise mode is responsible. ACSM evidence category B. Milder forms of exercise (*e.g.*, tai chi and yoga) have shown mixed results. ACSM evidence category C (123).
- ACSM and American Diabetes Association (ADA) recommend that, in addition to aerobic training, adults with Type 2 diabetes mellitus should undertake moderate-to-vigorous resistance training at least 2–3 d · wk^{-1}. ACSM evidence category B, ADA B level recommendation (123).
- Medication dosage adjustments to prevent exercise-associated hypoglycemia may be required by individuals using insulin or certain insulin secretagogues. Most other medications prescribed for concomitant health problems do not affect exercise, with the exception of β-blockers, diuretics, and statins. ACSM evidence category C. ADA C level recommendation (123).

Cancer

- Resistance training in adults with cancer should be done in a safe environment with the supervision of experts. It should target hypertrophy, BMD, strength, functional mobility, and body composition to improve quality of life (124).
- ACSM recommendations on resistance training to improve cancer-related fatigue, health-related quality of life, physical function, lymphedema, and bone health (125).
    - Cancer-related fatigue: Resistance only — 2×/week, 2 sets, 12–15 reps for major muscle groups at moderate intensity; combined aerobic and resistance — 3×/week for 30 minutes per session of moderate aerobic exercise plus 2×/week resistance training, 12–15 reps for major muscle groups at moderate intensity.

- Health-related quality of life: Resistance only — 2×/week, 2 sets, 8–15 reps for major muscle groups at moderate-to-vigorous intensity; combined aerobic and resistance — 2–3×/week for 20–30 minutes per session of moderate aerobic exercise plus 2×/week of resistance training, 2 sets, 8–15 reps for major muscle groups at moderate-to-vigorous intensity.
- Physical function: Resistance only — 2–3×/week, 2 sets, 8–12 reps for major muscle groups at moderate-to-vigorous intensity; combined aerobic and resistance — 3×/week for 20–40 minutes of moderate-to-vigorous aerobic exercise plus 2–3×/week of resistance training, 2 sets, 8–12 reps for major muscle groups at moderate-to-vigorous intensity.
- Lymphedema: Resistance only — 2–3×/week of progressive, supervised program for major muscle groups does not exacerbate lymphedema.
- Bone Health: resistance only — 2–3×/week of moderate-to-vigorous resistance training plus high impact training (3–4× bodyweight) for at least 12 months.

- Adults undergoing chemotherapy for breast cancer may improve muscle strength, reduce pain sensitivity, maintain body mass, and maintain cardiorespiratory fitness through participation in combined resistance training and HIIT (126). However, low-volume resistance training may increase muscle strength more than high-volume resistance training regardless of intensity and allow for gradual and personal progression (127).
- Adults with cancer undergoing chemotherapy and/or radiation, and who are survivors of cancer, benefit from exercise intervention to improve strength, fatigue, pain, and insomnia. However, physical symptoms, including nausea/vomiting, loss of appetite, constipation, and diarrhea, may not be influenced by exercise (128,129).
- Finally, advancement in exercise prescription for adults with cancer should include resistance training principles for healthy adults but be modified for the individual and specific limitations relating to their specific diagnosis and treatment (124).

REFERENCES

1. Stricker PR, Faigenbaum AD, McCambridge TM, Council on Sports Medicine and Fitness. Resistance training for children and adolescents. *Pediatrics*. 2020;145(6):e20201011.
2. Westcott WL. Resistance training is medicine: effects of strength training on health. *Curr Sports Med Rep*. 2012;11(4):209–16.
3. Keogh JWL, Winwood PW. The epidemiology of injuries across the weight-training sports. *Sports Med*. 2017;47(3):479–501.
4. Aasa U, Svartholm I, Andersson F, Berglund L. Injuries among weightlifters and powerlifters: a systematic review. *Br J Sports Med*. 2017;51(4):211–19.
5. Klimek C, Ashbeck C, Brook AJ, Durall C. Are injuries more common with CrossFit training than other forms of exercise? *J Sport Rehabil*. 2018;27(3):295–9.
6. Rønnestad BR, Mujika I. Optimizing strength training for running and cycling endurance performance: a review. *Scand J Med Sci Sports*. 2014;24(4):603–12.
7. Muniz-Pardos B, Gomez-Bruton A, Matute-Llorente A, et al. Swim-specific resistance training: a systematic review. *J Strength Cond Res*. 2019;33(10):2875–81.
8. Elkin JL, Kammerman JS, Kunselman AR, Gallo RA. Likelihood of injury and medical care between CrossFit and traditional weightlifting participants. *Orthop J Sports Med*. 2019;7(5):2325967119843348.
9. Lorenz T, Campello M. Biomechanics of skeletal muscle. In: Nordin M, Frankel VH, editors. *Basic Biomechanics of the Musculoskeletal System*. Philadelphia (PA): Lippincott Williams & Wilkins; 2001. p. 148–74.
10. Huxley HE. Fifty years of muscle and the sliding filament hypothesis. *Eur J Biochem*. 2004;271(8):1403–15.
11. MacDougall KB, Devrome AN, Kristensen AM, MacIntosh BR. Force–frequency relationship during fatiguing contractions of rat medial gastrocnemius muscle. *Sci Rep*. 2020;10(1):11575.
12. Duchateau J, Baudry S. Maximal discharge rate of motor units determines the maximal rate of force development during ballistic contractions in human. *Front Hum Neurosci*. 2014;8:234.
13. Garnett R, Stephens JA. Changes in the recruitment threshold of motor units produced by cutaneous stimulation in man. *J Physiol*. 1981;311:463–73.
14. Henneman E. Relation between size of neurons and their susceptibility to discharge. *Science*. 1957;126(3287):1345–7.
15. De Luca CJ, Erim Z. Common drive of motor units in regulation of muscle force. *Trends Neurosci*. 1994;17(7):299–305.
16. De Luca CJ, LeFever RS, McCue MP, Xenakis AP. Behaviour of human motor units in different muscles during linearly varying contractions. *J Physiol*. 1982;329:113–28.
17. De Luca CJ, LeFever RS, McCue MP, Xenakis AP. Control scheme governing concurrently active human motor units during voluntary contractions. *J Physiol*. 1982;329:129–42.
18. De Luca CJ, Hostage EC. Relationship between firing rate and recruitment threshold of motoneurons in voluntary isometric contractions. *J Neurophysiol*. 2010;104(2):1034–46.
19. Medler S. Mixing it up: the biological significance of hybrid skeletal muscle fibers. *J Exp Biol*. 2019;222(pt. 23):jeb200832.
20. Plotkin DL, Roberts MD, Haun CT, Schoenfeld BJ. Muscle fiber type transitions with exercise training: shifting perspectives. *Sports*. 2021;9(9):127.
21. Morales-López JL, Agüera E, Miró F, Diz A. Variations in fibre composition of the gastrocnemius muscle in rats subjected to speed training. *Histol Histopathol*. 1990;5(3):359–64.
22. Adams GR, Hather BM, Baldwin KM, Dudley GA. Skeletal muscle myosin heavy chain composition and resistance training. *J Appl Physiol*. 1993;74(2):911–5.
23. Anderson T, Kearney JT. Effects of three resistance training programs on muscular strength and absolute and relative endurance. *Res Q Exerc Sport*. 1982;53(1):1–7.
24. Ebben WP, Kindler AG, Chirdon KA, Jenkins NC, Polichnowski AJ, Ng AV. The effect of high-load vs. high-repetition training on endurance performance. *J Strength Cond Res*. 2004;18(3):513–7.
25. Liu Y, Cseresnyés Z, Randall WR, Schneider MF. Activity-dependent nuclear translocation and intranuclear distribution of NFATc in adult skeletal muscle fibers. *J Cell Biol*. 2001;155(1):27–39.
26. Gibala MJ, MacDougall JD, Tarnopolsky MA, Stauber WT, Elorriaga A. Changes in human skeletal muscle ultrastructure and force production after acute resistance exercise. *J Appl Physiol*. 1995;78(2):702–8.

27. Hather BM, Tesch PA, Buchanan P, Dudley GA. Influence of eccentric actions on skeletal muscle adaptations to resistance training. *Acta Physiol Scand*. 1991;143(2):177–85.
28. Ebbeling CB, Clarkson PM. Exercise-induced muscle damage and adaptation. *Sports Med*. 1989;7(4):207–34.
29. Higbie EJ, Cureton KJ, Warren GL III, Prior BM. Effects of concentric and eccentric training on muscle strength, cross-sectional area, and neural activation. *J Appl Physiol*. 1996;81(5):2173–81.
30. Sale DG. Neural adaptation to resistance training. *Med Sci Sports Exerc*. 1988;20(5 suppl l):S135–45.
31. Škarabot J, Balshaw TG, Maeo S, et al. Neural adaptations to long-term resistance training: evidence for the confounding effect of muscle size on the interpretation of surface electromyography. *J Appl Physiol*. 2021;131(2):702–15.
32. Pearcey GEP, Alizedah S, Power KE, Button DC. Chronic resistance training: is it time to rethink the time course of neural contributions to strength gain? *Eur J Appl Physiol*. 2021;121(9):2413–22.
33. Enoka RM. Neural adaptations with chronic physical activity. *J Biomech*. 1997;30(5):447–55.
34. Carolan B, Cafarelli E. Adaptations in coactivation after isometric resistance training. *J Appl Physiol*. 1992;73(3):911–17.
35. Häkkinen K, Kallinen M, Izquierdo M, et al. Changes in agonist-antagonist EMG, muscle CSA, and force during strength training in middle-aged and older people. *J Appl Physiol*. 1998;84(4):1341–9.
36. Stefanovic F, Ramanarayanan S, Karkera NU, Mujumdar R, Sivaswaamy Mohana P, Hostler D. Rate of change in longitudinal EMG indicates time course of an individual's neuromuscular adaptation in resistance-based muscle training. *Front Rehabil Sci*. 2022;3:981990.
37. Ohtsuki T. Decrease in human voluntary isometric arm strength induced by simultaneous bilateral exertion. *Behav Brain Res*. 1983;7(2):165–78.
38. Cirer-Sastre R, Beltrán-Garrido JV, Corbi F. Contralateral effects after unilateral strength training: a meta-analysis comparing training loads. *J Sports Sci Med*. 2017;16(2):180–6.
39. McNair PJ, Depledge J, Brettkelly M, Stanley SN. Verbal encouragement: effects on maximum effort voluntary muscle action. *Br J Sports Med*. 1996;30(3):243–5.
40. Yue G, Cole KJ. Strength increases from the motor program: comparison of training with maximal voluntary and imagined muscle contractions. *J Neurophysiol*. 1992;67(5):1114–23.
41. Paravlic AH, Slimani M, Tod D, Marusic U, Milanovic Z, Pisot R. Effects and dose–response relationships of motor imagery practice on strength development in healthy adult populations: a systematic review and meta-analysis. *Sports Med*. 2018;48(5):1165–87.
42. Spiering BA, Clark BC, Schoenfeld BJ, Foulis SA, Pasiakos SM. Maximizing strength: the stimuli and mediators of strength gains and their application to training and rehabilitation. *J Strength Cond Res*. 2023;37(4):919–29. doi:10.1519/JSC.0000000000004390
43. Bouguetoch A, Martin A, Grosprêtre S. Does partial activation of the neuromuscular system induce cross-education training effect? Case of a pilot study on motor imagery and neuromuscular electrical stimulation. *Eur J Appl Physiol*. 2021;121(8):2337–48.
44. Kraemer WJ, Adams K, Cafarelli E, et al. American College of Sports Medicine position stand. Progression models in resistance training for healthy adults. *Med Sci Sports Exerc*. 2002;34(2):364–80.
45. Wathen D, Roll F. Training methods and modes. In: Baechle TR, editor. *Essentials of Strength Training and Conditioning*. Champaign (IL): Human Kinetics; 1994. p. 403–15.
46. Conroy BP, Earle RW. Bone, muscle, and connective tissue adaptations to physical activity. In: Baechle TR, editor. *Essentials of Strength Training and Conditioning*. Champaign (IL): Human Kinetics; 1994. p. 435–46.
47. Narici MV, Hoppeler H, Kayser B, et al. Human quadriceps cross-sectional area, torque and neural activation during 6 months strength training. *Acta Physiol Scand*. 1996;157(2):175–86.
48. Deschenes MR, Kraemer WJ. Performance and physiologic adaptations to resistance training. *Am J Phys Med Rehabil*. 2002;81(11 suppl l):S3–16.
49. Aagaard P, Andersen JL, Dyhre-Poulsen P, et al. A mechanism for increased contractile strength of human pennate muscle in response to strength training: changes in muscle architecture. *J Physiol*. 2001;534(pt. 2):613–23.
50. Franchi MV, Atherton PJ, Maganaris CN, Narici MV. Fascicle length does increase in response to longitudinal resistance training and in a contraction-mode specific manner. *Springerplus*. 2016;5:94.
51. Street SF. Lateral transmission of tension in frog myofibers: a myofibrillar network and transverse cytoskeletal connections are possible transmitters. *J Cell Physiol*. 1983;114(3):346–64.
52. Bloch RJ, Gonzalez-Serratos H. Lateral force transmission across costameres in skeletal muscle. *Exerc Sport Sci Rev*. 2003;31(2):73–8.
53. McCall GE, Byrnes WC, Dickinson A, Pattany PM, Fleck SJ. Muscle fiber hypertrophy, hyperplasia, and capillary density in college men after resistance training. *J Appl Physiol*. 1996;81(5):2004–12.
54. Pallarés JG, Hernández-Belmonte A, Martínez-Cava A, Vetrovsky T, Steffl M, Courel-Ibáñez J. Effects of range of motion on resistance training adaptations: a systematic review and meta-analysis. *Scand J Med Sci Sports*. 2021;31(10):1866–81.
55. Ivey FM, Roth SM, Ferrell RE, et al. Effects of age, gender, and myostatin genotype on the hypertrophic response to heavy resistance strength training. *J Gerontol A Biol Sci Med Sci*. 2000;55(11):M641–8.
56. Kraemer WJ. Strength training basics: designing workouts to meet patients' goals. *Phys Sportsmed*. 2003;31(8):39–45.
57. Stamford B. Weight training basics part 2: a sample program. *Phys Sportmed*. 1998;26(3):91–2.
58. Knight KL. Knee rehabilitation by the daily adjustable progressive resistive exercise technique. *Am J Sports Med*. 1979;7(6):336–7.
59. Knight KL. Quadriceps strengthening with the DAPRE technique: case studies with neurological implications. *Med Sci Sports Exerc*. 1985;17(6):646–50.
60. Baker D, Wilson G, Carlyon R. Periodization: the effect on strength of manipulating volume and intensity. *J Strength Cond Res*. 1994:235–42.
61. American College of Sports Medicine. American College of Sports Medicine position stand. Progression models in resistance training for healthy adults. *Med Sci Sports Exerc*. 2009;41(3):687–708.
62. Ralston GW, Kilgore L, Wyatt FB, Baker JS. The effect of weekly set volume on strength gain: a meta-analysis. *Sports Med*. 2017;47(12):2585–601.
63. Schoenfeld BJ, Ogborn D, Krieger JW. Effects of resistance training frequency on measures of muscle hypertrophy: a systematic review and meta-analysis. *Sports Med*. 2016;46(11):1689–97.
64. Nóbrega SR, Scarpelli MC, Barcelos C, Chaves TS, Libardi CA. Muscle hypertrophy is affected by volume load progression models. *J Strength Cond Res*. 2023;37(1):62–7.
65. Wathen D. Load assignment. In: Baechle TR, editor. *Essentials of Strength Training and Conditioning*. Champaign (IL): Human Kinetics; 1994. p. 435–46.
66. Suchomel TJ, Nimphius S, Bellon CR, Stone MH. The importance of muscular strength: training considerations. *Sports Med*. 2018;48(4):765–85.
67. Brown LE. Nonlinear versus linear periodization models. *J Strength Cond Res*. 2001;23:42–4.

68. Kraemer WJ, Noble BJ, Clark MJ, Culver BW. Physiologic responses to heavy-resistance exercise with very short rest periods. *Int J Sports Med.* 1987;8(4):247–52.
69. Ratamess NA, Falvo MJ, Mangine GT, Hoffman JR, Faigenbaum AD, Kang J. The effect of rest interval length on metabolic responses to the bench press exercise. *Eur J Appl Physiol.* 2007;100(1):1–17.
70. Hannan AL, Hing W, Simas V, et al. High-intensity interval training versus moderate-intensity continuous training within cardiac rehabilitation: a systematic review and meta-analysis. *Open Access J Sports Med.* 2018;9:1–17.
71. Heinrich KM, Spencer V, Fehl N, Poston WSC. Mission essential fitness: comparison of functional circuit training to traditional army physical training for active-duty military. *Mil Med.* 2012;177(10):1125–30.
72. Heinrich KM, Becker C, Carlisle T, et al. High-intensity functional training improves functional movement and body composition among cancer survivors: a pilot study. *Eur J Cancer Care.* 2015;24(6):812–17.
73. Feito Y, Heinrich KM, Butcher SJ, Poston WSC. High-intensity functional training (HIFT): definition and research implications for improved fitness. *Sports.* 2018;6(3):76.
74. Alcaraz PE, Sánchez-Lorente J, Blazevich AJ. Physical performance and cardiovascular responses to an acute bout of heavy resistance circuit training versus traditional strength training. *J Strength Cond Res.* 2008;22(3):667–71.
75. Feito Y, Hoffstetter W, Serafini P, Mangine G. Changes in body composition, bone metabolism, strength, and skill-specific performance resulting from 16-weeks of HIFT. *PLOS One.* 2018;13(6):e0198324.
76. Hespanhol Junior LC, Pena Costa LO, Lopes AD. Previous injuries and some training characteristics predict running-related injuries in recreational runners: a prospective cohort study. *J Physiother.* 2013;59(4):263–9.
77. Wathen D. Exercise selection. In: Baechle TR, editor. *Essentials of Strength Training and Conditioning.* Champaign (IL): Human Kinetics; 1994. p. 416–30.
78. McHugh MP, Cosgrave CH. To stretch or not to stretch: the role of stretching in injury prevention and performance. *Scand J Med Sci Sports.* 2010;20(2):169–81.
79. Dent E, Morley JE, Cruz-Jentoft AJ, et al. International clinical practice guidelines for sarcopenia (ICFSR): screening, diagnosis and management. *J Nutr Health Aging.* 2018;22(10):1148–61.
80. Golshani K, Cinque ME, O'Halloran P, Softness K, Keeling L, Macdonell JR. Upper extremity weightlifting injuries: diagnosis and management. *J Orthop.* 2018;15(1):24–7.
81. Siewe J, Rudat J, Röllinghoff M, Schlegel UJ, Eysel P, Michael JWP. Injuries and overuse syndromes in powerlifting. *Int J Sports Med.* 2011;32(9):703–11.
82. Huebner M, Meltzer DE, Perperoglou A. Age-associated performance decline and sex differences in olympic weightlifting. *Med Sci Sports Exerc.* 2019;51(11):2302–8.
83. Huebner M, Perperoglou A. Sex differences and impact of body mass on performance from childhood to senior athletes in Olympic weightlifting. *PLoS One.* 2020;15(9):e0238369. doi:10.1371/journal.pone.0238369
84. Tøien T, Malmo T, Espedal L, Wang E. Maximal intended velocity enhances strength training-induced neuromuscular stimulation in older adults. *Eur J Appl Physiol.* 2022;122(12):2627–36.
85. Martins AD, Fernandes O, Pereira A, et al. The effects of high-speed resistance training on health outcomes in independent older adults: a systematic review and meta-analysis. *Int J Environ Res Public Health.* 2022;19(9):5390.
86. Borde R, Hortobágyi T, Granacher U. Dose–response relationships of resistance training in healthy old adults: a systematic review and meta-analysis. *Sports Med.* 2015;45(12):1693–720.
87. Karavirta L, Häkkinen K, Kauhanen A, et al. Individual responses to combined endurance and strength training in older adults. *Med Sci Sports Exerc.* 2011;43(3):484–90.
88. Clark LA, Russ DW, Tavoian D, et al. Heterogeneity of the strength response to progressive resistance exercise training in older adults: contributions of muscle contractility. *Exp Gerontol.* 2021;152:111437.
89. Hubal MJ, Gordish-Dressman H, Thompson PD, et al. Variability in muscle size and strength gain after unilateral resistance training. *Med Sci Sports Exerc.* 2005;37(6):964–72.
90. Markofski MM, Volpi E. Protein metabolism in women and men: similarities and disparities. *Curr Opin Clin Nutr Metab Care.* 2011;14(1):93–7.
91. Smith GI, Atherton P, Reeds DN, et al. No major sex differences in muscle protein synthesis rates in the postabsorptive state and during hyperinsulinemia-hyperaminoacidemia in middle-aged adults. *J Appl Physiol.* 2009;107(4):1308–15.
92. West DWD, Burd NA, Churchward-Venne TA, et al. Sex-based comparisons of myofibrillar protein synthesis after resistance exercise in the fed state. *J Appl Physiol.* 2012;112(11):1805–13.
93. Stupka N, Lowther S, Chorneyko K, Bourgeois JM, Hogben C, Tarnopolsky MA. Gender differences in muscle inflammation after eccentric exercise. *J Appl Physiol.* 2000;89(6):2325–32.
94. Roberts BM, Lavin KM, Many GM, et al. Human neuromuscular aging: sex differences revealed at the myocellular level. *Exp Gerontol.* 2018;106:116–24.
95. Roberts BM, Nuckols G, Krieger JW. Sex differences in resistance training: a systematic review and meta-analysis. *J Strength Cond Res.* 2020;34(5):1448–60.
96. Staron RS, Karapondo DL, Kraemer WJ, et al. Skeletal muscle adaptations during early phase of heavy-resistance training in men and women. *J Appl Physiol.* 1994;76(3):1247–55.
97. Simoneau JA, Bouchard C. Human variation in skeletal muscle fiber-type proportion and enzyme activities. *Am J Physiol.* 1989;257(4 pt. 1):E567–72.
98. Kissow J, Jacobsen KJ, Gunnarsson TP, Jessen S, Hostrup M. Effects of follicular and luteal phase-based menstrual cycle resistance training on muscle strength and mass. *Sports Med.* 2022;52(12):2813–19.
99. Yaping X, Huifen Z, Chunhong L, Fengfeng H, Huibin H, Meijing Z. A meta-analysis of the effects of resistance training on blood sugar and pregnancy outcomes. *Midwifery.* 2020;91:102839. doi:10.1016/j.midw.2020.102839
100. Thomas E, Gentile A, Lakicevic N, et al. The effect of resistance training programs on lean body mass in postmenopausal and elderly women: a meta-analysis of observational studies. *Aging Clin Exp Res.* 2021;33(11):2941–52.
101. Dahab KS, McCambridge TM. Strength training in children and adolescents. *Sports Health.* 2009;1(3):223–6.
102. Myer GD, Lloyd RS, Brent JL, Faigenbaum AD. How young is "too young" to start training?. *ACSMs Health Fit J.* 2013;17(5):14–23.
103. Zwolski C, Quatman-Yates C, Paterno MV. Resistance training in youth: laying the foundation for injury prevention and physical literacy. *Sports Health.* 2017;9(5):436–43.
104. Lauersen JB, Bertelsen DM, Andersen LB. The effectiveness of exercise interventions to prevent sports injuries: a systematic review and meta-analysis of randomised controlled trials. *Br J Sports Med.* 2014;48(11):871–7.
105. Lesinski M, Prieske O, Granacher U. Effects and dose–response relationships of resistance training on physical performance in youth athletes: a systematic review and meta-analysis. *Br J Sports Med.* 2016;50(13):781–95.
106. Faigenbaum A, Micheli L. *Youth Strength Training.* Indianapolis: American College of Sports Medicine; 2017.

107. Burke LM, Hawley JA, Wong SHS, Jeukendrup AE. Carbohydrates for training and competition. *J Sports Sci.* 2011;29(suppl 1):S17–27.
108. Henselmans M, Bjørnsen T, Hedderman R, Vårvik FT. The effect of carbohydrate intake on strength and resistance training performance: a systematic review. *Nutrients.* 2022;14(4):856.
109. Cermak NM, Res PT, de Groot LC, Saris WH, van Loon LJ. Protein supplementation augments the adaptive response of skeletal muscle to resistance-type exercise training: a meta-analysis. *Am J Clin Nutr.* 2012;96(6):1454–64.
110. Snijders T, Res PT, Smeets JSJ, et al. Protein ingestion before sleep increases muscle mass and strength gains during prolonged resistance-type exercise training in healthy young men. *J Nutr.* 2015;145(6):1178–84.
111. Hulmi JJ, Laakso M, Mero AA, Häkkinen K, Ahtiainen JP, Peltonen H. The effects of whey protein with or without carbohydrates on resistance training adaptations. *J Int Soc Sports Nutr.* 2015;12:48.
112. Pourabbas M, Bagheri R, Hooshmand Moghadam B, et al. Strategic ingestion of high-protein dairy milk during a resistance training program increases lean mass, strength, and power in trained young males. *Nutrients.* 2021;13(3):948.
113. McKenna CF, Salvador AF, Hughes RL, et al. Higher protein intake during resistance training does not potentiate strength, but modulates gut microbiota, in middle-aged adults: a randomized control trial. *Am J Physiol Endocrinol Metab.* 2021;320(5):E900–13.
114. Bonilla DA, Kreider RB, Petro JL, et al. Creatine enhances the effects of cluster-set resistance training on lower-limb body composition and strength in resistance-trained men: a pilot study. *Nutrients.* 2021;13(7):2303.
115. Vargas-Molina S, Petro JL, Romance R, et al. Effects of a ketogenic diet on body composition and strength in trained women. *J Int Soc Sports Nutr.* 2020;17(1):19.
116. Hevia-Larraín V, Gualano B, Longobardi I, et al. High-protein plant-based diet versus a protein-matched omnivorous diet to support resistance training adaptations: a comparison between habitual vegans and omnivores. *Sports Med.* 2021;51(6):1317–30.
117. Hackett DA, Johnson NA, Chow CM. Training practices and ergogenic aids used by male bodybuilders. *J Strength Cond Res.* 2013;27(6):1609–17.
118. Li J, Davies TB, Hackett DA. Self-reported training and supplementation practices between performance-enhancing drug-user bodybuilders compared with natural bodybuilders. *J Strength Cond Res.* 2023;37(5):1079–88. Published online September 22, 2022.
119. Pescatello LS, Franklin BA, Fagard R, et al. American College of Sports Medicine position stand. Exercise and hypertension. *Med Sci Sports Exerc.* 2004;36(3):533–53.
120. Lopes S, Afreixo V, Teixeira M, et al. Exercise training reduces arterial stiffness in adults with hypertension: a systematic review and meta-analysis. *J Hypertens.* 2021;39(2):214–22.
121. Pires NF, Coelho-Júnior HJ, Gambassi BB, et al. Combined aerobic and resistance exercises evokes longer reductions on ambulatory blood pressure in resistant hypertension: a randomized crossover trial. *Cardiovasc Ther.* 2020;2020:8157858.
122. Hanssen H, Boardman H, Deiseroth A, et al. Personalized exercise prescription in the prevention and treatment of arterial hypertension: a consensus document from the European association of preventive cardiology (EAPC) and the ESC council on hypertension. *Eur J Prev Cardiol.* 2022;29(1):205–15.
123. Colberg SR, Albright AL, Blissmer BJ, et al. Exercise and type 2 diabetes. American College of Sports Medicine and the American Diabetes Association: joint position statement. *Med Sci Sports Exerc.* 2010;42(12):2282–303.
124. Champ CE, Carpenter DJ, Diaz AK, Rosenberg J, Ackerson BG, Hyde PN. Resistance training for patients with cancer: a conceptual framework for maximizing strength, power, functional mobility, and body composition to optimize health and outcomes. *Sports Med.* 2023;53(1):75–89.
125. Campbell KL, Winters-Stone KM, Wiskemann J, et al. Exercise guidelines for cancer survivors: consensus statement from international multidisciplinary roundtable. *Med Sci Sports Exerc.* 2019;51(11):2375–90.
126. Mijwel S, Backman M, Bolam KA, et al. Highly favorable physiological responses to concurrent resistance and high-intensity interval training during chemotherapy: the OptiTrain breast cancer trial. *Breast Cancer Res Treat.* 2018;169(1):93–103.
127. Lopez P, Galvão DA, Taaffe DR, et al. Resistance training in breast cancer patients undergoing primary treatment: a systematic review and meta-regression of exercise dosage. *Breast Cancer.* 2021;28(1):16–24.
128. McGovern A, Mahony N, Mockler D, Fleming N. Efficacy of resistance training during adjuvant chemotherapy and radiation therapy in cancer care: a systematic review and meta-analysis. *Support Care Cancer.* 2022;30(5):3701–19.
129. Nakano J, Hashizume K, Fukushima T, et al. Effects of aerobic and resistance exercises on physical symptoms in cancer patients: a meta-analysis. *Integr Cancer Ther.* 2018;17(4):1048–58.

127 Wrestling

Thomas M. Howard

INTRODUCTION

- Wrestling is a contact sporting event that matches two competitors against each other physically and mentally. The origins of the sport date back to ancient Greek and Roman times circa 500 BC.
- In 2017, it was estimated that in the United States, 1.9 million participants aged 6 and older engage in the sport of wrestling (1).
- As the sport of wrestling has grown in popularity and as participation has increased, it has been noted that there are injuries and conditions that are unique to the sport.

WRESTLING STYLES (2)

- **Greco-Roman:** a style of wrestling that was developed and popularized in Europe.
  - Upper body throws are executed with the goal to touch the opponent's shoulders to the mat simultaneously.
  - Points are awarded for the skill of throwing.
  - At no time are the wrestlers allowed to use their own legs to gain advantage or contact their opponent's legs.
- **Freestyle:** a style used worldwide and in international wrestling meets.
  - This style of wrestling combines the use of the upper body and legs to execute maneuvers.
  - Points are awarded for exposure of the opponent's back to the mat, takedowns, and reversals.
  - Execution of a more difficult takedown with emphasis on exposure of the opponent's back to the mat will increase points awarded.
  - The main objective is to pin the opponent's shoulders to the mat for a 1-second count.
- **High school/collegiate:** This style of wrestling is most commonly seen in the United States.
  - Considered similar to freestyle because of the use of both upper body and legs
  - A major difference is that points are awarded for time advantage.
  - Also, a wrestler must ensure the safe return of their opponent to the mat after a throw or a takedown.
  - Emphasis is placed on pinning the opponent.

DEFINITION OF TERMS (3)

- **Takedown:** Points given to a wrestler when advantage is gained from a neutral position on feet. This may be achieved by a trip or throw. Depending on the style of wrestling, higher point values may be given for the more skillful maneuver to achieve the takedown.
- **Fall:** Also known as a *pin*. Determined by the referee when both shoulders are held to the mat for 1 second. The match is over at this time.
- **Time advantage:** This is popularly called "riding time". Time of control is recorded for both wrestlers and compared. A point is given to the wrestlers if their time is 1 or more minutes greater than their opponent's.
- **Sparring:** An activity participated in when both of the competitors are in a neutral position on their feet. Usually comprises grappling and blocking in an attempt to achieve a takedown.
- **Leg wrestling:** Term used to describe the use of legs while on the mat to attempt to control an opponent.
- **Injury timeout:** Amount of time allowed to a wrestler to attempt to recover from an illness or injury.
  - The time allotted is a maximum of 90 seconds throughout the match. Additionally, a competitor may have two timeouts during the match to tend to injuries as long as 90 seconds of total time is not taken.
- **Bleeding timeout:** Time allowed for the evaluation of a bleeding injury. This is different from an injury timeout. The amount of time is at the referee's discretion. Generally, blood timeout has no time limit, but an excessive bleeding injury may be a cause for disqualification as determined by the referee and athletic trainer or physician.

EPIDEMIOLOGY

- For the 2018–2019 season, the National Collegiate Athletic Association (NCAA) Injury Surveillance System (ISS) data conclude that collegiate wrestling has a relatively high rate of injury at 21.3 per 1000 athlete exposures for competition and 5.3 per 1000 athlete exposures for practice (4).

- Although injuries are common, there seems to be a consensus that most injuries are not serious on the basis of time lost (>7 days) or injuries that require surgery.
- The incidence of injury appears to be highest at the beginning of the season, compared with the latter part of the season.
- Contact with the opponent, as compared to contact with the mat, is the most common mechanism of injury and most injuries occur during takedowns and sparring.
- Comparison of the different weight classes has yielded no statistical difference in injury percentages.
  - However, the annual injury incidence is nearly five times higher among scholastic wrestlers (12–17 y/o), with approximately 30 injuries/1000 wrestlers/year compared to youth wrestlers at approximately 6.5 injuries/1000 wrestlers/year (5).
- The knee is the most commonly injured body part in both practice and competition, followed by the shoulder and ankle. The face and neck are the least injured.
  - Sprains are the most common type of injury both during practice and competition, with fractures being the least common.

MECHANISM OF INJURY (3)

- A direct blow from the mat or body contact may result in a laceration or contusion during a takedown or sparring. Potential serious injury may occur after a fall, especially if a competitor lands on an opponent after attempting a throw or other types of takedowns.
- Friction injuries may result in lacerations or abrasions. This can occur with continuous body contact or contact with the mat. This may later result in skin infections or bursitis.
- Sprains and strains may occur after a wrestler uses twisting or leverage maneuvers to gain advantage over an opponent.
- A competitor may also incur injury to his or her own person while attempting maneuvers.

HEAD INJURIES (2,3)

- Concussions occur with direct contact with a body part or contact with the mat or floor.
  - Concussions may occur with or without loss of consciousness and it is important to evaluate the athlete for any change in behavior or thinking or for physical signs and symptoms.
  - The competitor should be removed from play, evaluated by a trained medical professional who has experience in concussions, and returned to play dependent on the institution's concussion management protocol
  - The evaluation and treatment of concussion is discussed in depth in Chapter 49 of this text
- Lacerations and contusions occur frequently from direct blows from the mat and body parts, such as the head, elbow, and knee.
  - The most common areas are the bony areas around the orbits, zygoma, and scalp. Soft tissues around the mouth and ears are also potential sites of injury.
  - During the match, an injury timeout will be called to evaluate the area.
  - Treatment during the injury timeout may include using wound closure strips to provide temporary closure of the wound.
  - Dressing the wound may also be required at this time.
  - The match can continue as deemed by the referee depending on the severity of the injury.
  - After the match, lacerations should be cleaned and dressed properly.
    - Closure of wounds with heavy nylon sutures is recommended if necessary.
- Epistaxis may occur due to direct trauma to the nose from an opponent or the mat.
  - Blood timeout will be taken to determine the extent of the injury.
  - Direct pressure and ice may be applied to the nares to reduce the hemorrhage and a pledget or nose plug may be inserted to enable the wrestler to continue the match.
  - Several commercially available epistaxis products may also be considered, including those impregnated with hemostatic agents and devices using small balloons to tamponade bleeding. However, these devices are generally not intended for return to immediate sports participation.
  - If the hemorrhage continues even after the above treatments are implemented, then additional medical attention must be sought.
- Nasal fractures with associated epistaxis are treated as above, first to control bleeding, and then the athlete should be evaluated for nasal bone displacement, septal hematoma, and/or any septal deviation before considering return to play.
  - A protective facemask with proper nasal padding may be used to protect the nose from further injury during competition.
  - Maxillofacial injuries are discussed in further depth in Chapter 35 of this text.

EAR INJURIES (6–8)

- Auricular hematomas, also known as *cauliflower ear*, are a common injury for many competitive wrestlers. The advent of wearing properly fitted protective headgear has reduced but not eliminated the incidence of this injury. The pathogenesis of this injury is usually from a direct blow to the soft tissues of the auricle. Fluid collects between the auricular cartilage and the perichondrium, disrupting blood flow to the auricular cartilage.

- Treatment of auricular hematomas requires aspiration or incision and drainage. Without early aspiration, new auricular cartilage will form that is tightly encased. This can cause discomfort and eventual disfigurement. Compressive dressings are usually applied after aspiration. These dressings are worn for a period of 3–5 days before re-evaluation. Return to play is individualized based on pain and a discussion of the risks/benefits of continuing competition with possible fluid reaccumulating.
  - One technique described involves suturing the pressure dressing to the auricle with a resultant return to play in 24 hours with a low incidence of complications (6). This technique involves suturing dental roll on both sides of the pinna with 1.0 nonabsorbable suture.
  - A second technique involves aspiration followed by a collodion pressure dressing in the antihelix and an Ace wrap to ensure uniform pressure in the area of the hematoma (7). The athlete is then re-evaluated in 3–5 days. Earlier return to play is preceded by a careful discussion of risks and benefits.
  - A dry aspiration represents an organization of the hematoma and the early stages of formation of neocartilage consistent with cauliflower ear. Long-term management (otoplasty) is generally deferred until the completion of the wrestling season.

NECK AND BACK INJURIES (3)

- Neck injuries usually occur during takedowns, especially throws, or when a wrestler is diving for the opponent's legs and the head is the first part of the body that strikes the mat. This may cause injuries such as strains/sprains, stingers, disc injuries, degenerative joint disease, and even fractures or spinal cord injuries.
- The etiology of neck injuries is most commonly from hyperextension.
- A stinger is a neck injury in which the participant has transient burning or shooting pain or paresthesia in an arm directly related to neck or shoulder trauma. This may be from traction on the brachial plexus or from cervical nerve root impingement. Wrestling is second only to football in regard to stinger injuries.
- If a cervical fracture or spinal cord injury is suspected, then prompt medical attention should be sought.
- Acute back strains occur most often during takedowns and throws. Mechanisms that may lead to back injury include torsional movements, exertion against resistance, and hyperextension while in the standing position or hyperflexion while on the mat with an opponent.
- Chronic or recurrent back pain is not unusual in wrestlers and may include spondylolysis, spondylolisthesis, or sacroiliac dysfunction.
- Neck and back injuries are discussed further in Chapters 49 and 50 of this text.

CHEST INJURIES (3)

- Chest wall injuries may occur in a variety of ways including direct blows, compression, and exertion against resistance, and strains from torsion or twisting movements.
  - These mechanisms may cause rib contusions/fractures, costochondral separations, and abdominal wall strains.
  - Competitors often present with pain on breathing and moving or point tenderness.
  - If a rib fracture is suspected, evaluation should proceed to consider the possibility of a hemothorax or pneumothorax. Prompt medical attention must be sought if this is suspected including imaging with radiographs, ultrasound, or cross-sectional imaging.
  - Once severe intrathoracic injury has been excluded, musculoskeletal injuries may be treated with rest and analgesics including anti-inflammatory medications. Topical agents such as lidocaine patches may also be beneficial. Some clinicians consider local steroid injections to be beneficial as well though there is scant evidence to conclusively support their use in this setting.
  - Taping or padding of ribs may be instituted for comfort during training or competition once the initial symptoms have been treated, though caution should be used to ensure that athletes are using spirometry or other techniques to ensure deep breathing throughout the day.

SHOULDER AND ELBOW INJURIES

- Shoulder injuries comprise approximately 14% of all injuries and rank second to knee injuries (4).
- These injuries include acromioclavicular strain, shoulder dislocation, shoulder subluxation, and sternoclavicular strain.
  - Shoulder instability is also common in wrestlers.
- Shoulder injuries are described in depth in Chapters 51–54 of this text.
- The elbow may be injured when an outstretched arm contacts the mat in an attempt to break a fall. The elbow at this time will be hyperextended, leading to ligamentous injury or even possible dislocation or fracture.
- Olecranon bursitis is also common and results from direct trauma.
- Elbow injuries are described in depth in Chapters 56–58 of this text.

EXTREMITY INJURIES (4)

- Extremity injuries include injuries to fingers, thumbs, hands, and elbows.
- Of these, injuries to fingers are relatively common in wrestlers, including finger proximal interphalangeal dislocations or sprains and subluxation.
  - Sprains may be taped to the adjacent finger to allow use during competition.
  - Dislocations often needed splinted and padded to be functional.
  - Thumb injuries may be much more disabling.
    - Forceful adduction of the thumb during takedowns may damage the ulnar collateral ligament resulting in a *gamekeeper's thumb*.
    - The competitor may not have the grasp strength to be effective against an opponent.
    - Patient will need to be evaluated for possible thumb spica casting and may even need surgery.
- Hand and finger injuries are discussed further in Chapters 59 and 60 of this text.

KNEE INJURIES (4,5)

- The most common body part injured, knee injuries composed 21% of all injuries in a recent study. The most common of these injuries are strains/sprains, and meniscal/cruciate tears, as well as fractures, subluxation, and bursitis.
  - Collateral ligament injury is the most common type of injury, accounting for over 30% of knee injuries.
  - Cruciate ligament injury conversely is much less common (approximately 5%).
- Takedowns and leg wrestling are the most common etiologies of knee ligament damage.
- The lead leg used for defense and initiating takedowns is the most vulnerable knee.
- Wrestlers tend to have a predilection to injure the lateral meniscus or to have isolated lateral/medial collateral sprains as compared to other sports. Etiologies such as overuse, torsion, hyperextension, and shearing all have additive effects toward injury.
- Prepatellar bursitis is a common injury because of time spent on the knees while wrestling on the mat or performing takedowns.
- Knee injuries are described in depth in Chapters 63–66 of this text.

SKIN INFECTIONS (2–4)

- Skin infections are conditions that are rather unique to the sport of competitive wrestling and may be due to various bacteria, viruses, and fungi.
  - Modes of transmission include person-to-person contact on exposed skin, especially abraded skin, and contact with poorly disinfected wrestling mats or equipment.
  - According to recent NCAA ISS reports, skin infections are associated with at least 17% of the time-loss injuries in wrestling (4).
- All participating competitors are subject to entire body examinations at the time of weigh-in that should include the hair on the scalp and in the pubic area.
  - If an abraded area or an infectious skin condition cannot be adequately protected, the participant can be medically disqualified. Adequately protected is deemed where skin conditions are diagnosed as noninfectious and treated as per guidelines stipulated by a governing body such as the NCAA and are able to be covered with a bandage that will withstand the competition
- Documentation of a competitor's condition will be made available with diagnosis, culture results, and current medical therapy. The decision of the physician or athletic trainer is considered final.
- Bacterial infections of the skin include folliculitis, impetigo, furuncle/carbuncle, cellulitis, erysipelas, staphylococcal disease, hidradenitis suppurativa, and community-acquired methicillin-resistant *Staphylococcus aureus* (MRSA).
  - Competitors **must not have any new bacterial skin lesions for at least 48 hours** prior to medical examination.
  - **No moist or draining lesions at the time of the match** are allowed and **72 hours of antibiotic therapy must be completed** prior to an athlete being cleared to compete.
- *Pediculosis*- and scabies-infected participants must have been treated with the proper medication and examined before being allowed to participate in any competition
- Viral infections include herpes *gladiatorum*, herpes *zoster*, molluscum *contagiosum*, and *verruca*.
  - *Herpes gladiatorum* has received much attention because of the contagiousness with close skin-to-skin contact and the potential for morbidity.
    - Wrestlers must be free of systemic illness at the time of competition.
    - Competitors **must have been treated for at least 120 hours**, with proper antiviral therapy before and at the time of the event.
    - **No new active blisters or lesions may develop within 72 hours of the medical examination** and **dry lesions must be covered with an impermeable bandage.**
    - It is recommended that wrestlers with a history of recurrent herpes gladiatorum or labials be on prophylactic antiviral therapy after consultation with a team of physicians (9).
  - *Herpes zoster* infections must have crusted over lesions, and the patient cannot be systemically ill at the time of the competition.

- *Molluscum* lesions must be removed by the time of the competition.
  - **Localized lesions may be covered with a permeable membrane** followed by stretch tape.
- Verrucae-infected wrestlers are allowed to compete under the following conditions:
  - Lesions on the face must be adequately covered by a mask.
  - Solitary lesions on the face must be removed before the match to allow participation.
  - Verrucae on the hands must be covered.

- Fungal infections such as tinea have also come under scrutiny because of their high mode of transmission.
- *Tinea corporis:* **A minimum of 72 hours of topical fungicidal medication**, such as clotrimazole
- *Tinea capitis* infections must be treated with **a minimum of 2 weeks of systemic antifungal therapy.**
  - Treated lesions may be examined with a KOH preparation at the discretion of the examining provider.
  - Lesions should be washed with a fungal shampoo followed by an antifungal cream before being covered with a gas-permeable dressing and stretch tape.
  - A competitor will be disqualified if the lesion cannot be covered adequately.
- There is controversy about the spread of infection among teams during outbreaks.
  - Stanforth et al. reported on the prevalence of positive MRSA surface cultures in training rooms and wrestling facilities and suggested that teams with recurrent or widespread infections should thoroughly evaluate procedures for mat maintenance in cleaning and disqualifications of infectious wrestlers (10).
  - Anderson reported on the Minnesota experience of a herpes gladiatorum outbreak in 2007 favoring more aggressive management of cases and restriction of infected athletes as more important (9).
  - It is clear that properly cleaned facilities and identification and restriction of infected athletes are important.
- Dermatologic conditions are discussed further in Chapter 32 of this text.

WEIGHING IN (2,3)

- Competitors are placed into separate categories based on their body weight called weight classes. These are predetermined in advance by the governing body for the league/organization.
  - Currently, the NCAA guidelines have 10 weight classes ranging from 125 lb to heavyweight (183–235 lb)
  - US high-school participants compete in 14 different weight classes ranging from 103 to 275 lb.
  - At the beginning of the season, each wrestler is weighed, and a minimum weight for the competitor is established. Wrestlers are encouraged to lose weight slowly not losing more than 1.5% body weight in a 7-day period and a competitor must certify by November 1st in a weight class.
  - This examination is performed by a physician or certified athletic trainer and the minimum wrestling weight is established by a comparison of several different factors including skinfold measurements of triceps, subscapular areas, and abdomen which are measured to calculate the body fat percentage.
  - From this examination, wrestlers are certified for a minimal weight class they may wrestle for the season. They may compete at this weight class or in a higher weight class if desired.
  - At no time after this is a competitor allowed to wrestle at a weight class below the certified weight.
- During the season, wrestlers may attempt to use many methods to lose weight to make their respective weight classes.
  - These include vigorous exercise before weigh-in to lose water weight, use of saunas and plastic garments and self-imposed dehydration and fasting, and some athletes may even use weight-loss pills or diuretics. However, due to the risks they pose to athlete health and safety, all of these methods are forbidden!
    - The acute effects of these methods may be loss of strength and stamina, hypovolemia, heat exhaustion or heat stroke, and electrolyte imbalances.
  - The temperature of the practice room can be no higher than 80 degrees Fahrenheit.
- It is important for coaches, trainers, and physicians to properly educate the competitors on the dangers of rapid weight loss. Adequate counseling on nutrition and emphasis on conditioning during the season is paramount.
  - Long-term effects of continued rapid weight loss with weight gain include the following: chronically compromised cardiac and renal blood flow, neuropsychiatric disorders, such as depression, and anxiety, and disordered eating behaviors such as bulimia and anorexia nervosa may become prevalent.
    - Other sequelae may include decreased growth and maturation, especially in younger wrestlers.
  - The NCAA attempts to dissuade competitors from the practice of rapid weight loss and gain by decreasing the time between weighing in and the actual match.
  - By NCAA rules, competitors must weigh in no more than an hour before dual, triangular, and quadrangular matches.
  - In multiteam tournaments, wrestlers must be weighed no more than 2 hours before the first match.

REFERENCES

1. The Outdoor Foundation. *Outdoor Participation Report*. Washington (DC): The Outdoor Foundation; 2018.
2. Kiningham R. Wrestling. In: Madden CC, Putukian M, Mccarty E, Young C, editors. *Netter's Sports Medicine*. 3rd ed. Philadelphia (PA): Elsevier; 2023.
3. National Collegiate Athletic Association. 2021–22 *and* 2022–23 *Wrestling Rules*. Indianapolis, IA: National Collegiate Athletic Association; 2021.
4. Powell JR, Boltz AJ, Robison HJ, Morris SN, Collins CL, Chandran A. Epidemiology of injuries in National Collegiate Athletic Association men's wrestling: 2014–2015 through 2018–2019. *J Athl Train*. 2021 Jul 1;56(7):727–33.
5. Myers RJ, Linakis SW, Mello MJ, Linakis JG. Competitive wrestling-related injuries in school aged athletes in U.S. Emergency Departments. *West J Emerg Med*. 2010 Dec;11(5):442–9.
6. Schuller DE, Dankle SD, Strauss RH. A technique to treat wrestlers' auricular hematoma without interrupting training or competition. *Arch Otolaryngol Head Neck Surg*. 1989 Feb;115(2):202–6.
7. Brickman K, Adams DZ, Akpunonu P, Adams SS, Zohn SF, Guinness M. Acute management of auricular hematoma: a novel approach and retrospective review. *Clin J Sport Med*. 2013 Jul;23(4):321–3.
8. Krogmann RJ, Jamal Z, King KC. Auricular hematoma. In: *StatPearls* [Internet]. Treasure Island (FL): StatPearls Publishing; 2023 Jan. Available from: https://www.ncbi.nlm.nih.gov/books/NBK531499/
9. Anderson BJ. Managing herpes gladiatorum outbreaks in competitive wrestling: the 2007 Minnesota experience. *Curr Sports Med Rep*. 2008;7(6):323–7.
10. Stanforth B, Krause A, Starkey C, Ryan TJ. Prevalence of community-associated methicillin-resistant *Staphylococcus aureus* in high school wrestling environments. *J Environ Health*. 2010;72(6):12–6.

SECTION VII

Special Populations

The Pediatric Athlete

128

Thomas Swaffield, Christina Master, and Terry Adirim

EPIDEMIOLOGY

- According to the National Council of Youth Sports, 60 million children and adolescents are registered to participate in organized sports programs (1).
- In 2020, 54.1% of children aged 6–17 years participated in sports during the past 12 months (2).
- Non-Hispanic White children (60.4%) were more likely to have participated in sports compared with non-Hispanic Black (42.1%), Hispanic (46.9%), and non-Hispanic Asian (51.4%) children (2).
- More than 3.5 million kids under age 14 receive medical treatment for sports injuries each year with an estimated 2 million injuries, 500,000 doctor visits, and 30,000 hospitalizations each year in high school athletes (3).
- Twenty-five to thirty percent of these injuries occur during participation in organized sports and 40% occur in unorganized sports (4).
- Early sports specialization may be associated with increased risk of injuries and burnout (4,5).
- Musculoskeletal injuries are the most common injuries in youth sports (6).
- Growth and development of complex motor skills during childhood and adolescence are risk factors for injuries sustained in youth sports and recreation (7,8).

GENERAL CONSIDERATIONS

Growth, Development, and Sports Participation

- Neurodevelopment maturation is a complex, continuous process, encompassing multiple domains: physical, neuromotor, cognitive, perceptual-motor, language, visual, auditory, and psychological (see Table 128.1).
- Important factors to consider for sports participation and readiness in the youth athletes include attention to their neurodevelopment levels and adaptive abilities to meet the demands of a specific sport (9). Notably:
  - Social comparison is developed by age 6.
  - The competitive nature of sport is not understood till age 9.
  - Most children are mature enough to participate in most sports by 12.
- Currently, there is no evidence that enables the prediction of future athletic performance, and there is no firm guidance as to when to determine when a child is ready for sport... common sense should guide decisions (9).
- Regular physical activity does not appear to have any adverse effects on growth. In addition, appropriately designed resistance training programs do not appear to have a negative effect on physeal health, growth, or cardiovascular health in the youth athlete (10).
- The American Academy of Pediatrics (AAP) recommends rest from competitive sports, sport-specific training, and practice by taking 1–2 days off per week. This allows for physical and psychological recovery. The AAP also emphasizes the importance for appropriate fluid and caloric intake to optimize energy availability for recovery and growth (10).

Preseason Medical Evaluation

- The preparticipation physical examination is considered best practice in the care of the athletes, as it may prevent injury by identifying medical conditions that can be exacerbated by sports participation and musculoskeletal issues that can be addressed and rehabilitated before sports participation. It also provides information that can be used in a shared-decision-making process with the athlete and family regarding risk in sport (11).
- The primary objectives for this evaluation include the detection of conditions that may be life-threatening or disabling, or that predispose to injury. In addition, the identification of musculoskeletal problems requiring rehabilitation prior to participation is a priority. This examination also meets both legal and insurance requirements for participation in youth sports.
- Other important objectives include review of general health, including psychological health, counseling on health-related issues, and assessment of fitness level for specific sports, and identifying any issues requiring medical follow-up (2).
- Ideally, this evaluation should be conducted within the context of the medical home where the athlete's previous medical history is well-known and documented, enabling continuity of care in follow-up.

Table 128.1 Pediatric Developmental Milestones

	Skills Attainment	
	Cognitive	**Motor**
Toddler 9–30 mo	• Receptive understanding. • First words. • Follows commands. • Follows more than one command. • Begins to attend briefly.	• Stands without support. • Can walk sideways. • Jump from last stair to floor. • Walk upstairs alternating a forward foot. • Run, jump in place, and throw a large ball overhead.
Preschool 24–36 mo 4 yr	• Speaks in sentences. • Parallel play. • Concrete thinking. • Can remember basic information, count to 10, name colors, understand similarities and differences. • Focuses on own performance.	• Full arm swing. • Hop up to three times. • Throw a ball with forearm extension. • Catches a ball with fixed outstretched arm. • Can stand on one foot for up to 5 s. • Broad jump about 1 foot. • Hop up to six times, skip on one foot. • Climb a jungle gym. • Catch a ball (direct and bounced). • Throws overhand. • Kick a ball forward and agilely move backward and forward.
Early Middle Years 5 yr 6 yr	• Increase in expressive language. • Doubling of words. • Still does not fully understand coordinated team efforts leading to swarming behavior in team sports. • Increasing intelligibility and increasing sentence length, use of future tense.	• Runs well. • One-foot skip, hop on one foot up to nine times. • Catch a ball with both hands. • Can somersault. • Age 6 and younger, still naturally farsighted, and this may lead to limited ability in tracking objects and judging speed of moving objects. • Most can hit a target with a small ball, ride a bicycle, jump up to 1 foot, and broad jump up to 3 feets.
Middle Years 7–10 yr	• Most can begin to participate in team sports. • More mature comprehension of instructions. • Alert to events in the sports environment. • Analytic thinking, *e.g.*, can learn and play by rules, knows right from wrong. • Longer attention spans, but still easily distracted. • Developing sense of confidence, can give complex directions to others. • Begins to compare their performance with others.	• Most can ride a bicycle, pitch, and bat • Improved manual dexterity and motor planning. • Can learn soccer and baseball. • Can integrate sensory and motor input to estimate time of arrival of a ball so for example can catch a fly ball, hit a tennis ball.

Data from Patel DR, Soares N, Wells K. Neurodevelopmental readiness of children for participation in sports. *Transl Pediatr.* 2017;6(3):167–73.

- There is currently not sufficient evidence to warrant across-the-board preparticipation screening with electrocardiograms to prevent sudden cardiac death (12–14).
- Universal preinjury baseline testing for concussions is also not currently indicated based on the evidence (15).
- The preparticipation physical evaluation is further detailed in Chapter 18.

Strength Training

- Strength training for children and adolescents, when properly supervised, is considered safe and efficacious (10).
- Strength training is often recommended to improve physical literacy, injury rehabilitation, injury prevention, general health and fitness (10).
- Studies have shown that when properly structured, strength training can increase strength in preadolescents and adolescents with an emphasis on technique and adequate supervision (10).
- Childhood strength gains are primarily attributed to increase in motor neuron recruitment without muscle hypertrophy (10).
- "Training age" and "resistance training skill competency" (RTSC) are new concepts that aid in the design of resistance training programs for youth. Training age refers to the time spent in formalized training. RTSC refers to the amount of weight lifted, quality of the movement, and emotional maturity of the athlete. Understanding these concepts allows for the formation of developmentally appropriate training regimens (Table 128.2) (10).

Relative Energy Deficiency in Sport

- Relative Energy Deficiency in Sport (RED-S) terminology was introduced in 2014 and refers to how energy imbalance can lead to abnormal physiological function of organ systems (16).
- RED-S refers to impaired function of metabolism, menstrual cycle, bone mineral density, immunity, protein synthesis, and cardiovascular health.

Table 128.2 Pediatric Strength Training Guidelines

	American Academy of Pediatrics Recommendations for Youth Resistance Training
Topic	**Recommendation**
Youth with specific past medical history	Obtain consultation prior to initiating resistance training program for youth with uncontrolled hypertension, uncontrolled seizure disorders, cardiovascular conditions, or history of treatment with an anthracycline chemotherapeutic agent.
Youth with congenital cardiac disease	Obtain pediatric cardiology consultation prior to initiating resistance training program for youth with complex congenital cardiac disease.
Comprehensive fitness program	Integrate aerobic and resistance training with other skill-related fitness into a developmentally appropriate exercise training program.
Youth with obesity	Start with basic body weight resistance exercises in the context of a more aerobically based program, with the goal to encourage successful physical activity in the short and long terms.
Warm-up and cool down	Include dynamic warm-up exercises and cool down with less intense static stretching
Nutrition	Ensure adequate hydration and nutrition to optimize performance, recovery, and growth.
Resistance training skill competency (RTSC)	Assess RTSC and provide feedback on exercise technique to minimize risk and maximize benefit from resistance training. RTSC focuses on starting with minimal load and advancing as technique improves. RTSC should also consider training age and emotional maturity of the youth athlete.
Comprehensive resistance training program	All muscle groups of the upper body, lower body, and core should be included in the exercise program. Multijoint activities, such as squats and weightlifting exercises, are encouraged. Adding sport-specific exercises may complement the basic exercises.
Reduce overuse injuries	Account for time spent in resistance training as part of the total training program. This includes time spent in resistance training at school and community-based programs as part of the total training volume.
Evaluate for overuse injuries	Assess any symptom of illness or sign of injury or overuse from resistance training or sport before allowing youth to resume training.
Supervision	Incorporate weightlifting exercises into a resistance training program under the direction of a qualified professional. Progress in weight lifted as RTSC improves.
Performance enhancing substances	Educate youth about the risks involved with performance enhancing substances to discourage the use of such substances.
Resistance training program safety	Increase safety of youth resistance training programs by using professionals who are qualified, trained, and aware of the unique aspects of youth athletes. Licensed physical education teachers, certified fitness professionals, high school coaches, and strength and conditioning specialists may serve this role.
Technique and supervision	Any resistance training program involving children and adolescents should involve supervision by a qualified professional and emphasize proper technique.

Data from Stricker PR, Faigenbaum AD, McCambridge TM. Resistance training for children and adolescents. *Pediatrics*. 2020;145(6):e20201011. doi:10.1542/peds.2020-1011

- The medical complications observed in RED-S are a result of low energy availability. Energy availability is defined as dietary energy intake minus exercise energy expenditure divided by fat-free mass (17).
- RED-S is thought to be highly prevalent in athletes, although underreported due to difficulties in diagnosis. Estimated prevalence in low energy availability ranges from 14% to 63% (18). Data suggests that the prevalence of low energy availability in females across different sports is 44.8% in gymnastics, 33.3% in soccer, 22% in ballet dances, and 20% in volleyball players (18).
- Bone mineral density (BMD) declines as the number of missed menstrual cycles accumulates, and the loss of BMD may not be fully reversible. Stress fractures occur more commonly in physically active women with menstrual irregularities and/or low BMD, with a relative risk for stress fracture (16).
- Screening for RED-S can be challenging because its health consequences are not always readily apparent. Optimal screening times for RED-S occur at the preparticipation physical exam and annual health checkups (16).
- RED-S is further explained in Chapter 12, Nutrition, and Chapter 131, The Female Athlete.

Pain Management in the Pediatric Athlete

- Pain in the youth athlete can be influenced by several factors. While injuries can produce pain, pain response can be affected by optimism, catastrophizing, family dynamics, coaches, and peers (19).
- Acute pain is typically a nociceptive (pain from damage to nonneural tissue resulting in inflammation) or neuropathic (pain from injury to the peripheral nervous system) type of pain. Acute pain generally is limited and lasts for 6 weeks or less.
- Chronic pain is when pain persists beyond the typical course of an acute disease. It is considered to be pain that persists for more than 12 weeks and tends to involve nociplastic type of

pain (pain from altered nociception in the absence of tissue damage).

- Treatments for acute pain in youth athletes should initially focus on nonpharmacologic modalities. These may include protection, rest, ice, and compression. A gentle range of motion exercises can also help begin rehabilitation. Nonsteroidal anti-inflammatory drugs (NSAIDs) can be used as needed if pain is persistent and should be prescribed at the lowest effective dose for the shortest period of time. In youth athletes, dosing for pain medication regimens is based on weight and age. NSAIDs, in addition to acetaminophen, have been shown to be more effective for pain control than either alone. Opioid medications should be avoided in youth athletes; however, if pain persists despite the above recommendations, a 3-day prescription of a short acting opioid should be sufficient for most injuries (19).
- Treatments for chronic pain follow similar guidelines as acute pain, with the addition element of considering psychosocial modalities, such as cognitive behavioral therapy (19).

SPORT-RELATED CONCUSSION IN THE PEDIATRIC ATHLETE

Concussion Incidence

- Based on the 2019 Youth Risk Behavior Survey, a nationally representative sample of youth in the United States, an estimated 18% of middle school students and 14% of high school students reported one or more concussions in the previous year (20).
- From the National Health Interview Survey in 2020, 6.8% of children 17 years and younger had ever had symptoms of a concussion, and 3.9% had ever been diagnosed with a concussion by a healthcare provider, with boys (4.7%) and non-Hispanic White children (5.2%) more likely to have ever had a diagnosis of concussion (21).
- From the Adolescent Brain Cognitive Development Study of over 11,000 9- and 10-year-olds, 1.1% sustained a concussion during a 1-year follow-up period. A previous history of concussion was associated with 5.5 greater odds sustaining another concussion (22).

Concussion Management and Return to Play

- The current international guidelines for sport concussion management are reflected in the consensus statement of the Fifth International Conference on Concussion in Sport, held in Berlin, Germany in October 2017 (15).
- Any pediatric athlete suspected of having suffered a concussion should be immediately removed from that game or activity with no return to that activity that same day (15).
- Removal from play as soon as a concussion is suspected results in faster recovery compared to continuing to play with a concussion, even without another brain injury (23,24).
- There is evidence that 24–48 hours of relative rest or activity modification to give the brain the opportunity to recover is warranted. Limiting screen time during the first 48 hours results in quicker symptom recovery (25). The optimal time frame for returning to light symptom-limited aerobic physical activity (26,27) and school (28) with accommodations appears to be approximately 48 hours after injury (29). There does not appear to be benefit to prolonged physical or cognitive rest.
- For students, returning to learning should include accommodations for cognitive, visual, and executive function deficits, which may include reduced workload, breaks as needed for symptoms, extra time for assignments, no testing initially, with a gradual return to full school workload (30,31).
- Concussion symptoms are myriad and may be classified as somatic (headache, pressure in head, neck pain, nausea, vomiting, sensitivity to light, and sensitivity to noise), visio-vestibular (vision problems, hearing problems/ringing, balance problems, or dizziness), cognitive (do not feel right, confusion, feeling like in a fog, difficulty concentrating, difficulty remembering), sleep-related (feeling slowed down, drowsiness, fatigue/low energy, trouble falling asleep), and emotional (more emotional than usual, irritable, sadness, nervous/anxious) (32–34).
- Vision and vestibular deficits are common after concussion in children and should be assessed for with a visio-vestibular examination (35). These deficits can impact a child's ability to return to learning and activities and should be accounted for in academic accommodations (36).
- A return-to-play process is used to return athletes back to sports, including contact and collision sports, advancing from initial 48 hours of modified cognitive and physical activity through stages including light aerobic exercise then sport-specific exercise followed by noncontact training drills (15). Each step should take 24 hours, but it may take more if concussion symptom provocation occurs. In all 50 states in the United States, there are state laws mandating that children be evaluated by a clinician experienced in concussion diagnosis and management and determined to be clinically recovered before being cleared to advance to full-contact practice and, finally, full return to game play (37,38).
- There are currently no blood tests approved for use to support the diagnosis of concussion in children. The diagnosis of concussion remains clinical in nature, based on subjective patient-reported symptoms on standardized concussion symptom scales and supported by clinical examination, including visio-vestibular assessment (39). Additional tools, including computerized neurocognitive testing and/or the King-Devick test, a rapid-number naming test, may be used to support the diagnosis of concussion, but are not essential. Preinjury baseline testing is currently not indicated (15) nor a practical use of limited resources in youth sports.
- Most children will recover from a concussion within a month after injury, but up to 30% of children may have persisting symptoms beyond this time frame (40). Risk factors

for concussion symptoms persisting longer than 28 days included female sex, age 13 years or older, migraine history, prior concussion with symptoms lasting longer than 1 week, headache, sensitivity to noise, fatigue, answering questions slowly, and four or more errors on the Balance Error Scoring system tandem stance (40).

- For children with persisting concussion symptoms beyond 28 days, additional rehabilitative interventions may be useful, with emerging evidence to support active rehabilitative aerobic (41), vestibular (42,43), and vision (44–46) interventions.
- Mood and emotional dysregulation, including anxiety, depression, and even suicidality (47–50), may occur after concussion and should be screened for during any assessment for concussion, with appropriate referrals for further support.
- Primary prevention of concussion is primarily achieved through policy and rule changes in sport with the goal of protecting young athletes (51–53). There is currently conflicting evidence as to the utility of protective headgear in sports such as soccer and girls' lacrosse to mitigate the risk of concussion (54,55) and are currently not universally recommended.
- There is no consensus regarding when a youth athlete with a history of multiple concussions should be restricted from further participation in contact sports. Since our understanding of the longterm sequelae of repeat concussions and repetitive head impact exposure is still evolving, the approach to this difficult clinical scenario requires the utmost care. A conservative approach with shared-decision-making is appropriate, and decisions should be made on an individual basis (56–58).

FRACTURES IN THE PEDIATRIC ATHLETE

Physeal Fractures

- The physis is the weakest structure in the growing skeleton, making it more susceptible to injury than the surrounding muscles, tendons, and ligaments.

Salter-Harris Classification

- The Salter-Harris classification is the most widely used method of describing physeal fractures (59):
  - Type I: Through the physis, resulting in separation of the epiphysis from the metaphysis.
  - Type II: Through the physis and metaphysis. The separate metaphyseal fragment is known as the Thurston-Holland fragment.
  - Type III: Through the physis and epiphysis, involving the articular surface.
  - Type IV: Through the metaphysis, across the physis, through the epiphysis, and involving the articular surface.
  - Type V: Crush injury to the physis as a result of compression injuries.
- Type I fractures have the best prognosis, with minimal risk for growth arrest. These are more common in younger patients.
- This is the most common type of Salter-Harris fracture. In Type II fractures, growth arrest may occur, especially at specific sites, such as the distal femoral physis.
- In Type III fractures, growth arrest is rare, but since the joint surface is involved, anatomic reduction must be maintained to ensure articular cartilage congruity and prevent future joint degeneration.
- In Type IV fractures, there is concern for both growth arrest and articular cartilage congruity. As a complication, a longitudinally malreduced Type IV fracture has the potential to form a transphyseal bony bar with asymmetric growth or growth deformity.
- Type V fractures are usually diagnosed retrospectively after growth arrest or angular deformity has occurred.
- Salter-Harris fractures can usually be diagnosed with plain films, but magnetic resonance imaging (MRI) and computed tomography (CT) are sometimes used to more accurately delineate physeal injuries (59).

Apophyseal Avulsion Injuries

- Apophyses are growth plates that add shape and contour, rather than length, to a bone. They are often sites for muscle attachment.
- Apophyseal avulsions typically occur as a result of violent contraction of the attached muscle (60).
- The pelvis is a common site for avulsion fractures. Avulsion fractures of the anterior superior iliac spine (ASIS) and anterior inferior iliac spine (AIIS) occur with forceful contraction of the sartorius or rectus femoris. Typically, the hip will be in extension with the knee flexed, which occurs during sprinting, jumping, or kicking (60).
- Diagnosis of avulsion fractures can be made with plain radiographs. Treatment is conservative, including symptom-limited weight bearing until pain free, followed by rehabilitation and gradual return to activities.
- Recovery from an avulsion injury of the AIIS injury is typically more prolonged than that of an ASIS injury.
- Abrupt contraction of the abdominal muscles or tensor fascia lata (muscle of the iliotibial band), as with a rapid direction change, can lead to avulsion of the iliac crest. Direct trauma can also fracture the iliac crest apophysis. This commonly occurs when an athlete is tackled in football. Plain radiographs may not be as useful for diagnosis in this injury because displacement may be minimal. MRI may be helpful in diagnosing iliac crest avulsion. Treatment is conservative and includes protected weight-bearing until the athlete is not in pain followed by rehabilitation and progressive return to activity (60).
- Other sites of avulsion injury in the hip and pelvis include the greater trochanter (gluteus medius), lesser trochanter (iliopsoas), and ischial tuberosity (adductors, hamstrings). Diagnosis and treatment are similar to that mentioned for ASIS and AIIS injuries.

- Tibial tubercle avulsions typically occur when an athlete is landing or jumping, as a result of a violent contraction of the quadriceps. Excessive bleeding and swelling can cause anterior compartment syndrome, so a careful neurovascular examination is essential. Diagnosis can be made with plain radiographs. Long leg cast immobilization with the knee in extension for 3–4 weeks is adequate treatment for nondisplaced fractures. Open reduction with internal fixation (ORIF) is required if there is significant displacement of the fracture fragment.
- Avulsions of the medial epicondyle are common in throwing athletes. The athlete typically reports feeling a snap or pop during the throwing motion. Anteroposterior (AP) radiographs will typically demonstrate the avulsion. However, the fragment tends to move anterior and distal, thus obtaining internal oblique radiographs at 45° may improve accuracy when measuring maximal displacement (61). Nondisplaced or minimally displaced fractures can be treated with immobilization. Absolute indications for surgery include incarcerated fragments, open fracture, and ulnar nerve entrapment. There is no definitive agreement regarding absolute displacement distance requiring surgery (ranges reported from 2 to 10 mm) (61).
- Vertebral end-plate fractures are an avulsion of the ring apophysis of the vertebra. If the avulsion is from the posterior inferior portion of the vertebra, the apophyseal attachment of the associated disc and the apophysis can be displaced into the vertebral canal, causing neurologic symptoms. This injury can be difficult to distinguish from disc herniation. Plain radiographs can show the separated bony fragment, and MRI can demonstrate marrow edema. For symptomatic displacement of the apophysis into the vertebral canal, treatment is operative removal of the disc and bony fragment. Without neurologic symptoms, initial treatment is conservative management.

Torus Fractures

- Torus or buckle fractures are compressive fractures that lead to failure of the bone at the junction of the metaphysis and diaphysis.
- This type of injury only occurs in children and is due to the porous nature of their bones.
- Torus fractures have no disruption of the bone cortex, are stable, and heal well. They can be treated with splinting or casting for 3 weeks.

Greenstick Fractures

- The greenstick fracture only occurs in children, and it refers to an incomplete fracture in the shaft of a long bone. There is disruption of one cortex of the bone and bending of the other, which occurs due to the pliable nature of pediatric bones (62).
- Greenstick fractures with minimal angulation can be treated with immobilization.
- Surgical intervention may be required for fractures with significant angulation.

Complete Fractures

- Complete fractures are fractures through both cortices that are often displaced and/or angulated, requiring closed reduction or ORIF.

Wrist/Forearm Fractures

- Wrist and forearm fractures are some of the most common fractures in children.
- Most of these fractures can be treated with casting or splinting but may require reduction or ORIF.
- Carpal navicular or scaphoid fractures can occur in children with open growth plates and have a high rate of nonunion.

Supracondylar Fractures

- Supracondylar fractures are common among 3- to 11-year-old children.
- Supracondylar factures are one of the pediatric fractures with the highest risk of complications, including neurovascular complications and compartment syndrome.
- These fractures are usually sustained from a fall on an outstretched hand, but can also occur as a result of direct trauma to a flexed elbow. A thorough neurovascular examination is imperative if a supracondylar fracture is suspected.
- The diagnosis can typically be made with plain lateral radiographs of the elbow. Any child with a supracondylar fracture should be referred for evaluation by a pediatric orthopedist because many require surgical fixation (63).

OVERUSE INJURIES

- Overuse injuries have become more common in children with the growth of competitive youth sports programs.
- The risks of overuse are more serious in the pediatric/adolescent athlete because the growing bones of the young athlete cannot handle as much stress as the mature bones of adults (64).
- The American Academy of Pediatrics (AAP) recommends encouraging athletes to incorporate 1–2 d · wk of rest from competitive athletics, sports-specific training, and competitive practice to allow for children and adolescents to recover both physically and psychologically; limiting yearly participation time, limits on sport-specific repetitive movements (*e.g.*, pitch count limits), and scheduled rest periods are additionally recommended. The AAP also emphasizes that the focus of sports participation should be on fun, skill acquisition, safety, and sportsmanship (10).
- Risk factors for overuse injuries are often divided into **intrinsic** and **extrinsic** factors.

Intrinsic Risks for Overuse Injuries

- Intrinsic factors are defined as biological characteristics and psychosocial traits that predispose an individual to overuse injuries.
- Some issues specific to immature skeletons contribute to the risk for overuse injuries in children. For instance, children have growth cartilage in several areas of the skeleton, and it is particularly susceptible to injury from repetitive stress.
- Growth cartilage is found at the physes (epiphysis and apophysis).
- In addition, as children experience growth spurts, there are rapid changes in bone length, which can lead to a relative inflexibility of the muscle-tendon units that cross joints. This may predispose the growing athlete to muscular, joint, and physeal injuries.
- Abnormalities in alignment may also predispose an athlete to overuse injuries. Pes planus or cavus, overpronation, patellofemoral malalignment, tibial torsion, femoral anteversion, and leg length discrepancies may be related to increased risk for overuse injuries in athletes (64).

Extrinsic Risk Factors for Overuse Injury

- Extrinsic factors are defined as external forces, such as sport type, biomechanical sport-specific stressors, and sporting environment.
- Improper training technique can contribute to the risk for overuse injury.
- Increasing intensity, duration, or frequency of training too quickly can lead to overuse injury.
- In runners, injury may also result from persistently running in the same direction around the track or on the same side of the street due to angulation of the running surface.
- In addition, parental and coaching pressures to increase the intensity of a child's training can contribute to injuries.
- Improperly fitting or worn-out equipment may increase the risk of injury. For example, using worn-out running shoes or adult-sized weight-training equipment may predispose the pediatric athlete to overuse injury.
- Year-round participation in the same sport may increase the risk of overuse injury (64).

Common Overuse Injuries

Traction Apophysitis

- A traction apophysitis occurs where a muscle group attaches to a secondary center of ossification.
- It is caused by repetitive stress at these sites that can lead to pain and swelling.
- The diagnosis of apophysitis can usually be made on physical examination. In nonclassic cases, radiographs may help rule out other conditions.
- Osgood-Schlatter disease is an apophysitis at the patella tendon insertion on the tibial tubercle. It is associated with inflexibility of the quadriceps and hamstrings. Jumping and kicking activities exacerbate Osgood-Schlatter disease; therefore, it is commonly diagnosed in basketball and soccer players. Treatment involves relative rest, as well as quadriceps stretching. A knee strap may alleviate direct pressure on the tibial tubercle (65).
- Sinding-Larsen-Johansson syndrome is an apophysitis at the patella tendon origin on the inferior pole of the patella and is similar in cause and treatment to Osgood-Schlatter disease.
- Apophysitis of the medial epicondyle of the elbow is common in throwing athletes. It is often termed "little league elbow." Traction on the medial epicondyle occurs as a result of the valgus stress placed on the elbow during the throwing motion.
- Treatment includes relative rest followed by progressive strengthening and gradual return to throwing activities. Most athletes will need to rest from throwing for 6 weeks (65). The athlete's throwing frequency, effort, and technique should be evaluated, and any errors should be corrected. Pitch counts should be monitored closely to ensure that the volume of effort does not exceed an age-appropriate level.
- Sever disease, or calcaneal apophysitis, is a condition resulting in pain at the site of the Achilles tendon insertion on the calcaneus. This is associated with growth spurts and occurs mainly in active 8- to 15-year-olds.
- Treatment includes application of cold packs to the area, bilateral heel lifts in shoes while playing to reduce strain on the Achilles tendon insertion site, and relative rest followed by gradual return to play (65).
- Iselin disease is an apophysitis of the insertion site of the peroneus brevis tendon on the lateral aspect of the base of the fifth metatarsal.
- This condition may appear on x-ray as a widening of the apophysis on the inferior lateral base of the fifth metatarsal. This has an orientation parallel to the fifth metatarsal diaphysis. This parallel, rather than perpendicular, orientation helps differentiate this condition from Jones fractures and completed stress fractures. Typical rehabilitation includes rest, ice, and occasionally a CAM walking boot for 4 weeks (65).

Pelvis Apophysitis

- Apophysitis of the pelvis/hip usually affects 14- to 18-year-old runners, sprinters, dancers, soccer players, and ice hockey players. Adolescents with excessively tight hip and thigh muscles are more prone to this overuse condition.
- The apophyses most commonly affected are the ASIS, AIIS, ischial tuberosity, greater trochanter, lesser trochanter, and iliac crest (65).
- Differentiating between this and apophyseal avulsion injury is both clinical (slow onset of dull pain in the groin or side of the hip that worsens with activity rather than an acute or traumatic onset of pain) and radiologic. Both x-ray and ultrasound should show a symmetric width of the affected apophysis relative to the asymptomatic side.

- Differentiating pelvic apophysitis from muscle strain can be challenging, but is also managed similarly with relative rest, ice, gentle stretching, and gradual progression of activity as the symptoms resolve.

Patellofemoral Pain

- Musculoskeletal, biomechanical, and psychological factors can all play a role in patellofemoral pain. The most common causes of patellofemoral pain are typically associated with overuse, patellofemoral malalignment, muscle imbalance, and trauma (66).
- Important elements of the history include if there was an injury, location of the pain, and to consider hip pathology that may present as knee pain.
- Physical exam should assess for patellar tracking and patellar stability in addition to assessment of hip strength and lower extremity flexibility.
- Physical therapy remains the primary treatment with a focus on vastus medialis oblique muscle strengthening and stretching the quadriceps. Bracing and taping may also be helpful (57).

Osteochondritis Dissecans

- Osteochondritis dissecans (OCD) is a focal idiopathic abnormality of subchondral bone, with risk for instability and disruption of adjacent articular cartilage. This can result in early osteoarthritis if not recognized (67). There are several theories regarding the etiology of OCD lesions, none of which are universally accepted. However, there is some evidence that the summative effects of frequent sport participation from the prepubescent years transitioning to adolescence may be associated with knee OCD rather than direct trauma (67).
- Common sites for OCD in children include the knee, ankle, and elbow.
- OCD lesions are usually noted on plain radiographs, although MRI may be needed to identify early or subtle lesions. MRI is also used to assess the stability of the fragment and viability of subchondral bone.
- In general, younger patients and patients with stable lesions have the best prognosis. Skeletally immature athletes with an intact articular cartilage surface have the potential for healing, if impact activity is restricted (66).
- OCD in the knee is most often found on the lateral aspect of the medial femoral condyle but may also be found on the lateral femoral condyle or trochlea (67). Patients usually complain of vague knee pain with activity and intermittent swelling. If the affected fragment has detached from the underlying bone, creating a loose body, there may be complaints of locking and catching. If the fragment is stable, a period of rest and a gradual return to activity with physical therapy to improve leg strength may be adequate for treatment. If the articular cartilage is disrupted or a loose body is present, a surgical referral is indicated.
- The capitellum of the elbow is a common site for OCD lesions in throwing athletes and gymnasts. In young patients with stable lesions, treatment includes rest, physical therapy, and instruction in proper throwing technique. If the affected fragment is unstable, surgical referral is indicated.

OCD of the Talus

- Osteochondral lesions (OCL) are thought to be primarily due to trauma or repetitive microtrauma (68). A subset of OCLs are OCDs, which are classified as nontraumatic lesions in children or adolescents. The majority of lesions are located at the middle third of the medial talar rim in the anterior-posterior orientation (69).
- Most patients report diffuse ankle pain, typically with swelling or blocking.
- Radiographically, these lesions are best seen on mortise view with plantarflexion or dorsiflexion of the ankle. MRI or CT scan may be necessary for further characterization of the OCL.
- Conservative treatment includes rest, immobilization for 4–6 weeks with toe-touch weight-bearing, and NSAIDs as needed for pain (69).
- For nonresolution of symptoms with conservative treatment, surgical intervention may be necessary.

Scheuermann Disease

- Scheuermann disease is a common adolescent condition that causes a rigid painful thoracic kyphosis, loss of anterior vertebral body height, and wedging of the vertebral bodies (70).
- Most patients have tightness of the hamstrings, gluteals, and lumbodorsal fascia.
- The etiology is unclear, but a developmental or mechanical overuse cause has been suggested (71).
- Diagnosis can be made with plain radiographs of the thoracic spine, which demonstrate anterior wedging of at least three consecutive vertebral bodies, herniation of disc into vertebral end-plates (Schmorl nodes), and narrow disc spaces.
- Treatment includes physical therapy for strength and flexibility. Bracing may be used for a period of 9–12 months, if kyphosis with Cobb angle >60° is present and the patient is skeletally immature (70).

Stress Fractures

- Stress fractures occur when there is an accumulation of damage from repetitive stresses that outstrips the bone's ability to repair and remodel.
- Stress fractures are most commonly found in the lower extremities but can also be found in the spine and upper extremity.
- Stress fractures may be diagnosed with plain radiographs but single photon emission CT (SPECT), CT, or MRI may be needed.
- Many stress fractures are similar in the adult and pediatric populations; only stress fractures specific to the pediatric population are discussed here.

Spondylolysis

- The term "spondylolysis" refers to a stress fracture of the pars interarticularis of the spine.
- If there is a fracture of both pars, then it may become unstable, and forward displacement of one vertebra on another may result, which is termed as spondylolisthesis.
- Athletes participating in sports that require repetitive hyperextension, such as gymnastics or football, may be at increased risk for spondylolysis.
- Most patients complain of low back pain, which is worse with extension and is relieved by rest.
- Spondylolysis can often be diagnosed with plain radiographs and is best seen on lateral and oblique views. It can, however, occur without changes on plain radiographs. In this case, SPECT, MRI, or CT can be used to detect the abnormality (70).
- Treatment includes activity restriction until the patient is asymptomatic followed by a gradual return to activity. A program of core/lumbar strengthening and hamstring flexibility should also be instituted. Some practitioners recommend bracing at diagnosis, whereas others recommend bracing only if the patient continues to have pain, despite adequate rest.
- Prognosis is best in cases where only SPECT scan is positive, and there is not yet plain radiographic evidence of disease. In cases where radiographic evidence of spondylolysis is present, the likelihood of healing is lower.
- If spondylolisthesis has occurred, there is no chance for healing.
- Conservative therapy, similar to that for spondylolysis, is the most widely recommended treatment for spondylolisthesis.
- The role of surgery is controversial. In cases where neurologic compromise is evident or slipping of the vertebra progresses, surgical stabilization is recommended (70).

Proximal Humeral Physeal Stress Fracture

- The proximal humeral stress fracture is often referred to as "little league shoulder," although it is also seen in other overhead athletes, such as tennis or volleyball players.
- The throwing motion places torsion and distraction forces on the proximal humerus which, when done repetitively, can result in proximal humeral stress fracture. AP internal and external rotation views of the shoulder with comparison views of the opposite shoulder on radiograph can demonstrate widening, sclerosis, or cystic changes of the affected physis.
- Treatment involves cessation of throwing or other overhead activities until the child is asymptomatic, usually about 3 months. At that time, progressive return to activity is allowed. Throwing mechanics should be evaluated, and parents and coaches should be warned not to encourage excessive throwing. Age-appropriate pitch counts should be followed (61).

Distal Radius Physeal Stress Fracture

- Distal radius physeal stress fracture is a Salter-Harris Type V stress fracture that typically occurs in gymnasts.
- It is caused by the frequent upper extremity weight-bearing activities that gymnasts perform.
- Chronic, dull, dorsal, or radial-sided wrist pain is the most common symptom initially.
- The diagnosis may be made with plain radiographs by comparing the affected side to the nonpainful side. Abnormal widening of the physis, "beaking" of the epiphysis, and cystic changes on the metaphyseal side of the bone may be noted on the affected radius; however, MRI may be needed to make the diagnosis if plain radiographs are normal.
- Treatment includes rest until the athlete is asymptomatic, usually 6–8 weeks. Immobilization may be helpful (61).
- When pain has completely resolved, a gradual return to upper extremity weight-bearing is permitted. Attention to technique errors upon return to sport may help prevent reinjury.

Lunatomalacia (Kienböck Disease)

- Kienböck disease is a painful, unilateral condition of the wrist that radiates up the forearm in 20- to 40-year-olds. It involves collapse of the lunate from vascular insufficiency and avascular necrosis after single or repetitive microfractures of the bone. These fractures are thought to occur during recurrent compression of the lunate from loads to the wrist while in extremes of flexion and/or extension.
- Negative ulnar variance has historically been associated with this condition; however, the role of this finding in perpetuating disease is now more debated (72).
- Radiographic findings may be normal initially and progress to demonstrating total lunate collapse and fragmentation. Advanced imaging with MRI or CT scan can be helpful for staging.
- If not corrected surgically, this may progress to severe wrist disability and chronic pain.

ANATOMIC VARIANTS

- Several anatomic variants may predispose the pediatric athlete to pain and injury.

Discoid Lateral Meniscus

- Higher incidence in the Asian population (73).
- Symptoms can include snapping, pain, and limited mobility (74).
- Meniscal tears are a risk for young athletes.
- Some discoid menisci are not diagnosed until they are torn, in which case the athlete tends to complain of pain, swelling, and mechanical symptoms.
- Diagnosis can often be made on clinical examination. Patients may present with effusion, a lack of terminal extension, anterolateral bulging at full flexion, a positive McMurray test, or joint-line tenderness (74).

- MRI can also be used to diagnose meniscal tears and discoid lateral menisci. Arthroscopy may be necessary to confirm the diagnosis (74).
- A torn discoid lateral meniscus requires surgery. If a discoid lateral meniscus is found incidentally, surgery is not usually indicated.

Tarsal Coalition

- Tarsal coalition is a bony or fibrocartilaginous connection of two or more tarsal bones.
- It is estimated that one out of every hundred people may have a tarsal coalition
- The most common examples are calcaneonavicular and talocalcaneal coalitions. They are often bilateral. These can result in a rigid flat foot.
- Symptomatic patients typically complain of vague pain that is insidious in onset. The diagnosis of calcaneonavicular coalition can usually be made on the oblique view of the plain radiograph, but CT scan may be necessary to provide a more detailed view of the anatomy or to see talocalcaneal coalition. MRI may be helpful in identifying a fibrous or cartilaginous coalition.
- Plain radiographs may demonstrate an elongated anterior process of the calcaneus "anteater sign" in a calcaneonavicular coalition, or "talar beaking" on lateral radiographs in a talocalcaneal coalition.
- Conservative therapy includes rest, immobilization, rigid shoe inserts, and anti-inflammatory medication.
- In patients who fail conservative therapy, surgical resection of the coalition can be performed.

Accessory Ossicles

- Accessory ossicles are often the result of unfused ossification centers and are frequently congenital. They may also be the result of prior trauma
- Common in the foot, the accessory navicular is an accessory ossicle at the proximal medial navicular bone into which a portion of the posterior tibialis tendon inserts (75).
- Athletes involved in sports that stress the posterior tibialis tendon with running and jumping, such as basketball, may develop accessory navicular pain. Flexible flat feet (excessive foot pronation) are often present in them.
- Diagnosis can be made on the external oblique radiograph of the foot, though, often, it is an incidental finding on radiographs; for those difficult to diagnose, CT or MRI may be used.
- Treatment is typically conservative, with rest, shoe inserts, ice, nonsteroidal antiinflammatory drugs, and rarely, immobilization. Excision can be performed if conservative therapy fails.
- The os trigonum is another common accessory ossicle that is found posterior to the talus.
- Sports that involve repetitive plantarflexion, such as ballet or soccer, can lead to impingement of the os trigonum between the posterior tibia and calcaneus (75).
- An os trigonum can usually be seen on lateral radiograph of the ankle.
- Conservative therapy is usually effective. This includes physical therapy for strengthening and flexibility, relative rest, anti-inflammatory medication, and, sometimes, a steroid injection. Surgical excision can be performed if conservative therapy fails.

THE OSTEOCHONDROSES

- The osteochondroses are a group of chronic disorders that involve the epiphyses or apophyses.
- They begin as an avascular necrosis of the epiphyseal center followed by eventual repair and replacement of the ossification center.

Panner Disease

- Panner disease is an osteochondrosis of the capitellum associated with repetitive trauma from throwing. It involves variations in the normal ossification of the capitellum of the humerus (76,77).
- This condition typically affects children between 5 and 11 years of age, a younger age group than that which is typically affected by OCD of the capitellum.
- The athlete complains of pain at the lateral aspect of the elbow with activity and may have swelling.
- Fragmentation of the capitellum is noted on the radiograph of the elbow.
- This is a self-limiting disease and can be treated conservatively with activity modification.

Legg-Calve-Perthes Disease

- Legg-Calve-Perthes disease, an osteochondrosis of the hip, is a rare childhood condition.
- Symptoms include knee, groin, or anterior thigh pain and limping after activity.
- AP and frog lateral radiographs of the hip confirm the diagnosis.
- There are four stages of the condition: initial/necrosis, fragmentation, reossification, and healed (78).
- The main goal of treatment is to maintain range of motion and prevent deformity of the femoral head by keeping it contained in the acetabulum.
- Orthopedic referral is indicated.

Freiberg Disease

- Freiberg disease is an osteochondrosis of the metatarsal head.
- It usually affects adolescents.
- Forefoot pain is the typical complaint.
- Flattening of the metatarsal head and fragmentation of the epiphysis can be seen on plain radiographs. However, MRI or

bone scan may be necessary for diagnosis early in the disease process.

- With early diagnosis, conservative therapy, including relative rest, padding of the affected metatarsal head, and orthotics, may be successful. With failure of conservative therapy, surgical referral should be made.

Kohler Disease

- Kohler disease is a unilateral avascular necrosis of the navicular bone occurring in children less than the age of 10.
- This disease presents as a painful limp with shifting of weight to the lateral aspect of the foot. The navicular is the last bone in the foot to ossify, which may make it more vulnerable to compressive damage during weight-bearing.
- Radiographically, the appearance of the navicular bone in Kohler disease may be normal to completely collapsed (the opposite, asymptomatic side may have the same radiologic appearance).
- Prognosis is typically complete recovery within 1–3 years with conservative treatment, including control of pain and swelling, reduced strenuous activity, and longitudinal arch supports and/or medial heel wedges and/or 4–6 weeks of immobilization in a walking cast.

SAFETY AND OTHER CONSIDERATIONS

Heat and Cold Illness

- Children have a larger body surface area to body mass ratio than adults, making children more likely to gain heat from the environment in hot conditions and lose it in cold environments. Heat loss in children is even more apparent in water because of the high thermal conductivity of water (79,80).
- Compared to adults exercising at a given level, children have increased heat production per kilogram of body mass. This leads to faster increases in body temperature in warm weather, but can be protective when exercise is performed in cold environments (81).
- Another disadvantage for children exercising in warm environments is that the sweating rate in children is lower than in adults. This is particularly important when the temperature of the environment exceeds the skin temperature. In this type of environment, sweat evaporation from the skin is the only means for cooling the body.
- Children do not adapt to extremes of temperature as effectively as adults when exposed to a high climatic heat stress with the adaptation of adolescents falling in between children and adults. Even in relatively moderate summer temperatures, children demonstrate evidence of heat strain when participating in outdoor free play (82).
- Overall, evidence supporting the claim that children remain at higher risk for heat illness than adults is stronger in the pediatric population less than 4 years of age. It does not translate as well to the older youth athlete. Thus, despite the perceived inferior thermoregulatory mechanisms in children, current evidence fails to indicate clinically significant differences in the thermoregulatory mechanisms between children and adults. Thus, Rowland concludes that there is minimal convincing evidence to suggest children are at greater risk of heat illness exercising in high ambient temperature than adults (83).
- Data from the CDC-funded National High School Sports-Related Injury Surveillance Study indicates that exertional heat illness (EHI) occurred at an estimated rate of 1.20 cases per 100,000 athlete exposures, occurring mostly in August and distributed widely across the United States. Up to one third of the practice-related cases occurred >2 hours into the practice and one-third of all cases occurred when a medical professional was not onsite. The rate in football was 11.4 times higher than observed in all other sports (84). Recommendations to limit football practice to 3 hours appear to have an impact in lowering rates of EHI (85).
- Considerable effort has been made over the past several years to reduce heat injury in sports. The National Athletic Trainers' Association has developed heat acclimatization guidelines designed specifically to prevent deaths in high school football players (86).
- Other effective measures to prevent heat illness in children participating in sports includes acclimatization, adequate hydration and rehydration, limiting practice time, and providing adequate recovery between practices (87).
- Written emergency action plans are recommended for all athletic environments where children are participating in sports. If a child exhibits any neurologic dysfunction during a sporting event in the heat, on-site whole-body rapid cooling should be initiated without delay while emergency medical services are activated. The removal of clothing and equipment and cold or ice-water immersion should be performed emergently in these circumstances. Rectal temperature should be checked when feasible, but this should not delay cooling. Cooling should commence and continue until the rectal temperature is <39°C or there is apparent clinical neurologic improvement (87).
- Regarding cold stress and hypothermia, there are aspects by which children withstand hypothermia better than adults. Children are less likely to sustain fatal arrhythmias while hypothermic, and there appears to be some level of neuroprotection that occurs when children are exposed to hypoxia while hypothermic, which has been exploited clinically with therapeutic hypothermia interventions in certain settings (88).
- However, children are also more susceptible to environmental cold than adults, due to the higher surface area to body mass ratio, which is implicated in heat illness in children.
- Two types of environmental cold injuries may occur: freezing and nonfreezing. Frostbite is a freezing injury, categorized by the depth of the freezing injury. Hypothermia represents a nonfreezing injury that can occur even when temperatures are above freezing. Rewarming is the main principle in the treatment of both of these cold injuries.

- Rewarming areas affected by frostbite by monitored immersion in warm water is the consensus recommendation, with the water heated to approximately 98–101°F (37–39°C). Close observation for infection and considering tetanus prophylaxis depending on immunization status is warranted.
- Children with hypothermia may initially present with fatigue progressing to confusion, slurred speech, and motor incoordination. Rewarming can occur via passive methods (removing the child from cold, removing wet clothing, and wrapping them in blanket to allow their body to rewarm itself), active external rewarming (wrapping them in heated blanket), and active internal rewarming (administration of warm intravenous or peritoneal fluid). Prompt recognition and treatment are critical (89).

Hydration

- Children should be well hydrated (normal body weight and light-colored urine) prior to starting any physical activity (90).
- During activity, children should be encouraged to drink 120 mL (5 oz) of water every 20 minutes. Older, heavier children will require 250 mL (9 oz) every 30 minutes (79).
- For activities lasting longer than 1 hour, a 6% carbohydrate solution with sodium and chloride should be used.
- Beverages should be cold to improve palatability.
- Lightweight clothing should be worn to facilitate sweat evaporation.
- Weighing before and after a session can provide a good indication of hydration status.

Sun Exposure

- Exposure to ultraviolet (UV) radiation during childhood increases the risk of skin cancer in adulthood (91); therefore, prevention of UV sun exposure due to sports participation is critical.
- Sunscreen labeled as "broad-spectrum" will block both UVB and UVA rays. Sunscreen with sun protection factor (SPF) of 15 (or higher up to 50) should be applied 15–30 minutes prior to sun exposure to reduce the risk for sunburn and should be reapplied every 2 hours and after swimming, sweating, or drying off with a towel (92).
- Avoid sunscreen containing oxybenzone due to potential hormonal effects. Zinc oxide and titanium dioxide are the inorganic physical sunscreens approved by the US Food and Drug Administration.
- Clothing and hats represent excellent barriers to UV radiation, with darker colors providing greater protection than lighter colors.
- Sunglasses that absorb 99%–100% of the full UV spectrum should be worn to protect the eyes from UV exposure, which is associated with an increased risk of cataracts.

Proper Equipment

- Children should be provided with appropriately sized and well-fitted equipment in good condition for sport participation according to the rules of play for a given sport.
- Youth football helmets should be reconditioned using an authorized reconditioner for recertification every 2 years (93) to meet National Operating Committee on Standards for Athletic Equipment.
- Padding for football, hockey, and soccer is made in children's sizes.
- Weight-training equipment can be found in sizes and with weight increments appropriate for children.
- Mouthguards should be worn to prevent dental injury for all contact sports where they are required.
- There is conflicting evidence for the use of headgear in sports such as girls' lacrosse (94) and soccer (54).

REFERENCES

1. National Council of Youth Sports Web site [Internet]. *National Council of Youth Sports* [cited 2023 Feb 12]. Available from: https://ncys.org
2. Black LI, Terlizzi EP, Vahratian A. Organized sports participation among children aged 6-17 years: United States, 2020. *NCHS Data Brief.* 2022;441:1–8.
3. Powell JW, Barber-Foss KD. Injury patterns in selected high school sports: a review of the 1995-1997 seasons. *J Athl Train.* 1999;34(3):277–84.
4. LaPrade RF, Agel J, Baker J, et al. AOSSM early sport specialization consensus statement. *Orthop J Sports Med.* 2016;4(4):2325967116644241. doi:10.1177/2325967116644241
5. Kliethermes SA, Marshall SW, LaBella CR, et al. Defining a research agenda for youth sport specialisation in the USA: the AMSSM Youth Early Sport Specialization Summit. *Br J Sports Med.* 2021;55(3):135–43.
6. Costa E Silva L, Teles J, Fragoso I, Fragoso I. Sports injuries patterns in children and adolescents according to their sports participation level, age and maturation. *BMC Sports Sci Med Rehabil.* 2022;14(1):35. doi:10.1186/s13102-022-00431-3
7. Adirim T, Cheng T. Overview of injuries in the young athlete. *Sports Med.* 2003;33(1):75–81.
8. Patel DR, Yamasaki A, Brown K. Epidemiology of sports-related musculoskeletal injuries in young athletes in United States. *Transl Pediatr.* 2017 Jul;6(3):160–6. doi:10.21037/tp.2017.04.08
9. Patel DR, Soares N, Wells K. Neurodevelopmental readiness of children for participation in sports. *Transl Pediatr.* 2017;6(3):167–73.
10. Stricker PR, Faigenbaum AD, McCambridge TM, Council on Sports Medicine and Fitness. Resistance training for children and adolescents. *Pediatrics.* 2020;145(6):e20201011. doi:10.1542/peds.2020-1011
11. Arnaoutis G, Kavouras SA, Angelopoulou A, et al. Fluid balance during training in elite young athletes of different sports. *J Strength Cond Res.* 2015 Dec;29(12):3447–52. doi:10.1519/JSC.0000000000000400
12. O'Connor DP, Knoblauch MA. Electrocardiogram testing during athletic preparticipation physical examinations. *J Athl Train.* 2010 May-Jun;45(3):265–72. doi:10.4085/1062-6050-45.3.265
13. Roberts WO, Asplund CA, O'Connor FG, Stovitz SD. Cardiac preparticipation screening for the young athlete: why the routine use of ECG is not necessary. *J Electrocardiol.* 2015 May-Jun;48(3):311–5. doi:10.1016/j.jelectrocard.2015.01.010

14. Petek BJ, Baggish AL. Pre-participation cardiovascular screening in young competitive athletes. *Curr Emerg Hosp Med Rep.* 2020 Sep;8(3):77–89. doi:10.1007/s40138-020-00214-5
15. McCrory P, Meeuwisse W, Dvořák J, et al. Consensus statement on concussion in sport-the 5th international conference on concussion in sport held in Berlin, October 2016. *Br J Sports Med.* 2017 Jun;51(11):838–47. doi:10.1136/bjsports-2017-097699
16. Dave SC, Fisher M. Relative energy deficiency in sport (RED - S). *Curr Probl Pediatr Adolesc Health Care.* 2022;52(8):101242. doi:10.1016/j.cppeds.2022.101242
17. Elliott-Sale KJ, Tenforde AS, Parziale AL, Holtzman B, Ackerman KE. Endocrine effects of relative energy deficiency in sport. *Int J Sport Nutr Exerc Metab.* 2018;28(4):335–49. doi:10.1123/ijsnem.2018-0127
18. Fredericson M, Kussman A, Misra M, et al. The male athlete triad—a consensus statement from the female and male athlete triad coalition part II: diagnosis, treatment, and return-to-play. *Clin J Sport Med.* 2021;31(4):349–66. doi:10.1097/JSM.0000000000000948
19. Herring SA, Kibler BW, Putukian M. Select issues in pain management for the youth and adolescent athlete. *Curr Sports Med Rep.* 2020;19(8):329–38. doi:10.1249/JSR.0000000000000741
20. Sarmiento K, Miller GF, Jones SE. Sports-related concussions and adverse health behaviors among middle and high school students. *Am J Sports Med.* 2023 Feb;51(2):503–10. doi:10.1177/03635465221141440
21. Black LI, Zablotsky B. Concussions and brain injuries in children: United States, 2020. *NCHS Data Brief.* 2021 Dec;423:1–8.
22. Cook NE, Iverson GL. Concussion among children in the United States general population: incidence and risk factors. *Front Neurol.* 2021 Nov 1;12:773927. doi:10.3389/fneur.2021.773927
23. Elbin RJ, Sufrinko A, Schatz P, et al. Removal from play after concussion and recovery time. *Pediatrics.* 2016 Sep;138(3):e20160910. doi:10.1542/peds.2016-0910
24. Asken BM, Bauer RM, Guskiewicz KM, et al. Immediate removal from activity after sport-related concussion is associated with shorter clinical recovery and less severe symptoms in collegiate student-athletes. *Am J Sports Med.* 2018 May;46(6):1465–74. doi:10.1177/0363546518757984
25. Macnow T, Curran T, Tolliday C, et al. Effect of screen time on recovery from concussion: a randomized clinical trial. *JAMA Pediatr.* 2021 Nov 1;175(11):1124–31. doi:10.1001/jamapediatrics.2021.2782
26. Leddy JJ, Haider MN, Ellis MJ, et al. Early subthreshold aerobic exercise for sport-related concussion: a randomized clinical trial. *JAMA Pediatr.* 2019 Apr 1;173(4):319–25. doi:10.1001/jamapediatrics.2018.4397
27. Leddy JJ, Master CL, Mannix R, et al. Early targeted heart rate aerobic exercise versus placebo stretching for sport-related concussion in adolescents: a randomised controlled trial. *Lancet Child Adolesc Health.* 2021 Nov;5(11):792–9. doi:10.1016/S2352-4642(21)00267-4
28. Vaughan CG, Ledoux AA, Sady MD, et al. Association between early return to school following acute concussion and symptom burden at 2 weeks postinjury. *JAMA Netw Open.* 2023 Jan 3;6(1):e2251839. doi:10.1001/jamanetworkopen.2022.51839
29. Thomas DG, Apps JN, Hoffmann RG, McCrea M, Hammeke T. Benefits of strict rest after acute concussion: a randomized controlled trial. *Pediatrics.* 2015 Feb;135(2):213–23. doi:10.1542/peds.2014-0966
30. Halstead ME, McAvoy K, Devore CD, et al. Returning to learning following a concussion. *Pediatrics.* 2013 Nov;132(5):948–57. doi:10.1542/peds.2013-2867
31. Grady MF, Master CL. Return to school and learning after concussion: tips for pediatricians. *Pediatr Ann.* 2017 Mar 1;46(3):e93–8. doi:10.3928/19382359-20170220-04
32. Lumba-Brown A, Teramoto M, Bloom OJ, et al. Concussion guidelines step 2: evidence for subtype classification. *Neurosurgery.* 2020 Jan 1;86(1):2–13. doi:10.1093/neuros/nyz332
33. Eagle SR, Manderino L, Collins M, et al. Characteristics of concussion subtypes from a multidomain assessment. *J Neurosurg Pediatr.* 2022 Apr;30:107–12. doi:10.3171/2022.3.PEDS2267
34. Howell DR, Kriz P, Mannix RC, Kirchberg T, Master CL, Meehan WP III. Concussion symptom profiles among child, adolescent, and young adult athletes. *Clin J Sport Med.* 2019 Sep;29(5):391–7. doi:10.1097/JSM.0000000000000629
35. Master CL, Bacal D, Grady MF, et al. Evaluation of the visual system by the primary care provider following concussion. *Pediatrics.* 2022;150(2):e2021056048. doi:10.1542/peds.2021-056048
36. Master CL, Bacal D, Grady MF, et al. Vision and concussion: symptoms, signs, evaluation, and treatment. *Pediatrics.* 2022;150(2):e2021056047. doi:10.1542/peds.2021-056047
37. Albano AW Jr, Senter C, Adler RH, Herring SA, Asif IM. The legal landscape of concussion: implications for sports medicine providers. *Sports Health.* 2016 Sep;8(5):465–8. doi:10.1177/1941738116662025
38. Bell JM, Master CL, Lionbarger MR. The clinical implications of youth sports concussion laws: a review. *Am J Lifestyle Med.* 2019 Mar;13(2):172–81. doi:10.1177/1559827616688883
39. Master CL, Mayer AR, Quinn D, Grady MF. Concussion. *Ann Intern Med.* 2018 Jul 3;169(1):ITC1–16. doi:10.7326/AITC201807030
40. Zemek R, Barrowman N, Freedman SB, et al. Clinical risk score for persistent postconcussion symptoms among children with acute concussion in the ED. *JAMA.* 2016 Mar 8;315(10):1014–25. Erratum in: *JAMA.* 2016 Jun 21;315(23):2624. doi:10.1001/jama.2016.1203
41. Leddy JJ, Kozlowski K, Donnelly JP, Pendergast DR, Epstein LH, Willer B. A preliminary study of subsymptom threshold exercise training for refractory post-concussion syndrome. *Clin J Sport Med.* 2010;20(1):21–7.
42. Schneider KJ, Meeuwisse WH, Nettel-Aguirre A, et al. Cervicovestibular rehabilitation in sport-related concussion: a randomised controlled trial. *Br J Sports Med.* 2014 Sep;48(17):1294–8. doi:10.1136/bjsports-2013-093267
43. Kontos AP, Eagle SR, Mucha A, et al. A randomized controlled trial of precision vestibular rehabilitation in adolescents following concussion: preliminary findings. *J Pediatr.* 2021 Dec;239:193–9. doi:10.1016/j.jpeds.2021.08.032
44. Scheiman MM, Talasan H, Mitchell GL, Alvarez TL. Objective assessment of vergence after treatment of concussion-related CI: a pilot study. *Optom Vis Sci.* 2017 Jan;94(1):74–88. doi:10.1097/OPX.0000000000000936
45. Gallaway M, Scheiman M, Mitchell GL. Vision therapy for post-concussion vision disorders. *Optom Vis Sci.* 2017 Jan;94(1):68–73. doi:10.1097/OPX.0000000000000935
46. Storey EP, Master SR, Lockyer JE, Podolak OE, Grady MF, Master CL. Near point of convergence after concussion in children. *Optom Vis Sci.* 2017 Jan;94(1):96–100. doi:10.1097/OPX.0000000000000910
47. Iverson GL, Gaudet CE, Karr JE. Examining suicidality in adolescents who have sustained concussions. *J Neurotrauma.* 2023;40(7-8):730–41. doi:10.1089/neu.2022.0233
48. Ledoux AA, Webster RJ, Clarke AE, et al. Risk of mental health problems in children and youths following concussion. *JAMA Netw Open.* 2022 Mar 1;5(3):e221235. doi:10.1001/jamanetworkopen.2022.1235
49. Ziminski D, Szlyk HS, Baiden P, et al. Sports- and physical activity-related concussion and mental health among adolescents: findings from the 2017 and 2019 Youth Risk Behavior Survey. *Psychiatry Res.* 2022 Jun;312:114542. doi:10.1016/j.psychres.2022.114542
50. Iverson GL, Greenberg J, Cook NE. Anxiety is associated with diverse physical and cognitive symptoms in youth presenting to a multidisciplinary concussion clinic. *Front Neurol.* 2021;12:811462. doi:10.3389/fneur.2021.811462

51. Yang YT, Baugh CM. US youth soccer concussion policy: heading in the right direction. *JAMA Pediatr.* 2016 May 1;170(5):413–4. doi:10.1001/jamapediatrics.2016.0338
52. Emery CA, Kang J, Shrier I, et al. Risk of injury associated with body checking among youth ice hockey players. *JAMA.* 2010 Jun 9;303(22):2265–72. doi:10.1001/jama.2010.755
53. Obana KK, Mueller JD, Saltzman BM, et al. Targeting rule implementation decreases concussions in high school football: a national concussion surveillance study. *Orthop J Sports Med.* 2021 Oct 15;9(10):23259671211031191. doi:10.1177/23259671211031191
54. McGuine T, Post E, Pfaller AY, et al. Does soccer headgear reduce the incidence of sport-related concussion? A cluster, randomised controlled trial of adolescent athletes. *Br J Sports Med.* 2020 Apr;54(7):408–13. doi:10.1136/bjsports-2018-100238
55. Herman DC, Caswell SV, Kelshaw PM, Vincent HK, Lincoln AE. Association of headgear mandate and concussion injury rates in girls' high school lacrosse. *Br J Sports Med.* 2022 Sep;56(17):970–4. doi:10.1136/bjsports-2021-105031
56. Ellis MJ, McDonald PJ, Cordingley D, Mansouri B, Essig M, Ritchie L. Retirement-from-sport considerations following pediatric sports-related concussion: case illustrations and institutional approach. *Neurosurg Focus.* 2016 Apr;40(4):E8. doi:10.3171/2016.1.FOCUS15600
57. Davis-Hayes C, Baker DR, Bottiglieri TS, et al. Medical retirement from sport after concussions: a practical guide for a difficult discussion. *Neurol Clin Pract.* 2018 Feb;8(1):40–7. doi:10.1212/CPJ.0000000000000424
58. Wilson JC, Patsimas T, Cohen K, Putukian M. Considerations for athlete retirement after sport-related concussion. *Clin Sports Med.* 2021 Jan;40(1):187–97. doi:10.1016/j.csm.2020.08.008
59. Cepela DJ, Tartaglione JP, Dooley TP, Patel PN. Classifications in brief: Salter-Harris classification of pediatric physeal fractures. *Clin Orthop Relat Res.* 2016;474(11):2531–7. doi:10.1007/s11999-016-4891-3
60. Calderazzi F, Nosenzo A, Galavotti C, Menozzi M, Pogliacomi F, Ceccarelli F. Apophyseal avulsion fractures of the pelvis. A review. *Acta Biomed.* 2018;89(4):470–6. doi:10.23750/abm.v89i4.7632
61. Watkins RA, De Borja C, Ramirez F. Common upper extremity injuries in pediatric athletes. *Curr Rev Musculoskelet Med.* 2022;15(6):465–73. doi:10.1007/s12178-022-09784
62. Caruso G, Caldari E, Sturla FD, et al. Management of pediatric forearm fractures: what is the best therapeutic choice? A narrative review of the literature. *Musculoskelet Surg.* 2021;105(3):225–34. doi:10.1007/s12306-020-00684-6
63. Marson BA, Ikram A, Craxford S, Lewis SR, Price KR, Ollivere BJ. Interventions for treating supracondylar elbow fractures in children. *Cochrane Database Syst Rev.* 2022;6(6):CD013609. doi:10.1002/14651858.CD013609.pub2
64. DiFiori JP, Benjamin HJ, Brenner J, et al. Overuse injuries and burnout in youth sports: a position statement from the American Medical Society for Sports Medicine. *Clin J Sport Med.* 2014;24(1):3–20. doi:10.1097/JSM.0000000000000060
65. Ridenour R, Hennrikus W. Overuse injuries in pediatric athletes. *Adv Pediatr.* 2020;67:171–82. doi:10.1016/j.yapd.2020.04.001
66. Herring SA, Bergfeld JA, Bernhardt DT. Selected issues for the adolescent athlete and the team physician: a consensus statement. *Med Sci Sports Exerc.* 2008;40(11):1997–2012. doi:10.1249/MSS.0b013e31818acdcb
67. Nissen CW, Albright JC, Anderson CN, et al. Descriptive epidemiology from the research in osteochondritis dissecans of the knee (ROCK) prospective cohort. *Am J Sports Med.* 2022;50(1):118–27. doi:10.1177/03635465211057103
68. Tileston K, Baskar D, Frick SL. What is new in pediatric orthopaedic foot and ankle. *J Pediatr Orthop.* 2022;42(5):e448–52. doi:10.1097/BPO.0000000000002134
69. Bruns J, Habermann C, Werner M. Osteochondral lesions of the talus: a review on talus osteochondral injuries, including osteochondritis dissecans. *Cartilage.* 2021;13(1_suppl l):1380S–401S. doi:10.1177/1947603520985182
70. DePaola K, Cuddihy LA. Pediatric spine disorders. *Pediatr Clin North Am.* 2020;67(1):185–204. doi:10.1016/j.pcl.2019.09.008
71. Sardar ZM, Ames RJ, Lenke L. Scheuermann's kyphosis: diagnosis, management, and selecting fusion levels. *J Am Acad Orthop Surg.* 2019;27(10):e462–72. doi:10.5435/JAAOS-D-17-00748
72. Daly CA, Graf AR. Kienböck disease: clinical presentation, epidemiology, and historical perspective. *Hand Clin.* 2022;38(4):385–92. doi:10.1016/j.hcl.2022.03.002
73. Kocher MS, Logan CA, Kramer DE. Discoid lateral meniscus in children: diagnosis, management, and outcomes. *J Am Acad Orthop Surg.* 2017;25(11):736–43. doi:10.5435/JAAOS-D-15-00491
74. Kim JH, Ahn JH, Kim JH, Wang JH. Discoid lateral meniscus: importance, diagnosis, and treatment. *J Exp Orthop.* 2020;7(1):81. doi:10.1186/s40634-020-00294-y
75. Vora BMK, Wong BSS. Common accessory ossicles of the foot: imaging features, pitfalls and associated pathology. *Singapore Med J.* 2018;59(4):183–9. doi:10.11622/smedj.2018046
76. Achar S, Yamanaka J. Apophysitis and osteochondrosis: common causes of pain in growing bones. *Am Fam Physician.* 2019 May 15;99(10):610–18.
77. Claessen FM, Louwerens JK, Doornberg JN, van Dijk CN, Eygendaal D, van den Bekerom MP. Panner's disease: literature review and treatment recommendations. *J Child Orthop.* 2015;9(1):9–17. doi:10.1007/s11832-015-0635-2
78. American Academy of Orthopedic Surgeons Web site [Internet]. *Ortho Info: Perthes Disease.* Last reviewed October 2019. [cited 2023 Feb 20]. Available from: https://www.orthoinfo.org/en/diseases--conditions/perthes-disease/
79. Notley SR, Akerman AP, Meade RD, McGarr GW, Kenny GP. Exercise thermoregulation in prepubertal children: a brief methodological review. *Med Sci Sports Exerc.* 2020 Nov;52(11):2412–22. doi:10.1249/MSS.0000000000002391
80. Sullivan JA, Anderson SJ, editors. *Care of the Young Athlete.* 1st ed. Rosemont (IL): American Academy of Orthopaedic Surgeons; 2000.
81. Smolander J, Bar-Or O, Korhonen O, Ilmarinen J. Thermoregulation during rest and exercise in the cold in pre- and early pubescent boys and in young men. *J Appl Physiol.* 1992;72(4):1589–94.
82. McGarr GW, Saci S, King KE, et al. Heat strain in children during unstructured outdoor physical activity in a continental summer climate. *Temperature (Austin).* 2020 Aug 12;8(1):80–9. doi:10.1080/23328940.2020.1801120
83. Rowland T. Thermoregulation during exercise in the heat in children: old concepts revisited. *J Appl Physiol (1985).* 2008 Aug;105(2):718–24.
84. Kerr ZY, Casa DJ, Marshall SW, Comstock RD. Epidemiology of exertional heat illness among U.S. high school athletes. *Am J Prev Med.* 2013 Jan;44(1):8–14. doi:10.1016/j.amepre.2012.09.058
85. Tripp BL, Eberman LE, Smith MS. Exertional heat illnesses and environmental conditions during high school football practices. *Am J Sports Med.* 2015 Oct;43(10):2490–5. doi:10.1177/0363546515593947
86. Casa DJ, Csillan D, Inter-Association Task Force for Preseason Secondary School Athletics Participants, et al. Preseason heat-acclimatization guidelines for secondary school athletics. *J Athl Train.* 2009;44(3):332–3.
87. Council on Sports Medicine and Fitness and Council on School Health, Bergeron MF, Devore C, Rice SG, American Academy of Pediatrics. Policy statement-climatic heat stress and exercising children and adolescents. *Pediatrics.* 2011;128(3):E741–7.
88. Singer D. Pediatric hypothermia: an ambiguous issue. *Int J Environ Res Public Health.* 2021 Oct 31;18(21):11484. doi:10.3390/ijerph182111484

89. Schimelpfenig SS, Jacobsen B. Pediatric environmental cold injuries. *Pediatr Rev.* 2022 Aug 1;43(8):449–57. doi:10.1542/PIR2020005179
90. Bergeron MF. Hydration in the pediatric athlete - how to guide your patients. *Curr Sports Med Rep.* 2015 Jul-Aug;14(4):288–93. doi:10.1249/JSR.0000000000000179
91. Balk SJ, Council on Environmental Health, Section on Dermatology. Ultraviolet radiation: a hazard to children and adolescents. *Pediatrics.* 2011;127(3):e791–817. doi:10.1542/peds.2010-3502
92. Sun Safety: Information for Parents About Sunburn and Sunscreen Web site [Internet]. Healthychildren.org; [cited 2023 Mar 27]. Available from: https://www.healthychildren.org/English/safety-prevention/at-play/Pages/Sun-Safety.aspx
93. National Operating Committee on Standards for Athletic Equipment Web site [Internet]. *National Operating Committee on Standards for Athletic Equipment*; [cited 2023 Mar 27]. Available from: https://nocsae.org/players-parents-coaches/recertification/
94. Caswell SV, Kelshaw PM, Lincoln AE, et al. The effects of headgear in high school girls' lacrosse. *Orthop J Sports Med.* 2020 Dec 29;8(12):2325967120969685. doi:10.1177/2325967120969685

129 The Geriatric Athlete

Ian R. Reynolds and Brian K. Unwin

INTRODUCTION

- Age-related physiological and physical changes may impact the older adult athlete, necessitating adaptations to training regimens and a realignment of goals, though rarely do these changes completely preclude individuals from meaningful participation.
- This chapter focuses on:
  - The aging demographic of the American population;
  - Normal physiologic and physical changes inherent to aging and their potential impact on the older adult athlete;
  - A general exercise prescription for older adults;
  - Common injuries inherent to the older adult athlete;
  - Medical considerations unique to the older adult athlete.

THE OLDER ATHLETE

- For purposes of discussion, an older athlete will be defined as an individual age 65 years or greater.
- By 2030, approximately 20% of all Americans (70 million) will be age 65 or older and will outnumber the pediatric population.
- The average 75-year-old has three chronic conditions and is on five prescription medications. Exercise has demonstrated positive effects in preventing several chronic diseases and is also an important tool to treat these same conditions (1).
- A sedentary lifestyle is the most prevalent modifiable risk factor for heart disease, a condition present in approximately 50% of individuals aged 55–64, and 65% of those aged 65–74, yet one-third of all men aged 75 or greater and half of all women of the same age report no or limited physical activity (2).
- The number of older adults participating in competitive events continues to increase, outpacing that of younger adults (3).
- For many older adults, the benefits and motivation of sports and athletics shift from competition and cardiovascular fitness to preserving physical, cognitive, and emotional functioning. Preserving function and socialization in late life helps mitigate the direct and indirect costs related to the chronic care of older adults (4,5).

PHYSICAL AND PHYSIOLOGIC CHANGES RELATED TO AGING

- Normal physiologic changes affect nearly every organ system, particularly cardiovascular, musculoskeletal, and pulmonary mechanisms. For the older adult athlete, these changes may manifest as reduced resistance capacity related to sarcopenia, decreased cardiac output from lower achievable maximal heart rate, reduced VO_{2max} in part from diminished pulmonary diffusing capacity, and a tendency toward lower extremity injury related to tendon and joint stiffening. These changes frequently intertwine with common medical comorbidities in older adults such as hypertension, diabetes, hyperlipidemia, and arthritis (see Fig. 129.1).
- The older adult may also cope with aging-associated syndromes such as dementia, depression, disability, falls, incontinence, and frailty. See Table 129.1 for a synopsis of these conditions (6).
- An appreciation of this intersection of normal aging changes, common medical comorbidities, and geriatric syndromes is crucial to assist the aging athlete. Examples of this include:
  - The older postmenopausal female runner who develops incontinence.
  - Delirium manifesting in an older athlete who has just completed a marathon.
  - An older adult athlete with refractory gastro-esophageal reflux that results in malnutrition.
  - The older golfer with hypertension and aortic valvular sclerosis who develops syncope.

PHYSIOLOGIC AND FUNCTIONAL BENEFITS OF EXERCISE

- Some of the physiologic effects of exercise are listed in Table 129.1.

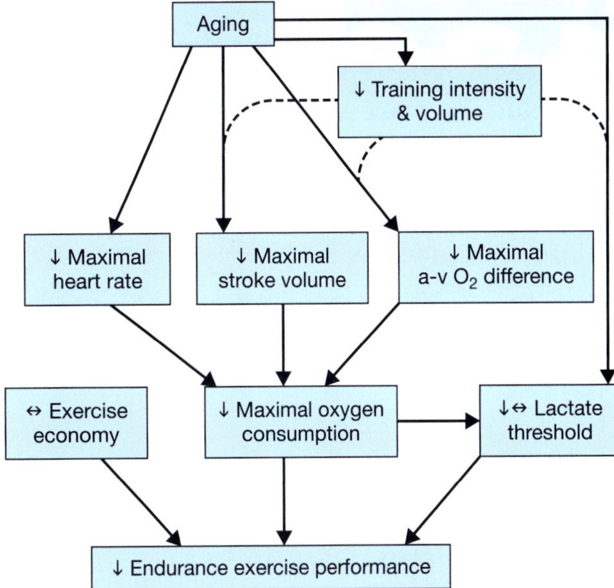

Figure 129.1: Factors and physiological mechanisms contributing to reductions in endurance exercise performance with advancing age in healthy adults. (Reprinted from Tanaka H, Seals DR. Endurance exercise performance in Masters athletes: age-associated changes and underlying physiological mechanisms. *J Physiol*. 2008;586:55–63. https://doi.org/10.1113/jphysiol.2007.141879.)

- Exercise improves body composition and improves the older adult's functional status in addition to imparting direct effects on the heart and muscular system.
  - Exercise increases high-density lipoprotein (HDL) cholesterol levels, lowers low-density lipoprotein (LDL) cholesterol levels, lowers blood pressure, improves insulin sensitivity, and decreases blood coagulability.
  - Direct effects on the heart musculature include increased myocardial oxygen supply, increased myocardial contractility, and electrical stability (6–8).
- Physical *inactivity* is a well-established risk factor for cognitive decline in later life and regular aerobic exercise seems to portend positive impacts on memory and recall, even if adopted in later life (9,10).
  - Exercise increases brain-derived neurotrophic factor (BDNF), a naturally occurring neurotrophic growth factor which has positive cerebrovascular effects within the central nervous system (7,11).
  - Exercise also reduces neurogenic oxidative stress (a pathogenesis postulated to contribute to the development of neurodegenerative disease) by mitigating reactive oxygen species through the induction and upregulation of antioxidant enzymes and by decreasing lipid peroxidation and protein oxidation (10).
  - At moderate intensity, late-life exercise has been shown to increase hippocampal volume, our brain memory storage hub, and to improve spatial memory (12).
  - Sustained exercise in later life improves cognitive processing speed and reaction time, and as such, has been thought to slow cognitive decline and prevent (or at least delay) the development of dementia (13,14).
- Over 20% of adults aged 60 and over suffer from a mental health or neurological disorder and of these, approximately 7% are related to depression and 3.8% are related to anxiety disorders (15).
- One-quarter of deaths from self-harm are among people aged 60 or above. Mood disturbances in later life are in part due to the unique challenges, experiences, and stressors that often accompany later life (such as changes in socioeconomic status, chronic disease states, or loss of a loved one) (15).
  - Physical activity has been shown to improve mental health outcomes throughout one's lifespan. Even low-intensity physical activity can positively impact overall mental health and well-being by improving self-esteem and decreasing anxiety levels (16).

AGE-ASSOCIATED REDUCTIONS IN ENDURANCE EXERCISE PERFORMANCE

- Master athletes are older adults who have strived to preserve or exceed their prior athletic performance and serve as a model to understand the limits to endurance performance with regards to aging.
- Peak athletic performance is maintained to approximately age 35, followed by a gradual decline to age 60, and an accelerated decline thereafter.
- The primary physiologic determinants to endurance exercise performance are exercise economy, lactate threshold, and maximal aerobic capacity (Fig. 129.1).
  - Exercise economy is the steady-state oxygen consumption that occurs during submaximal exercise below the lactate threshold. The exercise economy does not change in master athletes trained for endurance activities, which appears to be a product of the maintained distribution percentage of type I muscle fibers into older age (3).

Table 129.1 Common Conditions and Exercise Effect in Older Adults (6)

Aging-Related Physiologic Changes	Common Co-Morbid Conditions	Common Geriatric Syndromes	Exercise Effects
Cardiovascular: Decreased VO_{2max} Decreased maximal heart rate Decreased maximal cardiac output Rise in systolic blood pressure Widening pulse pressure Increased large artery stiffness Increased fibrosis Decreased innervation Valve fibrosis Myocyte dropout Skeletal muscle Sarcopenia; loss of Type I and II muscle fibers; decreased basal metabolic rate; decreased fiber volume; muscle denervation; decreased mitochondrial volume; increased collagen; decreased flexibility Pulmonary Lower maximal expiratory flows Stable total lung capacity Lower diffusing capacity Increased ventilation/perfusion mismatch (V/Q) Lower respiratory muscle strength Loss of lung elastic recoil Stiffer chest wall Increased airway reactivity Lower respiratory drive Declining PaO_2 to age 65 Bone, ligament, cartilage, meniscus, and tendon Bone: loss of mineral density; "tubularization" of diaphyseal bone Cartilage: chondromalacia; disuse activity with inactivity; Ligaments and tendons: stiffness; increased risk for complete failure; decreased vascularity; Meniscus: degeneration; subject to tears; less stress dissipation Renal Decreased renal blood flow and GFR Age-related glomerulosclerosis Impaired concentrating capacity Impaired sodium preservation Impaired response to vasopressin Decreased thirst perception Decreased total body water Decreased plasma renin and aldosterone production GI: Drug interaction Cholelithiasis Decreased anal sphincter pressure Delayed transit Decreased lower esophageal pressure Dysphagia Hematologic: Decreased hematopoietic response to stress Sensory: Presbyopia Presbycusis Cataracts	Anemia Arthritis Atrial fibrillation Cancer Chronic kidney disease Constipation COPD Diabetes Heart disease Hyperlipidemia Hypertension Osteoporosis Thyroid disorders Vascular disease	Delirium Dementia Depression Dizziness Falls Frailty Health illiteracy Iatrogenic injury Immune deficiency Impairments of IADLs and ADLs Incontinence Infection Insomnia Instability (Falls) Irritable bowels Polypharmacy Pressure ulcers Social isolation Syncope Temperature dysregulation	Cardiovascular: Increased VO_{2max}. No change in MHR. Increased stroke vol. Increase arterial-venous O_2 difference. Reduced mortality from cardiovascular disease and stroke. Decreased risk of: type 2 diabetes, high blood pressure, dyslipidemia, metabolic syndrome, colon and breast cancers. Moderate evidence for decreased risk of lung and endometrial cancers. Metabolic: Prevention of weight gain. Weight loss Weight maintenance after weight loss. Reduced abdominal obesity. Neuromuscular: Increased strength Increased Type I and II fibers. No change in the number of fibers. Increased muscle fiber size and area. Increased muscle oxidative capacity. Increased motor unit function. Fewer falls. Bone and Connective Tissue: Increased bone mass. Increased bone strength. Decreased bone reabsorption. Decreased risk of hip fracture. Mood: Effective in the treatment of depression Enhanced self-efficacy. Cognition: Suggestion of preserved cognition Function: Reduced falls. Improvements in ADL/IADLs. Improved quality of life. Improved sleep quality.

Permission from Micheo, W, Soto-Quijano, DA, Rivera-Tavarez, C, et al. Chapter 38: The geriatric runner. In: O'Connor FG, Wilder RP, Magrum E, editors. *Running Medicine*. Healthy Learning; 2017. p. 681.

- Lactate threshold also does not appear to change with advancing age in master athletes.
- The decrease in maximal aerobic capacity is the primary determinant of decreased endurance exercise performance (17).

PREPARTICIPATION SCREENING OF THE OLDER ATHLETE

- Responsibility for the preparticipation screening first begins with the athlete contacting a healthcare provider for assessment.
- Screening recommendations vary based on the individual's general health, medical comorbidities, and the desired level of activity.
- The clinician should have a clear understanding of the patient's exercise goal and plan for the development of endurance, strength, speed, flexibility, rest, and balance.
- Preparticipation cardiovascular screening includes assessment of:
  - Physical symptoms (fatigability, syncope, falls, dyspnea on exertion, and chest pain)
  - Family history (longevity, premature sudden death, heart disease in surviving relatives)
  - Personal history (heart murmur, hypertension, congenital and valvular heart disease, myocarditis, and Chagas disease)
  - Medications and over-the-counter agents
  - Health habits (alcohol, tobacco, and drug use)
  - Exercise history
  - Work history
  - Physical examination (postural vital signs, heart murmur, femoral pulses, findings of Marfan syndrome)
  - Laboratory findings (plasma glucose, hemoglobin A1C, and lipoprotein analysis).
- Medical evaluation and clearance of the older athlete should be tailored to the individual's characteristics and projected level of physical activity.
- Exercise stress testing may be performed when deemed appropriate (see Chapter 25 exercise stress testing); however, changes may be required in the exercise protocol and methodology in older adults (18,19) (see Table 129.2).
- The preparticipation assessment then focuses on problems identified in the health history.
- Assessment should consider case-by-case screening for common geriatric syndromes such as dementia, depression, and disablement.
- Vision and hearing are important to assess due to their roles in injury prevention, personal safety, and quality of life.
- Older athletes who wear glasses or contacts should consider wearing single-vision lenses to reduce their risk of outdoor falls (20).

Table 129.2 Special Considerations in Exercise Stress Testing for Older Adults

Special Considerations in Exercise Stress Testing for Older Adults
The initial workload should be light (*i.e.*, <3 METs) and workload increments should be small (*i.e.*, 0.5–1.0 MET) for those with low work capacities. The Naughton treadmill protocol is a good example of such a protocol.
A cycle ergometer may be preferable to a treadmill in those with: • Poor balance • Poor neuromotor coordination • Impaired vision • Impaired gait pattern • Weight-bearing limitations • Orthopedic problems Adding a treadmill handrail support may also be required, though note that this will reduce the accuracy of estimating peak MET capacity.
Treadmill workload may need to be adapted according to walking ability by increasing the grade, rather than the speed.
Older adults may exceed the age-predicted HR_{max} during a maximal exercise test. The HR_{max} equation 220-age may underpredict HR_{max} in older adults.
Prescribed medications may influence the ECG and hemodynamic responses to exercise.

Adapted from ACSM's Guidelines for Exercise Testing and Prescription, Eleventh Edition.

- Orthopedic examination should focus on upper and lower extremity joints for pain and limitation in range of motion.
- The neurologic exam should include an assessment of static balance (Romberg testing), and dynamic balance (observation of gait with walking, and ideally with running).
- Physical and occupational therapy can confer significant benefits to individuals with functional limitations, balance problems, and fall risks.

GENERAL EXERCISE PRESCRIPTION FOR THE OLDER RUNNER

- General recommendations for physical activity are presented in Table 129.3 (21).
- Modifications of these general recommendations are taken on a case-by-case basis for the needs of the individual athlete.
- It is important to emphasize the need for muscle-strengthening exercises in older athletes to preserve bone density and muscle mass.
  - Muscle-strengthening exercises should focus on core muscle groups (shoulders, back, chest, arms, abdomen, hips, and legs), and consist of one set of 8–12 repetitions per activity on two or more days a week.
  - More sets may offer additional benefits (21).
- Specific recommendations for balance exercises are presented in the Federal Exercise Guideline.

Table 129.3 General Exercise Prescription for the Older Runner (21)

Minimum activity to achieve health benefits:

- 150 min of moderate-intensity aerobic activity (*e.g.*, brisk walking) a week, plus muscle-strengthening activities at least 2 d a week

Or

- 75 min of vigorous-intensity aerobic activity (*e.g.*, jogging, running) a week, plus muscle-strengthening activities on at least 2 d a week

Or

- A combination of moderate- and vigorous-intensity aerobic activity equivalent to the above recommendations, plus muscle-strengthening exercises at least 2 d a week.

Increased activity for achieving increased health benefits:

- 300 min of moderate-intensity aerobic activity a week, plus muscle-strengthening activities at least 2 d a week.

Or

- 150 min of vigorous-intensity aerobic activity a week, plus muscle-strengthening activities on at least 2 d a week.

Or

- A combination of moderate- to vigorous-intensity aerobic activity equivalent to the above recommendations, plus muscle-strengthening activities on at least 2 d a week.

Physical Activity Guidelines for Americans, 2nd ed. (health.gov); 2018.

- Older adults at risk of falls should do balance training for 3 or more days a week.
  - Examples of these exercises include backwards walking, sideways walking, heel walking, toe-walking, and standing from a sitting position.
  - The exercises can increase in difficulty by progressing from holding onto a stable support (like furniture) while doing the exercises to doing them without support and then to eyes closed.
- Promotion of flexibility via stretching exercises is advised for all major muscle groups, as are warm-up and cool-down activities before all exercise events.
- Stretching should comprise three to five non-painful repetitions of a static stretch for each major muscle group, with each stretch lasting 10–30 seconds.
- A warm-up before moderate- or vigorous-intensity aerobic activity allows a gradual increase in heart rate and breathing at the beginning of the exercise session.
- A cool-down after activity allows a gradual decrease at the end of the episode.
- Time spent doing warm-up and cool-down may count toward meeting the aerobic activity guidelines if the activity is at least moderate intensity.
- The National Institute of Aging offers a free exercise guide for older adults. This guide includes general education, advice on goal setting, sample exercises, nutritional advice, and tracking tools (21).
- ACSM's Guidelines for Exercise Testing and Prescription has specific recommendations for advising older adults in safe exercise (22) (see Table 129.4).

COMMON INJURIES ENCOUNTERED IN OLDER ATHLETES

- Injuries are more common in older adult athletes compared to younger athletes, in part because of changes in biomechanics that accompany age.
- Gait changes common to the older adult athlete, including decreased leg stiffness, shorter stride length, and decreased knee and ankle excursion, can precipitate injuries.
- Older adult athletes are more likely to have experienced an injury in the past year (49% vs. 45%) and are more likely to experience multiple injuries in a given year (30% vs. 24%) (23).

Acute Traumatic Injuries

- Older adults have a lower incidence of acute traumatic injuries than younger adults due to greater experience and lower intensity of exercise performance (24).
- Acute skeletal fractures are uncommon when compared to the acute muscle sprains that older adults manifest within training and competition.
- The muscle-tendon junction is particularly vulnerable to injury, with the most common injuries involving the Achilles and quadriceps tendons.
  - These myotendinous injuries are attributable in part to decreased flexibility and increased muscle fatigue from participation in endurance sports.
  - Extrinsic factors such as training errors, training surface and incorrect shoe choice may also contribute to injury.

Chronic and Overuse Injuries

- Overuse injuries are common in older adult athletes, accounting for 70% of injuries in older athletes.
- These common injuries include stress fractures, focal cartilage injuries, plantar fasciitis, and degenerative meniscal tears.
- Approaches to treatment in the older adult are similar to that of a younger adult, except that healing and recovery are prolonged and that training and competition practices are possibly altered to a greater degree.

Osteoarthritis

- Physical activity itself does not necessarily contribute to the development of degenerative arthritis as an older adult.
- Potential mediating factors including age, sex, body mass index, body composition, and muscle strength that may contribute to its development (23).
- The development of osteoarthritis is more closely related to previous joint injury, training intensity, occupational

Table 129.4 FITT Recommendations for Older Adults

FITT	FITT Recommendations for Older Adults		
	Aerobic	**Resistance**	**Flexibility**
Frequency	$\geq$5 d · wk^{-1} for moderate intensity. $\geq$3 d · wk^{-1} for vigorous intensity. 3–5 d · wk^{-1} for a combination of moderate and vigorous-intensity.	$\geq$2 d · wk^{-1}	$\geq$2 d · wk^{-1}
Intensity	On a scale of 0–10 for the level of physical exertion: ➢ 5–6 for moderate intensity. ➢ 7–8 for vigorous intensity.	*Progressive weight training:* Light intensity (*i.e.* 40%–50% 1-RM) for beginners; progress to moderate-to-vigorous intensity (60%–80% 1-RM); alternatively, moderate (5,6) to vigorous (7,8) intensity on a 0–10 scale. *Power training:* Light-to-moderate loading (30%–60% of 1-RM)	Stretch to the point of feeling tightness or slight discomfort
Time	30–60 min · d^{-1} of moderate-intensity exercise; 20–30 min · d^{-1} of vigorous-intensity exercise Or An equivalent combination of moderate and vigorous exercise may be accumulated over the day.	*Progressive weight training:* 8–10 exercises involving the major muscle groups; $\geq$1 set of 10–15 repetitions for beginners, progress to 1–3 sets of 8–12 repetitions for exercise. *Power training:* 6–10 repetitions with high velocity	Hold stretch for 30–60 s
Type	Any modality that does not impose excessive orthopedic stress such as walking. Aquatic and stationary cycle exercise may be advantageous for those with limited tolerance for weight-bearing activity.	Progressive or power weight-training programs or weight-bearing calisthenics, stair climbing, and other strengthening activities that use the major muscle groups.	Any physical activities that maintain or increase flexibility using slow movements that terminate in static stretches for each muscle group rather than rapid ballistic movements.

1- RM: one repetition max.
Adapted from ACSM's Guidelines for Exercise Testing and Prescription, Eleventh Edition.

stresses, altered biomechanics, quadriceps muscle weakness, and incomplete rehabilitation (3,25).

- The evidence for using exercise as an effective treatment for osteoarthritis is well-established.
  - The MOVE! Weight Management Program consensus showed that both strengthening and aerobic exercise can reduce pain and improve function in individuals with hip and knee osteoarthritis (OA) (25).
  - These benefits are conferred through improved biomechanics and more stable loading of the knee over time (26).
- Various forms of conservative treatments can have positive impacts on modifiable risk factors affecting the exercising older adults with osteoarthritis.
- Treatment modalities include oral and topical medications (acetaminophen for mild OA, nonsteroidal anti-inflammatory medications for moderate-severe OA), ice massage (20 minutes, 5 days a week for 3 weeks), knee bracing, and isometric strengthening, and improved flexibility (27).

REHABILITATION AND RECOVERY

- The ideal strategy for injury recovery is injury prevention.
- Resistance training is vital to injury prevention.
- In a large meta-analysis, strength training was found to reduce the risk of overuse injury by 50% (28).
- In older athletes, strength training confers positive benefits to skeletal musculature at moderate to heavy weights with a dose of two to three sessions weekly at two to three sets per exercise with seven to nine repetitions per set (29).

NUTRITION

- Aging is associated with reductions in all components of energy expenditure (resting metabolic rate, thermic effect of food, and energy expenditure).
- Masters-level athletes may have unique nutritional needs, but little data exists on the nutritional needs of older athletes, and nutritional needs are determined by training intensity (30).
- Carbohydrate intake can be estimated as a percentage of total calories (45%–65%). Needs may also be estimated by grams per kilogram of body weight and level of training intensity.
  - For general training, 5–7 g · kg^{-1} · d^{-1} of carbohydrates are needed. Endurance athletes require 7–10 g · kg^{-1} · d^{-1}, and ultraendurance athletes need more than 10 g · kg^{-1} · d^{-1}. Thirty to Sixty grams of carbohydrates should be consumed for every hour of training.

- If training occurs daily, recovery from vigorous exercise is enhanced by 1.5 g/kg ingestion of carbohydrate immediately after exercise, and an additional carbohydrate feeding 2 hours later (31).

- Protein ingestion for older adults matches that of younger adults and should be greater than 1.2 $g \cdot kg^{-1} \cdot d^{-1}$.
  - Higher protein consumption should occur in resistance exercise (a daily target of 1.5–1.6 $g \cdot kg^{-1} \cdot d^{-1}$) and 1.6–1.8 $g \cdot kg^{-1} \cdot d^{-1}$ in endurance athletes.
  - Whole-food, high-quality protein sources are optimal and may be broadly distributed through the day.
- Fat intake should involve 20%–35% of total calories.
  - There is no demonstrated benefit to low-fat diets for athletes, and therefore the American Dietetic Association recommends that athletes do not restrict fat intake.
  - Monounsaturated and long-chain polyunsaturated fats ("heart healthy fats") are recommended.
- Little research on micronutrient intake has been performed on master-level athletes to determine optimal amounts.
  - Nutritional requirements for thiamine, riboflavin, choline, zinc and magnesium do not appear to be different in older vs. younger adults.
  - Further research is needed to address antioxidant requirements to offset the increased oxidative stress associated with aging.
  - No evidence suggests additional Vitamin C requirements in athletes, and the tolerable upper intake level (UL) is 2000 $mg \cdot d^{-1}$ for this vitamin.
  - Athletes taking supplements should adhere to the ULs of all vitamins and minerals to prevent toxicity.
  - Ideally, whole foods are the preferred source of micronutrients, but research has shown that athletes often do not meet Recommended Daily Allowances (RDAs) through their diet (31).

OSTEOPOROSIS

- Exercise is important in both the treatment and prevention of osteoporosis — defined as the bone mass loss of 2.5 standard deviations below that of a young adult female.
- Type I osteoporosis is a condition of postmenopausal women affecting trabecular bone. Fractures of the thoracic and upper-lumbar vertebrae and wrist are common with this condition.
- Type II osteoporosis affects both genders and is due to age-associated loss of cortical bone, such as the hip and femoral neck.
- Osteoporosis is either primary (due to aging), or secondary to an identifiable cause. Identification of secondary causes of osteoporosis is critical to prevent (and reverse) further bone loss.
- Prevention and treatment of osteoporosis is multi-faceted and includes weight-bearing exercises such as walking or running

FLUID REPLACEMENT

- Healthy older adults are generally adequately hydrated but have a blunted thirst response when deprived of water. This results in an increased risk of becoming dehydrated.
- Older adults also have an age-associated increase in plasma osmolality and are slower in achieving homeostasis after dehydration.
- Complicating this is that older adults are slower to excrete water and sodium following fluid loads, resulting in possible increases in blood pressure or the development of hyponatremia.
- Given sufficient time and access to fluids, older adults are able to appropriately rehydrate and should be encouraged to do so during and after exercise.
- Excessive fluid or sodium ingestion is inadvisable.
- Body weight changes can be used to calculate individual fluid replacement needs, with euhydration reflecting a weight within 1% of baseline readings. Urine specific gravity measurements of <1.020 likely reflect euhydration (32).

TEMPERATURE REGULATION

- Older adults deal with heat (and cold) challenges differently from younger adults in several ways.
- Heat stress in older adults results in higher core temperatures, heart rate and fluid losses, and lower sweating rates.
- Cold exposure is associated with blunted vasoconstrictor response and greater loss of heat in older adults.
- These observed physiologic phenomena are related to age, medical comorbidities, lifestyle choices, medications, acclimatization, and physical conditioning.
- Longitudinal studies of thermoregulation in aging athletes are lacking.
- Physicians should identify older athletes with these risk factors in common sense actions to reduce their risk of heat or cold-related injury (see Table 129.5) (33).

JOINT REPLACEMENT

- The rate of joint arthroplasty is expected to dramatically increase in the United States over the next 20 years due to the success of these procedures, and the demands of the "baby boomer" population.

Table 129.5 General Strategies for Prevention of Heat and Cold-Related Injuries (33)

Appropriate clothing for temperature
Adequate fluid intake and nutrition
Adequate sleep
Not running when acutely ill with viral illness or diarrhea
Avoidance of sunburn
Acclimatization for 10–14 d in the Heat
A running partner to monitor each other's wellbeing
Avoidance of temperature extremes
Recognition of early symptoms of heat/cold injury (clumsiness, stumbling, headache, nausea, dizziness, apathy, confusion, and altered consciousness)
Regular clinician monitoring of overall health and medication regimen.

American College of Sports Medicine Position Stand. Exertional heat illness during training and competition. *Med Sci Sports Exer.* 2007;39(3):556–72.

- Individuals decrease the number or intensity of athletic activities after joint replacement. However, there are no controlled studies evaluating appropriate athletic activities after joint replacement.
- Expert opinions from the American Association of Hip and Knee Surgeons (AAHKS), the Knee Society, and the Hip Society suggest imploring low-impact aerobic activities (including stationary cycling, dancing, golf, normal walking, speed walking and hiking). Skating, skiing, horseback riding, and weightlifting exercises are permissible if the patient has prior experience with these activities. Jogging, football, basketball, soccer, and volleyball are specifically not recommended (see Chapter 134: The Athlete with a Total Joint for further discussion).
- Stretching and strengthening of core muscles, along with back, hip and knee rehabilitation are felt to improve athletic performance after joint replacement (34).

SUMMARY

- Despite the physiologic changes that accompany aging, older adults remain capable of remaining physically active and should be encouraged to do so.
- Physical activity in older adulthood provides opportunities for continued physical health benefits, socialization, and improved mental health and well-being.
- Unique circumstances should be considered when counseling an older adult on physical activity, including fall risk, visual impairment, urinary incontinence, and joint replacement status.

REFERENCES

1. Tanaka H, Seals DR. Invited review: dynamic exercise performance in Masters athletes. Insight into the effects of primary human aging on physiological functional capacity. *J Appl Physiol.* 2003;95(5):2152–62.
2. Rodgers JL, Jones J, Bolleddu SI, et al. Cardiovascular risks associated with gender and aging. *J Cardiovasc Dev Dis.* 2019 Apr 27;6(2):19.
3. Tanaka H, Seals DR. Endurance exercise performance in Masters athletes: age associated changes and underlying physiological mechanisms. *J Physio.* 2008;586(1):55–63.
4. León-Guereño P, Galindo-Domínguez H, Balerdi-Eizmendi E, Rozmiarek M, Malchrowicz-Mośko E. Motivation behind running among older adult runners. *BMC Sports Sci Med Rehabil.* 2021 Oct 29;13(1):138.
5. Lee DC, Pate RR, Lavie CJ, Sui X, Church TS, Blair SN. Leisure-time running reduces all-cause and cardiovascular mortality risk. *J Am Coll Cardiol.* 2014 Aug 5;64(5):472–81.
6. Micheo W, Soto-Quijano DA, Rivera-Tavarez C, et al. Chapter 35: the geriatric runner. In: O'Connor FG, Wilder RP, editors. *Textbook of Running Medicine.* New York: McGraw-Hill Professional Publishing; 2001.
7. Spirduso WW, Clifford P. Replication of age and physical activity effects on reaction and movement time. *J Gerontol.* 1978 Jan;33(1):26–30.
8. Stessman J, Hammerman-Rozenberg R, Cohen A, Ein-Mor E, Jacobs JM. Physical activity, function, and longevity among the very old. *Arch Int Med.* 2009;169(16):1476–83.
9. Laurin D, Verreault R, Lindsay J, MacPherson K, Rockwood K. Physical activity and risk of cognitive impairment and dementia in elderly persons. *Arch Neurol.* 2001 Mar;58(3):498–504.
10. Radak Z, Hart N, Sarga L, et al. Exercise plays a preventive role against Alzheimer's disease. *J Alzheimers Dis.* 2010;20(3):777–83.
11. Blurton-Jones M, Kitazawa M, Martinez-Coria H, et al. Neural stem cells improve cognition via BDNF in a transgenic model of Alzheimer disease. *Proc Natl Acad Sci U S A.* 2009 Aug 11;106(32):13594–9.
12. Erickson KI, Voss MW, Prakash RS, et al. Exercise training increases size of hippocampus and improves memory. *Proc Natl Acad Sci U S A.* 2011 Feb 15;108(7):3017–22.
13. Middleton LE, Barnes DE, Li LY, et al. Physical activity over the life course and its association with cognitive performance and impairment in old age. *J Am Geriat Soc.* 2010;58:1322–6.
14. Rikli RE, Edwards DJ. Effects of a three-year exercise program on motor function and cognitive processing speed in older women. *Res Q Exerc Sport.* 1991 Mar;62(1):61–7.
15. *Mental Health of Older Adults.* 2017. https://www.who.int/news-room/fact-sheets/detail/mental-health-of-older-adults
16. Oswald F, Campbell J, Williamson C, Richards J, Kelly P. A scoping review of the relationship between running and mental health. *Int J Environ Res Public Health.* 2020 Nov 1;17(21):8059.
17. Jakovljevic DG. Physical activity and cardiovascular aging: physiological and molecular insights. *Exp Gerontol.* 2018;109:67–74.
18. Riebe D, Franklin BA, Thompson PD, et al. Updating ACSM's recommendations for exercise preparticipation health screening. *Med Sci Sports Exerc.* 2015;47(11):2473–9.
19. Borjesson M, Urhausen A, Kouidi E, et al. Cardiovascular evaluation of middle-aged/senior individuals engaged in leisure-time sport activities: position stand from the sections of exercise physiology and sports cardiology of the European Association of Cardiovascular Prevention and Rehabilitation. *Eur J Cardiovasc Prev Rehabil.* 2011;18(3):446–58.
20. Haran MJ, Cameron ID, Ivers RQ, et al. Effect on falls of single lens distance vision glasses to multifocal glasses wearers: VISABLE randomized controlled trial. *BMJ.* 2010;340:2265.
21. *Physical Activity Guidelines for Americans,* 2nd ed. (health.gov); 2018.
22. American College of Sports Medicine. *ACSM's Guidelines for Exercise Testing and Prescription.* 11th ed. Baltimore (MD): Wolters Kluwer; 2022. p. 177.

23. Wang BWE, Ramey DR, Schettler J, Hubert HB, Fries JF. Postponed development of disability in elderly runners: a 13-year longitudinal study. *Arch Intern Med.* 2002;162(20):2285–94.
24. Chen AL, Mears SC, Hawkins RJ. Orthopaedic care of the aging athlete. *J Am Acad Orthop Surg.* 2005;13(6):407–16.
25. Roddy E, Zhang W, Doherty M, et al. Evidence-based recommendations for the role of exercise in the management of osteoarthritis of the hip or knee--the MOVE consensus. *Rheumatology.* 2005;44(1):67–73.
26. Hafer JF, Kent JA, Boyer KA. Physical activity and age-related biomechanical risk factors for knee osteoarthritis. *Gait Posture.* 2019 May;70:24–9.
27. Castillo B, Sepúlveda F, Micheo W. Conservative management and rehabilitation in the older runner with knee osteoarthritis: an evidence-based review. *Am J Phys Med Rehabil.* 2019 May;98(5):416–21.
28. Lauersen JB, Bertelsen DM, Andersen LB. The effectiveness of exercise interventions to prevent sports injuries: a systematic review and meta-analysis of randomised controlled trials. *Br J Sports Med.* 2014 Jun;48(11):871–7.
29. Borde R, Hortobágyi T, Granacher U. Dose-response relationships of resistance training in healthy old adults: a systematic review and meta-analysis. *Sports Med.* 2015 Dec;45(12):1693–720.
30. Rosenbloom CA, Dunaway A. Nutrition recommendations for masters athletes. *Clin Sports Med.* 2007;26(1):91–100.
31. Desbrow B, Burd NA, Tarnopolsky M, Moore DR, Elliott-Sale KJ. Nutrition for special populations: young, female, and masters athletes. *Int J Sport Nutr Exerc Metab.* 2019;29(2):220–7.
32. American College of Sports Medicine, Sawka MN, Burke LM, Eichner ER, et al. American College of Sports Medicine position stand. Exercise and fluid replacement. *Med Sci Sports Exerc.* 2007;39(2):377–90.
33. American College of Sports Medicine, Armstrong LE, Casa DJ, Millard-Stafford M, et al. American College of Sports Medicine position stand. Exertional heat illness during training and competition. *Med Sci Sports Exerc.* 2007;39(3):556–72.
34. Healy WL, Sharma S, Schwartz B, Iorio R. Current concepts review: athletic activity after total joint arthroplasty. *J Bone Joint Surg Am.* 2008;90(10):2245–52.

The Transgender Athlete

130

Kathryn E. Ackerman

INTRODUCTION

- Sex and gender are multidimensional, complex constructs that are interrelated, but distinct. While most of the world's population falls into binary categories of sex (female or male) and gender (woman or man), and these categories typically have sex and gender alignment (*i.e.*, female woman and male man, cisgender), a minority of the population does not fall into such categories.
- Transgender and gender-diverse (TGD) people face significant challenges, with higher rates of mental health concerns, social isolation, negative self-image, substance abuse, physical health issues, educational barriers, poor access to health care, homelessness, and structural violence (1).
- Further, there is considerable debate and confusion regarding policies for TGD inclusion in sport, adding to the focus on, harassment of, and stress of TGD people, all of which can de-incentivize them from participating in physical activity (2). Regardless of changing political landscapes and policies, it is important for the sports medicine community to learn more about the TGD population and how to be a resource for information and appropriate medical care.

DEFINITIONS

- Please note that terminology evolves rapidly. The below terms and definitions are presently acceptable, but there may be other, preferred terms for individual people currently and in the future.
- **Biological sex:** A construct based on various anatomical and physiological traits (sex traits), including sex chromosomes, gonads, external genitalia, sex hormones, and secondary sex characteristics.
  - Typically "female" or "male."
  - Usually assigned at birth based on the appearance of external genitalia.
  - Sex traits are usually (but not always) unambiguous and correspond to the same sex.
  - There are some minority populations whose sex traits do not match the assigned sex at birth (ASAB), change over time, and/or do not correspond to a single sex (*e.g.*, intersex, differences in sexual development).
- **Gender:** A psychosocial construct involving gender identity and expression, as well as social/cultural aspects pertaining to characteristics and behaviors that are associated with sex traits.
  - Can change over time
  - **Cisgender:** gender identity that corresponds to ASAB
  - **Transgender:** gender identity that differs from ASAB
    - **Transgender woman/transfemme:** assigned male at birth (AMAB), but identifies and lives as a woman
    - **Transgender man/transmasculine:** assigned female at birth (AFAB), but identifies and lives as a man
  - **Gender diverse:** gender identity that differs from social/cultural expectations typical of their ASAB and does not fall within the binary of woman or man.
    - Includes those who are nonbinary, gender expansive, gender nonconforming, and others who do not identify as cisgender.
- **Gender transition:** The process of changing a person's social, physical, and/or legal identity characteristics consistent with their gender identity.
  - **Social transition:** The process of disclosing a gender identity to friends, family, and others that is different from the gender or sex assigned at birth (*i.e.*, "coming out") or a change in gender expression (*e.g.*, clothing, hair, make-up).
  - **Medical transition:** Using a hormone or medication to achieve physical characteristics of a different gender. This may include 'blockers,' typically a gonadotropin-releasing hormone analog to halt the progression of secondary sexual characteristics that do not align with gender identity. Typically, a medical transition consists of using hormones to induce a physical appearance more in keeping with one's gender identity.
  - **Legal transition:** Changing one's gender and/or name on legal identification documents (*e.g.*, birth certificate, driver's license, passport) (3).
- Further definitions can be found elsewhere (3,4).

PREVALENCE

- Because of differences in recognition and acceptance of TGD people in different countries and regions, global population estimates are difficult to determine.

- There are an estimated 1.6 million TGD people in the United States, including 0.5% (1.3 million) of the US adult population and 1.4% (300,000) of US youth ages 13–17 years (5).

MEDICAL CONSIDERATIONS

Diagnosis

- The 2013 *Diagnostic and Statistical Manual of Mental Disorders*, 5th edition (DSM-5), eliminated the diagnosis "gender identity disorder" and coined the term "gender dysphoria (GD)." This allows a diagnostic description (*i.e.*, GD) for the mental distress that some TGD people may experience when their gender identity is incongruent with their ASAB, but removes pathologizing gender/sex incongruence as a mental disorder (6). Some have recommended also removing GD from the next DSM to further minimize stigma.

Treatment

- As above, there are social, legal, medical, and surgical choices involved in gender affirmation, and each TGD person decides which of these to pursue. Not all TGD people desire medical and surgical treatment and of those who do, not all have access to these services for various reasons.
  - **Children:** Major medical societies, including the Endocrine Society, recommend against pubertal blockade and gender-affirming hormone treatment (GAHT) in *prepubertal (i.e., have not yet reached Tanner Stage 2 development)* children with gender incongruence (7). Thus, treatment primarily involves mental health services and social support.
  - **Adolescents:** If medical treatment criteria are met, pubertal suppression is often the first step and begins after puberty has already begun (*i.e.*, Tanner Stage 2 or 3 for birth-assigned females and 2 or higher for birth-assigned males) (8).
    - **Pubertal suppression:** In the United States, gonadotropin-releasing hormone analogs are often used, although in other countries, forms of progesterone may also be considered.
    - **GAHT:** It is recommended that an adolescent be supported by a multidisciplinary team of medical and mental health specialists to guide care.
      - Treatment goals are to induce physical changes that align with gender identity and eventually maintain hormone levels in the physiological range of the experienced gender.
      - Criteria for initiation include persistent, well-documented gender incongruence, mental capacity to make an informed decision, and adequate management of pertinent mental and medical health issues.
      - Sex hormones are provided in gradual, increasing doses.
      - Monitoring occurs every 3–6 months.
      - If under the age of 18 years, parental/guardian consent must be obtained.
  - **Adults:** Assessment of hormonal phase of gender transition, as well as coexisting medical conditions that may be affected by hormonal treatment, is needed prior to initiating GAHT.
    - **GAHT:** Similar mental and medical assessment as above, with additional attention to medical comorbidities.
  - **GAHT for transgender women** (7)**:** Goal is to suppress testosterone and give estrogen to promote female secondary sex characteristics.
    - **Feminization via estrogens:**
      - 17-β-estradiol is the most commonly prescribed estrogen (transdermal patch changed every 3–5 days, daily topical gel, or daily oral pill). The dosage depends on the route of administration.
      - The parenteral estrogens estradiol valerate and cypionate can be given intramuscularly every 2 weeks. Many people use this in a lower dose subcutaneously on a weekly basis.
      - Ethinyl estradiol is no longer recommended because of higher venous thrombotic event (VTE) risk.
      - Treatment with conjugated estrogens is challenging to monitor as commercial estradiol assays cannot detect their levels.
      - **Estrogen treatment risks:**
        - VTE
        - Breast cancer
        - Coronary artery disease (CAD)
        - Cerebrovascular disease (CVD)
        - Cholelithiasis
        - Hypertriglyceridemia
    - **Testosterone suppression:**
      - Preferred treatments:
        - Spironolactone: 100–300 mg/daily orally.
        - Cyproterone acetate (CPA): A progestin with antiandrogen properties; unavailable in the United States, but commonly used in other countries; dosage is 25–100 mg/daily orally.
      - Alternative treatments:
        - GnRH agonist:
          - Suppresses testosterone production by inhibiting gonadotropin secretion
          - Delivery: injection, implant
          - More expensive than both spironolactone and CPA, and thus not a preferred treatment
    - Monitoring should occur with every dosage modification. A typical monitoring schedule is ~4 times

per year for the first year and 1–2 times per year thereafter.
  - Treatment is generally lifelong.
- **GAHT for transgender men:** Goal is to stop menses and enable male secondary sex characteristics. This is obtained via administration of testosterone as monotherapy.
  - **Masculinization: testosterones**
    - Testosterone enanthate or testosterone cypionate are the most commonly prescribed testosterone formulations (intramuscular or subcutaneous).
      - Subcutaneous is not presently approved by the Food and Drug Administration in the United States but is utilized commonly in the United States and elsewhere.
    - Testosterone gel can also be used, though virilization may be slower due to inconsistent absorption and variable serum testosterone concentrations.
      - Some recommend switching to gels once masculinization is complete to avoid supraphysiologic concentrations of testosterone.
    - Other testosterone types and delivery methods exist, with oral testosterone undecanoate and subcutaneous testosterone pellets increasingly popular options.
    - **Testosterone treatment risks:**
      - Erythrocytosis (hematocrit >50%)
      - Liver dysfunction
      - CAD
      - CVD
      - Hypertension
      - Breast or uterine cancer
    - Alkylated androgens (*e.g.*, 17-α-methyl testosterone), dihydrotestosterone, and compounded testosterone should not be utilized.
  - Monitoring should occur with every dosage modification. A typical monitoring schedule is ~4 times per year for the first year and 1–2 times per year thereafter.
  - Treatment is generally lifelong.

Other Treatments

- In addition to or instead of GAHT, transgender men and women may engage in additional practices/treatments. Examples include:
  - **Gender-affirming surgery**
    - Masculinizing procedures:
      - **Top surgery:** mastectomy, chest wall reconstruction
      - **Bottom surgery:** hysterectomy, salpingo-oophorectomy, vaginectomy, phalloplasty, metoidioplasty, scrotoplasty, testicular prosthetic insertion
        - *Patients are generally only considered eligible after >1 year of GAHT* (7).
    - Feminizing procedures:
      - **Top surgery:** breast augmentation
      - **Bottom surgery:** penectomy, orchiectomy, clitoroplasty, labiaplasty, vaginoplasty
        - *Patients are generally only considered eligible after >1 year of GAHT* (7).
- **Hair removal**
- **Facial surgery**
- **Binding** (to minimize appearance of breasts in birth-assigned females)
- **Tucking** (to minimize appearance of genitals in birth-assigned males)

FEMALE VERSUS MALE SPORTS PERFORMANCE

- There are myriad **physiological contributors** to sports performance success. These include, but are not limited to:
  - Muscle force and power production
  - Anthropometric characteristics
  - Cardiorespiratory function
  - Metabolic factors
- **The above factors generally differ significantly between females and males**, partially because:
  - Many **genes are expressed differently** in the two sexes (the case for ~6500 genes).
  - **Androgens have significant influence** over such physiological contributors.
  - In utero, and more profoundly during puberty and beyond, testosterone exposure is greater in males versus females. **Testosterone increases by 2000% in males at puberty**, with 15 times greater testosterone concentrations in males versus females thereafter.
- Sports performances differ between females and males depending on developmental stage and sport.
  - Prepubertal differences exist but are much more pronounced after puberty.
  - At the adult, elite level, the performance gap is ~10%–50% between the sexes depending on the sport (9).

Differences in Sports Performance After Initiation of GAHT

- No longitudinal sports performance studies have been performed in transgender athletes.
- A systematic review of 24 studies examining the effects of **testosterone-suppressing GAHT on physiological parameters** that could influence sports performance in transwomen found:
  - **Hemoglobin/hematocrit concentrations dropped to levels comparable to those of cisgender women** (after 4 months of GAHT).

- **Strength, lean body mass, and muscle area dropped** (after 12 months of GAHT), **but not to the levels of cisgender women** (even after 36 months of GAHT) (10).

TRANSGENDER SPORT INCLUSION POLICIES

- To date, TGD sport inclusion policies differ by state, country, specific sport, and participation level. Policies are rapidly changing; it is therefore important for practitioners to be aware of the latest rules that may impact the TGD athletes to whom they provide care. Below are some examples that illustrate the range of regulations presently.
- **National Collegiate Athletic Association (NCAA)** (11)
  - Beginning in February 2025, The NCAA limited competition in women's sports categories to only AFAB athletes, aligning with US Executive Order 14201 (12). The NCAA policy permits TGD athletes AMAB to practice with women's teams and receive medical care.
- **United State Olympic and Paralympic Committee (USOPC)** (13)
  - In July 2025, the USOPC acknowledged that it had updated its eligibility rules and was banning transgender women from participation in Olympic women's sports by complying with federal expectations.
- **International Olympic Committee (IOC)** (14)
  - In 2021, the IOC published a framework intended to support governing bodies in the creation of policies, emphasizing the need to balance inclusion of trans athletes, fairness, and harm prevention.
  - Deferred policy development to each sport's corresponding international federation.
- **International Sport Federations**
  - At the publication of this chapter, numerous sports organizations are actively changing their TGD inclusion policies. Present policies range from testosterone cutoff levels in TGD women to testing all women participants for absence of the SRY gene. (The SRY gene encodes the male sex-determining region Y protein typically located on the Y chromosome).

PREPARTICIPATION EXAMINATION CONSIDERATIONS

- As with any patient, it is important to respect the privacy of TGD athletes.
- Learning an athlete's ASAB and their pronouns allows the sports medicine provider an opening to discuss pertinent TGD-related topics (*e.g.*, sports policies, medications, therapeutic use exemptions [TUEs], uniform concerns, locker room questions, gender and ASAB privacy issues).
- Being familiar with the athlete's stage of transition and providing a safe venue to discuss possible medical, surgical, and mental health side effects is important.
- Otherwise the preparticipation examination should be conducted as suggested by the ACSM-endorsed *Preparticipation Physical Evaluation*, 5th ed. (15).

THERAPEUTIC USE EXEMPTIONS

- TUEs are required for athletes being treated with substances on the prohibited substance list. A TUE can only be granted to an athlete eligible to compete in their respective sport, as determined by the appropriate governing body. To obtain a TUE, a medical report must be included in the application (16).
- Policies and the prohibited substance list are frequently updated. Thus, providers involved in the treatment and medical management of transgender athletes must consult the most recent policies. The following discussion outlines TUE considerations for commonly utilized GAHT at the time of publication (16):
  - Transgender females:
    - Estrogen: not a prohibited substance.
    - Spironolactone: requires a TUE.
    - GnRH analogues: only prohibited in athletes participating in a male category. Thus, if a transgender woman is eligible to compete in the "female" category in their respective sport, a TUE is not required.
  - Transgender men:
    - All forms of testosterone are prohibited substances and require a TUE.

FUTURE DIRECTIONS

- As our understanding of the biology and needs of TGD athletes expands, policies, treatments, and best practices are likely to change.
- Additional research, in the form of well-controlled, longitudinal studies, is needed to better understand the effects of gender-affirming care at different stages of the lifespan on physiology, as well as the implications for specific sporting disciplines.

REFERENCES

1. Kuper LE, Mathews S, Lau M. Baseline mental health and psychosocial functioning of transgender adolescents seeking gender-affirming hormone therapy. *J Dev Behav Pediatr*. 2019;40(8):589–96.
2. Kroshus E, Ackerman KE, Brown M, et al. Improving inclusion and well-being of trans and gender nonconforming collegiate student-athletes: foundational concepts from the National Collegiate athletic

association Summit on gender identity and student-athlete participation. *Br J Sports Med.* 2023;57(10):564–70.

3. National Academies of Sciences E, Medicine, Division of B, Social S, Education, Committee on National S, et al. The National Academies Collection: Reports funded by National Institutes of Health. In: Becker T, Chin M, Bates N, editors. *Measuring Sex, Gender Identity, and Sexual Orientation. The National Academies Collection: Reports funded by National Institutes of Health.* Washington (DC): National Academies Press (US); 2022. Copyright 2022 by the National Academy of Sciences. All rights reserved.
4. Transathlete.com Powered by @TheChrisMosier. Available from: https://www.transathlete.com. Accessed August 11, 2025.
5. Herman JL, Flores AR, O'Neill KK. *How Many Adults and Youth Identify as Transgender in the United States?* UCLA School of Law, Williams Institute; 2022.
6. American Psychiatric Association. *Diagnostic and Statistical Manual of Mental Disorders.* 5th ed. American Psychiatric Association; 2022.
7. Hembree WC, Cohen-Kettenis PT, Gooren L, et al. Endocrine treatment of gender-dysphoric/gender-incongruent persons: an endocrine society clinical practice guideline. *J Clin Endocrinol Metab.* 2017;102(11):3869–903.
8. Coleman E, Radix AE, Bouman WP, et al. Standards of care for the health of transgender and gender diverse people, version 8. *Int J Transgend Health.* 2022;23(suppl 1):S1–259.
9. Hilton EN, Lundberg TR. Transgender women in the female category of sport: perspectives on testosterone suppression and performance advantage. *Sports Med.* 2021;51(2):199–214.
10. Harper J, O'Donnell E, Sorouri Khorashad B, McDermott H, Witcomb GL. How does hormone transition in transgender women change body composition, muscle strength and haemoglobin? Systematic review with a focus on the implications for sport participation. *Br J Sports Med.* 2021;55(15):865–72.
11. NCAA announces transgender student-athlete participation policy change. Available from: https://www.ncaa.org/news/2025/2/6/media-center-ncaa-announces-transgender-student-athlete-participation-policy-change.aspx. Accessed August 11, 2025.
12. Executive Order 14201—Keeping Men Out of Women's Sports. Available from: https://www.presidency.ucsb.edu/documents/executive-order-14201-keeping-men-out-womens-sports. Accessed August 11, 2025.
13. U.S. Olympic officials change policy, ban transgender women from women's competitions; 2025. Available from: https://www.nytimes.com/athletic/6509733/2025/07/22/usopc-olympics-transgender-policy/
14. International Olympic Committee. IOC framework on Fairness, inclusion and Non-Discrimination on the basis of gender identity and sex variations. Available from: https://stillmed.olympics.com/media/Documents/News/2021/11/IOC-Framework-Fairness-Inclusion-Non-discrimination-2021.pdf?_ga=2.161647740.1701831780.1662638218-1095681707.1646126407. Accessed August 11, 2025.
15. *American Academy of Family Physicians, American Academy of Pediatrics, American Medical Society for Sports Medicine, American Orthopedic Society for Sports Medicine, and American Osteopathic Academy of Sports Medicine. Preparticipation Physical Evaluation.* 5th ed. Elk Grove (IL): American Academy of Pediatrics; 2019.
16. *TUE Physician Guidelines – Transgender Athletes.* WADA; 2022. Available from: https://www.wada-ama.org/en/resources/therapeutic-use-exemption/tue-physician-guidelines-transgender-athletes

131 The Female Athlete

Denise Torbert and Rochelle M. Nolte

INTRODUCTION

- In 1971, there were fewer than 300,000 girls participating in high school athletics, compared to 3.7 million boys. Title IX was passed in 1972, mandating nondiscrimination in all extracurricular activities and varsity athletics that received federal funding. In 2018, there were 3.4 million girls involved in high school sports compared to 4.5 million boys (1).
- Benefits of exercise for women include improved physical and mental health, improved sleep and physical function, improved pregnancy outcomes, and quality of life. Despite this, less than 20% of U.S. women achieve the recommended amount of leisure-time physical activity (2).
- Pregnant women should get 30 minutes of light to moderate activity at least 5 $d \cdot wk^{-1}$. The majority of women are insufficiently active during pregnancy, with a higher prepregnancy body mass index (BMI) being a risk factor for an even lower level of physical activity (3).
- The syndrome of relative energy deficiency in sport (RED-S) refers to impaired physiologic function caused by relative energy deficiency and includes, but is not limited to, impairments of metabolic rate, menstrual function, bone health, immunity, protein synthesis, and cardiovascular health described in the context of low energy availability (LEA) (4–6).

ANATOMY AND PHYSIOLOGY

- Peak height velocity usually occurs at age 10–11 in girls (during Tanner Stage 3), compared to age 12–16 in boys (7).
- Menarche occurs during Tanner Stage 4, and girls usually only grow an additional few centimeters in height after menarche.
- Epiphyseal fusion is complete at age 13.81 with 95% CI 11.40–16.62 in girls compared to 16.62 with 95% CI 14.20–18.24 in boys (8).
- Women, on average, have a wider pelvis, more narrow shoulders, an increased carrying angle at the elbow, and an increased Q angle at the knee compared to men (9).
- Women have about 2/3 the skeletal muscle mass of their male counterparts, with 6%–12% higher body fat on average (10).
- Girls do not have as much androgenic stimulation of the bone marrow as boys during adolescence, leading to a lower hematocrit by about 12% (7).
- Women have a smaller blood volume, smaller thoracic cavity, smaller lung volume, smaller left ventricular mass, lower stroke volume, lower cardiac output, lower aerobic capacity, and lower max anaerobic threshold than their male counterparts (8,9).

EXERCISE IN PREGNANCY

- The ideal time to start a family may coincide with peak performance for an athlete or any professional with a physically/technically demanding career. Managing a woman's fertility and optimizing her health before, during, and after pregnancy so she can achieve her professional and personal goals should be an ongoing aspect of care throughout her career.
- There are physiological changes associated with pregnancy that affect cardiorespiratory and musculoskeletal function.
- Fatigue is a common complaint in pregnancy, but there have been no studies on the rate of fatigue in elite athletes, or any trials on the effect of exercise on fatigue in pregnancy (11).
- Blood pressure usually falls slightly during pregnancy secondary to decreased peripheral vascular resistance, reaching a nadir in the second trimester, and then slowly rises to prepregnancy levels by term.
- Cardiac output increases by 30%–50% during pregnancy, secondary to a 10–15 $beats \cdot min^{-1}$ increase in heart rate and an increase in stroke volume (3,12).
- Blood volume increases by almost 50% at term.
- A dilutional anemia develops in the second trimester with an increase in plasma volume. This is partially corrected at term due to an increase in red cell mass in the third trimester.
- Progesterone is a potent respiratory stimulant, leading to an increased respiratory rate early in pregnancy (13).
- Relaxin facilitates chest wall adaptation so that the shape, but not the volume, of the thoracic cavity changes throughout pregnancy (13).
- Hormonal changes increase pelvic and joint laxity in pregnancy.

- The enlarging uterus and breasts with an increased lumbar lordosis and subsequent anterior pelvic rotation on the femur change the center of gravity.
- There are biomechanical changes to gait in pregnancy and the early postpartum period (11).
- More than 25% of pregnant women experience a fall, with a significant number of them sustaining an injury. The specific underlying postural and balance changes that arise during pregnancy and what mitigation strategies should be used to address this risk are not known (14).
- Pregnant women should get 30 minutes of moderate aerobic activity at least 5 days every week provided there are no contraindications. Pelvic floor muscle training should also be performed daily as well as an additional 2–3 days of resistance training using lighter weights and more repetitions (15,16).
- There is not enough evidence to have specific guidelines for women with twin or triplet pregnancies (15).
- Women meeting physical activity guidelines have 29% lower odds of gaining above the Institute of Medicine (IOM) recommended amount of weight during pregnancy than do inactive women (11).
- A decline in exercise from prepregnancy levels was significantly related to higher gestational weight gain (11).
- In the United States, 42%–57% of women gain more than the IOM recommended amount of weight during pregnancy (11).
- Pregnant patients are at risk of having preexisting obesity, hypertension, or Type 2 diabetes as all of these conditions have been increasing in the general population over the past few decades.
- Excessive maternal weight gain during pregnancy is associated with gestational diabetes, an increased risk of retained maternal weight/overweight or obesity, prolonged labor, preeclampsia, cesarean delivery, infants who are large for gestational age, and a subsequent increased risk of childhood obesity (3).
- Moderate intensity aerobic exercise throughout pregnancy is known to result in lower caesarean and instrumental delivery rates, a lower incidence of gestational diabetes and hypertension, decreased maternal weight gain, a lower incidence of urinary incontinence, a decreased incidence of lumbosacral pain, and improvements in prenatal mental health and quality of life. It also appears that vigorous intensity exercise completed into the third trimester is safe for most healthy pregnancies (16–21).
- Prenatal physical activity should be considered a front-line therapy for reducing the risk of pregnancy complications and enhancing maternal physical and mental health (16).
- Encouraging pregnant women to get the recommended amount of physical activity can lead to improved pregnancy outcomes and help to optimize maternal-fetal health.
- Exercise is safe throughout all trimesters, with no evidence that the cardiovascular effects of moderate intensity activity have any adverse effects on the mother or fetus in a healthy pregnancy (21,22).
- Exercise in pregnancy is not associated with miscarriage, stillbirth, neonatal death, preterm birth, preterm/premature rupture of membranes, neonatal hypoglycemia, low birth weight, birth defects, induction of labor, or birth complications (16,21,23).
- The quality of evidence on elite athletes exercising at >90% VO_{2max} in pregnancy is limited; however, a recent study of 42 elite and world class runners found no significant adverse maternal-fetal outcomes despite maintaining a training volume 2.5–3 times the evidence-based published recommendations (21,24).
- Light to moderate resistance training has no adverse health effects during pregnancy, but studies on strenuous strength training in pregnancy are sparse.
- There are some recommended restrictions on activity for all women during pregnancy. As there is not a large body of research on elite athletes during pregnancy, some questions about the effect of intense physical activity on the fetus remain unanswered.
- Activities that have a risk of trauma or falling should be avoided during pregnancy.
- During neural tube development in the first trimester, it is recommended to avoid a core temperature of >39°C/103°F. Exercising in pregnancy at 60%–70% of VO_{2max} in a controlled environment for up to 60 minutes does not raise the core temperature above 38°C. What temperature is reached when elite athletes exercise at >90% of VO_{2max} in the first trimester has not been studied (11,23).
- Exertion at altitudes up to 2500 m appears to be safe, but no study has explored the limits of exercise and altitude exposure in pregnancy, and there is a theoretical risk of decreased fetal oxygen saturation with high-intensity training at higher altitudes (11,16).
- Pregnant women should be cautioned to avoid SCUBA diving as the fetus is at increased risk of decompression illness, secondary to the inability of the fetal pulmonary circulation to filter bubble formation (25).
- Exercise in the supine position should be avoided when the uterus is large enough to obstruct the inferior vena cava, causing symptoms.
- Motionless standing can also lead to episodes of postural hypotension as pregnancy progresses and should be avoided if symptoms develop.
- Large increases in intra-abdominal pressure and the Valsalva maneuver during weight training may decrease blood flow to the fetus and harm the pelvic floor, but research is limited.
- There is no evidence to support improved outcomes with bed rest in twin or higher-order pregnancies (26).
- Bed rest may be associated with worse outcomes in patients with preeclampsia and preterm premature rupture of membranes (27,28).

- Contraindications to exercise listed in previous guidelines have been inconsistent, and frequently based on expert opinion. Recommendations continue to evolve as more evidence on physically active pregnant women becomes available (27).
- Some prior "contraindications," such as hypertension, obesity, and a history of a sedentary lifestyle, are in fact conditions that can be improved with exercise (27).
- The evidence on contraindications to exercise in pregnancy remains incomplete, but the following recommendations are based on a systematic review of the available evidence and recommendations from advisory organizations (27).
- Women with absolute contraindications should be discouraged from participating in moderate to vigorous physical activity, but should continue activities of daily living.
- There is no evidence that bed rest improves outcomes over continuing light activity and activities of daily living
- Absolute contraindications to aerobic exercise during pregnancy include the following (28):
  - Severe respiratory disease
  - Severe heart disease
  - Untreated, symptomatic, or severe arrhythmias
  - Placental abruption
  - Vasa previa
  - Uncontrolled Type 1 diabetes mellitus
  - Intrauterine growth restriction in current pregnancy
  - Active preterm labor
  - Severe preeclampsia
  - Cervical insufficiency
  - Preterm premature rupture of membranes
  - Placenta previa after 28 weeks
- Women with relative contraindications should have the condition addressed and optimized and discuss the potential risks and benefits of exercising with a physician, perhaps modifying, rather than eliminating exercise (27).
- Relative contraindications to aerobic exercise during pregnancy:
  - Mild/well-controlled respiratory disorders
  - Mild/well-controlled congenital or acquired heart disease
  - Well-controlled Type 1 diabetes
  - Mild preeclampsia
  - Symptomatic severe eating disorder
  - Multiple nutrient deficiencies/chronic undernutrition
  - Anemia
  - Poorly controlled hyperthyroidism
  - Heavy smoker with presence of comorbidities
- All women, regardless of baseline fitness, should monitor for the following warning signs to terminate exercise while pregnant:
  - Vaginal bleeding
  - Dyspnea prior to exertion
  - Dizziness
  - Headache
  - Chest pain
  - Muscle weakness
  - Calf pain or swelling
  - Preterm labor
  - Decreased fetal movement
  - Amniotic fluid leakage
- There are currently no definitive guidelines for elite athletes who would like to continue to train at a high level during pregnancy. These women should establish an ongoing relationship with a physician throughout their athletic career and participate in shared decision making with regard to their athletic and family goals.

OSTEOPOROSIS

- Osteoporosis is characterized by microarchitectural deterioration of bone tissue, leading to enhanced skeletal fragility, low bone mass, and an increased risk for fracture. It currently impacts 10.2% of adults over the age of 50 years with an estimated increase to 13% by 2030 (29).
- The incidence of low bone mass and osteoporosis in the female athlete is unknown. There is some controversy about whether the criteria for osteoporosis are appropriate to use when evaluating adolescents and young women with low bone mass, because they were developed to assess postmenopausal women (23).
- The World Health Organization has established diagnostic criteria for osteoporosis based on bone density measurements.
  - Osteoporosis is defined as a bone mineral density (BMD) greater than 2.5 standard deviations (SD) below the mean BMD of a young adult woman at her peak bone mass (T-score) (29).
  - Osteopenia is defined as a BMD between 1.0 and 2.5 SD below the mean.
  - A BMD within 1 SD of the mean is considered normal.
- The standard method of diagnosing osteoporosis is by dual x-ray absorptiometry (DEXA), which is used to measure bone density at various places, usually the hip, spine, and distal radius. These measurements are used to generate the previously mentioned T-score and an age-matched Z-score (30).
- The U.S. Preventive Services Task Force currently recommends routine screening for osteoporosis with a DEXA scan in women aged 65 years or women less than 65 years with greater than 8.4% fracture risk using the Fracture Risk Assessment Tool (29).
- Nonmodifiable risk factors for osteoporosis (30) include:
  - Age
  - Sex

  - Race
  - Family history of osteoporosis
  - Past history of low-trauma fracture
- Modifiable risk factors for osteoporosis (30) include:
  - Low body weight
  - Low calcium intake
  - Tobacco use
  - Excessive alcohol use
  - Lack of weight-bearing exercise
  - Low muscle mass
  - Estrogen deficiency (including history of oligomenorrhea, amenorrhea, and delayed menarche)
- Pharmacologic treatments for pre- and postmenopausal decreased BMD and osteoporosis include bisphosphonates, selective estrogen receptor modulators, and calcitonin. These antiresorptive agents are indicated for the prevention and treatment of postmenopausal osteoporosis (31).

PELVIC FLOOR DYSFUNCTION

- The pelvic floor muscles form the floor of the abdominal cavity, and the levator hiatus is the largest potential hernia portal in the body.
- The pelvic floor muscles provide structural support to the pelvic organs, and contraction of the pelvic floor muscles can prevent incontinence of urine, flatus, or stool.
- Pelvic floor dysfunction can manifest as urinary incontinence (UI), anal incontinence (AI), pelvic organ prolapse (POP), dysfunction of urination or defecation, sexual dysfunction, or pelvic floor pain syndromes.
- The most common type of UI is stress urinary incontinence (SUI), which is the involuntary loss of urine related to increased intra-abdominal pressure with activities such as sneezing, coughing, running, jumping, or heavy lifting.
- Risk factors for SUI include anything that increases intra-abdominal pressure and anything that could weaken the pelvic floor muscles, including strenuous work, exercise, pregnancy, and vaginal childbirth.
- Prevalence of SUI in the general female population is usually reported to be 25%–45%. In female athletes, it varies from 28% in university varsity athletes to 80% in teenaged nulliparous trampolinists. Athletes involved in high-impact activities such as gymnastics, trampolining, basketball, volleyball, or long-distance running are at increased risk for SUI (32,33).
- There are few studies reporting on AI, but one prevalence study found a higher incidence in women who exercised more than 8 $h \cdot wk^{-1}$ (34).
- There is scant literature on POP, but one study of 116 nulliparous female US Military Academy cadets found that those who attended paratrooper training were significantly more likely to demonstrate stage II POP than those who did not (35).
- Up to 30% of pregnant women and women with pelvic floor dysfunction may not be able to correctly contract their pelvic floor muscles based on initial assessment of women presenting for treatment (36).
- First-line management of UI is usually bladder training and pelvic floor muscle training (PFMT). Cure rates (defined as <2 g of leakage on pad tests) for stress urinary incontinence treated with PFMT vary between 44% and 70% (36).
- Pregnant continent women who perform PFMT are 62% less likely to experience UI in late pregnancy and have a 29% lower risk of UI in 3–6 months postpartum (36).
- Prenatal PFMT significantly shortens the first and second stages of labor without increasing the risk of episiotomy, instrumental vaginal delivery, or perineal lacerations (37).

RELATIVE ENERGY DEFICIENCY IN SPORT

- The syndrome of RED-S refers to impaired physiologic function caused by relative energy deficiency and includes, but is not limited to, impairments of metabolic rate, menstrual function, bone health, immunity, protein synthesis, and cardiovascular health described in the context of LEA (4–6).
  - Prevention of RED-S.
  - Increase awareness with education programs that should target individuals beyond athletes and coaches, be gender specific, involve significant others, and include changes to sports regulations, policy measures, and the health care system (38).
- Screening for RED-S:
  - The Relative Energy Deficiency in Sport Clinical Assessment Tool (RED-S CAT) was developed to assist with screening athletes for RED-S (39) (Fig. 131.1).
  - Any female athlete with positive screening on a clinical assessment tool, such as the Low Energy Availability in Females Questionnaire (LEAF-Q) (39) or RED-S CAT (39) (Fig. 131.1), should be evaluated, starting with a thorough history and physical examination.
- Treatment for RED-S:
  - Nonpharmacologic: nutritional education, including early involvement of an appropriately trained expert (*i.e.*, sports dietician) to optimize nutritional and matched exercise practices; cognitive behavioral therapy (40,41)
  - Supplementation (42):
    - Vitamin D 600–800 $IU \cdot d^{-1}$
    - Calcium 1000 $mg \cdot d^{-1}$ for ages 19–50, 1300 $mg \cdot d^{-1}$ for ages 9–18
  - Pharmacologic (43):
    - The use of combined oral contraceptives for the intention of regaining menses or improving BMD in RED-S is not recommended.

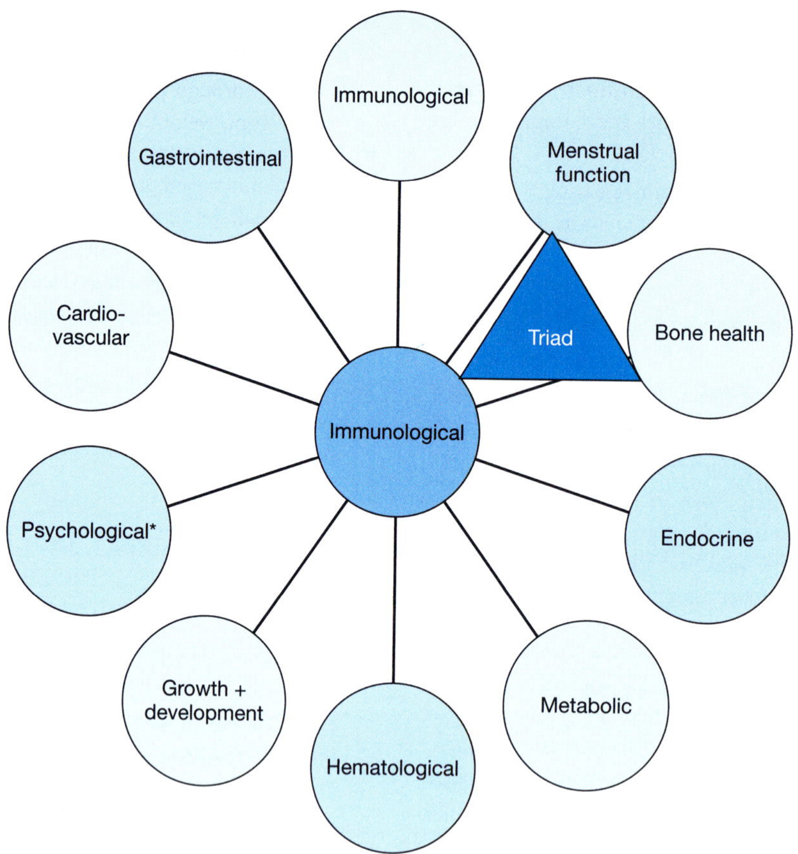

Figure 131.1: Health consequences of relative energy deficiency in sport (RED-S) showing an expanded concept of the female athlete triad to acknowledge a wider range of outcomes and potential performance effects of RED-S. *Please refer to original article for detailed clarification regarding the Psychological element of RED-S. (Reprinted from Figure 1 of Mountjoy M, Sundgot-Borgen J, Burke L, et al. International Olympic Committee (IOC) consensus statement on relative energy deficiency in sport (RED-S): 2018 update. *Int J Sport Nutr Exerc Metab*. 2018;28:316–331.)

        - Short-term use of transdermal estradiol (E2) therapy with cyclic oral progestin can be used to restore menses and bone health, but should not be relied upon for contraception.
        - Recombinant parathyroid hormone 1–34 (rPTH) has been shown to increase BMD in severe anorexia nervosa, but is contraindicated for use in patients with open growth plates.
- Low energy availability (LEA)
    - A mismatch between an athlete's energy intake and expenditure.
    - Persistent LEA could impair sport performance through a variety of indirect mechanisms (impaired recovery leading to premature reduction in physical, psychologic, and mental capacity and impairment of optimal muscle mass and function) (44), decreased neuromuscular performance (45), and training recovery (46).
    - Energy availability (EA) = Energy intake (EI) (kcal) – Exercise energy expenditure (EEE) (kcal)/fat-free mass (FFM) (kg)
    - Optimal EA for women for healthy physiological function is typically achieved at 45 kcal · kg^{-1} FFM · d^{-1} (47). Systems are substantially affected at an EA of <30 kcal · kg^{-1} FFM · d^{-1}, making it a targeted threshold for LEA (48).
- Measurement of EA:
    - No standardized or reference protocol.
    - The greatest challenge is to gain an accurate record of energy intake from self-report (48,49). In LEA, accurate data are often challenging due to the temporal dissociation of energy expenditure and matched eating as well as dietary habits that often coexist with LEA (high fiber intake, use of stimulants, and low-energy-density food consumption) (50).
- RED-S components:
    - The female athlete triad, as it was classically viewed, falls within this expanded view and involves menstrual function, bone health, and LEA, such as disordered eating or excessive exercise (35).
    - Menstrual function:
        - Pregnancy is the most common cause of amenorrhea in sexually active women and must be excluded.
        - Primary amenorrhea is diagnosed in females with secondary sexual characteristics without menarche at the age of 15 or 3 years post-thelarche (51).

- Athletes who begin intensive training before puberty, especially gymnasts and ballet dancers, are at risk of developing primary amenorrhea. Athletes who associate more stress with their sport and competition are more likely to be amenorrheic (52).
- Disruption of gonadotropin-releasing hormone (GnRH) pulsatility at the hypothalamus, followed by alterations of LH and FSH release from the pituitary and decreased estradiol and progesterone levels, also identified as functional hypothalamic amenorrhea (FHA) (43).
- Frequency of menstrual disturbances has been shown to be affected by the severity of the energy deficit, though a specific threshold of EA below which menstrual abnormalities occur has not been established (43).
- Evaluation of a patient with amenorrhea should include a thorough medical history, including pubertal milestones in the patient and other female relatives, a thorough menstrual history in patients presenting with secondary amenorrhea, a training and dietary history, medications (including over-the-counter medications such as diuretics, laxatives, ipecac, herbals, or supplements), a thorough family history, and psychological screening for evidence of increased stress, depression, anxiety, obsessive or compulsive personality traits, or symptoms of an eating disorder (52,53).
- A thorough physical exam should include vital signs, height, weight, body fat, arm span, Tanner stage, any characteristics of chromosomal anomalies, any traits of androgen excess, funduscopic examination and visual field confrontation, evaluation for galactorrhea, palpation of the thyroid, and a pelvic examination. Imaging studies may include computed tomography or magnetic resonance imaging to rule out a pituitary adenoma if indicated (52).
- A lack of any pubertal development can indicate hypothalamic, pituitary, or gonadal failure. An interruption of normal pubertal development can indicate ovarian failure or pituitary failure, as happens with a pituitary neoplasm.
- Normal breast and pubic development in the absence of menstrual periods can indicate an abnormality of the reproductive organs.
- Laboratory testing for primary amenorrhea is shown in Figure 131.2 and secondary amenorrhea in Figure 131.3.
- In hypothalamic amenorrhea, the pulsatile GnRH is abnormal. Rarely, this can be caused by a tumor, trauma, or a developmental defect. More commonly, it is thought that psychological and/or physical stress

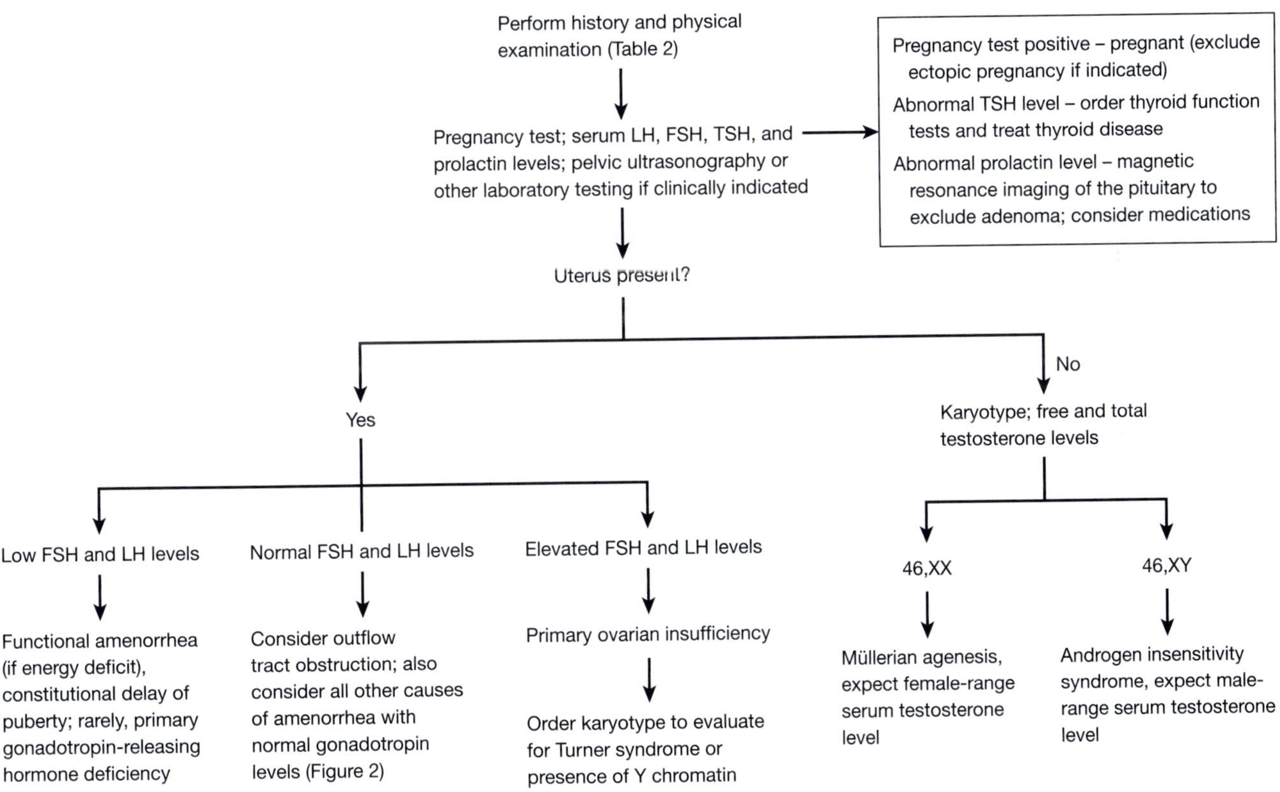

Figure 131.2: Laboratory evaluation of primary amenorrhea FSH, follicle-stimulating hormone; hCG, human chorionic gonadotropin; LH, luteinizing hormone; TSH, thyroid-stimulating hormone. Please refer to original article for additional referenced tables and figures not reprinted here. (Reprinted from Figure 1 of Klein DA, Poth MA. Amenorrhea: an approach to diagnosis and management. *Am Fam Physician*. 2013;87(11):784.)

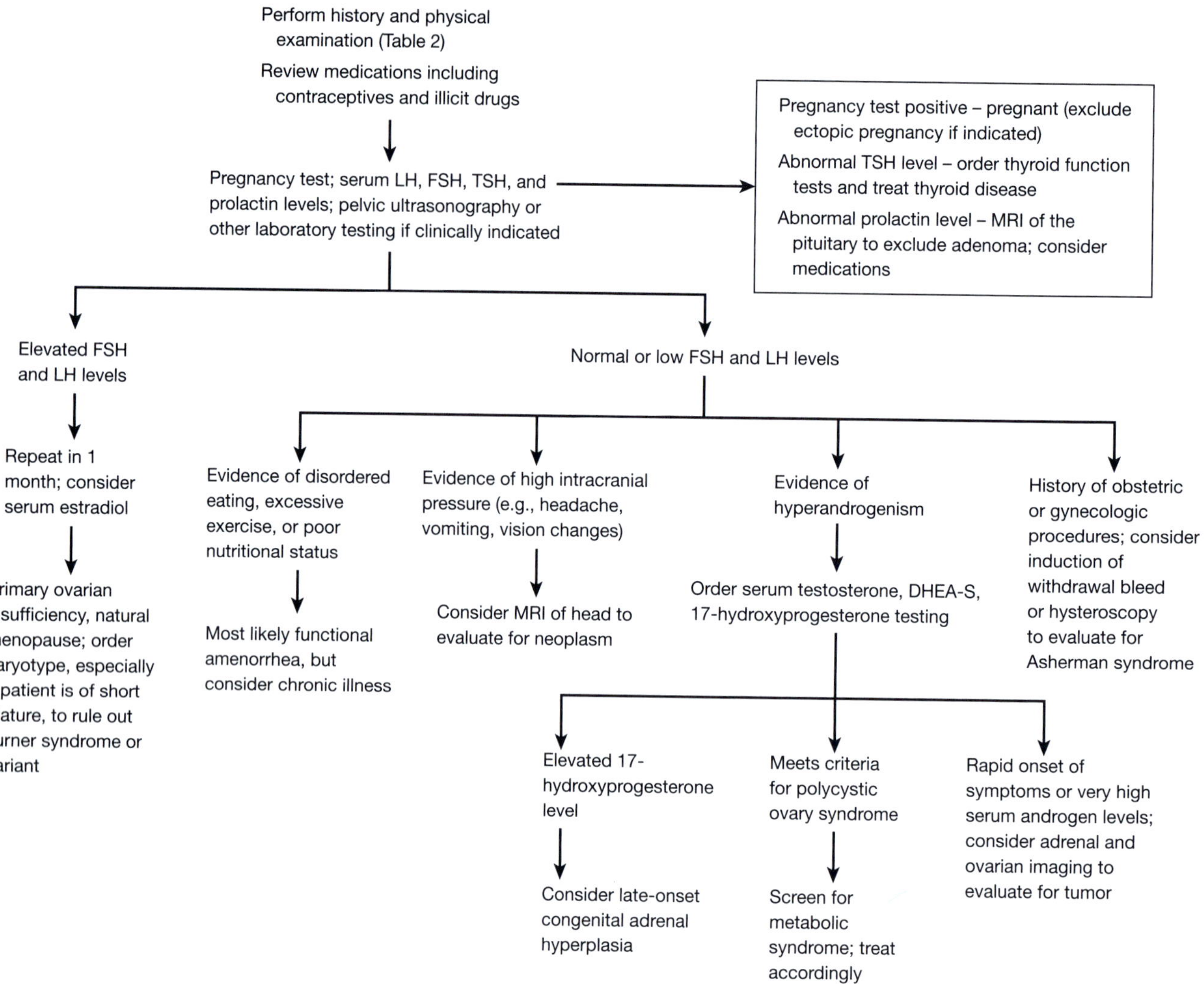

Figure 131.3: .Laboratory evaluation of secondary amenorrhea FSH, follicle-stimulating hormone; hCG, human chorionic gonadotropin; LH, luteinizing hormone; TSH, thyroid-stimulating hormone. Please refer to original article for additional referenced tables and figures not reprinted here. (Reprinted from Figure 2 of Klein DA, Poth MA. Amenorrhea: an approach to diagnosis and management. *Am Fam Physician*. 2013;87(11):784.)

affects neurohormones that regulate GnRH, leading to hypothalamic amenorrhea (54).

- Exercise-related amenorrhea can be considered a subset of hypothalamic amenorrhea, which also includes amenorrhea related to anorexia nervosa, weight loss, and psychological stress. It is, however, a diagnosis of exclusion. The recommended primary treatment is correcting the energy deficit by increasing caloric intake to the point that there is a spontaneous return of menses. This has also been associated with an increase in bone mass (54).

- Bone health/low BMD:
  - LEA leads to decreased BMD because bone growth and development are dependent on mechanical, nutritional, and hormonal influence.
  - Women and girls with an energy deficit resulting from decreased caloric intake are at risk of having decreased BMD.
  - Athletes in specific sports are at increased risk for low BMD, including jockeys, runners, swimmers, and cyclists (55).
  - Anatomical areas with less bone loading and/or trabecular versus cortical bone content, such as lumbar spine and radius versus total hip are at greater risk for low BMD.
  - BMI < 17.5 kg · m^{-2}, <85% body weight for adolescents, or >10% weight loss in 1 month are all associated with increased risk for low BMD (56).
- Nonpharmacologic measures used in the prevention and treatment of decreased BMD include the following: Ensuring adequate caloric intake to meet energy needs and maintaining regular menses if premenopausal, weight-bearing exercise, and decreasing tobacco and alcohol use (57).
- It is thought that the primary problem in the young female athlete is decreased bone formation rather than premature

bone loss, so the antiresorptive treatments may not address the problem of adolescent osteopenia/osteoporosis and are not indicated in this population. There is also the concern of possible teratogenic effects if bisphosphonates are used in women of childbearing age (58).

- Adequate nutrition and weight-bearing exercise during the adolescent years are important for achieving peak bone mass. On average, 92% of the total-body BMD is attained by age 18, and 99% is attained by age 26 (58).
- Different sites appear to mature at different ages. Peak bone mass appears to be complete by age 16 in the femoral neck, whereas the bone mass in the lumbar spine appears to increase into the third decade (58).
- Although amenorrhea is associated with osteopenia, using oral contraceptive pills to induce menses has not been shown to increase bone mass in the absence of improved nutrition and calcium intake. In fact, some studies have shown that oral contraceptives may actually cause a further decrease in BMD in adolescent athletes (52,59).
- When assessing overall bone health, vitamin D levels need to be checked, because insufficient and deficient levels have potential negative impact on athletes' health and ability to maximally train (60).
- Eating disorders and disordered eating (61):
  - Eating disorders are characterized by disturbances in eating behavior, body image, emotions, and relationships. Tables 131.1–131.3 exhibit diagnostic criteria of eating disorders.
  - Anorexia nervosa is an extreme version of restrictive eating behavior in which an individual continues to starve, even though it may be or is 15% or more below ideal body weight.
  - Bulimia nervosa has cycles of recurrent binge eating with a feeling of loss of control followed by inappropriate compensatory behavior. These behaviors occur, on average, at least once a week for 3 months. Self-evaluation is unduly influenced by body shape and weight.
  - Binge-eating disorder: Similar to bulimia nervosa in frequency, sense of loss of control, and eating behaviors, but lack a compensatory behavior component.
  - Other specified feeding or eating disorder (OSFED) is also included in the *Diagnostic and Statistical Manual of Mental Disorders*, 5th Edition (DSM-V) and includes patients who have eating disorders but do not meet the exact diagnostic criteria of anorexia nervosa or bulimia nervosa (Table 131.4).
  - Disordered eating includes the entire spectrum of abnormal eating behaviors that may not fit any of the DSM-V criteria for eating disorders.
- Disordered eating can have devastating effects on psychological well-being, skeletal health, and other physiologic problems such as dehydration, electrolyte disturbances, thermoregulatory and cardiac disturbances, loss of muscle mass, and decreased performance in addition to other medical complications.
- Disordered eating can lead to an energy deficit that contributes to menstrual irregularity and an increased risk of stress fractures and decreased BMD.
- Risk factors for disordered eating include the following:
  - Chronic dieting
  - Low self-esteem
  - Family dysfunction
  - Physical abuse
  - Biologic factors
  - Perfectionism
  - Lack of nutrition knowledge
  - An emphasis on body weight for performance or appearance

Table 131.1 Diagnostic Criteria for Anorexia Nervosa

A. Restriction of energy intake relative to requirements leading to a significantly low body weight in the context of age, sex, developmental trajectory, and physical health. Significantly low weight is defined as a weight that is less than minimally normal or, for children and adolescents, less than minimally expected.
B. Intense fear of gaining weight or becoming fat, or persistent behavior that interferes with weight gain, even though at a significantly low weight.
C. Disturbance in the way in which one's body weight or shape is experienced, undue influence of body weight or shape on self-evaluation, or persistent lack of recognition of the seriousness of the current low body weight.

Restricting Type: During the last 3 mo, the individual has not engaged in recurrent episodes of binge-eating or purging behavior (*i.e.*, self-induced vomiting or the misuse of laxatives, diuretics, or enemas). This subtype describes presentations in which weight loss is accomplished primarily through dieting, fasting, and/or excessive exercise.

Binge-Eating/Purging Type: During the last 3 mo, the individual has regularly engaged in recurrent episodes of binge-eating or purging behavior (*i.e.*, self-induced vomiting or the misuse of laxatives, diuretics, or enemas).

Specify current severity:
Mild: BMI > 17
Moderate: BMI 16–16.99
Severe: BMI 15–15.99
Extreme: BMI < 15

Source: American Psychiatric Association. *Diagnostic and Statistical Manual of Mental Disorders*. 5th ed. Arlington (VA): American Psychiatric Association; 2013.

Table 131.2 Diagnostic Criteria for Bulimia Nervosa

A. Recurrent episodes of binge eating. An episode of binge eating is characterized by both:
 Eating, in a discrete period of time (*e.g.*, within any 2-h period), an amount of food that is definitely larger than what most individuals would eat during a similar period of time and under similar circumstances
 A sense of lack of control over eating during the episodes (*e.g.*, a feeling that one cannot stop eating or control what or how much one is eating)
B. Recurrent inappropriate compensatory behavior to prevent weight gain, such as self-induced vomiting; misuse of laxative, diuretics, enemas, or other medications; fasting; or excessive exercise.
C. The binge eating and inappropriate compensatory behaviors both occur, on average, at least once a week for 3 months.
D. Self-evaluation is unduly influenced by body shape and weight.
E. The disturbance does not occur exclusively during episodes of anorexia nervosa.

Specify current severity:
Mild: An average of 1–3 episodes of inappropriate compensatory behaviors per week
Moderate: An average of 4–7 episodes of inappropriate compensatory behaviors per week
Severe: An average of 8–13 episodes of inappropriate compensatory behaviors per week
Extreme: An average of 14 or more episodes of inappropriate compensatory behaviors per week

Source: American Psychiatric Association. *Diagnostic and Statistical Manual of Mental Disorders*. 5th ed. Arlington (VA): American Psychiatric Association; 2013.

- Pressure to lose weight from parents, coaches, judges, and peers
- A drive to win at any cost
- Self-identity as an athlete only (no identity outside of sports)
- A sudden increase in training
- Exercising through injury
- Overtraining (especially when undernourished)
- A traumatic event such as an injury or loss of a coach
- Vulnerable times such as an adolescent growth spurt, entering college, retiring from athletics, and postpartum depression

- Treatment for disordered eating requires a multidisciplinary team, including a physician or other health care provider, mental health counselor, and a nutritionist.
  - Treatment includes the following:
    - Recognition of the problem
    - Identification and resolution of psychosocial precipitants
    - Stabilization of medical and nutritional conditions
    - Reestablishment of healthy eating patterns
    - Removal from sport if diagnosis of anorexia nervosa or bulimia nervosa

Table 131-3 Binge-Eating Disorder: Diagnostic Criteria

A. Recurrent episodes of binge eating. An episode of binge eating is characterized by both of the following:
 1. Eating, in a discrete period of time (e.g., within any 2-h period), an amount of food that is definitely larger than what most people would eat in a similar period of time under similar circumstances.
 2. A sense of lack of control over eating during the episodes (e.g., a feeling that one cannot stop eating or control what or how much one is eating).
B. The binge-eating episodes are associated with three (or more) of the following:
 1. Eating much more rapidly than normal.
 2. Eating until feeling uncomfortably full.
 3. Eating large amounts of food when not feeling physically hungry.
 4. Eating alone because of feeling embarrassed by how much one is eating.
 5. Feeling disgusted with oneself, depressed, or very guilty afterward.
C. Marked distress regarding binge eating is present.
D. The binge eating occurs, on average, at least once a week for 3 mo.
E. The binge eating is not associated with the recurrent use of inappropriate compensatory behavior as in bulimia nervosa and does not occur exclusively during the course of bulimia nervosa or anorexia nervosa.

Specify current severity:
The minimum level of severity is based on the frequency of episodes of binge eating (see below). The level of severity may be increased to reflect other symptoms and the degree of functional disability.
Mild: 1–3 binge-eating episodes per week.
Moderate: 4–7 binge-eating episodes per week.
Severe: 8–13 binge-eating episodes per week.
Extreme: 14 or more binge-eating episodes per week.
Unspecified

Source: American Psychiatric Association. *Diagnostic and Statistical Manual of Mental Disorders*. 5th ed. Arlington (VA): American Psychiatric Association; 2013.

Table 131-4 Other Specified Feeding or Eating Disorder: Diagnostic Criteria

This category applies to presentations in which symptoms characteristic of a feeding and eating disorder that cause clinically significant distress or impairment in social, occupational, or other important areas of functioning predominate but do not meet the full criteria for any of the disorders in the feeding and eating disorders diagnostic class. The other specified feeding or eating disorder category is used in situations in which the clinician chooses to communicate the specific reason that the presentation does not meet the criteria for any specific feeding and eating disorder. This is done by recording "other specified feeding or eating disorder" followed by the specific reason (e.g., "bulimia nervosa of low frequency").

Examples of presentations that can be specified using the "other specified" designation include the following:

1. Atypical anorexia nervosa: All of the criteria for anorexia nervosa are met, except that despite significant weight loss, the individual's weight is within or above the normal range. Individuals with atypical anorexia nervosa may experience many of the physiological complications associated with anorexia nervosa (Moskowitz and Weiselberg 2017; Peebles et al. 2010; Sawyer et al, 2016).
2. Bulimia nervosa (of low frequency and/or limited duration): All of the criteria for bulimia nervosa are met, except that the binge eating and inappropriate compensatory behaviors occur, on average, less than once a week and/or for less than 3 mo.
3. Binge-eating disorder (of low frequency and/or limited duration): All of the criteria for binge-eating disorder are met, except that the binge eating occurs, on average, less than once a week and/or for less than 3 mo.
4. Purging disorder: Recurrent purging behavior to influence weight or shape (e.g., self-induced vomiting; misuse of laxatives, diuretics, or other medications) in the absence of binge eating.
5. Night eating syndrome: Recurrent episodes of night eating, as manifested by eating after awakening from sleep or by excessive food consumption after the evening meal. There is awareness and recall of the eating. The night eating is not better explained by external influences such as changes in the individual's sleep-wake cycle or by local social norms. The night eating causes significant distress and/or impairment in functioning. The disordered pattern of eating is not better explained by binge-eating disorder or another mental disorder, including substance use, and is not attributable to another medical condition or to an effect of medication.

Source: Reprinted with permission from the *Diagnostic and Statistical Manual of Mental Disorders*, 5th ed. Text Revision (Copyright © 2022). American Psychiatric Association.

- Endocrine
  - Disruption of the hypothalamic-pituitary-gonadal axis, alterations in thyroid function, changes in appetite-regulating hormones (decreased leptin/oxytocin, increased ghrelin, peptide YY, and adiponectin), decreased insulin/insulin-like growth factor (IGF-1), increased growth hormone resistance, and elevations in cortisol (54)
- Metabolic
  - LEA has been correlated with decreased resting metabolic rate (RMR) in female endurance athletes (50).
  - Moderate energy deficiency associated with significantly decreased RMR and severe energy deficiency associated with significant decrease in leptin, T3, IGF-1 and an increase in ghrelin (62).
- Hematological
  - Iron deficiency: potential reduction in appetite, decreased metabolic fuel availability, and impaired metabolic efficiency, which leads to an increase in energy expenditure during exercise and rest (63).
- Cardiovascular
  - Early atherosclerosis has been associated with hypoestrogenism and FHA in young female athletes.
  - In more severe LEA, such as anorexia nervosa, changes include valve abnormalities, pericardial effusion, severe bradycardia, hypotension, and arrhythmias, including QTc prolongation (64).
- Gastrointestinal
  - Altered sphincter tone, delayed gastric emptying, and constipation (65)
- Growth and development
  - Linear growth retardation has been reported in female adolescents with severe anorexia nervosa, with studies demonstrating partial to complete catch up growth after recovery (66).
  - Amenorrheic athletes have demonstrated disorderly GH secretory patterns, decreased GH and IGF-1 secretory response to exercise accompanied by increased interpulse GH levels, and decreased IGF-1 and IGFBP-1 ratios (67).
- Immunological
  - Increased number of infections, lowered immunoglobulin A secretion rates, bodily aches, and headache (68)
- Psychological
  - Negative effects correlate with LEA.
  - Adolescent females with FHA have a higher incidence of mild depressive traits, psychosomatic disorders, and decreased ability to cope with stress (69).

CONCLUSION

- This chapter provides a brief overview of select musculoskeletal and medical issues that impact the female athlete. It is by no means all-encompassing as the body of research in female athlete care continues to expand.
- Significant advances have been made in multiple areas over the last several years, including the exploration of RED-S and its components as well as exercise in pregnancy.

- In addition, the number of female athletes participating in all levels of sport and activity continues to grow. Women are also staying active later in life, supporting the need for knowledge of topics not traditionally associated with athletes, such as pelvic floor dysfunction and osteoporosis outside of RED-S/female athlete triad concerns.
- Other topics commonly discussed with respect to female athletes, including noncontact anterior cruciate ligament injuries, patellofemoral pain, and shoulder injuries, are covered in other chapters within this text.

REFERENCES

1. National Federation of State High School Associations. *High School Sports Participation Increases for 29th Consecutive Year*. Indianapolis: National Federation of State High School Associations; 2018.
2. Blackwell, DACT. *State Variation in Meeting the 2008 Federal Guidelines for Both Aerobic and Muscle-Strengthening Activities through Leisure-Time Physical Activity Among Adults Aged* 18-64: *United States*, 2010-2015. US Department of Health and Human Services; 2018.
3. Barakat AJ. Exercise and pregnancy. In: Mountjoy M, editor. *Handbook of Sports Medicine and Science: The Female Athlete*. Hoboken, NJ: John Wiley and Sons; 2014. p. 110–9.
4. Mountjoy M, Sundgot-Borgen J, Burke L, et al. The IOC consensus statement: beyond the female athlete triad-relative energy deficiency in sport (RED-S). *Br J Sports Med*. 2014;48(7):491–7.
5. Mountjoy M, Sundgot-Borgen J, Burke L, et al. Authors' 2015 additions to the IOC consensus statement: relative energy deficiency in sport (RED-S). *Br J Sports Med*. 2015;49(7):417–20.
6. Mountjoy M, Sundgot-Borgen J, Burke L, et al. International Olympic Committee (IOC) consensus statement on relative energy deficiency in sport (RED-S): 2018 update. *Int J Sport Nutr Exerc Metab*. 2018;28(4):316–31.
7. Marcdante SA. Overview and assessment of adolescents. In: Marcdante KJ, Kliegman RM, Schuh AM, editors. *Nelson Essentials of Pediatrics*. 9th ed. Philadelphia, PA: Elsevier; 2023. p. 281–7.
8. Boeyer MEA. Early maturity as the new normal: a centruy-long study of bone age. *Clin Orthop Rela Res*. 2018;476:2112–22.
9. Hiort O. Normal and variant sex development. In: Legato MJ, editor. *Principles of Gender-specific Medicine: Gender in the Genomic Age*. 3rd ed. London: Elsevier; 2017. p. 1–16.
10. Lundsgaard AF. Exercise physiology in men and women. In: Legato MJ, editor. *Principles of Gender-specific Medicine: Gender in the Genomic Age*. 3rd ed. London: Elsevier; 2017. p. 525–42.
11. Bo KE. Exercise and pregnancy in recreational and elite athletes: 2016 evidence summary from the IOC expert group meeting, Lausanne. Part 1 – exercise in women planning pregnancy and those who are pregnant. *Brit J of Sports Med*. 2016;50:571–89.
12. Chu AK. Exercise considerations before, during, and after pregnancy. In: Frank R, editor. *The Female Athlete*. St. Louis: Elsevier; 2022. p. 311–17.
13. LoMauro AA. Respiratory physiology in pregnancy and assessment of pulmonary function. In: *Best Practice and Research Clinical Obstetrics and Gynaecology*. December; 2022; 85(Pt A):3–16.
14. Goossens N, Massé-Alarie H, Aldabe D, Verbrugghe J, Janssens L. Changes in static balance during pregnancy and postpartum: a systematic review. *Gait Posture*. 2022;96:160–72.
15. Nagpal M. Physical activity throughout pregnancy is key to preventing chronic disease. *Reproduction*. 2022;160:R111–8.
16. Mottola MF, Davenport MH, Ruchat SM, et al. 2019 Canadian guideline for physical activity throughout pregnancy. *Br J Sports Med*. 2018;52(21):1339–46.
17. Beetham KS, Giles C, Noetel M, et al. The effects of vigorous intensity exercise in the third trimester of pregnancy: a systematic review and meta-analysis. *BMC Pregnancy Childbirth*. 2019;18:281–98.
18. Davenport M, Ruchat SM, Sobierajski F, et al. Impact of prenatal exercise on maternal harms, labour and delivery outcomes: a systematic review and meta-analysis. *Br J Sports Med*. 2019;53(2):99–107.
19. Davenport M, McCurdy AP, Mottola MF, et al. Impact of prenatal exercise on both prenatal and postnatal anxiety and depressive symptoms: a systematic review and meta-analysis. *Br J Sports Med*. 2018;52(21):1376–85.
20. Cai C, Busch S, Wang R, Sivak A, Davenport MH. Physical activity before and during pregnancy and maternal mental health: A systematic review and meta-analysis of observational studies. *J Affect Disord*. 2022;309:393–403.
21. Darroch F, Schneeberg A, Brodie R, et al. Effect of pregnancy in 42 elite to world-class runners on training and performance outcomes. *Med Sci Sports Exerc*. 2023;55(1):93–100.
22. Davies G, Artal R. It's time to treat exercise in pregnancy as therapy. *Br J Sports Med*. 2019;53(2):81.
23. Team Physician Consensus Statement. Female athlete issues for the team physician: a consensus statement-2017 update. *Med Sci Sports Exer*. 2018;50(5):1113–22.
24. Bø K, Artal R, Barakat R, et al. Exercise and pregnancy in recreational and elite athletes: 2016 evidence summary from the IOC expert group meeting, Lausanne. Part 2 – the effect of exercise on the fetus, labour and birth. *Brit J of Sports Med*. 2016;50:1297–305.
25. Reid R, Lorenzo M. SCUBA diving in pregnancy. *J Obst Gynaecol Canada*. 2018;40(11):1490–6.
26. Da Silva Lopes K, Takemoto Y, Ota E, et al. Bed rest with and without hospitalisation in multiple pregnancy for improving perinatal outcomes (Review). *Cochrane Database Syst Rev*. 2017;3:1–51.
27. Meah DM. Why can't I exercise during pregnancy? Time to revisit medical "absolute" and "relative" contraindications: systematic review of evidence of harm and a call to action. *Brit J Sports Med*. 2020;54: 1395–404.
28. Roman A, Watters N, Moses D, Reisner J. Maternal activity level in patients with preterm premature rupture of membranes: a prospective observational cohort study. *Am J Obstet Gynecol*. 2018:S414–15.
29. Harris K, Zagar CA, Lawrence KV. Osteoporosis: common questions and answers. *Am Fam Physician*. 2023;107(3):238–46.
30. White L. Osteoporosis prevention, screening and diagnosis: ACOG recommendations. *Amer Fam Phys*. 2022;106(5):587–8.
31. Hauk L. Treatment of low BMD and osteoporosis to prevent fractures: updated guideline from the ACP. *Amer Fam Phys*. 2018;97(5):352–3.
32. Bø K, Nygaard IE. Is physical activity good or bad for the female pelvic floor: a narrative review. *Sports Med*. 2020;50(3):471–84.
33. Bø K. Exercise and plevic floor dysfunction in female elite athletes. In: Mountjoy M, editor. *Handbook of Sports Medicine and Science: The Female Athlete*. Incorporated: John Wiley & Sons; 2014.
34. Vitton V, Baumstarck-Barrau K, Brardjanian S, Caballe I, Bouvier M, Grimaud JC. Impact of high-level sport practice on anal incontinence in a healthy young female population. *J Womens Health*. 2011;20(5):757–63.
35. Larsen W, Yavorek T. Pelvic prolapse and urinary incontinence in nulliparous college women in relation to paratrooper training. *Int Urogynecol J*. 2007;18(7):769–71.
36. Woodley S, Lawrenson P, Boyle R, et al. Pelvic floor muscle training for prevention and treatment of urinary and faecal incontinence in antenatal and postnatal women (Review). *Cochrane Database Syst Rev*. 2017;12:1–212.

37. Du Y, Xu L, Ding L, Wang Y, Wang Z. The effect of antenatal pelvic floor muscle training on labor and delivery outcomes: a systematic review with meta-analysis. *Int Urogynecol J*. 2015;26(10):1415–27.
38. De Bruin APK. Athletes with eating disorder symptomatology, a specific population with specific needs. *Curr Opin Psychol*. 2017;16:148–53.
39. Mountjoy M, Sundgot-Borgen J, Burke L, et al. The IOC relative energy deficiency in sport clinical assessment tool (RED-S CAT). *Br J Sports Med*. 2015;49(21):1354.
40. Melin A, Tornberg AB, Skouby S, et al. The LEAF questionnaire: a screening tool for the identification of female athletes at risk for the female athlete triad. *Br J Sports Med*. 2014;48(7):540–5.
41. Cialdella-Kam L, Guebels CP, MAddalozzo GF, Manore MM. Dietary intervention restored menses in female athletes with exercise-associated menstrual dysfunction with limited impact on bone and muscle health. *Nutrients*. 2014;6(8):3018–39.
42. US Preventive Services Task Force, Grossman DC, Curry SJ, et al. Vitamin D, calcium, or combined supplementation for the primary prevention of fractures in community-dwelling adults. US preventive Services Task Force recommendation statement. *JAMA*. 2018;319(15):1592–9.
43. Gordon CM, Ackerman KE, Berga SL, et al. Functional hypothalamic amenorrhea: an endocrine society clinical practice guideline. *J Clin Endocrinol Metab*. 2017;102(5):1413–39.
44. Fogelholm M. Effects of bodyweight reduction on sports performance. *Sports Med*. 1994;18(4):249–67.
45. Tornberg ÅB, Melin A, Koivula FM, et al. Reduced neuromuscular performance in amenorrheic elite endurance athletes. *Med Sci Sports Exerc*. 2017;49(12):2478–85.
46. Woods AL, Garvican-Lewis LA, Lundy B, Rice AJ, Thompson KG. New approaches to determine fatigue in elite athletes during intensified training: resting metabolic rate and pacing profile. *PLoS One*. 2017;12(3):e0173807–17.
47. Loucks AB, Kiens B, Wright HH. Energy availability in athletes. *J Sports Sci*. 2011;29(suppl 1):S7–15.
48. Burke L, Deakin V. *Clinical Sports Nutrition*. 5th ed. North Ryde, Australia: McGraw-Hill Education Australia; 2015.
49. Burke LM, Lundy BL, Fahrenholtz L, Melin A. Pitfalls of conducting and interpreting estimates of energy availability in free-living athletes. *Int J Sport Nutr Exerc Metab*. 2018;28(4):350–63.
50. Melin A, Tornberg ÅB, Skouby S, et al. Low energy density and high fiber intake are dietary concerns in female endurance athletes. *Scand J Med Sci Sports*. 2016;26(9):1060–71.
51. Klein DA, Paradise SL, Reeder RM. Amenorrhea: a systematic approach to diagnosis and management. *Am Fam Physician*. 2019;100(1):39–48.
52. Bruckner P, Fricker P. Endocrinologic conditions. In: Fields KB, Fricker PA, editors. *Medical Problems in Athletes*. Oxford (UK): Blackwell Science; 1998.
53. Klein DA, Poth MA. Amenorrhea: an approach to diagnosis and management. *Am Fam Physician*. 2013;87(11):784.
54. Allaway HCM, Southmayd EA, De Souza MJ. The physiology of functional hypothalamic amenorrhea associated with energy deficiency in exercising women and in women with anorexia nervosa. *Horm Mol Biol Clin Investig*. 2016;25(2):91–119.
55. Wilson G, Hawken MB, Poole I, et al. Rapid weight loss impairs simulated riding performance and strength in jockeys: implications for making weight. *J Sports Sci*. 2014;32(4):383–91.
56. De Souza MJ, Nattiv A, Joy E, et al. 2014 female athlete triad coalition consensus statement on treatment and return to play of the female athlete triad: 1st international conference held in San Francisco, CA, may 2012, and 2nd international conference held in Indianapolis, IN, may 2013. *Clin J Sports Med*. 2014;24(2):97–119.
57. Ackerman KE, Nazem T, Chapko D, et al. Bone microarchitecture is impaired in adolescent amenorrheic athletes compared with eumenorrheic athletes and nonathletic controls. *J Clin Endocrinol Metab*. 2011;96(10):3123–33.
58. Meier DE. Osteoporosis and other disorders of skeletal aging. In: Cassel CK, Cohen HJ, Larson EB, et al, editors. *Geriatric Medicine*. 3rd ed. New York (NY): Springer-Verlag; 1997.
59. Klibanski A, Biller BM, Schoenfeld DA, Herzog DB, Saxe VC. The effects of estrogen administration on trabecular bone loss in young women with anorexia nervosa. *J Clin Endocrinol Metab*. 1995;80(3):898–904.
60. Ahmed I, Amarnani R, Fisher C. The metabolic crossroad of the adolescent athlete: achieving peak bone mass during athletic development. *Br J Sports Med*. 2022;56(23):1330–1.
61. American Psychiatric Association. *The Diagnostic and Statistical Manual of Mental Disorders*. 5th ed. Arlington, VA: Text Revision (DSM-5-TR); 2013.
62. Koehler K, Souza MJ, Williams NI. Less-than-expected weight loss in normal-weight women undergoing caloric restriction and exercise is accompanied by preservation of fat-free mass and metabolic adaptations. *Eur J Clin Nutr*. 2017;71(3):365–71.
63. Petkus DL, Murray-Kolb LE, De Souza MJ. The unexplored crossroads of the female athlete triad and iron deficiency: a narrative review. *Sports Med*. 2017;47(9):1721–37.
64. Spaulding-Barclay MA, Stern J, Mehler PS. Cardiac changes in anorexia nervosa. *Cardiol Young*. 2016;26(4):623–8.
65. Norris ML, Harrison ME, Isserlin L, Robinson A, Feder S, Sampson M. Gastrointestinal complications associated with anorexia nervosa: a systematic review. *Int J Eat Disord*. 2016;49(3):216–37.
66. Modan-Moses D, Yaroslavsky A, Novikov I, et al. Stunting of growth as a major feature of anorexia nervosa in male adolescents. *Pediatrics*. 2003;111(2):270–6.
67. Waters DL, Qualls CR, Dorin R, Veldhuis JD, Baumgartner RN. Increased pulsatility, process irregularity and nocturnal trough concentrations of growth hormone in amenorrheic compared to eumenorrheic athletes. *J Clin Endocrinol Metab*. 2001;86(3):1013–19.
68. Drew MK, Vlahovich N, Hughes D, et al. A multifactorial evaluation of illness risk factors in athletes preparing for the summer Olympic games. *J Sci Med Sport*. 2017;20(8):745–50.
69. Bomba M, Gambera A, Bonini L, et al. Endocrine profiles and neuropsychologic correlates of functional hypothalamic amenorrhea in adolescents. *Fertil Steril*. 2007;87(4):876–85.

132 The Athlete With Intellectual Disabilities

Connie Hsia and James Lynch

TERMINOLOGY

- *Intellectual disability* is a disorder characterized by significant limitations both in intellectual functioning (reasoning, learning, problem-solving) and in adaptive behavior, which covers a range of everyday social and practical skills (1).
  - Adaptive skill areas are those daily living skills needed to live, work, and play in the community. They include communication, self-care, home living, social skills, leisure, health and safety, self-direction, functional academics, community use, and work.
  - Adaptive skills are assessed in the person's typical environment across all aspects of an individual's life. A person with limits in intellectual functioning who does not have limits in adaptive skill areas may not be diagnosed as having intellectual disability (1).
- Intellectual disability is a common developmental disorder that affects approximately 6.5–7.5 million Americans.
- Definition of *intellectual disability*, according to the *Diagnostic and Statistical Manual of Mental Disorders, Fifth Edition* (2), includes deficits in intellectual functions, deficits in adaptive functioning, and onset of these deficits during the developmental period.
- Additionally, the definition of intellectual disability, according to the American Association on Intellectual and Developmental Disabilities, states that "This disability originates during the developmental period, which is defined operationally as before the individual attains age 22" (1).
- In 2007, the American Association on Mental Retardation changed its name to the American Association on Intellectual and Developmental Disabilities.
- US Public Law 111-256 (Rosa's Law) was passed in 2010, mandating replacement of the term "mental retardation" with "intellectual disability" in all federal laws.
- Medical and research literature now use both "intellectual developmental disorder" and "intellectual disability."

PHYSIOLOGIC CONSIDERATIONS

- Athletes with intellectual disabilities may have a variety of health-related issues that impact their participation in competitive athletics. With such a diverse population of athletes, there is no unifying list of diagnoses or conditions; however, there are some important points for the sports medicine team to consider.
- Epidemiologic studies of organized athletics for intellectually disabled athletes reveal some patterns and conditions that are more prevalent in this population. Generally speaking, intellectually disabled athletes, as compared to general population athletes, have:
  - A higher prevalence of hearing and visual impairment
  - Decreased measures of strength and endurance
  - Decreased agility, balance, speed, flexibility, and reaction time
  - Higher rates of obesity (half of all with intellectual disability)
  - Lower peak heart rate
  - Lower peak oxygen uptake (3–5)
- Using preparticipation screening exam data for Special Olympics athletes, the incidence of sports-significant abnormalities detected is roughly 40%.
  - The most common categories of problems detected among intellectually disabled athletes are neurologic (16%), ophthalmologic (15%), musculoskeletal (6%), and medical (5%).
  - The most common diagnoses are seizure disorder and vision loss (6).
- As a comparison, the incidence of sports-significant abnormalities detected among nondisabled athletes is historically 1%–3%.

PREPARTICIPATION EVALUATION

- The goal in performing a preparticipation physical evaluation (PPE) is to promote the health and safety of the athlete in training and competition.

- The *PPE: Preparticipation Physical Evaluation, Fifth Edition* monograph was updated in 2019 by all major American sports medicine societies. The authors stress that PPE for the athlete with special needs should be similar to any athlete without physical or cognitive disability (7).
  - The PPE should address the particular concerns of the athlete with special needs.
  - The health care provider should:
    - Be aware of common problems associated with different disabilities
    - Be able to diagnose abnormalities that may endanger the athlete
    - Provide support and encourage physical activity
- The preparticipation history has been shown to be helpful in detecting 88% of medical conditions and 67% of musculoskeletal conditions detected during the PPE (7,8).
- Careful attention to the neurologic, musculoskeletal, and cardiopulmonary examination is essential, in particular with the athlete with an intellectual disability.

INJURY AND ILLNESS PATTERNS

- Injury rates for individuals with intellectual disabilities are less than those reported for physically disabled and general population athletes.
- Epidemiologic data have been reported for state, national, and international events (9–12).
  - Studies have shown that 3%–4% of all athletes are treated at Special Olympics events.
  - Track and field, followed by softball, account for more sports injuries than other events.
  - The most commonly injured site is the knee.
  - Injury rates calculated per 1000 participant-hours are:
    - 0.4 for Special Olympics athletes
    - 2.0 for special education high school students in organized contact sports
    - These rates can be compared to the following non-disabled adult athletes' injury rates (per 1000 participant-hours):
      - 0.03 for swimming
      - 2.9 for badminton
      - 3.65 for soccer
      - 4.1 for football
      - 4.7 for ice hockey
- Frequently encountered injuries and illnesses are listed in Table 132.1.
- In a study of Special Olympics injuries in Texas, athletes with Down syndrome had a relative risk of injury or illness 3.2 times greater than the other athletes (6).

Table 132-1 Intellectually Disabled Athletics: Sport Injuries and Illnesses (11)

Summer Sports		Winter Sports	
Injuries	Illnesses	Injuries	Illnesses
Abrasion	Heat related	Abrasion	Respiratory
Strain	Gastrointestinal	Strain	Dehydration
Sprain	Seizure	Sprain	Behavioral
Contusion	Headache	Contusion	Gastrointestinal
Epistaxis	Asthma	Laceration	Dermatologic
Laceration	Diabetes control	Blister	Canker sores
Blister	Sunburn	Fracture	Gingivitis
Nail avulsion	Conjunctivitis		
Fracture	Dermatitis		
	Insect bite		

Used with permission from O'Connor FG. *Sports Medicine: Just the Facts*. New York (NY): McGraw-Hill; 2005:581–6.

DOWN SYNDROME

- The athlete with Down syndrome (trisomy 21) requires special consideration due to well-described conditions associated with increased risk in athletics.
- Down syndrome is the most common human chromosomal abnormality.
  - Its incidence is estimated at 1 in 600–800 live births.
  - Up to 30% of Special Olympics athletes have Down syndrome.
  - Phenotypically, Down syndrome can vary greatly, but frequent common findings include intellectual disability, orthopedic issues, cardiac anomalies, vision problems, epilepsy, and obesity (13).
- National Health Interview Survey data of children with Down syndrome in the United States from 1997–2005 revealed the following general health information:
  - Children with Down syndrome were more than twice as likely as children in the general population to have seizures, recent food allergy, frequent diarrhea, or three or more ear infections.
  - Children with other causes of intellectual disability had higher risks for frequent severe headaches and seizures than did children with Down syndrome (14).
- Cardiac anomalies are prevalent in roughly 50% of persons with Down syndrome as compared to about 1% in the general population.
  - Endocardial cushion defects make up the majority of these, most of which are surgically repaired at a young age.
  - Isolated ventricular septal defects, atrial septal defects, and patent ductus arteriosus compose another 20%

of the congenital heart disease associated with Down syndrome.

  - Pulmonary hypertension is also more common in individuals with Down syndrome (15).
  - With or without cardiac malformations, athletes with Down syndrome have been found to have lower cardiovascular fitness levels than their peers due to average lower peak heart rates (13).
- Persons with Down syndrome have a high prevalence of vision and eye health problems. Many eye problems are undetected secondary to infrequent examinations. Down syndrome is associated with an increased frequency of keratoconus, cataract, high refractive error, glaucoma, strabismus, and macular disease.
  - In studies screening Down syndrome athletes, about 20% were observed to have significant uncorrected refractive errors (>1 diopter).
  - About one-third to one-half of Down syndrome athletes screened prior to participation are observed to have a pathology sufficient to affect vision (16,17).
- Due in part to inherent ligamentous laxity, the musculoskeletal system is a frequent cause of disability in Down syndrome athletes. The major areas of concern include the neck, hips, knees, and feet.
  - Cervical spine instability is the most significant musculoskeletal issue for the athlete with Down syndrome.
    - Atlantoaxial instability (AAI), which affects 10%–30% of individuals with Down syndrome, denotes laxity of the articulation between C1 (atlas) and C2 (axis).
    - AAI is due to odontoid abnormalities or laxity of the transverse ligament that holds the odontoid process in place against the inner aspect of the arch of the atlas (18).
    - Although atlantoaxial dislocation can be a significant cause of cord compromise, approximately 98% of AAI cases are asymptomatic (19).
      - Symptoms of AAI include neck pain, cervical deformity, fatigability, abnormal gait, clumsiness, or altered sensation.
      - Neurologic signs include sensory deficits, spasticity, hyperreflexia, clonus, and extensor-plantar reflex.
    - Radiographic evaluation is necessary to detect AAI. Lateral cervical spine radiographs in flexion, extension, and neutral will allow for examination of the atlanto-dens interval, which is measured from the anterior aspect of odontoid to the posterior surface of anterior arch of atlas.
    - In the early 1980s, the Special Olympics and the American Academy of Pediatrics (AAP) began recommending cervical spine radiographic screening of Special Olympians with Down syndrome before participation in "high-risk" sports (20).
    - The high-risk sports included pentathlon, diving (either as a sport or in swimming starts), butterfly swimming stroke, high jump, gymnastics, soccer, judo, snowboarding, and alpine skiing.
    - However, evidence shows that performing routine screening radiographs on asymptomatic children does not predict increased risk of spine issues nor future risk of developing such. Currently, the AAP and the Special Olympics do not require screening radiographs for participation of athletes with Down Syndrome. Rather, screening questions are asked as part of the preparticipation exam to determine risk. If the athlete has signs or symptoms of spinal cord compression or AAI, clearance for sport is then determined by a neurologist, neurosurgeon, or other qualified physician (20,21).
- Acquired hip instability is seen in about 5% of persons with Down syndrome.
  - The natural history of this condition is to progress from acute dislocation to recurrent dislocation, then eventually to fixed dislocation.
  - If treated nonoperatively, caution should be used to modify sports participation to avoid complete hip dislocation (22).
- Patellofemoral dislocation occurs in 4%–8% of persons with Down syndrome.
  - Progression to fixed dislocations may occur but may do well with nonoperative management.
  - No restriction is necessary for asymptomatic instability.
  - A neoprene knee brace with patellar window and activity restriction may be helpful for an athlete with symptoms (22).
- Foot deformities are very common in athletes with Down syndrome due to generalized ligamentous laxity.
  - Athletes with Down syndrome are prone to pes planovalgus, metatarsus primus varus, and bunions.
  - Surgery is rarely necessary because these conditions are well tolerated in athletes with Down syndrome with appropriately fitting shoes (22).
- Life expectancy for individuals with Down syndrome has increased from 12 years of age in 1949, to 35 years of age in 1982, to 55 years of age currently. Hence, there are many older persons with Down syndrome participating in athletics now (23).
- Several health-related changes are associated with aging in athletes with Down syndrome. The following conditions apply to adults with Down syndrome:
  - 40% will develop hypothyroidism.
  - 46%–57% have mitral valve prolapse.
  - 50% have sleep apnea.
  - 70% have conductive hearing loss.
  - 70% over the age of 65 years have visual impairments.
  - Alzheimer disease increases with age from rates of 10% for ages 30–39 years up to 55% for ages 50–59 years (23).

SPECIAL OLYMPICS

- It would be difficult to discuss athletics for those with intellectual disabilities without a general understanding of the Special Olympics.
- Special Olympics International is a nonprofit, international program developed in the 1960s to provide athletic opportunities for people with intellectual disabilities. The first Special Olympics competition was held in 1968.
    - Mission: "to provide year-round sports training and athletic competition in a variety of Olympic-type sports for children and adults with intellectual disabilities, giving them continuing opportunities to develop physical fitness, demonstrate courage, experience joy and participate in sharing of gifts, skills and friendship with their families, other Special Olympics athletes and the community" (20).
    - Provides opportunities for over 2 million athletes to develop physical fitness and to experience camaraderie in 30 different sports programs in almost 180 countries.
    - Athlete's Oath: "Let me win. But if I cannot win, let me be brave in the attempt" (20).
- To be eligible to participate, an individual must be at least 8 years old, and:
    - Be identified by a professional agency as having an intellectual disability
    - Have a cognitive delay determined by standardized measures
    - Have significant learning or vocational problems due to cognitive delays that require special instruction (24)
    - For many athletes, Special Olympics is a path to empowerment, competence, acceptance, joy, and community (20)

EVENT COVERAGE

- Coverage of events for intellectually disabled athletes, such as Special Olympics events, frequently relies on volunteers who may or may not have experience with past events.
- As with any other athletic event, systematic planning can help ensure success. Some considerations are outlined below (11).
    - Know the minimal medical facility requirements. Special Olympics requires the following for large competitions (20).
        - A qualified emergency medical technician (EMT) must be in attendance or readily available at all times.
        - A licensed medical professional must be on site or on call at all times.
        - First aid areas must be clearly identified, adequately equipped, and staffed by a qualified EMT for the entire event.
        - An ambulance with advanced cardiac life support capabilities must be readily available at all times.
    - Estimated crowd attendance must be factored into planning.
    - Seizure precautions should be followed in all activities where there might be a risk of severe injury if a convulsion were to occur, such as in swimming, diving, skiing, or equestrian, for example.
    - Environmental concerns such as adequate shelter, water, and restrooms must be addressed while accounting for the climate and time of day. Fluids must be provided, and drinking breaks encouraged.
    - Preparticipation screening results may assist in planning for unique issues and identifying specific athletes at increased risk.
    - Medical records should be readily available to medical staff. Medical conditions, allergies, medications, and emergency contact information should be located in a central location or on identification badges or race bibs.
    - For monocular athletes, eye protection with polycarbonate lenses should be worn, especially for missile-type sports.
    - Supplies and equipment needed are comparable to other community sporting events. Automated external defibrillators (AEDs) and antiepileptic injectable medications are recommended per Special Olympics guidelines. Some requirements vary by state and may require medical staff to know the location of the closest AED. As with other events, it is important to know local policies.
    - Most care will involve general first aid. Advanced emergency care by trained providers will usually involve initial stabilization and rapid transport of those who require more than basic first aid.

CONCLUSION

- Athletes with intellectual disabilities have a variety of health-related issues that impact their participation in sports.
- Knowledge of illness and injury patterns in athletes with intellectual disabilities allows the sports medicine physician to effectively provide care for these athletes.
- Preparticipation evaluation for the athlete with special needs should be similar to any athlete without intellectual or physical disability but must consider specific conditions that are more prevalent in this population.

REFERENCES

1. Schalock RL. *Intellectual Disability: Definition, Classification, and Systems of Supports*. 12th ed. Silver Spring (MD): American Association on Intellectual and Developmental Disabilities; 2021.
2. American Psychiatric Association Task Force on DSM-V. *Diagnostic and Statistical Manual of Mental Disorders: DSM-V-TR*. 5th ed. Washington (DC): American Psychiatric Association; 2013.

3. Durstine JL, Moore GE, Painter PL, Roberts SO. *ACSM's Exercise Management for Persons with Chronic Diseases and Disabilities.* 3rd ed. Champaign (IL): Human Kinetics; 2009:359–67.
4. Murphy NA, Carbone PS, American Academy of Pediatrics Council on Children With Disabilities. Promoting the participation of children with disabilities in sports, recreation, and physical activities. *Pediatrics.* 2008;121(5):1057–61.
5. Patel DR, Greydanus DE. Sport participation by physically and cognitively challenged young athletes. *Pediatr Clin North Am.* 2010;57(3):795–817.
6. McCormick DP, Ivey FM Jr, Gold DM, Zimmerman DM, Gemma S, Owen MJ. The preparticipation sports examination in Special Olympics athletes. *Tex Med.* 1988;84(4):39–43.
7. Bernhardt DT, Roberts WO, editors. *PPE: Preparticipation Physical Evaluation Monograph.* 5th ed. Washington (DC): American Academy of Pediatrics; 2019:179–91.
8. Birrer RB. The Special Olympics athlete: evaluation and clearance for participation. *Clin Pediatr.* 2004;43(9):777–82.
9. Batts KB, Glorioso JE Jr, Williams MS. The medical demands of the special athlete. *Clin J Sport Med.* 1998;8(1):22–5.
10. McCormick DP, Niebuhr VN, Risser WL. Injury and illness surveillance at local special olympic games. *Br J Sports Med.* 1990;24(4):221–4.
11. O'Connor FG. *Sports Medicine: Just the Facts.* New York (NY): McGraw-Hill; 2005:581–6.
12. Ramirez M, Yang J, Bourque L, et al. Sports injuries to high school athletes with disabilities. *Pediatrics.* 2009;123(2):690–6.
13. Sanyer ON. Down syndrome and sport participation. *Curr Sports Med Rep.* 2006;5(6):315–8.
14. Schieve LA, Boulet SL, Boyle C, Rasmussen SA, Schendel D. Health of children 3 to 17 years of age with Down syndrome in the 1997-2005 National Health Interview Survey. *Pediatrics.* 2009;123(2):e253–60.
15. National Association for Child Development Web site [Internet]. *Congenital heart disease in children with Down syndrome*; [cited 2022 Oct 15]. Available from: http://downsyndrome.nacd.org/heart_disease.php
16. Gutstein W, Sinclair SH, North RV, Bekiroglu N. Screening athletes with Down syndrome for ocular disease. *Optometry.* 2010;81(2):94–9.
17. Woodhouse JM, Adler P, Duignan A. Vision in athletes with intellectual disabilities: the need for improved eyecare. *J Intellect Disabil Res.* 2004;48(Pt 8):736–45.
18. Cope R, Olson S. Abnormalities of the cervical spine in Down's syndrome: diagnosis, risks, and review of the literature, with particular reference to the Special Olympics. *South Med J.* 1987;80(1):33–6.
19. Hankinson TC, Anderson RC. Craniovertebral junction abnormalities in Down syndrome. *Neurosurgery.* 2010;66(3 suppl l):32–8.
20. Medical Form Instructions. *International Special Olympics Web site* [Internet]. Washington (DC): Special Olympics International; [cited 2023 Sep 21]. https://medform.specialolympics.org/
21. Bull MJ, Trotter T, Santoro SL, et al. Health supervision for children and adolescents with Down syndrome. *Pediatrics.* 2022;149(5):e2022057010.
22. Winell J, Burke SW. Sports participation of children with Down syndrome. *Orthop Clin North Am.* 2003;34(3):439–43.
23. Barnhart RC, Connolly B. Aging and Down syndrome: implications for physical therapy. *Phys Ther.* 2007;87(10):1399–406.
24. Platt LS. Medical and orthopaedic conditions in special olympics athletes. *J Athl Train.* 2001;36(1):74–80.

The Adaptive Athlete

133

Paul F. Pasquina, Tawnee L. Sparling, and Xiaoning (Jenny) Yuan

INTRODUCTION

- There are an estimated 61 million adults living with disability in the Unites States (1), with varying incidence, prevalence, and costs data across different conditions (2).
- The Americans with Disabilities Act defines "disability" as any physical or mental impairment that substantially limits at least one or more major life activity (3).
- Disability is associated with multiple negative determinants of health, including lower education, higher poverty, lower employment, and discriminatory societal attitudes.
  - These factors magnify underlying impairments leading to decreased activity, and higher rates of obesity, cardiovascular disease, morbidity, and mortality (4).
  - Athletes with disabilities are at a higher risk for sexual, physical, and emotional abuse than their able-bodied counterparts (5).
- While improved technology creates greater opportunities for adaptive sports (6,7), limited access and lack of awareness remain significant barriers to adaptive sports participation (8).
  - Individual counseling, however, can enhance physical activity and an active lifestyle (9).
- There are currently 28 Paralympic sports that have been sanctioned by the International Paralympic Committee (10).

Physical Benefits of Adaptive Sports

- Physical activity can provide multiple benefits including improvements in both mental health and quality of life (11), especially for children and adolescents (12).
- Athletes with disabilities demonstrate increased exercise endurance, muscle strength, cardiovascular efficiency, and flexibility; improved balance; and better motor skills compared with individuals with disabilities who do not participate in athletics.
- Physical activity and participation in sport are proven to prevent and manage diseases such as heart disease, stroke, hypertension, diabetes, obesity, and some cancers.
- In addition to physical benefits, the psychological benefits of exercise and adaptive sports participation include improved self-image, body awareness, motor development, mood, and quality of life (13).
- Individuals with disabilities who engage in sports and athletics have fewer cardiac risk factors, higher high-density lipoprotein cholesterol, and are less likely to smoke cigarettes than those who are not active (14).
- Individuals with amputations who participate in athletics have improved proprioception, body image, and proficiency in prosthetic use (15,16).
- Athletes with paraplegia are less likely to be hospitalized, have fewer pressure ulcers, and are less susceptible to infections than nonactive individuals with paraplegia (17).

Epidemiology

- The incidence, location, and nature of musculoskeletal injuries appear to be disability and sport dependent.
  - Lower extremity (LE) injuries are more common in ambulatory athletes (visually impaired, amputee, cerebral palsy), whereas upper extremity (UE) injuries are more frequent in athletes who use a wheelchair (18).
  - A 3-year, cross-disability prospective study found the injury rate of disabled athletes to be 9.30/1000 athlete exposures (19) — an injury rate less than what has been reported in college football (12.0–15.0/1000) and college soccer (9.8/1000), but higher than that reported in men's and women's college basketball (7.0/1000 and 7.3/1,000, respectively) (20,21).
  - A prospective study of intercollegiate wheelchair basketball demonstrated an increased incidence of injuries per 1000 athlete-exposures for females (13.1) versus males (12.2), with a greater relative risk of injury of 2.01 for females and 1.53 for males when compared to nondisabled basketball players (22).
  - Wheelchair users are at a significant increased risk of UE entrapment neuropathies, like carpal tunnel syndrome (CTS), with a reported prevalence rate of between 50% and 73%; however, it appears that wheelchair athletes have a lower prevalence than nonathletes (23,24).
  - However, with regard to winter sports, disabled athletes appear to have a lower incidence of injuries than able-bodied skiers (25).
  - Injury data from the Summer and Winter Paralympic Games demonstrate a higher incidence proportion of both injuries and illness compared to the Olympic Games (26).

PREPARTICIPATION ASSESSMENT (27)

- Preparticipation examination (PPE) should be performed in a systematic, comprehensive fashion similar to that performed for able-bodied athletes.
- Sports medicine practitioners be cautioned not to be overly focused on the athlete's impairment/disability such that they may overlook common medical issues.
- Sports medicine practitioners who are not familiar with certain impairments should solicit assistance from practitioners with more experience. This often requires a team approach. For example, a physician specializing in sports medicine may have little experience in spinal cord injuries (SCIs), whereas an SCI specialist may have even less experience in sports medicine. Together, however, they can jointly assess an individual and clear him or her safely for participation.
- The specific elements required in the PPE are determined by the sport, the level of participation, the athletic organization, the clinical indications, and the athlete. The PPE should provide information to guide the athlete, athletic trainer, coach, and team physician toward safe participation, activity limitations, and disability-specific training.
- Practitioners should avoid mass screening stations for individuals with disabilities in favor of private office setting visits, although mass screenings may be needed at Special Olympic events (28).
- It is recommended that the PPE be performed by a medical team that is involved in the longitudinal care of the athlete because knowledge of baseline functioning is essential.
  - Baseline assessment of cognition is especially important for athletes with a history of brain injury (29).
- Additional elements to the history should include the athlete's goals, predisability health, present level of training, sports participation, medications and supplements used, presence of impairments, past and family cardiopulmonary history, level of functional independence for mobility and self-care, and needs for adaptive equipment.
- Special attention should be paid to the athlete's mental health, stressors, and safety, including history of abuse (30).
- The objectives of the examination include the following:
  - Identify conditions that may require further medical evaluation before the athlete enters into training, require close supervision during training, and may predispose to injury.
  - Determine the athlete's general health to assess fitness level and performance.
  - Counsel on health-related issues and methods for safe participation.
  - Provide referral for identified conditions that require further evaluation and/or monitoring to physician's familiar with the disability and the management of the identified conditions.
- The elements of the disability and sports-specific physical examination are tailored for the individual.
  - Sensory deficits, neurologic deficits, joint stability and range of motion (ROM), muscle strength, flexibility, skin integrity, medications, and adaptive equipment needs must be assessed.
  - During the musculoskeletal examination of an athlete who uses a wheelchair, evaluate the stability, flexibility, and strength of the commonly injured sites (*e.g.*, shoulder, hand and wrist, and LEs) as well as the trunk.
- Special attention should be paid during the PPE to skin breakdown on insensate pressure areas as well as sites that come in contact with orthotics/prosthetics.
- Also, a careful history of heat/cold injuries and changes in neurologic function should be solicited.
- During the musculoskeletal examination of an individual who has had an LE amputation, assess the stability, flexibility, and strength of the trunk, as well as the hip girdle and the unaffected and affected LE with or without the prosthesis.
- For individuals with UE amputations, the stability, flexibility, and strength of the shoulder girdle must be assessed in the unaffected and affected extremity with and without prosthesis, in addition to a trunk and LE evaluation.
- For the athlete with brain injury, stroke, or multiple sclerosis, it is prudent to assess the limitations of the unaffected and affected areas based on mobility and sports-specific tasks.
- Cardiovascular and pulmonary examinations can identify conditions that can cause cardiopulmonary collapse or disease progression. Suggested guidelines for cardiovascular screening of the athlete are available from the American College of Sports Medicine, American Heart Association, and American College of Cardiology.
- Careful evaluation of the athlete's wheelchair, prosthetics, orthotics, and assistive/adaptive devices should also be performed prior to competition. This is usually facilitated by consultation with the individual's orthotist, prosthetist, or other health care specialists with experience in this area.
- A PPE is performed upon entry into sports and should be repeated at least every 2–3 years. An interim examination prior to each sport season may be necessary if the athlete's health condition changes.

INJURIES AND COMPLICATIONS BY CAUSE OF DISABILITY

- Athletes with disabilities are subject to many of the same injuries that affect their able-body counterparts, however, there are unique challenges that impact their sports performance, sport longevity, and more broadly, their health and quality of life

- Challenges for individuals with SCI often include somatic and autonomic nervous system dysfunction, resulting in sensory/motor deficits, spasticity, reduced peak pulmonary and cardiac function, and impaired temperature regulation (31).
- There is certainly an overlap between the categories of diagnoses resulting in disability. For example, many patients with SCIs are wheelchair users. For the purposes of this discussion, the following conditions will be considered: wheelchair use, major limb loss, and SCI.

WHEELCHAIR USE

- Wheelchair athletes are at significant risk for a multitude of unique musculoskeletal and medical problems. Therefore, preventive strategies have been proposed for several common conditions (32).
- Given the degree to which wheelchair users rely on their upper limbs for mobility and activities of daily living, the importance of recognizing, treating, and preventing upper limb injuries is magnified when compared with the able-bodied population.
  - Because relative rest of the upper limb may be impossible or nearly impossible in this population, other measures should be considered. These may include splinting and orthotic prescriptions, admission to an inpatient setting if rest is required, or home modifications or additional assistance (33).

Shoulder Injuries

- Wheelchair users are at increased risk for shoulder pathology, including pain, rotator cuff injuries, subacromial bursitis, acromioclavicular joint abnormalities, coracoacromial ligament thickening, subacromial spurs, distal clavicle osteolysis, and impingement syndrome (34,35).
- Factors contributing to the increased risk in this population include repetitive motion, increased pressure in the shoulder joint during wheelchair propulsion, and muscle imbalances in the shoulder girdle due to weakness (34).
- In wheelchair users, upper limb injuries, including shoulder injuries, are particularly disabling due to the fact that these patients rely on their upper limbs for weight bearing, transfers, and ambulation in addition to all of the demands placed on the upper limbs in the able-bodied population.
- Despite increases in repetitive use and high-intensity activity, wheelchair athletes do not have a higher incidence of shoulder pain than nonathletic wheelchair users. In fact, participation in athletic competition appears to be protective from shoulder pain (36). This is likely due to increased strength and endurance in the athletic population.
- Shoulder complaints among wheelchair users can be reduced by appropriate wheelchair design and the use of ideal propulsion techniques.

Elbow Injuries

- The elbow is a very common site of ulnar nerve entrapment, representing the second most common upper limb nerve entrapment syndrome.
- Wheelchair users are at an increased risk for ulnar neuropathy at the elbow (37). There is no evidence to suggest that wheelchair athletes are at a greater risk as compared with nonathlete wheelchair users.
- Symptoms of ulnar neuropathy at the elbow include numbness and tingling in the fifth digit and the ulnar half of the fourth digit, weakness and atrophy in the hand intrinsic muscles, and pain and tenderness in the ulnar groove. Diagnosis of ulnar neuropathy is made based on history, physical examination, and electrodiagnostic testing.
- Other sources of elbow pain that are reported in wheelchair users are lateral epicondylitis, osteoarthritis, and olecranon bursitis.
- Treatment of elbow pain and injuries in wheelchair users must be tailored to the individual needs of the patient, keeping in mind that many wheelchair users will be nonmobile if they are required to restrict weight bearing or otherwise limit activity involving their upper limb.

Wrist Injuries

- The carpal tunnel is the most common site of nerve entrapment in able-bodied and disabled persons.
- Long-term wheelchair users have a prevalence of CTS of 49%–73% (38).
- Symptoms of CTS include numbness and tingling in the radial three digits and the radial half of the fourth digit, weakness in thumb abduction, clumsiness, wrist pain, and nocturnal paresthesias. Diagnosis is based on history, physical examination, and electrodiagnostic testing.
- Wheelchair users with symptoms and physical examination findings of CTS have lower functional status as compared with wheelchair users without CTS (38).
- In addition to CTS, wheelchair users are at increased risk for other wrist overuse injuries and syndromes, including ulnar nerve entrapment in the Guyon canal (37), osteoarthritis, tendinitis, and de Quervain tenosynovitis (33).

Upper and Lower Limb Fractures

- Individuals with disabilities, particularly those with reduced ambulation, have a greater risk of low bone mineral density, osteopenia, osteoporosis, and fracture.
- Measures to reduce low bone mineral density include early weight-bearing activities after injury (tilt table or standing), functional electrical stimulation (FES), vitamin D, and calcium supplementation, as well as the use of bisphosphonates (32).

- One study reported that 9.4% of elite-level athletes with physical disabilities reported a history of a sports-related fracture (39).
- Wheelchair athletes may be at greater risk for upper limb fractures due to repetitive falls associated with many wheelchair sports, propulsion requiring positioning the hand in a location that is susceptible to injury from nearby wheelchairs or collisions, and relatively high speeds achieved during certain wheelchair sports.
- Fractures should be treated as in the able-bodied population.
- Restricted upper limb weight bearing in a wheelchair user may result in immobility of the athlete.

LIMB LOSS

Skin Complications

- Following amputation and prosthetic fitting, the skin of the distal portion of the residual limb becomes a weight-bearing surface where it had not previously been such. As a result, the distal residual limb is at increased risk for skin breakdown and other skin disorders.
- Verrucous hyperplasia is a wart-like lesion that may develop at the distal end of the residual limb. It may occur as a result of proximal residual limb constriction from a socket or wrap that causes decreased pressure in the distal residual limb. Prevention consists of equal distribution of pressure through the residual limb, as in a total contact socket (40).
- Skin breakdown may occur when pressure is applied disproportionately to a pressure-sensitive area of skin on the residual limb, such as the tibial tubercle in a transtibial amputee. The risk may be compounded by the fact that many amputees may have impaired sensation in the residual limb, and sweating with athletic activity can increase moisture at the skin-socket interface and make skin breakdown more likely.
- Skin breakdown can be particularly disabling for individuals who rely on weight bearing through the residual limb for ambulation. If restricted weight bearing is required, ambulation will not be possible.
- Prevention of skin breakdown involves prosthetic socket design that distributes pressure equally throughout the entire circumferential surface of the residual limb and reduces pressure over pressure-sensitive skin.
  - In addition, silicone liners, padded sleeves, socks, and additional padding can be preventive.

Heterotopic Ossification

- Heterotopic ossification (HO) is the formation of bone in tissues that are not normally ossified. It has been traditionally reported to occur following traumatic brain injury (TBI), SCI, burns, and total arthroplasty.
- Recently, HO has been reported to occur at high rates in the residual limbs of individuals with traumatic amputation (41).
  - HO in residual limbs may increase the risk of skin breakdown or cause pain with weight bearing.
- Following TBI, SCI, burns, and arthroplasty, HO typically develops around major joints, thus restricting ROM and limiting mobility. In contrast, following amputation, HO occurs in injured tissues in the residual limb and may not be in the vicinity of a joint.
- Recognition of HO in residual limbs allows for modifications in the design of a prosthetic socket to accommodate for the ectopic bone. Furthermore, monitoring for skin breakdown should be increased in amputees with HO.
- Surgical excision of HO may be required if conservative measures fail to restore adequate levels of function.

Neuroma

- A neuroma occurs at the distal end of a resected nerve in the residual limb of an amputee. When a neuroma is exposed to pressure, it creates paresthesias, dysesthesias, and radiating pain in the phantom distribution of the resected nerve.
- When a neuroma occurs at or near a weight-bearing structure, it can create severe pain with ambulation and weight bearing, limiting an athlete's ability to train and compete.
- Treatment may involve prosthetic modifications to relieve pressure on the neuroma, oral medications including antiepileptic and tricyclic antidepressants, and injection of corticosteroids and local anesthetic into the neuroma. Surgical excision may be necessary if conservative treatments fail.

SPINAL CORD INJURY

Thermoregulation (31)

- Following SCIs, there is disruption of neuroregulatory systems that are involved in the control of body temperature. Below the level of the lesion, athletes with SCI have impaired shivering to produce heat and impaired sweating and vasodilation to dissipate heat. Athletes with tetraplegia are at greater risk compared with those with paraplegia (42).
- Paraplegic and tetraplegic athletes are expected to see greater increases in body temperature with exertion and greater decreases in temperature with exposure to cold weather.
- Prevention of temperature-related injuries requires heightened awareness and monitoring, use of appropriate clothing and equipment, availability of rehydration, and avoidance of extremes of temperature when possible.
- Frostbite is of particular concern during cold weather events. Athletes with SCIs have impaired sensation and require frequent visual monitoring to prevent cold injuries.

Autonomic Dysreflexia (31)

- Patients with SCIs at the level of T6 and above are at risk for autonomic dysreflexia (AD), a potentially serious condition that occurs when sympathetic outflow in response to a noxious stimulus is unregulated due to the interruption of neural pathways after SCI.
- Symptoms include paroxysmal hypertension, bradycardia, facial flushing, and headache.
- If blood pressure continues to increase without treatment, stroke or death may occur.
- Common noxious stimuli that lead to AD include tight clothing, urinary or fecal retention, renal or bladder stones, pressure ulcers, infections, or intra-abdominal pathology (*e.g.*, appendicitis).
- Treatment involves sitting the patient upright, loosening clothing, and identifying and eliminating the noxious stimulus.
- For acute blood pressure control, chewable nifedipine or nitropaste can be used.
- "Boosting" describes the practice of intentionally inducing AD in order to improve athletic performance (43). This dangerous practice should be discouraged and may be life threatening.

Skin Breakdown

- Following SCI, insensate skin leads to a risk of skin breakdown or pressure ulcer.
- Regardless of the level of the injury, the skin over the sacrum, coccyx, and ischial tuberosities is frequently insensate. These areas represent the highest risk for skin breakdown in athletes with SCI.
- Specific athletic events may result in an increased risk of skin breakdown in additional areas. For example, wheelchair racers may have an increased risk of skin breakdown if the medial surface of the arm and forearm rubs against the wheelchair during propulsion. This may require customized equipment and padding to prevent skin breakdown in activity-specific, high-risk skin areas.
- Athletic wheelchairs commonly sacrifice pressure relief for higher performance.
- Pressure ulcers can be a significant cause of morbidity and mortality in the SCI population. Therefore, prevention of skin breakdown is of paramount importance in this population, which should cause the athlete and caregivers to increase vigilance in monitoring for this condition, changing position frequently, and limiting time in the wheelchair as much as possible. This is particularly important when an athlete is transitioning to a new piece of equipment (*e.g.*, a new wheelchair).
- At the first sign of skin breakdown or pressure ulcer, weight bearing and athletic activities should be modified or restricted to prevent further injury.

Heterotopic Ossification

- Following SCI, HO may occur below the level of the injury, and the most common site of HO after SCI is the hip, though the knee, elbow, and shoulder may also be affected, depending on the level of injury.
- Diagnosis of HO may be made by x-rays, bone scan, or trends in alkaline phosphatase levels.
  - The initial presentation may mimic deep venous thrombosis or joint infection, and diagnostic testing is often required to exclude these other diagnoses.
- Prevention of HO involves frequent ROM exercises. Pharmacologic prophylaxis may be considered in high-risk populations and may consist of nonsteroidal anti-inflammatory drugs or bisphosphonates.
- Extensive HO in athletes may limit participation by limiting ROM, causing pain, or contributing to skin breakdown.
- Surgical excision may be required if conservative and adaptive treatments are not successful.

Spasticity

- Spasticity is a velocity-dependent increase in muscle tone that occurs after injury to the upper motor neuron. It is a common complication of SCI that may limit athletic participation by interfering with voluntary movements and restricting ROM.
- An increase in spasticity may be an indicator of a systemic or otherwise asymptomatic condition. For example, infections, intra-abdominal pathology (*e.g.*, appendicitis), skin breakdown, or bladder distension may have few symptoms that are sensed by a patient with SCI. Therefore, a sudden increase in spasticity should lead to a search for underlying pathology.
- Treatment for spasticity consists of oral medications, including baclofen, dantrolene, tizanidine, and benzodiazepines; injectable medications such as botulinum toxin; and intrathecal medications such as baclofen.
  - If spasticity is resistant to conservative treatment, surgery for tendon lengthening may improve hygiene, activities of daily living, and functional activities, including participation in athletics.

Osteopenia and Osteoporosis

- Osteopenia and osteoporosis are nearly universal complications of SCI.
- Decreased weight bearing predisposes to low bone mineral density; however, many risk factors are independent of alterations in weight bearing. These risk factors include severity of the injury, spasticity, and time since injury (44).
- Osteoporosis results in increased fracture risk in athletes with SCI.

- Because of impaired sensation below the level of the injury, athletes with SCI may not immediately complain of pain after a fracture.
  - Increased spasticity or AD may both be warning signs that a more serious injury has occurred.
- Prevention of osteoporosis should include calcium and vitamin D supplementation for all athletes with SCI. In addition, early activity and weight bearing (standing and tilt table), FES, and bisphosphonates may also be used for prevention (32).

Orthostatic Hypotension

- Orthostatic hypotension occurs in most patients with SCI.
- Symptoms include light-headedness and dizziness upon moving from supine to seated or upright position, and syncope may occur if uncorrected.
- Orthostatic hypotension occurs after SCI because of decreased sympathetic efferent activity in the vasculature below the level of the injury and also because of decreased reflex vasoconstriction. The result is venous pooling in dependent areas (lower limbs or abdomen) that occurs with changes in position (45).
- Prevention includes the use of lower limb compression stockings and abdominal binders, maintenance of hydration, and salt supplementation.
  - If these measures are insufficient, pharmacologic treatment with midodrine, fludrocortisone, or ephedrine may be helpful (45).
- In athletes with SCI, nonpharmacologic prevention should be attempted before the use of pharmacologic agents is considered.

Acute Mountain Sickness (46)

- Acute mountain sickness involves a constellation of symptoms (headache, nausea, weakness, shortness of breath) and occurs with exposure to high altitudes. Incidence increases with increasing altitude.
- In many winter sports, competition at high altitudes increases the risk of acute mountain sickness.
- Acute mountain sickness is thought to be caused by alterations in the blood-brain barrier and cerebral vasculature that occur at high altitudes.
- Given their altered neurophysiology and anatomy, athletes with SCI may be at increased risk for acute mountain sickness.
- Acetazolamide may be used as prophylaxis, and treatment, in high-risk scenarios. Treatment may additionally include return to low altitude, or dexamethasone (see Chapter 48 on environmental illness).

REFERENCES

1. Centers for Disease Control and Prevention, *Disability Impacts All of Us*. Accessed 2022 Nov 11. https://www.cdc.gov/ncbddd/disabilityandhealth/infographic-disability-impacts-all.html
2. Lo J, Chan L, Flynn S. A systematic review of the incidence, prevalence, costs, and activity and work limitations of amputation, osteoarthritis, rheumatoid arthritis, back pain, multiple sclerosis, spinal cord injury, stroke, and traumatic brain injury in the United States: a 2019 update. *Arch Phys Med Rehabil.* 2021 Jan;102(1):115–31. doi:10.1016/j.apmr.2020.04.001
3. Americans with Disabilities Act National Networks. What is the definition of disability under the ADA? Accessed 2022Nov 12. https://adata.org/faq/what-definition-disability-under-ada
4. Blauwet CA, Iezzoni LI. From the Paralympics to public health: increasing physical activity through legislative and policy initiatives. *Pharm Manag PM R.* 2014 Aug;6(8 suppl):S4–10. doi:10.1016/j.pmrj.2014.05.014
5. Sacks H, Wu M, Carter C, Karamitopoulos M. Parasport: effects on musculoskeletal function and injury patterns. *J Bone Joint Surg Am.* 2022 Oct 5;104(19):1760–8. doi:10.2106/JBJS.21.01504
6. De Luigi AJ, Cooper RA. Adaptive sports technology and biomechanics: prosthetics. *Pharm Manag PM R.* 2014 Aug;6(8 Suppl):S40–57. doi:10.1016/j.pmrj.2014.06.011
7. Cooper RA, De Luigi AJ. Adaptive sports technology and biomechanics: wheelchairs. *Pharm Manag PM R.* 2014 Aug;6(8 Suppl):S31–9. doi:10.1016/j.pmrj.2014.05.020
8. Martin Ginis KA, Ma JK, Latimer-Cheung AE, Rimmer JH. A systematic review of review articles addressing factors related to physical activity participation among children and adults with physical disabilities. *Health Psychol Rev.* 2016 Dec;10(4):478–94. doi:10.1080/17437199.2016.1198240
9. van der Ploeg HP, Streppel KR, van der Beek AJ, et al. Counselling increases physical activity behaviour nine weeks after rehabilitation. *Br J Sports Med.* 2006 Mar;40(3):223–9. doi:10.1136/bjsm.2005.021139
10. International Paralympic Committee. *Paralympic Sports.* Accessed 2022 Nov 11. https://www.paralympic.org/sports
11. World Health Organization. Recommendation for physical activity for adults living with disability. Accessed 2022 Nov 12. https://www.who.int/news-room/fact-sheets/detail/physical-activity
12. Carbone PS, Smith PJ, Lewis C, LeBlanc C. Promoting the participation of children and adolescents with disabilities in sports, recreation, and physical activity. *Pediatrics.* 2021 Dec 1;148(6):e2021054664. doi:10.1542/peds.2021-054664
13. Diaz R, Miller EK, Kraus E, Fredericson M. Impact of adaptive sports participation on quality of life. *Sports Med Arthrosc Rev.* 2019 Jun;27(2):73–82. doi:10.1097/JSA.0000000000000242
14. Dearwater SR, LaPorte RE, Robertson RJ, Brenes G, Adams LL, Becker D. Activity in the spinal cord-injured patient: an epidemiologic analysis of metabolic parameters. *Med Sci Sports Exerc.* 1986;18(5):541–4.
15. Wetterhahn KA, Hanson C, Levy CE. Effect of participation in physical activity on body image of amputees. *Am J Phys Med Rehabil.* 2002;81(3):194–201.
16. Deans S, Burns D, McGarry A, Murray K, Mutrie N. Motivations and barriers to prosthesis users participation in physical activity, exercise and sport: a review of the literature. *Prosthet Orthot Int.* 2012 Sep;36(3):260–9. doi:10.1177/0309364612437905

17. Stotts KM. Health maintenance: paraplegic athletes and nonathletes. *Arch Phys Med Rehabil.* 1986;67(2):109–14.
18. Ferrara MS, Peterson CL. Injuries to athletes with disabilities: identifying injury patterns. *Sports Med.* 2000;30(2):137–43.
19. Ferrara MS, Buckley WE. Athletes with disabilities injury registry. *Adapt Phys Act Q (APAQ).* 1996;13:50–60.
20. Buckley WE. Five year overview of sport injuries: the NAIRS model. *J Phys Educ Recreat Dance.* 1982;17:36–40.
21. Buckley WE, Powell JP. NAIRS: an epidemiological overview of the severity of injury in college football. *J Athl Train.* 1982;18:279–82.
22. Kasitinon D, Royston A, Wernet L, Garner D, Richard J, Argo LR. Health-related incidents among intercollegiate wheelchair basketball players. *Pharm Manag PM R.* 2021 Jul;13(7):746–55. doi:10.1002/pmrj.12474
23. Boninger ML, Robertson RN, Wolff M, Cooper RA. Upper limb nerve entrapments in elite wheelchair racers. *Am J Phys Med Rehabil.* 1996;75(3):170–6.
24. Burnham RS, Steadward RD. Upper extremity peripheral nerve entrapments among wheelchair athletes: prevalence, location, and risk factors. *Arch Phys Med Rehabil.* 1994;75(5):519–24.
25. Laskowski ER, Murtaugh PA. Snow skiing injuries in physically disabled skiers. *Am J Sports Med.* 1992;20(5):553–7.
26. Fagher K, Dahlström Ö, Jacobsson J, Timpka T, Lexell J. Prevalence of sports-related injuries and illnesses in paralympic athletes. *Pharm Manag PM R.* 2020 Mar;12(3):271–80. doi:10.1002/pmrj.12211
27. Hawkeswood JP, O'Connor R, Anton H, Finlayson H. The preparticipation evaluation for athletes with disability. *Int J Sports Phys Ther.* 2014 Feb;9(1):103–15.
28. Seidenberg PH, Eggers JL. Mass screenings at mass participation events: MedFest at Special Olympics. *Curr Sports Med Rep.* 2015 May–Jun;14(3):176–81. doi:10.1249/JSR.0000000000000164
29. Weiler R, Blauwet C, Clarke D, et al. Concussion in para sport: the first position statement of the Concussion in Para Sport (CIPS) Group. *Br J Sports Med.* 2021 Nov;55(21):1187–95. doi:10.1136/bjsports-2020-103696
30. Swartz L, Hunt X, Bantjes J, Hainline B, Reardon CL. Mental health symptoms and disorders in Paralympic athletes: a narrative review. *Br J Sports Med.* 2019 Jun;53(12):737–40. doi:10.1136/bjsports-2019-100731
31. Cruz S, Blauwet CA. Implications of altered autonomic control on sports performance in athletes with spinal cord injury. *Auton Neurosci.* 2018 Jan;209:100–4. doi:10.1016/j.autneu.2017.03.006. .
32. Dutton RA. Medical and musculoskeletal concerns for the wheelchair athlete: a review of preventative strategies. *Curr Sports Med Rep.* 2019 Jan;18(1):9–16. doi:10.1249/JSR.0000000000000560
33. Paralyzed Veterans of America Consortium for Spinal Cord Medicine. Preservation of upper limb function following spinal cord injury: a clinical practice guideline for health-care professionals. *J Spinal Cord Med.* 2005;28(5):434–70.
34. Heyward OW, Vegter RJK, de Groot S, van der Woude LHV. Shoulder complaints in wheelchair athletes: a systematic review. *PLoS One.* 2017 Nov 21;12(11):e0188410. doi:10.1371/journal.pone.0188410
35. Brose SW, Boninger ML, Fullerton B, et al. Shoulder ultrasound abnormalities, physical examination findings, and pain in manual wheelchair users with spinal cord injury. *Arch Phys Med Rehabil.* 2008;89(11):2086–93.
36. Fullerton HD, Borckardt JJ, Alfano AP. Shoulder pain: a comparison of wheelchair athletes and nonathletic wheelchair users. *Med Sci Sports Exerc.* 2003;35(12):1958–61.
37. Groah SL, Lanig IS. Neuromusculoskeletal syndromes in wheelchair athletes. *Semin Neurol.* 2000;20(2):201–8.
38. Yang J, Boninger ML, Leath JD, Fitzgerald SG, Dyson-Hudson TA, Chang MW. Carpal tunnel syndrome in manual wheelchair users with spinal cord injury: a cross-sectional multicenter study. *Am J Phys Med Rehabil.* 2009;88(12):1007–16.
39. Patatoukas D, Farmakides A, Aggeli V, et al. Disability-related injuries in athletes with disabilities. *Folia Med.* 2011 Jan–Mar;53(1):40–6. doi:10.2478/v10153-010-0026-x
40. Kuiken TA, Miller L, Lipschutz R, Huang ME. Rehabilitation of people with lower limb amputation. In: Braddom RL, editor. *Physical Medicine and Rehabilitation.* Philadelphia (PA): Elsevier; 2007.
41. Potter BK, Burns TC, Lacap AP, Granville RR, Gajewski D. Heterotopic ossification in the residual limbs of traumatic and combat-related amputees. *J Am Acad Orthop Surg.* 2006;14(10 Spec No.):S191–7.
42. Price MJ, Campbell IG. Effects of spinal cord lesion level upon thermoregulation during exercise in the heat. *Med Sci Sports Exerc.* 2003;35(7):1100–7.
43. Harris P. Self-induced autonomic dysreflexia ("boosting") practised by some tetraplegic athletes to enhance their athletic performance. *Paraplegia.* 1994;32(5):289–91.
44. Jiang SD, Dai LY, Jiang LS. Osteoporosis after spinal cord injury. *Osteoporos Int.* 2006;17(2):180–92.
45. Krassioukov A, Eng JJ, Warburton DE, Teasell R. Spinal Cord Injury Rehabilitation Evidence Research Team. A systematic review of the management of orthostatic hypotension after spinal cord injury. *Arch Phys Med Rehabil.* 2009;90(5):876–95.
46. Dicianno BE, Aguila ED, Cooper RA, et al. Acute mountain sickness in disability and adaptive sports: preliminary data. *J Rehabil Res Dev.* 2008;45(4):479–87.

135 The Athlete With Cancer

Jason M. Matuszak and Tracey O'Connor

INTRODUCTION

- Cancer can strike individuals in the prime of their lives, and athletes are no exception.
- With advances in screening, diagnosis, and management, people increasingly survive cancer and return to activities that are important to them. As of 2022, there are an estimated 18 million cancer survivors in the United States (1).
- Physical activity has been linked to reduced risk of multiple types of cancer, with strong evidence demonstrating reduced risks of bladder, breast, colon, endometrial, esophageal adenocarcinoma, renal, and gastric cancers; moderate evidence of a reduced risk for lung cancers; and limited evidence for reduced risk in hematologic, head and neck, ovarian, pancreatic, and prostate cancers (2).
- Exercise training and testing are generally safe in a cancer patient or survivor (3) has benefits to survivorship, health, and general well-being (2).
- Inverse relationship between the amounts of physical activity and both cancer-specific and all-cause mortality for breast, colorectal, and prostate cancer (2).
- An extensive analysis of the benefits of exercise for cancer prevention was completed as part of the 2018 Physical Activity Guidelines Advisory Committee Summary Report.
- American College of Sports Medicine (ACSM) published a Consensus Statement on Exercise Guidelines for Cancer Survivors (3) (ACSM infographic).
  - "Designed to advance exercise recommendations beyond public health guidelines and toward prescriptive programs specific to cancer type, treatments, and/or outcomes" (3).
  - Specific doses of aerobic and resistance training, alone or in combination, can improve anxiety and depressive symptoms, fatigue, physical functioning, and health-related quality of life (3).
- Sports medicine physicians are ideally positioned to:
  - Educate athlete about cancer risk;
  - Screen for detectable cancers;
  - Evaluate musculoskeletal pain for potential malignant causes;
  - In conjunction with an athlete and their health care team, develop an exercise program/prescription;
  - Educate on the benefits of exercise in the cancer patient and in cancer prevention.

ATHLETES POTENTIALLY AT INCREASED RISK OF CANCER

- Environmental/skin exposure.
  - Many sports are played outdoors, and, as such, there is sun exposure. Multiple studies have shown an increased risk of skin cancer in outdoor sports, including aquatic and traditionally winter sports (4–6).
  - Athletes demonstrate a general lack of awareness of risk of skin cancer in some outdoor sports (7,8).
  - Evidence of increased hazard ratio (approx. 20% higher relative risk) of melanoma in physically active people (9).
  - Radiation exposure may be higher for athletes who travel frequently by airplane and who have undergone multiple x-rays or, especially, computed tomography scans (10–13).
- There appears to be an association between skin exposure to talc and certain cancers (14,15). Athletes may have frequent, recurrent, and persistent skin exposure to talc in various athletic powders either to control perspiration or for improved handling of sports equipment (*e.g.*, gymnastics, racquet sports, baseballs, etc.).
- Skin exposure to trihalomethanes or other carcinogens in swimming pool water has been suggested to be a risk factor for cancer (16).
- Drugs or ergogenic aids that may predispose for cancer.
  - Anabolic steroids have traditionally been implicated in hepatoma, and studies show there are sex hormone receptors in liver cancer cells (17,18).
  - Growth hormone and insulin-like growth factor 1 may affect cancer development and progression and have been associated with the development of several types of cancer (19).
  - Growth hormone
    - Evidence shows that individuals with acromegaly have pathologically increased tumor risk.

        - Supplementation for medical or ergogenic reasons may lead to increases in colorectal cancer, second tumors in previous cancer patients taking growth hormone, and in primary tumors as a result of the anabolic effects and resulting abnormal proliferation of malignant cells (17,18,20–22).
    - Erythropoietin (EPO) may lead to angiogenesis and inhibit apoptosis of abnormal cells.
    - Oral contraceptive pills may increase the risk of breast cancer, especially when started before the age of 20 (23,24). Early menarche has also been implicated, and some have theorized that this is an effect of increased estrogen.
    - Some supplements, including creatine and chromium, are being evaluated for carcinogenicity.
- Other risky behaviors.
    - Tobacco use — lung, oropharyngeal cancers (25,26).
    - Sexually transmitted diseases that increase the risk of cancer (26).
    - Human papillomavirus — cervical cancer, penile cancer.
- Prolonged strenuous exercise.
    - Possible immune suppression and increased oxidative stress associated with prolonged strenuous exercise have been hypothesized to lead to increased risk of cancer.
    - In vitro and animal studies suggest an increased incidence of DNA damage as a result of strenuous exercise; however, strenuous exercise has also been demonstrated to shrink tumor size (27–29).
    - Human data remain incomplete and inconclusive at this time.
    - One study of world-class Norwegian athletes showed a threefold increased risk of thyroid cancer in female athletes (30).

FINDING CANCER IN ATHLETES

Screening

- There is no age- or sport-specific recommendations for primary cancer screening for athletes above or beyond normal age-related cancer screenings.
- A history of night sweats, fatigue, unintentional weight loss, decreasing performance, treatment-resistant pain, nonhealing injuries, and recurrent infections suggest the need for further investigation.
- Social history should be reviewed for risk factors for cancer, such as tobacco, environmental exposures, or anabolic steroid use.
- A family history of malignancy is important, particularly in cancers that have a strong genetic link.
- Screening for testicular cancer with genital exam is not recommended during the routine preparticipation evaluation of athletes (PPE). (31) Breast cancer screening with breast examination is not recommended during routine PPE (31).

Malignancy as Musculoskeletal Pain

- Cancer can present as musculoskeletal pain and should be considered in the differential diagnosis, especially when certain warning signs are seen, including pain unrelieved by rest, unrelenting pain, night pain, or pain that does not improve despite appropriate treatment. It should also be considered when there are constitutional symptoms that suggest malignancy (32).
- Cancers that commonly present as musculoskeletal pain.
    - Metastases (most often from breast, lung, thyroid, kidney, and prostate)
        - Bone is the third most common site of metastases after lungs and liver (32).
        - More common than primary tumors of the bone.
        - More likely to cause significant clinical disease due to pain, pathologic fractures, hypercalcemia, and bone marrow replacement (33).
- Solitary primary musculoskeletal tumors, including osteosarcoma, chondrosarcoma, Ewing sarcoma, giant cell tumors, and rhabdomyosarcoma (Table 135.1)
- Cancers originating in the blood and bone marrow include leukemia, lymphoma, and multiple myeloma.

PREPARTICIPATION EVALUATION FOR THE ATHLETE PARTICIPATING WITH CANCER

- Given the large health benefits associated with physical activity in the cancer patient and survivor, barriers preventing activity should be eliminated to the greatest extent possible.
- Despite the documented benefits of exercise, only 25%–30% of cancer survivors are reported to be physically active (defined as meeting the public health exercise guidelines) (34).
- Barriers identified include lack of awareness of safety and value of exercise in the cancer patient, uncertainty of the safety or suitability of a particular exercise in a specific patient, and lack of awareness of available programs or methods of making referrals (35).
- A comprehensive pre-exercise evaluation will allow for an assessment of physical fitness and cancer-specific considerations to individualize the exercise program, requiring this assessment likely creates an unnecessary barrier to activity and is deemed unnecessary to begin a low-intensity aerobic, resistance, and flexibility program in most survivors (3).
- National Comprehensive Cancer Network offers a triage approach to preparticipation evaluation considerations of the athlete or active persons with cancer (3).
    - No comorbidities.
        - No further pre-exercise medical evaluation.
    - Peripheral neuropathy or other conditions affecting the limbs (*e.g.*, arthritis, osteoporosis, lymphedema).
        - Pre-exercise evaluation with modification of exercises based on evaluation.

Table 135.1 Malignant Solid Tumors of the Musculoskeletal System

Tumor	Population Notes	Radiographic/Disease Notes
Primary osteosarcoma	<30 y of age; male predominance	60% in the knee; also consider in hip, pelvis, shoulder "Moth-eaten" or "sunburst" appearance Codman's triangle
Chondrosarcoma	>20 y of age	Hip, pelvis, femoral diaphysis, ribs, and proximal humerus Pathologic fracture
Ewing sarcoma	<30 y of age; male 2:1 predominance	Pelvis, femur, humerus; lucency/lysis; "onion-skin layering"
Giant cell tumors	20–40 y of age; female predominance	Lytic; "soap bubble lesion" Nonsclerotic, sharply defined borders Pathologic fracture Epiphyseal predilection
Rhabdomyosarcomas	90% < 20 y of age	Enlarging, painful, soft tissue mass Most occur in areas naturally lacking significant skeletal muscle (head, neck, genitourinary tract)
Multiple myeloma	>50 y of age	Spine or ribs Mechanical back pain Bence-Jones protein Lytic, punched out lesions

  - Thoracic/abdominal surgery, ostomy, cardiopulmonary diseases, or other systemic manifestations.
    - Pre-exercise evaluation and clearance by physician.
- Understand that athletes undergoing active cancer treatment can feel profoundly different over short periods of time. They should remain flexible with their exercise programs to their changing conditions.
- Cancer treatments may result in different complications. Chemotherapy, radiation, and hormone therapy can all have side effects that affect an individual's ability to participate in activities. The profile of the specific agents should be understood prior to starting an exercise program. Effects can be seen with loss of exercise tolerance, muscle strength and endurance, alterations in body composition, impaired flexibility, tissue elasticity, and joint range of motion of joints (3).
- If surgery has already been performed, evaluate for possible site-specific or regional complications (*i.e.*, wound integrity, lymphedema of the arm or leg with lymph node dissection).
- Cardiac complications can be seen with a number of chemotherapy agents, and these may place the athlete at a higher risk for arrhythmias or cardiomyopathy. There is some evidence to show that stress testing or submaximal stress testing can be used to determine the ability to start an exercise program (36).
- Resistance training can be safely undertaken by athletes with active cancer and cancer survivors. Consideration should be given for fracture risk with osteoporosis related to cancer treatment or bony metastases. Also, care must be taken when performing resistance training with abdominal wounds or an ostomy following cancer surgery to decrease the risk of herniation by avoiding excessive intra-abdominal pressure (37,38).
- Flexibility training may be undertaken safely. Avoid excessive intra-abdominal pressure for athletes with ostomies (38).
- Using ergogenic aids for cancer in athletes.
  - It is important to be aware of regular restrictions for the use of ergogenic aids for athletes in competition.
  - Androgen receptor agonists, including anabolic androgenic steroids and nonsteroidal agonists (selective androgen receptor modulators), can help with cancer cachexia (39).
  - Growth hormone use may lead to an increased risk of second cancer (18,21).
  - EPO is considered for anemia related to cancer treatment.

THE BENEFITS OF EXERCISE IN THE CANCER PATIENT

- Exercise training is generally safe for cancer survivors, and every survivor should "avoid inactivity" and programs may include both aerobic and resistance training with certain training methods, improving different symptoms faced by survivors (Table 135.2) (3). Specific exercise guidance is illustrated in Figure 135.1.
- Exercise in the cancer survivor generally improves health, quality of life, and mental health outcomes (3). The benefits of exercise are illustrated in Table 135.3.

Table 135.2 Impact of Exercise on Cancer Symptomatology

Symptom	Aerobic Only	Aerobic + Resistance	Resistance Only	Notes
Anxiety	X	X	-	
Depression	X	X	-	
Fatigue	X	X	X	
Health-related quality of life	-	X	-	
Lymphedema	-	-	-	May be beneficial in supervised settings
Physical function	X	X	-	
Bone Health	-	-	X	Resistance + impact training is likely beneficial
Sleep	X	-	-	
Cardiotoxicity	-	-	-	
Chemotherapy-induced peripheral neuropathy	-	-	-	
Cognitive function	-	-	-	
Falls	-	-	-	
Nausea	-	-	-	
Pain	-	-	-	
Sexual function	-	-	-	
Treatment tolerance	-	-	-	

X, moderate to strong evidence; -, limited to no evidence.
Adapted from Table 2 of Campbell KL, Winters-Stone KM, Wiskemann J, et al. Exercise guidelines for cancer survivors: consensus statement from International Multidisciplinary Roundtable. *Med Sci Sports Exerc*. 2019 Nov;51(11):2375–90.

- Physical activity is generally well tolerated during and following cancer treatment.
- Exercise is safe both during and after most types of cancer treatments, including life-threatening treatments, such as bone marrow transplant, with attention to infection risk among those immunocompromised due to treatment (*e.g.*, care to avoid spread of infection through the use of equipment at public gyms) (38).
- Exercise before and after a breast cancer diagnosis has been associated with a decreased risk of recurrence and/or death from breast cancer in observational studies (40–42). Two reported observational studies suggest that exercise after a colon cancer diagnosis may reduce the risk of colon cancer–specific and overall mortality (43,44).
- Exercise programs and cancer-related fatigue (CRF)
  - Fatigue is a common symptom in patients with cancer and is nearly universal in those undergoing cytotoxic chemotherapy, radiation therapy, bone marrow transplantation, or treatment with biologic agents (45). Patients perceive CRF to be the most distressing symptom they suffer, more distressing even than nausea and vomiting or pain, which can often be managed with medications (46,47).
  - Current research evidence suggests that both aerobic and resistance exercise programs are beneficial at improving CRF. Recent evidence suggests that greater benefits may be seen when exercise programs are implemented in the survivorship phase rather than the active treatment phase (48,49).
  - In a randomized controlled trial, a 12-week supervised aerobic exercise program versus usual care in 122 lymphoma patients was shown to offer significant benefit for symptoms of CRF and cardiorespiratory fitness, lean body mass, and depression (50).
  - In prostate cancer patients, both resistance and aerobic exercise was found to significantly attenuate CRF over the short term. Only resistance exercise, however, was found to significantly improve CRF in the long term (51).
- The pediatric athlete and cancer
  - Despite purported benefits of physical activity, childhood cancer survivors spend significantly more time sedentary and less time in moderate-to-vigorous physical activity (52).
  - Limitations on bodily functions, including fatigue, physical weakness, and reduced lung capacity related to treatment, were identified by childhood cancer survivors as barriers to participation, especially with team sports and school physical education. These effects were further positively or negatively modified by social support and personal factors, such as motivation, acceptance, or anxiety (53).
  - Childhood cancer survivors may show increased cardiac morbidity and mortality throughout life (54).
  - Childhood cancer survivors with decreased bone mineral density were able to increase their bone mineral density if they were compliant with a physical activity program promoting bone health (55).

Effects of Exercise on Health-Related Outcomes in Those with Cancer

What can exercise do?

- **Prevention of 7 common cancers***
  Dose: 2018 Physical Activity Guidelines for Americans: 150-300 min/week moderate or 75-150 min/week vigorous aerobic exercise
- **Survival of 3 common cancers****
  Dose: Exact dose of physical activity needed to reduce cancer-specific or all-cause mortality is not yet known; Overall more activity appears to lead to better risk reduction

**bladder, breast, colon, endometrial, esophageal, kidney and stomach cancers*
***breast, colon and prostate cancers*

Overall, avoid inactivity, and to improve general health, aim to achieve the current physical activity guidelines for health (150 min/week aerobic exercise and 2x/week strength training).

Outcome	Aerobic Only	Resistance Only	Combination (Aerobic + Resistance)
Strong Evidence	**Dose**	**Dose**	**Dose**
Cancer-related fatigue	**3x**/week for **30** min per session of moderate intensity	**2x**/week of **2** sets of **12-15** reps for major muscle groups at moderate intensity	**3x**/week for **30** min per session of moderate aerobic exercise, plus **2x**/week of resistance training 2 sets of 12-15 reps for major muscle groups at moderate intensity
Health-related quality of life	**2-3x**/week for **30-60** min per session of moderate to vigorous	**2x**/week of **2** sets of **8-15** reps for major muscle groups at a moderate to vigorous intensity	**2-3x**/week for **20-30** min per session of moderate aerobic exercise plus **2x**/week of resistance training **2** sets of **8-15** reps for major muscle groups at moderate to vigorous intensity
Physical Function	**3x**/week for **30-60** min per session of moderate to vigorous	**2-3x**/week of **2** sets of **8-12** reps for major muscle groups at moderate to vigorous intensity	**3x**/week for **20-40** min per session of moderate to vigorous aerobic exercise, plus **2-3x**/week of resistance training **2** sets of **8-12** reps for major muscle group at moderate to vigorous intensity
Anxiety	**3x**/week for **30-60** min per session of moderate to vigorous	Insufficient evidence	**2-3x**/week for **20-40** min of moderate to vigorous aerobic exercise plus **2x**/week of resistance training of **2** sets, **8-12** reps for major muscle groups at moderate to vigorous intensity
Depression	**3x**/week for **30-60** min per session of moderate to vigorous	Insufficient evidence	**2-3x**/week for **20-40** min of moderate to vigorous aerobic exercise plus **2x**/week of resistance training of **2** sets, **8-12** reps for major muscle groups at moderate to vigorous intensity
Lymphedema	Insufficient evidence	**2-3x**/week of progressive, supervised program for major muscle groups does not exacerbate lymphedema	Insufficient evidence
Moderate Evidence			
Bone health	Insufficient evidence	**2-3x**/week of moderate to vigorous resistance training plus high-impact training (sufficient to generate ground reaction force of **3-4** times body weight) for at least **12** months	Insufficient evidence
Sleep	**3-4x**/week for **30-40** min per session of moderate intensity	Insufficient evidence	Insufficient evidence

Citation: bit.ly/cancer_exercise_guidelines

Moderate intensity (40%-59% heart rate reserve or VO_2R) to vigorous intensity (60%-89% heart rate reserve or VO_2R) is recommended.

MOVING THROUGH CANCER | Exercise is Medicine® | AMERICAN COLLEGE of SPORTS MEDICINE®

Figure 135.1: Specific exercise guidance from American College of Sports Medicine. (Reprinted from https://acsm.org/wp-content/uploads/2025/02/Effects-of-Exercise-on-Health-Related-Outcomes-in-Those-with-Cancer-PDF.pdf.)

Table 135.3 Level of Supporting Evidence for Benefit of Physical Activity on Lifetime Risk of Cancer

Cancer Type	Evidence Grade
Bladder	Strong
Breast	Strong
Colon	Strong
Endometrial	Strong
Esophageal	Strong
Gastric	Strong
Renal	Strong
Lung	Moderate
Hematologic	Limited
Head and Neck	Limited
Ovarian	Limited
Pancreatic	Limited
Prostate	Limited
Brain	Limited
Thyroid	No effect — Moderate evidence
Rectal	No effect — Limited evidence

Evidence grade is strength of evidence in the literature regarding the association.
Adapted from 2018 Physical Activity Guidelines Advisory Committee. *2018 Physical Activity Guidelines Advisory Committee Scientific Report*. Washington (DC): US Department of Health and Human Services; 2018.

- Exercise interventions in pediatric oncology patients are feasible and safe (56).
  - No adverse events reported.
  - Positive effects on the immune system, body composition, sleep, activity levels, and aspects of physical functioning.
- Exercise interventions resulted in improvements in strength and global quality of life of adolescents and young adults with cancer (57).
  - In acute lymphocytic leukemia, studies demonstrate improved physical fitness and positive effects for body composition, flexibility, muscle strength, and health-related quality of life (58).
- Most studies showing benefits on exercise related to survivorship and prevention exclude pediatric populations.

EXERCISE FOR THE PREVENTION OF CANCER

- Physical activity and exercise are important health behaviors in the prevention and management of many acute and chronic diseases (59). Physical activity has a prominent place in many cancer control and exercise science guidelines, including the American Cancer Society's guidelines for cancer prevention (60) and survivorship (61).
- 2018 Physical Activity Guidelines evidence regarding exercise/physical activity for cancer prevention (62) is illustrated in Table 135.3.
- Bladder cancer
  - Strong evidence demonstrates that greater amounts of physical activity are associated with reduced risk of developing bladder cancer.
  - Moderate evidence indicates a dose-response relationship of physical activity on the prevention of bladder cancer.
  - Limited evidence that effects of physical activity on bladder cancer risk are less for men than women.
- Breast cancer
  - Strong evidence that multiple types of physical activity are associated with a decreased risk of breast cancer.
  - Strong evidence of a dose-response relationship for increasing physical activity with decreased risk of breast cancer with moderate evidence this relationship is true regardless of BMI and limited evidence this relationship does not vary by race/ethnicity.
- Colon cancer
  - Strong evidence of dose-response relationship with increasing physical activity with decreased risk of colon cancer.
  - Strong evidence the protective effects are seen in both men and women and moderate evidence that weight status does not affect the associations.
  - Strong evidence that the association was true for both proximal and distal colon cancer.
- Endometrial cancer
  - Strong evidence of greater amounts of physical activity associated with lower risk of endometrial cancer.
  - Moderate evidence of a dose-response relationship.
  - Moderate evidence of a greater risk reduction in women with a body mass index (BMI) greater than 25 $kg \cdot m^{-2}$ compared with women with BMI less than 25 $kg \cdot m^{-2}$.
- Esophageal cancer
  - Strong evidence that greater amounts of physical activity are associated with lower risk of developing adenocarcinoma of the esophagus (limited evidence greater amounts of physical activity are NOT associated with a lower risk of developing squamous cell carcinoma).
  - Limited evidence of a dose-response relationship.
- Gastric cancer
  - Strong evidence demonstrates greater amounts of physical activity are associated with lower risk of gastric cancer.
  - Moderate evidence of dose-response relationship and moderate evidence this is true for both cardia and noncardia adenocarcinoma.
- Renal cancer
  - Strong evidence that greater amounts of physical activity are associated with reduced risk of developing renal cancer with limited evidence the effects were similar for men

and women and that the effects did not vary by weight status.
  - Limited evidence of a dose-response relationship.
- Lung cancer
  - Moderate evidence greater amounts of physical activity associated with lower risk of lung cancer with limited evidence the relationship does not vary by age or by cancer histology.
  - Limited evidence that a greater risk reduction is seen in females than in males and in those with a BMI less than 25 kg · m^{-2} than in those with a higher BMI.
  - Limited evidence of dose-response relationship.
  - Moderate evidence a greater risk reduction for current and former smokers than in never smokers.
- Hematologic cancers
  - Limited evidence greater amounts of physical activity associated with reduced risk of lymphoma and myeloma, but not leukemia.
- Head and neck cancers
  - Limited evidence suggests greater amounts of physical activity associated with lower risk of head and neck cancer
  - Limited evidence the relationship does not vary by age, sex, BMI, or smoking status.
  - Limited evidence the relationship may vary by type of head and neck cancer.
- Ovarian cancer
  - Limited evidence of a weak relationship between greater levels of physical activity and lower risk of ovarian cancer.
  - Limited evidence suggests NO dose-response effect.
- Pancreatic cancer
  - Limited evidence greater amounts of physical activity associated with lower risk of pancreatic cancer.
  - Limited evidence of NO dose-response effect.
  - Limited evidence the relationship does not vary by sex.
- Prostate cancer
  - Limited evidence of a weak relationship between greater levels of physical activity with a lower risk of prostate cancer.
- Brain cancer
  - Limited evidence of increased physical activity associated with a decreased risk of glioma and meningioma.
- Thyroid
  - Moderate evidence greater amounts of physical activity are NOT associated with risk of thyroid cancer.
- Rectal
  - Limited evidence greater amounts of physical activity are NOT associated with risk of rectal cancer.
- Other cancers
  - Indeterminate as to whether there is an association between the amount of physical activity with liver, gallbladder, small intestine, or soft tissue cancers, or melanoma.

REFERENCES

1. Miller KD, Nogueira L, Devasia T, et al. Cancer treatment and survivorship statistics, 2022. *CA Cancer J Clin.* 2022;72:409–36. DOI:10.3322/caac.21731
2. McTiernan A, Friedenreich CM, Katzmarzyk PT, 2018 Physical Activity Guidelines Advisory Committee, et al. Physical activity in cancer prevention and survival: a systematic review. *Med Sci Sports Exerc.* 2019 Jun;51(6):1252–61. DOI:10.1249/MSS.0000000000001937
3. Campbell KL, Winters-Stone KM, Wiskemann J, et al. Exercise guidelines for cancer survivors: Consensus statement from International Multidisciplinary Roundtable. *Med Sci Sports Exerc.* 2019 Nov;51(11):2375–90. DOI:10.1249/MSS.0000000000002116
4. Andersen PA, Buller DB, Walkosz BJ, et al. Environmental cues to UV radiation and personal sun protection in outdoor winter recreation. *Arch Dermatol.* 2010;146(11):1241–7.
5. Haley A, Nichols A. A survey of injuries and medical conditions affecting competitive adult outrigger canoe paddlers on O'ahu. *Hawaii Med J.* 2009;68(7):162–5.
6. Walkosz BJ, Buller DB, Andersen PA, et al. Increasing sun protection in winter outdoor recreation a theory-based health communication program. *Am J Prev Med.* 2008;34(6):502–9.
7. De Castro-Maqueda G, Gutierrez-Manzanedo JV, Ponce-González JG, Fernandez-Santos JR, Linares-Barrios M, De Troya-Martín M. Sun protection habits and sunburn in elite aquatics athletes: surfers, windsurfers and olympic sailors. *J Cancer Educ.* 2020 Apr;35(2):312–20. DOI:10.1007/s13187-018-1466-x
8. Wysong A, Gladstone H, Kim D, Lingala B, Copeland J, Tang JY. Sunscreen use in NCAA collegiate athletes: identifying targets for intervention and barriers to use. *Prev Med.* 2012 Nov;55(5):493–6. DOI:10.1016/j.ypmed.2012.08.020
9. Patel AV, Friedenreich CM, Moore SC, et al. American College of sports medicine roundtable Report on physical activity, sedentary behavior, and cancer prevention and control. *Med Sci Sports Exerc.* 2019 Nov;51(11):2391–402. DOI:10.1249/MSS.0000000000002117
10. Agredano YZ, Chan JL, Kimball RC, Kimball AB. Accessibility to air travel correlates strongly with increasing melanoma incidence. *Melanoma Res.* 2006;16(1):77–81.
11. Downs NJ, Schouten PW, Parisi AV, Turner J. Measurements of the upper body ultraviolet exposure to golfers: non-melanoma skin cancer risk, and the potential benefits of exposure to sunlight. *Photodermatol Photoimmunol Photomed.* 2009;25(6):317–24.
12. Friedberg W, Copeland K, Duke FE, O'Brien K 3rd, Darden EB Jr. Radiation exposure during air travel: guidance provided by the federal aviation administration for air carrier crews. *Health Phys.* 2000;79(5):591–5.
13. Kim JN, Lee BM. Risk factors, health risks, and risk management for aircraft personnel and frequent flyers. *J Toxicol Environ Health B Crit Rev.* 2007;10(3):223–34.
14. Berge W, Mundt K, Luu H, Boffetta P. Genital use of talc and risk of ovarian cancer: a meta-analysis. *Eur J Cancer Prev.* 2018;27(3):248–57. DOI:10.1097/CEJ.0000000000000340
15. O'Brien KM, D'Aloisio AA, Shi M, Murphy JD, Sandler DP, Weinberg CR. Perineal talc use, douching, and the risk of uterine cancer. *Epidemiology.* 2019 Nov;30(6):845–52. DOI:10.1097/EDE.0000000000001078
16. Panyakapo M, Soontornchai S, Paopuree P. Cancer risk assessment from exposure to trihalomethanes in tap water and swimming pool water. *J Environ Sci.* 2008;20(3):372–8.
17. Bain J. The many faces of testosterone. *Clin Interv Aging.* 2007;2(4):567–76.

18. Tentori L, Graziani G. Doping with growth hormone/IGF-1, anabolic steroids or erythropoietin: is there a cancer risk? *Pharmacol Res.* 2007;55(5):359–69.
19. De Santi M, Baldelli G, Brandi G, GSMS-SItI Working Group on Movement Sciences for Health Italian Society of Hygiene preventive Medicine and Public Health, WDPP Working Group Doping Prevention Project, WDPP, Working Group Doping Prevention Project. Use of hormones in doping and cancer risk. *Ann Ig.* 2019 Nov-Dec;31(6):590–4. DOI:10.7416/ai.2019.2319
20. Gullett NP, Hebbar G, Ziegler TR. Update on clinical trials of growth factors and anabolic steroids in cachexia and wasting. *Am J Clin Nutr.* 2010;91(4):1143S–7S.
21. Ogilvy-Stuart AL, Gleeson H. Cancer risk following growth hormone use in childhood: implications for current practice. *Drug Saf.* 2004;27(6): 369–82.
22. Ogilvy-Stuart AL, Shalet SM. Tumour occurrence and recurrence. *Horm Res.* 1992;38(suppl 1):50–5.
23. Hunter DJ, Colditz GA, Hankinson SE, et al. Oral contraceptive use and breast cancer: a prospective study of young women. *Cancer Epidemiol Biomarkers Prev.* 2010;19(10):2496–502.
24. Iodice S, Barile M, Rotmensz N, et al. Oral contraceptive use and breast or ovarian cancer risk in BRCA1/2 carriers: a meta-analysis. *Eur J Cancer.* 2010;46(12):2275–84.
25. Connolly GN, Orleans CT, Blum A. Snuffing tobacco out of sport. *Am J Public Health.* 1992;82(3):351–3.
26. Nattiv A, Puffer JC, Green GA. Lifestyles and health risks of collegiate athletes: a multi-center study. *Clin J Sport Med.* 1997;7(4):262–72.
27. Bacurau AVN, Belmonte MA, Navarro F, et al. Effect of a high-intensity exercise training on the metabolism and function of macrophages and lymphocytes of walker 256 tumor bearing rats. *Exp Biol Med.* 2007;232(10):1289–99.
28. Barnard RJ, Ngo TH, Leung PS, Aronson WJ, Golding LA. A low-fat diet and/or strenuous exercise alters the IGF axis in vivo and reduces prostate tumor cell growth in vitro. *Prostate.* 2003;56(3):201–6.
29. Poulsen HE, Weimann A, Loft S. Methods to detect DNA damage by free radicals: relation to exercise. *Proc Nutr Soc.* 1999;58(4):1007–14.
30. Robsahm TE, Hestvik UE, Veierød MB, et al. Cancer risk in Norwegian world class athletes. *Cancer Causes Control.* 2010;21(10):1711–9.
31. American Academy of Pediatrics, American Academy of Family Physicians, American College of Sports Medicine, American Medical Society for Sports Medicine, & American Osteopathic Academy of Sports Medicine. In: *Preparticipation Physical Evaluation.* (5th ed.). American Academy of Pediatrics; 2019.
32. Bruera ED, Portenoy RK. *Cancer Pain Assessment and Management.* Cambridge (UK): Cambridge University Press; 2003.
33. Orr FW, Kostenuik P, Sanchez-Sweatman OH, Singh G. Mechanisms involved in the metastasis of cancer to bone. *Breast Cancer Res Treat.* 1993;25(2):151–63.
34. Gjerset GM, Fosså SD, Courneya KS, Skovlund E, Thorsen L. Exercise behavior in cancer survivors and associated factors. *J Cancer Surviv.* 2011;5(1):35–43.
35. Schmitz KH, Campbell AM, Stuiver MM, et al. Exercise is medicine in oncology: Engaging clinicians to help patients move through cancer. *CA Cancer J Clin.* 2019 Nov;69(6):468–84. DOI:10.3322/caac.21579
36. May AM, van Weert E, Korstjens I, et al. Monitoring training progress during exercise training in cancer survivors: a submaximal exercise test as an alternative for a maximal exercise test? *Arch Phys Med Rehabil.* 2010;91(3):351–357.
37. De Backer IC, Schep G, Backx FJ, Vreugdenhil G, Kuipers H. Resistance training in cancer survivors: a systematic review. *Int J Sports Med.* 2009;30(10):703–12.
38. Schmitz KH, Courneya KS, Matthews C, et al. American College of Sports Medicine roundtable on exercise guidelines for cancer survivors. *Med Sci Sports Exerc.* 2010;42(7):1409–26.
39. Burckart K, Beca S, Urban RJ, Sheffield-Moore M. Pathogenesis of muscle wasting in cancer cachexia: targeted anabolic and anticatabolic therapies. *Curr Opin Clin Nutr Metab Care.* 2010;13(4):410–416.
40. Friedenreich CM, Gregory J, Kopciuk KA, Mackey JR, Courneya KS. Prospective cohort study of lifetime physical activity and breast cancer survival. *Int J Cancer.* 2009;124(8):1954–62.
41. Holmes MD, Chen WY, Feskanich D, Kroenke CH, Colditz GA. Physical activity and survival after breast cancer diagnosis. *JAMA.* 2005;293(20):2479–86.
42. Irwin ML, Smith AW, McTiernan A, et al. Influence of pre- and post-diagnosis physical activity on mortality in breast cancer survivors: the health, eating, activity, and lifestyle study. *J Clin Oncol.* 2008;26(24): 3958–64.
43. Meyerhardt JA, Giovannucci EL, Holmes MD, et al. Physical activity and survival after colorectal cancer diagnosis. *J Clin Oncol.* 2006;24(22): 3527–34.
44. Meyerhardt JA, Heseltine D, Niedzwiecki D, et al. Impact of physical activity on cancer recurrence and survival in patients with stage III colon cancer: findings from CALGB 89803. *J Clin Oncol.* 2006;24(22):3535–41.
45. Berger AM, Abernethy AP, Atkinson A, et al. NCCN clinical practice guidelines cancer-related fatigue. *J Natl Compr Canc Netw.* 2010;8(8): 904–31.
46. Hinds PS, Quargnenti A, Bush AJ, et al. An evaluation of the impact of a self-care coping intervention on psychological and clinical outcomes in adolescents with newly diagnosed cancer. *Eur J Oncol Nurs.* 2000;4(1):6–19, discussion 18–9.
47. Vogelzang NJ, Breitbart W, Cella D, et al. Patient, caregiver, and oncologist perceptions of cancer-related fatigue: results of a tripart assessment survey. The fatigue coalition. *Semin Hematol.* 1997;34(3 suppl 2):4–12.
48. Cramp F, Daniel J. Exercise for the management of cancer-related fatigue in adults. *Cochrane Database Syst Rev.* 2008;2:CD006145.
49. Speck RM, Courneya KS, Mâsse LC, Duval S, Schmitz KH. An update of controlled physical activity trials in cancer survivors: a systematic review and meta-analysis. *J Cancer Surviv.* 2010;4(2):87–100.
50. Courneya KS, Sellar CM, Stevinson C, et al. Randomized controlled trial of the effects of aerobic exercise on physical functioning and quality of life in lymphoma patients. *J Clin Oncol.* 2009;27(27):4605–4612.
51. Segal RJ, Reid RD, Courneya KS, et al. Randomized controlled trial of resistance or aerobic exercise in men receiving radiation therapy for prostate cancer. *J Clin Oncol.* 2009;27(3):344–51.
52. Götte M, Basteck S, Beller R, et al. Physical activity in 9-15 year-old pediatric cancer survivors compared to a nationwide sample. *J Cancer Res Clin Oncol.* 2023;149(8):4719–29. DOI:10.1007/s00432-022-04392-5
53. Larsen EH, Mellblom AV, Larsen MH, et al. Perceived barriers and facilitators to physical activity in childhood cancer survivors and their parents: a large-scale interview study from the International PACCS Study. *Pediatr Blood Cancer.* 2023;70(1):e30056. DOI:10.1002/pbc.30056
54. von Scheidt F, Pleyer C, Kiesler V, et al. Left Ventricular Strain analysis during submaximal Semisupine bicycle exercise stress Echocardiography in childhood cancer survivors. *J Am Heart Assoc.* 2022 Jul 19;11(14):e025324. DOI:10.1161/JAHA.122.025324
55. Jung R, Zürcher SJ, Schindera C, et al. Effect of a physical activity intervention on lower body bone health in childhood cancer survivors: a randomized controlled trial (SURfit). *Int J Cancer.* 2023;152(2): 162–71. DOI:10.1002/ijc.34234
56. Baumann FT, Bloch W, Beulertz J. Clinical exercise interventions in pediatric oncology: a systematic review. *Pediatr Res.* 2013 Oct;74(4):366–74. DOI:10.1038/pr.2013.123

57. Munsie C, Ebert J, Joske D, Ackland T. A randomised controlled trial investigating the ability for supervised exercise to reduce treatment-related decline in adolescent and young adult cancer patients. *Support Care Cancer.* 2022 Oct;30(10):8159–71. DOI:10.1007/s00520-022-07217-w
58. Braam KI, van der Torre P, Takken T, Veening MA, van Dulmen-den Broeder E, Kaspers GJ. Physical exercise training interventions for children and young adults during and after treatment for childhood cancer. *Cochrane Database Syst Rev.* 2016 Mar 31;3(3):CD008796. DOI:10.1002/14651858.CD008796.pub3
59. Courneya KS, Friedenreich CM. Physical activity and cancer: an introduction. *Recent Results Cancer Res.* 2011;186:1–10.
60. Kushi LH, Byers T, Doyle C, et al. American Cancer Society guidelines on nutrition and physical activity for cancer prevention: reducing the risk of cancer with healthy food choices and physical activity. *CA Cancer J Clin.* 2006;56(5):254–314, quiz 313–4.
61. Doyle C, Kushi LH, Byers T, et al. Nutrition and physical activity during and after cancer treatment: an American Cancer Society guide for informed choices. *CA Cancer J Clin.* 2006;56(6):323–53.
62. 2018 Physical Activity Guidelines Advisory Committee. *2018 Physical Activity Guidelines Advisory Committee Scientific Report.* Washington (DC): US Dept of Health and Human Services; 2018.

Human Immunodeficiency Virus and Sports

136

Ryan Flowers and Robert J. Dimeff

PATHOPHYSIOLOGY

Definition (1)

- Human immunodeficiency virus (HIV) is a human retrovirus that targets and infects a cluster of differentiation (CD) 4^+ T-helper cells. It replicates within the $CD4^+$ cells and causes cell death.
- Acquired immunodeficiency syndrome (AIDS) is a chronic illness with an average natural history of >10 years. It is the result of a progressively immunocompromised state due to quantitative and functional defects in $CD4^+$ T-helper cells. The decline in $CD4^+$ cells results in decreased function of the immune system and the development of opportunistic infections and various malignancies.

Natural History (1–5)

- Following a 10- to 28-day incubation period after exposure to HIV, the individual may develop an acute and self-limited viral-like syndrome, followed by seroconversion.
- Seroconversion may occur with the development of the viral syndrome.
- Signs and symptoms of acute (primary) HIV infection in descending order of prevalence include fever, fatigue, myalgia, skin rash, headache, pharyngitis, cervical adenopathy, arthralgia, night sweats, and diarrhea.
- After seroconversion, a clinical latency period occurs that may last over 10 years. During this time, the infected person has normal immune and exercise function.
- When the patient becomes immunocompromised, symptoms may include weight loss, night sweats, fatigue, muscle or joint pain, painful or swollen glands, lymphadenopathy, and fever. Antibodies may be detected within 1 year of infection.
- AIDS is defined as the acquisition of opportunistic infections ranging from mild candidiasis to life-threatening *Pneumocystis carinii* pneumonia *or* a drop in $CD4^+$ count less than 200 cells · μL^{-1}. Malignancies such as lymphoma and Kaposi sarcoma may develop. Muscle wasting occurs through mechanisms that are still not completely understood. Approximately 50% of people develop AIDS within 10 years of becoming infected with HIV and many will then die within 2 years of symptom onset.
- Diagnosis and staging is defined by the CDC, ranging from stage 0 to stage 3.

EPIDEMIOLOGY

Worldwide and USA Specific (see Online Addendum Chapter 136, Human Immunodeficiency Virus and Sports)

Athletics (7–11)

- The incidence and prevalence of HIV/AIDS in athletes are unknown, but there are several high-profile elite and professional athletes who have acquired HIV, including Earvin "Magic" Johnson in 1991 (competed in National Basketball Association [NBA] and 1992 Summer Olympics with HIV), Greg Louganis (competed in 1988 Olympics with HIV), and Ji Wallace (competed in 2020 Olympics with HIV) who attribute their infection to personal behaviors unrelated to sports participation.
- Tommy Morrison (professional boxing) was banned from sports after testing positive for HIV in 1996. He was reinstated in 2006 after apparently becoming HIV-negative and has subsequently fought professionally. Controversy regarding his true testing and disease status continues to exist.
- Several professional athletes have died from AIDS contracted from nonsports activities including sexual activity, drug abuse, and blood transfusion. Prominent HIV-positive athletes include Bill Goldsworthy (National Hockey League [NHL]), Jerry Smith (National Football League [NFL]), Alan Wiggins (Major League Baseball [MLB]), Esteban DeJesus (boxing), Tim Richmond (NASCAR driver), Robert McCall, Rudy Galindo, Robert Wagenhoffer, and John Curry (figure skating), Glenn Burke (MLB), and Arthur Ashe and Michael Westphal (professional tennis).

- Fears of the widespread dissemination of HIV throughout professional sports have been fueled by reports such as in 1991 when two Canadian physicians announced a woman who had died of AIDS had disclosed that she had sexual intercourse with 30–70 different hockey players in the NHL.
- HIV-positive athletes have participated in intercollegiate sports, the 2011 Ironman World Championship, and the Ironman Scotland.

TRANSMISSION AND TESTING (SEE ONLINE ADDENDUM CHAPTER 136, HUMAN IMMUNODEFICIENCY VIRUS AND SPORTS)

Mandatory Testing in Sports

- The American College of Sports Medicine, National Collegiate Athletic Association (NCAA), Canadian Academy of Sport and Exercise Medicine, CDC, International Federation of Sports Medicine, International Olympic Committee, and the World Health Organization do not recommend mandatory screening of athletes for HIV. Any testing that is performed must be accompanied by pre- and posttest counseling, incorporate confidentiality measures, address the frequency of testing, and adhere to local and federal law.
- The 1993 survey of NCAA institutions concerning HIV/AIDS policies found that routine HIV testing for athletes occurred in 4% of institutions and only two were mandatory (28). Updated recommendations from the NCAA in 2014 maintain that mandatory testing of collegiate athletes is not indicated (19). Athletes who wish to be tested should be provided assistance in obtaining such services and encouraged to do so to help modify behavior, reduce the risk of transmission, and initiate therapy when indicated.
- None of the four major professional sports leagues in North America (NFL, NBA, MLB, or NHL) have adopted mandatory HIV testing, but they do recommend routine screening for athletes engaging in high-risk behaviors. In the NFL, the New York Giants and the Philadelphia Eagles reportedly tested players and personnel in 1991 and 1992 despite some of the players being unaware of the testing (8).
- In 1988, the Nevada Boxing Commission mandated HIV testing for all boxers fighting in Nevada, and a positive result would disqualify a boxer from fighting. Numerous boxing commissions followed the lead, and currently, boxers with a positive HIV test are not allowed to box in the United States, although several have fought in other countries (17).
- Governing organizations of some sports require preparticipation screening for blood-borne pathogens (BBPs), including the International Federation of Associated Wrestling Styles, International Boxing Federation, International Amateur Boxing Association, and various state boxing commissions. These organizations have not provided any evidence-based rationale for their requirement (14).
- The International Climbing and Mountaineering Federation (UIAA) does not recommend mandatory HIV testing or widespread screening, but voluntary testing is encouraged in the setting of high-risk behaviors. Athletes with confirmed HIV status should not be banned from participation in climbing or climbing competitions due to the very low risk for transmission (29).

TREATMENT

- Refer to Online Addendum Chapter 136, HIV

HIV AND EXERCISE

- See Online Addendum Chapter 136, Human Immunodeficiency Virus and Sports for additional detailed information on the impact of aerobic and resistance exercise on the athlete with HIV

Exercise Recommendations for HIV-Positive Athletes (1,17,78,145)

- Moderate exercise is beneficial to the physical and psychological well-being of the HIV-positive patient, but strenuous exercise may be detrimental according to findings in some studies. Although the exercise demands of high-level and professional athletes may be safe and beneficial, the possible psychological stress must be assessed on an individual basis.
- A complete physical exam should be performed to assess the overall health and status of HIV infection before beginning an exercise program. Measurements of lymphocyte levels, $CD4^+$ levels, $CD4^+$:$CD8^+$ ratio, and viral load should be obtained. Cardiopulmonary exercise testing with gas exchange measurements should be considered before determining an exercise prescription, especially in patients with low $CD4^+$ counts or high viral loads. HIV-positive individuals should begin exercising while healthy and attempt to maintain their exercise program. Exercise may help manage their illness and improve their quality of life.
- There are currently no specific guidelines for the optimum mode, intensity, frequency, and duration of exercise in relation to disease status. For healthy, asymptomatic, HIV-positive individuals, unrestricted exercise is acceptable. Avoidance of overtraining should be emphasized. Stress related to competition should be minimized. Moderate exercise (40%–60% $\dot{V}O_{2max}$) or heavy aerobic exercise (60%–80% $\dot{V}O_{2max}$) can be recommended depending on patient preference and motivation. An exercise program prescription should include 30–60 minutes of aerobic exercise most days

of the week with resistance training 2–5 days · wk^{-1} depending on the routine.

- For individuals with advanced HIV infection with mild to moderate symptoms or lower $CD4^+$ counts (<200 cells · μL^{-1}), competition, restrictive training schedules, and exhaustive exercise should be avoided. Physical activity and moderate exercise training should be encouraged under close supervision.
- Athletes with frank AIDS may remain active on a symptom-related basis but should avoid strenuous exercise and reduce or stop training during acute illness.

Recommendations and Restrictions for the HIV-Positive Athlete (1,17,28,146,147)

- The most widely used recommendations regarding restriction of the HIV-positive athletes from competition come from the American Academy of Pediatrics (AAP) and the NCAA.
- AAP recommendations: Athletes infected with HIV should be allowed to participate in all competitive sports. Physicians should respect the right to confidentiality including not disclosing infection status to participants or to staff of athletic programs. Physicians should counsel the known HIV-positive athlete on the theoretical risk of infecting others during sports involving blood exposure, especially wrestling and boxing. In these circumstances, physicians should encourage the HIV-positive athlete to consider another sport.
- The NCAA recommendations state that HIV-positive student-athletes should be allowed to participate in intercollegiate athletics based on the individuals health status. The athlete should be allowed to play if asymptomatic with no evidence of immunodeficiency. However, the intensity of training and the stress of competition should be considered to prevent the deterioration of the athlete's health status. Despite this recommendation, a number of NCAA institutions may restrict HIV-positive athletes from participating in selected sports.
- HIV-positive boxers are not allowed to box in any US state or territory, are stripped of their title, and must relinquish any championship belt. While not specifically barred from participation in the four major professional sports in North America, given the demands of training and competition on overall health, adverse effects of therapy, and theoretical risk of transmission, most experts recommend against continued participation.

PREVENTION

- Physicians should educate athletes about risky behaviors and consider HIV testing on a voluntary basis. Education should include discussions on abstinence, safe sex, and the use of shared needles or personal items such as razors, clippers, and earrings that may be contaminated with blood. Participation in the Mathare Youth Soccer Association in Kenya, which emphasizes education and sports participation, has been shown to decrease high-risk behavior such as unprotected sexual activity and drug abuse (148). Researchers in the Dominican Republic trialed the Grassroot Soccer curriculum, a 10-hour HIV prevention intervention, and demonstrated improvements in knowledge, attitude, and communication around HIV that remained significant at a four-month follow-up (149).
- Multiple studies out of Africa have demonstrated the need and potential benefit of HIV education and improved access to care for STIs/HIV, including the use of HIV self-testing kits, among athletes in multiple sports (150,151).
- The International Olympic Committee and Joint United Nations Programme on HIV/AIDS joined forces and started a campaign through the implementation of a toolkit aimed at education and awareness of HIV/AIDS (152).
- Coaches and athletic trainers should receive training in universal precautions and prevention of HIV transmission. The Occupational Safety and Health Administration (OSHA) has standards concerning occupational exposure to bloodborne pathogens, which are applicable to the athletic training room.
- Athletes with skin wounds and potentially infectious skin lesions should be securely covered with bandages and wraps before competition.
- Athletes participating in sports with extensive skin-to-skin contact (*i.e.*, wrestling) should be excluded from matches or practice when skin wounds or lesions are contagious or cannot be securely covered.
- Ambu bags and oral airways should be available for use for cardiopulmonary resuscitation.
- Athletic trainers and health care personnel should use disposable, preferably sterile, examination gloves when treating athletes who are bleeding. Hands should be washed after glove removal.
- Immediate treatment is indicated when an athlete sustains a laceration or wound with substantial bleeding. The blood should be washed off thoroughly with soap and water. Emergency care should not be delayed if gloves are not available. A bulky towel may be used to cover the wound until an off-the-field location is reached and gloves can be used for definitive treatment. The athlete should be allowed to return only after the bleeding is controlled and the wound has been securely covered or wrapped.
- Small amounts of dried blood on uniforms or equipment does not constitute a risk for transmission and does not warrant changing; however, if uniforms or equipment appear wet with blood, or if blood has penetrated both sides of the uniform fabric, it should be changed at the next stoppage of play.
- After each practice or game, any uniforms or equipment soiled with blood should be laundered using standard laundry cycles.

- Disposable towels or absorbent cleaning material should be used to clean environmental surfaces. Clean with soap and water, a germicide registered with the Environmental Protection Agency, or a 1/100 dilution of bleach in tap water (one cup of bleach to 4 gallons of water).
- Receptacles should be available for uniforms soiled with bodily fluids. Sharps containers should be used for needles or scalpel blades.
- Rules forbidding activities such as biting, scratching, fighting, or other unsportsmanlike behaviors that may lead to bloody contact should be strictly enforced (10,146).
- The National Athletic Trainers Association provides similar recommendations for preventing the spread of communicable and infectious diseases in secondary school sports (153).

ETHICAL AND LEGAL IMPLICATIONS

Mandatory Testing

- The proposed testing policy should be ethically acceptable purpose. Protection of the HIV-positive and uninfected athletes from transmission is an ethical purpose. The use of test results for discrimination against HIV-positive athletes is unethical.
- Because HIV transmission on the playing field has never been documented and the risk is theoretically low, mandatory testing remains unnecessary.
- Mandatory testing does violate the individual rights of the athlete, but the question for the professional athlete is if this intrusion is permitted under the collective bargaining agreement of that profession.
- Arguments in favor of permitting violations of the right to privacy cite existing exceptions to HIV testing without consent, including criminal justice settings, life insurance underwriting, defense department and military recruits, immigrants to the United States, State Department foreign service personnel, and the Federal Bureau of Prisons for prison inmates.
- A professional team player contract defines the consequences of failure to maintain physical fitness or pass the preseason medical exam, which may include suspension or termination. Proponents of mandatory testing argue that the acceptance of their contract negates any invasion of privacy. It can be argued that the player's privacy is no more violated by HIV testing than by other routine medical tests required by team and league policies. It can also be argued that the team owner should know the overall health status of a player who may be signed to a long-term, multimillion-dollar contract.
- Professional boxers and other combative sports athletes are subjected to mandatory HIV testing to theoretically protect others who may be exposed to blood during training and competition; this has yet to be contested in court. The Association of Boxing Commissions and Combative Sports provides a list of applicable combative sports by state, including professional and amateur MMA, kickboxing, Muay Thai, and wrestling. Individual state commissions include different sports and carry different requirements, ranging from testing within 1 month to 1 year, or not at all. The necessity for HIV testing may also vary state-by-state according to professional versus amateur status (17,154).
- Most law theorists conclude that mandatory testing is both unethical and illegal (8).

Competition Exclusion (8,18)

- Courts have ruled that without sufficient medical reason, an HIV-positive athlete cannot be excluded from sports participation (School Board of Nassau County, Florida vs Arline, 480. U.S. 273 [1987]).
- The Americans with Disabilities Act and the Rehabilitation Act of 1973 do not allow discrimination against people who have contagious diseases who are otherwise qualified to participate. Concern regarding the potentially harmful effects of competition on the immune system of the HIV-positive athlete has not been viewed as legally valid grounds for exclusion from sanctioned athletic events.
- Courts have permitted schools to prohibit HIV-positive students from school-sponsored contact sports because of the perceived risk of transmission (Doe vs Dolton Elementary School District Number 148, 694F supp. 440 [1988]) and have upheld the decision to exclude an HIV-positive athlete from contact karate (Montalov vs Radcliffe, 167F. 3d 873 [fourth Cir. 1999], cert. Denied, 120 S Ct. 48 1999).
- Ruben Palacio won the World Boxing Organization Featherweight World Championship in 1993 after 12 years in boxing. On the eve of his first title defense, he was subjected to mandatory HIV testing and tested positive. They stripped him of his title and refused to allow him to compete. Other boxers have suffered a similar fate, being forced to retire from their sport.
- In cases in which HIV-positive individuals fail to disclose their status to sexual partners, the courts have ruled in favor of the plaintiff and have fined and sentenced the HIV-positive individual to prison. Canadian Football League Saskatchewan Roughriders player Trevis Smith, who played professional football while he was HIV positive, was convicted of sexual assault and sentenced to 6 years in prison for failure to disclose his HIV status to a sexual partner. If an athlete fails to disclose their HIV-positive status and infects another player on the playing field, it is not known how the court may respond.

SUMMARY

- The total number of people living with HIV-AIDS continues to increase worldwide, although the number of new cases is decreasing and death rates have declined significantly.

- The incidence of HIV among athletes is unknown. Males comprise the majority of new HIV diagnoses over the age of 13 years, with the highest incidence in those 25–34 years of age. MSM are at 44 times greater risk of HIV infection than men having sex with women, accounting for more than two-thirds of new cases.
- There have been no documented cases or reports of HIV transmission through athletic venues or during sporting events, either between athletes or athletes and health providers; however, the CDC reported two cases of transmission during bloody fistfights. Athletes are at higher risk for transmission through personal behaviors from nonathletic activities than through athletic activities. Male collegiate athletes demonstrate higher risk behaviors compared to male nonathletes. The risk among professional athletes is unknown, but anecdotal evidence suggests their celebrity status may lead to higher risks. The theoretical risk to the athletic healthcare provider is based on data on health care professionals exposed to HIV by needlestick and is estimated at 0.3%.
- The proposed testing policy should be ethically acceptable purpose. Protection of the HIV-positive and uninfected athletes from transmission is an ethical purpose. The use of test results for discrimination against HIV-positive athletes is unethical.
- HIV status does not currently preclude participation in professional or collegiate sports, with the exception of combat sports (*e.g.*, professional and amateur MMA, boxing, kickboxing, karate, Muay Thai, and wrestling) as named and whose medical screening is governed by individual state commissions.
- The American College of Sports Medicine, National Collegiate Athletic Association (NCAA), Canadian Academy of Sport and Exercise Medicine, CDC, International Federation of Sports Medicine, International Olympic Committee, and the World Health Organization do not recommend mandatory screening of athletes for HIV. Any testing that is performed must be accompanied by pre- and posttest counseling, incorporate confidentiality measures, address the frequency of testing, and adhere to local and federal law.
- None of the four major professional sports leagues in North America (NFL, NBA, MLB, or NHL) have adopted mandatory HIV testing, but they do recommend routine screening for athletes engaging in high-risk behaviors.
- Professional boxers and other combative sports athletes are subjected to mandatory HIV testing to theoretically protect others who may be exposed to blood during training and competition. An athlete with a positive or reactive test result is restricted from participation.
- There are no published data on the effects of long-term intense training and competition on an elite, highly competitive HIV-positive student-athlete. There are also currently no specific guidelines for the optimum mode, intensity, frequency, and duration of exercise in relation to the disease status.
- Athletes with frank AIDS may remain active on a symptom-related basis but should avoid strenuous exercise and reduce or stop training during acute illness.
- The Americans with Disabilities Act and the Rehabilitation Act of 1973 do not allow discrimination against people who have contagious diseases who are otherwise qualified to participate. Concern regarding the potentially harmful effects of competition on the immune system of the HIV-positive athlete has not been viewed as legally valid grounds for exclusion from sanctioned athletic events.
- Courts have ruled that without sufficient medical reason, an HIV-positive athlete cannot be excluded from sports participation. If an athlete fails to disclose their HIV-positive status and infects another player on the playing field, it is not known how the court may respond.

REFERENCES

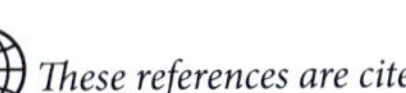
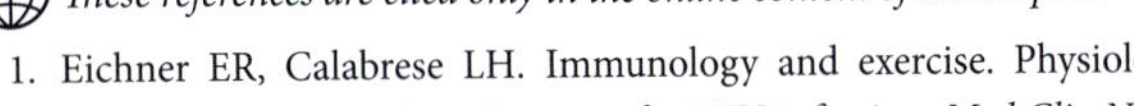
These references are cited only in the online content of the chapter.

1. Eichner ER, Calabrese LH. Immunology and exercise. Physiology, pathophysiology, and implications for HIV infection. *Med Clin North Am*. 1994;78(2):377–88. 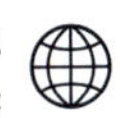
2. Centers for Disease Control and Prevention (CDC). *Diagnoses of HIV Infection in the United States and Dependent Areas, 2020.* HIV Surveillance Report; 2022:33. [cited 2022 Dec 12]. Available from: http://www.cdc.gov/hiv/library/reports/hiv-surveillance.html 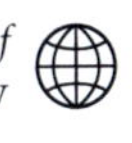
3. Dominguez KL, Smith D, Vasavi T, et al. *Updated Guidelines for Antiretroviral Postexposure Prophylaxis after Sexual, Injection Drug Use, or Other Nonoccupational Exposure to HIV-United States.* Centers for Disease Control and Prevention; 2016. [cited 2022 Dec 13]. Available from: https://stacks.cdc.gov/view/cdc/38856 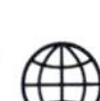
4. Infectious diseases, bloodborne pathogens, and universal precautions. In: Prentice WE, editor. *Principles of Athletic Training: A Guide to Evidence-Based Clinical Practice.* 16th ed. McGraw Hill; 2018. [cited 2022 Nov 11]. Available from: https://accessphysiotherapy-mhmedical-com.foyer.swmed.edu/content.aspx?bookid=2429§ionid=189098180
5. *HIV and AIDS: The basics.* National Institutes of Health; [cited 2023 Feb 16]. Available from: https://hivinfo.nih.gov/understanding-hiv/fact-sheets/hiv-and-aids-basics
6. Web site of CDC. *HIV/AIDS* [Internet]. [cited 2022 Nov 7]. Available from: https://www.hiv.gov/hiv-basics/overview/data-and-trends/global-statistics 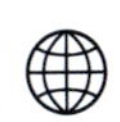
7. Martinez J. *A History of Athletes with HIV/AIDS.* Complex; Published April 17, 2020. [cited 2022 Nov 7]. Available from: https://www.complex.com/sports/2013/12/athletes-with-hiv-aids
8. Johnston JL. Is mandatory HIV testing of professional athletes really the solution? *Health Matrix Clevel.* 1994;4(1):159–203. 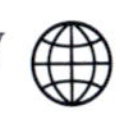
9. Laird R. *Personal Communication.* October 8, 2011.
10. Mast EE, Goodman RA, Bond WW, Favero MS, Drotman DP. Transmission of blood-borne pathogens during sports: risk and prevention. *Ann Intern Med.* 1995;122(4):283–5. 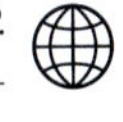
11. Smith D. *Athletes Who Live With HIV/AIDS—#WorldAidsDay.* Compete Magazine; Published December 1, 2021. [cited 2022 Oct 28]. Available from : https://competenetwork.com/athletes-who-live-with-hiv-aids-worldaidsday/

12. Mesquita Soares TC, Galvão De Souza HA, De Medeiros Guerra LM, et al. Morphology and biochemical markers of people living with HIV/AIDS undergoing a resistance exercise program: clinical series. *J Sports Med Phys Fit.* 2011;51(3):462–6.
13. Dorman JM. Contagious diseases in competitive sport: what are the risks? *J Am Coll Health.* 2000;49(3):105–9.
14. McGrew C, MacCallum DS, Narducci D, et al. AMSSM position statement update: blood-borne pathogens in the context of sports participation. *Clin J Sport Med.* 2020;30(4):283–90.
15. Farinatti PT, Borges JP, Gomes RD, Lima D, Fleck SJ. Effects of a supervised exercise program on the physical fitness and immunological function of HIV-infected patients. *J Sports Med Phys Fit.* 2010;50(4):511–8.
16. Gerberding JL. Management of occupational exposures to blood-borne viruses. *N Engl J Med.* 1995;332(7):444–51.
17. Feller A, Flanigan TP. HIV-infected competitive athletes. What are the risks? What precautions should be taken? *J Gen Intern Med.* 1997;12(4):243–6.
18. Brown LS Jr, Drotman DP, Chu A, Brown CL Jr, Knowlan D. Bleeding injuries in professional football: estimating the risk for HIV transmission. *Ann Intern Med.* 1995;122(4):273–4.
19. *NCAA Publications* - 2014-15 *NCAA Sports Medicine Handbook.* [cited 2022 Nov 19]. Available from: http://www.ncaapublications.com/p-4374-2014-15-ncaa-sports-medicine-handbook.aspx
20. Nattiv A, Puffer JC. Lifestyles and health risks of collegiate athletes. *J Fam Pract.* 1991;33(6):585–90.
21. Kokotailo PK, Koscik RE, Henry BC, Fleming MF, Landry GL. Health risk taking and human immunodeficiency virus risk in collegiate female athletes. *J Am Coll Health.* 1998;46(6):263–8.
22. Hurt CB, Nelson JAE, Hightow-Weidman LB, Miller WC. Selecting an HIV test: a narrative review for clinicians and researchers. *Sex Transm Dis.* 2017;44(12):739–46. doi:10.1097/OLQ.0000000000000719.
23. Greenwald JL, Burstein GR, Pincus J, Branson B. A rapid review of rapid HIV antibody tests. *Curr Infect Dis Rep.* 2006;8(2):125–31.
24. Center for Biologics Evaluation and Research. *Oraquick advance rapid HIV-1/2 antibody test.* U.S. Food and Drug Administration. [cited 2023 May 27]. Available from: https://www.fda.gov/vaccines-blood-biologics/approved-blood-products/oraquick-advance-rapid-hiv-12-antibody-test
25. *FDA approved HIV tests.* Centers for Disease Control and Prevention. [cited 2022 Nov 15]. Available from: https://www.cdc.gov/hiv/testing/laboratorytests.html
26. National Center for HIV/AIDS, Viral Hepatitis, and TB Prevention (U.S.), Association of Public Health Laboratories, Division of HIV/AIDS Prevention. *2018 quick reference guide: Recommended laboratory HIV testing algorithm for serum or plasma specimens.* Centers for Disease Control and Prevention. [cited 2022 Nov 15]. Available from: https://stacks.cdc.gov/view/cdc/50872

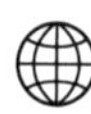

27. Gallant JE, Hoffmann DJ. *CD4 Cell Count.* Johns Hopkins HIV Guide; 2007. [Internet]. [cited 2022 Nov 7]. Available from: http://www.hopkinsguides.com/hopkins/ub/view/Johns_Hopkins_HIV_Guide/545031/all/CD4_Cell_Count
28. McGrew CA, Dick RW, Schniedwind K, Gikas P. Survey of NCAA institutions concerning HIV/AIDS policies and universal precautions. *Med Sci Sports Exerc.* 1993;25(8):917–21.
29. Schöffl V, Morrison A, Küpper T. Risk of transmission of blood borne infections in climbing—consensus statement of UIAA Medcom. *Int J Sports Med.* 2011;32(3):170–3.
30. Eggleton JS, Nagalli S. Highly active antiretroviral Therapy (HAART) [Updated 2022 Jul 4]. In: *StatPearls* [Internet]. Treasure Island (FL): StatPearls Publishing; [cited 2023 May 11].
31. Sabin CA, Philips AN. Should HIV treatment be started at a CD4 cell count above 350 cells/microl in asymptomatic HIV-1 infected patients? *Curr Opin Infect Dis.* 2009;22(2):191–7.
32. US Preventive Services Task Force, Owens DK, Davidson KW, Krist AH, et al. Preexposure prophylaxis for the prevention of HIV infection: US preventive services task force recommendation statement. *JAMA.* 2019;321(22):2203–13. doi:10.1001/jama.2019.6390

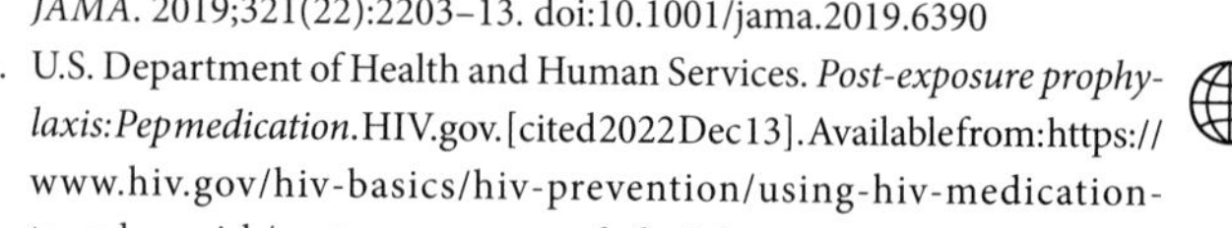
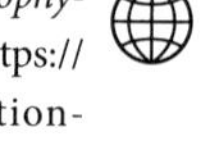

33. U.S. Department of Health and Human Services. *Post-exposure prophylaxis: Pep medication.* HIV.gov. [cited 2022 Dec 13]. Available from: https://www.hiv.gov/hiv-basics/hiv-prevention/using-hiv-medication-to-reduce-risk/post-exposure-prophylaxis/

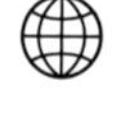

34. Goldschmidt R, Chu C. HIV infection in adults: initial management. *Am Fam Physician.* 2021;103(7):407–16. Gale OneFile: Health and Medicine. [cited 2023 Mar 21]. Available from: link.gale.com/apps/doc/A655652535/HRCA?u=txshracd2621&sid=bookmark-HRCA&xid=95be07ca

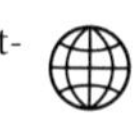

35. Armstrong W, Calabrese L, Taege A. HIV update 2002: delaying treatment to curb rising resistance. *Cleve Clin J Med.* 2002;69(12):995–9.

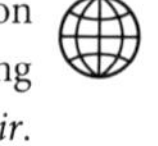

36. Rodríguez-Arenas MA, Jarrín I, del Amo J, et al. Delay in initiation of HAART, poorer virologic response, and higher mortality among HIV-infected injecting drug users in Spain. *AIDS Res Hum Retrovir.* 2006;22(8):715–23.

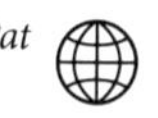

37. Das S. Insulin resistance and diabetes in HIV Infection. *Recent Pat Anti-Infect Drug Discov.* 2011;6(3):260–8.
38. Jellin JM, ed. *Prescriber's Letter.* Vol. 10(4); 2003. 23 p.

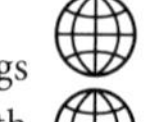
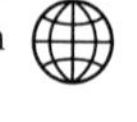

39. Rhoads MP, Lanigan J, Smith CJ, Lyall EG. Effect of specific ART drugs on lipid changes and the need for lipid management in children with HIV. *J Acquir Immune Defic Syndr.* 2011;57(5):404–12.
40. Stringer WW, Sattler FR. Metabolic syndromes associated with HIV: mitigating the side effects of drug therapy. *Phys Sportsmed.* 2001;29(12):19–26.

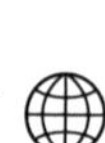

41. Knapp PE, Storer TW, Herbst KL, et al. Effects of a supraphysiological dose of testosterone on physical function, muscle performance, mood, and fatigue in men with HIV-associated weight loss. *Am J Physiol Endocrinol Metab.* 2008;294(6):E1135–43.

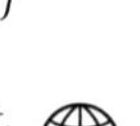

42. Moyle G, Moutschen M, Martínez E, et al. Epidemiology, assessment, and management of excess abdominal fat in persons with HIV infection. *AIDS Rev.* 2010;12(1):3–14.

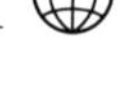

43. Benedini S, Terruzzi I, Lazzarin A, Luzi L. Recombinant human growth hormone: rationale for use in the treatment of HIV-associated lipodystrophy. *BioDrugs.* 2008;22(2):101–12.

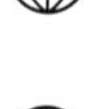

44. Field CJ, Johnson I, Pratt VC. Glutamine and arginine: immunonutrients for improved health. *Med Sci Sports Exerc.* 2000;32(7 Suppl):377–88.

45. Dröge W, Holm E. Role of cysteine and glutathione in HIV infection and other diseases associated with muscle wasting and immunologic dysfunction. *FASEB J.* 1997;11(13):1077–89.

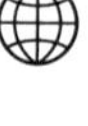

46. Sakkas GK, Mulligan K, Dasilva M, et al. Creatine fails to augment the benefits from resistance training in patients with HIV infection: a randomized, double-blind, placebo controlled-study. *PLoS One.* 2009;4(2):e4605.

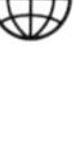

47. Balasubramanyam A, Coraza I, Smith EO, et al. Combination of niacin and fenofibrate with lifestyle changes improves dyslipidemia and hypoadiponectinemia in HIV patients on antiretroviral therapy: results of "heart positive," a randomized, controlled trial. *J Clin Endocinol Metab.* 2011;96(7):2236–47.

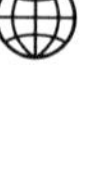

48. Leyes P, Martínez E, Forga Md T. Use of diet, nutritional supplements and exercise in HIV-infected patients receiving combination antiretroviral therapies: a systematic review. *Antivir Ther.* 2008;13(2):149–59.

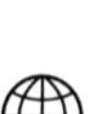
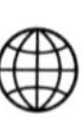

49. Eichner ER. Exercise immunology reconsidered. *Curr Sports Med Rep.* 2020;19(9):341–2.

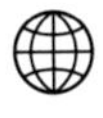
50. Minuzzi LG, Carvalho HM, Brunelli DT, et al. Acute hematological and inflammatory responses to high-intensity exercise tests: impact of duration and mode of exercise. *Int J Sports Med.* 2017;38(7):551–9.

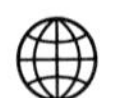
51. Peake JM, Neubauer O, Walsh NP, Simpson RJ. Recovery of the immune system after exercise. *J Appl Physiol.* 2017;122(5):1077–87.

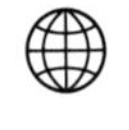
52. Rooney BV, Bigley AB, Emily EC, Laughlin M, Pedlar C, Simpson RJ. Human lymphocytes egress peripheral blood within minutes after cessation of acute dynamic exercise. *Brain Behav Immun.* 2017;66(1):e30.

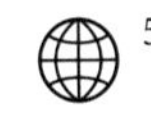
53. Plakida AL. Changes in immunological parameters in ultramarathon runners depending on the duration of the load. *J Sports Med Phys Fit.* 2021;61(2):261–8.

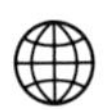
54. Mackinnon LT. Chronic exercise training effects on immune function. *Med Sci Sports Exerc.* 2000;32(7):369–76.

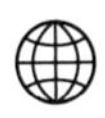
55. Morgado JP, Monteiro CP, Matias CN, et al. Long-term swimming training modifies acute immune cell response to a high-intensity session. *Eur J Appl Physiol.* 2018;118(3):573–83.

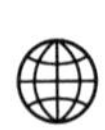
56. Shaw DM, Merien F, Braakhuis A, Dulson D. T-cells and their cytokine production: the anti-inflammatory and immunosuppressive effects of strenuous exercise. *Cytokine.* 2018;104:136–42.

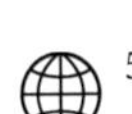
57. Souza D, Vale AF, Silva A, et al. Acute and chronic effects of interval training on the immune system: a systematic review with meta-analysis. *Biology.* 2021;10(9):868.

58. Forte P, Branquinho L, Ferraz R. The relationships between physical activity, exercise, and sport on the immune system. *Int J Environ Res Publ Health.* 2022;19(11):6777.

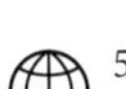
59. Khammassi M, Ouerghi N, Said M, et al. Continuous moderate-intensity but not high-intensity interval training improves immune function biomarkers in healthy young men. *J Strength Cond Res.* 2020;34(1):249–56.

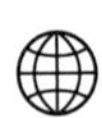
60. Walsh NP, Oliver SJ. Exercise, immune function and respiratory infection: an update on the influence of training and environmental stress. *Immunol Cell Biol.* 2016;94(2):132–9.

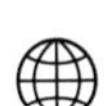
61. Padilha CS, Von Ah Morano AE, Krüger K, Rosa-Neto JC, Lira FS. The growing field of immunometabolism and exercise: key findings in the last 5 years. *J Cell Physiol.* 2022;237(11):4001–20.

62. Rumpf C, Proschinger S, Schenk A, et al. The effect of acute physical exercise on NK-cell cytolytic activity: a systematic review and meta-analysis. *Sports Med.* 2021;51(3):519–30.

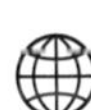
63. Llavero F, Alejo LB, Fiuza-Luces C, et al. Exercise training effects on natural killer cells: a preliminary proteomics and systems biology approach. *Exerc Immunol Rev.* 2021;27:125–41.

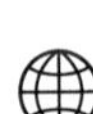
64. dos Santos L, Andreatta MV, Curty VM, Marcarini WD, Ferreira LG, Barauna VG. Effects of blood flow restriction on leukocyte profile and muscle damage. *Front Physiol.* 2020;11:572040.

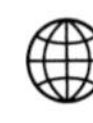
65. Docherty S, Harley R, McAuley JJ, et al. The effect of exercise on cytokines: implications for musculoskeletal health—a narrative review. *BMC Sports Sci Med Rehabil.* 2022;14(1):5.

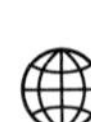
66. Salimans L, Liberman K, Njemini R, Kortekaas Krohn I, Gutermuth J, Bautmans I. The effect of resistance exercise on the immune cell function in humans: a systematic review. *Exp Gerontol.* 2022;164:111822.

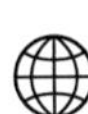
67. Baker JM, Nederveen JP, Parise G. Aerobic exercise in humans mobilizes HSCs in an intensity-dependent manner. *J Appl Physiol.* 2017;122(1):182–90.

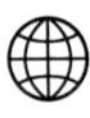
68. Schlabe S, Vogel M, Boesecke C, et al. Moderate endurance training (marathon-training)—effects on immunologic and metabolic parameters in HIV-infected patients: the 42 KM cologne project. *BMC Infect Dis.* 2017;17(1):550.

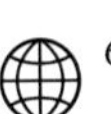
69. Maduagwu SM, Gashau W, Balami A, et al. Aerobic exercise improves quality of life and CD4 cell counts in HIV seropositives in Nigeria. *J Hum Virol.* 2017;5(3):00151.

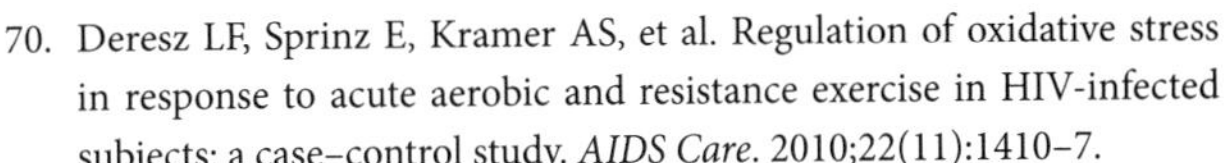
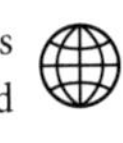
70. Deresz LF, Sprinz E, Kramer AS, et al. Regulation of oxidative stress in response to acute aerobic and resistance exercise in HIV-infected subjects: a case–control study. *AIDS Care.* 2010;22(11):1410–7.

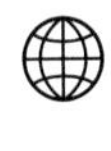
71. Lopez J, Richardson E, Tiozzo E, et al. The effect of exercise training on disease progression, fitness, quality of life, and mental health in people living with HIV on antiretroviral therapy: a systematic review. *JCTR.* 2015;1(3):129–39.

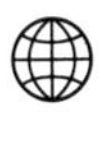
72. Ullum H, Palmø J, Halkjaer-Kristensen J, et al. The effect of acute exercise on lymphocyte subsets, natural killer cells, proliferative responses, and cytokines in HIV-seropositive persons. *J Acquir Immune Defic Syndr.* 1994;7(11):1122–33.

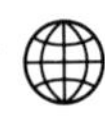
73. Ceccarelli G, Pinacchio C, Santinelli L, et al. Physical activity and HIV: effects on fitness status, metabolism, inflammation and immune-activation. *AIDS Behav.* 2020;24(4):1042–50.

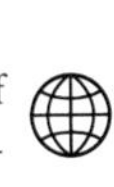
74. Erlandson KM, Wilson MP, MaWhinney S, et al. The impact of moderate or high-intensity combined exercise on systemic inflammation among older persons with and without HIV. *J Infect Dis.* 2021;223(7):1161–70.

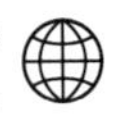
75. Pedro RE, Candido N, Guariglia DA, et al. Exercise improves cytokine profile in HIV-infected people: a randomized clinical trial. *Cytokine.* 2017;99:18–23.

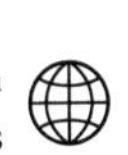
76. Ibeneme SC, Omeje C, Myezwa H, et al. Effects of physical exercises on inflammatory biomarkers and cardiopulmonary function in patients living with HIV: a systematic review with meta-analysis. *BMC Infect Dis.* 2019;19(1):359.

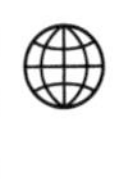
77. Ibeneme SC, Irem FO, Iloanusi NI, et al. Impact of physical exercises on immune function, bone mineral density, and quality of life in people living with HIV/AIDS: a systematic review with meta-analysis. *BMC Infect Dis.* 2019;19(1):340.

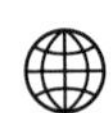
78. Stringer WW. Mechanisms of exercise limitation in HIV+ individuals. *Med Sci Sports Exerc.* 2000;32(7 Suppl):412–421.

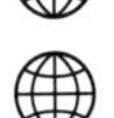
79. Fillipas S, Cherry CL, Cicuttini F, Smirneos L, Holland AE. The effects of exercise training on metabolic and morphological outcomes for people living with HIV: a systematic review of randomised controlled trials. *HIV Clin Trials.* 2010;11(5):270–82.

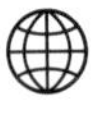
80. O'Brien KK, Tynan AM, Nixon SA, Glazier RH. Effectiveness of aerobic exercise for adults living with HIV: systematic review and meta-analysis using the Cochrane Collaboration protocol. *BMC Infect Dis.* 2016;16:182.

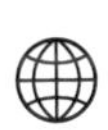
81. Briggs BC, Ryan AS, Sorkin JD, Oursler KK. Feasibility and effects of high-intensity interval training in older adults living with HIV. *J Sports Sci.* 2021;39(3):304–11.

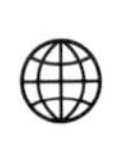
82. Ortmeyer HK, Ryan AS, Hafer-Macko C, Oursler KK. Skeletal muscle cellular metabolism in older HIV-infected men. *Physiol Rep.* 2016;4(9):e12794.

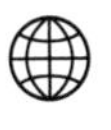
83. Jankowski CM, Wilson MP, MaWhinney S, et al. Blunted muscle mitochondrial responses to exercise training in older adults with HIV. *J Infect Dis.* 2021;224(4):679–83.

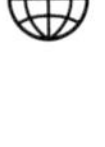
84. Irving BA, Lanza IR, Henderson GC, Rao RR, Spiegelman BM, Nair KS. Combined training enhances skeletal muscle mitochondrial oxidative capacity in-dependent of age. *J Clin Endocrinol Metab.* 2015;100(4):1654–63.

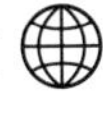
85. Erlandson KM, MaWhinney S, Wilson M, et al. Physical function improvements with moderate or high-intensity exercise among older adults with or without HIV infection. *AIDS.* 2018;32(16):2317–26.

86. Hand GA, Lyerly GW, Jaggers JR, Dudgeon WD. Impact of aerobic and resistance exercise on the health of HIV-infected persons. *Am J Lifestyle Med.* 2009;3(6):489–99.

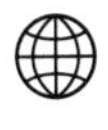
87. LaPerriere A, Fletcher MA, Antoni MH, Klimas NG, Ironson G, Schneiderman N. Aerobic exercise training in an AIDS risk group. *Int J Sports Med.* 1991;12(1):53–7.

88. Lindegaard B, Hansen T, Hvid T, et al. The effect of strength and endurance training on insulin sensitivity and fat distribution in human immunodeficiency virus-infected patients with lipodystrophy. *J Clin Endocrinol Metab.* 2008;93(10):3860–9.
89. O'Brien K, Nixon S, Tynan AM, Glazier R. Aerobic exercise interventions for adults living with HIV/AIDS. *Cochrane Database Syst Rev.* 2010;2010:CD001796.
90. Oursler KK, Sorkin JD, Smith BA, Katzel LI. Reduced aerobic capacity and physical functioning in older HIV-infected men. *AIDS Res Hum Retrovir.* 2006;22(11):1113–21.
91. Poton R, Polito MD. The effects of aerobic training on the CD4 cells, VO_2max, and metabolic parameters in HIV-infected patients: a meta-analysis of randomized controlled trials VO_2max, and metabolic parameters in HIV-infected patients—a meta-analysis of randomized controlled trials. *J Sports Med Phys Fit.* 2020;60(4):634–42.
92. Pérez-Moreno F, Cámara-Sánchez M, Tremblay JF, Riera-Rubio VJ, Gil-Paisán L, Lucia A. Benefits of exercise training in Spanish prison inmates. *Int J Sports Med.* 2007;28(12):1046–52.
93. Pavone RM, Burnett KF, LaPerriere A, Perna FM. Social cognitive and physical health determinants of exercise adherence for HIV-1 seropositive, early symptomatic men and women. *Int J Behav Med.* 1998;5(3):245–58.
94. Petróczi A, Hawkins K, Jones G, Naughton DP. HIV patient characteristics that affect adherence to exercise programmes: an observational study. *Open AIDS J.* 2010;4:148–55.
95. Bessa A, Lopez JC, DI Masi F, Ferry F, Costa E Silva G, Martins Dantas EH. Lymphocyte CD4+ cell count, strength improvements, heart rate and body composition of HIV-positive patients during a 3-month strength training program. *J Sports Med Phys Fit.* 2017;57(7-8):1051–6.
96. O'Brien K, Tynan AM, Nixon S, Glazier RH. Effects of progressive resistive exercise in adults living with HIV/AIDS: systematic review and meta-analysis of randomized trials. *AIDS Care.* 2008;20(6):631–53.
97. Poton R, Polito M, Farinatti P. Effects of resistance training in HIV-infected patients: a meta-analysis of randomised controlled trials. *J Sports Sci.* 2017;35(24):2380–9.
98. Anandh V, Ivor D'SA, Jagatheesan A, et al. Effect of progressive resistance training on cardio vascular fitness, quality of life and CD4 count in people with HIV/AIDS. *Biomedicine.* 2013;33(4):555–9.
99. Alves TC, Santos AP, Abdalla PP, et al. Resistance training with blood flow restriction: impact on the muscle strength and body composition in people living with HIV/AIDS. *Eur J Sport Sci.* 2021;21(3):450–9.
100. Nielsen JL, Aagaard P, Prokhorova TA, et al. Blood flow restricted training leads to myocellular macrophage infiltration and upregulation of heat shock proteins, but no apparent muscle damage. *J Physiol.* 2017;595(14):4857–73.
101. Pedro RE, Guariglia DA, Peres SB, Moraes SM. Effects of physical training for people with HIV-associated lipodystrophy syndrome: a systematic review. *J Sports Med Phys Fit.* 2017;57(5):685–94.
102. Zanetti HR, Lopes LTP, Gonçalves A, et al. Effects of resistance training on muscle strength, body composition and immune-inflammatory markers in people living with HIV: a systematic review and Meta-analysis of randomized controlled trials. *HIV Res Clin Pract.* 2021;22(5):119–27.
103. Souza PM, Jacob-Filho W, Santarém JM, Silva AR, Li HY, Burattini MN. Progressive resistance training in elderly HIV-positive patients: does it work? *Clinics.* 2008;63(5):619–24.
104. Lox CL, McAuley E, Tucker RS. Aerobic and resistance exercise training effects on body composition, muscular strength, and cardiovascular fitness in an HIV-1 population. *Int J Behav Med.* 1996;3(1):55–69.
105. Gomes Neto M, Conceição CS, Oliveira Carvalho V, Brites C. Effects of combined aerobic and resistance exercise on exercise capacity, muscle strength and quality of life in HIV-infected patients: a systematic review and meta-analysis. *PLoS One.* 2015;10(9):e0138066.
106. Shephard RJ. Physical impairment in HIV infections and AIDS: responses to resistance and aerobic training. *J Sports Med Phys Fit.* 2015;55(9):1013–28.
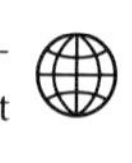
107. Robinson FP, Quinn LT, Rimmer JH. Effects of high-intensity endurance and resistance exercise on HIV metabolic abnormalities: a pilot study. *Biol Res Nurs.* 2007;8(3):177–85.
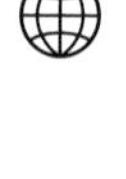
108. O'Brien KK, Tynan AM, Nixon SA, Glazier RH. Effectiveness of Progressive Resistive Exercise (PRE) in the context of HIV: systematic review and meta-analysis using the Cochrane Collaboration protocol. *BMC Infect Dis.* 2017;17(1):268.
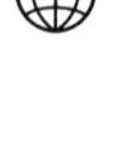
109. Gomes-Neto M, Saquetto MB, Alves IG, Martinez BP, Vieira JPB, Brites C. Effects of exercise interventions on aerobic capacity and health-related quality of life in people living with HIV/AIDS: systematic review and network meta-analysis. *Phys Ther.* 2021;101(7):pzab092.
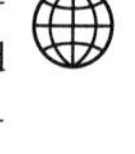
110. Ghayomzadeh M, Earnest CP, Hackett D, et al. Combination of resistance and aerobic exercise for six months improves bone mass and physical function in HIV infected individuals: a randomized controlled trial. *Scand J Med Sci Sports.* 2021;31(3):720–32.
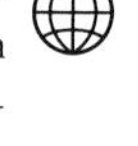
111. Pérez Chaparro CGA, Zech P, Schuch F, Wolfarth B, Rapp M, Heiβel A. Effects of aerobic and resistance exercise alone or combined on strength and hormone outcomes for people living with HIV. A meta-analysis. *PLoS One.* 2018;13(9):e0203384.
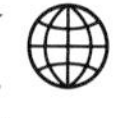
112. Hand GA, Phillips KD, Dudgeon WD, William Lyerly G, Larry Durstine J, Burgess SE. Moderate intensity exercise training reverses functional aerobic impairment in HIV-infected individuals. *AIDS Care.* 2008;20(9):1066–74.
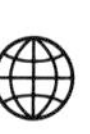
113. Fillipas S, Oldmeadow LB, Bailey MJ, Cherry CL. A six-month, supervised, aerobic and resistance exercise program improves self-efficacy in people with human immunodeficiency virus: a randomised controlled trial. *Aust J Physiother.* 2006;52(3):185–90.
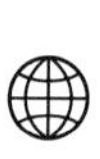
114. Dolan SE, Frontera W, Librizzi J, et al. Effects of a supervised home-based aerobic and progressive resistance training regimen in women infected with human immunodeficiency virus: a randomized trial. *Arch Intern Med.* 2006;166(11):1225–31.
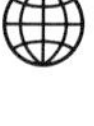
115. Dudgeon WD, Phillips KD, Durstine JL, et al. Individual exercise sessions alter circulating hormones and cytokines in HIV-infected men. *Appl Physiol Nutr Metab.* 2010;35(4):560–8.
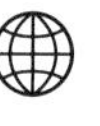
116. Miller TL, Somarriba G, Kinnamon DD, Weinberg GA, Friedman LB, Scott GB. The effect of a structured exercise program on nutrition and fitness outcomes in human immunodeficiency virus-infected children. *AIDS Res Hum Retrovir.* 2010;26(3):313–9.
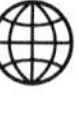
117. Miller TL. A hospital-based exercise program to improve body composition, strength, and abdominal adiposity in 2 HIV-infected children. *AIDS Read.* 2007;17(9):450–8. 450-2, 455, 458.
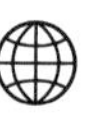
118. Cade WT, Reeds DN, Mittendorfer B, et al. Blunted lipolysis and fatty acid oxidation during moderate exercise in HIV-infected subjects taking HAART. *Am J Physiol Endocrinol Metab.* 2007;292(3):E812–9.
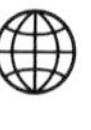
119. Mutimura E, Stewart A, Crowther NJ, Yarasheski KE, Cade WT. The effects of exercise training on quality of life in HAART-treated HIV-positive Rwandan subjects with body fat redistribution. *Qual Life Res.* 2008;17(3):377–85.
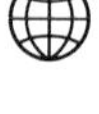
120. Yarasheski KE, Cade WT, Overton ET, et al. Exercise training augments the peripheral insulin-sensitizing effects of pioglitazone in HIV-infected adults with insulin resistance and central adiposity. *Am J Physiol Endocrinol Metab.* 2011;300(1):E243–51.
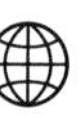
121. Terry L, Sprinz E, Stein R, Medeiros NB, Oliveira J, Ribeiro JP. Exercise training in HIV-1-infected individuals with dyslipidemia and lipodystrophy. *Med Sci Sports Exerc.* 2006;38(3):411–7.

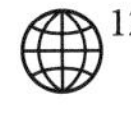
122. Quiles NN, Piao L, Ortiz A. The effects of exercise on lipid profile and blood glucose levels in people living with HIV: a systematic review of randomized controlled trials. *AIDS Care.* 2020;32(7):882–9.

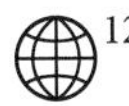
123. Rodrigues KL, Borges JP, Lopes GdO, et al. Influence of physical exercise on advanced glycation end products levels in patients living with the human immunodeficiency virus. *Front Physiol.* 2018;9:1641.

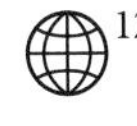
124. Zanetti HR, Gonçalves A, Teixeira Paranhos Lopes L, et al. Effects of exercise training and statin use in people living with human immunodeficiency virus with dyslipidemia. *Med Sci Sports Exerc.* 2020;52(1):16–24.

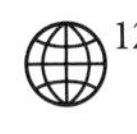
125. Zanetti HR, da Cruz LG, Lourenço CL, et al. Nonlinear resistance training enhances the lipid profile and reduces inflammation marker in people living with HIV: a randomized clinical trial. *J Phys Act Health.* 2016;13(7):765–70.

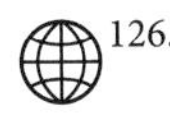
126. Anyanwu EG, Onuchukwu CL. Does plantar lipoatrophy affect dynamic balance in HIV infected persons?. *Gait Posture.* 2021;86:101–5.

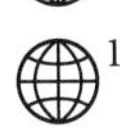
127. Volino-Souza M, de Oliveira GV, Barros-Santos E, et al. Near-infrared spectroscopy-derived muscle oxygen saturation during exercise recovery and flow-mediated dilation are impaired in HIV-infected patients. *Microvasc Res.* 2020;130:104004.

128. Borges J, Soares P, Farinatti P. Autonomic modulation following exercise is impaired in HIV patients. *Int J Sports Med.* 2012;33(4):320–4.

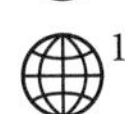
129. Quiles N, Taylor B, Ortiz A. Effectiveness of an 8-week aerobic exercise program on autonomic function in people living with HIV taking anti-retroviral therapy: a pilot randomized controlled trial. *AIDS Res Hum Retrovir.* 2020;36(4):283–90.

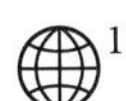
130. Quiles N, Garber C, Ciccolo J. Resting autonomic function in active and insufficiently active people living with HIV. *Int J Sports Med.* 2018;39(1):73–8.

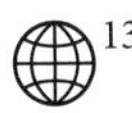
131. Chisati EM, Constantinou D, Lampiao F. Effects of maximal strength training on bone mineral density in people living with HIV and receiving anti-retroviral therapy: a pilot study. *BMC Sports Sci Med Rehabil.* 2020;12:67.

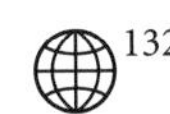
132. Santos WR, Santos WR, Paes PP, et al. Impact of strength training on bone mineral density in patients infected with HIV exhibiting lipodystrophy. *J Strength Cond Res.* 2015;29(12):3466–71.

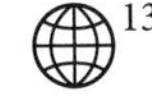
133. Bonato M, Bossolasco S, Galli L, et al. Moderate aerobic exercise (Brisk Walking) increases bone density in cART-treated persons. *J Int AIDS Soc.* 2012;15(4):49–50.

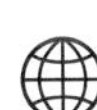
134. Patterson AJ, Sarode A, Al-Kindi S, et al. Evaluation of dyspnea of unknown etiology in HIV patients with cardiopulmonary exercise testing and cardiovascular magnetic resonance imaging. *J Cardiovasc Magn Reson.* 2020;22(1):74.

135. Brazier A, Mulkins A, Verhoef M. Evaluating a yogic breathing and meditation intervention for individuals living with HIV/AIDS. *Am J Health Promot.* 2006;20(3):192–5.

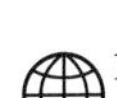
136. Cade WT, Reeds DN, Mondy KE, et al. Yoga lifestyle intervention reduces blood pressure in HIV-infected adults with cardiovascular disease risk factors. *HIV Med.* 2010;11(6):379–88.

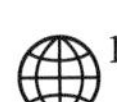
137. Dunne EM, Balletto BL, Donahue ML, et al. The benefits of yoga for people living with HIV/AIDS: a systematic review and meta-analysis. *Complement Ther Clin Pract.* 2019;34:157–64.

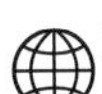
138. Kuloor A, Kumari S, Metri K. Impact of yoga on psychopathologies and quality of life in persons with HIV: a randomized controlled study. *J Bodyw Mov Ther.* 2019;23(2):278–83.

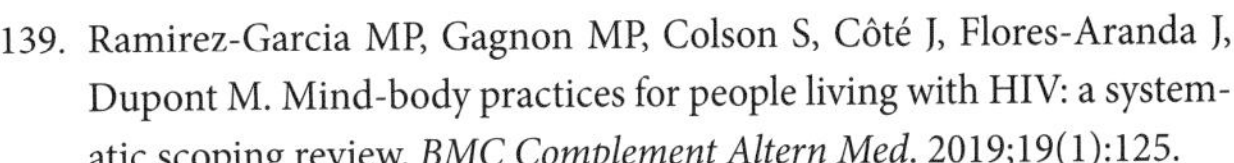
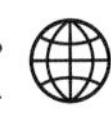
139. Ramirez-Garcia MP, Gagnon MP, Colson S, Côté J, Flores-Aranda J, Dupont M. Mind-body practices for people living with HIV: a systematic scoping review. *BMC Complement Altern Med.* 2019;19(1):125.

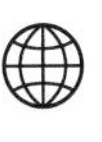
140. Jiang T, Hou J, Sun R, et al. Immunological and psychological efficacy of meditation/yoga intervention among People Living With HIV (PLWH): a systematic review and meta-analyses of 19 randomized controlled trials. *Ann Behav Med.* 2021;55(6):505–19.

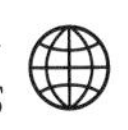
141. Nicholas PK, Kemppainen JK, Canaval GE, et al. Symptom management and self-care for peripheral neuropathy in HIV/AIDS. *AIDS Care.* 2007;19(2):179–89.

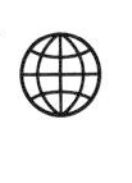
142. Tumusiime DK, Stewart A, Venter FWD, Musenge E. The effects of a physiotherapist-led exercise intervention on peripheral neuropathy among people living with HIV on antiretroviral therapy in Kigali, Rwanda. *SAJPA.* 2019;75(1):1328.

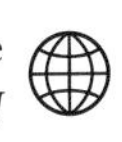
143. Jaggers JR, Hand GA, Dudgeon WD, et al. Aerobic and resistance training improves mood state among adults living with HIV. *Int J Sports Med.* 2015;36(2):175–81.

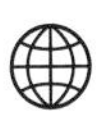
144. Ahmad B, Glufke K, Grau M, et al. Influence of endurance training and marathon running on red cell deformability in HIV patients. *Clin Hemorheaol.* 2014;57(4):355–66.

145. Grace JM, Semple SJ, Combrink S. Exercise therapy for human immunodeficiency virus/AIDS patients: guidelines for clinical exercise therapists. *J Exerc Sci Fit.* 2015;13(1):49–56.

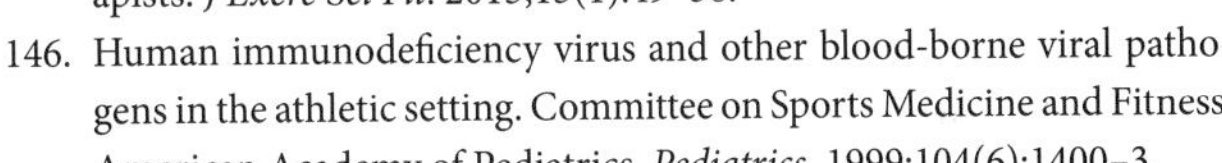
146. Human immunodeficiency virus and other blood-borne viral pathogens in the athletic setting. Committee on Sports Medicine and Fitness. American Academy of Pediatrics. *Pediatrics.* 1999;104(6):1400–3.

147. *NCAA Guideline 2h: Blood-Borne Pathogens and Intercollegiate Athletics.* Indianapolis (IN): National Collegiate Athletic Association; August 2000.

148. Delva W, Michielsen K, Meulders B, et al. HIV prevention through sport: the case of the Mathare Youth Sport Association in Kenya. *AIDS Care.* 2010;22(8):1012–20.

149. Kaufman ZA, Welsch RL, Erickson JD, Craig S, Adams LV, Ross DA. Effectiveness of a sports-based HIV prevention intervention in the Dominican Republic: a quasi-experimental study. *AIDS Care.* 2012;24(3):377–85.

150. Hershow R, Gannett K, Merrill J, et al. Using soccer to build confidence and increase HCT uptake among adolescent girls: a mixed-methods study of an HIV prevention programme in South Africa. *Sport Soc.* 2015;18(8):1009–22.

151. Vrana-Diaz CJ, Stevens DR, Ndeche E, Korte JE. HIV self-testing knowledge and attitudes at sports-based HIV prevention tournaments in Nairobi, Kenya. *J HIV AIDS Soc Serv.* 2019;18(2):180–96.

152. Doupe A. *UNAIDS. Together for HIV and AIDS prevention a toolkit for the sports community.* [cited 2023 Feb 20]. Available from: https://data.unaids.org/publications/irc-pub06/ioc_toolkit_20dec05_en.pdf

153. *Official statement from the National Athletic Trainers' Association on Communicable and Infectious Diseases in Secondary School Sports.* National Athletic Trainers Association. [cited 2022 Nov 14]. Available from: https://www.nata.org/sites/default/files/communicableinfectiousdiseasessecondaryschoolsports.pdf

154. Brown S, Bowler S, Hagen D, Alexander H, Gentile F. *Medical requirements by commission.* Association of Boxing Commissions. [cited 2023 Jun 15]. Available from: https://www.abcboxing.com/medical-requirements-by-commission/.

Index

Note: Page numbers with "f ", "t", and "b" denotes figures, tables, and boxes, respectively and those preceded by an "e" indicate material in online chapters.

A

E

F

O

P

U

V

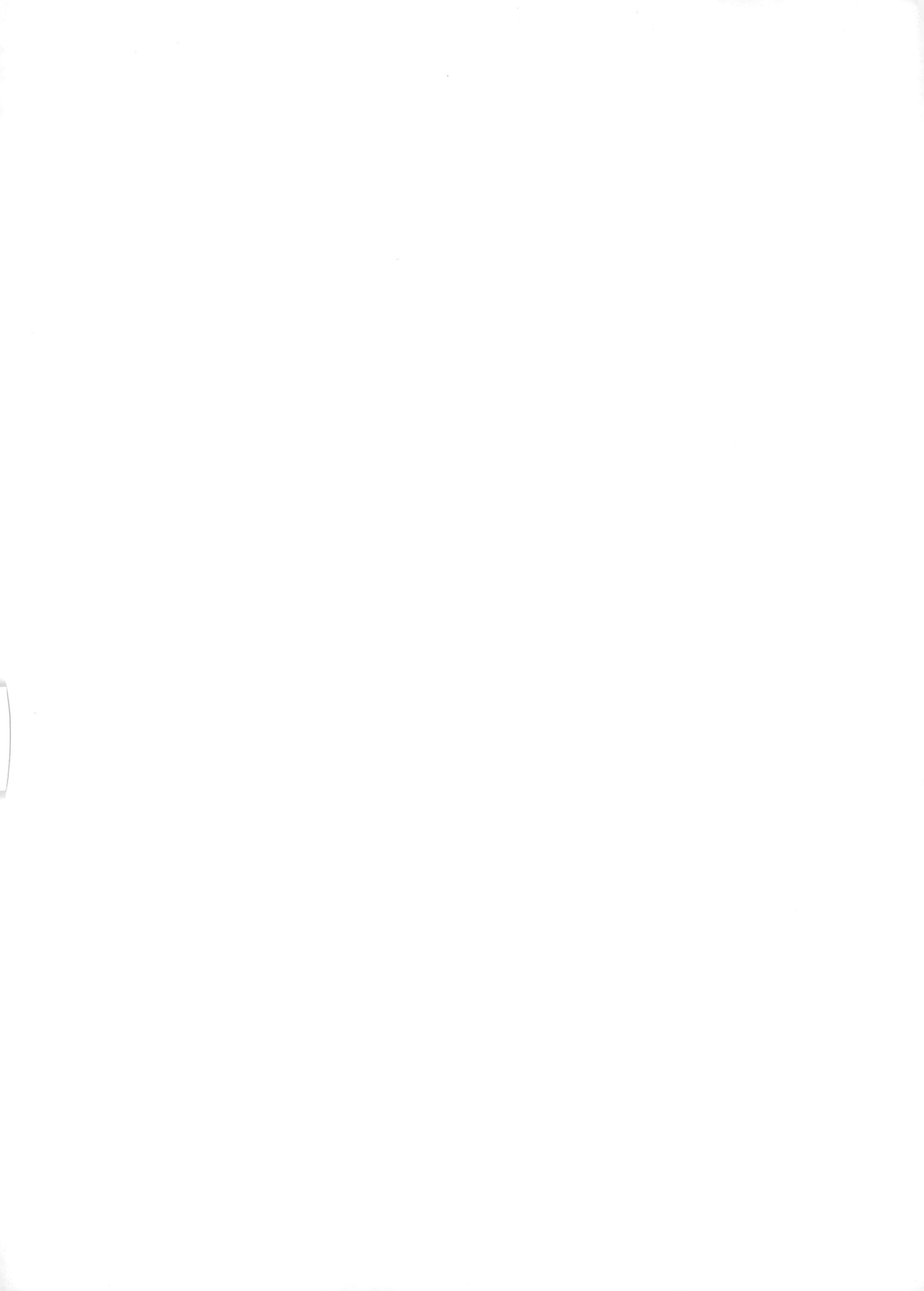